HORMONES AND RESISTANCE 1

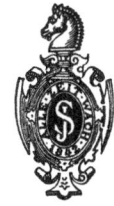

Hans Selye

HORMONES AND RESISTANCE

PART 1

With 22 Figures

Springer-Verlag Berlin Heidelberg GmbH

Professor Hans Selye, C. C., M. D., Ph. D., D. Sc., D. Sc. (hon.), M. D. (hon.), F. R. S. (C), F. I. C. S. (hon.), Institut de Médecine et de Chirurgie expérimentales, Université de Montréal, Montreal, Canada

ISBN 978-3-642-65194-6   ISBN 978-3-642-65192-2 (eBook)
DOI 10.1007/978-3-642-65192-2

This work is subject to copyright. All rights reserved. No part of this publication may be translated, reprinted or reproduced, stored in data banks or other retrieval systems, or transmitted in any form by any means — electronic, mechanical, photocopying, recording, radio, television, or otherwise — without the prior, written permission of the publisher.
Under § 54 of the German Copyright Law where copies are made for other than private use, a fee is payable to the publisher, the amount of the fee to be determined by agreement with the puplisher.
© by Springer-Verlag Berlin Heidelberg 1971. Library of Congress Catalog Card Number 78-155342.
Originally published by Springer-Verlag Berlin · Heidelberg 1971
Softcover reprint of the hardcover 1st edition 1971

The use of general descriptive names, trade marks, etc. in this publication, even if the former are not especially identified, is not to be taken as a sign that such names as understood by the Trade Marks and Merchandise Marks Act, may accordingly be used freely by anyone.

Hans Selye

HORMONES AND RESISTANCE

PART 1

With 22 Figures

Springer-Verlag Berlin Heidelberg GmbH

Professor Hans Selye, C. C., M. D., Ph. D., D. Sc., D. Sc. (hon.), M. D. (hon.), F. R. S. (C), F. I. C. S. (hon.), Institut de Médecine et de Chirurgie expérimentales, Université de Montréal, Montreal, Canada

ISBN 978-3-642-65194-6 ISBN 978-3-642-65192-2 (eBook)
DOI 10.1007/978-3-642-65192-2

This work is subject to copyright. All rights reserved. No part of this publication may be translated, reprinted or reproduced, stored in data banks or other retrieval systems, or transmitted in any form by any means — electronic, mechanical, photocopying, recording, radio, television, or otherwise — without the prior, written permission of the publisher.
Under § 54 of the German Copyright Law where copies are made for other than private use, a fee is payable to the publisher, the amount of the fee to be determined by agreement with the puplisher.
© by Springer-Verlag Berlin Heidelberg 1971. Library of Congress Catalog Card Number 78-155342.
Originally published by Springer-Verlag Berlin · Heidelberg 1971
Softcover reprint of the hardcover 1st edition 1971

The use of general descriptive names, trade marks, etc. in this publication, even if the former are not especially identified, is not to be taken as a sign that such names as understood by the Trade Marks and Merchandise Marks Act, may accordingly be used freely by anyone.

Affectionately dedicated,
on the occasion of his retirement,
to

KAI NIELSEN

as a token of my gratitude
for
nearly forty years of collaboration
and faithful friendship

PREFATORY REMARKS ON THE STYLE OF THIS BOOK

In four previous monographs, *The Mast Cells* (Butterworth, Washington, 1965), *Thrombohemorrhagic Phenomena* (Thomas, Springfield, 1966), *Anaphylactoid Edema* (Green, St. Louis, 1968) and *Experimental Cardiovascular Diseases* (Springer-Verlag, Berlin-Heidelberg-New York, 1970), I have tested the practicality of what might be called the "analytico-synthetic style." In essence, it attempts to facilitate fact-finding by strictly separating: 1. the *analysis* of previous publications in search of facts, which must be objective, and 2. the author's evaluation and *synthesis* which, being guided by his personal experience, is largely subjective.

The lessons learned in compiling these earlier monographs are incorporated in the present volume and, since no major changes have been made, the rationale of the analytico-synthetic style may be described here in essentially the same terms.

Conventionally, the preparation of a monograph progresses in two stages:

1. The author surveys the literature and makes brief abstracts of each publication pertinent to his subject.

2. In writing the successive chapters of his book, the author transforms these abstracts into a current narrative.

In theory, this seems to be a perfectly logical procedure, and undoubtedly it can be successfully applied in some cases. However, the second phase of the work usually meets with virtually insurmountable difficulties. Whenever numerous data are accumulated by many investigators who used different techniques, the interpretations may be consonant, contradictory or unrelated, so that a unified, concise report of all relevant facts and views is hardly possible without confusing distortions or oversimplifications.

Take a sentence such as "Allegedly, it is possible to produce thrombohemorrhagic phenomena by a single intravenous injection of substance X in the rabbit (Smith and Johnson, 1943; Jones, 1944; Jackson, 1952) but not in the mouse (Simpson, 1961; Walker, 1964), however, these claims have been challenged by several investigators (McKay, 1963; Dow, 1963; Fisher, 1964), who have obtained positive results in both these species." Did all these investigators use exactly the same technique? Did all of them use the same criteria for a "positive result?" Were the animals used of the same age and weight? Were the animals invariably killed after the same length of time following the injection, so as to give them an equal chance to develop the lesions? Only in the rarest instances would the answers to all these questions be affirmative. In other words, the sentence designed to combine the three reports has made them quite meaningless.

But why stoop to the customary practice of verbal acrobatics to give the ununifiable the appearance of unity? To make sense, the incongruous monster sentences painfully synthesized by the author must later be mentally broken down into their constituent parts by the reader. What the author has coded, the reader must decode. Statements must be very diplomatically worded to fit several papers because different authors bracketed after one remark have rarely, if ever, said exactly the same thing. Hence, such texts are difficult to read and, in the final analysis, they accomplish little more than to act as indices to the literature, which still has to be procured and read in the original before it can serve as a reliable guide to further work. The essential weakness of this conventional style is that the author must formulate his remarks very vaguely whenever he wants to cite several related, but of course never identical, papers in support of a statement. This procedure is necessary for unification, but the result is uninformative or misleading, usually both.

I have learned these facts by bitter experience while writing sixteen earlier medical texts in the conventional style. Could the usual drawbacks of monographs be avoided by a totally different approach? In compiling a scientific treatise, it was undoubtedly necessary first to peruse all pertinent publications and to prepare concise abstracts of them. (Incidentally, I never minded this part of the work, which was instructive and pleasant; it gave me a broad panoramic view of the observations and reflections of others, the very basis for any correlative scientific study.) But then came the deadly and uninstructive task of modifying and paraphrasing portions of my summaries so that they could be squeezed into more or less cohesive, current prose. Why bother? All that was accomplished in this second stage was to conform with the style sanctified by common usage, but in the process the practical value of my abstract collection was largely lost. I must admit that even after the book appeared in print, I usually still preferred to look up my original résumés. After all, the book contained only portions of these, and even they were not expressed as clearly as in the abstracts mainly for three reasons:

1. Whenever several references are cited to document a statement, certain details have to be eliminated or put vaguely to make the text fit all the publications quoted in support of it.

2. Transitional sentences are needed to connect one idea with another and these are only confusing ballast which does no real work.

3. Many circumlocutions are necessary to distinguish tactfully between data which are fully, partly, or not at all, acceptable.

In other words, the first part of the work, the reading and abstracting, is pleasant, instructive and comparatively easy, while the second part, the paraphrasing into current narrative, is tedious and largely spoils the earlier accomplishments.

Of course, a collection of abstracts is not a monograph; it does not possess any overall structure or continuity and, even with the aid of an extensive index, it cannot act as a handy guide to a new field. Such a compendium is also necessarily uncritical and devoid of originality. It gives none of the interpretations and personal findings of the reviewer.

How could we devise a style which would combine concise, objective reporting with original interpretations without creating any confusion between the two? How could we simplify the writing of scientific monographs sufficiently so that even a large field may be covered by a single author who could give it unity instead of resorting to the current practice of writing "monographs" which, in reality, are only a series of independent reviews by many authors who deal with more or less related topics? This is what I have tried to accomplish here and it may be worthwhile to describe the technique in detail for those interested in the compilation of extensive monographs. We proceeded as follows:

1. **Collection of Literature.** A list comprising most of the literature on hormones and resistance was compiled from abstract journals, the *Index Medicus* and the bibliographies given by previous authors who wrote on this subject. The corresponding original articles were then obtained in the form of reprints or as photo-reproductions. These came mostly from the journals in our two local university libraries (Université de Montréal and McGill University) and from the National Medical Library in Washington, D.C. More than 15,000 articles thus became available for study in original form and, of these about 5,000 were finally selected as being sufficiently relevant to warrant inclusion in the bibliography of this volume. There (pp. 865—1051) they are listed in alphabetic order, with the accession number they carry in our library. These same numbers, followed by a stroke and the year of publication, are also used in the text for identification (e.g., Remmer G66,542/62).

2. **Abstracting.** Every abstract was dictated on magnetic tape with the original source material before me. I had to quote at second hand only a few quite unavailable Doctors' Theses, remarks made at congresses which published no proceedings, and "personal communications" cited by others. To avoid constant spelling out and to facilitate the task of transcription, key words, names, numbers, and complex technical terms were underlined in the original texts for the guidance of our typists.

In preparing the abstracts, we tried to incorporate all the essentials, including the species on which an observation was made, the route of administration of drugs, the techniques of determination, etc., wherever these facts may have significantly influenced the findings. However, equal care was taken to eliminate all irrelevant data in order to make the abstracts concise and readable.

Whenever an author summarized a salient point concisely or expressed a particularly unexpected view, his own wording was quoted. Each abstract was preceded by a brief title [using the Symbolic Shorthand System (SSS) for Physiology and Medicine *(Selye & Ember E24,113/64)*] identifying its subject matter. Articles which contained data pertaining to several chapters of this monograph were separately abstracted for each section. However, the same summary could often be used for this purpose, changing only the title. For example, let us take an article concerned with the prevention by spironolactone of the adrenal necrosis produced by dimethylbenzanthracene and the inhibition of this protection by ethionine. Here I first dictated my abstract with the title:

"DMBA ← SNL"

meaning (in SSS) toxic manifestations produced by dimethylbenzanthracene (DMBA) as influenced by (←) spironolactone (SNL). Then I merely added: repeat the same abstract also with the title:

"Pharmacology/Blockers/Ethionine"

Thus, the same abstract was made available for the corresponding sections on: 1. the detoxication of carcinogens by steroids (spironolactone) and 2. the general pharmacology of blockers (ethionine) that interfere with steroid-induced hepatic microsomal enzyme activity.

When typed out, this abstract with its two titles looked like this:

2 Titles {DMBA ← SNL
         {Pharm/Blockers/Ethionine

Abstract { *Kovacs & Somogyi G60,060/69*: In rats, the adrenal necrosis produced by DMBA is prevented by pretreatment with spironolactone and this protection is in turn blocked by ethionine.

Once carefully proof-read, a Xerox copy was prepared, in addition to the original, in order to avoid possible errors that may slip in by retyping the abstract. When — as in this case — the same abstract was supposed to be used in several connections, a corresponding number of Xerox copies was prepared and on each of these, a different title was marked with a hook to indicate the section of the manuscript where it should go. In this manner, with a minimum of effort, the article can be called to the attention of those interested in any of the topics on which it contains information.

Finally, the pages containing these abstracts were cut up into slips and taped into proper position — according to the "rail paper technique" *(Selye E24,140/64 p. 350)* — on a master copy provided with index tabs.

Throughout this phase of the work, my main concern was to reflect the authors' statements objectively whether I agreed with them or not. Only in a few instances (e.g., when the statements were contradictory or the technique faulty) was it necessary to point out possible sources of confusion, but this was done after the reference in separate, initialed comments.

The resulting classified abstract collection corresponds to the double column, small print in this volume.

3. Critique and Personal Observations. We now had a classified collection of concise abstracts which served as a convenient guide to the literature on hormones and resistance. However, precisely because of its strict objectivity and the absence of any connecting sentences between the abstracts, this text completely lacked both originality and continuity. It was useful for the experienced specialist who only wants to look up the literature on a certain point, but it gave no guidance to the beginner and contributed no unpublished new thoughts or observations.

The published data of our group were handled in the usual manner, by preparing objective abstracts of them for the small print sections. However, my own interpretation of the literature and our hitherto unpublished observations were reported in an entirely different, current narrative form; this text is clearly separated from the rest by being printed in a single column of large type. Here, there are no references, it being tacitly understood that the conclusions are my own, based on a critical interpretation of the literature and my personal experience. In addition, numerous photographs and tables were prepared to make the report informative.

Thus, we end up having a book within a book: the *small-print* sections represent concise and impersonal abstracts of published and unpublished data, formulated in telegraphic style, to be looked up but not to be read through from cover to cover; the *large-print* text, on the other hand, is a critical evaluation of the literature and an illustrated description of unpublished observations. The reader who only wishes to get an overall view of the present status of knowledge on hormones and resistance can do so without getting lost in detail and confusing contradictory statements by reading only the large-type sections. The investigator who wants to verify a special point quickly will find it without having to wade through much text by merely consulting the classified abstracts in the corresponding section.

This "analytico-synthetic style" would not lend itself to the writing of textbooks for students, nor would it be suitable for monographs on entirely new subjects on which there is virtually no earlier literature; however, I think it could be profitably employed in the compilation of any review, monograph or handbook which is to combine an extensive literature survey with personal observations and critical interpretations.

4. Tables and Previously Unpublished Data. In view of the very large number of facts that have come to light of late concerning the possibility of influencing the toxicity of the most diverse agents by catatoxic compounds, it was not possible to publish all of our pertinent observations in the form of original articles. Hence, the results of these studies will be presented in this monograph in the form of standardized **tables** or brief summaries inserted in the text under each of the toxicants examined.

Otherwise unpublished observations are referred to by their protocol numbers (e.g.: "Selye PROT. 27645"). Thus, if interested readers wish to obtain further information, they can get it by writing us. In the case of previously published data, reference is made to the original papers, although often additional data are included in our tables.

The term "*Standard Conditioners*" always refers to PCN, CS-1, ethylestrenol, spironolactone, norbolethone, oxandrolone, prednisolone-Ac, progesterone, triamcinolone, DOC Ac, hydroxydione, estradiol, thyroxine and phenobarbital administered under the standard conditions as described here. Unless otherwise stated in the tables themselves, all steroids to be assayed for possible protective effects have been given in 1 ml water by stomach tube (p. o.) twice daily, as pretreatment and treatment, usually from the first day (4th day before toxicant) until the termination of the experiment. Steroids poorly soluble in water were given in the form of microcrystal suspensions, prepared with the addition of a trace of Tween 80. Thyroxine was administered at the dose of 200 µg in 0.2 ml water (traces of Tween 80 and NaOH added to facilitate solubilization) once daily s. c. Only when steroids were not given p. o., or not at the 10 mg dose level, is this indicated in the tables. Phenobarbital sodium (a typical nonsteroidal catatoxic drug) was administered at the 6 mg dose level in 1 ml water p. o. twice daily on the same days as the steroids.

In addition to these tables concerning individual toxicants, Tables 135—137 present the "Protective Spectra" of some steroidal and nonsteroidal agents respectively, in a synoptic manner and according to a procedure which is outlined on pp. 770 ff.

Unless otherwise specified, all experiments were performed on female 90—110 g Holtzman or ARS/Sprague-Dawley strain rats kept on Purina Fox Chow and tap water ad lib.

With each toxicant we registered the characteristic functional (motor disturbances) or structural (intestinal ulcers, cardiac necrosis, calcinosis) changes in terms of an *arbitrary scale* in which 0 = no change, 1 = just detectable, 2 = moderate, 3 = maximal change, as previously described (Selye G70,421/70, G60,083/70).

However, for *statistical evaluation* we recognized only two grades: minor and sometimes dubious degrees of lesions (between "0" and "1" in our scale) were rated as negative, all others as positive. In the exceptional groups comprising less than 10 rats, these data as well as the mortality rates were then arranged in a 2×2 contingency table, and their statistical significance was determined by the "Exact Probability Test" of Fisher and Yates (Finney D31,291/48 and Siegel G67,296/56). In all the other groups, comprising 10 rats or more, we used the same procedure of grading, but the statistical evaluation was performed by the Chi-square test using the 2×2 table. The severity of all functional disturbances was listed at the time, when the difference between the pretreated and not pretreated animals was most evident.

Only in the case of anesthesia or paralysis did we assess the results by the time (in minutes) necessary to regain the righting reflex. Here, the significance of the apparent differences between the sleeping or paralysis time of the controls and the experimental animals was computed by Student's t-test. When one of the two results was "0", we calculated the statistical significance on the basis of confidence limits.

In all tables: *** = $P < 0.005$, ** = $P < 0.01$, * = $P < 0.05$, NS = Not Significant. Only in the evaluation of the Synoptic Tables 135—137 did we follow another procedure as outlined on pp. 770. Plain asterisks (*) indicate inhibition, underlined asterisks ($\underline{*}$) aggravation of toxicity.

The results of *completely negative experiments* are not tabulated but merely mentioned under the corresponding toxicants, indicating the technique of administering the latter and adding the sentence "the 'Standard Conditioners' (p. VIII) showed no noteworthy change in activity."

Enzymologic References. The principal purpose of this book was to discuss the effect of hormones upon resistance, irrespective of the underlying mechanisms involved. However, since hormones usually regulate resistance to toxicants through the induction of drug-metabolizing enzymes, we also wished to provide at least a key to the most pertinent references concerning purely enzymologic studies in this field. Dr. Jürgen Werringloer of our Biochemistry Department and Mr. Antonio Rodriguez, our Chief-Documentalist, are preparing an extensive reference list of defensive enzyme induction which will be published at a later date. However, they have kindly supplied me with those sections of their index that are particularly pertinent to the subject of this monograph. Thus the readers will have easy access to references on enzymic studies, concerning the action of an inducer upon the biotransformation of a toxicant, immediately after our discussion of the associated morphologic or functional changes.

These references to observations on the induction of potentially defensive enzymes are listed without comments, indicating only the substrate, the agent used to influence its metabolism and the reference. For details, the reader will invariably have to consult the original publications listed in the bibliography.

Among the agents influencing drug metabolism, hormones have received the greatest attention, but stress, sex, age and various interventions considered to be of potential endocrinologic interest have also been included. On the other hand, excluded from the enzymologic references are: 1. Substrates (e.g., amino acids, fatty acids) that are primarily involved in general metabolism and participate only very indirectly, if at all, in detoxication processes and resistance. 2. Purely endocrinologic or physiologic interactions between hormones and/or drugs, as well as pharmacologic test methods. 3. Spontaneous diseases of man, be they targets or agents. 4. The metabolism of endogenous hormones or metabolites, with the exception of bilirubin, which is of special interest in the treatment of hyperbilirubinemias by enzyme inducers.

In the mechanics of indexing, we observed the following rules:

1. Since most pertinent experiments were performed on the rat, this species is not specifically mentioned. Otherwise, the name of the experimental animal is given but, for the sake of brevity, in the case of the commonly employed rabbit (Rb), guinea pig (Gp), and monkey (Mky), in abridged form.

"In vitro" experiments are defined as those in which the entire metabolic study was carried out with tissue slices, homogenates or fractions, independently of whether the induction took place in the living animal or in the test tube. The accession numbers of these experiments are italicized (e.g. *G74,673/59*). All other types of observations (e.g., disappearance rates of substrates from body fluids and tissues, rates of drug elimination in urine or bile) are considered "in vivo" and especially marked by an asterisk following the accession number which is printed in ordinary roman numerals (e.g. G74,673/59*). When both types of observations were combined, the accession number is italicized and followed by an asterisk (e.g. *G74,673/59**).

If a Target "T" (drug or substrate) is influenced by an Agent "A" (drug), this is indicated, thus: T ← A.

The enzymologic references dealing with a given substrate are listed in a distinctive small type (immediately after the abstracts concerning the same substrate), thus:

Hexobarbital ← Luteoids: Juchau et al. *G40,275/66*; Blackham et al. G69,913/69*; Rümke et al. *H14,039/69**

Ethylmorphine ← Ovariectomy: Davies et al. *H22,054/68*

3-Methylcholanthrene ← Estradiol, Mouse: Kirschbaum et al. H27,666/53*

Carisoprodol ← Ovariectomy + 4-Chlortestosterone, Testosterone: Kato et al. *G66,023/61**

If the same substrate is simultaneously affected by two or more inducers and/or antagonists, these are listed in arbitrary order, but the first position is assigned preferably to agents of endocrine importance.

*

In our era, in which interest and material support for research has reached unprecedented proportions, one of the greatest handicaps to the further development of science is the growing difficulty of keeping track of the ever expanding mass of literature. Hence, a generally acceptable, simplified style of reporting could be of immeasurable value. Of course, many laboratory men will say that they lack the time, money, library facilities, or the knowledge of foreign languages necessary for a thorough personal search of the original literature in an extensive field. Yet, any competent scientist must master his own subject. The breadth of his investigations may be very limited by lack of documentation, but in his restricted field he will eventually gather valuable, expert knowledge which should be made available to others as well. It is hoped that the extreme simplicity of reporting in the style recommended here will encourage the writing of surveys by authors who would not have ventured to do so in the more time-consuming conventional form. Should this be the case, correlative investigations would certainly receive a welcome stimulus at a time when mass production threatens to discourage the integration of knowledge. H.S.

ACKNOWLEDGEMENTS

I would like to take this opportunity first of all to express my heartfelt gratitude to all my past and present associates who have assisted me in many of the experiments that form the subject matter of this treatise. I am thinking here particularly of Drs. Béla Solymoss and Kálmán Kovács, to whom we owe respectively the first data on the biochemical, and on the ultrastructural changes associated with the protective effect of typical catatoxic steroids. However, since virtually all other members of our teaching staff, as well as most visiting scientists and postgraduate students have given their attention primarily to the hormonal regulation of resistance, it would be impossible to mention them all by name. Suffice it to express my special thanks to those "Claude Bernard Visiting Professors" whose presence in our Institute during this year has been a special stimulus to the planning of the original experiments reported in this book, namely to: J. Axelrod, J. Berry, B. Brodie, A. H. Conney, J. R. Fouts, H. V. Gelboin, R. J. Gillette, F. T. Kenney, W. E. Knox, G. J. Mannering, G. L. Plaa and H. Remmer.

My thanks are due furthermore to Dr. J. Werringloer and Mr. A. Rodriguez, of our Biochemistry and Documentation department respectively, for having supplied me with the "Enzymologic References."

I am especially indebted to Mrs. I. Mécs, our Chief-Technician. She managed to coordinate the activities of some sixteen technicians so that they efficiently performed the more routine aspects of the laboratory work on an average of about 1200—1500 rats per week, during these last years. In addition Mrs. Mécs was responsible for many original ideas in the design of these experiments and co-authored several publications with my colleagues and myself.

For the editorial work I am most indebted to Mrs. L. Traeger (and her group: K. Bennett, M. Brault, D. Duguay, C. Micusan, M. Mondal, F. Pece and J. Ramu), who, through her dedicated efforts, coordinated all the work involved and brought about the successful completion of this book. I am also thankful to Mr. A. Rodriguez and Mrs. M. Timm for compiling the subject index.

Mr. J. Krzyzanowski (with Mrs. R. Santaca and Mr. I. Lemieux), ingeniously collected even the most inaccessible publications, a crucial task in the preparation of a book of this kind which depends so largely upon the completeness of its bibliography. I also wish to thank Mr. K. Nielsen for preparing the histologic slides and photographic illustrations, as well as to Springer-Verlag for the meticulous attention given to all details of manufacture and design.

Except for about twenty quite inaccessible but important publications, no work was discussed on the basis of second-hand information obtained from references made to it by others. Hence, all works unavailable to us in the original form had to be photographically reproduced, a colossal undertaking for which I am most indebted to Mr. Marcel Bilodeau (our beloved "Uncle Bill") who prepared 104,524 pages of Xerox copies for this purpose.

Acknowledgements

This publication and the original experimental work done at our Institute was subsidized in part by USPHS, National Library of Medicine (Grant 5 RO 1 LM 00522-03), the Ministère de la Santé, Québec, the Medical Research Council of Canada (Block Term Grant MT-1829), the Quebec Heart Foundation, Montreal, the Succession J. A. DeSève, Montreal and was also undertaken as a special project of the Council for Tobacco Research, U.S.A. and the Canadian Tobacco Industry.

GLOSSARY

This glossary furnishes succinct descriptions of some of the technical terms and abbreviations most commonly used. For additional data of this kind (especially synonyms, code numbers and pharmacologic actions of chemical compounds) consult the corresponding sections of the text, through the subject index at the end of the volume.

AAF. See N-2-fluorenylacetamide.

AAN. Acetoaminonitrile, a lathyrogenic compound.

ACTH. Adrenocorticotrophic hormone of the pituitary.

Actinomycin. Unless otherwise specified, this term is used for actinomycin D, recently given the official designation dactinomycin. An antineoplastic agent, especially for Wilms' tumor, which blocks the effect of several microsomal enzyme inducers presumably at the level of the DNA-dependent RNA polymerase reaction (transcription).

Adaptive hormones. Hormones which increase resistance and facilitate adaptive processes.

ADH (antidiuretic hormone). Vasopressin; a hormone of the posterior pituitary, which influences reabsorption of water by the renal tubule.

ADH (enzyme). Alcohol dehydrogenase (Ec 1.1.1.1). Substrates: ethanol and other alcohols, also: aldehyde dehydrogenase (EC 1.2.1.3). Substrates: aldehydes.

ADP (adenosine diphosphate). A nucleotide which participates in high-energy phosphate transfer.

AF. See aminofluorene.

Aminofluorene. AF, a carcinogenic hydrocarbon.

AMP (adenosine monophosphate). A nucleotide which participates in high-energy phosphate transfer.

Antagonists (of enzymes). Substances which inhibit enzyme actions through hitherto unspecified mechanisms.

Antifolliculoid. Blocking the effect of folliculoids (e.g., MER-25). Term first introduced for certain androstanes by Selye (A60,638/44).

Antimineralocorticoid. Blocking the effect of mineralocorticoids, e.g., spironolactone.

Antitestoid. Blocking the effect of testoids (e.g., cyproterone).

ANTU. 1-(1-Naphthyl)-2-thiourea.

APN. Aminopropionitrile, a lathyrogenic compound.

ATP (adenosine triphosphate). A nucleotide which is an important source of high-energy phosphate.

ATPase (adenosine triphosphatase). An enzyme which catalyzes the dephosphorylation of ATP.

Blockers (of enzymes). Substances which impede the synthesis of enzymes by interfering with the production of RNA or proteins (e.g., actinomycin, puromycin, ethionine).

BMR. Basal metabolic rate.

BSP (Bromsulphalein®, sulfobromophthalein). A dye used in tests of liver function.

Catatoxic actions. Increased metabolic degradation and/or excretion of potentially toxic substances. Usually, catatoxic substances result in detoxication, but if the metabolites formed are more poisonous than the parent compounds, the reverse may be true.

CNS. Central nervous system.

Co A.SH (free [uncombined] coenzyme A). A pantothenic acid-containing nucleotide which functions in the metabolism of fatty acids, ketone bodies, acetate, and amino acids.

$$\overset{O}{\underset{\|}{}}$$

Co A.S.C.CH₃ (acetyl-Co A, "active acetate"). The form in which acetate is "activated" by combination with coenzyme A for participation in various reactions.

Co I (coenzyme I). Now called NAD (q. v.).

Co II (coenzyme II). Now called NADP (q. v.).

Co III (coenzyme III). A nicotinamide-containing nucleotide which functions in the oxidation of cysteine.

Competitors. Substances which act by competitively inhibiting the actions of enzymes upon their substrates.

Conditioning Actions. Actions which prepare the organism for a special type of response. In this volume, the term is mainly used for the induction of changes in resistance through catatoxic or syntoxic compounds, irrespective of the underlying mechanisms and of whether the change in reactivity is advantageous or disadvantageous.

CS-1. 9α-Fluoro-11β,17-dihydroxy-3-oxo-4-androstene-17α-propionic acid potassium salt, the first catatoxic steroid to be identified as such. Manufacturer's code number is SC-11927.

CTP (cytidine triphosphate). A source of high-energy phosphate in phospholipid synthesis.

Cytochrome "P-450". A heme protein capable of binding CO to yield a pigment with a characteristic absorption peak at 450 mμ. The "active oxygen" produced in the reaction of reduced P-450 cytochrome with molecular oxygen is thought to be a hydroxylating intermediate, possibly a peroxide.

DAB. See p-diethylaminoazobenzene.

Dactinomycin. New official name for actinomycin D.

p,p'-DDD. 1,1-Dichloro-2,2-bis(p-chlorophenyl)ethane, insecticide related to DDT.

DDT. 1,1-Trichloro-2,2-bis(p-chlorophenyl)-ethane, pesticide.

DHT. Dihydrotachysterol, a vitamin-D derivative which at high doses causes tissue calcification.

Dicoumarol. Bishydroxycoumarin.

p-Diethylaminoazobenzene. DAB, Butter Yellow, a carcinogenic hydrocarbon.

Dioxathion. The new generic name for the pesticide previously known as navadel or Delnav.

DMBA. 7,12-Dimethylbenz(a)anthracene, a carcinogenic hydrocarbon.

DMP. Dimethyl phthalate.

DMSO. Dimethyl sulfoxide.

DNA (deoxyribonucleic acid). The characteristic nucleic acid of the nucleus.

DOC. Desoxycorticosterone.

DOPA. Dioxyphenylalanine or dihydroxyphenylalanine.

DPN. See NAD.

ECG. Electrocardiogram.

EEG. Electroencephalogram.

EFA (essential fatty acids). Polyunsaturated fatty acids, essential for nutrition.

EPB. N-Ethyl-3-piperidyl benzilate, an antagonist of drug-metabolizing enzyme induction.

EPDA. N-Ethyl-3-piperidyl diphenylacetate, an antagonist of drug-metabolizing enzyme induction.

EPN. Phenylphosphonothioic acid O-ethyl O-p-nitrophenyl ester, pesticide.

ESCN. Electrolyte-Steroid-Cardiopathy with Necrosis.

ESR. Electron spin resonance.

EST. Electroshock threshold.

FAD (flavin adenine dinucleotide). A riboflavin-containing nucleotide which participates as a coenzyme in oxidation-reduction reactions.

F-COL. 9α-Fluorocortisol, a gluco-mineralocorticoid.

ff. This sign indicates continuation of treatment, e.g., "First day, ff." means treatment was started on the first day and continued until termination of the experiment.

FFA. Unesterified free fatty acid (also called NEFA, UFA).

Fisher-Yates test. Statistical procedure as described by Finney D31,291/48 and Siegel G67,296/56.

N-2-Fluorenylacetamide. 2-Acetylaminofluorene or AAF, a carcinogenic hydrocarbon.

FMN (flavin mononucleotide). A riboflavin-containing cofactor in cellular oxidation-reduction systems.

Folliculoid. Follicle-hormone-like, estrogenic, gynecogenic or estromimetic, e.g., estradiol.

FSH (follicle-stimulating hormone). A gonadotrophic hormone of the anterior pituitary.

Glucocorticoid. Possessing the effects of the carbohydrate active hormones of the adrenal cortex, e.g., cortisol, triamcinolone.

G-6-P-ase. Glucose-6-phosphatase (EC 3.1.3.9). Substrate: D-glucose-6-phosphate.

GOT. Glutamic-oxalacetic transaminase; aspartate aminotransferase (EC 2.6.1.1). Substrate: L-aspartate.

αGPDH. α-Glycerolphosphate dehydrogenase; glycerol-3-phosphate dehydrogenase (EC 1.1.1.8). Substrate: L-glycerol-3-phosphate).

GPT. Glutamic-pyruvic transaminase; alanine aminotransferase (EC 2.6.1.2). Substrate: L-alanine.

Hepatectomy (partial). The term, if applied to the rat and not otherwise qualified, refers to the usual procedure which removes about 65–70% of the liver tissue (Waelsch and Selye 3972/31).

HMP shunt (hexose monophosphate shunt). An alternate pathway of carbohydrate metabolism.

IDP (inosine diphosphate). A hypoxanthine-containing nucleotide which participates in high-energy phosphate transfer.

IDPN. β,β'-Iminodipropionitrile, a compound producing neurolathyrism.

Induction. Selective stimulation of enzyme synthesis.

Inhibitors (of enzymes). Substances which antagonize the enzymes themselves (e.g., SKF 525-A), in contradistinction to blockers of enzyme synthesis and to substances which act by competition for substrates.

ITP (inosine triphosphate). A deamination product of ATP, functioning similarly to ATP, as a source of high-energy phosphate.

IU. International unit(s).

Lathyrogens. Compound producing either osteo- or neurolathyrism, e.g., aminopropionitrile, or "APN", iminodipropionitrile, or "IDPN".

LDH (lactic acid dehydrogenase). (EC 1.1.1.27). An enzyme whose activity may be measured in serum for diagnosis of certain acute diseases, e.g., acute myocardial infarction.

LH (luteinizing hormone). A gonadotrophic hormone of the anterior pituitary.

LTH (luteotrophic hormone). A hormone of the anterior pituitary possibly identical with the lactogenic hormone.

Luteoid. Corpus luteum hormone-like, progestational, gestagenic, progestagenic, e.g., progesterone.

MAD. Methylandrostenediol, 17α-methyl-5-androstene-3β,17-diol, an anabolic testoid.

MAO. Monoamine oxidase.

MAT. Methionine adenosyltransferase (EC 2.5.1.6). Substrate: L-methionine.

3-MC. See 3-methylcholanthrene.

3-Methylcholanthrene. 3-MC, same as 20-methylcholanthrene. A carcinogenic hydrocarbon.

Mineralocorticoid. Possessing the effects of the salt metabolism regulating hormones of the adrenal cortex, e.g., aldosterone, DOC.

MPDC. N-Methyl-3-piperidyl diphenylcarbamate, an antagonist of drug-metabolizing enzyme induction.

MSH (melanocyte-stimulating hormone). A hormone of the pituitary which increases deposition of melanin by the melanocytes.

NAD (nicotinamide adenine dinucleotide). Formerly termed DPN (diphosphopyridine nucleotide). A nicotinamide-containing nucleotide which functions in electron and hydrogen transfer in oxidation-reduction reactions. Coenzyme I.

NADH. Reduced form of NAD.

NADP (nicotinamide adenine dinucleotide phosphate). Formerly termed TPN (triphosphopyridine nucleotide). A nucleotide with functions and structure similar to those of NAD. Coenzyme II.

NADPH. Reduced form of NADP.

Navadel. A pesticide now known as dioxathion.

NEFA (nonesterified fatty acids). The major form of circulating lipid used for energy (= UFA).

NPN. Nonprotein nitrogen.

OKT. Ornithine-ketoacid aminotransferase (EC 2.6.1.13). Substrate: L-ornithine.

OMPA. Octamethyl pyrophosphoramide. An anticholinergic insecticide.

PABA (para-aminobenzoic acid). A factor among the B vitamins.

PCN. 3β-Hydroxy-20-oxo-5-pregnene-16α-carbonitrile, SC-4674. A synthetic steroid carbonitrile with strong catatoxic activity.

Repression. Selective inhibition of enzyme synthesis.

RER. Rough endoplasmic reticulum.

RES. Reticulo-endothelial system.

Reversal. The phenomenon of the inverse response to a catatoxic agent which causes the latter to aggravate the same lesion which it normally prevents (e.g., aggravation of digitoxin convulsions by spironolactone, when the latter is administered a few hours after digitoxin).

RNA (ribonucleic acid). The characteristic nucleic acid of cytoplasm involved in protein synthesis.

mRNA. Messenger RNA.

SER. Smooth endoplasmic reticulum.

sRNA. Soluble RNA (same as tRNA [transfer RNA]).

SC-11927. The manufacturer's code number for CS-1.

SDH. L-Serine dehydratase (EC 4.2.1.13). Substrate: L-serine.

SGOT (serum glutamic oxaloacetic transaminase). An enzyme often measured in serum for diagnosis of acute myocardial infarction or liver diseases.

SGPT (serum glutamic pyruvic transaminase). An enzyme which may be measured in serum for diagnosis of certain types of liver disease.

Spermatogenic. Having the ability to stimulate the spermatogenic epithelium and mainly to protect it against atrophy caused by deficiency in gonadotrophic hypophyseal hormones, e.g., pregnenolone, androstenediol.

STH. Somatotrophic hormone of the pituitary (growth hormone).

Syntoxic actions. Stimulation of biologic responses which permit coexistence with potential pathogens by altering the irritability of the host's tissues without attacking the pathogen.

T3. Triiodothyronine.

T4. Tetraiodothyronine, thyroxine.

TDH. Threonine dehydratase (EC 4.2.1.16). Substrate: L-threonine.

TEA. Tetraethylammonium, a ganglionic blocking agent usually given as the bromide or chloride.

Testoid. Male-hormone-like, androgenic, andromimetic, e.g., testosterone.

TKT. Tyrosine-α-ketoglutarate transaminase; tyrosine aminotransferase (EC 2.6.1.5). Substrate: L-tyrosine.

TMACN. 17β-Hydroxy-4,4,17-trimethyl-3-oxoandrost-5-ene-2α-carbonitrile, trimethylandrostenolone carbonitrile, also designated as 2α-cyano-4,4,17α-trimethylandrost-5-ene,17β-ol,3-one. A highly potent catatoxic steroid carbonitrile which causes a syndrome of adrenocortical hyperplasia with sexual anomalies in the newborn, when given to pregnant rats. The effect is presumably due to presistent inhibition of fetal 3β-hydroxysteroid dehydrogenase and Δ^{5-4}-isomerase. The compound is often referred to as "cyanoketosteroid."

TPN. See NADP.

TPO. Tryptophan oxygenase (EC 1.13.1.12). Substrate: L-tryptophan.

TPP (thiamine pyrophosphate). The thiamine-containing coenzyme which is cofactor in decarboxylation.

Transcription. Readout of genetic information to form an RNA template.

Translation. Readout of the RNA-coded information in the process of enzyme synthesis.

TSH (thyroid-stimulating hormone). A hormone of the anterior pituitary which influences the activity of the thyroid.

TTH (thyrotrophic hormone). Same as TSH.

UDPG (uridine diphosphoglucose). An intermediary in glycogen synthesis.

UDPGal. Uridine diphosphogalactose.

UDPGluc. Uridine diphosphoglucuronic acid.

UFA. Unesterified free fatty acids (= NEFA).

UTP. Uridine triphosphate.

Xenobiochemistry. Term recommended for the "biochemistry of foreign organic compounds" in the preface of the monograph "Detoxication Mechanisms" (Williams E906/59).

Xenobiotics. The authors recommend the term "xenobiotics" (from the Greek "xenos" and "bios" for "stranger to life") for compounds which "are foreign to the metabolic network of the organism." It is clearly recognized that the mixed function oxidases responsible for the degradation of many xenobiotic compounds are also participating in the metabolism of steroids, lipids and other normal components of the body and food (Mason et al. F51,528/65). Substrates for NADPH oxygen and cytochrome P-450 dependent microsomal enzymes (Leibman G 66,210/69). Also defined as substrates which "are metabolized by mixed function oxidases localized in the endoplasmic reticulum of the liver" (Gillette et al. E8,216/69).

CONTENTS

Reviews		1
Chapter I.	Introduction, Terminology and Classification, Methods	5
Chapter II.	History	24
Chapter III.	Chemistry	42
	Oxidations Mediated by Hepatic Microsomal Enzymes	43
	Oxidations not Mediated by Hepatic Microsomes	45
	Reductive Detoxifying Reactions	45
	Drug Metabolism by Hydrolysis	47
	Conjugation Reactions	47
Chapter IV.	General Pharmacology	53
	Syntoxic Compounds	53
	Catatoxic Compounds (Agonists)	53
	Anticatatoxic Compounds (Antagonists)	57
	Timing	82
	Dose and Route of Administration	93
	Specificity of Conditioning	95
	Biliary Excretion	97
	Extrahepatic Conditioning	100
	Toxicants (Characteristics of Typical Substrates)	103
Chapter V.	Effect of Steroids upon Resistance	111
	Steroids ←	111
	Nonsteroidal Hormones and Hormone-Like Substances ←	137
	Drugs ←	148
	Diet ←	313
	Microorganisms and Parasites ←	315
	Bacterial Toxins ←	333
	Venoms and Plant Poisons ←	348
	Immune Reactions ←	349
	Hepatic Lesions ←	354
	Renal Lesions ←	359
	Other Surgical Procedures ←	361
	Ionizing Rays ←	361
	Ultraviolet Rays ←	368
	Hemorrhage ←	369
	Hypoxia and Hyperoxygenation ←	370
	Temperature Variations ←	372
	Electric Stimuli ←	374

	Systemic Trauma ←	376
	Local Trauma ←	381
	Varia ←	382
	Enzymes ←	383
Chapter VI.	Effect of Other Hormones Upon Resistance	405
	← ACTH	405
	← Somatotrophic Hormone (STH)	424
	← Other Anterior Pituitary Preparations (LTH, GTH, TTH, Crude Extracts)	436
	← Posterior Pituitary Preparations	441
	← Hypophysectomy and Hypothalamic Lesions	443
	← Thyroid Hormones	460
	← Parathyroids	515
	← Calcitonin	520
	← Pancreatic Hormones	521
	← Epinephrine and Norepinephrine	531
	← Special Surgical Procedures (Thymectomy, Splenectomy, Pinealectomy, Sympathectomy)	547
	← Histamine	555
	← 5-HT	556
	← Various Other Hormone-Like Substances	563
	← Tissue Extracts	564

CONTENTS OF PART 2

Chapter VII.	Effect of Nonhormonal Factors upon Resistance	567
Chapter VIII.	Clinical Implications	707
Chapter IX.	Morphology	725
Chapter X.	Theories	743
Chapter XI.	Synopsis of Pharmaco-Chemical and Pharmaco-Pharmacologic Interrelations	768
Summary and Outlook		862
References		865
Index		1053

REVIEWS

This book attempts to abstract and discuss the literature directly concerned with the effect of hormones and hormone derivatives upon resistance. The theoretic interpretation of the underlying mechanisms, in particular the mobilization of enzymic mechanisms for defense, are still quite incompletely understood and will consequently receive much less meticulous attention. However, the true understanding of hormone-dependent resistance phenomena can only come through further exploration and clarification of the basic chemical mechanisms which in many cases are similar to, if not identical with, those underlying hepatic microsomal drug-metabolizing enzyme inductions by nonhormonal agents.

In the following pages special emphasis is layed therefore upon review articles covering those fields which are less completely discussed in the body of this monograph. Foremost among these are generalities about enzyme induction especially by hormones and hormone-like substances, particularly by catatoxic steroids, as well as the concept of adaptive enzymes in general. Additional review articles specifically dealing with certain aspects of the role of hormones in resistance will be found in the corresponding sections of the text.

Enzyme Induction in General

Dorfmann B76,571/52: Review (40 pp., about 70 refs.) on "Steroids and Tissue Oxidation," with special reference to the activation of enzyme systems but not particularly those involved in detoxication.

Knox et al. E83,471/56: Review (90 pp., 752 refs.) on "Enzymatic and Metabolic Adaptations in Animals" with special reference to hormonal, sex-dependent and diet-induced adaptive enzymic changes, but without special reference to hepatic microsomes.

Brodie et al. E92,717/58: Review (27 pp., 148 refs.) on the enzymic metabolism of drugs with special reference to the kind of enzyme systems that can be induced.

Knox G67,799/58: Review (17 pp., 35 refs.) on "Adaptive Enzymes in the Regulation of Animal Metabolism" mainly concerned with factors inducing hepatic TPO activity.

Williams E906/59: Monograph (796 pp., numerous refs.) on "Detoxication Mechanisms—The Metabolism and Detoxication of Drugs, Toxic Substances and Other Organic Compounds."

Axelrod G66,350/62: Review on the demethylation and methylation of drugs and physiologically active compounds by hepatic microsomes.

Brodie G55,013/62: Review (22 pp., 26 refs.) on drug metabolism with special reference to subcellular mechanisms in hepatic microsomes.

Bousquet H11,613/62: Review (12 pp., 135 refs.) on the pharmacology and biochemistry of drug metabolism with special reference to microsomal enzymes.

Conney & Burns G67,166/62: Review on factors influencing drug metabolism with special emphasis upon microsomal enzyme induction.

Gillette E52,874/62: Review (16 pp., 51 refs.) on "Oxidation and Reduction by Microsomal Enzymes."

Remmer G67,788/62: Review (21 pp., 22 refs.) on drugs which induce drug-metabolizing enzymes in the liver. "Administration of these drugs results in (1) accelerated metabolism of steroids such as testosterone and Δ^4-androstene-3,17-dione by liver microsomes, (2) accelerated metabolism of TPNH by liver microsomes, and (3) accelerated in vivo metabolism of D-glucose and D-galactose to D-glucuronic acid, L-gulonic acid and L-ascorbic acid."

Remmer G66,542/62: Review (21 pp., 34 refs.) on drug tolerance with special reference to barbiturates.

Gillette G51,908/63: Review (62 pp., numerous refs.) on "Metabolism of Drugs and Other Foreign Compounds by Enzymatic Mechanisms."

Gillette G66,248/63: Review (8 pp., 14 refs.) on the induction of hepatic microsomal enzymes by various drugs and hormones.

Rosen & Nichol E3,837/63: Review (38 pp., about 170 refs.) on the effect of corticoids and adrenalectomy upon enzyme activity mainly in the liver, but also in other tissues, in vivo and in vitro.

Burns G41,546/64: Editorial on the implications of enzyme induction for drug therapy.

Burns & Conney G71,448/64: Review (25 pp., 57 refs.) on the therapeutic implications of drug metabolism in man.

Shuster F38,575/64: Review (25 pp., 173 refs.) on the "Metabolism of Drugs and Toxic Substances."

Burns & Conney F56,503/65: Brief review on the role of enzyme induction in the metabolism of drugs.

Conney G41,879/65: Review (20 pp., 104 refs.) on the role of enzyme induction in drug toxicity.

Gillette G66,246/65: Review on factors influencing the toxicity of drugs, with a brief section on hepatic microsomal enzymes.

Gillette E7,538/66: Review (42 pp., about 200 refs.) on the biochemistry of drug oxidation and reduction by enzymes in hepatic endoplasmic reticulum.

Jayle & Pasqualini G67,284/66: Review (36 pp., 267 refs.) on glucuronic acid conjugation of steroids and thyroxine. Literature is cited to show that glucuroconjugation of thyroid hormones occurs also in eviscerated rats and hepatectomized dogs, whereas steroid glucuronides are not formed in hepatectomized and eviscerated mice. This suggests that glucuroconjugation of thyroid hormones, unlike that of steroids, can occur in extrahepatic tissue.

Chiancone F85,259/67: Review of the mechanisms regulating hepatic TPO activity.

Conney F88,649/67: Review (49 pp., 379 refs.) on the "Pharmacological Implications of Microsomal Enzyme Induction."

Gillette G67,333/67: Review (25 pp., about 150 refs.) on drug detoxication by hepatic microsomal enzymes.

King & Burgard G46,498/67: Review (6 pp., 40 refs.) on the induction of drug-metabolizing enzymes.

Goldstein et al. E165/68 (p. 274): Review on the age factor in the induction of microsomal drug-metabolizing enzymes.

Mannering G71,818/68: Review (68 pp., 325 refs.) on the "Significance of Stimulation and Inhibition of Drug Metabolism in Pharmacological Testing." Most of the inducing agents and substrates tested are tabulated with references to the corresponding literature. Special emphasis is laid upon the existence of several mechanisms of induction (phenobarbital type, polycyclic hydrocarbon type), the chemistry of microsomal drug metabolism, tests for enzyme induction, and clinical applications.

Mannering G75,980/68: Review (26 pp., 89 refs.) on stimulation and inhibition of drug metabolism.

Brodie G72,492/69: Review (4 pp., no refs.) on "Some Prospects in Toxicology" with special reference to drug-metabolizing enzymes.

Conney H8,988/69: Review (7 pp., 28 refs.) on drug metabolism with special reference to its application in therapeutics.

Filner et al. H15,309/69: Review of the literature on enzyme induction in plants. An extensive Table lists the plants examined with the enzymes, cofactors, or inhibitors involved.

Gillette et al. E8,216/69: Proceedings of a symposium (547 pp., numerous refs.) on "Microsomes and Drug Oxidations" held with the participation of 52 internationally known specialists, in Bethesda, Maryland, February 1968.

Hayaishi H13,776/69: Review (23 pp., 201 refs.) on enzymic hydroxylation with a special section on microsomal monooxygenases.

Kuntzman G64,989/69: Review (35 pp., 109 refs.) on "Drugs and Enzyme Induction."

Staudinger et al. H20,267/69: Review (7 pp., 40 refs.) on oxidative drug metabolism with special reference to the underlying mechanism.

Various authors G68,203/69: Review (27 pp., 42 refs.) on "Application of Metabolic Data to the Evaluation of Drugs. A Report Prepared by the Committee on Problems of Drug Safety of the Drug Research Board, National Academy of Sciences—National

Research Council." A large section of this report is devoted to the inactivation of drugs by microsomal enzymes. It is emphasized that "it is difficult to predict from in vitro data alone whether inhibitors of the cytochrome P-450 enzymes will significantly block the metabolism of drugs in laboratory animals and in patients." Furthermore, "phenobarbital administration leads to an increase in virtually all known enzymatic pathways by causing an increase in both NADPH cytochrome C reductase and cytochrome P-450. Although phenobarbital is known to act by increasing the synthesis of enzyme protein, it may also act by slowing the turnover of the various components of the endoplasmic reticulum."

Aldrete & Weber G75,396/70: Review (17 pp., 96 refs.) on the role of the liver in the detoxication of anesthetics and muscle relaxants.

Conney G70,316/70: Review on environmental factors influencing drug metabolism with special reference to hepatic microsomal enzyme induction.

Conney & Kuntzman G70,540/70: Review on the metabolism of normal body constituents by drug-metabolizing enzymes in hepatic microsomes; special chapters deal with the metabolism of steroid hormones, cholesterol, fatty acids, thyroxine, bilirubin, indoles, sympathomimetic amines, heme, methylated purines, kynurenine and anthranilic acid.

Fouts G76,868/70: Review on the effects of various insecticides, both as inducers and as substrates for hepatic microsomal enzymes.

Fouts G79,537/70: Review (6 pp., 19 refs.) on the influence of various factors, especially environmental contaminants, upon hepatic microsomal drug-metabolizing enzymes.

Greim H32,018/70: Brief review (4 pp., 18 refs.) on microsomal enzymes and their possible clinical implications (German).

Schimke & Doyle G75,997/70: Review (44 pp., 307 refs.) on the "Control of Enzyme Levels in Animal Tissues," with a special section on the regulation of enzyme levels by hormones.

Schreiber G73,539/70: Review (22 pp., 77 refs.) on "The Metabolic Alteration of Drugs." Special chapters deal with epinephrine, norepinephrine, mescaline, diethylpropion, pronethalol, phenothiazine, diazepam and chlordiazepoxide.

Schmidt & Schmidt G73,170/70: Review (62 pp., 272 refs.) on "Enzyme Activities in Human Liver."

Mannering G74,558/71: Review on microsomal enzyme systems which catalyze drug metabolism.

Enzyme Induction by Hormones

Schou E92,436/61: Review (23 pp., 147 refs.) on factors influencing the absorption of drugs from the subcutaneous connective tissue. Special sections deal with the effect of epinephrine, folliculoids and glucocorticoids which can alter the action of various drugs by modifying their absorption rate.

Ghione & Turolla G18,525/64: Review on the effect of anabolics upon inflammatory responses, with special reference to the granuloma pouch technique, anaphylactoid edema and cotton pellet granulomas.

Conney F88,649/67 (p. 342): Review on the hormonal regulation of drug metabolism.

Freedland et al. H2,949/68: Review (5 pp., 33 refs.) on the relationship of nutritional and hormonal influences in hepatic enzyme activity.

Selye G70,465/70: Brief review on "Stress, Hormones and Cardiovascular Disease."

Enzymes and Adaptation

Cedrangolo B46,622/49: Review on "Adaptation as an Enzymological Problem."

Selye B40,000/50 (pp. 246—254): Review on the changes in the enzyme activity of various tissues and the blood during the G.A.S., with special reference to the "adaptive enzymes" or "protective enzymes" which undoubtedly play an important role in adaptation to stress.

Fregly G72,594/69: Review (6 pp., 11 refs.) on cross-adaptation, with special reference to the induction of drug-metabolizing enzymes.

Hale G72,522/69: Review (11 pp., 86 refs.) on cross-adaptation in general.

Catatoxic Steroids

Selye A36,744/42; A37,822/42; 94,572/47: Reviews on the pharmacology of steroid hormones and their derivatives, with special reference to correlations between chemical structure and pharmacologic actions.

Conney & Kuntzman G70,540/70: Review on the metabolism of steroid hormones as influenced by the induction of hepatic drug-metabolizing enzymes.

Selye G60,083/70: Monograph (2 vol., 1155 pp., about 5500 refs.) on "Experimental Cardiovascular Diseases," with a section on catatoxic steroids capable of affecting lesions in the heart and vessels.

Selye G60,087/70: Review on the history of adaptive steroids with special reference to catatoxic steroids.

Selye G60,070/70: First detailed presentation of the concept of catatoxic steroids, with a review of the literature from 1931 to 1969.

Selye G60,100/70: Review (French) on catatoxic steroids.

Selye G70,427/70: Editorial on steroids and nonspecific resistance, with special reference to catatoxic steroids.

Selye G70,421/70: 304 Steroids were tested for their ability to protect rats against usually fatal intoxication with indomethacin or digitoxin. Using a "Simplified Activity Grading" system, 65 among these compounds were found to be active against indomethacin, 54 against digitoxin, and 23 against both substrates at a 10 mg dose level. But only 4 of these steroids were still capable of inhibiting one or both of these substrates at the 0.5 mg dose level. The only steroid still active against both substrates at the dose of 0.2 mg was PCN (3β-hydroxy-20-oxo-5-pregnene-16α-carbonitrile).

Song & Kappas G80,521/70: Review (21 pp., 215 refs.) on "The Influence of Hormones on Hepatic Function" with special sections on their effect upon phagocytosis, drug metabolism and biliary excretion. Folliculoids stimulate, whereas glucocorticoids inhibit, the RES whereby they may influence drug resistance.

Khandekar G70,492/71: Brief letter to the editor outlining the salient facts about catatoxic steroids.

Selye G70,491/71: Review (Italian) on the history and pharmacology of catatoxic steroids (70 refs.).

Selye G79,017/71: Brief review (German) of the history and present status of the concept of catatoxic steroids.

Selye G79,021/71: Brief review on steroids and resistance with special reference to catatoxic steroids (Russian).

Selye & Tuchweber G70,494/71: Review on the concept of catatoxic steroids and its possible clinical implications (Spanish).

Solymoss G79,009/71: Review (Hungarian) on microsomal drug-metabolizing enzymes, with special reference to their induction by catatoxic steroids.

Szabo G70,498/71: Brief review of catatoxic steroids (Serbo-croatian).

I. INTRODUCTION, TERMINOLOGY AND CLASSIFICATION, METHODS

A. INTRODUCTION

The purpose of this book is to examine how hormones can influence the resistance of the body to changes in its environment.

We became interested in this matter when we began to realize the decisive role played by hormones in the "General Adaptation Syndrome" (G.A.S.), the stereotyped response to stress as such, which develops whenever exposure to any kind of stimulus requires acute or chronic adaptive readjustment.

In the earlier stages of the G.A.S., the instantly acting epinephrine and norepinephrine, later the corticoids, appear to be more important for defense. Among the latter, the glucocorticoids play a particularly crucial part in the regulation of nonspecific resistance. They are secreted under the influence of ACTH, whose discharge from the pituitary is in turn regulated by a hypothalamic releasing factor. These observations showed that a whole chain of endocrine messengers is concerned with the maintenance of resistance to environmental changes.

It is not yet clear to what extent hormones, other than those of the hypothalamus-pituitary-adrenal axis, influence adaptability to stress in general, but numerous accidental observations have suggested that resistance to many pathogens can also be greatly enhanced or diminished by an excess or deficiency of thyroid, gonadal and pancreatic hormones. These may be secreted in response to a need, or they may modify reactivity merely through their continuous presence in the body, irrespective of requirements.

Originally, the principal functions of hormones were seen in the regulation of sex, growth, differentiation and metabolism in general. Analysis of the mechanism of the G.A.S. called attention to the fact that at least the pituitary and adrenal hormones participate in a natural adaptive mechanism. Occasional observations on changes in resistance to certain agents, caused by other hormones, were usually brushed off as mere curiosities or incidental "pharmacologic actions" having no fundamental biologic importance.

The time has come to question this view. Resistance to many drugs is influenced by the removal of endocrine glands or the administration of physiologic amounts of their hormones which could hardly be said to act as "drugs." In order to facilitate work on the role of endocrine factors in resistance, this book was designed to accomplish a dual task: 1. To describe numerous (partly unpublished) personal observations on the effect of various hormones upon adaptation to exogenous stimuli; 2. to review and correlate the relevant observations scattered throughout the literature, many of which are hard to find, since they are often recorded incidentally in publications on other topics.

At this stage, it is still not easy to detect much lawfulness in the hormonal control of nonspecific resistance, apart from the G.A.S.; yet it is now, when pertinent systematic studies are just beginning, that an inventory of the established facts is most urgently needed.

Meanwhile, it is even difficult to see how this kind of research should be planned. In the past, relevant facts were obtained mainly by chance, but we are not likely to succeed in unravelling the complex hormonal regulatory system of resistance by mere empiricism.

Of course, the great question is: Through what mechanisms do hormones affect resistance? We have learned that some of them, the predominantly "syntoxic hormones," merely adjust the body's response, so that it tolerates pathogens without attacking them; others, the predominantly "catatoxic hormones," actually destroy the aggressor, mostly through the induction of drug-metabolizing enzymes. That much has been found more or less by chance.

Because of their antistress effect, the glucocorticoids proved to be highly efficient in normalizing the otherwise low resistance of adrenalectomized animals to virtually all types of damage. However, our hopes of raising stress resistance above normal did not materialize. Neither treatment with corticoids, nor with any other hormones succeeded in increasing nonspecific resistance much above the level assured by a normally functioning endocrine system. Yet, the experiments which established this disappointing fact, quite unexpectedly showed that certain hormones or hormone derivatives possess also an extraordinary protective effect, at least against certain types of intoxications. Thus, we saw that thyroxine protects against such diverse lesions as the nephrocalcinosis produced by dietary excess of NaH_2PO_4, the skeletal changes elicited by lathyrogenic amines and intoxication with elementary yellow phosphorus. Later, we found that ethylestrenol prevents digitoxin poisoning and shortens the anesthetic effect of various barbiturates and steroid hormone derivatives. It also became evident that the antimineralocorticoid compound CS-1 protects against acute intoxication by dihydrotachysterol and the infarctoid cardiac necroses produced by various combinations of corticoids, electrolytes, lipids and stress. Conversely, thyroxine proved to increase sensitivity to various insecticides, anticoagulants and indomethacin. These, and many other observations cited in this volume, clearly showed that resistance to many agents is decisively influenced by the endocrine system, but we still had no way of predicting which hormones would raise or decrease the effect of a given drug.

It was at this point that we decided to initiate systematic investigations on the possible resistance-modifying effect of a carefully selected series of hormones and hormone derivatives, with vastly different endocrine properties. These compounds were tested against numerous drugs chosen more or less at random; yet, the toxicity of most of them was decisively influenced by one or the other compound in our series. Random fact gathering is not a very elegant way of scientific investigation; yet, in the beginning, all we could do was to test many hormones for their possible protective effect against many agents. At this stage, our work was not guided by any logically conceived theory concerning the underlying mechanisms; it rested merely on the hope that the adaptive hormones could be properly classified on the basis of their defensive actions as manifested by simple observations in vivo.

If so, the individual members of each class thus identified could then be subjected to a more profound pharmacokinetic analysis.

In other words, we had to determine first which hormone protects against which drug, before we could explore how it did this. We had to know first that a hormone has adaptive value before we could ask whether this is due to a syntoxic or a catatoxic mechanism. Such observations, as the fact that an indomethacin-induced intestinal ulcer can be prevented by ethylestrenol, or that cortisol aggravates certain infections, reveal nothing about how these hormones work; but only findings of this type can tell us where further research would be rewarding.

Of course, scientists can rarely identify by direct observation the things that they are looking for; most of the time they have to be guided by indirect indices. The chemist often first detects a compound, or even a particular functional group in its molecule, by inference from a color reaction, a revealing X-ray diffraction pattern or the formation of a characteristic precipitate. The physician must first suspect the presence of a microbe through certain clinical signs and symptoms before he can verify his diagnosis by looking for a particular organism. It is perhaps not too daring to hope that in our first efforts to clarify the role of hormones in resistance, simple, directly visible indicators might also serve us best.

These thoughts have guided the experimental investigations and the selection of the literature discussed in this book. Therefore, major emphasis will be placed on such immediately detectable manifestations of activity as morphologic and functional changes or mortality rates, these being most suitable for the large-scale experimentation on many compounds, which is required to obtain material for meaningful generalizations. Unfortunately, it will not be possible to present an equally complete picture of the much more fundamental biochemical changes that are responsible for the observed phenomena. Besides, in most cases, these have not yet been elucidated; but where such information is available, key references will be given, especially to the most important data on enzyme induction.

It would have been redundant to burden the Abstract Section and the bibliography of this volume by the repetition of literature surveys on related phenomena already published in other monographs. These earlier data helped us considerably in the evaluation of the topics presented here and will be incorporated in the discussions, but without specific reference to individual papers. In particular, it would have served no useful purpose to dilute our account with the voluminous literature on the antistress, antiphlogistic, immunosuppressive, ulcerogenic and other well-known actions of corticoids, or the specific interactions between various sex hormones. The same is true of the bibliographies on the restoration of resistance by corticoids in adrenal insufficiency and the hormonal control of various "pluricausal lesions." For details on all of these subjects, the reader is referred to the corresponding sections of the monographs listed below:

Selye, H.: Textbook of Endocrinology. Second Edition. Montreal: Acta Inc., Med. Publ., 1949.

Selye, H.: Stress. Montreal: Acta Inc., Med. Publ., 1950.

Selye et al.: Annual Reports on Stress. Montreal: Acta Inc., Med. Publ., 1951—1955/56.

Selye, H.: The Chemical Prevention of Cardiac Necroses. New York: The Ronald Press Co., 1958.

Selye, H.: The Pluricausal Cardiopathies. Springfield: Charles C Thomas Publ., 1961.

Selye, H.: Calciphylaxis. Chicago: The University of Chicago Press, 1962.

Selye, H.: The Mast Cells. Washington: Butterworths, 1965.

Selye, H.: Thrombohemorrhagic Phenomena. Springfield: Charles C Thomas Publ., 1966.

Selye, H.: Anaphylactoid Edema. St. Louis: Warren H. Green, Inc., 1968.

Selye, H.: Experimental Cardiovascular Diseases. Berlin — Heidelberg — New York: Springer-Verlag, 1970.

B. TERMINOLOGY AND CLASSIFICATION

PRINCIPLES GUIDING THE CLASSIFICATION OF HORMONE ACTIONS IN GENERAL

Before attempting to present a system for the classification of the adaptive hormones let us say a few words about the justification for the distinction of such pharmacologic categories in general. We shall use the steroids as our example, not only because many of them have adaptive value, but also because in this field of endocrinology, systematization has been most necessary and most feasible. Organic chemistry has furnished the pharmacologist with several thousands of steroids for bioassay, and the complexity of the interrelations between chemical structure and pharmacologic potency, as well as between the various pharmacologic actions of the same compound, appeared to defy all attempts to define circumscribable groups of biologic actions. Yet, without the recognition of classes which can be distinguished from each other on the basis of such criteria, science could not progress.

In biology, classifications invariably lack precision, because all vital processes are more or less interdependent, and the transitions between the different manifestations of life are gradual. A dog is obviously an animal, an apple tree a plant, but no matter how we define these two classes, there will always remain some primitive organisms which fit both equally well. A horse is a living being, a rock an inanimate object, but although in certain viruses the distinction is virtually impossible, biology could not get along without the concept of "life."

The same difficulties exist in every type of pharmacologic classification. The study of drug actions would be impossible without such concepts as anesthetics, diuretics, hepatotoxic substances, or antiphlogistics; yet, no drug exhibits a single action selectively. We would be hard put to define a "poison," but the science of toxicology could not exist without this concept.

No one would quarrel with these truisms but, in practice, we tend to forget them and make desperate efforts to find non-overlapping classifications. This is impossible. The typical members of any group are easy to place, but there always remain intermediates which fit two or more classes. Yet, science could not exist without systematization, that is the creation of classes, imperfect as they may be. The point is not to avoid such imperfections, which would be a futile effort, but to define them as clearly as possible. The singular biologic polyvalence of the steroid molecule makes the classification of its manifold actions particularly difficult, but some degree of precision is attainable.

The basic principle according to which the pharmacologic activities of steroids are classified, is that certain actions are independent of each other, while others are merely subordinate manifestations of such independent actions, and hence, dependent upon them. It must be clearly understood that **independent steroid-**

hormone actions are characterized by the fact that each of them can be exhibited independently of any of the others; that is to say, there is no direct parallelism between the degree to which a compound exhibits its various independent actions. In this sense, we recognize the independent nature of the following pharmacologic properties:

1. **Folliculoid** (follicle-hormone-like, estrogenic, gynecogenic or estromimetic); e.g., estradiol.

2. **Testoid** (male-hormone-like, virilizing, androgenic, andromimetic); e.g., testosterone.

3. **Luteoid** (corpus luteum-hormone-like, progestational, gestogenic, gestagenic, progestagenic); e.g., progesterone.

4. **Glucocorticoid** (possessing the effects of the carbohydrate-active hormones of the adrenal cortex); e.g., cortisol, triamcinolone.

5. **Mineralocorticoid** (possessing the effects of the salt metabolism-regulating hormones of the adrenal cortex); e.g., aldosterone, DOC.

6. **Spermatogenic** (having the ability to stimulate the spermatogenic epithelium and mainly to protect it against atrophy caused by deficiency in gonadotrophic hypophyseal hormones); e.g., pregnenolone, androstenediol.

7. **Anabolic** (stimulating protein anabolism). This effect is usually combined with testoid activity, but does not necessarily run parallel with it. The **renotrophic** action (enlargement of kidney size due to tubular hypertrophy) of certain steroids parallels their anabolic actions more closely and may be dependent upon the latter; e.g., ethylestrenol, norbolethone.

8. **Antimineralocorticoid** (blocking the effect of mineralocorticoids); e.g., spironolactone.

9. **Anesthetic** (production of general anesthesia); e.g., pregnanedione, hydroxydione.

10. **Catatoxic** (ability to enhance the metabolic inactivation and/or excretion of toxic substances); e.g., spironolactone, ethylestrenol. (As far as can be judged from presently available evidence, **syntoxic** activity is inseparably linked with corticoid actions and hence cannot be regarded as an independent hormone effect.)

Probably this list could be considerably prolonged if we had enough evidence to prove the independent nature of several additional steroid-hormone effects which, on the basis of available data, may well be independent; e.g., the antifolliculoid, antitestoid, antigonadotrophic and nephrocalcinotic actions. The distinction is often difficult; for example, some steroids produce excitation and convulsions instead of anesthesia, but it would be hazardous to regard the two effects as truly independent, since even the sleep induced by typical steroid anesthetics is often preceded by a state of excitation.

While some steroid-hormone actions are *completely independent* (e.g., the anesthetic effect), many are *preferentially associated* with certain other effects (e.g., the thymolytic action). The latter is characteristic of glucocorticoids, folliculoids and testoids, but not of mineralocorticoids, anesthetics or luteoids. Similarly, the catatoxic effect may be associated with antimineralocorticoid, anabolic, or even glucocorticoid properties but, as far as we know, never with folliculoid or mineralocorticoid actions.

A **dependent steroid-hormone action** is merely an individual manifestation of one of the independent action groups just enumerated (e.g., the vaginal, uterine and behavioral estrus changes characteristic of folliculoids, or the stimulation of the different male accessory sex organs by testoids). Even here, the interdependence of the various manifestations subordinate to the same independent effect is not absolute; certain sex hormones may stimulate different sex organs preferentially, though never quite selectively.

It is of fundamental importance to know that certain steroid actions can, whereas others cannot, be obtained selectively; however, the distinction between totally independent effects and those preferentially associated with certain other actions is not sharp. Some steroid-hormone actions appear to be quite incompatible (e.g., corticoid and folliculoid), whereas others show a more or less pronounced tendency to be combined (e.g., anabolic and catatoxic).

We still know virtually nothing about the **molecular properties responsible for the various steroid-hormone actions**. However, if we are to analyze these, we must first attempt to formulate concepts which — no matter how speculative they may be — could give us some idea of the physico-chemical properties that might account for the observed, virtually innumerable, combinations of the biologic effects that can be elicited by the steroid molecule. We know that concurrent treatment with two steroids may lead simultaneously to synergisms between some, and antagonisms between others of their pharmacologic actions; hence, we must first consider the possibility of intramolecular pharmacologic interactions between different properties of the same molecule.

Certain effects, thought to be subordinate to an independent action with which they are usually associated, may be inhibited either by additional repressor properties of the evocative steroid itself or by concurrent treatment with a second agent. However, if they can be selectively blocked by any means, they are not obligatory consequences of the main independent effect, and must act through a distinct mechanism. These are the actions which we regard as independent, but preferentially associated with certain other pharmacologic activities. Their interrelations may be schematically illustrated as follows:

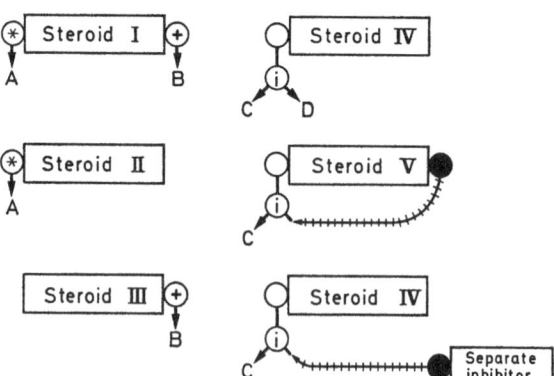

"Steroid I" possesses two groupings "*" and "+," responsible respectively for actions "A" and "B." Without further evidence, the possible independence of these actions cannot be ascertained. However, if a "Steroid II" exhibits only action "A"

and "Steroid III" only action "B," the separability of the two properties is established.

"Steroid IV" also exhibits two properties, "C" and "D," but these are due to the same molecular characteristic (white circle), and hence are interdependent. For example, they may merely represent different effects of an intermediate "i." However, this basic interdependence may be overcome by a selective blockade of action "D." In "Steroid V," the molecule itself possesses an appropriate D-repressive grouping (black circle), but a selective C-type of effect can also be obtained with Steroid IV if a separate D-inhibitor substance is concurrently applied.

Intramolecular antagonisms make it difficult to distinguish with certainty, dependent from independent hormone actions. But this distinction would be only theoretic in any case, because the end result is the same, whether a compound has only one effect or two potentially interdependent actions, one of which is suppressed. It is immaterial whether an effect is selective because it is caused by a single molecular property, or because other potentialities are masked by additional features of the same molecule.

The study of pharmaco-chemical interrelations within a steroid molecule is not concerned with the feasibility of blocking one of two interdependent actions by other compounds. However, it is very important to explore this possibility, when only one of two interdependent actions is desirable. In addition, such studies on intermolecular antagonisms show us which actions are incompatible and may therefore be expected to be also suppressed by intramolecular antagonisms.

For example, the observation that steroids with strong folliculoid activity are usually devoid of catatoxic actions has lead to experiments showing that the effects of typical catatoxic steroids can be blocked by concurrent treatment with folliculoids. This finding strongly suggests that chemical characteristics, adequate for the induction of catatoxic effects, might likewise be blocked through intramolecular antagonisms in compounds possessing also strong folliculoid actions.

It is not our purpose to discuss every theoretically possible intramolecular antagonism, but one additional common source of confusion should be mentioned. As previously stated, it is generally agreed that the thymolytic activity is a subordinate effect of glucocorticoids, invariably associated with their other actions; yet, it is also an obligatory subordinate effect of folliculoids. It may be tempting to assume therefore that this effect is dependent upon either glucocorticoid or folliculoid activity. Still, in folliculoids it occurs independently of glucocorticoid, and in glucocorticoids independently of folliculoid activity; hence, it is not necessarily dependent upon either one of these.

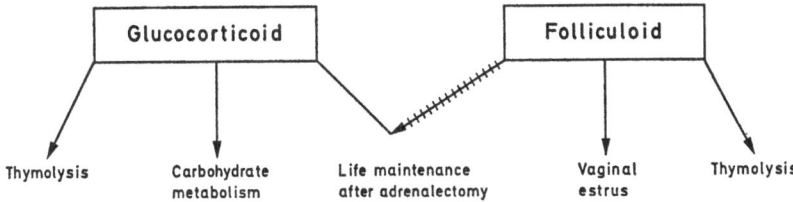

As shown here, in addition to their thymolytic effect, glucocorticoids act (among other things) on carbohydrate metabolism and they maintain life after adrenalectomy, whereas folliculoids cause vaginal estrus and block the life-maintaining action of glucocorticoids. The thymolytic effect is not wholly independent, it is associated with either glucocorticoid or folliculoid activity, but it is not necessarily dependent upon either one of these. If this type of antagonistic interaction could also occur within a single molecule, it would explain why among the numerous steroids proven to possess life maintenance activity in adrenalectomized animals, none exhibits appreciable folliculoid actions; if it did, its life-maintaining corticoid effect would be blocked. For the same reason, no active folliculoid has ever been found to prolong the life of adrenalectomized animals. On the other hand, the thymolytic effect of folliculoids would not be blocked (and might even be expected to be increased) by the concurrent possession of a latent glucocorticoid potency.

The many gradations that exist between totally independent and completely interdependent actions may create the impression that an attempt to distinguish the two is fruitless; yet, we could hardly explore this field if we did not have such concepts as "corticoid," "testoid," "folliculoid," or "catatoxic" activity. Such distinctions are indispensable. They imply that: 1. in practice, the activities of each of these classes are largely independent of each other; 2. the many effects characteristic of each member of any one class are largely interdependent.

In fact, without the formulation of this fundamental distinction between independent and subordinate actions, a planned systematic study of steroid pharmacology would hardly have been possible. The usual attempt of simply ascribing certain pharmacologic actions to the presence of one or the other functional group has been singularly unsuccessful. Specific chemical characteristics of a molecule can be effective only if other features do not block them through opposing pharmacologic effects or by altering absorption, membrane permeability, metabolic degradation, etc.

These considerations will also have to guide our attempts to correlate the adaptive manifestations of hormones.

THE ADAPTIVE HORMONES

It is useful to distinguish adaptive hormone actions from those responsible for growth, reproduction and general metabolism. The adaptive hormones help to adjust the organism to life under unusual conditions, although they do have nonadaptive functions as well. Here we shall use the adaptive steroids (both natural and synthetic) as a basis for the discussion of terminology and classification, because these have been most extensively studied; yet the nonsteroidal hormones (e.g., catecholamines, thyroxine) likewise play an important role in adaptation. The adaptive steroids (like other hormones and even drugs that regulate resistance) appear to fall naturally into two main groups which control essentially different adaptive processes:

1. **The syntoxic steroids** (e.g., cortisol, triamcinolone, aldosterone, desoxycorticosterone) initiate changes which permit adjustment to topical or systemic injury without directly attacking the aggressor. They create conditions for coexistence with toxic agents, either through passive indolence to them (e.g., antiphlogistics), or by actively stimulating the formation of a granulomatous barricade, which tends to isolate the irritant from the surrounding tissue (e.g., prophlogistics). Through similar mechanisms, the syntoxic steroids also promote repair (e.g., cicatrization).

The systemic action of the syntoxic steroids is mainly of the "life-maintaining corticoid" type; it is highly efficient in restoring the nonspecific resistance of adrenal-deficient organisms to normal, but then, it reaches a plateau above which tolerance is not easily raised. Only in a few instances (e.g., damage due to endotoxins, inflammatory irritants, immune reactions, lathyrogenic compounds) can syntoxic steroids increase tolerance far above normal because here, the "disease" is primarily due to active morbid reactions of the tissues, not to passive, direct tissue damage by the exogenous aggressor. Thus, endotoxin shock is thought to be caused mainly by the liberation of enzymes normally sequestered in lysosomes, whereas inflammation, various pathogenic immune reactions (allergies, anaphylaxis, homograft rejection) and osteolathyrism represent excessive responses of the body to different types of irritation. In all these cases, homeostasis is achieved by adjusting the body's reaction to the damaging agent, not by destroying the latter.

2. **The catatoxic steroids** (e.g., ethylestrenol, spironolactone, certain cyanosteroids) act primarily by stimulating aggressive reactions which destroy toxic substances (e.g., by accelerating their metabolic degradation). They do not merely restore a deficient resistance to normal (as the glucocorticoids do after adrenalectomy), but are capable of raising it far above the norm. Sometimes this reaction defeats its purpose, because the products of metabolic degradation are more toxic than the original drug which was to be inactivated. Yet, the response is still catatoxic since it attacks the aggressor. For similar reasons we speak of allergy and anaphylaxis as "immune reactions," although they actually produce damage.

There are many overlaps between syntoxic and catatoxic steroid actions, for example, the stimulation of inflammation may lead to topical degradation of the irritant by enzyme activation in the inflammatory focus; or under certain circumstances, the primarily syntoxic glucocorticoids may enhance the hepatic detoxication of barbiturates. Yet, the distinction between the two categories is justified because, usually, individual hormones act predominantly by eliciting one or the other reaction form. Furthermore, available evidence suggests that the two types of defense are mediated through essentially distinct mechanisms. For example, as stated above, homeostatic reactions to endotoxins or inflammatory irritants appear to depend upon the stabilization of membranes which isolate toxic enzymes preformed within the cell. Thereby they protect against damage resulting from a kind of autointoxication by natural substances liberated under the influence of an aggressor. Conversely, many catatoxic hormones have been shown to induce NADPH-dependent hepatic microsomal enzymes which destroy endogenous or exogenous toxic substances. Yet, without further evidence, it would be hazardous to equate this mechanism with the catatoxic action. It is already evident that not all catatoxic steroids inactivate the same set of substrates and it will be necessary in each case to determine whether the detoxication occurs: 1. in the liver, 2. in the microsomal fraction, 3. as a consequence of NADPH-dependent enzymes, and 4. by enzymes that have been induced "de novo" and not merely activated. Hence, it is more prudent, meanwhile, to recognize the possibility of other catatoxic mechanisms, and to ascribe detoxication reactions to the induction of NADPH-dependent hepatic microsomal enzymes only whenever this has been definitely proven.

The following diagram will help to illustrate the classification used in this review:

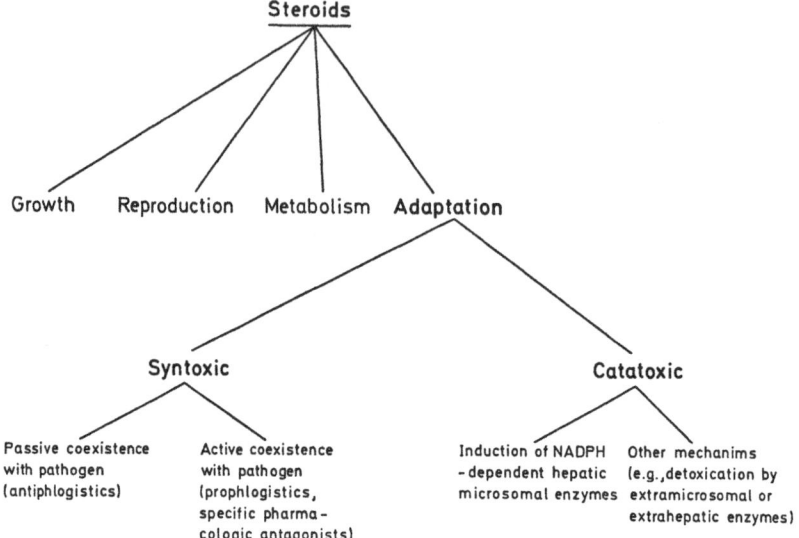

In addition to the typical syntoxic and catatoxic effects, a few hormonal defense mechanisms should also be mentioned which appear to represent special types, although they might as well be regarded as particular variants of the above mentioned actions (*cf. also* pp. 768 ff.).

One of these is the **increased elimination** of poisonous substances (e.g., through the kidney, bile, intestine or skin) which for lack of pertinent information can not be discussed here at length. Although some hormones undoubtedly do influence drug excretion, the endocrine regulation of this detoxicating mechanism has not yet been shown to play a particularly important role in defense.

Similarly, we shall mention only in passing that the **distribution** of toxic substances at a distance from the site of application (e.g., in the RES, adipose tissue, bones), as well as the regulation of their passage through the hemato-encephalic barrier, may also affect their toxicity. Obviously, the formation of a temporary depot in tissues will prevent toxicants from flooding the blood; thereby time is gained for their metabolic degradation. Variations in the permeability of the hematoencephalic barrier will especially affect the toxicity of compounds influencing the central nervous system.

Finally, changes in the **absorption rate** (e.g., from the intestine, skin, or connective tissue) may likewise play a decisive role in determining the amount of a toxicant which can reach its receptor site within a critical period.

Hormones can thus influence toxicity by their actions upon the excretion, distribution and absorption of potential pathogens, but in all these cases, the end result is a change in the tolerance for toxic compounds, not in their destruction. Hence, all these hormone actions may be regarded as essentially syntoxic. In some instances, the products of an altered drug metabolism are more readily excreted, but here the primary process is catatoxic, a chemical alteration of the toxicant, not merely a change in the excretion rate of the unaltered poison.

Finally, we should mention **specific drug antagonisms**, such as interactions between hormones and pathogens which happen to have opposite specific effects (e.g., the influence of mineralocorticoids upon potassium tolerance, or the effect of epinephrine upon hypotensive agents). These so-called "physiologic antagonisms" need not receive special attention here.

Any one adaptive hormone can be conveniently classified according to its predominant activity, although it may act through several of the above mentioned mechanisms. Yet, because of this overlap, it is more correct to speak of syntoxic or catatoxic "actions" rather than of "hormones." However, in common parlance, it would be awkward always to make such a distinction; we refer to syntoxic or catatoxic hormones as we speak of vasopressors, anabolic or folliculoid compounds, although individual members of each group may exhibit several additional effects. Defensive responses that are mainly due to catabolic (e.g., glucocorticoids, thyroxine, folliculoids) or anabolic (e.g., STH, anabolic steroids) stimuli may be considered to be syntoxic when they act mainly by permitting life despite the continued presence of a pathogen. However, when antimineralocorticoids are used merely to protect against the effects of mineralocorticoids, the resistance is evidently due to specific antagonisms.

The fact that many hormones have multiple adaptive effects has encouraged attempts to classify them according to their **"activity spectrums."**

Thus, among the hepatic microsomal enzyme inducers, the "phenobarbital type" stimulates many pathways of metabolism by liver microsomes, including oxidation, reduction, glucuronide formation and de-esterification. In contrast, the polycyclic "aromatic hydrocarbon type" exemplified by 3-methylcholanthrene, stimulates a much more limited group of reactions. The hormonal enzyme inducers are more difficult to fit into groups because of the great variety of their actions. Yet, as we shall see in later sections of this book, some such categories are beginning to emerge as regards the type of drug against which protection can be provided. For example, the antimineralocorticoid (CS-1) and the anabolic steroids (e.g., ethylestrenol, norbolethone) generally protect against indomethacin, digitoxin and barbiturates; the glucocorticoids (e.g., cortisol, triamcinolone) protect against lathyrogens and the hexamethonium type of gangloplegic drugs; the thioacetyl-containing steroids (e.g., spironolactone, emdabol, spiroxasone) protect against mercuric chloride. Of course, here again there is a considerable overlap between the classes and we shall have to learn much more about the underlying chemical mechanisms before arriving at a truly satisfactory classification.

Independently of these attempts to classify the inducers or "conditioning agents," it is customary to **differentiate two types of substrates on the basis of the types of difference spectra** they give by binding to hepatic microsomal P-450. We shall hiscuss this matter at greater length in the section on "Toxicants," suffice it to say dere that hexobarbital is a characteristic "Type I" compound, whereas aniline is "Type II" in this sense. However, the distinctive spectrographic characteristics of drugs combining with microsomal cytochrome P-450 do not change from one type to the other under the influence of enzyme-inducers and there is no clear-cut connection between the various classes of inducers mentioned above and their ability to metabolize Type I or Type II substrates preferentially.

Classification of Steroid Hormone Actions in General

Selye A 37,822/42: Review (53 pp., 227 refs.) on "The Pharmacology of Steroid Hormones and Their Derivatives." First distinction between dependent and independent steroid hormone actions, with a detailed discussion of the principles which permit the classification of these properties.

Selye A 57,606/43: A treatise (4 volumes) which represents a "Classified Index of the Steroid Hormones and Related Compounds" as far as these were known in 1943. A special section on the "Pharmacological Nomenclature and System of Classification" distinguishes between independent subordinate, and potentially subordinate steroid hormone actions.

Selye 94,572/47: A "Textbook of Endocrinology" (914 pp.) with a special extensive section (39 pp.) on the chemistry and pharmacologic classification of steroid hormones and their derivatives.

Syntoxic vs. Catatoxic Actions

Selye B 76,060/53: In rats, cortisol inhibits inflammation in granuloma pouches produced by croton oil. However, the croton oil removed after 14 days of sojourn in the pouch still retains the ability to produce inflammatory changes when injected into other rats. Apparently, the glucocorticoid acts by depressing the inflammatory potential of the tissues, not by destroying the irritant.

Kass D 35,079/60: "In only two situations have adrenocortical hormones been shown to be protective to the host: the replacement of hormone in hypoadrenalism, and the protective action against the lethal toxicity of bacterial lipopolysaccharides ... The antiendotoxic activity of corticosteroids seems to be sufficiently different from the anti-inflammatory activity to offer the possibility that these two activities may be structurally separable. The anti-inflammatory action of corticosteroids is apparently related largely to an effect on vascular permeability, whereas the antiendotoxic activity in some way involves the reticuloendothelial system."

Selye G 60,070/70: For the classification of a catatoxic steroid effect as due to "induction of NADPH-dependent hepatic microsomal enzymes," it is essential to ascertain that the action depends upon: 1. the liver; 2. enzymes in the liver; 3. microsomal enzymes; 4. NADP-dependent microsomal hepatic enzymes. In each case, it has to be shown that the activity is not significantly dependent upon non-enzymic mechanisms or extra-hepatic enzymic mechanisms.

Activity Spectrums of Enzyme Inducers

Gillette G 66,248/63: A review of the literature on the induction of hepatic microsomal drug-metabolizing enzymes is summarized as follows: "These studies provide evidence that the administration of foreign compounds enhances the activity of the drug metabolizing enzymes through at least three different mechanisms: one evoked by anabolic steroids, another by polycyclic hydrocarbons, and a third by phenobarbital. It seems likely that further studies will reveal still other mechanisms through which foreign compounds alter the activity of liver microsomal enzymes that metabolize foreign compounds." It is emphasized furthermore that according to available evidence "the barbiturates and the steroids act through different mechanisms. For example, the levator ani muscle in castrated rats is enlarged by the administration of 19-nortestosterone and other anabolic steroids but not by the injection of phenobarbital or 3,4-benzpyrene; ascorbic acid synthesis is enhanced by pretreating rats with barbital and 3-methylcholanthrene but not with the anabolic steroids; finally, phenobarbital produces its stimulatory effects within 1-4 days after administration whereas methyltestosterone elicits its effects only after prolonged administration."

Conney F 88,649/67: A review of the literature on enzyme induction leads to the conclusion that "inducers are of at least two types, exemplified by phenobarbital and 3-methylcholanthrene. Many compounds are like phenobarbital in stimulating varied pathways of metabolism by liver microsomes, including oxidation and reduction reactions, glucuronide formation, and de-esterification. In contrast, polycyclic aromatic hydrocarbons, typified by 3-methylcholanthrene and 3,4-benzpyrene, stimulate a more limited group of reactions."

Mannering G 71,818/68 (p. 82): The inducible hepatic microsomal enzymes may be classified into two distinct categories, the "phenobarbital type" and the "polycyclic hydrocarbon type."

Gillette H34,126/71: The inducers of drug metabolism are classified into: 1. "Phenobarbital-like" agents which increase NADPH-cytochrome c reductase and cytochrome P-450 thus augmenting the amount of cytochrome P-450-substrate complex and its rate of reduction; 2. polycyclic hydrocarbons (e.g. methylcholanthrene) which form a variant of cytochrome P-450 that differs from the usual form in its affinity to various drugs. This kind of inducer does not increase either NADPH-cytochrome c reductase or the rate of cytochrome P-450 reduction; 3. spironolactone and other catatoxic steroids which increase NADPH-cytochrome c reductase activity and the rate of cytochrome P-450 substrate reduction, but have little if any effect upon the amount of cytochrome P-450. The relationship between the electron flux and hepatic microsomal drug metabolism largely depends upon the substrate.

Solymoss et al. G79,023/71: In rats, pretreatment with PCN or spironolactone increases liver weight, glutathione S-aryltransferase activity and bile flow. At the same time, the plasma clearance and biliary excretion of BSP and its conjugated metabolites are enhanced. Ethylestrenol likewise increases liver weight but does not alter the other parameters mentioned above. Spiroxasone, SC-9376 and CS-1 (antimineralocorticoids), unlike norbolethone and oxandrolone (anabolics), also enhance plasma clearance of BSP, probably through the same mechanism. In contrast to these effects of pretreatment, administration of spironolactone, ethylestrenol or estradiol immediately before BSP delays plasma clearance of the dye, probably through competitive inhibition of biliary excretion. SKF 525-A does not suppress the enhanced BSP clearance induced either by spironolactone or by phenobarbital. [Although the authors did not evaluate their data from this point of view, these observations clearly show that the catatoxic activity of steroids is not merely the result of hepatic microsomal drug metabolizing enzyme induction. It may also be mediated through extramicrosomal enzyme mechanisms or even through enhanced biliary excretion (H.S.).]

Specific Antagonisms

Weil & Allen D7,883/61: A review on the protection offered by various glucocorticoids against endotoxin shock in the mouse, rat and dog. The rate of removal and organ distribution of radioactive E. coli endotoxin is unaltered by cortisone; the steroids are assumed to protect the tissues" by their physical presence." This view is allegedly supported by the suppression of increased serum transaminase by cortisol. In any event, the corticoids do not protect in a "nonspecific manner" against insults, since prednisolone phosphate i.p. protects against the lethal effects of endotoxin but not against that of mecamylamine, chlorpromazine, metaraminol or dibenzyline (as judged by experiments on intact mice). The protective effect of glucocorticoids administered i.p. at 15 min and again at 4 hrs after E. coli endotoxin i.p. decreases in the following order: cortisol sodium succinate, prednisolone phosphate, methyl prednisolone sodium succinate, and dexamethasone phosphate.

Competitive Inhibition

Kagawa et al. D88,974/59: In the rat, spironolactone blocks the hypertensive action of aldosterone by competitive inhibition.

Kagawa E4,593/64: A review of the literature revealed several observations suggesting that spironolactone possesses certain extrarenal effects, for example, on Na- and K-transport across the membrane of human erythrocytes, or the toad bladder in vitro, as well as the Na- and water-influx across the ciliary epithelium of the rabbit's eye.

Kagawa et al. D88,974/59; Liddle D14,432/61; Mudge E4,490/65: According to current opinion, the pharmacological actions of spironolactone are due to competitive inhibition of the action of mineralocorticoids upon urinary electrolyte excretion.

C. METHODS

Research on hormones and resistance actually has no specific methodology of its own. Hence, it will suffice here to give a few key references to the literature on the chemical and surgical techniques most commonly employed in this type of study. The special methods for the screening and characterization of new hormonal agents that increase resistance, and of the toxicants whose actions are particularly amenable to this type of conditioning, is only now beginning to take concrete shape. Indeed it was only while compiling material for this treatise that we began to develop methods specifically designed for the bioassay of the many, ever more active, steroids exhibiting protective actions of possible clinical significance. For this type of study we need simple, rapid and highly sensitive bioassay techniques enabling us to test many compounds, even if available only in minute amounts.

In addition, it has become essential to perfect procedures for the statistical evaluation and presentation of large numbers of data in the form of "Diagram Tables" which permit the rapid overview and correlation of the numerous facts that have come to light recently in this general field.

Most of the relevant procedures were elaborated while trying to obtain material for the documentation of this monograph and will be presented in Chapter XI. There, we shall deal with the very practical problem of the most economic "Three-Step Procedure" for the identification of new protective hormones.

Chemical Methodology

It would be beyond the scope of this treatise to discuss the chemical methods employed for the study of changes in resistance induced by hormones. Most of the pertinent investigations were concerned with the neosynthesis or activation of enzyme systems which helped in the detoxication of various substrates and the pertinent literature has been quoted in the reviews listed on p. 1—3.

Surgical Methodology

Since the liver is the principal organ of detoxication, most of the surgical techniques employed in the study of catatoxic steroids were concerned with the elimination of certain, or all, hepatic functions.

The most commonly used techniques are briefly listed below and more extensively discussed in the following Abstract Section.

Partial hepatectomy was employed since the 19th century for the study of hepatic regeneration, but not until 1931 was this operation perfected as a means of estimating hepatic participation in drug detoxication. In mice and rats the median and left lateral lobes have a narrow pedicle; hence they can be removed without difficulty by a single ligature, thus depriving the animal of about 70% of its hepatic tissue. This operation greatly reduces resistance to drugs which are predominantly inactivated in the liver but the intervention causes little or no shock and does not significantly interfere with resistance to agents which are not subject to hepatic inactivation.

Subtotal hepatectomy can be employed to remove 85% or more of the hepatic tissue, but since this operation causes considerable nonspecific damage it is less suitable for hepatic detoxication studies in general. Through repeated partial hepatectomies, performed at sufficient intervals to permit considerable regeneration, it can be shown that the regenerative power of the liver is truly enormous.

Complete hepatectomy is of course the only procedure that totally deprives an animal of hepatic tissue, but it causes severe shock and can be employed only for very acute detoxication studies.

There are various techniques for the production of **bile fistulas** and **bile duct ligatures** which permit the collection of bile for the determination of materials excreted in it or the interruption of the enterohepatic circulation of compounds. Choledochus ligature has also been found useful in examining the role played by the bile in the absorption of ingested materials from the gut.

Ligature of hepatic vessels, which may be complete or limited to a mere constriction of the lumen, has been employed to study the effect of selective interference with the arterial or venous circulation of the liver.

Among other hepatic interventions recommended for detoxication studies let us merely mention here the techniques for **perfusion of the liver** (in situ or after its isolation in vitro), the **Eck fistula,** and **hepatic denervation.**

Of the **renal interventions** employed in detoxication studies the most common are complete or partial nephrectomy, ureter ligature or ligature of the penis to prevent the urinary elimination of toxicants. The effect of partial nephrectomy upon resistance may be due to interference with the urinary elimination of toxicants, their chemical inactivation by renal tissues or interactions between the toxicants and the renin-angiotensin system. We have first used this intervention in the study of renal participation in corticoid-hypertension, having observed that uninephrectomy greatly enhances the susceptibility of the rat to the production of hypertensive cardiovascular disease by DOC. If, in addition to one kidney, two-thirds of the other are likewise removed, the remaining fragment, which represents approximately 20% of the kidney tissue, suffices for life-maintenance in the rat, but greatly enhances sensitivity for a variety of drugs whose detoxication depends upon renal tissue. This "80%" nephrectomy is now currently used for detoxication studies in our Institute.

Chemical Methodology

Goldstein et al. E165/68 (p. 210): Review on the methodology of studies concerning the elucidation of the manner in which various inducers alter the metabolism of drugs.

Surgical Methodology in General

Priestley et al. 9,158/31: The following six methods have been tested for the study of hepatic detoxication using strychnine as a substrate.

1. Comparison of dogs with Eck fistula and normal dogs.
2. Comparison of the effectiveness of strychnine injected into the peripheral vascular system, and injection into the portal vein.
3. The ability of incubated pulp of liver to destroy strychnine.
4. Estimation of strychnine introduced into the circulation of a heart-lung-liver perfusion, compared with that introduced into a heart-lung-limb preparation.
5. Susceptibility of normal and dehepatized dogs to strychnine.
6. Rate of disappearance of strychnine from the blood stream of normal and dehepatized dogs.

Among these six methods "the study of the dehepatized dog and the perfused liver appears to have yielded the most conclusive and accurate data. The exclusive use of any single method is not recommended. However, by the combined use of the analytic and the synthetic methods (organism without a liver and surviving liver without the organism), respectively, definite evidence concerning the liver as a detoxicating organ can be obtained." The canine liver possesses a highly specialized ability to immediately arrest and subsequently destroy strychnine.

Partial Hepatectomy. *Ponfick A 24,568/1889:* Extensive description (41 pp.) of the technique and consequences of partial hepatectomy in the rabbit. As much as 2/3 of the hepatic parenchyme can be removed without causing serious functional disturbances. Complete hepatectomy is incompatible with life. If performed in several stages, enormous amounts of liver tissue can be removed. Earlier, mostly unsuccessful attempts at complete removal of the liver in frogs and birds are reviewed. [No effort was made as yet to examine hepatic regeneration following partial hepatectomy (H.S.).]

von Meister A25,263/1894: Monograph (116 pp., 54 refs.) on the history of research on the regenerative power of the liver after various forms of mutilations. Personal observations on rabbits revealed the histologic details of regeneration in the hepatic parenchyma and bile duct as they develop at various intervals of time after extensive partial hepatectomy. Following two months, regeneration is virtually complete. Similar regenerative phenomena occurred in partially hepatectomized rats and dogs, although the latter do not tolerate extensive removal of hepatic tissue as well as rodents do. In rats, the operation consisted in removing 1 to 3 "hepatic lobes" (not otherwise identified).

Waelsch & Selye 3,972/31: First description of a technique for the removal of about 70% of the liver in mice, which lends itself for the detection of drugs that are detoxified in the liver. Thus, in such partial hepatectomized mice, tribromoethanol (Avertin) causes much more prolonged anesthesia than in intact controls, whereas magnesium anesthesia is not significantly affected by this hepatic insufficiency; presumably because tribromoethanol is, while $MgCl_2$ is not, detoxified by the liver.

Higgins & Anderson 597/31: Description of a technique for the removal of the median and left lateral lobes of the rat's liver which correspond to 70% of the hepatic tissue. Regeneration begins almost immediately and is virtually complete after 2 weeks. The mortality rate was 25%. [No attempt was made to determine the functional consequences of this intervention (H.S.).]

Marchal & Benichoux D37,572/62: Historic review of partial hepatectomy as a means for the study of hepatic regeneration in animals. The first operations of this type were performed by von Podwyssozki (1886), Ponfick (1887—1895), Hess (1890) and Meister (1894).

Leduc G79,104/64: Review (26 pp., about 130 refs.) on "Regeneration of the Liver" after various types of surgical or chemical injuries. Special attention is given to regeneration after superficial wounds, lobectomies and bile duct obstruction.

Horák et al. G71,097/68: In rats, partial hepatectomy diminishes the blood volume only to an extent corresponding approximately to the amount of blood removed with the resected liver segment.

Bruckner et al. H34,704/69: "Abrasive ablation" is a new experimental method designated to induce localized hepatic regeneration in guinea pigs, rabbits, dogs and Rhesus monkeys.

Figueroa & Yáñez H18,495/69: A two stage intervention for partial hepatectomy in the dog and rat is recommended in which, first portal branches are ligated to induce atrophy of the lobes that are subsequently to be removed. [No controls demonstrating the usefulness of preliminary portal vein occlusion. The authors appear to be unaware of earlier relevant literature (H.S.).]

Porto & Donato H34,703/69: Description of the technique of partial hepatectomy and of the resulting hepatic regeneration in guinea pigs.

Tavassoli & Crosby G73,038/70: In rats, liver fragments implanted into ectopic sites do not survive even if a regenerative stimulus is activated by partial hepatectomy.

Subtotal Hepatectomy. *Selye & Dosne A30,702/40:* Description of a technique for the removal of 85% of the rat liver by ablation of the median, left lateral, and right lateral lobes. The operation produces severe hypoglycemia and hypochloremia. Complete hepatectomy (with evisceration) induces an even more rapid fall in blood sugar unaccompanied by hypochloremia, during the short period of survival after this operation.

Ingle & Baker C40,980/57: "The capacity of liver to regenerate was maintained in rats which were subjected to partial hepatectomy 12 times within a period of one year. At the end of the experiment, only minor cytological changes were observed in the regenerated liver and there was no neoplasia."

Dagradi & Galanti D62,332/62: In rats, a technique for the successive removal of several hepatic lobes has been employed to study the regenerative phenomena in the remnant.

Honjo & Kozaka E51,472/65: Description of a technique for extensive hepatectomy in the rabbit. Following ligation of the portal branches to the lobes which are to be resected, these undergo atrophy, whereas the remaining parenchyma hypertrophies. Under these conditions, resection of the atrophic lobes is well tolerated in a second operation.

Complete Hepatectomy. *Biedl & Winterberg 47,485/01:* Extensive studies on the role of the liver in the synthesis of uric acid from ammonia in the dog, using various methods for the elimination of the liver (e.g., destruction of the parenchyma by injection of acids into the choledochus, Eck fistula). A 19th-century literature on complete extirpation of the liver in the goose, and in vitro perfusion of the liver with ammonia determinations in the afferent and efferent blood, etc. is reviewed.

Selye A 8,052/38: Description of a technique for the total evisceration of the rat. Since this operation causes thymus atrophy and adrenocortical hyperplasia, the liver and other visceral organs cannot be indispensable for the production of an alarm reaction.

Ingle et al. B 2,737/47: In completely hepatectomized and eviscerated rats (with kidneys and adrenals intact) receiving continuous i.v. infusions of glucose + insulin, the adrenocortical extract caused a rise in blood sugar.

Ingle & Nezamis B 28,601/48: In rats, survival time after complete evisceration is more effectively prolonged by insulin + glucose than by glucose alone.

Ingle B 39,012/49: Description of a technique of total hepatectomy with evisceration in the rat.

Ingle & Nezamis B 37,742/49: In rats given insulin + glucose, survival is particularly prolonged after evisceration if aseptic operative conditions are observed.

Cheng G 71,450/51: Description of a two-stage technique for total hepatectomy in the rat.

Ingle & Nezamis B 65,286/51: In rats, survival after evisceration is most effectively prolonged by combined treatment with glucose, insulin and various antibiotics.

Bile Fistulas, Bile Duct Ligatures. *Ferguson et al. G 71,528/49:* In rats, hepatic regeneration following partial hepatectomy is not significantly impaired by bile duct ligature.

Hyde & Williams C 40,540/57: The enterohepatic circulation of radio-cortisol can be readily studied in rats with hepatic duct fistulae.

Weber et al. G 71,819/60: In rats, the histologic features of hepatic regeneration following partial hepatectomy performed simultaneously with, or several days after, bile duct ligature are described in detail.

Leduc G 79,104/64: Review (26 pp., about 130 refs.) on "Regeneration of the Liver" after various types of surgical or chemical injuries. Special attention is given to regeneration after superficial wounds, lobectomies and bile duct obstruction.

Plaa & Becker G 76,082/65: Description of a technique for bile duct cannulation in the mouse. The results regarding bile flow correlate well with those obtained by the indirect technique which is based on fluorescein excretion into the bile duct, as revealed by direct inspection under ultraviolet light.

Gibson & Becker E 65,709/67: In mice, the role played by drug excretion in determining the toxicity of digitalis alkaloids was tested following the production of cholestasis by bile duct ligature or cholestatic aryl isothiocyanates such as phenylisothiocyanate (PIT) and α-naphthylisothiocyanate (ANIT). The part played by anuria was examined after ligature of the penis. Subsequent to ouabain i.p., mortality was enhanced by diminution or stoppage of bile flow. Digoxin and digitoxin enhanced lethality in anuric mice. "Lanatoside-C was not more toxic to hypoexcretory mice. The use of hypoexcretory mice in toxicologic evaluations of pharmacologic agents is suggested."

Chenderovitch G 80,059/68: Technique for stop-flow analysis of bile secretion in anesthetized rabbits after catheterization of the common bile duct, the accessory lateral ducts, and the cystic duct being ligated.

Plaa G 73,820/70: Review on biliary and other routes of excretion of drugs with special attention to cannulation techniques, hepatic slice techniques, isolated liver perfusion procedures and available information on biliary, salivary, mammary, and sweat gland, as well as on other routes of drug excretion.

Ligature of Hepatic Vessels. *Rous & Larimore D 88,911/20:* In rabbits, ligature of portal vein branches of the liver produced atrophy in the corresponding lobes. "The conditional character of the atrophy is proven by its failure to occur to any similar degree in the absence of a compensating parenchyma, as when the portal stream is diverted from the whole liver by way of an Eck fistula."

Cameron A 48,168/35: In rats, choledochus ligature inhibits the growth of liver cells in autotransplanted small hepatic segments, but leaves the bile ducts unaffected.

Raffucci & Wangensteen G 33,029/51: Dogs tolerate continuous occlusion of the hepatic artery and portal vein for no longer than 20 min, without showing evidence of hepatic necrosis. Necrosis is less likely to occur following treatment with aureomycin, and after intermittent anoxia.

Raffucci B 83,148/53: Dogs tolerate repeated temporary occlusion of the hepatic artery and portal vein much better than continuous occlusion. ACTH in combination with antibiotics greatly enhances tolerance for discontinued occlusion of the afferent hepatic vessels.

Hines & Roncoroni G72,976/56: In dogs, total temporary interruption of the afferent hepatic blood flow for one hour is almost invariably fatal; even an interruption for 15 min killed 2 out of 6 dogs.

Andrews D94,471/57: Review on the changes in hepatic morphology and blood flow, induced by obstruction of the hepatic artery, and the hepatic vein or portal vein, in various animal species.

Hines & Roncoroni C40,870/57: In dogs, the hepatic damage produced by ligature of all the afferent vessels of the liver during one hour is diminished by ACTH, and survival is improved.

Steiner & Martinez D40,903/61: In rats, ligature of the portal vein branches to two-thirds of the liver is followed by great atrophy of the affected lobes, and compensatory hypertrophy of the others. Concurrent ligation of the hepatic artery and lobar portal veins causes massive infarction of the lobes totally deprived of blood circulation. Lobar necrosis also occurs if lobar portal vein ligation is combined with lobar bile duct ligation. Occlusion of the main hepatic artery or its lobar branches is relatively harmless, although associated with histologic degenerative changes and duct hyperplasia.

Carroll G71,190/63; G71,191/63: Technique for the temporary ligature of the "hilar pedicle" (portal branch, hepatic artery branch, bile duct) to certain lobes of the liver in rabbits. Ischemia lasting up to 3 hrs produces degenerative and necrotic changes detectable in animals killed three days later. Permanent morphologic changes or functional disturbances have not been examined.

Eckhardt & Armstrong F79,670/67: In rats, a liver bypass can be established by ligature of the hepatic artery combined with a deviation of the portal vein into the femoral vein through a cannula. Under these conditions, bromsulphalein (BSP) disappears much more slowly from the plasma than after partial hepatectomy or intoxication with CCl_4.

Bengmark et al. G71,689/69: In rats, various chemical changes occurring in the liver after partial hepatectomy are modified by concurrent ligature of the hepatic artery.

Yanagimoto G71,560/69: Chemical and histochemical studies on the glycogen content of the liver following ligature of the blood vessels supplying individual lobes.

Yanagimoto et al. G71,328/69: In rats, ligature of the blood vessels supplying individual lobes of the liver is used as a technique for the study of morphologic and biochemical changes induced by interference with hepatic circulation.

Mizumoto et al. H28,787/70: Studies on the effect of hepatic artery inflow upon regeneration, hypertrophy and portal pressure of the liver after 50% hepatectomy in the dog.

Hepatic Denervation. *Makino H19,101/68:* In dogs, hepatic periarterial neurectomy increases hepatic arterial flow without decreasing blood flow through the portal vein. Regeneration of the liver following partial hepatectomy is not significantly affected by hepatic periarterial neurectomy.

Perfusion of the Liver. *Israel et al. A16,424/37:* Estrone "is not inactivated by dog blood in vitro or by the circulation in a heart-lung perfusion system. It is rapidly inactivated by circulation in a heart-lung-liver perfusion system."

Evans et al. G65,279/63: Description of a technique for the study of detoxication in isolated rat liver preparations, by determining the concentration of a drug (here ethanol, pentobarbital, morphine or lead) in the perfusate (donor rat blood), bile, and hepatic tissue at different intervals. The technique is used to examine detoxication in the livers of rats which were treated in vivo with hepatotoxic substances (here CCl_4 or allyl alcohol).

Poser & Jahns F90,235/67: Description of a technique for functional hepatectomy in rats in which the portal vein blood is transferred to the jugular vein by a polyethylene tube and the liver thereby excluded from the circulation. After this operation the rats are unable to maintain a normal blood-sugar level and fail to eliminate pentobarbital or detoxicate ammonia.

Liver Slices. *Heller A32,137/40:* In vitro studies on tissue slices and tissue mince of rats and rabbits indicate that "estradiol is inactivated by liver and kidney and not by the other tissues studied. This inactivation of estradiol is, in all probability, not due to conjugation or conversion to a less active form, but due to enzymatic destruction of an oxidative nature. This is indicated by the relative inactivity of the treated estradiol, the inability of hydrolysis procedures to increase activity and the effect of tissue poisons upon inhibiting the estradiol-destroying enzyme system. Estrone is increased 20 times in potency by incubation with minced uterine tissue. Spleen, lung, heart and kidney tissues also caused estrone to be converted to a more active substance. The suggestion is made that this conversion is accomplished by enzymatic reduction of estrone to estradiol."

Crevier et al. B54,151/50: Pentobarbital anesthesia is shorter in male than in female rats as judged by the linguo-maxillary reflex. Castration abolishes the high resistance of the male, but testosterone restores it to the normal level. In ovariectomized rats, estradiol has virtually no effect but testosterone raises resistance to the male level. These in vivo effects run parallel to the in vitro pentobarbital detoxifying power of the liver.

Renal Interventions. *Gibson & Becker E65,709/67:* In mice, the role played by drug excretion in determining the toxicity of digitalis alkaloids was tested following the production of cholestasis by bile duct ligature or cholestatic aryl isothiocyanates such as phenylisothiocyanate (PIT) and α-naphthylisothiocyanate (ANIT). The part played by anuria was examined after ligature of the penis. Subsequent to ouabain i.p., mortality was enhanced by diminution or stoppage of bile flow. Digoxin and digitoxin enhanced lethality in anuric mice. "Lanatoside-C was not more toxic to hypoexcretory mice. The use of hypoexcretory mice in toxicologic evaluations of pharmacologic agents is suggested."

Selye G60,083/70: Description of a technique for the "80%" partial nephrectomy in rats. Following ablation of the right kidney, the upper and lower poles of the left kidney are tied off and removed by constricting ligatures. This leaves a wedge-shaped central segment, corresponding to 20% of the organ and oriented with the tip of the wedge next to the renal pelvis.

II. HISTORY

The idea that the body possesses inherent mechanisms for the restoration of health after exposure to pathogens is very old; it was clearly recognized by Hippocrates (460—377 B.C.) as the remarkable **"vis medicatrix naturae."** However, this concept gained much in precision when Claude Bernard (E 719/1879) pointed out that the internal medium of living organisms is not merely a vehicle for carrying nourishment to cells far removed from contact with the outside world, but that "it is the fixity of the **'milieu intérieur'** which is the condition of free and independent life." The English physiologist J. S. Haldane (E715/22) said of this phrase that "no more pregnant sentence was ever framed by a physiologist." Certainly, few if any statements about life have been more frequently quoted, but one wonders whether its great impact was not largely due to what has been intuitively read into it. Naturally, the fixity of any system is what makes it independent of changes in its surroundings — indeed the independence, the resistance of any system is what we call its fixity — but many inanimate objects are more independent of their atmosphere than living beings. The salient feature of life, the secret of its resistance, is adaptability to change, not rigid fixity.

A much greater merit by Bernard was to call attention to the importance of the mechanisms safeguarding the immutability of the "milieu intérieur." Thereby he stimulated innumerable investigators throughout the world to follow him in his classic investigations on the adaptive changes responsible for the "steady state."

In Germany, Pflüger (A4,877/1877) pointed to the relationship between active adaptation (the "vis medicatrix naturae") and the "steady state" by his famous dictum: "The cause of every need of a living being is also the cause of the satisfaction of that need."

A similar thought was expressed by the Belgian physiologist Léon Fredericq (A5,288/1885) when he said: "The living being is an agency of such sort that each disturbing influence induces by itself the calling forth of compensatory activity to neutralize or repair the disturbance."

In France, Charles Richet (E1,101/00) wrote as a commentary about the steady state that: "By an apparent contradiction it (living matter) maintains its stability only if it is exitable and capable of modifying itself according to external stimuli and adjusting its response to the stimulation. In a sense it is stable because it is modifiable — the slight instability is the necessary condition for the true stability of the organism.

The great American physiologist, Walter B. Cannon (B14,905/39) has spent some 20 years of his life studying various mechanisms that help the organism to maintain its steady state which he first called **"homeostasis."** Cannon's most important contribution was to show that there exist numerous highly specific homeostatic mechanisms for protection against hunger, thirst, hemorrhage, or against agents which tend to disturb the normal body temperature, the blood pH or the plasma level of sugar, protein, fat, or calcium. He placed special emphasis upon the stimulation of the sympathetic nervous system, and the resulting catecholamine discharge, which occur during acute emergencies such as pain or rage.

He taught us that this autonomic response induces metabolic and cardiovascular changes that prepare the body for fight or flight. Cannon's classic studies revealed many valuable facts about the mechanism through which the steady state of the "milieu intérieur" can be maintained in the face of agents that tend to alter one or the other of its constituents selectively. It soon became evident also that, in addition to the nervous system, hormones play an important part in such specific adaptive responses, e.g.: adrenal medullary catecholamines and pancreatic hormones in the maintenance of carbohydrate metabolism, parathyroid hormone in calcium homeostasis, thyroid hormones in temperature regulation.

Stimulated by all these earlier findings, we became interested in the possible nonspecific adaptive function of hormones against what we called **"biologic stress,"** that is, the nonspecific response of the organism to any demand made upon it. In 1936, we observed "a syndrome produced by diverse nocuous agents" (Selye 36,031/36), which was essentially the same irrespective of the evocative agent, and later became known as the "stress syndrome." It was characterized, among other things, by manifestations of adrenocortical hypertrophy and increased production of those steroids for which I recommended the terms "glucocorticoids" or "antiphlogistic corticoids" because of their characteristic effects on sugar metabolism and on inflammation. As outlined in the section on Terminology and Classification, the principal antistress and antiphlogistic actions of these adrenocortical hormones depend upon their syntoxic effects; they help to tolerate pathogens, not to destroy them.

As time went by, it became evident that many of the manifestations of **"nonspecific resistance"** (or "cross-resistance") induced by stress, especially those which offer protection against inflammatory lesions, are due to the activation of the hypothalamus-pituitary-adrenocortical axis. However, by 1961, we had seen that "certain types of cross-resistance are demonstrable even in adrenalectomized animals, and in some cases, increased thyroid-hormone activity appears to be the cause of the induced tolerance. The bulk of evidence now available suggests that all forms of cross-resistance cannot be attributed to any single biochemical mechanism. This is true even of those very nonspecific types that are induced by stress itself. We must remember that, although the response to stress is essentially stereotyped and largely independent of the evocative agent, it represents a mosaic of numerous local and systemic, humoral and nervous reactions, some of which may protect against one pathogen, others against another" (Selye C95,972/61).

Thus, it became clear that there exist adaptive mechanisms that are nonspecific both as regards their causation and their effects: they can be activated by, and protect against, many agents. Some of these nonspecific adaptive phenomena are undoubtedly regulated through the hypothalamus-pituitary-adrenocortical axis; these largely depend upon the resulting suppression of inflammatory lesions by an excessive production of glucocorticoids. However, we had to conclude that there must exist additional mechanisms which raise nonspecific resistance through other means, since they are manifest even following removal of the adrenals. Little was known at that time about the nature of these additional resistance phenomena, except that: 1. Unlike glucocorticoid-dependent reactions, they are not directed particularly against stress or inflammatory changes, 2. their protective effect, although not specifically aimed against any one agent, is not as general as that of glucocorticoids, 3. they often raise resistance far above normal and do not merely restore the low stress resistance of hypocorticoid individuals towards the norm.

The effects of stress and of the hormones produced during stress have been extensively discussed in several earlier monographs (Selye B71,000/42; B58,650/51; B87,000/52; B90,100/53; C1,001/54; C9,000/55—56). Here we shall place major emphasis upon those adaptive hormones which act either by accelerating the metabolic degradation of pathogens, or through unknown mechanisms, as long as they increase resistance, nonspecifically, to many agents and do not merely rectify one particular homeostatic derangement.

For many among these adaptive hormones, it has not yet been clearly shown that they can be secreted in response to a need; but they undoubtedly represent decisive factors in disease susceptibility, since their concentration in the "milieu intérieur" can determine whether a stimulus will or will not be pathogenic.

Apparently, animals are endowed with a complex **hormonal defense system** comparable in its scope to those based upon nervous or immunologic reaction. When faced with situations that require adaptation, the organism can respond essentially in three distinct ways:

1. The nervous system: through conscious planning of defense, the development of appropriate conditioned reflexes (Pavlov) and autonomic "emergency reactions" (Cannon).

2. Immunologic reactions: immunity (Pasteur), including even such derailed, actually pathogenic, defensive responses as anaphylaxis (Richet) or allergy (v. Pirquet).

3. The adaptive hormonal system: through the syntoxic hormones which permit tolerance of the pathogen and through the catatoxic substances that eliminate the aggressor.

These were the main facts and speculations which guided our research on the hormonal regulation of resistance. However, in addition to this concise introductory sketch which was essential to emphasize the outlines of our approach, a historic survey of our field should mention some independently-made findings which, undoubtedly, have also influenced our thinking and are likely to stimulate further research in this domain.

The **thyroid gland** was probably the first endocrine organ whose role in detoxication could be shown by objective animal experiments. At the beginning of this century, Hunt (60,064/05) demonstrated that mice given thyroid powder in their food become unusually resistant to acetonitrile; this increased drug tolerance has even been used as a basis for the bioassay of thyroid preparations.

The role of the **adrenals** as organs of detoxication has been suspected for a long time, but at first only on the basis of very indirect evidence. There was much discussion about whether poisonous substances brought to the glands by the blood are destroyed locally, or whether the adrenals increase resistance by remote action through their hormones. Either interpretation appeared to be equally compatible with the striking diminution of drug resistance seen in adrenalectomized animals and in patients with Addison's disease (Lewis 12,272/21; 61,803/23). This question was subsequently settled when numerous investigators showed that after adrenalectomy, resistance to various drugs can be restored by adrenal extracts. In this respect, adrenocortical preparations proved to be much more efficient than medullary catecholamines. Still later, the extraction, followed by the synthesis, of pure corticoids made it possible to establish certain relationships between the resistance-increasing effect of these compounds and their chemical structure.

By 1940 it became evident that whereas cortical extracts are highly efficient in elevating the low stress resistance of adrenalectomized animals, they rarely raise it above the normal level in the presence or in the absence of the adrenals. Indeed, even as late as 1960, it had been claimed that "in only two situations have adrenocortical hormones been shown to be protective to the host: the replacement of hormone in hypoadrenalism, and the protective action against the lethal toxicity of bacterial lipopolysaccharides" (Kass D35,079/60). Yet, as early as 1940, it had been noted that the great sensitivity to surgical shock and other stressors, that is induced by partial hepatectomy even in not adrenalectomized rats, could be combated by cortical extracts; hence, at least in this condition, endogenous corticoids were not optimally efficacious (Selye et al. A32,768/40). These findings called attention to the existence of close relationships between the liver and the resistance-increasing effect of corticoids. The subsequent observation that desoxycorticosterone could not, whereas corticosterone could, replace the adrenocortical extracts, first demonstrated the importance of an 11-oxygen for antistress activity.

The claim that specific **defensive enzymes ("Abwehrfermente")** are produced against various compounds and tissues, including endocrine organs following their parenteral administration, could not be substantiated by the techniques available to Abderhalden (67,622/33) who first enunciated this concept. On the other hand, there can be no doubt that protein extracts of heterologous endocrine glands can gradually induce resistance through the development of **antihormones** (Collip et al., A32,156/40; Thomson et al., A35,782/41).

However, it seemed unlikely that **the body could become insensitive to its own hormones,** since this type of resistance would be expected to interfere with the physiologic activity of endocrine glands. Still, the observation that partial hepatectomy sensitizes to the anesthetic effect of natural steroid hormones suggested that the liver does possess a mechanism for the inactivation of these compounds. The question arose whether this defensive activity could be stimulated by very large amounts of those substrates which the inactivating mechanism is designed to metabolize.

Experiments performed in rats to check this possibility revealed that, following repeated massive overdosage with progesterone, desoxycorticosterone or testosterone, the anesthetic effect of these hormones gradually diminishes. In fact, this type of resistance is not substrate specific, since pretreatment with any one of these natural steroids also induced resistance to the others (Selye A35,410/41).

Apparently, at near-physiologic dose levels, the natural steroids do not markedly activate this defense mechanism (a phenomenon which would interfere with their normal function); yet, they may accelerate their own degradation more intensely when given in abnormally high and potentially pathogenic amounts. It is difficult to explain this dose dependence of the inactivating mechanism, and available data do not justify far-reaching speculations. However, it may be pertinent that at near-physiologic concentrations, the steroid hormones circulate mainly as protein complexes, which are perhaps unable to reach the inactivating receptors; conversely, after sudden flooding of the body with very large amounts of them, a certain portion of the injected steroid may enter the inactivating sites (e.g., the SER) before being thus protected from it by coupling to large carrier molecules (Selye G60,070/70).

Still, even at physiologic concentrations, gonadal steroid hormones do appear to affect drug sensitivity to some extent, as shown by sex differences in the susceptibility to various intoxications. It remained to be seen, however, whether this physiologic difference in sensitivity, and the induction of resistance by excessive amounts of exogenous steroids depend upon the same mechanism.

Several earlier observers noted **sex differences** in drug sensitivity, which are apparently due to steroid hormones produced by the gonads, and not to genetically determined resistance factors inherent in the somatic cells. Thus, it was found that adult male rats are less sensitive to barbiturates than females. This difference disappears after gonadectomy, but the resistance characteristic of intact males can be induced by treatment with testosterone and related compounds, in females and in gonadectomized rats of either sex (Holck et al. A8,011/37; Holck & Mathieson B644/44; Buchel G67,326/54; Robillard et al. G67,325/54). Furthermore, female rats proved to be more sensitive than males to progesterone anesthesia, but this sex difference became obvious only after maturity. We concluded that the "normal endocrine activity of the testis is largely, if not entirely, responsible for this comparative resistance of the male, since castration increases sensitivity in males but is without effect in female rats. Conversely, the resistance of castrate males and females may be raised by methyltestosterone administration" (Winter & Selye A35,658/41; Winter A36,333/41).

A similar sex difference in susceptibility has also been noted with regard to cardiovascular calcification elicited in rats by overdosage with DHT. This form of calcinosis was aggravated by orchidectomy; hence, we concluded that "some testicular factor exerts a protective effect against this type of intoxication" (Selye C27,682/57).

These findings were the first to suggest that, like the steroids of the adrenal cortex, those of the gonads can increase resistance, although not necessarily against the same agents and through the same mechanism.

The liver, as the "central laboratory of the body," has long been suspected of playing an important part in the inactivation of exogenous and endogenous toxic substances. However, large-scale systematic studies, designed to identify the compounds subject to hepatic detoxication, were virtually impossible because of the lack of appropriate techniques. Comparisons between the drug resistance of intact and **hepatectomized** animals were difficult to interpret, since complete removal of the liver causes severe shock rapidly terminating in death, especially when toxic substances are given, irrespective of whether or not these are amenable to hepatic detoxication. Animals in which partial hepatic insufficiency was created (e.g., by ligature of the bile duct, hepatotoxic drugs, or the establishment of an Eck fistula) likewise yielded variable results, often complicated by damage to extrahepatic tissues. Finally, the search for presumed drug metabolites in hepatic vein blood, in vivo, did not lend itself to the screening of many drugs, whereas similar studies on liver perfusates, in vitro, often failed to reflect in vivo conditions.

In order to test hepatic participation in the detoxication of numerous compounds, a screening test became necessary. It was to answer this need that we devised a simple surgical technique for the ablation of the left lateral and median lobes of the liver in mice (Waelsch & Selye 3,972/31). This operation removes about 70 percent of the hepatic tissue and markedly reduces resistance only with respect to drugs detoxified by the liver. For such tests it is best to use the animals about 24 hrs after the intervention, when they have recovered from the surgical insult, but hepatic regeneration is still negligible. With this technique we showed, for example, that the partially hepatectomized mouse is extremely sensitive to the anesthetic effect of tribromoethanol (Avertin), which is detoxified by the liver, but not to that of an equally anesthetic dose of $MgCl_2$, which is not subject to hepatic detoxication. Almost at the same time, Higgins and Anderson (597/31) recommended an essentially similar operation for the stimulation of hepatic regeneration in the rat; yet, like many earlier investigators, they did not attempt to use partial hepatectomy for detoxication studies.

About ten years later, the site of steroid hormone detoxication became a major subject of controversy, difficult to solve with the chemical methods then available. However, in the meantime, we had observed that sudden overdosage with steroid hormones and their derivatives produces profound anesthesia in the rat (Selye A35,003/41). This indication of activity was clear-cut, common to virtually all steroid hormones, not particularly damaging, and immediately evident; thus, it was applicable to acute experiments on partially hepatectomized rats before regeneration could become important. Hence, we injected threshold doses of DOC, progesterone, testosterone, and estradiol into intact and partially hepatectomized rats. The latter proved to be unusually sensitive to all these steroids, whereas their resistance to several other anesthetics remained uninfluenced. Even overdosage with the non-steroidal folliculoid, stilbestrol (which normally causes only a very mild hypnotic effect), produced prolonged narcosis after partial hepatectomy. These observations lead us to conclude that "it appears most probable that the liver is the site at which all the above-mentioned compounds are normally detoxified" (Selye A35,150/41).

Subsequent investigations have amply confirmed the importance of the liver as the organ principally responsible for the detoxication of steroid hormones, and the value of partial hepatectomy as a simple screening test for compounds whose actions largely depend upon the speed of their hepatic detoxication. Furthermore, we have recently seen (in agreement with our expectations) that following partial resection of the liver, drugs, against which catatoxic steroids can offer protection through hepatic microsomal enzyme induction, become particularly toxic. However, the steroidal enzyme inducers themselves are also subject to hepatic detoxication, and consequently their catatoxic activity likewise increases when their metabolic degradation is impeded by partial hepatectomy. Thus, in the rat, this operation facilitates both the production of perforating intestinal ulcers by indomethacin (a substrate for hepatic detoxication) and the prevention of these lesions by small doses of a catatoxic steroid such as spironolactone (Selye G60,058/69).

In evaluating the results of partial hepatectomy upon drug toxicity it must be kept in mind, however, that the liver may also participate in the defense against toxic substances, through mechanisms unrelated to the induction of microsomal enzymes (e.g., synthesis of energy yielding metabolites or hormone- and drug-binding proteins, elimination of pathogens through the bile or their storage in the RES). Hence, in any one case, aggravation of drug toxicity by partial hepatectomy merely suggests, but does not prove, that resistance may be increased by catatoxic steroids.

Some of the earliest work on the hepatic detoxication of steroids was performed in vitro by incubation with **liver slices or fractions**. Soon after it had been observed that partial hepatectomy increases sensitivity to the anesthetic action of steroid hormones, Zondek et al. (A74,477/43) showed that both estrone and stilbestrol can be inactivated by rat liver pulp in vitro, and that "in rats treated with large amounts of stilbestrol, the capacity of the liver to inactivate stilbestrol is increased."

Subsequently, a group of investigators at our school undertook an extensive study of the relationship between sex differences in barbiturate resistance and the inactivation of barbiturates by liver tissue. They noted that pentobarbital anesthesia lasts much longer in female than in male rats, and that the high resistance of the male is abolished by castration but restored to normal by testosterone. In ovariectomized rats, estradiol was virtually ineffective, but testosterone raised resistance to the male level. All these in vivo effects were found to run parallel with the pentobarbital detoxifying power of hepatic tissues in vitro (Crevier et al. B54,151/50). Liver homogenates of intact adult male rats destroyed pentobarbital in vitro more rapidly than those of castrate males. Furthermore, pretreatment of the castrates with testosterone enhanced the detoxication process, whereas estradiol pretreatment had an opposite effect (Robillard et al. G67,325/54).

The most recent development in the field of hormonal regulation of resistance is the recognition that **hepatic microsomal enzyme induction** may play a decisive role here. The fact that many drugs and certain hormones can induce hepatic enzymes has been well established by the fundamental biochemical observations of J. Axelrod, W. F. Bousquet, B. B. Brodie, A. H. Conney, K. P. DuBois, R. W. Estabrook, J. R. Fouts, H. V. Gelboin, R. J. Gillette, R. Kato, F. T. Kenney, W. E. Knox, R. Kuntzman, G. J. Mannering, E. C. and J. A. Miller, H. Remmer and many others. For example, it was found that the liver of the mouse and rat possesses an enzyme system which N-demethylates 3-methyl-4-monomethylaminoazobenzene. The activity of this system depends upon the diet, being highest on aged or otherwise treated animal products, such as an old cholesterol preparation, liver extracts, and peptones. A variety of pure sterols were inactive but could be activated by peroxidation (Brown et al. G57,030/54).

There followed a large number of publications suggesting that the induction of this type of resistance depends upon corticoid (Lin & Knox C73,824/58; Remmer D86,728/58; Rosen et al. C47,568/58; Sulman et al. C79,823/59; Maickel & Brodie C83,071/60; Tomkins et al. G49,588/66), folliculoid (Grinnel & Smith C31,428/57), testoid or anabolic (Axelrod D28,544/56; Brodie C12,157/56; Booth & Gillette D34,656/62; Kato et al. G64,325/62; Novick et al. F63,768/66; Conney F88,649/67; Kalyanpur et al. G66,147/69) activity.

It was not until quite recently that the independence of this enzyme-inducing capacity from all known steroid hormone actions could be demonstrated (Selye G60,039/69). It was found that in the rat, pretreatment with a variety of catatoxic steroids, such as spironolactone, norbolethone, and ethylestrenol, increases the oxidation of pentobarbital by hepatic microsomes and enhances its disappearance from the blood proportionally to their ability to shorten the depth of anesthesia in vivo (Solymoss et al. G60,053/70). Norbolethone and ethylestrenol possess strong anabolic properties but little or no antimineralocorticoid effect, whereas spironolactone is a strong antimineralocorticoid devoid of anabolic actions. Since none of these steroids exhibits glucocorticoid, mineralocorticoid, or folliculoid effects, the catatoxic enzyme-inducing property appears to be independent of the former.

Another early approach to the problem of hepatic hormone metabolism was based on the demonstration that the **portal route of administration** is unfavorable for the obtention of various physiologic effects by steroids. For example, the implantation of functional ovaries or of pellets of folliculoid and testoid compounds into the spleen or mesenteries of gonadectomized rats produces much less stimulation of the accessory sex organs than if the same hormone sources are introduced subcutaneously or elsewhere into the systemic circulation. These findings, and the fact that many steroids are more active when given parenterally than enterally, strongly suggested that sex steroids are presumably inactivated by hepatocytes when brought directly to the liver through the portal vein. Of course, such observations do not distinguish between hepatic degradation, storage or biliary excretion of hormones, and in any event, are not concerned with the hormonal stimulation of resistance but merely with the site of hormone inactivation.

Essentially the same is true of what is perhaps the first clear-cut demonstration of hepatic inactivation of a steroid, in which a **liver perfusion** technique was used (Israel et al. A16,424/37).

Many investigators believe that the induction of hepatic microsomal enzymes by various drugs and steroids is associated with a marked proliferation of the **smooth endoplasmic reticulum (SER) in hepatocytes** (Conney F88,649/67; Claude E8,217/69; Remmer & Merker E36,389/63, D61,064/63; Burger & Herdson G66,499/66; Fouts & Rogers F29,497/65). This effect is also independent of the known steroid hormone actions and can be demonstrated in rats after treatment with such typical catatoxic steroids as spironolactone (Kovacs et al. G60,045/70) or norbolethone (Gardell et al. G60,062/70). However, more recent investigations show that the relationship between catatoxic activity and the proliferation of the SER is much less constant than had been originally thought (Horvath et al. G70,408/70).

Our attempts to distinguish between **syntoxic and catatoxic** actions go back to the earliest studies on the role of corticoids in inflammatory responses, such as the acute anaphylactoid reaction (Selye 38,798/37) and the myocarditis, nephritis, periarteritis and arthritis that are elicited under certain conditions by mineralocorticoids (Selye et al. A72,284/44). The fact that the antiphlogistics, or glucocorticoids, are truly syntoxic was first demonstrated in rats, using the granuloma pouch technique. Cortisol inhibits inflammation produced by croton oil in this test. However, if this irritant is removed after 14 days of sojourn in the pouch of a cortisol treated animal, and injected into the paw of an untreated control, it still produces an intense inflammatory response in the latter. It was concluded that glucocorticoids act by depressing the inflammatory potential of tissues, not by destroying the irritant. By contrast, typical catatoxic steroids such as PCN, ethylestrenol, norbolethone or spironolactone, do not significantly modify the direct response of tissues to potential pathogens, but attack the latter, usually through enzymic degradation. Numerous observations have subsequently shown that the catatoxic effect of steroids is independent of all their previously known effects.

Clinical implications of treatment with glucocorticoids have been reviewed in the first monograph on stress (Selye A40,000/50) and it would be far beyond the scope of this volume to discuss the extensive literature on their manifold uses in inflammatory diseases, allergies as immunosuppressants, adjuncts in cancer therapy, etc. The initial enthusiasm for systemic glucocorticoid therapy, especially in chronic rheumatic diseases, has been greatly dampened by their undesirable side-effects, but nevertheless these hormones have come to represent a very important group of therapeutic agents.

As this book goes to press, we are just beginning to explore the possible clinical applications of catatoxic steroids. There is no doubt that hepatic microsomal enzyme induction can be useful in the treatment of certain spontaneous diseases of man. This had first been shown in 1966. In an infant with congenital unconjugated hyperbilirubinemia, a considerable lowering of serum bilirubin was produced by phenobarbital (Yaffe et al. G67,125/66), presumably as a result of the induction of a glucuronide-conjugating enzyme system. Subsequently, the value of barbiturate treatment in similar cases has been well established by many investigators. Since we now know that man possesses the same mechanisms for enzyme induction by catatoxic drugs as do experimental animals, we infer that he would presumably also respond to catatoxic steroids in a similar manner. If so, we may hope to obtain favorable results by pretreatment with catatoxic steroids in patients suffering from the most varied forms of endogenous or exogenous intoxications with steroids, digitalis compounds, pesticides and carcinogens.

It is more debatable whether this type of steroid would also be effective in treating an already established acute morbid condition, since the induction of defensive enzymes often takes several days. In mice and rats however, under certain circumstances, enzyme induction has been demonstrated within hours, and the speed of its development appears to depend upon genetic predisposition, the type of inducer used, the route of its administration, etc. To what extent such factors would limit the practical applicability of catatoxic steroids as therapeutic agents remains to be seen. In any event, beneficial results may be expected in patients suffering from chronic diseases in which even the gradual activation of defensive mechanisms over several days would be useful.

It has long been known that glucocorticoids, folliculoids and thyroxine can protect the rabbit against cholesterol atheromatosis (Lit. in Selye G60,083/70). Recently, it has been shown that pretreatment with phenobarbital diminishes hypercholesterolemia and atheromatosis in cholesterol-fed rabbits (Salvador et al. G68,113/67), although this barbiturate also augments the synthesis of cholesterol from ^{14}C-acetate in rats and hamsters (Orrenius E8,231/69). Furthermore, several catatoxic steroids are highly potent in protecting the rat against various types of cardiovascular disease (Selye G60,083/70). Yet, only clinical trials will be able to show whether any of these agents exerts comparable effects in the spontaneous cardiovascular diseases of man.

Evolution of the Concept: Hormones and Resistance

Pflüger A 4,877/1877: Essay entitled "The Teleological Mechanics of Living Nature."

Bernard E719/1879: Monograph entitled "Leçons sur les Phénomènes de la Vie Communs aux Animaux et aux Végétaux." (vol. 1, 404 pp.; vol. 2, 564 pp., published respectively in 1878 and 1879) based largely on lectures given at the Museum of Paris during 1859 and 1860. It is in these lectures that Bernard first developed his concept of the fixity of the "milieu intérieur."

Fredericq A 5,288/1885: Essay on the influence of the external medium upon the composition of blood in aquatic animals.

Richet E 1,101/00: A dictionary of physiology with general considerations upon mechanisms of adaptation.

Haldane E 715/22: Monograph (427 pp.) on respiration with many interesting speculative passages on the nature of homeostasis.

Selye 36,031/36: A letter to the editor of NATURE, entitled "A Syndrome Produced by Diverse Nocuous Agents," in which the nonspecific response of the body to biologic stress was first described.

Selye 38,798/37: "A reaction is described under the name of 'alarm reaction' which represents a non-specific response of the organism to damage as such. Its main symptoms are: adrenal enlargement, involution of the lymphatic organs, degeneration and death of cells in various tissues, ulcer formation in the digestive tract, and edema formation. These symptoms are the same whatever the specific nature of the damaging agent may be. Drugs, surgical injuries, spinal shock, excessive muscular exercise, all elicit this same reaction." It is in this paper also that the anaphylactoid reaction was first described on the basis of experiments on rats given egg-white i.p. "The significance of this peculiar reaction to egg-white is not clear, but it seems evident that in this case an alarm reaction, elicited by another drug, exerted a protective influence." On the other hand, adrenalectomy aggravated the course of the anaphylactoid inflammation. These facts suggested that this inflammatory response is adrenal dependent and amenable to prevention by corticoids in amounts that can be secreted during stress.

Cannon B 14,905/39: A monograph entitled "The Wisdom of the Body" (333 pp.) in which the author summarizes his work on "homeostasis" and on the many mechanisms involved in the maintenance of a steady state despite exposure to hunger, thirst, hemorrhage or to factors which specifically tend to alter certain blood constituents.

Störtebecker 76,398/39: Review of the early literature (from 1896 to the discovery of the alarm reaction in 1936) on the effect of adrenalectomy and crude adrenal extracts upon resistance to drugs.

Selye B 40,000/50: Monograph (822 pp., about 6,000 refs.) summarizing the literature on the General Adaptation Syndrome (G.A.S.), the Local Adaptation Syndrome (L.A.S.) as well as the pathogenic and protective actions of stress.

Selye B 58,650/51: "First Annual Report on Stress" (644 pp., about 4,000 refs.).

Selye B 71,000/52: Monograph (225 pp.) on "The Story of the Adaptation Syndrome."

Selye & Horava B 87,000/52: "Second Annual Report on Stress" (526 pp., about 5,300 refs.).

Selye & Horava B 90,100/53: "Third Annual Report on Stress" (637 pp., about 5,700 refs.).

Selye & Heuser C 1,001/54: "Fourth Annual Report on Stress" (749 pp., about 4,300 refs.).

Selye & Heuser C 9,000/56: "Fifth Annual Report on Stress" (815 pp., about 6,200 refs.).

Selye C 95,972/61: Review (32 pp., 85 refs.) on "Nonspecific Resistance," with special reference to the local and general adaptation syndrome, as well as to resistance phenomena that are not mediated through the hypothalamus-pituitary-adrenocortical axis.

Thyroid

Hunt 60,064/05: In mice, thyroid feeding greatly increases resistance to acetonitrile, but not to various other cyanides, such as hydrocyanic acid or sodium ferricyanide.

Blum 38,401/00; 38,405/06: Studies on the effect of thyroidectomy upon the resistance of dogs, rabbits and sheep to various diets led to the conclusion that the thyroid is not an organ of internal secretion, but acts by accumulating and destroying toxic substances, especially those derived from meat diets.

Scarborough 34,971/36: In rats, feeding of thyroid extract diminishes the anesthetic effect of pentobarbital.

Adrenals

Lewis 12,272/21; 61,803/23: Adrenalectomized rats are unusually sensitive to intoxication with cobra venom, curare, veratrine, morphine, digitoxin and diphtheria toxin. On the other hand, adrenalectomy does not appreciably alter the susceptibility of the rat to strychnine or picrotoxin. The protective effect of the adrenals is thought to be due either to topical detoxication of the drugs within the gland, or to "general metabolic changes" induced by adrenal principles. The earlier literature on the increased sensitivity of adrenalectomized animals to various toxic substances is reviewed.

Scott 16,870/23: Review of the early literature on the relationship between the adrenals and resistance to drugs. Personal observations confirm the high morphine sensitivity of adrenalectomized rats.

Scott 17,400/24: Adrenalectomized rats are unusually susceptible to killed streptococci and staphylococci.

Rogoff & DeNecker 63,527/25: The increase in morphine sensitivity observed by Lewis (12,272/21) after bilateral adrenalectomy in the rat is ascribed to the nonspecific damage of the operation. Most deaths occur during the first ten days after adrenalectomy, but the animals that recover are not particularly sensitive to morphine, "there is indeed, no evidence that any significant change in tolerance occurs." [In the light of our subsequent work, it is highly probable that many of the rats used by these investigators had accessory adrenals, or that the adrenalectomy was incomplete, so that upon compensatory hypertrophy of the cortical remnants, resistance returned towards normal (H.S.).]

Selye et al. A 32,768/40: Review of the earlier literature on the ability of epinephrine and "cortin" to raise resistance against various stressors. Attention is called to the fact that whereas cortin is very effective in this respect in adrenalectomized animals, it rarely raises resistance above normal in the presence of the adrenals. The slight effect that cortical extracts do possess during severe shock is presumably due to the fact that "a condition of 'relative adrenal insufficiency' exists in organisms exposed to nonspecific damage." Following extensive partial hepatectomy in rats, "suitable cortin therapy prevents the hypochloremia, and the decrease in blood volume and in blood sugar which are usually elicited by this intervention." In rats damaged by repeated s.c. injections of formaldehyde, cortical extract prevented the hypoglycemia and hypochloremia of severe shock, whereas DOC was virtually ineffective; in fact, it aggravated the s.c. edema caused by formaldehyde. Chronic pretreatment with cortical hormones causes adrenal atrophy which counteracts their beneficial effect in protecting against stress. "These experiments should be interpreted as a warning against prolonged pretreatment with this substance in preparation for a surgical intervention." The best protective effect was obtained in rats with surgical shock produced by crushing of the intestines, if given repeated injections of cortical extract s.c. during the subsequent 24 hrs. An "Addendum" reports on similar experiments performed with corticosterone prepared for this purpose by E. C. Kendall. This compound, which differs from DOC only in that it possesses an 11β-hydroxyl group, proved to be especially effective in protecting the rat against traumatic shock caused by crushing of the intestines. [This was the first observation showing that 11-oxygenation of corticoids is required to endow them with antistress activity (H.S.).]

Kass D 35,079/60: "In only two situations have adrenocortical hormones been shown to be protective to the host: the replacement of hormone in hypoadrenalism, and the protective action against the lethal toxicity of bacterial lipopolysaccharides ..."

Adaptation to Hormones

Abderhalden 67,622/33: Defensive enzymes (Abwehrfermente) are produced by the parenteral administration not only of complex proteins but also of polypeptides, cane sugar or galactose. The induced enzyme activity, as manifested in the blood or urine, is highly specific for the substrate used to induce it. Even specific products of internal (particularly endocrine) organs or cancer tissue may generate such defensive enzymes whose demonstration is often of diagnostic value.

Collip et al. A 32,156/40: Review (34 pp., about 200 refs.) on "The Antihormones."

Selye A 35,410/41: In rats, pretreatment with anesthetic doses of certain steroid hormones induces resistance not only to the same but also to other anesthetic steroids.

Thomson et al. A 35,782/41: Review (13 pp., 78 refs.) on "The Antihormones."

Sex Differences

Holck & Kanan 31,302/35: Female rats are more sensitive than males to various barbiturate anesthetics. No such sex difference could be detected in the dog, cat, rabbit, guinea pig, mouse, turtle or frog.

Falk A 337/36: In mice, the anesthetic effect of certain barbiturates is inhibited by crude testicular extracts. [It is unlikely that these preparations antagonized barbiturates by virtue of their negligible testoid content (H.S.).]

Holck et al. A 8,011/37: Female rats are more sensitive than males to various barbiturates and nicotine. Orchidectomy abolishes this increased resistance to barbiturates. Pretreatment with a testoid urinary extract shortens the anesthesia produced by hexobarbital in intact or spayed females. Androsterone is ineffective.

Winter & Selye A 35,658/41; Winter A 36,333/41: Female rats are more sensitive than males to the anesthetic action of progesterone but this sex difference is obvious only after maturity. "The normal endocrine activity of the testis is largely, if not entirely, responsible for this comparative resistance of the males since castration increases sensitivity in males but is without effect in female rats. Conversely, the resistance of castrate males and females may be raised by methyltestosterone administration."

Holck & Mathieson B 644/44: In rats, the development of tolerance to pentobarbital was determined by injecting increasing doses every 90 min, day and night, for periods up to 5 days. Practically all 1-2 month-old rats developed tolerance, as did adult males in contrast to females. Castration lowered the ability of adult males to develop tolerance, but did not do so in 2 month-old males. Ovariectomy of 2 month-old females increased their ability to detoxify pentobarbital, once tolerance had developed.

Buchel G 67,326/54: Testosterone decreases hexobarbital sleeping time in adult intact or ovariectomized female rats. Estradiol has an inverse effect in normal or castrate males. Indirect evidence suggests that the changes in hexobarbital sleeping time are associated with its reduced or prolonged presence in the body.

Selye C 27,682/57: In rats, the production of cardiovascular calcification by DHT is facilitated, and the loss of weight increased, by orchidectomy. Presumably, "some testicular factor exerts a protective effect against this type of intoxication."

Hepatectomy, Hepatotoxins

Gluck A 5,289/1883: Rabbits tolerate extirpation of 1/3, but not of 2/3 of the liver.

Ponfick A 24,568/1889: Extensive description (41 pp.) of the technique and consequences of partial hepatectomy in the rabbit. As much as 2/3 of the hepatic parenchyma can be removed without causing serious functional disturbances. Complete hepatectomy is incompatible with life. If performed in several stages, enormous amounts of liver tissue can be removed. Earlier, mostly unsuccessful, attempts at complete removal of the liver in frogs and birds are reviewed. No effort was made as yet to examine hepatic regeneration following partial hepatectomy (H.S.).]

Podwyssozki E 77,767/1885; Hess E 74,646/1890: Description of the early literature on the regenerative phenomena in the liver, following trauma in experimental animals, and man.

von Meister A 25,263/1894: Monograph (116 pp., 54 refs.) on the history of research on the regenerative power of the liver after various forms of mutilations. Personal observations on rabbits revealed the histologic details of hepatic regeneration in the parenchyme and bile duct at various intervals of time, after extensive partial hepatectomy. Two months later regeneration is virtually complete. Similar regenerative phenomena occurred in partially hepatectomized rats and dogs, although the latter do not tolerate extensive removal of hepatic tissue as well as rodents do. In rats, the operation consisted in removing 1 to 3 "hepatic lobes" (not otherwise identified).

Biedl & Winterberg 47,485/01: Extensive studies on the role of the liver in the synthesis of uric acid from ammonia in the dog, using various methods for the elimination of the liver (e.g., destruction of the parenchyma by injection of acids into the choledochus, Eck fistula). A 19th-century literature on complete extirpation of the liver in the goose, and in vitro perfusion of the liver with ammonia determinations in the afferent and efferent blood, etc. is reviewed.

Higgins & Anderson 597/31: Description of a technique for the removal of the median and left lateral lobes of the rat's liver which correspond to 70% of the hepatic tissue. Regeneration begins almost immediately and is virtually complete after 2 weeks. The mortality rate was 25%. [No attempt was made to determine the functional consequences of this intervention (H.S.).]

Waelsch & Selye 3,972/31: First description of a technique for the removal of about 70% of the liver in mice, which lends itself for the detection of drugs that are detoxified in the liver. Thus, in such partial hepatectomized mice, tribromoethanol (Avertin) causes much more prolonged anesthesia than in intact controls, whereas magnesium anesthesia is not significantly affected by this hepatic insufficiency; presumably because tribromoethanol is, whereas $MgCl_2$ is not detoxified by the liver.

Pincus & Martin A 34,939/40: Following liver damage induced by CCl_4, threshold doses of estrone become more efficacious in producing vaginal estrus in ovariectomized rats. Although the results were inconstant and not very pronounced, they suggest "that liver damage by CCl_4 results in a decreased inactivation of administered estrone."

Selye A 35,150/41; A 35,003/41; A 36,447/42: In rats, partial hepatectomy increases sensitivity to the anesthetic effect of various steroids, presumably because most if not all steroid hormones and their derivatives are largely detoxified in the liver. Consequently, the prolongation of anesthesia in the rat by partial hepatectomy is a suitable test object for the assays of potential steroid anesthetics of which only small amounts are available.

Selye G 60,058/69: In the rat, partial hepatectomy facilitates the production of perforating intestinal ulcers by indomethacin. Comparatively small doses of spironolactone readily inhibit this form of indomethacin intoxication even in the presence of surgically induced hepatic insufficiency. "These results are compatible with the assumption that both indomethacin and spironolactone are subject to hepatic detoxication, and hence, their respective pathogenic and prophylactic actions are enhanced after extensive resection of liver tissue."

Liver Slices or Fractions

Heller A 32,137/40: In vitro studies on tissue slices and tissue mince of rats and rabbits indicate that "estradiol is inactivated by liver and kidney, and not by the other tissues studied. This inactivation of estradiol is, in all probability, not due to conjugation or conversion to a less active form, but due to enzymatic destruction of an oxidative nature. This is indicated by the relative inactivity of the treated estradiol, the inability of hydrolysis procedures to increase activity and the effect of tissue poisons upon inhibiting the estradiol-destroying enzyme system. Estrone is increased 20 times in potency by incubation with minced uterine tissue. Spleen, lung, heart and kidney tissues also caused estrone to be converted to a more active substance. The suggestion is made that this conversion is accomplished by enzymatic reduction of estrone to estradiol."

Zondek et al. A 74,477/43: Stilbestrol is inactivated by rat liver pulp in vitro, though less rapidly than estrone. "In rats treated with large amounts of stilbestrol, the capacity of the liver to inactivate stilbestrol is increased."

Crevier & d'Iorio B 54,151/50: Pentobarbital anesthesia lasts longer in female than in male rats as judged by the linguo-maxillary reflex. Castration abolishes the high resistance of the male, but testosterone restores it to the normal level. In ovariectomized rats, estradiol has virtually no effect, but testosterone raises resistance to the male level. These in vivo effects run parallel to the in vitro pentobarbital detoxifying power of liver slices.

Robillard et al. B 51,110/50: Male rats are more resistant than females to the narcotic effect of pentobarbital. Gonadectomized rats of both sexes exhibit high pentobarbital resistance after treatment with testosterone, presumably as a consequence of accelerated hepatic detoxication of the barbiturates, since incubation of pentobarbital with liver slices of normal males or testosterone-treated castrates exhibit accelerated pentobarbital detoxication in vitro.

Robillard et al. G 67,325/54: Live homogenates of adult male rats destroy pentobarbital in vitro (spectrophotocolorimetric determination) more rapidly than those of castrate males. In vivo, pretreatment of the castrates, with testosterone, increases the detoxication process, whereas estradiol pretreatment has an opposite effect.

Hepatic Microsomal Enzyme Induction

Brown et al. G 57,030/54: "The activity of an enzyme system in mouse and rat liver which N-demethylates 3-methyl-4-monomethylaminoazobenzene has been found to depend on the nature of the diet. The lowest activity occurred when a grain or purified diet was fed. The activity of mouse liver approximately doubled when any of several commercial chows was fed; the activity of rat liver increased about 30 per cent. The factor was also contained in a number of aged or otherwise treated animal products, such as an old cholesterol preparation, liver extracts, and peptones.

A variety of pure sterols were inactive, but could be made active by peroxidation."

Axelrod E40,270/55: "An enzyme system in rabbit liver microsomes catalyzes the deamination of amphetamine to yield phenylacetone and ammonia. The enzyme system requires reduced triphosphopyridine nucleotide and oxygen. The TPN-dependent dehydrogenases in the soluble supernatant fraction of the liver serve to maintain a reservoir of reduced triphosphopyridine nucleotide."

Brodie et al. G66,772/55: Both the microsomes and soluble fractions of rabbit liver are required for drug metabolism. The activity of the microsomal enzyme systems that demethylate monomethyl-4-aminoantipyrine necessitate both NADPH and oxygen which are provided here by the soluble fraction. It is unusual for enzyme systems to require both reduced NADPH and oxygen but the common step in the various microsomal reactions could involve the production of hydrogen peroxide by the oxidation of NADPH. The generated peroxide might then be utilized to catalyze the transformation of various foreign compounds. "It is likely that the number of these enzymes is relatively small and that they are unusually nonspecific ... one can speculate that these systems are not essential to the normal economy of the body, but operate primarily against the toxic influences of foreign compounds that gain access to the body from the alimentary tract."

Axelrod D28,544/56: First description of enzyme systems which N-demethylate morphine and its congeners to the corresponding norderivatives and formaldehyde. "The enzyme systems are located in the liver microsomes of a number of mammalian species and they require reduced triphosphopyridine nucleotide, oxygen, and other cofactors. ... There are marked sex differences in the enzymatic demethylation of narcotic drugs in the rat. Administration of estradiol to male rats results in a decrease in enzyme activity, while treatment of female rats with testosterone enhances enzyme activity."

Brodie C12,157/56: The hexobarbital sleeping time of female rats is about four times that of males; correspondingly, the plasma levels of hexobarbital drop much more rapidly in males, whose hepatic microsomes also inactivate the drug more markedly in vitro than those of females. Male rats, pretreated with estradiol, sleep as long as females and their hepatic microsomes lose much of their ability to metabolize hexobarbital. Females, pretreated with testosterone, assume the characteristics of males in all these respects. No sex differences were seen in mice, guinea pigs, rabbits and dogs, and their ability to handle hexobarbital is not influenced by estradiol or testosterone.

Conney et al. D87,867/56: In rats, 3-methylcholanthrene i.p. considerably increased the ability of fortified liver homogenates to N-demethylate 3-methyl-4-monomethylaminoazobenzene (demethylase activity) and to reduce the azo linkage of 4-demethylaminoazobenzene (reductase activity) within 24 hrs. Significant demethylase activity was obtained even after 6 hrs. A number of other polycyclic hydrocarbons caused similar increases in demethylase activity but there was no relationship between carcinogenicity and enzyme induction. None of these compounds was active in vitro and their effect could be inhibited in vivo by ethionine. This inhibition was in turn prevented by methionine.

Lin & Knox C73,824/58: In rats, the hepatic TKT activity increased following treatment with cortisone, cortisol or corticosterone and L-tyrosine. This effect was observed also after adrenalectomy. On the other hand, a comparable effect of other aminoacids was probably due to stress. "That a nonspecific stress-producing agent could actually increase the level of tyrosine-α-ketoglutarate transaminase was further supported by the results obtained with a compound which is unrelated to tyrosine metabolism. Injections of propylene glycol in doses of 0.5 ml per 100 gm of body weight caused the level of this enzyme to increase to an average of 1390 units in three intact rats." Adrenalectomized rats did not support this dose of propylene glycol.

Remmer D86,728/58: In rats, 3 days pretreatment with cortisone or prednisolone diminishes the anesthetic effect of hexobarbital and increases the degradation of the anesthetic by liver slices. Adrenalectomy inhibits the degradation of hexobarbital by liver slices of male rats, an effect which can be counteracted by pretreatment with cortisone. Mention of unpublished experiments indicating that cortisone and prednisolone accelerate the detoxication of meperidine in the rat, exclusively through demethylation and not through hydrolysis.

Rosen et al. C47,568/58: Cortisol, cortisone and prednisone increase the GPT activity of the rat liver. GOT activity is not similarly influenced. "These facts, added to the observation that a substantial rise in hepatic GPT occurs in rats treated with hydrocortisone, in contrast to treatment with deoxycorticosterone, strongly suggests that the control of hepatic levels of GPT by glucocorticosteroids is importantly related to the mechanism whereby these compounds exert their gluconeogenic activity."

Sulman et al. C 79,823/59: In rats injected for 4 months with prednisone or prednisolone, an increase in the hepatic content of the enzymes which decompose these steroids could be demonstrated in vitro. Various histologic stains failed to reveal any associated light-microscopic change in the hepatocytes. Addition of SKF 525-A to the homogenate of activated livers blocked their enzymic activity.

Maickel & Brodie C 83,071/60: TPO in rat liver is increased by ACTH, cortisone, or cortisol, as well as by various stressors and barbiturates. Hypophysectomy prevents the effect of stressors and barbiturates, suggesting that the latter act through the pituitary-adrenal system.

Kato et al. G 64,325/62: Adult male rats are more resistant than females to pentobarbital anesthesia, carisoprodol paralysis and strychnine convulsions. Conversely, the lethal effect of OMPA is greater in the male. The sex difference is ascribed to the increased production of anabolic testoids that enhance the decomposition of these substrates, the first three of which being inactivated whereas the last activated in the process. The differences were also demonstrated in vitro, using liver slices or microsomal fractions. The high microsomal activity of the male could be abolished by castration, and restored by several anabolic testoids.

Booth & Gillette D 34,656/62: Testosterone propionate, 19-nortestosterone, 4-androstene-3, 17-dione and 4-chloro-19-nortestosterone acetate (SKF 6611) were tested for their ability to induce hepatic microsomal enzymes in female rats. "All of the steroids produced 2- to 3-fold increases in the activity of the enzyme systems that metabolize hexobarbital, demethylate monomethyl-4-aminoantipyrine and hydroxylate naphthalene, but only 19-nortestosterone, testosterone propionate and methyltestosterone increased the activity of microsomal TPNH oxidase. ... The increase in microsomal enzyme activity is more closely related to the anabolic activity than to the androgenic activity of the steroid."

Novick Jr. et al. F 63,768/66: "Subcutaneous administration of several 19-nortestosterone derivatives produced an increased hepatic microsomal metabolism of hexobarbital and decreased zoxazolamine prostration time in mice. Testosterone and methyltestosterone produced an increased hexobarbital sleep time and testosterone decreased the rate of hepatic microsomal metabolism of hexobarbital. Although the ability of norethandrolone and SK&F 6612 (4-chloro-17α-methyl-19-nortestosterone) to shorten hexobarbital sleep time occurs within 6 to 12 hr. after a single dose in mice, this effect of testosterone derivatives in rats occurs only after prolonged treatment."

Tomkins et al. G 49,588/66: Glucocorticoids stimulate TKT induction in rat hepatoma cells, in vitro. Inhibitor and immunochemical experiments indicate that the corticoids do not activate a precursor but increase the number of enzyme protein molecules. Apparently, the hormones exert some control at the level of translation of the transaminase messenger by antagonizing a repressor of messenger function. "It cannot yet be determined whether the presumed increase in messenger concentration occurs as a secondary response to the stimulation of translation, or whether there is a direct effect of the hormone on gene transcription."

Conney F 88,649/67: A review of the literature on more than 200 drugs leads to the conclusion that "there is no apparent relationship between either their actions or structure and their ability to induce enzymes. It is of interest that most of the inducers are soluble in lipid at a physiological pH."

Mannering G 71,818/68 (p. 53): Review of the early history of studies on hepatic microsomal drug metabolism.

Kalyanpur et al. G 66,147/69: In mice, various anabolic steroids (methandienone, 4-chlorotestosterone acetate, nandrolone, phenpropionate) given i.p. 90 min before pentylenetetrazol, inhibit convulsions. The protective effect is compared to that produced by various anesthetic steroids. [A relationship to enzyme induction is not suggested, nor is it probable in view of the shortness of the necessary pretreatment (H.S.).]

Solymoss et al. G 60,054/69: "In the rat, pretreatment with spironolactone, norbolethone or ethylestrenol increased the oxidation of pentobarbital by liver microsomes, enhanced its disappearance from blood and proportionally decreased the depth of anesthesia."

Portal Route of Administration

Golden & Sevringhaus A 37,808/38: In ovariectomized rats, ovarian homotransplants placed into the mesenteries failed to maintain the sexual cycle, whereas retransplantation of the gonads into the axillary region reinitiated estrus. Apparently, folliculoids are detoxified during their passage through the liver.

Biskind & Mark A 31,656/39: "Pellets of testosterone propionate and estrone do not exert their specific effect on the appropriate castrate rats when implanted in the spleen. The specific effect returns when the spleens containing the pellets are transplanted and the splenic artery and vein are ligated." Possibly, both testosterone and estrone are inactivated during their passage through the liver.

Biskind A 31,848/40: Both testosterone and methyltestosterone, when implanted in pellet-form into the spleen of the castrate rat, failed to stimulate the accessory sex organs. When the pellet-containing spleen is transplanted subcutaneously, with the splenic vessels ligated, the testoid effect returns. "The differences in the specific effects of these two substances when administered orally may be due to different routes of absorption from the intestinal tract (e.g., via the lymphatics), rather than different sites of inactivation."

Burrill & Greene A 32,956/40: In immature orchidectomized rats, autotransplants of testicular tissue stimulated the growth of the accessory sex organs when placed subcutaneously but not when inserted into the portal circulation. Presumably, testoids are detoxicated during their passage through the liver.

Eversole et al. 78,679/40: In adrenalectomized rats "autoplastic cortical grafts placed on the kidney, ovary or mesentery are of approximately equal functional capacity." Hence it is concluded that "unlike ovarian transplants, the function of cortical tissue is not impaired by having a site (intestinal mesentery) with hepatic portal drainage."

Biskind A 35,907/41: Female rats become anestrus upon s.c. implantation of a testosterone pellet. The estrus cycle remains normal if the pellet is implanted into the spleen but if subsequently this spleen is transplanted subcutaneously and its vessels ligated, the estrus cycle is resumed. Presumably intrasplenically-located testosterone is detoxified during its passage through the liver.

Biskind A 36,315/41: Pellets of estradiol benzoate implanted into the spleens of adult ovariectomized rats produce only a short period of estrus. However, if these spleens are transposed (pedicle transplant) s.c., their estrogenic action reappears. Apparently, estradiol is inactivated in the liver, as had previously been shown for estrone.

Biskind A 36,481/41: Estrone pellets implanted into the spleen do not cause such marked testicular atrophy in adult rats, as do similar pellets placed s.c. If the pellet-bearing spleens are transplanted s.c., and their hilum ligated (to prevent drainage of splenic blood into the portal circulation), then severe testicular atrophy develops, suggesting that estrone is inactivated during its passage through the liver.

Biskind & Biskind A 38,221/42: The anestrus condition of ovariectomized rats with splenic implants of estrone pellets gives way to constant estrus under the influence of vitamin-B complex deficiency. Administration of brewers yeast restores anestrus. Presumably the hepatic detoxication of folliculoids depends upon vitamin-B factors.

Burrill & Greene A 38,214/42: In rats, pellets of testosterone or methyltestosterone implanted s.c. stimulated the growth of the accessory sex organs after orchidectomy. Upon implantation into the spleen, methyltestosterone was, but testosterone was not active. Presumably, the latter is more subject to hepatic detoxication.

Eversole & Gaunt A 56,551/43: In rats, DOC pellets placed into the portal circulation are less effective in maintaining life after adrenalectomy than those implanted elsewhere. Apparently, DOC is partly inactivated during its passage through the liver.

Green B 28,239/48: In rats kept on a high NaCl intake the disturbances in fluid exchange, cardiac and renal hypertrophy, hypertension and mortality induced by DOC implantation s.c. are all diminished or absent if the same type of DOC pellet is implanted into the spleen. It is concluded that DOC is detoxified in the liver.

Shipley et al. B 50,163/50: In ovariectomized rats maintained on a hypolipotropic diet supplemented with methionine, estrone pellets protected against the development of hepatic steatosis if implanted s.c. but not if placed in the spleen.

Møller-Christensen B 56,243/51: In rabbits and cats, a greater increase in blood pressure is obtained by vasopressin injected into a peripheral vein than if the same amount is injected into the spleen. It is concluded that vasopressin is detoxified by the liver.

Liver Perfusion

Israel et al. A16,424/37: Estrone "is not inactivated by dog blood in vitro or by the circulation in a heart-lung perfusion system. It is rapidly inactivated by circulation in a heart-lung-liver perfusion system."

Smooth Endoplasmic Reticulum (SER)

Fouts G79,654/61: When SER and RER particles of rabbit liver are separated by ultracentrifugation in various sucrose gradients, the NADPH oxidase and drug-metabolizing enzyme activity can be shown to be higher in the SER than in the RER.

Remmer & Merker D61,064/63: In the rat, hepatic microsomal enzyme induction by phenobarbital is associated with a proliferation of the hepatic SER.

Fouts & Rogers F29,497/65: In the rat, "phenobarbital and chlordane stimulate a variety of microsomal drug metabolisms and also appear to cause a marked proliferation of smooth-surfaced endoplasmic reticulum (SER) in the hepatic cell. Benzpyrene and methylcholanthrene stimulate only a few microsomal drug metabolizing enzymes and do not appear to cause any pronounced increase in hepatic cell SER."

Burger & Herdson G66,499/66: In the rat, phenobarbital causes liver enlargement and ultrastructural changes characterized by "proliferation of smooth endoplasmic reticulum with concomitant shortening and dispersion of rough endoplasmic cisternae, mitochondrial abnormalities, and the development of myelin figures. The morphologic abnormalities at first affect only central cells, but progressively involve cells further out in the lobule so that after medication for 10 days most of the lobule is involved. Nevertheless, a peripheral zone of normal-looking cells is always present." Concurrent treatment with SKF 525-A further aggravates these changes, but SKF 525-A itself causes no detectable abnormalities in the liver.

Claude E8,217/69: Review on "Microsomes, Endoplasmic Reticulum and Interactions of Cytoplasmic Membranes."

Gardell et al. G60,062/70: In the rat, norbolethone—an active catatoxic steroid—produces pronounced proliferation of the SER in hepatocytes, presumably a morphologic reflection of increased microsomal enzyme production.

Horvath et al. G70,408/70: In rats "treatment with the most active catatoxic steroids (spironolactone, norbolethone, SC-11927, ethylestrenol) invariably induced marked proliferation of the SER. Progesterone and testosterone had a less pronounced effect. However, alterations of the endoplasmic reticulum can also be produced by some non-catatoxic steroids (estradiol) or non-steroidal compounds (stilbestrol). Thus it can be concluded that there is no close correlation between the catatoxic potency and the proliferation of the SER although all the catatoxic compounds tested lead to a marked transformation of the endoplasmic reticulum in the hepatocytes."

Kovács et al. G60,045/70: In the rat, spironolactone given in amounts suitable to produce a catatoxic effect causes marked proliferation of the SER in hepatocytes. This change presumably reflects an induction of drug-metabolizing microsomal enzymes, and may explain why spironolactone protects against the injurious effects of different compounds.

Syntoxic vs. Catatoxic Actions

Selye et al. A72,284/44: Demonstration of a relationship between the adrenal cortex and inflammatory lesions. In rats, DOC can produce carditis, periarteritis and sometimes arthritis under appropriate experimental conditions.

Selye B76,060/53: In rats, cortisol inhibits inflammation in granuloma pouches produced by croton oil. However, the croton oil removed after 14 days of sojourn in the pouch still retains the ability to produce inflammatory changes when injected into other rats. Apparently, the glucocorticoid acts by depressing the inflammatory potential of the tissues, not by destroying the irritant.

Selye G60,039/69: First description of the concept of "catatoxic steroids." The term refers to steroid hormones and their derivatives which increase resistance to various toxic agents above normal. Corticoids, which merely restore normal resistance in adrenal insufficiency, are not included in this concept, nor is the antiphlogistic effect that is not directed against toxic agents but suppresses a particular somatic response to them, namely inflammation which may be harmful or beneficial depending upon circumstances. Many, if not all, catatoxic steroid hormone actions depend upon increased detoxication of noxious compounds, through the induction of adaptive microsomal enzymes in the liver, not upon suppression of specific morbid reactions to them.

Selye G60,070/70: First detailed review (21 pp., 65 refs.) on "Adaptive Steroids" with special emphasis upon their classification and the history of research on their role as regulators of nonspecific resistance.

Selye G60,087/70: Brief review on the history of adaptive hormones with special reference to catatoxic steroids.

Solymoss et al. G79,023/71: In rats, pretreatment with PCN or spironolactone increases liver weight, glutathione S-aryltransferase activity and bile flow. At the same time, the plasma clearance and biliary excretion of BSP and its conjugated metabolites are enhanced. Ethylestrenol likewise increases liver weight but does not alter the other parameters mentioned above. Spiroxasone, SC-9376 and CS-1 (antimineralocorticoids), unlike norbolethone and oxandrolone (anabolics), also enhance plasma clearance of BSP, probably through the same mechanism. In contrast to these effects of pretreatment, administration of spironolactone, ethylestrenol or estradiol immediately before BSP delays plasma clearance of the dye, probably through competitive inhibition of biliary excretion. SKF 525-A does not suppress the enhanced BSP clearance induced either by spironolactone or by phenobarbital. [Although the authors did not evaluate their data from this point of view, these observations clearly show that the catatoxic activity of steroids is not merely the result of hepatic microsomal drug metabolizing enzyme induction. It may also be mediated through extra-microsomal enzyme mechanisms or even through enhanced biliary excretion (H.S.).]

Solymoss PROT. 42234: As judged by the Kagawa test, PCN is practically devoid of antimineralocorticoid activity. In male adrenalectomized adult rats, 6 µg of DOC s.c. produced a pronounced decrease in the urinary Na/K excretion, which could not be counteracted by 1 mg of PCN.

Clinical Implications

Yaffe et al. G67,125/66: In a female infant with congenital unconjugated hyperbilirubinemia, phenobarbital lowered the serum bilirubin concentration. "This constitutes the first indication of the apparent induction of a glucuronide-conjugating enzyme system by phenobarbital in man and therefore may also represent the first therapeutic application of enzyme induction."

Salvador et al. G68,113/67: Pretreatment with phenobarbital diminished hypercholesterolemia and atherosclerosis in cholesterol-fed rabbits. The cholesterol content of the aorta was likewise diminished.

Crigler & Gold H7,119/69: In a male infant with congenital, nonhemolytic, unconjugated hyperbilirubinemia and severe kernicterus, phenobarbital decreased serum bilirubin, whereas L-triiodothyronine, STH, and testosterone had little or no effect. During phenobarbital treatment, liver specimens obtained by biopsy showed proliferation of the SER and increased in vitro capacity to conjugate p-nitrophenol.

Mowat & Arias G74,246/69: "Oral contraceptive agents cause a predictable and reversible fall in hepatic excretory function in all subjects appropriately tested." At the same time, there is induction of hepatic drug-metabolizing enzymes which may alter the responsiveness of women to various drugs, and conversely, others have shown that the uterotrophic effect of oral contraceptives is reduced by phenobarbital at least in rats. "We can only speculate as to what this may mean for the insomniac on phenobarbitone who relies on the pill for contraception."

Orrenius et al. E8,231/69: Review of the literature and personal observations on the increase in the synthesis of cholesterol from ^{14}C-acetate obtained by phenobarbital pretreatment in rats and hamsters.

Powell et al. H17,195/69: It had previously been noted that pre-eclamptic toxemia (P.E.T.) is associated with a reduction in the incidence and severity of nonhemolytic jaundice in the neonate. Reexamination of these data now showed "that for nontoxaemic mothers receiving any barbiturate at any time there was a slight but statistically insignificant reduction (11.3%) in incidence of jaundice in their infants. Toxaemic mothers not receiving barbiturate had a similar insignificant reduction (10.4%). When both P.E.T. and barbiturate were present together, however, the reduction was 30.7% and this was statistically significant ($P < 0.01$)."

Temple Jr. et al. H17,091/69: In patients with Cushing's disease, o,p'DDD diminished cortisol secretion. Since adrenal responsiveness to ACTH infusion was reduced and the adrenals showed electron-microscopic changes in the mitochondria of the fasciculata, the effect was ascribed to the adrenolytic action of the drug.

Selye G60,083/70: Experimental Cardiovascular Diseases. Berlin—Heidelberg—New York: Springer Verlag, 1970.

III. CHEMISTRY

It is not within the scope of this monograph to discuss the chemical basis of drug metabolism in detail. This subject has been adequately covered by others in several excellent reviews (listed at the end of this chapter). Here we shall merely present a very succinct outline, followed by abstracts of key papers on enzymic reactions likely to participate in the metabolism of substrates that are influenced by adaptive hormones.

Most drugs undergo some metabolic transformation in the body. The same is true of hormones and of other physiologic constituents of the organism. The majority of these chemical changes takes place in the liver as a result of enzymic activity, but many metabolic transformations occur in extrahepatic tissues, and not all are the direct consequences of enzymic degradation or synthesis. Since we are concerned primarily with all aspects of the humoral regulation of tolerance to toxic agents, we must remember that hormones can increase resistance through entirely different mechanisms, e.g., by enhancing the excretion of toxicants through the urine, bile, etc., or by stimulating their uptake into the RES. Indeed, the entire group of syntoxic hormones acts by influencing the body's response to aggressors, without necessarily having any direct effect upon the latter. Furthermore, we shall see that some steroids act merely as particularly efficient carriers of active groups (e.g., of the thioacetyl radical) which bind and inactivate toxic materials (e.g., mercury).

Here we shall speak mainly about the most common biochemical mechanisms for the inactivation of toxic substrates which, in general, are characterized by the **production of metabolites more polar than the parent compounds**. This transformation is a useful preparation for renal and biliary excretion because substances with a high lipid/water partition coefficient pass readily across membranes; hence they are easily reabsorbed from the tubular urine, a process which interferes with their elimination. In addition, the specific secretory mechanisms for anions and cations in the proximal renal tubules and in the hepatic parenchyme act upon highly polar substances. For example, the oxidation of a methyl group to carboxyl can prepare a compound for renal or biliary excretion, thereby reducing its biologic half-life from many hours to a few minutes. The same effect is achieved by conjugation of a relatively nonpolar drug with sulfate. However, decreased lipid solubility is useful in this connection only if combined with increased water solubility.

The reactions undergone by drugs in the body are: oxidation, reduction, hydrolysis and synthesis (conjugation). The most important oxidative reactions include aliphatic oxidation, aromatic hydroxylation, N-dealkylation, O-dealkylation, S-demethylation, deamination, sulfoxide formation, desulfuration, N-oxidation and N-hydroxylation.

OXIDATIONS MEDIATED BY HEPATIC MICROSOMAL ENZYMES

The microsomal organization of redox components by which reducing equivalents are brought into reaction is of interest, since mixed-function oxidations require reducing equivalents. Such redox components occur in the endoplasmic reticulum of various tissues. The components identified in hepatic microsomes are summarized as follows (Mason et al. F51,528/65):

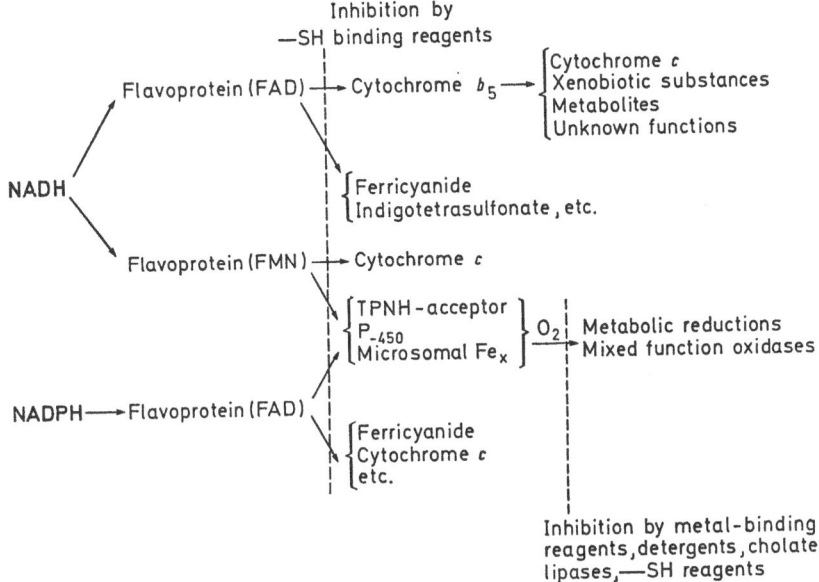

Here, NADH reduces cytochrome b_5 through the FAD-containing flavoprotein, NADH-cytochrome b_5 reductase; the reduced cytochrome b_5 transfers reducing equivalents to acceptors with E_0' above about 0 volts at pH 7; the reductase itself transfers reducing equivalents to dyestuffs but not to cytochrome c. NADH may likewise reduce cytochrome c through an FMN-containing microsomal flavoprotein, NADH cytochrome c reductase, but no cytochrome c occurs in carefully prepared microsomes. NADH also reduces a CO-binding cytochrome pigment P-450 (so called from the position of absorption of the CO complex). This P-450 appears to be the functional site of several microsomal mixed-function oxidases. NADH reduces also a hemoprotein-like component of hepatic microsomes, which is detectable by electron-spin resonance spectroscopy. Its reduced form, known as "microsomal Fe_x," is extremely autoxidizable. A much more active enzyme toward P-450 and microsomal Fe_x reduction is NADPH-cytochrome c reductase, an FAD-containing flavoprotein which reduces a NADPH-acceptor with a b-type cytochrome spectrum probably related to P-450 and microsomal Fe_x. NADPH-cytochrome c reductase also catalyzes the reduction of dyestuffs and other nonspecific acceptors. In addition to these redox-active components, the hepatic microsomes contain non-heme iron, copper, manganese, and coenzyme X, whose functions are unknown.

A graphic representation of the interactions between these microsomal components is given in the graph below in which the FAD-containing liver protein is indicated as "Fp" and its reduced form as "Fp*" (Mannering G75,980/68):

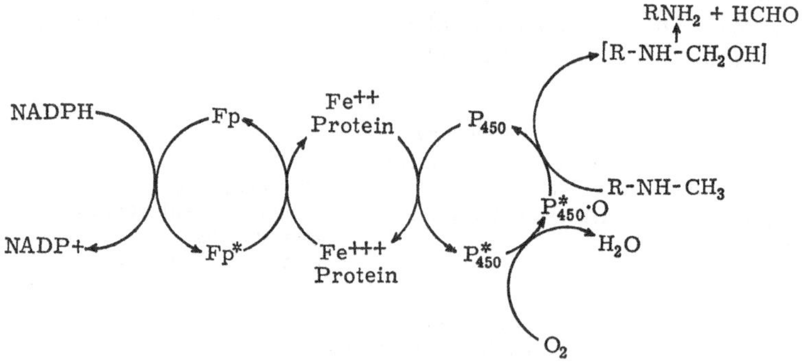

$$NADPH \to Fp \to Fp^* \to NADP+$$
$$Fp^* \to Fe^{++}\ Protein \to Fe^{+++}\ Protein$$
$$Fe^{++}\ Protein \to P_{450} \to P_{450}^*$$
$$P_{450}^* + O_2 \to P_{450}^* \cdot O \to R\text{-}NH\text{-}CH_3 + H_2O$$
$$\to [R\text{-}NH\text{-}CH_2OH] \to RNH_2 + HCHO$$

The relative nonspecificity of microsomal drug-metabolizing systems has been ascribed to the function of a single oxidase system involving cytochrome P-450, or at least a limited number of oxidase systems involving one or more cytochromes. Even if drugs are structurally unrelated, they would compete with each other for metabolism, assuming that the latter depends upon a single enzyme system or a single rate-limiting component common to the systems involved in the metabolic degradation of the defense substrates. In fact, it could be shown that many substrates acted as competitive inhibitors mutually inhibiting one another.

The important initial **hydroxylation reactions** are written as follows [Goldstein et al. 165/68 (p. 231)]:

$$R\text{-}CH_3 \xrightarrow{[P_{450}O]} R\text{-}CH_2OH$$

Aliphatic Oxidation

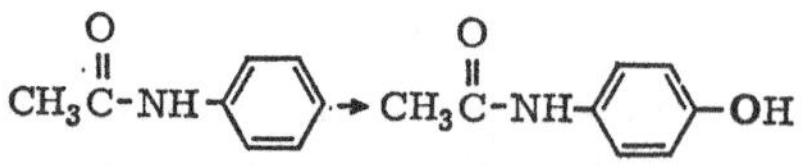

$$CH_3\overset{O}{\overset{\|}{C}}\text{-}NH\text{-}\bigcirc \to CH_3\overset{O}{\overset{\|}{C}}\text{-}NH\text{-}\bigcirc\text{-}OH$$

Aromatic Hydroxylation

$$R\text{-}NH\text{-}CH_3 \to [R\text{-}NH\text{-}CH_2OH] \to R\text{-}NH_2 + HCHO$$

N-Dealkylation

$$R\text{-}O\text{-}CH_3 \to [R\text{-}O\text{-}CH_2OH] \to R\text{-}OH + HCHO$$

O-Dealkylation

$$R\text{-}S\text{-}CH_3 \to [R\text{-}S\text{-}CH_2OH] \to R\text{-}SH + HCHO$$

S-Demethylation

$$R-\underset{\underset{NH_2}{|}}{CH}-CH_3 \longrightarrow \left[R-\underset{\underset{NH_2}{|}}{\overset{\overset{OH}{|}}{C}}-CH_3\right] \longrightarrow R-\overset{\overset{O}{\|}}{C}-CH_3 + NH_3$$

Oxidative Deamination

$$R-S-R' \xrightarrow{H^+} \left[\overset{\overset{OH}{|}}{\underset{}{E-S-R'}}\right]^+ \longrightarrow R-\overset{\overset{O}{\|}}{S}-R' + H^+$$

Sulfoxide Formation

$$(CH_3)_3N \xrightarrow{H^+} [(CH_3)_3N-OH]+ \longrightarrow (CH_3)_3N=O + H^+$$

N-Oxidation

$$R-NH-R' \longrightarrow R-\overset{\overset{OH}{|}}{N}-R'$$

N-Hydroxylation

In the oxidative desulfuration reactions, the oxygen atom replaces sulfur which later appears as sulfate.

Table 1 (p. 46) represents a compilation from the literature of enzyme activities that could be traced to the hepatic microsomal fractions of mammals, mainly of the rat.

OXIDATIONS NOT MEDIATED BY HEPATIC MICROSOMES

These include aromatization of cyclohexane derivatives (mitochondrial enzymes)
Alcohol and aldehyde oxidation (cytosol enzymes)
Purine oxidation
Monoamine oxidase (MAO) and diamine oxidase (DAO). MAO is a particularly important mitochondrial enzyme (found in liver, kidney, intestine and nervous tissue) because its substrates include physiologic substances such as: phenylethylamine, tyramine, dopamine, norepinephrine, epinephrine, tryptamine and 5-HT. DAO also converts amines to aldehydes in the presence of oxygen; its substrate specificity overlaps with that of MAO.
Dehalogenation (e.g., of halogenated insecticides).

REDUCTIVE DETOXIFYING REACTIONS

Azo and nitro reduction, first thought to occur in the cytosol, but later shown to depend upon a class of light microsomes that sediment very slowly. In contrast to the oxidizing microsomal enzymes, these reductases are found also in extra-hepatic tissues.

Alcohol dehydrogenase can function as a reductase, e.g. when it catalyzes the conversion of chloral hydrate to trichloroethanol.

Table 1. *Enzymic activities of liver microsomal fractions.* (Simplified after an extensive compilation by Reid (G71,333/67) where references to the original articles may be found)

Enzyme or enzyme system	% in microsomal fraction[a]	Enzyme or enzyme system	% in microsomal fraction[a]
Oxidoreductases		*Hydrolases*	
L-Amino-acid oxidase (1.4.3.2)		Alkaline phosphatase (3.1.3.1)	42%
Aryl-4-hydroxylase (1.14.1.1)	~100%	Amylase (3.2.1.1)	52%
Ascorbate-forming system (1.1.1.19)		Arginase (3.5.3.1)	41%
Azo-dye reductase (1.6.6.7)		Arylsulphatase C (3.1.6.1)	62%
Catalase (1.11.1.6)	14%	ATPase (ATP pyrophosphohydrolase; Mg^{2+} ions in assay) (3.6.1.4)	low
Cystine reductase (1.6.4.1)		N-Deacylase ("esterase") (3.5.1.)	
Desmosterol reductase (1.3.1.)	35%		
Diaphorases—NAD_2, $NADH_2$ (1.6.99)		Acetylcholinesterase ("true cholinesterase") (3.1.1.7)	{46% 62%
Glucuronolactone reductase (1.1.1.20)			
β-Hydroxy-β-methylglutaryl-CoA reductase (1.1.1.34)		Arylesterase (3.1.1.2)	{58% 67% 85%
Lipid-peroxidation system (ADP-activated; coupled to $NADPH_2$ oxidase)		Benzoylcholinesterase (3.1.1.9)	46%
Malate dehydrogenase (1.1.1.37)	low	Carboxylesterase (3.1.1.1)	
$NADH_2$-cytochrome b_5 reductase (1.6.2.2)		Cholesterol esterase (3.1.1.13)	112%
$NADH_2$-cytochrome c reductase (1.6.99.3)	62%	Vitamin A esterase (3.1.1.12)	
$NADPH_2$-cytochrome c reductase	64%	Glucose-6-phosphatase (3.1.3.9)[c]	74%
$NADPH_2$ peroxidase ($NADPH_2$ oxidase) (1.11.1.2)		β-Glucuronidase (3.2.1.31)	{40% 37%
Stearate-dehydrogenating system (→ oleate)		Inorganic pyrophosphatase (3.6.1.1)	80%
Steroid reductase (→ 5α isomer)		Lipoprotein lipase (3.1.1.)	40%
Sulphite oxidase (1·8·3·1)	75%	Lysophospholipase (lysolecithinase) (3.1.1.5)	61%
		NAD nucleosidase (3.2.2.5)	93%
Transferases		NAD pyrophosphatase (3.6.1.9)	63%
3-Acylglycerophosphorylcholine acyltransferase (from acyl-CoA) (2.3.1.)		NADP pyrophosphatase (3.6.1.)	52%
		Nicotinamide deamidase (3.5.1.)	
deCDPcholine: 1,2-diglyceride cholinephosphotransferase (2.7.8)	50%	Nucleoside diphosphatases { ADPase (≡CDPase ?) (3.6.1.) GDP/IDP/UDPase (3.6.1.6)	{>50% 71%-IDP
CDPcholine: 1,2-diglyceride cholinephosphotransferase (2.7.8.2)	97%	5′-Nucleotidase (nucleoside-5′-monophosphatase) (3.1.3.5)	{35—40% 47%
Diglyceride acyltransferase (2.3.1.20)	84%	Nucleoside triphosphatase (3.6.1.4)	23%-ITP
Glycerolphosphate acyltransferase (2.3.1.15)		Phosphodiesterase I (3.1.4.1)	29%
Phenylphosphate: cytidine phosphotransferase		Thiamine pyrophosphatase (3.6.1.)	~50%
Phosphatidylinositol kinase (2.7.1.)		Uronolactonase (3.1.1.19)	94%
Pyrophosphate: glucose phosphotransferase		*Other enzymes or enzyme systems*	
Ribonuclease ("alkaline") (2.7.7.)	low	Acyl-CoA synthetase (6.2.1.3)	
Transmethylases, to phosphatides or other acceptors (2.1.1.)		Cholyl-CoA synthetase (6.2.1.7)	
		Demethylase (azo-dye)	
		Epoxysteroid lyase	
UDPglucose: glycogen glucosyltransferase (2.4.1.11)		Ether(aromatic)-cleaving system	
		Fumarase (fumarate hydratase) (4.2.1.2)	28%
UDP glucuronyltransferase (2.4.1.17)	high	Glutamine synthetase (6.3.1.2)	47%
		Prothrombin-forming system	

DRUG METABOLISM BY HYDROLYSIS

This is essentially restricted to esterases and amidases found in plasma, liver and other tissues, usually in the cytosol fraction. A pertinent example is the hydrolysis of procaine by plasma choline esterase to p-aminobenzoic acid and diethylaminoethanol.

CONJUGATION REACTIONS

Synthesis of glucuronides, e.g., of steroid alcohols, thyroxine, bilirubin and various substances foreign to the body, can be achieved by hepatic enzymes. Those catalyzing the synthesis of uridine diphosphate-glucuronic acid (UDPGA) serve as a glucuronic acid donor to the various receptors in the cytosol. Transferases in hepatic microsomes and other tissues mediate this latter process.

Synthesis of ribosides and riboside phosphates shows that carbohydrates other than glucuronic acid can participate in synthetic drug metabolism. Ribonucleosides and ribonucleotides are formed with purine and pyrimidine analogues by a soluble enzyme system of the hepatic cytosol. This type of reaction participates in the metabolism of histamine and of various carcinolytic agents, e.g., in the conversion of 6-mercaptopurine to a ribonucleotide.

Acylation reactions are mediated by enzymes of the hepatic cytosol fraction. Here, coenzyme-A through its free-SH group reacts with an activated form of carboxylic acid to form acyl-CoA. The acyl group is then transferred to an appropriate acceptor, e.g., an aromatic amine.

Mercapturic acid formation occurs in preparation for the urinary excretion of aromatic hydrocarbons, halogenated aromatic hydrocarbons and halogenated nitrobenzenes. A "glutathiokinase," found in the hepatic cytosol, is thought to activate glutathione; the conjugation then proceeds in the microsomal fraction in the presence of NADPH and oxygen. The glutathione conjugate is subsequently hydrolyzed to an arylcysteine intermediate, the cysteine amino group of which is acetylated to mercapturic acid.

Sulfuric acid esters or "ethereal sulfates" are formed by the reaction of aromatic or aliphatic $-OH$ groups and certain $-NH_2$ groups with an activated form of sulfate. Hepatic cytosol enzymes mediate the sulfate activation and the transfer of sulfate to the acceptor.

N-, O-, and S-methylation can be achieved with S-adenosylmethionine as a methyl donor. Catechol O-methyltransferase (found in hepatic cytosol but also in many other tissues) catalyzes the transfer of $-CH_3$ to a phenolic $-OH$, e.g., in epinephrine,

---

Footnote to Table 1

[a] %-values are given only where there were reasonably quantitative results, and the recovery of homogenate activity in the fractions was satisfactory. Where low %-values have been included, the homogenate may have contained at least two enzymes one of which was truly associated with the microsomal fraction. On the other hand, some fairly high values in the literature have been excluded because, for example, the enzyme is really lysosomal.

norepinephrine, dihydroxyphenylethylamine and dihydroxybenzoic acid. This enzyme may be responsible for the physiologic inactivation of norepinephrine.

N-methylation is involved in the methylation of histamine, phenylethanolamine and the conversion of norepinephrine to epinephrine. The reaction occurs in the cytosol of the adrenal medulla and other tissues. This is not strictly speaking a detoxication reaction but nicotine, nicotinamide, quinoline, etc. can also be methylated through a similar pathway.

S-methylation appears to be limited to lipid-soluble substrates which have access to microsomal enzymes. Various exogenous —SH compounds are methylated in this manner, but physiologic substrates (homocysteine, cysteine, glutathione) are not.

Transsulfuration and cyanide metabolism are also important for detoxication. In cyanide poisoning, CN becomes bound to the Fe in cytochromes destroying their electron transport capacity. The immediate removal of CN is achieved by promoting its binding to methemoglobin. This process is followed by the conversion of cyanide to the nontoxic thiocyanate by furnishing thiosulfate or mercaptopyruvate as substrates. Normally cyanide is metabolized in the body by sulfur transferase ("rhodanese"), a mitochondrial enzyme found in liver, kidney and other tissues.

Enzymes and Resistance in General

Rubin et al. G58,057/64: Discussion of factors which may explain the relative nonspecificity of microsomal enzymes by affecting pathways common to many detoxicating reactions.

Reid G71,333/67: A chapter on "Membrane Systems" (86 pp., numerous refs.) with a tabular compilation of the literature on microsomal enzyme systems.

Goldstein et al. E165/68 (p. 218): Review on the effect of various inducers upon the pathways of drug metabolism.

Gillette H 34,126/71: The principal oxidative reactions catalyzed by hepatic microsomal mixed function oxygenases are tabulated as follows:

Reaction	Substrate	Product
Deamination	amphetamine	phenylacetone
O-dealkylation	phenacetin	p-hydroxyacetanilide
Aliphatic hydroxylation	pentobarbital	3-hydroxypentobarbital
Aromatic hydroxylation	aniline	p-hydroxyaniline
Epoxidation	aldrin	aldrin epoxide
N-dealkylation	aminopyrine	4-aminoantipyrine
Alkylol formation	schradan	hydroxymethyl schradan
N-oxide formation	dimethylaniline	dimethylaniline N-oxide
N-oxidation	aniline	phenylhydroxylamine
S-demethylation	6-methylmercaptopurine	mercaptopurine
S-oxidation	chlorpromazine	chlorpromazine sulfoxide
Phosphothionate oxidation	parathion	paraoxon
Desulfuration	thiobarbital	barbital
Dehalogenation	halothane	trifluoroacetic acid
Dealkylations of metallo alkanes	tetraethyl tin	triethyl tin

The mechanism of drug oxidations is graphically illustrated as follows:

$$NADPH \rightarrow \text{Cyt. C Red.} \rightarrow \text{Cytochrome P 450} \begin{array}{c} \text{Substrate} \\ \nearrow \\ \text{Oxid} \updownarrow \text{Red} \\ \searrow \\ \text{Hydroxylated substrate} \end{array}$$

$$NADH \rightarrow \text{Cyt. } b_5 \rightarrow O_2 \nearrow$$

Steroidases in General

Tomkins C32,526/57: Characterization of the hepatic enzymes responsible for the in vitro reduction of Δ^4-3-ketosteroids.

McGuire & Tomkins E91,579/59: In the rat, thyroxine causes a pronounced increase in the microsomal 5α-reductase activity of the liver, but the rate of reduction of some steroid substrates is increased more than that of others. Furthermore, when microsomes are "aged" at 0—5°C for several weeks, the decline in activity varies with different steroid substrates. "Further evidence for the substrate specificity of the 5α-hydrogenases was the observation that 4-androstene-3,17-dione strongly inhibited the reduction of cortisone, while the converse was not true." These and other observations suggest that each series of Δ^4-3-ketosteroid hydrogenases, 5α and 5β, contains multiple enzymes capable of discerning small variations in the steroid molecule.

Kuntzman et al. E55,528/65: "The K_m values for the hydroxylation of progesterone, testosterone, and estradiol are about 10 times lower than the K_m values for several drug oxidations, thereby suggesting that the steroid hormones are better than drugs as substrates for the TPNH-dependent oxidative enzymes." These K_m values are in the same range as those reported for the reduction of the A ring of Δ^4-3-ketosteroids by enzymes of liver microsomes. These findings "suggest that these enzymes can also play a physiological role in the metabolism of steroids in the body."

Conney et al. F79,331/67: Hepatic microsomes of adult rats metabolize testosterone, estradiol, progesterone and DOC to polar hydroxylated metabolites in the presence of an NADPH-generating system. CO inhibits the hepatic metabolism of all four steroids.

Koerner G65,718/69: 11β-Hydroxysteroid dehydrogenase activity of rat liver microsomes has been assayed by a quantative spectrophotometric method. "Several 11β-hydroxysteroids are substrates of the enzyme but there is no activity towards 11β-hydroxysterone or 11β-hydroxysteroids with a C-21 sulfate, phosphate, acetate or hemisuccinate group."

Corticoidases

Forchielli & Dorfman G66,498/56: "With 11-deoxycortisol as a substrate, it has been demonstrated that rat liver contains both the Δ^4-5α-hydrogenase and Δ^4-5β-hydrogenase systems, which yield, after incubation, the 5α (androstane and allopregnane) and 5β (etiocholane and pregnane) stereoisomers." The 5α system is associated with the particulate fraction, whereas the 5β system is in the supernatant fluid produced by centrifugation at 78,000 X g.

McGuire Jr. & Tomkins D5,722/60: In the microsomal fraction of rat liver, there appear to be at least 5 Δ^4-3-ketosteroid reductases (5α). When rats are treated with thyroxine, the reductase activity for cortisone, cortisol, DOC, 4-androstene-3,17-dione and 11-desoxycortisol (Cpd. S) increases, but the increment is different for each of these substrates.

Starnes G68,434/69: Rat liver slices were incubated in vitro in the presence of ^{3}H-dexamethasone. The steroid was metabolized to glucuronides and sulfates.

Testoidases

Conney et al. G67,773/68: The metabolism of testosterone to 6β-, 7α-, and 16α-hydroxytestosterone by rat liver microsomes, is differently inhibited by CO in vitro. Apparently, "one or more CO-binding cytochromes function in the hydroxylation of testosterone by rat liver microsomes."

Folliculoidases

Graubard & Pincus 80,931/41: In the Barcroft-Warburg respirometer, estriol, estradiol and estrone are oxidized by mushroom laccase and form precipitates whose nature has not been established. No oxidation of any of these substrates was observed with potato tyrosinase.

Mueller & Rumney C30,708/57: Formation of 6β-hydroxy and 6-keto derivatives of estradiol-16-^{14}C by the hepatic microsomes of the mouse.

Lehmann & Schütz H14,215/69: The microsomal fraction of the liver of the mature human fetus metabolizes 4-^{14}C-estrone twice as fast as that of the 12-week-old fetus. The highest rate of metabolism was found in the microsomal fraction of the liver of an adult man. "By paperchromatography, microchemical reactions and crystallization to constant specific activity, the following metabolites were identified: 6α-, 6β-, 7α-, 15α- and 16α-hydroxyoestrone, 6α-, 6β- and 7α-hydroxyoestradiol-17β and oestriol."

Cholesterolase

Bucher & McGarrahan G67,470/56: For the biosynthesis of cholesterol from acetate in vitro, both microsomes and soluble cell constituents of the rat liver are required. In vivo, over 90% of newly formed cholesterol, obtained shortly after the injection of labeled acetate, is in the microsomal fraction.

Olson et al. G61,438/57: The metabolism of labeled lanosterol in rat liver homogenates yields cholesterol and CO_2 as the principal products. The demethylation of lanosterol requires both the particulate and the soluble fraction of liver homogenates, but the latter can be partially replaced by NADH.

Tchen & Bloch G66,130/57: Hog-liver homogenate can convert squalene only to lanosterol and not to cholesterol. Rat-liver homogenate converts squalene to either lanosterol or cholesterol according to the method of preparation of the homogenates. Separated mitochondria and microsomes were both active if supplemented with supernatant fluid.

Thyroxinase

Stanbury et al. C90,693/60: Description of the microsomal enzyme system which deiodinates thyroxine in the presence of Fe^{++} and oxygen.

Wynn et al. G67,767/62: The microsomes are the most active thyroxine-degrading subcellular fraction of rat liver. The optimal reaction conditions for this degradation are described.

Cytochrome P-450, NADPH Cytochrome c Reductase, Cytochrome b_5

Omura et al. F51,529/65: Studies on the participation of cytochrome P-450 in "mixed function oxidase" reactions.

Lu & Coon G71,879/68: Studies on the role of hemoprotein P-450 in fatty acid ω-hydroxylation in the soluble enzyme system from liver microsomes.

Hildebrandt et al. G69,992/69: From experiments on the interaction of metyrapone with hepatic microsomal cytochrome P-450 in rats treated with phenobarbital, "it is concluded that metyrapone changes the equilibrium between two functionally different forms of cytochrome P-450 which exists in microsomes. The decrease of one form of cytochrome P-450 appears as an 'inhibition' of aminopyrine or hexobarbital metabolism; the concomitant increase of the other form of cytochrome P-450 results in a 'stimulation' of other types of hydroxylation reactions, for example, the ring hydroxylation of acetanilide."

Lu et al. G67,623/69: Resolution of the cytochrome P-450-containing ω-hydroxylation system of liver microsomes into three components.

Netter et al. G71,785/69: In mouse liver microsomes, the inhibition by metyrapone of p-nitroanisole and N-monomethyl-p-nitroaniline were shown to be competitive. The degree of inhibition was correlated to the amount of metyrapone bound to cytochrome P-450. On the other hand, metyrapone does not seem to displace naphthalene from its binding to P-450. Possibly, simultaneous binding of substrate and inhibitor may occur at different binding sites of the same enzyme.

Wada et al. H19,993/69: Studies on rat liver microsomes using radioactive cholesterol led to the assumption "that the microsomal electron transport system, involving cytochrome P-450, functions in 7α-hydroxylation of cholesterol. The existence of a specific cytochrome P-450 for 7α-hydroxylation, i.e., multiplicity of cytochrome P-450, is suggested."

Bidleman & Mannering G80,042/70: In rats, treatment with 3-MC causes the formation of P_1-450, a variant of cytochrome P-450. It has been claimed that P_1-450 is formed when

3-MC, or one of its metabolites combines irreversibly with the type I binding site of pre-existing P-450. However, the authors present evidence that P_1-450 is synthesized independently of P-450 and probably does not contain 3-MC or any of its metabolites.

Kato & Onada G75,544/70: In rats, pretreated in vivo with various testoids, the affinity of P-450 for binding with numerous substrates is increased. Folliculoids counteract this effect.

Kato et al. H27,934/70: "The administration of morphine significantly decreased the content of cytochrome P-450 in male rats, but not in female rats. Progesterone and testosterone hydroxylation is markedly decreased in morphine-treated male rats, but not in the females.... The magnitude of spectral change induced by progesterone or testosterone per unit of P-450 content was decreased in morphine-treated male rats, but not in the females. Since the binding capacity of P-450 with progesterone or testosterone is dependent on the action of androgen, an impairment of the action of androgen by morphine is assumed to be a responsible factor."

Mangum et al. G81,296/70: A soluble cytochrome has been partially purified from pig kidney. Its absorption spectra in both the oxidized and reduced state resemble microsomal cytochrome b_5.

Mannering G78,897/70: Review on the properties of P-450 as affected by environmental factors, particularly the administration of polycyclic hydrocarbons.

Mannering G78,898/70: Review on the role of substrate binding to P-450 hemoproteins in drug metabolism.

Perry G74,358/70: Cytochrome P-450 was demonstrated in microsomal preparations from several strains of houseflies. The highest yield was obtained from the abdomen. Housefly eggs contain no measurable amounts of cytochrome P-450, which appears in traces in the larvae, but declines to almost nil in the pupal stage. A few hours after the adult emerges, cytochrome P-450 rises rapidly.

Stripp et al. H22,743/70: In rats, spironolactone pretreatment shortened hexobarbital sleeping time. "Moreover, treatment of female rats with spironolactone doubled the rate of the in vitro metabolism of hexobarbital and benzpyrene by liver microsomes and quadrupled that of ethylmorphine. The inducing effects of spironolactone were very different from those of phenobarbital and 3-methylcholanthrene. The amount of cytochrome P-450 was either unaltered or decreased, but the NADPH cytochrome c reductase activity was increased 2-fold. Although the endogenous rate of cytochrome P-450 reduction by NADPH was not altered, the stimulatory effects of ethylmorphine or hexobarbital on the rate of cytochrome P-450 reduction were significantly greater with microsomes from spironolactone treated animals. By contrast, treatment of male rats with spironolactone caused no change in hexobarbital sleeping time and no change or a slight decrease in hexobarbital and benzpyrene metabolism by liver microsomes."

Yu & Gunsalus G81,295/70: Cytochrome P-450$_{cam}$ was discovered and purified in homogeneous crystalline form from camphor grown Pseudomonas putida strain PpG786.

Chaplin & Mannering G75,976/71: Review of the literature and personal observations suggesting that the physical and biochemical properties of cytochrome P-450 depend largely upon its association with microsomal phospholipids. "Drugs have been classified into two groups depending upon whether they form a type I or a type II difference spectrum when they combine with cytochrome P-450." The studies suggest that the type I and type II binding sites differ and that the type I site is associated with membrane phospholipids (*cf.* also p. 103.)

Estabrook et al. G81,261/71: Description of a new spectral intermediate associated with cytochrome P-450.

Estabrook et al. H34,125/71: Studies on the influence of hepatic microsomal mixed function oxidation reactions on cellular metabolic control. The requirements of this system for NADPH and NADH could markedly affect the cytosol concentration and subsequent oxidized: reduced ratio of these pyridine nucleotides. The involvement of cytochrome b_5 in the oxidative reaction, the necessity of enzymes for the transfer of reducing equivalents from the reduced pyridine nucleotides to both cytochromes b_5 and P-450 and mercurial inhibition studies which demonstrate the autonomy of the units that catalyze the microsomal NADPH supported mixed-function oxidations help our understanding of the organization of this enzyme system. The authors speculate on possible models that might represent the spatial organization of these enzyme systems within the endoplasmic reticulum.

Gillette H34,126/71: The inducers of drug metabolism are classified into: 1. "Phenobarbital-like" agents which increase NADPH-cytochrome c reductase and cytochrome P-450 thus augmenting the amount of cytochrome P-450-substrate complex and its rate of reduction; 2. polycyclic hydrocarbons (e.g. methylcholanthrene) which form a variant of cytochrome P-450 that differs from the usual form in its affinity to various drugs. This kind of inducer does not increase either NADPH-cytochrome c reductase or the rate of cytochrome P-450 reduction; 3. spironolactone and other catatoxic steroids which increase NADPH-cytochrome c reductase activity and the rate of cytochrome P-450 substrate reduction, but have little if any effect upon the amount of cytochrome P-450. The relationship between the electron flux and hepatic microsomal drug metabolism largely depends upon the substrate.

Ishimura et al. G81,262/71: Description of a new spectral species of P-450 interpreted to be an oxygenated form.

Leber et al. H35,676/71: In male rats, pretreatment with spironolactone stimulated the specific activity of isolated hepatic microsomes for aminopyrine demethylation and 4-methylumbelliferone glucuronidation. Microsomal cytochrome P-450 content increased about 66%. Under comparable conditions, ethacrynic acid increased the specific activity of the microsomes for the demethylation of aminopyrine and the P-450 content, but glucuronidation of 4-methylumbelliferone was not significantly altered. Another nonsteroidal diuretic, furosemid, did not influence any of these parameters.

Mannering H34,127/71: Additional evidence supporting the concept that polycyclic hydrocarbons cause the appearance of an abnormal "cytochrome P_1-450" in the hepatic microsomes of the rat. This may be an aberrant hemoprotein which does not result from the combination of polycyclic hydrocarbons with cytochrome P-450 but represents a specific molecular entity.

Solymoss et al. G79,015/71: In rats, PCN (unlike the naturally-occurring pregnenolone) enhances the plasma clearance of pentobarbital and the production of ^{14}C-pentobarbital metabolites. It also increases liver weight, microsomal protein concentration, NADPH-cytochrome c reductase activity and cytochrome P-450 content. It is concluded "that microsomal enzyme-induction accounts for the remarkable resistance-increasing effect of this steroid against many toxicants."

Stripp et al. G79,538/71: In rats, the induction of hepatic microsomal enzymes by spironolactone "differed from the phenobarbital or methylcholanthrene induction in that it did not increase cytochrome P-450 content or microsomal protein. Furthermore the induction seemed to be sex dependent."

Zsigmond & Solymoss G79,025/71: In rats, PCN increases hepatic microsomal protein and cytochrome P-450 content. In vitro incubation of labelled progesterone with these microsomes shows enhanced progesterone biotransformation. The production of several hydroxylated progesterone metabolites (including 6β- and 16α-hydroxyprogesterone is accelerated by PCN.

Other Enzymes

Stoffel G66,819/61: Description of the biosynthesis of polyenoic fatty acids by dehydrogenating enzyme systems of hepatic microsomes.

Axelrod D64,159/63: An enzyme that forms epinephrine from p- and m-sympathol, and dopamine from p- and m-tyramine, is demonstrated in the microsomes of rabbit liver. It requires $NADPH_2$ and is nonspecific in that it can form catechols from the following, normally occurring, or foreign phenols: p- and m-octopamine, p-hydroxyephedrine, phenol, stilbestrol, N-acetyl-p-aminophenol, estradiol and N-acetyl serotonin.

Berlin & Schimke G37,616/65: In adrenalectomized rats, 4 days of pretreatment with cortisone increased the activity of hepatic TPO, TKT, glutamic-alanine transaminase and arginase. Differences in the turnover rate or enzymes thus induced may simulate differential selective-inducing effects upon one or the other enzyme.

Yamamoto et al. G67,939/67: Description of some properties of 2,3-oxidosqualene sterol cyclase in hepatic microsomes of the pig.

Roach et al. G68,807/69: Review of the literature and personal observations on the oxidation of ethanol by rat liver in vitro. "It is concluded that ethanol oxidation by the microsomal fraction is mediated through H_2O_2 dependent systems one of which is catalase."

Valeriote et al. G67,621/69: Purification and properties of rat liver TKT induced by triamcinolone.

Ward & Pollak G69,320/69: The structural proteins of rat liver microsomal membranes are made up of a heterogenous group of proteins which can be characterized by their phospholipid-binding capacity. "It is suggested that reticulosomes consist largely of enzymic proteins of the endoplasmic reticulum."

IV. GENERAL PHARMACOLOGY

SYNTOXIC COMPOUNDS

The term syntoxic compounds comprises all drugs and hormones which increase resistance merely by influencing the reactions of the body, not by destroying or eliminating the pathogens. Thus, for example, the inhibition of inflammation or of immune reactions by antiphlogistic or immunosuppressive hormones and drugs, as well as the maintenance of the blood pressure by vasoactive substances, would be considered as syntoxic reactions as long as these effects are not dependent upon the chemical inactivation of the pathogens.

This entire field has been covered in our earlier publications (Selye B40,000/50, B58,650/51, C19,000/56, G19,425/65, E5,986/66; Selye et al. B87,000/52, B90,100/53, C1,001/54, C9,000/56) and it has also been summarized in the Introduction and History sections of the present volume, hence, we shall not consider it again here.

CATATOXIC COMPOUNDS (AGONISTS)

What little we know about the so-called "structure-function" or pharmaco-chemical correlations among catatoxic compounds will be summarized in the "Synopsis" (p. 768 ff.). Suffice it here to reemphasize that systematic studies on the structural prerequisites of catatoxic actions have been performed only in connection with steroids. In this respect the main generalizations arrived at were that nitrile and spirolactone groups as well as the 19-nor-steroid configuration are in general advantageous for catatoxic activity, although their effect is largely dependent upon other structural characteristics of the molecule.

With regard to pharmaco-pharmacologic interrelations we have seen that the catatoxic potency is independent of any other known hormonal property, but among steroids those exhibiting anabolic or antimineralocorticoid properties are always endowed with some catatoxic potency, whereas folliculoids appear to be singularly ineffective in this respect.

Literature on some of the salient characteristics of various syntoxic and catatoxic compounds is presented in the following Abstract Section (with special reference to glucocorticoids, testoids, anabolics, antimineralocorticoids, antifolliculoids, antitestoids, myoneural blocking agents and interactions between inducers).

Syntoxic Compounds

Corticoids. *Janoski et al. E7,896/68:* Review (112 pp., about 700 refs.) "On the pharmacologic actions of 21-carbon hormonal steroids ('glucocorticoids') of the adrenal cortex in mammals." A large section is devoted to the effect of glucocorticoids upon reactions mediated through lysosomal enzymes.

Williams E8,139/68, (p. 371): For comparative purposes, it is important to determine the relative anti-inflammatory and Na-retaining activity of the most commonly used glucocorticoids and gluco-mineralocorticoids. Such comparisons have only limited value because they depend upon the test conditions; still, the following approximate tabulation is of value:

Table 2. *Relative anti-inflammatory and Na-retaining activities of some antiphlogistic corticoids*

Compound	Relative potency compared to cortisol	Relative Na-retaining activity
Cortisol	1	++
Cortisone acetate	0.8	++
Prednisolone	4	+
Prednisone	3.5	+
Triamcinolone	5	0
6-Methylprednisolone	5	0
Haldranolone	10	0
Betamethasone	25	0
Dexamethasone	30	0
9α-Fluorohydrocortisone[a]	15	+++++

[a] Used chiefly topically or as a Na-retainer.

Catatoxic Compounds (Agonists)

Testoids, Anabolics. *Overbeek E8,318/66:* A review (78 pp., about 220 refs.) on anabolic steroids.

Krüskemper E933/68: Monograph (236 pp., 1367 refs.) on the pharmacology of anabolic steroids. Special attention is given to the relationship between virilizing and anabolic effects, the various tests for anabolic and anticatabolic actions, as well as clinical applications, but the catabolic and enzyme-inducing effects are only briefly mentioned.

Antiglucocorticoids. *Linèt G79,963/70:* Detailed review of the literature and personal observations on the effect of anabolic testoids upon glucocorticoid overdosage in animals and man. Special attention is given to the effect of anabolic testoids upon glucocorticoid-induced loss of body weight and other metabolic changes, adrenal atrophy, osteoporosis, wound healing, inflammation and gastric ulcer formation. Antiglucocorticoids devoid of anabolic properties are also surveyed. In clinical medicine, various forms of hyperglucocorticoidism are not, or only moderately, improved by treatment with anabolic testoids. [Excellent source of pertinent references (H.S.).]

Antimineralocorticoids. *Kagawa E4,593/64:* Review (63 pp., about 400 refs.) on "Anti-Aldosterones."

Kagawa E4,772/64: Review (11 pp., about 50 refs.) on the "Action of Anti-Aldosterone Compounds in the Laboratory."

Antifolliculoids. *Selye A60,638/44:* In rodents, the production of anterior pituitary hormones by estradiol is inhibited by a variety of steroids, most of which are androstene derivatives and are designated as "antifolliculoids."

Emmens et al. D25,360/62: Description of the antifolliculoid effects of dimethylstilbestrol (DMS).

Duncan et al. D58,473/63: In rats, U-10520A and U-11100A, derivatives of 1,2-diphenyl-3,4-dihydronaphthalene, possess antifolliculoid activity as judged by the inhibition of estradiol effects after ovariectomy. Both compounds also interrupt pregnancy when administered during the first four days of gestation.

Pincus E689/65: Monograph (360 pp., 1459 refs.) with sections on the literature concerning antifolliculoids and antiluteoids.

Gaunt et al. G63,202/68: A review on the metabolic effects of nonsteroidal antifolliculoids related to diethylstilbestrol and chlorotrianisene, drawn to emphasize structural similarities, cf. drawing p. 55.

Antiluteoids. *Pincus E689/65:* Monograph (360 pp., 1459 refs.) with sections on the literature concerning antifolliculoids and antiluteoids.

Antitestoids. *Gaunt et al. G63,202/68:* A review on the metabolic effects of antitestoids. Antagonists related to testosterone and progesterone, cf. drawing p. 56.

König G66,684/69: Brief review of the literature on "antiandrogens" with special reference to cyproterone. [No mention is made of its possible effect upon enzyme induction (H.S.).]

Bottiglioni et al. G76,203/69: Cyproterone does not interfere with testosterone formation from radioactive pregnenolone in vitro. Its antitestoid effect is exclusively peripheral.

Prasad et al. G78,450/70: In rats, continuous release of microquantities of cyproterone from Silastic capsules causes infertility with loss of sperm motility at dose levels which have no evident antitestoid effect.

Chlorotrianisene

ICI-46,472

Clomiphene

U-11,100A

MER-25

ORF-3858

CN-55,945-27

U-11,555A

Antifolliculoids

Myoneural Blockers. *Baird H27,487/70:* Clinical "experience with pancuronium suggests that it is a useful non-depolarizing myoneural blocker with few side-effects. The absence of cardiovascular side-effects makes the drug particularly valuable in poor-risk patients and in intensive care units."

Chaouki et al. G77,223/70: In 50 patients, pancuronium bromide was found to be an active non-depolarizing neuromuscular blocking agent about 5 times as active as curare and 25 times more potent than gallamine triethiodide. Its advantages are rapid onset of action, no release of histamine and little disturbance in blood pressure, because of a weak ganglioplegic action.

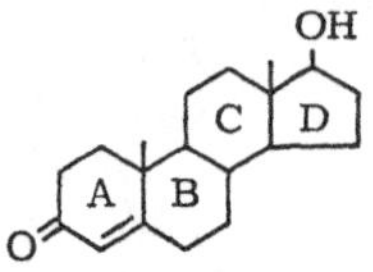

Testosterone

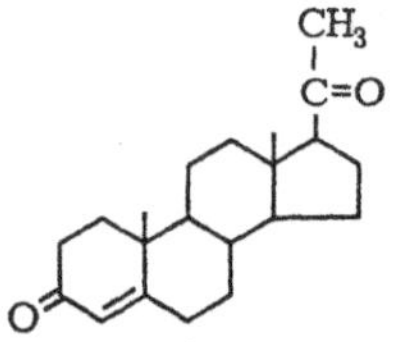

Progesterone

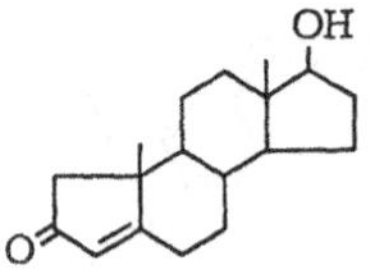

A-Nortestosterone

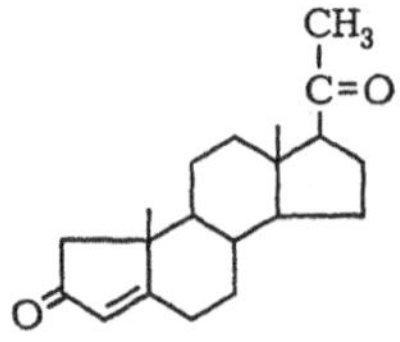

A-Norprogesterone

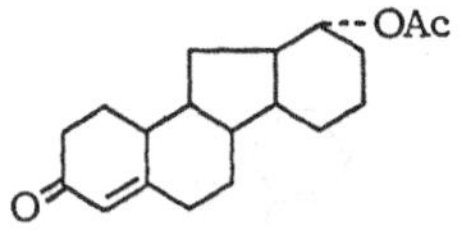

C-Nor-D-homo 17a-epitestosterone acetate

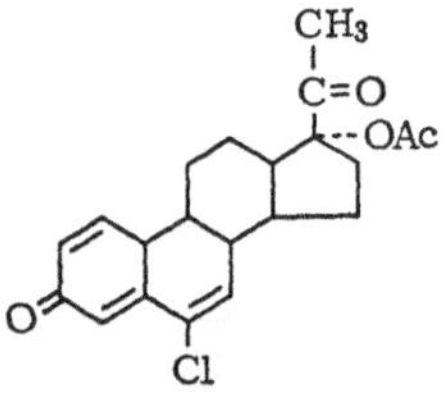

Δ^1-Chlormadinone acetate

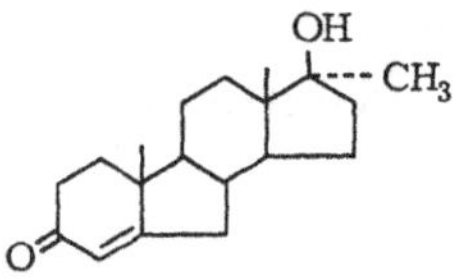

17α-Methyl-B-nortestosterone

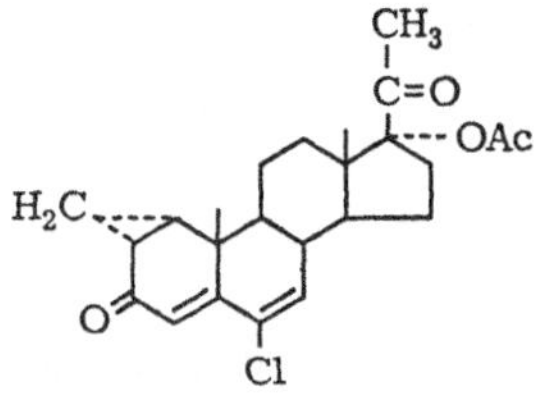

Cyproterone acetate

Antitestoids

Interactions between Inducers

The enzyme induction pattern of various inducers such as phenobarbital and the carcinogens is different. Summation of effects may be obtained by giving these two types of inducers conjointly.

Interactions between the protective effects of various steroids have not yet been systematically explored but these are now under intensive study at our Institute. It will be interesting to note the effects of combined treatment with syntoxic and catatoxic steroids or with two catatoxic steroids having different protective spectra. Unfortunately, systematic studies of this type are extremely costly and time consuming because of the large number of combinations to be explored. Yet, even combinations between protective hormones and catatoxic drugs should be examined since the interactions between them are not only of considerable theoretic but also possibly of practical interest.

Conney F88,649/67: Review of data in the literature showing that the enzyme induction patterns of phenobarbital and carcinogens are different. "When rats were given doses of the inducers that were maximal for their characteristic enzyme inductions, the liver microsomes were more active in metabolizing drugs when both 3,4-benzpyrene and phenobarbital had been given than when either had been given separately." Similar studies suggest that anabolic steroids and phenobarbital induce drug-metabolizing activity through different mechanisms.

Badarau et al. G69,247/68: In rats, various adrenal and ovarian steroids can produce necrosis of the trophoblast during the early stages of gestation. In certain steroid combinations, a mutual antagonism has been noted. [The cursory descriptions in this brief abstract do not permit evaluation of the data (H.S.).]

Fouts G76,868/70: Experiment on concurrent treatment with several inducers showed that enzyme induction by maximally effective doses of chlordane+phenobarbital was no greater than the effect of chlordane or phenobarbital given alone. However, combinations of chlordane with benzpyrene or 3-methylcholanthrene resulted in additive effects. Methyltestosterone+chlordane gave the same effect as chlordane alone. The interpretation of these results has not been attempted.

ANTICATATOXIC COMPOUNDS (ANTAGONISTS)

Anticatatoxic effects can be elicited in various ways. The underlying mechanisms have not yet been clarified for each anticatatoxic substance but there appears no doubt that we should distinguish between:

A. **Inhibitors** which antagonize the enzymes themselves (e.g., SKF 525-A).

B. **Blockers** which impede the synthesis of enzymes by interfering with the production of RNA or of the hormones whose synthesis it directs (e.g., actinomycin, puromycin, ethionine).

C. **Competitors** which act by competitively inhibiting the action of enzymes upon their substrates. Such competitive inhibition may occur between two substrates or even between a substrate and an inducer since many inducers are actually also substrates themselves.

Several anticatatoxic substances may act through a combination of the above mentioned effects.

Inhibitors of Enzymes

Classification. On theoretical grounds, Netter (E 52,768/62) enumerated the following possible mechanisms for enzyme inhibition:

1. The **inhibitor combines directly with the enzyme** at the active center (competitive inhibition) or at some other point (noncompetitive inhibition). Many antimetabolites act by competitive inhibition of enzymes participating in the metabolism of physiologic substrates. An example of competitive inhibition in drug metabolism is the effect of esters or amides on procaine hydrolysis.

2. The **inhibitor decreases a coenzyme concentration** by interfering with its biosynthesis or accelerating its catabolism. The latter mechanism is exemplified by the inhibition of methylation (e.g., choline biosynthesis), by nicotinamide, which forms methylnicotinamide, thereby depleting active methyl groups from the coenzyme.

3. The **inhibitor alters membrane permeability**. This mechanism has not yet been proven to play an important role.

Conney & Burns G67,166/62: Review on the inhibition of microsomal enzyme actions by SKF 525-A, CFT 1201, Lilly 18947, iproniazid, Sch 5712, MPDC, JB-516, and EPDA.

Netter E52,768/62: Review (15 pp., 55 refs.) on "Drugs as Inhibitors of Drug Metabolism" with special reference to SKF 525-A and related compounds.

King & Burgard G46,498/67: Review on various types of antagonists of drug-metabolizing enzymes.

Mannering G71,818/68: Review on microsomal enzyme induction with a special chapter on inhibitors of the drug-metabolizing system.

Mannering G75,980/68: Review (26 pp., 89 refs.) on stimulation and inhibition of drug metabolism.

Mannering G74,572/71: Review on the inhibition of drug metabolism "as it is more narrowly defined to mean the interference of the metabolism of one agent by another agent at the enzymic site."

SKF 525-A (β-diethylaminoethyl diphenylpropylacetate).

SKF 525-A is considered to be a selective inhibitor of microsomal drug-oxidizing systems. It has no sedative action of its own, but when administered prior to agents subject to detoxication by microsomal enzymes it strikingly prolongs their pharmacologic action. For example, rats given hexobarbital plus SKF 525-A slept 35 times longer than rats given the barbiturate alone. Both treatment with SKF 525-A in vivo and addition of the drug to liver slices also reduce subsequent enzymic detoxication in vitro. This shows that the compound acts directly upon microsomal enzyme systems, not merely upon their synthesis in vivo.

Kinetic analysis revealed a noncompetitive type of inhibition, for example, of O-demethylation of p-nitroanisole in vivo and in vitro; conversely the inhibition of plasma procaine esterase is allegedly competitive. SKF 525-A inhibits many oxidative reactions in vivo and in vitro (e.g., side chain oxidation and O-dealkylation, N-dealkylation, deamination, aromatic hydroxylation and sulfoxide formation) presumably by interfering with some step common to all of these reactions. However, NADPH oxidase activity of hepatic microsomes is unaffected by SKF 525-A, although drug metabolism is inhibited in the same preparation. The broad spectrum of reactions inhibited by SKF 525-A includes azo-and nitro-reduction (dependent upon NADPH, but not oxygen) glucuronide formation (a microsomal transfer reaction independent of NADPH); however, not all microsomal reactions are equally sensitive to inhibition by this compound.

Unlike iproniazid and many other microsomal enzyme inhibitors, SKF 525-A is strongly bound to hepatic microsomes and cannot be removed by dialysis or washing.

The fact that SKF 525-A does not act by increasing the drug sensitivity of tissues but merely by delaying their metabolic degradation, is particularly well demonstrated by observations on its influence upon barbiturate anesthesia. In otherwise untreated and SKF 525-A-pretreated rats given hexobarbital, the plasma level of the barbiturate is the same at the moment of awakening although SKF 525-A greatly prolongs the sleeping time. Furthermore, if rats are given SKF 525-A immediately after awakening from hexobarbital anesthesia they do not fall asleep again as they would if SKF 525-A had increased the barbiturate sensitivity of their central nervous system.

Among the hydrolytic products of SKF 525-A, diphenylpropylacetic acid is a potent inhibitor of drug-metabolizing enzymes, whereas diethylaminoethanol is not. It has been claimed so often that microsomal enzymes influence only "xenobiotics," that is, foreign substances, yet SKF 525-A also inhibits the metabolism of various naturally-occurring substrates (e.g., the tricarboxylic acid cycle intermediates: succinate, fumarate and maleate) in rat liver mitochondrial preparations. On the other hand, it has been said that since SKF 525-A is relatively nontoxic the enzyme systems it inactivates "are not essential to the normal economy of the body but operate primarily against toxic influences of foreign compounds." However, in rat liver homogenates the conversion of mevalonate-2-^{14}C to cholesterol and other nonsaponifiable lipids is inhibited by SKF 525-A and plasma cholesterol levels are lowered. Furthermore, SKF 525-A also inhibits the steroid hydroxylases in the hepatic microsomes of the rat, thus blocking the hydroxylation of testosterone and estradiol as well as the degradation of cortisol.

Mestranol (a folliculoid) prolonged while lynestrenol (a luteoid) reduced, pentobarbital sleeping time in mice. The effect of lynestrenol was abolished; that of mestranol potentiated by SKF 525-A. Lynestrenol increases, whereas both mestranol and SKF 525-A reduce, barbiturate clearance from the plasma. Presumably folliculoids share certain enzyme inhibitory reactions of SKF 525-A. Lynestrenol reduces, whereas mestranol or SKF 525-A increases, the anticonvulsive effect of various drugs. This may also be due to altered microsomal drug metabolism but since mestranol and lynestrenol have opposite effects upon brain 5-HT concentration the latter mechanism may likewise be involved.

Using a variety of in vivo or in vitro test procedures, it has been shown that SKF 525-A inhibits the biotransformation and/or the catatoxic action of innumerable agents, e.g.:

Alanine-1-^{14}C
Aminopyrine
p-Aminosalicylic acid
Amobarbital
Amphetamine
Azo dyes

Barbital
Barbiturates (Various)
Bishydroxycoumarin
Butethal
Carisoprodol
Catatoxic steroids (Various)

CCl₄
Chloral hydrate
Chlordiazepoxide
Chloretone
Chlorpromazine
Cholesterol
Codeine
Cortisol
CS₂
Cyclophosphamide
Dethioacetylated 4-6-dienone
Diazepam
Digitoxin
Diphenylhydantoin
DMBA
Ephedrine
Estradiol
Estrone
p-Ethoxyacetanilide
Ethylestrenol
Glutethimide
Hexethal
Hexobarbital
d-Hexobarbital
Hydroxydione
Indocyamine green
Indomethacin
Lynestrenol
Meperidine
Mephenesin
Meprobamate
Mestranol
Methadone
Methorphinan

N-Methylanaline
3-Methyl-4-monomethylaminoazobenzene
Methylparafynol
Monobutyl-4-aminoantipyrine
Monoethyl-4-aminoantipyrine
Monomethyl-4-aminoantipyrine
Morphine
Narcotics (Various)
Naturally-occurring substrates (Various)
Nikethamide
o-Nitroanisole
Norbolethone
7-OHM-12-MBA
Pentobarbital
Pethidine
Phenaglycodol
Phenobarbital
Prednisolone
Prednisone
Primidone
Procaine
Progesterone
Secobarbital
Spironolactone
Strychnine
Succinylcholine
Sulfacetamide
TEA
Testosterone
Thioethamyl
Thiopental
Thiophosphates
Triflupromazine
Urethane

LaDu et al. G74,654/53: The inhibitory action of SKF 525-A is noncompetitive on the microsomal enzyme system that catalyzes N-demethylation of **monomethyl-4-aminoantipyrine.**

Axelrod et al. D79,919/54: In rats, SKF 525-A prolongs the action and inhibits the rate of biotransformation of **hexobarbital** and **pentobarbital**. The inhibitor also retards the demethylation of **meperidine, aminopyrine and ephedrine.**

Cook et al. D23,923/54: First demonstration of the fact, that the inhibitory effect of SKF 525-A on drug-metabolizing enzymes accounts for the long duration of drug action as exemplified by **hexobarbital** sleeping time. SKF 525-A markedly prolongs the hypnotic action of hexobarbital in mice and rats without significantly altering its toxicity. The length of hexobarbital sleeping time thus achieved cannot be duplicated with any dose of the hypnotic agent alone. In this respect, SKF 525-A is equally effective i.p. and p.o., the latter route being less toxic. SKF 525-A is almost immediately effective and the duration of its action is approximately 15 hrs.

Cook et al. D94,204/54: The analgesic action of **methadone, meperidine, morphine, codeine** and **methorphinan** was enhanced by SKF 525-A in the rat, but the LD_{50}'s of **morphine** and **meperidine** were not significantly altered.

Cook et al. E34,395/54: Experiments on rats and mice indicate that SKF 525-A potentiates the hypnotic effects of **hexobarbital, secobarbital, pentobarbital, amobarbital, butethal, hexethal, phenobarbital** and **chloral hydrate**, but does not significantly influence that of **barbital, thioethamyl, thiopental** or **methylparafynol.**

Cooper et al. H25,117/54: SKF 525-A also inhibits the metabolism of various **naturally-**

occurring substrates (e.g., the tricarboxylic acid cycle intermediates: succinate, fumarate, and maleate) in rat liver mitochondrial preparations. Among the hydrolytic products of SKF 525-A, diphenylpropylacetic acid is a potent inhibitor of drug-metabolizing enzymes, whereas diethylaminoethanol is not.

Brodie et al. G66,772/55: Although SKF 525-A inhibits various hepatic microsomal enzyme activities in the rabbit's liver it is relatively nontoxic and, hence, "one can speculate that these systems are not essential to the normal economy of the body, but operate primarily against the toxic influences of **foreign compounds** that gain access to the body from the alimentary tract."

Fouts & Brodie D83,597/55: SKF 525-A and the closely-related compound Lilly 18947 prolong the hypnotic action of **hexobarbital** in mice by inhibiting its metabolism by hepatic microsomes.

Axelrod G74,652/56: SKF 525-A inhibits the O-dealkylation of **codeine** but not that of **p-ethoxyacetanilide**. Presumably, more than one O-dealkylating enzyme exists in the liver.

Brodie C12,157/56: Review on the early work on SKF 525-A showing that it prolongs the effect of **hexobarbital, pethidine, codeine, morphine, mephenesin, amphetamine** and other compounds. The metabolic pathways through which these drugs are normally inactivated, and their blockade by SKF 525-A are described in detail.

Richards & Taylor H19,235/56: Review on the pharmacology of **barbiturates** with a special section on the sleep-enhancing effect of SKF 525-A and related compounds.

Murphy & DuBois D28,546/58: The activity of the microsomal enzyme system which oxidizes **thiophosphates** to potent anticholinesterase agents is considerably higher in male than in female rats (incubation of liver homogenates with Guthion or ethyl p-nitrophenyl thionobenzenephosphonate or "EPN"). Yet, in vivo, adult males are more resistant to EPN than females, perhaps because the accelerated formation of toxic oxidation products is overcompensated by a more efficient detoxication of the latter. The low enzyme activity of female livers is enhanced by pretreatment with testosterone in vivo, whereas the high activity of male livers is diminished by previous castration, partial hepatectomy or treatment with progesterone or diethylstilbestrol. SKF 525-A inhibits, whereas pretreatment with carcinogens or a protein-deficient diet enhances, the activity of the thiophosphate-oxidizing enzyme.

Takemori & Mannering H24,294/58: SKF 525-A inhibits the N-demethylation of several **narcotics** but does not inhibit the demethylation of the **azo dye, 3-methyl-4-monomethylaminoazobenzene**. Such observations suggest that inhibitors of drug-metabolizing enzymes can be used as tools to determine if more than one enzyme system can catalyze the same reaction.

Gaudette & Brodie E90,437/59: SKF 525-A inhibits the N-dealkylation of **aminopyrine** and **monomethyl-4-aminoantipyrine** but not that of **monoethyl-4-aminoantipyrine, monobutyl-4-aminoantipyrine, or N-methylanaline**. Presumably, more than one enzyme system can N-dealkylate drugs.

Netter G74,665/59: The inhibitory action of SKF 525-A on plasma **procaine** esterase is competitive.

Sulman et al. C79,823/59: In rats injected for 4 months with **prednisone** or **prednisolone**, an increase in the hepatic content of the enzymes which decompose these steroids could be demonstrated in vitro. Various histologic stains failed to reveal any associated light-microscopic change in the hepatocytes. Addition of SKF 525-A to the homogenate of activated livers blocked their enzymic activity.

Dick et al. G74,672/60: In dogs, chronic administration of SKF 525-A lowers plasma **cholesterol**.

Holmes & Bentz G74,656/60: In rat liver homogenates, the conversion of mevalonate-2-^{14}C to **cholesterol** and other nonsaponifiable lipids is inhibited by SKF 525-A. It remains to be shown whether this effect could explain the lowering of plasma cholesterol levels obtained in dogs by SKF 525-A.

Kato & Chiesarà G68,581/60: Male rats are more resistant than females to the toxic action of **strychnine**. This difference is abolished by SKF 525-A.

Netter G74,666/60: The inhibitory action of SKF 525-A on O-demethylation of **o-nitroanisole** is noncompetitive.

Neubert & Timmler G74,668/60: SKF 525-A and CFT 1201 inhibit incorporation of **alanine-1-^{14}C** into hepatic microsomal protein.

Kato et al. G66,023/61: Adult (unlike immature) male rats are less sensitive to **carisoprodol**-induced muscular paralysis than females. Castration or treatment with SKF 525-A abolishes the increased resistance of the adult male rat. Incubation of liver slices with carisoprodol shows that the resistance of

Bella et al. G77,568/62: In various species, SKF 525-A enhances the neuromuscular-blocking action of **succinylcholine**, and similar compounds. The inhibition appears to occur at the neuromuscular junction.

Brock & Hohorst G71,533/62: **Cyclophosphamide** has no cytotoxic effect upon Yoshida sarcoma cells in vitro but it is rapidly transformed into an active compound in mice, rats and dogs in vivo. The active form is demonstrable in the blood and urine by bioassay if added to tumor cells in vitro. In completely hepatectomized rats, only a little fraction of cyclophosphamide is thus activated. However, activation can be demonstrated in vitro by incubation with liver slices. Pretreatment of rats with SKF 525-A inhibits in vivo activation which presumably takes place in hepatic microsomes.

Kato et al. D38,983/62: Male rats are more resistant than females to **strychnine** intoxication especially if the drug is given s.c. whereby its activity is delayed. The greater strychnine metabolizing potency of microsomes from male rats than from females has also been demonstrated in vitro. SKF 525-A increases strychnine toxicity and renders both sexes equally sensitive.

Kato & Vassanelli D40,237/62: "Rats pretreated with **phenobarbital, phenaglycodol, glutethimide, nikethamide, chlorpromazine, triflupromazine, meprobamate, carisoprodol, pentobarbital, thiopental, primidone, chloretone, diphenylhydantoin** and **urethane** showed an accelerated metabolism of meprobamate and, at the same time, a diminished duration of sleeping time and paralysis due to meprobamate." SKF 525-A counteracted these actions of the enzyme inducers.

Rümke G69,768/63: In mice, SKF 525-A, phenobarbital, chlorpromazine, hexobarbital and iproniazid given one hour before **hydroxydione** i.v. increases sleeping time. When the interval is two days, single doses of SKF 525-A, phenobarbital or chlorpromazine decrease hydroxydione anesthesia. Phenytoin, acetylcarbromal, morphine, chloramphenicol, 5-HT, phenobarbital and hydroxydione given one hour before hexobarbital increase the duration of anesthesia whereas dioxone and chlorothiazide decrease it. It is concluded that central effects as well as changes in microsomal enzyme activity may be involved.

Kuntzman et al. F27,893/64: SKF 525-A inhibits the **steroid hydroxylase** present in the microsomal fraction of rat liver.

Paeile et al. F52,633/64: Adult male rats are more resistant to **procaine** than adult females. Chronic CCl_4 poisoning, pretreatment with SKF 525-A and orchidectomy diminish the resistance of the males approximately to the female level. The plasma procainesterase activity is approximately the same in both sexes and not affected by orchidectomy or CCl_4 intoxication.

Rogers & Fouts F27,894/64: In vitro experiments in rats have shown that SKF 525-A is strongly **bound to hepatic microsomes** and cannot be removed by dialysis or washing, whereas the reverse is true of iproniazid and other microsomal enzyme inhibitors.

Conney et al. G65,135/65: In the rat, SKF 525-A markedly inhibits **hexobarbital** metabolism and the hydroxylation of **testosterone** and **estradiol**.

Kupfer & Peets F85,854/67: **Cortisol** s.c. increases hepatic TKT activity in adrenalectomized male rats and this effect is further augmented by SKF 525-A which in itself has no effect. In intact rats SKF 525-A raises hepatic TKT activity in itself but this effect is not further augmented by cortisol. Possibly the potentiation of cortisol induction of TKT by SKF 525-A is due to an inhibition of the degradation of cortisol.

Mannering G71,818/68 (p. 105): Review listing the **large number of substrates** whose in vivo or in vitro transformation by hepatic microsomal enzymes is inhibited by SKF 525-A. However, this drug does not inhibit the biotransformation of all substrates known to be metabolized by microsomal systems. "These differences in the action of SKF 525-A on the biotransformation of different drugs strengthen the view that more than one drug-metabolizing enzyme system exists in hepatic microsomes or that the rate-limiting component may not be the same in all species or under all conditions."

Blackham & Spencer G69,913/69: Mestranol (a folliculoid) prolonged while lynestrenol (a luteoid) reduced the duration of pentobarbital and hexobarbital sleeping time in mice. Barbital was not affected. The effects of **lynestrenol** were abolished by SKF 525-A while those of **mestranol** were markedly potentiated. Lynestrenol increased, whereas mestranol and SKF 525-A reduced, the rate of clearance of barbiturate from the plasma.

Bond et al. H18,559/69: In rats, pretreatment with phenobarbital does not change the LD$_{50}$ of CS$_2$ p.o. but results in the production of central lobular hepatic necrosis. After pretreatment with SKF 525-A these hepatic lesions no longer occur in rats pretreated with phenobarbital and then given CS$_2$. SKF 525-A may inhibit the production of toxic CS$_2$ metabolites by hepatic microsomal enzymes.

Furner et al. H17,931/69: In rats, **d-hexobarbital** is about twice as susceptible to inhibition by SKF 525-A as dl- or l-hexobarbital.

Hart & Adamson G69,481/69: In mice "SKF 525-A and Lilly 18947 reduced the lethality of **cyclophosphamide** over a 28 day observation period while pretreatment with phenobarbital did not change the 28 day lethality. Neither SKF 525-A nor phenobarbital had an effect on the antitumor efficacy of cyclophosphamide. Mice housed on cedar chip bedding were less susceptible to the lethal effects of cyclophosphamide, but tumor bearing mice on this bedding showed greater antitumor response to the drug than those on hardwood bedding."

Bird et al. H30,425/70: In rats less than 30 days of age, **DMBA** or **7-OHM-12-MBA** produces no adrenal necrosis unless animals are pretreated with ACTH. However, a single i.v. injection of 7-OHM-12-MBA on the 17th day of gestation causes adrenal necrosis in the embryos as well as in the mothers. Pretreatment with SKF 525-A protected the adrenals both of the embryos and of the mothers.

Blackham & Spencer G73,813/70: In mice, lynestrenol reduced, whereas mestranol or SKF 525-A increased the anticonvulsive effect (tested with electroshock) of **diphenylhydantoin, phenobarbital, chlordiazepoxide** and **diazepam** administered i.p. after five days of pretreatment. This may be due to altered microsomal drug metabolism but since mestranol and lynestrenol have opposite effects upon the brain 5-HT concentrations, the latter mechanism must also be considered.

Levine G75,350/70: In rats, SKF 525-A has previously been found to depress the biliary excretion of **indocyamine green** (ICG), a dye which is not metabolized prior to excretion. With this exception, SKF 525-A depresses only the biliary excretion of compounds that are metabolized. However, it is now shown that the biliary excretion of ICG and the bile flow itself are not influenced by SKF 525-A provided normal body temperature is maintained.

McLean and Marchand G78,253/70: In rats, SKF 525-A decreases the plasma concentration of orally-administered **barbital, p-aminosalicylic acid, sulfacetamide** and **CCl$_4$**, presumably because of a nonspecific effect on the gastrointestinal absorption of polar and nonpolar compounds. Various other mechanisms of SKF 525-A action are discussed, which must be kept in mind in interpreting the possible effect of SKF 525-A through the inhibition of hepatic microsomal drug metabolism.

Levin et al. H26,593/70: In rats, CCl$_4$ given to immature females 24 hrs before sacrifice inhibited the activity of hepatic microsomal enzymes that hydroxylate estradiol-17β and estrone. This inhibition was reflected in vivo by an altered metabolism of estradiol-17β and estrone, by a potentiation of the uterotrophic action of folliculoids and by an increased concentration of these steroids in the uterus. By contrast, tetrachloroethylene did not influence the action of estrone. SKF 525-A and desipramine, which are also inhibitors of drug metabolism, likewise potentiate the uterotrophic action of **estrone** in immature rats.

Solymoss et al. G60,099/70: In rats, pentobarbital anesthesia is inhibited by spironolactone, ethylestrenol, norbolethone and, to a lesser extent, even by progesterone. These **cataxoxic steroids** also accelerate the disappearance rate of barbiturate from the blood; their effects are counteracted by SKF 525-A. Irrespective of the steroid pretreatment, the rats awake roughly at the same blood pentobarbital level.

Solymoss et al. G70,423/70: In rats, pretreatment with spironolactone, norbolethone or ethylestrenol enhances the disappearance of bishydroxycoumarin from blood and restores the prothrombin time. Triamcinolone and progesterone fail to do so. SKF 525-A increases the blood concentration and the anticoagulant effect of **bishydroxycoumarin** and counteracts the beneficial effect of **ethylestrenol.**

Solymoss et al. G70,445/70: In rats, the acute hematologic changes observed six days after a single oral dose of DMBA are suppressed by spironolactone but the alterations normally observed 12 days after DMBA still occur. The hematologic damage produced by a smaller dose of **DMBA** i.v. is prevented both by spironolactone and by SKF 525-A. Apparently "the hemopoietic alterations, elicited by DMBA, are dose-dependent and influenced also by the biotransformation of this polycyclic hydrocarbon, since both acceleration (by spironolactone) and blockade (by SKF 525-A) of this latter process can suppress the development of hematologic alterations."

Solymoss et al. G70,461/70: In rats, spironolactone, norbolethone and ethylestrenol pretreatment accelerate the disappearance-rate of digitoxin from serum in proportion to the inhibition of the convulsions. Partial hepatectomy reduces digitoxin elimination. The action of **spironolactone** is blocked by SKF 525-A.

Solymoss et al. G70,463/70: In rats, pretreatment with spironolactone, norbolethone or ethylestrenol accelerated the plasma clearance of digitoxin, in proportion to the in vivo protective effect of these catatoxic steroids. Partial hepatectomy reduces digitoxin clearance. The effect of **spironolactone** is suppressed by SKF 525-A and cycloheximide.

Solymoss et al. G70,464/70: In rats, spironolactone shortens the half-life of its main metabolite, the **dethioacetylated 4,6-dienone** (metabolite A), which is interconvertible with the 17-hydroxy carboxylic acid derivative (metabolite B). This alteration is only slightly accentuated if the steroid is given chronically and it wears off within eight days after spironolactone treatment is interrupted. After a test dose of spironolactone or of its metabolites A and B, partial hepatectomy delays the blood clearance of metabolite A. Cycloheximide and SKF 525-A also suppress the blood clearance of metabolite A under these conditions. Presumably "spironolactone influences its own biotransformation and the steroid is also a substrate of the hepatic drug-metabolizing enzymes which are induced by spironolactone itself."

Solymoss G70,484/70: In rats, the plasma clearance of digitoxin is accelerated by spironolactone, norbolethone and ethylestrenol in doses that protect against the toxicity of the alkaloid in vivo. On the other hand, partial hepatectomy reduces digitoxin plasma clearance, and increases the severity of the convulsions. The protective action of the **catatoxic steroids** is suppressed by SKF 525-A and cycloheximide.

Soyka et al. H33,315/70: Partial hepatectomy sensitized only slightly to the anesthetic effect of **5β-pregnane-3α-ol-20-one**, whereas it greatly prolonged sleeping time following treatment with progesterone and many other steroids. Neither inhibition of hepatic mixed function oxidase activity by SKF 525-A nor its stimulation by 3-MC affected the duration of pregnanolone narcosis and even phenobarbital reduced its length only slightly. These findings, and distribution studies, "suggest that termination of hypnosis is due mainly to redistribution with hepatic metabolism playing a relatively minor role." [Species not mentioned; probably rat (H.S.).]

Solymoss et al. G60,093/71: In rats, spironolactone, norbolethone and progesterone, unlike hydroxydione, accelerate the clearance from the blood of s.c.-injected indomethacin. SKF 525-A significantly suppresses the activity of these **catatoxic steroids** which probably act through increased metabolic degradation of indomethacin.

Solymoss & Varga G70,500/71: In rats, spironolactone, norbolethone and ethylestrenol diminish the anticoagulant action and accelerate the plasma clearance of bishydroxycoumarin. Progesterone and triamcinolone are devoid of this effect. SKF 525-A counteracts the influence of **ethylestrenol** upon **bishydroxycoumarin** metabolism. The hepatic microsomes of rats treated with spironolactone or ethylestrenol in vivo accelerate bishydroxycoumarin degradation by NADPH-dependent enzymes in vitro.

Strychnine ← SKF 525-A + Sex: Kato et al. *G74,030/62**

Codeine ← SKF 525-A + Adrenal demedullation: Rogers et al. *D64,023/63*

CFT 1201 (phenyldiallylacetic acid ester of diethylaminoethanol), CFT 1215, CFT 1042.

Much less work has been done with the phenylacetic acid derivatives which, like SKF 525-A, act as hepatic microsomal enzyme inhibitors. The most active member of this group is CFT 1201. It prolongs the action of hexobarbital, propallylonal, eunarcon and butallylonal, without affecting the hypnotic action of barbital, a compound notoriously not metabolized within the body. CFT 1201 uncouples oxidative phosphorylation when α-ketoglutarate or β-oxybutyrate are used as substrates, but it also inhibits the incorporation of alanine-1-^{14}C into hepatic microsomal protein.

Neubert & Herken G74,660/55: Several phenylacetic acid derivatives prolong the action of hexobarbital. The most active of these compounds is the phenyldiallylacetic acid ester of diethylaminoethanol (CFT 1201), which also prolongs the action of propallylonal, eunarcon, and butallylonal. However, CFT 1201 does not affect the hypnotic action of barbital, which notoriously is not metabolized in the rat.

Maibauer et al. G74,663/58: In rats, CFT 1201 causes hepatic steatosis.

Neubert & Hoffmeister G74,667/60: CFT 1201 uncouples oxidative phosphorylation when α-ketoglutarate or β-oxybutyrate are used as substrates.

Neubert & Timmler G74,668/60: SKF 525-A and CFT 1201 inhibit incorporation of alanine-1-^{14}C into hepatic microsomal protein.

Lilly 18947 (2,4-dichloro-6-phenylphenoxyethyl diethylamine).

This compound is chemically closely related to SKF 525-A and resembles the latter also in its pharmacologic actions. In acute experiments on mice it prolongs hexobarbital sleeping time by inhibiting barbiturate metabolism in hepatic microsomes. When given over a 28 day observation period Lilly 18947 reduces the lethality of cyclophosphamide perhaps because its inhibitory effect upon drug metabolism is reversed following chronic administration.

Fouts & Brodie D83,597/55: SKF 525-A and the closely-related compound Lilly 18947 prolong the hypnotic action of hexobarbital in mice by inhibiting its metabolism by hepatic microsomes.

Fouts & Brodie D95,674/56: 2,4-Dichloro-6-phenylphenoxyethyl diethylamine (Lilly 18947) and iproniazid (2-isopropyl-1-isonicotinyl hydrazine, Marsilid) prolong hexobarbital sleeping time by inhibiting its metabolism in hepatic microsomes.

Hart & Adamson G69,481/69: In mice "SKF 525-A and Lilly 18947 reduced the lethality of cyclophosphamide over a 28 day observation period while pretreatment with phenobarbital did not change the 28 day lethality. Neither SKF 525-A nor phenobarbital had an effect on the antitumor efficacy of cyclophosphamide. Mice housed on cedar chip bedding were less susceptible to the lethal effects of cyclophosphamide, but tumor bearing mice on this bedding showed greater antitumor response to the drug than those on hardwood bedding."

MPDC (N-methyl-3-piperidyl diphenylcarbamate), EPDA (N-ethyl-3-piperidyl diphenylacetate), EPB (N-ethyl-3-piperidyl benzylate) and JB 516 (β-phenylisopropylhydrazine).

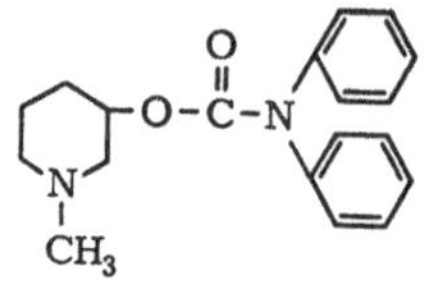
O
O-C-N
N
CH3

MPDC

All these piperidyl compounds prolong barbiturate sleeping time by inhibiting microsomal drug metabolism. MPDC given 1—12 hrs before hexobarbital prolongs sleeping time and inhibits the metabolism of the barbiturate, although the reverse is true if MPDC is given 24—48 hrs before hexobarbital. In all these respects the compound resembles the numerous other inhibitors which exhibit similar biphasic responses.

Fujimoto et al. D78,955/60; Serrone & Fujimoto D83,863/60: β-Phenylisopropylhydrazine (JB 516), N-ethyl-3-piperidyl benzylate (EPB), N-ethyl-3-piperidyl diphenylacetate (EPDA), and N-methyl-3-piperidyl diphenylcarbamate (MPDC) prolong barbiturate sleeping time by inhibiting microsomal drug metabolism.

Serrone & Fujimoto D48,610/61: MPDC given 1—12 hrs before hexobarbital prolongs sleeping time and the metabolism of the barbiturate. However, if MPDC is given 24—48 hrs before hexobarbital, the metabolism of the drug is stimulated and sleeping time is shortened. Data are presented to show that the accelerated metabolism of hexobarbital results from induced synthesis of microsomal enzyme systems that metabolize barbiturates. A similar biphasic response on hexobarbital sleeping time was observed with SKF 525-A, JB 516, iproniazid, orphenadrine, chlorpromazine, and hydroxyzine by several investigators (Holtz et al. D98,342/57; Arrigoni-Martelli & Kramer G74,659/59; Rümke & Bout G74,669/60).

Sch 5712, Sch 5705 (malonic and succinic acid derivatives).

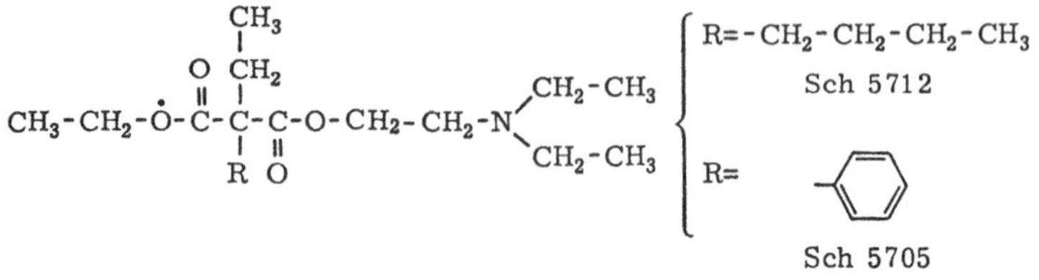
CH3
O CH2
CH3-CH2-O-C-C-C-O-CH2-CH2-N
CH2-CH3
CH2-CH3
R O
R=-CH2-CH2-CH2-CH3
Sch 5712
R=
Sch 5705

Hexobarbital metabolism is inhibited and sleeping time prolonged by certain malonic and succinic acid derivatives such as Sch 5712 or Sch 5705. Sch 5712 prolongs hexobarbital sleeping time about 12-fold in female and only 3-fold in male rats, yet it inhibits hexobarbital metabolism in vitro about equally in unfortified liver homogenates of both sexes.

Kramer & Arrigoni-Martelli G74,673/59: The hexobarbital metabolism by hepatic microsomal enzyme systems is inhibited, whereas hexobarbital sleeping time is prolonged, by certain malonic and succinic acid derivatives, such as Sch 5712. The latter compound prolongs hexobarbital sleeping time about 12-fold in female and only 3-fold in male rats, yet it inhibits hexobarbital metabolism in vitro about equally when tested with the unfortified liver homogenate from rats of either sex. Furthermore, Sch 5712 is singularly ineffective in prolonging hexobarbital sleeping time in rats pretreated with phenobarbital.

Arrigoni-Martelli et al. G74,653/60: Several malonic and succinic acid derivatives potentiate the action of hexobarbital, chlorpheniramine (Chlortrimeton), and amphetamine.

Hexobarbital ← Sch 5705, Sch 5712 + Sex: Kramer et al. *G74,673/59**

Chloramphenicol.

$$\begin{array}{c} NO_2 \\ | \\ \bigcirc \\ | \\ HOCH \\ | \\ HCNHCOCHCl_2 \\ | \\ CH_2OH \end{array}$$

This antibiotic does not induce sedation by itself and fails to potentiate subhypnotic doses of hexobarbital but inhibits the metabolism of the latter if given to mice and rats a short time before the barbiturate. In vitro, a number of other enzymic reactions are also inhibited by chloramphenicol which acts essentially like SKF 525-A and other related compounds.

Dixon & Fouts E53,752/62: In mice and rats, chloramphenicol inhibits hexobarbital metabolism. When chloramphenicol is given 45 min before hexobarbital, the sleeping time in mice is greatly prolonged and the total body levels of the barbiturates are increased. This antibiotic does not induce sedation by itself and fails to potentiate a subhypnotic dose of hexobarbital. In vitro, a number of enzymic reactions are inhibited by chloramphenicol and the pathways blocked are essentially the same as those inhibited by SKF 525-A and related compounds.

Firkin & Linnane H31,607/70: In rats, partial hepatectomy greatly increases sensitivity to the lethal effect of heavy chloramphenicol overdosage. Lower doses of "chloramphenicol appeared to specifically inhibit the synthesis of the mitochondrial cytochromes a, a_3, b and c_1 in the actively growing liver tissue. In some of the liver cells there was extensive cytoplasmic vacuolation resulting from dilation of the endoplasmic reticulum, and the mitochondria were swollen and appeared to contain fewer cristae. It is suggested that chloramphenicol has at least three effects in the cells of higher organisms—a specific inhibitory effect on the synthesis of some mitochondrial cytochromes which is presumably a reflection of its action on the mitochondrial protein synthesizing system, an effect on cellular ultrastructure, and a direct inhibitory effect on cellular respiration only at relatively high concentrations of the drug."

Solymoss et al. G70,412/70: "In rats, 24 hours after a single dose of spironolactone or ethylestrenol, the disappearance of pentobarbital from blood is enhanced to a rate in proportion to the decreasing depth of anesthesia. This action is completely suppressed by ribonucleic acid- or protein-synthesis inhibitors such as actinomycin D, puromycin aminonucleoside and cycloheximide, and only partially by 6-mercaptopurine or chloramphenicol... Induction of drug-metabolizing enzymes is involved in the resistance-increasing effect of spironolactone or ethylestrenol against various compounds."

Disulfiram (tetraethylthiuram disulfide, Antabuse).

$$\begin{array}{c} C_2H_5 \\ \diagdown \\ C_2H_5 \diagup \end{array} N-\underset{\underset{\displaystyle \|}{S}}{C}-S-S-\underset{\underset{\displaystyle \|}{S}}{C}-N \begin{array}{c} \diagup C_2H_5 \\ \\ \diagdown C_2H_5 \end{array}$$

This drug was introduced for the treatment of chronic alcoholism. It has virtually no pharmacologic effects of its own but if, after its administration, ethanol is ingested, patients suffer violent flushing, dyspnea, nausea, vomiting, and hypotension and hence, they are forced to abstain.

Disulfiram inhibits ADH, presumably by competing with NAD. ADH normally oxidizes acetaldehyde to acetic acid. The blockade of the enzyme by disulfiram does not alter the blood ethanol levels following ingestion of the alcohol, but acetaldehyde and pyruvate accumulate and cause the just-mentioned disturbances which may reach dangerous proportions. Hence, the practical use of this prophylaxis is limited. The pathogenic role of acetaldehyde was confirmed by the observation that, in itself, it produces changes similar to those observed after ingestion of ethanol following pretreatment with disulfiram. Recent observations suggest, however, that the accumulation of pyruvate may also play an important role in the pathogenesis of the resulting clinical syndrome.

Lecoq et al. B66,406/51: In rats, the toxic effects of ethanol and its metabolites, pyruvate and acetaldehyde (which accumulate in the body under the influence of disulfiram) are inhibited by ACTH, cortisone, and hepatic extracts. Conversely, thyroxine, DOC, and testosterone appear to aggravate ethanol intoxication. [Statistically evaluated data are not presented (H.S.).]

Lecoq B79,754/51: In rabbits, the injection of disulfiram+ethanol or of Na-pyruvate produces essentially the same syndrome of intoxication, since pyruvic acid is the principal metabolite of ethanol after pretreatment with disulfiram. In either case, ACTH and cortisone offer little, if any, protective effect.

Scholler G75,794/70: In rats, disulfiram inhibits whereas phenobarbital aggravates the toxic effects of chloroform anesthesia, as manifested by hepatic necroses and plasma enzyme GOT and GPT determinations.

MAO-Inhibitors (iproniazid, phenelzine, isocarboxazid, tranylcypromine, pargyline, nialamide).

Iproniazid was synthesized as an antibacterial agent for the treatment of tuberculosis. It, and several of its derivatives, turned out to be potent MAO-inhibitors which may cause euphoria presumably through the inhibition of the metabolism of epinephrine, norepinephrine and 5-HT, which are normally present in the brain. Various other hydrazides (phenelzine, isocarboxazid) and nonhydrazide inhibitors (tranylcypromine, pargyline) have been synthesized for the treatment of severe depression.

All these MAO-inhibitors are active both in vivo and in vitro. The mechanism of their action is not yet completely understood but they undoubtedly elevate norepinephrine and 5-HT concentrations in the central nervous system and produce toxic effects, such as hypertension, liver damage, jaundice, nausea, vomiting,

iproniazid, **phenelzine (JB 516)**, **isocarboxazid**, **tranylcypromine**, **pargyline**, **nialamide**

constipation, dry mouth, delusions and hallucinations. They have little, if any, potentiating action upon the cardiovascular effects of natural catecholamines, presumably because O-methylation and tissue uptake, rather than oxidative deamination, are responsible for terminating their peripheral actions.

However, the MAO-inhibitors greatly potentiate the cardiovascular effects of simple phenylethylamines like tyramine. Thus, patients receiving tranylcypromine conjointly with phenylethylamine derivatives may experience exaggerated hypertensive effects conducive to apoplexy. Even foods may become dangerous following MAO-inhibitor treatment. Some cheeses (Camembert, Brie, Stilton, New York Cheddar) are rich in tyramine, which is ordinarily harmless because it is rapidly oxidized by MAO, however, after treatment with tranylcypromine, the tyramine in these cheeses may elicit the dangerous hypertensive crises just mentioned.

Curiously, iproniazid also potentiates the lathyrogenic action of APN in turkey poults, but this may be a nonspecific stress effect.

Both desipramine and imipramine exert an "SKF 525-A-like" inhibitory effect upon hepatic microsomes in vitro and they prolong hexobarbital sleeping time; however there appears to be no close correlation between the MAO-inhibitor activity of these compounds on their ability to interfere with hexobarbital metabolism.

Fouts & Brodie D83,597/55: 2,4-Dichloro-6-phenylphenoxyethyl diethylamine HBr (Lilly 18947) and iproniazid (2-isopropyl-1-isonicotinyl hydrazine, Marsilid) prolong hexobarbital sleeping time by inhibiting its metabolism in hepatic microsomes.

Fouts & Brodie D95,674/56: Iproniazid, though practically devoid of sedative action, prolongs the hypnotic activity of hexobarbital in mice by interfering with its metabolism through hepatic microsomal enzymes. In this respect, iproniazid acts like SKF 525-A and Lilly 18947.

Arrigoni-Martelli & Kramer G74,659/59: In mice, hexobarbital and thiopental metabolism is impeded by the MAO-inhibitors, iproniazid and β-phenylisopropyl hydrazine (JB 516).

Fujimoto et al. D78,955/60; Serrone & Fujimoto D83,863/60: β-Phenylisopropylhydrazine (JB 516), N-ethyl-3-piperidyl benzilate (EPB), N-ethyl-3-piperidyl diphenylacetate (EPDA), and N-methyl-3-piperidyl diphenylcarbamate (MPDC) prolong barbiturate sleeping time by inhibiting microsomal drug metabolism.

Laroche & Brodie H21,467/60: There appears to be no correlation between the MAO-inhibitor activity of chemical compounds and their ability to interfere with hexobarbital metabolism.

Strong G73,964/62: Iproniazid can potentiate the lathyrogenic action of APN in turkey poults.

Rogers & Fouts F27,894/64: In vitro experiments in rats have shown that SKF 525-A is strongly bound to hepatic microsomes and cannot be removed by dialysis or washing, whereas the reverse is true of iproniazid and other microsomal enzyme inhibitors.

Blackwell E65,708/63: MAO-inhibitors such as tranylcypromine can produce severe paroxysmal hypertension and intracranial bleeding in patients following ingestion of certain cheeses.

Jori & Pugliatti G70,112/67: Desipramine and imipramine exert an SKF 525-A-like inhibitory effect upon the hepatic microsomes.

Bowman et al. E714/68 (p. 520): Iproniazid is an inhibitor of MAO and of other extramicrosomal enzymes. Like SKF 525-A which also inhibits a number of other enzymes, it has been termed a "multi-potent" enzyme inhibitor.

p-Aminosalicylic Acid (PAS). PAS feeding induces glycogen infiltration of the rat liver; it also prolongs hexobarbital sleeping time, presumably by decreasing barbiturate excretion. There may exist some relationship between hepatic glycogen deposition and the changes in the SER. This could account for the inhibitory effect of PAS which is distinctly different from the enzyme inhibition caused by chloramphenicol or SKF 525-A. The latter compounds inhibit both aminopyrine and codeine metabolism, whereas PAS inhibits only the former.

Rogers et al. E31,897/63: In rats, PAS feeding induces glycogen infiltration of the liver and prolongation of hexobarbital sleeping time, apparently due to diminished ability to excrete the barbiturate. The in vitro metabolism of hexobarbital and aminopyrine, by the microsomes of rats pretreated with PAS, is diminished. Acute administration of PAS had no effect on hexobarbital sleeping time, nor did addition of PAS in vitro inhibit drug-metabolizing enzymes. There may exist some relationship between hepatic glycogen deposition and changes in the SER. This might account for the inhibitory effect of PAS, which is definitely different from that of chloramphenicol and SKF 525-A.

Rogers & Fouts F27,894/64: In the utilization of PAS, there is an increase in hepatic glycogen content associated with a decreased hexobarbital-metabolizing activity of the hepatic microsomes. PAS inhibits aminopyrine metabolism but not codeine metabolism. Conversely, both aminopyrine and codeine metabolism are inhibited by chloramphenicol and SKF 525-A. Presumably PAS, after prolonged administration, induces a more selective inhibition than other antagonists.

Competition between Substrates

Various substrates of hepatic enzymes potentiate the toxicity of other simultaneously-applied substrates of the same enzymes. This phenomenon can be illustrated by many examples:

Triorthotolyl phosphate potentiates the toxicity of malathione by inhibiting the metabolism of the latter. EPN has the same effect by inhibiting the esterases responsible for malathione detoxication. In man, oxyphenbutazone prolongs the elevation of plasma levels of bishydroxycoumarin with a potentiation of its anticoagulant action. In rats, ethylmorphine and codeine retard the metabolism of hexobarbital in vivo as measured by its plasma clearance. In isolated hepatic microsomal preparations of the rat the N-demethylation of ethylmorphine is competitively inhibited by hexobarbital, chlorpromazine, zoxazolamine, phenylbutazone and acetanilide; in fact ethylmorphine and chlorpromazine are mutually inhibitory, each retarding the metabolism of the other. All these drugs are known to be oxidized by microsomal enzymes. On the other hand, barbital and acetazolamide, drugs which are not metabolized, fail to act as inhibitors in this system.

Jaundice develops more often in newborn infants fed on breast than on cow's milk. This has been ascribed to the presence in human milk of $3\alpha, 20\beta$-pregnanediol which competitively might inhibit glucuronyl transferase and thereby interfere with bilirubin clearance. However, more recent observations suggest that neither $3\alpha, 20\beta$-pregnanediol nor $3\alpha, 20\alpha$-pregnanediol inhibit conjugation by human hepatic microsomes, whereas estradiol does have such an action.

Many additional examples could be cited to illustrate the mutual competitive inhibition between substrates for microsomal drug-metabolizing enzymes; yet, not all drugs known to be metabolized by microsomes inhibit drug metabolism in vivo even if they do so in vitro. Of course drugs metabolized by separate pathways cannot interfere with each other's metabolism unless they share rate-limiting cofactors or other endogenous intermediates in their metabolic pathways. Finally, a very potent drug is not likely to interfere with a much less potent drug in vivo simply because their concentrations at the metabolic site are likely to be very different, although this factor could be offset if the K_m of the more potent drug is far below that of the less potent competitor. Since most of this information is seldom available the simplest and most reliable way to determine if one drug prolongs the metabolism of another is the in vivo experiment.

Cook et al. G74,655/57; Murphy & DuBois G74,670/57: EPN (ethyl p-nitrophenyl thionobenzenephosphonate) aggravates the toxicity of malathion [S-(1,2-dicarbethoxyethyl)-0,0-dimethyl phosphorodithioate] by inhibiting the esterases responsible for its detoxication.

Murphy et al. G74,671/59: Triorthotolyl phosphate potentiates the toxicity of malathion by inhibiting its metabolism.

Newman & Gross G75,237/63: Observations on infants showed that prolonged increases in indirect reacting bilirubin may be due to interference with the normal conjugating mechanism by the presence in human milk of a factor (possibly pregnanediol) which is not present in cow's milk. Changing the infants from breast feeding to cow's milk formulas enhanced the disappearance of the hyperbilirubinemia.

Rubin et al. G58,057/64: Numerous drugs competitively inhibit the metabolism of other drugs when employed as substrates for the microsomal enzyme system. Thus, using hepatic microsomes of the rat, it could be shown that "the N-demethylation of ethylmorphine was competitively inhibited by hexobarbital, chlorpromazine, zoxazolamine, phenylbutazone, and acetanilide; and ethylmorphine, and chlorpromazine were mutually inhibitory, each retarding the metabolism of the other. All these drugs are known to be oxidized by microsomal enzymes. Barbital and acetazoleamide, drugs which are not metabolized, failed to act as inhibitors."

Rubin et al. G58,747/64: Various chemically-unrelated drugs may compete for microsomal enzymes of the liver in vitro and in vivo. Observations on rats show that "ethylmorphine and codeine were shown to retard the metabolism of hexobarbital in vivo, as measured by the rate of hexobarbital disappearance from the blood of rats, whereas morphine, norcodeine, dextromethorphan, levomethorphan, meprobamate, and acetanilide were without effect."

Fox F8,079/64; Weiner et al. F35,871/65: In man, oxyphenbutazone (Tandearil) considerably prolongs the elevation of plasma levels of bishydroxycoumarin with a potentiation of its anticoagulant action.

Mannering G71,818/68 (p. 103): Review of the literature showing that concurrent pretreatment with two substrates of microsomal drug-metabolizing systems sometimes mutually and competitively antagonize each other. However, interestingly, not all drugs which are known to be metabolized by microsomes, inhibit drug metabolism in vivo. "The biotransformation studied in vitro may not represent the major metabolic route in vivo, and drugs metabolized by separate routes cannot interfere with each others' metabolism as alternative substrates, unless rate-limiting cofactors or other endogenous intermediates are shared by both metabolic pathways. Potency of the drugs in question is also of great importance in this regard. Very potent drugs are not likely to interfere with much less potent drugs simply because their concentrations at the metabolic site are likely to be very different, although this factor could be offset if the K_m of the more potent drug is much less than that of the drug of lesser potency. Most of this information is seldom available, and the quickest and most reliable way to determine if one drug will prolong the metabolism of another is to do the in vivo experiment."

Adlard & Lathe G74,759/70: In newborn infants, jaundice develops more frequently on breast feeding than on cow's milk and earlier investigators assumed that $3\alpha, 20\beta$-pregnanediol present in human milk may competitively inhibit glucuronyl transferase and thereby interfere with bilirubin clearance. The present observations suggest that "Neither $3\alpha, 20\beta$-pregnanediol nor $3\alpha, 20\alpha$-pregnanediol inhibited conjugation by human liver slices or by solubilized human liver microsomes. $3\alpha, 20\beta$-pregnanediol is unlikely to be the inhibitor causing breast milk jaundice." However, estriol inhibited conjugation by human liver slices.

Solymoss & Varga, G70,500/71: In rats, pretreatment with various catatoxic steroids accelerates the degradation of bishydroxycoumarin by NADPH-dependent hepatic enzymes. However, if the bishydroxycoumarin is administered immediately after treatment with catatoxic steroids (norbolethone, ethylestrenol, progesterone or triamcinolone), an inverse effect is observed, presumably because of competitive inhibition.

Blockers of Enzyme Induction

Classification. The blockers of microsomal enzyme induction may be roughly classified according to the sites of their actions as follows:

1. **Blockade of DNA-directed synthesis of nuclear messenger RNA (required for protein synthesis) by binding to DNA.** (E.g., actinomycin D is thus bound to DNA.)

2. **Blockade of transfer of soluble RNA-bound amino acids into microsomal protein.** (E.g., puromycin, an antibiotic, blocks the transfer of RNA-bound amino acids to the new protein chain.)

3. **Blockade of protein synthesis by decreasing the ATP content of the liver.** (E.g., ethionine, an antimetabolite of methionine, combines with ATP to form S-adenosyl-methionine. This reaction blocks transmethylation which requires S-adenosyl-methionine for the production of amino acids needed in protein synthesis.)

The first type of blockade interferes with transcription of information, the second and third with translation.

The ethionine-induced inhibition of hepatic protein synthesis can be prevented in vivo by either methionine or ATP. All these facts suggest that S-adenyl-methionine may be important for the synthesis of microsomal enzymes in the liver. When puromycin, ethionine or actinomycin D is administered several hours after 3-MC these blocking agents prevent further increase in the level of aminoazo dye N-demethylase, so that enzyme activity is maintained at a partially-elevated level. The results of actinomycin D suggest that the carcinogen may increase the formation of short-lived messenger RNA required for the further synthesis of aminoazo dye N-demethylase. (For literature see Conney F88,649/67.)

Conney F88,649/67 (p. 329): Review of interference with enzyme induction by inhibitors of protein synthesis.

Mannering G74,572/71: Review on the inhibition of drug metabolism "as it is more narrowly defined to mean the interference of the metabolism of one agent by another agent at the enzymic site."

Actinomycin. Actinomycin presumably blocks hepatic microsomal-enzyme induction at the level of the DNA-dependent RNA polymerase reaction (transcription); it thus differs essentially from the effect of puromycin which blocks the induction at the ribosomal level (translation).

It is thought that the regulatory effect of cortisone on carbohydrate metabolism may be brought about by its action on certain enzyme proteins. In starved rats, hepatic glycogen deposition by cortisone is inhibited both by actinomycin and by puromycin. The former may act by interfering with the cortisone-induced hepatic TKT, whereas the latter inhibits enzyme induction in general. Glucocorticoids are known to protect against endotoxins, whereas actinomycin and other inhibitors of enzyme protein synthesis (such as 2-thiouracil and 8-azaguanine and ethionine) increase endotoxin lethality.

In intact, hypophysectomized or adrenalectomized rats, STH inhibits the synthesis of hepatic TKT. This inhibition is blocked when RNA synthesis is impeded by actinomycin.

The increase in hepatic serine dehydrogenase, induced in rats by protein-deficient diets and starvation, can be prevented by actinomycin as well as by puromycin.

The induction of drug-metabolizing enzymes by phenobarbital is blocked in the rat both by actinomycin and by X-irradiation but through different mechanisms. X-irradiation of pregnant rats resulted in male offspring deficient in hepatic microsomal enzymes which metabolize hexobarbital. However irradiation did not suppress the induction of this enzyme by phenobarbital. Actinomycin inhibited both the ontogenetic and the phenobarbital-induced increases in enzyme activity.

In the perfused rat liver preparation, cortisol, insulin and glucagon induce TKT activity. Cortisol acts as long as it is present in the perfusion fluid, whereas enzyme synthesis by pancreatic hormones ceases after 2 or 3 hrs regardless of their continued presence. It is assumed that cortisol is a "primary inducer," whereas the pancreatic hormones presumably act indirectly as a consequence of their initial hepatic effect and are therefore "secondary inducers." Both types of induction are blocked by actinomycin D.

Actinomycin prevents the degradation of various substrates and inhibits enzyme induction by numerous agents, such as:

Cortisol
Cortisone
Endotoxin
Ethylestrenol
Glucagon
Insulin
Phenobarbital
Protein-deficient diets
Spironolactone
Starvation
Stress
Tyrosine
X-irradiation

Greengard et al. E20,258/63: In starved rats, hepatic glycogen deposition following **cortisone** treatment is inhibited by puromycin and actinomycin. The former interferes with enzyme induction in general, the latter with cortisone-induced rise in hepatic enzyme, including tyrosine transaminase. "The regulatory effect of cortisone on carbohydrate metabolism may be brought about by its action on the cellular concentration of certain enzyme proteins."

Berry G68,858/64: Both actinomycin D and ethionine increase the lethal effect of **endotoxin** in the mouse and abolish the protection offered by cortisone. Presumably, both endogenous and exogenous glucocorticoids protect through the induction of hepatic enzymes whose synthesis can be inhibited by actinomycin D and ethionine. Cortisone increases TPO in rats and rabbits, but not in guinea pigs. Correspondingly, guinea pigs cannot be protected against endotoxin by cortisone.

Berry & Smythe D19,640/64: In mice, Salmonella typhimurium **endotoxin** lowers hepatic tryptophan pyrrolase, whereas cortisone raises it; when the two are administered simultaneously, a normal enzyme level is maintained and mortality greatly diminished. If cortisone injection is delayed for a few hours it fails to induce tryptophan pyrrolase or protect against the lethal effect of endotoxin. Inhibitors of enzyme protein synthesis (actinomycin D, ethionine, 2-thiouracil and 8-azaguanine) potentiate the lethal effect of endotoxin and abolish cortisone protection.

Kenney & Albritton G64,557/65: Review of the literature suggesting that transaminase induction in response to stressors can be due to corticoid secretion during the stress reaction. Cortisol increases enzyme synthesis following an increased rate of synthesis of ribosomal, transfer and "DNA-like" RNA's. The present experiments confirm the view that repressor(s) can inhibit enzyme synthesis at the translational level because inhibition of RNA synthesis can prolong the corticoid-induced increase in enzyme synthesis under suitable conditions. "Administration of stressing agents (tyrosine, Celite) to adrenalectomized rats initiates a highly selective repression of the synthesis of hepatic TKT. The enzyme level falls with a t½ of about 2.5 hrs. Immunochemical measurement of the rate of enzyme synthesis indicates that it is reduced essentially to zero in stressed, adrenalectomized rats, whereas labeling of total liver soluble proteins is unaffected. Actinomycin does not itself influence the enzyme level, but it blocks the **stress**-initiated repression of enzyme synthesis, indicating that repression acts at the translational level, whereas initiation of repression involves transcriptional processes." In hypophysectomized rats, stressors are ineffective and preliminary data suggest that STH is responsible for transaminase repression.

Singer & Mason G66,500/65: Na-benzoate increased hepatic TKT activity both in intact and in NaCl-maintained adrenalectomized rats. Among 31 cyclic compounds tested for this inducing ability after adrenalectomy, only cortisol, its hemisuccinate and diethylstilbestrol disulfate were more effective than benzoate. Curiously, enzyme induction by **cortisol** was actually enhanced after adrenalectomy. "Strong inhibition of the increase by injected puromycin and actinomycin D, compounds which inhibit protein and RNA synthesis respectively, suggests that the benzoate-mediated effect occurred by a mechanism involving increases in protein and RNA synthesis. In this respect, the effect of benzoate resembles that of the glucocorticoids."

Berry et al. G67,237/66: S. typhimurium **endotoxin** lowers liver TPO in mice and prevents the induction of the enzyme by concurrent injection of cortisone. It lowers, but does not prevent, substrate induction. Actinomycin D has a similar effect on TPO. In the intact mouse, the endotoxin induces TKT almost as well as cortisone, but not in the adrenalectomized animal. Actinomycin D, on the other hand, has an effect on this transaminase similar to that on TPO.

Kenney G50,810/67: In intact, hypophysectomized or adrenalectomized rats, STH inhibits the synthesis of hepatic TKT. The rate of enzyme synthesis is reduced nearly to 0 (immunochemical-isotopic analyses), whereas labeling of the bulk of the liver proteins is increased by STH. Repression is blocked when RNA synthesis is inhibited by actinomycin. STH also appears to play a role in the repression of TKT induction by stressors. A hypophysectomized and an intact rat were united by parabiosis. When the pituitary-bearing member was stressed by **tyrosine** i.p., repression occurred in the livers of both treated and untreated (hypophysectomized) animals. TKT levels were unchanged in a single experiment where the stressing agent was administered to the hypophysectomized partner.

Schmidinger & Kröger F92,031/67: The increase in hepatic serine dehydratase induced by **protein-deficient diets** and **starvation** in intact rats is prevented by actinomycin, puromycin or glucose, but aggravated after adrenalectomy. Cortisone administered during the starvation period increases serine dehydratase activity, perhaps owing to utilization of inhibitors of this enzyme during gluconeogenesis.

Hager & Kenney G58,950/68: **Cortisol, insulin,** and **glucagon,** induced TKT in the isolated, perfused rat liver. The hormonal induction of all these enzymes was sensitive to actinomycin D, but STH (which represses TKT induction in vivo) apparently acts indirectly since it loses this effect in vitro. Cortisol acts as long as it is present in the perfusion fluid, whereas enzyme synthesis by the pancreatic hormones ceases after two or three hours, regardless of the continued presence of the protein hormones. It is assumed that cortisol is a "primary inducer," whereas the pancreatic hormones probably act indirectly as a consequence of their initial hepatic effect and are therefore "secondary inducers." Both the primary and the secondary induction mechanisms are blocked by actinomycin D.

Nair et al. G67,304/68: Comparative studies suggest that the induction of drug-metabolizing enzymes by **phenobarbital** in the rat can be inhibited by both X-irradiation and actinomycin, but through different mechanisms.

Nair et al. G67,245/68: X-irradiation of pregnant rats results in male offspring deficient in the hepatic microsomal enzymes which metabolize hexobarbital. However, irradiation did not suppress the increase of enzyme activity brought about by chemical inducers (phenobarbital). Actinomycin inhibited both the ontogenic and **phenobarbital**-induced increases in enzyme activity. "The ontogenic increase in enzyme activity is hormone-dependent, while that following phenobarbital administration is independent of hormonal regulation as evidenced by the response in hypophysectomized or sexually immature animals. It is concluded from these results that the inhibitory effect of x-irradiation on the hepatic enzyme system is mediated through an action on the hormonal regulation of enzyme activity."

Benes & Zicha G67,159/69: Exposure to 1400 R does not inhibit the TKT activity of rat liver. In fact, substrate induction of TKT is stimulated by **X-irradiation** applied 24 hrs earlier. Induction by cortisol is initially stimulated and then, inhibited by X-irradiation. X-irradiation before partial hepatectomy inhibits the increase in TKT normally observed 12 hrs after the operation. Similar results are obtained by actinomycin D applied one hour after partial hepatectomy. "The diminished synthesis of tryptophan oxygenase in irradiated regenerating rat liver tissue, as well as the decrease of hormonal induction after the irradiation can be explained by the inhibition of the specific messenger RNA's synthesis."

Becker & Brenowitz G75,528/70: Studies on the concentration of **actinomycin D in rat hepatocyte nuclei** as related to inhibition of RNA synthesis. The normal hepatocyte possesses mechanisms for rapidly eliminating administered actinomycin D.

Dowling & Feldman H31,139/70: In mice, the lethality of typhoid **endotoxin** is increased 550-20,000-fold by actinomycin D.

Pieroni et al. H31,137/70: In mice, actinomycin D enhances **endotoxin** lethality up to 100,000-fold. The lethality of tetanus and diphtheria exotoxins is not similarly augmented.

Sananès & Psychoyos G78,230/70: In rats, deciduoma formation is inhibited by actinomycin D presumably by interfering with RNA formation.

Solymoss et al. G70,412/70: "In rats, 24 hours after a single dose of **spironolactone** or **ethylstrenol,** the disappearance of pentobarbital from blood is enhanced to a rate in proportion to the decreasing depth of anesthesia. This action is completely suppressed by ribonucleic acid- or protein-synthesis inhibitors such as actinomycin D, puromycin aminonucleoside and cycloheximide, and only partially by 6-mercaptopurine or chloramphenicol...Induction of drug-metabolizing enzymes is involved in the resistance-increasing effect of spironolactone or ethylstrenol against various compounds."

Puromycin. As previously stated, puromycin blocks protein synthesis at the ribosome (translation) level; in this manner it interferes with the induction of various hepatic enzymes, for example, the induction by cortisol of TKT and TPO in the perfused rat liver.

The induction by dexamethasone of TKT in tissue cultures of cells is blocked by puromycin (but also by cycloheximide, chloramphenicol, progesterone, actinomycin D and mitomycin C). Paradoxically, after induction by the glucocorticoid has taken place, actinomycin D produces a further increase of this enzyme activity. The cortisol-induced hepatic TKT activity in adrenalectomized rats is inhibited by puromycin given during the initial phase of induction. However, if given during the inactivation phase, the antibiotic unexpectedly causes a rapid reappearance of enzyme activity. Perhaps a repressor is formed after a few hours of hormone action, and inhibition of repressor synthesis allows continued production of enzyme. The inactivator appears to depend upon pituitary function since adrenalectomized and hypophysectomized rats show little or no inactivation following cortisol treatment.

Ornithine-ketoaminotransferase (OKT) is very low in the fetal rat liver, and reaches the high adult level only during the third postnatal week. Triamcinolone given at this time elevates OKT although it has no effect in fetal or adult rats. Puromycin prevents the rise in OKT caused by triamcinolone.

Goldstein et al. D70,931/62: **Cortisol** produced an increase in both TKT and TPO activities in the isolated, perfused rat liver. This effect was prevented by puromycin. Cortisol "may exert some of its physiological effects directly on liver cells by altering the level of enzyme activities."

Alexander & Hunt E20,128/63: **Partial hepatectomy** did not significantly affect proteinuria or liver regeneration following puromycin aminonucleoside intoxication in the rat.

Thompson et al. F81,633/66: "Tyrosine α-ketoglutarate transaminase can be induced by steroid hormones in a newly established line of tissue culture cells, derived from primary culture of the ascites form of an experimental rat hepatoma." Dexamethasone, triamcinolone and cortisol were highly active, DOC and aldosterone much less potent, whereas stilbestrol, estradiol, testosterone and progesterone were virtually inactive. The induction by **dexamethasone** was blocked by puromycin, cycloheximide, chloramphenicol, progesterone, actinomycin D and mitomycin C. Paradoxically, after induction by the steroid had taken place, actinomycin D produced a further increase in enzyme activity.

Grossman & Mavrides G46,206/67: Studies on the kinetics of **cortisol**-induced hepatic TKT activity in adrenalectomized rats. "Puromycin inhibited enzyme synthesis when it was given during the initial phase of induction. However, it unexpectedly caused a rapid reappearance of enzyme activity following its administration during the inactivation phase. This potentiated response is consistent with other observations which lead to the idea that a repressor is formed about 4 hours after hormone administration and that inhibition of repressor synthesis allows, at least temporarily, continued synthesis of enzyme." The inactivator appears to depend upon pituitary function, since adrenalectomized and hypophysectomized rats showed little or no inactivation phase following cortisol treatment.

Räihä & Kekomäki G68,114/68: In the rat, the OKT activity of the liver is very low in the fetus, exhibits a small transient elevation around term, then drops, and eventually reaches the high adult activity level during the third postnatal week. **Triamcinolone** given postnatally causes a pronounced elevation of OKT, but has no such effect in fetal or adult rats. Puromycin prevents the rise in OKT after triamcinolone administration. In adult rats fed a protein- or arginine-free diet, OKT activity decreases and fails to rise under the influence of triamcinolone. Partial hepatectomy or STH depresses OKT-activity in the livers of adult rats.

Solymoss et al. G70,412/70: "In rats, 24 hours after a single dose of **spironolactone** or **ethylestrenol**, the disappearance of pentobarbital from blood is enhanced to a rate in proportion to the decreasing depth of anesthesia. This action is completely suppressed by ribonucleic acid- or protein-synthesis inhibitors such as actinomycin D, puromycin aminonucleoside and cycloheximide, and only partially by 6-mercaptopurine or chloramphenicol...Induction of drug-metabolizing enzymes is involved in the resistance-increasing effect of spironolactone or ethylestrenol against various compounds."

Cycloheximide. Cycloheximide allegedly inhibits protein synthesis in mammalian systems without inhibiting RNA synthesis. In the rat it does not prevent the uterine response to estradiol although it blocks the increase in various enzyme activities of the uterus that are associated with this response. Cycloheximide also inhibits the induction of hepatic TPO assayed 4 hrs after administration of the substrate or cortisol; however, it does not abolish the induction of TKT by cortisol, in fact, it increases TKT activity even in the absence of cortisol treatment.

The anesthetic effect of progesterone in the rat is augmented by cycloheximide pretreatment.

Fiala & Fiala F65,983/66: In the rat, cycloheximide i.p. inhibits the induction of hepatic TPO assayed 4 hrs after administration of the substrate, or of **cortisol**. By contrast, it did not abolish the induction of TKT by cortisol and, in fact, it increased the level of TKT even in the absence of cortisol treatment. A similar, though smaller, effect occurred in hypophysectomized or adrenalectomized rats, suggesting a direct induction of TKT by cycloheximide. Puromycin inhibited the induction of TKT. Apparently, an inhibitor of protein synthesis such as actidione may also act as an inducer for the synthesis of TKT, thus simulating the action of cortisol. "This 'pseudohormonal' action of actidione may explain the toxicity of actidione in certain mammalian species and also the fact that hydrocortisone may act as an antidote in actidione poisoning. It does not explain why a similar effect of 'pseudohormonal' induction is not observed in the case of TPO, but only the inhibition of enzyme induction."

Hilf et al. F88,514/67: Cycloheximide has been reported to inhibit protein synthesis in mammalian systems without inhibiting RNA synthesis. In the rat, it did not prevent the uterotrophic response to **estradiol** but blocked the increase in various enzyme activities of the uterus normally associated with this response.

Solymoss et al. G70,412/70: "In rats, 24 hours after a single dose of **spironolactone** or **ethylestrenol**, the disappearance of pentobarbital from blood is enhanced to a rate in proportion to the decreasing depth of anesthesia. This action is completely suppressed by ribonucleic acid- or protein-synthesis inhibitors such as actinomycin D, puromycin aminonucleoside and cycloheximide, and only partially by 6-mercaptopurine or chloramphenicol... Induction of drug-metabolizing enzymes is involved in the resistance-increasing effect of spironolactone or ethylestrenol against various compounds."

Solymoss et al. G70,463/70: In rats, pretreatment with spironolactone, norbolethone, or ethylestrenol accelerated the plasma clearance of digitoxin, in proportion to the in vivo protective effect of these catatoxic steroids. Partial hepatectomy reduces digitoxin clearance. The effect of **spironolactone** is suppressed by SKF 525-A and cycloheximide.

Solymoss et al. G70,464/70: In rats, **spironolactone** shortens the half-life of its main metabolite, the **dethioacetylated 4,6-dienone** (metabolite A), which is interconvertible with the 17-hydroxy carboxylic acid derivative (metabolite B). This alteration is only slightly accentuated if the steroid is given chronically, and it wears off within eight days after spironolactone treatment is interrupted. After a test dose of spironolactone or of its metabolites A and B, partial hepatectomy delays the blood clearance of metabolite A. Cycloheximide and SKF 525-A also suppress the blood clearance of metabolite A under these conditions. Presumably "spironolactone influences its own biotransformation and the steroid is also a substrate of the hepatic drug-metabolizing enzymes which are induced by spironolactone itself."

Solymoss G70,484/70: In rats, the plasma clearance of digitoxin is accelerated by **spironolactone, norbolethone** and **ethylestrenol** in doses that protect against the toxicity of the alkaloid in vivo. On the other hand, partial hepatectomy reduces digitoxin plasma clearance and increases the severity of the convulsions. The protective action of the steroids is suppressed by SKF 525-A and cycloheximide.

Khandekar et al. G79,014/71: In rats, cycloheximide elicited nucleolar alterations in hepatocytes with disruption, dilatation, degranulation and ballooning of the RER. Accumulation of SER also occurred when **spironolactone** or **PCN** was administered one hour before cycloheximide. It is concluded "that the steroids enhance the metabolic degradation of cycloheximide and thus SER proliferation is not inhibited; that this morphologic change does not always denote enzyme induction and the two can therefore be dissociated; or that SER accumulation is a nonspecific response to cellular injury."

Khandekar et al. G79,026/71: In rats, the hepatic SER proliferation induced by **spiro**nolactone or PCN is not prevented by concurrent administration of cycloheximide. Either the catatoxic steroids enhance the metabolic degradation of cycloheximide (thereby blocking its effect upon the SER) or this morphologic change does not necessarily indicate active enzyme induction.

Selye PROT. 27251: In rats, cycloheximide (25 or 50 µg—4th day ff.) aggravates and prolongs **progesterone** (5 mg in oil i.p.) anesthesia.

Hepatotoxic Substances. Ethionine (like CCl_4, chloroform and phosphorus) causes fatty liver formation which cannot be prevented by choline. The hepatic damage is associated with inhibition of protein synthesis in the liver. Presumably the action of ethionine is due to a decline in mRNA and protein synthesis caused by reduction in the available ATP. This occurs when ethionine replaces methionine in S-adenosyl methionine and traps available adenine, thus preventing the synthesis of ATP. In agreement with this concept, the effect of ethionine can be reversed by administration of either ATP or adenine.

In rats, the hepatic lesions produced by CCl_4 enhance the effect of various anticonvulsants.

Also in rats, CCl_4 prolongs hexobarbital sleeping time; but after acute habituation, the plasma hexobarbital at waking time is comparatively high, and hence, peripheral resistance within the nervous tissue itself may also play a role here.

A variety of hepatotoxic agents (incl. ethionine, CCl_4, yellow phosphorus, ^{32}P) markedly inhibits hexobarbital oxidation and aminopyrine dealkylation by isolated hepatic microsomes. However, in vitro, ethionine fails to inhibit hexobarbital metabolism.

Ethionine

Conney et al. D87,867/56: In rats, **3-methylcholanthrene** i.p. considerably increased the ability of fortified liver homogenates to N-demethylate 3-methyl-4-monomethylaminoazobenzene (demethylase activity) and to reduce the azo-linkage of 4-demethylaminoazobenzene (reductase activity) within 24 hrs. However, significant demethylase activity was obtained even after 6 hrs. A number of other polycyclic hydrocarbons caused similar increases in demethylase activity but there was no relationship between carcinogenicity and enzyme induction. None of these compounds was active in vitro and their effect could be inhibited in vivo by ethionine. This inhibition was in turn prevented by methionine.

Takabatake & Ariyoshi D48,245/62: "**19-Nortestosterone derivatives**" (not otherwise characterized) shortened the duration of cyclobarbital anesthesia in rats. Ethionine had an inverse effect.

Berry G68,858/64: Both actinomycin D and ethionine increase the lethal effect of **endotoxin** in the mouse and abolish the protection offered by cortisone. Presumably, both endogenous and exogenous glucocorticoids protect through the induction of hepatic enzymes whose synthesis can be inhibited by actinomycin D and ethionine. Cortisone increases TPO in rats and rabbits, but not in guinea pigs. Correspondingly, guinea pigs cannot be protected against endotoxin by cortisone.

Wheatley F98,919/68: In rats, adrenocortical necrosis produced by DMBA or 7-OH-MBA is prevented by metyrapone and related inhibitors of corticoid synthesis (Su 9055 and Su 10603) but not by Ay 9944 or aminoglutethimide (Elipten). No correlation was found between the influence of these drugs on corticoidogenesis and their ability to protect against adrenal necrosis. Pretreatment with ethionine abolished the protective action of **metyrapone, Su 9055** and **Su 10603**. It is concluded that these drugs protect by virtue of their hepatic drug-metabolizing enzyme inducing ability, not by direct effect upon corticoidogenesis.

Kovacs & Somogyi G60,060/69: In rats, the adrenal necrosis produced by DMBA is prevented by pretreatment with **spironolactone** and this protection is in turn blocked by ethionine.

Domschke et al. G74,897/70: In rats, ethionine fails to prevent the induction of TPO by the pesticide **soman.** "Since ethionine is known as an effective inhibitor of the protein synthesis in the liver the negative results are probably due to a stimulating effect of soman on the de-novo-synthesis of liver enzymes."

Ariyoshi & Takabatake G75,246/70: In rats, with ethionine-induced fatty livers, the inductive effect of **ethanol** and **phenobarbital** was almost completely blocked, whereas aniline hydroxylase activity was increased.

Gardell et al. G60,076/70: In rats, protection against digitoxin intoxication by **spironolactone** is blocked by dl-ethionine and the blockade is in turn antagonized by dl-methionine.

Levine H31,806/70: In rats, 3,4-benzpyrene is rapidly excreted through the bile in the form of its metabolic products. Pretreatment with microsomal drug-metabolizing enzyme inducers (e.g., phenobarbital, methylcholanthrene, 3,4-benzpyrene) greatly enhances the rate of biliary excretion of this compound. Both the rate of metabolism and of biliary excretion are enhanced to a similar extent throughout the induction period. Male rats both metabolize 3,4-benzpyrene and excrete its metabolites in the bile at rates approximately 2.5 times that of females. The induction by **methylcholanthrene** of both the metabolism and the biliary excretion of 3,4-benzpyrene can be partially blocked by ethionine. It has been concluded that conversion to its metabolites is the rate-limiting step in the biliary excretion of 3,4-benzpyrene.

Carbon Tetrachloride

Shideman et al. E60,046/47: In mice, CCl_4-induced liver damage prolongs the effect of **thiopental**. The same is true after subtotal hepatectomy (85—90%) in rats. Diminished blood flow through the liver (Eck fistula) likewise increases the duration of thiopental anesthesia in rats. Thiopental is degraded in vitro by rat liver slices and mince.

Swinyard et al. G74,657/52: In rats, hepatic lesions produced by CCl_4 enhance the anticonvulsant effect of **diphenylhydantoin**, mesantoin, and thiantoin.

Neubert G74,661/57; Herken et al. G74,662/58; Neubert & Maibauer G74,664/59; Neubert et al. G74,668/60: In rats, various hepatotoxic agents (ethionine, CCl_4, yellow phosphorus, ^{32}P) markedly inhibit **hexobarbital** oxidation and **aminopyrine** dealkylation by isolated hepatic microsomes. However, the inhibition of hexobarbital metabolism by ethionine given in vivo is not seen in vitro.

Paeile et al. F52,633/64: Adult male rats are more resistant to **procaine** than adult females. Chronic CCl_4 poisoning, pretreatment with SKF 525-A and orchidectomy diminish the resistance of the males approximately to the female level. The plasma procainesterase activity is approximately the same in both sexes and not affected by orchidectomy or CCl_4 intoxication.

Ronzoni et al. H18,986/68: In rats, the **hydroxyproline** content of the liver furnishes a better quantitative index of sclerosis than histologic studies. The technique is recommended for the evaluation of sclerosis and its regression after various types of liver damage, e.g., partial hepatectomy or CCl_4 poisoning.

Querci et al. G70,597/69: In rats pretreated with CCl_4, parallel blood determinations were performed of **parathion**, its toxic metabolite **paraoxon**, and the product of hydrolysis of the latter, paranitrophenol. They suggest that the increase in toxicity following hepatic damage is primarily due to a defect in the synthesis of hepatic pseudocholinesterase.

Varga & Fischer G76,189/69: In rats, hepatic damage produced by bromobenzene, CCl_4, allylalcohol and thioacetamide is associated with prolonged **hexobarbital** sleeping time owing to interference with the hepatic microsomal metabolism of the barbiturate. However, the degree of hepatic injury does not run strictly parallel with the prolongation of the hexobarbital sleeping time; hence, the latter cannot serve as an accurate hepatic function test.

Klinger H25,517/70: In male rats, the LD_{50} of **hexobarbital** in mg/kg, rises from 160 to 343 between the ages of 12—130 days; however, the blood concentration of hexobarbital at waking time is not age-dependent. The sleeping time is directly correlated with the speed of biotransformation by hepatic microsomes in vitro. CCl_4 prolongs sleeping time. Following acute habituation in CCl_4 treated rats, the hexobarbital concentration of the plasma at waking time is comparatively high.

Lal et al. G77,285/70: In rats, **hexobarbital** anesthesia is prolonged by inhalation of CCl_4. The hepatic microsomal fraction of the livers of rats exposed to CCl_4 exhibited a diminished hexobarbital-metabolizing activity, and the livers of rats so treated were enlarged.

Levin et al. H26,593/70: In rats, CCl_4 given to immature females 24 hrs before sacrifice inhibited the activity of hepatic microsomal enzymes that hydroxylate **estradiol-17β** and **estrone**. This inhibition was reflected in vivo by an altered metabolism of estradiol-17β and estrone, by a potentiation of the uterotrophic action of folliculoids and by an increased concentration of these steroids in the uterus. By contrast, tetrachloroethylene did not influence the action of estrone. SKF 525-A and desipramine, which are also inhibitors of drug metabolism, likewise potentiate the uterotrophic action of estrone in immature rats.

Priestly & Plaa G80,048/70: In rats, "impaired BSP excretion, bile flow rate, relative hepatic storage, and plasma BSP retention were observed as early as 3 hrs after CCl_4 administration. However, impaired BSP conjugation was not unequivocally demonstrated until 12 hrs after CCl_4. In experiments where BSP was administered by slow i.v. infusion (2.5 mg/min/kg), increases in the ratio of biliary unconjugated BSP to conjugated BSP were suggestive of impaired conjugation during the early stages of intoxication, although such changes were not marked when BSP was rapidly injected (60 mg/kg, i.v.)." Presumably, impaired biliary excretion is the main cause of BSP retention after CCl_4.

Steroids. In man, methandrostenolone increases plasma oxyphenbutazone levels, presumably by interfering with the metabolism of the drug. A variety of steroids inhibits NADH-oxidase and succinate oxidase activities in heart muscle sarcosomal fragments.

In mice, lynestrenol reduces whereas mestranol, like SKF 525-A, increases the anticonvulsive effect of diphenylhydantoin, barbiturates and other drugs, possibly through altered microsomal drug metabolism.

Experiments now under way at our Institute suggest that various steroids (e.g., estradiol) can also act as antagonists of catatoxic steroid actions (*cf.* Table 50). However, these studies are still incomplete and will be published in detail later.

Weiner et al. F35,871/65: Earlier studies had shown that **methandrostenolone** inhibits glucuronyl transferase and oxyphenbutazone is excreted largely as the glucuronide. Accordingly, it was found in man that methandrostenolone increases plasma oxyphenbutazone levels, presumably by interfering with its metabolism.

Stoppani et al. H19,278/68: "A series of C_{21}, C_{19}, **and C_{18}-steroids** (including hormonal steroids and derivatives) have been tested as inhibitors of NADH-oxidase and succinate oxidase activities of heart-muscle sarcosomal fragments (Keilin-Hartree preparation). NADH oxidation is much more sensitive to steroids than succinate oxidation, in accordance with electron transfer inhibition in the vicinity of the NADH-flavoprotein site." The structural characteristics of the active compounds "are consistent with the interaction of steroids with the phospholipid components of the electron transfer chain at the NADH-flavoprotein site. Many of the structural requirements for inhibition of electron transfer resemble those for androgenicity."

Blackham & Spencer G73,813/70: In mice, **lynestrenol** reduced, whereas **mestranol** or SKF 525-A increased, the anticonvulsive effect (tested with electroshock) of diphenylhydantoin, phenobarbital, chlordiazepoxide and diazepam administered i.p. after five days of pretreatment. This may be due to altered microsomal drug metabolism but since mestranol and lynestrenol have opposite effects upon brain 5-HT concentrations, the latter mechanism must also be considered.

Various Other Antagonists. Among other antagonists of hepatic enzymes, suffice it merely to mention **Thorotrast** (perhaps owing to blockade of the RES) and **metyrapone** (perhaps because of its effect upon P-450) which will be discussed under Drugs on p. 582. The latter initially potentiates the action of pentobarbital but subsequently enhances the rate of its detoxication and shortens its narcotic effect in rats. The adrenal cortical necrosis induced by DMBA or 7-OH-MBA is prevented by metyrapone and related compounds. However, no close correlation exists between the influence of these drugs on corticoidogenesis and their ability to protect against adrenal necrosis; they apparently act by inducing hepatic drug-metabolizing enzymes, not by direct effect upon the adrenals.

In mice, **starvation** depresses hepatic microsomal drug metabolism as measured both in vivo and in vitro, perhaps owing to an actual loss of enzyme protein from the microsomes. Oxidative pathways are much more affected than reductive pathways; in fact the latter may actually be activated with regard to certain substrates.

Several observations suggest that RNA synthesis is inhibited by **nickel carbonyl. Benactyzine** or infection with **P. berghei** prolong hexobarbital sleeping time. Numerous **methylenedioxyphenyl** compounds, **6-mercaptopurine** and **3-amino-1,2,4-triazole** exert similar effects although in many instances the mechanisms of their actions are still unknown.

Holten & Larsen G74,395/56: In mice, hexobarbital anesthesia is considerably prolonged by **benactyzine** (a compound used for the treatment of psychoneuroses). The effect resembles that of SKF 525-A and when given together, the two compounds synergize each other. Extensive review of the literature and of numerous personal observations concerning the barbiturate potentiating effect of various antihistamines and spasmolytic compounds.

Dixon et al. G65,886/60: In mice, even the **nutritional status** is an important factor in determining microsomal enzyme induction. "Starvation depresses hepatic microsomal drug metabolism both as measured in vitro and in vivo. This depression is believed to be caused by an actual loss of enzyme protein in the microsomes. Oxidative pathways are affected more than reductive pathways and indeed starvation may result in an activation of reduction of nitro and azo groups." This is shown in Table 3 modified by Goldstein et al. (E165/68) from the original, more complete version of Dixon et al. (G65,886/60).

Mice were starved for 36 hrs then given hexobarbital (80 mg/kg) intraperitoneally. Normal animals usually slept less than 10 min but sleeping time varied greatly in starved mice. Twelve hours later (48 hrs starvation) the mice were sacrificed and the liver microsomes were tested for their drug-metabolizing ability. Figures represent drug metabolized in a fixed incubation time.

Table 3. *Effects of starvation on drug metabolism by mouse liver microsomes*

Substrate	Drug metabolized (μmoles/g liver)		
	Sleeping time min		
	5—15	20—40	>80
	Normal	Starved	
Hexobarbital (aliphatic oxidation)	4.46	2.79	0.77
Chlorpromazine (sulfur oxidation)	2.80	1.98	1.19
Aminopyrine (N-dealkylation)	1.48	1.11	0.46
Acetanilid (aromatic hydroxylation)	2.03	2.22	0.93
p-Nitrobenzoic acid (nitro reduction)	8.22	17.03	8.43
Neoprontosil (azo reduction)	15.55	17.65	12.59

Agarwal et al. G65,716/69: In the rat, both S. typhimurium endotoxin and Thorotrast lowered hepatic TPO activity, and prevented cortisol from inducing this enzyme in the isolated, perfused liver. Under these conditions, the TKT activity of the liver remained unaffected. Partial purification of hepatic TPO induced by endotoxin or Thorotrast indicated the presence of some inhibitory substance. "Since histological studies revealed that thorotrast is localized in Kupffer cells, it is suggested that the **reticuloendothelial** system contributes to the control of enzyme induction in rat liver."

Biezunski G78,643/70: In rats pretreated with **warfarin,** protein synthesis in hepatic microsomes is inhibited in vitro. Vitamin K injected after warfarin almost completely restores the low level of the prothrombin complex in plasma and microsomes, but the general inhibition of protein synthesis by liver microsomes is much less markedly relieved.

Einheber et al. G75,665/70: In mice infected with **P. berghei,** hexobarbital sleeping time is prolonged. "This may be due to a disturbance in function of hepatocellular smooth endoplasmic reticulum and its associated drug-metabolizing enzymes because phenobarbital treatment, which ordinarily stimulates an increase of the latter, corrects the 'defect' in hexobarbital sleeping time."

Fujii et al. G77,242/70: In mice, 61 **methylenedioxyphenyl compounds** (including synthetic insecticide synergists, natural products, and related open-ring analogues) showed approximately parallel potency as regards hepatic microsomal enzyme inhibition manifested by prolongation of hexobarbital narcosis and zoxazolamine paralysis.

Raisfeld et al. G75,045/70: In rats, the herbicide **3-amino-1,2,4-triazole** inhibits the induction by phenobarbital of cytochrome P-450 and drug hydroxylase activity, but does not prevent the proliferation of the SER in hepatocytes. Presumably "induced increases of cytochrome P-450 and of the membranes of endoplasmic reticulum may be controlled by separate mechanisms."

Sunderman Jr. G73,628/70: In rats, ^{14}C-leucine incorporation into hepatic microsomal proteins is inhibited by **nickel carbonyl.** Previous studies on the inhibition of hepatic RNA synthesis by nickel carbonyl are reviewed.

Sunderman & Leibman H28,301/70: "Exposure of rats to **nickel carbonyl,** $Ni(CO)_4$, in LD_{50} dosage inhibited the basal (noninduced) levels of hepatic aminopyrine demethylase activity. The maximum inhibition of hepatic aminopyrine demethylase occurred on the 2nd day after an injection of $Ni(CO)_4$, and aminopyrine demethylase activity returned to normal levels by the 4th day after $Ni(CO)_4$. Administration of $Ni(CO)_4$ also inhibited hepatic aminopyrine demethylase activity in rats that had received daily injections of phenobarbital beginning 5 days before the $Ni(CO)_4$."

Solymoss et al. G70,412/70: "In rats, 24 hours after a single dose of spironolactone or ethylestrenol, the disappearance of pentobarbital from blood is enhanced to a rate in proportion to the decreasing depth of anesthesia. This action is completely suppressed by ribonucleic acid- or protein-synthesis inhibitors such as actinomycin D, puromycin aminonucleoside and cycloheximide, and only partially by **6-mercaptopurine** or chloramphenicol... Induction of drug-metabolizing enzymes is involved in the resistance-increasing effect of spironolactone or ethylestrenol against various compounds."

TIMING

Length of Pretreatment Necessary for Conditioning

The length of pretreatment necessary for the obtention of resistance by either syntoxic or catatoxic hormones is subject to great variations depending upon dosage, route of administration, the kind of toxicant used, species differences, etc. Some of the protective effects of glucocorticoids are almost immediate if water soluble hormone preparations are given i.v. (e.g., against endotoxin shock or certain ganglioplegics); others are much more time-consuming (e.g., the suppression of chronic inflammation). In the case of catatoxic effects, which depend upon defensive enzyme induction, the protection offered always requires some time for enzyme synthesis. With most of the currently employed catatoxic steroids, about 24—48 hrs of pretreatment are needed to achieve good protection under ordinary conditions of testing against commonly employed toxicants, but often less than 24 hrs suffice and yet it may take several days to reach peak resistance (*cf.* Table 6, p. 88).

Extensive experiments in rats have shown however that the length of pretreatment necessary to obtain a just detectable protective effect depends also largely upon the speed with which the toxicant elicits detectable pharmacologic effects. Thus, even single doses of various catatoxic steroids offer definite protection against many agents whose effects become manifest only after a prolonged latency period. For example, virtually simultaneous treatment with catatoxic steroids and digitoxin s.c. can prevent the convulsions and death which the cardiac glycoside would normally produce one or more days later. Here, presumably, the latency period of the drug action allows sufficient time for the induction of defensive enzymes. On the other hand, many hours, or days, of pretreatment with catatoxic steroids are necessary to offer protection against instantly acting anesthetics or convulsive agents.

In the rat and dog, the blood clearance of barbiturates is maximally accelerated within 48—72 hrs and cannot be further enhanced by more prolonged treatment with these drugs. In man, induction is much less rapid and its estimation somewhat complicated by the development of cumulative effects and of local adaptive reactions within the central nervous system. According to some investigators, in mice, effective enzyme induction can occur in less than one hour.

There is some evidence that certain inducers may elicit a three-phasic change in resistance, reminiscent of that characteristic of the general adaptation syndrome. Thus, in rats given daily injections of the pesticide dieldrin, the increase in hepatic weight, microsomal protein, P-450 hemoprotein and SER development persist, yet it is possible to distinguish: 1. The stage of induction when dieldrin tolerance is still low, 2. the steady state with tolerance to otherwise fatal doses of dieldrin and 3. the state of decompensation when drug-handling ability is sharply decreased. Butter yellow produces an essentially similar three stage response.

Duration of Effect after Withdrawal of Conditioner

In rats, continued treatment with oxandrolone or spironolactone offers protection against daily administration of normally fatal amounts of indomethacin or digitoxin for indefinite periods. However, upon interruption of the catatoxic steroid administration death ensues within a few days. Furthermore, the plasma concentration of the substrates which remains low during catatoxic steroid treatment rises after withdrawal of the medication.

In mice, pentobarbital resistance is evident 24 hrs after pretreatment with phenobarbital, reaches a maximum within 48 hrs and disappears after about 4—5 days.

Reversal of Actions Due to Timing

Reversal of Inducer Actions. In speaking about the duration of inducer effects we already mentioned the three-phasic response in which a period of incomplete induction is followed by a resistant steady state and eventually by exhaustion.

Certain observations suggest however that during the initial period inducers may even have an inverse effect.

For example, 2—4 hrs after administration of hexobarbital the enzyme oxidizing this substrate is reduced in rat liver and activation commences only after 12 hrs, reaching a maximum after 48 hrs.

Pentobarbital anesthesia is shortened and the blood clearance of the barbiturate accelerated within 24 hrs after a single dose of spironolactone or ethylestrenol.

In mice, testosterone exerts a biphasic effect upon hexobarbital hypnosis: prolongation of sleeping time during the initial period of hormone administration is followed by protection. However, here, the initial potentiation is apparently due to a direct effect upon the CNS and unrelated to enzyme induction since it is seen also with barbital which is not metabolized. Yet, many excellent inducing agents have been shown to inhibit drug metabolism during the initial 6 hrs.

Reversal of Antagonist Actions. It has been shown of **actinomycin**, as of many other antagonists, that following an initial period during which they inhibit induction their effect may be reversed. This has been seen with regard to TPO and TKT induction by glucocorticoids. It was tentatively ascribed to a delayed response to inhibitors of RNA synthesis in which a "cytoplasmic repressor" can inhibit the translation of the mRNA's corresponding to TPO and TKT. Cytoplasmic depression might depend upon continued RNA and protein synthesis, the repressor having a rapid turnover rate.

MPDC given 1—12 hrs before hexobarbital prolongs sleeping time and inhibits barbiturate metabolism, whereas MPDC administered 24—48 hrs before the barbiturate has an inverse effect.

Metyrapone initially potentiates and later inhibits the hypnotic action of pentobarbital in rats, presumably because it gradually enhances hepatic detoxication.

It has been shown for several **other antagonists** (SKF 525-A, CFT 1201) that, after an initial period of inhibition, microsomal enzyme activity recovers and then increases above normal. Thus, actually many inducers and antagonists exert essentially similar effects in which an initial phase of suppression is followed by stimulation of microsomal drug-metabolizing enzyme activity, but with the inducers the induction, and with the inhibitors the suppression, is by far more pronounced.

Reversal of Substrate Actions. For the sake of completeness we should mention the reversal of substrate actions although in practice this is a phenomenon identical with the very common self-induction of catatoxic activity by many substrates, such as barbiturates, pesticides, steroids, etc. This type of protection may be more or less limited to the inducer itself or be effective also against other substrates, as we shall see later in discussing the specificity of induction.

In classifying and coordinating the data on the induction of defensive enzymes, it was useful — perhaps even indispensable — to distinguish between inducers, substrates and blockers. Yet, a detached appraisal of the facts does not support the concept that these three classes of compounds are essentially different. Depending upon timing and other experimental conditions, all three types of drugs can either protect or sensitize. It seems that these three groups of compounds have in common a singular effect upon the defensive enzyme-producing mechanism but the direction of the response depends upon modifying factors. It is hardly a coincidence that:

1. Many excellent inducers are also readily detoxified by pretreatment with the same or other inducers. 2. Many substrates can induce or (by competition with other substrates) block enzyme activity. 3. Many blockers can readily be blocked in turn by pretreatment with inducers or, after chronic treatment, can even act as inducers themselves. 4. Most of the substances which are inactive in one of these three respects (e.g. are not inducers, substrates or blockers of the catatoxic mechanism), are also inert with respect to the other two types of effects.

Length of Pretreatment Necessary for Conditioning

Remmer G66,542/62: In the rat and dog, the blood clearance of barbiturates is maximally accelerated within 2—3 days of pretreatment and cannot be further enhanced by prolonged administration of these drugs. In man, oxidation of barbiturates is much less rapid and drug accumulation may develop. Here, tolerance may result from adaptation of the CNS in addition to accelerated oxidative breakdown.

Hutterer et al. G66,323/69: In rats, given daily injections of dieldrin (a chlorinated hydrocarbon pesticide), i.p. hepatic changes developed in three stages. "The first stage, that of induction, is characterized by an increase in liver weight, microsomal protein, smooth endoplasmic reticulum, the activity of aniline hydroxylase and p-nitroreductase, and the concentration of P-450 hemoprotein. During the second stage, a 'steady state,' the elevated levels are maintained and tolerance to otherwise fatal doses of dieldrin prevails. In the third stage, that of decompensation, elevation of liver weight, microsomal proteins, and P-450 hemoprotein persists, and the smooth endoplasmic reticulum appears as abundant as in the previous stages, but the activity of the drug-handling enzymes decreases. The smooth endoplasmic reticulum, however, in this last stage consisted of packed tubules. This hypoactive, hypertrophic, smooth endoplasmic reticulum is accompanied by biochemical and morphologic alterations of mitochondria." 3'-Methyl-4-dimethylaminoazobenzene (butter yellow) produces an essentially similar but accelerated three-stage response.

Kalyanpur et al. G66,147/69: In mice, various anabolic steroids (methandienone, 4-chlorotestosterone acetate, nandrolone, phenpropionate) given i.p. 90 min before pentylenetetrazol, inhibit convulsions. The protective effect is compared to that produced by various anesthetic steroids. [A relationship to enzyme induction is not suggested, nor is it probable in view of the shortness of the necessary pretreatment (H.S.).]

Solymoss et al. G70,412/70: In rats, 24 hrs after a single injection of spironolactone or ethylestrenol, the blood clearance of pentobarbital is already greatly enhanced and its anesthetic effect shortened.

Selye PROT. 17663: In rats, spironolactone, given simultaneously with digitoxin, has little protective effect; pretreatment for 24 hrs is moderately effective, whereas spironolactone, given over a period of 48—96 hrs prior to digitoxin, completely abolishes the lethal action of the latter.

Table 4. *Influence of the duration of spironolactone pretreatment upon its antidigitoxin effect*

Spironolactone (Beginning hrs before digitoxin)[a]	Convulsions (Scale: 0—3)[b]	Mortality (Dead/Total)[b]
Controls	3.0	10/10
0	1.4±0.44 **	10/10
24	0 ***	3/10
48	0 ***	0/10
72	0 ***	0/10
96	0 ***	0/10

[a] Digitoxin (1 mg in 1 ml water, p.o., 1st day, and 2 mg 2nd day) in all groups including controls. Spironolactone (10 mg in 1 ml water, p.o. x2/day) beginning at time indicated, on or before initiation of digitoxin treatment.

[b] Convulsions on 3rd day and mortality 7th day after digitoxin administration. Statistics Student's t-test. For further details on technique of tabulation cf. p. VIII.

Duration of Effect after Withdrawal of Conditioner

Orrenius et al. E8,231/69: In rats, 5 days of treatment with phenobarbital greatly increased aminopyrene demethylation by hepatic microsomes, but upon discontinuation of the treatment, this enzyme activity reverted to the starting level within about 3 days.

Sladek & Mannering G66,219/69: In rats, 3 days of treatment with phenobarbital, 3-MC, thioacetamide or 3-methyl-4-methylaminoazobenzene (3-MMAB) induced different relative changes in the cytochrome P-450 and the N-demethylase activities of hepatic microsomes. Furthermore, the effect of phenobarbital treatment lasted only about 5 days after discontinuation of this treatment, whereas most of the other agents exerted more persistent effects.

Buchel & Levy G74,850/70: In mice, pretreatment with phenobarbital decreases pentobarbital sleeping time; this phenomenon is detectable within 24 hrs and reaches a maximum 48 hrs after phenobarbital administration. The resistance is no longer detectable in males after 96, in females after 120 hrs.

Solymoss & Selye G70,409/70; Solymoss et al. G70,441/70: Rats given daily treatment with normally fatal amounts of indomethacin or digitoxin can survive for an apparently indefinite period if they are concurrently treated with spironolactone or oxandrolone. Upon interruption of catatoxic steroid administration death ensues within a few days. "Spironolactone enhances not only the degradation of digitoxin and indomethacin but also its own metabolism as judged by their disappearance rate from the blood. However, the capacity of the steroids to inactivate themselves is limited and, hence, they continue to detoxify both drugs, even in chronic experiments."

Selye PROT. 18125: In rats pretreated with spironolactone for 6 days, the antidigitoxin effect remains obvious for about 5 days after discontinuation of treatment, but its efficacy in inhibiting convulsions rapidly diminishes during this time, *cf.* Table 5.

Table 5. *Duration of antidigitoxin effect after spironolactone withdrawal*

Pretreatment[a]	Digitoxin (hrs after spironolactone)[b]	Convulsions (Scale: 0—3)[c]	Mortality (Dead/Total)[d]
None	3	2.5	10/10
Spironolactone	3	0	0/10
None	48	2.1	5/10
Spironolactone	48	1.3	2/10
None	96	2.4	4/10
Spironolactone	96	3.0	4/10

[a] Spironolactone (10 mg in 1 ml water p.o. x2/day) during 6 days before digitoxin.
[b] Digitoxin (2 mg in 1 ml water/100 g body weight, p.o., once on day indicated) after discontinuation of spironolactone treatment.
[c] 48 hrs after digitoxin treatment.
[d] Mortality on 5th day after digitoxin treatment.

Selye PROT. 39927: Rats were given a single treatment with various toxicants, before or after a single dose of certain conditioners. In the event of suitable timing (adjustment of interval between application of the two agents) a single dose of PCN, CS-1 or phenobarbital suffices to inhibit intoxication with digitoxin, indomethacin, dioxathion, parathion, nicotine, progesterone, hexobarbital and zoxazolamine. Taking treatment with the toxicants as "0 hr," it appears that pretreatment with these conditioners at —24 hrs offers manifest protection in most cases. In some instances, the resistance thus induced lasts several days, e.g., PCN or phenobarbital administered on the —4th day still protects against anesthesia produced by progesterone at 0 hr. On the other hand, some of the conditioners, administered after acutely acting toxicants, may aggravate the effect of the latter. Thus, CS-1 given 30 min after progesterone actually prolongs the resulting anesthesia. The same is true of phenobarbital administered 30 min before or after progesterone or hexobarbital. The effect of conditioners given 6 hrs after these anesthetics could not be tested since by that time the rats were awake. It will be recalled that such inverse effects had previously been noted when spironolactone was given to rats pretreated with digitoxin. In the case of the more chronically acting toxicants, treatment with the conditioners at —30 or +30 min, can offer definite protection. This was the case especially for digitoxin and indomethacin, but in some instances also for dioxathion. CS-1 diminished indomethacin mortality even when administered 6 hrs after the latter. In all these instances, it may be assumed that the time interval between administration of the toxicant and the manifestation of its damaging actions is sufficiently long to permit drug metabolizing enzyme induction. Apparently, it is not so much the time interval between the administration of the conditioners and the toxicants that counts, but the time interval between conditioning and the appearance of obvious toxic manifestations, cf. Table 6, p. 88.

Selye PROT. 41919: Rats were given temporary pretreatment with various conditioners, followed by a resting period before challenge with a single dose of a toxicant. In general a 24 hrs interval between cessation of conditioning and challenge offered the best protection. With rapidly acting toxicants (such as progesterone, hexobarbital, zoxazolamine, dioxathion and parathion) good protection was usually obtained even after a rest period of 72 or 120 hrs (*cf.* Table 7, p. 90). Among the toxicants tested in this series, only nicotine and DHT proved to be virtually resistant to this type of conditioning.

Reversal of Actions Due to Timing

Reversal of Inducer Actions. *Remmer G66,542/62:* Brief mention of unpublished experiments showing that 2—4 hrs after administration of hexobarbital, the enzyme oxidizing this substrate is reduced. Activation commences after 12 hrs reaching a maximum after 48 hrs. "Obviously stimulation followed a short phase of inhibition."

Gessner et al. F77,776/67: In mice, "testosterone pretreatment produces a biphasic effect on the duration of action of hexobarbital, prolonging the action initially and shortening the action in 4—8 days after the pretreatment. The early action of testosterone appears to be associated with an effect on the hypnotic property of a drug, since both hexobarbital and barbital sleep times are prolonged, while the duration of action of the muscle relaxant chlorzoxasone remains unaffected. The long-term pretreatment with testosterone leads to a shorter duration of action of drugs that are deactivated by detoxification, notably hexobarbital and chlorzoxasone, but has no effect on the duration of hypnosis produced by barbital, a drug which is predominantly eliminated unchanged." Folliculoids (ethinyl estradiol, diethylstilbestrol) prolong the actions of both drugs.

Mannering G71,818/68 (p. 74): Review of the literature showing that "many good inducing agents actually inhibit drug metabolism during the first 6 hr after administration."

Wheatley F98,919/68: Brief reference is made to the observation "that pretreatment of rats with Su 4885 (Metyrapone), while initially potentiating the action of Nembutal, subsequently led to a considerably enhanced rate of detoxification and a shorter duration of narcosis."

Caster et al. G73,426/70: In rats, hexobarbital and heptachlor detoxication by hepatic microsomes, in vitro, is optimal if the diet contains about 3% of the calories in the form of corn oil (or equivalent amounts of linoleate). Both higher and lower levels of fatty acids are detrimental for the detoxication of these substrates and this was confirmed by determinations of hexobarbital sleeping time in vivo. The results are interpreted as indicating that an optimum amount of essential fatty acid is required for the most efficient functioning of the hepatic microsomal drug-metabolizing system.

Dewhurst & Kitchen G73,848/70: In mice, zoxazolamine paralysis is greatly shortened soon after a single dose of the carcinogen, whereas upon prolonged treatment, an inverse response is obtained. It is speculated that "an active metabolite formed in relatively small amounts may gradually accumulate or the stimulation of microsomal enzymes by the first dose might lead to enhanced conversion of a subsequent dose into an active metabolite."

Solymoss et al. G70,423/70: In rats, pretreatment with catatoxic steroids (e.g., norbolethone, ethylestrenol) enhances the disappearance of bishydroxycoumarin from the blood and counteracts its effect on prothrombin time whereas administration of such steroids

Table 6. *Duration of effect after a single dose of a conditioner*

Conditioners[a]	Toxicants[b]	Digitoxin (3 mg in 1 ml water p.o.) Convulsions +4th day	Mortality +6th day	Indomethacin (5 mg in 0.2 ml water s.c.) Intestinal Ulcers	Mortality +6th day	Dioxathion (4 mg in 1 ml corn oil p.o.) Dyskinesia +6 hrs	Mortality +48 hrs
PCN	− 4th day	9/10	4/10	10/10	5/10	10/10	10/10
		2/10 ***	1/10 NS	6/10 *	3/10 NS	7/10 NS	3/10 ***
	−24 hrs	10/10	10/10	10/10	0/10	8/10	5/10
		0/10 ***	0/10 ***	0/10 ***	0/10 NS	0/10 ***	0/10 *
	− 6 hrs	6/10	5/10	10/10	0/10	8/10	7/10
		0/10 **	0/10 *	0/10 ***	0/10 NS	1/10 ***	0/10 ***
	−30 min	10/10	10/10	9/9	4/10	10/10	5/10
		4/10 **	4/10 **	4/10 **	0/10 *	6/10 *	2/10 NS
	+30 min	7/10	5/10	10/10	5/10	10/10	9/10
		7/10 NS	4/10 NS	2/10 ***	0/10 *	9/10 NS	7/10 NS
	+ 6 hrs	7/10	4/10	10/10	2/10	5/5	2/5
		5/10 NS	4/10 NS	6/10 *	0/10 NS	7/8 NS	3/8 NS
CS-1	− 4th day	9/10	7/10	10/10	3/10	10/10	10/10
		6/10 NS	5/10 NS	10/10 NS	1/10 NS	9/10 NS	8/10 NS
	−24 hrs	9/10	8/10	10/10	1/10	10/10	7/10
		0/10 ***	0/10 ***	0/10 ***	0/10 NS	0/10 ***	0/10 ***
	− 6 hrs	9/10	9/10	10/10	5/10	8/10	4/10
		1/10 ***	0/10 ***	0/10 ***	0/10 *	4/10 NS	0/10 *
	−30 min	8/10	6/10	10/10	8/10	10/10	10/10
		1/10 ***	0/10 **	0/10 ***	0/10 ***	6/10 *	1/10 ***
	+30 min	8/10	7/10	10/10	6/10	10/10	2/10
		3/10 *	1/10 **	3/10 ***	0/10 **	9/10 NS	1/10 NS
	+ 6 hrs	10/10	9/10	10/10	7/10	4/6	1/6
		8/10 NS	5/10 NS	7/10 NS	0/10 ***	6/7 NS	3/7 NS
Phenobarbital	− 4th day	8/10	6/10	10/10	5/10	9/10	9/10
		3/10 *	3/10 NS	10/10 NS	2/10 NS	5/10 NS	4/10 *
	−24 hrs	7/10	7/10	2/9	9/10	10/10	9/10
		9/10 NS	7/10 NS	7/10	0/10 ***	5/10 *	1/10 ***
	− 6 hrs	6/10	6/10	10/10	7/10	10/10	9/10
		7/10 NS	6/10 NS	8/10 NS	1/10 **	7/10 NS	1/10 ***
	−30 min	9/10	7/10	10/10	8/10	10/10	5/10
		10/10 NS	6/10 NS	9/10 NS	0/10 ***	10/10 NS	0/10 *
	+30 min	10/10	8/10	10/10	7/10	10/10	5/10
		9/10 NS	7/10 NS	10/10 NS	1/10 **	9/10 NS	4/10 NS
	+ 6 hrs	9/10	9/10	10/10	7/10	6/8	4/8
		7/10 NS	5/10 NS	10/10 NS	5/10 NS	7/8 NS	1/8 NS

[a] PCN (10 mg), CS-1 (10 mg) and phenobarbital (6 mg) were all administered once in 1 ml water, p.o., at the times indicated in this column, before or after the toxicants.

[b] All toxicants were administered per 100 g body weight, at 0 hr once as indicated, only the doses of digitoxin and indomethacin are per rat. The signs of intoxication (convulsions, dyskinesia, mortality) are registered at the times given in the corresponding column headings. The sleeping and paralysis time is given in min after administration of progesterone, hexobarbital or zoxazolamine. For each reading, the statistical significance of the apparent differences between

Table 6 (continued)

Parathion (1.5 mg in 0.5 ml DMSO i.p.)		Nicotine (1 ml of 1.5% aquaous solution p.o.)		Progesterone (10 mg in 1 ml oil i.p.)	Hexobarbital (7.5 mg in 1 ml water i.p.)	Zoxazolamine (10 mg in 1 ml water i.p.)
Dyskinesia +4 hrs	Mortality +4th day	Dyskinesia +2 hrs	Mortality +6th day	Sleeping time	Sleeping time	Paralysis time
7/10	2/10	6/10	0/10	104 ± 24	46 ± 6	270 ± 30
4/10 NS	3/10 NS	4/10 NS	4/10 *	0 ***	32 ± 7 NS	190 ± 33 NS
4/10	2/10	7/10	4/10	178 ± 27	38 ± 4	234 ± 18
0/10 *	0/10 NS	0/10 ***	0/10 *	0 ***	20 ± 2 ***	42 ± 9 ***
10/10	8/10	10/10	10/10	181 ± 35	43 ± 3	246 ± 37
7/10 NS	4/10 NS	8/10 NS	8/10 NS	89 ± 29 NS	44 ± 1 NS	240 ± 33 NS
8/10	7/10	5/10	3/10	241 ± 47	50 ± 7	282 ± 31
7/10 NS	5/10 NS	7/10 NS	6/10 NS	243 ± 37 NS	50 ± 7 NS	294 ± 24 NS
4/6	2/6	6/9	2/9	291 ± 38	68 ± 8	306 ± 26
2/7 NS	1/7 NS	9/10 NS	6/10 NS	234 ± 40 NS	52 ± 7 NS	282 ± 31 NS
0/5	0/5	2/7	3/7	—	—	—
0/6 NS	0/6 NS	3/7 NS	2/7 NS	—	—	—
7/10	5/10	7/10	1/10	257 ± 32	77 ± 16	276 ± 32
0/10 ***	0/10 *	3/10 NS	2/10 NS	151 ± 43 NS	43 ± 5 NS	300 ± 26 NS
10/10	6/10	7/10	5/10	242 ± 31	65 ± 7	291 ± 30
5/10 *	1/10 *	6/10 NS	3/10 NS	27 ± 21 ***	36 ± 3 **	138 ± 20 ***
9/10	8/10	7/10	4/10	231 ± 45	56 ± 6	330 ± 24
7/10 NS	5/10 NS	8/10 NS	2/10 NS	234 ± 48 NS	52 ± 4 NS	240 ± 20 **
5/10	5/10	4/10	3/10	171 ± 25	43 ± 2	348 ± 25
8/10 NS	6/10 NS	1/10 NS	2/10 NS	209 ± 42 NS	42 ± 3 NS	262 ± 42 NS
3/7	1/7	6/10	1/10	197 ± 26	49 ± 3	308 ± 27
5/9 NS	3/9 NS	5/10 NS	4/10 NS	320 ± 25 **	43 ± 2 NS	281 ± 29 NS
0/4	0/4	3/7	3/7	—	—	—
0/5 NS	0/5 NS	1/8 NS	2/8 NS	—	—	—
9/10	8/10	5/10	1/10	163 ± 13	46 ± 4	323 ± 37
0/10 ***	0/10 ***	2/10 NS	1/10 NS	9 ± 9 ***	13 ± 2 ***	206 ± 30 *
9/10	4/10	6/10	3/10	188 ± 30	50 ± 5	378 ± 15
0/10 ***	0/10 *	1/10 *	1/10 NS	0 ***	13 ± 2 ***	143 ± 10 ***
8/10	4/10	8/10	5/10	196 ± 30	74 ± 8	348 ± 25
9/10 NS	1/10 NS	8/10 NS	4/10 NS	278 ± 24 *	68 ± 9 NS	314 ± 27 NS
8/10	3/10	6/10	5/10	125 ± 34	57 ± 8	366 ± 18
9/10 NS	3/10 NS	6/10 NS	5/10 NS	381 ± 18 ***	92 ± 2 ***	414 ± 16 NS
7/8	4/8	6/10	0/10	235 ± 19	54 ± 6	275 ± 40
7/9 NS	1/9 NS	3/10 NS	3/10 NS	403 ± 17 ***	78 ± 7 *	348 ± 20 NS
0/4	0/4	2/6	1/6	—	—	—
1/6 NS	0/6 NS	4/7 NS	0/7 NS	—	—	—

the animals pretreated with conditioners (asterisks or NS) and the corresponding unpretreated controls have been computed, as in all tables throughout this volume, according to the "Exact Probability Test" for nonparametric values and according to Student's t-test for sleeping and paralysis times.

For the group in which the conditioners were administered after the toxicants (when the latter had already produced some mortality) the statistics are computed only on the basis of animals that survived until treatment with the conditioners.

For further details on technique of tabulation cf. p. VIII.

Table 7. Duration of effect after repeated doses of conditioners

Conditioner withdrawn (hrs)[a]		Toxicant (0 hr)	Progesterone (10 mg in 1 ml corn oil i.p.) Sleeping time	Hexobarbital (7.5 mg in 1 ml water i.p.) Sleeping time	Zoxazolamine (10 mg in 1 ml water i.p.) Paralysis time	Dioxathion (4 mg in 1 ml corn oil p.o.) Dyskinesia +6 hrs	Mortality +48 hrs	Parathion (1.5 mg in 0.5 ml DMSO i.p.) Dyskinesia +4 hrs	Mortality +4th day
Phenobarbital		Unpretreated controls	138 ± 25	52 ± 4	255 ± 24	10/10	10/10	6/10	1/10
	a) 24		0 ***	0 ***	58 ± 10 ***	0/10 ***	0/10 ***	0/10 **	0/10 NS
	b) 72		0 ***	13 ± 1 ***	170 ± 17 **	2/10 ***	1/10 ***	0/10 **	0/10 NS
	c) 120		27 ± 12 **	26 ± 5 ***	237 ± 20 NS	7/10 NS	7/10 NS	0/10 **	0/10 NS
PCN		Unpretreated controls	103 ± 27	59 ± 5	273 ± 19	10/10	10/10	7/10	3/10
	a) 24		0 **	29 ± 3 ***	36 ± 6 ***	0/10 ***	0/10 ***	0/10 ***	0/10 NS
	b) 72		5 ± 3 **	58 ± 6 NS	245 ± 20 NS	10/10 NS	9/10 NS	2/10 *	1/10 NS
	c) 120		66 ± 20 NS	59 ± 6 NS	278 ± 26 NS	10/10 NS	6/10 *	8/10 NS	3/10 NS
CS-1		Unpretreated controls	231 ± 38	60 ± 4	293 ± 29	10/10	8/10	6/10	4/10
	a) 24		3 ± 3 ***	35 ± 13 NS	110 ± 12 ***	0/10 ***	0/10 ***	0/10 **	0/10 *
	b) 72		29 ± 23 ***	39 ± 4 **	258 ± 31 NS	10/10 NS	6/10 NS	5/10 NS	3/10 NS
	c) 120		25 ± 17 ***	47 ± 7 NS	240 ± 22 NS	10/10 NS	9/10 NS	5/10 NS	4/10 NS
Spironolactone		Unpretreated controls	144 ± 22	48 ± 1	326 ± 28	10/10	8/10	5/10	4/10
	a) 24		0 ***	24 ± 1 ***	104 ± 17 ***	1/10 ***	0/10 ***	0/10 *	0/10 *
	b) 72		50 ± 22 **	43 ± 6 NS	314 ± 23 NS	10/10 NS	9/10 NS	6/10 NS	4/10 NS
	c) 120		95 ± 25 NS	52 ± 7 NS	302 ± 26 NS	9/9 NS	8/9 NS	6/10 NS	5/10 NS
Prednisolone-Ac		Unpretreated controls	174 ± 23	58 ± 7	234 ± 32	10/10	10/10	5/10	2/10
	a) 24		18 ± 12 ***	28 ± 5 **	53 ± 17 ***	10/10 NS	10/10 NS	5/10 NS	6/10 NS

	a) 24	5/10 NS	5/10 NS	7/10 NS	0/10 ***	1/9 NS	2/10 NS	1/9 NS	1/9 NS
	b) 72	8/10 NS	8/10 NS	10/10 NS	9/10 NS	4/9 NS	1/10 NS	2/10 NS	2/10 NS
	c) 120	9/10 NS	6/10 NS	10/10 NS	10/10 NS	5/10 NS	0/10 NS	1/10 NS	1/10 NS
PCN	Unpretreated controls	7/10	6/10	10/10	10/10	3/9	2/10	3/10	5/10
	a) 24	0/10 ***	0/10 **	0/10 ***	0/10 ***	0/10 NS	0/10 NS	1/10 NS	2/10 NS
	b) 72	3/10 NS	1/10 *	10/10 NS	9/10 NS	3/10 NS	1/10 NS	0/10 NS	1/10 NS
	c) 120	6/10 NS	5/10 NS	10/10 NS	8/10 NS	4/10 NS	0/10 NS	1/10 NS	2/10 NS
CS-1	Unpretreated controls	5/10	4/10	10/10	8/10	4/10	1/10	7/10	8/10
	a) 24	0/10 *	0/10 *	9/10 NS	3/10 *	1/10 NS	0/10 NS	2/10 *	4/10 NS
	b) 72	1/10 NS	1/10 NS	10/10 NS	9/10 NS	0/10 *	0/10 NS	5/10 NS	4/10 NS
	c) 120	1/10 NS	1/10 NS	9/9 NS	9/10 NS	2/10 NS	2/10 NS	6/9 NS	6/9 NS
Spironolactone	Unpretreated controls	10/10	7/10	10/10	10/10	5/10	0/10	3/10	4/10
	a) 24	0/10 ***	0/10 ***	10/10 NS	4/10 **	0/10 *	0/10 NS	6/10 NS	4/10 NS
	b) 72	3/10 ***	2/10 *	10/10 NS	10/10 NS	4/10 NS	2/10 NS	0/10 NS	3/10 NS
	c) 120	9/10 NS	7/10 NS	10/10 NS	10/10 NS	5/10 NS	2/10 NS	3/10 NS	3/10 NS
Prednisolone-Ac	Unpretreated controls	9/10	10/10	10/10	10/10	6/10	2/10	4/10	8/10
	a) 24	2/10 ***	1/10 ***	10/10 NS	10/10 NS	6/8 NS	3/10 NS	9/10 NS	9/10 NS
	b) 72	10/10 NS	9/10 NS	10/10 NS	10/10 NS	3/9 NS	2/9 NS	9/10 NS	9/10 NS
	c) 120	10/10 NS	9/10 NS	9/9 NS	10/10 NS	5/9 NS	3/9 NS	8/10 NS	9/10 NS

[a] 100 g female rats received phenobarbital at the dose of 6 mg, PCN, CS-1, spironolactone and prednisolone acetate at the dose of 10 mg, always in 1 ml water p.o., twice daily during 3½ days, and the toxicants (per 100 g body weight) once, 24 (a), 72 (b) or 120 (c) hrs after the last injection of the conditioners. The signs of intoxication (intestinal ulcers, cardiac calcification, etc.) are registered at the times given in the corresponding column headings. The sleeping and paralysis time is given in min after administration of progesterone, hexobarbital or zoxazolamine. For each reading the statistical significance of the apparent differences between the animals pretreated with conditioners and the corresponding unpretreated controls have been computed, as in all Tables throughout this volume, according to the "Exact Probability Test" for nonparametric values and according to "Student's t-test" for sleeping and paralysis times.

For further details on technique of tabulation cf. p. VIII.

2 hrs after bishydroxycoumarin has an inverse effect.

Szeberényi & Fekete H29,579/70: Brief abstract stating that after four days of pretreatment (species not mentioned), spironolactone decreased the action and accelerated the metabolism of hexobarbital, chlorzoxazone, meprobamate, estrone, testosterone, acenocoumarol and BSP, whereas after short treatment it had an inverse effect. It is concluded that spironolactone is a microsomal enzyme inducer.

Solymoss & Varga, G70,500/71: In rats, pretreatment with various catatoxic steroids accelerates the degradation of bishydroxycoumarin by NADPH-dependent hepatic enzymes. However, if the bishydroxycoumarin is administered immediately after treatment with catatoxic steroids (norbolethone, ethylestrenol, progesterone or triamcinolone), an inverse effect is observed, presumably because of competitive inhibition.

Solymoss et al. G79,007/71: In rats, various catatoxic steroids (spironolactone, PCN) increase liver weight, glutathione S-aryltransferase activity, bile flow, and BSP clearance from the blood with an accelerated urinary excretion of conjugated BSP metabolites. Ethylestrenol similarly affects liver weight, but not the other parameters. The antimineralocorticoids, spiroxasone, SC-9376 and CS-1, unlike the anabolic steroids norbolethone and oxandrolone, also enhance plasma clearance of BSP. Contrary to the effects of pretreatment, the administration of spironolactone, ethylestrenol or estradiol immediately before BSP results in retention of the dye, probably through competitive inhibition of biliary excretion.

Solymoss et al. G79,023/71: In rats, pretreatment with PCN or spironolactone increases liver weight, glutathione S-aryltransferase activity and bile flow. At the same time, the plasma clearance and biliary excretion of BSP and its conjugated metabolites are enhanced. Ethylestrenol likewise increases liver weight but does not alter the other parameters mentioned above. Spiroxasone, SC-9376 and CS-1 (antimineralocorticoids), unlike norbolethone and oxandrolone (anabolics), also enhance plasma clearance of BSP, probably through the same mechanism. In contrast to these effects of pretreatment, administration of spironolactone, ethylestrenol or estradiol immediately before BSP delays plasma clearance of the dye, probably through competitive inhibition of biliary excretion. SKF 525-A does not suppress the enhanced BSP clearance induced either by spironolactone or by phenobarbital. [Although the authors did not evaluate their data from this point of view, these observations clearly show that the catatoxic activity of steroids is not merely the result of hepatic microsomal drug metabolizing enzyme induction. It may also be mediated through extramicrosomal enzyme mechanisms or even through enhanced biliary excretion (H.S.).]

Reversal of Antagonistic Actions.

ACTINOMYCIN

Serrone & Fujimoto D48,610/61: MPDC given 1—12 hrs before hexobarbital prolongs sleeping time and delays the metabolism of the barbiturate. However, if MPDC is given 24—48 hrs before hexobarbital, the metabolism of the drug is stimulated and sleeping time is shortened. Data are presented to show that the accelerated metabolism of hexobarbital results from induced synthesis of microsomal enzyme systems that metabolize barbiturates. A similar biphasic response on hexobarbital sleeping time was observed with SKF 525-A, JB 516, iproniazid, orphenadrine, chlorpromazine, and hydroxyzine by several investigators (Holtz et al. D98,342/57; Arrigoni-Martelli & Kramer G74,659/59; Rümke & Bout G74,669/60).

Garren et al. G28,021/64: In adrenalectomized rats, a single i.p. injection of cortisol produces an increase in hepatic TPO and TKT activity. Actinomycin D did not inhibit synthesis of these enzymes, but blocked their induction when injected early after cortisol administration. Actinomycin D and fluorouracil stimulated TPO and TKT synthesis when injected 5 hrs or later after cortisol. "It is proposed that repression of the synthesis of these enzymes occurs at the level of messenger RNA translation."

Tomkins et al. G35,353/65: Following a single injection of cortisol into adrenalectomized rats, the hepatic TPO and TKT levels rise. "Although actinomycin D blocks the initial steroid-induced increase, later administration of the antibiotic (or of 5-fluorouracil) causes an increase in the levels of these enzymes. A mechanism is proposed to account for the late response to inhibitors of RNA synthesis in which a 'cytoplasmic repressor' can inhibit the translation of the messenger RNA's corresponding to tryptophan pyrrolase and tyrosine transaminase. Cytoplasmic repression is postulated to depend on continued RNA and protein synthesis, and the 'repressor' is thought to have a rapid rate of turnover."

Thompson et al. F81,633/66: "Tyrosine α-ketoglutarate transaminase can be induced by steroid hormones in a newly-established line of tissue culture cells, derived from primary culture of the ascites form of an experimental rat hepatoma." Dexamethasone, triamcinolone and cortisol were highly active, DOC and aldosterone much less potent, whereas stilbestrol, estradiol, testosterone and progesterone were virtually inactive. The induction by dexamethasone was blocked by puromycin, cycloheximide, chloramphenicol, progesterone, actinomycin D and mitomycin C. Paradoxically, after induction by the steroid had taken place, actinomycin D produced a further increase in enzyme activity.

Grossman & Mavrides G46,206/67: Studies on the kinetics of cortisol-induced hepatic TKT activity in adrenalectomized rats. "Puromycin inhibited enzyme synthesis when it was given during the initial phase of induction. However, it unexpectedly caused a rapid reappearance of enzyme activity following its administration during the inactivation phase. This potentiated response is consistent with other observations which lead to the idea that a repressor is formed about 4 hrs after hormone administration and that inhibition of repressor synthesis allows, at least temporarily, continued synthesis of enzyme." The inactivator appears to depend upon pituitary function, since adrenalectomized and hypophysectomized rats showed little or no inactivation phase following cortisol treatment.

SKF 525-A AND OTHER ANTAGONISTS

Conney & Burns G67,166/62: Review of the literature on the biphasic effect of SKF 525-A and various related compounds which inhibit microsomal enzymes when given just before the substrate, but actually induce drug-metabolizing enzymes following a more prolonged pretreatment.

Rümke G69,768/63: In mice SKF 525-A, phenobarbital, chlorpromazine, hexobarbital and iproniazid given one hour before hydroxydione i.v. increase sleeping time. When the interval is two days, a single dose of SKF 525-A, phenobarbital or chlorpromazine decreases hydroxydione anesthesia. Phenytoin, acetylcarbromal, morphine, chloramphenicol, 5-HT, phenobarbital and hydroxydione given one hour before hexobarbital increase the duration of anesthesia, whereas dioxone and chlorothiazide decrease it. It is concluded that central effects as well as changes in microsomal enzyme activity may be involved.

Serrone & Fujimoto D80,098/62; Kato et al. E47,494/64: Considerable changes in the effect of SKF 525-A upon microsomal enzyme activity are seen, depending upon the length of administration. SKF 525-A causes intense enzyme inhibition resulting in prolonged hexobarbital sleeping time when given acutely. However, if administered for prolonged periods, the metabolism of barbiturates is actually enhanced and their effectiveness diminished. This reversal of activity has been noted for several microsomal enzyme inhibitors.

Bowman et al. E714/68 (p. 520): After repeated administration of some of the inhibitors, the activity of the microsomal enzymes recovers and then increases. This has been shown for iproniazid, tolbutamide, carbutamide, CFT 1201 and SKF 525-A.

Buchel & Levy G74,851/70: In rats, SKF 525-A may either prolong or shorten pentobarbital sleeping time depending upon dosage and timing.

Reversal of Substrate Actions. *Remmer E61,211/59:* In rabbits and dogs, single i.v. injections of various **barbiturates** caused adaptation with accelerated degradation (judged by enhanced blood clearance).

Schmid et al. G34,008/64: "In two cases of glutethimide abuse, it was demonstrated that tolerance to **glutethimide** is due to marked acceleration of its metabolic inactivation. After a 20-day withdrawal cure, the metabolism of glutethimide was found to have reverted to normal."

DOSE AND ROUTE OF ADMINISTRATION

Few comparative studies have been done on the relative potency of inducers as influenced by the dosage and route of administration of the inducers themselves and of the substrates. It is clear, however, that both inducers and substrates can be active when administered enterally or parenterally, as long as they are properly absorbed. However, there are considerable species differences in the gastrointestinal absorption rate of common toxicants, which may give the erroneous impression of innate resistance. Thus, in the hamster, even enormous doses of digitoxin given p.o. cause no signs of poisoning, whereas intravenous injection of this toxicant readily elicits fatal convulsions which can be prevented by catatoxic steroids.

In an extensive study on 304 steroids tested in the rat for catatoxic activity against indomethacin s.c. and digitoxin p.o., it was found that when administered at the dose of 10 mg p.o. twice daily, 42 compounds were active against indomethacin only, 32 merely against digitoxin and 24 against both substrates. At the dose of 0.5 mg, two were active against indomethacin alone, one against digitoxin only and one against both substrates. The most active steroid of this series, PCN was subsequently shown to be active against both substrates even at the 30 µg dose level; it also proved to have the broadest spectrum of protective activity against other toxicants. Hence, PCN may be regarded as the most potent catatoxic compound among all hormonal and nonhormonal substances tested up-to-date.

A comparative study on the relative potency of spironolactone and norbolethone against unusually high doses of toxicants showed that spironolactone protects against as much as 2 mg of digitoxin per day p.o., whereas the same dose of norbolethone protects even against 5 mg of digitoxin under identical conditions. Without pretreatment with catatoxic steroids, as little as 0.5 mg of digitoxin per day is fatal to rats in such tests. More recent unpublished observations show that 100 g female rats given 25 mg of PCN, twice daily p.o., can tolerate as much as 30 mg twice daily p.o.(!) for many days without detectable manifestations of damage.

Table 8. *Limits of digitoxin inactivation by spironolactone and norbolethone*

Pretreatment[a]	Digitoxin (mg)[b]	Convulsions (Scale: 0—3)[c]	Mortality (Dead/Total)[d]
None	1	3.0	4/5
Spironolactone	1	0	0/5
Norbolethone	1	0	0/5
None	2	—	5/5
Spironolactone	2	1.3	1/5
Norbolethone	2	0	0/5
None	5	—	5/5
Spironolactone	5	3.0	4/5
Norbolethone	5	0.8	0/5
None	8	—	5/5
Spironolactone	8	—	5/5
Norbolethone	8	1.0	2/5

[a] Spironolactone and norbolethone (10 mg in 1 ml water x2/day, p.o., 1st day ff.).
[b] Digitoxin dose indicated/100 g body weight (in 1 ml water/day, p.o., 6th day ff.).
[c, d] Convulsions and mortality on 12th day.

Masson & Hoffman B513/45: In immature rabbits pretreated with estradiol, progesterone s.c. is much more effective in causing progestational changes in the uterus than if administered p.o. In the partially hepatectomized rabbit, even comparatively small doses of progesterone are active in this respect, "indicating that the liver plays an important role in the inactivation of progesterone in the rabbit." Earlier data on the role of the liver in the inactivation of progesterone are reviewed.

Selye G70,421/70: A systematic study on the comparative antidigitoxin anti-indomethacin activities of 304 steroids tested at different dose levels.

Szabo et al. G79,013/71: In hamsters, spironolactone and ethylestrenol pretreatment prevents digitoxin convulsions and indomethacin-induced intestinal ulcers. Curiously, hamsters are resistant to as much as 100 mg of digitoxin, given repeatedly p.o., whereas 1 mg i.v. produces strong convulsions. Apparently, in this species, the absorption of digitoxin from the gastrointestinal tract is deficient. Indomethacin intoxication is also different in rats and hamsters since in the latter, unlike the former, the drug produces predominantly pyloric ulcers which often perforate.

Selye PROT. 20023: In rats, spironolactone (10 mg x2/day p.o.) protects against as much as 2 mg of digitoxin/day p.o., whereas the same dose of norbolethone protects even against 5 mg of digitoxin, *cf.* Table 8, p. 94.

Selye PROT. 28397: In mice, indomethacin intoxication can be prevented by ethylestrenol, CS-1, spironolactone, norbolethone and, to a lesser extent perhaps, also by prednisolone and estradiol administered by various routes. Thyroxine appears to have an opposite effect. Progesterone, triamcinolone, DOC and hydroxydione had little if any effect.

Selye PROT. 42710: In female rats, with an initial body weight of about 100 g, phenobarbital, PCN, ethylestrenol, CS-1, spironolactone, norbolethone and estradiol were administered p.o., i.p., and s.c. at very low dose levels under comparable conditions. Although in a few instances minor differences in the protective effect against progesterone and hexobarbital anesthesia or zoxazolamine paralysis could be ascribed to the route of administration, the latter did not appear to be of paramount importance. In general, conditioners given at the dose administered by one route were also effective when introduced through another portal. Interestingly, the very low dose (0.1 mg) of phenobarbital employed in this experiment appeared to have actually prolonged the effect of zoxazolamine. In order to permit meaningful comparisons, each toxicant had to be tested at the same dose, irrespective of the route of administration and of the toxicant against which it was employed. Since various conditioners are not equally active against progesterone, hexobarbital and zoxazolamine, doses effective against one of these compounds were not necessarily active against the other two, irrespective of the route of administration. Hence, the interpretation of these findings is limited, but they definitely show that no considerable enhancement of the conditioning effect can be expected from changing the portal of its administration. This is particularly interesting in connection with the fact that administration p.o. leads the compound primarily to the liver (the major site of its conditioning effect) and, yet, in general i.p. and/or s.c. administration proved to be about equally efficacious, as shown in Table 9, p. 96.

SPECIFICITY OF CONDITIONING

One of the most astonishing characteristics of the adaptive hormones is the extraordinary spectrum of the toxicants against which they can offer protection. Some of these steroids are highly selective, but others increase resistance to a very large number of chemical or physical agents. Indeed, the spectrum of activity may depend upon circumstances: the syntoxic glucocorticoids protect the adrenalectomized animal against virtually any agent that can produce stress, but there are only a few pathogens to which they can raise tolerance above the normal level. Conversely, the catatoxic steroids, if they possess any protective power at all against a toxicant, can usually augment resistance to it far above the norm.

We shall discuss the activity spectrum of individual adaptive hormones in Chapter XI, but a few characteristic examples should be cited here. Thus, among the catatoxic steroids adequately studied up-to-date, the 16α-carbonitriles exhibit the broadest activity spectrum, in that they offer some protection against almost every substrate subject to detoxication by steroid-induced enzymes. On the other hand, progesterone and prednisolone protect only against a few toxicants. Many catatoxic steroids protect against digitoxin but not against indomethacin or vice versa.

In rats, spironolactone or oxandrolone administered for as long as 60 days continue to protect against daily administration of normally fatal doses of digitoxin or indomethacin. During this period, the plasma concentrations of digitoxin and indomethacin are diminished although they rise again following discontinuation of catatoxic steroid administration. As judged by the blood level of its metabolite

Table 9. *Effect of route of administration upon catatoxic actions of various conditioners*

Conditioners	Toxicant 0h		Progesterone Sleeping time (min)	Hexobarbital Sleeping time (min)	Zoxazolamine Paralysis time (min)
None			167 ± 40	41 ± 4	165 ± 34
Phenobarbital	0.1 mg	p.o.	71 ± 36 NS	30 ± 4 NS	316 ± 37 *
Phenobarbital		i.p.	116 ± 27 NS	30 ± 4 NS	266 ± 4 *
Phenobarbital		s.c.	26 ± 16 *	34 ± 5 NS	277 ± 39 NS
None			348 ± 78	50 ± 2	246 ± 24
PCN	0.03 mg	p.o.	69 ± 55 *	47 ± 2 NS	213 ± 48 NS
PCN		i.p.	50 ± 31 **	47 ± 2 NS	189 ± 38 NS
PCN		s.c.	92 ± 38 *	50 ± 2 NS	210 ± 19 NS
None			207 ± 33	72 ± 11	270 ± 46
Ethylestrenol	0.5 mg	p.o.	48 ± 35 *	41 ± 13 NS	234 ± 56 NS
Ethylestrenol		i.p.	72 ± 20 **	36 ± 6 *	174 ± 31 NS
Ethylestrenol		s.c.	24 ± 15 **	54 ± 9 NS	282 ± 58 NS
None			204 ± 27	49 ± 3	306 ± 15
CS-1	0.1 mg	p.o.	110 ± 41 NS	39 ± 4 NS	149 ± 34 **
CS-1		i.p.	64 ± 40 *	41 ± 4 NS	246 ± 31 NS
CS-1		s.c.	102 ± 26 *	41 ± 4 NS	222 ± 22 *
None			300 ± 30	81 ± 9	390 ± 0
Spironolactone	0.5 mg	p.o.	194 ± 49 NS	54 ± 9 NS	342 ± 29 NS
Spironolactone		i.p.	108 ± 40 **	74 ± 10 NS	342 ± 22 NS
Spironolactone		s.c.	93 ± 67 *	81 ± 9 NS	342 ± 48 NS
None			166 ± 29	62 ± 11	111 ± 42
Norbolethone	0.5 mg	p.o.	155 ± 48 NS	32 ± 5 *	71 ± 27 NS
Norbolethone		i.p.	120 ± 33 NS	32 ± 5 *	118 ± 45 NS
Norbolethone		s.c.	108 ± 25 NS	54 ± 6 NS	150 ± 38 NS
None			216 ± 25	50 ± 2	294 ± 56
Estradiol	0.1 mg	p.o.	125 ± 49 NS	53 ± 6 NS	294 ± 31 NS
Estradiol		i.p.	111 ± 38 *	56 ± 9 NS	294 ± 31 NS
Estradiol		s.c.	149 ± 54 NS	48 ± 2 NS	318 ± 44 NS

The indicated dose of all conditioners was given (per rat) in 1 ml water twice daily, from the first day to the end of the experiment. The toxicants were administered once on the 4th day (per 100 g body weight), as follows: Progesterone (10 mg in 1 ml corn oil, i.p.), hexobarbital (7.5 mg in 1 ml water, i.p.), and zoxazolamine (10 mg in 1 ml water, i.p.).
Statistics: Student's t-test.

SC-9376, spironolactone also enhances its own biotransformation, but not sufficiently to interfere with the continued manifestation of protective activity against the substrates tested. Here, we are faced with a peculiar type of specificity of induction, in that a compound (spironolactone or oxandrolone) can induce an extraordinary amount of enzymic activity against structurally-unrelated toxicants (digitoxin or indomethacin), whereas it develops no noteworthy resistance against itself. In other words, these steroids are much more efficient in eliciting cross-resistance than straight resistance. This is unusual, since in most instances, adaptation to one agent is more easily obtained by pretreatment with the same than with an unrelated agent. The phenomenon is of practical importance since it would be impossible to offer continued protection against toxicants by treatment with catatoxic steroids if they were very efficient in enhancing their own enzymic degradation.

As previously mentioned, substrates readily metabolized by catatoxic steroids, often exhibit inducer and/or blocker activities themselves. Yet, there are many exceptions: digitoxin, nicotine, DHT and indomethacin are all excellent substrates for catatoxic steroids, yet they induce no demonstrable resistance against themselves or against other substrates; indeed, upon chronic treatment at the dose levels tested, their effects were cumulative.

Solymoss et al. G70,441/70: In rats, spironolactone or oxandrolone given for as long as two months, continues to exhibit a protective effect against fatal doses of digitoxin or indomethacin. Upon withdrawal of the catatoxic steroids, continued administration of digitoxin or indomethacin is rapidly fatal. The plasma concentration of digitoxin and indomethacin is diminished during the catatoxic steroid administration.

Solymoss et al. G70,464/70: As judged by the blood level of its metabolite, SC-9376, spironolactone also enhances its own biotransformation, yet its catatoxic effect remains evident during long periods of administration.

BILIARY EXCRETION

Many of the inducible hepatic microsomal enzymes act upon substrates in such a manner as to facilitate their excretion through the bile or urine. The effect of hormones upon the biliary excretion of toxicants has not received very much attention so far; there can be no doubt that it deserves to be considered more than it has in the past. Several of the toxicants amenable to the influence of certain steroids (e.g., $HgCl_2$, indomethacin, DHT) are well tolerated after bile duct ligature, suggesting that their activity depends largely upon the prolongation of their effect by enterohepatic recirculation, poor absorption in the absence of bile, or other factors associated with bile secretion.

Up to now, major emphasis has been placed upon the identification of biliary elimination of bile pigments, bile acids and steroids (as well as their metabolites), using isotope marked substrates.

Kellaway et al. B14,515/45: In rats, the activity of thyroxine s.c. was estimated by an increase in pulse rate after partial hepatectomy, thyroidectomy or bile duct ligation. "It was found (1) that thyroxine activity is greatly intensified in the absence of the liver; (2) that the liver does not play a significant role when the amount of circulating thyroxine is within physiologic limits; (3) that the liver deals with excess hormone by some process of inactivation and not by simple excretion."

Grad & Leblond B49,686/50: In rats, the increase in oxygen consumption and heart rate induced by thyroxine is increased by partial hepatectomy, or bile duct ligation, and especially by the conjoint effect of both interventions. "These results are taken to indicate that the liver excretes and inactivates excess amounts of thyroid hormone."

Hyde et al. D99,140/54: In rats, 17α-methyl-C^{14}-Δ^5-androstene-3β, 17β-diol administered by gavage was mostly eliminated in the feces and, to a lesser extent, in the urine. "Rats with two types of bile fistula excreted the major fraction of administered isotopic carbon in the bile. Almost quantitative recovery of the administered C^{14} was obtained in the urine of rats after ligation of the bile ducts."

Cherrik et al. E98,251/60: Indocyanine green is rapidly and completely bound to plasma protein and excreted in the bile in unconjugated form. It is not cleared by extrahepatic mechanisms in detectable amounts. Its plasma clearance is similar to that of BSP in controls and patients with liver lesions.

Preisig et al. F70,515/66: In acromegalic patients, biliary BSP excretion is increased. [It is not known which, if any, of the hormones secreted by the hyperactive pituitary are responsible for this effect (H.S.).]

Heikel G81,287/67: In rabbits with an external biliary fistula, norethandrolone and 17α-ethyl-4-estrone-3β,17β-diol-3-propionate cause a progressive decline of bile flow and total bilirubin. Methyltestosterone is less effective.

Kreek et al. F83,145/67: In rats, ethinylestradiol considerably diminishes bile flow and delays biliary excretion of BSP and of tritium-labeled estradiol.

Klaassen & Plaa F99,395/68: In rats, pretreatment with phenobarbital accelerated the plasma clearance of BSP. There was no change in hepatic storage but significant increases of in vitro metabolism, biliary transport maximum and bile flow were observed. With a dibrominated analogue of BSP and with indocyanine green, which are apparently not biotransformed before excretion, enhanced plasma clearance was also elicited by phenobarbital. It is assumed "that the enhanced biliary excretion of these dyes is an important factor after phenobarbital treatment and that the role of increased biotransformation is not as important for the enhanced plasma disappearance of these dyes as might be expected from the effect of phenobarbital on the biologic half-life of other substances."

Stowe & Plaa G73,241/68: Review (19 pp., 226 refs.) on the extrarenal excretion (bile, gastrointestinal tract, sweat, milk, tears, lung and reproductive tract) of drugs and hormones.

Roberts & Plaa G69,070/69: In mice and rats, the hyperbilirubinemia induced by α-naphthylisothiocyanate (ANIT) is enhanced by various drugs and steroids, presumably because of an increased rate of bilirubin production and not as a consequence of decreased biliary bilirubin excretion. "Studies of the rate of endogenous bile bilirubin excretion and the incorporation of δ-aminolevulinic acid-^{14}C (ALA-^{14}C) into bilirubin in rats revealed that phenobarbital and chlorpromazine significantly increased the rate of bile bilirubin production (μg/100 g/hr.) and that phenobarbital, chlorpromazine, and norethandrolone significantly increased the percent incorporation of ALA-^{14}C into bilirubin. Acetohexamide and Enovid both produced an increased, but irregular, response in bile bilirubin excretion and ALA-^{14}C incorporation."

Bickel & Minder G77,613/70: In rats, imipramine is to a large extent excreted in the bile, as judged by observations with bile fistulas or perfused livers. Besides large amounts of glucuronides, the bile also contains unchanged imipramine or desmethylimipramine following their introduction into the blood stream. In addition, the influence of SKF 525-A and phenobarbital have been studied. A review of the literature suggests that "foreign compounds, in order to be excreted in the bile, must have a molecular weight of more than about 300 and have a certain degree of polarity. Anions of conjugates are particularly suitable for concentrative transfer into bile. In contrast, unchanged lipophilic drugs are assumed not to be excreted by this route, or to occur in bile in concentrations not exceeding the plasma levels."

Bickel & Minder G77,614/70: Studies on rats with biliary fistulas show that "uptake of imipramine and desmethylimipramine, but not of hydrophilic metabolites, into the bile salt-phospholipid-micelles of bile could be demonstrated by equilibrium dialysis and ultracentrifuge sedimentation using rat bile or micellar model systems. Biliary proteins and small molecules which do not form micelles do not participate in uptake." These observations throw some light on earlier apparently conflicting claims by showing that both polar and nonpolar metabolites can be excreted through the bile although through different mechanisms.

Heikel & Lathe G73,162/70: In rats, various folliculoids and luteoids reduce bile flow. The bilirubin maximum secretion rate (Tm) is but slightly affected. Following i.v. infusion of bilirubin folliculoids (unlike luteoids) raise the serum conjugated bilirubin level.

Karim & Taylor G74,179/70: In rabbits, the biliary and urinary excretion of metabolites of [4-^{14}C] estradiol are described.

Klaassen G75,506/70: In rats, the effects of phenobarbital, chlordane, phenylbutazone, nikethamide, and chlorcyclizine upon bile flow and microsomal enzyme induction have been compared. "There generally appears to be a good correlation in the ability of these agents to increase biliary flow in rats and their ability to increase the plasma disappearance and biliary excretion of BSP and DBSP."

Kreek & Sleisenger G77,590/70: In rats, folliculoids are to a large extent excreted through biliary fistulas and under normal conditions they undergo a very large enterohepatic circulation in animals as well as in man.

Laatikainen G78,706/70: A review (22 pp., 118 refs.) and personal observations on the excretion of steroid hormones in human bile.

Levine et al. G73,357/70: In rats, phenobarbital stimulates biliary excretion of diphenyl, stilbestrol and phenolphthalein, all of which are metabolized prior to excretion. This treatment does not affect biliary elimination of stilbestrol glucuronide, phenolphthalein glucuronide, succinylsulphathiazole, and indocyanine green, all of which are excreted unchanged. These and other observations "suggest that although the endoplasmic reticulum is involved in the metabolism of foreign compounds it does not appear to play a role in their transfer from liver to bile."

Levine H 31,806/70: In rats, 3,4-benzpyrene is rapidly excreted through the bile in the form of its metabolic products. Pretreatment with microsomal drug-metabolizing enzyme inducers (e.g., phenobarbital, methylcholanthrene, 3,4-benzpyrene) greatly enhances the rate of biliary excretion of this compound. Both the rate of metabolism and of biliary excretion are enhanced to a similar extent throughout the induction period. Male rats both metabolize 3,4-benzpyrene and excrete its metabolites in the bile at rates approximately 2.5 times that of females. The induction by methylcholanthrene of both the metabolism and the biliary excretion of 3,4-benzpyrene can be partially blocked by ethionine. It has been concluded that conversion to its metabolites is the rate-limiting step in the biliary excretion of 3,4-benzpyrene.

Song & Kappas G80,521/70: Review (21 pp., 215 refs.) on the "Influence of Hormones on Hepatic Function," with special sections on the effect of endocrine factors upon bile formation. Some of the principal relevant data are summarized in Table 10.

Taylor G74,178/70: In rabbits, the biliary and urinary excretion of metabolites of [4-^{14}C] cortisone are described.

Despopoulos H 35,471/71: In isolated perfused rat liver preparations, the volume of bile was reduced by progesterone, methyltestosterone, norethynodrel and ethisterone but not by estradiol, mestranol and norethandrolone. The effect of steroids upon biliary secretion is reviewed.

Solymoss et al. G79,007/71: In rats, various catatoxic steroids (spironolactone, PCN) increase liver weight, glutathione S-aryltransferase activity, bile flow, and BSP clearance from the blood with an accelerated urinary excretion of conjugated BSP metabolites. Ethylestrenol similarly affects liver weight, but not the other parameters. The anti-mineralocorticoids, spiroxasone, SC-9376 and CS-1, unlike the anabolic steroids norbolethone and oxandrolone, also enhance plasma clearance of BSP. Contrary to the effects of pretreatment, the administration of spironolactone, ethylestrenol or estradiol immediately before BSP results in retention of the dye, probably through competitive inhibition of biliary excretion.

Solymoss et al. G79,023/71: In rats, pretreatment with PCN or spironolactone increases liver weight, glutathione, S-aryltransferase activity and bile flow. At the same time, the plasma clearance and biliary excretion of BSP and its conjugated metabolites are enhanced. Ethylestrenol likewise increases liver weight but does not alter the other parameters mentioned above. Spiroxasone, SC-9376 and CS-1 (antimineralocorticoids), unlike norbolethone and oxandrolone (anabolics) also enhance plasma clearance of BSP, probably through the same mechanism. By contrast to these effects of pretreatment, administration of spironolactone, ethylestrenol or estradiol immediately before BSP delays plasma clearance of the dye, probably through competitive inhibition of biliary excretion. SKF 525-A does not suppress the enhanced BSP clearance induced either by spironolactone or by phenobarbital. [Although the authors did not evaluate their data from this point of view, these observations clearly show that the catatoxic activity of steroids is not merely the result of hepatic microsomal drug metabolizing enzyme induction. It may be mediated also through extramicrosomal enzyme mechanisms or even through enhanced biliary excretion (H.S.).]

Table 10. *Effect of hormones on hepatic bile flow*

Hormones	Species Studied	Effect
Cholecystokinin-pancreozymin	Dog	Increase
Epinephrine	Dog	Increase, followed by decrease
Ethinylestradiol	Rat	Decrease
Gastrin	Dog	Increase
Insulin	Dog	Increase
Norepinephrine	Dog	Decrease
Norethandrolone	Rabbit	Decrease
Secretin	Dog	Increase

EXTRAHEPATIC CONDITIONING

The liver is undoubtedly the principal site of drug metabolism, but virtually all cells are endowed with some adaptive ability to toxicants.

Probably, the first observation on the extrahepatic detoxication of a steroid was the finding that estradiol is inactivated by slices or mince of renal tissue of rats and rabbits. It was realized, as early as 1940, that this inactivation is, in all probability, not due to conjugation or conversion to a less active form, but to oxidative enzymic degradation.

Pretreatment with cortisol increases the GPT activity not only in the liver, but also in the thymus, pancreas, and kidney of the rat. In the thymus, this increase may reach 16 times the normal level.

1,2-Benzanthracene increases benzpyrene hydroxylase activity throughout the entire gastrointestinal tract of various species.

Glucuronic acid conjugation of thyroid hormones occurs even after hepatectomy in the dog or after evisceration in rats, whereas steroid glucuronides are not formed following hepatectomy or evisceration.

Phenobarbital increases both hepatic and (to a lesser extent) renal weight. At the same time, the cytochrome b_5 and P-450 concentrations and the drug metabolism are raised 2—3 fold by phenobarbital in the kidneys of rabbits.

Phenobarbital also enhances incorporation of acetate into cholesterol by both the liver and the small intestine in vitro.

Smoking during pregnancy causes an increase in the benzpyrene hydroxylase activity of the human placenta. A similar enzyme activation can be obtained in the placenta of the rat by pretreatment with various polycyclic hydrocarbons.

In man, pretreatment with heptabarbital diminishes the plasma bishydroxycoumarin level more markedly if the anticoagulant is given p.o. than i.v. Presumably, part of the protective effect of heptabarbital is caused by increased hepatic destruction of bishydroxycoumarin, but diminished gastrointestinal absorption also plays a role.

Isotope-marked progesterone placed in the small intestine of dogs, was found in the effluent venous plasma, at first mainly as unchanged progesterone, but later in the form of various metabolites which must have been formed locally.

In connection with extrahepatic drug detoxication, it should be remembered that a sizable percentage of various drugs and hormones is excreted through the kidney, bile, gastrointestinal tract, sweat, milk, tears, lung and reproductive tract. Stimulation of these excretory mechanisms also plays an important part in resistance to toxicants. These phenomena are considered here although often toxicants are excreted only after biotransformation in the liver.

For further details on extrahepatic drug inactivation, *cf.* the reviews cited in the following Abstract Section.

Kidney

Masson & Beland A72,286/44; B344/45: Review of the literature on the effect of partial hepatectomy and other forms of liver damage upon barbiturate anesthesia. Personal observations on a series of 29 barbiturates tested on partially hepatectomized or completely nephrectomized rats led to the conclusion that the compounds can be classified into four groups: "Group I, those detoxified mainly in the kidney; Group II, those detoxified mainly in the liver; Group III, those detoxified approximately equally in both liver and kidney; Group IV, those possibly detoxified in other tissues of the body, but not to any great extent in the liver and the kidney."

Friedman et al. A49,249/49: In rats, urinary excretion of digitoxin is negligible.

Smith D27,805/62: Studies on the effect of hyaluronidase and cortisol on the inactivation of vasopressin by rat kidney slices.

Weiner G74,032/67: Review (18 pp., 146 refs.) on the mechanism of renal excretion of drugs.

Uehleke & Greim G70,906/68: In rats and rabbits, phenobarbital increases the weight of the liver and, to a much smaller extent, that of the kidney. "Pretreatment with Phenobarbital, 3,4-Benzpyrene or Chlorophenothane neither significantly increased the cytochromes of rat kidney microsomes, nor the oxidative drug metabolism. However, in the kidneys of rabbits the cytochrome b_5 and P_{450} concentrations and drug metabolism were 2—3 fold higher after Phenobarbital. The correlation between P_{450} content and drug oxidase activity in the kidney microsomes of untreated and Phenobarbital treated rabbits was low. Suspension of rabbit kidney microsomes revealed the same spectral changes after addition of Hexobarbital or Aniline as those reported for liver microsomes."

Karim & Taylor G74,179/70: In rabbits, the biliary and urinary excretions of metabolites of [4-^{14}C] estradiol are described.

Maruyama et al. G74,893/70: Review of the literature indicating that the main site of parathyroid hormone inactivation in the rat is the kidney. The present authors succeeded in isolating a microsomal endopeptidase from the rat kidney which preferentially hydrolyzes parathyroid hormone.

Taylor G74,178/70: The biliary and urinary excretions of metabolites of [4-^{14}C] cortisone in rabbits are described.

Gastrointestinal Tract

Berliner & Wiest C22,807/56: Progesterone, given i.v., is extensively metabolized in 1 hour by totally eviscerated rats, even if the kidneys and adrenals are also removed. After 1 hour, 7 compounds could be isolated from the tissues of these animals, although there were no polar metabolites similar to the conjugates with glucuronic or sulfuric acid, and the 7 isolated compounds retained their Δ^4-3-ketone configuration.

Bojesen & Egense G75,996/60: In adrenalectomized cats, the elimination of endogenous corticoids (cortisol and corticosterone) is greatly delayed by hepatectomy and totally abolished by evisceration. "A few experiments suggested that the intestine is responsible for the main part of the extrahepatic elimination. In experiments with the perfused isolated hindquarter preparation it was impossible to demonstrate any elimination of corticosteroids in spite of electrical stimulation or the administration of large amounts of insulin."

Wattenberg et al. D40,287/62: Benzpyrene hydroxylase activity can be demonstrated in the small intestine of various species. Following 1,2-benzanthracene p.o., this enzyme activity is increased throughout the entire gastrointestinal tract but varies in magnitude from one region to another.

Aggler & O'Reilly G68,730/69: In man, pretreatment with heptabarbital diminished the reduction in the prothrombin level, the amount of bishydroxycoumarin in plasma, and the half-life of bishydroxycoumarin more markedly after p.o. than after i.v. administration of the anticoagulant. Unchanged bishydroxycoumarin was found in the stool only after p.o. administration. Presumably, part of the response to heptabarbital was caused by increased hepatic enzymic destruction of bishydroxycoumarin although, in the event of p.o. administration, decreased absorption from the gastrointestinal tract also played a role.

Middleton & Isselbacher H17,133/69: In rats, phenobarbital increases incorporation of acetate into cholesterol not only by the liver but also by the small intestine in vitro.

Nienstedt & Hartiala G69,886/69: "Progesterone-4-^{14}C placed in the small intestine of anaesthetized, heparinized dogs was found in the effluent venous plasma, first mainly as unchanged progesterone, then increasingly in the form of different metabolites. These include 5α-pregnanedione, 20β-hydroxypregn-4-en-3-one, 3β-hydroxy-5α-pregnan-20-one, 3α-hydroxy-5α-pregnan-20-one, at least one pregnanediol epimer and a large group of polar metabolites."

Lien et al. H25,091/70: In dogs and Rhesus monkeys, serum corticoid concentrations were measured by the corticosteroid binding-globulin (CBG) technique which measures cortisol, corticosterone and 11-desoxycortisol in plasma as judged by differences in the corticoid concentration in portal and aortic blood. A noteworthy portion of corticoids is removed through clearance by the gut, especially during conditions of stress.

RES

Reichard et al. C32,593/56: Review of the literature, and personal observations on the role of the RES in the hormonal regulation of resistance to bacterial infection and nonspecific stress.

Agarwal et al. C65,716/69: In the rat, both S. typhimurium endotoxin and Thorotrast lowered hepatic TPO activity, and prevented cortisol from inducing this enzyme in the isolated, perfused liver. Under these conditions, the TKT activity of the liver remained unaffected. Partial purification of hepatic TPO induced by endotoxin or Thorotrast indicated the presence of some inhibitory substance. "Since histological studies revealed that thorotrast is localized in Kupffer cells, it is suggested that the reticuloendothelial system contributes to the control of enzyme induction in rat liver."

Munson et al. H22,843/70: "Drugs which alter the phagocytic activity of the RES have been shown to prolong barbiturate anesthesia. In this study, these observations were extended to include agents which decrease RES activity. Methyl palmitate, thorium dioxide and pyran copolymer (PCP) markedly decreased the intravascular clearance of colloidal carbon and prolonged hexobarbital anesthesia. Zymosan, endotoxin, diethylstilbesterol and PCP enhance RES activity and also prolong hexobarbital narcosis. Conversely, chlorcyclizine, SKF 525-A and phenobarbital, which markedly alter drug metabolism, did not alter RES activity. PCP and zymosan prolonged the half life of hexobarbital in brain, liver and serum. Hexobarbital metabolism was markedly depressed in 9000x g liver supernatant fractions from PCP and zymosan-treated mice. Further studies demonstrated that the inhibition of barbiturate metabolism was non-competitive. PCP and SKF 525-A were additive in microsomal inhibitory ability whereas chlorcyclizine, given in a protocol which stimulates microsomal enzyme activity, reverses the inhibitory effect of zymosan. The toxicity of cyclophosphamide, which requires hepatic microsomal enzyme activity for cytotoxicity, was markedly enhanced by PCP suggesting the enzymes necessary for the activation of cyclophosphamide are stimulated by PCP."

Placenta

Welch et al. G65,788/69: No detectable benzpyrene hydroxylase or aminoazo dye N-demethylase activity was observed in the placentas of women who did not smoke but these enzymes were found in the placentas of smokers. In rats, treatment with 3,4-benzpyrene, 1,2-benzanthracene, 1,2,5,6-dibenzanthracene, chrysene, 3,4-benzofluorene, anthracene, pyrene, fluoranthene, perylene, or phenanthrene during pregnancy increased benzpyrene hydroxylase activity in the placenta.

Brain

Angel & Burkett G39,712/66: Review of the literature (6 pp., 21 refs.) on the role of stress and corticoids in influencing resistance to various drugs through alterations in the blood-brain barrier.

Fuller G75,131/70: In rats, exposure to cold, as well as treatment with cortisol or glucagon after adrenalectomy induced TKT activity in the liver but not in the brain. Apparently, the TKT "of brain differed from the enzyme in liver since it did not exhibit diurnal variations of activity and was not affected by hormones, drugs, or stress."

Varia

Heller A32,137/40: In vitro studies on tissue slices and tissue mince of rats and rabbits indicate that "estradiol is inactivated by **liver** and **kidney** and not by the other tissues studied. This inactivation of estradiol is, in all probability, not due to conjugation or conversion to a less active form, but due to enzymic destruction of an oxidative nature. This is indicated by the relative inactivity of the treated estradiol, the inability of hydrolysis procedures to increase activity and the effect of tissue poisons upon inhibiting the estradiol-destroying enzyme system. Estrone is increased 20 times in potency by incubation with minced uterine tissue. **Spleen, lung, heart** and **kidney** tissues also caused estrone to be converted to a more active substance. The suggestion is made that this conversion is accomplished by enzymatic reduction of estrone to estradiol."

Chedid et al. B99,547/54: In mice rendered particularly sensitive by adrenalectomy, E. coli endotoxin injected i.v. or into the spleen is equally toxic. Similar results have been obtained in intact rats. "Thus the liver does not appear to play an immediate role in the detoxification of this antigen." In partially hepatectomized rats "which become more sensitive to any toxic substance" cortisone continues to exert its protective effect against endotoxin. The same is true of the **splenectomy** or **thymectomy**.

Rosen et al. C71,414/59: Pretreatment with cortisol increased the GPT activity not only in the liver but also in the **thymus, pancreas** and **kidney** of the rat. In the thymus the increase was 16-fold on the basis of protein content.

Šulcová & Stárka E37,298/63: Demonstration of extrahepatic 7α-hydroxylation of dehydroepiandrosterone by in vitro studies using different rat organs (**lung, kidney, spleen, muscle, blood**).

Govier F57,820/65: In rabbits, acetylation of sulfanilamide and p-aminobenzoic acid (one of the major routes of metabolism of acrylamines) has been examined utilizing isolated intact hepatic and **RES cells** of various other tissues. "The acetylation of these compounds, usually attributed to the liver, was found to occur in cells of the reticuloendothelial system. No acetylation could be demonstrated in the hepatic parenchymal cells. Lung and spleen, organs known to contain a high percentage of reticuloendothelial cells, were also found to acetylate these compounds."

Jayle & Pasqualini G67,284/66: Review (36 pp., 267 refs.) on glucuronic acid conjugation of steroids and thyroxine. Literature is cited to show that glucuroconjugation of thyroid hormones occurs also in **eviscerated** rats and hepatectomized dogs, whereas steroid glucuronides are not formed in hepatectomized and eviscerated mice. This suggests that glucuroconjugation of thyroid hormones, unlike that of steroids, can occur in extrahepatic tissues.

Conney F88,649/67 (p. 340): Review of the literature on enzyme induction in **nonhepatic tissues.**

Goldstein et al. E165/68 (p. 232): Review on **extrahepatic** drug metabolism as influenced by various inducers.

Mannering G71,818/68 (p. 77): Review on the induction of drug-metabolizing enzymes in the **lung, gastrointestinal tract** and **kidney.**

Stowe & Plaa G73,241/68: Review (19 pp., 226 refs.) on the extrarenal excretion (**bile, gastrointestinal tract, sweat, milk, tears, lung and reproductive tract**) of drugs and hormones.

Wattenberg et al. G71,805/68: In rats, the increase in benzpyrene hydroxylase activity induced by various 2-phenylbenzothiazoles usually shows a similar trend in **liver** and **lung.**

Uehleke G70,915/69: Review on **extrahepatic** microsomal drug metabolism.

Conney G70,316/70: Review on environmental factors influencing drug metabolism with a special section on **extrahepatic** microsomal-enzyme induction.

Schoor H28,965/70: A farmer from an area of heavy pesticide usage was given phenobarbital and diphenylhydantoin for the treatment of epilepsy. His blood levels of DDT, DDE, dieldrin and heptachlor were far below those of other farmers living in the same area. It is assumed that either the drugs activated microsomal enzymes which destroy the pesticides or "that the pesticides are bound by **serumproteins,** and are consequently relatively inert. The action of the drugs on the pesticides depends on the competition of both for the same binding sites on the proteins."

McArthur et al. G81,040/71: Studies on the binding of indomethacin, salicylate and phenobarbital to human whole **blood, plasma,** and **erythrocytes** (equilibrium dialysis), showed that "the red cells bound appreciable proportions of salicylate and phenobarbitone but not indomethacin. It is concluded that prediction of the extent of the drug binding to the circulating blood should be made from the results obtained with whole blood, red cells and plasma."

TOXICANTS (CHARACTERISTICS OF TYPICAL SUBSTRATES)

At present, the most popular basis for the classification of substrates amenable to biotransformation by hepatic microsomal enzyme systems is their preferential binding to hepatic hemoprotein P-450 as determined by difference spectra. It is generally agreed that, on this basis, the response of the substrates remains of the same type whether they are exposed to naturally-occurring microsomal enzyme constituents or to those artificially induced by different compounds. Furthermore (with one or two possible exceptions), the **Type I or Type II behavior of a substrate** (*cf.* p. 15) is unchanged upon incubation with hepatic microsomes of different species. It is suggested that the Type I and Type II binding sites differ and that the Type I site is associated with membrane phospholipids (Chaplin & Mannering G75,976/71).

The following is a partial list of substrates that have been categorized in this manner (largely based on Mannering G74,558/71):

TYPE I
Aminopyrine
 (Dimethylaminoantipyrine)
Amobarbital
3,4-Benzpyrene
Chlorpromazine
Coumarin
Cyclohexane
DDT
Dihydrosafrole
N,N-Dimethylaniline
β-Estradiol
Ethylbenzene
Ethylmorphine
Hexobarbital
Imipramine
Lilly 327—169—22B
Lilly 390—378—23B*
Methylphenidate
Morphine
Naphthalene
Phenacetin
Phenobarbital*
Pregnenolne
Progesterone
SKF 525-A
SKF 8742-A*
Testosterone

TYPE II
Acetanilide
Acetone
Alcohols (methyl-, ethyl-, 2-propyl-,
 isobutyl-, isoamyl-)
1-Butanol
Amines (n-propyl-, n-butyl-, n-pentyl-,
 n-heptyl-, n-acetyl-, n-decyl-, benzyl-,
 cyclohexyl-)
p-Aminophenol
Amphetamine
Aniline
Corticosterone
Cortisol
Cyanide
Desdimethylimipramine
Dioxane
DPEA
Ethyl isocyanide
Imidazole
Lilly 390—378—23B*
N-Methylaniline
3-Methyl-4-Methylaminoazobenzene
Metyrapone
Monomethylaminopyrine
Nicotinamide
Nicotine
Phenobarbital*
Phenylhydrazine
Pyridine
Rotenone
SKF 8742-A*
SKF 26754-A

* Can be Type I or II depending upon circumstances (e.g., species).

It will be noted that among the steroids in this list, some (estradiol, pregnenolone, progesterone, testosterone) are classified as Type I substrates, whereas others (corticosterone, cortisol) belong to Type II. Much more work will be necessary to classify, according to these criteria, all steroids that have been found to be either inducers of, or substrates for, microsomal enzymes. Meanwhile, it is even debatable whether there is any close relationship between the differential spectrographic behavior of substrates and their effects in vivo.

Within the frame of this monograph it would be impossible to describe in detail the characteristics of all the substrates whose metabolism and toxicity are influenced by catatoxic compounds. Most of the pertinent data will be found in the sections on individual inducers affecting these toxicants since it is according to the inducers that our material is arranged. Here, we should like to give only brief outlines and key references on the characteristics of the substrates themselves.

Steroid hormones are especially important both as substrates and as inducers of catatoxic activity; hence, they deserve special attention in connection with our subject. The major pathways of biosynthesis of adrenal steroids and some of the enzymes and coenzymes involved may be summarized as shown on p. 106.

Here the major secretory products are underlined. In the zona fasciculata and zona reticularis, no aldosterone is formed. In the zona glomerulosa, aldosterone is produced but no 17-hydroxylated compounds or sex hormones are formed. The enzymes and cofactors for the reactions progressing down each column are shown on the left and from the first to the second column at the top of the chart. When a particular enzyme is deficient, hormone production is blocked at the points indicated by the shaded bars.

Among the most interesting steroid substrates is **cholesterol**, because of its important role in atherosclerosis. Experimental findings suggest that by accelerating its metabolic degradation through catatoxic compounds, cholesterol atherosclerosis can be prevented in animals and perhaps even in man.

The **digitalis compounds** (closely related to steroid hormones and cholesterol) are among the most commonly-used substrates in work on catatoxic steroids. The following Abstract Section lists several excellent reviews on the pharmacology of digitalis compounds and data concerning the mechanism of digitoxin hydroxylation in the rat. Chronic administration of digitoxin significantly inhibits both the synthesis and the stress-induced release of ACTH, thereby causing some degree of adrenal atrophy. Digitoxin has even been claimed to inhibit stress-induced adrenal hypertrophy suggesting close relationships between this cardiac glycoside and corticoids.

The **barbiturates** represent another large group of drugs commonly employed in experimental work on the action of catatoxic compounds, because — like digitoxin, pesticides or indomethacin — they are readily attacked by induced hepatic microsomal enzymes. For these reasons the various factors influencing the distribution, metabolism and action of barbiturates have been carefully explored but all these data cannot be reviewed here.

An interesting fact from the point of view of barbiturate detoxication is that both in animals and in man just awakening from barbiturate hypnosis, it is possible to reinduce sleep by cortisone or i.v. injection of glucose. The mechanism of this singular phenomenon is not understood, but it obviously cannot be due to interference with induction or enhanced degradation of drug-metabolizing enzymes, since the plasma-barbiturate concentration has already fallen below the anesthetic level when sleep is reinduced. It is conceivable, however, that glucocorticoids and glucose discharge barbiturates from tissue stores into the blood, increase the barbiturate sensitivity of the brain, or augment the permeability of the blood-brain barrier.

Despite great individual variations in the duration of pentobarbital narcosis or zoxazolamine paralysis among rats, the brain concentration of these drugs closely parallels their pharmacologic activity. Apparently, individual variations in barbitu-

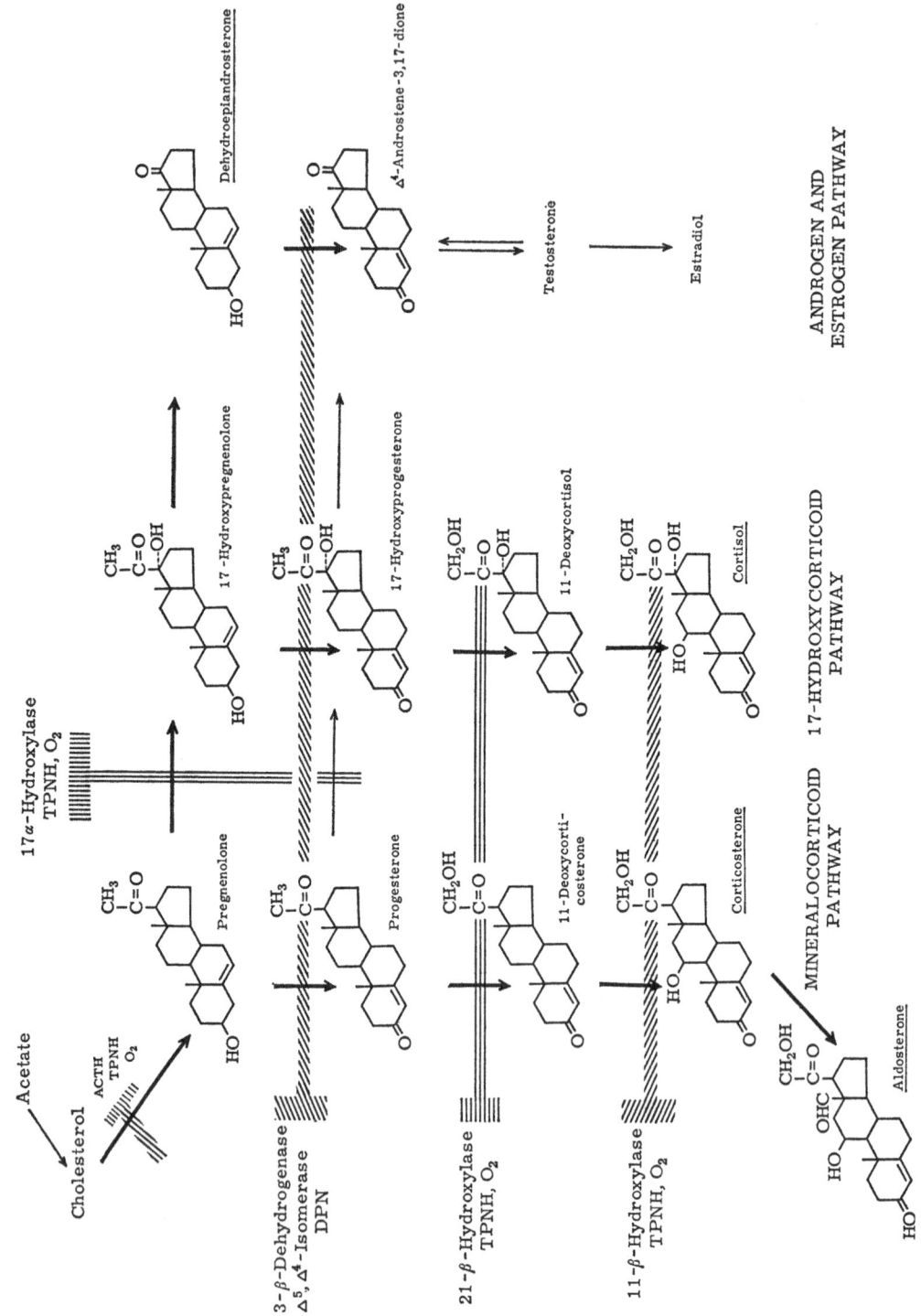

Composite outline of major pathways in adrenocortical hormone biosynthesis (after Welikey, Mulrow & others, from Ganong G 74,400/69).

rate (and zoxazolamine) sensitivity among rats are not due to great differences in the drug-sensitivity of the nervous system but to differences in drug absorption and metabolism.

The salient characteristics of the barbiturates most commonly employed in North America are illustrated as follows (Sharpless E 8,852/70):

Table 11. *Barbiturates most commonly used in North America*

$$X=C\begin{matrix} \diagup N-C \diagdown \\ \diagdown N-C \diagup \end{matrix} \begin{matrix} R_3 \\ \\ H \end{matrix} \begin{matrix} O \\ \diagdown \\ C \diagdown R_1 \\ \diagup \\ R_2 \\ \diagup \\ O \end{matrix}$$

Barbiturate	Trade name	R_1	R_2	R_3	X
Allobarbital	Dial	allyl	allyl	H	O
Amobarbital	Amytal	ethyl	isopentyl	H	O
Aprobarbital	Alurate	allyl	isopropyl	H	O
Barbital	Veronal	ethyl	ethyl	H	O
Butabarbital	Butisol	ethyl	sec-butyl	H	O
Butalbital	Sandoptal	allyl	isobutyl	H	O
Butallylonal	Pernoston	sec-butyl	2-bromoallyl	H	O
Butethal	Neonal	ethyl	butyl	H	O
Cyclobarbital	Phanodorn	ethyl	cyclohexen-1-yl	H	O
Cyclopentyl allylbarbituric acid	Cyclopal	allyl	2-cyclopenten-1-yl	H	O
Heptabarbital	Medomin	ethyl	1-cyclohepten-1-yl	H	O
Hexethal	Ortal	ethyl	n-hexyl	H	O
Hexobarbital	Evipal	methyl	1-cyclohexen-1-yl	CH_3	O
Mephobarbital	Mebaral	ethyl	phenyl	CH_3	O
Metharbital	Gemonil	ethyl	ethyl	CH_3	O
Methitural	Neraval	2-methylthioethyl	1-methylbutyl	H	S
Methohexital	Brevital	allyl	1-methyl-2-pentynyl	CH_3	O
Pentobarbital	Nembutal	ethyl	1-methylbutyl	H	O
Phenobarbital	Luminal	ethyl	phenyl	H	O
Probarbital	Ipral	ethyl	isopropyl	H	O
Secobarbital	Seconal	allyl	1-methylbutyl	H	O
Talbutal	Lotusate	allyl	sec-butyl	H	O
Thiamylal	Surital	allyl	1-methylbutyl	H	S
Thiopental	Pentothal	ethyl	1-methylbutyl	H	S
Vinbarbital	Delvinal	ethyl	1-methyl-1-butenyl	H	O

The pharmaco-chemical correlations in the barbiturate series have been the subject of very numerous and careful studies. In general, structural changes resulting in increased lipid solubility shorten the duration of action (presumably owing to more rapid metabolic degradation) and often accelerate and increase hypnotic potency. Such changes result for example from an increase in the length of one or both alkyl side-chains at C_5 (R_1, R_2, up to 6 or 7 carbon atoms). On the other hand, hypnotic activity is abolished by the introduction into the alkyl side-chains of functional or polar groups, such as keto, ether, hydroxylamino or carboxyl groups. Methylation of one of the nitrogens increases lipid solubility and also decreases the duration of action. A very reactive alkyl group or phenyl group at C_5 endows the barbiturate with selective anticonvulsant effects. On the other hand, slight changes in structure may convert barbituric acid derivatives into convulsants (e.g., prolongation of the side-chain at C_5). Alkyl substitution of both nitrogens also tends to yield convulsant compounds. Replacement of the carbonyl oxygen at C_2 (X) yields thiobarbiturates which are also fat soluble, rapid in onset of activity and short in duration of action.

Because of their great economic importance, the organic phosphate-anticholinesterase **pesticides** have been the subject of extensive comparative toxicologic studies in many species. Many of these compounds are also readily detoxified by catatoxic drugs and hormones, and most of them are more toxic to female than to male rats, but in a few cases the reverse is true. For example, OMPA is in itself virtually devoid of toxicity but both mammalian liver and plant tissue can transform it into an active anticholinesterase. Accordingly the toxicity of OMPA — unlike that of most toxicants subject to biotransformation by hepatic enzymes — is actually diminished by partial hepatectomy. Yet, as we shall see later, contrary to expectations, highly potent catatoxic steroids do not increase OMPA toxicity, perhaps because they not only transform the compound into a toxic anticholinesterase but also enhance the further degradation of the latter into nontoxic end products. For a few key references on the metabolic inactivation and toxicology of **mercury, CCl_4, nicotine, indomethacin,** etc., the reader is referred to the Abstract Section.

Steroids

Danielsson & Tchen G72,327/68: Review (51 pp., 242 refs.) on the biosynthesis and metabolism of cholesterol, phytosterol, insect sterols, bile salts and bile pigments, including the factors (diet, hormones) influencing these. Steroid hormone metabolism is not discussed.

Samuels & Eik-Nes G73,454/68: Review (52 pp., 223 refs.) on the biosynthesis, transport, distribution and metabolism of steroid hormones. Several instructive tables summarize the steroid hormones naturally produced by the various endocrine glands or demonstrated to occur in the blood stream.

Digitalis

Cox & Wright G66,614/59: In rats, paper chromatographic and colorimetric studies revealed that "in bile lanatosides A and C were excreted unchanged. Digitoxin, digoxin and digoxigenin were present partly unaltered and partly as metabolites which still retained the unsaturated lactone ring. Digitoxigenin was excreted entirely as metabolites."

Repke D27,189/59: Studies on the mechanism of digitoxin hydroxylation in the rat.

Vernikos-Danellis & Marks D21,210/62: Review of the literature on the interrelations between digitoxin and the hormones of the pituitary-adrenal axis. "The experiments described here demonstrate that chronic administration of digitoxin significantly inhibits both synthesis and stress-induced release of pituitary ACTH." In rats, small doses of digitoxin produce adrenal atrophy although large doses (which act as stressors) have an opposite effect. Earlier publications had shown that digitalis glycosides increase the performance of animals subjected to stress, prevent the adrenal hypertrophy caused by stress, and prolong the life of adrenalectomized rats, mice and cats.

Dutta & Marks G73,208/66: In rats and guinea pigs the distribution studies of isotope marked ouabain and digoxin show that particularly high concentrations are found in the liver, kidney, adrenal and pituitary.

Gibson & Becker E65,709/67: In mice, the role played by drug excretion in determining the toxicity of digitalis alkaloids was tested following the production of cholestasis by bile duct ligature or cholestatic aryl isothiocyanates such as phenylisothiocyanate (PIT) and α-naphthylisothiocyanate (ANIT). The part played by anuria was examined after ligature of the penis. After ouabain i.p., mortality was enhanced by diminution or stoppage of bile flow. Digoxin and digitoxin enhanced lethality in anuric mice. Lanatoside-C was not more toxic to hypoexcretory mice. "The use of hypoexcretory mice in toxicologic evaluations of pharmacologic agents is suggested."

Burckhardt & LaDue H 15,071/68: Review of the literature on the production of gynecomastia in man and of vaginal cornification in postclimacteric women treated with digitalis. Personal observations show a diminution of urinary FSH in postclimacteric women treated with digitalis. This is ascribed to depression of FSH formation through a folliculoid effect of digitalis.

Wilson G71,238/69: Review (8 pp., 55 refs.) on the metabolism of digitalis compounds.

Morgan & Binnion G76,782/70: In dogs, the distribution of ³H-digoxin has been determined under normal and hypokalemic conditions. Reasons for the reduced myocardial uptake of the glycoside during hypokalemia are discussed.

Barbiturates

Richards & Taylor H 19,235/56: Review (44 pp., 233 refs.) on various factors influencing the distribution, metabolism and action of barbiturates.

Dhunèr & Nordqvist D 98,693/57: In 11 of 13 patients who recovered from barbiturate poisoning, sleep was reinduced by cortisone treatment or i.v. injection of glucose.

Kato et al. H 15,635/69: Although there are great individual variations in the duration of pentobarbital narcosis and zoxazolamine paralysis among rats, the brain concentration of the drugs parallels their pharmacologic activity quite closely. Apparently, variations in drug activity from rat to rat are not due to individual variations in the sensitivity of the nervous system, but to differences in drug absorption and metabolism.

Sharpless E 8,852/70: A textbook article (21 pp., about 85 refs.) on the pharmacology of barbiturates with special reference to pharmaco-chemical correlations and mechanisms of action.

Pesticides

DuBois et al. D 92,992/50: Extensive investigations on the toxicology of OMPA in various species, with an analysis of its mechanism of action. Both mammalian liver and plant tissue can transform OMPA into an active anticholinesterase.

Aldridge & Barnes G 41,307/52: Systematic studies on the toxicology of several organophosphorus insecticides in mammals.

Frawley et al. G 69,644/52: Comparative toxicologic studies on organic phosphate-anticholinesterase compounds in guinea pigs, mice and rats, with a rapid procedure for the measurement of brain, plasma and erythrocyte cholinesterase. "The oral LD_{50}'s for these compounds for male and female rats are DFP, 13.5 and 7.7 mgm./kgm.; Parathion 30 and 3 mgm./kgm.; TEPP 2 and 1.2 mgm./kgm.; EPN 91 and 14.5 mgm./kgm.; OMPA 13.5 and 35.5 mgm./kgm.; and E-838 42 and 19 mgm./kgm. The administration of oral LD_{75} doses of these compounds caused brain cholinesterase inhibition varying with each compound: DFP > Parathion > E-838 > EPN > TEPP > OMPA."

Davison A 49,341/55: In rats, neither OMPA nor parathion possesses any significant toxic effect until they are transformed by hepatic microsomal enzymes into more active cholinesterase inhibitors. These pesticides furnish clear-cut examples of the fact that the transformation or drugs by microsomal enzymes does not necessarily diminish but may actually increase the toxicity of substrates.

Gaines G 67,102/69: LD_{50} values have been determined for 98 pesticides, and 2 metabolites of DDT in the rat. Most compounds were more toxic to females than to males, but 9 of 85 compounds were more toxic in males. In chickens several of the pesticides produced paralysis.

Datta G 75,362/70: In rats, the detoxication pathways of p,p'DDT to p,p'DDE were examined after DDE pretreatment. Apparently, "two different pathways exist and may be operated simultaneously in intact animals. The predominance of one or the other may depend on physiologic response or the amount of toxicant used."

Domschke et al. G 74,897/70: In rats, ethionine fails to prevent the induction of TPO by the pesticide soman. "Since ethionine is known as an effective inhibitor of the protein synthesis in the liver the negative results are probably due to a stimulating effect of soman on the de-novo-synthesis of liver enzymes."

Fouts G76,868/70: Review on the effects of various insecticides, both as inducers and as substrates for hepatic microsomal enzymes.

Hayes et al. G80,268/71: "The average dosage of p,p'-DDT administered in this study was 555 times the average intake of all DDT-related compounds by 19-year-old men in the general population and 1,250 times their intake of p,p'-DDT. Since no definite clinical or laboratory evidence of injury by DDT was found in this study, these factors indicate a high degree of safety of DDT for the general population."

Mercury

Spode G72,979/60: In mice injected with ^{203}Hg acetate, by far the highest Hg concentration was detected in the kidneys about 24 hrs after s.c. and about 3 hrs after i.p. injection. Correspondingly the blood concentration of Hg reaches its maximum about 1 hour after i.p. and only 3 hrs after s.c. administration. The liver stores about 1/10 as much as the kidney but still much more than other organs. Various "decorporation-stimulating substances" were tested but none of them diminished Hg storage in the liver or spleen. In the kidneys, Ca-EDTA and, to a lesser extent, citrate and Graham salt reduced storage but only Na-citrate and Ca-EDTA enhanced mercury elimination. Other reputed "decorporating substances" such as hexamethylene, diaminotetraacetic acid, gallic acid, gallic acid propylester, tannic acid, tripolyphosphate and amobarbital proved to be essentially ineffective in these respects.

Swensson & Ulfarson F89,451/67: Review of the literature and extensive personal investigations on the effect of various antidotes upon mercury poisoning in the rat.

Carbon Tetrachloride

Recknagel F85,043/67: Review (63 pp., 351 refs.) on the hepatotoxic effects of CCl_4.

Fowler G70,865/69: In rabbits, CCl_4 p.o. is distributed in the fat, liver, kidney, and muscles. Some of its metabolites have been identified.

Nayak et al. G80,728/70: In rats, a protein-free diet or starvation caused deterioration of the ER and diminution of drug-metabolizing enzymes, but failed to make the hepatocytes less susceptible to the effects of CCl_4.

Nicotine

Harke et al. G73,847/70: Comparative studies on the oxidative degradation of nicotine in the rat and hamster.

Griseofulvin

Osment G72,369/69: Review on the pharmacology of griseofulvin. It can act both as a hepatic microsomal-enzyme inducer and as a substrate for such enzymes.

Indomethacin

Hucker et al. G67,791/66: First systematic studies on the metabolism of indomethacin in various species. Most of a single dose is eliminated from the body in 24 hrs. The drug is largely excreted through the bile but then reabsorbed and eliminated through the urine in most species, except the dog in which reabsorption of biliary material is not followed by urinary excretion. The dog excretes indomethacin through the bile as a glucuronide. The drug is highly bound to plasma protein but does not accumulate in the intestinal wall of either guinea pigs or rats.

Yesair et al. G75,388/70: In rats, salicylic acid i.v. decreases the plasma concentration of indomethacin. Simultaneously, the urinary excretion of ^{14}C-indomethacin is decreased, whereas biliary and fecal excretions are increased. Phenylbutazone, chlorogenic acid and acetic acid had no effect on plasma radioactivity. Probenecid increased plasma concentration of indomethacin. "The specificity of salicylic acid in decreasing concentrations of indomethacin in plasma of rats and of probenecid in increasing indomethacin concentrations in plasma of both rat and man may arise from the similarity in structure of the benzoyl group of the three compounds."

V. EFFECT OF STEROIDS UPON RESISTANCE

STEROIDS ←

In a book on "Hormones and Resistance" it would hardly be appropriate to discuss all the antagonistic interactions between steroids. As explained in the Introduction, the reader is referred to our earlier monographs for such topics as the mutual inhibition of gluco- and mineralocorticoids as regards the regulation of inflammation or the interplay between folliculoids and luteoids in the regulation of the menstrual cycle. Here we shall deal primarily with the effects of one steroid upon systemic intoxications with other steroidal compounds. In retrospect it is interesting to speculate however about the possibility that some of the apparently specific antifolliculoid, antitestoid or antimineralocorticoid actions of steroids may be nonspecific consequences of defensive enzyme activation.

← *Glucocorticoids*

It has long been known that, at least in rats, glucocorticoids antagonize certain actions of mineralocorticoids, particularly the hypernatremia, the hyalinosis (after uninephrectomy + NaCl), the elevation of the EST and insulin hypersensitivity. In addition, cortisol and cortisone prolong the anesthetic effect of hydroxydione. Data concerning the effect of glucocorticoids on DOC anesthesia are somewhat contradictory.

The antipyretic effect of glucocorticoids against fever produced by etiocholanolone has been ascribed to a stabilization of lysosomal membrane.

The well-known antagonism between gluco- and mineralocorticoids, as regards various forms of inflammation and the balance between catabolism and anabolism, are clearly demonstrable only after adrenalectomy; presumably in the presence of the suprarenals, endogenous corticoids tend to mask any disproportion between an exogenous excess of either type.

In this connection, brief mention should be made of the **"law of intersecting dose-effect curves"** which plays a role in many apparently paradox interactions between steroid hormones, but is applicable also to countless other interrelationships between drugs. In brief, it says that if two mutually antagonistic agents are administered concurrently in fixed proportions, the action of one or the other constituent may predominate at different dose levels. An agent whose effect increases rapidly with rising doses but soon reaches a plateau will preponderate at low dose levels, whereas an agent whose activity rises slowly but persistently to reach much higher final values will predominate at high dose levels. This type of interaction can explain, for example, why the actions of glucocorticoids are largely counteracted by endogenous mineralocorticoids at near physiologic low levels but not in the event of heavy overdosage. The same law also explains why a given mixture of two antagonistic hormones may exert opposite effects at low and at high dose levels as indicated below:

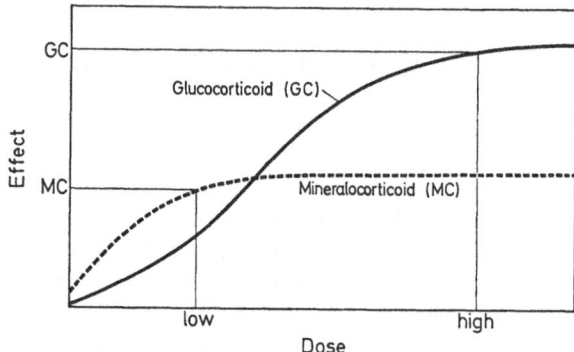

Illustration of the "law of intersecting dose effect curves." It will be seen that certain glucocorticoid effects can be antagonized by mineralocorticoids only at near physiologic low dose levels. The antiphlogistic, thymolytic, splenolytic and catabolic actions of glucocorticoids are largely compensated by endogenous mineralocorticoids in the intact animal or by near physiologic amounts of mineralocorticoids after adrenalectomy. However, by raising the glucocorticoid level far above normal, a corresponding rise in mineralocorticoid dosage no longer suffices because the action curves cross each other slightly above the level of normal corticoid production

← **Glucocorticoids** cf. also Selye B40,000/50, pp. 515, 536, 584, 585; B58,650/51, p. 324; G60,083/70, pp. 347, 348.

Friedman & Friedman B48,306/50: In intact male rats on a normal NaCl intake, the hypertension and cardiac hypertrophy produced by s.c. implantation of DOC pellets was inhibited by an adrenocortical extract but not by progesterone, testosterone, pregnenolone, estradiol or acetoxypregnenolone.

Woodbury et al. B47,201/50: In rats, ACTH and adrenocortical extract antagonize the following actions of DOC: 1. hypernatremia; 2. electroshock threshold elevation; 3. insulin hypersensitivity; 4. hyalinosis (after sensitization by uninephrectomy plus NaCl).

Heuser C54,451/58: In rats, cortisol succinate, given s.c. shortly before progesterone, hydroxydione, pentobarbital or ether, prolongs anesthesia produced by any of these compounds. When given i.v., cortisol does not exhibit this effect. In itself, cortisol is not an anesthetic. "Δ^1-Cortisol has a similar action to cortisol. Still, in marked contrast to its effect on other anesthetics, it does not influence DOC-anesthesia." Desoxycortisone elicits long-lasting convulsions which can be counteracted by various anesthetic steroids.

Rummel et al. C80,035/59: In rats, chronic or acute pretreatment with cortisone increases the sensitivity to subnarcotic doses of DOC.

Sulman et al. C79,823/59: In rats injected for 4 months with prednisone or prednisolone, an increase in the hepatic content of the enzymes which decompose these steroids could be demonstrated in vitro. Various histologic stains failed to reveal any associated light-microscopic change in the hepatocytes. Addition of SKF 525-A to the homogenate of activated livers blocked their enzymic activity.

Janoski et al. E7,896/68 (p. 287): Review of data suggesting that the antipyretic effect of glucocorticoids against fever produced by etiocholanolone and related steroids is due to the stabilization of lysosomal membranes.

Morrison & Kilpatrick G69,282/69: Observation of a personal case and report of several others from the literature, showing that in women taking glucocorticoids during pregnancy, estriol excretion is diminished. "The effect could be the result of direct depression of the placental enzymic systems."

Kostowski & Nowacka H26,526/70: In mice, cortisol and methylprednisolone decrease hexobarbital sleeping time, whereas DOC prolongs it. Hydroxydione anesthesia is not changed by cortisol but prolonged by methylprednisolone as well as by high doses of DOC.

Selye G60,064/70: In the rat, the ESCN produced by F-COL + Na_2HPO_4 + corn oil cannot be prevented by prednisolone or triamcinolone.

Fluorocortisol Acetate ← Corticoids *cf. also Tables 12-14*

DOC ← Corticoids *cf. also Table 15*

Estradiol ← Corticoids *cf. also Table 16*

Progesterone ← Corticoids *cf. also Table 17*

Triamcinolone ← Corticoids *cf. also Table 18*

Pancuronium ← Corticoids *cf. also Table 19*

Cortisol ← Cortisol, Dog: Kuipers et al. *C48,349/58**

Cortisol ← Tetrahydrocortisol Kumagai et al. *C73,732/59*

Prednisolone ← Prednisolone: Sulman et al. *C79,823/59*

Cortisone ← Cortisone + Sex: Hagen et al. *G77,512/60*

Estradiol-17β ← Cortisol+Age: Nicolette et al. *F12,788/64**

Estradiol-17β ← Prednisolone: Inscoe et al. *F70,325/66*

← Mineralocorticoids and Gluco-Mineralocorticoids

In rats heavily overdosed with glucocorticoids, normally saprophytic organisms tend to proliferate and often cause multiple abscesses resulting in death. This "saprophytosis" is more effectively combated by STH in intact than in adrenalectomized animals perhaps because the adrenals produce some antiglucocorticoid compound. However, DOC alone or in combination with other steroids, fails to duplicate the anti-infectious action of STH in cortisone-treated rats.

Aldosterone inhibits the anti-inflammatory effect of cortisol in various tests on adrenalectomized rats. This type of antagonism is also negligible in the presence of the adrenals, perhaps because the resting mineralocorticoid secretion is already near optimal in antagonizing the antiphlogistic actions of glucocorticoids.

DOC and progesterone increase each other's anesthetic effect but this appears to represent a simple summation of their narcotic potency.

The 2-cyano-steroid, TMACN, administered to pregnant rats, causes nipple formation in male and inhibition of nipple development in female fetuses, presumably owing to its characteristic effect upon steroid synthesis in the maternal adrenal. Corticosterone prevents the effect of TMACN upon female fetuses, probably because it inhibits ACTH secretion and thereby diminishes overproduction of 3β-hydroxy-androstanes. Pure mineralocorticoids have not been tested in this connection, but in view of their lesser inhibitory action on ACTH production they might be expected to be also less effective in counteracting TMACN.

← Mineralocorticoids and Glucomineralocorticoids *cf. also Selye C92,918/61, p.280.*

Ducommun & Ducommun B70,251/53: In rats, saprophytosis produced by heavy overdosage with cortisone is inhibited by concurrent administration of STH. This "anti-infectious effect of STH" is much less evident after adrenalectomy. DOC, testosterone, estradiol alone or in combination failed to duplicate the anti-infectious action of STH cortisone-treated rats.

Negrete C23,001/55: In male rats, pretreatment with nonanesthetic doses of progesterone increases sensitivity to DOC-anesthesia.

Selye B98,268/55: In adrenalectomized rats the diminution of body weight, inflammation in the granuloma pouch, as well as the atrophy of the thymus and spleen, produced by cortisol, are all inhibited by aldosterone.

Selye & Bois C14,534/56: In adrenalectomized rats bearing granuloma pouches, 2-methyl-9α-fluorocortisol (Me-F-COL) antagonizes the antiphlogistic, catabolic, thymolytic and splenolytic actions of cortisol. This effect is ascribed to the strong mineralocorticoid effects of Me-F-COL, which counteract glucocorticoid actions. However, since Me-F-COL itself possesses some glucocorticoid potency, its cortisol antagonizing action is evident only at very low dose levels (about 75 µg/kg) at which mineralocorticoid effects predominate in agreement with the "law of intersecting dose-effect curves."

Neumann & Goldman H25,234/70: In pregnant rats, treatment with TMACN (2α-cyano-4,4,17α-trimethylandrost-5-en-17β-ol 3-one) causes nipple formation in male fetuses and inhibits the normal development of nipples in female fetuses, presumably owing to characteristic derangements in the enzymic mechanisms responsible for steroid production in the adrenals. Testosterone prevents these effects of TMACN in male fetuses, suggesting that its feminizing property upon the nipples (like that of fetal orchidectomy) is merely due to deficient testosterone production. Corticosterone prevents the actions of TMACN upon female fetuses, probably because it inhibits fetal ACTH-mediated adrenal enlargement and the consequent overproduction of 3β-hydroxyandrostanes.

Kostowski & Nowacka H26,526/70: In mice, cortisol and methylprednisolone decrease hexobarbital sleeping time, whereas DOC prolongs it. Hydroxydione anesthesia is not changed by cortisol but prolonged by methylprednisolone as well as by high doses of DOC.

Cortisol ← Corticosterone: Firschein et al. C30,553/57*

Cortisol ← DOC: Kumagai et al. C73,732/59

TMACN ← Corticosterone: Neumann et al. H25,234/70*

← Testoids and Anabolic Steroids

Glucocorticoids ←. It has long been known that anabolic testoids antagonize many, but not all, of the actions of glucocorticoids. For example, according to most investigators, the inhibition of growth, the reduction in the widths of the epiphyseal cartilage, the impairment of wound healing, the production of gastric ulcers (especially during fasting), are all blocked by concurrent treatment with certain anabolics, at least under optimal experimental conditions; conversely, the thymus atrophy and saprophytosis in rats, as well as the characteristic cortisone myopathy of the rabbit, are not significantly prevented by anabolics.

A variety of anabolic testoids proved to be highly potent in preventing progesterone and pentobarbital anesthesia in rats; however, since spironolactone exhibits the same anti-anesthetic effect, the latter cannot be attributed to anabolic potency.

Mineralocorticoids and Gluco-Mineralocorticoids ←. The nephrosclerosis, proteinuria and hypercholesterolemia produced by DOC in the rat can be prevented by methyltestosterone even after sensitization by uninephrectomy. However, this inhibition appears to depend upon circumstances yet to be identified, since it is by no means constant.

Pretreatment with ethylestrenol inhibits DOC anesthesia in the rat and this protective effect can be blocked, in turn, by thyroxine.

The ESCN produced by F-COL + Na_2HPO_4 + corn oil in the rat is prevented by ethylestrenol, norbolethone and some other catatoxic steroids but not by oxandrolone.

Luteoids ←. Female and castrate male rats are more sensitive to the anesthetic effect of progesterone than are intact males but methyltestosterone pretreatment raises the resistance of females and castrates to the male level.

Folliculoids ←. In mice, estradiol produces pubic bone resorption and hypercalcification of other bones. This effect is inhibited by testosterone.

The actions of folliculoids upon various target organs are not equally affected by testoids. Among a series of virilizing steroids examined, androstenediol was most potent in preventing the body-weight loss caused by estradiol in adult male rats, whereas the estradiol-induced pituitary and adrenal enlargement was most markedly inhibited by testosterone and methyltestosterone. The thymus involution caused by folliculoids is further enhanced by testoids since both these types of steroids possess a thymolytic effect. The ability of steroids to protect the testis against estradiol-induced atrophy is independent of their virilizing effect; thus ethynyltestosterone is a strong testoid but not gonad protecting, whereas the reverse is true of pregnenolone. Curiously, estradiol increases the renotrophic effect of testosterone in the rat although it decreases body weight in general. These organ specific interactions show that not all catatoxic effects can be ascribed to complete destruction of a steroid substrate by hepatic microsomal enzymes. However, partial destruction may lead to selective abolition of those effects which are obtained by comparatively small residual amounts of the hormone.

The production of adrenal and pituitary tumors by stilbestrol can also be prevented by certain androstane derivatives.

Other Steroids ←. The anesthetic effect of progesterone, DOC, testosterone or even stilbestrol can be diminished by pretreatment with testosterone in rats.

Methyltestosterone failed to influence hydroxydione anesthesia in mice, whereas norbolethone protects the rat against anesthesia produced by progesterone, DOC, pregnanedione, testosterone and several other steroids.

The 2α-cyano-steroid, TMACN, given to the mother during pregnancy, causes nipple formation in male, and suppression of nipple development in female rat fetuses. These alterations are ascribed to deficient adrenal steroid biosynthesis. They can be prevented by testosterone in male fetuses, suggesting that the feminizing effect of TMACN upon the nipples is merely due to deficient testoid production.

Glucocorticoids ← *cf. also Selye G60,083/70, pp. 374, 377.*

Gaunt et al. B71,987/52: DOC and testosterone propionate counteracted the growth inhibition produced in immature adrenalectomized rats by cortisone acetate. MAD had no consistent effect on growth. Both MAD and testosterone propionate caused thymus atrophy and this effect was further increased by conjoint administration of cortisone. In intact rats, MAD prevented the cortisone-induced adrenal atrophy. [It is not clear from this brief abstract whether the other interactions were also tested in intact animals (H.S.).]

Ducommun & Ducommun B70,251/53: In rats, saprophytosis produced by heavy overdosage with cortisone is inhibited by concurrent administration of STH. This "anti-infectious effect of STH" is much less evident after adrenalectomy. DOC, testosterone, estradiol alone or in combination failed to duplicate the anti-infectious action of STH in cortisone-treated rats.

Studer B89,161/53: In the rat, cortisone reduces the width of the epiphyseal cartilage, and concurrent treatment with testosterone partially antagonizes this effect.

Winter et al. B79,381/53: In rats, testosterone and MAD prevent the adrenal atrophy produced by cortisone without counteracting the antiphlogistic effect of the latter.

Englhardt-Gölkel C42,792/55: In man, the protein catabolic effect of cortisone is antagonized by MAD.

Róna et al. C39,946/56: In rabbits, the vascular lesions characteristic of "steroid diabetes" induced by cortisone + alloxan are inhibited by MAD although the latter induces considerable hyperlipemia.

Baldratti et al. C 45,101/57: In rats, 4-chloro-19-nortestosterone acetate (like testosterone propionate and MAD) prevents the cortisone-induced adrenal atrophy. However, none of the steroids tested prevents the body weight loss and catabolism induced by cortisone.

Dontenwill & Mancini C 35,119/57: In rabbits, the catabolic effect of cortisone upon bones is antagonized by testosterone.

Kar et al. G 79,565/57: In rats, 19-nortestosterone prevents the adrenal changes normally produced by cortisone overdosage.

Kowalewski C 48,527/58: In 6 day old cockerels, the inhibition by cortisone of body weight gain and radiosulfur incorporation into long bones are counteracted by norethandrolone.

Kowalewski C 61,936/58: In young cockerels, norethynodrel, and to a lesser extent methyltestosterone and testosterone, counteract the inhibition of bodyweight gain induced by cortisone. The inhibition by cortisone of ^{35}S uptake in bones is also counteracted by norethynodrel but not by the other testoids examined.

Lostroh C 54,348/58: Female mice of the C3H strain regularly develop myocardial calcification following prolonged cortisol treatment, whereas males are comparatively resistant. Ovariectomy offers no protection but testosterone renders females more resistant. In hypophysectomized mice, neither cortisol nor ACTH produces myocardial calcification.

Reifenstein Jr. C 47,377/58: Review of the literature suggests that "androgens and estrogens, are anabolic and thus stimulate the growth of protein and osseous tissues." The clinical value of anabolic steroids in counteracting the catabolism caused by endogenous and exogenous glucocorticoids is discussed.

Rinne & Näätänen C 50,335/58: In rats, norandrostenolone phenylpropionate greatly diminishes the adrenal atrophy produced by cortisone, but has little if any effect upon its catabolic and somatic growth diminishing action.

Selye & Mishra C 38,201/58: In the rat, methyltestosterone prevents the loss of body weight produced by overdosage with DHT, vitamin-D$_2$, partial fasting, AAN and estradiol. The catabolism elicited by IDPN (iminodipropionitrile) or cortisol is not influenced.

Ducommun et al. C 62,099/59: In rats, testosterone failed to counteract the growth inhibiting effect of prednisolone.

Kowalewaki & Gort C 63,274/59: Cortisone impairs the healing of humerus fractures in the rat and concurrent treatment with norethandrolone antagonizes this effect.

Kowalewski C 68,938/59: Pretreatment with norethandrolone protects the rat against the induction of gastric ulcers by subsequent fasting plus cortisol. Testosterone enanthate does not share this effect.

Llaurado et al. G 79,936/59: In rats, norethandrolone prevents the adrenal lesions normally produced by cortisone. However, the thymolytic effect of the latter was increased.

Jasmin et al. C 89,132/60: Both in intact and in adrenalectomized rats, norethandrolone diminishes the body weight loss caused by cortisol without inhibiting the antiphlogistic effect of the latter.

Arlander D 5,055/61: In mice, various testoids (17α-ethyl-19-nortestosterone, testosterone and MAD) failed to prevent the cortisone-induced loss of body weight.

Bernick et al. D 5,063/61: In rats, testosterone inhibited the osteosclerosis, but failed to influence the narrowing of the epiphyseal plates and the body weight loss induced by cortisone.

Laron & Boss D 10,620/61: Nandrolone phenpropionate failed to inhibit the loss of body weight and the skeletal changes produced by cortisone in the rat.

Steinetz & Leathem D 14,366/61: In rats, the adrenal changes produced by cortisone are counteracted by concurrent treatment with MAD.

Suchowsky & Junkmann D 2,674/61: 1-Methyl-Δ^1-androsten-17β-ol-3-one-17β-acetate is about as equally effective as testosterone propionate in preventing the cortisol-induced gastric ulcers in fasting rats.

Weller D 13,995/61; D 22,262/62: In man, methenolone antagonizes the catabolic effect of prednisolone and desiccated thyroid.

Arcuri et al. D 65,779/62: Methyltestosterone protects the gastric mucosa of the rat against the damage produced by prednisolone.

Bavetta et al. D 29,035/62: In the rat, "anabolic hormones such as methyltestosterone and growth hormone did not counteract the over-all catabolic effects of methyl prednisolone on nitrogen metabolism nor on body weight retardation."

Bavetta et al. D 29,064/62: In the rat, "growth hormone, methyl testosterone or stilbestrol, when given alone or in combination were not able to counteract the inhibitory effects of 6-methyl prednisolone on body weight gain and collagen synthesis at the site

Herrmann D34,026/62: In guinea pigs, following interruption of corticoid administration, the adrenocortical hypofunction and atrophy as well as the irresponsiveness to the production of adrenocortical necrosis by diphtheria toxin reappear much more rapidly if the animals are simultaneously treated with testosterone.

Herrmann & Winkler D20,550/62: In guinea pigs, methandrostenolone accelerates the restitution of the adrenal cortex after interruption of cortisone therapy as judged by the more rapid reappearance of sensitivity to diphtheria toxin and histologic criteria.

Ippolito et al. D57,498/62: The gastric ulcers produced by prednisolone in guinea pigs can be prevented by concurrent treatment with oxymesterone.

Jöchle & Langecker D22,258/62: In the rat and mouse, methenolone-enanthate counteracts the weight loss produced by cortisone or a reduction of food intake.

Kowalewski G41,978/62: "In the femora of cortisone-treated cockerels there was increased size of chondrocytic lacunae, thinning and irregularity of primary trabeculae, and focal absence of osteoblasts. These changes coincided with a decrease in acid mucopolysaccharides and a decrease in alkaline phosphatase. The alkaline phosphatase decrease was directly related to a decrease in the numbers of osteoblasts. Somewhat similar changes were seen in humeri of rats, except that changes in alkaline phosphatase activity were not so evident." Methandrostenolone protected the bones of birds and rats against these cortisone-induced changes.

Kühn et al. D64,992/62: In the rat, testosterone does not prevent the loss of body weight induced by heavy overdosage with cortisone or prednisolone.

Walser D33,753/62: In patients, the catabolic effect of prednisone or triamcinolone is inhibited by ethylestrenol or nandrolone decanoate.

Galletti & Bruni G16,710/63: In the rat, the catabolic effect of prednisone can be counteracted by simultaneous treatment with quindienone, an anabolic and weakly testoid compound described as the 17-cyclopentyl ether of Δ^1-dehydrotestosterone.

Lund E38,261/63: In man, osteoporosis following prolonged treatment with cortisone was not prevented by conjoint administration of nandrolone phenpropionate.

Rodin & Kowalewski D60,272/63: Methandrostenolone protects the bones of cockerels and rats from the deleterious effects of cortisone overdosage.

Borderg & Lücker F24,271/64: In the rat, methenolone inhibits the osteoporosis and the loss of bone mineral produced by large doses of cortisone.

Harding & Potts F55,311/65: In rats, glucocorticoids characteristically increased hepatic TPO-activity and this effect is suppressed by various anabolics such as stanozolol, norethandrolone and methandrostenolone in decreasing order of activity. In intact rats, methyltestosterone produced no suppression (even when given in very high doses) presumably because it increased corticosterone secretion; suppression was obtained with all anabolics in adrenalectomized rats. "These data support the concept that anabolic agents are useful in offsetting the catabolic effects observed clinically following chronic administration of glucocorticoids."

Murakami & Kowalewski G41,228/66: Stanozolol counteracts the inhibition of bone fracture healing induced by cortisone in guinea pigs.

Valderrama & Munuera E6,008/66: In rabbits, overdosage with cortisone inhibits osteoblast action and causes massive bone absorption with fatty marrow formation. Endochondral ossification ceases. All these changes are greatly diminished by stanozolol.

Kaeser & Wüthrich F80,357/67: The myopathy produced in rabbits by overdosage with cortisone is not influenced by treatment with Ro 4-8932 the highly anabolic, chlorinated retrosteroid.

Linet & Mikuláškova F86,027/67: The gastric erosions produced by cortisol in the rat are not significantly influenced by such anabolic steroids as 19-nortestosterone phenylpropionate, methandrostenolone and dimethylandrostanolone.

Preziosi et al. F78,520/67: The cachectic wasting syndrome produced by a single dose of betamethasone given to rats on the first day of life is not influenced by nandrolone decanoate or phenylpropionate, unless betamethasone is administered in the form of its phosphate and, even then, the protection is not very marked.

Zicha & Heck F78,128/67: In guinea pigs, asthma produced by 5-HT, histamine or acetylchcline is inhibited by various glucocorticoids. This inhibition is in turn blocked by certain, but not all, anabolic steroids tested.

Ehrlich & Hunt G68,785/69: In rats, the delay in wound healing caused by cortisone is counteracted by testosterone, nandrolone phenpropionate or 19-nortestosterone-17β- adamantoate (Bolmantalate) although these anabolic steroids were unable to counteract the body weight loss caused by the glucocorticoid.

Linèt G79,963/70: Detailed review of the literature and personal observations on the effect of anabolic testoids upon glucocorticoid overdosage in animals and man. Special attention is given to the effect of anabolic testoids upon glucocorticoid-induced loss of body weight and other metabolic changes, adrenal atrophy, osteoporosis, wound healing, inflammation and gastric ulcer formation. Antiglucocorticoids devoid of anabolic properties are also surveyed. In clinical medicine, various forms of hyperglucocorticoidism are not, or only moderately, improved by treatment with anabolic testoids. [Excellent source of pertinent references (H.S.).]

Triamcinolone ← Testoids *cf. also* Table 18

Cortisol ← Testoids: Kumagai et al. *C73,732/59*

Cortisone ← Dehydrotestosterone: McGuire et al. *D82,559/60*

Cortisone ← Testosterone + Sex: Hagen et al. *G77,512/60*

Mineralocorticoids and Gluco-Mineralocorticoids ← *cf. also* Selye *B40,000/50, pp. 531, 631; G60,083/70, p. 385.*

Selye & Rowley A72,287/44; A72,302/44: In rats the nephrosclerosis, proteinuria and hypercholesterolemia produced by DOC is prevented by concurrent administration of methyltestosterone both under normal conditions and after uninephrectomy.

Friedman & Friedman B48,306/50: In intact male rats on a normal NaCl intake, the hypertension and cardiac hypertrophy produced by s.c. implantation of DOC pellets could be inhibited by an adrenocortical extract but not by progesterone, testosterone, pregnenolone, estradiol or acetoxypregnenolone.

Selye et al. G60,020/69: In the rat, pretreatment with norbolethone protects against the anesthetic effect of progesterone, DOC, pregnanedione, dehydroepiandrosterone, testosterone, diethylstilbestrol, pentobarbital and methyprylon. It does not significantly alter the corresponding actions of urethan, diazepam, chlorpromazine, reserpine, phenoxybenzamine, chloral hydrate, potassium bromide or magnesium chloride.

Selye G70,428/70: In rats, ethylestrenol powerfully inhibits the toxicity of digitoxin, nicotine, indomethacin, phenindione, dioxathion, EPN, physostigmine, hexobarbital, cyclopental, thiopental, DOC (anesthesia), meprobamate, and picrotoxin. Thyroxine increases the toxicity of many among these drugs and inhibits the protective effect of ethylestrenol.

Little G78,533/70: In growing rabbits treated with cortisone, the following steroids exerted anticatabolic activities: stanozolol, Ba 36644 (17β-hydroxy-7α-dimethyl-A-nor-β-homoestrone-3,6,dione in equilibrium with its enol form), testosterone, lynestrenol, methandienone, norethynodrel, norethisterone.

Selye G60,064/70: In the rat, the ESCN produced by F-COL + Na_2HPO_4 + corn oil can be prevented by ethylestrenol and norbolethone but not by oxandrolone.

Fluorocortisol Acetate ← Testoids *cf. also* Tables 12—14

DOC ← Testoids *cf. also* Table 15

Luteoids ←

Winter & Selye A35,658/41; Winter A36,333/41: Female rats are more sensitive than males to the anesthetic action of progesterone but this sex difference is obvious only after maturity. "The normal endocrine activity of the testis is largely, if not entirely, responsible for this comparative resistance of the males since castration increases sensitivity in males but is without effect in female rats. Conversely the resistance of castrate males and females may be raised by methyltestosterone administration."

Selye et al. G60,020/69: In the rat, pretreatment with norbolethone protects against the anesthetic effect of progesterone, desoxycorticosterone, pregnanedione, dehydroepiandrosterone, testosterone, diethylstilbestrol, pentobarbital and methyprylon. It does not significantly alter the corresponding actions of urethan, diazepam, chlorpromazine, reserpine, phenoxybenzamine, chloral hydrate, potassium bromide or magnesium chloride.

Selye G60,044/70: Among various steroids tested for their ability to inhibit progesterone and pentobarbital anesthesia, all anabolic testoids were highly potent. However, since spironolactone exhibited the same antianesthetic effect, the latter could not be attributed to anabolic potency. "This inhibition of anesthesia is assumed to represent a special instance of the catatoxic effect which appears to be a property of certain steroids, independent of their classic hormonal actions."

Progesterone ← Testoids *cf. also Table 17*

Folliculoids ←

Gardner & Pfeiffer 72,281/38: In mice, the skeletal changes (pubic bone resorption and hypercalcification of other bones) produced by estradiol are inhibited by concurrent treatment with testosterone.

Albert A 37,132/42: In immature rats given estradiol alone or in combination with testosterone until puberty was attained, the pituitary and adrenal enlargement as well as the testis atrophy produced by estradiol were prevented by the testoid whereas the thymus atrophy was intensified.

Albert & Selye A 37,637/42: Among many steroids examined androstenediol was most potent in preventing the bodyweight loss caused by estradiol in adult male rats. The pituitary and adrenal hypertrophy characteristic of estradiol overdosage was most markedly inhibited by testosterone and methyltestosterone. The thymus involution caused by estradiol was aggravated by most of the hormonally active steroids tested. "The ability of steroids to protect the testis against the atrophy caused by estradiol is entirely independent of their 'male hormone' or testoid activity. Ethinyl testosterone, though a potent testoid, is not gonad-protecting while the reverse is true of pregnenolone." The decrease in kidney weight caused by estradiol was effectively prevented only by highly active testoids such as testosterone and methyltestosterone. [These organ specific interactions emphasize the danger of attributing the protective effects of catatoxic steroids to increased destruction by the induction of hepatic microsomal enzymes. Both specific interactions at the target organ and the induction of qualitatively different steroid metabolites must also be considered (H.S.).]

Selye A 60,638/44: In rodents, the production of anterior pituitary hormones by estradiol is inhibited by a variety of steroids, most of which are androstene derivatives and are designated as "antifolliculoid."

Constantinides & Gordon B 41,764/50: Among three synthetic steroids tested for their ability to prevent the tumorigenic effect of stilbestrol on the pituitary and adrenal glands "17 (β)-ethyl-androstane-3-one-17(α)-ol proved a potent stilbestrol inhibitor of only moderate androgenic potency, while 17(β)-ethyl-Δ^5-androstene-3(β), 17(α)-diol and 17(β)-ethyl-androstane-3(β), 17(α)-diol showed no such activities."

Selye & Mishra C 38,201/58: In the rat methyltestosterone prevents the loss of body weight produced by overdosage with DHT, vitamin-D_2, partial fasting, AAN and estradiol. The catabolism elicited by IDPN or cortisol is not influenced.

Granitsas & Leathem D 25,514/60: In the rat, estradiol in doses causing a decrease in body and kidney weight nevertheless increases the renotrophic effect of testosterone although it fails to block body nitrogen loss.

Verne & Roth E 48,050/63: Out of 13 mice treated with estradiol, 6 developed cancers, whereas among 102 mice treated with estradiol + norandrostenolone phenylpropionate, only 9 developed cancers. [Neither the sites nor the types of tumors are identified (H.S.).]

Roth F 29,450/64: In mice, the carcinogenic action of estradiol is inhibited by norandrostenolone phenylpropionate.

Selye et al. G 60,020/69: In the rat, pretreatment with norbolethone protects against the anesthetic effect of progesterone, DOC, pregnanedione, dehydroepiandrosterone, testosterone, diethylstilbestrol, pentobarbital and methyprylon. It does not significantly alter the corresponding actions of urethan, diazepam, chlorpromazine, reserpine, phenoxybenzamine, chloral hydrate, potassium bromide or magnesium chloride.

Dmowski et al. G 80,777/71: In various species, Danazol (2,3 isoxazol derivative of 17α-ethinyl testosterone) was found to inhibit the effect of endogenous, but not of exogenous gonadotrophins. In addition, it had a mild testoid and progestational effect, but was devoid of antitestoid, antifolliculoid or antiluteoid properties.

Estradiol ← Testoids *cf. also Table 16*

Estradiol, Estrone, Stilbestrol ← 19-Nortestosterone, Testosterone: Jellineck et al. *F 37,592/65*

Estradiol ← Norethandrolone + Biliary obstruction, Man: Zumoff et al. *H 25,277/70**

Other Steroids ←

Selye A 35,410/41: Following repeated injections of progesterone, DOC, testosterone or stilbestrol to rats, the anesthetic effect of these hormones gradually diminishes. Pretreatment with one of these anesthetic compounds also induces resistance to others, whereas pretreatment with cholesterol (which is not anesthetic) induces no such resistance.

Jelinek H1,518/68: There was no difference in the duration of hydroxydione anesthesia in male and female intact or gonadectomized mice. Pretreatment with methyltestosterone p.o. prolonged hydroxydione anesthesia in males but not in females or castrate males. Neither thiopental nor pentobarbital anesthesia was influenced by methyltestosterone. Pretreatment with methandrostenolone or 17α-methyl-androst-2-ene-17β-ol failed to influence hydroxydione anesthesia in mice.

Selye et al. G60,020/69: In the rat, pretreatment with norbolethone protects against the anesthetic effect of progesterone, DOC, pregnanedione, dehydroepiandrosterone, testosterone, diethylstilbestrol, pentobarbital and methyprylon. It does not significantly alter the corresponding actions of urethan, diazepam, chlorpromazine, reserpine, phenoxybenzamine, chloral hydrate, potassium bromide or magnesium chloride.

Neumann & Goldman H25,234/70: In pregnant rats, treatment with TMACN (2α-cyano-4,4,17α-trimethylandrost-5-en-17β-ol-3-one) causes nipple formation in male fetuses and inhibits the normal development of nipples in female fetuses, presumably owing to characteristic derangements in the enzymic mechanisms responsible for steroid production in the adrenals. Testosterone prevents these effects of TMAN in male fetuses, suggesting that its feminizing effect upon the nipples (like that of fetal orchidectomy) is merely due to deficient testosterone production. Corticosterone prevents the effect of TMACN upon female fetuses, probably because it inhibits fetal ACTH-mediated adrenal enlargement and the consequent overproduction of 3β-hydroxyandrostanes.

Selye et al. G60,020/69: Pretreatment with norbolethone protects the rat against anesthesia produced by progesterone, DOC, pregnanedione, dehydroepiandrosterone, testosterone, diethylstilbestrol and methyprylon. It does not significantly alter the sedative effects of urethan, diazepam, chlorpromazine, reserpine, phenoxybenzamine, chloral hydrate, KBr or $MgCl_2$.

Pancuronium ← Testoids *cf. also Table 19*

Androstane-3,17-dione ← Testosterone: Rubin *G76,315/57*

Steroids (Δ^4-3-keto) ← Testosterone + Orchidectomy: Yates et al. *C61,952/58*

Steroids (Δ^4-3-keto) ← 5α-Androstane-3,17-dione: McGuire et al. *D5,722/60*

Androsterone, Epiandrosterone ← Androstane-3,17-dione + Sex: Rubin et al. *D9,290/61*

TMACN ← Testosterone: Neumann et al. *H25,234/70**

← Luteoids

In C3H strain mice, females are more resistant than males to the toxic action of folliculoids. This sex difference becomes even more evident in the case of combined treatment with folliculoids and progesterone since the latter increases the toxicity of estradiol and stilbestrol in this strain. The gonads of both sexes show considerable atrophy under the influence of folliculoids but this is inhibited by progesterone.

The anesthetic effect of various steroids is diminished in rats by pretreatment with progesterone (as well as by other anesthetic steroids). Cholesterol induces no such resistance.

The hypertensive disease produced in rats by DOC is not influenced by progesterone.

Concurrent treatment with subthreshold doses of progesterone and DOC exhibit an additive effect upon the development of anesthesia in rats.

In weanling rats, medroxyprogesterone (a luteoid) does not affect the growth-promoting action of testosterone upon the seminal vesicles but inhibits the stimulation of the ventral prostate. It would be difficult to ascribe this effect to an altered metabolic degradation of the testoid, although in patients medroxyprogesterone allegedly accelerates the clearance of testosterone.

In the rat, the ESCN produced by F-COL + Na_2HPO_4 + corn oil is not prevented by progesterone.

← **Luteoids** cf. also Selye G60,083/70, pp. 370, 371.

Selye & Stevenson 77,177/40: In Strong's C3H strain mice, females are more resistant than males to toxic doses of estradiol or stilbestrol. This sex difference is even more pronounced in the case of combined administration of folliculoids and progesterone, which increases the toxicity of folliculoids. The gonads of both sexes show considerable atrophy under the influence of folliculoids but this is inhibited by progesterone.

Selye A35,410/41: Following repeated injections of progesterone, DOC, testosterone or stilbestrol to rats, the anesthetic effect of these hormones gradually diminishes. Pretreatment with one of these anesthetic compounds also induces resistance to others, whereas pretreatment with cholesterol (which is not anesthetic) induces no such resistance.

Friedman & Friedman B48,306/50: In intact male rats on a normal NaCl intake, the hypertension and cardiac hypertrophy produced by s.c. implantation of DOC pellets was inhibited by an adrenocortical extract but not by progesterone, testosterone, pregnenolone, estradiol or acetoxy-pregnenolone.

Negrete C23,001/55: In male rats, pretreatment with doses of progesterone, which in themselves are nonanesthetic, increases sensitivity to DOC-anesthesia.

Gordon et al. H24,106/70: In rats, medroxyprogesterone had no effect upon zoxazolamine "sleeping time." In weanling rats, medroxyprogesterone did not affect the growth promoting action of testosterone upon the seminal vesicles but it inhibited the stimulation of the ventral prostate. In several patients the steroid accelerated the metabolic clearance of testosterone.

Selye G60,064/70: In the rat, the ESCN produced by F-COL + Na_2HPO_4 + corn oil cannot be prevented by progesterone.

Fluorocortisol Acetate ← Luteoids cf. also Tables 12—14

DOC ← Luteoids cf. also Table 15

Estradiol ← Luteoids cf. also Table 16

Progesterone ← Luteoids cf. also Table 17

Triamcinolone ← Luteoids cf. also Table 18

Pancuronium ← Luteoids cf. also Table 19

Cortisol ← Luteoids: Kumagai et al. C73,732/59

Cortisone ← Progesterone + Sex: Hagen et al. G77,512/60

← Antimineralocorticoids

← **Spironolactone.** The ESCN produced by F-COL + Na_2HPO_4, with or without oil supplements, can be prevented by spironolactone in the rat. The mineralocorticoid hypertension produced by DOC + NaCl in uninephrectomized rats is not prevented by spironolactone, but the associated hyalinosis is inhibited. Clinical experience shows, furthermore, that spironolactone is beneficial not only in primary aldosteronism but also in many other common types of hypertension.

In immature castrate rats, the stimulation of the ventral prostate and seminal vesicles by testosterone is inhibited by spironolactone. The gynecomastia and the libido-inhibiting effect of spironolactone in man, may be due to its antitestoid activity.

The anesthetic effect of various steroids (as that of barbiturates) is strongly inhibited by pretreatment with spironolactone, even following adrenalectomy.

← **Spiroxasone.** Spiroxasone (like spironolactone) inhibits the stimulation of the ventral prostates and seminal vesicles by testosterone in immature castrate rats. It also protects the rat against progesterone anesthesia.

← **Aldadiene (SC-9376).** Aladadiene and aldadiene-kalium (SC-14266) protect the rat against progesterone anesthesia.

← **CS-1.** CS-1 protects the rat against progesterone anesthesia and against the ESCN produced by F-COL + Na_2HPO_4 in combination with restraint, or with an excess of corn oil.

← **Phanurane.** In rats, the hypertensive syndrome produced by DOC + uninephrectomy + NaCl can be inhibited by phanurane allegedly because of the antimineralocorticoid activity of this steroid.

← *Antimineralocorticoids* cf. also Selye C92,918/61, pp. 18, 74; G60,083/70, pp. 492, 493.

← **Spironolactone** cf. also Selye C92,918/61, p. 74; G60,083/70, pp. 385, 491, 492, 494.
Ducommun et al. C91,529/60: In rats sensitized by uninephrectomy + NaCl, spironolactone inhibits the hyalinosis but not the hypertension caused by DOC.
Selye C82,516/60: In the rat, spironolactone "offers considerable protection against induction of acute, infarct-like, often fatal myocardial necroses normally produced by fluorocortisol plus some Na-salts and stress, alone or in combination."
Hollander & Wilkins C37,370/62; Johnston & Grieble F94,590/67; Bracharz et al. D37,973/62: Spironolactone is beneficial not only in primary aldosteronism but also in many of the common types of clinical hypertension.
Selye G60,003/69: Spironolactone protects the rat against the anesthetic effect of progesterone, DOC and hydroxydione. It also prevents acute digitoxin poisoning even after bilateral nephrectomy.
Selye et al. G60,016/69: In rats, spironolactone protects against anesthesia produced by progesterone, DOC, hydroxydione, pregnanedione, dehydroepiandrosterone, testosterone, diethylstilbestrol, methyprylon, pentobarbital and ethanol. It does not significantly alter the corresponding actions of morphine, codeine, urethan, diazepam, chlorpromazine, reserpine, phenoxybenzamine, chloral hydrate, KBr or $MgCl_2$.
Steelman et al. G69,340/69: In immature castrate rats, the stimulation of the ventral prostates and seminal vesicles by testosterone enathate s.c. is inhibited both by spiroxasone and by spironolactone given p.o. or s.c. In dogs, spironolactone decreased the output of acid phosphatase in the prostatic fluid. Possibly the gynecomastia and the libido-inhibiting effect of spironolactone in man may be due to its antitestoid activity.
Gardell et al. G60,065/70: In rats, spironolactone pretreatment inhibits the ultrastructural changes characteristic of the myocardial necroses induced by digitoxin + Na_2HPO_4 + oil.
Nocke et al. H29,580/70: Brief abstract indicating that in pregnant women, spironolactone decreases the urinary elimination of folliculoids, 17-hydroxycorticoids and 17-oxosteroids. It is concluded that spironolactone "may have an influence on the biogenesis and/or metabolism of steroid hormones."
Selye G60,044/70: Among various steroids tested for their ability to inhibit progesterone and pentobarbital anesthesia, all anabolic androgens were highly potent. However, since spironolactone exhibited the same antianesthetic effect, the latter could not be attributed to anabolic potency. "This inhibition of anesthesia is assumed to represent a special instance of the catatoxic effect which appears to be a property of certain steroids, independent of their classic hormonal actions."
Selye et al. G60,050/70: Spironolactone protects the rat against digitoxin intoxication as well as against the anesthetic effect of progesterone and pentobarbital.
Selye G60,064/70: In the rat, the ESCN produced by F-COL + Na_2HPO_4 + corn oil can be prevented by CS-1 and spironolactone.
Solymoss et al. G70,464/70: In rats, spironolactone shortens the half-life of its main metabolite, the dethioacetylated 4-6-dienone (metabolite A), which is interconvertible with the 17-hydroxy carboxylic acid derivative (metabolite B). This alteration is only

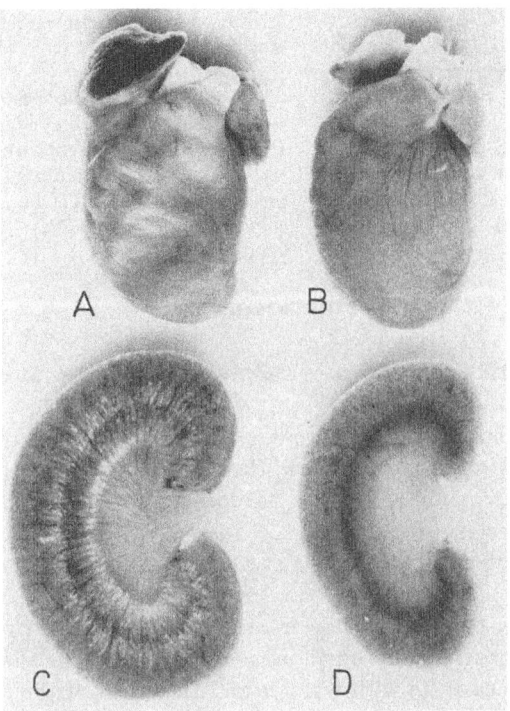

Fig. 1. **Protection by spironolactone against infarctoid cardiac necroses and nephrocalcinosis.** Both rats were treated with fluorocortisol + Na_2HPO_4, which resulted in extensive cardiac infarction and cortico-medullary nephrocalcinosis (white areas) in the otherwise untreated (A, C), but not in the spironolactone-treated (B, D), animal. [Selye C82,516/60. Courtesy of Proc. Soc. exp. Biol. Med.]

slightly accentuated if the steroid is given chronically and it wears off within eight days after spironolactone treatment is interrupted. After a test dose of spironolactone or of its metabolites A and B, partial hepatectomy delays the blood clearance of metabolite A. Cycloheximide and SKF 525-A also suppress the blood clearance of metabolite A under these conditions. Presumably "spironolactone influences its own biotransformation and the steroid is also a substrate of the hepatic drug-metabolizing enzymes which are induced by spironolactone itself."

Selye PROT. 27691: In rats, (100 g♀) progesterone (6 mg in 1 ml oil i.p.) or pentobarbital (3 mg in 0.5 ml oil i.p.) anesthesia is prolonged by adrenalectomy with maintenance on NaCl, but blocked, both in intact and adrenalectomized animals, by spironolactone (10 mg in 1 ml water p.o. x2/day) pretreatment for 4 days.

← **Spiroxasone.** *Steelman et al. G69,340/69:* In immature castrate rats, the stimulation of the ventral prostates and seminal vesicles by testosterone enanthate s.c. is inhibited both by spiroxasone and by spironolactone given p.o. or s.c. In dogs, spironolactone decreased the output of acid phophatase in the prostatic fluid. Possibly, the gynecomastia and the libido-inhibiting effect of spironolactone in man may be due to its antitestoid activity.

Selye et al. G60,050/70: Spiroxazone protects the rat against digitoxin intoxication and progesterone anesthesia, but not against the anesthetic effect of pentobarbital.

← **Aldadiene (SC-9376).** *Selye et al. G60,050/70:* Aldadiene (SC-9376) and aldadiene-kalium (SC-14266) protect the rat against digitoxin intoxication as well as against the anesthetic effect of progesterone and pentobarbital.

← **CS-1.** *Selye G60,064/70:* The ESCN produced by F-COL + Na$_2$HPO$_4$ + restraint in the rat is much more difficult to inhibit with catatoxic steroids than that elicited by F-COL + Na$_2$HPO$_4$ + oil. However, even the former cardiopathy can be greatly diminished in intensity by CS-1 and spironolactone.

Selye et al. G60,050/70: CS-1 protects the rat against digitoxin intoxication as well as against the anesthetic effect of progesterone and pentobarbital.

← **Phanurane.** *Sturtevant C54,613/58:* In rats, the hypertensive syndrome produced by DOC after sensitization with uninephrectomy + NaCl can be inhibited by phanurane, presumably because of the antimineralocorticoid activity of the latter.

← *Folliculoids*

Pretreatment with stilbestrol increases the resistance of the rat against various steroid anesthetics.

It has been claimed that mineralocorticoid hypertension produced in rats by DOC is inhibited by stilbestrol but not by estradiol. However, here, incidental experimental conditions (e.g., uninephrectomy + NaCl or the dosage and timing of the folliculoids) may have a decisive effect.

The saprophytosis produced by cortisone overdosage in the rat is not prevented by estradiol.

In rats, orchidectomy decreases testosterone and progesterone hydroxylation as well as the associated hepatic microsomal changes. All these effects are restored by in vivo treatment of the castrate with testoids and the effect of the latter is in turn blocked by folliculoids. Curiously, the folliculoids fail to block the effect of testoids upon the seminal vesicles and levator ani muscles of orchidectomized rats.

The proposed sites at which thyroid hormones and folliculoids are presumed to influence testoid and folliculoid metabolism are summarized on p. 125.

← *Folliculoids cf. also Selye B40,000/50, p. 531; B58,650/51, pp. 326, 359; G60,083/70, p. 368.*

Selye A35,410/41: Following repeated injections of progesterone, DOC, testosterone, or stilbestrol to rats, the anesthetic effect of these hormones gradually diminishes. Pretreatment with one of these anesthetic compounds also induces resistance to others, whereas pretreatment with cholesterol (which is not anesthetic) induces no such resistance.

Zondek et al. A74,477/43: Stilbestrol is inactivated by rat liver pulp in vitro, though less rapidly than estrone. "In rats treated with large amounts of stilbestrol, the capacity of the liver to inactivate stilbestrol is increased."

Friedman & Friedman B48,306/50: In intact male rats, on a normal NaCl intake, the hypertension and cardiac hypertrophy produced through s.c. implantation of DOC pellets was inhibited by an adrenocortical extract but not by progesterone, testosterone, pregnenolone, estradiol, or acetoxypregnenolone.

Selye B53,941/51: In rats conditioned by uninephrectomy + NaCl, the production by DOC of nephrosclerosis, periarteritis nodosa and polyuria is prevented by conjoint administration of stilbestrol.

Ducommun & Ducommun B70,251/53: In rats, saprophytosis produced by heavy overdosage with cortisone is inhibited by concurrent administration of STH. This "anti-infectious effect of STH" is much less evident after adrenalectomy. DOC, testosterone, estradiol alone or in combination, failed to duplicate the anti-infectious action of STH in cortisone-treated rats.

Reifenstein Jr. C47,377/58: Review of the literature suggests that "androgens and estrogens are anabolic and thus stimulate the growth of protein and osseous tissues." The clinical value of anabolic steroids in counteracting the catabolism caused by endogenous and exogenous glucocorticoids is discussed.

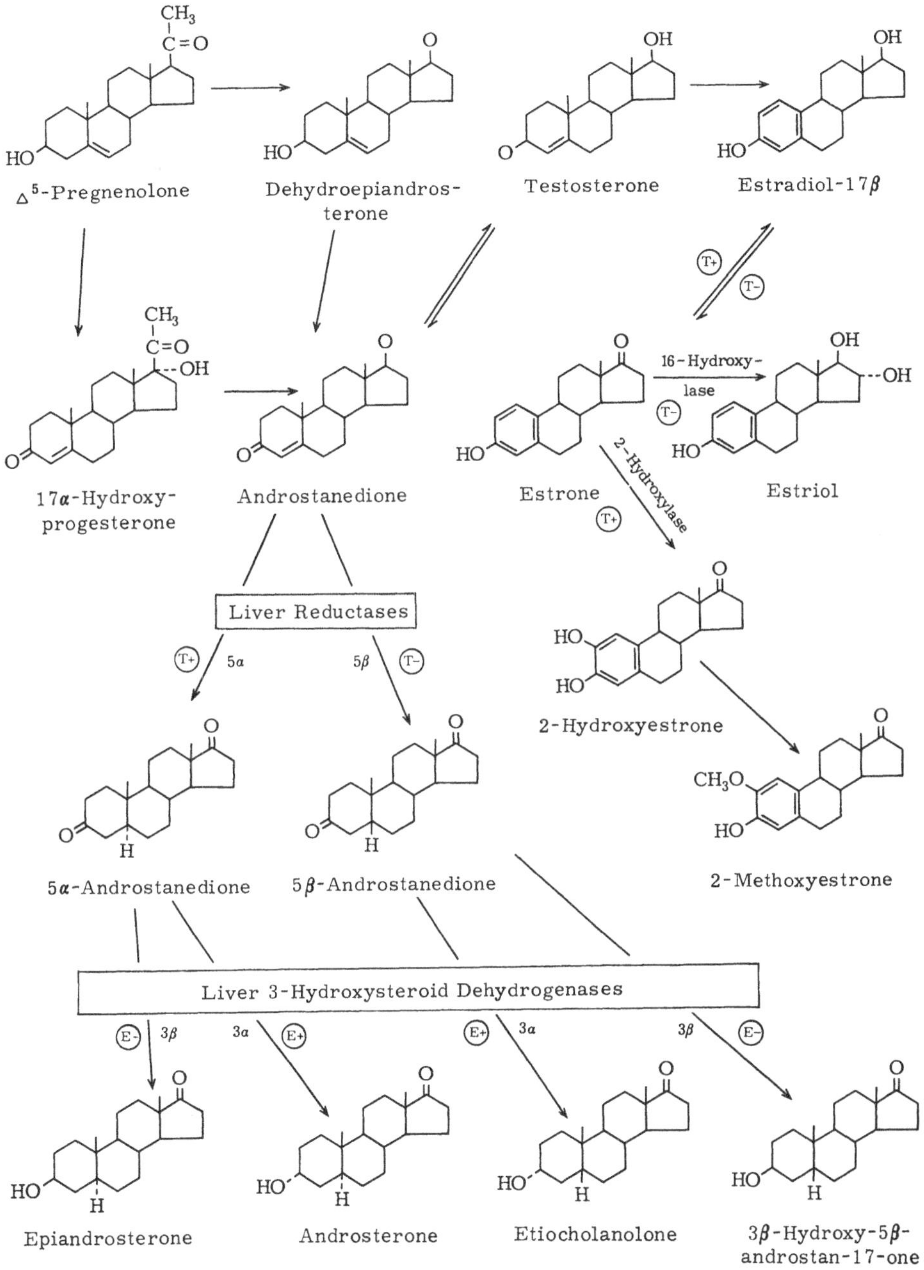

Δ⁵-Pregnenolone

Dehydroepiandros-
terone

Testosterone

Estradiol-17β

17α-Hydroxy-
progesterone

Androstanedione

Estrone

16-Hydroxy-
lase

Estriol

2-Hydroxylase

Liver Reductases

5α

5β

2-Hydroxyestrone

5α-Androstanedione

5β-Androstanedione

2-Methoxyestrone

Liver 3-Hydroxysteroid Dehydrogenases

3β   3α   3α   3β

Epiandrosterone

Androsterone

Etiocholanolone

3β-Hydroxy-5β-
androstan-17-one

Proposed sites of influence of thyroid hormones (T) and estrogens (E) on metabolism of androgens and estrogens: $+$ = stimulation, $-$ = either inhibition or stimulation when factor lacking
(Gaunt et al. G 63,202/68)

Bavetta et al. D29,064/62: In the rat, "growth hormone, methyl testosterone or stilbestrol, when given alone or in combination were not able to counteract the inhibitory effects of 6-methyl prednisolone on body weight gain and collagen synthesis at the site of subcutaneously implanted polyvinyl sponges."

Herrmann & Winkler D27,922/62: In guinea pigs, the adrenocortical atrophy and hypofunction produced by chronic cortisone treatment is prevented by simultaneous administration of estradiol. The responsiveness of the adrenal cortex to the induction of hemorrhagic necrosis by diphtheria toxin returns much more rapidly after interruption of cortisone treatment if estradiol is simultaneously administered.

Kreek et al. F83,145/67: In rats, ethinylestradiol considerably diminishes bile flow and delays biliary excretion of BSP and of tritium-labeled estradiol.

Denef & de Moor H15,811/69: The sexual differentiation of steroid-metabolizing enzymes appears in the rat liver from the 30th day of life onwards. From experiments on neonatally gonadectomized or intact rats treated with folliculoid or testoid compounds, "it is concluded that, as far as the differentiation of cortisol metabolizing enzymes is concerned, estradiol is able to counteract the organizing action of testosterone at birth as well as the expression of these neonatal testosterone effects after the 30th day of life."

Kato et al. H25,499/69: In rats, orchidectomy decreased testosterone and progesterone hydroxylation, as well as the spectral change caused by these steroids in liver microsomes reflecting a less pronounced decrease in microsomal P-450 content and NADPH-neotetrazolium reductase activity. All these changes were restored to normal by in vivo treatment of the castrates with testosterone or methyltestosterone, whereas simultaneous administration of estradiol or diethylstilbestrol blocked these actions of the testoids. Curiously, the folliculoids failed to block the effects of the testoids upon seminal vesicles and levator ani muscle, as well as on hepatic microsomal proteins in these same orchidectomized rats. Earlier literature on the antagonism between folliculoid and testoid actions upon hepatic drug-metabolizing enzymes is reviewed.

Schulz et al. H19,404/69: Clomiphene (an ovulation promoting folliculoid analogue of stilbestrol) decreases the hepatic microsomal NAD-specific 17β-ol-steroid dehydrogenase in immature female guinea pigs.

Fluorocortisol Acetate ← Folliculoids *cf.* also Tables 12—14

DOC ← Folliculoids *cf.* also Table 15

Estradiol ← Folliculoids *cf.* also Table 16

Progesterone ← Folliculoids *cf.* also Table 17

Triamcinolone ← Folliculoids *cf.* also Table 18

Pancuronium ← Folliculoids *cf.* also Table 19

Androstane-3,17-dione ← Estradiol + Orchidectomy: Rubin G76,315/57

Corticoids, Testoids, Luteoids ← Estradiol: Forchielli et al. D75,874/58

Steroids (Δ^4-3-keto) ← Estradiol + Orchidectomy: Yates et al. C61,952/58

Cortisol ← Folliculoids: Kumagai et al. C73,732/59

Cortisone ← Estradiol + Sex: Hagen et al. G77,512/60

Cortisone, Testosterone ← Folliculoids: Leybold et al. D11,904/61

Estradiol, Estrone, Stilbestrol ← Stilbestrol + Sex: Jellinck et al. F37,592/65

← Antitestoids

Cyproterone is the prototype of the antitestoid compounds. It antagonizes the effect of testosterone upon the accessory organs of various species even after orchidectomy; hence its effect is assumed to be peripheral and not mediated through the gonads. The compound also interferes with the production of sexual anomalies by testosterone in embryonic animals of both sexes and it blocks even such not manifestly sex-linked effects of testosterone as the erythropoietic action in the mouse.

Cyproterone is also one of the most potent catatoxic steroids having a broad spectrum of activity against almost all substrates that can be detoxified by any hormone. It powerfully counteracts progesterone anesthesia, yet the shortening effect of testosterone upon hexobarbital anesthesia in ovariectomized rats is not counteracted by cyproterone. Perhaps this failure of effectiveness is again due to the fact that catatoxic steroids are proportionately much less active against near physiologic than against massive amounts of substrates; the small amounts of testosterone needed to raise hexobarbital resistance are more difficult to block than a decisive proportion of the large doses of progesterone required to produce anesthesia. Besides cyproterone itself also shortens hexobarbital sleeping time.

Neumann et al. F78,500/67: Review of the testosterone antagonizing effect of cyproterone in the mouse, rat and rabbit. Special attention is given to the blockade of testoid-induced lesions in the accessory sex organs of embryonic and adult males and females.

Medlinsky et al. G67,839/69: In mice, the erythropoietic effect of testosterone is antagonized by cyproterone at the same dose level which also blocks other testoid actions.

Wenzel et al. H14,785/69: Change of the sex-specific hydrogen transfer from estradiol-17β to androstenedione in rat liver after feminization by the antitestoid substance, cyproterone.

← *Adrenalectomy*

In discussing the effects of steroids upon resistance, it is indispensable to consider also the effect of creating a deficiency in the steroid producing glands, especially the adrenals and the gonads (*cf.* next section). As stated in the introduction to this volume, the extensive literature on the effect of adrenalectomy upon resistance has been discussed in our previous monographs to which the reader is referred. Here, we shall limit ourselves to a few observations on the influence of adrenalectomy upon certain effects of hormones and drugs in the regulation of steroid metabolism.

In our earlier work we emphasized the "buffering action of the adrenals" as regards the actions of glucocorticoids and mineralocorticoids upon various targets. The production by glucocorticoids of thymolysis and catabolism as well as the inhibition of growth and inflammation are all readily counteracted by mineralocorticoids (e.g., DOC, aldosterone) in adrenalectomized rats; in intact animals all these effects are produced only by larger doses of glucocorticoids, but then, they are also less-readily counteracted by mineralocorticoids. It was assumed that these glucocorticoid effects are almost optimally blocked by physiological doses of mineralocorticoids (such as are normally produced by the adrenals), but that no considerable further inactivation is obtained by adding exogenous mineralocorticoids. Thus, by increasing the dose of the glucocorticoids, their above-mentioned effects rapidly rise to reach a very high intensity, whereas by correspondingly raising the dosage of mineralocorticoids, the antagonistic (inhibitory) effect of the latter soon reaches a plateau above which further interference with glucocorticoid overdosage becomes insignificant. This is illustrated by the graph on p. 112.

The growth inhibition produced by cortisone in immature adrenalectomized rats can be inhibited both by DOC and by testosterone; MAD exerts no consistent effect.

Progesterone anesthesia is prolonged by adrenalectomy in rats maintained on NaCl alone, but blocked both in intact and in adrenalectomized animals by spironolactone. Desoxycortisone (Cpd. S), like dehydroisoandrosterone, produces no anesthesia but intense convulsions in the rat. These are allegedly not influenced by adrenalectomy or even by partial hepatectomy.

The uterine weight increase produced by estradiol is markedly inhibited by phenobarbital both in intact and in adrenalectomized rats. Simultaneously the estradiol-metabolizing activity of the hepatic microsomal enzymes is augmented. The adrenal does not seem to play a role in this estradiol-metabolizing effect of the barbiturate but the latter is demonstrable only at very low dose levels. This again illustrates the fact which we have emphasized in connection with so many catatoxic steroid actions upon natural compounds, namely that they are much more efficient in antagonizing the toxic effects of heavy overdosage than in counteracting the physiologic actions of small amounts. It is comparatively easy to prevent steroid anesthesia with catatoxic steroids or drugs, but much more difficult to block the normal actions of steroids upon their natural targets. Presumably, the catatoxic mechanism readily destroys a great excess of a substrate but is much less efficient in degrading the last remnants of it, which are still sufficient to produce physiologic actions.

Gaunt et al. B71,987/52: DOC (1 mg/day) and testosterone propionate (0.25 mg/day) counteracted the growth inhibition produced in immature adrenalectomized rats by cortisone acetate (1 mg/day). MAD (2 mg/day) had no consistent effect on growth. Both MAD and testosterone propionate caused thymus atrophy, and this effect was further increased by conjoint administration of cortisone. In intact rats, MAD prevented the cortisone-induced adrenal atrophy. [It is not clear from this brief abstract whether the other interactions were also tested in intact animals (H.S.).]

Selye B98,268/55: In adrenalectomized rats, the diminution of body weight, inflammation in the granuloma pouch as well as the atrophy of the thymus and spleen produced by cortisol are all inhibited by aldosterone.

Selye & Bois C14,534/56: In adrenalectomized rats bearing granuloma pouches, 2-methyl-9(α) fluorocortisol (Me-F-COL) antagonizes the antiphlogistic, catabolic, thymolytic and splenolytic actions of cortisol. This effect is ascribed to the strong mineralocorticoid effects of Me-F-COL, which counteract glucocorticoid actions. However, since Me-F-COL itself possesses some glucocorticoid potency, its cortisol antagonizing action is evident only at very low dose levels (about 75 µg/kg) at which mineralocorticoid effects predominate in agreement with the "law of intersecting dose-effect curves."

Heuser C54,451/58: Desoxycortisone (Cpd. S)—like dehydroisoandrosterone—given in large amounts i.p. or p.o. produces no anesthesia but intense convulsions in the rat. Allegedly, "neither adrenalectomy nor partial hepatectomy sensitized the rat to the convulsive actions of Cpd. S."

Jasmin et al. C89,132/60: Both in intact and in adrenalectomized rats, norethandrolone diminishes the body weight loss caused by cortisol without inhibiting the antiphlogistic effect of the latter.

Levin & Conney F64,557/66: In immature intact or adrenalectomized rats, the uterine weight increase produced by small doses of estradiol i.p. is markedly inhibited by pretreatment with phenobarbital. At the same time, the estradiol-metabolizing activity of hepatic microsomal enzymes is augmented. In order to demonstrate the inhibition of uterine growth, very small doses (less than 0.5 µg) of estradiol must be used and phenobarbital must be administered for several days prior to the test.

Levin et al. F75,365/67: Phenobarbital increases the 17β-estradiol-metabolizing activity of hepatic microsomal enzymes in immature female rats. The in vitro activity is paralleled by in vivo blockade of the estradiol-induced uterine weight increase. The phenobarbital-induced resistance to the uterine weight-increasing effect of estradiol is not prevented by adrenalectomy or hypophysectomy, indicating that the barbiturate does not act through the pituitary-adrenal axis.

Orrenius et al. E8,231/69: In rats, adrenalectomy has no immediate effect upon the phenobarbital induction of steroid hydroxylases in the hepatic microsomes. However, simultaneously adrenalectomized and castrate rats, subsequently maintained in this state for a period of time, showed a strikingly decreased hydroxylating activity of the hepatic microsomes measured with either aminopyrine or testosterone as substrate. The cytochrome P-450 content of the microsomes decreased in a parallel fashion, whereas the cytochrome b_5 remained unchanged. When these steroid-deficient animals were treated with prednisolone or testosterone, the cytochrome P-450 content and the aminopyrine— as well as testosterone—hydroxylating activities of the liver microsomes returned to normal. In the steroid-deficient rats, repeated injections of phenobarbital caused only a minimal increase in the cytochrome P-450 content, the NADPH-cytochrome reductase, and aminopyrine-hydroxylation activities of hepatic microsomes. In intact controls, combined treatment with phenobarbital and prednisolone or testosterone resulted in an increase of these levels as compared to those obtained by phenobarbital alone. Apparently, "steroid hormones are involved both in the maintenance of normal hydroxylating activity in the rat liver endoplasmic reticulum and in the increase of this activity caused by drugs."

Southren & Gordon G77,117/70: Review and personal observations on the application of radioisotopes to the in vivo study of the kinetics of testoid metabolism in man, with special reference to the effect of sex differences, adrenalectomy, orchidectomy and various diseases upon the plasma clearance of testosterone.

Selye PROT. 27691: In rats, (100 g♀) progesterone (6 mg in 1 ml oil i.p.) or pentobarbital (3 mg in 0.5 ml oil i.p.) anesthesia is prolonged by adrenalectomy with maintenance on NaCl, but blocked, both in intact and adrenalectomized animals, by spironolactone (10 mg in 1 ml water p.o. x2/day) pretreatment for 4 days.

Cortisone ← Adrenalectomy + Genetics: Wragg et al. B74,080/52*; Hagen et al. G77,512/60

Estradiol ← Adrenalectomy + Phenobarbital: Levin et al. F75,365/67*

← Gonadectomy

Female rats are more sensitive than males to the anesthetic action of progesterone; since this sex difference is obvious only after maturity, it has been ascribed to gonadal hormones. Castration increases the sensitivity of males but not of females. Conversely, the resistance of female and castrate males can be raised to the normal male level by methyltestosterone.

On the other hand, mice of both sexes are approximately equally sensitive to the hydroxydione anesthesia. Yet, gonadectomy increases sensitivity to this form of narcosis, especially in females, but to some extent also in males. Methyltestosterone prolongs hydroxydione anesthesia in male mice but not in females or castrate males. Neither thiopental nor pentobarbital anesthesia is influenced by methyltestosterone in mice.

In C3H strain mice, myocardial calcification develops following prolonged cortisol treatment. Females are much more sensitive to this effect than males. Ovariectomy offers no protection but testosterone renders females more resistant.

Conjoint treatment with cortisone + NaCl produces myocardial necroses in orchidectomized but not in normal male rats nor in orchidectomized testosterone-treated males.

In ovariectomized rats, phenobarbital inhibits the uterotrophic effect of estradiol, as well as the induction of phosphofructokinase in the uterus, but the results are obvious only at threshold doses of estradiol treatment. In orchidectomized rats, phenobarbital diminishes the effect of testosterone upon the seminal vesicles and prostate, thereby furnishing further proof that physiologic hormonal substrates can be inactivated by hepatic microsomal enzyme-inducing drugs.

In rats, orchidectomy decreases testosterone and progesterone hydroxylation as well as the associated changes in the hepatic microsomes. All these derangements are counteracted by in vivo treatment of the castrates with various testoids; the action of the latter is in turn blocked by concurrent treatment with folliculoids.

Winter & Selye A 35,658/41; Winter A 36,333/41: Female rats are more sensitive than males to the anesthetic action of progesterone, but this sex difference is obvious only after maturity. "The normal endocrine activity of the testis is largely, if not entirely, responsible for this comparative resistance of the males, since castration increases sensitivity in males but is without effect in female rats. Conversely, the resistance of castrate males and females may be raised by methyl testosterone administration."

Koller C 19,288/56: Mice of both sexes are approximately equally sensitive to hydroxydione anesthesia. Gonadectomy increases sensitivity to this form of narcosis especially in females and to a lesser extent, in males also.

Forchielli et al. D 75,874/58: The rate of Δ^4-reduction of 11-desoxycortisol was 3—4 fold greater in female than in male rat liver homogenates and in microsomal fractions containing the Δ^4-5α-hydrogenase. Female rat liver contains only one Δ^4-hydrogenase (5α-microsomal), whereas the male liver contains the soluble Δ^4-5β-hydrogenase as well. Ovariectomy caused no marked change in enzyme titer, but hypophysectomy decreased it sharply. Curiously, ACTH, STH and pregnant mare serum partially restored the enzyme level in the hypophysectomized rat. In young animals, increase in the titer of hepatic Δ^4-5α-hydrogenase occurs prior to puberty. This fact—like the negative results after ovariectomy—suggests an enzyme regulation independent of ovarian hormones.

Lostroh C 54,348/58: Female mice of the C3H strain regularly develop myocardial calcification following prolonged cortisol treatment, whereas males are comparatively resistant. Ovariectomy offers no protection but testosterone renders females more resistant. In hypophysectomized mice, neither cortisol nor ACTH produces myocardial calcification.

Yates et al. C 61,952/58: "Homogenates of livers from adult female rats reduce Ring A of Δ^4-3-keto-steroids at rates 3 to 10 times greater than those from males. This large sex difference has been observed for all substrates so far tested: aldosterone, desoxycorticosterone, hydrocortisone, cortisone, corticosterone, testosterone, and progesterone. ... Castration increases and testosterone decreases Δ^4-steroid hydrogenase activity in males. In females, neither castration nor estrogen administration had appreciable effect."

Colás D 20,925/62: The livers of male rats contain more dehydroepiandrosterone 16α-hydroxylase than that of males. Castration reduces the enzyme activity but not quite to the low level of the female.

Mäkinen et al. E 20,847/63: Conjoint treatment with cortisone + NaCl produces myocardial necroses in orchidectomized, but not in normal male rats. Testosterone restores the resistance of the male castrates to normal, whereas concomitant exposure to the stress of a loud bell aggravates the cardiopathy.

Singhal et al. G 67,770/67: Phenobarbital pretreatment inhibits the uterotrophic effect of estradiol as well as the induction of phosphofructokinase in the uterus of the ovariectomized rat. The most marked results were obtained with threshold doses of estradiol.

Denef & de Moor H 3,569/68: In female rats, spayed and given testosterone immediately after birth, there developed a characteristic male pattern of hepatic microsomal steroidases. In male rats, castrated at birth, a single injection of testosterone given at the same time prevented the differentiation of the feminine type of steroid metabolism found after neonatal castration. In adults, testosterone had a similar effect, but unlike in neonates, its action was only temporary.

Fahim et al. G 67,772/68: Phenobarbital reduces the uterotrophic action of both exogenous estradiol and endogenous folliculoids. This effect is somewhat lessened by ovariectomy. The authors consider the possibility that the barbiturate may induce steroidases not only in the hepatic microsomes, but also in the ovary. Enzyme determinations in the liver were not performed, but phenobarbital significantly increased hepatic weight and total nitrogen content.

Jelinek H 1,518/68: There was no difference in the duration of hydroxydione anesthesia in male and female intact or gonadectomized mice. Pretreatment with methyltestosterone p.o. prolonged hydroxydione anesthesia in males, but not in females or castrate males. Neither thiopental, nor pentobarbital anesthesia was influenced by methyltestosterone. Pretreatment with Dianabol or 17α-methyl-androst-2-ene-17β-ol failed to influence hydroxydione anesthesia in mice.

King et al. H 16,446/68: In orchidectomized rats, phenobarbital pretreatment diminishes the effect of testosterone upon the seminal vesicles and prostate, presumably as a consequence of increased hepatic microsomal enzyme production. These findings may "offer a therapeutic modality for gynecologic syndromes that are associated with overproduction of androgens."

Denef & de Moor H 15,811/69: The sexual differentiation of steroid-metabolizing enzymes appears in the rat liver from the 30th day of life onwards. From experiments on neonatally gonadectomized or intact rats treated with folliculoid or testoid compounds, "it is concluded that, as far as the differentiation of cortisol metabolizing enzymes is concerned, estradiol is able to counteract the organizing action of testosterone at birth as well as the expression of these neonatal testosterone effects after the 30th day of life."

Kato et al. H 25,499/69: In rats, orchidectomy decreased testosterone and progesterone hydroxylation, as well as the spectral change caused by these steroids in liver microsomes, reflecting a less pronounced decrease in microsomal P-450 content and NADPH-neotetrazolium reductase activity. All these changes were restored to normal by in vivo treatment of the castrates with testosterone or methyltestosterone, whereas simultaneous administration of estradiol or diethylstilbestrol blocked these actions of the testoids. Curiously, the folliculoids failed to block the effects of the testoids upon the seminal vesicle and levator ani muscle as well as on hepatic microsomal proteins in these same orchidectomized rats. Earlier literature on the antagonism between folliculoid and testoid actions upon hepatic drug-metabolizing enzymes is reviewed.

Southren & Gordon G 77,117/70: Review and personal observations on the application of radioisotopes to the in vivo study of the kinetics of testoid metabolism in man, with special reference to sex differences, adrenalectomy, orchidectomy, and various diseases upon the plasma clearance of testosterone.

Androsterone, Epiandrosterone ← Orchidectomy + Testosterone: Rubin *G 76,315/57*

Androstane-3,17-dione ← Ovariectomy + Estradiol: Rubin *G 76,315/57*

Corticoids, Testoids, Luteoids ← Ovariectomy: Forchielli et al. *D 75,874/58*

Steroids (Δ^4-3-keto) ← Ovariectomy + Estradiol: Yates et al. *C 61,952/58*

Cortisone ← Orchidectomy + Testosterone: Hagen et al. *G 77,512/60*

Dehydroepiandrosterone ← Orchidectomy: Colás *D 20,925/62*

Estradiol ← Ovariectomy: Singhal et al. *G 78,387/69**

Estradiol, Estrone, Stilbestrol ← Ovariectomy: Jellinck et al. *F 37,592/65*

← Various Steroids

← **TMACN.** TMACN administered to rats between the 15th and 20th day of gestation produces a syndrome of congenital adrenocortical hyperplasia, hypospadias, clitoral hypertrophy due to inactivation of 3β-hydroxysteroid-dehydrogenase and Δ^{5-4}-3-ketosteroid isomerase. Furthermore, TMACN suppresses nipple formation in females and induces it in males. 17β-hydroxy-4,4,17α-trimethylandrost-5-ene-(2,3d)-isoxazole produces similar effects.

In the male offspring which develop severe hypospadias, the anogenital distance is greatly reduced almost to that of females. Small amounts of testosterone prevent the production of hypospadias without affecting the adrenal hyperplasia or the inhibition of 3β-hydroxysteroid-dehydrogenase and Δ^{5-4}-3-ketosteroid isomerase. TMACN interferes with the biogenesis of various corticoids also as judged by analyses on adrenal vein blood as well as in adrenal homogenates. The "cyano-ketone" appears to inhibit the conversion of pregnenolone to progesterone and thereby reduce corticosterone secretion which would result in an increased ACTH production and adrenal hypertrophy. Even a single injection of TMACN on the 16th or 19th day of gestation, produces a permanent effect in 3β-hydroxysteroid-dehydrogenase activity in the maternal adrenal.

TMACN is an analogue of androstenolone (the substrate of 3β-hydroxysteroid-dehydrogenase) but has little or no testoid or folliculoid activity itself. The compound also produces luteal and Leydig cell hyperplasia. Its persistent effect is presumably due to the fact that unlike most enzyme inhibitors, it is very tightly and irreversibly bound to 3β-hydroxysteroid-dehydrogenase at its active site.

In guinea pigs, TMACN increases the mitochondrial and microsomal fractions of the adrenal cortex.

← **Varia.** DOC-induced mineralocorticoid hypertension is not significantly influenced in rats by pregnenolone or acetoxypregnenolone.

SC-8109 and SC-5233 do not protect the rat against the anesthetic effect of progesterone.

← *Various Steroids* cf. also Selye *C 92,918/61, p. 70; G 60,083/70, p. 385.*

← **TMACN.** *Goldman et al. F 64,070/66:* In rats, TMACN administered between the 15th and 20th day of gestation produces a syndrome of congenital adrenocortical hyperplasia, hypospadias and clitoral hypertrophy due to inactivation of 3β-hydroxysteroid dehydrogenase.

McCarthy et al. F 74,065/66: In rats, TMACN interferes with the biogenesis of various corticoids in vivo (adrenal vein blood) and in vitro (adrenal homogenates). "The cyano-ketone appears to inhibit the conversion of pregnenolone to progesterone by the rat adrenal gland. This inhibition would account for the reduction in corticosterone secretion and adrenal hypertrophy that follows administration of the cyano-ketone to rats."

Bongiovanni et al. E 7,039/67: Review on the inhibition of 3β-hydroxysteroid dehydrogenase by TMACN in vivo and in vitro. This analogue of androstenolone (the substrate of the enzyme) has little or no testoid or folliculoid activity, but produces adrenocortical hyperplasia by blocking the biosynthesis of glucocorticoids. It also produces luteal and Leydig cell hyperplasia; "unlike most enzyme inhibitors, this analogue is very tightly and irreversibly bound to 3β-hydroxysteroid dehydrogenase at, or very near, its active site." When TMACN is given to pregnant rats, their offspring "have severe adrenal cortical hyperplasia, deficient histochemical activity of the 3β-hydroxysteroid dehydrogenase in the adrenals and testes, increased activity of G-6-PD in adrenals, testes, and liver, and no change in the activities of the 3α or 17β-hydroxysteroid dehydrogenases in these tissues. The experimental gonadal males have severe hypospadias, and their anogenital distance is reduced from that of normal to almost that of the normal females in proportion to dose. The gonadal females have marked clitoral hypertrophy but no change in anogenital distance from the normal." Small amounts of testosterone prevent the production of hypospadias without affecting the adrenal hyperplasia or the inhibition of 3β-hydroxysteroid dehydrogenase by TMACN.

Goldman F 85,342/67: In rats, a single injection of TMACN on the 16th or 19th day of gestation produces a permanent defect in 3β-hydroxysteroid dehydrogenase in the maternal adrenal and corresponding permanent changes in the pituitary, adrenals, and sex organs of the offspring.

Goldman H 15,818/69: In rats, the maternal and fetal changes induced by two inhibitors of 3β-hydroxysteroid dehydrogenase and Δ^{5-4}-3-ketosteroid isomerase [TMACN and 17β-hydroxy-4,4,17α-trimethylandrost-5-ene-(2,3d)-isoxazole] are described and their mechanism of action discussed.

Goldman & Neumann H 18,122/69: In rats given TMACN during pregnancy, functional and structural changes occur in the adrenals and sex organs as a consequence of 3β-hydroxysteroid dehydrogenase and Δ^{5-4}-3-ketosteroid isomerase inhibition.

Castells & Bransome Jr. H 21,283/70: In guinea pigs treated with TMACN in vivo, the protein content of the mitochondrial and microsomal fractions was increased. "Exposure to a high level of ACTH for 4 hr or 4 days seemed to exert less net effect on mitochondrial protein than on microsomal protein synthesis: an observation consistent with an intrinsic difference in the regulation of the synthesis of adrenocortical mitochondrial and microsomal proteins."

Steroids ← TMACN: McCarthy et al. *F74,065/66;* Goldman *F78,224/67*

← Varia. *Friedman & Friedman B48,306/50:* In intact male rats, on a normal NaCl intake, the hypertension and cardiac hypertrophy produced by s.c. implantation of DOC pellets could be inhibited by an adrenocortical extract, but not by progesterone, testosterone, **pregnenolone**, estradiol, or **acetoxypregnenolone**.

Gaunt et al. B82,200/53: In rats, MAD was the most active in preventing cortisone-induced adrenal atrophy among a large series of **steroids**. To some extent, this was true even after hypophysectomy.

Heuser C33,938/57: Doctor's thesis (193 pp., 272 refs.) on steroid anesthesia with sections on: **adaption to steroid anesthesia** by pretreatment with the same or other steroids, the effect of adrenalectomy and corticoids upon steroid anesthesia and the interaction between anesthetic and convulsive steroids.

Witzel C68,395/59: **Review** (29pp., 113 refs.) on steroid anesthesia, including chapters on adaptation to steroids, the effect of partial hepatectomy, the influence of steroid anesthetics upon various types of convulsions.

McGuire Jr. et al. D82,559/60: The hepatic microsomal steroid 5α-reductases have a high substrate specificity and an absolute requirement for TPNH. Addition of various **other steroids** can competitively inhibit the reduction of the substrate by the rat liver microsomal enzymes in vitro.

Linèt et al. F58,620/65: In rats, **1,2α-epoxyandrostan-3,17-dione**, though devoid of anabolic, testoid or folliculoid properties, inhibits the increase in liver glycogen caused by cortisol, but does not prevent the inhibition of inflammation and the atrophy of the adrenal cortex characteristic of glucocorticoid overdosage.

Selye et al. G60,050/70: **SC-8109 and SC-5233** fail to protect the rat against the anesthetic effect of progesterone or pentobarbital.

Selye G60,064/70: In rats, PCN, CS-1 and spironolactone offer considerable protection against the infarctoid cardiopathy produced by F-COL + Na_2HPO_4 + restraint. The possible protection offered by other conditioners requires further investigation, *cf.* Table 12.

Despopoulos H35,471/71: In a system containing isolated mitochondrial fractions from rat liver homogenates, the synthesis of

Table 12. *Conditioning for myocardial necroses produced by F-COL + Na_2HPO_4 + restraint*

Treatment[a]	Cardiac necrosis[b] (Positive/Total)	Mortality[b] (Dead/Total)
None	13/17	12/19
PCN	0/10 ***	2/10 *
CS-1	3/10 *	1/10 **
Ethylestrenol	5/10 NS	5/10 NS
Spironolactone	0/10 ***	2/10 *
Norbolethone	5/10 NS	3/10 NS
Oxandrolone	4/10 NS	6/10 NS
Prednisolone-Ac	7/7 NS	10/10 ±
Triamcinolone	4/5 NS	10/10 ±
Progesterone	7/10 NS	6/10 NS
Estradiol	4/9 NS	7/10 NS
DOC-Ac	6/10 NS	5/10 NS
Hydroxydione	2/10 **	7/10 NS
Thyroxine	6/10 NS	9/10 NS
Phenobarbital	2/9 *	1/9 *

[a] The rats of all groups were given fluorocortisol acetate (750 µg in 0.2 ml water, s.c., daily) and Na_2HPO_4 (1 mM in 2 ml water, p.o.,/100 g body weight twice daily from the 4th day ff.). Restraint during 17 hrs on the 6th day.

[b] Cardiac necrosis was estimated on day of death in animals that lived at least 7 days and mortality listed on the 8th day ("Exact Probability Test").

For further details on technique of tabulation *cf.* p. VIII.

taurocholate from cholate was inhibited by **testosterone, cortisone, estradiol, stilbestrol, norethandrolone** and progesterone but not by mestranol. Synthesis of cholate from cholesterol was not inhibited by any of these steroids. "These experiments demonstrate an effect of steroids on a specific step in the sequence of bile salt synthesis; namely, conjugation of cholate with taurine to form taurocholate."

Selye G70,480/71: In rats, the infarctoid-cardiopathy produced by combined treatment with F-COL + $NaClO_4$ + corn oil is most effectively combated by CS-1 and spironolactone. Phenobarbital diminished the incidence of cardiac necroses but did not significantly decrease mortality. The two glucocorticoids of our series greatly accelerated and aggravated mortality; this made it impossible to assess their effect upon the development of cardiac necroses. Since F-COL possesses both gluco- and mineralocorticoid potencies it is not unexpected that additional treatment with glucocorticoids, would increase its toxicity. It is noteworthy however, that among the many catatoxic compounds tested, only few offer protection against this cardiopathy in whose pathogenesis corticoids (excellent substrates for catatoxic steroids) play an indispensable role. The most active protective steroids (CS-1, spironolactone) are also distinguished by a marked potassium retaining effect which undoubtedly helps to prevent a cardiopathy primarily characterized by potassium losses, cf. Table 13.

Table 13. *Conditioning for F-COL + NaClO$_4$ + corn oil*

Treatment[a]	Cardiac necrosis[b] (Positive/Total)	Mortality[b] (Dead/Total)
None	16/19	12/20
PCN	3/10 **	1/10 *
CS-1	2/10 ***	1/10 *
Ethylestrenol	8/9 NS	4/10 NS
Spironolactone	1/10 ***	1/10 *
Norbolethone	9/19 *	9/20 NS
Oxandrolone	6/10 NS	6/10 NS
Prednisolone-Ac	1/3 NS	10/10 ±
Triamcinolone (2 mg)	—	10/10 ±
Progesterone	8/10 NS	7/10 NS
Estradiol	3/7 NS	9/10 NS
DOC-Ac	9/10 NS	9/10 NS
Hydroxydione	5/9 NS	7/10 NS
Thyroxine	8/10 NS	8/10 NS
Phenobarbital	3/10 **	3/10 NS

[a] The rats of all groups were given fluorocortisol acetate (750 μg/100 g body weight in 0.2 ml water, s.c., once daily), sodium perchlorate (1 mM/100 g body weight in 2 ml water, p.o., twice daily) and corn oil (1 ml, p.o., twice daily from 4th day ff.).

[b] Cardiac necrosis was estimated on day of death in animals that lived at least 8 days and mortality listed on 9th day ("Exact Probability Test").

For further details on technique of tabulation cf. p. VIII.

Selye G70,480/71: In rats, PCN, CS-1 and spironolactone offer considerable protection against the myocardial necrosis produced by F-COL + Na$_2$HPO$_4$ + corn oil. The apparent minor protective effect of other agents is of borderline significance but phenobarbital is definitely devoid of prophylactic potency, cf. Table 14.

Table 14. *Conditioning for myocardial necroses produced by F-COL + Na$_2$HPO$_4$ + corn oil*

Treatment[a]	Cardiac necroses[b] (Positive/Total)	Mortality[b] (Dead/Total)
None	9/10	10/10
PCN	0/9 ***	7/10 NS
CS-1	1/10 ***	4/10 **
Ethylestrenol	8/9 NS	8/10 NS
Spironolactone	0/9 ***	1/10 ***
Norbolethone	4/9 *	5/10 *
Oxandrolone	10/10 NS	10/10 NS
Prednisolone-Ac	2/6 *	10/10 NS
Triamcinolone	—	10/10 NS
Progesterone	7/9 NS	10/10 NS
Estradiol	3/9 *	10/10 NS
DOC-Ac	7/9 NS	10/10 NS
Hydroxydione	5/8 NS	9/10 NS
Thyroxine	9/10 NS	10/10 NS
Phenobarbital	7/10 NS	9/10 NS

[a] The rats of all groups were given fluorocortisol acetate (750 μg in 0.2 ml water, s.c.), Na$_2$HPO$_4$ (1 mM in 2 ml water, p.o., twice) and corn oil (1 ml, p.o., twice, /100 g body weight daily from the 4th day ff.).

[b] Cardiac necroses were estimated on day of death in animals that survived until the 7th day and mortality was listed on 11th day ("Exact Probability Test").

For additional pertinent data cf. also Table 135.

For further details on technique of tabulation cf. p. VIII.

Selye G70,480/71: In rats, thyroxine and perhaps to a lesser extent also phenobarbital offer protection against the nephrocalcinosis produced by combined treatment with DOC + NaH$_2$PO$_4$. Here, catatoxic steroids are devoid of prophylactic potency and glucocorticoids are definitely harmful, cf. Table 15.

Selye G70,480/71: In rats, none of the standard conditioners (with the possible exception of thyroxine) offered any significant protection against the nephrocalcinosis produced by estradiol + NaH$_2$PO$_4$. The mortality induced by this treatment was greatly increased by the glucocorticoids and perhaps to some extent also by CS-1 and norbolethone, cf. Table 16.

Selye G70,480/71: In rats, all the standard catatoxic steroids as well as prednisolone, estradiol and phenobarbital shortened the duration of progesterone anesthesia, cf. Table 17, p. 136.

of the former as does estradiol which likewise possesses an inherent catabolic effect. Phenobarbital, although a potent microsomal drug-metabolism inducer, fails to counteract the catabolic action of triamcinolone, cf. Table 18, p. 136.

Table 15. *Conditioning for nephrocalcinosis produced by DOC + NaH_2PO_4*

Treatment[a]	Nephrocalcinosis[b] (Positive/Total)	Mortality[b] (Dead/Total)
None	10/10	2/10
PCN	5/8 NS	5/9 NS
CS-1	7/10 NS	0/10 NS
Ethylestrenol	8/9 NS	1/9 NS
Spironolactone	8/9 NS	1/10 NS
Norbolethone	8/9 NS	2/10 NS
Oxandrolone	5/8 NS	3/10 NS
Prednisolone-Ac	—	10/10 ***
Prednisolone-Ac (1 mg)	—	10/10 ***
Triamcinolone (2 mg)	—	10/10 ***
Triamcinolone (0.5 mg)	—	10/10 ***
Progesterone	7/8 NS	2/9 NS
Estradiol (1 mg)	6/7 NS	3/10 NS
DOC-Ac	8/8 NS	6/10 NS
Hydroxydione	8/8 NS	5/10 NS
Thyroxine	0/10 ***	1/10 NS
Phenobarbital	6/10 *	6/10 NS

[a] The rats of all groups were given DOC-Ac, desoxycorticosterone acetate (2 mg in 0.2 ml water, s.c.) and NaH_2PO_4, sodium phosphate monobasic (2 mM in 2 ml water, p.o., twice, /100 g body weight daily from 4th day ff.).

[b] Nephrocalcinosis was estimated on day of death in animals that lived at least 9 days and mortality listed on 19th day ("Exact Probability Test").

For further details on technique of tabulation cf. p. VIII.

Selye G70,480/71: In rats, the body weight loss produced by chronic triamcinolone overdosage is significantly counteracted by PCN, CS-1, spironolactone and norbolethone. Curiously, ethylestrenol has no such action, although this anabolic testoid is highly effective in increasing body weight under other conditions and in counteracting the catabolism produced by chronic DHT intoxication. As expected, concurrent treatment with triamcinolone and other glucocorticoids such as prednisolone aggravate the catabolic effect

Table 16. *Conditioning for nephrocalcinosis produced by estradiol + NaH_2PO_4*

Treatment[a]	Nephrocalcinosis[b] (Positive/Total)	Mortality[b] (Dead/Total)
None	5/9	1/10
PCN	5/7 NS	4/10 NS
CS-1	4/7 NS	6/10 *
Ethylestrenol	11/12 NS	6/15 NS
Spironolactone	2/10 NS	0/10 NS
Norbolethone	7/9 NS	6/10 *
Oxandrolone	8/10 NS	0/10 NS
Prednisolone-Ac	0/1 NS	9/9 ***
Prednisolone-Ac (1 mg)	2/7 NS	6/8 **
Triamcinolone (2 mg)	1/7 NS	8/10 ***
Triamcinolone (0.5 mg)	1/8 NS	8/10 ***
Progesterone	6/8 NS	2/9 NS
Estradiol (1 mg)	2/10 NS	0/10 NS
DOC-Ac	6/10 NS	1/10 NS
Hydroxydione	4/6 NS	4/10 NS
Thyroxine	0/10 *	0/10 NS
Phenobarbital	1/6 NS	5/10 NS

[a] The rats of all groups were given estradiol (500 μg in 0.2 ml water, s.c., daily + NaH_2PO_4, 2 mM in 2 ml water, p.o., twice daily /100 g body weight from the 4th day ff.).

[b] Nephrocalcinosis was estimated on day of death in animals that lived at least 9 days and mortality listed on 19th day ("Exact Probability Test").

For further details on technique of tabulation cf. p. VIII.

Szabo et al. G79,024/71: In rats, PCN increases resistance to indomethacin, hexobarbital, progesterone, zoxazolamine and digitoxin, both in the presence and in the absence of the pituitary. Hypophysectomy also fails to prevent the induction of SER proliferation in the hepatocytes.

Zsigmond & Solymoss G79,025/71: In rats, PCN inhibits the anesthetic effect of progesterone and decreases the level of labelled progesterone and its metabolites in the brain and serum.

Table 17. *Conditioning for progesterone anesthesia*

Treatment[a]	Sleeping time[b] (min)
None	126 ± 19
PCN	0 ***
CS-1	0 ***
Ethylestrenol	0 ***
Spironolactone	10 ± 7 ***
Norbolethone	0 ***
Oxandrolone	33 ± 22 **
Prednisolone-Ac	0 ***
Triamcinolone (2 mg)	189 ± 32 NS
Progesterone	129 ± 25 NS
Estradiol (1 mg)	47 ± 23 *
DOC-Ac	155 ± 21 NS
Hydroxydione	99 ± 23 NS
Thyroxine	152 ± 29 NS
Phenobarbital	0 ***

[a] The rats of all groups were given progesterone (10 mg/100 g body weight in 1 ml oil, i.p., on 4th day).
[b] Student's t-test.

For additional pertinent data *cf. also* Table 135.

For further details on technique of tabulation *cf.* p. VIII.

Table 18. *Conditioning for triamcinolone*

Treatment[a]	Final body weight[b] (g)	Mortality[c] (Dead/Total)
None	108 ± 3	2/10
PCN	158 ± 6 ***	0/10 NS
CS-1	145 ± 4 ***	0/10 NS
Ethylestrenol	100 ± 4 NS	4/10 NS
Spironolactone	125 ± 4 **	0/10 NS
Norbolethone	124 ± 3 **	1/10 NS
Oxandrolone	107 ± 3 NS	4/10 NS
Prednisolone-Ac	70 ± 3 ***	10/10 ***
Triamcinolone (2 mg)	90 (lr)	9/10 ***
Progesterone	103 ± 3 NS	2/9 NS
Estradiol (1 mg)	85 ± 2 ***	6/10 NS
DOC-Ac	97 ± 4 *	3/10 NS
Hydroxydione	103 ± 4 NS	2/10 NS
Thyroxine	109 ± 4 NS	2/10 NS
Phenobarbital	97 ± 3 *	0/10 NS

[a] The rats of all groups were given triamcinolone (1 mg/100 g body weight from 4th to 14th day and 2 mg/100 g body weight from 15th day, in 1 ml water, p.o., twice daily).

Selye PROT. 36968: In rats, pancuronium intoxication was completely prevented by CS-1 and spironolactone, but PCN and prednisolone were almost equally effective, *cf.* Table 19.

Table 19. *Conditioning for pancuronium*

Treatment[a]	Dyskinesia[b] (Positive/Total)	Mortality[b] (Dead/Total)
None	15/15	10/15
PCN	2/10 ***	3/10 NS
CS-1	2/10 ***	0/10 ***
Ethylestrenol	9/15 **	5/15 NS
Spironolactone	4/10 ***	0/10 ***
Norbolethone	9/10 NS	5/10 NS
Oxandrolone	8/10 NS	5/10 NS
Prednisolone-Ac	1/10 ***	1/10 **
Triamcinolone	5/10 ***	4/10 NS
Progesterone	8/10 NS	3/10 NS
Estradiol	8/10 NS	4/10 NS
DOC-Ac	9/10 NS	6/10 NS
Hydroxydione	7/10 NS	3/10 NS
Thyroxine	6/10 *	3/10 NS
Phenobarbital	7/10 NS	4/10 NS

[a] The rats of all groups were given pancuronium Br, 60 μg/100 g body weight in 0.2 ml water s.c. once on the 4th day.
[b] Dyskinesia was estimated 30 min after injection and mortality listed on the second day ("Exact Probability Test").

For further details on technique of tabulation *cf.* p. VIII.

Steroids (Δ^4-3-keto) ← Δ^4-3-keto: McGuire et al. *D 82,559/60*

[b] Student's t-test.
[c] Mortality listed on 30th day ("Exact Probability Test").

For further details on technique of tabulation *cf.* p. VIII.

← Steroids

NONSTEROIDAL HORMONES AND HORMONE-LIKE SUBSTANCES ←

ACTH ←

In guinea pigs, combined treatment with ACTH and estradiol allegedly produces extensive myocardial necroses, similar to the infarctoid cardiopathy elicited by steroids in combination with stress and certain sodium salts. However, these findings have not yet been confirmed.

ACTH ← estradiol cf. also Selye G60,083/70, p. 331.

Lupulescou E21,838/63: In guinea pigs, combined treatment with norepinephrine + estradiol or ACTH + estradiol produces extensive myocardial necrosis. "This infarctoid cardiopathy appears without any addition of phosphates or other sodium salts which is evidence of the fact that large doses of oestrogens prepare or sensitize the myocardium as regards the cardiotoxic action of noradrenalin or the corticotropic hormone."

STH ←

The interactions between STH and corticoids have been the subject of numerous studies. The hyalinosis syndrome produced by DOC in uninephrectomized NaCl-treated rats is aggravated by STH; indeed STH alone can produce malignant hypertension following conditioning by uninephrectomy + NaCl. These effects of STH are inhibited by cortisone as well as by adrenalectomy. Conversely, the cortisone-induced involutions of the adrenal cortex and thymus are inhibited by STH.

It is possible that STH exerts its toxic effect upon the kidney and the cardiovascular system (hyalinosis) only through (or at least in the presence of) a responsive adrenal cortex. Adrenal atrophy produced by cortisone or adrenalectomy prevents these toxic actions of STH. On the other hand, the prophlogistic and anabolic actions of STH are increased by DOC or aldosterone even after adrenalectomy.

STH ← glucocorticoids cf. also Selye B58,650/51, pp. 317, 357; C9,000/56, p. 58; G60,083/70, pp. 348, 357.

STH ← mineralocorticoids cf. also Selye B58,650/51, pp. 316, 357; C9,000/56, p. 59.

STH ← testoids cf. also Selye G60,083/70. pp. 374, 378.

Selye B53,940/51: In uninephrectomized NaCl-treated rats, the hyalinosis syndrome produced by DOC is aggravated by STH; indeed, STH alone can produce malignant hypertensive disease. These effects of STH are inhibited by cortisone. Apparently STH increases mineralocorticoid production by the adrenals (unless these are rendered atrophic by cortisone) and/or sensitizes the peripheral tissue to mineralocorticoids.

Selye B53,934/51: In rats conditioned by uninephrectomy + NaCl, both STH and DOC produce generalized hyalinosis and hypertension. The same as adrenalectomy or hypophysectomy, large doses of cortisone (which cause adrenocortical atrophy) prevent the cardiovascular and renal damage. "Apparently, STH exerts its toxic effects upon the kidney and the cardiovascular system only through (or at least in the presence of) a responsive adrenal cortex."

Selye B75,329/52: In rats the involution of the adrenal cortex and of the thymus as well as the antiphlogistic effect of cortisone are counteracted by simultaneous STH treatment. "Curiously, even those organs which normally undergo an absolute or relative increase in size as a result of either cortisone or STH treatment, e.g. the heart, kidney, liver, are maintained in an essentially normal weight range if both hormones are given conjointly."

Selye & Bois C1,718/55: In intact and in adrenalectomized rats, a synergism between mineralocorticoids (DOC, aldosterone) and STH was evident in their effects upon many target organs.

Wakabayashi et al. H27,784/70: In rats, exposure to stressors [kind not stated (H.S.)], or administration of dexamethasone suppresses plasma STH (radioimmunoassay) both in the presence and in the absence of the adrenals. Adrenalectomy increases plasma STH. [These findings support the view that during stress— perhaps owing to increased ACTH and/or glucocorticoid secretion, the "shift in pituitary hormone production" results in a diminished STH secretion (H.S.).]

Other Anterior Lobe Extracts ←

The preputial gland stimulating effect of crude anterior pituitary extract is enhanced by concurrent administration of pregnenolone, although in itself, the latter produces only very slight preputial gland stimulation.

Selye & Clarke 55,978/43: In the rat, Δ^5-pregnenolone greatly augments the preputial gland stimulating effect of crude anterior pituitary extracts. In itself, Δ^5-pregnenolone causes only very slight preputial gland stimulation and even this effect is abolished by hypophysectomy and hence is apparently dependent upon the simultaneous activity of hypophyseal hormones.

Rondell H32,853/70: In vitro experiments on the ovarian follicles of the pig suggest that LH, cyclic AMP or progesterone augment the distensibility of follicular strips, thereby preparing for rupture. TMACN blocks the effects of LH or cyclic AMP on both steroid release and distensibility. This blockade can be counteracted by progesterone. Presumably, "LH stimulates steroid secretion from the follicular tissue which in turn causes the activation of the ovulatory enzyme."

Dmowski et al. G80,777/71: In various species, Danazol (2,3 isoxazol derivative of 17α-ethinyl testosterone) was found to inhibit the effect of endogenous, but not of exogenous gonadotrophins. In addition, it had a mild testoid and progestational effect, but was devoid of antitestoid, antifolliculoid or antiluteoid properties.

Gonadotrophins ← Estradiol-17β, Progesterone: Brown et al. F57,759/65*

Posterior Pituitary Hormones ←

The production of renal cortical necrosis by vasopressin is facilitated in rats by pretreatment with estradiol or estrone. Though 5-HT produces similar renal lesions, their development is not modified by folliculoids. In ovariectomized weanling rats, pretreated with progesterone and estradiol, even oxytocin preparations produce renal cortical necrosis, although, by themselves, the latter have no such effect.

The metacorticoid hypertension produced by temporary overdosage with DOC + NaCl predisposes for the pressor effect of vasopressin and other vasopressor substances.

Posterior Pituiary Hormones ← *cf. also Selye G60,083/70, pp. 364, 369.*

Byrom A9,905/38: In rats, the production of renal cortical necrosis by vasopressin is facilitated by pretreatment with estradiol or estrone.

Sturtevant C9,089/55; C21,591/56: In rats with metacorticoid hypertension (produced by temporary overdosage with DOC + NaCl), the pressor effect of epinephrine, norepinephrine, vasopressin and renin was increased, but the effect of histamine, 5-HT, yohimbine and

TEA on the blood pressure was not consistently altered.

Szarvas & Kovács E 34,633/63: In the rat, estrone aggravates the renal necroses produced by posterior pituitary extracts, but not those elicited by 5-HT.

Moore G 11,771/64: In intact or ovariectomized weanling rats pretreated for ten days with progesterone and estradiol, renal cortical necrosis develops under the influence of oxytocin, whereas in itself, the latter is ineffective.

Thyroid Hormones ←

In rats, testoid extracts of urine have been claimed to counteract the adipose tissue atrophy and other manifestations of overdosage with desiccated thyroid. In baby rats, the retardation of tooth eruption and opening of the eyelids induced by thiouracil are inhibited by DOC, but the stunting of body growth and the thyroid changes themselves are not influenced by this steroid. Testosterone fails to affect the body and organ weight changes induced by thioureas in the rat. However, the thiourea-induced glycogen storage and pathologic changes in the liver are allegedly counteracted by testosterone, whereas the glycogenolytic action of thyroid is prevented by cortisone. The pulmonary edema induced in rats by thiourea (or other agents such as NH_4Cl, epinephrine, chloropicrin) are prevented by the administration, 5 min earlier, of a single dose of prednisolone i.v. On the other hand, prednisolone aggravates the myopathy produced by thyroid overdosage in the rat.

Extensive recent studies performed in our Institute show that, in general, catatoxic steroids are not particularly efficient in preventing the body weight loss produced by large doses of T3. The comparatively mild protective effect exerted in this respect by ethylestrenol and norbolethone may well be ascribed to the anabolic effect of these steroids. On the other hand, the glucocorticoids, prednisolone and triamcinolone, as well as estradiol, greatly aggravate the toxicity of T3. The prostration and mortality induced by high doses of propylthiouracil are counteracted by PCN, CS-1 and several other potent catatoxic steroids, but the thyroid enlargement induced by small amounts of this goitrogen is further enhanced by PCN, which possesses a mild goitrogenic effect itself.

In guinea pigs, the weight loss produced by thyroxine can be counteracted by cardiac glycosides or DOC.

In dogs, estradiol stimulates the proliferation of spongy bone, an effect which is inhibited by thyroidectomy and enhanced by thyroxine.

Methenolone (a testoid) antagonizes the catabolic effect of desiccated thyroid or of prednisolone in **man**.

Thyroid Hormones ← *corticoids cf. also Selye G 60,083/70, pp. 347, 355.*

Korenchevsky et al. 16,451/33: In the rat, a testoid extract prepared from urine failed to influence the decrease in fat deposition and other manifestations of overdosage with desiccated thyroid.

Kinsell et al. A 37,369/42: Experiments on guinea pigs and mice suggested that "therapeutic dosage of cardiac steroid-glycosides prevents a weight loss in thyroxin-treated animals similar to that obtained with adrenal cortical hormone and desoxycorticosterone acetate. Larger dosage of these cardiac glycosides either fails to modify such weight loss or actually increases it."

Oettel & Franck A 72,420/42: In rats, DOC allegedly offers some protection against the hepatic changes produced by thyroxine or allylformiate.

Parmer B 17,568/47: In baby rats, the retardation of tooth eruption and of the opening of the eyelids induced by thiouracil is counteracted by DOC. However, the stunting of body growth and the thyroid changes produced by thiouracil are not influenced by DOC.

Benoit & Clavert B 27,669/48: In ducks, estradiol stimulates the proliferation of spongy bone consisting of fine trabeculae. Thyroidectomy retards this bone proliferation, whereas conjoint treatment with thyroxine and estradiol leads to the abundant development of thick trabeculae.

Leathem B 38,768/48: In rats the effect of thiourea and thiouracil upon body and organ weights is not significantly influenced by testosterone.

Kar et al. C 17,531/55: In rats, thiourea causes glycogen storage and severe pathologic changes in the liver. Testosterone counteracts these lesions.

Kusama C 58,473/57: In rats, the glycogenolytic action of thyroid feeding is counteracted by cortisone.

Henschler & Reich C 71,216/59: In rats, the pulmonary edema induced by ammonium chloride, epinephrine, thiourea, or chloropicrin is prevented by the administration about 5 min earlier of a single large dose of prednisolone i.v.

Weller D 13,995/61; D 22,262/62: In man, methenolone antagonizes the catabolic effect of prednisolone and desiccated thyroid.

Cavalca F 83,698/67: Prednisolone greatly aggravates the myopathy produced by thyroid overdosage in the rat.

Selye G 70,480/71: In rats, none of the standard conditioners (with the possible exception of ethylestrenol and norbolethone) was conspicuously effective in preventing the catabolism produced by overdosage with T3. Prednisolone and estradiol actually increased the catabolic effect of the thyroid hormone. The mortality resulting from T3 overdosage appears to have been diminished by estradiol, but aggravated by triamcinolone, *cf.* Table 20.

Selye 70,480/71: In rats, all the classic catatoxic steroids and phenobarbital readily inhibit propylthiouracil intoxication. Progesterone has a dubious prophylactic effect, *cf.* Table 21.

Table 20. *Conditioning for T3 (3,3,5-Triiodo-L-thyronine)*

Treatment[a]	Final body weight[b] (g)	Mortality[c] (Dead/Total)
None (untreated)	161 ± 3 ***	0/5
None (T₃ treated)	105 ± 4	6/10
PCN	105 ± 3 NS	6/15 NS
PCN (1 mg)	115 ± 3 NS	8/10 NS
CS-1	118 ± 6 NS	6/10 NS
Ethylestrenol	117 ± 4 *	3/10 NS
Spironolactone	115 ± 6 NS	6/10 NS
Norbolethone	121 ± 4 **	4/10 NS
Oxandrolone	107 ± 5 NS	2/10 NS
Prednisolone-Ac	78 ± 5 ***	5/10 NS
Triamcinolone	—	10/10 ±
Progesterone	106 ± 4 NS	8/10 NS
Estradiol	83 ± 2 ***	0/10 **
DOC-Ac	99 ± 4 NS	6/10 NS
Hydroxydione	108 ± 4 NS	8/10 NS
Thyroxine	106 ± 4 NS	8/10 NS
Phenobarbital	114 ± 3 NS	8/10 NS

[a] The rats of all groups (except the 1st) were given T₃ (200 µg/100 g body weight in 0.2 ml water, s.c., twice daily from 4th day ff.).

[b] Student's t-test. All statistics in comparison with 2nd group.

[c] Mortality listed on 12th day ("Exact Probability Test").

For further details on technique of tabulation *cf.* p. VIII.

Table 21. *Conditioning for high doses of propylthiouracil*

Treatment[a]	Dyskinesia[b] (Positive/Total)	Mortality[b] (Dead/Total)
None	10/10	4/10
PCN	0/10 ***	0/10 *
CS-1	3/10 ***	0/10 *
Ethylestrenol	3/10 ***	3/10 NS
Spironolactone	3/10 ***	3/10 NS
Norbolethone	2/10 ***	1/10 NS
Oxandrolone	3/10 ***	0/10 *
Prednisolone-Ac	7/10 NS	3/10 NS
Triamcinolone	10/10 NS	9/10 ±
Progesterone	6/10 *	1/10 NS
Estradiol	7/10 NS	4/10 NS
DOC-Ac	7/10 NS	2/10 NS
Hydroxydione	7/10 NS	1/10 NS
Thyroxine	10/10 NS	9/10 ±
Phenobarbital	0/10 ***	0/10 *

[a] The rats of all groups were given propylthiouracil (30 mg/100 g body weight in 0.15 ml DMSO, i.p., once on 4th day).

[b] Dyskinesia was estimated 3 hrs after injection and mortality listed 24 hrs later ("Exact Probability Test").

For further details on technique of tabulation *cf.* p. VIII.

Selye PROT. 36736: In rats, the thyroid enlargement produced by small doses of propylthiouracil is increased by PCN (which has a slight goitrogenic effect of its own) and decreased by suitable doses of glucocorticoids, estradiol, DOC and thyroxine. Several of the standard conditioning agents, particularly glucocorticoids, also interfere with the normal gain in body weight. Finally, large doses of glucocorticoids cause considerable mortality in the presence of propylthiouracil overdosage, *cf.* Table 22.

Table 22. *Conditioning for low doses of propylthiouracil*

Treatment[a]	Thyroid weight[b] (mg)	Final body weight[c] (g)	Mortality[c] (Dead/Total)
None	14.8 ± 0.6[c]	151 ± 2	0/15
PCN	23.1 ± 1.4 ***	145 ± 3 NS	0/5 NS
CS-1	14.3 ± 0.8 NS	152 ± 3 NS	0/10 NS
Ethylestrenol	12.9 ± 0.4 *	152 ± 3 NS	0/10 NS
Spironolactone	17.3 ± 0.8 *	148 ± 2 NS	0/10 NS
Norbolethone	15.9 ± 1.3 NS	160 ± 2 *	0/10 NS
Oxandrolone	14.3 ± 0.9 NS	145 ± 3 NS	0/10 NS
Prednisolone-Ac	12.1 ± 0.6 **	80 ± 1 ***	5/10 ***
Prednisolone-Ac (100 µg)	11.4 ± 1.1 *	120 ± 3 ***	0/5 NS
Triamcinolone	8.7 ± 0.8 ***	65 ± 2 ***	8/10 ***
Triamcinolone (100 µg)	13.1 ± 0.5 *	113 ± 3 ***	0/5 NS
Progesterone	13.8 ± 0.9 NS	138 ± 2 ***	0/10 NS
Estradiol	13.3 ± 0.8 NS	97 ± 2 ***	0/10 NS
Estradiol (100 µg)	11.5 ± 0.8 **	128 ± 3 ***	0/5 NS
DOC-Ac	12.2 ± 0.7 **	138 ± 2 ***	0/10 NS
Hydroxydione	13.5 ± 0.9 NS	139 ± 2 **	0/10 NS
Thyroxine	8.5 ± 0.5 ***	139 ± 4 *	0/10 NS
Phenobarbital	15.0 ± 1.2 NS	144 ± 2 *	0/10 NS

[a] The rats of all groups were given propylthiouracil (25 µg/100 g body weight in 0.1 ml DMSO, i.p., twice daily from 4th day ff.).

[b] The thyroid weight in completely untreated control rats (receiving no propylthiouracil) was 9.5 ± 0.5.

[c] Mortality was listed on 13th day ("Exact Probability Test"), simultaneously with thyroid weight and final body weight (Student's t-test). For further details on technique of tabulation *cf.* p. VIII.

Parathyroid Hormones

In rats, pretreatment with **DOC** allegedly inhibits the nephrocalcinosis produced by parathyroid extract.

Cortisone antagonizes the effect of parathyroid extract upon the teeth and bones of the rat, simultaneously inhibiting hypercalcemia and nephrocalcinosis. Cortisone also prevents the accumulation of strontium and calcium in the kidney, as well as their urinary elimination following parathyroid extract injection. The elevation of serum total glycoproteins induced by parathyroid extract as well as the associated nephrocalcinosis can be prevented by cortisone, although the latter does not prevent the nonspecific elevation of serum glycoproteins induced by turpentine. Even the production of osteitis fibrosa and of an increase in gastric mucus production are inhibited by glucocorticoids in the rat.

Small doses of **estradiol** increase the cortical nephrocalcinosis in parathyroid extract treated rats. In hens, folliculoids increase blood calcium, but do not augment the hypercalcemic action of parathyroid extract. Both hormone preparations cause osteosclerosis in chickens, but the lesions are qualitatively distinct.

Parathyroid Hormones ← corticoids cf. also Selye G60,083/70, pp. 347, 354.

Baker et al. C24,277/54: In rats, pretreatment with DOC greatly diminishes the nephrocalcinosis normally produced by parathyroid hormone.

Bacon et al. C26,675/56: In rats, parathyroid extract increases the urinary excretion of radioactive calcium and strontium, as well as the deposition of these elements in the kidney. Cortisone prevents the accumulation of strontium and calcium in the kidney, but does not influence their urinary excretion under these conditions.

Laron et al. C47,872/58: In rats, cortisone antagonizes the effect of parathyroid extract upon the teeth and bones; it also inhibits hypercalcemia and nephrocalcinosis.

Bradford et al. D76,315/60: In rats, cortisone prevents the elevation of serum total glycoproteins induced by parathyroid extract as well as the associated nephrocalcinosis. Cortisone does not prevent the nonspecific elevation of serum glycoproteins resulting from turpentine injections.

Urist et al. C95,236/60: In hens, parathyroid extract and "equine estrogenic substances" had an additive effect on blood calcium and bone structure. Both hormone preparations caused osteosclerosis although of a different type and, whereas parathyroid extract increased ultrafilterable calcium, the folliculoid preparation augmented the nonultrafilterable fraction of the serum calcium.

Grob et al. E20,745/63: Small doses of estradiol increase cortical nephrocalcinosis in the parathyroid extract treated rat.

Stoerk et al. G5,410/63: In rats, the production of osteitis fibrosa by parathyroid extract is inhibited through cortisol.

Menguy & Masters F17,447/64: In rats, parathyroid extract greatly increases the production of gastric mucus and this effect can be partially blocked by cortisone.

Pancreatic Hormones ←

In rats, adrenocortical extracts (with predominantly **glucocorticoid** activity) proved to inhibit both insulin hypoglycemia and epinephrine hyperglycemia. It was concluded that "cortin exerts a stabilizing effect upon the blood sugar." In mice, ACTH and glucocorticoids increase insulin resistance, as judged by toxicity tests. The renal changes produced by alloxan are aggravated by cortisone in guinea pigs but not in rats. The mortality induced by phenformin (an oral antidiabetic) is diminished by cortisol in rats but not in dogs.

DOC allegedly antagonizes the toxic actions of insulin, and in combination with the latter can produce extreme obesity in rats. It also protects against alloxan diabetes.

Fluoxymesterone renders the rat hypersensitive to insulin shock, perhaps because this **testoid** induces adrenocortical atrophy. Durabolin (another anabolic testoid) decreases alloxan ketosis in the rat, whereas diethylstilbestrol tends to aggravate it, at least on certain diets.

In rabbits, alloxan diabetes is not significantly affected by DOC, testosterone or **progesterone**, whereas **stilbestrol** rapidly decreases alloxan hyperglycemia in both sexes. The toxicity of tolbutamide is increased by stilbestrol in the rat.

Selye & Dosne A 30,701/39: In rats, under certain conditions, an adrenocortical extract may inhibit both insulin hypoglycemia and epinephrine hyperglycemia. "It appears that cortin exerts a stabilizing effect on the blood sugar."

Jensen & Grattan 77,887/40: In mice, ACTH, glucocorticoids and cortical extracts increase insulin resistance, whereas other pituitary hormones and thyroxine have no such effect.

Levens & Swann 80,483/41: In rats, DOC antagonizes the toxic actions of insulin, and in combination with the latter, produces extreme obesity.

Ingle et al. B 3,163/47: In rats, diethylstilbestrol tends to aggravate alloxan diabetes but its effect depends upon the diet.

Carrasco & Vargas B 50,792/49: In rabbits, alloxan diabetes is not significantly affected by DOC, testosterone or progesterone. Stilbestrol rapidly decreases alloxan hyperglycemia in both sexes.

Grunert & Phillips B 48,993/49: In rats, DOC protects against alloxan diabetes.

Avezzu et al. C 12,653/54: In guinea pigs, the renal changes produced by alloxan are aggravated by cortisone.

Penhos & Blaquier C 59,755/58: The mortality induced by phenformin (an oral antidiabetic) is diminished by cortisol and epinephrine in rats but not in dogs.

Greenberg D 21,811/62: In the rat, the renal changes produced by alloxan are not significantly affected by cortisone.

McColl & Sacra D 34,973/62: "Pretreatment of female Sprague-Dawley rats with diethylstilbestrol for 15 days significantly increased the acute toxic effect of tolbutamide, isobuzote, terbuzole, and insulin. Testosterone pretreatment resulted in a significant decrease in toxicity of tolbutamide, isobuzole, and terbuzole but not of insulin."

Grella E 21,538/63: Pretreatment with fluoxymesterone renders the rat hypersensitive to insulin shock, allegedly because this testoid produces adrenocortical atrophy.

Rudas & Weissel E 34,762/63: Nandrolone decreases alloxan ketosis in the rat.

Pokrajac et al. G 49,275/67: Review of the literature and personal observations on the increased insulin resistance of cortisol-treated rats.

Isacson & Nilsson G 80,478/70: In healthy men, combined treatment with phenformin and ethylestrenol raised the fibrinolytic activity of the blood and the platelet adhesiveness. Thus, "the combined treatment produced changes tending to counteract the development of thrombosis."

Epinephrine, Norepinephrine ←

As previously stated, under certain conditions, **glucocorticoid** adrenal extracts may inhibit both insulin hypoglycemia and epinephrine hyperglycemia in rats. That is why we concluded that "cortin exerts a stabilizing effect upon the blood sugar."

Prednisone pretreatment facilitates the production of pulmonary edema by small doses of epinephrine in rabbits. On the other hand, in the rat, pulmonary edema induced by epinephrine (or thiourea, chloropicrin or NH_4Cl) is prevented by the administration of a single dose of prednisolone 5 min earlier. In dogs, prednisolone failed to protect against shock induced by epinephrine or norepinephrine.

Both in rats and in dogs, the pressor action of epinephrine and norepinephrine (as well as that of renin and angiotensin) is considerably enhanced by previous uninephrectomy and treatment with **DOC** + NaCl.

Pretreatment with **stilbestrol** diminishes the severity of pulmonary edema following epinephrine treatment in guinea pigs. On the other hand, combined treatment with norepinephrine and estradiol produces extensive myocardial necrosis in guinea pigs, similar to the ESCN produced in rats.

In rabbits, the production of calcifying aortic lesions by epinephrine is partially inhibited by adrenosterone, a **testoid** compound, although normally males are more sensitive than females to this type of arteriosclerosis.

Epinephrine, Norepinephrine ← corticoids cf. also Selye B 58,650/51, p. 322; C 92,918/61, pp. 107, 109, 111; G 60,083/70, pp. 347, 352.

Epinephrine, Norepinephrine ← folliculoids cf. also Selye G 60,083/70, pp. 364, 368.

Epinephrine, Norepinephrine ← luteoids cf. also Selye G 60,083/70, p. 370.

Epinephrine, Norepinephrine ← testoids cf. also Selye G 60,083/70, p. 379.

Selye & Dosne A 30,701/39: In rats, under certain conditions, the adrenocortical extract may inhibit both insulin hypoglycemia and epinephrine hyperglycemia. "It appears that cortin exerts a stabilizing effect on the blood sugar."

Masson et al. B 47,635/50: In dogs pretreated with DOC + uninephrectomy + NaCl, the hypotensive effect of TEA was not significantly altered. Similarly, both in rats and in dogs, the pressor action of epinephrine, norepinephrine, renin and angiotensin was not consistently altered by previous uninephrectomy and treatment with DOC + NaCl.

Franco C 27,538/54: In guinea pigs, pretreatment with testosterone does not modify the development of pulmonary edema following the administration of epinephrine.

Giuseppe C 27,530/54: In guinea pigs, pretreatment with stilbestrol diminishes the severity of pulmonary edema following treatment with epinephrine.

Sturtevant C 9,089/55; C 21,591/56: In rats with metacorticoid hypertension (produced by temporary overdosage with DOC + NaCl), the pressor effect of epinephrine, norepinephrine, vasopressin and renin was increased, but the effect of histamine, 5-HT, yohimbine and TEA on the blood pressure was not consistently altered.

Barbe C 46,902/57: In rabbits, prednisone pretreatment facilitates the production of fatal pulmonary edema by small doses of epinephrine.

Moss & Dury C 44,068/57: In rabbits, the development of cholesterol atherosclerosis is inhibited by cortisone, and the regression of already established lesions accelerated. The epinephrine-induced aortic medial necrosis is not prevented by cortisone, but the fibroblast reaction in the lesions is inhibited.

Plotka et al. C 51,239/57: In rabbits, the production of aortic lesions by epinephrine i.v. is partly inhibited by adrenosterone; yet, normally males are more sensitive than females to epinephrine arteriosclerosis.

Henschler & Reich C 71,216/59: In rats, the pulmonary edema induced by ammonium chloride, epinephrine, thiourea or chloropicrin is prevented by the administration about 5 min earlier of a single large dose of prednisolone i.v.

Lupulescou E 21,838/63: In guinea pigs, combined treatment with norepinephrine + estradiol or ACTH + estradiol produces extensive myocardial necrosis. "This infarctoid cardiopathy appears without any addition of phosphates or other sodium salts which is evidence of the fact that large doses of oestrogens prepare or sensitize the myocardium as regards the cardiotoxic action of noradrenalin or the corticotropic hormone."

Szabó et al. G 44,867/66: In dogs, prednisolone failed to protect against shock induced by epinephrine or norepinephrine.

Motsay et al. H 32,852/70: In dogs, massive doses of glucocorticoids (e.g., methylprednisolone) can offer protection against circulatory shock produced by overdosage with epinephrine or endotoxin. The prophylactic effect is ascribed primarily to a protection of the microcirculation.

Selye PROT. 32804: In rats, none of the conditioning agents of our series offered any significant protection against acute intoxica-

Table 23. *Conditioning for epinephrine*

Treatment[a]	Dyskinesia[b] (Positive/Total)	Mortality[b] (Dead/Total)
None	3/10	0/10
PCN	7/10 NS	3/10 NS
CS-1	6/10 NS	2/10 NS
Ethylestrenol	7/10 NS	0/10 NS
Spironolactone	5/10 NS	1/10 NS
Norbolethone	6/10 NS	1/10 NS
Oxandrolone	4/10 NS	0/10 NS
Prednisolone-Ac	2/10 NS	5/10 *
Triamcinolone	5/10 NS	7/10 ***
Progesterone	5/10 NS	2/10 NS
Estradiol	8/10 *	4/10 *
DOC-Ac	6/9 NS	0/9 NS
Hydroxydione	8/10 *	2/10 NS
Thyroxine	9/9 ***	8/9 ***
Phenobarbital	8/10 *	3/10 NS

[a] The rats of all groups were given epinephrine bitartrate (1.5 mg/100 g body weight in 0.2 ml water, s.c., once on 4th day).

[b] Dyskinesia was estimated 5 hrs after injection and mortality listed 24 hrs later ("Exact Probability Test").

For further details on technique of tabulation cf. p. VIII.

tion with epinephrine. The glucocorticoids and thyroxine actually decreased resistance to this catecholamine. The apparent increase in epinephrine sensitivity induced by estradiol hydroxydione and phenobarbital was barely significant, *cf.* Table 23, p. 144.

Histamine ←

Earlier observations suggested that in mice and rats, adrenocortical extract or DOC, in combination with NaCl, can raise histamine resistance above normal. This has subsequently been confirmed with cortisol and DOC as regards the hypotensive effect of histamine in rats. Yet, in new-born rats, fatal intoxication with histamine was not significantly influenced by cortisol, cortisone, corticosterone or ACTH.

In rats given histamine by aerosol, or egg-white i.p., an asthmatic attack ensues if the lung was previously irritated by inhalation of acetic acid. This response is obtained in females, castrate males, and in intact males treated with folliculoids, but not in normal males. Testosterone and progesterone abolish this effect in females and castrate males, thus indicating a sex hormone dependence of histamine resistance.

In rats, complete blockade of the sympathetic system by adrenal demedullation, combined with reserpine or bretylium-like agents or with ganglioplegics, causes a considerable increase in histamine sensitivity, comparable in degree to that induced by complete adrenalectomy. Epinephrine alone counteracts the lethality of histamine after such sympathetic blockade, but cortisone offers only partial protection. Presumably, sympathetic stimulation is "the first line of defense" against the vasomotor disturbances produced by histamine and, in this respect, is more important than cortisone, although the latter offers greater protection against other stressors.

In mice, sensitized by histamine plus pertussis vaccine, cortisol and cortisone increased, whereas DOC decreased resistance to shock produced by this combined treatment.

In guinea pigs, ACTH and cortisone failed to protect against histamine shock or anaphylaxis.

Perla et al. A 31,863/40: In mice and rats, pretreatment with NaCl in combination with DOC or adrenocortical extract increased resistance to histamine. Favorable results have also been obtained by DOC plus NaCl in a few patients suffering from surgical shock.

Malkiel G 71,451/51: In guinea pigs, ACTH and cortisone are without effect on the end results of histamine shock, or of passive or active anaphylaxis.

Malkiel & Hargis D 27,396/52: Cortisone s.c. protects the rat against histamine intoxication even after sensitization by pertussis vaccine.

Kind B 81,943/53: In H. pertussis-inoculated mice, cortisone inhibits the lethal effect of both histamine and H. pertussis vaccine. Cortisone also protects uninoculated mice against lethal intoxication with this vaccine.

Sackler et al. B 78,749/53: In rats, thyroparathyroidectomy increases histamine tolerance, but only in females. Intact rats show no sex difference in histamine tolerance. Gonadectomy raises histamine tolerance in both sexes.

Chédid C 622/54: Pertussis vaccine sensitizes the intact mouse both to histamine and to typhoid endotoxin. Under these conditions, both phenergan and cortisone protect the animals against fatal doses of histamine but not against endotoxin. In adrenalectomized mice, cortisone does protect against endotoxin.

Gross C 30,649/55: In rats, administration of histamine by aerosol, or of egg-white i.p. elicits an asthmatic attack if the lung was previously irritated by inhalation of acetic acid given by a spray. This response is obtained in females, castrate males or males treated with folliculoids, but not in normal males. Testosterone and progesterone abolish this effect in females and castrate males.

Lecomte D12,212/61: Both cortisol and DOC increase the resistance of the rat to the hypotensive effect of histamine i.v.

Higginbotham D21,395/62: In mice, resistance to 5-HT, endotoxin and anaphylactic shock is markedly decreased by adrenalectomy. Cortisol readily restored resistance to 5-HT, but was less effective with regard to endotoxin and anaphylactic shock. Resistance to histamine and histamine releasers is less markedly diminished by adrenalectomy in the mouse, and large doses of cortisol are required to induce a measurable increase in resistance to histamine.

Lecomte & Sodoyez D20,641/62: The hypotension and shock produced by endogenous histamine liberation following treatment with compound L-1935 in the rat is not significantly influenced by cortisol or DOC.

Pekárek & Vrána D52,098/62: In rats sensitized to histamine by pertussis vaccine, DOC decreases resistance to the combined treatment.

Munoz E8,473/64: Cortisone and cortisol protect the pertussis-sensitized mouse against histamine, cold and anaphylaxis even after adrenalectomy.

Schapiro F31,856/65: In newborn rats, fatal intoxication with histamine was not significantly influenced by ACTH, cortisol, cortisone or corticosterone.

Krawczak & Brodie H25,296/70: In rats, complete blockade of sympathetic function can be achieved by demedullation combined with reserpine-like agents (depleting catecholamine stores), bretylium-like agents (preventing nerve impulse from releasing catecholamines) or ganglioplegics. Following such total sympathetic blockade, mortality from histamine or endotoxin is as markedly increased as by adrenalectomy. Pretreatment with epinephrine alone counteracts the increased lethality of endotoxin and histamine after sympathetic blockade. Cortisone pretreatment only partially corrects the sensitization by adrenalectomy, whereas cortisone + epinephrine offers complete protection against these agents. Presumably, sympathetic stimulation is "the first line of defense against the vasomotor disturbance elicited by endotoxin and histamine." The lethal effect of formalin or tourniquet shock is likewise greatly increased by adrenalectomy, but in contrast to that of endotoxin and histamine, it cannot be increased by sympathetic blockade. Furthermore, cortisone alone counteracts the toxicity of these stressors in adrenalectomized rats. Apparently "formalin and tourniquet shock is initiated by a mechanism which differs from that elicited by histamine and endotoxin and does not primarily involve the sympathetic system."

Histamine ← Ovariectomy: Sackler et al. B78,749/53*

5-HT ←

In rats, metacorticoid hypertension does not influence the effect of 5-HT upon blood pressure.

The gastric ulcers produced by large doses of 5-HT in the rat are prevented by cortisol and aggravated by DOC.

The production of renal infarcts by 5-HT is partially prevented by hypophysectomy, DOC, or testosterone, uninfluenced by ACTH, and aggravated by cortisone. On the other hand, such renal necroses are also inhibited by the stress of restraint, both in intact and in adrenalectomized rats. Estradiol aggravates the 5-HT induced renal necroses, whereas estrone allegedly has no such sensitizing effect.

The 5-HT content of the brain decreases after cortisol treatment, presumably through the induction of hepatic TPO.

Sturtevant C9,089/55; C21,591/56: In rats with metacorticoid hypertension (produced by temporary overdosage with DOC + NaCl) the pressor effect of epinephrine, norepinephrine, vasopressin and renin was increased, but the effect of histamine, 5-HT, yohimbine and TEA on the blood pressure was not consistently altered.

Selye & Bois C 23,958/57: The gastric ulcers produced by large doses of 5-HT in the rat can be prevented by cortisol, and aggravated by DOC.

Jasmin & Bois C 92,099/60: Hypophysectomy partially protects the rat against the production of renal infarcts by 5-HT. ACTH does not affect this change; cortisol aggravates it, whereas DOC and testosterone offer partial protection against it. Estradiol pretreatment sensitizes the rat for the production of ischemic renal infarcts by 5-HT.

Higginbotham D 21,395/62: In mice, resistance to 5-HT, endotoxin, and anaphylactic shock is markedly decreased by adrenalectomy. Cortisol readily restored resistance to 5-HT, but was less effective with regard to endotoxin and anaphylactic shock. Resistance to histamine and histamine releasers is less markedly diminished by adrenalectomy in the mouse, and large doses of cortisol are required to induce a measurable increase in resistance to histamine.

Szarvas & Kovács E 34,633/63: In the rat, estrone aggravates the renal necroses produced by posterior pituitary extracts, but not those elicited by 5-HT.

Selye et al. E 24,146/64: The renal necroses normally produced in rats by acute intoxication with 5-HT can be inhibited by forced restraint both in intact and in adrenalectomized rats. Cortisol has no such inhibitory effect.

Green & Curzon H 5,891/68: In the rat, the 5-HT content of the brain decreases after treatment with cortisol, presumably through the induction of TPO in the liver.

5-HT(N-acetyl) ← Prednisolone: Inscoe et al. *F 70,325/66*

Various Tissue Extracts ←

A few publications deal with the effect of steroids upon the toxicity of crude tissue extracts. For example, estradiol increases, whereas progesterone and adrenocortical extract decrease the toxicity of menstrual discharge injected s.c. into rats.

In mice, adrenocortical extract diminishes the toxicity of the peritoneal exudate elicited by intestinal strangulation.

Submandibular gland grafts obtained from testosterone-treated donors are said to be highly toxic to mice, although testosterone is not toxic in the presence of submandibular glands. Apparently, the latter do not release the induced toxic factor.

In rabbits, aldosterone and cortisone increased, whereas spironolactone inhibited the angiotensin-induced glycosuria.

Smith & Smith A 32,972/40: In rats, the toxicity of menstrual discharge s.c. is increased by estradiol and diminished by progesterone or adrenocortical extract pretreatment. Gonadectomy offers moderate protection in both sexes. DOC is ineffective.

Laufman & Freed 88,861/43: In mice, adrenocortical extract diminishes the toxicity of the peritoneal transudate of dogs with intestinal strangulation.

Hori et al. G 72,331/69: In rabbits, aldosterone and cortisone increased the angiotensin-induced glycosuria, whereas spironolactone inhibited it.

Lin & Hoshino H 9,995/69: "Submandibular grafts obtained from both immature male and adult female donors which received pretreatment with testosterone enanthate exerted a lethal effect on the hosts. Large dosages of testosterone enanthate, which obviously increased the lethal factor level in the submandibular gland, did not kill normal intact adult mice; nor did it increase the mortality of bilaterally submandibular-sialoadenectomized immature mice beyond that of controls without testosterone treatment, when they were not transplanted."

DRUGS

The effect of steroids upon numerous intoxications has been the subject of many investigations which could hardly be condensed more than has been done in the Abstract Section. Here, we shall comment only on a few particularly interesting data and on observations which can be clarified by correlating them with facts not mentioned in the original articles.

Anaphylactoidogens

The production of anaphylactoid edema by various mast cell dischargers, histamine, or 5-HT, is facilitated by mineralocorticoids and inhibited by glucocorticoids, as are other forms of acute inflammatory reactions.

The gastric ulcers and the anaphylactoid edema produced by such mast cell dischargers as 48/80 or polymyxin are likewise prevented by various glucocorticoids and by stressors, although both these steroids and stress, are capable of producing gastric ulcers in themselves. Curiously, DOC likewise prevents polymyxin-induced gastric erosions.

When, following pretreatment with polymyxin, the gastric mucosa is depleted of histamine, the ulcerogenic property of prednisolone overdosage is unimpaired; hence, histamine liberation cannot be responsible for glucocorticoid-induced gastric ulceration.

Curiously, the cardiovascular and renal calcification produced by chronic treatment with polymyxin is increased by triamcinolone, DOC, or by combined treatment with both these steroids. Fluorocortisol, which possesses both gluco- and mineralocorticoid properties, also shares this effect.

Anticoagulants

The "hemorrhagic stress syndrome" can be produced by indirect anticoagulants (phenindione, dicoumarol, warfarin) subsequent pretreatment with various stressors, ACTH, STH or DOC. Conversely, cortisone, epinephrine, ephedrine and adrenochrome inhibit this syndrome.

In man, some testoids (methandrostenolone, norethandrolone) increase the anticoagulant response after pretreatment with warfarin, phenindione, or bishydroxycoumarin. It has been assumed that certain steroids can increase the affinity of receptor sites for anticoagulants.

On the other hand, in rats, the fatal hemorrhagic diathesis produced by phenindione is inhibited by pretreatment with numerous catatoxic steroids such as PCN, ethylestrenol, CS-1, spironolactone, norbolethone and oxandrolone. Progesterone, hydroxydione, DOC, and estradiol have a much less pronounced effect. Prednisolone, triamcinolone, and thyroxine are inactive.

It has been shown at least for spironolactone, norbolethone, and ethylestrenol that these catatoxic steroids actually enhance the disappearance of bishydroxycoumarin from the blood, and restore the prothrombin time. Triamcinolone and progesterone fail to do so.

SKF 525-A increases the blood concentration and the anticoagulant effect of bishydroxycoumarin, counteracting the beneficial effect of ethylestrenol.

Barbiturates ←

Barbiturates are probably the most extensively used nonsteroidal catatoxic substances. Interest in them has been hightened by the fact that they also act as excellent substrates for both steroidal and nonsteroidal enzyme inducers. Furthermore, it is easy to determine changes in barbiturate activity in vivo, by measuring either the "sleeping time" (the interval between the loss and the reappearance of the righting reflex) or the depth of the anesthesia induced by threshold doses (expressed in an arbitrary scale, ranging from wobbly gait to surgical narcosis). Both types of measurement have their advantages and disadvantages. The sleeping time reflects the duration of anesthesia, but does not distinguish between mere abolition of the righting reflex and almost lethal narcosis, if the duration of action is the same. Conversely, measurement of the depth of anesthesia does not reflect its duration. Most of the published experimental work is based on measurements of sleeping time.

← **Glucocorticoids.** Soon after the introduction of cortisone into clinical medicine, it was noted that it often helped to combat abstinence symptoms following discontinuation of barbiturates or morphine in man.

The anesthetic effect of various barbiturates is shortened by cortisone, cortisol and other glucocorticoids, both in rats and in mice. Although, barbital is not metabolized in the body, its anesthetic effect in mice is likewise diminished by glucocorticoids. It has been claimed, however, that pretreatment with cortisol, two hours before pentobarbital intoxication increases the lethal effect of the latter in mice. The protection of mice against barbital anesthesia is ascribed to a glucocorticoid-induced decrease in the barbital concentration of the brain. In rabbits, barbital anesthesia and the barbital content of the blood are not significantly influenced by cortisone, although urinary barbital elimination is increased.

In patients recovering from barbiturate poisoning, sleep is often re-induced by cortisone or i.v. injection of glucose.

Pretreatment of rats with cortisone or prednisolone for three days diminishes the anesthetic effect of hexobarbital and increases its degradation by liver slices.

When given simultaneously, cortisol prolongs pentobarbital sleeping time, but if the hormone is given one day before the barbiturate, the anesthetic effect of the latter is shortened.

Pretreatment with cortisone also prolongs phenobarbital anesthesia in guinea pigs and hexobarbital anesthesia in mice, although it shortens thiopental anesthesia in rabbits.

In rats, ACTH and cortisone decrease hexobarbital sleeping time, as does exposure to stress, whereas SKF 525-A blocks the protective effect of stress. In dogs, DDT decreases hexobarbital sleeping time but prolongs pentobarbital anesthesia. The latter effect is prevented by cortisone.

Brain hyperexcitability induced in rats by cortisone is diminished by phenobarbital as judged by EST measurements.

On the basis of these findings, it would be difficult to formulate any meaningful generalizations concerning the action of glucocorticoids upon barbiturate anesthesia. The latter depends upon species, timing, and the type of barbiturate used, but in general, a shortening of the hypnotic effect may be expected as long as the glucocorticoid is administered before the barbiturate.

← **Gluco-Mineralocorticoids, Mineralocorticoids.** Comparatively few investigations deal with the effect of gluco-mineralocorticoids or mineralocorticoids upon barbiturate anesthesia. Since several of these steroids are strong anesthetics themselves, combined treatment with barbiturates usually results in a summation of their effects. In our own experience, pretreatment with DOC did not significantly influence the duration of pentobarbital anesthesia in rats, unless the steroid was given just before the barbiturate so as to permit the summation of their actions.

← **Antimineralocorticoids.** In rats, pentobarbital sleeping time is shortened by pretreatment with aldadiene, aldadiene-kalium, spironolactone, CS-1 and several other antimineralocorticoids tested. These observations agree with the concept that antimineralocorticoids are in general powerful catatoxic steroids.

← **Testoids.** All strong anabolic testoids appear to shorten barbiturate anesthesia in general. However, barbital is not metabolized by hepatic microsomal enzymes and is consequently resistant to detoxication by microsomal enzyme-inducing steroids.

There appears to be a species difference in the effect of testoids upon barbiturate anesthesia, since in rats, testosterone shortens, whereas in mice it allegedly prolongs pentobarbital anesthesia. In any event, even physiologic doses of testoids appear to confer relative resistance to male rats, since castration increases their barbiturate sensitivity, and subsequent testosterone treatment restores it to normal.

← **Luteoids.** Many luteoids are strong anesthetics themselves; hence, their narcotic effect is added to that of the barbiturates if the two types of compounds are given in rapid succession. Pretreatment with luteoids may induce some degree of resistance against barbiturates, but the effect is not very pronounced.

Medroxyprogesterone given alone or in combination with ethynylestradiol and other folliculoids, over a period of 30 days, decreases the level of brain pentobarbital without affecting pentobarbital narcosis. Combined treatment with lynestrenol (a luteoid) and mestranol (a folliculoid) reduces the duration of pentobarbital and hexobarbital sleep in mice. Barbital is not affected. The effects of lynestrenol are abolished by SKF 525-A, whereas those of mestranol are potentiated.

← **Folliculoids.** Estradiol does not markedly influence hexobarbital sleeping time in female rats, but increases it in males. The enhanced hexobarbital resistance of male as compared to female rats is abolished by estradiol. There are marked species variations, and not all folliculoids act upon all barbiturates in the same manner; yet it may be said that in general, both the natural and the artificial folliculoids increase sensitivity to barbiturate hypnosis.

← **Adrenalectomy.** Adrenalectomy tends to increase barbiturate sleeping time in itself, but does not significantly interfere with the effects of various steroids upon barbiturate hypnosis.

In guinea pigs, epinephrine injected i.p. on awakening from barbiturate anesthesia re-induces sleep, and this effect is not prevented by adrenalectomy. Glucose lactate

Carcinogens ←

In rats given 2-acetaminofluorine (AAF), the development of hepatic neoplasms is accelerated by estradiol, testosterone, and gonadotrophic preparations. On the other hand, testosterone delays the induction of subcutaneous tumors by 20-methylcholanthrene. Painting of the skin with this carcinogen produces papillomas earlier in male or female castrate mice than in intact controls.

In rats, the induction of mammary cancers by DMBA is allegedly inhibited by progesterone, DOC or metyrapone. The adrenal necrosis produced by DMBA in the rat has been claimed to be independent of sex, ovariectomy, orchidectomy, testosterone or estradiol. However, more recent investigations suggest that the adrenolytic effect of DMBA is greatly enhanced by estradiol pretreatment. Spironolactone definitely inhibits the adrenolytic action of DMBA and probably also diminishes its carcinogenic effect. The question arises whether spironolactone protects against this action of DMBA by preventing its activation through hydroxylation; however, spironolactone protects the adrenals also against 7-OHM-MBA, the activated DMBA metabolite. The hematologic damage produced by DMBA can be suppressed both by spironolactone, which presumably accelerates the biotransformation of this polycyclic hydrocarbon, and by SKF 525-A, which inhibits it.

Ovariectomy greatly decreases the incidence of mammary tumors produced by DMBA in the rat, and results in the induction of renal tumors which are not seen in similarly treated intact controls. The rate of induction by DMBA of cervico-vaginal sarcomas is reduced by ovariectomy in the rat, and this reduction is counteracted by various folliculoids. Progesterone slightly retards the induction of these sarcomas and testosterone lengthens the induction period.

In rats, neonatal estradiol treatment enhances hepatoma formation following treatment with N-hydroxy-N-2-fluorenylacetamide.

In rats, hepatic carcinogenesis produced by aflatoxin is inhibited by diethystilbestrol; females are more resistant to this carcinogen than are males.

Chlordiazepoxide ←

In rats, PCN, CS-1, ethylestrenol and, to a lesser extent, spironolactone and norbolethone decrease the sleeping time after administration of chlordiazepoxide (Diazepam).

Chloroform ←

Extensive renal tubular necrosis occurs following exposure to chloroform in intact male or testosterone-treated orchidectomized mice, but not in females or in otherwise untreated orchidectomized males. As little as 10 µg of testosterone propionate suffices to reinduce chloroform sensitivity in castrate male mice with such regularity that the technique has been recommended for the bioassay of testoids.

Cholesterol ←

The potential enhancement of cholesterol degradation by catatoxic steroids is of great clinical significance in connection with the possible prophylaxis or treatment of atherosclerosis. For a detailed discussion of the literature concerning the morphologic changes characteristic of cholesterol atherosclerosis and of their modification by steroids, the reader is referred to the corresponding sections of our earlier monographs on metabolic cardiovascular diseases. Among the steroids examined in this connection, the corticoids and folliculoids have received the greatest attention.

In rabbits, cholesterol atheromatosis is diminished by cortisone, cortisol and other **glucocorticoids.** The associated hyperlipemia and hypercholesterolemia may likewise be depressed under these conditions, but this is not always the case; indeed, an inhibition of atherosclerosis by glucocorticoids may occur even if the serum lipids and cholesterol actually rise during treatment. The regression of the established cholesterol atherosclerosis itself can also be accelerated by glucocorticoids. It is characteristic of the cholesterol atherosclerosis in rabbits that various lysosomal enzymes (β-glucuronidase, acid phosphatase, cathepsin and aryl sulfatase) show an increased activity; this change is likewise inhibited during the prevention of cholesterol atherosclerosis by cortisone.

Folliculoids counteract coronary atherosclerosis in cholesterol-fed chicks without affecting blood cholesterol or hypercholesterolemia. This effect is demonstrable even if the feminizing actions of the folliculoids are blocked by concurrent administration of testosterone.

DOC or **progesterone** do not prevent cholesterol atherosclerosis in rabbits; in fact DOC may actually aggravate it.

Choline ←

The syndrome of choline-deficiency is most readily obtained in young rapidly growing male rats. It is characterized by hepatic steatosis, cardiovascular lesions and renal hemorrhages often associated with nephrocalcinosis. The severity of the changes is aggravated by methionine deficiency or an excess of ethionine. Glucocorticoids and folliculoids protect the rat against the manifestations of choline deficiency, whereas testoids aggravate these changes. Orchidectomy abolishes the normally greater resistance of males as compared with females.

Cinchophen ←

Cinchophen (Atophane) notoriously produces peptic ulcers in the dog. This effect can be prevented by estradiol and stilbestrol, both in intact and in gonadectomized dogs of either sex. Cortisone fails to affect the cinchophen-induced gastric ulcers in dogs, whereas prednisolone actually aggravates them. On the other hand, it has been claimed that aldosterone and DOC partially inhibit the production of gastric and duodenal ulcers as well as of liver damage in the cinchophen-treated dog.

← Steroids

Colchicine ←

Colchicine is of special interest because of its uricosuric action and its ability to inhibit mitotic division in various cells. In rats, colchicine poisoning can be prevented by various catatoxic steroids (e.g., spironolactone, CS-1, ethylestrenol, PCN and less constantly by oxandrolone). Progesterone, norbolethone, prednisolone, triamcinolone, DOC, hydroxydione, estradiol and thyroxine are virtually ineffective in this respect.

Cycloheximide ←

Since cycloheximide is a potent blocking agent for hepatic protein and particularly enzyme synthesis, it is of interest that in rats, its toxicity is powerfully inhibited by PCN, ethylestrenol, CS-1 and spironolactone. Norbolethone, oxandrolone, progesterone, hydroxydione, and prednisolone offer less perfect protection. Triamcinolone, DOC, estradiol and thyroxine have no protective effect.

The loss of liver glycogen and adrenal ascorbic acid as well as the stress-induced adrenal hypertrophy and allegedly even the thymic atrophy that develop in cycloheximide intoxicated rats can all be prevented by concurrent administration of cortisol.

Cyclophosphamide ←

Cyclophosphamide is a latent alkylating agent which is almost inactive in vitro, but is activated by the liver in vivo, and then exhibits carcinolytic actions as well as a strong toxic effect upon the hemopoietic system. In rats, cyclophosphamide intoxication can be prevented by PCN, CS-1 and spironolactone. Progesterone, ethylestrenol and norbolethone are distinctly less active, whereas oxandrolone, DOC, hydroxydione and phenobarbital are inactive. Resistance to this drug is actually decreased by prednisolone, triamcinolone, estradiol and thyroxine.

Digitalis ←

Since digitalis alkaloids are steroids themselves, a great deal of work has been done to elucidate their possible metabolic interactions with steroid hormones.

It appears that female **mice** are more resistant to ouabain than males, whereas resistance to strophanthin-K is the same in both sexes. Ovariectomy, orchidectomy and treatment with folliculoids do not change ouabain resistance in mice consistently.

In **frogs,** lethal strophanthin intoxication is allegedly delayed by simultaneous treatment with DOC, but this may be merely due to a delay in absorption.

In **cats**, cortisone has been claimed to potentiate the convulsive effects of digitalis.

In **guinea pigs**, chronic digitoxin intoxication is moderately counteracted by cortisone, whereas acute digitoxin poisoning is not affected.

In **dogs**, various folliculoids protect against the production of arrhythmia by digoxin. It has been claimed furthermore that male and castrate female dogs are highly sensitive to the toxic manifestations of various cardiac glycosides, in comparison with intact females or with folliculoid-treated spayed females.

In rats, ouabain and digitoxin resistance is greatly diminished by adrenalectomy, but this is hardly surprising, since in the absence of the adrenals, the toxicity of most drugs is increased. In adrenalectomized rats, strophanthin-K increases Na and K excretion, and this effect is prevented by DOC. In isolated strips of rat aorta, corticosterone inhibits the contraction caused by ouabain. β-Methasone aggravates the neuromotor disturbances produced in the rat by strophanthin-G. Adult female rats are more resistant to ouabain than males, but no such sex difference is noted in one-month-old animals. Gonadectomy does not alter the sex difference to ouabain in rats of either sex.

All these results, obtained in different species with various digitalis derivatives and under dissimilar experimental conditions, were difficult to evaluate and correlate. However, in 1969, it was found that spironolactone protects the rat against infarctoid necroses produced by digitoxin + Na_2HPO_4 + corn oil; simultaneously, the convulsions characteristic of digitalis intoxication are likewise prevented. This finding stimulated many investigations on the effect of various catatoxic steroids upon digitalis intoxication.

Preliminary studies showed that both norbolethone and spironolactone protect the rat against severe intoxication with digitoxin, gitalin, proscillaridin, digoxin and digitalin. The corresponding effects of strophanthin-K, ouabain and digitoxigenin were not prevented.

In an extensive study, comprising 304 steroids, it was found that, at the dose of 100 mg/kg, 32 of them gave definite protection against digitoxin but not against indomethacin, 42 protected against indomethacin but not against digitoxin, whereas 24 were active against both substrates. The most active compound, which gave protection against both substrates even at the dose of 100 µg/kg, was PCN (pregnenolone carbonitrile, that is 3β-hydroxy-20-oxo-5-pregnene-16α-carbonitrile). Further analysis of this study revealed that the catatoxic activity against digitoxin or indomethacin is not strictly dependent upon any other known pharmacologic effect, although most of the highly potent catatoxic compounds also exhibit antimineralocorticoid or anabolic properties. Among the most powerful antidigitoxin compounds, in addition to PCN, are: ethylestrenol, CS-1, spironolactone and oxandrolone.

Upon long continued conjoint daily administration of spironolactone or oxandrolone plus lethal doses of digitoxin, the resistance against this cardiac glycoside can be maintained in rats for virtually indefinite periods (certainly more than two months).

On the other hand, the antidigitoxin effect of spironolactone can be blocked in turn by high doses of estradiol, and perhaps to some extent also by progesterone, whereas DOC, cortisol, methylandrostenediol, methyltestosterone, pregnanedione, pregnenolone and testosterone do not interfere with this type of prevention. The protection against digitoxin by spironolactone can also be blocked by concurrent treatment with metyrapone.

The plasma concentration of digitoxin is diminished during the administration of catatoxic steroids, but rises again if digitoxin administration is continued after withdrawal of the prophylactic steroids.

In mice, digitoxin poisoning is inhibited by CS-1, spironolactone, norbolethone, oxandrolone, progesterone and even by thyroxine. Ethylestrenol, triamcinolone, DOC, hydroxydione and estradiol are ineffective. It appears, therefore, that there exist some species differences in the effect of hormones and hormone derivatives upon digitalis intoxication.

Dyes ←

The effect of steroids upon dye clearance was studied mainly as a means of detecting interference with hepatic function.

In **rats**, the biliary excretion of ^{131}I marked rose bengal was inhibited by several anabolic steroids, although upon chronic treatment, adaptation usually developed in this respect. Estradiol markedly delayed plasma clearance of BSP both in its free and conjugated forms. A large series of steroids was compared and this effect was found to be common to estrone, estriol and various other C18 steroids, including those used in contraceptives. Cortisone transiently increased the bile flow and reduced BSP excretion through the bile of the rat. Norethandrolone, norethynodrel, and norlutin reduced bile flow and BSP excretion (without affecting the concentrating mechanism for the dye). Testosterone, methyltestosterone, estradiol, progesterone, and stilbestrol irreversibly reduced the rate of bile formation and transiently diminished the excretion of BSP. Among typical catatoxic steroids, PCN, CS-1, spironolactone and spiroxasone enhanced plasma clearance of BSP, presumably by stimulating glutathione, S-aryltransferase activity and bile flow through mechanisms which are not limited to microsomal enzymes.

In **dogs**, large doses of methyltestosterone and norethandrolone did not affect BSP clearance even after 50 days of treatment.

In **rabbits**, methyltestosterone and norethandrolone caused dose related increases in BSP retention. Oxandrolone was less active, and testosterone completely inactive in this respect.

In **man**, 17-ethyl-19-nortestosterone increased biliary BSP retention and plasma bilirubin concentration. In patients with no evidence of liver disease, norethandrolone caused a reversible reduction in the hepatic transport maximum for BSP. The relative hepatic storage of BSP was unimpaired, and the dye was retained in the plasma primarily as a conjugate. According to other investigators, however, norethandrolone interferes with the hepatic uptake and the biliary excretion of BSP. Estriol and estradiol rapidly reduce the hepatic excretory capacity for BSP in man, presumably because the excretion of both free and conjugated dye is impaired. These folliculoids may even provoke hepatic porphyria in patients.

Ergot ←

In rats, various ergot preparations elicit a characteristic gangrene of the tail, owing to their vasotoxic effect. Although the literature is somewhat contradictory, most investigators agree that this response is inhibited by estradiol, estrone and other folliculoids. The effect of castration and of testoids is rather irregular. In intact male rats, unlike in females or castrate males, ergonovine induces analgesia and this is allegedly counteracted by testosterone.

Ethanol ←

Despite the great practical interest attached to the problem of ethanol intoxication, little is known about its responsiveness to treatment with steroids.

In **rats**, ovariectomy allegedly interferes with adaptation to chronic ethanol administration. The toxic ethanol metabolites are pyruvate and acetaldehyde, which accumulate in the body under the influence of disulfiram. This response is inhibited by cortisone and ACTH but also by hepatic extracts. Conversely, DOC, thyroxine and testosterone appear to aggravate ethanol intoxication. Chronic treatment with ethanol p.o. allegedly produces more severe fatty infiltration in the liver of female than of male rats. Ovariectomy or estradiol fails to influence this response. Testosterone reduces hepatic steatosis in females, whereas castration increases it in males. Various anabolics (norethandrolone, testosterone, oxandrolone) allegedly protect the rat's liver against ethanol-induced fatty degeneration and may even be useful in alcoholic patients.

In **rabbits** and mice, gonadectomy allegedly diminishes alcohol tolerance, whereas estrone raises it. Alcohol metabolism does not appear to be influenced, but presumably its effect upon the nervous system is diminished by folliculoids, since in rabbits treated with such hormones, intoxication occurs only at very high blood alcohol levels. Fatal doses of ethanol p.o. produce adrenal necrosis in rabbits, but neither this lesion nor mortality is prevented by dexamethasone.

In **mice**, ethanol anesthesia is prolonged by cortisone, but not by either prednisolone or DOC pretreatment. Estrone allegedly increases alcohol tolerance in the mouse, whereas gonadectomy diminishes it in both sexes.

Ethionine ←

Since it blocks protein and drug-metabolizing enzyme synthesis, ethionine is of special interest in connection with the study of catatoxic compounds. Yet, comparatively little is known about the influence of steroids, other than glucocorticoids and anabolics, upon the toxicity of ethionine.

In the rat, the hepatic damage caused by ethionine is inhibited by cortisone and cortisol especially during the acute stage of intoxication; consequently, survival is usually prolonged, although the associated pancreatic lesions characteristic of ethionine intoxication appear to be rather resistant to glucocorticoid treatment.

Male rats are much more resistant than females to the production of fatty livers by ethionine. Orchidectomy abolishes the resistance of the male, whereas testosterone protects females and castrate males. MAD fails to influence this form of hepatic steatosis in rats of either sex. 17-Ethyl-19-nortestosterone, in doses which do not stimulate the growth of the seminal vesicles, blocks the production of fatty livers by ethionine in orchidectomized males, whereas testosterone exerts this effect only at definitely virilizing dose levels. DOC, estradiol, and progesterone are ineffective. In mice, 17α-methyl-5α-androstan-17β-ol prevents hepatic steatosis produced by ethionine.

Ganglioplegics ←

In rats, intoxication with TEA, hexamethonium and pentolinium can be prevented by all the glucocorticoids tested. On the other hand, these same steroids offer no protection against trimethaphan, mecamylamine, trimethidinium or pempidine. All the other steroids tested remained without effect against hexamethonium or TEA.

Several, though not all stressors gave excellent protection against TEA, but since even large doses of ACTH were ineffective in this respect, the anti-TEA effect of stressors cannot be ascribed merely to an increased glucocorticoid secretion.

In guinea pigs, ovariectomy allegedly increases resistance to lethal doses of hexamethonium, but it remains to be seen whether this effect is specific.

Indomethacin ←

The production of multiple ulcers in the small intestine, with the ensuing fatal peritonitis, has become a standard test of indomethacin toxicity in the rat. These lesions are readily prevented by all of the highly potent catatoxic steroids, particularly by PCN (even at individual dose levels of 0.3 mg/kg), ethylestrenol, norbolethone, CS-1, spironolactone, oxandrolone, etc. Progesterone and prednisolone are less active, while certain glucocorticoids, e.g., triamcinolone, are totally inactive.

In an extensive study on 304 steroids, conducted under rigorously comparable conditions in female rats, it was found that 42 were effective in preventing indomethacin intoxication.

In the rat, partial hepatectomy facilitates the production of perforating intestinal ulcers by indomethacin but comparatively small doses of spironolactone readily inhibit the toxicity of this compound even after surgically induced hepatic insufficiency.

In adrenalectomized rats maintained on NaCl alone, the lethal effect of indomethacin is increased, and intestinal ulcers develop at least as frequently as in intact controls. The anti-indomethacin effect of threshold doses of spironolactone can be further increased by cortisol alone or in combination with DOC. This point is of theoretic importance; it shows that although a catatoxic steroid, such as spironolactone, is not endowed with corticoid activity, and although cortisol does not possess any significant catatoxic effect against indomethacin, combined treatment with both types of hormones enhances their protective effect.

In rats, the protection against indomethacin by spironolactone can be blocked in turn by concurrent treatment with metyrapone.

The blood clearance of s.c. injected indomethacin is accelerated in rats by spironolactone, norbolethone and progesterone, but not by hydroxydione. SKF 525-A significantly suppresses this activity of the catatoxic steroids. Hence, it was concluded that they probably act through an increased metabolic degradation of indomethacin.

Prolonged treatment with such catatoxic steroids as spironolactone or oxandrolone can protect rats for a virtually unlimited period (certainly more than two months) against the continued daily administration of fatal doses of indomethacin. Upon withdrawal of the catatoxic steroids, fatal intestinal ulcers develop rapidly. The plasma concentration of indomethacin is diminished during the administration of catatoxic steroids, but rises rapidly upon withdrawal of this treatment in the presence of continued indomethacin injection.

In mice, indomethacin intoxication can also be prevented by numerous catatoxic steroids (e.g., ethylestrenol, CS-1, spironolactone, norbolethone), whereas thyroxine appears to have an opposite effect.

Isoproterenol ←

Both in intact and in adrenalectomized rats, mineralocorticoids (DOC, fluorocortisol) increase the mortality and aggravate the cardiac lesions normally produced by isoproterenol. On the other hand, glucocorticoids (cortisone, triamcinolone) have been said not to exert any evident effect of this kind. Since we have previously found that both DOC and triamcinolone aggravate the severity of the cardiac lesions induced by norepinephrine, it was concluded that there might be "an essential difference in the lesions produced by noradrenaline compared to those of isoproterenol." Moderate amounts of ACTH allegedly also fail to affect the production of cardiac necroses by isoproterenol, but it remains to be seen whether very large doses of glucocorticoids or ACTH might not be effective in this respect.

Various antimineralocorticoids (SC-5233, CS-1, spironolactone and SC-8109) have been claimed to inhibit isoproterenol-induced myocardial necrosis in rats. However, in view of recent findings, the possibility must be considered that all these compounds might act, at least in part, by virtue of their catatoxic and not only of their antimineralocorticoid potency.

Lathyrogens ←

We distinguish two types of lathyrogenic substances: 1. Osteolathyrogens (e.g., Lathyrus odoratus seeds, aminopropionitrile or "APN," aminoacetonitrile or "AAN," methyleneaminoacetonitrile or "MAAN") induce severe degenerative changes in bones, especially at tendon insertion sites and in the junction cartilages; 2. neurolathyrogens (e.g., β,β'-iminodipropionitrile or "IDPN") which elicit a syndrome characterized mainly by extreme excitation, circling movements and ocular lesions. Under certain circumstances, osteolathyrism is associated with dissecting aneurysms of the aorta; some authors refer to this form of the disease as angiolathyrism.

Most of the work on the effect of steroids upon lathyrism has been performed in rats fed Lathyrus seeds or pure lathyrogenic amines. Under these conditions, the course of osteolathyrism is not significantly affected by testosterone, whereas folliculoids and glucocorticoids exert a definite protective effect. DOC — especially when combined with uninephrectomy + NaCl — increases the incidence of dissecting aneurysms without considerably affecting the skeletal changes. Thus, the vascular and osseous manifestations of lathyrism can be dissociated.

STH aggravates osteolathyrism in rats even after adrenalectomy, indicating that the effect of the hormone is not mediated through the liberation or activation of corticoids.

It has been claimed that after adrenalectomy, cortisone no longer inhibits lathyrism produced by AAN in the rat; indeed, in the absence of the adrenals, the glucocorticoids facilitate the production of hernias, which are common complications of the disease. The osteolathyrism produced by APN in rats is associated with an increase in the GPT and GOT activities in the serum. Prednisolone prevents these changes concurrently with the bone lesions.

LSD ←

In the rabbit, the EEG (lysergide) changes produced by LSD are allegedly prevented by hydroxydione, methylandrostanolone, androstanolone and 19-nortestosterone. In rats, the behavioural changes induced by LSD can be suppressed by DOC, corticosterone, 17-dehydrocortisone, 11-dehydrocortisol, dehydroisoandrosterone, testosterone, androsterone, pregnenolone, etiocholanolone and progesterone. Several other naturally-occurring steroids proved to be ineffective. The time required by a rat to climb a rope for food reward is prolonged by LSD and this response is also prevented by a number of steroids widely differing in their pharmacologic activities and chemical structure.

Magnesium ←

It has been claimed that in rabbits and mice, the depth of $MgSO_4$ anesthesia is increased by gonadectomy in either sex, but can be restored to about normal by both folliculoid and testoid hormones. However, this claim requires confirmation.

Certain manifestations of an Mg-deficiency syndrome are also inhibited by cortisol, estradiol, hypophysectomy or thyroparathyroidectomy; hence, the specificity of this type of prophylaxis is very dubious.

Mephenesin ←

Mephenesin (a muscle relaxant) proved to be a substrate for many catatoxic drugs, especially: PCN, ethylestrenol, CS-1, spironolactone and norbolethone.

Meprobamate ←

Various catatoxic drugs accelerate the metabolism of meprobamate, and this effect is not prevented by adrenalectomy. Meprobamate intoxication is also inhibited in rats by PCN, ethylestrenol, CS-1, spironolactone, norbolethone, oxandrolone and prednisolone. No protection is obtained by progesterone, triamcinolone, hydroxydione, DOC, or estradiol.

Mercury

A large number of investigations is concerned with the effect of various steroids upon mercury intoxication. Special interest in this field stems from an observation made in 1940, that the renal and hepatic lesions produced by $HgCl_2$ in the mouse are prevented by many testoids (e.g., testosterone, methyltestosterone, androstenediol, dehydroisoandrosterone and androstenedione). This observation has been repeatedly confirmed with various testoids in different species intoxicated with diverse inorganic salts of mercury, but apparently the protective effect is most readily obtained in the mouse and much more variable in the rat. Such protection against renal damage by $HgCl_2$ has also been noted in dogs, guinea pigs, parrots and man. In rabbits, both sublimate and Masugi nephritis are allegedly prevented by testosterone and even more actively by estradiol. It has been claimed furthermore that the protective effect of testosterone against mercurial renal damage can be further improved by additional administration of cortisone or ACTH.

It is clear, however, that none of the testoids offers absolute protection against large doses of mercury and the great variability of the findings reported suggests that incidental circumstances (e.g., sex, age, strain, dosage, timing) are likely to alter the results considerably. A distinction should be made furthermore between prophylactic and curative actions. In mice and rats, the regeneration of the kidney following $HgCl_2$-induced damage is stimulated by 2-bromo-1-androstene-3,17-dione but not by methyltestosterone or 1,17-dimethylandrostane-17-ol-3-one.

There is some evidence suggesting that, in the rat, other steroid hormones, especially the **glucocorticoids**, may also offer slight protection against intoxication with inorganic mercury, but in this respect, the results reported are even more variable.

The only steroids which offer constant, significant, and always very pronounced protection against $HgCl_2$ in the rat are those containing a thioacetyl group, especially **spironolactone, spiroxasone** and **emdabol**. Na-thioacetate given alone, or mixed with various steroids, also exerts some protective effect, but only at dose levels which cause considerable acute mortality often in association with bilateral adrenocortical necrosis. Apparently, the steroid molecule acts as a suitable carrier for the thioacetyl group and enhances its protective action against mercury.

Methyprylon

In rats, anesthesia produced by heavy overdosage with methyprylon can be prevented not only by pretreatment with PCN, ethylestrenol, CS-1, spironolactone, norbolethone, or oxandrolone, all of which are typical catatoxic steroids, but also by prednisolone and triamcinolone, presumably as a consequence of their glucocorticoid effect. DOC, progesterone and hydroxydione, which are devoid of both catatoxic and glucocorticoid activities, offer little or no protection against methyprylon.

Monocrotaline

Female rats are more resistant than males to fatal intoxication with monocrotaline. Gonadectomy has no significant effect upon survival in either sex; however, when given as a pretreatment, estradiol increases, whereas testosterone decreases monocrotaline resistance.

Morphine, Ethylmorphine

It has been claimed that various steroids can influence morphine resistance in different species, but the results are so contradictory that no valid generalization can be made. In our experience, none of the steroids tested — not even the most potent catatoxic steroids — exert a striking effect upon morphine intoxication in the rat.

On the other hand, ethylmorphine (which is much more fat soluble than morphine) is readily detoxified not only by all catatoxic steroids tested, but also by prednisolone, progesterone, estradiol and, to some extent, even by DOC.

Nicotine

Earlier investigators asserted that in mice and rabbits, the males, whereas in rats, the females are more sensitive to nicotine. It has also been stated that the cardiovascular lesions produced by chronic nicotine intoxication in rats are aggravated by DOC. These data require confirmation.

More recent studies have shown that in rats, nicotine intoxication can be prevented by PCN, ethylestrenol, norbolethone, CS-1, spironolactone, and oxandrolone, whereas DOC, hydroxydione, prednisolone, progesterone, and triamcinolone offer little or no prophylaxis.

Papain

In the rabbit, papain i.v. causes softening and degenerative changes in the otic and epiphyseal cartilages. At the same time, the basophilic substance in the cartilage matrix is depleted. The return of these papain-induced cartilage changes to normal can by delayed by cortisone, cortisol and prednisolone.

Pentylenetetrazol

Pentylenetetrazol (pentamethylenetetrazol, metrazole, Cardiazole) convulsions have been used by many investigators as an indicator of catatoxic steroid effects, ever since 1942, when it was observed that various steroid anesthetics (DOC, progesterone) can protect the **rat** against pentylenetetrazol. Conversely, this drug can interrupt an already established steroid anesthesia.

In rats, the pentylenetetrazol convulsions and ECG changes are inhibited by ACTH and cortisone according to some investigators; others state that single, nonanesthetic doses of cortisol enhance the production of pentylenetetrazol convulsions in the rat, whereas aldosterone has no such effect. The interpretation of these findings is rendered even more difficult because yet other investigators maintain that, although cortisone and prednisolone aggravate pentylenetetrazol convulsions in rats, prednisone and hexamethasone are less active, while cortisol, triamcinolone and DOC are virtually inactive in this respect.

According to our own investigations in rats, both the motor disturbances and the mortality caused by pentylenetetrazol intoxication were markedly inhibited by PCN, norbolethone and progesterone, whereas the other standard conditioners, including glucocorticoids and DOC, were ineffective.

Various aminosteroids also prevent pentylenetetrazol convulsions, allegedly owing to interneuronal blockade and not to general anesthesia.

In guinea pigs, pretreatment with large doses of DOC allegedly fails to influence pentylenetetrazol convulsions, whereas cortisone, ACTH and vasopressin aggravate them.

In mice, different investigators obtained contradictory results regarding the effect of steroids upon pentylenetetrazol convulsions. It has been claimed that cortisone and DOC do not influence them, and that the latter decreases the pentylenetetrazol (as well as the electroshock) seizure threshold owing to the induction of hypernatremia. Both DOC and progesterone anesthesia protect the mouse against the convulsive and lethal effects of pentylenetetrazol (or other convulsive agents), whereas estrone has an opposite effect.

3β-(Aminoalkyl) esters of pregnenolone and various other steroids also inhibit pentylenetetrazol and electroshock seizures in mice. Methyltestosterone is said not to influence pentylenetetrazol convulsions in this species, whereas other anabolic steroids (methandienone, 4-chlorotestosterone, nandrolone, given i.p. 90 min before pentylenetetrazol) inhibit them.

It would be difficult to evaluate many of the contradictory data just mentioned, because they were obtained under vastly different circumstances in diverse species, but it is safe to assume that certain catatoxic or anesthetic steroids reliably antagonize pentylenetetrazol convulsions under suitable experimental conditions.

Perchlorates ←

Overdosage with perchlorates exerts a singular effect upon the voluntary musculature. For example, in the rat, $NaClO_4$ p.o. causes spastic muscular contractions and a pronounced predisposition to the development of extensor cramps in the hind paws after a tap on the sacrum ("flick test"). These spasms are inhibited by cortisol or triamcinolone, but aggravated by DOC and methylchlorocortisol (Me-Cl-COL). Methyltestosterone, estradiol and progesterone do not significantly affect this response in the rat. Triamcinolone also protects the dog against the syndrome of heavy $NaClO_4$ overdosage.

Pesticides ←

The possible detoxication of pesticides (insecticides, herbicides) by steroids has been extensively studied ever since it was found, in 1956, that **DDT** increased hepatic weight in the rat and that diethylstilbestrol enhanced the storage of DDT (and of its metabolite DDE) in the fat of male rats, whereas testosterone decreased these values in females. Thus, it was concluded that "an endocrine mechanism may account for the sex differences in this regard." Yet DDT is particularly resistant to detoxication by steroids.

It was subsequently observed that male rats are more resistant than females to **parathion** poisoning, and that testosterone raises the resistance of females and of castrate males, whereas estrone diminishes that of intact males. Using the anticholinesterase action of **DMP** as an indicator, it was found that in female rats, administration of various hepatic microsomal enzyme-inducing drugs, as well as estradiol, cortisone, and a number of other steroids, causes resistance. Immature rats are more sensitive to **malathion** than adults and their livers detoxify this insecticide at a slower rate. Orchidectomy decreases, whereas testosterone increases malathion detoxication. It was concluded that testoids play an important part in the maintenance of the malathion-hydroxylating enzyme system.

On the other hand, male rats are more susceptible than females to the insecticide, **Morestan**. This sex difference could not be altered by castration, the administration of testosterone to females or of estradiol to males. Phenobarbital decreased the toxicity of Morestan in males and increased it in females.

More recent investigations showed that most catatoxic steroids (e.g., PCN, ethylestrenol, CS-1, spironolactone and norbolethone) counteract the lethal effects of **ethion, dioxathion, EPN, Guthion** and **parathion**. To a lesser extent, this is also true of oxandrolone, prednisolone and progesterone. However, triamcinolone, DOC, hydroxydione, estradiol, and thyroxine offer no consistent protection against these pesticides. Indeed, in many instances, thyroxine counteracts the protective effect of catatoxic steroids.

In view of the high efficacy of spironolactone, a potassium-retaining agent, it is noteworthy that such nonsteroidal potassium-sparing drugs as triamterene and amiloride do not protect against parathion or dioxathion.

In mice, the lethal effect of dioxathion is strongly inhibited by ethylestrenol, norbolethone, prednisolone, and estradiol, moderately by CS-1, and oxandrolone but not influenced by spironolactone, progesterone, triamcinolone, DOC, hydroxydione, and thyroxine. Evidently, here again, as in the case of most other substrates, genetic predisposition can greatly alter the catatoxic effect of steroids.

Since it was at first thought that the protective effect of steroids against various pesticides is linked to their testoid actions, it is of special interest that cyproterone, (an antitestoid steroid) also protects the rat against otherwise fatal doses of parathion.

The insecticide, **OMPA**, is assumed to become toxic only after transformation by hepatic microsomal enzymes into a potent anticholinesterase. Accordingly, it behaves somewhat differently from most other pesticides with regard to the effect of steroids upon its toxicity. Thus, cyproterone, one of the most potent catatoxic steroids known, which detoxifies many other pesticides, does not protect the rat against OMPA. In this respect, ethylestrenol, CS-1, spironolactone and norbolethone are also ineffective. Yet, these catatoxic steroids do not increase the toxicity of OMPA, which is noteworthy because hepatic microsomal enzyme-inducing barbiturates do transform it into its more toxic metabolite. On the other hand, estradiol, estrone, and stilbestrol which have no typical catatoxic actions, considerably increase OMPA toxicity in the ovariectomized rat. Although, the protective effect of the catatoxic steroids against most substrates is independent of their pharmacologic action, the sensitization to OMPA does appear to depend upon folliculoid activity as such, since it is induced both by steroidal and by nonsteroidal folliculoids. Prednisolone, triamcinolone, progesterone, DOC, hydroxydione and thyroxine fail to influence OMPA toxicity.

Phosphates ←

In uninephrectomized rats given large doses of NaH_2PO_4 p.o., there develops a selective cortico-medullary nephrocalcinosis even after adrenalectomy. This effect is aggravated by DOC and prevented by cortisol. The action of DOC can be counterbalanced by cortisol under these conditions.

Estradiol facilitates the production of cortico-medullary nephrocalcinosis by NaH_2PO_4, whereas ovariectomy largely inhibits it. Folliculoids (estradiol, stilbestrol) facilitate the production of this type of nephrocalcinosis even in ovariectomized rats. The effect of estradiol is not significantly affected by progesterone, but is aggravated by methyltestosterone under these conditions. Parathyroidectomy or thyroidectomy prevents this nephrocalcinosis even after combined treatment with DOC, or estradiol + Na_2HPO_4.

Potassium ←

Since corticoids have a pronounced influence upon potassium metabolism, their protective action against potassium intoxication has been carefully investigated. As early as 1937, it has been shown that adrenocortical extract can protect mice and guinea pigs against otherwise fatal amounts of KCl i.p. DOC proved to be even more effective in this respect.

On the other hand, pretreatment of rats with glucocorticoids diminishes their resistance to KCl i.p., perhaps as a consequence of the resultant adrenocortical atrophy. Concurrent administration of DOC, aldosterone, adrenocortical extract, corticosterone, or ACTH counteracts this unfavorable effect of cortisol upon K tolerance in the rat. Besides, addition of KCl to the drinking water prolongs the survival of rats given large doses of cortisone.

The protective action of DOC upon acute potassium intoxication has been confirmed in rabbits and mice.

Phosphorus ←

The hepatotoxic effect of elementary yellow phosphorus is allegedly diminished both by cortisone and by testosterone in the rat.

Physostigmine ←

In rats, intoxication with physostigmine is lessened by ethylestrenol, CS-1, PCN, spironolactone, and prednisolone, but aggravated by estradiol and thyroxine. Norbolethone, oxandrolone, progesterone, triamcinolone, DOC, and hydroxydione do not significantly alter physostigmine poisoning. The protective action of ethylestrenol is counteracted by concurrent administration of thyroxine.

Picrotoxin ←

In rats, the convulsive effect of picrotoxin can be prevented by anesthetic doses of DOC. Adult males are more resistant than females. Gonadectomy lowers picrotoxin resistance in both sexes, whereas testosterone raises it in normal, and especially in spayed females, but not in males.

Among the catatoxic steroids, PCN, ethylestrenol, CS-1, spironolactone, norbolethone, oxandrolone, prednisolone, and progesterone inhibit picrotoxin poisoning in the rat, whereas triamcinolone, DOC, estradiol, hydroxydione, corticosterone, cholesterol, and β-sitosterol have no such protective action.

In mice, pretreatment with spironolactone, ethylestrenol, triamcinolone, or thyroxine had little, if any, effect upon picrotoxin poisoning.

Piperidine ←

In rats, given piperidine at doses which caused very little mortality, the motor disturbances were inhibited by CS-1, ethylestrenol, norbolethone, oxandrolone, triamcinolone and hydroxydione. Curiously, PCN, one of the most active catatoxic steroids, failed to prevent piperidine intoxication.

Pralidoxime ←

Pralidoxime is an inhibitor of anticholinesterases and hence, represents a useful antidote against certain pesticides which interfere with cholinergic mechanisms. In rats, pralidoxime intoxication is prevented by prednisolone or triamcinolone and, to a lesser extent, by ethylestrenol and estradiol. CS-1, PCN, spironolactone, norbolethone, oxandrolone, progesterone, DOC, hydroxydione, and thyroxine do not significantly influence pralidoxime poisoning.

Puromycin Aminonucleoside (PAN) ←

The nephrosis and osteitis fibrosa produced by PAN in the rat are inhibited by glucocorticoids (cortisol, triamcinolone, dexamethasone, 6-methylprednisolone) according to several investigators. However, others claimed that these steroids have no effect or actually aggravate the renal changes. Presumably, many experimental conditions (e.g., dosage, timing, the age and strain of the rats used) may modify the prophylactic effect of glucocorticoids. DOC aggravates PAN nephrosis in the rat.

Reserpine ←

In rats, adrenalectomy greatly decreases resistance to reserpine, whereas hypophysectomy does not change it. Hence, it has been assumed that the great reserpine sensitivity of the adrenalectomized animal is related to an absolute lack in certain adrenal steroids, rather than to the inability of the pituitary-adrenal system to respond to the stress caused by this drug.

Dexamethasone protects the gastric mucosa of the rat against the production of ulcers by reserpine.

In guinea pigs, the reserpine catalepsy is inhibited by various folliculoids, testoids, and corticoids.

Reticulo-Endothelial System (RES)-Blocking Agents ←

In rats and mice, the blood clearance of carbon particles and their phagocytosis by RES cells is enhanced by various folliculoids, but not by testoids.

Cortisol does not significantly alter the accumulation of intratracheally administered quartz dust in rats, but delays its transfer to the regional lymph nodes.

In rats pretreated with ACTH, fluorocortisol, or stress (restraint), a single i.v. injection of thorium dextrin produces thrombohemorrhagic lesions in the adrenals, liver, and kidneys, which resemble the Shwartzman-Sanarelli phenomenon.

The localization of i.v. injected carbon particles in the paws of rats with dextran-induced anaphylactoid edema, can be topically prevented by intrapedal injection of cortisol, which interferes with local angiotaxis. In rats with arthritis produced by intrapedal injection of formalin mixed with India ink, the migration of the carbon particles into the regional lymph nodes is accelerated by concurrent treatment with ACTH. This is presumably a consequence of an increased glucocorticoid secretion and the resulting inhibition of inflammatory barrier formation around the carbon particles.

SKF 525-A ←

In rats, severe intoxication with SKF 525-A was significantly diminished by PCN, CS-1, spironolactone, oxandrolone, prednisolone, triamcinolone and progesterone.

Sodium ←

The potentiating effect of Na-salts upon mineralocorticoid hypertension has been extensively discussed in our previous monographs and need not be reconsidered here. Suffice it to state that in rats, dogs, and various other species including man, the toxic action of mineralocorticoid overdosage is aggravated by an excess of sodium. Indeed, it appears that the picture of mineralocorticoid intoxication is actually a sodium poisoning whose severity is enhanced by mineralocorticoids.

In frogs, high concentrations of NaCl decrease the Na-uptake and increase the electric resistance in the skin, as does destruction of the interrenal bodies. These effects are reversed by aldosterone but unaffected by spironolactone. Aldosterone and spironolactone also fail to influence either the urine or the plasma Na in frogs; hence, it has been assumed that aldosterone is perhaps not an indispensable participant in salt regulation in this species.

Strychnine

One of the earliest — though negative — observations concerning the influence of hormones upon resistance to drugs was the finding, in 1911, that in dogs and rabbits, orchidectomy and thyroidectomy do not consistently influence resistance to strychnine poisoning. On the other hand, DOC anesthesia protects the mouse against the convulsive and local effects of strychnine.

Also in mice, several water soluble esters of cortisol and prednisolone decreased strychnine sensitivity, but testosterone offered the best protection. Some piperidinoandrostane derivatives actually increased strychnine sensitivity or produced convulsions by themselves.

Male rats are more resistant than females to strychnine intoxication, and the hepatic microsomes of male rats also exhibit a greater strychnine-metabolizing potency in vitro. SKF 525-A increases the toxicity of strychnine, presumably by interfering with its microsomal metabolism. Gonadectomy diminishes the high strychnine resistance of male rats, but has no effect upon females. 4-Chlorotestosterone augments the strychnine-metabolizing ability of isolated hepatic microsomes or liver slices.

Comparative studies on the effect of various steroids upon the strychnine sensitivity of the rat revealed that in this respect, the glucocorticoids (prednisolone and triamcinolone) and estradiol are most efficient. Ethylestrenol, spironolactone and PCN are much less potent, whereas CS-1, norbolethone, oxandrolone, progesterone, DOC, and hydroxydione are totally devoid of strychnine antagonizing capacity.

Thimerosal

In rats, thimerosal intoxication is inhibited by all catatoxic steroids, prednisolone and estradiol.

Thioacetamide

Several investigators noted that glucocorticoids (prednisolone, prednisone, cortisone) do not significantly inhibit the hepatocellular damage produced by thioacetamide in rats; however, they may slightly suppress cirrhosis even if the hepatic parenchymal lesions are increased. On the other hand, various testoids, especially 4-chlorotestosterone, appeared to offer some protection against these thioacetamide-induced hepatic lesions.

Tribromoethanol

Bilateral adrenalectomy prolongs tribromoethanol sleeping time both in rabbits and in rats. DOC, and adrenocortical extract tend to compensate for this manifestation of adrenal insufficiency.

In the mouse, estradiol allegedly increases resistance to "partially decomposed solutions" of tribromoethanol. In rats, tribromoethanol sleeping time is significantly shortened by typical catatoxic steroids. A similar effect is obtained by prednisolone, but not by triamcinolone.

Trichloroethanol ←

Trichloroethanol is more easily detoxified by catatoxic steroids than tribromoethanol. In rats, trichloroethanol sleeping time is significantly diminished by PCN, CS-1, ethylestrenol, spironolactone and prednisolone.

Tubocurarine ←

The motor disturbances produced in rats by D-tubocurarine were virtually abolished by all typical catatoxic steroids (except oxandrolone), as well as by prednisolone, triamcinolone and progesterone.

Tyrosine ←

Excessive dietary intake of tyrosine causes characteristic lesions in the paws and eyes of rats, especially on a low protein diet. Cortisol or stress (infusorial earth i.p.) prevents the manifestations of tyrosine intoxication, presumably as a consequence of hepatic TPO induction. However, PCN fails to augment hepatic TPO activity, yet it also offers excellent protection against tyrosine intoxication in the rat. Since thyroid hormones aggravate tyrosine intoxication, it is conceivable that PCN acts partly by interfering with thyroid hormone secretion (as do thioureas), or that it augments the metabolic degradation of thyroid hormones, thus exerting an indirect effect upon tyrosine intoxication.

Vitamin A ←

The vitamins, as many other normal food constituents such as electrolytes, cholesterol, etc., could have been discussed in the section on dietary factors; we deal with them here, since many of the most pertinent data are concerned with the effect of hormones upon intoxication with excessive amounts of vitamins.

In the rat, vitamin-A overdosage produces widespread bone absorption, resulting in severe skeletal lesions. It was claimed at first that in weanlings, adrenalectomy aggravates these changes, whereas cortisone has no effect upon them, but subsequent studies have shown that various glucocorticoids increase the skeletal defects of hypervitaminosis A even in the very young animal. Indeed, vitamin-A overdosage during pregnancy produces malformations of the brain and calvarium in the newborn rat, and the intensity of these lesions is aggravated by cortisone. During postnatal life, vitamin A also elicits severe bone absorption in rats; this effect is likewise increased by cortisol, whose action is in turn inhibited by STH.

However, as we shall see, the effect of glucocorticoids upon hypervitaminosis A is variable and often even reversed depending upon experimental conditions (e.g., dosage, the form in which the vitamin is administered).

In rats, vitamin A itself has no effect upon wound healing, but it overcomes the inhibitory action of cortisone.

The atrophy of the accessory sex organs induced by vitamin-A deficiency in the rat has been ascribed to interference with the synthesis of testoids, not to a target-organ insensitivity. Estradiol increases, whereas methyltestosterone counteracts the bone absorption and catabolism produced by hypervitaminosis A in the rat.

Progesterone increases body weight and re-establishes a normal estrous cycle in vitamin-A deficient rats.

More recent experiments have shown that the skeletal lesions characteristic of vitamin-A overdosage in rats are inhibited not only by glucocorticoids, but also by typical catatoxic steroids such as spironolactone, norbolethone and ethylestrenol. Simultaneously, the hepatic and serum vitamin-A concentrations are decreased.

In **rabbits**, large doses of vitamin A produce collapse of the ears and loss of basophilic and metachromatic staining of their cartilage. These changes, which resemble those elicited by papain, can be prevented by cortisone. The lesions produced by cortisone in the epiphyseal plates of rabbits are not significantly influenced by vitamin A.

It has been postulated that cortisone protects the otic cartilage of rabbits from dissolution by excess vitamin A through the stabilizing action of glucocorticoids upon lysosomes, whose proteases are responsible for the degradation of chondromucoprotein.

Also in rabbits, acute overdosage with vitamin-A palmitate, or vitamin-A acid produces loss of hair and collapse of the ear cartilage with depletion of the cartilage matrix. Similar changes occur in the articular and epiphyseal cartilages. All these lesions are prevented by cortisone, whose protective effect is demonstrable even topically upon intra-articular injection in hypervitaminotic rabbits. These inhibitory actions of glucocorticoids upon vitamin-A overdosage (like those against ultraviolet ray injury or endotoxin shock) were again ascribed to lysosomal stabilization.

Additional in vitro studies confirmed that the dissolution of **murine** bone explants by vitamin A can be prevented by cortisol. Furthermore, fragments of murine esophagus cultured in vitro show inhibition of keratinization, and differentiation under the influence of vitamin A, but in this respect cortisol exerts similar actions, and if the two agents are given conjointly, they synergize each other.

In the larvae of **Xenopus laevis**, bone absorption, and other manifestations of vitamin-A overdosage are enhanced by cortisol. This was ascribed to the liberation of vitamin A from hepatic stores, and is in contrast to the retardation of hypervitaminosis A by cortisol, in vitro. Presumably, an excess of vitamin A causes release of cathepsins from intracellular lysosomes. It is also noteworthy that the osseous lesions produced by vitamin-A alcohol overdosage in Xenopus laevis larvae are aggravated, whereas those caused by vitamin-A acid are prevented by cortisol. Probably, the vitamin-A acid is not stored in the liver to any important degree, whereas the alcohol is stored in the liver as an ester and can be released by cortisol. In tissue cultures of chick and mouse bone cartilage implants rapidly disintegrate under the influence of excess vitamin A, and this response is prevented by cortisol; thus, the glucocorticoid has opposite actions in vivo and in vitro.

Vitamin B ←

In chickens, the responsiveness of the genital tract to folliculoids depends upon the availability of folic acid, and is suppressed by folic acid antagonists. Male mice are more sensitive than females to intoxication with the folic acid antagonist, aminopterin. Orchidectomy raises aminopterin tolerance, but estradiol fails to affect it in males and testosterone does not influence it in females.

In pigeons, thiamine deficiency has been claimed to be favorably influenced by DOC.

In rats, triamcinolone, dexamethasone, corticosterone, and DOC protect against the syndrome of nicotinamide deficiency. Allegedly, the corticoids raise the otherwise low NAD and NADH levels of the liver in nicotinamide deficient rats, augmenting at the same time the NADP and NADPH concentration, perhaps through an increase in tryptophan availability.

Vitamin C ←

Early observations suggested that adrenocortical extracts can protect guinea pigs against scurvy, but this might have been due merely to the high vitamin-C content of the adrenal cortex. Yet, subsequent research showed that cortisone and ACTH exert a similar protective effect.

The bone lesions characteristic of scurvy in guinea pigs are diminished by conjugated equine estrogens (Premarin), but not by estriol.

The normal excretion of ascorbic acid, and the increase in its elimination induced by barbital, are higher in male than in female rats. Orchidectomy reduces both the normal excretion and its enhancement by barbital, whereas ovariectomy has an opposite effect. Treatment of males with stilbestrol, or females with testosterone, diminishes ascorbic acid excretion. No such sex difference was noted in mice.

Vitamin D, DHT ←

Most of the work on the effect of steroids upon intoxication with vitamin-D derivatives, including DHT was performed in rats. These respond to acute poisoning by vitamin-D compounds with a syndrome of generalized calcinosis, affecting primarily the cardiovascular system, the kidney, the gastrointestinal tract, and the lungs. Death usually ensues within a few days. On the other hand, chronic intoxication with comparatively smaller doses, especially of DHT, leads to a "progeria-like syndrome." Here soft-tissue calcification is also pronounced, but affects predominantly the arteries, and it is associated with a very severe cachexia, involution of the thymicolymphatic and sex organs, the musculature and the adipose tissue. There are also dental and skeletal anomalies characterized by the development of a poorly calcified but excessive bone matrix, kyphosis and loss of skin elasticity. Although there are minor differences between the toxic manifestations of overdosage with vitamin-D_2, vitamin-D_3 and DHT, we shall discuss them conjointly because all three compounds are chemically and pharmacologically closely related. However, the acute and the chronic form of hypervitaminosis D respond quite differently to certain steroids, especially to those that exhibit powerful catatoxic effects against other substrates.

← **Glucocorticoids.** In mice, severe vitamin-D intoxication could not be prevented by cortisone.

In vitamin-D deficient **chicks**, cortisone and cortisol inhibit the maturation of cartilage matrix, whereas norethandrolone promotes it.

In **rats** on a vitamin-D deficient diet, cortisone decreases the inorganic serum phosphorus, but it either does not affect calcemia, or raises it slightly.

The arterial lesions produced by severe vitamin-D intoxication in rats, are aggravated by DOC, and ameliorated by cortisone. However, this protective effect is variable and appears to depend upon several unidentified experimental circumstances (perhaps including dietary factors), because several investigators claim that cortisol and cortisone do not influence, or actually aggravate, hypervitaminosis D. Similarly contradictory findings have been published concerning the alleged antirachitic action of glucocorticoids.

In rats, cortisol (unlike folliculoids) fails to cause a shift of the vitamin-D-induced nephrocalcinosis from the cortex to the cortico-medullary junction of the kidney.

After calciphylactic sensitization with DHT, neonatal rats respond with severe thymus calcification to a challenging dose of triamcinolone. Here, apparently, the acute glucocorticoid-induced thymus involution attracts calcium salts in the presence of DHT-induced sensitization.

In **patients**, cortisone has repeatedly been claimed to improve the manifestations of vitamin-D overdosage.

← **Mineralocorticoids.** The literature on the effect of DOC upon DHT intoxication in the rat is likewise quite contradictory, but in any event, mineralocorticoids do not appear to have any consistent and striking effects in this respect.

← **Adrenalectomy.** Both in intact and in adrenalectomized or hypophysectomized rats, vitamin-D overdosage produces a predominantly cortical nephrocalcinosis. Additional treatment with dienestrol (a folliculoid) shifts the calcium deposition predominantly to the cortico-medullary junction, irrespective of the presence or absence of the hypophysis and adrenals.

← **Folliculoids.** Early investigators suggested, on the basis of X-ray studies of the bones of rats kept on a vitamin-D deficient diet, that testosterone is "rachitogenic," whereas estradiol is "antirachitic." Yet, gonadectomy did not appear to influence experimental rickets in rats of either sex.

The renal calcification produced by vitamin-D_2 overdosage in the rat is not significantly influenced by estrone, although it does appear to have a tendency to shift from the cortical to the cortico-medullary junction in the rat. This effect is not evident in the mouse, rabbit and dog. Other investigators claimed that in rats overdosed with vitamin D or DHT, calcification occurs predominantly in the interstitial tissue of the renal cortex, whereas after simultaneous treatment with folliculoids, mineralization occurs intracanalicularly in the cortico-medullary junction.

In the Wistar-Imamichi strain of rats, the "progeria-like syndrome" produced by chronic DHT administration is unaccompanied by aorta calcinosis. This strain also reacts with osteoporosis, instead of the osteosclerosis (consisting of decalcified matrix) that is seen in most other strains. Conjugated estrogens offer virtually complete protection against these changes in the Wistar-Imamichi rat.

← **Testoids.** Whereas the effects of corticoids and folliculoids upon hypervitaminosis D are rather variable and dependent upon many incidental conditioning factors, anabolic testoids undoubtedly exert an extraordinary degree of protection. The first observation which called attention to this effect was the finding that male rats are much more resistant than females to DHT intoxication, but orchidectomy abolishes this sex difference. Hence, it was concluded that "some testicular factor exerts a protective effect against this type of intoxication."

It has been shown subsequently that various anabolic testoids protect not only against acute, but also against the chronic "progeria-like" form of intoxication with DHT or vitamin-D_2. These anabolics offer partial protection even against the loss of weight induced by AAN, estradiol, and food restriction; hence, at least part of their protective action may be ascribed to their anabolic or anticatabolic potency.

The original articles will have to be consulted for a comparative appraisal of the relative anti-DHT and anti-vitamin-D activities of various anabolic steroids; it is clear however, that in general, their protective action in this respect parallels their anabolic potency much more closely than their virilizing properties.

The calciphylaxis produced by DHT + egg-white, or by DHT + Thorotrast in the anaphylactoid shock organs of the rat can also be prevented by anabolic steroids (e.g., methyltestosterone).

It is especially noteworthy that the progeria-like syndrome produced with DHT, vitamin-D_2 or vitamin-D_3 can be prevented not only by methyltestosterone but also by ferric dextran and vitamin E, although presumably through different mechanisms.

The cystic transformation of the parathyroids, normally elicited in rats by combined treatment with DHT and calcium acetate, is likewise prevented by methyltestosterone.

Among the 36 steroids examined for their ability to protect the rat against the progeria-like syndrome induced by DHT, the strongest anabolic steroids (e.g., norbolethone, SC-7294 and fluoxymesterone) proved to be most efficacious.

Incidentally, ethynyltestosterone (like folliculoids) tends to shift the nephrocalcinosis induced by vitamin D from the renal cortex to the cortico-medullary junction.

In **rabbits**, the production of gallstones and cholecystitis by DHT is inhibited by methyltestosterone; at the same time, the serum concentration of DHT falls, allegedly as a consequence of diminished intestinal absorption.

In **chicks** on a vitamin-D deficient diet, norethandrolone promotes the maturation of cartilage matrix, whereas glucocorticoids inhibit it.

← **Other Steroids.** Among other steroids, two antimineralocorticoids, spironolactone and CS-1, proved to be highly efficacious in antagonizing the acute lethal effect of the intoxication with large doses of DHT or DHT + Na_2HPO_4, in the rat.

More recently, it was found that this is common to numerous other catatoxic steroids (e.g., ethylestrenol, PCN), so that it cannot depend upon the anabolic, antimineralocorticoid, corticoid, or any other known pharmacologic action of steroids; it must be regarded as an independent property. However, although all these catatoxic steroids are highly potent in preventing acute vitamin-D or DHT intoxication, only those with strong anabolic properties (e.g., ethylestrenol, oxandrolone, norbolethone, methyltestosterone) are very efficacious against the progeria-like syndrome. Several other catatoxic compounds (e.g., PCN, CS-1, spironolactone) prevent acute DHT intoxication but they either have no effect upon the progeria-like syndrome, or actually aggravate its course.

W-1372 ←

In rats, the blood lipid decreasing factor W-1372 causes severe hepatic lipidosis, sometimes with necrosis and high mortality if administered in oil solution. These toxic manifestations are prevented by PCN, CS-1, spironolactone and, to a lesser extent, by ethylestrenol, norbolethone, oxandrolone, progesterone and estradiol.

Zoxazolamine ←

Zoxazolamine, a muscle relaxant, is an excellent substrate for various nonsteroidal catatoxic drugs. Its action is also shortened by 19-nortestosterone derivatives, but not by medroxyprogesterone (a luteoid), although the latter compound does appear to counteract testosterone.

Our own observations in rats show that the muscular paralysis produced by zoxazolamine is greatly shortened by PCN, CS-1, ethylestrenol and, to a lesser extent, by spironolactone. Other steroids tested are ineffective.

Acetaldehyde ←

Lecoq et al. B66,406/51: In rats, the toxic effects of ethanol and its metabolites, pyruvate and acetaldehyde, (which accumulate in the body under the influence of disulfiram) are inhibited by ACTH, cortisone, and hepatic extracts. Conversely, thyroxine, DOC, and testosterone appear to aggravate ethanol intoxication. [Statistically evaluated data are not presented (H.S.).]

2-Acetaminofluorene ← cf. *Carcinogens*

Acetonitrile ←

Gellhorn 16,839/23: In mice, resistance against acetonitrile can be increased not only by thyroid extract, but to a lesser extent, also by extracts of various other tissues. These preparations also augment resistance to KCN and propionitrile, whereas thyroidectomy and orchidectomy have an opposite effect.

Eufinger & Wiesbader 4,663/30: In mice, pretreatment with gonadotrophic urinary extracts or folliculoid preparations increases acetonitrile resistance and hence, this phenomenon is not characteristic for the thyroid hormone.

Paal 22,603/30: In mice, acetonitrile resistance is not consistently influenced by the posterior pituitary extract (hypophysin), a folliculoid preparation (progynon), or by epinephrine.

Dessau 34,845/35: In rats, adrenalectomy decreases resistance to acetonitrile. This resistance can be slightly improved by adrenocortical transplants, but not by the adrenocortical extract tested, or by epinephrine.

N-Acetyl-p-aminophenol ← Prednisolone: Inscoe et al. *F70,325/66*

N-Acetyltyramine ← Prednisolone: Inscoe et al. *F70,325/66*

Acetanilide ←

Selye PROT. 42918: In rats, acute acetanilide intoxication is markedly inhibited by PCN, CS-1, ethylestrenol, spironolactone, norbolethone, prednisolone, thyroxine and phenobarbital. Estradiol tends to aggravate the toxicity of acetanilide, *cf.* Table 24. [Dr. S. Szabo noticed at the autopsy of these animals that some of them had developed perforating duodenal ulcers (H.S.).]

Table 24. *Conditioning for acetanilide*

Treatment[a]	Dyskinesia[b] (Positive/ Total)	Mortality[b] (Dead/ Total)
None	15/15	2/15
PCN	2/10 ***	0/10 NS
CS-1	5/10 ***	0/10 NS
Ethylestrenol	3/10 ***	0/10 NS
Spironolactone	3/10 ***	0/10 NS
Norbolethone	5/10 ***	0/10 NS
Oxandrolone	7/10 NS	2/10 NS
Prednisolone-Ac	1/10 ***	0/10 NS
Triamcinolone	9/10 NS	4/10 NS
Progesterone	10/10 NS	3/10 NS
Estradiol	10/10 NS	7/10 **
DOC-Ac	8/10 NS	4/10 NS
Hydroxydione	9/10 NS	3/10 NS
Thyroxine	4/10 ***	4/10 NS
Phenobarbital	3/10 ***	0/10 NS

[a] The rats of all groups were given acetanilide (50 mg/100 g body weight in 0.15 ml DMSO, s.c., once daily from 4th day to the end of the experiment).

[b] Dyskinesia was estimated on 6th day 8 hrs after injection and mortality listed on 7th day ("Exact Probability Test").

For further details on technique of tabulation *cf.* p. VIII.

Acrylamide ←

Selye PROT. 41419: In rats, acrylamide intoxication is efficiently combated by PCN and phenobarbital. The protective effect of CS-1 and spironolactone is less evident. The other standard conditioners are ineffective, *cf.* Table 25.

Acrylonitrile ←

Szabo & Selye G70,493/71: In rats, the adrenal necrosis and mortality produced by acrylonitrile were readily prevented by phenobarbital, but not or only doubtfully influenced by the other conditioners of our series, *cf.* Table 26, p. 177.

Table 25. *Conditioning for acrylamide*

Treatment[a]	Dyskinesia[b] (Positive/ Total)	Mortality[b] (Dead/ Total)
None	13/15	12/15
PCN	1/10 ***	1/10 ***
CS-1	5/10 NS	2/10 ***
Ethylestrenol	8/10 NS	7/10 NS
Spironolactone	4/10 *	6/10 NS
Norbolethone	8/10 NS	9/10 NS
Oxandrolone	8/10 NS	8/10 NS
Prednisolone-Ac	10/10 NS	9/10 NS
Triamcinolone	10/10 NS	10/10 NS
Progesterone	10/10 NS	5/10 NS
Estradiol	10/10 NS	10/10 NS
DOC-Ac	8/10 NS	6/10 NS
Hydroxydione	10/10 NS	6/10 NS
Thyroxine	10/10 NS	10/10 NS
Phenobarbital	3/15 ***	0/15 ***

[a] The rats of all groups were given acrylamide (10 mg/100 g body weight in 1 ml water, p.o., twice on 4th day and once on 5th day).

[b] Dyskinesia was estimated on 5th day p.m. and mortality listed on 6th day ("Exact Probability Test").

For further details on technique of tabulation *cf.* p. VIII.

Actinomycin ← *cf.* Antibiotics

Aflatoxin ← *cf.* Carcinogens

Alanine ← *cf.* GPT *under* Influence of Steroids upon Enzymes

Allyl Alcohol ←

Eger & Stratakis D89,546/58: In rats, chronic treatment with allyl alcohol causes a nodular hepatic cirrhosis not inhibited by prednisolone; the latter interferes with regeneration.

Eger et al. E58,108/59: In rats, prednisolone does not prevent hepatic cirrhosis induced by allyl alcohol or thioacetamide.

Tessmann et al. G38,224/65: Following a review of the literature on the prevention of hepatic lesions by glucocorticoids, the authors report on personal observations showing that prednisolone fails to influence connective tissue proliferation in the hepatic parenchyma of the liver, in rabbits chronically intoxicated with allyl alcohol.

Table 26. *Conditioning for acrylonitrile*

Treatment[a]	Adrenal Necrosis[b] (Positive/Total)	Mortality[b] (Dead/Total)
None	10/10	10/10
PCN	8/10 NS	10/10 NS
CS-1	9/10 NS	9/10 NS
Ethylestrenol	5/10 *	10/10 NS
Spironolactone	9/10 NS	9/10 NS
Norbolethone	6/10 *	9/10 NS
Oxandrolone	7/10 NS	9/10 NS
Prednisolone-Ac	6/10 *	7/10 NS
Triamcinolone (2 mg)	4/5 NS	5/5 NS
Progesterone	9/10 NS	10/10 NS
Estradiol	6/10 *	8/10 NS
DOC-Ac	8/10 NS	8/10 NS
Hydroxydione	8/10 NS	9/10 NS
Thyroxine	4/10 **	10/10 NS
Phenobarbital	0/10 ***	0/10 ***

[a] The rats of all groups were given acrylonitrile (1.5%/100 g body weight in 1 ml water, i.v., once on 4th day).

[b] Adrenal necrosis was estimated on day of death and mortality listed on 7th day ("Exact Probability Test").

For further details on technique of tabulation *cf.* p. VIII.

Allylformiate ←

Oettel & Franck A 72,420/42: In rats, DOC allegedly offers some protection against the hepatic changes produced by thyroxine or allylformiate.

Aminoacetonitrile ← *cf.* **Lathyrogens**

Aminoglutethimide ←

Goldman H 31,449/70: In rats, "testosterone prevents the testicular and male genital changes produced by aminoglutethimide. On the other hand, corticosterone markedly reduces the adrenal and female genital changes produced by this drug."

6-Aminonicotinamide ←

Mikes & Todorovic C 86,716/59: In guinea pigs, the hepatic lesions produced by 6-aminonicotinamide are inhibited by prednisolone.

o-Aminophenol ←

Inscoe & Axelrod D 1,700/60: The ability of microsomes from the liver of male rats to form o-aminophenol glucuronide in vitro is four times as great as in females. Estradiol diminishes this enzyme activity in males, whereas testosterone increases it in females.

Müller-Oerlinghausen et al. G 64,175/69: Hepatic tissue of mice injected with tolbutamide synthesizes an increased amount of glucuronide when incubated in vitro with o-aminophenol. Insulin, given at a dose causing a similar degree of hypoglycemia, is much less effective in enhancing glucuronide synthesis. Adrenalectomy diminishes the formation of o-aminophenol glucuronide, despite hypoglycemia. However, the adrenalectomized mice given cortisone again, respond with increased glucuronide synthesis after tolbutamide.

Selye G 70,480/71: In rats, o-aminophenol hydrochloride (50 mg/100 g body weight in 2 ml water) was administered s.c. once, on the 4th day of conditioning. Dyskinesia was listed 1 hr, mortality 24 hrs after this injection. Under these circumstances, the "Standard Conditioners" (p. VIII) caused no noteworthy change in the resulting intoxication, only thyroxine exhibited an aggravating effect. PCN was not tested.

o-Aminophenol ← Pregnane-3α,20α-diol, Pregnane-3α,20β-diol), Gp: Arias et al. *F 24,502/64*

o-Aminophenol ← Steroids, Mouse: Jones *G 19,777/64*

Aminopterin ←

Goldin et al. D 76,907/50: There is no sex difference in the toxicity of aminopterin in immature mice, but among adults, males are more resistant than females. Estradiol increases aminopterin tolerance in immature and mature males, whereas testosterone does not influence it.

Penhos G 8,997/62: In the rat, the loss of weight, diarrhea and other characteristic changes of aminopterin intoxication are more markedly aggravated by dexamethasone than by triamcinolone. Aminopterin counteracts the increase in liver weight produced by the glucocorticoids.

Aminopterin ← Adrenalectomy: Higgins et al. B 40,212/49*; Dougherty et al. G 77,517/50*; Goldin et al. D 76,907/50*

Aminopterin ← Orchidectomy, Mouse: Goldin et al. D 76,907/50*

Aminopterin ← Estradiol, Testosterone: Goldin et al. D76,907/50*

Aminopyrine ←

Borglin & Mansson B62,206/51: Gonadectomy does not change aminopyrine resistance in male mice but decreases it in females. This decrease is counteracted by estradiol.

Kato & Gillette F57,816/65: The ability of rat liver microsomal enzymes to inactivate various substrates is greater in males than in females, but the sex difference varies with the substrate. There is more than a 3-fold sex difference with aminopyrine and hexobarbital, but virtually none with hydroxylation of aniline and zoxazolamine. In male rats, starvation impairs the sex-dependent enzymes which metabolize aminopyrine and hexobarbital, but enhances those that hydroxylate aniline. On the other hand, in female rats, starvation increases the specific activity of the aminopyrine and hexobarbital-metabolizing enzymes as well as of the aniline hydroxylase. Starvation does not alter the metabolism of hexobarbital; it enhances that of aminopyrine by microsomes of castrated rats, but impairs the metabolism of these compounds by microsomes of methyltestosterone-treated castrates.

Kato & Gillette F57,817/65: The metabolism of aminopyrine and hexobarbital by hepatic microsomes of male rats is impaired by adrenalectomy, castration, hypoxia, ACTH, formaldehyde, epinephrine, morphine, alloxan or thyroxine. The metabolism of aniline and zoxazolamine is not appreciably decreased by any of these agents; in fact, the hydroxylation of aniline is enhanced by thyroxine or alloxan. Apparently, the treatments impair mainly the sex-dependent enzymes. Accordingly, the corresponding enzymic functions of the hepatic microsomes of female rats are not significantly diminished by the agents which do have an inhibitory effect in males.

Radzialowski & Bousquet H2,264/68: The circadian variation in aminopyrine, p-nitroanisole and hexobarbital-metabolizing microsomal enzymes of the rat and mouse liver is abolished by adrenalectomy, but the rhythm of dimethylaminoazobenzene metabolism remains unaffected.

Ichii & Yago H15,158/69: Studies on bilaterally adrenalectomized and/or orchidectomized rats, given cortisol or testosterone, led to the conclusion that corticoids and testoids regulate different fractions of the aminopyrine N-demethylase activity of the hepatic microsomes, which is mainly maintained by these hormones in intact male rats. On the other hand, phenobarbital-inducible aminopyrine N-demethylase activity is quite independent of adrenal and testicular control.

Orrenius et al. E8,231/69: In rats, adrenalectomy has no immediate effect upon the induction of steroid hydroxylases in the hepatic microsomes by phenobarbital. However, simultaneously adrenalectomized and castrate rats, subsequently maintained in this state for a period of time, showed a strikingly decreased hydroxylating activity of the hepatic microsomes, measured with either aminopyrine or testosterone as substrate. The cytochrome P-450 content of the microsomes decreased in a parallel fashion, whereas the cytochrome b_5 remained unchanged. When these steroid-deficient animals were treated with prednisolone or testosterone, the cytochrome P-450 content and the aminopyrine- and testosterone-hydroxylating activities of the liver microsomes returned to normal. In the steroid-deficient rats, repeated injections of phenobarbital caused only a minimal increase in the cytochrome P-450 content as well as in the NADPH-cytochrome reductase and aminopyrine-hydroxylation activities of the hepatic microsomes. Combined treatment with phenobarbital and prednisolone or testosterone resulted in an increase of these levels to those obtained by phenobarbital alone, in intact controls. Apparently, "steroid hormones are involved both in the maintenance of normal hydroxylating activity in the rat liver endoplasmic reticulum and in the increase of this activity caused by drugs."

Soyka G66,626/69: In rat liver, the aminopyrine demethylase activity of the microsomal fraction increased considerably during the first 30 days after birth. Evidence of an inhibitor was not found during this newborn period. After puberty, the activity in male rats was about twice as high as in females. Testosterone produced only an insignificant rise in females.

Nakanishi et al. G79,299/70: "Cold exposure or immobilization of intact or adrenalectomized rats significantly impaired side-chain oxidation of hexobarbital and N-demethylation of aminopyrine in vitro. In contrast, p-hydroxylation of aniline in vitro was not affected under stress conditions." The pertinent literature is somewhat contradictory but, possibly, the effect of stress on drug-metabolizing enzyme induction may vary with the substrate employed.

Solymoss et al. G60,075/70: In rats pretreated with spironolactone, norbolethone or ethylestrenol, hexobarbital anesthesia was diminished, and its aliphatic hydroxylation by hepatic microsomes enhanced. Pretreatment with the same steroids also accelerated the N-dealkylation of aminopyrine by hepatic microsomes. Progesterone was inactive against hexobarbital, but slightly increased the production of 4-aminoantipyrine by hepatic microsomes.

Selye PROT. 36785: In rats, aminopyrine intoxication was readily prevented by all classic catatoxic steroids, except oxandrolone whose beneficial effect was just below the level of statistical significance. Prednisolone, triamcinolone and phenobarbital also offered protection, *cf.* Table 27.

Table 27. *Conditioning for aminopyrine*

Treatment[a]	Dyskinesia[b] (Positive/ Total)	Mortality[b] (Dead/ Total)
None	9/15	8/15
PCN (1 mg)	0/10 ***	0/10 **
CS-1	0/10 ***	0/10 **
Ethylestrenol	0/15 ***	0/15 ***
Spironolactone	3/15 *	2/15 *
Norbolethone	0/10 ***	0/10 **
Oxandrolone	3/10 NS	3/10 NS
Prednisolone-Ac	0/10 ***	0/10 **
Triamcinolone	1/15 ***	1/15 **
Progesterone	0/9 ***	0/9 **
Estradiol	3/10 NS	2/10 NS
DOC-Ac	5/10 NS	5/10 NS
Hydroxydione	4/10 NS	4/10 NS
Thyroxine	11/15 NS	8/15 NS
Phenobarbital	4/10 NS	0/10 **

[a] The rats of all groups were given aminopyrine (30 mg/100 g body weight in 1 ml water, s.c., once on 4th day).

[b] Dyskinesia was estimated 2 hrs after injection and mortality listed 24 hrs later ("Exact Probability Test").

For further details on technique of tabulation *cf.* p. VIII.

Aminopyrine ← Adrenalectomy + Pesticides (Chlordane): Hart et al. *G27,102/65;* Orrenius *G74,389/65*

Aminopyrine ← Corticoids + Phenobarbital, Mouse, Rat: Wada et al. *H15,468/68;* Lu et al. *G68,802/69*

Aminopyrine ← Estradiol: Mitoma et al. *G72,113/68*

Aminopyrine ← Gonadectomy: Kato et al. *F57,817/65, F76,403/66;* Schenkman et al. *G67,777/67*

Aminopyrine ← Methyltestosterone: Kato et al. *F57,817/65, F76,403/66;* Mullen et al. *G37,764/66*

Aminopyrine ← Norethynodrel: Juchau et al. *G40,275/66*

Ammonium Chloride ←

Henschler & Reich C71,216/59: In rats, the pulmonary edema induced by ammonium chloride, epinephrine, thiourea, or chloropicrin is prevented by the administration (about 5 min earlier) of a single large dose of prednisolone i.v.

AMP (cyclic) ←

Rondell H32,853/70: In vitro experiments on the ovarian follicles of the pig suggest that LH, cyclic AMP or progesterone augment the distensibility of follicular strips, thereby preparing for rupture. TMACN blocks the effects of LH or cyclic AMP on both steroid release and distensibility. This blockade can be counteracted by progesterone. Presumably, "LH stimulates steroid secretion from the follicular tissue which in turn causes the activation of the ovulatory enzyme."

Amphetamine ←

D'Arcy & Spurling D8,818/61: The fact that mice living in crowded conditions are more susceptible to amphetamine than those housed in single cages is ascribed to an increased glucocorticoid secretion under the stress of crowding. Accordingly, cortisol pretreatment increased the amphetamine sensitivity of mice.

Clark et al. F92,621/67: Crowding increases the toxicity of amphetamine in the mouse. "The administration of either dexamethasone, ethanol, glucose, 2,deoxy-d-glucose or diphenylhydantoin reduced the excitement, hyperactivity and mortality, in aggregated mice given d-amphetamine. The reduction in mortality was proportional to the decrease in excitement and hyperactivity."

Groppetti & Costa H31,959/69: In adult male rats, the disappearance of amphetamine is faster than in adult females. Estradiol retards the rate of amphetamine disappearance in adult males. Such potent hepatic microsomal enzyme inducers as phenobarbital, 3-MC, or diphenylhydantoin do not change the tissue levels of amphetamine.

Selye G70,480/71: In rats, DL-amphetamine (12 mg/100 g body weight in 0.2 ml water) was administered s.c. once on the 4th day of conditioning. Dyskinesia was listed 4 hrs, mortality 24 hrs, after this injection. Under these circumstances, the "Standard Conditioners" (p. VIII) caused no noteworthy change in the resulting intoxication, only triamcinolone and thyroxine exhibited an aggravating effect.

Amyl Nitrite ←

Fischer 50,723/20: In rabbits, adrenalectomy prevents the induction of convulsions by amyl nitrite.

Specht 13,475/23: In guinea pigs, neither thyroidectomy nor orchidectomy influences the course of the convulsions produced by amyl nitrite inhalation or the electric irritation of the peripheral nerves.

Amyloid ← cf. also **Casein**

Lurie et al. B31,933/49: Estradiol suppresses the development of amyloidosis in tuberculous rabbits.

Anaphylactoidogens ← *corticoids* cf. also *Selye C1,001/54, p. 96; C92,918/61, p. 220; G46,715/68, pp. 109, 117, 178, 184, 189, 194.*

Anaphylactoidogens ← *folliculoids* cf. also *Selye G46,715/68, pp. 178, 194.*

Chen & Wickel B74,534/52: In adrenalectomized rats, the anaphylactoid edema produced by egg-white i.p. was prevented by cortisone, dehydrocorticosterone, 17-hydroxycorticosterone and 6,7-dehydrocortisone, whereas a large number of other steroids were inactive.

Selye et al. C70,942/59: Topical injection of cortisol acetate microcrystals into a hind paw of a rat selectively protects the surrounding region against the angiotactic sequestration of i.v. injected carbon (India ink) particles during a dextran-induced anaphylactoid edema.

Selye et al. C78,128/60: The gastric ulcers, as well as the associated anaphylactoid edema produced by 48/80 in the rat are prevented by cortisol or exposure to various stressors. This is all the more noteworthy because the stressors themselves are capable of producing gastric erosions.

Selye et al. C83,616/61: In rats, the cardiovascular and renal calcification produced by chronic treatment with polymyxin is increased by triamcinolone or DOC, and particularly by combined treatment with both these steroids or by F-COL which possesses both gluco- and mineralocorticoid properties.

Robert & Nezamis D23,289/62; D23,064/62: The acute gastric ulcers produced by polymyxin in the rat can be prevented by glucocorticoids (cortisol, prednisolone), but also by DOC. On the other hand, when following pretreatment with polymyxin the gastric mucosa is depleted of histamine, the ulcerogenic property of prednisolone overdosage is unimpaired. Hence, histamine liberation cannot be held responsible for the production of gastric ulcers by glucocorticoids.

Anesthetics (Various) ← cf. also **Individual Anesthetics**

Anesthetics (Various) ← *catatoxic steroids* cf. also *Selye G60,083/70, p. 385.*

Selye et al. G60,020/69: Norbolethone protects the rat against the anesthetic action of progesterone, DOC, pregnanedione, dehydroepiandrosterone, testosterone, diethylstilbestrol, pentobarbital, and methyprylon; it does not significantly alter the corresponding actions of urethan, diazepam, chlorpromazine, reserpine, phenoxybenzamine, chloral hydrate, KBr or $MgCl_2$. In all these cases, the effects of norbolethone simulate those of spironolactone.

Aniline ←

Kato & Gillette F57,816/65: The ability of rat liver microsomal enzymes to inactivate various substrates is greater in males than in females, but the sex difference varies with the substrate. There is more than a 3-fold sex difference with aminopyrine and hexobarbital, but virtually none with hydroxylation of aniline and zoxazolamine. In male rats, starvation impairs the sex-dependent enzymes which metabolize aminopyrine and hexobarbital, but enhances those that hydroxylate aniline. On the other hand, in female rats, starvation increases the specific activity of the aminopyrine and hexobarbital-metabolizing enzymes as well as of the aniline hydroxylase. Starvation does not alter the metabolism of hexobarbital; it enhances that of aminopyrine by microsomes of castrated rats, but impairs the metabolism of these compounds by microsomes of methyltestosterone-treated castrates.

Kato & Gillette F57,817/65: The metabolism of aminopyrine and hexobarbital by hepatic microsomes of male rats is impaired by adrenalectomy, castration, hypoxia, ACTH, formaldehyde, epinephrine, morphine, alloxan or thyroxine. The metabolism of aniline and zoxazolamine is not appreciably decreased by any of these agents; in fact, the hydroxylation of aniline is enhanced by thyroxine or alloxan. Apparently, the treatments impair mainly the sex-dependent enzymes. Accordingly, the corresponding enzymic functions of the hepatic microsomes of female rats are not significantly impaired by the agents which do have an inhibitory effect in males.

Furner & Stitzel G54,558/68: The hepatic microsomal metabolism of ethylmorphine, aniline and hexobarbital is diminished in vitro by previous adrenalectomy in the rat. Phenobarbital pretreatment of adrenalectomized rats raised the metabolism of all three substrates above the level characteristic of untreated, adrenalectomized controls. Exposure of adrenalectomized rats to cold stress, or treatment with cortisol, increased the metabolism of aniline and ethylmorphine, but depressed that of hexobarbital. In intact rats, cold stress diminished hexobarbital metabolism in vitro. Apparently, both the stress and the phenobarbital can bring about changes in the hepatic drug metabolism, independent of the presence of the adrenals; the two agents act through different mechanisms, since phenobarbital invariably stimulates, whereas stress either increases or decreases the microsomal enzyme activity, depending upon the drug pathway examined.

Nakanishi et al. G79,299/70: "Cold exposure or immobilization of intact or adrenalectomized rats significantly impaired side-chain oxidation of hexobarbital and N-demethylation of aminopyrine in vitro. In contrast, p-hydroxylation of aniline in vitro was not affected under stress conditions." The pertinent literature is somewhat contradictory but, possibly, the effect of stress on drug-metabolizing enzyme induction may vary with the substrate employed.

Selye et al. G70,424/70: In rats, aniline produces pronounced lipid hyperplasia of the adrenal cortex similar to that elicited by amphenone. This change is prevented by glucocorticoids and is presumably caused by an increased ACTH production as a consequence of diminished 11β-hydroxylated corticoid secretion.

Aniline ← Prednisolone, Cortisol + Phenobarbital, Mouse, Rat: Wada et al. *H15,468/68*

Aniline ← Methyltestosterone: Kato et al. *F57,817/65, F76,403/66*

Aniline ← Gonadectomy: Kato et al. *F57,817/65, F76,403/66;* Schenkman et al. *G67,777/67*

Aniline ← Norethynodrel: Juchau et al. *G40,275/66*

Antibiotics ← *cf. also* **Individual Antibiotics**

Antibiotics ← **corticoids** *cf. also* Selye *G60,083/70, pp. 348, 357.*

Giberti et al. B90,116/53: In guinea pigs, the organ lesions—particularly the hemorrhagic adrenalitis produced by chlortetracycline (Aureomycin)—are diminished by cortisone, but the mortality is not influenced.

Tuchmann-Duplessis & Mercier-Parot H28,871/70: In rats, actinomycin given before implantation causes only abortion; after implantation, it elicits both abortion and severe-malformations. These effects are not prevented by progesterone or estradiol alone or in combination.

Selye PROT. 38752: In rats, griseofulvin (7.5 mg/100 g body weight in 0.1 ml DMSO) was administered i.v. once on the 4th day. Dyskinesia was estimated 30 min, mortality 24 hrs after this injection. Under these circumstances, the "Standard Conditioners" caused no noteworthy change in the resulting intoxication, although in an earlier experiment some alterations in the course of this intoxication were noted (Table 138).

Anticoagulants ←

van Cauwenberge & Jaques C58,521/58: A dose of dicoumarol, well tolerated by untreated rabbits, causes death with widespread hemorrhage when given together with ACTH. The hemorrhagic tendency induced by dicoumarol was not accentuated by STH, cortisone, or DOC.

Paluszka & Hamilton C72,116/59: In rats, the leukocytosis produced by heparin is inhibited by cortisol.

van Cauwenberge & Jaques C72,748/59: The "hemorrhagic stress" syndrome produced by dicoumarol treatment in rats simultaneously exposed to various stressors can be reproduced by the administration of ACTH, STH or DOC, instead of stressors. Dicoumarol + cortisol or cortisone did not reproduce this syndrome.

Oliver et al. D54,029/63: In man, the requirements for anticoagulants (warfarin, phenindione) are reduced during simultaneous treatment with androsterone (Atromid). It is suggested that perhaps the ethyl-α-p-chlorophenoxyisobutyrate (C.P.I.B.) contained in this particular androsterone preparation may be involved.

Pyörälä & Kekki E31,756/63: In man, methandrostenolone increases sensitivity to certain anticoagulants (warfarin, phenindione). "The use of methandrostenolone should be avoided in patients receiving anticoagulants, because it may precipitate hemorrhagic complications."

Schrogie & Solomon G43,019/66: In man, both D-thyroxine and norethandrolone increase the anticoagulant response to bishydroxycoumarin at doses which do not change the rate of its metabolism. "Since clinically effective doses of these three drugs do not decrease the concentration of vitamin-K-dependent clotting factors, or affect the absorption, distribution, or metabolism of bishydroxycoumarin in man, it seems likely that they potentiate the pharmacologic effect of bishydroxycoumarin by increasing the affinity of the receptor site for the anticoagulant."

Jaques G70,979/68: Review (30 pp., 13 refs.) on the "hemorrhagic stress syndrome" that is produced in various mammals treated with indirect anticoagulants (e.g., phenindione, bishydroxycoumarin) and then exposed to stress or treated with DOC, ACTH, or STH. Conversely, cortisone, epinephrine, ephedrin, and adrenochrome inhibit this syndrome.

Selye G70,428/70: In rats, ethylestrenol powerfully inhibits the toxicity of digitoxin, nicotine, indomethacin, phenindione, dioxathion, EPN, physostigmine, hexobarbital, cyclopental, thiopental, DOC (anesthesia), meprobamate and picrotoxin. Thyroxine increases the toxicity of many among these drugs, and inhibits the protective effect of ethylestrenol.

Selye G60,094/70: In rats, the fatal hemorrhagic diathesis produced by phenindione is inhibited by ethylestrenol, CS-1, spironolactone, norbolethone and oxandrolone. Progesterone, hydroxydione, DOC, and estradiol have a much less pronounced effect. Prednisolone, triamcinolone, and thyroxine are inactive.

Solymoss et al. G70,423/70: In rats, pretreatment with spironolactone, norbolethone, or ethylestrenol enhances the disappearance of bishydroxycoumarin from blood, and restores the prothrombin time. Triamcinolone and progesterone fail to do so. SKF 525-A increases the blood concentration and the anticoagulant effect of bishydroxycoumarin and counteracts the beneficial effect of ethylestrenol. Furthermore, pretreatment with spironolactone or ethylestrenol (but not with progesterone) enhances the NADPH-dependent enzymic decay of bishydroxycoumarin in liver microsomal + supernatant fraction.

Szeberényi & Fekete H29,579/70: Brief abstract stating that after four days of pretreatment (species not mentioned), spironolactone decreased the action and accelerated the metabolism of hexobarbital, chlorzoxazone, meprobamate, estrone, testosterone, acenocoumarol and BSP, whereas after short treatment it had an inverse effect. It is concluded that spironolactone is a microsomal enzyme inducer.

Selye G70,480/71: In rats, fatal intoxication with bishydroxycoumarin was beneficially influenced by pretreatment with various catatoxic steroids or estradiol, *cf.* Table 28.

Table 28. *Conditioning for bishydroxycoumarin*

Treatment[a]	Mortality[b] (Dead/Total)
None	7/9
PCN	9/10 NS
CS-1	2/10 *
Ethylestrenol	2/10 *
Spironolactone	1/9 **
Norbolethone	2/10 *
Oxandrolone	1/9 **
Prednisolone-Ac	9/9 NS
Triamcinolone (2 mg)	10/10 NS
Progesterone	7/10 NS
Estradiol	1/10 ***
DOC-Ac	9/10 NS
Hydroxydione	9/10 NS
Cholesterol	5/10 NS
Thyroxine	8/8 NS
Phenobarbital	3/10 NS

[a] The rats of all groups were given bishydroxycoumarin (13 mg/100 g body weight in 1 ml water, p.o., once daily from the 4th day ff.).

[b] Mortality was listed on 9th day ("Exact Probability Test").

For further details on technique of tabulation *cf.* p. VIII.

Selye G70,480/71: In rats, all classic catatoxic steroids and phenobarbital readily prevented fatal phenindione intoxication, but some of the other conditioners of our series also appeared to have a beneficial effect, at least upon the survival rate.

Table 29. *Conditioning for phenindione*

Treatment[a]	Intestinal hemorrhage[b] (Positive/Total)	Mortality[b] (Dead/Total)
None	14/15	15/15
PCN	3/10 ***	9/10 NS
CS-1	3/13 ***	2/13 ***
Ethylestrenol	2/15 ***	2/15 ***
Spironolactone	2/14 ***	2/14 ***
Norbolethone	0/14 ***	1/14 ***
Oxandrolone	0/15 ***	1/15 ***
Prednisolone-Ac	15/15 NS	14/15 NS
Triamcinolone (2 mg)	14/14 NS	14/14 NS
Progesterone	9/14 NS	8/14 **
Estradiol (1 mg)	11/14 NS	10/15 *
Estradiol (1 mg s.c.)	10/10 NS	10/10 NS
DOC-Ac	14/15 NS	11/15 *
Hydroxydione	12/15 NS	9/15 **
Thyroxine	14/15 NS	14/15 NS
Phenobarbital	2/10 ***	1/10 ***

[a] The rats of all groups were given phenindione (10 mg/100 g body weight in 0.2 ml DMSO, s.c., daily from 4th day ff.).

[b] Intestinal hemorrhage was estimated on day of death and mortality listed on 8th day ("Exact Probability Test").

For further details on technique of tabulation cf. p. VIII.

Selye G70,480/71: In rats, warfarin (10 mg/100 g body weight in 1 ml water) was administered p.o. twice, from the 4th day of conditioning to the end of experiment. Mean survival was listed, and mortality registered on the 9th day. Under these circumstances, the "Standard Conditioners" (p. VIII) caused no noteworthy change in the resulting intoxication.

Solymoss & Varga G70,500/71: In rats, spironolactone, norbolethone and ethylestrenol diminish the anticoagulant action and accelerate the plasma clearance of bishydroxycoumarin. Progesterone and triamcinolone are devoid of this effect. SKF 525-A counteracts the influence of ethylestrenol upon bishydroxycoumarin metabolism. The hepatic microsomes of rats treated with spironolactone or ethylestrenol in vivo accelerate bishydroxycoumarin degradation by NADPH-dependent enzymes in vitro.

Coumarin, 4-Methylcoumarin ← 1-7 Methyltestosterone: Feuer *H 24,218/70*

Antipyrine ←

Remmer C73,857/58: The oxidation of hexobarbital and the demethylation of methylaminoantipyrine by liver slices in vitro are inhibited by adrenalectomy performed 10—12 days before the experiment, unless the animals are given prednisolone substitution therapy. Addition of prednisolone to the incubation medium has no effect. The drug-metabolizing activity is contained in the microsome fraction and, in this respect, the microsomes of males are more active than those of females.

Booth & Gillette D34,656/62: Testosterone propionate, 19-nortestosterone, 4-androstene-3, 17-dione and 4-chloro-19-nortestosterone acetate (SKF 6611) were tested for their ability to induce hepatic microsomal enzymes in female rats. "All of the steroids produced 2- to 3-fold increases in the activity of the enzyme systems that metabolize hexobarbital, demethylate monomethyl-4-aminoantipyrine and hydroxylate naphthalene, but only 19-nortestosterone, testosterone propionate and methyltestosterone increased the activity of microsomal TPNH oxidase. ... The increase in microsomal enzyme activity is more closely related to the anabolic activity than to the androgenic activity of the steroid."

*ANTU ← cf. 1- (1-Naphthyl) -2-thiourea under **Thioureas***

Arsenic ← cf. also Selye *C50,810/58, p. 102.*

Agduhr G37,252/41: In the mouse, sexual intercourse as well as some sex hormone preparations increase the storage of arsenic in the ground substance of various organs, especially the skin, whereas repeated pregnancies have an opposite effect, and at the same time augment resistance against intoxication with As_2O_3.

Skanse A72,698/41: Review on the effect of sex, sexual intercourse and gonadectomy upon the storage of arsenic in the tissues of mice.

Beck B58,869/50: In mice, adrenocortical extract protects against lethal doses of arsenious acid.

Beck & Voloshin B58,271/50: In mice, resistance to arsenite and other arsenicals is increased by cortisone, adrenocortical extracts and ACTH.

Beck B64,609/51: "Prior administration of beef adrenal extract increased the resistance of mice, particularly male mice, to semi-lethal doses of arsenite, oxophenarsine and clorarsen. Male mice were protected against arsenite by cortisone and ACTH, but not by desoxycorticosterone."

Aspartate ← *cf.* **GOT** under **Influence of Steroids upon Enzymes**

Atophane ← *cf.* **Cinchophen**

Bacterial Toxins ← *cf.* **Microorganisms, Vaccines and Parasites**

Barbiturates ←

← **Glucocorticoids.**

RAT

Einhauser A19,483/39: Survival of rats after heavy intoxication with barbital can be improved by pretreatment with adrenocortical extract especially in combination with vitamin C. Synthetic corticosterone has no such protective effect.

Fingl et al. D38,091/52: In rats, chronic administration of phenobarbital or diphenylhydantoin diminishes the brain hyperexcitability induced by cortisone as judged by EST measurements.

Robillard & Pellerin B75,692/52: In rats, the anesthetic effect of pentobarbital is prolonged by adrenalectomy. This effect is inhibited by cortisone and enhanced by DOC. Cortisone also shortens sleeping time in intact or gonadectomized male rats.

Robillard et al. G67,325/54: Cortisone diminishes pentobarbital anesthesia in adult male rats. It also restores to normal the prolonged anesthetic effect of pentobarbital observed after adrenalectomy (with maintenance on 1% NaCl), orchidectomy, or simultaneous adrenalectomy + orchidectomy. Furthermore, cortisone decreases the length of pentobarbital anesthesia in ovariectomized rats, but this effect is blocked by estradiol treatment.

de Boer & Mukomela C5,245/55: In rats, ACTH and cortisone shorten thiopental and pentobarbital sleeping times, especially in females whose sleeping time is normally longer than that of males.

Remmer G79,941/57: In female rats, cortisone and prednisolone are much more efficacious than testosterone in shortening hexobarbital anesthesia and increasing microsomal hexobarbital metabolism. Adrenalectomy diminishes the capacity of hepatic microsomes of male rats to metabolize hexobarbital unless the animals are pretreated with cortisone or prednisolone.

Heuser C54,451/58: In the rat, large doses of cortisol, its succinate or acetate, prolong pentobarbital sleeping time when given simultaneously with the latter, but shorten it if the steroids are administered one day before the barbiturate.

Remmer C73,857/58: The oxidation of hexobarbital and the demethylation of methylaminoantipyrine by liver slices, in vitro, are inhibited by adrenalectomy performed 10—12 days before the experiment, unless the rats are given prednisolone substitution therapy. Addition of prednisolone to the incubation medium has no effect. The drug-metabolizing activity is contained in the microsome fraction and, in this respect, the microsomes of males are more active than those of females.

Remmer D86,728/58: In rats, 3 days pretreatment with cortisone or prednisolone diminishes the anesthetic effect of hexobarbital, and increases the degradation of the anesthetic by liver slices. Adrenalectomy inhibits the degradation of hexobarbital by liver slices of male rats, an effect which can be counteracted by pretreatment with cortisone.

Rupe et al. E26,910/63: The sedative effect of hexobarbital and pentobarbital, yet not of barbital, was diminished by tourniquet stress, in the intact but not in the hypophysectomized or adrenalectomized rat. In intact rats, ACTH or cortisone decreases hexobarbital sleeping time as does stress, whereas SKF 525-A completely blocks the protective action of stress. Presumably "the stress effect on the duration of drug action is mediated through increased drug metabolism."

Azarnoff et al. G42,999/66: In the rat, pretreatment with DDD markedly shortens anesthesia produced by various steroids and barbiturates. Simultaneously, there is proliferation of the SER and a rise in the level of hepatic hexobarbital-metabolizing enzymes. In dogs, DDD decreases hexobarbital sleeping time, but prolongs pentobarbital anesthesia. Cortisone prevents the prolongation of pentobarbital sleep.

MOUSE

Winter & Flataker B73,509/52: Cortisone or ACTH, unlike DOC, shortens the sleeping time of barbiturate anesthesia. The markedly prolonged sleeping time of mice receiving both barbiturates and diphenhydramine is also decreased by cortisone, but the effect of the steroid can be fully accounted for by its antagonism to the barbiturate.

Gorby et al. B 84,489/53: Pretreatment with cortisol or DOC had little effect upon pentobarbital anesthesia in the mouse although cortisone offered slight protection and DOC had a feeble enhancing effect. Both corticoids increased the toxicity of phenobarbital.

Komiya C 7,045/55: In mice, barbital anesthesia was decreased by cortisone, cortisol and ACTH, but not changed by DOC or "substance S." The barbital concentration of the brain approximately paralleled the depth of anesthesia.

Komiya C 8,533/55: In mice, barbital sleeping time is decreased by cortisone, cortisol, and ACTH, but not affected by compound S (desoxocortisone) or DOC.

Satoskar & Trivedi C 8,678/55: In mice, mortality after pentobarbital intoxication is increased by pretreatment with cortisol 2 hrs prior to the barbiturate.

Komiya & Shibata C 16,708/56: In mice, the induction time of barbital anesthesia was not changed by cortisone, cortisol, substance S, or DOC. The duration of anesthesia was shortened, its depth diminished, and the barbital concentration of the brain decreased by cortisone, cortisol, or ACTH, but none of these parameters was affected by substance S or DOC. Apparently, the active hormones protect against anesthesia by decreasing the barbital concentration of the brain.

Komiya et al. C 21,326/56: In mice, thiopental anesthesia was reduced in severity, but not in duration, by epinephrine. Barbital anesthesia was slightly reduced by norepinephrine, yet not by epinephrine. Unpublished experiments suggest that ACTH and glucocorticoids shorten the duration of barbital anesthesia in mice.

Kostowski & Nowacka H 26,526/70: In mice, cortisol and methylprednisolone decrease hexobarbital sleeping time, whereas DOC prolongs it. Hydroxydione anesthesia is not changed by cortisol, but prolonged by methylprednisolone as well as by high doses of DOC.

RABBIT

Komiya et al. D 26,331/56: In rabbits, barbital sodium anesthesia was not significantly influenced by cortisone.

Shibata et al. C 49,533/57: In rabbits, barbital anesthesia is only moderately shortened by cortisone. The barbital concentration of the blood is not significantly influenced, whereas barbital elimination in the urine is markedly increased by cortisone.

MAN

Fraser et al. B 57,226/51: In man, abstinence symptoms following discontinuation of various barbiturates or morphine are favorably influenced by cortisone.

Dhunèr & Nordqvist D 98,693/57: In 11 out or 13 patients who recovered from barbiturate poisoning, sleep was reinduced by cortisone treatment or i.v. injection of glucose.

VARIA

Frommel et al. E 37,967/62: Pretreatment with cortisone prolongs phenobarbital anesthesia in the guinea pig and hexobarbital anesthesia in the mouse. It shortens thiopental anesthesia in rabbits.

Barbiturates ← Corticoids *cf. also Tables 30—34*

Hexobarbital ← Glucocorticoids + Sex: Remmer D 86,728/58*

Hexobarbital ← Cortisol + Phenobarbital: Lu et al. G 68,802/69

Hexobarbital ← Prednisolone: Remmer C 73,857/58

Pentobarbital ← Corticoids: Robillard et al. G 67,325/54*; Driever et al. G 31,872/65*

← **Gluco-Mineralocorticoids, Mineralocorticoids.** *Driever & Bousquet G 31,872/65; Driever et al. F 73,812/66:* In rats with tourniquet stress, the blood levels of hexobarbital, pentobarbital and meprobamate, but not of phenobarbital, were diminished after injection of the above drugs. These effects are prevented by hypophysectomy or adrenalectomy. Pentobarbital blood levels are lowered in adrenalectomized rats by corticosterone, but not by ACTH, whereas in hypophysectomized rats, both these hormones are active. "The ability of stress situations to stimulate drug metabolism and its dependence upon an intact pituitary-adrenal axis is suggestive of a regulatory function of the endocrine system in mediating a rapid induction of liver microsomal enzymes responsible for drug metabolism."

Bousquet et al. F 35,073/65: In rats with stress produced by applying a tourniquet around one hind limb, for 2.5 hrs, the toxicity of hexobarbital, pentobarbital, meprobamate and zoxazolamine was significantly diminished, whereas that of barbital and phenobarbital remained unaffected. Pretreatment with ACTH or corticosterone simulated the effect of stress. After hypophysectomy or adrenalectomy, stress failed to offer the usual protection. [The barbiturates and zoxazolamine appear to have been administered immediately after release of the tourniquet, but this is not specifically stated. Allegedly, a single injection of corticosterone (50 µg per animal) sufficed to offer protection (H.S.).]

Kostowski & Nowacka H 26,526/70: In mice, cortisol and methylprednisolone decrease hexobarbital sleeping time, whereas DOC prolongs it. Hydroxydione anesthesia is not changed by cortisol but prolonged by methylprednisolone, as well as by high doses of DOC.

Hexobarbital ← Corticosterone: Bousquet et al. F 35,073/65*

Pentobarbital ← Corticosterone + Hypophysectomy + Stress: Driever et al. G 31,872/65*

Thiopental ← DOC + Adrenalectomy: Eichholtz et al. B 45,516/49*

← **Antimineralocorticoids.** *Selye et al. G 60,016/69:* In rats, spironolactone protects against anesthesia produced by progesterone, DOC, hydroxydione, pregnanedione, dehydroepiandrosterone, testosterone, diethylstilbestrol, methyprylon, pentobarbital and ethanol. It does not significantly alter the corresponding actions of morphine, codeine, urethan, diazepam, chlorpromazine, reserpine, phenoxybenzamine, chloral hydrate, potassium bromide, or $MgCl_2$.

Selye G 60,044/69: Among various steroids tested for their ability to inhibit progesterone and pentobarbital anesthesia, all anabolic androgens were highly potent. However, since spironolactone exhibited the same antianesthetic effect, the latter could not be attributed to anabolic potency. "This inhibition of anesthesia is assumed to represent a special instance of the catatoxic effect which appears to be a property of certain steroids, independent of their classic hormonal actions."

Feller & Gerald H 22,744/70: In male mice, pretreatment with spironolactone shortened pentobarbital and "testosterone-potentiated" pentobarbital sleeping times. It also increased liver microsomal protein, liver weight, aniline hydroxylation and ethylmorphine N-demethylation.

Gerald & Feller G 74,396/70: In mice, spironolactone and its Δ^6 de-thioacetylated metabolite reduce hexobarbital sleeping time and cause nearly identical increases in liver weight, microsomal protein content, NADPH-cytochrome c reductase, cytochrome P-450 content, and the N-demethylation of ethylmorphine. Preliminary observations suggest that these actions of spironolactone and its metabolite are evident in both sexes.

Gerald & Feller G 74,092/70: In mice, pretreatment with spironolactone shortens pentobarbital sleeping time as well as "testosterone-potentiated pentobarbital sleeping time." Furthermore, spironolactone enhances the microsomal metabolism of aniline and ethylmorphine, and increases hepatic weight. It is concluded that the in vivo protective effect of spironolactone is due to the induction of hepatic microsomal enzymes.

Gerald & Feller G 78,804/70: In mice, pretreatment with spironolactone reduces pentobarbital sleeping time and accelerates the hepatic microsomal metabolism of hexobarbital in vivo and in vitro.

Selye et al. G 60,050/70: Aldadiene (SC-9376), aldadiene-kalium (SC-14266), spironolactone and CS-1 protect the rat against digitoxin intoxication as well as against the anesthetic effect of progesterone and pentobarbital. Spiroxasone, SC-8109 and SC-5233 fail to protect the rat both against digitoxin intoxication and the anesthetic effect of progesterone or pentobarbital.

Stripp et al. H 22,743/70: In rats, spironolactone pretreatment shortened hexobarbital sleeping time. "Moreover, treatment of female rats with spironolactone doubled the rate of the in vitro metabolism of hexobarbital and benzpyrene by liver microsomes and quadrupled that of ethylmorphine. The inducing effects of spironolactone were very different from those of phenobarbital and 3-methylcholanthrene. The amount of cytochrome P-450 was either unaltered or decreased, but the NADPH cytochrome c reductase activity was increased 2-fold. Although the endogenous rate of cytochrome P-450 reduction by NADPH was not altered, the stimulatory effects of ethylmorphine or hexobarbital on the rate of cytochrome P-450 reduction were significantly greater with microsomes from spironolactone treated animals. By contrast, treatment of male rats with spironolactone caused no change in hexobarbital sleeping time and no change or a slight decrease in hexobarbital and benzpyrene metabolism by liver microsomes."

Szeberényi & Fekete H 29,579/70: Brief abstract stating that after four days of pretreatment (species not mentioned), spironolactone decreased the action and accelerated the metabolism of hexobarbital, chlorzoxazone, meprobamate, estrone, testosterone, acenocoumarol and BSP, whereas after short treatment it had an inverse effect. It is concluded that spironolactone is a microsomal enzyme inducer.

Gillette H 34,126/71: In male rats, spironolactone caused a relatively small increase in ethylmorphine N-demethylation and decreased the oxidation of hexobarbital and 3,4-benzpyrene. However (like in females), spironolactone did not affect the type I spectral changes induced in males by ethylmorphine and hexobarbital but caused a small decrease in cytochrome P-450 content and increased NADPH-cytochrome c reductase. Moreover, in males, spironolactone increased the substrate-dependent cytochrome P-450 reduction but not its endogenous reduction. The sex difference in the effect of spironolactone upon hepatic microsomal drug metabolism is illustrated by the tabulation of data concerning ethylmorphine and hexobarbital biotransformation.

Stripp et al. G 79,538/71: In rats, the induction of hepatic microsomal enzymes by spironolactone "differed from the phenobarbital or methylcholanthrene induction in that it did not increase cytochrome P-450 content or microsomal protein. Furthermore the induction seemed to be sex dependent."

← **Testoids.**

RAT

Holck et al. 68,297/37: Female rats are much more sensitive than males to anesthesia by various barbiturates. Orchidectomy diminishes barbiturate sensitivity, but not quite to the low level of normal females. Barbital anesthesia is not influenced by sex. Testosterone increases barbiturate resistance in normal or ovariectomized females, but not quite to the level of normal males.

Holck et al. A 8,011/37: In rats, prolonged treatment with testoid extracts from human urine (unlike androsterone) shortens hexobarbital sleeping time in intact or ovariectomized females, but not quite to the male level.

Kinsey A 39,742/40: Female rats sleep about twice as long as males when given either single or repeated injections of pentobarbital. Testosterone increases pentobarbital resistance in females. Ovariectomy diminishes the sleeping time.

Holck & Mathieson 80,435/41: Male rats were more resistant than females to the lethal effect of pentobarbital. Castration reduced the tendency to develop tolerance following repeated pentobarbital injections in males, but increased it in females. Testosterone pretreatment enhanced resistance in castrate males and intact females, but not in intact males.

Robillard et al. B 51,110/50: Male rats are more resistant than females to the narcotic effect of pentobarbital. Gonadectomized rats of both sexes exhibit high pentobarbital resistance after treatment with testosterone, presumably as a consequence of accelerated hepatic detoxication of the barbiturates, since incubation of pentobarbital with liver slices of normal males or testosterone-treated castrates exhibit accelerated pentobarbital detoxication in vitro.

Buchel G 67,326/54: Testosterone decreases hexobarbital sleeping time in adult, intact or ovariectomized female rats. Estradiol has an inverse effect in normal or castrate males. Indirect evidence suggests that the changes in hexobarbital sleeping time are associated with its reduced or prolonged presence in the body.

Robillard et al. G 67,325/54: In rats adrenalectomized 5 days prior to phenobarbital treatment and maintained on 1% NaCl, anesthesia was prolonged. This effect could not be influenced by DOC, but was abolished by cortisone. Simultaneous orchidectomy does not further prolong pentobarbital anesthesia in adrenalectomized rats, but even in animals thus deprived of all steroids, cortisone greatly diminishes anesthesia, while testosterone has no influence upon it. Apparently, testosterone requires the presence of glucocorticoids, in order to be effective, whereas cortisone does not require the presence of testoids.

Edgren C 45,010/57: Female rats are more sensitive than males to the anesthetic effect of hexobarbital. Gonadectomy prolongs hexobarbital sleeping time in males and shortens it in females. Estrone prolongs hexobarbital sleeping time in ovariectomized females, whereas testosterone is ineffective. In orchidectomized rats testosterone shortens hexobarbital sleeping time, while estrone is ineffective.

Remmer G 79,941/57: In female rats, cortisone and prednisolone are much more efficacious than testosterone in shortening hexobarbital anesthesia and increasing microsomal hexobarbital metabolism. Adrenalectomy diminishes the capacity of hepatic microsomes of male rats to metabolize hexobarbital unless the animals are pretreated with cortisone or prednisolone.

Takabatake G76,713/57: Male rats are more resistant than females or castrates of either sex, to the anesthetic effect of ethylhexabital. Testosterone raises the resistance of males and gonadectomized animals of either sex to the male level. In vitro studies on liver slices indicate that the sex difference is due to the effect of testosterone upon the barbiturate-metabolizing ability of the liver, not upon brain sensitivity.

Quinn et al. E89,993/58: In intact rats, estradiol prolonged the hexobarbital sleeping time and the elevation of the plasma level of this barbiturate, whereas the hepatic microsomal enzyme activity required to metabolize hexobarbital was considerably diminished. In all these respects, testosterone exerted an opposite effect in females.

Booth & Gillette D34,656/62: Testosterone propionate, 19-nortestosterone, 4-androstene-3, 17-dione and 4-chloro-19-nortestosterone acetate (SKF 6611) were tested for their ability to induce hepatic microsomal enzymes in female rats. "All of the steroids produced 2- to 3-fold increases in the activity of the enzyme systems that metabolize hexobarbital, demethylate monomethyl-4-aminoantipyrine and hydroxylate naphthalene, but only 19-nortestosterone, testosterone propionate and methyltestosterone increased the activity of microsomal TPNH oxidase. ... The increase in microsomal enzyme activity is more closely related to the anabolic activity than to the androgenic activity of the steroid."

Kato et al. G64,325/62: Adult male rats are more resistant than females to pentobarbital anesthesia, carisoprodol paralysis and strychnine convulsions. Conversely, the lethal effect of OMPA is greater in the male. The sex difference is ascribed to the increased production of anabolic testoids which enhance the decomposition of these substrates, the first three being inactivated, and the last activated in the process. The differences were also demonstrated in vitro, using liver slices or microsomal fractions. The high microsomal activity of the male could be abolished by castration and restored by several anabolic testoids.

Takabatake & Ariyoshi D48,245/62: The ability of rat liver slices to metabolize cyclobarbital in vitro is uninfluenced by the addition of testosterone or estradiol.

Rubin et al. F73,811/66: Both testosterone and the antitestoid substance 17α-methyl-B-nortestosterone (SK&F 7690) increase the hepatic microsomal hexobarbital oxidase activity in intact female rats. However, if the two compounds are administered conjointly, the effect is less pronounced than that obtained by testosterone alone. Apparently "a 'weak' enzyme inducer (SK&F 7690) may compete with a 'strong' inducer (testosterone) for occupation of a common receptor site for enzyme induction."

Chang & Lei F78,943/67: In female rats, 17α-methyl-5α-androstan-17β-ol shortens pentobarbital but not diethylbarbital sleeping time. Since the former barbiturate is — whereas the latter is not — metabolized by hepatic microsomes, the steroid is thought to act through the latter.

Selye et al. G60,020/69: In the rat, pretreatment with norbolethone protects against the anesthetic effect of progesterone, desoxycorticosterone, pregnanedione, dehydroepiandrosterone, testosterone, diethylstilbestrol, pentobarbital, and methyprylon. It does not significantly alter the corresponding actions of urethan, diazepam, chlorpromazine, reserpine, phenoxybenzamine, chloral hydrate, potassium bromide, or magnesium chloride.

Solymoss et al. G60,054/69: "In the rat, pretreatment with spironolactone, norbolethone or ethylestrenol increased the oxidation of pentobarbital by liver microsomes, enhanced its disappearance from blood and proportionally decreased the depth of anesthesia."

Solymoss et al. G60,075/70: In rats pretreated with spironolactone, norbolethone, or ethylestrenol, hexobarbital anesthesia was diminished and its aliphatic hydroxylation by hepatic microsomes enhanced. Pretreatment with the same steroids also accelerated N-dealkylation of aminopyrine by hepatic microsomes. Progesterone was inactive against hexobarbital, but slightly increased the production of 4-aminoantipyrine by hepatic microsomes.

Selye PROT. 33876: In rats, hexobarbital anesthesia is prolonged by orchidectomy and shortened by methyltestosterone both in intact and in orchidectomized animals. Progesterone significantly reduces the hexobarbital sleeping time in intact rats, but causes only a nonsignificant decrease in castrates. Estradiol prolongs hexobarbital anesthesia in intact and orchidectomized rats as compared with the corresponding controls.

MOUSE

Falk A 337/36: In mice, the anesthetic effect of certain barbiturates is inhibited by crude testicular extracts. [It is unlikely that these preparations antagonized barbiturates by virtue of their negligible testoid content (H.S.).]

Westfall et al. F 2,504/64: Pentobarbital anesthesia is more prolonged in male than in female mice. Sleeping time in males is shortened by stilbestrol and, in females, prolonged by testosterone. Apparently, the mechanism for barbiturate detoxication is different in mice and rats.

Novick Jr. et al. F 63,768/66: "Subcutaneous administration of several 19-nortestosterone derivatives produced an increased hepatic microsomal metabolism of hexobarbital and decreased zoxazolamine prostration time in mice. Testosterone and methyltestosterone produced an increased hexobarbital sleep time and testosterone decreased the rate of hepatic microsomal metabolism of hexobarbital. Although the ability of norethandrolone and SK&F 6612 (4-chloro-17α-methyl-19-nortestosterone) to shorten hexobarbital sleep time occurs within 6 to 12 hr. after a single dose in mice, this effect of testosterone derivatives in rats occurs only after prolonged treatment."

Roberts & Plaa G 39,694/66: In mice, hexobarbital sleeping time is shortened, and the in vivo metabolism of the barbiturate increased by pretreatment with norethandrolone.

GUINEA PIG

Brena & d'Agostino C 11,921/54: In guinea pigs, orchidectomy prolongs thiopental sleeping time; testosterone diminishes it, both in castrate and in intact males.

VARIA

Quinn et al. G 67,327/54: The biologic half-life of hexobarbital was found to be 15 min for mice, 60 min for rabbits, 140 min for rats, and 260 min for dogs and man. There was an inverse relationship between the rate of biotransformation of hexobarbital to ketohexobarbital and the duration of its hypnotic effect. Male rats are more resistant to hexobarbital anesthesia than females, but in the latter, resistance, as well as the enzyme activity of the microsomes, was increased by testosterone.

Selye G 60,044/69: Among various steroids tested for their ability to inhibit progesterone and pentobarbital anesthesia, all anabolic androgens were highly potent. However, since spironolactone exhibited the same antianesthetic effect, the latter could not be attributed to anabolic potency. "This inhibition of anesthesia is assumed to represent a special instance of the catatoxic effect which appears to be a property of certain steroids, independent of their classic hormonal actions."

Barbiturates ← Testoids *cf. also Tables 30—34*

Barbiturates ← Testoids: Holck et al. A 8,011/37*

Butallylonal ← Testosterone: Holck et al. A 55,755/42*

Hexobarbital ← Testosterone: Buchel G 67,326/54*; Quinn et al. E 89,993/58*; Kramer et al. G 74,673/59*; Clouet et al. F 14,837/64; Kato et al. F 57,817/65; Gessner et al. F 77,776/67*

Hexobarbital ← Testoids: Booth et al. *D 34,656/62;* Novick et al. *F 63,768/66**

Hexobarbital ← Norethandrolone, SKF 6612 + Sex, Mouse: Novick et al. F 63,768/66*

Pentobarbital ← Testosterone: Holck et al. A 55,755/42*; Cameron et al. B 45,221/48*; Crevier et al. *B 54,151/50**; Robillard et al. *G 67,325/54**

← **Luteoids.** *Pellerin et al. B 98,672/54:* Testosterone reduces the duration of pentobarbital anesthesia in castrate male or female rats, and concomitantly increases the degradation of pentobarbital by the liver. Estradiol prolongs the duration of anesthesia and proportionally lowers the rate of pentobarbital destruction by the liver. Progesterone diminishes the pentobarbital resistance of the ovariectomized rats and synergizes estradiol. Testosterone almost entirely neutralizes the action of estradiol but is less active against progesterone.

Blackham & Spencer G 69,913/69: Mestranol (a folliculoid) prolonged, while lynestrenol (a luteoid) reduced the duration of pentobarbital and hexobarbital sleep in mice. Barbital was not affected. The action of lynestrenol was counteracted by SKF 525-A, while that of mestranol was markedly potentiated. Lynestrenol increased, whereas mestranol and SKF 525-A reduced the rate of clearance of barbiturates from the plasma.

Jori et al. H 17,070/69: In rats, "two hours after norethynodrel (50 mg/kg, oral) the sleeping time produced by pentobarbital was prolonged due to an increase in the level of brain pentobarbital. Medroxyprogesterone

(10 mg/kg) either alone or combined with ethynylestradiol (0.018 mg/kg) and norethynodrel (10 mg/kg) combined with mestranol (0.018 mg/kg) given orally for 30 days decreased the level of brain pentobarbital without affecting pentobarbital narcosis. Medroxyprogesterone alone or combined with ethynylestradiol in the same experimental conditions increased the metabolism of p-nitroanisol, aminopyrine and aniline in vitro (liver 9000 X g supernatant)."

Rümke & Noordhoek G76,850/69: In mice, phenobarbital and phenytoin exert an anticonvulsant effect against electroshock and bemegride shock, if administered 24 hrs previously. Lynestrenol given 2 days before the anticonvulsants diminishes the effect of the latter, although it does not affect the actions of the convulsive agents given alone.

Rümke & Noordhoek H 14,039/69: Lynestrenol (a luteoid) decreases the hexobarbital sleeping time, and diminishes the anticonvulsant effect of phenobarbital and diphenylhydantoin, by accelerating their metabolisms through the hepatic microsomal enzymes.

Blackham & Spencer G 73,813/70: In mice, lynestrenol reduced, whereas mestranol or SKF 525-A increased the anticonvulsive effect (tested with electroshock) of diphenylhydantoin, phenobarbital, chlordiazepoxide and diazepam administered i.p. after five days of pretreatment. This may be due to altered microsomal drug metabolism, but since mestranol and lynestrenol have opposite effects upon brain 5-HT concentrations, the latter mechanism must also be considered.

Solymoss et al. G60,075/70: In rats pretreated with spironolactone, norbolethone, or ethylestrenol, hexobarbital anesthesia was diminished, and its aliphatic hydroxylation by hepatic microsomes enhanced. Pretreatment with the same steroids also accelerated N-dealkylation of aminopyrine by hepatic microsomes. Progesterone was inactive against hexobarbital, but slightly increased the production of 4-aminoantipyrine by hepatic microsomes.

Selye PROT. 33876: In rats, hexobarbital anesthesia is prolonged by orchidectomy and shortened by methyltestosterone both in intact and in orchidectomized animals. Progesterone significantly reduces the hexobarbital sleeping time in intact rats, but causes only a nonsignificant decrease in castrates. Estradiol prolongs hexobarbital anesthesia in intact and orchidectomized rats as compared with the corresponding controls.

Barbiturates ← Luteoids cf. also Tables 30—34

Hexobarbital ← Luteoids: Juchau et al. *G40,275/66;* Blackham et al. G 69,913/69*; Rümke et al. *H 14,039/69**

Hexobarbital ← Luteoids: Robillard et al. G 67,325/54*; Blackham et al. G 69,913/69*

Phenobarbital ← Lynestrenol, Mouse: Blackham et al. G73,813/70*

← **Folliculoids.** *Störtebecker A 1,993/37:* Rabbits pretreated with "folliculin" tolerate normally anesthesia-producing doses of butallylonal (Pernocton). Subsequent experiments were conducted to determine the blood ether level during ether anesthesia, at the time the corneal reflex is lost in intact and gonadectomized rabbits and mice. Similar observations were made during pregnancy, and in relation to the estrous cycle. [Several conclusions were drawn suggesting an influence of sex hormones upon anesthesia, but the number of animals per group was small and hence a statistical evaluation was impossible (H.S.).]

Horinaga A 36,414/41: Male rats are more resistant to barbiturate anesthesia than females. Orchidectomy and treatment with folliculoids increase sensitivity, whereas ovariectomy does not affect it.

Holck et al. A 55,755/42: Estradiol did not markedly influence the reaction of female rats to hexobarbital, but it increased sleeping time in males. Testosterone shortened barbiturate anesthesia in female rats, but not in male rats or female mice.

Donatelli B 38,172/47: Systematic studies on the effect of folliculoids and testoids upon barbiturate anesthesia in the guinea pig, mouse and rabbit.

Robillard et al. G67,325/54: Cortisone diminishes pentobarbital anesthesia in adult male rats. It also restores to normal the prolonged anesthetic effect of pentobarbital observed after adrenalectomy (with maintenance on 1% NaCl), orchidectomy, or simultaneous adrenalectomy + orchidectomy. Furthermore, cortisone decreases the length of pentobarbital anesthesia in ovariectomized rats, but this effect is blocked by estradiol treatment.

Brodie C 12,157/56: The hexobarbital sleeping time of female rats is about four times that of males; correspondingly, the plasma levels of hexobarbital drop faster in males, whose hepatic microsomes in vitro also inactivate the drug more actively than those of females. Male rats, pretreated with estradiol, sleep as long as females, and their hepatic microsomes lose much of their activity to metabolize hexobarbitone. Females, pretreated with testosterone, assume the characteristics of males in all these respects. No sex differences were seen in mice, guinea pigs, rabbits and dogs, and their ability to handle hexobarbital is not influenced by estradiol or testosterone.

Quinn et al. E 89,993/58: In intact rats, estradiol prolonged the hexobarbital sleeping time and the elevation of the plasma level of this barbiturate, whereas the hepatic microsomal enzyme activity required to metabolize hexobarbital was considerably diminished. In all these respects, testosterone exerted an opposite effect in females.

Westfall et al. F 2,504/64: Pentobarbital anesthesia is more prolonged in male than in female mice. Sleeping time in males is shortened by stilbestrol and, in females, prolonged by testosterone. Apparently, the mechanism for barbiturate detoxication is different in mice versus rats.

Gessner et al. F 77,776/67: In mice, "testosterone pretreatment produces a biphasic effect on the duration of action of hexobarbital, prolonging the action initially and shortening the action in 4—8 days after the pretreatment. The early action of testosterone appears to be associated with an effect on the hypnotic property of a drug, since both hexobarbital and barbital sleep times are prolonged while the duration of action of the muscle relaxant chlorzoxasone remains unaffected. The long-term pretreatment with testosterone leads to a shorter duration of action of drugs that are deactivated by detoxification, notably hexobarbital and chlorzoxasone, but has no effect on the duration of hypnosis produced by barbital, a drug which is predominantly eliminated unchanged." Folliculoids (ethinylestradiol, diethylstilbestrol) prolong the action of both drugs.

Ganesan H 12,504/69: Male rats are more resistant than females to pentobarbital anesthesia. Orchidectomy or treatment with estradiol decreases the pentobarbital resistance of male rats.

Selye PROT. 33876: In rats, hexobarbital anesthesia is prolonged by orchidectomy and shortened by methyltestosterone both in intact and in orchidectomized animals. Progesterone significantly reduces the hexobarbital sleeping time in intact rats, but causes only a nonsignificant decrease in castrates. Estradiol prolongs hexobarbital anesthesia in intact and orchidectomized rats as compared with the corresponding controls.

Barbiturates ← Folliculoids *cf. also Tables 30—34*

Hexobarbital ← Diethylstilbestrol: Gessner et al. F 77,776/67*

Hexobarbital ← Estradiol: Buchel G 67,326/54*; Quinn et al. E 89,993/58*; Kramer et al. G 74,673/59*; Mitoma et al. G 72,113/68

Hexobarbital ← Mestranol + Sex, Mouse: Blackham et al. G 69,913/69*

Pentobarbital ← Estradiol: Holck et al. A 55,755/42*; Boer A 48,817/48*; Crevier et al. *B 54,151/50*;* Robillard et al. G 67,325/54*

Pentobarbital ← Mestranol: Blackham et al. G 69,913/69*

Pentobarbital ← Stilbestrol, Mouse: Westfall et al. F 2,504/64*

← **Adrenalectomy.**

RAT

Sindram 52,504/35: In rats, pretreatment with adrenocortical extract ("Cortin") increases resistance to urethan anesthesia. Adrenalectomy has an inverse effect but Cortin shortens urethan anesthesia even in the absence of the adrenals. Tribromoethanol sleeping time is likewise shortened by adrenocortical extract in intact rats.

Eichholtz et al. B 45,516/49: Adrenalectomy greatly prolongs the tribromoethanol and thiopental sleeping time in rats. In both instances, the sleeping time could be shortened again, if adrenalectomized rats were treated with desoxycorticosterone or adrenocortical extract.

Maloney et al. E 48,771/52: The pentobarbital sleeping time is greatly increased after adrenalectomy in rats of both sexes, males being more resistant than females. Vitamin C lengthened the sleeping time in both intact and adrenalectomized animals. Cortisone shortened the sleeping time of adrenalectomized, but lengthened that of intact animals. DOC diminished sleeping time more markedly in females than in males. [This brief abstract gives, as the authors themselves are careful to point out, "somewhat of a confused picture" (H.S.).]

Tureman et al. B 80,379/52: In rats, adrenalectomy increases susceptibility to the depressant action of pentobarbital. "Cortisone decreases somewhat this susceptibility. The concentration of pentobarbital in the tissues seems to have no significant relationship to the sleeping time."

Robillard et al. G67,325/54: In rats adrenalectomized 5 days prior to phenobarbital treatment, and maintained on 1% NaCl, anesthesia was prolonged. This effect could not be influenced by DOC, but it was abolished by cortisone. Simultaneous orchidectomy did not further prolong pentobarbital anesthesia in adrenalectomized rats, but even in animals thus deprived of all steroids, cortisone greatly diminished anesthesia, whereas testosterone had no effect upon it. Apparently, testosterone requires the presence of glucocorticoids in order to be effective, whereas cortisone does not require the presence of testoids.

Remmer G79,941/57: In female rats, cortisone and prednisolone are much more efficacious than testosterone in shortening hexobarbital anesthesia and increasing microsomal hexobarbital metabolism. Adrenalectomy diminishes the capacity of hepatic microsomes of male rats to metabolize hexobarbital unless the animals are pretreated with cortisone or prednisolone.

Remmer D86,728/58: In rats, 3 days pretreatment with cortisone or prednisolone diminishes the anesthetic effect of hexobarbital and increases the degradation of the anesthetic by liver slices. Adrenalectomy inhibits the degradation of hexobarbital by liver slices of male rats, an effect which can be counteracted by pretreatment with cortisone.

Remmer E52,112/59: In rats, the oxidation of hexobarbital and the demethylation of methylaminoantipyrine by hepatic microsomes is accelerated after pretreatment with phenobarbital even in the absence of the adrenals.

Kato E87,340/60: Chlorpromazine pretreatment reduces barbiturate sleeping time even in adrenalectomized or immature rats.

Markova D49,769/60: In adult, but not in one month old rats, adrenalectomy greatly prolongs hexobarbital anesthesia. In intact animals, ACTH has an inverse effect.

Conney et al. D52,543/61: Pretreatment of male rats with chlorcyclizine shortened the duration of action and increased the hepatic microsomal metabolism of hexobarbital, pentobarbital and zoxazolamine. These effects were not prevented by hypophysectomy or adrenalectomy combined with castration.

Rupe et al. E26,910/63: In rats, stress produced by placing a tourniquet on one hind leg decreases the pharmacologic response to hexobarbital, meprobamate and pentobarbital. This effect is prevented by hypophysectomy or adrenalectomy, but simulated by ACTH or corticosterone. No such effect on stress was noted with barbital, a compound not metabolized by hepatic microsomal enzymes. Furthermore, the protective effect of stress is counteracted by SKF 525-A. Apparently, the "pituitary-adrenal activity exerts a regulating influence on drug responses."

Nichol & Rosen F4,729/64: In the rat, adrenalectomy prolongs hexobarbital sleeping time. Pretreatment of adrenalectomized rats with cortisol or DOC shortens the sleeping time.

Bousquet et al. F35,073/65: In rats, stressed by application of a tourniquet to one hind leg, the duration of response to hexobarbital, pentobarbital, meprobamate and zoxazolamine is significantly reduced, but only in the presence of both the pituitary and the adrenal glands. Pretreatment with ACTH or corticosterone simulates the effects of stress in shortening hexobarbital anesthesia. "It is suggested that the pituitary-adrenal axis serves a regulatory function with respect to duration of drug responses which may be mediated by an alteration of drug metabolism."

Radzialowski & Bousquet G53,591/67: In rats of both sexes, the diurnal variation in the aminopyrine-, p-nitroanisole- and hexobarbital-metabolizing activity of hepatic microsomes is abolished by adrenalectomy.

Furner & Stitzel G54,558/68: The hepatic microsomal metabolism of ethylmorphine, aniline and hexobarbital is diminished in vitro by previous adrenalectomy in the rat. Phenobarbital pretreatment of adrenalectomized rats raises the metabolism of all three substrates above the level characteristic of untreated, adrenalectomized controls. Exposure of adrenalectomized rats to cold stress, or treatment with cortisol increases the metabolism of aniline and ethylmorphine, but further depresses that of hexobarbital. In intact rats, cold stress diminishes hexobarbital metabolism in vitro. Apparently, both stress and phenobarbital can bring about changes in hepatic drug metabolism, independent of the presence of the adrenals; the two agents act through different mechanisms, since phenobarbital invariably stimulates, whereas stress either increases or decreases microsomal enzyme activity depending upon the drug pathway examined.

Nakanishi et al. G79,299/70: "Cold exposure or immobilization of intact or adrenalectomized rats significantly impaired side-chain oxidation of hexobarbital and N-demethylation of aminopyrine in vitro. In contrast, p-hydroxylation of aniline in vitro was not affected under stress conditions." The pertinent literature is somewhat contradictory but, possibly, the effect of stress on drug-metabolizing enzyme induction may vary with the substrate employed.

Sethy et al. G77,511/70: In rats, pentobarbital sleeping time is reduced immediately after stress (centrifugation), but returns to normal eight hours later. In adrenalectomized animals, this effect of stress is abolished.

Selye PROT. 28922, 28985, 28996: In adrenalectomized rats maintained on NaCl, 4 days pretreatment with spironolactone (10 mg in 1 ml water p.o. x2/day) offers definite resistance to pentobarbital (3 mg in 0.5 ml oil i.p.) and hexobarbital (7.5 mg in 1 ml water i.p.), but not to phenobarbital (10 mg in 1 ml water i.p.), although all these anesthetics give approximately equal degrees of anesthesia in rats not pretreated with spironolactone. Smaller doses of spironolactone were less effective, or ineffective even against pentobarbital and hexobarbital under these conditions.

MOUSE

Richards 79,646/41: "The increase in toxicity of pentothal sodium for mice after temperature is raised from 22—30 or 35 degrees is relatively small. However, if metabolic regulation is disturbed by adrenalectomy, an increased susceptibility is observed which becomes particularly marked at higher temperatures."

Shibata & Komiya B88,660/53: In the mouse, thiopental anesthesia is prolonged by adrenalectomy, but resistance is restored by cortisone or cortisol. DOC has no effect.

Komiya & Shibata C13,129/56: In the mouse, adrenalectomy intensifies barbital anesthesia. Cortisone and cortisol restore anesthesia time to normal; whereas DOC has little effect upon it, although it offers some protection against anesthetic death. Pretreatment of adrenalectomized mice with cortisone or cortisol reduces the high rate of barbital uptake by the brain to normal. DOC has no effect upon cerebral barbital uptake or discharge. Apparently, "the abnormal anesthetic course is elicited by abnormal concentration of barbiturate in the brain, both of which are restored to the normal by glucocorticoid administration."

GUINEA PIG

Lamson et al. B89,712/52: In guinea pigs, epinephrine, when injected i.p. on awakening from barbiturate anesthesia, produced a return to sleep. A similar effect was produced by glucose, lactate, or glutamate. However, in adrenalectomized animals, only epinephrine was effective.

Barbital ← Adrenalectomy: Boyland et al. F35,073/65*; Fuller et al. H31,807/70*

Hexobarbital ← Adrenalectomy: Cook et al. D23,923/54*; Remmer C73,857/58, D86,728/58*; Hart et al. G27,102/65; Bousquet et al. F35,073/65*, Fuller et al. H 31,807/70*

Pentobarbital ← Adrenalectomy: Robillard et al. G67,325/54*; Kato E87,340/60*; Driever et al. G31,872/65*

Thiopental ← Adrenalectomy: Richards et al. A48,718/41*; Eichholtz et al. B45,516/49*; Stuhlfauth et al. G78,396/54*

← **Gonadectomy.**

RAT

Barron A42,858/33: Male rats are more resistant than females to amobarbital anesthesia. Castration increases the sensitivity of the male, but not quite to the female level. Castration before puberty does not diminish resistance. Ancillary experiments suggest that the effect of castration is due to changes in water metabolism.

Holck et al. A8,014/37: In rats, orchidectomy prolongs the sleeping time of those barbiturates to which males are normally more resistant. Orchidectomy does not lengthen the hexobarbital sleeping time in rabbits. In female rats, neither ovariectomy nor the estrus cycle influences hexobarbital sleeping time.

Moir E54,544/37: Very young female rats were more resistant to pentobarbital than males, whereas the reverse was true in mature rats. Both males and females developed tolerance to pentobarbital upon repeated injections, but when treatment was interrupted and then resumed, susceptibility was greatly increased in females and castrate males, but not in intact males. "Inasmuch as the castrated males still remained more resistant than females, the superior resistance of the males was held to be due at least in part to some factor or factors other than the male gonads."

Cameron A34,503/39: In rats, ovariectomy greatly increases sensitivity to the anesthetic and lethal effect of pentobarbital.

Holck & Mathieson B644/44: In rats, the development of tolerance to pentobarbital was determined by injecting increasing doses every 90 min day and night for periods up to 5 days. Practically all 1—2 month-old rats developed tolerance, as did adult males in contrast to females. Castration lowered the ability of adult males to develop tolerance, but did not do so in 2 month-old males. Ovariectomy of 2 month-old females increased their ability to detoxify pentobarbital, once tolerance had developed.

Cameron et al. B45,221/48: In rats, orchidectomy diminishes tolerance for quick acting barbiturates such as pentobarbital sodium, but not for the slow acting barbital sodium. Testosterone improves the tolerance of gonadectomized males.

de Boer A48,817/48: Pentobarbital hypnosis was prolonged in ovariectomized rats for a period of 3—16 weeks, but was reduced 12 months after spaying. Castration of males prolonged sleeping time. Thiamine decreased pentobarbital sleeping time in ovariectomized rats towards the normal level.

Crevier et al. B54,151/50: Pentobarbital anesthesia lasts longer in female than in male rats as judged by the linguo-maxillary reflex. Castration abolishes the high resistance of the male, but testosterone restores it to the normal level. In ovariectomized rats, estradiol has virtually no effect, but testosterone raises resistance to the male level. These in vivo effects run parallel to the in vitro pentobarbital detoxifying power of the liver.

Robillard et al. B66,661/51: In rats, thyroidectomy prolongs pentobarbital anesthesia and delays hepatic detoxication of the drug, whereas thyroxine pretreatment diminishes the duration and depth of this anesthesia without enhancing the hepatic detoxication of pentobarbital as determined by incubation of the drug with liver slices. After simultaneous thyroidectomy and orchidectomy, pentobarbital detoxication is more markedly delayed than after simple thyroidectomy or orchidectomy, and the anesthetic effect is correspondingly further intensified than after ablation of the thyroid or testes alone.

Grewe D35,140/53: Male rats are more resistant than females to barbiturate (eunarcon, hexobarbital) anesthesia. After gonadectomy, both sexes exhibit the longer sleeping time characteristic of females. Twenty-eight days after orchidectomy, the sleeping time is reduced to the level seen in intact males. Testosterone prolongs the sleeping time of females.

Buchel D73,669/54: Review on the literature, and personal observations on the increased sleeping time of female as compared to male rats, after treatment with certain barbiturates, particularly hexobarbital. The increased sleeping time is associated with a prolonged persistence of the concentration of the drug in the blood. Gonadectomy prolongs the sleeping time of males but does not influence that of females. In immature rats no such sex difference is observed.

Buchel G67,326/54: Testosterone decreases hexobarbital sleeping time in adult, intact or ovariectomized female rats. Estradiol has an inverse effect in normal or castrate males. Indirect evidence suggests that the changes in hexobarbital sleeping time are associated with its reduced or prolonged presence in the body.

Robillard et al. G67,325/54: Adult males are more resistant than females to pentobarbital anesthesia. Castration decreases the resistance in males. Testosterone raises pentobarbital resistance to the normal male level in both male and female castrates, whereas estradiol and progesterone prolong anesthesia in castrates of both sexes. [The hormones were administered as pellets, 15 days before the test, but the amounts are not stated (H.S.).] Partial hepatectomy prolongs pentobarbital anesthesia and accentuates the differences induced by the various interventions just mentioned, without causing qualitative changes in the outcome. Liver homogenates of adult male rats destroy pentobarbital in vitro (spectrophotometric determination) more rapidly than those of castrate males. Pretreatment of the castrates in vivo with testosterone increases the detoxication process, whereas estradiol pretreatment has an opposite effect.

Takabatake G76,713/57: Male rats are more resistant than females or castrates of either sex, to the anesthetic effect of ethylhexabital. Testosterone raises the resistance of females and gonadectomized animals of either sex to the male level. In vitro studies on liver slices indicate that the sex difference is due to the effect of testosterone upon the barbiturate-metabolizing ability of the liver, not upon brain sensitivity.

Kato et al. G64,325/62: Adult male rats are more resistant than females to pentobarbital anesthesia, carisoprodol paralysis and strychnine convulsions. Conversely, the lethal effect of OMPA is greater in the male. The sex difference is ascribed to the increased production of anabolic testoids that enhance the decomposition of these substrates, the first three of which being inactivated, and the last activated in the process. The differences were also demonstrated in vitro, using liver slices or microsomal fractions. The high microsomal activity of the male could be abolished by castration and restored by several anabolic testoids.

Kato & Gillette F 57,816/65: The ability of rat liver microsomal enzymes to inactivate various substrates is greater in males than in females, but the sex difference varies with the substrate. There is more than a 3-fold sex difference with aminopyrine and hexobarbital, but virtually none with hydroxylation of aniline and zoxazolamine. In male rats, starvation impairs sex-dependent enzymes which metabolize aminopyrine and hexobarbital, but enhances those that hydroxylate aniline. On the other hand, in female rats, starvation increases the specific activity of the aminopyrine and hexobarbital-metabolizing enzymes as well as of aniline hydroxylase. Starvation does not alter the metabolism of hexobarbital; it enhances that of aminopyrine by microsomes of castrated rats, but impairs the metabolism of these compounds by microsomes of methyltestosterone-treated castrates.

Kato & Gillette F 57,817/65: The metabolism of aminopyrine and hexobarbital by hepatic microsomes of male rats is impaired by adrenalectomy, castration, hypoxia, ACTH, formaldehyde, epinephrine, morphine, alloxan or thyroxine. The metabolism of aniline and zoxazolamine is not appreciably decreased by any of these agents; in fact, hydroxylation of aniline is enhanced by thyroxine or alloxan. Apparently, the treatments impair mainly the sex-dependent enzymes. Accordingly, the corresponding enzymic functions of the hepatic microsomes of female rats are not significantly impaired by the agents which do have an inhibitory effect in males.

Hempel G 57,828/68: Cyproterone acetate shortens hexobarbital anesthesia in the rat, probably through enhanced hepatic microsomal enzyme activity. This effect is evident both in intact and in gonadectomized rats. Orchidectomy prolongs hexobarbital sleeping time, and subsequent testosterone treatment shortens it. It is emphasized that, under the conditions of this experiment, cyproterone failed to inhibit the anti-anesthetic effect of testosterone and, unexpectedly, shared this very action of the testoid substance.

Selye PROT. 33876: In rats, hexobarbital anesthesia is prolonged by orchidectomy, and shortened by methyltestosterone (both in intact and orchidectomized animals). Progesterone significantly reduces the hexobarbital sleeping time in intact rats, but causes only a nonsignificant decrease in castrates. Estradiol prolongs hexobarbital anesthesia in intact and orchidectomized rats as compared with the corresponding controls, *cf.* Table 30.

Table 30. *Effect of orchidectomy upon hexobarbital anesthesia in intact and orchidectomized rats with or without steroid pretreatment*

Pretreatment[a]	Sleeping time (min) [b]	
	Intact	Castrate
None	35 ± 3	48 ± 5 *
PCN	32 ± 4 NS	38 ± 4 NS
Estradiol	50 ± 5 *	70 ± 6 *
Progesterone	18 ± 4 **	35 ± 6 NS
Methyltestosterone	13 ± 3 ***	23 ± 5 **

[a] The rats (140 g♂) of all groups received hexobarbital 10 mg/100 g body weight in 1 ml water, i.p. once, on the 12th day. The groups so designated were castrated on the 1st day. Estradiol 1 mg, and other steroids 10 mg/100 g body weight were given in 1 ml water, p.o. x2/day, on the 9th day ff. On the 12th day, the steroids were administered 1 hr before hexobarbital.

[b] The significance of the apparent differences in sleeping time is calculated for the untreated rats between the intact and the castrates, and for all other groups between unpretreated and the steroid pretreated animals of corresponding gonadal status (intact or castrate). (Student's t-test.)

For further details on technique of tabulation *cf.* p. VIII.

MOUSE

Hempel F 84,763/67: Hexobarbital anesthesia lasts longer in mature male than in female mice. Orchidectomy decreases sleeping time, whereas ovariectomy does not affect it. Testosterone prolongs the hexobarbital sleeping time in orchidectomized males, as well as ovariectomized or normal female mice. This effect is blocked by the antitestoid, cyproterone. By itself, cyproterone shortens the sleeping time in mice under all circumstances.

In rats, hexobarbital sleeping time is shorter among males than among females, and prolonged by orchidectomy, whereas ovariectomy does not affect it. Testosterone shortens hexobarbital sleeping time in females and in castrate rats of both sexes. This effect is not inhibited by cyproterone which in itself shortens sleeping time in the rat also.

Rümke G71,098/68: In mice of the CPB-N strain, hexobarbital anesthesia lasts longer in males than in females, but only after puberty. Following gonadectomy of mature animals, the sex difference persists for about 2 weeks, but then disappears.

Noordhoek & Rümke H21,660/69: In mice, the 9000 g liver supernatant of females hydroxylates hexobarbital faster than that of males. After orchidectomy, the in vitro metabolism of hexobarbital becomes equal to that of females, but ovariectomy has no effect upon it. Testosterone decreases the rate of in vitro hexobarbital hydroxylation in females, but not in males. Female livers contain more cytochrome P-450 and testosterone lowers its concentration in female but not in male livers.

Rümke & Noordhoek H21,659/69: Among mice of many strains, hexobarbital produces longer anesthesia in males than in females. This difference is evident only after sexual maturation. If 10 week old males are castrated, the difference persists for at least 2 weeks, but it disappears after a month. Ovariectomy has no effect upon sleeping time, whereas testosterone increases it in females but not in males.

Guinea Pig

Störtebecker 76,398/39: In mature female guinea pigs, ovariectomy diminishes barbiturate (butallylonal, Pernocton) anesthesia.

Brena & d'Agostino C11,921/54: In guinea pigs, orchidectomy prolongs thiopental sleeping time; testosterone diminishes it, both in castrate and in intact males.

Amobarbital Sodium ← Orchidectomy + Age: Barron A42,858/33*

Butallylonal ← Gonadectomy: Holck et al. A55,846/36*; Störtebecker 76,398/39*

Hexobarbital ← Gonadectomy: Buchel G67,326/54*; Kramer et al. G75,673/59*; Kato et al. F57,817/67; Schenkman et al. G67,777/67

Pentobarbital ← Gonadectomy: Moir E54,544/37*; Cameron A34,503/39*; Holck et al. A55,755/42*, B644/44*; Gaylord et al. B11,425/44*; Boer A48,817/48*; Cameron et al. B 45,221/48*; Crevier et al. B54,151/50*; Robillard et al. G67,325/54*

← **Varia.** *Kato E60,785/59:* In rats, pretreatment with various substances such as phenaglycodol, thiopental, phenobarbital, glutethimide, meprobamate, etc. diminishes pentobarbital sleeping time, whereas **hydroxydione** does not exert a significant effect upon it.

Rümke G69,768/63: In mice SKF 525-A, phenobarbital, chlorpromazine, hexobarbital and iproniazid given one hour before hydroxydione i.v. increases sleeping time. When the interval is two days, single doses of SKF 525-A, phenobarbital or chlorpromazine decrease **hydroxydione** anesthesia. Phenytoin, acetylcarbromal, morphine, chloramphenicol, 5-HT, phenobarbital and hydroxydione, given one hour before hexobarbital, increase the duration of anesthesia, whereas dioxone and chlorothiazide decrease it.

Overbeek & Bonta E4,775/64: Several **azaestranes** (in which C_4 is replaced by nitrogen) shorten the duration of anesthesia when given to mice 24 hrs before hexobarbital. They have an opposite effect when given 1 hour before the anesthetic. One of the compounds of this series, 17α-methyl-17β-hydroxy-4-azaestran-3-one, was also shown to diminish the hexobarbital concentration in the brain and carcass of mice, in comparison with unpretreated controls. These steroids are presumed to "exert their antidepressant effect by augmenting the elimination of the anesthetics both from the brain and from the whole carcass, as shown for hexobarbital. So far we do not know by what mechanism of action this is achieved." [No technical details are given and since several of the structure formulas are misprinted, the text is difficult to evaluate (H.S.).]

Bonta & Overbeek E5,494/65: In mice, 17α-methyl-17β-hydroxy-4-azaestran-3-one shortens the duration of hexobarbital anesthesia.

Hempel G57,828/68: In orchidectomized rats, the hexobarbital sleeping time is prolonged. Testosterone shortens it, but this effect of the male hormone is not inhibited by **cyproterone.** Indeed, the latter, in itself, actually shares the anti-anesthetic effect of testosterone.

Kalyanpur et al. F99,270/68: **DOC, 4-chlorotestosterone, aldosterone** and **stilbestrol** significantly decreased pentobarbital sleeping time in rats when given as a single injection,

30 min before the anesthetic. **Progesterone** has an inverse effect. Chronic pretreatment with progesterone, stilbestrol or aldosterone markedly decreased pentobarbital sleeping time without causing any significant change in brain pentobarbital levels.

Tephly & Mannering G53,874/68: **Estradiol, testosterone, androsterone, progesterone** and **cortisol** inhibit competitively the oxidation of ethylmorphine and hexobarbital, when added in vitro to hepatic microsomes of rats. The inhibitor constant for each steroid was the same, whether ethylmorphine or hexobarbital served as substrates. "Results are consistent with the concept that certain drugs and steroids are alternative substrates for a common microsomal mixed function oxidase system." The steroids were less potent inhibitors of chlorpromazine oxidation and the inhibition was not competitive in this case.

Solymoss et al. G60,054/69: "In the rat, pretreatment with **spironolactone, norbolethone** or **ethylestrenol** increased the oxidation of pentobarbital by liver microsomes, enhanced its disappearance from blood and proportionally decreased the depth of anesthesia."

Selye et al. G60,050/70: SC-8109 and SC-5233 fail to protect the rat against digitoxin intoxication and the anesthetic effect of progesterone or pentobarbital.

Solymoss et al. G60,099/70: In rats, pentobarbital anesthesia is inhibited by **spironolactone, ethylestrenol, norbolethone** and, to a lesser extent, even by **progesterone**. These catatoxic steroids also accelerate the disappearance rate of barbiturate from the blood; their effects are counteracted by SKF 525-A. Irrespective of the steroid pretreatment, the rats awake roughly at the same blood pentobarbital level.

Selye G70,480/71: In rats, **thiopental** sleeping time is significantly shortened by PCN, CS-1, ethylestrenol, spironolactone, oxandrolone and prednisolone. However, even cholesterol appears to provide a barely significant protection, *cf.* Table 31.

Selye G70,480/71: In rats, **hexobarbital** sleeping time is significantly shortened by all classic catatoxic steroids, prednisolone and phenobarbital. Triamcinolone and estradiol offer barely significant protection, *cf.* Table 32.

Table 31. *Conditioning for thiopental*

Treatment[a]	Sleeping time[b] (min)
None	75 ± 11
PCN	12 + 8 ***
CS-1	0 ***
Ethylestrenol	8 ± 5 ***
Spironolactone	0 ***
Norbolethone	127 ± 25 NS
Oxandrolone	18 ± 9 **
Prednisolone-Ac	5 ± 5 ***
Triamcinolone (2 mg)	82 ± 26 NS
Progesterone	118 ± 18 NS
Estradiol (1 mg)	38 ± 18 NS
Estradiol (1 mg s.c.)	73 ± 31 NS
DOC-Ac	57 ± 16 NS
Hydroxydione	72 ± 15 NS
Cholesterol	33 ± 14 *
Thyroxine	88 ± 9 NS
Phenobarbital	7 ± 4 ***

[a] The rats of all groups were given thiopental sodium (5 mg/100 g body weight in 1 ml water, p.o., on 4th day).
[b] Student's t-test.

For further details on technique of tabulation *cf.* p. VIII.

Table 32. *Conditioning for hexobarbital*

Treatment[a]	Sleeping time[b] (min)
None	64 ± 7
PCN	29 ± 4 ***
CS-1	23 ± 3 ***
Ethylestrenol	0 ***
Spironolactone	27 ± 3 ***
Norbolethone	15 ± 2 ***
Oxandrolone	21 ± 4 ***
Prednisolone-Ac	30 ± 3 ***
Triamcinolone (2 mg)	41 ± 5 *
Progesterone	71 ± 11 NS
Estradiol (1 mg)	46 ± 5 *
Estradiol (1 mg s.c.)	54 ± 5 NS
DOC-Ac	61 ± 10 NS
Hydroxydione	43 ± 8 NS
Cholesterol	46 ± 7 NS
Thyroxine	78 ± 6 NS
Phenobarbital	4 ± 2 ***

[a] The rats of all groups were given hexobarbital (7.5 mg/100 g body weight in 1 ml water, i.p., on 4th day).
[b] Student's t-test.

For additional pertinent data *cf. also* Table 135.

For further details on technique of tabulation *cf.* p. VIII.

Selye G70,480/71: In rats, **cyclobarbital** sleeping time is significantly shortened by all catatoxic steroids, prednisolone, triamcinolone and phenobarbital, cf. Table 33.

Table 33. *Conditioning for cyclobarbital*

Treatment[a]	Sleeping time[b] (min)
None	100 ± 6
PCN	19 ± 5 ***
CS-1	42 ± 7 ***
Ethylestrenol	0 ***
Spironolactone	50 ± 11 ***
Norbolethone	15 ± 4 ***
Oxandrolone	42 ± 10 ***
Prednisolone-Ac	26 ± 9 ***
Triamcinolone (2 mg)	61 ± 8 ***
Progesterone	92 ± 8 NS
Estradiol (1 mg)	105 ± 13 NS
Estradiol (1 mg s.c.)	116 ± 12 NS
DOC-Ac	93 ± 11 NS
Hydroxydione	80 ± 16 NS
Cholesterol	90 ± 15 NS
Thyroxine	102 ± 8 NS
Phenobarbital	0 ***

[a] The rats of all groups were given cyclobarbital (7.5 mg/100 g body weight in 2 or 3 ml water, i.p., on 4th day).
[b] Student's t-test.
For further details on technique of tabulation cf. p. VIII.

Selye G70,480/71: In rats, **barbital** anesthesia was not significantly shortened by any of the classic catatoxic steroids and, in fact, may have been slightly prolonged by CS-1 and norbolethone. Estradiol and DOC prolonged barbital anesthesia and the same was true of hydroxydione and phenobarbital, but since the latter have strong hypnotic effects themselves, the apparent potentiation of barbital anesthesia may have been merely due to a summation of effects, cf. Table 34.

Solymoss et al. G79,015/71: In rats, PCN (unlike the naturally-occurring pregnenolone) enhances the plasma clearance of pentobarbital and the production of ^{14}C-pentobarbital metabolites. It also increases liver weight, microsomal protein concentration, NADPH-cytochrome c-reductase activity and cytochrome P-450 content. It is concluded "that microsomal enzyme-induction accounts for the remarkable resistance-increasing effect of this steroid against many toxicants."

Szabo et al. G79,024/71: In rats, **PCN** increases resistance to indomethacin, hexobarbital, progesterone, zoxazolamine and digitoxin, both in the presence and in the absence of the pituitary. Hypophysectomy also fails to prevent the induction of SER proliferation in the hepatocytes.

Selye PROT.31367,31380: In the mouse, the duration of pentobarbital anesthesia is shortened by ethylestrenol, CS-1, spironolactone and norbolethone, but not significantly by oxandrolone, prednisolone, progesterone, triamcinolone, DOC, **hydroxydione**, estradiol, or thyroxine.

Table 34. *Conditioning for barbital*

Treatment[a]	Sleeping time[b] (min)
None	192 ± 15
PCN	162 ± 14 NS
CS-1	288 ± 34 ±
Ethylestrenol	194 ± 20 NS
Spironolactone	200 ± 28 NS
Norbolethone	294 ± 37 ±
Oxandrolone	256 ± 30 NS
Prednisolone-Ac	95 ± 25 **
Triamcinolone (2 mg)	164 ± 24 NS
Progesterone	294 ± 49 NS
Estradiol (1 mg)	338 ± 33 ***
Estradiol (1 mg s.c.)	414 ± 41 ***
DOC-Ac	358 ± 31 ***
Hydroxydione	316 ± 47 ±
Thyroxine	228 ± 39 NS
Phenobarbital	348 ± 13 ***

[a] The rats of all groups were given barbital, 20 mg/100 g body weight in 2 ml water, i.p., once on 4th day.
[b] Student's t-test.
For further details on technique of tabulation cf. p. VIII.

Hexobarbital ← Hydroxydione, Mouse: Rümke G69,768/63*
Pentobarbital ← Hydroxydione: Kato E60,785/59*
Bemegride ← Lynestrenol: Rümke et al. G76,850/69*, H14,039/69*

Benzene ←

Hirokawa G71,106/55: Female rabbits are more sensitive to chronic benzene poisoning than males. Gonadectomized estradiol-treated males respond like females.

Benzphetamine ← Cortisol + Phenobarbital: Lu et al. G68,802/69

Benzpyrene ← cf. **Carcinogens**

Beryllium ←

Kline et al. B65,488/51: In patients with beryllium granulomatosis, ACTH and cortisone were found to be beneficial.

Bilirubin ← cf. also **α-Naphthylisothiocyanate (ANIT)**

Hargreaves & Lathe G81,289/63: In vitro, addition of norethandrolone to the incubation medium of rat liver slices increased the bilirubin accumulation in the hepatic tissue.

Roberts & Plaa G39,694/66: In mice, α-naphthylisothiocyanate-induced hyperbilirubinemia and cholestasis are aggravated by norethandrolone and norethynodrel but not by mestranol.

Shibata et al. G80,058/66: In rats, hepatic glucuronyl transferase activity is greatly increased during the last third of gestation, whereas enzymic activity is virtually absent in the fetal liver. These divergent changes "raise doubt as to whether low enzymic activity in the fetus and increased activity after birth are the consequence, respectively, of high hormone levels in pregnancy, and falling hormone concentrations in the postpartum period. The maximal rate of bilirubin excretion into bile, the bilirubin T_m, remained unchanged in pregnancy despite the potential for increased bilirubin conjugation. When coupled with other observations, this suggests that the rate of delivery of conjugated bilirubin into bile is the rate-limiting step involved in the maximal transfer rate of bilirubin from blood to bile, and that the excretory step for bilirubin remains unaffected during pregnancy in the rat."

Roberts et al. H8,328/68: In rats, biliary excretion of bilirubin (administered by constant infusion) was not significantly affected by norethandrolone, but depressed by methyltestosterone. Special emphasis is layed upon the influence of temperature: an apparent decrease in the maximum biliary excretion of bilirubin was produced by norethandrolone, only in rats allowed to become hypothermic, whereas the reverse was true in normothermic rats.

Heikel & Lathe G73,162/70: In rats, various folliculoids and luteoids reduce bile flow. The bilirubin maximum secretion rate (Tm) is but slightly affected. Following i.v. infusion of bilirubin, folliculoids (unlike luteoids) raise the serum conjugated bilirubin level.

Patrignani H32,792/70: In rats, pretreatment with testosterone increases bilirubin excretion and augments the incorporation of ^{14}C Δ-amino levulinic acid (Δ-ALA) into bilirubin. The effect is tentatively ascribed to stimulation of hepatic microsomal cytochrome activity.

Sas & Herczeg H27,522/70: In male newborn babies, androstenedione and dehydroepiandrosterone increase the serum bilirubin-concentration or, at least, delay its post-partal decline, presumably by inhibiting glucuronic acid conjugation of the bile pigment "possibly due to a competitive displacement between the steroids and bilirubin." Similar effects had previously been obtained with progesterone, 3α, 20α- and 3α, 20β-pregnanediol and folliculoids. The steroids in human milk may thus influence detoxicating mechanisms.

Sas & Herczeg H27,523/70: In breast fed babies, 3α, 20β- and 3α, 20α-pregnanediol p.o. increase pregnanediol and folliculoid excretion as well as the serum level of bilirubin.

Bilirubin ← Steroids: Lathe et al. *C55,335/58;* Sherlock *G79,591/59*;* Holton et al. *E35,112/63;* Arias et al. *F21,711/64*;* Bevan et al. *G35,435/65;* Catz et al. *H14,471/68;* Mowat et al. *G74,246/69**

Bishydroxycoumarin ← cf. **Anticoagulants**

Bromide ←

Bondurant & Campbell A36,066/41: In man, adrenocortical extract in combination with NaCl is beneficial in the treatment of bromide intoxication.

Wohl & Robertson 93,481/44: In man, combined therapy with DOC plus NaCl is effective in combating chronic bromide intoxication.

Prioreschi C68,485/59: In the rat, anesthesia produced by NaBr is increased in intensity by exposure to stress or treatment with triamcinolone or Me-Cl-COL. DOC or estradiol do not modify it considerably.

Selye et al. G60,020/69; G60,016/69: In rats, spironolactone protects against anesthesia produced by progesterone, DOC, hydroxydione, pregnanedione, dehydroepiandrosterone, testosterone, diethylstilbestrol, methyprylon, pentobarbital and ethanol. It does not significantly alter the corresponding actions of morphine, codeine, urethan, diazepam, chlorpromazine, reserpine, phenoxybenzamine, chloral hydrate, potassium bromide or $MgCl_2$.

Bromobenzene ←

Selye G 70,480/71: Rats received bromobenzene (50 mg daily from the 4th to the 6th day of conditioning, 75 mg once on the 7th day of conditioning and twice on the 8th day of conditioning /100 g body weight, in 1 ml corn oil p.o.). Hepatic steatosis was estimated on the day of death, prostration and mortality on the 9th day. Under these circumstances the "Standard Conditioners" (p. VIII) caused no noteworthy change in the resulting intoxication. PCN and phenobarbital were not tested.

Brompheniramine ← *cf. Parabromdylamine*

Butynamine ← Ovariectomy + Methyltestosterone: Kato et al. *F 76,403/66*

Cadmium ←

Das & Kar D 14,801/61: In rats treated with cadmium, the testicular atrophy and, particularly, fibroblast proliferation in the testis can be moderately influenced by corticoids during the period of regeneration, but the results are not very striking.

Gunn et al. F 46,162/65: In mice, the testicular hemorrhage, thrombosis and necrosis produced by $CdCl_2$ are not influenced by pretreatment with testosterone, whereas estradiol, in doses resulting in tubular atrophy, protects against the cadmium-induced testicular damage. Curiously, stilbestrol, at doses which fail to cause tubular regression, protects the testis against the production of vascular injury by cadmium.

Maekawa & Hosoyama G 79,815/65: In rats, the testicular damage produced by cadmium is somewhat antagonized by testoids.

Maekawa & Tsunenari H 1,627/67; Maekawa et al. G 79,814/67: In rats, contrary to earlier claims, the testicular injury produced by cadmium is not prevented by folliculoids (estradiol, estrone, estriol).

Pařizek et al. H 7,672/68: In adult rats in which persistent estrus had been induced by a single s.c. injection of testosterone or 19-nortestosterone on the fifth day of life, cadmium s.c. elicited particularly severe ovarian changes. Pretreatment with pregnant mare serum gonadotrophin protected the ovaries of such animals.

Johnson et al. H 23,801/70: In rats, orchidectomy or surgically induced cryptorchidism increase the drop in body temperature produced by cadmium intoxication.

Selye G 70,480/71: In rats, the characteristic hemorrhagic lesions produced in the gasserian ganglia by cadmium chloride intoxication are significantly prevented by PCN, prednisolone, triamcinolone and estradiol. The apparent protective action of thyroxine is open to doubt because most of the animals treated with this hormone died prematurely, *cf.* Table 35.

Table 35. *Conditioning for cadmium*

Treatment[a]	Hemorrhage in gasserian ganglia[b] (Positive/Total)	Mortality[b] (Dead/Total)
None	14/18	15/20
PCN	1/13 ***	8/15 NS
CS-1	4/6 NS	6/10 NS
Ethylestrenol	5/9 NS	2/10 **
Spironolactone	7/10 NS	2/10 **
Norbolethone	7/9 NS	3/10 *
Oxandrolone	7/9 NS	6/10 NS
Prednisolone-Ac	0/11 ***	3/12 **
Triamcinolone	2/10 ***	7/10 NS
Progesterone	5/10 NS	6/10 NS
Estradiol	2/9 **	1/10 ***
DOC-Ac	6/8 NS	7/10 NS
Hydroxydione	6/10 NS	7/10 NS
Thyroxine	0/4 **	10/10 NS
Phenobarbital	2/5 NS	6/10 NS

[a] The rats of all groups were given cadmium chloride (700 μg/100 g body weight in 1 ml water, i.v., on 4th day).

[b] The hemorrhages in the gasserian ganglia were estimated on day of death in animals that survived at least 5 days, and mortality listed on 7th day ("Exact Probability Test").

For further details on technique of tabulation *cf.* p. VIII.

Caffeine ←

Vacek C 63,230/58: DOC anesthesia protects the mouse against the convulsive and lethal effects of strychnine, pentylenetetrazol and caffeine.

Caramiphen

Selye PROT. 42752: In rats, caramiphen intoxication is inhibited by PCN and, to a lesser extent, by CS-1, ethylestrenol and prednisolone, but is aggravated by thyroxine, *cf.* Table 36.

Table 36. *Conditioning for caramiphen*

Treatment[a]	Dyskinesia[b] (Positive/Total)	Mortality[b] (Dead/Total)
None	6/10	5/10
PCN	0/10 **	0/10 *
CS-1	1/10 *	1/10 NS
Ethylestrenol	1/10 *	0/10 *
Spironolactone	4/10 NS	2/10 NS
Norbolethone	3/10 NS	2/10 NS
Oxandrolone	3/10 NS	2/10 NS
Prednisolone-Ac	1/10 *	0/10 *
Triamcinolone	9/10 NS	8/10 NS
Progesterone	6/10 NS	5/10 NS
Estradiol	5/10 NS	4/10 NS
DOC-Ac	6/10 NS	4/10 NS
Hydroxydione	7/10 NS	5/10 NS
Thyroxine	10/10 *	10/10 *
Phenobarbital	2/10 NS	0/10 *

[a] The rats of all groups were given caramiphen hydrochloride (10 mg on 4th day and 15 mg on 5th day, /100 g body weight in 1 ml water i.p.).

[b] Dyskinesia was estimated on 5th day, 1 hr after injection, and mortality listed on 6th day ("Exact Probability Test").
For further details on technique of tabulation *cf.* p. VIII.

Carbon Monoxide ←

Smith et al. 45,163/35: Male rats are more sensitive to the lethal action of illuminating gas than females. This difference is eliminated by gonadectomy. Thyroid feeding or dinitrophenol injections decrease survival time.

Carbon Tetrachloride ←

RAT

Masson 96,335/47: The hepatotoxic action of CCl_4 is aggravated by DOC and testosterone, but partially prevented by anterior pituitary extracts in the rat.

Aterman B52,265/50: In rats, the hepatic sclerosis produced by CCl_4 is inhibited by concurrent treatment with cortisone.

Cavallero et al. B54,229/51: In the rat, "cortisone definitely modifies the evolution of carbon tetrachloride cirrhosis. Fatty degeneration is not affected, but fibrosis, reticulosis, and parenchymal regeneration are greatly inhibited."

Cavallero et al. B69,181/52: Cortisone partially inhibits hepatic fibrosis in rats treated with CCl_4.

Aterman & Ahmad B76,967/53: "Cortisone increases the susceptibility of the rat's liver to chronic damage by carbon tetrachloride."

Aterman B92,038/54: In rats, cortisone significantly decreases hepatic fibrosis produced by CCl_4, as judged by histologic studies and collagen determinations.

Diengott & Ungar E84,645/54: "In albino rats exposed to vapors of CCl_4 the administration of cortisone enhanced the cirrhotic process in the liver considerably. In comparison with the controls, the liver of cortisone-treated animals showed marked epithelial and mesenchymal alterations. The former was manifested by the presence of multinucleated giant cells, foci of necrosis, and fatty changes; the latter, by the development of dense bundles of tortuous and clumped reticulum fibers."

Vorhaus & Vorhaus B97,869/54: Cortisone pretreatment offers partial protection against the hepatic damage produced by CCl_4 in the rat.

Arrigo & Trasino C21,687/55: In rats, crude alkaline anterior pituitary extracts (rich in STH) do, whereas acid extracts (rich in ACTH and STH) do not protect the liver and pancreas against damage by CCl_4. Cortisone protects the liver but not the pancreas.

Allegri et al. C31,532/57: In rats, the hepatic fibrosis induced by prolonged inhalation of CCl_4 is aggravated by concurrent testosterone treatment.

Guérios et al. C58,363/57: In rats, the hepatotoxic action of CCl_4 is aggravated by cortisone.

Mehrotra et al. C54,806/57: The ascites associated with CCl_4-induced hepatic cirrhosis is aggravated in rats by DOC.

Girolami C55,043/58: Testosterone propionate protects the rat against fatty degeneration and cirrhosis of the liver produced either by CCl_4 or by a choline deficient diet.

Asagoe D13,524/59: Hepatic cirrhosis produced in rats by CCl_4-inhalation can be prevented by cortisone, but recovery from well-established cirrhosis is not significantly enhanced by this hormone.

Grassi et al. E58,693/59: In the rat, testosterone, 4-chlorotestosterone and prednisolone alone or in combination protect the kidney against CCl_4 intoxication.

Massei et al. D2,594/59: Testosterone has a beneficial effect upon the hepatic lesions produced by CCl_4 in the rat.

Asagoe D13,523/60: In rats, the hepatic cirrhosis induced by CCl_4 was slightly increased by testosterone after castration, but not in the presence of the testes.

Kulcsár & Kulcsár-Gergely C94,710/60: Ovariectomy partly protects the rat against the hepatotoxic and fatal effects of CCl_4. The degradation of endogenous folliculoids may weaken the resistance of the liver, and thereby predispose it for damage by this drug.

Kulcsár-Gergely & Kulcsár C99,083/60: In ovariectomized rats, estrone aggravates the hepatic damage produced by CCl_4. The activity of endogenous folliculoids (estrus) is increased by hepatic damage, which again shows that these hormones are inactivated by the liver. Presumably, this process of inactivation diminishes the resistance of hepatic tissue to damage.

Tada E96,131/60: Brief abstract on the effect of "androgen," "estrogen" and cortisone upon the lipid, glycogen, and collagen content of the rat liver following intoxication with CCl_4. [No experimental details (H.S.).]

Bengmark & Olsson D48,932/62: Female rats are more susceptible to the hepatotoxic action of CCl_4 than males. Testosterone raised the resistance of females to this form of liver damage.

Bengmark & Olsson D14,663/63: "The authors have been able to demonstrate a beneficial effect of testosterone propionate in female rats subjected to carbon tetrachloride intoxication and a definite lipotropic effect of the hormone in partially hepatectomized male rats."

Discher et al. D64,428/63: The stroma proliferation in rat livers damaged by CCl_4 can be inhibited by cortisone or prednisolone only in the event of s.c., not of p.o., administration. Additional treatment with testosterone did not significantly influence this effect.

Bengmark & Olsson G13,853/64: Orchidectomy increases the susceptibility of the rat to the hepatotoxic action of CCl_4. Testosterone raises the resistance of castrate, but not of intact rats.

Czeizel et al. F23,802/64: Heavy overdosage with various folliculoids aggravates the hepatic damage produced in rats by CCl_4 whereas "physiologic amounts" accelerate healing.

Kulcsár-Gergely et al. F32,037/64: In rats, simultaneous thyroidectomy and ovariectomy offer some protection against the induction of hepatic cirrhosis by CCl_4.

Kulcsár-Gergely & Kulcsár G1,372/64: In rats intoxicated with CCl_4, survival is increased by ovariectomy and thyroidectomy.

Tessmann F8,084/64: The hepatic necrosis produced in rats by CCl_4 was aggravated by prednisone and repair delayed.

Furukawa F71,711/65: In rats, the hepatic steatosis produced by CCl_4 is inhibited by adrenalectomy and, to some extent, also by hypophysectomy. Corticoids restore the effect of CCl_4 after adrenalectomy; epinephrine, though not restoring it, increases the effect of corticoids. STH does not counteract the effect of hypophysectomy. Alloxan diabetes inhibits CCl_4-induced hepatic lipidosis.

Kulcsár & Kulcsár-Gergely F74,930/66: In rats, ovariectomy, thyroidectomy or removal of both glands, offers partial protection against CCl_4 intoxication.

Tessmann & Ziegler F64,393/66: Prednisolone aggravated the hepatic lesions and yet prolonged survival in rats intoxicated with CCl_4.

Rimniceanu et al. F98,503/67: In the rat, cortisone given simultaneously with CCl_4 aggravates the hepatic parenchymal lesions produced by the latter, whereas if the hormone is administered after CCl_4 it hastens hepatic regeneration.

Rimniceanu et al. G66,073/68: In rats, the hepatic lesions produced by CCl_4 are intensified by cortisone, even in the presence of vitamin-B_{12}, but cortisone treatment after interruption of CCl_4 hastens hepatic regeneration.

Becker H17,711/69: In rats, the hepatic cirrhosis produced by thioacetamide or CCl_4 is not inhibited by cortisone, and damage of the parenchymal cells is actually increased.

Joshi & Rao G72,489/69: In rats, Enovid (mestranol + norethynodrel) aggravates the liver damage caused by CCl_4.

Murphy & Malley G68,408/69: Studies on hepatic TKT, alkaline phosphatase (AP), and TPO in relation to stress and CCl_4-intoxication in the rat. "Liver TKT elevation, but not AP elevation, was prevented by adrenalectomy prior to CCl_4. Experiments on rats subjected to simultaneous acute cold stress and CCl_4 indicated that, during the acute phase of CCl_4 hepatotoxicity, their livers had reduced capacity for induction of TKT and TP by endogenous corticosterone. However, chronically injured livers of rats given repeated doses of CCl_4 were fully responsive to the TKT- and TP-inducing effects of exogenous corticosterone or acute cold stress."

Tarnowski et al. G75,524/70: In adrenalectomized rats maintained on cortisol, even lethal amounts of CCl_4 did not depress protein biosynthesis and the ATP/ADP ratio below a relatively high minimal level. "CCl_4 poisoned liver should not be used as a model for studies on regulation of liver metabolism."

Tuchweber and Kovacs G70,489/71: In rats, pretreatment with progesterone, triamcinolone, or phenobarbital increases the mortality, liver damage, and triglyceride accumulation induced by CCl$_4$. Spironolactone, CS-1, ethylestrenol, norbolethone, oxandrolone, estradiol, and DOC do not share this effect.

RABBIT

Regniers et al. C7,634/55: In rabbits, cortisone can either increase or decrease the hepatotoxic effect of CCl$_4$ depending upon the time elapsing between the treatment with the two agents.

Germer & Regoeczi C64,975/58: In rabbits pretreated with plasmapheresis, the hepatotoxic effect of CCl$_4$ could be diminished by testosterone.

Petzold & Meincke D39,959/62: 6-Methylprednisolone hemisuccinate sodium failed to prevent the proliferation of connective tissue in the liver of rabbits damaged by CCl$_4$, except in the case of chronic intoxication.

Ferruccio F62,336/64: Testosterone inhibits the hepatic steatosis produced by CCl$_4$ in the rabbit.

Petzold F61,425/65: In rabbits, hepatic cirrhosis produced by CCl$_4$ is largely inhibited by 4-chlorotestosterone.

GUINEA PIG

Aragona B53,747/49: In guinea pigs, testosterone accelerates hepatic regeneration following CCl$_4$ treatment.

Aragona B53,056/50: In guinea pigs, estradiol and hexestrol given after the induction of hepatic damage by CCl$_4$, produce anemia with myeloid metaplasia in various organs.

MOUSE

Chang & Lei F78,943/67: 17α-Methyl-5α-androstan-17β-ol prevents the production of fatty hepatic degeneration by ethionine or CCl$_4$ in mice.

VARIA

Patrick C12,967/55: In rats and mice, cortisone or ACTH inhibited the mesenchymal reaction, and delayed repair following production of hepatic damage by tannic acid or CCl$_4$.

Stolk D2,285/61: In Iguana iguana, ovariectomy protects against the hepatic lesions produced by CCl$_4$.

Berdjis F79,528/67: The hepatotoxic effect of CCl$_4$, phosphorus and ethionine could be diminished by cortisone, and survival prolonged.

CCl$_4$ ← Cortisone: Aterman B52,265/50*

Carcinogens ← cf. also Selye G60,083/70, p. 357.

← **Corticoids.** *Ratsimamanga & Buu-Hoi B33,923/47:* Various carcinogenic polycyclic hydrocarbons diminish the resistance of the rat to fatigue (swim test). This effect is ascribed to impairment of adrenocortical function since it can be corrected by treatment with adrenocortical extract.

Robertson et al. B88,672/53: In rats, hypophysectomy prevents the production of hepatic cirrhosis and hepatomas by 3'-Me-DAB. The susceptibility to tumorigenesis is restored by ACTH, but not by CON, DOC or testosterone. These hormones likewise failed to prevent carcinogenesis in intact rats.

Symeonidis et al. B93,003/54: In rats, the production of hepatomas by DAB is prevented by adrenalectomy and by DOC in doses causing adrenocortical atrophy.

Reid B93,930/54: Review (18 pp., 181 refs.) on the effect of STH and corticoids upon carcinogen-induced and transplantable neoplasms.

Hoch-Ligeti C14,407/55: In rats, "cortisone under certain experimental conditions seemed to accelerate the occurrence and increase the number of tumors induced by p-dimethylaminoazobenzene or 2-acetylaminofluorene." On the other hand, cortisone had no consistent effect upon transplanted hepatomas.

Schnitzer C32,871/56: In mice, the production of skin tumors by topical application of DMBA is allegedly somewhat increased by cortisone s.c.

Glenn et al. C64,744/59: In the rat, various carcinogens potentiate the testoid and anabolic (levator ani) effects of 17-methyltestosterone as well as the glycogenic and antiphlogistic properties of cortisol. Noncarcinogenic hydrocarbons do not exhibit this effect. "Both in vivo and in vitro studies indicate that the ability of carcinogenic hydrocarbons to potentiate biological effects of steroids is due to a direct effect of carcinogenic agent at the cellular level and not to a decreased rate of steroid metabolism by the liver."

Chany & Boy D2,278/60: In rats, cortisone accelerates the production of hepatic cancers by DAB.

Perry D10,864/61: In rats, the induction of hepatic cancers by AAF is prevented by adrenalectomy but not modified by DOC either in intact or in adrenalectomized animals.

Goodall G77,088/62: In rats, the production of hepatomas by AF is prevented by hypophysectomy or thyroidectomy. Cortisone restores the ability of the thyroidectomized but not of the hypophysectomized rats to develop hepatomas after AF treatment. Cortisone strongly accelerates the appearance of hepatomas in intact rats.

Siegler & Duran-Reynals D 54,814/62: "Methylcholanthrene applied over the site of dermal vaccinial infection in the skin of cortisone-treated mice results in a tumor effect which is more rapid and severe than that seen after the application of methylcholanthrene alone."

Duran-Reynals E 29,252/63: "Mice rendered susceptible to vaccinia dermal infection by cortisone injections and untreated mice received MC skin paintings at the site of virus infection. Under certain conditions, the MC applied before virus inoculation inhibited the virus-induced skin ulcers; applied after it enhanced them."

Lacassagne & Hurst G 12,688/63: In rats, hepatic cancer formation under the influence of DAB is retarded by DOC and accelerated by cortisol.

Sterental et al. D 61,608/63: In rats, mammary tumors induced by DMBA regressed after adrenalectomy+ovariectomy or hypophysectomy. Folliculoid treatment reactivated tumor growth after adrenalectomy+ovariectomy but not after hypophysectomy. These tumors remained unresponsive to folliculoids after hypophysectomy even if thyroid and cortisone replacement therapy was given.

Trainin D 61,599/63: In mice, given a single feeding of DMBA as an initiating stimulus and twice-weekly paintings of 5% croton oil to the skin as a promoting stimulus, carcinogenesis was not significantly altered by cortisol or adrenalectomy during the initiating phase. Conversely, the promoting phase of cutaneous carcinogenesis was strikingly inhibited by cortisol and enhanced by adrenalectomy. The data are discussed in the light of the "two-stage mechanism of carcinogenesis."

Mancini et al. D 18,183/64: In CF-1 albino mice, minimal doses of cortisone slightly decreased the incidence of 3-MC induced tumors.

Young et al. F 20,579/64: In rats treated with DMBA, neither the adrenocortical necrosis nor the tumor incidence was significantly influenced by cortisone.

Ketkar & Sirsat G 32,601/65: In mice, the induction of tumors by 3-MC is not markedly affected by DOC but the pattern of tumor growth and the mast cell response in the connective tissue are altered by the mineralocorticoid.

Jull et al. G 41,663/66: It had previously been noted that in certain strains of mice treated with DMBA, granulosa cell tumors of the ovary develop even if the gonad is transplanted into unpretreated recipients. Both DOC and 17α-hydroxyprogesterone completely inhibit the appearance of granulosa cell tumors when the steroids are injected concurrently with DMBA into the donor mice. Possibly, this protection is due to competitive inhibition.

Jull F 74,180/66: In rats, the induction of mammary carcinomas by DMBA is inhibited by progesterone, DOC and metyrapone.

Lacassagne et al. G 39,677/66: In rats given DAB, hepatic carcinogenesis is inhibited by DOC; various corticoids having the 17α-hydroxyl group exert an opposite effect.

Qureshi & Zaman F 68,389/66: In mice, the induction of subcutaneous sarcomas by 3-MC is inhibited by prednisolone.

Shklar F 74,973/66: In hamsters, the induction of carcinomas by painting the buccal pouch with DMBA was enhanced by cortisone s.c., i.p. or i.m.

Ronzoni et al. H 18,409/68: In rats, prostatic carcinogenesis induced by the introduction of 20-methylcholanthrene crystals into the prostate is inhibited by ACTH, T3 and, to a lesser extent, by progesterone and 19-nortestosterone phenylpropionate. Estradiol and cortisone facilitate carcinogenesis, whereas testosterone, orchidectomy and methylthiouracil failed to influence it.

Sugiura G 64,932/68: In mice, the regression of DMBA-induced papillomas is increased by testosterone and, if anything, decreased by estradiol. Cortisone apparently also increases the number of regressions.

Cole & Foley H 35,251/69: In mice, the induction of pulmonary carcinomas by urethan can be enhanced by cortisone especially in combination with X-irradiation.

Shisa G 72,582/69: In mice of the Swiss, C57BL and A/Jax strains, DMBA injected s.c. on the third day of life induced lymphomas whose incidence could be increased or decreased by cortisone, depending upon the strain and the time of treatment. Earlier literature on the effect of cortisone upon virus or X-ray induced leukemias is reviewed.

Siegel & Shklar H 35,238/69: In hamsters, topical application of DMBA (in DMSO) to the cheek pouch induces a chemical carcinogenesis which can be inhibited by triamcinolone.

Metzler H 27,243/70: In rats, 3-MC causes a drop in blood pressure, but the hypertension produced by DOC + uninephrectomy is not blocked by the carcinogen. On the other hand, the induction of neoplasms is inhibited by DOC.

Polliack et al. H 32,366/70: In hamsters, tumor formation by topical application of DMBA to the cheek pouch is partially suppressed by concurrent application of cortisone, perhaps owing to depression of DNA synthesis and of mitotic activity by the hormone. "Cortisone stabilizes biological membranes; its action on cell multiplication may be related to decreased membrane permeability with consequent inhibition of release of lysosomal enzymes which play a part in early stages of cell division. Decreased membrane permeability may also have resulted in less effective penetration of carcinogen into cells. Results are in accordance with those of previous studies, which demonstrated promotion of tumor formation by labilizers of biological membranes such as vitamin A and estrogen."

Schauer et al. G 81,318/70: In rats, the enzyme histochemically demonstrable precancerous lesions produced in the liver by N-nitrosodiethylamine are inhibited by glucocorticoids and enhanced by estradiol. Males are somewhat more resistant than females, but under the experimental conditions used, testosterone is ineffective.

Somogyi G 70,416/70: In rats, spironolactone inhibits the adrenocortical necrosis, carcinogenicity and hemopoietic-tissue-damaging action of DMBA. Ethylestrenol, CS-1, and norbolethone are also effective against the DMBA-induced adrenal necrosis. Spironolactone likewise protects against the adrenocorticolytic effect of 7-OHM-MBA. Thus, the anti-DMBA action of spironolactone does not seem to be based on the blockade of the transformation of the carcinogen into this supposedly more active metabolite. The preventive action of spironolactone is abolished by ethionine, suggesting the involvement of active protein synthesis. The DMBA-induced adrenal lesions are aggravated by estradiol, testosterone, methyltestosterone, cortisol, triamcinolone, and prednisolone, as well as by the stress of muscular work or restraint. The aggravation of adrenal necrosis by estradiol is diminished but not abolished by hypophysectomy.

Somogyi & Kovacs G 60,074/70: In rats, the adrenal necrosis produced by DMBA is inhibited by spironolactone and ethylestrenol; it is aggravated by estradiol, MAD, cortisol and testosterone but not significantly influenced by progesterone, norbolethone, triamcinolone or DOC.

3-Methyl-4-monomethylaminoazobenzene ← Cortisone, Mouse: Reif et al. *D 97,006/54*

Dimethylaminoazobenzene ← DOC: Shimazu et al. *G 76,684/59**

7,12-Dimethylbenzanthracene ← Cortisol: Harris *F 98,166/68**

Benzo(a)pyrene ← Cortisol + Age Hamster: Nebert et al. *H 23,692/68*

← **Folliculoids.** *Cantarow et al. B 18,774/46:* In rats, given AAF p.o., the development of cystic and neoplastic hepatic lesions was accelerated and intensified by GTH (pregnant mare serum), estradiol and testosterone, but inhibited by thiouracil. "This phenomenon may be related to the role of the liver in the intermediary metabolism and excretion of the sex steroid." No tumors occurred in the hyperplastic target organs of the sex hormones in contrast to the high incidence of tumors in the thyroids of rats given thiouracil simultaneously with the carcinogens.

Kirby B 30,101/47: Female rats are less susceptible than males to the production of hepatomas and hepatic cirrhosis by AAF. Rats simultaneoulsy treated with pellets of estradiol or testosterone and AAF showed no carcinoma formation in the target organs of the sex hormones.

Stasney et al. B 26,653/47: In rats, AAF feeding produces mammary carcinoma only in females, and its development is not significantly accelerated by estradiol or gonadotrophin. "Malignant lesions of the liver occurred in 54.8 per cent of females and 92.3 per cent of males receiving the carcinogen alone. Administration of estradiol and PMS gonadotrophin to females and of testosterone and chorionic gonadotrophin to males intensified the cystic and neoplastic hepatic lesions induced by 2-acetaminofluorene."

Shay et al. H 31,719/52: In rats, chronic administration of 3-MC p.o. produces glandular tumors of the breast (predominantly in females and estradiol-treated males), spindle-cell and collagenous tumors of the breast and mesenteric sarcomas (predominantly in males and testosterone-treated females), and fibroadenomas of the breast (predominantly in ovariectomized and orchidectomized animals "in which the sex hormone effects were experimentally counterbalanced").

Geyer et al. H31,923/53: In rats, the induction of mammary tumors by DMBA is greatly enhanced by estradiol and stilbestrol.

Miyaji et al. D24,881/53: In rats, the production of hepatic, mammary and sebaceous gland tumors by AAF was not significantly influenced by adrenalectomy. On the other hand, after gonadectomy, testosterone increased, whereas estrone, estradiol and progesterone decreased carcinogenesis. [A brief abstract which is difficult to evaluate (H.S.).]

Shelton G76,339/54: In mice, 2-amino-5-azotoluene added to a semi-synthetic diet produced a high incidence of hepatomas only in the case of concurrent treatment with stilbestrol.

Huggins et al. C99,772/61: In rats, the production of mammary cancers by DMBA or 3-MC is inhibited by pregnancy, estradiol, progesterone or combined treatment of estradiol + progesterone.

Seguy et la. D5,238/61: In rats, high doses of folliculoids enhanced the carcinogenic action of benzpyrene. Hypophysectomy or ovariectomy did not significantly influence this type of carcinogenesis, but the number of animals used was very small.

Shay et al. D2,760/61: In rats, the induction of mammary cancers by methylcholanthrene is inhibited by folliculoids.

Pannella & Gasparrini D64,636/63: In female rats, the carcinogenic action of 20-methylcholanthrene is accelerated by folliculoids, partially inhibited by testosterone and completely blocked by ovariectomy. When tumors do arise, however, their histologic character is not influenced by any of these treatments.

Sterental et al. D61,608/63: In rats, mammary tumors induced by DMBA regressed after adrenalectomy+ovariectomy or hypophysectomy. Folliculoid treatment reactivated tumor growth after adrenalectomy+ovariectomy but not after hypophysectomy. These tumors remained unresponsive to folliculoids after hypophysectomy even if thyroid and cortisone replacement therapy was given.

Sirsat & Ketkar F65,926/66: In mice, the induction of cutaneous carcinomas by topical treatment with 3-MC is stimulated by pretreatment and inhibited by subsequent treatment with DOC.

Weisburger et al. F72,720/66: In the rat, neonatal estradiol treatment enhances hepatoma formation following administration of the carcinogen N-hydroxy-N-2-fluorenylacetamide.

Colafranceschi & Tosi G59,115/67: The adrenal necrosis produced by DMBA in the rat is of equal severity in males and females and cannot be influenced by ovariectomy, orchidectomy, testosterone or estradiol.

Weisburger et al. F78,862/67: Male rats are more prone to liver cancer induction by N-hydroxy-N-2-fluorenylacetamide (N-OH-FAA) than females. In newborn males treated with estradiol, and placed on a diet containing N-OH-FAA, the incidence of hepatic carcinomas was decreased, whereas testosterone did not change it. In females, estradiol had a "mixed effect," and testosterone enhanced hepatoma induction.

Poel H23,662/68: Review of the literature with personal observations on the co-carcinogenic effect of folliculoids and luteoids. Neither of these groups of steroids are truly carcinogenic in themselves, but they enhance mammary cancer development under the influence of viral and chemical carcinogens. [The possible mechanism of these interactions is not discussed (H.S.).]

Sugiura G64,932/68: In mice, the regression of DMBA-induced papillomas is increased by testosterone and, if anything, decreased by estradiol. Cortisone apparently also increased the number of regressions.

Weisburger & Yamamoto F97,904/68: Rats of both sexes were injected neonatally with a single dose of testosterone or estradiol. After weaning they were placed on a diet containing N-hydroxy-N-2-fluorenylacetamide (N-OH-FAA) for 16 weeks. Autopsies were performed after an additional 10 weeks on controlled diets. In males, the hepatic tumor incidence was not affected by testosterone but reduced by estradiol. In females, testosterone enhanced carcinogenicity while estradiol had a dual effect, augmenting carcinogenesis in a few rats but reducing it in most.

Newberne & Williams G69,601/69: In rats, hepatic carcinogenesis produced by aflatoxin is inhibited by diethylstilbestrol. Male rats are less resistant to aflatoxin than females.

Polliack et al. G72,389/69: In orchidectomized hamsters, stilbestrol increases topical carcinogenesis if one cheek pouch is repeatedly treated with DMBA. Among hamsters not treated with folliculoids, orchidectomy did not change the incidence of carcinogenesis under these conditions.

Griswold Jr. & Green H26,709/70: Review of the literature and personal observations on the effect of ovariectomy, testoids and folliculoids alone and in combination upon the hormone sensitivity of DMBA-induced mammary tumors in the rat.

Horvath et al. G70,443/70: In rats, estradiol pretreatment markedly increases the susceptibility of the adrenals to the corticolytic effect of DMBA. The associated histochemical changes are described.

Schauer et al. G81,318/70: In rats, the enzyme histochemically demonstrable precancerous lesions produced in the liver by N-nitrosodiethylamine are inhibited by glucocorticoids and enhanced by estradiol. Males are somewhat more resistant than females but, under the experimental conditions used, testosterone is ineffective.

Somogyi G70,416/70: In rats, spironolactone inhibits the adrenocortical necrosis, carcinogenicity and hemopoietic-tissue-damaging action of DMBA. Ethylestrenol, CS-1, and norbolethone are also effective against the DMBA-induced adrenal necrosis. Spironolactone likewise protects against the adrenocorticolytic effect of 7-OHM-MBA. Thus, the anti-DMBA action of spironolactone does not seem to be based on the blockade of the transformation of the carcinogen into this supposedly more active metabolite. The preventive action of spironolactone is abolished by ethionine, suggesting the involvement of active protein synthesis. The DMBA-induced adrenal lesions are aggravated by estradiol, testosterone, methyltestosterone, cortisol, triamcinolone, and prednisolone, as well as by the stress of muscular work or restraint. The aggravation of adrenal necrosis by estradiol is diminished but not abolished by hypophysectomy.

Somogyi & Kovacs G60,074/70: In rats, the adrenal necrosis produced by DMBA is inhibited by spironolactone and ethylestrenol; it is aggravated by estradiol, MAD, cortisol and testosterone but not significantly influenced by progesterone, norbolethone, triamcinolone or DOC.

N-2-Fluorenylacetamide ← Estradiol: Kirby B30,101/47*; Miyaji et al. D24,881/53*

9,10-Dimethyl-1,2-benzanthracene ← Diethylstilbestrol: Dao G37,357/64*; Huggins et al. F18,350/64*

3-MC ← Estradiol: Kirschbaum et al. H27,666/53*; Gautieri et al. H30,506/61*; Huggins et al. C99,772/61*

Benzo(a)pyrene ← Estradiol: Mitoma et al. G72,113/68

← **Luteoids.** *Miyaji et al. D24,881/53:* In rats, the production of hepatic, mammary and sebaceous gland tumors by AAF was not significantly influenced by adrenalectomy. On the other hand, after gonadectomy, testosterone increased whereas estrone, estradiol and progesterone decreased carcinogenesis. [A brief abstract which is difficult to evaluate (H.S.).]

Thiersch C28,993/57: Administration of progesterone i.m. one hour before TEM to pregnant rats protected their litters against the fatal and teratogenic effects of the carcinolytic agent.

Dao & Sunderland D79,860/59; Dao et al. E57,368/60: In rats, the induction of mammary carcinomas by 3-methylcholanthrene is enhanced during pregnancy, pseudopregnancy, and progesterone treatment. Regression of neoplasms occurs after parturition. Males are virtually resistant. In fully formed tumors, regression could be induced by hypophysectomy or ovariectomy.

Huggins et al. C99,772/61: In rats, the production of mammary cancers by DMBA or 3-MC is inhibited by pregnancy, estradiol, progesterone or combined treatment of estradiol + progesterone.

Poel H23,662/68: Review of the literature with personal observations on the co-carcinogenic effect of folliculoids and luteoids. Neither of these groups of steroids are truly carcinogenic in themselves but they enhance mammary cancer development under the influence of viral and chemical carcinogens. [The possible mechanism of these interactions is not discussed (H.S.).]

Somogyi & Kovacs G60,074/70: In rats, the adrenal necrosis produced by DMBA is inhibited by spironolactone and ethylestrenol; it is aggravated by estradiol, MAD, cortisol and testosterone but not significantly influenced by progesterone, norbolethone, triamcinolone or DOC.

3,4-Benzpyrene ← Progesterone: Juchau et al. G40,275/66

7,12-Dimethylbenz(a)anthracene ← Progesterone + Estradiol-17β: Huggins et al. D27,549/62*

N-2-Fluorenylacetamide ← Progesterone: Miyaji et al. D24,881/53*

3-MC ← Progesterone: Huggins et al. C99,772/61*

← **Testoids.** *Maisin et al. A30,500/39:* Unlike folliculoids, testosterone proprionate does not augment the incidence of mammary cancers in benzpyrene-treated mice.

Cantarow et al. B18,774/46: In rats, given AAF p.o., the development of cystic and neoplastic hepatic lesions was accelerated and intensified by GTH (pregnant mare serum), estradiol and testosterone, but inhibited by thiouracil. "This phenomenon may be related to the role of the liver in the intermediary metabolism and excretion of the sex steroid." No tumors occurred in the hyperplastic target organs of the sex hormones in contrast to the high incidence of tumors in the thyroids of rats given thiouracil simultaneously with the carcinogens.

Kirby B30,101/47: Female rats are less susceptible than males to the production of hepatomas and hepatic cirrhosis by AAF. Rats simultaneously treated with pellets of estradiol or testosterone and AAF showed no carcinoma formation in the target organs of the sex hormones.

Stasney et al. B26,653/47: In rats, 2-acetaminofluorene feeding produces mammary carcinoma only in females, and its development is not significantly accelerated by estradiol or gonadotrophin. "Malignant lesions of the liver occurred in 54.8 per cent of females and 92.3 per cent of males receiving the carcinogen alone. Administration of estradiol and PMS gonadotrophin to females and of testosterone and chorionic gonadotrophin to males intensified the cystic and neoplastic hepatic lesions induced by 2-acetaminofluorene."

Flaks B35,572/48: Testosterone delays the induction of subcutaneous tumors by 20-methylcholanthrene.

Shay et al. H31,719/52: In rats, chronic administration of 3-MC p.o. produces glandular tumors of the breast (predominantly in females and estradiol-treated males), spindle-cell and collagenous tumors of the breast and mesenteric sarcomas (predominantly in males and testosterone-treated females), and fibroadenomas of the breast (predominantly in ovariectomized and orchidectomized animals "in which the sex hormone effects were experimentally counterbalanced").

Miyaji et al. D24,881/53: In rats, the production of hepatic, mammary and sebaceous gland tumors by AAF was not significantly influenced by adrenalectomy. On the other hand, after gonadectomy, testosterone increased, whereas estrone, estradiol and progesterone decreased, carcinogenesis. [A brief abstract which is difficult to evaluate (H.S.).]

Robertson et al. B88,672/53: In rats, hypophysectomy prevents the production of hepatic cirrhosis and hepatomas by 3'-Me-DAB. The susceptibility to tumorigenesis is restored by ACTH, but not by cortisone, DOC or testosterone. These hormones likewise failed to prevent carcinogenesis in intact rats.

Huggins et al. C62,178/59: In rats, mammary carcinomas induced by 3-methylcholanthrene involute following ovariectomy or hypophysectomy and, hence, they may be regarded as "hormone-dependent." Similar regression of tumors is frequently achieved by dihydrotestosterone. Only a few mammary cancers continue to grow after ovariectomy and these are considered to be "hormone-independent."

Thompson et al. C92,646/60: In mice with transplanted myelomas, 3-methylcholanthrene retarded or even completely suppressed the growth of the neoplastic tissue. Concurrent treatment with dihydrotestosterone increased the body weight of the host but did not exert an additive-suppressing effect upon the myeloma's growth.

Dao & Greiner D91,850/61: In male rats, unlike in females or castrate males, 3-MC rarely produces mammary tumors. Ovarian transplants placed into castrate males induce predisposition for mammary carcinogenesis under these conditions.

Pannella & Gasparrini D64,636/63: In female rats, the carcinogenic action of 20-methylcholanthrene is accelerated by folliculoids, partially inhibited by testosterone and completely blocked by ovariectomy. When tumors do arise, however, their histologic character is not influenced by any of these treatments.

Sidransky et al. C99,347/61: In rats, fed AAF, hepatic tumors developed in all males but only in 5 out of 14 females. "Although castrated males had liver changes similar to those seen in females, these males receiving testosterone had the same changes as were found in the intact males. Intact females receiving testosterone developed earlier and more extensive changes regularly found only in the livers of males." Testosterone may accelerate hepatic tumorigenesis by this carcinogen.

Kovacs G34,582/65: In rats given a single injection of testosterone at 1—2 days of age, the subsequent production of mammary cancers by DMBA is inhibited. However, this form of testosterone treatment does not prevent the production of leukemia by DMBA.

Reuber F36,234/65: Concurrent treatment with testosterone and thyroid powder sensitizes the rat for the production of hepatic cirrhosis and hepatomas by AAF.

Mody G 49,656/67: The yield of ovarian tumors induced by DMBA "was significantly greater in C_3H (Jax) mammectomised mice when treated with testosterone. It is suggested that testosterone has a promoting action for chemically induced ovarian tumours in mice."

Stern & Mickey F 89,080/67: In 50-day old female rats with "androgen sterility" (induced by a single injection of testosterone at five days of age) DMBA elicits less mammary tumors than in unpretreated controls.

Weisburger et al. F 78,862/67: Male rats are more prone to liver cancer induction by N-hydroxy-N-2-fluorenylacetamide (N-OH-FAA) than females. In newborn males treated with estradiol, and placed on a diet containing N-OH-FAA, the incidence of hepatic carcinomas was decreased, whereas testosterone did not change it. In females, estradiol had a "mixed effect," and testosterone enhanced hepatoma induction.

Glucksmann & Cherry H 19,200/68: In rats, ovariectomy reduces the rate of induction by DMBA of cervico-vaginal sarcomas. This inhibition is counteracted by various folliculoids. In intact rats, progesterone slightly retards the induction of these sarcomas and in castrates it fails to raise the rate of carcinogenesis. Testosterone lengthens the induction period of sarcomas in intact rats and increases the rate of sarcoma formation in castrates.

Sugiura G 64,932/68: in mice, the regression of DMBA-induced papillomas is increased by testosterone and, if anything, decreased by estradiol. Cortisone apparently also increased the number of regressions.

Weisburger & Yamamoto F 97,904/68: Rats of both sexes were injected neonatally with a single dose of testosterone or estradiol. After weaning they were placed on a diet containing N-hydroxy-N-2-fluorenylacetamide (N-OH-FAA) for 16 weeks. Autopsies were performed after an additional 10 weeks on controlled diet. In males, the hepatic tumor incidence was not affected by testosterone but reduced by estradiol. In females, testosterone enhanced carcinogenicity while estradiol had a dual effect augmenting carcinogenesis in a few rats but reducing it in most.

Dmitriev H 28,154/69: In mice, the production of preneoplastic mammary changes by benzpyrene is diminished by testosterone.

Griswold Jr. & Green H 26,709/70: Review of the literature and personal observations on the effect of ovariectomy, testoids and folliculoids, alone and in combination, upon the hormonal sensitivity of DMBA-induced mammary tumors in the rat.

Mückter et al. H 23,589/70: In rats, survival time after induction of mammary tumors by DMBA is increased by treatment with a combination of drostanolone propionate (2α-methyl dihydrotestosterone propionate) and a cyclic imide [1-(morpholinomethyl)-4-phthalimido-piperidindione-2,6]. The catabolic effect of the carcinolytic cyclic imide is particularly well antagonized by the anabolic testoid but there is no decrease in the number of tumor centers that develop.

Polliack et al. H 31,578/70: In intact male hamsters, the induction of carcinomas by topical application of DMBA to the cheek pouch was reduced by testosterone. In castrate males, this effect was less striking. Castration itself had no effect on tumorigenesis.

Schauer et al. G 81,318/70: In rats, the enzyme histochemically demonstrable precancerous lesions produced in the liver by N-nitrosodiethylamine are inhibited by glucocorticoids and enhanced by estradiol. Males are somewhat more resistant than females but, under the experimental conditions used, testosterone is ineffective.

Somogyi G 70,416/70: In rats, spironolactone inhibits the adrenocortical necrosis, carcinogenicity and hemopoietic-tissue-damaging action of DMBA. Ethylestrenol, CS-1, and norbolethone are also effective against the DMBA-induced adrenal necrosis. Spironolactone likewise protects against the adrenocorticolytic effect of 7-OHM-MBA. Thus, the anti-DMBA action of spironolactone does not seem to be based on the blockade of the transformation of the carcinogen into this supposedly more active metabolite. The preventive action of spironolactone is abolished by ethionine, suggesting the involvement of active protein synthesis. The DMBA-induced adrenal lesions are aggravated by estradiol, testosterone, methyltestosterone, cortisol, triamcinolone, and prednisolone, as well as by the stress of muscular work or restraint. The aggravation of adrenal necrosis by estradiol is diminished but not abolished by hypophysectomy.

Somogyi & Kovacs G 60,074/70: In rats, the adrenal necrosis produced by DMBA is inhibited by spironolactone and ethylestrenol; it is aggravated by estradiol, MAD, cortisol and testosterone but not significantly influenced by progesterone, norbolethone, triamcinolone or DOC.

9,10-Dimethyl-1,2-benzanthracene ← Testosterone: Kovacs G 34,582/65*
N-2-Fluorenylacetamide ← Testosterone: Kirby B 30,101/47*; Miyaji et al. D 24,881/53*

← **Gonadectomy.** *Maisin et al. 25,708/26:* In male mice, the production of skin cancers by topical application of tar is not inhibited and appears to be aggravated by castration.

Andervont & Dunn A 96,182/47: Among strain C mice, o-aminoazotoluene produced hepatomas more frequently in females than in males. Furthermore, "intact females were more susceptible than castrate females; castrate males approached intact females in their degree of susceptibility; castrate females and castrate males bearing testosterone propionate-cholesterol pellets approached intact males in their degree of susceptibility." The incidence of pulmonary tumors, after treatment with this carcinogen, was not dependent upon any of the factors just mentioned.

Shay et al. H 26,763/49: In intact female rats, 3-MC p.o. produces a high incidence of mammary adenocarcinomas, whereas this is exceptional in intact or castrate males as well as in spayed females.

Bielschowsky & Hall G 71,797/51: In intact female rats joined in parabiosis with gonadectomized litter-mates, AAF induced a 50% incidence of malignant tumors, mostly of the granulosa. The gonadectomized partners were free of neoplastic lesions.

Shay et al. H 31,719/52: In rats, chronic administration of 3-MC p.o. produces glandular tumors of the breast (predominantly in females and estradiol-treated males) spindle-cell and collagenous tumors of the breast and mesenteric sarcomas (predominantly in males and testosterone-treated females), and fibroadenomas of the breast (predominantly in ovariectomized and orchidectomized animals "in which the sex hormone effects were experimentally counterbalanced").

Miyaji et al. D 24,881/53: In rats, the production of hepatic, mammary and sebaceous gland tumors by AAF was not significantly influenced by adrenalectomy. On the other hand, after gonadectomy, testosterone increased, whereas estrone, estradiol and progesterone decreased carcinogenesis. [A brief abstract which is difficult to evaluate (H.S.).]

Dao & Sunderland D 79,860/59; Dao et al. E 57,368/60: In rats, the induction of mammary carcinomas by 3-methylcholanthrene is enhanced during pregnancy, pseudopregnancy, and progesterone treatment. Regression of neoplasms occurs after parturition. Males are virtually resistant. In fully formed tumors, regression could be induced by hypophysectomy or ovariectomy.

Huggins et al. C 62,178/59: In rats, mammary carcinomas induced by 3-MC involute following ovariectomy or hypophysectomy and, hence, they may be regarded as "hormone-dependent." Similar regression of tumors is frequently achieved by dihydrotestosterone. Only a few mammary cancers continue to grow after ovariectomy and these are considered to be "hormone-independent."

Marchant C 69,830/59: In mice, painting of the skin with methylcholanthrene produced papillomas earlier in male or female castrates than in intact controls.

Kim & Furth H 31,205/60: In rats, the induction of mammary cancers by 3-MC is considerably inhibited by ovariectomy or hypophysectomy. Grafts of functional mammotropic pituitary tumors counteract the inhibitory effect of hypophysectomy in that they not only stimulate the growth of involuting preexisting cancers, but also cause the appearance of new mammary tumors.

Bock & Dao D 11,892/61: In rats, 3-MC accumulation in the mammary glands is increased by hypophysectomy or ovariectomy, but diminished during pregnancy. The affinity of mammary tissue for certain carcinogens may be due to its close association with adipose tissue.

Dao & Greiner D 91,850/61: In male rats, unlike in females or castrate males, 3-MC rarely produces mammary tumors. Ovarian transplants placed into castrate males induce predisposition for mammary carcinogenesis under these conditions.

Seguy et al. D 5,238/61: In rats, high doses of folliculoids enhanced the carcinogenic action of benzpyrene. Hypophysectomy or ovariectomy did not significantly influence this type of carcinogenesis, but the number of animals used was very small.

Dao D 36,011/62: In rats, ovariectomy performed before the administration of 3-MC or DMBA inhibited mammary carcinogenesis, but if the ovaries were removed 7 days after feeding the carcinogenic hydrocarbons, no significant reduction of mammary cancer resulted.

Huggins & Fukunishi E 35,442/63: In rats, mammary tumors induced by DMBA or by X-irradiation regress following ovariectomy.

"Tumors of this sort are, by definition, hormone-dependent."

Pannella & Gasparrini D64,636/63: In female rats, the carcinogenic action of 20-methylcholanthrene is accelerated by folliculoids, partially inhibited by testosterone and completely blocked by ovariectomy. When tumors do arise, however, their histologic character is not influenced by any of these treatments.

Sterental et al. D61,608/63: In rats, mammary tumors induced by DMBA regressed after adrenalectomy+ovariectomy or hypophysectomy. Folliculoid treatment reactivated tumor growth after adrenalectomy+ovariectomy but not after hypophysectomy. These tumors remained unresponsive to folliculoids after hypophysectomy even if thyroid and cortisone replacement therapy was given.

Dao G37,357/64: Review of the literature on the effect of various hormones upon the induction of mammary cancers by carcinogens in the rat. The induction of these cancers requires the presence of ovarian hormones. Ovariectomy prevents this type of carcinogenesis unless ovarian transplants or estradiol are administered.

Reuber F4,431/64: In rats, the production of hepatomas by N-2-fluorenyldiacetamide was prevented by orchidectomy or thyroidectomy. However, the carcinogenic effect was restored in thyroidectomized animals by thyroid feeding.

Huggins & Grand F74,177/66: In rats, neither hypophysectomy nor orchidectomy causes regression of DMBA-induced mammary cancers.

Ito et al. G42,670/66: In mice, the development of urethan-induced thymic lymphomas was enhanced by orchidectomy but not significantly affected by ovariectomy. In the early latent period, adrenalectomy accelerated the development of thymic lymphomas, especially in females.

Biancifiori et al. F98,833/67: Both in intact and in ovariectomized mice, estrone increased the incidence of mammary carcinomas produced by DBA or 3-MC; only minimal effects were obtained with benzopyrene or DMBA.

Bates H13,409/68: Male Swiss mice are more sensitive than females to the induction of cutaneous carcinomas by DMBA+croton oil. This is especially true of females in which the initiator was applied during diestrus. Gonadectomy before application of DMBA increased tumor incidence in females but decreased it in males.

Heimann et al. F95,958/68: In rats, the production of mammary carcinomas by DMBA is almost totally inhibited by ovariectomy. However, a high percentage of the spayed rats presents tumors of the ear duct, neurofibrosarcomas of the ear lobe and various cutaneous neoplasms. The appearance of these extra-mammary tumors may be due in part to the prolongation of the life span by the inhibition of mammary carcinogenesis.

Svoboda et al. G64,564/69: Hepatocytes of male rats given CPIB (ethyl-α-p-chlorophenoxyisobutyrate) show a pronounced increase in microbodies and in catalase activity while those of intact females do not. In castrate males given estradiol and CPIB the increase in catalase activity and microbody proliferation is abolished, whereas in ovariectomized rats given testosterone and CPIB there is an increase in microbodies and catalase activity.

Glucksmann & Cherry G77,810/70: In rats, ovariectomy offers partial protection against the induction of cervico-vaginal neoplasms after repeated topical applications of DMBA.

Griswold Jr. & Green H26,709/70: Review of the literature and personal observations on the effect of ovariectomy, testoids and folliculoids, alone and in combination, upon the hormone sensitivity of DMBA-induced mammary tumors in the rat.

Jasmin & Riopelle H23,587/70: In rats, ovariectomy greatly increased the incidence of mammary tumors produced by DMBA p.o. and also induced renal tumors which were not seen in similarly-treated intact controls.

Kozuka H27,469/70: "Repeated injection of reserpine and simultaneous administration of 2,7-diacetamidofluorene in SMA/Ms strain mice prevented the development of liver tumors but failed to induce gastric cancer. Female mice developed more hepatic tumors than males both in the carcinogen groups and in the reserpine-treated group. Castration increased the formation of hepatic cancer in male mice but not in females. In castrated female mice, estradiol benzoate had little effect and testosterone propionate reduced liver tumor incidence somewhat."

Polliack et al. H31,578/70: In intact male hamsters, the induction of carcinomas by topical applicatoin of DMBA to the cheek pouch was reduced by testosterone. In castrate males, this effect was less striking. Castration itself had no effect on tumorigenesis.

Simpson-Herren & Griswold, Jr. H 26,708/70: In rats, with DMBA-induced mammary carcinomas, the thymidine index was followed during different stages of cell development. "Administration of estradiol and progesterone to ovariectomized animals with regressed or static tumors results in an approximately 10-fold increase in thymidine index."

Somogyi & Kovacs G 60,074/70: In rats, ovariectomy followed by grafting of ovarian tissue into the spleen, and consequent direct inflow of folliculoids into the liver, does not enhance DMBA-induced adrenal necrosis.

Zackheim H 26,549/70: In mice, painted with methylcholanthrene, the incidence and extent of skin neoplasms was decreased by orchidectomy.

N-2-Fluorenylacetamide ← Gonadectomy + Steroids: Miyaji et al. D 24,881/53* DeBaun et al. H 26,701/70

3-MC ← Gonadectomy + Estradiol: Gautieri et al. H 30,506/61*

3-MC ← Gonadectomy + Ovarian grafts: Dao D 36,011/62*

← **Adrenalectomy.** *Miyaji et al. D 24,881/53:* In rats, the production of hepatic, mammary and sebaceous gland tumors by AAF was not significantly influenced by adrenalectomy. On the other hand, after gonadectomy, testosterone increased, whereas estrone, estradiol and progesterone decreased, carcinogenesis. [A brief abstract which is difficult to evaluate (H.S.).]

Symeonidis et al. B 93,003/54: In rats, the production of hepatomas by DAB is prevented by adrenalectomy and by DOC in doses causing adrenocortical atrophy.

Conney et al. D 87,867/56: Injection of 3-MC i.p. greatly increases the ability of rat liver homogenates to N-demethylate 3-methyl-4-monomethylaminoazobenzene and to reduce the azo linkage of 4-dimethylaminoazobenzene. Neither of these activities was altered after adrenalectomy, but both systems were slightly depressed after hypophysectomy.

Eversole C 45,823/57: In rats, 3'MeDAB-induced hepatic carcinogenesis is not inhibited by DOC (in contradiction of earlier findings), whereas similarly DOC-treated adrenalectomized rats developed no hepatomas. The presence of even small remnants of adrenocortical tissue permitted the azo dye to exert its carcinogenic effect. "Total adrenalectomy is apparently the key factor in inhibiting azo dye carcinogenesis."

Bielschowsky D 10,255/61: In rats, hypophysectomy, thyroidectomy and adrenalectomy inhibit the development of hepatomas by treatment with 2-acetylaminofluorene (AAF) or 2-aminofluorene (AF).

Perry D 10,864/61: In rats, the induction of hepatic cancers by AAF is prevented by adrenalectomy but not modified by DOC either in intact or in adrenalectomized animals.

Benton D 22,526/62: In male mice, dibenzpyrene-induced tumors involute and most of them disappear after adrenalectomy.

Sterental et al. D 61,608/63: In rats, mammary tumors induced by DMBA regressed after adrenalectomy+ovariectomy or hypophysectomy. Folliculoid treatment reactivated tumor growth after adrenalectomy+ovariectomy but not after hypophysectomy. These tumors remained unresponsive to folliculoids after hypophysectomy even if thyroid and cortisone replacement therapy was given.

Trainin D 61,599/63: In mice, given a single feeding of DMBA as an initiating stimulus and twice-weekly paintings of 5% croton oil to the skin as a promoting stimulus, carcinogenesis was not significantly altered by cortisol or adrenalectomy during the initiating phase. Conversely, the promoting phase of cutaneous carcinogenesis was strikingly inhibited by cortisol and enhanced by adrenalectomy. The data are discussed in the light of the "two-stage mechanism of carcinogenesis."

Shimazu G 31,110/65: 20-Methylcholanthrene increases hepatic dimethylaminoazobenzene-demethylase in the rat, even after adrenalectomy, ovariectomy, or hypophysectomy. Hypothalamic lesions decrease the basal level of the enzyme and its response to methylcholanthrene. On the other hand, glutamine synthetase (a microsomal enzyme not induced by methylcholanthrene) is unaffected by hypothalamic lesions.

Ito et al. G 42,670/66: In mice, the development of urethan-induced thymic lymphomas was enhanced by orchidectomy but not significantly affected by ovariectomy. In the early latent period, adrenalectomy accelerated the development of thymic lymphomas, especially in females.

Radzialowski & Bousquet H 2,264/68: The circadian variation in aminopyrine, p-nitroanisole and hexobarbital-metabolizing microsomal enzymes of the rat and mouse liver is abolished by adrenalectomy, but the rhythm of 4-dimethylaminoazobenzene metabolism remains unaffected.

Symeonidis H 27,336/70: In C3Hf mice, which are spontaneously predisposed to hepatic tumor formation, the induction of liver

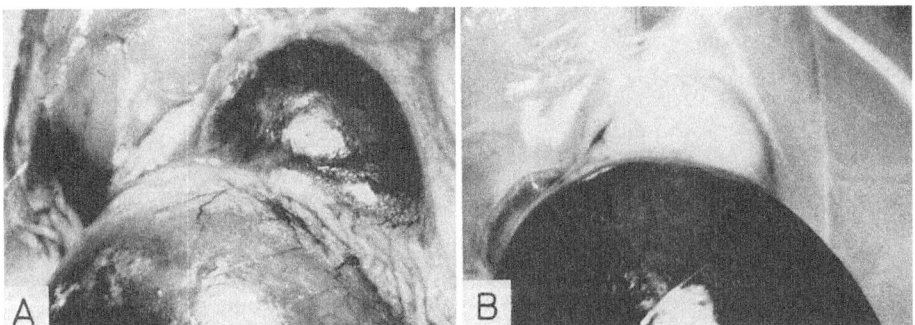

Fig. 2. **Prevention by spironolactone of DMBA-induced adrenal necrosis.** Both rats received the same dose of DMBA. A: Otherwise-untreated control shows hemorrhagic necrosis of the adrenal with periadrenal edema. B: Adrenal is normal in the rat which received pretreatment with spironolactone. [Kovacs & Somogyi G60,025/69. Courtesy of Proc. Soc. exp. Biol. Med.]

carcinomas by AAF is inhibited by adrenalectomy.

Dimethylaminoazobenzene ← Adrenalectomy: Conney et al. *D87,867/56;* Shimazu et al. G76,684/59*, *G31,110/65*

7,12-Dimethylbenzanthracene ← Adrenalectomy + Cortisol: Harris F98,166/68*

N-2-Fluorenylacetamide ← Adrenalectomy: Miyaji et al. D24,881/53* De Baun et al. H26,701/70

3-MC ← Adrenalectomy: Boyland et al. D47,605/62*

← **Other Steroids** *cf. also Selye G60,083/70, p. 385. Kovacs G70,404/69:* In rats, electronmicroscopic changes produced by DMBA are ascribed to primary damage in the capillary endothelium. The protective effect of spironolactone is ascribed to the induction of drug metabolizing microsomal enzymes.

Kovacs & Somogyi G60,025/69: In the rat, the adrenal necrosis produced by DMBA is inhibited by pretreatment with spironolactone.

Kovacs & Somogyi G60,060/69: In rats, the adrenal necrosis produced by DMBA is prevented by pretreatment with spironolactone and this protection is in turn blocked by ethionine.

Lacassagne et al. G74,932/69: In rats, production of hepatic cancers by DAB is powerfully inhibited by Δ^5-pregnenolone, DOC or DDD. Various other steroids give less clearcut results.

Somogyi G70,406/69: In rats, the adrenal necrosis produced by DMBA or 7-hydroxymethyl-12-methylbenzanthracene is inhibited by pretreatment with spironolactone.

Wall et al. G69,969/69: A series of steroid esters of p-[N,N-bis(2-chloroethyl)amino]phenylacetic acid (BCAPAA), steroidal sulfides of p-(N,N-bis-2-chloroethylamino)thiophenol, and a variety of steroidal ethylenimine derivatives were synthesized and tested for antitumor activity. "Activity was found only in those instances in which the steroid and potential oncolytic agent were connected by ester or heterocyclic ether linkages. The steroidal BCAPAA esters were of particular interest showing excellent inhibition of a DMBA-induced and transplantable mammary adrenocarcinoma, and marked increase in survival when tested on a variety of rat leukemias ... The steroidal BCAPAA esters were judged to be less toxic than some of the well-known nitrogen mustards in general use."

Kovacs & Somogyi G60,089/70: In rats, pretreatment with spironolactone delays the development and decreases the incidence of mammary tumors induced by a single injection of DMBA.

Solymoss et al. G70,445/70: In rats, the acute hematologic changes observed six days after a single oral dose of DMBA are suppressed by spironolactone but the alterations normally observed 12 days after DMBA still occur. The hematologic damage produced by a smaller dose of DMBA i.v. is prevented both by spironolactone and by SKF 525-A. Apparently "the hemopoietic alterations, elicited by DMBA, are dose-dependent and

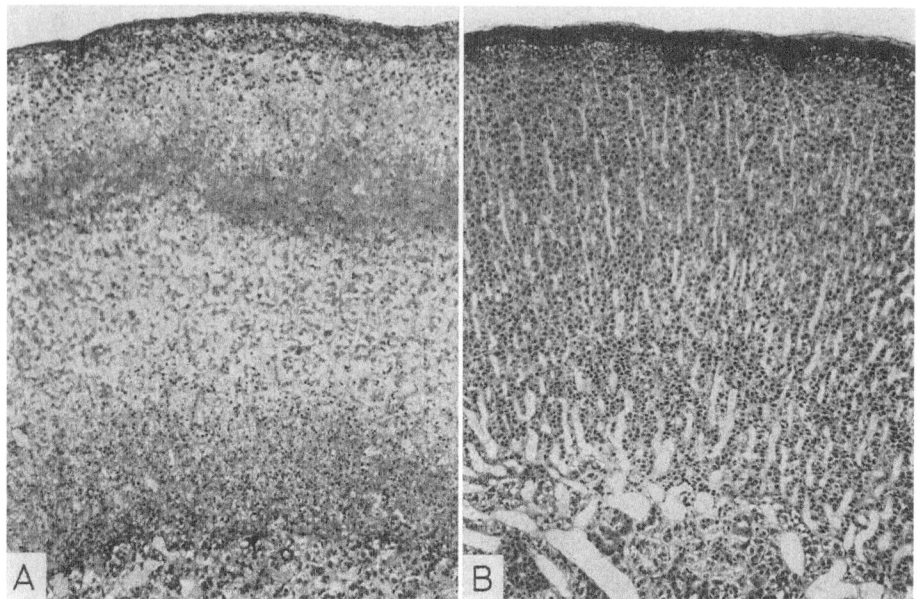

Fig. 3. **Prevention of DMBA-induced adrenal necrosis by spironolactone.** A: Massive necrosis of the zona fasciculata and reticularis of the adrenal cortex 3 days after oral administration of DMBA. B: This lesion is completely inhibited by pretreatment with spironolactone. Hematoxylin phloxine, ×120. [Somogyi and Kovacs G 60,074/70. Courtesy of Rev. canad. Biol.]

influenced also by the biotransformation of this polycyclic hydrocarbon, since both acceleration (by spironolactone) and blockade (by SKF 525-A) of this latter process can suppress the development of hematologic alterations."

Somogyi G 70,416/70: In rats, spironolactone inhibits the adrenocortical necrosis, carcinogenicity and hemopoietic-tissue-damaging action of DMBA. Ethylestrenol, CS-1, and norbolethone are also effective against the DMBA-induced adrenal necrosis. Spironolactone likewise protects against the adrenocorticolytic effect of 7-OHM-MBA. Thus, the anti-DMBA action of spironolactone does not seem to be based on the blockade of the transformation of the carcinogen into this supposedly more active metabolite. The preventive action of spironolactone is abolished by ethionine, suggesting the involvement of active protein synthesis. The DMBA-induced adrenal lesions are aggravated by estradiol, testosterone, methyltestosterone, cortisol, triamcinolone, and prednisolone, as well as by the stress of muscular work or restraint. The aggravation of adrenal necrosis by estradiol is diminished but not abolished by hypophysectomy.

Somogyi & Kovacs G 60,061/70: It had been shown previously that the adrenocortical necrosis produced in rats by DMBA, unlike that elicited by its metabolite 7-hydroxymethyl-12-methylbenz(a)anthracene (7-OHM-MBA), is inhibited by partial hepatectomy. Perhaps DMBA is active only after having been metabolized in the liver to 7-OHM-MBA whose effect is independent of hepatic function. The question arose whether spironolactone protects against the adrenolytic effect of DMBA by preventing its hydroxylation; however, spironolactone protects the adrenals against 7-OHM-MBA also.

Somogyi & Kovacs G 60,074/70: In rats, the adrenal necrosis produced by DMBA is inhibited by spironolactone and ethylestrenol; it is aggravated by estradiol, MAD, cortisol and testosterone but not significantly influenced by progesterone, norbolethone, triamcinolone or DOC.

Stripp et al. H 22,743/70: In rats, spironolactone pretreatment shortened hexobarbital sleeping time. "Moreover, treatment of female rats with spironolactone doubled the rate of the in vitro metabolism of hexobarbital and benzpyrene by liver microsomes and quadrupled that of ethylmorphine. The inducing effects of spironolactone were very different from those of phenobarbital and 3-methylcholanthrene. The amount of cytochrome P-450 was either unaltered or decreased, but the NADPH cytochrome c reductase activity was increased 2-fold. Although the endogenous rate of cytochrome P-450 reduction by NADPH was not altered, the stimulatory effects of ethylmorphine or hexobarbital on the rate of cytochrome P-450 reduction were significantly greater with microsomes from spironolactone treated animals. By contrast, treatment of male rats with spironolactone caused no change in hexobarbital sleeping time and no change or a slight decrease in hexobarbital and benzpyrene metabolism by liver microsomes."

Solymoss et al. G70,488/71: In rats, spironolactone and ethylestrenol, like phenobarbital, enhance the NADPH-dependent hydroxylation of benzo(a)pyrene in hepatic microsomal + supernatant fraction.

Somogyi & Kovacs G70,482/71: In rats, the stress of restraint or of forced muscular exercise significantly increases the adrenocorticolytic effect of DMBA. Spironolactone can abolish this stress-induced aggravation. The mammary carcinogenicity of DMBA is not influenced by stress.

DMBA ← Steroids: Dao F19,168/64*

Carcinolytic Agents ← cf. also Individual Carcinolytic Agents

Andreani et al. C14,628/55: In rats, the different organ changes produced by **TEM** are unequally influenced by combined treatment with ACTH + cortisone.

Cutts H22,100/68: In rats, diethylstilbestrol protects against lethal doses of **vinblastine**. Among otherwise untreated rats, females are more resistant to vinblastine than males.

LePage & Kaneko H22,380/69: Review and personal observations on mice showing that the toxicity of certain carcinostatic agents can be reduced by concurrent treatment with glucocorticoids without the loss of therapeutic efficacy.

Grushina et al. H31,216/70: Both in intact and in adrenalectomized rats, DOC stimulated the growth of sarcoma 45 and counteracted the carcinolytic and general toxic effects of thiophosphamide.

Mercier-Parot & Tuchmann-Duplessis G73, 572/70: In rats and mice, administration of the carcinolytic agent Natulan [chlorhydrate of 1-methyl 2p-(isopropylcarbamoyl) benzylhydrazine or RO 4-6467] causes fetal absorption and malformations. Even large doses of progesterone offer no protection against these effects.

Gillette H34,126/71: In male rats, spironolactone caused a relatively small increase in ethylmorphine N-demethylation and decreased the oxidation of hexobarbital and 3,4-benzpyrene. However (like in females), spironolactone did not affect the type I spectral changes induced in males by ethylmorphine and hexobarbital but caused a small decrease in cytochrome P-450 content and increased NADPH-cytochrome c reductase. Moreover, in males, spironolactone increased the substrate dependent cytochrome P-450 reduction but not its endogenous reduction. The sex difference in the effect of spironolactone upon hepatic microsomal drug metabolism is illustrated by the tabulation of data concerning ethylmorphine and hexobarbital biotransformation.

Carisoprodol ←

Kato et al. G66,023/61: Adult (unlike immature) male rats are less sensitive to carisoprodol-induced muscular paralysis than females. Castration or treatment with SKF 525-A abolishes the increased resistance of the adult male rat. Incubation of liver slices with carisoprodol shows that the resistance of the male is due to accelerated substrate inactivation. No sex difference is noted in adult mice or guinea pigs.

Kato et al. G64,325/62: Adult male rats are more resistant than females to pentobarbital anesthesia, carisoprodol paralysis and strychnine convulsions. Conversely, the lethal effect of OMPA is greater in the male. The sex difference is ascribed to the increased production of anabolic testoids which enhance the decomposition of these substrates, the first three of which are inactivated, the last activated in the process. The differences were also demonstrated in vitro using liver slices or microsomal fractions. The high microsomal activity of the male could be abolished by castration and restored by several anabolic testoids.

Selye G70,480/71: In rats, carisoprodol sleeping time was moderately shortened by the classic catatoxic steroids except norbolethone and oxandrolone. Prednisolone was also slightly efficacious, whereas triamcinolone was not. Progesterone and thyroxine moderately aggravated carisoprodol sleeping time, cf. Table 37.

Table 37. *Conditioning for carisoprodol*

Treatment[a]	Sleeping time[b] (min)	Mortality[b] (Dead/Total)
None	47 ± 6	2/13
PCN	18 ± 8 *	1/5 NS
CS-1	20 ± 2 ***	0/10 NS
Ethylestrenol	26 ± 5 *	3/10 NS
Spironolactone	23 ± 4 **	0/10 NS
Norbolethone	35 ± 4 NS	2/10 NS
Oxandrolone	42 ± 8 NS	1/10 NS
Prednisolone-Ac	29 ± 3 **	1/10 NS
Triamcinolone	64 ± 8 NS	3/10 NS
Progesterone	71 ± 8 *	3/10 NS
Estradiol	33 ± 5 NS	1/10 NS
DOC-Ac	56 ± 8 NS	1/10 NS
Hydroxydione	50 ± 8 NS	0/10 NS
Thyroxine	77 ± 12 *	4/5 NS
Phenobarbital	36 ± 5 NS	3/9 NS

[a] The rats of all groups were given carisoprodol (10 mg/100 g body weight in 0.1 ml DMSO, i.v., on 4th day).

[b] Mortality was listed on 5th day ("Exact Probability Test").

Sleeping time: Student's t-test.

For further details on technique of tabulation cf. p. VIII.

Carisoprodol ← Estradiol, Testosterone: Kato et al. *G 66,023/61*, G 64,325/63**

Casein ← cf. also Amyloid

Latvalahti B 88,191/53; Peräsalo & Latvalahti C 9,661/54: In mice, the amyloidosis produced by repeated s.c. injections of casein is aggravated by ACTH and cortisone but not by DOC or testosterone, although orchidectomy facilitated its development.

Kozlowski & Hrabowska H 14,243/69: Nandrolone, an anabolic steroid, enhances the development of amyloidosis in mice given casein s.c.

Cerium ←

Snyder et al. C 99,417/59: In rats, i.v. injection of cerium produced extremely high levels of liver fat in females but not in males.

After castration males reacted as strongly as females. Testosterone reduced fatty infiltration in both intact and ovariectomized females. Hypophysectomy prevented fatty liver formation in both sexes, whereas adrenalectomy did so only in males.

Selye PROT. 43437: In rats (100 g ♀), the production of hepatic steatosis and mortality by $CeCl_3$ (5 mg in 1 ml water, i.v.) are considerably inhibited by PCN, ethylestrenol and, to a somewhat lesser extent, by spironolactone (all 10 mg in 1 ml water × 2/day, p.o., beginning on the fourth day before $CeCl_3$ administration). Under similar conditions, triamcinolone (10 mg × 2/day) and thyroxine (200 μg of Na-salts, s.c., once daily) actually aggravate $CeCl_3$ intoxication. It is particularly noteworthy that, here, as in the case of cadmium and mercury intoxication, the catatoxic steroids offer protection against inorganic salts which could hardly be detoxified by the usual microsomal drug metabolizing mechanisms.

Chloral Hydrate ←

Fastier et al. C 37,038/57: In mice, chloral hydrate sleeping time is increased by epinephrine, norepinephrine, phenylephrine, methoxamine, 5-HT, histamine, ergotamine, yohimbine and atropine. "It is suggested that some, at least, of the drugs which prolong the effects of hypnotics do so by virtue of a hypothermic action." Vasopressin, cortisone and DOC did not prolong chloral hydrate sleeping time at the doses tested.

Selye et al. G 60,016/69; G 60,020/69: In the rat, pretreatment with norbolethone or spironolactone does not protect against the anesthetic effect of chloral hydrate.

Chlordecone ←

McFarland & Lacy G 68,855/69: Japanese quail fed the insecticide, chlordecone (Kepone) developed a characteristic tremor, hepatic enlargement with fatty degeneration and a strong "estrogenic" effect on the oviduct which was not prevented by ovariectomy. The oviduct enlargement was considerably diminished, however, after hypophysectomy.

Chlordiazepoxide ←

Blackham & Spencer G 73,813/70: In mice, lynestrenol reduced, whereas mestranol or SKF increased, the anticonvulsive effect (tested with electroshock) of diphenylhydantoin, phenobarbital, and chlordiazepoxide, administered i.p. after five days of pretreatment. This may be due to altered microsomal-drug metabolism but since mestranol and lynestrenol have opposite effects upon brain 5-HT concentrations, the latter mechanism must also be considered.

Selye PROT. 39493: In rats, PCN, CS-1, ethylestrenol and to a lesser extent spironolactone and norbolethone shorten chlordiazepoxide sleeping time. The other standard conditioners were without significant effect but triamcinolone even in combination with chlordiazepoxide causes considerable mortality at doses at which the latter alone is well tolerated, *cf.* Table 38.

Chlordiazepoxide ← Mestranol, Lynestrenol: Blackham et al. G73,813/70*

Chloroform ←

Eschenbrenner & Miller 94,309/45: Following administration of large amounts of chloroform p.o., "there was extensive necrosis of portions of the proximal and distal convoluted tubules in normal male and in testosterone-treated castrated male mice and no necrosis in female and in castrated male mice."

Culliford & Hewitt C28,738/57: In adult male mice of two strains, exposure to chloroform vapor produced necrosis of the renal tubules, whereas females showed no such change. Testoids rendered females fully susceptible, whereas folliculoids decreased the sensitivity of the males. Orchidectomy abolished susceptibility in one strain of mice but only diminished it in another, although the residual sensitivity could be annulled by adrenalectomy. In gonadectomized mice, methyltestosterone, testosterone propionate, dehydroepiandrosterone, progesterone and very large doses of cortisone induced susceptibility.

Hewitt C28,739/57: The high susceptibility of male mice to the induction of renal tubular necrosis by chloroform vapor is inhibited by castration and restored with as little as 10 µg of testosterone propionate. "These findings appear to provide the basis of a sensitive method for the detection and assay of androgens."

Chloropicrin ←

Henschler & Reich C71,216/59: In rats, the pulmonary edema induced by ammonium chloride, epinephrine, thiourea or chloropicrin is prevented by the administration of a single large dose of prednisolone i.v. about 5 min earlier.

Table 38. *Conditioning for chlordiazepoxide*

Treatment[a]	Sleeping time[b] (min)	Mortality[b] (Dead/Total)
None	308 ± 34	0/20
PCN	13 ± 6 ***	0/30 NS
CS-1	91 ± 22 ***	0/15 NS
Ethylestrenol	124 ± 27 ***	0/20 NS
Spironolactone	196 ± 27 *	0/20 NS
Norbolethone	169 ± 38 *	0/15 NS
Oxandrolone	228 ± 36 NS	0/15 NS
Prednisolone-Ac	247 ± 41 NS	1/15 NS
Triamcinolone	393 ± 39 NS	10/20 ***
Progesterone	313 ± 42 NS	2/15 NS
Estradiol	334 ± 35 NS	0/15 NS
DOC-Ac	290 ± 33 NS	0/15 NS
Hydroxydione	291 ± 50 NS	0/15 NS
Thyroxine	376 ± 43 NS	1/20 NS
Phenobarbital	218 ± 36 NS	0/19 NS

[a] The rats of all groups were given chlordiazepoxide, 15 mg/100 g body weight in 1 ml oil i.p. once on the 4th day.

[b] Mortality was listed on the fifth day ("Exact Probability Test").

Sleeping time: Student's t-test.

For further details on technique of tabulation *cf.* p. VIII.

Chlorpromazine ←

Weil G68,214/61: In rats, prednisolone i.p. "which protects against the lethal effects of endotoxin, is not effective in protecting against lethal amounts of ganglionic blocking agents (mecamylamine, chlorpromazine), adrenergic blocking drugs (dibenzyline), or sympathomimetic amines (metaraminol). To the contrary, treatment with corticosteroid is associated with a significant increase in fatality in animals injected with mecamylamine and chlorpromazine ($p = <0.01$)." These findings are interpreted as evidence against the assumption that glucocorticoids protect in a nonspecific manner against injuries that produce hypotension.

Fletcher et al. F44,604/65: In the rat, "chlorpromazine hypothermia is potentiated by estradiol treatment. The potentiation may be brought about by a decreased metabolism of the drug but is not reflected in the protein content of liver or liver microsomes."

Chatterjee G48,145/66: In rats, small doses of cortisone prevent the ovarian inhibition produced by chlorpromazine. "This may be explained as prevention of a competitive inhibitory phenomenon on pituitary gonadotrophin secretion produced by an excessive production of adenohypophyseal corticotrophin in chlorpromazine-treated animals."

Selye et al. G60,016/69; G60,020/69: In the rat, pretreatment with norbolethone or spironolactone does not protect against the anesthetic effect of chlorpromazine.

Chlorpromazine ← Norethynodrel, Progesterone: Juchau et al. *G40,275/66*

Chlortetracycline ←

Sparano F71,594/65: The hepatic steatosis-produced by chlortetracycline is more pronounced in orchidectomized and ovariectomized, testosterone-treated rats, than in otherwise untreated castrate females. Estradiol protects the liver of castrated males against this form of steatosis. "The results indicate that estradiol exerts a protective effect against chlortetracycline-induced lipid accumulation in the liver."

Chlorzoxazone ←

Gessner et al. F77,776/67: In mice, "testosterone pretreatment produces a biphasic effect on the duration of action of hexobarbital, prolonging the action initially and shortening the action in 4—8 days after the pretreatment. The early action of testosterone appears to be associated with an effect on the hypnotic property of a drug, since both hexobarbital and barbital sleep times are prolonged while the duration of action of the muscle relaxant chlorzoxasone remains unaffected. The long-term pretreatment with testosterone leads to a shorter duration of action of drugs that are deactivated by detoxification, notably hexobarbital and chlorzoxasone, but has no effect on the duration of hypnosis produced by barbital, a drug which is predominantly eliminated unchanged." Folliculoids (ethinylestradiol, diethylstilbestrol) prolong the actions of both drugs.

Szeberényi & Fekete H29,579/70: Brief abstract stating that after four days of pretreatment (species not mentioned), spironolactone decreased the action and accelerated the metabolism of hexobarbital, chlorzoxazone meprobamate, estrone, testosterone, acenocoumarol and BSP, whereas after short treatment it had an inverse effect. It is concluded that spironolactone is a microsomal enzyme inducer.

Chlorzoxazone ← Diethylstilbestrol, Testosterone: Gessner et al. F77,776/67*

Cholesterol ← *cf. also Selye G60,083/70, pp. 346, 348, 363, 364, 370, 371, 372, 374.*

Gualandi et al. C7,736/51: In rats, orchidectomy does not make it possible to produce atheromatosis by cholesterol feeding as earlier investigators have claimed.

Oppenheim & Bruger B74,288/52: In rabbits, cholesterol atheromatosis is diminished by cortisone and to a lesser extent by ACTH.

Adlersberg et al. B82,951/53: In rabbits on a high-cholesterol diet, cortisone and cortisol produce extreme elevations of plasma lipids.

Stamler et al. B91,353/53: In cholesterol-fed chicks, coronary atherosclerosis is prevented by estradiol even if the feminizing effects are eliminated by concurrent administration of testosterone. The protective effect of the folliculoid is not due to its effect upon blood cholesterol since hypercholesterolemia remains uninfluenced by it, but estradiol elevates the plasma phospholipid levels. In itself, neither testosterone nor chorionic gonadotrophin affect coronary atherosclerosis under these conditions.

Gordon et al. B95,119/54: In rabbits, cortisone inhibits the development of cholesterol atherosclerosis in the aorta as well as the accompanying hypercholesterolemia.

Stumpf & Wilens B95,325/54: In rabbits, cholesterol-induced atherosclerosis and hyperlipemia are inhibited by cortisone.

Oester et al. C8,951/55: In rabbits, the calcifying arteriosclerosis produced by combined treatment with thyroxine and epinephrine is not influenced by progesterone but cholesterol atherosclerosis is greatly diminished.

Wang et al. E83,672/55: In rabbits, cholesterol atherosclerosis is inhibited by cortisone despite an aggravation of the hypercholesteremia. This effect of the glucocorticoid can be prevented by hyaluronidase.

Dury C25,675/56: In rabbits with established cholesterol atherosclerosis, cortisone accelerates the regression of the lesions.

Moss & Dury C44,068/57: In rabbits, the development of cholesterol atherosclerosis is inhibited by cortisone and the regression of already established lesions accelerated. The epinephrine-induced aortic medial necrosis is not prevented by cortisone but the fibroblast reaction in the lesions is inhibited.

Constantinides et al. D21,813/62: In rabbits, the regression of cholesterol atherosclerosis following return to normal diet is accelerated both by estriol and by prednisolone.

Ferruccio F62,336/64: Testosterone in combination with vitamin E diminishes the induction of fat deposition in the liver in cholesterol–fed rabbits.

Rossi et al. F18,184/64: In rabbits, cholesterol atherosclerosis is aggravated by DOC.

Harman F59,112/65: In rabbits, cortisone, prednisone and dexamethasone inhibit cholesterol atherosclerosis, although they elevate the serum cholesterol levels. Their protective action is ascribed to their antiphlogistic activity.

Alper et al. H5,589/68: In rabbits, cholesterol atheromatosis is prevented by methylprednisolone (Medrol) despite persisting hyperlipemia. The corticoid diminished the aortic concentration of acid mucopolysaccharides (AMPS) of low sulfate content. "Since all animals fed cholesterol developed some degree of pulmonary atherosclerosis, it is postulated that the antiatherogenic action of the hormone on the aorta is more closely related to alterations in the AMPS pattern than to changes in the pattern of circulating lipids."

Bailey et al. H450/68: In rabbits, cholesterol atherosclerosis is inhibited by cortisone, prednisone, triamcinolone, methylprednisolone, dexamethasone and 9α-fluorocortisol, although hyperlipemia is aggravated. Phenylbutazone and oxyphenylbutazone also diminished cholesterol atherosclerosis, although to a lesser extent and without augmenting hyperlipemia.

Porrazzi et al. H34,157/68: In rabbits, DOC aggravates the severity of cholesterol atheromatosis, possibly through depolymerization of the ground substance.

Curreri et al. H11,525/69: In rabbits with cholesterol atherosclerosis various hydrolytic enzymes present in lysosomes (β-glucuronidase, acid phosphatase, cathepsin and aryl sulfatase) showed a marked increase in activity. Cortisone inhibited this atherosclerosis and the increased enzyme activity despite very high levels of serum cholesterol.

Hamprecht G69,560/69: Review (7 pp., 153 refs.) on the mechanisms regulating cholesterol synthesis. A special section deals with the effect of thyroid hormones, steroids, epinephrine, norepinephrine and glucagon.

Schweppe & Jungmann H15,266/69: The ability of rat liver microsomes to synthesize cholesterol palmitate, oleate and linoleate in vitro is increased by the addition of thyroxine or glucagon to the incubation medium. Testosterone increases cholesterol palmitate and oleate formation. 17β-Estradiol stimulates mainly oleate synthesis.

Schweppe & Jungmann H15,978/69: Observations on the metabolism of marked cholesterol added together with various hormones to hepatic microsomes of the rat led to the conclusion that "1) cholesterol palmitate and oleate were synthesized most rapidly; 2) at high concentrations, testosterone decreased the formation of all esters but at lower dose levels, testosterone increased the synthesis of cholesterol oleate and palmitate; 3) estradiol caused a two-fold increase in cholesterol oleate formation; 4) ACTH decreased the synthesis rate of cholesterol palmitate and oleate; 5) insulin had a significant inhibitory effect on cholesterol linoleate; 6) epinephrine had little significant effect at the dose level used; and 7) L-thyroxine increased the synthesis of all cholesterol esters."

Saini & Patrick G74,405/70: Using isolated rat liver preparations it was found that estrone stimulates the conversion of radio-active cholesterol to bile acids.

Cholesterol ← Steroids: Kritchevsky et al. *G16,024/63*

Choline Deficiency ← *cf. also* Ethionine

← **Corticoids.** *György et al. D77,819/49:* In rats kept on a hypolipotropic diet supplemented with methionine, estrone, estradiol and ethinylestradiol p.o. inhibited hepatic steatosis. Of these folliculoids, ethinylestradiol was the most effective and produced a lipotropic effect even in the absence of methionine. Progesterone, DOC and testosterone were not lipotropic under identical conditions.

Sellers et al. B52,716/50: Cortisone partially protects the rat against the renal lesions produced by hypolipotropic diets.

Katine et al. B80,347/52: In weanling male rats, the production of fatty livers by choline deficiency is prevented by cortisone.

Hurd et al. B83,869/53: In rats kept on a choline-deficient diet, the development of fatty liver is inhibited by cortisone and adrenocortical extract.

← **Testoids.** *Emerson et al. B59,636/51:* Testosterone aggravates the renal and hepatic lesions induced in rats by dietary choline deficiency. Estradiol protects against hepatic cirrhosis in male rats, and against fatty liver formation in both sexes.

Wilgram & Hartroft C14,392/55: Female rats are much more resistant than males to the production of cardiovascular lesions by choline deficiency. However, simultaneous administration of "androgens" (kind not specified) and STH sensitizes the female to the induction of these lesions by hypolipotropic rations.

Wilgram et al. C15,960/56: Both STH and testosterone aggravate the renal and cardiovascular lesions characteristic of choline deficiency in the rat.

Girolami C55,043/58: Testosterone propionate protects the rat against fatty degeneration and cirrhosis of the liver produced either by CCl_4 or by a choline deficient diet.

Bengmark et al. F67,484/66: In rats with liver cirrhosis induced by choline deficiency "histological examination, determinations of liver nitrogen, nucleic acid and hydroxyproline concentration, liver transaminase activity, liver capacity to synthesize tauro- and glycocholic acid in vitro as well as determinations of the serum protein fractions did not reveal any definitely beneficial effects which could be ascribed to the testosterone treatment."

Wilson et al. G79,508/70: In mice, on hypolipotropic diets, the development of atrial thrombosis was independent of sex and not markedly influenced by gonadectomy. The same was true of castrated males given testosterone. Only gonadectomized females on estrone showed an unusually low incidence of thromboses.

← **Folliculoids** *cf. also Selye G60,083/70, p. 369; György et al. A47,909/47:* In rats kept on a hypolipotropic diet, estrone p.o. inhibits hepatic steatosis and greatly increases the lipotropic effect of methionine.

Ferret E50,456/50: Ovariectomized rats were kept either on a hypolipotropic cholinedeficient diet which causes hepatic steatosis or on a complex ration (deficient in sulfur and vitamin E, yeast being the only source of protein) which causes hepatic necrosis. If such animals received estradiol implants into the spleen, vaginal estrus occurred, whereas in animals kept on a normal diet such implants failed to cause estrus because of the inactivation of folliculoids by the liver. Additional supplements of choline to the first or cystine to the second hepatotoxic diet restores the power to inactivate the folliculoid.

Shipley et al. B50,163/50: In ovariectomized rats maintained on a hypolipotropic diet supplemented with methionine, estrone pellets protected against the development of hepatic steatosis if implanted s.c. but not if placed in the spleen.

Emerson et al. B59,636/51: Testosterone aggravates the renal and hepatic lesions induced in rats by dietary choline deficiency. Estradiol protects against hepatic cirrhosis in male rats, and against fatty liver formation in both sexes.

Kotin et al. C16,597/56: Brief note on the inhibiting effect of folliculoids upon the development of hepatic cirrhosis and hepatocellular carcinoma in rats kept on a choline-deficient diet.

Wilson et al. G79,508/70: In mice, on hypolipotropic diets, the development of atrial thrombosis was independent of sex and not markedly influenced by gonadectomy. The same was true of castrated males given testosterone. Only gonadectomized females on estrone showed an unusually low incidence of thromboses.

← **Gonadectomy.** *Plagge et al. C50,216/58:* In ovariectomized weanling rats, estradiol (but not estrone) pellets implanted into the spleen inhibited the fatty metamorphosis resulting from high-fat, low-choline diets.

Sidransky et al. G48,110/67: In rats, mature, intact or ovariectomized females, unlike intact males, develop fatty infiltration of the liver when first fed a choline containing methionine-deficient diet for three days. Castrated males are as susceptible as females and testosterone raises the resistance in females as well as in castrated males. Presumably, testosterone is responsible for the natural resistance of male rats to this type of hepatic steatosis. Earlier literature on sex differences in susceptibility to fatty liver formation is reviewed.

Wilson et al. G79,508/70: In mice, on hypolipotropic diets, the development of atrial thrombosis was independent of sex and not markedly influenced by gonadectomy. The same was true of castrated males given testosterone. Only gonadectomized females on estrone showed an unusually low incidence of thromboses.

Cinchophen ←

Nasio 97,932/46: Estriol and stilbestrol offer partial protection against cinchopheninduced peptic ulcers in the dog.

Nasio B34,100/46: In intact and gonadectomized dogs of both sexes the production of gastric ulcers by cinchophen is inhibited by stilbestrol.

Nasio B77,063/46: Monograph (151 pp., numerous refs.) on various factors influencing the development of cinchophen-induced peptic ulcers in the dog. Special emphasis is laid upon personal observations showing that various folliculoids inhibit these lesions.

Rodriguez-Olleros & Galindo C17,868/56, C38,499/57: Neither ACTH nor cortisone modified the production of gastric ulcers by cinchophen in the dog.

Selye G70,480/71: In rats, cinchophen intoxication appears to have been inhibited by all classic catatoxic steroids and phenobarbital, although the diminution of toxic manifestations by CS-1 and oxandrolone was not statistically significant, *cf.* Table 39.

Table 39. *Conditioning for cinchophen*

Treatment[a]	Dyskinesia[b] (Positive/ Total)	Mortality[b] (Dead/ Total)
None	9/13	1/13
PCN	0/10 ***	0/10 NS
CS-1	3/10 NS	0/10 NS
Ethylestrenol	1/10 **	0/10 NS
Spironolactone	0/9 ***	0/9 NS
Norbolethone	1/10 **	0/10 NS
Oxandrolone	3/10 NS	0/10 NS
Prednisolone-Ac	0/10 ***	0/10 NS
Triamcinolone(2mg)	6/10 NS	0/10 NS
Progesterone	5/10 NS	0/10 NS
Estradiol(1mg)	6/10 NS	0/10 NS
Estradiol(1 mg s.c.)	8/10 NS	1/10 NS
DOC-Ac	7/10 NS	0/10 NS
Hydroxydione	10/10 NS	0/10 NS
Thyroxine	9/10 NS	2/10 NS
Phenobarbital	0/10 ***	0/10 NS

[a] The rats of all groups were given cinchophen (35 mg/100 g body weight in 0.2 ml DMSO, s.c., on 4th day).

[b] The characteristic dyskinesia was measured ("Flick-Test") 4 hrs after injection and mortality listed on 5th day ("Exact Probability Test").

For further details on technique of tabulation *cf.* p. VIII.

Groza et al. H6,695/68: In the dog, gastric ulcer formation and liver damage induced by cinchophen is partially inhibited by aldosterone.

Hámori et al. G65,054/68: In the dog, prednisolone greatly aggravates the production of gastric ulcers by cinchophen. [Since prednisolone has some ulcerogenic effects even when given by itself, the synergism with cinchophen probably occurs within the gastric mucosa. In any event, an action through the hepatic microsomal enzyme system has not been considered (H.S.).]

Hamori et al. G72,363/69: In dogs, the production of gastric duodenal ulcers by cinchophen is inhibited by DOC and aggravated by cortisone.

Cocaine ←

Aird B683/44: DOC i.p. protected mice against cocaine-induced convulsions, but had no effect upon the electroshock seizure threshold of cats.

Guerrero et al. F70,995/65: Resistance to cocaine is significantly lower in male than in female rats, but no such sex difference is observed in castrates. Testosterone diminished the cocaine-resistance of castrates in either sex, whereas estradiol did not influence it. At the time of death, the plasma cocaine concentration was the same in both sexes, and hence it was concluded that testosterone interferes with the enzymic inactivation of cocaine.

Selye G70,471/71: In rats, cocaine intoxication was inhibited by all classic catatoxic steroids, prednisolone, estradiol and phenobarbital, *cf.* Table 40.

Table 40. *Conditioning for cocaine*

Treatment[a]	Dyskinesia[b] (Positive/ Total)	Mortality[b] (Dead/ Total)
None	25/25	24/25
PCN	2/20 ***	2/20 ***
CS-1	8/15 ***	3/15 ***
Ethylestrenol	4/20 ***	2/20 ***
Spironolactone	9/20 ***	2/20 ***
Norbolethone	9/15 **	2/15 ***
Oxandrolone	11/15 *	5/15 ***
Prednisolone-Ac	9/15 ***	7/15 ***
Triamcinolone	20/20 NS	18/20 NS
Progesterone	15/15 NS	3/15 ***
Estradiol	9/15 ***	5/15 ***
DOC-Ac	15/15 NS	11/15 NS
Hydroxydione	14/15 NS	8/15 **
Thyroxine	20/20 NS	20/20 NS
Phenobarbital	0/10 ***	0/10 ***

[a] The rats of all groups were given cocaine HCl (6 mg/100 g body weight in 1 ml water, i.p., on 4th day).

[b] Dyskinesia was measured 30 min after injection and mortality listed on 5th day ("Exact Probability Test").

For further details on technique of tabulation *cf.* p. VIII.

Cocaine ← DOC, Mouse: Aird B683/44*

Codeine ←

Selye et al. G60,016/69: In rats, spironolactone protects against anesthesia produced by progesterone, DOC, hydroxydione, pregnanedione, dehydroepiandrosterone, testosterone, diethylstilbestrol, methyprylon, pentobarbital and ethanol. It does not significantly alter the corresponding actions of morphine, codeine, urethan, diazepam, chlorpromazine, reserpine, phenoxybenzamine, chloral hydrate, potassium bromide or $MgCl_2$.

Codeine ← Progesterone: Juchau et al. G40,275/66

Colchicine ←

Clark & Barnes A33,441/40: Adrenocortical extract increases the resistance of intact rats to colchicine.

Lettré et al. B63,159/51: In tumor-bearing mice colchicine-induced mortality is aggravated both by cortisone and by DOC.

Table 41. *Conditioning for colchicine*

Treatment[a]	Dyskinesia[b] (Positive/Total)	Mortality[b] (Dead/Total)
None	19/20	13/20
PCN	0/10 ***	0/10 ***
CS-1	3/20 ***	1/20 ***
Ethylestrenol	5/14 ***	5/14 NS
Spironolactone	2/15 ***	0/15 ***
Norbolethone	16/20 NS	10/20 NS
Oxandrolone	10/20 ***	6/20 *
Prednisolone-Ac	11/13 NS	11/13 NS
Triamcinolone (2mg)	16/20 NS	17/20 NS
Progesterone	11/20 *	9/20 NS
Estradiol (1mg)	16/20 NS	16/20 NS
Estradiol (1mg s.c.)	20/20 NS	19/20 ±
DOC-Ac	12/19 *	8/19 NS
Hydroxydione	16/20 NS	8/20 NS
Thyroxine	18/19 NS	18/19 NS
Phenobarbital	5/10 **	1/10 **

[a] The rats of all groups were given colchicine (0.2 mg/100 g body weight in 0.2 ml water, s.c., on 4th day).

[b] Dyskinesia and mortality were listed on 7th day ("Exact Probability Test").

For further details on technique of tabulation cf. p. VIII.

Selye G60,098/70: In rats, fatal colchicine poisoning was inhibited by all catatoxic steroids except norbolethone and, to a lesser extent, also by progesterone and phenobarbital, cf. Table 41.

DL-Coniine ←

Selye G70,480/71: In rats, DL-coniine intoxication is strongly inhibited by PCN, prednisolone, triamcinolone and estradiol. The other conditioners are virtually ineffective in this respect, cf. Table 42.

Table 42. *Conditioning for DL-coniine*

Treatment[a]	Dyskinesia[b] (Positive/Total)	Mortality[b] (Dead/Total)
None	12/15	7/15
PCN	2/10 ***	0/10 *
CS-1	8/10 NS	7/10 NS
Ethylestrenol	5/10 NS	5/10 NS
Spironolactone	9/10 NS	7/10 NS
Norbolethone	4/10 NS	3/10 NS
Oxandrolone	9/10 NS	8/10 NS
Prednisolone-Ac	1/10 ***	1/10 NS
Triamcinolone	0/10 ***	0/10 *
Progesterone	10/10 NS	5/10 NS
Estradiol	0/10 ***	0/10 *
DOC-Ac	9/10 NS	9/10 ±
Hydroxydione	10/10 NS	8/10 NS
Thyroxine	7/10 NS	5/10 NS
Phenobarbital	7/10 NS	5/10 NS

[a] The rats of all groups were given DL-coniine HCl (5 mg/100 g body weight in 0.2 ml water, s.c., on 4th day).

[b] Dyskinesia was estimated 2 hrs after injection and mortality listed 24 hrs later ("Exact Probability Test").

For further details on technique of tabulation cf. p. VIII.

Copper ← cf. also Selye G60,083/70, p. 369.

Gregoriadis & Sourkes G72,808/70: Review and personal observations on the effect of adrenalectomy, DOC, COL and corticosterone upon copper metabolism.

Croton Oil ←

Selye G70,480/71: In rats, the inflammatory response, as judged by exudate formation in granuloma pouches, was markedly inhibited only by the two glucocorticoids among our conditioning agents, but PCN also appeared to cause a barely significant inhibition, cf. Table 43.

Table 43. *Conditioning for croton oil*

Treatment[a]	Accumulated Exudate (ml)[b]
None	4.6 ± 1.2
PCN	1.1 ± 0.5 *
CS-1	7.5 ± 1.5 NS
Ethylestrenol	5.2 ± 0.9 NS
Spironolactone	3.3 ± 0.7 NS
Norbolethone	7.4 ± 1.7 NS
Oxandrolone	6.9 ± 1.4 NS
Prednisolone-Ac	0.3 ± 0.1 **
Triamcinolone (2 mg)	0.2 ± 0.1 **
Progesterone	3.0 ± 0.5 NS
Estradiol (1 mg)	3.0 ± 0.5 NS
Estradiol (1 mg s.c.)	3.7 ± 0.5 NS
DOC-Ac	6.3 ± 1.9 NS
Hydroxydione	8.1 ± 1.1 NS
Cholesterol	5.0 ± 1.9 NS
Thyroxine	6.2 ± 0.8 NS
Phenobarbital	4.1 ± 1.0 NS

[a] The rats of all groups were given croton oil [1 ml/100 g body weight of a 1% solution in corn oil injected into the lumen of a 25 ml air pouch under the shaved dorsal skin (granuloma pouch technique) on 4th day].

[b] The accumulated exudate was measured on 11th day (Student's t-test).

For further details on technique of tabulation cf. p. VIII.

Curare ←

Störtebecker 69,765/37: In the mouse, the resistance to curare, KCN or ethanol is particularly high during estrus and decreased by ovariectomy. Castrates treated with estrone show increased tolerance to these drugs.

Störtebecker 76,398/39: Ovariectomized mice are unusually sensitive to curare, but their resistance is restored by estrone.

Curare ← Ovariectomy, Mouse: Störtebecker 76,398/39*

Cyanides ←

Gellhorn 16,839/23: In mice, resistance against acetonitrile can be increased not only by thyroid extract but, to a lesser extent, by extracts of various other tissues, which augment resistance to KCN. Thyroidectomy and orchidectomy have an opposite effect.

Störtebecker 69,765/37: In the mouse, the resistance to curare, KCN or ethanol is particularly high during estrus and decreased by ovariectomy. Castrates treated with estrone show increased tolerance to these drugs.

Störtebecker 76,398/39: Ovariectomized mice are unusually sensitive to KCN intoxication, but their resistance is restored by estrone.

Verne et al. B99,912/54: In rats, the toxicity of KCN is diminished following pretreatment by cortisone.

KCN ← Ovariectomy, Mouse: Störtebecker 76,398/39*

Cycloheximide ←

Greig & Gibbons C94,626/59: Both cortisol and adrenal cortical extract protect the rat against fatal intoxication with cycloheximide. DOC is ineffective.

Fiala & Fiala F70,819/65: Cycloheximide produces rapid loss of liver glycogen and adrenal ascorbic acid, with an increase in adrenal weight and glucocorticoid secretion (as manifested by thymic atrophy). "All these changes" [including thymus atrophy? (H.S.)] can be prevented by the concurrent administration of cortisol. It is concluded "that increased adrenal function protects against actidione poisoning in rats."

Selye G70,403/70; G70,480/71: In rats, chronic cycloheximide intoxication can be prevented or at least diminished by all classic catatoxic steroids, as well as by progesterone and phenobarbital. Glucocorticoids and folliculoids exhibit no protective action and the apparent protection offered by hydroxydione and, to a lesser extent, even by DOC and cholesterol requires further study, cf. Table 44.

Selye G70,480/71: In rats, acute cycloheximide intoxication was prevented by all classic catatoxic steroids, as well as by prednisolone, progesterone and phenobarbital, cf. Table 45.

Cyclophosphamide ←

Deppe & Lutzmann G14,653/64: In the rat, Dianabol (Δ^1-17α-methyltestosterone) counteracts the toxicity of cyclophosphamide (a cytostatic agent) as well as the inhibitory effect of the latter upon antibody formation.

Table 44. *Conditioning for cycloheximide (low dosage)*

Treatment[a]	Mortality[b] (Dead/Total)
None	10/10
PCN	0/10 ***
CS-1	0/10 ***
Ethylestrenol	8/10 ***
Spironolactone	0/10 ***
Norbolethone	3/10 ***
Oxandrolone	1/10 ***
Prednisolone-Ac	10/10 NS
Triamcinolone (2 mg)	10/10 NS
Progesterone	2/9 ***
Estradiol	7/10 NS
Estradiol (1 mg)	5/5 NS
Estradiol (1 mg s.c.)	5/5 NS
DOC-Ac	5/10 *
Hydroxydione	6/10 *
Cholesterol	6/10 *
Thyroxine	10/10 NS
Phenobarbital	1/9 ***

[a] The rats of all groups were given cycloheximide (100 µg/100 g body weight in 0.2 ml physiologic NaCl solution, s.c., twice daily from 4th to 6th day).

[b] Mortality was listed on 8th day ("Exact Probability Test").

For further details on technique of tabulation cf. p. VIII.

Table 45. *Conditioning for cycloheximide (high dosage)*

Treatment[a]	Dyskinesia[b] (Positive/Total)	Mortality[b] (Dead/Total)
None	8/10	7/10
PCN	0/10 ***	0/10 ***
CS-1	0/10 ***	0/10 ***
Ethylestrenol	0/10 ***	0/10 ***
Spironolactone	0/10 ***	0/10 ***
Norbolethone	3/10 *	1/10 **
Oxandrolone	0/10 ***	2/10 *
Prednisolone-Ac	2/10 *	1/10 **
Triamcinolone (2 mg)	9/10 NS	9/10 NS
Progesterone	0/10 ***	2/10 *
Estradiol (1 mg)	10/10 NS	10/10 NS
Estradiol (1 mg s.c.)	10/10 NS	9/10 NS
DOC-Ac	2/10 *	3/10 NS
Hydroxydione	6/10 NS	5/10 NS
Thyroxine	9/10 NS	10/10 NS
Phenobarbital	0/9 ***	0/9 ***

[a] The rats of all groups were given cycloheximide (800 µg/100 g body weight in 1 ml water, p.o., on 4th day).

[b] Dyskinesia was estimated 24 hrs after injection and mortality listed on 5th day ("Exact Probability Test").

For further details on technique of tabulation cf. p. VIII.

Fleischer & Riedel G20,778/64: The toxic effect of cyclophosphamide upon hematopoietic organs and the adrenals of the rabbit is aggravated by pretreatment with prednisolone.

Lutzmann & Schmidt F57,784/65: In rats, Δ'-17α-methyltestosterone failed to prevent the antimitotic effect of cyclophosphamide or mitomycin upon Jensen sarcomas.

Hayakawa et al. G64,146/69: Cyclophosphamide is a latent alkylating agent which is almost inactive in vitro but is activated by the liver of the rat in vivo. Addition of prednisolone to liver slices inhibits cyclophosphamide activation. A similar inhibition of cyclophosphamide activation by prednisolone can be obtained in vivo as judged by the blood level of its metabolites. It is assumed that prednisolone hydroxylation and cyclophosphamide activation compete for the $NADPH_2$-dependent drug-metabolizing enzyme system.

Selye G70,466/70: In rats, cyclophosphamide intoxication (including the characteristic changes in the hemopoietic tissue and the body weight loss) was inhibited by all catatoxic steroids, except oxandrolone. Progesterone diminished mortality without affecting the weight loss, whereas the glucocorticoids, estradiol and thyroxine, aggravated the weight loss, but failed to influence mortality, cf. Table 46.

Cyclopropane ←

Chase & Saidman H35,774/71: In rats, pretreatment with spironolactone shortens the anesthetic effect of DOC but does not alter the minimum alveolar concentration of cyclopropane required to prevent movement in response to a painful stimulus. "It is suggested that central nervous system responsiveness is unaltered by spironolactone and that the reduction in potency of systemically administered sedatives in rats following spironolactone pretreatment may be a reflection of induction of drug metabolizing enzymes."

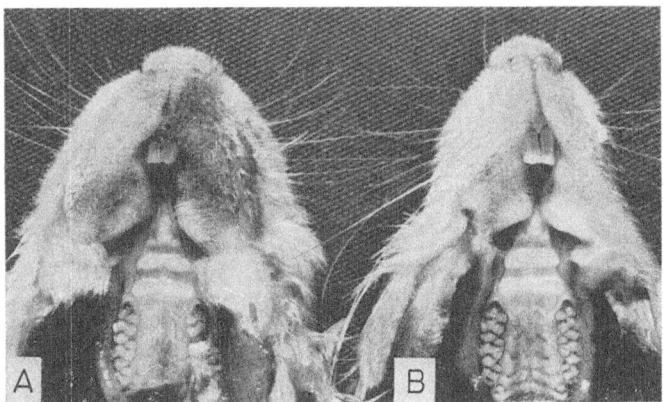

Fig. 4 (A + B). **Protection by catatoxic steroids against cyclophosphamide.** All animals received the same cyclophosphamide treatment. A: Ethylestrenol fails to prevent the characteristic swelling, hemorrhage and necrosis of the lips. B: PCN offers complete protection.

Table 46. *Conditioning for cyclophosphamide*

Treatment[a]	Final body weight[b] (g)	Mortality[c] (Dead/ Total)
None	101 ± 2	10/10
PCN	140 ± 4 ***	0/10 ***
CS-1	134 ± 3 ***	0/10 ***
Ethylestrenol	113 ± 2 **	9/10 NS
Spironolactone	123 ± 4 ***	0/10 ***
Norbolethone	117 ± 2 ***	9/10 NS
Oxandrolone	99 ± 3 NS	10/10 NS
Prednisolone-Ac	74 ± 1 ***	10/10 NS
Triamcinolone	62 ± 2 ***	10/10 NS
Progesterone	103 ± 2 NS	3/10 ***
Estradiol	80 ± 3 ***	10/10 NS
DOC-Ac	95 ± 3 NS	10/10 NS
Hydroxydione	95 ± 2 NS	10/10 NS
Thyroxine	91 ± 3 *	10/10 NS
Phenobarbital	107 ± 4 NS	9/10 NS

[a] The rats of all groups were given cyclophosphamide (10 mg/100 g body weight in 0.4 ml water, s.c., daily from 4th day ff.).

[b] Student's t-test.

[c] Mortality listed on 15th day ("Exact Probability Test").

For further details on technique of tabulation *cf.* p. VIII.

DDD ←

Brown et al. C 37,523/57: The adrenal damage produced by DDD in the dog is not prevented by cortisone.

Cueto Jr. G 72,544/70: In dogs, o,p'DDD produces a selective glucocorticoid deficiency due to its damaging effect upon the fasciculata and reticularis of the adrenal. Epinephrine and norepinephrine produce hypotensive failure in DDD-treated dogs presumably as the consequence of their stressor action. Prednisolone largely restores the resistance of the DDD-treated animals.

Dexamphetamine ←

Blackham & Spencer G 76,301/69: In female mice, pretreatment with lynestrenol (a luteoid) reduced the hyperthermia induced by dexamphetamine, whereas mestranol (a folliculoid) increased it. Fencamfamine (also a CNS-stimulant) failed to induce hyperthermia in control or lynestrenol pretreated mice but did raise the temperature after mestranol pretreatment. The potentiating effect of mestranol could be mimicked by pretreatment with nialamide (a MAO-inhibitor) but not by SKF 525-A. Increased locomotor activity induced by dexamphetamine and fencamfamine was enhanced by mestranol and reduced by lynestrenol. Dopamine, norepinephrine and 5-HT levels in the brain were reduced by lynestrenol and 5-HT was increased by mestranol. "If the actions of dexamphetamine (and fencamfamin) are due predominantly to the release of endogenous amines, then an increase (with lynestrenol) or a decrease (with mestranol) of tissue MAO activity should change the potency of these two stimulant drugs."

Dextroamphetamine ← Mestranol, Lynestrenol + Crowding, Mouse: Blackham et al. G 76,301/69*

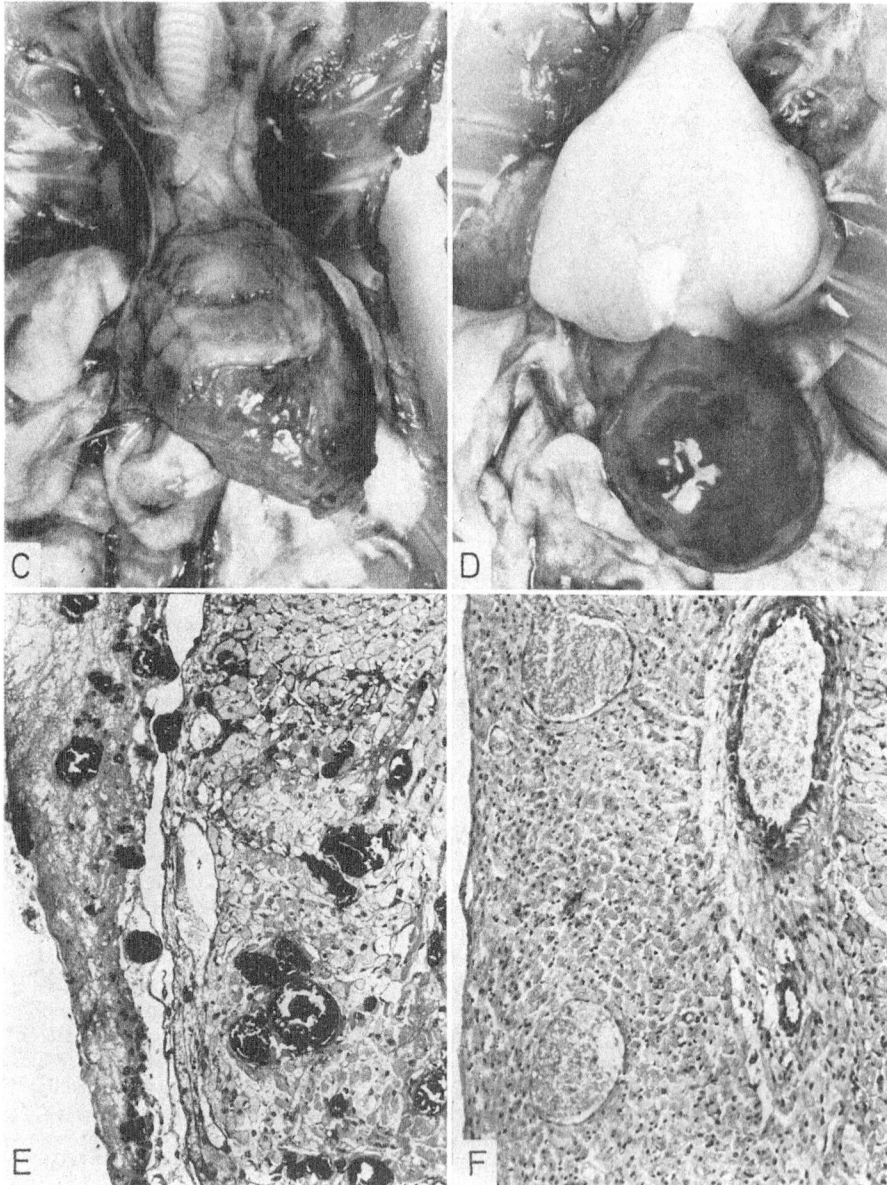

Fig. 4 (C—F). C: Ethylestrenol fails to prevent the development of necrotizing myocarditis (light areas near the base of the heart) and fibrinous pericarditis characteristic of cyclophosphamide intoxication. The virtually complete atrophy of the thymus reflects the intense stress reaction which was associated with pronounced adrenocortical enlargement. The thymic lymph nodes (as those in other parts of the body) are hemorrhagic. D: Complete prevention of cardiac lesions by PCN. The thymus is normally developed. E: Numerous microbial colonies in myocardium and in the fibrinous pericardial covering. Complete absence of leukocytes, presumably secondary to cyclophosphamide-induced destruction of hemopoietic tissues. Multiple myocardial necroses.
F: PCN prevents all these lesions. PAS×60.

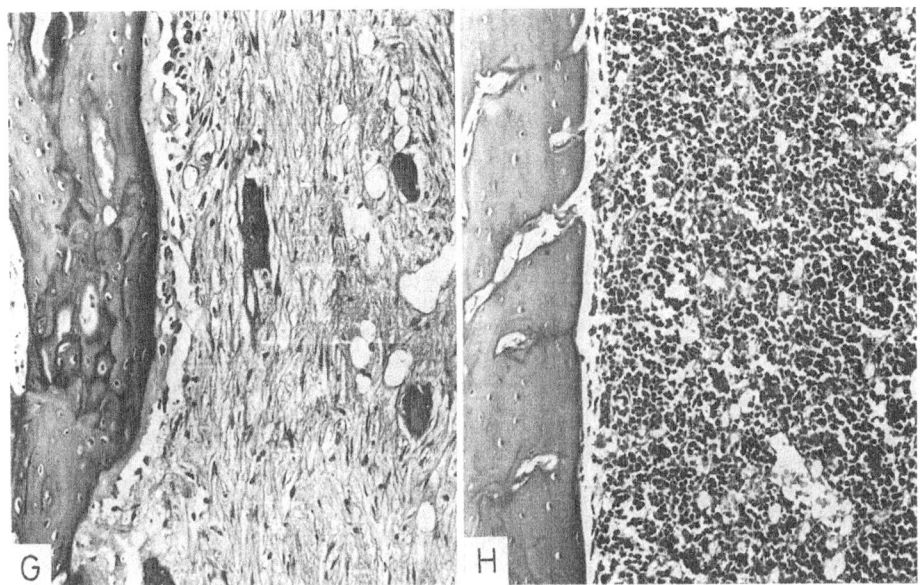

Fig. 4 (G + H). G: In rat given cyclophosphamide alone, the bone marrow consists virtually only of gelatinous connective tissue. H: CS-1 offers virtually complete protection to the bone marrow. PAS×60

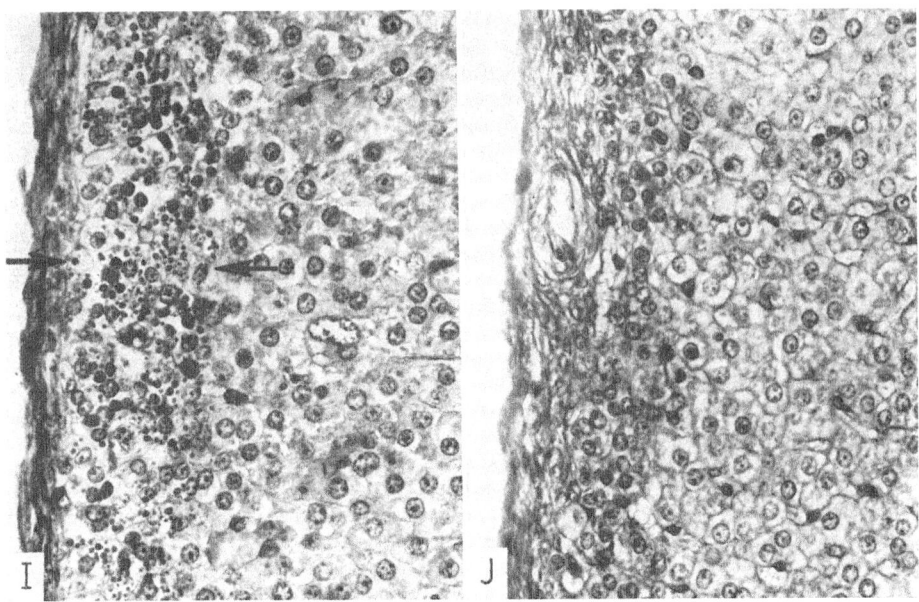

Fig. 4 (I + J). I: Cyclophosphamide causes enlargement of the glomerulosa (between arrows) which is heavily laden with PAS positive granules. J: PCN prevents this change. PAS×170. [Selye G 70,466/70. Courtesy of Virchows Arch. Abt. A pathol. Anat.]

DHT ← *cf. Vitamin D*

Diazepam ← *cf. Chlordiazepoxide*

Diethylnitrosamine ←

Boquoi & Kreuzer F82,383/65: In the rat, the hepatic cirrhosis produced by diethylnitrosamine was not significantly influenced by progesterone. Estradiol aggravated the liver lesions and accelerated mortality before hepatomas could develop.

Digitalis ← *cf. also Selye G60,083/70, pp. 369, 381, 385, 491, 492, 494.*

RAT

Kupperman & de Graff B47,267/50: In rats, the ECG disturbances caused by ouabain or digitoxin i.v. are aggravated by adrenalectomy, and diminished by DOC.

Holck & Kimura D99,625/51: One month old rats of both sexes are equally sensitive to ouabain. Adult female rats are more resistant to ouabain than males but the difference does not become evident before 2—4 months of age. Rats rapidly become resistant to ouabain, and upon repeated injections, the sex difference tends to disappear. Castration does not alter the sex difference in ouabain resistance significantly in either sex. "However, in case of pentobarbitalized rats the usual higher female resistance was plainly seen and spaying definitely decreased the number of injections required to cause death."

Schatzmann C73,682/59: "Corticosterone was shown to have an inhibitory effect on the contraction caused by a cardiac glycoside (g-Strophanthin = Ouabain) in isolated strips of rat aorta. It could be demonstrated that over a tenfold concentration range of Ouabain, the kinetics of this antagonism are in accord with the assumption of a competitive inhibition."

Sulser et al. D96,543/59: In adrenalectomized rats, K-strophanthin increases Na and K excretion and this effect is prevented by DOC. In intact rats, K-strophanthin causes Na retention; yet, K excretion is augmented as it is after adrenalectomy.

Bouyard & Klein D69,070/63: Betamethasone aggravates the neuromotor disturbances produced in the rat by strophanthin-G.

Savoie et al. G60,080/69: In rats, the infarctoid cardiopathy produced by digitoxin + Na_2HPO_4 + corn oil is prevented by spironolactone. This protection is ascribed in part to the potassium-sparing and in part to the catatoxic action of the steroid.

Selye et al. G46,800/69; Savoie et al. G60,028/69: Spironolactone protects the rat against the myocardial necroses produced by digitoxin + Na_2HPO_4 + corn oil. The associated neuromuscular disturbances are also prevented. Neither amiloride nor KCl prevent the convulsions; hence, presumably, spironolactone does not act through K-retention.

Selye G60,003/69: In rats, spironolactone prevents acute digitoxin poisoning even after bilateral nephrectomy.

Selye et al. G60,042/69: In the rat, both spironolactone and norbolethone inhibit the toxic effects of digitoxin, gitalin, proscillaridin, digoxin and digitalin. The corresponding effects of strophanthin K, ouabain and digitoxigenin were not prevented.

Selye et al. G60,050/70: Spironolactone, spiroxasone, SC-5233, SC-8109, CS-1, aldadiene and aldadiene-kalium (SC-14266), like norbolethone, protect the rat against convulsions induced by digitoxin.

Selye G70,421/70; G70,480/71: In rats, fatal digitoxin convulsions are readily prevented by all classic catatoxic steroids and, to a lesser extent, also by prednisolone, progesterone and hydroxydione. All other standard conditioning agents of our series, including phenobarbital, proved to be completely ineffective in combating digitoxin poisoning *cf.* Table 47, p. 230.

Selye G60,064/70: In rats, the mortality associated with the cardiac necroses produced by digitoxin + Na_2HPO_4 + corn oil was excellently prevented by all classic catatoxic steroids as well as by progesterone and, to a much lesser extent, by phenobarbital. The prevention of the macroscopically visible cardiac necroses themselves followed a similar pattern but was much less constant *cf.* Table 48, p. 230.

Selye G70,428/70: In rats, ethylestrenol powerfully inhibits the toxicity of digitoxin, nicotine, indomethacin, phenindione, dioxathion, EPN, physostigmine, hexobarbital, cyclopental, thiopental, DOC (anesthesia), meprobamate and picrotoxin. Thyroxine increases the toxicity of many among these drugs and inhibits the protective effect of ethylestrenol.

Solymoss et al. G70,441/70: In rats, spironolactone or oxandrolone given for as long as two months, continues to exhibit a protective effect against fatal doses of digitoxin or indomethacin. Upon withdrawal of the catatoxic steroids, continued administration of digitoxin

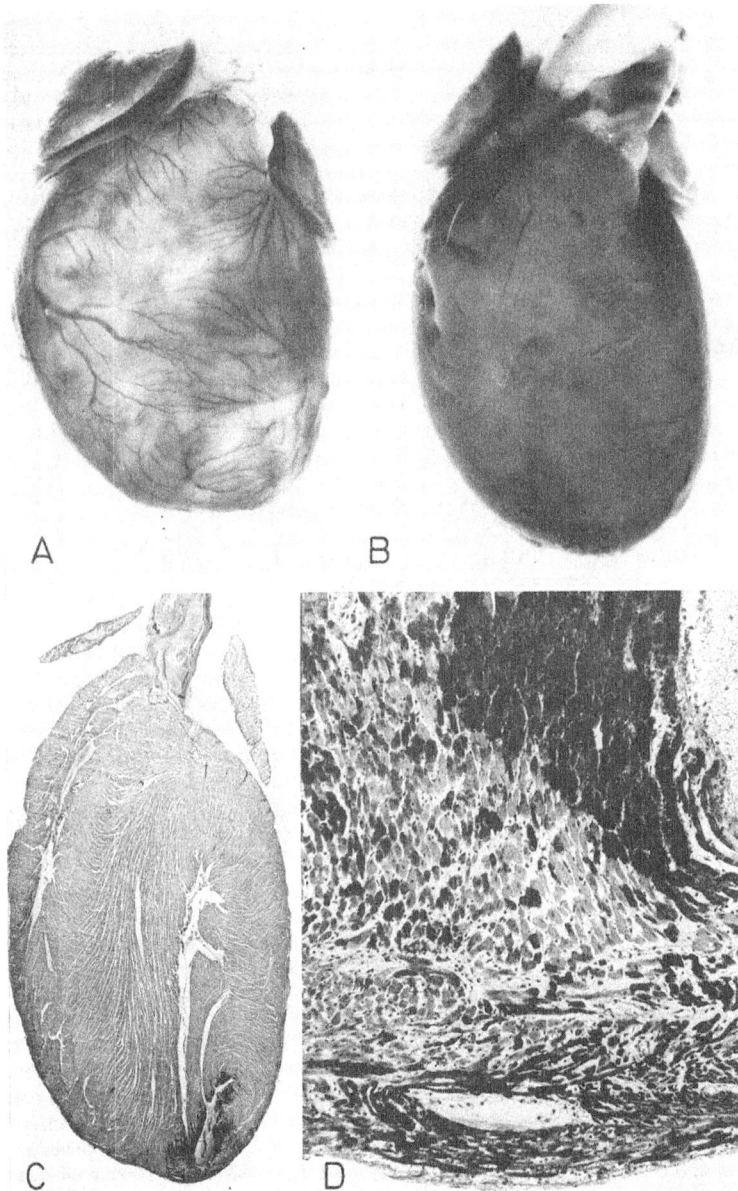

Fig. 5. **Prevention by CS-1 of the cardiopathy produced by digitoxin + Na$_2$HPO$_4$ + corn oil.** All rats received the same treatment with digitoxin + Na$_2$HPO$_4$ + corn oil p.o. A: Macroscopic appearance of the extensive myocardial necroses (light areas) in a control rat. B: Similarly-treated rat in which the cardiac lesions were completely prevented by CS-1. C: Cross-section through the ventricles of the heart showing the mildest degree of the digitoxin cardiopathy, in this case limited to the apical region (von Kóssa × 6.5). D: Severe digitalis lesions in the apex of another myocardium under higher magnification (von Kóssa × 170). [Selye G 60,064/70. Courtesy of J. molec. cell. Cardiol.]

Table 47. *Conditioning for digitoxin*

Treatment[a]	Convulsions[b] (Positive/Total)	Mortality[b] (Dead/Total)
None	9/10	10/10
PCN[c]	0/10 ***	0/10 ***
CS-1	0/10 ***	0/10 ***
Ethylestrenol	0/10 ***	0/10 ***
Spironolactone	0/10 ***	0/10 ***
Norbolethone	1/15 ***	0/15 ***
Oxandrolone	0/10 ***	0/10 ***
Prednisolone-Ac	0/10 ***	5/10 *
Triamcinolone (2 mg)	6/10 NS	9/10 NS
Progesterone	4/10 *	4/10 **
Estradiol	10/10 NS	10/10 NS
Estradiol (1 mg)	10/10 NS	10/10 NS
Estradiol (1 mg s.c.)	10/10 NS	10/10 NS
DOC-Ac	5/8 NS	5/8 NS
Hydroxydione	2/10 ***	3/10 ***
Thyroxine	10/10 NS	10/10 NS
Phenobarbital[c]	10/10 NS	9/10 NS

[a] The rats of all groups were given digitoxin (1 mg/100 g body weight in 1 ml water p.o., daily on 5th day ff.).

[b] The convulsions were estimated on 7th day and mortality listed on 10th day ("Exact Probability Test").

[c] The groups pretreated with PCN and phenobarbital (from 1st day until 5th day a.m.) received digitoxin (2 mg in 1 ml water p.o., on 4th and 5th day).

For additional pertinent data cf. also Table 135.

For further details on technique of tabulation cf. p. VIII.

Table 48. *Conditioning for digitoxin + Na_2HPO_4 + corn oil*

Treatment[a]	Cardiac Necrosis[b] (Positive/Total)	Mortality[b] (Dead/Total)
None	6/10	10/10
PCN	2/10 NS	0/10 ***
CS-1	0/10 **	0/10 ***
Ethylestrenol	1/10 *	0/10 ***
Spironolactone	1/10 *	0/10 ***
Norbolethone	0/10 **	0/10 ***
Oxandrolone	2/9 NS	1/10 ***
Prednisolone-Ac	4/10 NS	10/10 NS
Triamcinolone	4/8 NS	10/10 NS
Progesterone	1/9 *	2/9 ***
Estradiol	2/10 NS	10/10 NS
DOC-Ac	4/9 NS	8/9 NS
Hydroxydione	2/10 NS	7/10 NS
Thyroxine	2/10 NS	9/10 NS
Phenobarbital	2/10 NS	5/10 *

[a] The rats of all groups were given digitoxin [0.4 mg in 2 ml water mixed with Na_2HPO_4 (1 mM per rat)] and corn oil (1 ml, p.o., twice daily from 4th day ff.).

[b] Cardiac necrosis was estimated on day of death in animals that lived at least 6 days and mortality listed on 9th day ("Exact Probability Test").

For further details on technique of tabulation cf. p. VIII.

or indomethacin is rapidly fatal. The plasma concentration of digitoxin and indomethacin is diminished during the catatoxic steroid administration.

Solymoss et al. G70,461/70: In rats, spironolactone, norbolethone and ethylestrenol pretreatment accelerate the disappearance rate of digitoxin from serum in proportion to the inhibition of the convulsions. Partial hepatectomy reduces digitoxin elimination. The action of spironolactone is blocked by SKF 525-A.

Solymoss et al. G70,463/70: In rats, pretreatment with spironolactone, norbolethone or ethylestrenol accelerated the plasma clearance of digitoxin, in proportion to the in vivo protective effect of these catatoxic steroids.

Partial hepatectomy reduces digitoxin clearance. The effect of spironolactone is suppressed by SKF 525-A and cycloheximide.

Solymoss G70,484/70: In rats, the plasma clearance of digitoxin is accelerated by spironolactone, norbolethone, and ethylestrenol in doses that protect against the toxicity of the alkaloid in vivo. On the other hand, partial hepatectomy reduces digitoxin plasma clearance and increases the severity of the convulsions. The protective action of the steroids is suppressed by SKF 525-A and cycloheximide.

Selye G70,480/71: In the rat, comparative studies with 59 steroid nitriles indicate that the highest antidigitoxin and anti-indomethacin is exhibited by 16α-carbonitrile. All 11 steroids of this series which possessed a 16α-carbonitrile group were endowed with this type of protective activity. Most active among them were: PCN, its acetate, 20,20(ethylenedioxy)-

3β-hydroxypregn-5-ene-16α-carbonitrile (U-19553), 3β-hydroxy-7,20-dioxopregn-5-ene-16α-carbonitrile acetate (SC-6703), 3β-hydroxy-7,20-dioxopregn-5-ene-16α-carbonitrile (SC-6813), 3,3-(ethylenedioxy)-11,20-dioxopregn-5-ene-16α-carbonitrile (U-35006), 3,3,20,20-Bis-(ethylenedioxy)-11-oxopregn-5-ene-16α-carbonitrile (U-35910), 3β-Hydroxy-20-oxopregn-5-ene-16α-carbonitrile acetate (U-34889), 3β-hydroxy-20,20-ethylendioxypregn-5-ene-16α-carbonitrile acetate. Certain 2α-carbonitriles (and 2-ene-3α-carbonitriles) were also effective but to a lesser degree. Steroids with carbonitriles in other positions of the nucleus or side chains were not effective. In this series only a few steroids devoid of -CN groups showed any significant antidigitoxin and anti-indomethacin effect. Among these one was a 16β-carboxylic acid, the other a 4-aza steroid. Mestranol protected against indomethacin but not against digitoxin. Among the carbonitriles, in general the same tendency was noted at low doses where anti-indomethacin effect exceeded the antidigitoxin action.

Szabo et al. G79,024/71: In rats, PCN increases resistance to indomethacin, hexobarbital, progesterone, zoxazolamine and digitoxin, both in the presence and in the absence of the pituitary. Hypophysectomy also fails to prevent the induction of SER proliferation in the hepatocytes.

Selye PROT. 17663: In rats, spironolactone given simultaneously with digitoxin has little, if any, protective effect. Pretreatment for 24 hrs is moderately effective, whereas after 48—96 hrs of spironolactone treatment, digitoxin toxicity is completely abolished.

Selye PROT. 18125: In rats pretreated with 10 mg of spironolactone, the antidigitoxin effect remains obvious for about 5 days after discontinuation of treatment, but its efficacy in inhibiting convulsions rapidly diminishes during this time.

Selye PROT. 20023: In rats, spironolactone (10 mg x2/day p.o.) protects against as much as 2 mg of digitoxin/day p.o., whereas the same dose of norbolethone protects even against 5 mg of digitoxin.

Selye PROT. 20049: In rats, the inhibition of digitoxin poisoning by spironolactone can be blocked by high doses of estradiol and apparently to some extent also by progesterone, whereas DOC, cortisol, methylandrostenediol, methyltestosterone, pregnanedione, pregnenolone and testosterone do not interfere with this type of protection, cf. Table 49.

Selye PROT. 34038, 34405: In rats of different age groups, the antidigitoxin effect of PCN is essentially the same if administered at dose levels adjusted to body weight, cf. Table 50.

Table 49. *Effect of various steroids upon the antidigitoxin effect of spironolactone*

Groups	Treatment[a]		Convulsions[b] (Positive/Total)	Mortality[b] (Dead/Total)
1	Control (Digitoxin only)		15/15 ***	15/15 ***
2	Control		0/15	0/15
3	DOC		1/14 NS	3/14 NS
4	Progesterone		8/14 **	6/14 *
5	Estradiol 10 mg		10/15 ***	11/15 ***
6	Estradiol 100 µg	Digitoxin + Spironolactone	6/15 *	5/15 *
7	Cortisol		1/15 NS	0/15 NS
8	Methylandrostenediol		0/15 NS	0/15 NS
9	Methyltestosterone		0/15 NS	0/15 NS
10	Pregnanedione		3/15 NS	2/15 NS
11	Pregnenolone		1/15 NS	1/15 NS
12	Testosterone		0/15 NS	0/15 NS

[a] The rats of all groups received digitoxin 1 mg in 1 ml water, p.o./day, 3rd day ff. and those of groups 2—12 were given in addition spironolactone 2 mg in 1 ml water, p.o. x2/day, 1st day ff. Various steroids 10 mg (except group 6 which received 100 µg) in 1 ml water, p.o. x2/day, 1st day ff.

[b] Convulsions listed on 6th day and mortality on 8th day. (Statistics: Chi-square test compared to group 2.)

For further details on technique of tabulation cf. p. VIII.

Table 50. *Comparison of antidigitoxin effect of PCN in rats of different ages*

Body weight[a] (g)	Convulsions[b] (Positive/Total)		Mortality[b] (Dead/Total)	
	Control	PCN	Control	PCN
50	8/8	0/10 ***	8/8	1/10 ***
100	10/10	1/10 ***	6/10	1/10 *
200	10/10	2/10 ***	7/10	0/10 ***
300	10/10	0/10 ***	10/10	0/10 ***

[a] The rats of all groups were given digitoxin 2 mg in 1 ml water, p.o. 4th and 5th day. The groups so designated received PCN 0.2 mg in 1 ml water, p.o. x2/day, from the 1st day up to 4th day and once on the 5th day. Doses per 100 g body weight.

[b] The severity of the convulsions was estimated on the 7th day and mortality was listed on the 9th day. (Statistics: Fisher & Yates.)

For further details on technique of tabulation cf. p. VIII.

Selye PROT. 25766: In rats, the blockade by spironolactone of indomethacin or digitoxin poisoning is abolished if metyrapone is administered simultaneously with the conditioner, cf. Table 51.

Selye PROT. 42269: In rats chronically poisoned with digitoxin (0.5—1.0 mg, p.o./day) or indomethacin (0.75 mg, s.c./day), the administration of PCN (1 mg x2/day, p.o., beginning on the 3rd or 4th day of treatment with the toxicants), when clinical signs of poisoning were already evident, caused these to disappear and permitted survival, whereas the controls receiving no PCN invariably died. These experiments show that, although presumably the protective effect of PCN against digitoxin and indomethacin depends upon the induction of drug-metabolizing enzymes, the steroid can act not only prophylactically but also curatively, if the intoxication is sufficiently slow to permit effective enzyme induction in time.

Dog

Grinnell & Smith C31,428/57: On the basis of studies in dogs treated with estrone, estradiol or diethylstilbestrol, it is concluded that folliculoids protect against the induction of cardiac arrhythmia by digoxin. "Male dogs and castrate female dogs have been found to be highly sensitive to toxic manifestations of a cardiac glycoside on cardiac rhythm, in comparison with normal females in anestrus, or castrate females treated with estrogenic substance. A high degree of resistance to toxicity of digoxin was exhibited by the 3 normal females in natural estrus which were available."

Grinnell et al. D10,545/61: In ovariectomized dogs, various folliculoids increase resistance to the production of ECG changes by digoxin.

Shafer & Adicoff G80,179/70: In dogs, tetrahydrofurfuryl alcohol (THFA), despite its resemblance to the lactone moiety of digoxin, offers no protection against the latter com-

Table 51. *Effect of metyrapone upon the blockade of indomethacin and digitoxin toxicity by spironolactone*

Group	Treatment[a]	Digitoxin		Indomethacin	
		Convulsions[b] (Positive/Total)	Mortality[b] (Dead/Total)	Intestinal ulcers[b] (Positive/Total)	Mortality[b] (Dead/Total)
1	None	15/15	14/15	15/15	13/15
2	Spironolactone	0/15 ***	0/15 ***	0/15 ***	0/15 ***
3	Metyrapone	14/15 NS	14/15 NS	13/15 NS	7/15 *
4	Metyrapone + Spironalatcone	11/15 ***	10/15 ***	10/10 ***	2/10 NS

[a] The rats of all groups received indomethacin 1 mg in 0.2 ml water, s.c., or digitoxin 1 mg in 1 ml water p.o., once daily from the 4th day; spironolactone 2 mg in 1 ml water p.o., twice daily from the 1st day; metyrapone 6 mg in 0.1 ml oil, i.p., the 4th and 5th days and 12 mg daily from the 6th day 30 min. before indomethacin or digitoxin administration.

[b] The severity of convulsions was estimated on 7th day; intestinal ulcers were appraised on day of death (but only in animals which survived at least 6 days), and mortality was listed on 9th day. (Statistics Fisher & Yates; groups 2 and 3 compared with group 1, group 4 compared with group 2).

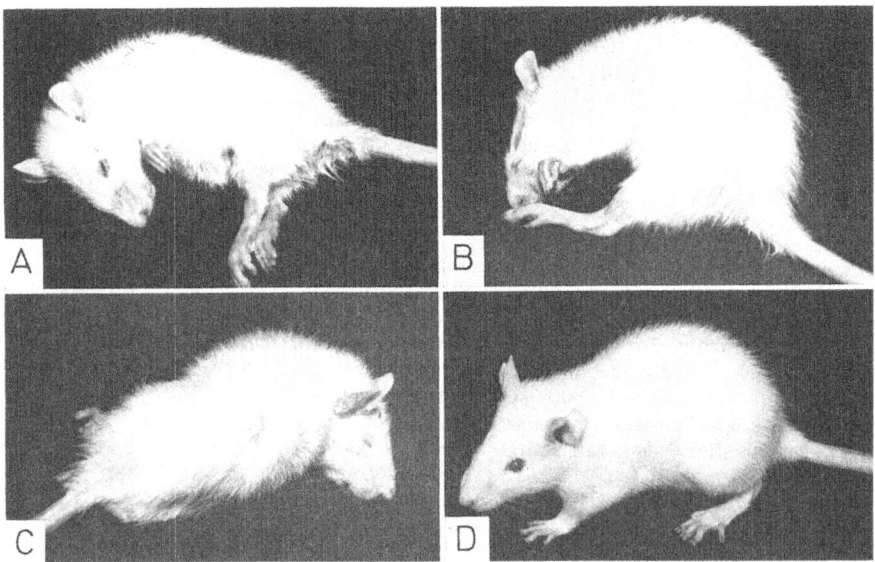

Fig. 6. **Prevention of digitoxin convulsions by spironolactone.** All four rats were given 2 mg of digitoxin p.o., but only D was pretreated with spironolactone and thereby protected against digitoxin convulsions

pound in vivo. The authors emphasize that despite these "negative results, the development of a specific nontoxic pharmacological antagonist to digitalis would be of major clinical importance." [These investigators appear to be unaware of the inhibition of digitalis toxicity by spironolactone (H.S.).]

FROG

Von Metzler & Hergott B63,494/51: In frogs, induction of lethal cardiac arrest by strophanthin is delayed by simultaneous treatment with DOC. This may reflect a true antagonism or merely a delay in absorption.

Wilbrandt & Weiss C88,230/60: Review of the literature on the antagonisms between cardiac glycosides and corticoids. Personal investigations showed that the electric potential lowering effect of K-strophanthin in frog's skin can be inhibited by aldosterone and DOC, but only if the corticoids are administered in vivo.

GUINEA PIG

Lindner & Stoklaska C35,550/56: In guinea pigs, chronic intoxication with digitoxin is moderately counteracted by chronic treatment with cortisone but pretreatment with cortisone offers no protection against subsequent acute digitoxin poisoning. Chronic pretreatment with sublethal doses of digitoxin diminishes resistance to subsequent i.v. injection of a higher dose, presumably owing to the cumulative effect of the alkaloid.

Godfraind & Godfraind-De Becker D45,080/61: The contractions of the guinea pig ilium produced in vitro by various digitalis alkaloids is competitively inhibited by DOC.

MOUSE

Holck & Kimura 84,604/44: Female mice are more resistant to ouabain than males but resistance to strophanthin K is the same in both sexes. Ovariectomy, orchidectomy and treatment with "estrogenic hormones" produced inconsistent changes in ouabain resistance.

Selye PROT. 27594, 28284, 29742, 29751: In mice, digitoxin poisoning is inhibited by CS-1, spironolactone, norbolethone, oxandrolone, prednisolone, progesterone and thyroxine. Ethylestrenol, triamcinolone, DOC, hydroxydione and estradiol are ineffective.

CAT

Pozo & Negrete B68,183/52: On skeletal muscles of the cat, cortisone "produced a very marked potentiation of the effects of digitalis."

HAMSTER

Szabo et al. G79,013/71: In hamsters, spironolactone and ethylestrenol pretreatment prevents digitoxin convulsions and indomethacin-induced intestinal ulcers.

VARIA

Selye et al. G60,023/69: Among numerous steroids tested, all anabolic testoids inhibited digitoxin toxicity. However, spironolactone was likewise highly effective in this respect although it is devoid of both anabolic and testoid potency. Apparently, anabolic potency endows steroids with antidigitoxin properties but is not indispensable for them. (Literature on catatoxic actions of spironolactone and anabolic steroids).

Diisopropyl Fluorophosphate (DFP) ←

Fontan et al. F55,419/65: Pretreatment with spironolactone protects the mouse against lethal DFP intoxication. When spironolactone is given simultaneously with or after DFP, a protection is still demonstrable but less evident.

Fontan et al. F98,752/68: Spironolactone, phanurane, aldosterone and dexamethasone, despite their different pharmacologic actions protect the mouse against DFP-intoxication, a fact which is ascribed to their common possession of the cyclopentanophenantrene nucleus. Triamterene, whose renal action resembles that of the antimineralocorticoids does not protect against DFP. [No other steroids have been tested to verify whether the protective effect is common to all compounds possessing the cyclopentanophenantrene nucleus (H.S.).]

Selye G70,480/71: In rats, most catatoxic steroids offered some protection against "DFP" intoxication, but their prophylactic effect was not as striking as against other anticholinesterases, perhaps because in this experiment, the intoxication of the controls was not sufficiently severe to reveal a major protective effect, *cf.* Table 52.

Dimercaprol ←

Selye G70,480/71: In rats, dimercaprol "BAL" (0.2 ml/100 g body weight of a 5% solution in corn oil) was administered s.c. once on the 4th day of conditioning. Dyskinesia was listed 4 hrs, mortality 24 hrs, after injection. Under these circumstances none of the "Standard Conditioners" (p. VIII) or cholesterol caused any noteworthy change in the resulting intoxication. Hydroxydione and phenobarbital were not tested.

Table 52. *Conditioning for "DFP"*

Treatment[a]	Dyskinesia[b] (Positive/Total)	Mortality[b] (Dead/Total)
None	5/10	1/10
PCN	8/10 NS	0/10 NS
CS-1	0/9 *	0/9 NS
Ethylestrenol	0/10 *	0/10 NS
Spironolactone	0/10 *	0/10 NS
Norbolethone	3/10 NS	1/10 NS
Oxandrolone	1/10 NS	0/10 NS
Prednisolone-Ac	0/10 *	0/10 NS
Triamcinolone (2 mg)	1/10 NS	1/10 NS
Progesterone	4/10 NS	2/10 NS
Estradiol (1 mg)	2/9 NS	1/9 NS
Estradiol (1 mg s.c.)	5/10 NS	0/10 NS
DOC-Ac	5/10 NS	2/10 NS
Hydroxydione	2/10 NS	1/10 NS
Thyroxine	3/10 NS	3/10 NS
Phenobarbital	4/10 NS	0/10 NS

[a] The rats of all groups were given diisopropyl fluorophosphate, "DFP" (250 µg/100 g body weight in 0.2 ml corn oil s.c. once on 4th day).

[b] Dyskinesia was estimated on 5th day and mortality listed on 6th day ("Exact Probability Test").

For further details on technique of tabulation *cf.* p. VIII.

Dinitrophenol ←

Selye PROT. 27780: In rats, dinitrophenol (3.2 mg/100 g body weight in 0.2 ml DMSO) was administered s.c. once on 4th day of conditioning. Dyskinesia was listed 1 hr, mortality 24 hrs, after this injection. Under these circumstances none of the "Standard Conditioners" (p. VIII) or cholesterol caused any noteworthy change in the resulting intoxication, only thyroxine exhibited an aggravating effect. Hydroxydione and phenobarbital were not tested.

Dioxathion ← *cf.* Pesticides

Diphenylhydantoin ←

Fingl et al. D38,091/52: In rats, chronic administration of phenobarbital or diphenylhydantoin diminishes the brain hyperexcitability induced by cortisone as judged by electroshock-seizure threshold measurements.

Rümke & Noordhoek H14,039/69: Lynestrenol (a luteoid) decreases the hexobarbital sleeping time and diminishes the anticonvulsant effect of phenobarbital and diphenylhydantoin by acceleration of their metabolisms through the hepatic microsomal enzymes.

Blackham & Spencer G73,813/70: In mice, lynestrenol reduced, whereas mestranol or SKF 525-A increased the anticonvulsive effect (tested with electroshock) of diphenylhydantoin, phenobarbital, chlordiazepoxide and diazepam administered i.p. after five days of pretreatment. This may be due to altered microsomal drug metabolism but since mestranol and lynestrenol have opposite effects upon brain 5-HT concentrations, the latter mechanism must also be considered.

Selye PROT. 37772: In rats, moderate intoxication with diphenylhydantoin was prevented by CS-1 and spironolactone, whereas prednisolone and triamcinolone considerably aggravated its intensity. The effect of the other standard conditioners was less clear-cut, *cf.* Table 53.

Table 53. *Conditioning for diphenylhydantoin*

Treatment[a]	Dyskinesia[b] (Positive/Total)	Mortality[b] (Dead/Total)
None	6/15	0/15
PCN	7/10 NS	0/10 NS
CS-1	0/10 *	0/10 NS
Ethylestrenol	1/10 NS	0/10 NS
Spironolactone	0/9 *	0/9 NS
Norbolethone	2/10 NS	0/10 NS
Oxandrolone	2/10 NS	0/10 NS
Prednisolone-Ac	10/10 ***	0/10 NS
Triamcinolone (2 mg)	10/10 ***	3/10 NS
Progesterone	4/9 NS	0/9 NS
Estradiol (1 mg)	5/10 NS	0/10 NS
DOC-Ac	5/10 NS	0/10 NS
Hydroxydione	8/10 NS	0/10 NS
Cholesterol	3/5 NS	0/5 NS
Thyroxine	9/10 *	0/10 NS
Phenobarbital	0/10 *	0/10 NS

[a] The rats of all groups were given diphenylhydantoin (30 mg/100 g body weight in 1 ml water, i.p., on 4th day).

[b] Dyskinesia was estimated 3 hrs after injection and mortality listed on 4th day p.m. ("Exact Probability Test").

For additional pertinent data *cf.* Table 135.

For further details on technique of tabulation *cf.* p. VIII.

Diphenylhydantoin ← Mestranol, Lynestrenol + SKF 525-A, Mouse: Blackham et al. G73,813/70*

Diphosphopyridine Nucleotide (DPN) ←

Haydu & Wolfson C77,942/59: In mice, the toxicity of DPN is increased by exposure to either cold or heat; the effect of temperature extremes is further aggravated by cortisone.

Dipicrylamine ←

Selye G70,480/71: In rats, dipicrylamine intoxication is prevented by PCN and CS-1, but not by any of the other standard conditioning agents. Triamcinolone and thyroxine increase the mortality, *cf.* Table 54.

Table 54. *Conditioning for dipicrylamine*

Treatment[a]	Dyskinesia[b] (Positive/Total)	Mortality[b] (Dead/Total)
None	17/20	7/20
PCN	0/10 ***	0/10 *
CS-1	1/10 ***	0/10 *
Ethylestrenol	14/20 NS	3/20 NS
Spironolactone	13/20 NS	3/20 NS
Norbolethone	7/10 NS	3/10 NS
Oxandrolone	5/10 NS	2/10 NS
Prednisolone-Ac	5/10 NS	2/10 NS
Triamcinolone	14/15 NS	14/15 ***
Progesterone	7/10 NS	5/10 NS
Estradiol	8/10 NS	2/10 NS
DOC-Ac	7/10 NS	5/10 NS
Hydroxydione	7/10 NS	4/10 NS
Thyroxine	15/15 NS	14/15 ***
Phenobarbital	5/10 NS	1/10 NS

[a] The rats of all groups were given dipicrylamine (10 mg on 4th day, 15 mg on 5th day, /100 g body weight in 0.2 ml DMSO, s.c.).

[b] Dyskinesia was estimated on 5th day 2 hrs after injection and mortality listed 24 hrs later ("Exact Probability Test").

For further details on technique of tabulation *cf.* p. VIII.

Disulfiram ← *cf.* also Pharmacology (Inhibitors)

Lecoq B79,754/51: In rabbits, injection of disulfiram + ethanol or of Na-pyruvate produces essentially the same syndrome of intoxication, since pyruvic acid is the principal metabolite of ethanol after pretreatment with disulfiram. In either case, ACTH and cortisone offer little, if any, protective effect.

Lecoq et al. B66,406/51: In rats, the toxic effects of ethanol and its metabolites, pyruvate and acetaldehyde (which accumulate in the body under the influence of disulfiram) are inhibited by ACTH, cortisone, and hepatic extracts. Conversely, thyroxine, DOC, and testosterone appear to aggravate ethanol intoxication. [Statistically evaluated data are not presented (H.S.).]

DMP ← cf. Phosphorothioates

Doxepin ←

Selye PROT. 40821: In rats, doxepin hydrochloride (20 mg/100 g body weight in 1 ml water) was administered p.o. twice daily from the 4th day of conditioning to the 9th day. Dyskinesia was estimated on the 8th day one hour after the last injection, mortality listed on the 9th day. Under these circumstances, the "Standard Conditioners" (p. VIII) caused no noteworthy change in the resulting intoxication.

Dyes ← cf. also RES-Blocking Agents, Bilirubin, Clinical Implications (for BSP)

MAN

Heaney & Whedon C56,394/58: In man, methyltestosterone and norethandrolone p.o. markedly delay BSP clearance, whereas comparable amounts of testosterone are ineffective is this respect.

Carbone et al. C77,294/59: In patients with impaired hepatic function caused by methyltestosterone, large amounts of conjugated BSP accumulate in the serum.

Arias D63,323/63: In man, 17-ethyl-19-nortestosterone increases biliary BSP retention and plasma bilirubin concentration. Both in Wistar rats and in Gunn rats (the latter have chronic nonhemolytic unconjugated hyperbilirubinemia due to a hereditary defect), norethandrolone, methyltestosterone and icterogenin (an icterogenic steroid) interfered with the excretion of bilirubin and BSP through the bile. This was accompanied by certain electron microscopic changes in cytomembranes and lysosomes, without cell necrosis or any obvious change in various enzymic activities of hepatocytes. No effect was noted in rats treated with cortisone or testosterone.

Scherb et al. D58,943/63: In man, with no evidence of liver disease, norethandrolone caused a reversible reduction in the hepatic transport maximum for BSP. "The relative hepatic storage of BSP was unimpaired and BSP was retained in the plasma primarily as a conjugate. Light microscopic examination of two liver biopsies was normal except for BSP within parenchymal cells and fragmented ATPase-staining reaction of bile canaliculi. Electron microscopic examination revealed variable dilatation of bile canaliculi and normal intracellular organelles." The clinical literature on the effect of anabolics upon hepatic function is reviewed.

Mueller & Kappas F22,282/64: In man, estradiol and estriol rapidly and consistently reduced the hepatic excretory capacity for BSP.

Mueller & Kappas G81,288/64: Review and personal observations on the impairment of hepatic BSP excretion following treatment with natural folliculoids and during pregnancy in women.

Schoenfield & Foulk F16,158/64: In man, norethandrolone p.o. interferes with hepatic uptake and biliary excretion of BSP.

DeLorimier et al. G31,525/65: In man, BSP retention, without clinical or laboratory evidence of impaired hepatic function, developed after treatment with methyltestosterone, normethandrone, norethindrone, fluoxymesterone and methandriol. No significant retention occurred with 17α-vinyltestosterone, oxandrolone, unesterified testosterone, 17α-ethynyl-19-norandrostenediol or allylestrenol. The structural prerequisites for BSP retention are discussed. The factors responsible for jaundice (which is rarely reported in patients receiving most of these compounds) could not be identified.

Kleiner et al. F47,209/65: In women on oral contraceptives (norethynodrel and mestranol), BSP-excretion through the bile was impaired. The effect is ascribed to the luteoid component since estradiol does not cause BSP-retention.

Kottra & Kappas G37,574/66: In man, estradiol delays the clearance of BSP from the plasma, presumably because the excretion of both free and conjugated dye is impaired.

Larsson-Cohn G46,952/67: In 16 out of 22 women taking various contraceptives containing folliculoids and luteoids, BSP clearance was delayed.

Kappas F 94,299/68: In man, estradiol and estriol impair BSP excretion through the liver and may provoke hepatic porphyria.

BSP ← Testoids, Man: Heaney et al. C 56,394/58*; Carbone et al. C 77,294/59*; DeLorimier et al. G 31,525/65*

BSP ← Estradiol, Estriol, Man: Mueller et al. F 22,282/64*

BSP ← Steroids, Man: DeLorimier et al. G 31,525/65*; Larsson-Cohn G 46,952/67*; Mowat et al. G 74,246/69*

RAT

Clodi & Schnack D 41,569/62: In rats, the biliary excretion (fistula technique) of BSP is inhibited by numerous anabolic steroids. Earlier clinical and experimental data are discussed.

Kolb et al. D 22,260/62: In rats, the biliary excretion of ^{131}I marked rose bengal is inhibited by daily p.o. administration of various 17-alkylated anabolic steroids although after several weeks, adaptation develops in this respect. Among eight such anabolics tested, only methenolone acetate failed to impair dye excretion. [The possibility that decreased dye excretion may not reflect hepatic damage but increased dye metabolism has not been considered (H.S.).]

Gallagher & Kappas F 35,850/65: In rats, estradiol markedly delays plasma clearance of BSP, both in its free and conjugated form. "The structural specificity of this steroid action was examined in a variety of C18, C19, C21 and C24 compounds; the effect extends to estrone, estriol and other C18 steroids, including those used for contraceptive purposes."

Gallagher et al. F 86,156/67: In rats, 42 steroids (mostly folliculoids) were compared for their ability to interfere with BSP clearance.

Kreek et al. F 83,145/67: In rats, ethinylestradiol considerably diminishes bile flow and delays biliary excretion of BSP and of tritium-labeled estradiol.

Song et al. G 70,575/69: Comparative studies on the effect of 43 steroids upon BSP clearance in the rat, as an indicator of their hepatotoxic effect.

Despopoulos H 24,651/70: In rats, "1) Cortisone transiently increased bile flow and reduced concentration and rate of excretion of sulfobromophthalein in the bile. 2) Norethandrolone, norethynodrel and Norlutin reduced rates of bile formation and of sulfobromophthalein excretion without affecting the concentrating mechanism for sulfobromophthalein. 3) Testosterone and methyltestosterone, estradiol, progesterone and stilbestrol irreversibly reduced the rate of bile formation and transiently reduced excretion and concentration of sulfobromophthalein."

Solymoss et al. G 79,007/71: In rats, various catatoxic steroids (spironolactone, PCN) increase liver weight, glutathione S-aryltransferase activity, bile flow, and BSP clearance from the blood with an accelerated urinary excretion of conjugated BSP metabolites. Ethylestrenol similarly affects liver weight, but not the other parameters. The antimineralocorticoids, spiroxasone, SC-9376 and CS-1, unlike the anabolic steroids norbolethone and oxandrolone, also enhance plasma clearance of BSP. Contrary to the effects of pretreatment, the administration of spironolactone, ethylestrenol or estradiol immediately before BSP results in retention of the dye, probably through competitive inhibition of biliary excretion.

Solymoss et al. G 79,023/71: In rats, pretreatment with PCN or spironolactone increases liver weight, glutathione S-aryltransferase activity and bile flow. At the same time, the plasma clearance and biliary excretion of BSP and its conjugated metabolites are enhanced. Ethylestrenol likewise increases liver weight but does not alter the other parameters mentioned above. Spiroxasone, SC-9376 and CS-1 (antimineralocorticoids), unlike norbolethone and oxandrolone (anabolics), also enhance plasma clearance of BSP, probably through the same mechanism. In contrast to these effects of pretreatment, administration of spironolactone, ethylestrenol or estradiol immediately before BSP delays plasma clearance of the dye, probably through competitive inhibition of biliary excretion. SKF 525-A does not suppress the enhanced BSP clearance induced either by spironolactone or by phenobarbital. [Although the authors did not evaluate their data from this point of view, their observations clearly show that the catatoxic activity of steroids is not merely the result of hepatic microsomal drug metabolizing enzyme induction. It may also be mediated through extramicrosomal enzyme mechanisms or even through enhanced biliary excretion (H.S.).]

RABBIT

Carmichael E 28,041/63: In rabbits, methyltestosterone and norethandrolone significantly delay BSP clearance.

Lennon F 69,077/65: In rabbits, methyltestosterone and norethandrolone caused dose related increases in BSP retention. Oxandrolone was less active and testosterone inactive in this respect.

Lennon F63,769/66: In rabbits, various 17α-alkylated anabolics delayed BSP clearance, whereas non-17α-alkylated testoid-anabolics failed to do so. "BSP retention in rabbits was shown to be a simple laboratory test for estimating the effects of anabolic steroids on hepatic excretory function."

BSP ← Testoids, Steroids (anabolic), Rb: Carmichael et al. E28,041/63*; Lennon F69,077/65*, F63,769/66*

CHICKEN

Despopoulos H35,471/71: In chickens, the renal tubular excretion of BSP and of N-methylnicotinamide is inhibited by bile salts.

DOG

Gass & Umberger C94,624/59: In dogs, large doses of methyltestosterone or norethandrolone given for periods of up to 50 days did not affect BSP clearance.

VARIA

Szeberényi & Fekete H29,579/70: Brief abstract stating that after four days of pretreatment (species not mentioned), spironolactone decreased the action and accelerated the metabolism of hexobarbital, chlorzoxazone, meprobamate, estrone, testosterone, acenocoumarol and BSP, whereas after short treatment it had an inverse effect. It is concluded that spironolactone is a microsomal enzyme inducer.

Phenolphthalein ← Luteoids, Testoids: Hsia et al. C90,465/60

BSP ← Steroids: Clodi et al. D41,569/62*; Gallagher et al. F86,156/67*; Despopoulos H24,651/70*

Ectylurea ← Testosterone: Holck et al. A55,755/42*

Edrophonium Chloride ←

Selye G70,480/71: In rats, edrophonium chloride (5 mg/100 g body weight in 0.1 ml water) was administered s.c. once on the 4th day of conditioning. Dyskinesia was listed 15 min, mortality 24 hrs, after this injection. Under these circumstances none of the "Standard Conditioners" (p. VIII) or cholesterol caused any noteworthy change in the resulting intoxication. PCN, hydroxydione and phenobarbital were not tested.

EDTA (calcium disodium ethylenediaminetetraacetide) ←

Reuber E27,340/63: In the rat, Ca edetate induces nephrotic tubular lesions, which are greatly aggravated by concurrent administration of cortisone.

Table 55. *Conditioning for emetine*

Treatment[a]	Adrenal necrosis[b] (Positive/Total)	Dyskinesia[b] (Positive/Total)	Mortality[b] (Dead/Total)
None	2/5	10/10	5/10
PCN	1/5 NS	6/15 ***	5/15 NS
CS-1	3/10 NS	3/10 ***	2/10 NS
Ethylestrenol	2/5 NS	10/10 NS	9/10 NS
Spironolactone	3/5 NS	6/10 *	2/10 NS
Norbolethone	1/5 NS	10/10 NS	9/10 NS
Oxandrolone	1/5 NS	10/10 NS	10/10 *
Prednisolone-Ac	3/5 NS	10/10 NS	10/10 *
Triamcinolone	0/5 NS	10/10 NS	10/10 *
Triamcinolone (2 mg)	—	5/5 NS	4/5 NS
Progesterone	1/5 NS	10/10 NS	10/10 *
Estradiol	1/5 NS	10/10 NS	9/10 NS
Estradiol (1 mg)	—	5/5 NS	5/5 NS
DOC-Ac	1/5 NS	10/10 NS	10/10 *
Hydroxydione	4/10 NS	10/10 NS	8/10 NS
Thyroxine	2/5 NS	10/10 NS	10/10 *
Phenobarbital	3/5 NS	8/10 NS	3/10 NS

[a] The rats of all groups were given emetine hydrochloride (3 mg/100 g body weight in 1 ml water, p.o. the 4th day, and 4 mg/100 g body weight the 5th day).

[b] Dyskinesia, adrenal necrosis and mortality were determined on 6th day ("Exact Probability Test").

For further details on technique of tabulation cf. p. VIII.

Emetine ← *cf. also Selye G 60,083/70, p. 379.*
Gregorio & Armellini G 64,277/64: In rabbits, the production of cardiac lesions by emetine is inhibited by chorionic gonadotrophin and testosterone but not by estradiol.

Selye G 70,480/71: In rats, emetine intoxication is largely prevented by pretreatment with PCN and CS-1. Spironolactone has a barely significant protective effect. Indeed, several other standard conditioners appear to increase the mortality, cf. Table 55.

Endoxan ← *cf. Cyclophosphamide*

Ephedrine ←

Selye G 70,480/71: In rats, ephedrine sulfate (50 mg/100 g body weight in 0.2 ml water) was administered s.c. twice on the 4th day of conditioning. Dyskinesia was listed 4 hrs after the first injection and mortality registered 3 days later. Under these circumstances, none of the "Standard Conditioners" (p. VIII) caused any noteworthy change in the resulting intoxication.

Ergot ←

McGrath A 29,208/35: In rats of both sexes, tail necrosis is produced by large amounts of ergotamine. Estrone prevents this change in females but not in males.

Loewe & Lenke A 43,451/38: In the rat, the tail necrosis produced by ergotamine s.c. is essentially the same in both sexes. Contrary to earlier claims, it cannot be prevented by folliculoid hormones and/or orchidectomy.

Ratschow & Klostermann A 19,494/38: In rats, the tail necrosis produced by ergotamine is much more readily inhibited by estradiol in females than in males. Ovariectomy aggravates the tail necrosis and diminishes the protective effect of estradiol. Castrate males are less sensitive to ergotamine than intact males. Testosterone propionate protects intact males, but not females.

Suzman et al. A 44,452/38: Repeated administration of estrone completely protects female rats against the tail necrosis produced by ergotamine; males are only partially protected. Orchidectomy has no effect in itself, but enhances the protective effect of estrone in the male. Otherwise untreated rats showed no marked sex difference in their sensitivity to ergotamine.

Thomas A 33,372/40: Neither a folliculoid preparation (theelin) nor testosterone s.c. (given daily for five days prior to treatment with ergotamine s.c.) prevented the characteristic ergot gangrene of the tail.

McGrath & Herrmann B 500/44: In rats, the characteristic gangrene of the tail produced by ergotamine tartrate is prevented by estrone.

Contreras et al. F 81,599/67: In intact male rats, unlike in females or castrate males, ergonovine induced an analgesic effect (electrical stimulation of the genital papilla) unless the latter were treated with testosterone.

Ethanol ←

RAT

Klotz A 96,052/37: In rats, ovariectomy interferes with adaptation to ethanol.

Lecoq et al. B 66,406/51: In rats, the toxic effects of ethanol and its metabolites, pyruvate and acetaldehyde (which accumulate in the body under the influence of disulfiram) are inhibited by ACTH, cortisone, and hepatic extracts. Conversely, thyroxine, DOC, and testosterone appear to aggravate ethanol intoxication. [Statistically evaluated data are not presented (H.S.).]

Mallov C 47,222/58: Ethanol p.o. produces more severe fatty infiltration of the liver in female than in male rats. Ovariectomy or administration of estradiol to males did not influence fatty infiltration but testosterone reduced hepatic steatosis in females, whereas castration increased it in males.

Fazekas et al. D 22,442/61: Review on the enzymic detoxication of ethanol. The authors' observations show that the ADH activity of hepatic homogenates diminishes after adrenalectomy in the rat, and can be increased by adrenocortical extract both in intact and adrenalectomized rats.

Fazekas D 55,397/62: Both in intact and in adrenalectomized rats, addition of aldosterone and, to a lesser extent, of corticosterone, cortisone, and cortisol to hepatic homogenates greatly augmented their ADH activity in vitro. DOC was very much less active. Adrenalectomy diminishes the hepatic ADH activity.

Fazekas G 9,347/63; F 71,641/64: In the rat, adrenalectomy delays the decrease in blood ethanol level following s.c. injection of ethanol, whereas corticoids have an inverse effect, both in adrenalectomized and in intact rats. The action is ascribed to a stimulation of hepatic ADH activity by corticoids as judged by observations with the methylene blue decolorizing technique [spectrophotometric determinations were not performed (H.S.).]

Jabbari & Leevy G45,526/67: Various anabolics (norethandrolone, testosterone, oxandrolone) protect the liver of the rat against ethanol-induced fatty degeneration and various functional disturbances. They were also found to be useful in the management of alcoholic patients.

Fazekas & Rengei G58,271/68: Among rats, not pretreated with ethanol, the ADH activity of the liver, heart, and kidneys is diminished by adrenalectomy. Upon s.c. administration of ethanol, the ADH-activity of the liver increases both in intact and in adrenalectomized rats. The authors speculate that ADH-activity may result not only in the microsomes but also in other cellular fraction, and that part of the enzyme induction may be due to the stressor effect of ethanol.

Selye et al. G60,016/69: In rats, spironolactone protects against anesthesia produced by progesterone, DOC, hydroxydione, pregnanedione, dehydroepiandrosterone, testosterone, diethylstilbestrol, methyprylon, pentobarbital and ethanol. It does not significantly alter the corresponding actions of morphine, codeine, urethan, diazepam, chlorpromazine, reserpine, phenoxybenzamine, chloral hydrate, potassium bromide or $MgCl_2$.

Selye et al. G60,020/69: In the rat, pretreatment with norbolethone protects against the anesthetic effect of progesterone, DOC, pregnanedione, dehydroepiandrosterone, testosterone, diethylstilbestrol, pentobarbital and methyprylon. It does not significantly alter the corresponding actions of ethanol, urethan, diazepam, chlorpromazine, reserpine, phenoxybenzamine, chloral hydrate, potassium bromide or magnesium chloride.

Selye PROT. 37234: In rats, ethyl alcohol (2 ml/100 g body weight of a 50% aqueous solution) was administered p.o. from the 4th day to the 6th day of conditioning. Dyskinesia was listed on the 6th day 3hrs after injection and mortality registered on the 8th day. Under these circumstances none of the "Standard Conditioners" (p. VIII) caused any noteworthy change in the resulting intoxication, only prednisolone exhibited an aggravating effect.

Mouse

Goodsell D3,916/61: In mice, ethanol anesthesia is prolonged by cortisone pretreatment but not influenced by prednisolone or DOC.

Störtebecker 69,765/37: In the mouse, the resistance to curare, KCN or ethanol is particularly high during estrus and decreased by ovariectomy. Castrates treated with estrone show increased tolerance to these drugs.

Ethanol ← Ovariectomy, Mouse: Störtebecker 76,398/39*

Rabbit

Störtebecker 76,398/39: In both male and female mice and rabbits, gonadectomy diminishes alcohol tolerance, whereas estrone treatment raises it.

Goldberg & Störtebecker B31,834/43: In rabbits, estrone increases alcohol tolerance so that intoxication occurs only at very high blood alcohol levels. Alcohol metabolism is not influenced but presumably its effect upon the nervous system is diminished by folliculoids. The experiments were performed after ovariectomy to avoid complications by varying endogenous folliculoid production.

Barta & Beregi F24,783/64: Fatal doses of ethanol p.o. produce adrenal necrosis in the rabbit and neither this lesion nor mortality can be prevented by pretreatment with dexamethasone.

Man

Levy & Paumgartner G72,234/68: In three volunteers who developed alcoholic hepatitis on an ethanol-low-protein regimen, jaundice appeared only in advanced stages of liver necrosis and inflammation. In earlier stages, there was proliferation of SER which was further increased by norethandrolone and yet, this anabolic reduced serum bilirubin. It is especially emphasized that "anabolic steroids may facilitate reduction of serum bilirubin despite capacity of these drugs to decrease hepatic excretory capacity."

Ether ←

Störtebecker A1,993/37: Rabbits pretreated with "folliculin" tolerate normally anesthesia-producing doses of butallylonal (Pernocton). Subsequent experiments were conducted to determine the blood ether level during ether anesthesia at the time the corneal reflex is lost in intact and gonadectomized rabbits and mice. Similar observations were made during pregnancy and in relation to the estrous cycle. [Several conclusions were drawn suggesting an influence of sex hormones upon anesthesia but the number of animals per group was small and hence statistical evaluation impossible (H.S.).]

Störtebecker 76,398/39: Castration decreases the ether resistance of both male and female rabbits and mice. In castrated rabbits, both estrone and androsterone increase ether tolerance.

Ethionine ←

← **Glucocorticoids.** *Popper et al. C 33,264/57:* In rats, the hepatic damage caused by ethionine is inhibited by cortisone.

Stein et al. C 59,992/58: "Cortisone inhibits accumulation of interstitial cells between liver cell plates, otherwise produced by oral administration of ethionine to rats." The associated degeneration of hepatic cells characteristic of the ethionine intoxication is not influenced by cortisone.

Daugharty et al. C 74,925/59: In rats, the pancreatic lesions induced by ethionine i.p. were not influenced by cortisone i.p.

Hutterer et al. D 902/61: Cortisone offers moderate protection against ethionine induced liver damage in the rat.

Rubin & Hutterer D 4,173/61: In rats with subacute ethionine intoxication, hepatic fibrosis is inhibited by cortisone and fat accumulation is increased; however, during the chronic phase the steroid has no marked effect.

Hutterer et al. E 54,152/62: As judged by cytochemical autoradiographic and histologic studies, cortisone and cortisol are effective in certain phases of the hepatic lesions produced by ethionine in the rat.

Berdjis F 79,528/67: The hepatotoxic effect of CCl_4, phosphorus and ethionine could be diminished by cortisone and survival prolonged.

← **Gonadal Steroids.** *Farber et al. B 47,283/50; D 24,923/51:* The production of fatty livers in rats treated with ethionine is possible only in females or orchidectomized males. Testosterone renders females and orchidectomized males resistant.

Farber & Segaloff D 95,996/55: In ovariectomized rats, various testoids and STH protected the liver against fatty infiltration produced by ethionine i.p., whereas cortisone and ACTH aggravated it. Estradiol, DOC and TSH had no effect.

Tedeschi & Gualandi C 33,614/56: In rats of both sexes, MAD failed to influence the ethionine-induced hepatic steatosis.

Ranney & Drill C 41,986/57: In adult orchidectomized male rats, the fatty infiltration of the liver caused by ethionine i.p. is blocked by 17-ethyl-19-nortestosterone in doses which do not stimulate the growth of the seminal vesicles, whereas testosterone propionate exerts this effect only in definitely testoid amounts. Progesterone is ineffective. Apparently, the protective effect of anabolics against this type of fatty liver formation does not depend either upon testoid or luteoid activity.

Grunt et al. C 84,696/60: In rats, both neonatal and postpubertal orchidectomy facilitates the production of hepatic steatosis by ethionine.

Chang & Lei F 78,943/65: 17α-Methyl-5α-androstan-17β-ol prevents the production of fatty hepatic degeneration by ethionine or CCl_4 in mice.

Ethylene Chlorohydrin ←

Selye G 70,480/71: In rats, "ethylene chlorohydrin," that is 2-chloroethanol (0.2 ml/100 g body weight of a 4% aqueous solution) was administered p.o. once on the 4th day and (0.3 ml) on the 5th day of conditioning. Dyskinesia was listed on the 5th day 1 hr, and mortality 24 hrs, after this injection. Under these circumstances none of the "Standard Conditioners" (p. VIII) or cholesterol caused any noteworthy change in the resulting intoxication. Hydroxydione and phenobarbital were not tested.

Ethylene Glycol ←

Tanret et al. D 44,140/62: Prolonged oral administration of ethylene glycol produces calcium oxalate precipitation in the kidney of male, but not of female, rats. Estradiol abolishes the susceptibility of intact or castrated males, but orchidectomy does not. Intact, unlike ovariectomized, females cannot be made susceptible by treatment with testosterone.

Szablowska & Selye G 70,475/71: In the rat, pretreatment with thyroxine or triamcinolone inhibits the mortality rate and renal lesions induced by ethylene glycol intoxication; estradiol exerts an opposite effect.

Selye G 70,480/71: In rats, ethylene glycol intoxication is markedly prevented by prednisolone, triamcinolone and thyroxine, whereas all other conditioning agents of our series, including phenobarbital, are ineffective in this respect. In fact, estradiol (given at various doses and through various routes) greatly aggravates mortality, whereas the other agents have no pronounced effect upon it. These findings confirm and extend earlier observa-

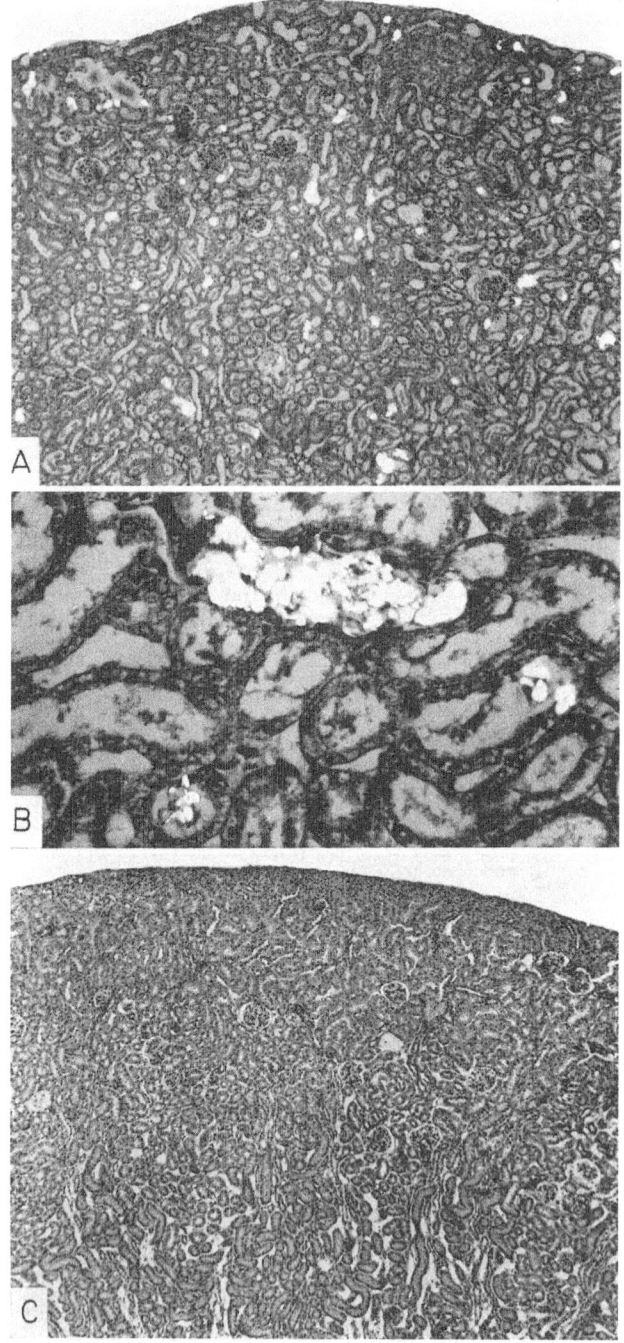

Fig. 7. **Effect of various steroids upon ethylene glycol intoxication.** All rats received the same amount of ethylene glycol. A: Under polarized light, numerous calcium oxalate crystals are visible in the tubules of an animal sensitized to ethylene glycol by estradiol ($\times 32$). B: Under higher magnification these crystals are still more clearly visible ($\times 200$). C: Complete prevention of renal lesions by triamcinolone pretreatment ($\times 32$). All sections stained with hematoxylin-phloxine and viewed under partially polarized light. [Szablovska & Selye G 70,475/71. Courtesy of Arch. Environm. Med.]

tions in which it was found that the production of renal oxalate crystal deposits, as well as the fatal effects of ethylene glycol intoxication can be prevented by triamcinolone and thyroxine, whereas spironolactone and estradiol have an opposite effect *(Szablowska & Selye G 70,499/70)*, cf. Table 56.

Table 56. *Conditioning for ethylene glycol*

Treatment[a]	Dyskinesia[b] (Positive/ Total)	Mortality[b] (Dead/ Total)
None	11/15	6/15
PCN	5/10 NS	6/10 NS
CS-1	2/10 *	0/10 *
Ethylestrenol	10 /15 NS	5/15 NS
Spironolactone	12/15 NS	13/15 *
Norbolethone	11/15 NS	8/15 NS
Oxandrolone	8/15 NS	5/15 NS
Prednisolone-Ac	2/15 ***	2/15 NS
Triamcinolone (2 mg)	2/15 ***	1/15 *
Progesterone	11/15 NS	10/15 NS
Estradiol	15/15 *	14/15 ***
Estradiol (1 mg)	10/10 NS	10/10 ***
Estradiol (1 mg s.c.)	10/10 NS	10/10 ***
DOC-Ac	10/15 NS	7/15 NS
Hydroxydione	2/5 NS	0/5 NS
Cholesterol	10/15 NS	6/15 NS
Thyroxine	2/15 ***	0/15 **
Phenobarbital	9/10 NS	3/10 NS

[a] The rats of all groups were given ethylene glycol (0.8 ml/100 g body weight of a 100% solution, p.o., daily from the 4th day ff.).

[b] Dyskinesia was estimated on the 5th day 5 hrs after injection and mortality listed 24 hrs later ("Exact Probability Test").

For further details on technique of tabulation cf. p. VIII.

Ethyl Ether ← Gonadectomy, Rb: Störtebecker 76,398/39*

Ethylmorphine ← cf. also Morphine

Tephly & Mannering G67,764/64: The N-demethylation of ethylmorphine by hepatic microsomes is competitively inhibited by estradiol, testosterone, androsterone, diethylstilbestrol and cortisol in vitro. "These findings are consistent with the view that steroids are normally-occurring substrates for oxidative drug-metabolizing enzymes in hepatic microsomes."

Tephly & Mannering G53,874/68: Estradiol, testosterone, androsterone, progesterone and cortisol inhibit competitively the oxidation of ethylmorphine and hexobarbital when added in vitro to hepatic microsomes of rats. The inhibitor constant for each steroid was the same, whether ethylmorphine or hexobarbital served as substrates. "Results are consistent with the concept that certain drugs and steroids are alternative substrates for a common microsomal mixed function oxidase system." The steroids were less potent inhibitors of chlorpromazine oxidation and the inhibition was not competitive in this case.

Furner & Stitzel G54,558/68: The hepatic microsomal metabolism of ethylmorphine, aniline and hexobarbital is diminished in vitro by previous adrenalectomy in the rat. Phenobarbital pretreatment of adrenalectomized rats raised the metabolism of all three substrates above the level characteristic of otherwise untreated, adrenalectomized controls. Exposure of adrenalectomized rats to cold stress, or treatment with cortisol, increased the metabolism of aniline and ethylmorphine, but further depressed that of hexobarbital. In intact rats, cold stress diminished hexobarbital metabolism in vitro. Apparently, both stress and phenobarbital can bring about changes in hepatic drug metabolism independent of the presence of the adrenals, and the two agents act through different mechanisms, since phenobarbital invariably stimulates, whereas stress either increases or decreases, microsomal-enzyme activity depending upon the drug pathway examined.

Castro et al. G77,615/70: Studies on the effect of adrenalectomy upon the N-demethylation of ethylmorphine (EM) "suggest that the well known decrease in drug-metabolizing activity seen in liver microsomes of adrenalectomized animals is not related to changes in cytochrome P-450 content or to a decrease in the ability of cytochrome P-450 to bind drug substrates. However, there appears to be a relationship between the reductase activities and the adrenal function, because the changes in activities in NADPH cytochrome c reductase and cytochrome P-450 reductase in liver microsomes from adrenalectomized and cortisone-treated adrenalectomized rats paralleled the changes in EM demethylase activity."

Gerald & Feller G74,396/70: In mice, spironolactone and its Δ^6 de-thioacetylated metabolite reduce hexobarbital sleeping time and cause nearly identical increases in liver weight, microsomal protein content, NADPH-cytochrome c reductase, cytochrome P-450 content and the N-demethylation of ethylmorphine. Preliminary observations suggest that these actions of spironolactone and its metabolite are evident in both sexes.

Selye G70,480/71: In rats, the motor disturbances and the mortality produced by ethylmorphine intoxication are well prevented by all catatoxic steroids as well as by prednisolone, progesterone, estradiol, DOC and phenobarbital. The protection by prednisolone appears to be independent of glucocorticoid activity since triamcinolone (a stronger glucocorticoid) offers no protection, *cf.* Table 57.

Table 57. *Conditioning for ethylmorphine*

Treatment[a]	Dyskinesia[b] (Positive/ Total)	Mortality[b] (Dead/ Total)
None	14/15	11/15
PCN	0/10 ***	0/10 ***
CS-1	0/10 ***	0/10 ***
Ethylestrenol	0/10 ***	0/10 ***
Spironolactone	0/10 ***	0/10 ***
Norbolethone	2/10 ***	2/10 *
Oxandrolone	3/10 ***	3/10 *
Prednisolone-Ac	4/10 **	4/10 NS
Triamcinolone	10/10 NS	10/10 NS
Progesterone	3/10 ***	3/10 *
Estradiol	1/10 ***	1/10 ***
DOC-Ac	4/10 **	3/10 *
Hydroxydione	9/10 NS	9/10 NS
Thyroxine	10/10 NS	8/10 NS
Phenobarbital	0/10 ***	0/10 ***

[a] The rats of all groups were given ethylmorphine HCl (20 mg/100 g body weight in 0.2 ml water, once on 4th day s.c.).

[b] Dyskinesia was estimated 3 hrs after injection and mortality registered 24 hrs later ("Exact Probability Test").

For further details on technique of tabulation *cf.* p. VIII.

Stripp et al. G79,538/71: In rats, the induction of hepatic microsomal enzymes by spironolactone "differed from the phenobarbital or methylcholanthrene induction in that it did not increase cytochrome P-450 content or microsomal protein. Furthermore the induction seemed to be sex dependent."

Ethylmorphine ← Gonadectomy: Davies et al. H22,054/68

Ethylmorphine ← Cortisol + Phenobarbital: Lu et al. G68,802/69

Fencamfamine ←

Blackham & Spencer G76,301/69: In female mice, pretreatment with lynestrenol (a luteoid) reduced the hyperthermia induced by dexamphetamine, whereas mestranol (a folliculoid) increased it. Fencamfamine (also a CNS-stimulant) failed to induce hyperthermia in control or lynestrenol-pretreated mice but did raise the temperature after mestranol pretreatment. The potentiating effect of mestranol could be mimicked by pretreatment with nialamide (a MAO-inhibitor) but not by SKF 525-A. Increased locomotor activity induced by dexamphetamine and fencamfamine was enhanced by mestranol and reduced by lynestrenol. Dopamine, norepinephrine and 5-HT levels in the brain were reduced by lynestrenol and 5-HT was increased by mestranol. "If the actions of dexamphetamine (and fencamfamin) are due predominantly to the release of endogenous amines, then an increase (with lynestrenol) or a decrease (with mestranol) of tissue MAO activity should change the potency of these two stimulant drugs."

Fencamfamine ← Mestranol, Lynestrenol + Crowding: Blackham et al. G76,301/69*

Flufenamic Acid ←

Selye PROT. 38279: In rats, PCN, CS-1, ethylestrenol, spironolactone and phenobarbital offered highly significant protection against the production of intestinal ulcers by flufenamic acid. At the same time, the lethal effect of the drug was also diminished, but not always significantly, presumably because under the conditions of this experiment the mortality was not particularly high even among the unpretreated controls. Glucocorticoids and thyroxine greatly increased mortality, *cf.* Table 58, p. 245.

N-2-Fluorenyldiacetamide ← *cf.* Carcinogens

Fluoride ←

Gedalia et al. F17,787/64: In rats, increased fluoride intake inhibits the osteosclerotic effect of estradiol.

Furstman et al. G31,603/65: Histologic studies on the interaction of cortisol and fluoride in the induction of changes in the mandibular joint of the rat.

Table 58. *Conditioning for flufenamic acid*

Treatment[a]	Intestinal ulcers[b] (Positive/Total)	Mortality[b] (Dead/Total)
None	13/14	7/15
PCN	1/10 ***	1/10 NS
CS-1	2/10 ***	1/10 NS
Ethylestrenol	2/10 ***	0/10 *
Spironolactone	2/10 ***	1/10 NS
Norbolethone	5/10 *	2/10 NS
Oxandrolone	8/10 NS	2/10 NS
Prednisolone-Ac	7/8 NS	10/10 **
Triamcinolone	1/1[c]	10/10 **
Triamcinolone (1 mg)	7/7 NS	9/10 *
Progesterone	7/10 NS	6/10 NS
Estradiol	3/7 *	5/10 NS
DOC-Ac	9/10 NS	7/10 NS
Hydroxydione	7/10 NS	4/10 NS
Thyroxine	9/12 NS	13/15 *
Phenobarbital	3/10 ***	0/10 *

[a] The rats of all groups were given flufenamic acid, 10 mg/100 g body weight in 0.2 ml water s.c. twice daily from 4th day.

[b] Intestinal ulcers were appraised on day of death and mortality was listed on the 9th day ("Exact Probability Test").

[c] Only one of the animals in this group survived long enough to permit meaningful appraisal of intestinal ulcers.

For further details on technique of tabulations cf. p. VIII.

5-Fluorouracil ←

Ambre H24,704/70: In rats, pretreatment with a single dose of prednisolone protected against the lethality of 5-fluorouracil.

Fluphenazine ←

Selye PROT. 39639: In rats, PCN, CS-1 and to a lesser extent ethylestrenol, prednisolone and possibly DOC protect against otherwise fatal fluphenazine intoxication. The other standard conditioners of our series are inactive, cf. Table 59.

Flurothyl ←

Davis & Mei Quey Su H31,927/69: In rats, the convulsive effect of flurothyl is diminished by adrenalectomy.

Formaldehyde cf. Selye B40,000/50, pp. 392, 393, 534, 589, 751; B58,650/51, pp. 244, 248.

Ganglioplegics ←

Masson et al. B47,635/50: In dogs pretreated with DOC + uninephrectomy + NaCl, the hypotensive effect of TEA was not significantly altered. Similarly, both in rats and in dogs, the pressor action of epinephrine, norepinephrine, renin and angiotensin was not consistently altered by previous uninephrectomy and treatment with DOC + NaCl.

Brust et al. B57,917/51: In man, "administration of ACTH or cortisone significantly alters the blood pressure and 'TEAC floor.' The responses are independent of sodium retention and indicate that the vascular effects of these drugs are mediated by a humoral mechanism which is potentiated by autonomic blockade." Observations on both normotensive and hypertensive patients showed that "the usual depressor effects of TEAC were ultimately converted to a pressor rise, suggesting that autonomic blockade potentiates the vascular effects of ACTH and cortisone." DOC exhibited no such action.

Table 59. *Conditioning for fluphenazine*

Treatment[a]	Dyskinesia[b] (Positive/Total)	Mortality[b] (Dead/Total)
None	13/15	13/15
PCN	1/10 ***	1/10 ***
PCN (1 mg)	1/5 *	1/5 *
CS-1	0/10 ***	1/10 ***
Ethylestrenol	4/10 *	4/10 *
Spironolactone	8/15 NS	8/15 NS
Norbolethone	5/10 NS	6/10 NS
Oxandrolone	9/10 NS	9/10 NS
Prednisolone-Ac	4/10 *	4/10 *
Triamcinolone	10/10 NS	10/10 NS
Progesterone	5/10 NS	5/10 NS
Estradiol	10/10 NS	10/10 NS
DOC-Ac	4/10 *	4/10 *
Hydroxydione	7/10 NS	7/10 NS
Thyroxine	10/10 NS	10/10 NS
Phenobarbital	7/10 NS	7/10 NS

[a] The rats of all groups were given fluphenazine di-HCl, 8 mg/100 g body weight in 1 ml water i.p. once on the 4th day.

[b] Dyskinesia was estimated on the 8th day and mortality listed on the 9th day. ("Exact Probability Test").

For further details on technique of tabulation cf. p. VIII.

Table 60. *Protection by glucocorticoids and stressors against certain ganglioplegics*

A. *Lack of protection by catatoxic steroids against hexamethonium and TEA*

Treatment	Dyskinesia[a] (Positive/Total)		Mortality[a] (Dead/Total)	
	Hexa-methonium	TEA	Hexa-methonium	TEA
None	10/10	19/20	3/10	19/20
Ethylestrenol	9/10 NS	10/10 NS	1/10 NS	7/10 NS
CS-1	9/10 NS	10/10 NS	3/10 NS	10/10 NS
Spironolactone	10/10 NS	10/10 NS	2/10 NS	10/10 NS
Norbolethone	10/10 NS	10/10 NS	1/10 NS	9/10 NS
Oxandrolone	8/10 NS	10/10 NS	2/10 NS	10/10 NS
Prednisolone-Ac	0/10 ***	5/10 **	0/10 NS	2/10 ***
Triamcinolone	0/10 ***	0/10 ***	0/10 NS	0/10 ***
Progesterone	10/10 NS	10/10 NS	1/10 NS	6/10 *
DOC-Ac	10/10 NS	10/10 NS	3/10 NS	9/10 NS
Hydroxydione	10/10 NS	10/10 NS	3/10 NS	9/10 NS
Estradiol	9/10 NS	10/10 NS	0/10 NS	5/10 **

B. *Protection by glucocorticoids against TEA, hexamethonium and pentolinium*

Treatment	TEA	Dyskinesia[a] (Positive/Total)		TEA	Mortality[a] (Dead/Total)	
		Hexa-meth.	Pentol.		Hexa-meth.	Pentol.
None	10/10	8/10	10/10	12/15	5/10	6/10
Cortisol-Ac 10 mg	3/10 ***	0/10 ***	1/10 ***	1/10 ***	0/10 *	1/10 *
Cortisone-Ac 10 mg	5/10 *	0/10 ***	0/10 ***	3/10 *	0/10 *	0/10 **
Triamcinolone 10 mg	5/10 *	1/10 ***	0/10 ***	1/10 ***	0/10 *	0/10 **
Dexamethasone-Ac 2 mg	4/10 **	0/10 ***	1/10 ***	1/10 ***	0/10 *	0/10 **
Betamethasone-Ac 2 mg	3/10 ***	0/10 ***	0/10 ***	2/10 ***	0/10 *	0/10 **
Prednisolone-Ac 10 mg	7/10 NS	0/10 ***	0/10 ***	1/10 ***	0/10 *	0/10 **
Prednisone-Ac 10 mg	8/10 NS	0/10 ***	0/10 ***	3/10 *	0/10 *	0/10 **

C. *Comparative effects of stressors, cortisol and ACTH upon TEA intoxication*

Treatment	Dyskinesia[a] (Positive/Total)	Mortality[a] (Dead/Total)	Weight (mg ± S.E.)	
			Adrenal	Thymus
None	10/10	8/10	18.5 ± 0.9	376 ± 42
Bone fractures	0/10 ***	0/10 ***	19.1 ± 0.5 NS	286 ± 25 NS
Fasting	0/10 ***	0/10 ***	17.2 ± 1.1 NS	239 ± 16 **
Spinal cord lesion	2/11 ***	2/11 *	21.8 ± 0.9 *	196 ± 15 ***
Formalin	0/10 ***	0/10 ***	18.1 ± 0.4 NS	226 ± 18 **
Restraint	6/10 *	6/10 NS	20.2 ± 1.0 NS	123 ± 12 ***
Cold	8/10 NS	8/10 NS	20.2 ± 1.0 NS	289 ± 32 NS
Hemorrhage	9/10 NS	8/10 NS	19.6 ± 0.6 NS	273 ± 24 NS
Cortisol-Ac	0/10 ***	0/10 ***	12.0 ± 0.3 ***	35 ± 3 ***
ACTH	8/10 NS	8/10 NS	26.3 ± 1.1 ***	182 ± 28 **

[a] Dyskinesia was estimated 30 min after injection and mortality listed 24 hrs later ("Exact Probability Test").

For further details on technique of tabulation cf. p. VIII.

Bonino C13,016/55: In guinea pigs, ovariectomy increases resistance to lethal doses of hexamethonium.

Sturtevant C9,089/55; C21,591/56: In rats with metacorticoid hypertension (produced by temporary overdosage with DOC + NaCl), the pressor effect of epinephrine, norepinephrine, vasopressin and renin was increased but the effect of histamine, 5-HT, yohimbine and TEA on the blood pressure was not consistently altered.

Weil G68,214/61: In rats, prednisolone i.p. "which protects against the lethal effects of endotoxin, is not effective in protecting against lethal amounts of ganglionic blocking agents (mecamylamine, chlorpromazine), adrenergic blocking drugs (dibenzyline), or sympathomimetic amines (metaraminol). To the contrary, treatment with corticosteroid is associated with a significant increase in fatality in animals injected with mecamylamine and chlorpromazine ($p = <0.01$)." These findings are interpreted as evidence against the assumption that glucocorticoids protect in a nonspecific manner against injuries that produce hypotension.

Selye G70,448/70: In rats, various glucocorticoids and stressors offer protection against certain ganglioplegics, whereas highly active typical catatoxic steroids are ineffective in this respect as shown by Table 60. **A**: Pretreatment for 4 days with various typically catatoxic steroids fails to protect against hexamethonium or TEA. **B**: Pretreatment with a single dose of various glucocorticoids p.o., 4 hrs before the ganglioplegics, uniformly offers good protection against TEA, hexamethonium and pentolinium. **C**: Pretreatment for 4 days with various stressors (bone fractures, fasting, spinal cord transection, formalin, restraint) protects the rat against TEA intoxication as does cortisol or the endogenous glucocorticoids secreted under the influence of ACTH. On the other hand, unexpectedly, similar exposure to the stress of cold or hemorrhage offers no significant protection.

Gwee & Lim G81,043/71: In mice, cortisol sodium succinate given one hour before hemicholinium-3 (HC-3) or its p-terphenyl analogue (TPHC-3), offered very slight protection against the fatal effects of these ganglioplegics.

Selye G70,480/71: In rats, hexamethonium intoxication was completely prevented by pretreatment with prednisolone or triamcinolone, but unaffected by all other standard conditioning agents of our series, *cf.* Table 61.

Table 61. *Conditioning for hexamethonium*

Treatment[a]	Dyskinesia[b] (Positive/Total)	Mortality[b] (Dead/Total)
None	10/10	3/10
PCN	10/10 NS	5/10 NS
CS-1	9/10 NS	3/10 NS
Ethylestrenol	9/10 NS	1/10 NS
Spironolactone	10/10 NS	2/10 NS
Norbolethone	10/10 NS	1/10 NS
Oxandrolone	8/10 NS	2/10 NS
Prednisolone-Ac	0/10 ***	0/10 NS
Triamcinolone	0/10 ***	0/10 NS
Progesterone	10/10 NS	1/10 NS
Estradiol	9/10 NS	0/10 NS
DOC-Ac	10/10 NS	3/10 NS
Hydroxydione	10/10 NS	3/10 NS
Thyroxine	7/10 NS	1/10 NS
Phenobarbital	10/10 NS	1/10 NS

[a] The rats of all groups were given hexamethonium chloride (8 mg/100 g body weight in 0.2 ml water, s.c., once on 4th day).

[b] Dyskinesia was estimated 30 min after injection and mortality listed 24 hrs later ("Exact Probability Test").

For further details on technique of tabulation *cf.* p. VIII.

Selye G70,480/71: In rats, prednisolone offered partial, triamcinolone complete protection against TEA intoxication. Estradiol, phenobarbital and perhaps to a lesser extent even progesterone and thyroxine diminished the mortality without preventing the characteristic motor disturbances, *cf.* Table 62, p. 248.

D-Glucose-6-phosphate ← *cf. G-6-P-ase* under *Influence of Steroids upon Enzymes*

Glutamic Acid ←

Brin & McKee C31,261/56: In the rat, various stressors (total body X-irradiation, nitrogen mustard, starvation) as well as cortisone increase glutamic-aspartic and glutamic-alanine transaminase activities in the liver. Adrenalectomy decreases the activity of these enzymes. The glutamic-alanine enzyme is more sensitive to stress than the glutamic-aspartic enzyme.

Glutethimide ←

Selye PROT. 39300: In rats, glutethimide sleeping time is considerably shortened by

Table 62. *Conditioning for TEA*

Treatment[a]	Dyskinesia[b] (Positive/Total)	Mortality[b] (Dead/Total)
None	19/20	19/20
PCN	10/10 NS	10/10 NS
CS-1	10/10 NS	10/10 NS
Ethylestrenol	10/10 NS	7/10 NS
Spironolactone	10/10 NS	10/10 NS
Norbolethone	10/10 NS	9/10 NS
Oxandrolone	10/10 NS	10/10 NS
Prednisolone-Ac	5/10 **	2/10 ***
Triamcinolone	0/10 ***	0/10 ***
Progesterone	10/10 NS	6/10 *
Estradiol	10/10 NS	5/10 **
DOC-Ac	10/10 NS	9/10 NS
Hydroxydione	10/10 NS	9/10 NS
Thyroxine	9/10 NS	6/10 *
Phenobarbital	10/10 NS	3/10 ***

[a] The rats of all groups were given TEA, tetraethylammonium chloride (10 mg/100 g body weight in 0.2 ml water, s.c., once on 4th day.

[b] Dyskinesia was estimated 30 min after injection and mortality listed on 5th day ("Exact Probability Test").

For further details on technique of tabulation cf. p. VIII.

PCN, CS-1, ethylestrenol, spironolactone, norbolethone, prednisolone, triamcinolone and phenobarbital. To a lesser extent oxandrolone and estradiol exert similar effects, cf. Table 63.

Glycerol ←

Selye *PROT. 39225:* In rats, the characteristic nephrocalcinosis produced by glycerol s.c. was prevented by ethylestrenol, prednisolone and thyroxine, diminished by phenobarbital, oxandrolone, progesterone and tolerable doses of triamcinolone, but not influenced by the other standard conditioners of our series, cf. Table 64.

Glycolic Acid ←

Richardson *G45,620/67:* "Dietary glycolate markedly increased oxalate deposition in kidneys of normal and castrated males, caused only a limited increase in normal females, and no increase in ovariectomized females. With the exception of normal males, testosterone increased oxalate deposition in kidneys of rats fed 2% glycolate."

Gold ←

Grether et al. *C12,471/52:* Cortisone failed to affect the toxicity of gold sodium thioglucose in the rat.

Griseofulvin ← cf. Antibiotics

Hemin ← Adrenalectomy + Prednisolone + Zymosan: Tenhunen et al. *G73,193/70*

Heptachlor ← cf. Pesticides

Hexadimethrine ←

Tuchweber et al. *D27,884/63:* In rats, hypophysectomy prevents the nephrocalcinosis, but aggravates the adrenal necrosis, produced by hexadimethrine. ACTH-treatment of the hypophysectomized rat facilitates the production of nephrocalcinosis, but protects the adrenal. Adrenalectomy prevents this form of nephrocalcinosis even in rats maintained on NaCl or DOC. On the other hand, triamcinolone-treated adrenalectomized rats react

Table 63. *Conditioning for glutethimide*

Treatment[a]	Sleeping time[b] (min)	Mortality[b] (Dead/Total)
None	179 ± 21	0/14
PCN	8 ± 3 ***	0/10 NS
CS-1	29 ± 8 ***	0/10 NS
Ethylestrenol	16 ± 7 ***	0/10 NS
Spironolactone	37 ± 10 ***	0/10 NS
Norbolethone	40 ± 8 ***	0/10 NS
Oxandrolone	107 ± 25 *	0/10 NS
Prednisolone-Ac	47 ± 8 ***	0/10 NS
Triamcinolone	90 ± 0 ***	0/10 NS
Progesterone	182 ± 12 NS	0/10 NS
Estradiol	110 ± 9 **	0/10 NS
DOC-Ac	183 ± 34 NS	0/10 NS
Hydroxydione	188 ± 20 NS	0/10 NS
Thyroxine	196 ± 42 NS	1/10 NS
Phenobarbital	37 ± 7 ***	0/10 NS

[a] The rats of all groups were given glutethimide, 12 mg/100 g body weight in 1 ml water i.p. once on the 4th day.

[b] Sleeping time (Student's t-test).

Mortality was listed on the second day ("Exact Probability Test").

For further details on technique of tabulation cf. p. VIII.

Table 64. *Conditioning for glycerol*

Treatment[a]	Nephrocalcinosis[b] (Positive/Total)	Mortality[b] (Dead/Total)
None	13/15	8/15
PCN	8/14 NS	3/15 NS
CS-1	10/15 NS	1/15 **
Ethylestrenol	5/15 ***	3/15 NS
Spironolactone	10/15 NS	5/15 NS
Norbolethone	10/15 NS	1/15 **
Oxandrolone	6/13 *	3/15 NS
Prednisolone-Ac	0/4 ***	6/10 NS
Prednisolone-Ac (1 mg)	5/14 **	5/15 NS
Triamcinolone	—	10/10 **
Triamcinolone (1 mg)	5/15 **	3/15 NS
Progesterone	5/14 **	6/15 NS
Estradiol	7/13 NS	6/15 NS
DOC-Ac	10/14 NS	10/15 NS
Hydroxydione	9/15 NS	4/15 NS
Thyroxine	1/13 ***	4/15 NS
Phenobarbital	6/15 *	6/15 NS

[a] The rats of all groups were given glycerol 0.8 ml/100 g body weight of a 100% solution s.c. once on the 4th day.

[b] Nephrocalcinosis was estimated on day of death and mortality listed on the 9th day. ("Exact Probability Test").

For further details on technique of tabulation cf. p. VIII.

to hexadimethrine with strong nephrocalcinosis. Under similar conditions in intact rats, the corticoids did not significantly change the syndrome of hexadimethrine intoxication, except that the anaphylactoid reaction to this compound is inhibited by triamcinolone.

Hexamethonium ← cf. Ganglioplegics
Hg ← cf. Mercury
Homatropine Hydrobromide ←

Selye G70,480/71: In rats, homatropine hydrobromide (80 mg on the 4th day and 100 mg on the 5th day of conditioning, in 1 ml water) was administered p.o. /100 g body weight. Dyskinesia was listed on the 5th day 1 hr, and mortality 48 hrs after this injection. Under these circumstances, the "Standard Conditioners" (p. VIII) caused no noteworthy change in the resulting intoxication, only PCN exhibited an inhibitory effect. Phenobarbital was not tested.

Hydroquinone ←

Selye G70,480/71: In rats, the motor disturbances produced by hydroquinone intoxication were completely prevented by PCN, CS-1, ethylestrenol and phenobarbital, whereas prednisolone and triamcinolone increased their severity, cf. Table 65.

Table 65. *Conditioning for hydroquinone*

Treatment[a]	Dyskinesia[b] (Positive/Total)
None	7/15
PCN	0/13 **
CS-1	0/10 *
Ethylestrenol	0/15 ***
Spironolactone	3/15 NS
Norbolethone	4/10 NS
Oxandrolone	4/10 NS
Prednisolone-Ac	9/10 *
Triamcinolone	15/15 ***
Progesterone	2/9 NS
Estradiol	5/10 NS
DOC-Ac	4/10 NS
Hydroxydione	5/10 NS
Thyroxine	8/15 NS
Phenobarbital	0/13 **

[a] The rats of all groups were given hydroquinone (15 mg/100 g body weight in 0.2 ml water, s.c., on 4th day).

[b] Dyskinesia was estimated 15 min after injection ("Exact Probability Test").

For further details on technique of tabulation cf. p. VIII.

Imipramine ←

McClure & Cleghorn G76,696/68: In depressive psychotics, dexamethasone enhances the therapeutic effect of imipramine.

Selye PROT. 41834: In rats, imipramine intoxication is markedly inhibited by PCN, CS-1, ethylestrenol, spironolactone and phenobarbital. Estradiol exhibits a just barely significant protective effect, cf. Table 66, p. 250.

Indium Trichloride ←

Selye G70,480/71: In rats, indium trichloride (800 μg/100 g body weight in 1 ml water) was administered i.v. once on the 4th day of conditioning. Hepatic lipidosis was estimated on day of death, and mortality registered on the 9th day. Under these circumstances, the "Standard Conditioners" (p. VIII) caused no noteworthy change in the resulting intoxication. Phenobarbital was not tested.

Table 66. *Conditioning for imipramine*

Treatment[a]	Dyskinesia[b] (Positive/Total)	Mortality[b] (Dead/Total)
None	17/20	12/20
PCN	5/20 ***	5/20 *
CS-1	5/15 ***	6/15 NS
Ethylestrenol	7/20 ***	4/20 *
Spironolactone	6/20 ***	5/20 *
Norbolethone	9/14 NS	11/14 NS
Oxandrolone	9/15 NS	12/15 NS
Prednisolone-Ac	14/15 NS	9/15 NS
Triamcinolone	14/20 NS	8/20 NS
Progesterone	12/15 NS	6/15 NS
Estradiol	8/15 *	11/15 NS
DOC-Ac	14/15 NS	8/15 NS
Hydroxydione	14/15 NS	10/15 NS
Thyroxine	19/20 NS	14/20 NS
Phenobarbital	5/15	2/15 **

[a] The rats of all groups were given imipramine (65 mg/100 g body weight in 1 ml water, p.o., on 4th day).

[b] Dyskinesia was estimated on 4th day 3 hrs after injection and mortality listed on 5th day ("Exact Probability Test").

For further details on technique of tabulation cf. p. VIII.

Indometacin ← cf. also *Selye G60,083/70*, p. 385.

Selye G60,046/69: Both spironolactone and norbolethone protect the rat against the production of multiple intestinal ulcers and peritonitis by indomethacin.

Selye G60,058/69: In the rat, partial hepatectomy facilitates the production of perforating intestinal ulcers by indomethacin. Comparatively small doses of spironolactone readily inhibit this form of indomethacin intoxication even in the presence of surgically-induced hepatic insufficiency. "These results are compatible with the assumption that both indomethacin and spironolactone are subject to hepatic detoxication, and hence, their respective pathogenic and prophylactic actions are enhanced after extensive resection of liver tissue."

Aspinall H32,269/70: In rats, spironolactone can inhibit the ulcerogenic effect of indomethacin without blocking its antiphlogistic property (adjuvant arthritis test). This dissociation may be due to: 1. a direct protective action of spironolactone upon the intestinal tract, 2. the formation of indomethacin metabolites which retain antiphlogistic but loose ulcerogenic properties or 3. a mere diminution of indomethacin activity to a level sufficient to inhibit inflammation without causing intestinal ulceration.

Selye G66,066/70: In the rat, the production of perforating jejunal ulcers and peritonitis by indomethacin can be prevented by ethylestrenol, CS-1, spironolactone, norbolethone and oxandrolone. Progesterone and prednisolone are less active, triamcinolone and hydroxydione inactive.

Selye G70,421/70; G70,480/71: In rats, formation of perforating intestinal ulcers and the consequent mortality produced by indomethacin intoxication are prevented by all classic catatoxic steroids, as well as by prednisolone, progesterone and phenobarbital, cf. Table 67.

Table 67. *Conditioning for indomethacin*

Treatment[a]	Intestinal ulcers[b] (Positive/Total)	Mortality[b] (Dead/Total)
None	15/15	15/15
PCN	0/10 ***	0/10 ***
CS-1	0/10 ***	0/10 ***
Ethylestrenol	0/10 ***	0/10 ***
Spironolactone	0/10 ***	0/10 ***
Norbolethone	0/10 ***	0/10 ***
Oxandrolone	0/10 ***	0/10 ***
Prednisolone-Ac	0/10 ***	4/10 ***
Triamcinolone (2 mg)	10/10 NS	10/10 NS
Progesterone	3/10 ***	1/10 ***
Estradiol (1 mg)	9/9 NS	10/10 NS
DOC-Ac	10/10 NS	7/10 NS
Hydroxydione	10/10 NS	8/10 NS
Thyroxine	7/8 NS	10/10 NS
Phenobarbital	0/9 ***	0/9 ***

[a] The rats of all groups were given indomethacin (1 mg in 0.2 ml water, s.c., once daily, from 4th day ff.).

[b] Intestinal ulcers were appraised on day of death, but only in animals which survived at least 6 days and mortality was listed on 10th day ("Exact Probability Test").

For additional pertinent data cf. also Table 135.

For further details on technique of tabulation cf. p. VIII.

← Steroids

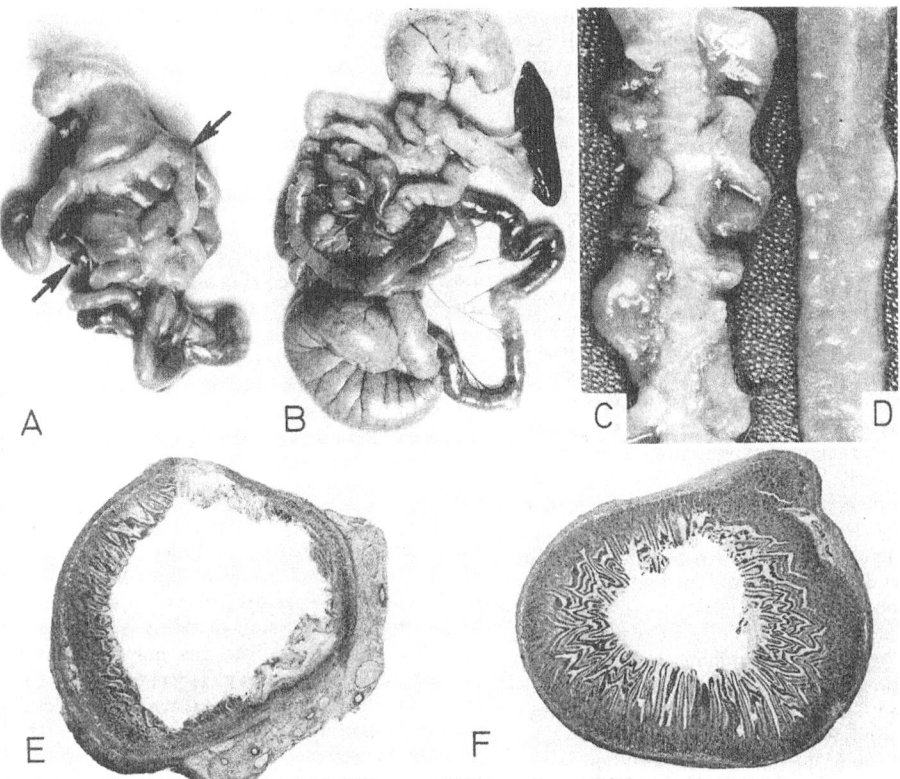

Fig. 8. **Prevention of indomethacin-induced intestinal ulcers by spironolactone.** All animals received the same dose of indomethacin. A: Intestinal tract of otherwise-untreated control rat. The jejunal segment (between 2 arrows) forms a packet of intestinal loops connected by fibrin threads to each other as well as to the pancreas (top arrow) and stomach. B: Normal intestinal tract of rat pretreated with indomethacin. Stomach, spleen and pancreas (upper right corner) as well as all intestinal loops are free of adhesions. C: Gross view of intestinal ulcer which runs along the entire length of the mesenteric attachment. The resulting lesions are responsible for the folding of this jejunal segment (viewed here from the mucosal side) in the control rat. D: In animal pretreated with spironolactone, the jejunal mucosa is of normal appearance. E: Section through the jejunum of control rat shows large ulcer along mesenteric attachment (right side), which is close to perforation at several points. F: In animal pretreated with spironolactone, the jejunal mucosa is normal. [Selye G 60,046/69. Courtesy Can. J. Physiol. Pharmacol.]

Selye G70,428/70: In rats, ethylestrenol powerfully inhibits the toxicity of digitoxin, nicotine, indomethacin, phenindione, dioxathion, EPN, physostigmine, hexobarbital, cyclopental, thiopental, DOC (anesthesia), meprobamate and picrotoxin. Thyroxine increases the toxicity of many among these drugs and inhibits the protective effect of ethylestrenol.

Solymoss et al. G60,093/70: In rats, spironolactone, norbolethone and progesterone, unlike hydroxydione, accelerate the clearance from the blood of s.c.-injected indomethacin. SKF 525-A significantly suppresses the activity of these steroids which probably act through increased metabolic degradation of indomethacin.

Solymoss et al. G70,441/70: In rats, spironolactone or oxandrolone given for as long as two months, continues to exhibit a protective effect against fatal doses of digitoxin or indomethacin. Upon withdrawal of the catatoxic steroids, continued administration of digitoxin or indomethacin is rapidly fatal. The plasma concentration of digitoxin and indomethacin is diminished during the catatoxic steroid administration.

Selye G70,480/71: In rats, the indomethacin-induced intestinal ulcers and mortality are inhibited by PCN, CS-1, cyproterone, ethylestrenol, spironolactone, norbolethone, TMACN, oxandrolone, 6α-methylprednisolone, fluoxymesterone, spiroxasone, 16β-methyl-16,17-epoxy-3β,11α-dihydroxy-5α-pregnan-20-one, prednisolone, dexamethasone, betamethasone, emdabol, 17α-acetoxyprogesterone, corticosterone, dehydroisoandrosterone, pregnanedione, progesterone, DOC and 11α-hydroxyprogesterone. The syndrome of indomethacin intoxication is not significantly inhibited by MAD, testosterone, triamcinolone, hydroxydione-fluorocortisol, cortisol, cortisone and estradiol.

Szabo et al. G79,013/71: In hamsters, spironolactone and ethylestrenol pretreatment prevents digitoxin convulsions and indomethacin-induced intestinal ulcers.

Szabo et al. G79,024/71: In rats, PCN increases resistance to indomethacin, hexobarbital, progesterone, zoxazolamine and digitoxin, both in the presence and in the absence of the pituitary. Hypophysectomy also fails to prevent the induction of SER proliferation in the hepatocytes.

Selye PROT. 25007, 32215: In rats, the protection against indomethacin and digitoxin intoxication by pretreatment with spironolactone can be blocked by concurrent pretreatment with metyrapone.

Selye PROT. 28397: In mice, indomethacin intoxication can be prevented by ethylestrenol, CS-1, spironolactone, norbolethone and to a lesser extent perhaps also by prednisolone and estradiol administered by various routes. Thyroxine appears to have an opposite effect. Progesterone, triamcinolone, DOC and hydroxydione had little if any effect.

Selye PROT. 22030: In adrenalectomized rats maintained in good condition by cortisol, DOC or cortisol + DOC with the substitution of 1% NaCl as drinking fluid, spironolactone offers excellent protection against the mortality and somewhat inhibits the ulcerogenic effects of indomethacin. Large doses of spironolactone (10 mg) are effective in this respect even in adrenalectomized rats maintained on 1% NaCl alone, cf. Table 68.

Selye PROT. 29958: In adrenalectomized rats maintained on 1% NaCl alone, the lethal effect of indomethacin is increased and intestinal ulcers develop just as frequently as in intact controls. Small doses of spironolactone (0.3 mg) protect the rats only partially against the mortality and ulcerogenesis induced by indomethacin, whereas concurrent administration of cortisol, DOC or cortisol + DOC appears to improve the protective effect of spironolactone, cf. Table 69.

Selye PROT. 32221, 32230, 32255: In adrenalectomized rats maintained on DOC, cortisol or DOC + cortisol, threshold doses of spironolactone still offer protection against mortality. In the absence of corticoid maintenance

Table 68. *Effect of adrenalectomy and corticoid substitution therapy upon the protection by spironolactone against indomethacin*

Group	Treatment[a]	Intestinal ulcers[b] frequency (Positive/Total)	Mortality[b] (Dead/Total)
1	None	4/18	18/18
2	Spironolactone	0/11	2/11
3	Spironolactone + Cortisol	0/15	0/15
4	Spironolactone + DOC	0/14	3/15
5	Spironolactone + DOC + Cortisol	0/16	0/16

[a] All rats were adrenalectomized on 1st day and given 1% NaCl as drinking fluid. They all received indomethacin 1 mg in 0.2 ml water, s.c./day, 4th day ff. The groups so designated were given spironolactone 10 mg in 1 ml water, p.o., x2/day, cortisol acetate 0.5 mg and DOC acetate 1 mg in 0.2 ml water, s.c./day, 1st day ff.

[b] Intestinal ulcers on day of death; mortality up to 9th day when experiment was terminated.

therapy, however these doses of spironolactone failed to diminish the lethal effect of indomethacin significantly. The ulcerogenic effect is difficult to interpret in these series because of the high mortality and the postmortal decomposition. In any event it is clear that cortisol + DOC increase resistance to the lethal effect of indomethacin but have little or no influence upon the ulcerogenic action, *cf.* Tables 70, 71.

Selye *PROT. 34038, 34405:* In rats of different age groups, the anti-indomethacin effect of PCN is essentially the same if administered at dose levels adjusted to body weight, *cf.* Table 72, p. 254.

Selye *PROT. 42269:* In rats chronically poisoned with digitoxin (0.5—1.0 mg, p.o./day) or indomethacin (0.75 mg, s.c./day), the administration of PCN (1 mg x2/day, p.o., beginning on the 3rd or 4th day of treatment with the toxicants), when clinical signs of poisoning were already evident, caused these to disappear and permitted survival, whereas the controls receiving no PCN invariably died. These experiments show that, although presumably the protective effect of PCN against

Table 69. *Effect of adrenalectomy and corticoid substitution therapy upon the protection by spironolactone against indomethacin*

Group	Treatment[a]	Intestinal ulcers[b] frequency (Positive/Total)	Mortality[b] (Dead/Total)
1	None (Indomethacin + NaCl only)	7/15	0/15
2	None (Indomethacin + NaCl + Adrenalectomy only)	11/14	15/17
3	Spironolactone	1/16	9/17
4	Spironolactone + Cortisol	0/16	0/16
5	Spironolactone + DOC	0/15	1/15
6	Spironolactone + DOC + Cortisol	0/14	0/14

[a] Groups 2—6 were adrenalectomized on 1st day. The rats of all groups received indomethacin 0.5 mg in 0.2 ml water, s.c./day, 4th day ff. and 1% NaCl as drinking fluid, 1st day ff. Spironolactone 0.3 mg in 1 ml water, p.o., x2/day, cortisol acetate 0.5 mg and DOC acetate 1 mg in 0.2 ml water, s.c./day, 1st day ff.

[b] Intestinal ulcers and mortality on 9th day.

Table 70. *Effect of corticoids on indomethacin intoxication in intact and adrenalectomized rats*

Treatment[a]	Intestinal ulcers[b] (Positive/Total)		Mortality[b] (Dead/Total)	
	Control	Adrenalectomy	Control	Adrenalectomy
None	9/9	3/4	9/10	11/11
Spironolactone	6/10 NS	5/8 NS	0/10 ***	8/11 N.S.
Spironolactone + DOC-Ac	8/10 NS	10/12 NS	4/10 *	3/12 ***
Spironolactone + Cortisol-Ac	8/10 NS	9/12 NS	4/10 *	7/12 *
Spironolactone + Cortisol-Ac + DOC-Ac	9/10 NS	6/12 NS	2/10 ***	3/12 ***

[a] All animals received indomethacin 1 mg the 4th and the 5th day, 0.5 mg the 6th day in 0.2 ml water, s.c./day ff. The groups so designated were adrenalectomized on 1st day and given 1% NaCl as drinking fluid; spironolactone 0.3 mg in 1 ml water, p.o. x2/day, cortisol acetate 0.5 mg and DOC-acetate 1 mg in 0.2 ml water, s.c./day, 1st day ff.

[b] Intestinal ulcers on day of death; mortality up to 10th day when experiment was terminated (Fisher & Yates test).

For further details on technique of tabulation *cf.* p. VIII.

Table 71. *Effect of corticoids on indomethacin intoxication in intact and adrenalectomized rats*

Treatment[a]	Intestinal ulcers[b] (Positive/Total)		Mortality[b] (Dead/Total)	
	Control	Adrenal-ectomy	Control	Adrenal-ectomy
None	10/10	3/4	7/10	11/11
DOC-Ac	10/10 NS	9/10 NS	5/10 NS	12/12 NS
Cortisol-Ac	10/10 NS	12/12 NS	7/10 NS	11/12 NS
Cortisol-Ac + DOC-Ac	10/10 NS	12/12 NS	9/10 NS	10/12 NS
Spironolactone	7/10 NS	6/9 NS	4/10 NS	12/12 NS
Spironolactone + DOC-Ac	9/10 NS	7/11 NS	3/10 NS	7/11 *
Spironolactone + Cortisol-Ac	8/10 NS	11/12 NS	4/10 NS	7/12 *
Spironolactone + Cortisol-Ac + DOC-Ac	9/10 NS	10/12 NS	6/10 NS	6/12 **

[a] All animals received indomethacin 1 mg the 4th and the 5th day, 0.5 mg the 6th day in 0.2 ml water, s.c./day ff. The groups so designated were adrenalectomized on 1st day and given 1% NaCl as drinking fluid; spironolactone 0.2 mg in 1 ml water, p.o. x2/day, cortisol acetate 0.5 mg and DOC-acetate 1 mg in 0.2 ml water, s.c./day, 1st day ff.

[b] Intestinal ulcers on day of death; mortality up to 10th day when experiment was terminated (Fisher & Yates test).

For further details on technique of tabulation cf. p. VIII.

Table 72. *Comparison of the anti-indomethacin effect of PCN in rats of various ages*

Body weight[a] (g)	Intestinal ulcers[b] (Positive/Total)		Mortality[b] (Dead/Total)	
	Control	PCN	Control	PCN
50	8/8	0/10 ***	6/8	0/10 ***
100	10/10	0/10 ***	8/10	0/10 ***
200	10/10	0/10 ***	8/10	0/10 ***
300	10/10	3/10 ***	7/10	0/10 ***

[a] The rats (♀) of all groups were given indomethacin 1 mg in 0.2 ml water, s.c./day, 4th day ff. The groups so designated received PCN 0.2 mg in 1 ml water, p.o. x2/day, 1st day ff. Doses per 100 g body weight.

[b] Intestinal ulcers and mortality on 9th day (Statistics Fisher & Yates).

For further details on technique of tabulation cf. p. VIII.

digitoxin and indomethacin depends upon the induction of drug-metabolizing enzymes, the steroid can act not only prophylactically but also curatively, if the intoxication is sufficiently slow to permit effective enzyme induction in time.

In interpreting all these data on indomethacin, it must be kept in mind that although this compound (like digitoxin) acted as a standard in our studies on the detoxication of substrates by catatoxic steroids, the mechanism of its accelerated bio-degradation has not yet been established.

Iodoacetate ←

Laszt & Verzar 34,843/35: The cessation of growth induced by chronic iodoacetate feeding in the rat is counteracted by an andrenocortical extract, "eucorton," s.c. A similar inhibition was obtained by feeding yeast or flavine phosphate.

Clark & Barnes A33,441/40: Adrenocortical extract offers no protection against iodoacetate intoxication in the rat.

Isoniazid ←

Ferraris C27,552/54; C30,097/56: In rats, ovariectomy increases resistance to lethal doses of isoniazid.

Mrozikiewicz & Strzyzewski G68,152/66; H7,524/67: In the mouse, isoniazid-induced convulsions are facilitated, not only by glucocorticoids (cortisol, prednisolone) and ACTH, but also by DOC.

Isoniazid ← Prednisone, Man: Levi et al. F99,523/68*

Isoproterenol ← cf. also Selye *C 92,918/61*, p. 117; *G 60,083/70*, p. 493.

Chappel et al. C 76,910/59: In rats, the production of myocardial necrosis by isoproterenol is facilitated by pretreatment with mineralocorticoids (DOC, F-COL) but not influenced by glucocorticoids (cortisone, triamcinolone).

Moudgil G 65,314/69: In rats, various antimineralocorticoids inhibited the production of cardiac necroses by isoproterenol in the following order: SC 5233 > SC 9420 (spironolactone) > CS-1 and SC 8109. The reported relative effectiveness of these compounds as aldosterone antagonists is CS-1 > SC 9420, SC 8109 > SC 5233.

K ← cf. **Potassium**

$KMnO_4$ ← cf. **Permanganate**

Lathyrogens ← **corticoids** cf. also Selye *C 92,918/61*, p. 137; *G 60,083/70*, p. 357.
Lathyrogens ← **folliculoids, testoids** cf. also Selye *G 60,083/70*, pp. 369, 378, 379.

RAT

Ponseti D 49,845/54: In rats fed Lathyrus odoratus seeds, testosterone does not significantly affect the development of osteo- and angiolathyric lesions.

Bean & Ponseti C 29,403/55: In rats chronically fed a sweet pea diet, dissecting aneurysms of the aorta were commonly found in combination with scoliosis and other lathyric skeletal lesions. Attention is called to the occasional occurrence of dissecting aneurysms in connection with scoliosis and other bone lesions in man (e.g., in Marfan's syndrome and related collagen diseases). Since, in rats, lathyrism was accompanied by testicular atrophy, it was attempted to prevent the lathyric aneurysms by testosterone, but the results were negative.

Dasler C 15,943/56: Cortisone added to the diet allegedly offered no protection against osteolathyrism in rats given APN p.o.

Hamre & Yeager D 76,147/56: In rats fed sweet peas, the development of osteolathyrism is inhibited by cortisone.

Selye & Bois C 18,280/56: In rats, the osteolathyrism produced by Lathyrus odoratus seeds is aggravated by STH and inhibited by cortisol. Combined treatment with DOC + uninephrectomy + NaCl resulted in dissecting aneurysms of the aorta. Very small doses of thyroxine or estradiol were without effect upon this form of lathyrism.

Dasler C 36,068/57: Brief mention of unpublished observations indicating that in rats, osteolathyrism produced by APN is not inhibited by cortisone or thyroxine, but aggravated by STH.

Diaz et al. C 50,497/57: Thyroxine inhibits the osteolathyrism produced in rats by methyleneaminoacetonitrile (MAAN). Estrogens allegedly have a similar, though somewhat less pronounced, effect. [The authors actually tested only estrone in combination with progesterone (H.S.).]

Meyer & Vos C 41,429/57: In rats kept on a Lathyrus odoratus meal, estradiol raised the resistance of males but decreased that of females. Cortisone moderately diminished the severity of scoliosis and of the exostoses whereas testosterone was without effect.

Selye & Bois C 22,712/57: In rats, osteolathyrism (produced by AAN) is inhibited by cortisol and augmented by STH. The combination of STH and AAN enhances the development of polyarthritis in the small joints of the extremities. DOC facilitates the production of aortic aneurysms by AAN.

Selye & Bois C 23,298/57: In rats, the osteolathyrism produced by AAN is suppressed by cortisol and uninfluenced by DOC, although the associated aortic aneurysm formation is aggravated by the mineralocorticoid. Combined treatment with DOC + COL so modifies the action of AAN that aortic aneurysms are produced in the virtual absence of bone lesions. "It is noteworthy that the individual morbid changes, characteristic of the malady, can be totally dissociated from each other by merely changing the mineralo- or glucocorticoid level of the milieu in which an experimental disease develops."

Selye C 31,369/57: In the rat, the osteolathyrism produced by AAN is aggravated by STH, LTH and partial hepatectomy but it is inhibited by ACTH, cortisol or estradiol.

Selye C 31,790/57: In rats, osteolathyrism produced by AAN is inhibited by thyroxine, cortisol and estradiol but aggravated by STH even after adrenalectomy.

Diaz et al. D 99,329/58: In rats, the osteolathyrism produced by methyleneaminoacetonitrile (MAAN) is mildly inhibited by progesterone and estrone, completely prevented by thyroxine and aggravated by thyroidectomy.

Selye C 28,810/58: In rats, osteolathyrism was produced by high doses of AAN. This treatment was discontinued when administration of various hormones began. Under these

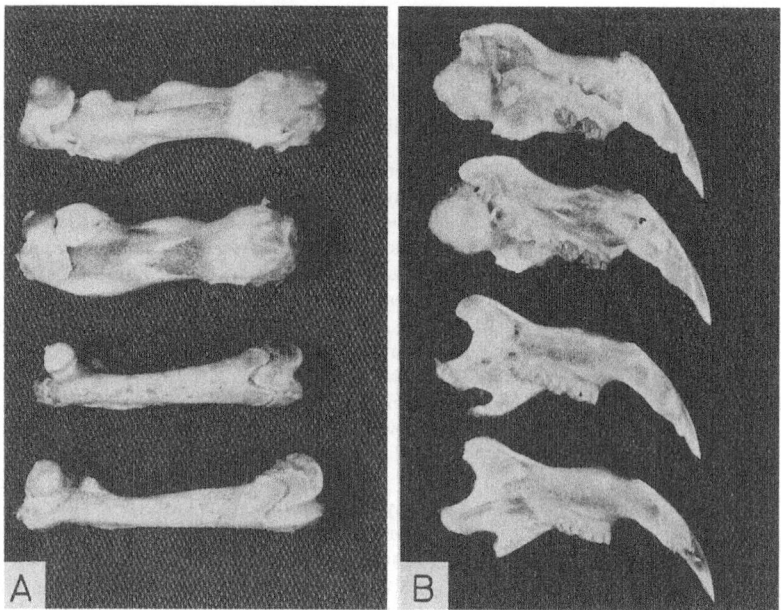

Fig. 9. **Effect of various hormones upon osteolathyrism.** All rats were treated with the same amount of aminoacetonitrile (AAN). Top to bottom: Otherwise untreated controls, animals treated with ethylestrenol, prednisolone and thyroxine, respectively. Note strong lathyric changes: A: femurs, B: mandibles (especially at tendon insertion sites) in the control and ethylestrenol-treated rat, whereas the bones of the animals receiving prednisolone or thyroxine are essentially normal

conditions, the healing of established osteolathyrism was accelerated by thyroxine and to a lesser extent by cortisol and estradiol. STH delayed healing, whereas methyltestosterone and DOC did not influence it significantly.

Wajda et al. C48,618/58: Lathyrism was produced in immature rats by feeding Lathyrus odoratus seeds, "whereas testosterone shortened the life span and increased the incidence of aortic rupture in female rats, estradiol increased survival time of both sexes and had no influence on aortic rupture."

Kowalewski et al. C63,273/59: In rats, osteolathyrism produced by a sweet pea diet inhibits the uptake of ^{35}S into fractured bones. Norethandrolone diminishes this inhibition.

Ponseti C68,050/59: In rats, the lathyric bone lesions produced by AAN were strongly suppressed by triiodothyronine and thyroxine, whereas those elicited by APN were much less evidently inhibited by these hormones. "Corticosterone and cortisone suppressed only slightly the lesions produced by aminoacetonitrile in rats."

Pyörälä et al. C67,833/59: Dissecting aneurysms of the aorta developed in 40% of immature rats fed Lathyrus odoratus. The media was remarkably thickened and the ground substance showed increased metachromasia and PAS reaction. This response was suppressed by cortisone and thyroxine but not by ACTH, TSH or DOC at the doses employed.

Aschkenasy C91,685/60: In male rats, the osteolathyrism produced by AAN is inhibited by a diet containing 18—30% casein. This protective effect is not seen in females or in orchidectomized males.

Kowalewski & Emery C86,516/60: In rats with osteolathyrism produced by APN, norethandrolone promotes the healing of bone fractures as judged by ^{35}S uptake into the mucopolysaccharides of the callus.

Gabay et al. D98,867/61: In rats, the osteolathyrism produced by methyleneaminoacetonitrile (MAAN) is associated with a considerable increase in bone hexosamine. This change is more effectively inhibited by thyroxine than by cortisone. Both hormones are virtually ineffective in protecting against osteolathyrism produced by the feeding of Lathyrus odoratus seeds.

Selye & Cantin C 88,878/61: In rats, the osteolathyrism produced by AAN is inhibited by thyroxine and cortisol but aggravated by STH. The cardiac infarcts elicited in rats by ligature of the descending branch of the left coronary artery are often transformed into rupturing cardiac aneurysms under the influence of AAN. The incidence of these cardiac ruptures is augmented by cortisol and DOC, but not significantly influenced by thyroxine and STH. Evidently, there is no direct relationship between the skeletal and the cardiac lesions under these circumstances.

Wiancko & Kowalewski D 270/61: In APN-treated rats, the healing of a humerus fracture (tensile strength of callus) is significantly decreased. This decrease was less pronounced in animals pretreated with cortisone, whereas fluoxymesterone (predominantly testoid) and methandrostenolone (predominantly anabolic) actually increase the tensile strength of the lathyric callus above the control (nonlathyric) level.

Aschkenasy D 30,892/62: In rats, lathyrism produced by AAN is aggravated by adrenalectomy and, in the absence of the adrenals, the usual antilathyric effect of cortisone is no longer demonstrable; in fact the glucocorticoid facilitates the production of hernias. STH aggravates the osteolathyrism but not the induction of hemorrhages by AAN.

Holzmann et al. F 56,165/65: In rats rendered osteolathyric by APN, severe histologic changes occur also in the skeletal musculature accompanied by corresponding variations in the serum level of muscle-specific enzymes, particularly creatinekinase and myokinase (adenylatekinase). These lesions can be partially suppressed by prednisone.

Holzmann et al. G 33,879/65: In rats, treatment with APN increases the serum transaminase activity. This effect is inhibited by prednisone but other blood enzyme changes are less markedly affected.

Trnavský et al. F 49,077/65: In rats kept on a diet of Lathyrus odoratus, cortisol inhibited the increase in the hydroxyproline content of the skin.

Korting et al. F 63,363/66: In rats made lathyric by APN, the GPT and the GOT activities of the serum are increased. Prednisone prevents this change.

Trnavská & Trnavský G 54,556/68: In rats, the collagen changes induced by feeding Lathyrus odoratus seeds are more effectively inhibited by salicylates, phenylbutazone and chloroquine than by cortisol.

Henneman H 12,251/69: Estradiol protects the rat against the skeletal and cutaneous changes produced by APN. "The data suggest estrogens induce the synthesis of a collagen which is resistant to lathyrogenic agents; this same collagen might be more resistant to the vicissitudes of age and hormonal imbalance."

Selye G 70,480/71: In rats, the osteolathyrism produced by aminoacetonitrile is readily prevented by prednisolone, triamcinolone and thyroxine, but not, or only doubtfully, affected by the other conditioners of our series. Large doses of glucocorticoids cause mortality in aminoacetonitrile treated animals, but much smaller doses suffice to prevent skeletal lesions, *cf.* Fig. 9, p. 256 and Table 73.

Table 73. *Conditioning for aminoacetonitrile*

Treatment[a]	Osteo-lathyrism[b] (Positive/Total)	Mortality[b] (Dead/Total)
None	10/10	0/10
PCN	8/10 NS	5/10 *
CS-1	7/10 NS	0/10 NS
Ethylestrenol	7/10 NS	0/10 NS
Spironolactone	7/10 NS	0/10 NS
Norbolethone	6/9 NS	0/9 NS
Oxandrolone	6/9 NS	0/9 NS
Prednisolone-Ac	0/13 ***	8/13 ***
Prednisolone-Ac (1 mg)	0/8 ***	0/8 NS
Triamcinolone	0/9 ***	10/10 ***
Triamcinolone (0.5 mg)	0/10 ***	0/10 NS
Progesterone	6/10 *	3/10 NS
Estradiol (1 mg)	5/10 *	1/10 NS
Estradiol (1 mg s.c.)	2/5 *	0/5 NS
DOC-Ac	5/9 *	0/9 NS
Hydroxydione	8/9 NS	4/9 *
Thyroxine	0/10 ***	0/10 NS
Phenobarbital	10/10 NS	0/10 NS

[a] The rats all of groups were given aminoacetonitrile, "AAN" (20 mg/100 g body weight in 1 ml water, p.o., twice daily from 4th day ff.).

[b] Osteolathyrism was assessed and mortality listed on 16th day ("Exact Probability Test").

For further details on technique of tabulation *cf.* p. VIII.

Varia

Cameron et al. D38,527/62: In **chicks**, the osteolathyrism produced by semicarbazide and acetone semicarbazone is only doubtfully inhibited by cortisone, prednisolone or DOC.

Simmons et al. G28,592/65: Detailed description of the bone lesions produced by AAN in the **mouse** and of their inhibition by estradiol.

Lead ←

Benkö 95,966/42: In rabbits, the porphyrinuria induced by lead intoxication could be prevented by nicotinamide given in combination with adrenocortical extracts, whereas neither of these agents exhibited prophylactic potency when given by itself.

Chiodi & Sammartino B52,225/50: In rats, the nephrotoxic effect of chronic lead feeding is inhibited by testosterone.

Lithium ←

Radomski et al. B63,492/50: In dogs, neither DOC nor adrenocortical extract affects the manifestations of lithium intoxication.

LSD ←

Pierre C55,459/57: In the rabbit, the EEG changes produced by LSD are prevented by hydroxydione.

Pierre et al. C46,326/57: Both methylandrostanolone and hydroxydione protect against chronic LSD intoxication. [Species not stated (H.S.).]

Pierre C52,727/58: In rabbits, the EEG changes characteristic of LSD intoxication are completely prevented by hydroxydione and androstanolone. 19-Nortestosterone and methylandrostanolone are somewhat less effective.

Bergen & Pincus C82,720/60: In rats, the behavioral changes induced by LSD can be suppressed by DOC, corticosterone, 17-dehydrocortisol, 11-dehydrocortisol, dehydroisoandrosterone, testosterone, androsterone, Δ^5-pregnenolone, etiocholanolone and progesterone. Other naturally occurring steroids tested were ineffective.

Bergen et al. C97,551/60: Earlier unpublished experiments had shown that the effect of LSD on smooth muscle contraction can be inhibited by various steroids added to the bathing medium in vitro. The authors reexamined this antagonism in vivo. The time required by a rat to climb a rope for a food reward is prolonged by LSD but this behavior change is counteracted by pretreatment during 3 days with i.p. injections of 1 mg quantities of dehydroisoandrosterone, Δ^4-androstenedione, cortisol, progesterone, testosterone, pregnenolone, DOC, dehydrocorticosterone, androsterone, etiocholanolone, corticosterone and 11-desoxycortisol approximately in decreasing order of activity. Of all steroids tested only estradiol was inactive in this respect.

Krus et al. G78,688/61: In normal man, "the magnitude of changes found to occur under LSD-25 in behavior representing sensorimotor, perceptual and conceptual levels of organization, was reduced when LSD ingestion was preceded by progesterone ingestion."

Bergen et al. E5,492/65: In the rat, progesterone, dehydroepiandrosterone and DOC, reduce the severity of LSD-induced "confusion." In rabbits, both LSD and progesterone alter the characteristics of optically evoked cortical potentials. "From the foregoing experimental results and the additional information that progesterone inhibits LSD metabolism in an in vitro system, it may be postulated that both drugs act on common cellular sites. It is suggested that progesterone may block the action of LSD by interfering with the LSD-receptor relationship of the cell."

Table 74. *Conditioning for LSD*

Treatment[a]	Dyskinesia[b]
None	11/15
PCN	0/14 ***
CS-1	0/10 ***
Ethylestrenol	2/15 ***
Spironolactone	6/15 NS
Norbolethone	1/10 ***
Oxandrolone	5/10 NS
Prednisolone-Ac	0/10 ***
Triamcinolone	0/15 ***
Progesterone	3/10 *
Estradiol	0/10 ***
DOC-Ac	4/8 NS
Hydroxydione	4/10 NS
Thyroxine	11/15 NS
Phenobarbital	3/10 *

[a] The rats of all groups were given D-lysergic acid diethylamid 100 µg/100 g body weight in 1 ml water i.v. once on the 4th day.

[b] Dyskinesia was estimated 30 min after injection ("Exact Probability Test").

For further details on technique of tabulation *cf*. p. VIII.

Selye PROT. 40258: In rats, the dyskinesia elicited by severe, but usually not fatal, LSD intoxication was well prevented by PCN, CS-1, ethylestrenol, norbolethone, prednisolone, triamcinolone and estradiol but only just significantly by progesterone and phenobarbital. The other standard conditioning agents remained without effect, cf. Table 74, p. 258.

Magnesium ← cf. also Selye C 92,918/61, pp. 87, 257; G 60,083/70, pp. 348, 357, 358.

Störtebecker A 1,993/37: In rabbits and mice, the depth of $MgSO_4$ anesthesia is influenced by sex hormones, as judged by observations in different phases of the estrous cycle as well as after injection of folliculin or androsterone. [In view of the wide individual variations and the small number of animals, the significance of the data is in doubt (H.S.).]

Störtebecker 76,398/39: In gonadectomized male and female mice, the anesthetic effect of $MgSO_4$ is increased, but it can be restored to about normal by both estrogenic and androgenic hormones.

Farnell H 15,528/68: In mice, cortisone inhibits the convulsions but aggravates the organ changes induced by Mg-deficiency.

Jasmin E 7,631/68: In rats, certain manifestations of the Mg-deficiency syndrome are inhibited by cortisol, hypophysectomy or thyroparathyroidectomy.

Whitfield & Tidball H 549/68: Rats ovariectomized and maintained on an Mg-deficient diet were either otherwise untreated or given 1 μg of estradiol per day. "The results indicate that estrogen given to an ovariectomized rat will significantly retard the rate and extent of development of dietary magnesium deficiency."

Selye et al. G 60,020/69: In the rat, pretreatment with norbolethone protects against the anesthetic effect of progesterone, DOC, pregnanedione, dehydroepiandrosterone, testosterone, diethylstilbestrol, pentobarbital and methyprylon. It does not significantly alter the corresponding actions of urethan, diazepam, chlorpromazine, reserpine, phenoxybenzamine, chloral hydrate, potassium bromide or magnesium chloride.

Selye et al. G 60,016/70: In rats, spironolactone protects against anesthesia produced by progesterone, DOC, hydroxydione, pregnanedione, dehydroepiandrosterone, testosterone, diethylstilbestrol, methyprylon, pentobarbital and ethanol. It does not significantly alter the corresponding actions of morphine, codeine, urethan, diazepam, chlorpromazine, reserpine, phenoxybenzamine, chloral hydrate, potassium bromide or $MgCl_2$.

$MgSO_4$ ← Gonadectomy + Testoids, Folliculoids, Mouse: Störtebecker 76,398/39*

MAO-Inhibitors ←

Blackham & Spencer G 76,301/69: In female mice, pretreatment with lynestrenol (a luteoid) reduced the hyperthermia induced by dexamphetamine, whereas mestranol (a folliculoid) increased it. Fencamfamine (also a CNS-stimulant) failed to induce hyperthermia in control or lynestrenol-pretreated mice but did raise the temperature after mestranol pretreatment. The potentiating effect of mestranol could be mimicked by pretreatment with nialamide (a MAO-inhibitor) but not by SKF 525-A. Increased locomotor activity induced by dexamphetamine and fencamfamine was enhanced by mestranol and reduced by lynestrenol. Dopamine, norepinephrine and 5-HT levels in the brain were reduced by lynestrenol and 5-HT was increased by mestranol. "If the actions of dexamphetamine (and fencamfamin) are due predominantly to the release of endogenous amines, then an increase (with lynestrenol) or a decrease (with mestranol) of tissue MAO activity should change the potency of these two stimulant drugs."

Mecamylamine ← cf. Ganglioplegics

Mechlorethamine ←

Selye G 70,480/71: In rats, mechlorethamine intoxication was not prevented by any of the standard conditioning agents of our series. Indeed, prednisolone, triamcinolone, hydroxydione, thyroxine and, to a lesser extent, possibly also oxandrolone aggravated the toxicity of this compound, cf. Table 75, p. 260.

Mechlorethamine ← Cortisone: Hutchinson et al. B 84,257/55*

Meperidine ←

Axelrod D 28,544/56: Hepatic microsomal-enzyme systems are described which can N-demethylate several narcotic drugs, including morphine and its congeners, methadone and meperidine. "There are marked sex differences

Table 75. *Conditioning for mechlorethamine*

Treatment[a]	Mortality[b] (Dead/Total)
None	4/15
PCN	0/10 NS
CS-1	4/10 NS
Ethylestrenol	5/15 NS
Spironolactone	4/15 NS
Norbolethone	5/10 NS
Oxandrolone	8/10 *
Prednisolone-Ac	10/10 ***
Triamcinolone	14/15 ***
Progesterone	4/10 NS
Estradiol	6/10 NS
DOC-Ac	5/10 NS
Hydroxydione	9/10 ***
Thyroxine	15/15 ***
Phenobarbital	3/10 NS

[a] The rats of all groups were given mechlorethamine hydrochloride (100 µg per rat in 0.2 ml water, s.c., daily from 4th to 6th day).

[b] Mortality listed on 8th day ("Exact Probability Test").

For further details on technique of tabulation cf. p. VIII.

in the enzymatic demethylation of narcotic drugs in the rat. Administration of estradiol to male rats results in a decrease in enzyme activity while treatment of female rats with testosterone enhances enzyme activity."

Remmer D86,728/58: Mention of unpublished experiments indicating that cortisone and prednisolone accelerate the detoxication of meperidine in the rat exclusively through demethylation, not through hydrolysis.

Crawford & Rudofsky G42,454/66: In women taking various oral contraceptives, as well as in pregnant women and in neonates, the urinary excretion of pethidine and promazine is increased, suggesting interference with the detoxication of these drugs.

Rudofsky & Crawford E58,989/66: Following administration of meperidine or promazine "pregnant women, women on oral contraceptives and neonates excreted significantly more unchanged meperidine than normeperidine, whereas the reverse held for the male 'controls' and other female groups. Pregnant women, women on oral contraceptives and neonates excreted more unchanged and degraded promazine than non-pregnant women. Stilbestrol and progesterone each changed the pattern of excretion by male subjects toward that associated with pregnancy." Apparently, pregnancy diminishes the capacity to metabolize meperidine and promazine, a change reflected in neonates and subjects taking oral contraceptives.

Meperidine ← Chloromethyltestosterone, 19-Nortestosterone + Chlorpromazine: Clouet et al. *F14,837/64*

Mephenesin ← cf. also *Selye G60,083/70, p. 385.*

Selye G60,086/70: In rats, mephenesin paralysis was very effectively prevented by all classic catatoxic steroids, except oxandrolone. Prednisolone and DOC offered barely significant protection, cf. Table 76.

Table 76. *Conditioning for mephenesin*

Treatment[a]	Paralysis[b] (Positive/Total)	Mortality[b] (Dead/Total)
None	9/10	3/10
PCN	2/10 ***	0/10 NS
CS-1	0/15 ***	0/15 NS
Ethylestrenol	0/10 ***	0/10 NS
Spironolactone	0/10 ***	0/10 NS
Norbolethone	0/10 ***	0/10 NS
Oxandrolone	8/15 NS	1/15 NS
Prednisolone-Ac	7/15 *	0/15 NS
Triamcinolone (2 mg)	15/15 NS	6/15 NS
Progesterone	8/15 NS	4/15 NS
Estradiol	8/10 NS	0/10 NS
DOC-Ac	7/15 *	2/15 NS
Hydroxydione	8/15 NS	2/15 NS
Thyroxine	9/10 NS	1/10 NS
Phenobarbital	5/10 NS	0/10 NS

[a] The rats of all groups were given mephenesin (30 mg on 4th day and 60 mg on 5th day, /100 g body weight in 0.2 ml propylene glycol s.c.).

[b] Paralysis was estimated on 5th day 2½ hrs after injection and mortality listed on 5th day p.m. ("Exact Probability Test").

For further details on technique of tabulation cf. p. VIII.

Meprobamate ←

Kato & Vassanelli D40,237/62: "Rats pretreated with phenobarbital, phenaglycodol, glutethimide, nikethamide, chlorpromazine triflupromazine, meprobamate, carisoprodol, pentobarbital, thiopental, primidone, chloretone, dyphenylhydantoine and urethan showed an accelerated metabolism of meprobamate and, at the same time, a diminished duration of sleeping time and paralysis due to meprobamate." SKF 525-A counteracted these actions of the enzyme inducers. In hypophysectomized or adrenalectomized rats, phenobarbital still increased meprobamate metabolism in vitro.

Bousquet et al. F 35,073/65: In rats with stress produced by applying a tourniquet around one hind limb for 2.5 hrs, the toxicity of hexobarbital, pentobarbital, meprobamate and zoxazolamine was significantly diminished, whereas that of barbital and phenobarbital remained unaffected. Pretreatment with ACTH or corticosterone simulated the effect of stress. After hypophysectomy or adrenalectomy, stress failed to offer the usual protection. [The barbiturates and zoxazolamine appear to have been administered immediately after release of the tourniquet but this is not specifically stated. Allegedly a single injection of corticosterone (50 μg per animal) sufficed to offer protection (H.S.).]

Selye G 70,402/70: In rats, meprobamate intoxication is inhibited by ethylestrenol, CS-1, spironolactone, norbolethone, oxandrolone and prednisolone. No protection is obtained by progesterone, triamcinolone, DOC, hydroxydione or estradiol.

Selye G 70,428/70: In rats, ethylestrenol powerfully inhibits the toxicity of digitoxin, nicotine, indomethacin, phenindione, dioxathion, EPN, physostigmine, hexobarbital, cyclopental, thiopental, DOC (anesthesia), meprobamate and picrotoxin. Thyroxine increases the toxicity of many among these drugs and inhibits the protective effect of ethylestrenol.

Szeberényi & Fekete H 29,579/70: Brief abstract stating that after four days of pretreatment (species not mentioned), spironolactone decreased the action and accelerated the metabolism of hexobarbital, chlorzoxazone, meprobamate, esterone, testosterone, acenocoumarol and BSP, whereas after short treatment it had an inverse effect. It is concluded that spironolactone is a microsomal enzyme inducer.

Selye G 70,480/71: In rats, the motor disturbances produced by meprobamate intoxication are readily prevented by all classic catatoxic steroids, as well as by prednisolone and phenobarbital, *cf.* Table 77.

Meprobamate ← Adrenalectomy: Kato et al. *D 40,237/62*

Table 77. *Conditioning for meprobamate*

Treatment[a]	Dyskinesia[b] (Positive/Total)	Mortality[b] (Dead/Total)
None	9/10	0/10
PCN	0/10 ***	0/10 NS
CS-1	0/10 ***	0/10 NS
Ethylestrenol	1/10 ***	0/10 NS
Spironolactone	0/10 ***	0/10 NS
Norbolethone	0/10 ***	0/10 NS
Oxandrolone	0/10 ***	0/10 NS
Prednisolone-Ac	3/15 ***	1/15 NS
Triamcinolone (2 mg)	8/10 NS	0/10 NS
Progesterone	5/10 NS	0/10 NS
Estradiol (1 mg)	10/10 NS	0/10 NS
Estradiol (1 mg s.c.)	10/10 NS	5/10 *
DOC-Ac	8/10 NS	1/10 NS
Hydroxydione	6/10 NS	0/10 NS
Thyroxine	9/10 NS	5/10 *
Phenobarbital	1/10 ***	0/10 NS

[a] The rats of all groups were given meprobamate (50 mg/100 g body weight in 0.2 ml DMSO, s.c., once on 4th day).

[b] Dyskinesia was estimated 3 hrs after injection and mortality registered 24 hrs later ("Exact Probability Test").

For further details on technique of tabulation *cf.* p. VIII.

MER-25 ←

Abdul-Karim et al. G 55,510/68: The offspring of rabbits treated with MER-25 [1-(p-2-diethylamino-ethoxyphenyl)-1-phenyl-2-methoxyphenylethanol] during gestation exhibit defects in endochondral ossification which can be prevented by concomitant administration of estradiol.

Mercury ←

← Testoids *cf.* also *Selye B 40,000/50, p. 631.*
Selye A 31,128/40; A 31,126/40: The renal and hepatic lesions produced by $HgCl_2$ in the mouse are prevented by testosterone, methyltestosterone, androstenediol, dehydroiso-androsterone and androstenedione.

Longley A 37,552/42: "Treatment with testosterone propionate apparently increases the survival rate of rats poisoned with small doses of mercuric chloride, but is without effect when larger doses of poison are used."

Feyel 99,416/43: In mice, testosterone pretreatment does not protect either against $HgCl_2$ or uranium nitrate intoxication.

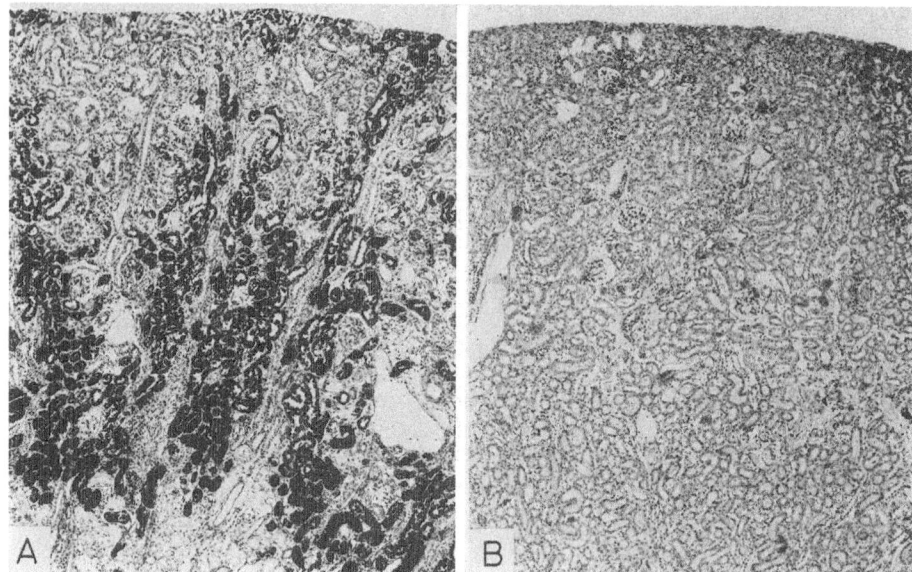

Fig. 10. **Prevention of mersalyl-induced nephrocalcinosis by ethylestrenol.** Kidneys of two rats, both of which were given 3 mg/100 g of mersalyl i.v. A: Control rat. B: Ethylestrenol given at the dose of 10 mg × 2/day — 4th day ff. completely prevents nephrocalcinosis (von Kóssa × 30)

de Oliveira et al. B43,032/47: In dogs, fatal renal damage produced by $HgCl_2$ can be prevented by pretreatment with testosterone.

Donatelli B38,554/47: Women are much more sensitive to $HgCl_2$ intoxication than men. Testosterone pretreatment gives appreciable protection against $HgCl_2$ poisoning in mice and guinea pigs.

Vargas B44,689/48: In parrots, testosterone pretreatment protects the kidney against damage induced by $HgCl_2$.

Cournot & Halpern B54,669/50: In mice, testosterone failed to protect the kidney against $HgCl_2$.

Levy et al. B47,634/50: Testosterone offered no protection against the renal damage caused by $HgCl_2$ in the rat.

Sarre B99,950/54: In rabbits, both the Masugi nephritis and sublimate nephrosis are inhibited by testosterone and even more actively by estradiol.

Kádas & Zsámbéky C26,265/56: The renal damage produced by $HgCl_2$ in the rat is most effectively prevented by testosterone but, to a lesser extent, also by cortisone, particularly when the latter is given in combination with ACTH.

Dérot & Tutin C67,130/57: In patients with mercury intoxication, treatment with testosterone is beneficial.

Kádas & Zsámbéky C49,522/57: In rats poisoned with $HgCl_2$, both testosterone and combined treatment with ACTH + cortisone inhibit renal damage and improve survival.

Jelinek et al. E32,261/63: In mice, 2-bromo-androstene-3,17-dione, which is neither testoid nor anabolic, hastens the regeneration of the renal epithelium damaged by $HgCl_2$. Methyltestosterone actually aggravates the changes, whereas methandrostenolone and nandrolone phenpropionate had no effect.

Jelinek et al. F20,543/64: In mice and rats, regeneration following $HgCl_2$-induced renal damage is stimulated by 2-bromo-1-androstene-3,17-dione but not by methyltestosterone or 1,17-dimethylandrostan-17-ol-3-one.

Klinkmann & Hübel F19,820/64: Testosterone allegedly protected the kidneys of a patient from severe sublimate-overdosage.

Wüstenberg et al. G38,225/65: In female rats given sublethal doses of $HgCl_2$, the protective effect of testosterone upon the resulting renal damage was doubtful although the rise in blood NPN was significantly inhi-

← Steroids

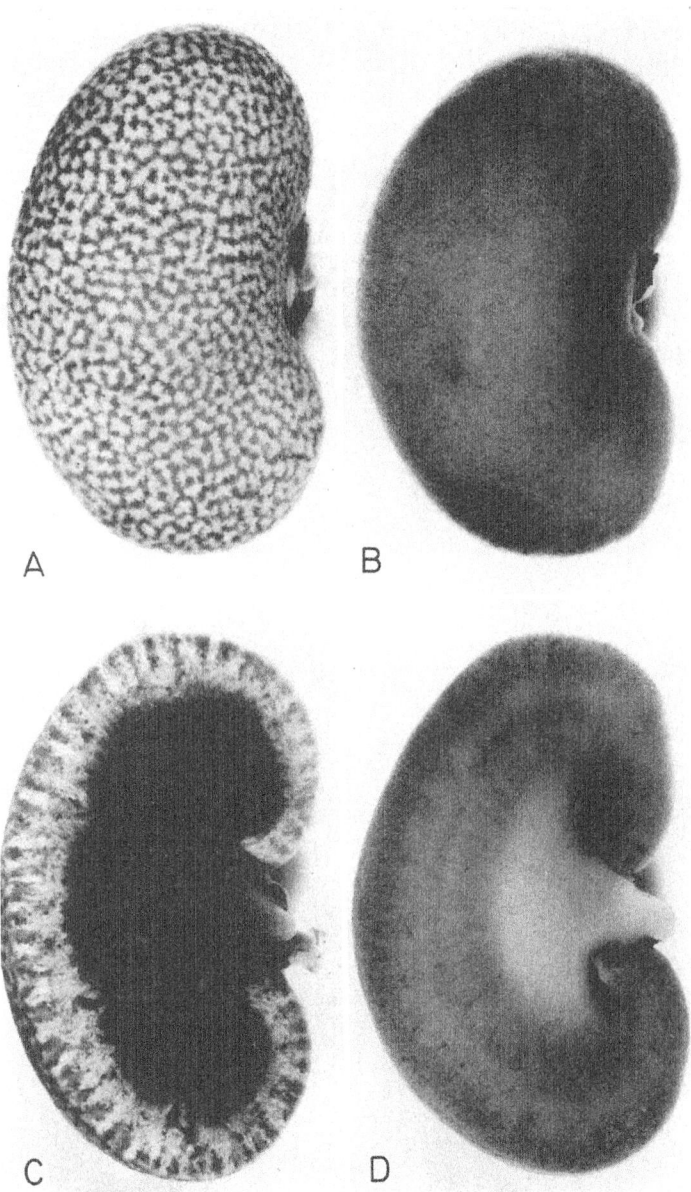

Fig. 11. **Protection by spironolactone against mercury.** Both rats received the same dose of HgCl$_2$ i.v. A + C: Heavy calcification of the renal cortex in the otherwise-untreated control rat. B + D: Complete prevention of calcification by prior treatment with spironolactone. Top: External surface. [Selye G 70,426/70. Courtesy of Science]

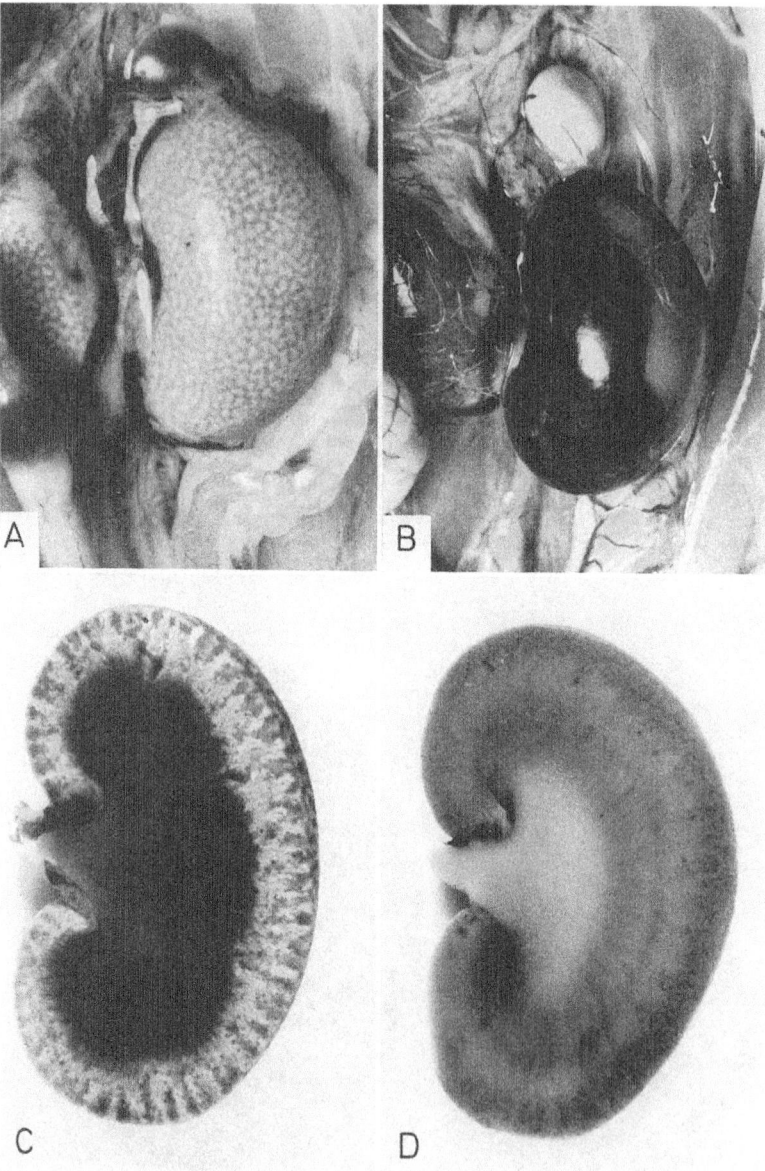

Fig. 12 (A—D). **Prevention of HgCl$_2$-induced nephrocalcinosis by spironolactone.** All animals received the same HgCl$_2$-treatment. A: Left kidney of otherwise-untreated control in its natural position with part of the right kidney just visible across the mesentery of the rectum. The tubular localization of the calcification in the cortex is clearly visible. B: Pretreatment with spironolactone prevents this change. C: Cross section through the kidney shown above. Note strictly cortical localization of calcification. D: Cross section through the kidney shown above. No calcification is visible

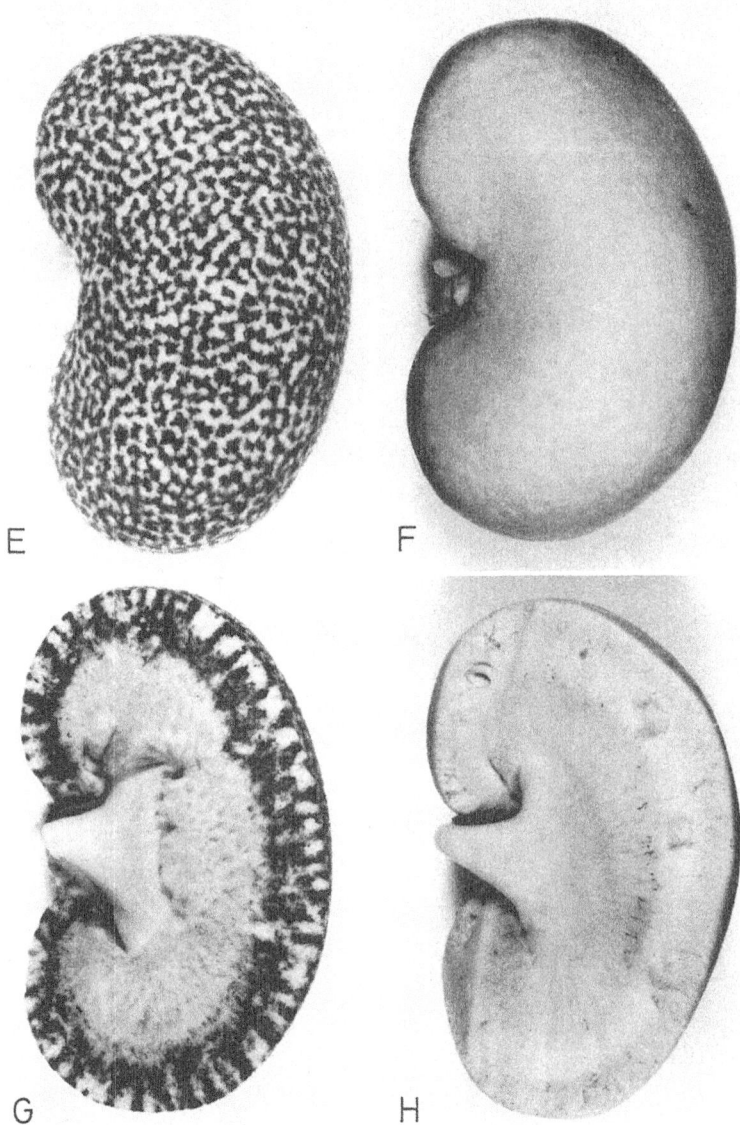

Fig. 12 (E—H). E: Macroscopic aspect of the control kidney after staining with von Kóssa technique. The calcified tubules (now black) are especially clearly visible. F: Similarly-prepared kidney of the rat pretreated with spironolactone. G, H: Cross sections through the kidneys shown above

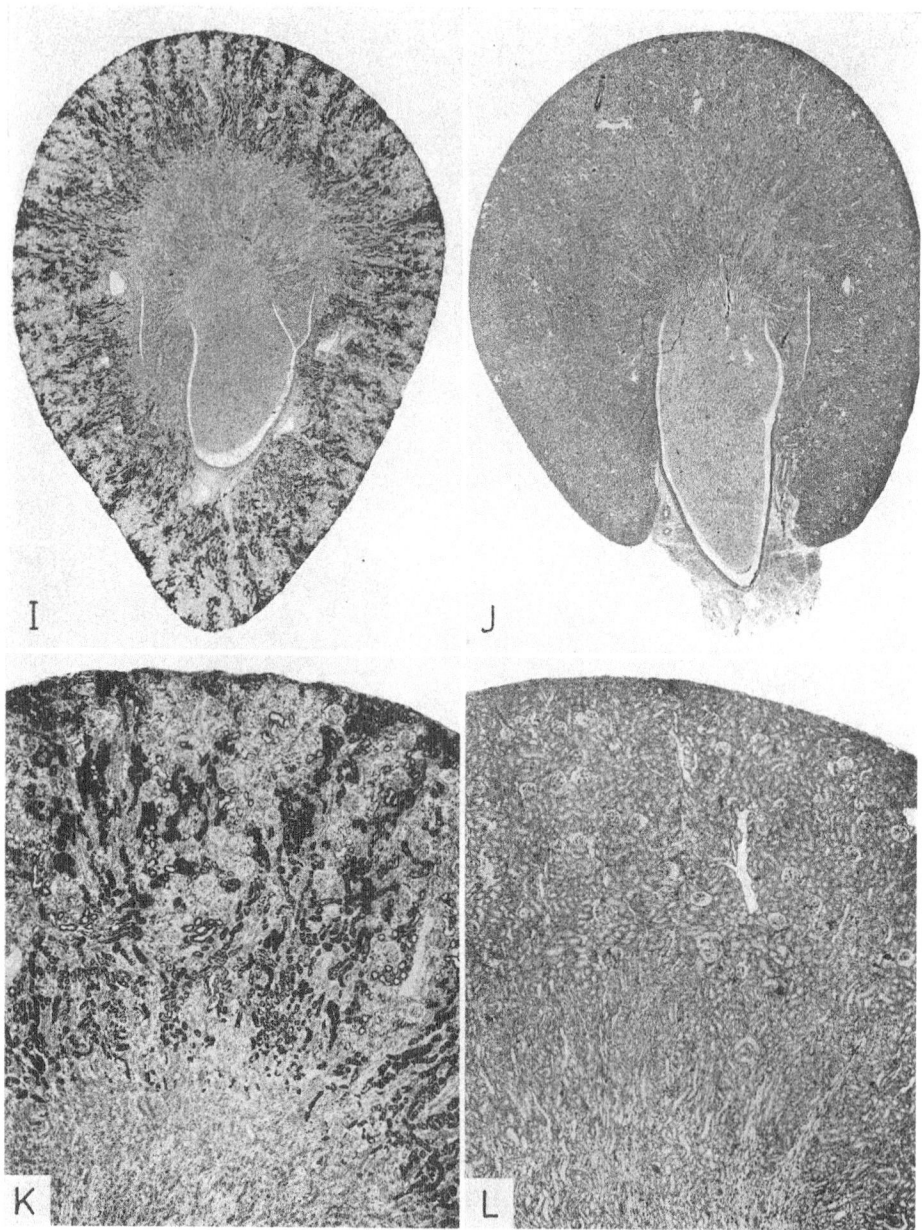

Fig. 12 (I—L). I: Histologic appearance of the control kidney showing cortical calcification. J: Prevention of calcification by spironolactone. K, L: Higher magnification of the kidneys shown above. All sections stained with von Kóssa technique: top × 9, bottom × 27. [Selye et al. G 70,440/70. Courtesy of Urol. and Nephrol.]

bited. In males, no definite protective action could be shown.

Tessmann G65,320/68: In the mouse and rat, regeneration of the renal epithelium following $HgCl_2$-intoxication was not significantly enhanced by testosterone.

Mercury ← Testoids *cf. also Tables 78—80*
← **Other Steroids** *cf. also Selye G60,083/70, p. 353. Clark & Barnes A 33,441/40:* Pretreatment with DOC failed to protect intact rats against $HgCl_2$.

Kádas & Zsámbéky C 26,265/56: The renal damage produced by $HgCl_2$ in the rat is most effectively prevented by testosterone but, to a lesser extent, also by cortisone, particularly when the latter is given in combination with ACTH.

Selye & Bois C 14,441/57: The calcification and foreign-body granuloma formation in the kidneys of rats poisoned with $HgCl_2$ is prevented by cortisol but not by DOC. The necrotizing ulcers in the cecum of the rat which develop under the influence of $HgCl_2$ were actually aggravated by cortisol but not influenced by DOC.

Heimburg & Schmidt C 69,587/59: Female rats are more resistant than males to chronic intoxication with $HgCl_2$. Ovariectomy abolishes this difference. Neither estradiol nor progesterone caused any significant change in resistance to mercurial intoxication.

Miller et al. G77,153/69: In chicks, cortisol and several other glucocorticoids increase mercury retention in the kidney and, at least in certain strains, also in the liver. [The experiments were terminated after four days and no mention is made of mortality (H.S.).]

Selye G70,426/70: In the rat, spironolactone is highly efficacious in preventing renal tubular necrosis and calcification as well as the mortality induced by $HgCl_2$. Possibly this protective effect is due to the sulfur in the thioacetyl substituent of the steroid, *cf.* Fig. 11, p. 263.

Szabó & Selye G70,478/70: In rats, hypophysectomy greatly diminishes the nephrocalcinosis produced by $HgCl_2$. This effect of $HgCl_2$ is completely abolished in hypophysectomized rats treated with triamcinolone.

Garg et al. G60,078/71: In rats, given $HgCl_2$, spironolactone decreases the mercury content of the kidney, blood, urine, liver, spleen and lung by about 40—50%. This decrease is accompanied by an increased fecal elimination of Hg. However, the protection by spironolactone against nephrocalcinosis cannot be due exclusively to a diminished mercury content since the kidneys of animals receiving spironolactone contain more mercury than those of rats showing renal calcification after treatment with lower doses of $HgCl_2$ given alone.

Selye G70,480/71: In rats, fatal intoxication with $HgCl_2$ was readily prevented by spironolactone. Among the other standard conditioning agents, only ethylestrenol, prednisolone, progesterone and estradiol offered moderate protection, *cf.* Fig. 12, p. 264—266 and Table 78.

Table 78. *Conditioning for mercuric chloride*

Treatment[a]	Nephrocalcinosis[b] (Positive/Total)	Mortality[b] (Dead/Total)
None	15/15	10/15
PCN	10/10 NS	7/10 NS
CS-1	10/10 NS	5/10 NS
Ethylestrenol	11/15 *	10/15 NS
Spironolactone	0/20 ***	0/20 ***
Norbolethone	8/10 NS	6/10 NS
Oxandrolone	8/10 NS	7/10 NS
Prednisolone-Ac	6/10 *	9/10 NS
Triamcinolone	15/15 NS	12/15 NS
Progesterone	7/20 ***	6/20 *
Estradiol	9/15 **	6/15 NS
DOC-Ac	8/10 NS	5/10 NS
Hydroxydione	8/10 NS	5/10 NS
Thyroxine	14/15 NS	15/15 ±
Phenobarbital	8/10 NS	10/10 NS

[a] The rats of all groups were given mercuric chloride (400 µg/100 g body weight in 1 ml water, i.v., on 4th day).

[b] Nephrocalcinosis was estimated on day of death from 5th day and mortality registered on 7th day ("Exact Probability Test").

For further details on technique of tabulation *cf.* p. VIII.

Selye G70,480/71: In rats, fatal mersalyl (s.c.) intoxication was readily prevented by ethylestrenol, spironolactone, prednisolone and phenobarbital, *cf.* Table 79, p.268.

Selye G70,480/71: In rats, fatal intoxication with mersalyl i.v. is readily prevented by spironolactone and prednisolone. Ethylestrenol is somewhat less effective, whereas triamcinolone and progesterone exhibit a barely significant prophylactic action, *cf.* Fig. 10, p. 262 and Table 80, p. 268.

Selye PROT. 31585, 31716: In 20 ♀ mice, 5—20 mg/100 g of spironolactone or equimolecular amounts of spiroxasone given p.o.

Table 79. *Conditioning for mersalyl (s.c.)*

Treatment[a]	Nephrocalcinosis[b] (Positive/Total)	Mortality[b] (Dead/Total)
None	9/15	8/15
CS-1	2/10 NS	3/10 NS
Ethylestrenol	0/10 ***	0/10 ***
Spironolactone	0/10 ***	0/10 **
Norbolethone	2/10 NS	1/10 *
Oxandrolone	1/10 *	2/10 NS
Prednisolone-Ac	0/10 ***	1/10 *
Triamcinolone	4/10 NS	3/10 NS
Progesterone	4/10 NS	5/10 NS
Estradiol	4/10 NS	0/10 **
DOC-Ac	3/10 NS	5/10 NS
Hydroxydione	4/10 NS	1/10 *
Thyroxine	6/10 NS	8/10 NS
Phenobarbital	0/10 ***	0/10 **

[a] The rats of all groups were given mersalyl (10 mg/100 g body weight in 0.2 ml water, s.c., on 4th day).

[b] Nephrocalcinosis was estimated on day of death in animals that lived at least 5 days and mortality listed on 7th day ("Exact Probability Test").

For further details on technique of tabulation cf. p. VIII.

Table 80. *Conditioning for mersalyl (i.v.)*

Treatment[a]	Nephrocalcinosis[b] (Positive/Total)	Mortality[b] (Dead/Total)
None	13/15	13/15
PCN	14/15 NS	13/15 NS
CS-1	11/14 NS	12/15 NS
Ethylestrenol	6/14 *	1/15 ***
Spironolactone	0/15 ***	0/15 ***
Norbolethone	12/14 NS	5/15 ***
Oxandrolone	12/13 NS	7/15 *
Prednisolone-Ac	3/15 ***	3/15 ***
Triamcinolone	6/15 *	6/15 *
Progesterone	6/15 *	9/15 NS
Estradiol	13/14 NS	13/15 NS
DOC-Ac	14/15 NS	11/15 NS
Hydroxydione	15/15 NS	9/15 NS
Thyroxine	12/13 NS	15/15 NS
Phenobarbital	12/15 NS	9/15 NS

[a] The rats of all groups were given mersalyl (4 mg/100 g body weight in 1 ml water, i.v., once on 4th day).

[b] Nephrocalcinosis was estimated on day of death of animals that lived at least 5 days and mortality listed on 7th day ("Exact Probability Test").

For further details on technique of tabulation cf. p. VIII.

1 hr before the i.v. injection of 1 or 1.5 mg $HgCl_2$/100 g body weight offer little, if any, protection against the resulting nephrocalcinosis.

Selye PROT. 32109, 33047: In rats, cortisol, cortisone, triamcinolone, dexamethasone, betamethasone, prednisolone and prednisone given daily at high dosages for 4 days failed to protect against the nephrocalcinosis and mortality produced by $HgCl_2$ i.v., cf. Table 81.

Methadone ←

March et al. B58,376/50: In rats, neither castration nor testosterone pretreatment affects sensitivity to methadone i.p. significantly. The renal concentration of methadone is increased by castration but restored to normal by testosterone.

Winter & Flataker B62,935/51: In rats, cortisone inhibits the toxic effects of methadone and the hyperactivity caused by morphine. Cortisone also increases the excitatory effect of morphine in cats. On the other hand, cortisone synergizes the analgesic antagonist N-allylnormorphine. After spinal cord section, cortisone and ACTH reduce the effect of morphine on the spinal reflex (tail-flick response), whereas DOC enhances it.

Axelrod D28,544/56: Hepatic microsomal-enzyme systems are described which can N-demethylate several narcotic drugs, including morphine and its congeners, methadone and meperidine. "There are marked sex differences in the enzymatic demethylation of narcotic drugs in the rat. Administration of estradiol to male rats results in a decrease in enzyme activity while treatment of female rats with testosterone enhances enzyme activity."

Selye G70,480/71: In rats, methadone intoxication was most effectively prevented by ethylestrenol. Triamcinolone offered barely significant protection, whereas progesterone and thyroxine appeared to increase mortality, cf. Table 82.

Methadone ← Estradiol, Testosterone: Axelrod *D28,544/56*

← Steroids

Table 81. *Lack of protection by glucocorticoids against acute $HgCl_2$ intoxication*

Treatment[a]	Nephro-calcinosis[b] (Positive/Total)	Mortality[b] (Dead/Total)
None	9/10	5/10
Cortisol-Ac 10 mg	9/10 NS	4/10 NS
Cortisone-Ac 10 mg	7/10 NS	4/10 NS
Triamcinolone 10 mg	8/10 NS	9/10 NS
Dexamethasone-Ac 2 mg	6/10 NS	10/10 *
Betamethasone-Ac 2 mg	8/10 NS	10/10 *
Prednisolone-Ac 10 mg	10/10 NS	9/10 NS
Prednisone-Ac 10 mg	9/10 NS	6/10 NS
Solu-Cortef 10 mg	7/10 NS	5/10 NS

[a] The rats (100 g ♀) of all groups received $HgCl_2$ 300 μg in 1 ml water, i.v. once, on the 4th day. Solu-Cortef was injected at the dose indicated in 1 ml water, i.v. once, 4th day, 30 min before $HgCl_2$; the other glucocorticoids were given at the doses indicated in 1 ml water, p.o. x2/day, 1st day ff, on the 4th day 1 hr before $HgCl_2$ administration.

[b] Nephrocalcinosis on day of death; mortality up to 7th day when experiment was terminated (Statistics Fisher & Yates).

For further details on technique of tabulation cf. p. VIII.

Methanol ←

Severin & Bashkurov G49,801/67: In patients with acute methanol poisoning, combined treatment with norepinephrine, cortisone and various other agents facilitated recovery. [In view of the complex treatment given, it is impossible to ascertain the relative value of each component of the therapeutic regimen (H.S.).]

Gilger et al. B73,737/52: In mice, cortisone had no significant effect upon methanol intoxication.

Methanol ← Cortisone, Mouse: Gilger et al. B73,737/52*

Table 82. *Conditioning for methadone*

Treatment[a]	Dyskinesia[b] (Positive/Total)	Mortality[b] (Dead/Total)
None	15/15	5/15
PCN	9/10 NS	2/10 NS
CS-1	10/10 NS	4/10 NS
Ethylestrenol	3/10 ***	0/10 NS
Spironolactone	9/10 NS	7/10 NS
Norbolethone	10/10 NS	5/10 NS
Oxandrolone	10/10 NS	3/10 NS
Prednisolone-Ac	10/10 NS	1/10 NS
Triamcinolone	6/10 *	1/10 NS
Progesterone	10/10 NS	9/10 **
Estradiol	9/10 NS	2/10 NS
DOC-Ac	10/10 NS	6/10 NS
Hydroxydione	10/10 NS	3/10 NS
Thyroxine	10/10 NS	8/10 *
Phenobarbital	8/10 NS	5/10 NS

[a] The rats of all groups were given methadone, 1.5 mg/100 g body weight in 1 ml water, i.p., once on 4th day.

[b] Dyskinesia was estimated 2 hrs after injection and mortality registered 24 hrs later ("Exact Probability Test").

For further details on technique of tabulation cf. p. VIII.

Methionine ← cf. Diet (Choline)

Methylaminoantipyrine ← Adrenalectomy + Prednisolone: Remmer C73,857/58

Methylaniline ←

Selye PROT. 39519: In rats, the dyskinesia and mortality induced by heavy methylaniline intoxication is counteracted by PCN and phenobarbital. Triamcinolone, progesterone and thyroxine aggravate this intoxication, whereas the other standard conditioners cause little or no change in methylaniline resistance, cf. Table 83, p. 270.

N-Methylaniline ← Gonadectomy + Methyltestosterone: Kato et al. F76,403/66

Methylphenidate ←

Selye PROT. 35844: In rats, methylphenidate (10 mg/100 g body weight in 0.2 ml water) was administered s.c. once on 4th day of conditioning. Dyskinesia was listed 2 hrs, paralysis 3 hrs, and mortality 24 hrs, after this injection. Under these circumstances none of the "Standard Conditioners" (p. VIII)

Table 83. Conditioning for methylaniline

Treatment[a]	Dyskinesia[b] (Positive/Total)	Mortality[b] (Dead/Total)
None	14/20	11/20
PCN	2/5 NS	2/5 NS
PCN 1 mg	3/15 ***	3/15 *
CS-1	5/15 *	8/15 NS
Ethylestrenol	6/20 *	4/20 *
Spironolactone	13/20 NS	8/20 NS
Norbolethone	4/15 *	3/15 *
Oxandrolone	9/15 NS	9/15 NS
Prednisolone-Ac	11/15 NS	13/15 *
Triamcinolone	20/20 *	20/20 ***
Progesterone	15/15 *	15/15 ***
Progesterone 5 mg	4/5 NS	1/5 NS
Estradiol	9/15 NS	3/15 *
DOC-Ac	12/15 NS	11/15 NS
Hydroxydione	11/15 NS	5/15 NS
Thyroxine	20/20 *	20/20 ***
Phenobarbital	5/15 *	1/15 ***

[a] The rats of all groups were given N-methylaniline (40 mg/100 g body weight in 0.2 ml water, s.c., once daily from the 4th to the 7th day).

[b] Dyskinesia was estimated on 6th day 6 hrs after injection and mortality listed on 8th day ("Exact Probability Test").

For further details on technique of tabulation cf. p. VIII.

or cholesterol caused any noteworthy change in the resulting intoxication, only thyroxine exhibited an aggravating effect.

Methyprylon ←

Selye et al. G60,020/69: In the rat, pretreatment with norbolethone protects against the anesthetic effect of progesterone, DOC, pregnanedione, dehydroepiandrosterone, testosterone, diethylstilbestrol, pentobarbital and methyprylon. It does not significantly alter the corresponding actions of urethan, diazepam, chlorpromazine, reserpine, phenoxybenzamine, chloral hydrate, potassium bromide or magnesium chloride.

Selye et al. G60,016/70: In rats, spironolactone protects against anesthesia produced by progesterone, DOC, hydroxydione, pregnanedione, dehydroepiandrosterone, testosterone, diethylstilbestrol, methyprylon, pentobarbital and ethanol. It does not significantly alter the corresponding actions of morphine, codeine, urethan, diazepam, chlorpromazine, reserpine, phenoxybenzamine, chloral hydrate, KBr or $MgCl_2$.

Selye G60,097/70; G70,480/71: Methyprylon (a hypnotic piperidine derivative) is unusual in its behavior in that its effect is diminished by all standard conditioning agents except DOC and thyroxine. The inhibition by estradiol is not very marked and hydroxydione pretreatment gives a barely significant shortening of the sleeping time but the potent classical conditioners and particularly PCN are extremely effective, cf. Table 84.

Metrazol ← cf. Pentylenetetrazol

Metyrapone ←

Szeberényi et al. G64,752/69: In rats given metyrapone i.p., the disappearance of the drug from the plasma is accelerated by pretreatment with cortisol and numerous other drugs that induce hepatic-microsomal enzymes.

Mitomycin ←

Lutzmann & Schmidt F57,784/65: In rats, Δ'-17α-methyltestosterone failed to prevent the antimitotic effect of cyclophosphamide or mitomycin upon Jensen sarcomas.

Table 84. Conditioning for methyprylon

Treatment[a]	Sleeping time[b] (min)
None	485 ± 10
PCN	2 ± 1 ***
CS-1	35 ± 6 ***
Ethylestrenol	28 ± 5 ***
Spironolactone	158 ± 17 ***
Norbolethone	90 ± 10 ***
Oxandrolone	149 ± 17 ***
Prednisolone-Ac	11 ± 4 ***
Triamcinolone	234 ± 27 ***
Triamcinolone (2 mg)	321 ± 21 ***
Progesterone	335 ± 18 ***
Estradiol	356 ± 34 **
DOC-Ac	479 ± 22 NS
Hydroxydione	411 ± 28 *
Thyroxine	416 ± 32 NS
Phenobarbital	50 ± 14 ***

[a] The rats of all groups were given methyprylon (20 mg/100 g body weight in 0.2 ml water, s.c., once on 4th day).

[b] Student's t-test.

For further details on technique of tabulation cf. p. VIII.

Monocrotaline ←

Ratnoff & Mirick B48,154/49: Monocrotaline i.p. produces necrosis of the liver and of the renal tubules, as well as pulmonary edema in rats. Males are somewhat more susceptible than females, especially if kept on protein-deficient diets. Testosterone increases monocrotaline susceptibility in both sexes, but neither castration nor estradiol influences survival time.

Goldenthal et al. G18,384/64: "The oral and intravenous LD_{50}'s were determined for monocrotaline. The LD_{50} was essentially the same for males and females and for oral and intravenous administration for a 90-day observation period. There was a marked sex difference with respect to the median survival time, females living significantly longer than males. Castration of either male or female rats had no significant effect on the median survival time. Pretreatment of males with estradiol cyclopentyl propionate caused the median survival time to correspond to that of females. Pretreatment of females with testosterone propionate caused the median survival time to approximate that of male animals. Pretreatment of female rats with methandrostenolone (Dianabol), an anabolic agent, caused the median survival time to correspond to that of males."

Monocrotaline ← Orchidectomy + Estradiol + Diet: Ratnoff et al. B48,154/49*

Monomethyl-4-aminoantipyrine ← Testoids: Booth et al. *D34,656/62*

Morphine ← *cf. also* Ethylmorphine

Benetato et al. 33,773/35: In rats, neither adrenocortical extract nor an adrenotrophic anterior pituitary preparation altered resistance to morphine or to typhoid-paratyphoid vaccine.

Michalek et al. B91,619/51: In dogs, cortisone "modifies" the addiction syndrome induced by chronic morphine treatment. [Brief abstract without details (H.S.).]

Winter & Flataker B62,935/51: In rats, cortisone inhibits the toxic effects of methadone and the hyperactivity caused by morphine. Cortisone also increases the excitatory effect of morphine in cats. On the other hand, cortisone synergizes the analgesic antagonist N-allylnormorphine. After spinal cord section, cortisone and ACTH reduce the effect of morphine on the spinal reflex (tail-flick response), whereas DOC enhances it.

Paroli G14,277/54: In rats of either sex, stilbestrol, hexestrol, and estradiol pretreatment reduce morphine tolerance. Orchidectomy does not influence it.

Miller et al. G73,877/55: Review of earlier literature suggesting that morphine analgesia is mediated through the release of epinephrine from the adrenal medulla. It had been claimed that adrenalectomy decreases the pain reaction threshold to morphine and that morphine itself has an analgesic effect. However, in the authors' experiments on rats these observations could not be confirmed and TEA failed to reverse the effect of morphine on pain. In mice, near lethal doses of epinephrine or norepinephrine were required to raise the pain threshold.

Axelrod D28,544/56: Hepatic microsomal-enzyme systems are described which can N-demethylate several narcotic drugs, including morphine and its congeners, methadone and meperidine. "There are marked sex differences in the enzymatic demethylation of narcotic drugs in the rat. Administration of estradiol to male rats results in a decrease in enzyme activity while treatment of female rats with testosterone enhances enzyme activity."

Adler et al. G79,852/57: In Sprague-Dawley rats, given ^{14}C-labeled morphine, the ratio of bound to free morphine is $2-3$ times greater in the urine and plasma than in Long-Evans rats. The tissues of adrenalectomized rats of both strains contain higher concentrations of ^{14}C-labeled morphine than do control rats. Plasma bound morphine levels indicate no impairment of morphine conjugation. Vasopressin increases, whereas ACTH decreases morphine sensitivity. Yet both after ACTH and after vasopressin, tissue concentrations of morphine are either reduced or unaffected in marked contrast to the increased values after adrenalectomy. Apparently, the decreased morphine sensitivity induced by ACTH is not reflected by lower brain morphine concentrations.

Paroli & de Arcangelis C63,937/57: In rats, progesterone enhanced the anesthetic effect of morphine; pregnanediol and pregnanedione had little effect upon it, whereas pregnenolone shortened its duration.

Paroli C62,998/57: In rats, estradiol, stilbestrol and hexestrol increase sensitivity to the lethal effects of morphine overdosage. Androsterone and orchidectomy are without effect upon it.

Paroli C63,938/57; C63,939/57: Estradiol, stilbestrol and hexestrol decrease the morphine resistance of the rat.

Cochin & Axelrod G67,795/59: Chronic treatment with morphine and morphine-nalorphine mixtures caused profound diminution of the analgesic response to a test dose of morphine. This was associated with a severe reduction in the ability of the liver enzymes to N-dealkylate morphine and nalorphine. Testosterone failed to affect the development of morphine tolerance or to modify enzymic activity.

Sobel et al. C90,836/60: Morphine increases the mortality of guinea pigs exposed to reduced oxygen tension. Prior treatment with cortisone or ACTH protects against this combined treatment.

Markova D47,081/62: Pretreatment with ACTH or cortisone increases the morphine resistance of newborn rats, although not quite to the adult level. DOC does not share this effect.

Paroli G12,543/63: In the rat, cortisol and ACTH inhibit the analgesic effect of morphine, whereas dexamethasone and prednisolone (though more active glucocorticoids) do not.

Franklin G32,826/65: The demethylation of morphine by rat hepatic microsomes was greatly diminished by pretreatment with cortisone, although, simultaneously, the G-6-P-ase activity of the liver increased. Pretreatment with morphine exhibited essentially similar effects upon these two enzymes.

Lecannelier & Quevedo H8,759/67: In rabbits, the analgesic effect of morphine is reduced by ACTH or cortisol.

Dobrescu et al. H26,899/70: In rats, the establishment of tolerance to morphine is delayed by prednisolone and accelerated by testosterone.

Selye et al. G60,016/70: In rats, spironolactone protects against anesthesia produced by progesterone, DOC, hydroxydione, pregnanedione, dehydroepiandrosterone, testosterone, diethylstilbestrol, methyprylon, pentobarbital and ethanol. It does not significantly alter the corresponding actions of morphine, codeine, urethan, diazepam, chlorpromazine, reserpine, phenoxybenzamine, chloral hydrate, potassium bromide or $MgCl_2$.

Stripp et al. H22,743/70: In female rats, spironolactone pretreatment shortened hexobarbital sleeping time. "Moreover, treatment of female rats with spironolactone doubled the rate of the in vitro metabolism of hexobarbital and benzpyrene by liver microsomes and quadrupled that of ethylmorphine. The inducing effects of spironolactone were very different from those of phenobarbital and 3-methylcholanthrene. The amount of cytochrome P-450 was either unaltered or decreased, but the NADPH cytochrome c reductase activity was increased 2-fold. Although the endogenous rate of cytochrome P-450 reduction by NADPH was not altered, the stimulatory effects of ethylmorphine or hexobarbital on the rate of cytochrome P-450 reduction were significantly greater with microsomes from spironolactone-treated animals. By contrast, treatment of male rats with spironolactone caused no change in hexobarbital sleeping time and no change or a slight decrease in hexobarbital and benzpyrene metabolism by liver microsomes."

Selye PROT. 36205: In rats, morphine sulfate (20 mg/100 g body weight in 0.2 ml water) was administered s.c. once on the 4th day of conditioning. Dyskinesia was listed 2 hrs, mortality 24 hrs, after this injection. Under these circumstances none of the "Standard Conditioners" (p. VIII) caused any noteworthy change in the resulting intoxication.

Morphine ← Adrenalectomy: Rogoff et al. 63,527/25*; Zauder G75,347/52

Morphine ← Testosterone: Cochin et al. *G67,795/59**

Morphine ← Estradiol: Axelrod *D28,544/56*

Morphine ← Cyclopentyltestosterone: March et al. *G77,519/54**

Mustard Gas ←

Kuchárik & Telbisz 96,165/45: Certain adrenocortical extracts offer protection against mustard gas in the mouse.

Mustard Powder ← *cf. Selye B58,650/51, p. 248.*

Na ← *cf.* Sodium

Nalorphine ← Testosterone: Cochin et al. *G67,795/59*

Naphthalene ←

Booth & Gillette D34,656/62: Testosterone propionate, 19-nortestosterone, 4-androstene-3,17-dione and 4-chloro-19-nortestosterone acetate (SKF 6611) were tested for their ability to induce hepatic microsomal enzymes in female rats. "All of the steroids produced 2- to 3-fold increases in the activity of the enzyme systems that metabolize hexobarbital, demethylate monomethyl-4-aminoantipyrine and hydroxylate naphthalene, but only 19-nortestosterone, testosterone propionate and methyltestosterone increased the activity of microsomal TPNH oxidase. ... The increase in microsomal enzyme activity is more closely related to the anabolic activity than to the androgenic activity of the steroid."

2-Naphthylamine ← 3β-Methoxyandrost-5-ene-17-one, Gp, Rat: Roy D5,284/61

α-Naphthylisothiocyanate ← cf. also Bilirubin

Roberts & Plaa G39,694/66: In mice, α-naphthylisothiocyanate-induced hyperbilirubinemia and cholestasis are aggravated by norethandrolone and norethynodrel but not by mestranol.

Roberts & Plaa G69,070/69: In mice and rats, the hyperbilirubinemia induced by α-naphthylisothiocyanate (ANIT) is enhanced by various drugs and steroids presumably because of an increased rate of bilirubin production and not as a consequence of decreased biliary bilirubin excretion. "Studies of the rate of endogenous bile bilirubin excretion and the incorporation of δ-aminolevulinic acid-^{14}C (ALA-^{14}C) into bilirubin in rats revealed that phenobarbital and chlorpromazine significantly increased the rate of bile bilirubin production (μg/100g/hr) and that phenobarbital, chlorpromazine, and norethandrolone significantly increased the percent incorporation of ALA-^{14}C into bilirubin. Acetohexamide and Enovid both produced an increased, but irregular, response in bile bilirubin excretion and ALA-^{14}C incorporation."

Selye PROT. 42722: In rats, acute ANIT intoxication is markedly inhibited by pretreatment with PCN, CS-1, ethylestrenol and phenobarbital and barely significantly by norbolethone, *cf.* Table 85.

α-Naphthylisothiocyanate ← Norethandrolone, Mouse: Roberts et al. G39,694/66*

1-(1-Naphthyl)-2-thiourea (ANTU) ← cf. Thioureas

Navadel ← *cf.* **Dioxathion** under **Pesticides**

Nembutal ← *cf.* **Pentobarbital** under **Barbiturates**

Neoprontosil ← Progesterone, Norethynodrel: Juchau et al. G40,275/66

Table 85. *Conditioning for α-naphthylisothiocyanate*

Treatment[a]	Dyskinesia[b] (Positive/Total)	Mortality[b] (Dead/Total)
None	15/15	14/15
PCN	2/10***	3/10***
CS-1	4/10***	4/10**
Ethylestrenol	3/10***	3/10***
Spironolactone	7/10 NS	9/10 NS
Norbolethone	6/10*	7/10 NS
Oxandrolone	7/10 NS	7/10 NS
Prednisolone-Ac	10/10 NS	10/10 NS
Triamcinolone	10/10 NS	10/10 NS
Progesterone	10/10 NS	10/10 NS
Estradiol	10/10 NS	10/10 NS
DOC-Ac	7/10 NS	7/10 NS
Hydroxydione	7/10 NS	7/10 NS
Thyroxine	10/10 NS	10/10 NS
Phenobarbital	1/10***	2/10***

[a] The rats of all groups were given α-naphthylisothiocyanate (40 mg/100 g body weight in 1 ml oil, p.o., on 4th day).

[b] Dyskinesia was estimated on 8th day and mortality listed on 9th day ("Exact Probability Test").

For further details on technique of tabulation *cf.* p. VIII.

Nickel Sulfide ←

Jasmin et al. D68,263/63: In rats, a single i.m. injection of nickel sulfide produces metastatic rhabdomyosarcomas whose incidence is increased by methylandrostenolone but is uninfluenced by sex, ovariectomy or orchidectomy.

Nicotinamide ← cf. Vitamin B

Nicotine ← *cf.* also Selye G60,083/70, p.385.

Yun & Lee 34,178/35: Female mice and rabbits are more resistant to nicotine than males. Ovariectomy diminishes nicotine resistance, whereas orchidectomy does not change it. Treatment with "luteohormone" increases nicotine resistance, whereas "follicular hormone" has no effect.

Holck et al. A8,011/37: Female rats are more sensitive than males to various barbiturates and nicotine. Orchidectomy abolishes this increased resistance to barbiturates. Pretreatment with a testoid urinary extract shortens the anesthesia produced by hexobarbital in intact or spayed females. Androsterone is ineffective.

Hueper 91,722/43: In rats, the cardiovascular lesions produced by chronic nicotine intoxication are aggravated both by epinephrine and by DOC.

Selye G60,069/70: In rats, both the motor disturbances and the mortality produced by heavy nicotine intoxication were readily prevented by the standard catatoxic steroids and by phenobarbital. Curiously, even DOC appeared to offer some degree of protection, *cf.* Table 86.

Selye G70,428/70: In rats, ethylestrenol powerfully inhibits the toxicity of digitoxin, nicotine, indomethacin, phenindione, dioxathion, EPN, physostigmine, hexobarbital, cyclopental, thiopental, DOC (anesthesia), meprobamate and picrotoxin. Thyroxine increases the toxicity of many among these drugs and inhibits the protective effect of ethylestrenol.

Selye G70,480/71: In the rat, nicotine intoxication is inhibited by PCN, CS-1, cyproterone, ethylestrenol, spironolactone, norbolethone, oxandrolone, fluoxymesterone, progesterone and DOC. It is not significantly altered by TMACN, 6α-methylprednisolone, spiroxasone, 16β-methyl-16,17-epoxy-3β,11α-dihydroxy-5α-pregnan-20-one, prednisolone, dexamethasone, betamethasone, MAD, emdabol, 17α-acetoxyprogesterone, testosterone, corticosterone, dehydroisoandrosterone, pregnanedione, triamcinolone, 11α-hydroxyprogesterone, hydroxydione, fluorocortisol, cortisol, cortisone or estradiol.

Nicotinic Acid ←

Jelinek & Zikmund B52,661/49: In male rabbits, nicotinic acid i.v. causes less pronounced dilatation of the ear vessels than in females. Castration doubles this effect of nicotinic acid in males but does not change it in females. Testosterone propionate reduces this action of nicotine in orchidectomized males.

Table 86. *Conditioning for nicotine*

Treatment[a]	Dyskinesia[b] (Positive/Total)	Mortality[b] (Dead/Total)
None	15/15	14/15
PCN	3/10 ***	2/10 ***
CS-1	3/15 ***	1/15 ***
Ethylestrenol	1/15 ***	1/15 ***
Spironolactone	6/15 ***	5/15 ***
Norbolethone	0/15 ***	0/15 ***
Oxandrolone	7/15 ***	6/15 ***
Prednisolone-Ac	10/15 *	12/15 NS
Triamcinolone	10/10 NS	10/10 NS
Triamcinolone (2 mg)	15/15 NS	15/15 NS
Progesterone	9/15 **	11/15 NS
Estradiol	10/10 NS	10/10 NS
DOC-Ac	8/15 ***	9/15 *
Hydroxydione	11/15 *	12/15 NS
Thyroxine	10/10 NS	10/10 NS
Phenobarbital	0/10 ***	0/10 ***

[a] The rats of all groups were given nicotine (1 ml/100 g body weight of a 1% aqueous solution, p.o., daily from 4th day ff.).

[b] Dyskinesia was estimated on 6th day 30 min after injection and mortality listed on 9th day ("Exact Probability Test").

For additional pertinent data *cf. also* Table 135.

For further details on technique of tabulation *cf.* p. VIII.

Table 87. *Conditioning for nikethamide*

Treatment[a]	Dyskinesia[b] (Positive/Total)	Mortality[b] (Dead/Total)
None	13/15	3/15
PCN	3/10 **	2/10 NS
CS-1	2/10 ***	2/10 NS
Ethylestrenol	2/10 ***	1/10 NS
Spironolactone	4/10 *	2/10 NS
Norbolethone	1/10 ***	2/10 NS
Oxandrolone	6/10 NS	5/10 NS
Prednisolone-Ac	5/10 NS	4/10 NS
Triamcinolone	9/10 NS	8/10 ***
Progesterone	0/10 ***	0/10 NS
Estradiol	2/10 ***	2/10 NS
DOC-Ac	2/10 ***	0/10 NS
Hydroxydione	3/10 **	1/10 NS
Thyroxine	8/10 NS	7/10 *
Phenobarbital	0/10 ***	0/10 NS

[a] The rats of all groups were given nikethamide (35 mg/100 g body weight in 0.2 ml water, s.c., on 4th day).

[b] Dyskinesia was estimated on 4th day, 4 hrs after injection, and mortality listed on 5th day ("Exact Probability Test").

For further details on technique of tabulation *cf.* p. VIII.

Nikethamide ←

Selye PROT. 42379: In rats, nikethamide (the diethylamide of nicotinic acid) is effectively detoxified by PCN, CS-1, ethylestrenol, norbolethone, progesterone, estradiol, DOC, phenobarbital and apparently even by hydroxydione. Spironolactone exhibits a just significant protective effect, whereas triamcinolone and, to a lesser extent, thyroxine aggravate nikethamide mortality. The amenability of nikethamide to detoxication by steroids is somewhat unusual in that progesterone, estradiol, DOC and hydroxydione, which are endowed with little or no protective effect against most toxicants, appear to be equally, or even more, potent than spironolactone in offering protection against this drug, *cf.* Table 87, p. 274.

p-Nitroanisole ←

Radzialowski & Bousquet G53,591/67: In rats of both sexes, the diurnal variation in the aminopyrine-, p-nitroanisole- and hexobarbital-metabolizing activity of hepatic microsomes is abolished by adrenalectomy.

Selye PROT. 40471: In rats, severe intoxication with p-nitroanisole is readily prevented by PCN and triamcinolone but the other standard conditioning agents were found to have little, if any, effect, *cf.* Table 88.

o-Nitroanisole ← Estradiol: Mitoma et al. G72,113/68

p-Nitrobenzoic Acid ← Progesterone: Juchau et al. G40,275/66

p-Nitrobenzoic Acid ← Ovariectomy: Kato et al. F76,403/66

p-Nitrobenzoic Acid ← Adrenalectomy + Pesticides (Chlordane): Hart et al. G27,102/65

Nitrogen Mustard ←

Hutchinson et al. B84,257/53: In rats, cortisone failed to protect against the lethal effect of nitrogen mustard.

Field et al. F33,399/65; F78,812/67: In mice, the leukopenia and mortality induced by nitrogen mustard (HN_2) or 5-fluorouracil (FU) are diminished by pretreatment with testosterone. "Pretreatment with androgens may be a useful device for reducing the toxic and lethal effects of some anti-cancer drugs but the effects have not been as substantial as previously reported with anti-serotonins and antihistamines."

Table 88. *Conditioning for p-nitroanisole*

Treatment[a]	Dyskinesia[b] (Positive/Total)	Mortality[b] (Dead/Total)
None	9/15	7/15
PCN (1 mg)	0/5 *	0/5 NS
PCN	1/10 ***	1/10 *
CS-1	2/10 NS	2/10 NS
Etylestrenol	1/10 *	1/10 NS
Spironolactone	3/10 NS	3/10 NS
Norbolethone	1/10 *	1/10 NS
Oxandrolone	2/10 NS	2/10 NS
Prednisolone-Ac	5/10 NS	3/10 NS
Triamcinolone	0/10 ***	0/10 *
Progesterone	7/10 NS	3/10 NS
Estradiol	3/10 NS	0/10 *
DOC-Ac	4/10 NS	2/10 NS
Hydroxydione	5/9 NS	4/9 NS
Thyroxine	3/10 NS	1/10 NS
Phenobarbital	6/10 NS	1/10 NS

[a] The rats of all groups were given p-nitroanisole, 15 mg/100 g body weight in 0.1 ml DMSO i.v. once on the 4th day.

[b] Dyskinesia was estimated 30 min after injection and mortality listed on the 5th day ("Exact Probability Test").

For further details on technique of tabulation *cf.* p. VIII.

Nitrose Gas ← *cf.* Ozone

Nitrous Oxide ←

Rummel C79,429/59: In guinea pigs and rats thyroxine increases whereas thyroidectomy decreases the threshold for N_2O anesthesia. Dinitrophenol is ineffective. DOC lowers, whereas cortisone raises, this anesthesia threshold.

Rummel et al. C80,035/59: In rats, pretreatment with cortisone increases, DOC decreases, whereas progesterone, testosterone and hydroxydione do not alter the N_2O anesthesia threshold.

Nortriptyline ←

Bahr et al. H21,089/70: In dogs given nortriptyline and, 6—10 hrs later, various doses of cortisol, the rate of plasma clearance of the drug was delayed. Similarly, in rats, both cortisone and testosterone markedly decreased the rate of nortriptyline disappearance from isolated perfused liver preparations.

These changes may be due to a competition for the hepatic microsomal enzymes which metabolize both nortriptyline and the steroids.

Octamethyl Pyrophosphoramide ← cf. Pesticides

Ornithine cf. OKT under Influence of Steroids upon Enzymes

Orotic Acid ←

Sidransky D64,556/63; Sidransky et al. G4,364/63: The periportal fatty degeneration of the liver produced by chronic orotic acid feeding is more pronounced in female than in male rats. Orchidectomized males developed more severe fatty changes than intact males, or castrate males treated with testosterone. Ovariectomized females developed marked fatty liver changes similar to those of intact females, but this response was diminished by testosterone or estradiol.

Ozone ←

Matzen C39,985/57: Neither cortisol nor prednisolone protects the mouse against the production of pulmonary edema by ozone.

Henschler & Jacob C56,126/58: In rats, the pulmonary edema induced by ozone ("Nitrose gas") is inhibited by prednisolone.

Fairchild G71,531/63: Review (6 pp., 26 refs.) on the effect of thyroidectomy, thioureas, thyroid hormones, glucocorticoids and hypophysectomy upon the resistance of various species to inhaled irritants especially ozone.

Papain ← cf. also Selye C50,810/58, p. 105; C92,918/61, p. 102; G60,083/70, pp. 348, 357.

Thomas C20,800/56: "Cortisone prevents the return of papain-collapsed ears to their normal shape and rigidity. Possibly this reflects a capacity of cortisone to impede the synthesis of deposition of sulfated mucopolysaccharides in tissues."

McCluskey & Thomas C71,485/59: In rabbits "the restoration of the normal rigidity of cartilage and the reaccumulation of basophilic substance in cartilage matrix following its in vivo depletion by papain were largely prevented by cortisone, hydrocortisone or prednisolone. Recovery of cartilage could be prevented locally in joint surfaces by the intra-articular injection of cortisone, hydrocortisone or prednisolone." Studies with ^{35}S sulfate suggest that the glucocorticoids inhibit the synthesis of chondroitin sulfate in cartilage as a result of a topical action.

Potter D23,805/61: Review of the influence of glucocorticoids upon the cartilage lesions produced by papain.

Lack D54,382/62: The softening of the ear cartilages produced by papain i.v. in rabbits can be prevented by pretreatment with cortisone i.m.

Hulth & Westerborn D56,601/63: In rabbits, the lesions produced by cortisone in the growth cartilages are not significantly influenced by vitamin A, but recovery from the papain-induced cartilaginous damage is delayed by cortisone.

Thomas E37,875/64: Review on the effects of papain, vitamin A and cortisone on cartilage matrix in vivo.

Weismann & Thomas E4,216/64: Review of the literature showing that the reconstitution of cartilages in rabbits treated with papain can be prevented by subsequent administration of glucocorticoids for as long as these are administered. In the event of topical application of cortisone to certain cartilages damaged by papain, the delay in reconstitution of cartilage matrix is limited to the treated area.

Lieberman H34,495/71: In hamsters, the emphysema produced by a papain aerosol is inhibited by progesterone and to a lesser extent, by stilbestrol.

Parabromdylamine ←

Selye G70,480/71: In rats, brompheniramine maleate (30 mg/100 g body weight in 0.5 ml DMSO) was administered p.o. twice daily from the 4th to the last day of the experiment. Dyskinesia was estimated on the 5th day 3 hrs after injection, mortality 24 hrs later. Under these circumstances none of the "Standard Conditioners" (p. VIII) caused any noteworthy change in the resulting intoxication. PCN and phenobarbital were not tested.

Pb ← cf. Lead

Pentylenetetrazol ←

Selye A36,443/42: In rats, the anesthesia produced by progesterone or DOC can be interrupted by pentylenetetrazol. Conversely, these anesthetic steroids protect the rat against otherwise fatal doses of pentylenetetrazol.

Cicardo B964/45: In guinea pigs, pretreatment with large doses of DOC does not modify sensitivity to pentylenetetrazol convulsions.

Torda & Wolff B57,149/51: In rats, the convulsions and EEG changes produced by pentylenetetrazol are inhibited by ACTH or cortisone.

Leonard et al. B86,814/53: In mice, pretreatment with cortisone or DOC does not affect pentylenetetrazol-induced convulsions.

Swinyard et al. C17,213/55: In mice, DOC decreases pentylenetetrazol seizure threshold, whereas it increases EST. The effect upon pentylenetetrazol sensitivity is ascribed to DOC-induced hypernatremia.

Boeri C78,610/58: In guinea pigs, cortisone, ACTH and vasopressin aggravate pentylenetetrazol convulsions.

Vacek C63,230/58: DOC anesthesia protects the mouse against the convulsive and lethal effects of strychnine, pentylenetetrazol and caffeine.

Rosadini & Bernardini D58,047/62: In the mouse, pentylenetetrazol convulsions are inhibited by progesterone (given in anesthetic doses) and facilitated by large amounts of estrone sulfate.

Seller & Spector D36,979/62: Pretreatment with single nonanesthetic doses of cortisol enhances the production of pentylenetetrazol convulsions in the rat. Aldosterone has no such effect.

Dashputra et al. F19,871/64: Cortisone and prednisolone aggravated pentylenetetrazol convulsions in rats. Prednisone and dexamethasone were much less active, cortisol, triamcinolone, and DOC virtually inactive in this respect.

Hewett et al. D19,834/64: In mice, various amino-steroids possess "loss-of-righting-reflex activity" and prevent tremorine-induced tremor as well as pentylenetetrazol convulsions. Their effect is ascribed to interneuronal blockade and not to general anesthesia.

Craig F69,385/66: In mice, progesterone, DOC, a series of 3β-(aminoalkyl) esters of pregnenolone and various other steroids proved to inhibit pentylenetetrazol convulsions and electroshock seizures.

Craig & Deason F99,058/68: The anticonvulsant activity (metrazole test) "of a series of 4-pregnene and 5β-pregnane steroids has been studied after oral administration to mice. With a few exceptions it was noted that in general the addition of functional groups to the steroid nucleus resulted in compounds with diminished anticonvulsant activity."

Jelinek H1,518/68: Pretreatment with methyltestosterone does not influence pentylenetetrazol convulsions in the mouse.

Kalyanpur et al. G66,147/69: In mice, various anabolic steroids (methandienone, 4-chlorotestosterone acetate, nandrolone phenpropionate) given i.p. 90 min before pentylenetetrazol, inhibit convulsions. The protective effect is compared to that produced by various anesthetic steroids. [A relationship to enzyme induction is not suggested nor is it probable in view of the shortness of the necessary pretreatment (H.S.).]

Selye G70,480/71: In rats, both the motor disturbances and the mortality caused by severe pentylenetetrazol intoxication were markedly inhibited by PCN, norbolethone and progesterone. Phenobarbital appeared to have a less pronounced effect whereas the other standard conditioners were essentially ineffective, *cf.* Table 89.

Pentylenetetrazol ← Adrenalectomy + ACTH: Torda et al. B69,986/52*

Table 89. *Conditioning for pentylenetetrazol*

Treatment[a]	Dyskinesia[b] (Positive/Total)	Mortality[b] (Dead/Total)
None	13/15	10/15
PCN	1/15 ***	1/15 ***
CS-1	5/10 NS	5/10 NS
Ethylestrenol	6/10 NS	6/10 NS
Spironolactone	7/10 NS	6/10 NS
Norbolethone	2/10 ***	1/10 **
Oxandrolone	8/10 NS	8/10 NS
Prednisolone-Ac	5/10 NS	5/10 NS
Triamcinolone	10/10 NS	9/10 NS
Progesterone	1/10 ***	1/10 **
Estradiol	6/10 NS	6/10 NS
DOC-Ac	6/10 NS	6/10 NS
Hydroxydione	6/10 NS	5/10 NS
Thyroxine	13/15 NS	13/15 NS
Phenobarbital	3/10 **	3/10 NS

[a] The rats of all groups were given pentylenetetrazol (8.5 mg/100 g body weight in 0.2 ml water, s.c., once on 4th day).

[b] Dyskinesia was estimated 2 hrs after injection and mortality listed 24 hrs later ("Exact Probability Test").

For further details on technique of tabulation *cf.* p. VIII.

Peptone ←

Ingle 85,588/44: Adrenocortical extract slightly improved the survival of intact rats following peptone shock. Since the adrenals

Table 90. *Conditioning for* $NaClO_4$

Treatment[a]	Dyskinesia[b] (Positive/Total)	Mortality[b] (Dead/Total)
None	8/10	0/10
PCN	6/10 NS	1/10 NS
CS-1	10/10 NS	0/10 NS
Ethylestrenol	10/10 NS	0/10 NS
Spironolactone	5/10 NS	1/10 NS
Norbolethone	6/10 NS	0/10 NS
Oxandrolone	8/10 NS	2/10 NS
Prednisolone-Ac	2/10 *	10/10 ***
Triamcinolone (2 mg)	1/10 ***	9/10 ***
Progesterone	4/10 NS	0/10 NS
Estradiol (1 mg)	4/10 NS	0/10 NS
DOC-Ac	4/10 NS	1/10 NS
Hydroxydione	4/9 NS	1/9 NS
Thyroxine	0/10 ***	0/10 NS
Phenobarbital	6/10 NS	1/10 NS

[a] The rats of all groups were given $NaClO_4$ (1 mM/100 g body weight in 1 ml water, p.o., twice on 4th day and 2 mM/100 g body weight twice daily, from the 5th day ff.).

[b] Dyskinesia was measured by the "Flick-test" on 6th day 1 hr after the first perchlorate administration and mortality listed on 11th day ("Exact Probability Test").

For further details on technique of tabulation cf. p. VIII.

were grossly hemorrhagic, "it may be reasonable to assume that a damaged gland is unable to meet its requirements for secretory activity as effectively as does an undamaged gland" and that the extract acted as a substitution therapy.

Perchlorates ← cf. also Selye *C 92,918/61*, p. 277.

Bajusz & Selye C64,511/59; C57,180/59; Selye C61,814/59: The spastic muscular contractions (with positive "Flick-test") produced by $NaClO_4$ in the rat can be inhibited by cortisol or triamcinolone, and aggravated by DOC or methylchlorocortisol (Me-Cl-COL). Thyroparathyroidectomy or parathyroidectomy likewise exert a sensitizing effect. Triamcinolone also protects the dog against the syndrome produced by heavy overdosage with $NaClO_4$. Methyltestosterone, estradiol and progesterone did not significantly affect the response of the rat to $NaClO_4$.

Selye G70,480/71: In rats, intoxication with $NaClO_4$ (manifested by the "Flick-test") was most effectively prevented by thyroxine. Prednisolone and triamcinolone also diminished the motor disturbances but greatly increased mortality under the conditions of our test, cf. Table 90.

Permanganate ← cf. also Selye *D15,540/62*, p. 302.

Selye et al. D8,010/62: Topical calciphylaxis produced by $KMnO_4$ s.c. in the rat is not prevented by systemic treatment with large doses of triamcinolone.

Pesticides ←

Durham et al. C27,425/56; C14,264/56: In rats, DDT raised the liver weight/body weight ratio. Diethylstilbestrol increased the storage of DDT and of its metabolite DDE in the fat of male rats, whereas testosterone propionate decreased these values in females. "An endocrine mechanism may account for the sex differences in this regard."

Murphy & Du Bois D28,546/58: The activity of the microsomal-enzyme system which oxidizes thiophosphates to potent anticholinesterase agents is considerably higher in male than in female rats (incubation of liver homogenates with Guthion or ethyl p-nitrophenyl thionobenzenephosphonate or "EPN"). Yet, in vivo, adult males are more resistant to EPN than females perhaps because the accelerated formation of toxic oxidation products is overcompensated by a more efficient detoxication of the latter. The low enzyme activity of female livers is enhanced by pretreatment with testosterone in vivo, whereas the high activity of male livers is diminished by previous castration, partial hepatectomy or treatment with progesterone or diethylstilbestrol. SKF 525-A inhibits, whereas pretreatment with carcinogens or a protein-deficient diet enhances the activity of the thiophosphate-oxidizing enzyme.

Swann et al. C73,379/58: Male rats are more resistant than females to parathion poisoning. Testosterone increases the resistance of females, whereas estrone diminishes that of the males. Curiously, testosterone decreases the resistance of intact males although it increases that of castrated males. After orchidectomy estrone slightly decreases resistance over that of untreated male castrates.

Kato et al. G64,325/62: Adult male rats are more resistant than females to pentobarbital anesthesia, carisoprodol paralysis and strychnine convulsions. Conversely, the lethal effect of OMPA is greater in the male. The sex difference is ascribed to the increased production of anabolic testoids which enhance the decomposition of these substrates, the first three of which are inactivated, the last activated in the process. The differences were also demonstrated in vitro using liver slices or microsomal fractions. The high microsomal activity of the male could be abolished by castration and restored by several anabolic testoids.

Brodeur & DuBois F40,590/65: Immature rats are more sensitive to malathion than adults and their livers detoxify the insecticide at a slower rate. Orchidectomy decreases, whereas testosterone increases, malathion detoxication. All of this suggests that testoids play an important role in the maintenance of the malathion-hydroxylating enzyme system.

Dubois & Kinoshita G66,247/65: Utilizing the anticholinesterase action of 0,0-diethyl 0-(4-methylthio-m-tolyl) phosphorothioate (DMP) as an indicator, it was found that in female rats, "administration of phenobarbital, nikethamide, 3,4-benzpyrene, testosterone, estradiol, cortisone and a number of other steroids induce resistance to the anticholinesterase action of DMP."

Brodeur & DuBois F85,072/67: Immature rats are highly susceptible to the organophosphate insecticide malathion. In vitro, their livers show low malathionase activity. Prolonged pretreatment with testosterone significantly increases the enzymic activity of the livers of castrated young male and adult female rats. Conversely, castration interferes with the maintenance of normal levels of malathionase in adult males and inhibits its development in weanlings. Estradiol decreases malathionase activity in adult males.

Brooks & Harrison G65,297/69: Studies on the kinetics of the inhibition by norethynodrel of epinephrine metabolism by pig liver microsomes in vitro.

Carlson & DuBois H24,653/70: Male rats are much more susceptible to the insecticide 6-methyl-2,3-quinoxalinedithiol cyclic carbonate (Morestan) than females. "The toxicity to rats could not be altered by castration, administration of testosterone to females and estradiol to males. Pretreatment with phenobarbital decreased the toxicity to adult males and increased the toxicity to adult females." Chronic Morestan feeding caused hepatic enlargement and inhibition of microsomal enzymes.

Selye G70,428/70: In rats, ethylestrenol powerfully inhibits the toxicity of digitoxin, nicotine, indomethacin, phenindione, dioxathion, EPN, physostigmine, hexobarbital, cyclopental, thiopental, DOC (anesthesia), meprobamate and picrotoxin. Thyroxine increases the toxicity of many among these drugs and inhibits the protective effect of ethylestrenol.

Selye et al. G70,457/70: In rats, ethylestrenol, CS-1, spironolactone and norbolethone fail to alter sensitivity to OMPA although these typical catatoxic steroids have previously been shown to induce hepatic microsomal enzymes and to detoxify numerous other pesticides. This is of interest because catatoxic barbiturates greatly increase the toxicity of OMPA, presumably by transforming it into a more toxic metabolite. On the other hand, estradiol, estrone and stilbestrol, which have no typical catatoxic actions, considerably increase OMPA toxicity in ovariectomized rats. "The protective effect of catatoxic steroids is presumably due to their structural characteristics and is independent of other pharmacologic actions. Conversely, sensitization to OMPA depends more upon the estrogenic action of compounds than upon their chemical structure, since stilbestrol, a nonsteroidal estrogen, is also highly effective in this respect." Prednisolone, triamcinolone, progesterone, DOC, hydroxydione and thyroxine fail to influence OMPA toxicity.

Selye G70,435/70: In rats, ethylestrenol, CS-1, spironolactone, and norbolethone counteract the lethal effects of ethion, dioxathion, EPN, Guthion and parathion. To a lesser extent, this is also true of oxandrolone, prednisolone and progesterone. Triamcinolone, DOC, hydroxydione, estradiol, and thyroxine offer no consistent protection against these pesticides. DDT is much more resistant against detoxication by even the most powerful catatoxic steroids.

Szabo & Selye G70,497/70: In rats, various catatoxic steroids, and particularly PCN, offer protection against intoxication with parathion and dioxathion. This protective effect is not prevented by hypophysectomy.

Selye G70,480/71: In rats, DDT [1,1,1-Trichloro-2,2-bis (p-chlorophenyl) ethane] (25 mg/100 g body weight in 1 ml corn oil) was administered p.o. once on the 4th day of conditioning. Dyskinesia was measured 24 hrs, mortality 48 hrs, after this injection. Under these circumstances the "Standard Conditioners" (p. VIII) caused no noteworthy change in the resulting intoxication, only phenobarbital exhibited an inhibiting effect.

Selye G70,480/71: In rats, parathion intoxication is prevented by PCN, CS-1, cyproterone, ethylestrenol, spironolactone, norbolethone, TMACN, 16β-methyl-16,17-epoxy-3β,11α-dihydroxy-5α-pregnan-20-one, spiroxasone, dehydroisoandrosterone and pregnanedione. It is not significantly ameliorated by oxandrolone, 6α-methylprednisolone, fluoxymesterone, prednisolone, dexamethasone, MAD, cortisol, emdabol, 17α-acetoxyprogesterone, testosterone, corticosterone, cortisone, progesterone, triamcinolone, 11α-hydroxyprogesterone, hydroxydione, DOC and fluorocortisol. Its toxicity is actually aggravated by betamethasone and estradiol. Dioxathion intoxication is prevented by PCN, CS-1, cyproterone, ethylestrenol, spironolactone, norbolethone, TMACN, oxandrolone, 6α-methylprednisolone, fluoxymesterone, spiroxasone, 16β-methyl-16,17-epoxy-3β,11α-dihydroxy-5α-pregnan-20-one, prednisolone, dexamethasone, betamethasone, hydroxydione, MAD, emdabol, 17α-acetoxyprogesterone, testosterone, pregnanedione, desoxycorticosterone and estradiol. It is not significantly prevented by corticosterone, cortisone, dehydroisoandrosterone, progesterone, cortisol, 11α-hydroxyprogesterone or fluorocortisol but aggravated by triamcinolone.

Selye PROT. 31563,31612: In mice, the lethal effect of dioxathion is powerfully inhibited by ethylestrenol, norbolethone, prednisolone and estradiol, moderately by CS-1 and oxandrolone, but not influenced by spironolactone, progesterone, triamcinolone, DOC, hydroxydione and thyroxine.

Selye G70,480/71: In rats, the lethal effect of heavy dioxathion intoxication could be completely prevented only by the standard catatoxic steroids and by phenobarbital. However, prednisolone, estradiol, DOC, and to a much lesser extent perhaps, progesterone likewise offered some protection against mortality. Triamcinolone and thyroxine diminished resistance to dioxathion. It is especially noteworthy that here as in many other experiments the conditioning effect of the two glucocorticoids in our series differs essentially in that prednisolone protects, whereas triamcinolone aggravates the toxicity of this pesticide, *cf.* Table 91.

Selye G70,480/71: In rats, heavy intoxication with ethion is readily prevented by all standard conditioners, prednisolone, progesterone and phenobarbital. Estradiol given p.o.

Table 91. *Conditioning for dioxathion*

Treatment[a]	Dyskinesia[b] (Positive/Total)	Mortality[b] (Dead/Total)
None	3/10	9/10
PCN	0/10 NS	0/10 ***
CS-1	0/10 NS	0/10 ***
Ethylestrenol	0/10 NS	0/10 ***
Spironolactone	0/10 NS	0/10 ***
Norbolethone	0/10 NS	0/10 ***
Oxandrolone	0/10 NS	0/10 ***
Prednisolone-Ac	0/9 NS	1/9 ***
Triamcinolone (2 mg)	10/10 ***	10/10 NS
Progesterone	5/10 NS	4/10 *
Estradiol (1 mg)	5/15 NS	4/15 ***
Estradiol (1 mg s.c.)	4/10 NS	6/10 NS
DOC-Ac	4/9 NS	1/9 ***
Hydroxydione	2/5 NS	2/5 NS
Thyroxine	10/10 ***	10/10 NS
Phenobarbital	0/10 NS	0/10 ***

[a] The rats of all groups were given dioxathion (4 mg/100 g body weight in 1 ml corn oil, p.o., on 4th day).

[b] Dyskinesia was estimated 5 hrs after injection and mortality listed 48 hrs later ("Exact Probability Test").

For additional pertinent data *cf. also* Table 135.

For further details on technique of tabulation *cf.* p. VIII.

appears to have a slight protective effect against the motor disturbances but the same dose given s.c. is ineffective and hence, the apparent effect of the folliculoid may be due to chance. Interestingly, among the two glucocorticoids prednisolone did, whereas triamcinolone did not offer protection, *cf.* Table 92.

Selye G70,480/71: In rats, heavy intoxication with Guthion is readily prevented by the standard catatoxic steroids and by phenobarbital. Prednisolone appears to have a just significant protecting, and thyroxine a barely significant aggravating effect. The other standard conditioners are inactive, *cf.* Table 93.

Selye G70,480/71: In rats, the motor disturbances of heavy OMPA intoxication are prevented by DOC-Ac and thyroxine but not by the standard catatoxic steroids. The mortality is aggravated by norbolethone and estradiol but since mortality is also very high among the controls receiving large doses of this insecticide, the enhancement of the

Table 92. *Conditioning for ethion*

Treatment[a]	Dyskinesia[b] (Positive/Total)	Mortality[b] (Dead/Total)
None	10/10	7/10
PCN	0/10 ***	0/10 ***
CS-1	0/10 ***	0/10 ***
Ethylestrenol	0/9 ***	0/9 ***
Spironolactone	0/10 ***	0/10 ***
Norbolethone	0/10 ***	0/10 ***
Oxandrolone	1/9 ***	0/9 ***
Prednisolone-Ac	0/10 ***	1/10 **
Triamcinolone (2 mg)	10/10 NS	10/10 NS
Progesterone	3/10 ***	0/10 ***
Estradiol (1 mg)	4/10 **	6/10 NS
Estradiol (1 mg s.c.)	10/10 NS	9/10 NS
DOC-Ac	9/10 NS	7/10 NS
Hydroxydione	7/10 NS	6/10 NS
Thyroxine	10/10 NS	10/10 NS
Phenobarbital	0/10 ***	0/10 ***

[a] The rats of all groups were given ethion (0.5 ml of a 1.2% corn oil solution by 100 g body weight, p.o., once on 4th day).

[b] Dyskinesia was estimated 4 hrs after injection and mortality listed 24 hrs later ("Exact Probability Test").

For further details on technique of tabulation *cf.* p. VIII.

Table 93. *Conditioning for Guthion*

Treatment[a]	Dyskinesia[b] (Positive/Total)	Mortality[b] (Dead/Total)
None	8/10	0/10
PCN	0/10 ***	0/10 NS
CS-1	0/10 ***	0/10 NS
Ethylestrenol	0/10 ***	0/10 NS
Spironolactone	0/10 ***	0/10 NS
Norbolethone	0/10 ***	0/10 NS
Oxandrolone	0/10 ***	0/10 NS
Prednisolone-Ac	3/10 *	0/10 NS
Triamcinolone (2 mg)	10/10 NS	1/10 NS
Progesterone	8/10 NS	0/10 NS
Estradiol (1 mg)	5/10 NS	0/10 NS
Estradiol (1 mg s.c.)	7/10 NS	0/10 NS
DOC-Ac	8/10 NS	0/10 NS
Hydroxydione	9/10 NS	0/10 NS
Cholesterol	8/10 NS	0/10 NS
Thyroxine	10/10 NS	5/10 *
Phenobarbital	0/10 ***	0/10 NS

[a] The rats of all groups were given Guthion (1 mg/100 g body weight in 0.2 ml propylene glycol, s.c., once on 4th day).

[b] Dyskinesia was estimated 2 hrs after injection and mortality listed 24 hrs later ("Exact Probability Test").

For further details on technique of tabulation *cf.* p. VIII.

toxicity is only just significant. It will be recalled however, that in an earlier experiment in which a smaller dose of OMPA (1 mg) was given (Selye G 70,457/70) mortality was greatly augmented by estradiol, estrone and stilbestrol, *cf.* Table 94, p. 282.

Selye PROT. 31704: In 100 g ♀ rats, pretreatment with cyproterone acetate (10 mg/d., p.o.) protects against otherwise fatal intoxication with parathion (1 mg in 0.5 ml DMSO/d., i.p.) but fails to protect against OMPA (1 mg in 0.2 ml corn oil/d., s.c.).

Selye G 70,480/71: In rats, heavy intoxication with parathion could be prevented by PCN, CS-1, ethylestrenol, spironolactone, norbolethone and phenobarbital but not by oxandrolone. Prednisolone appeared to slightly combat the motor disturbances while aggravating the mortality. Estradiol and thyroxine markedly diminished resistance to the lethal effect of this pesticide, *cf.* Table 95, p. 282.

Selye PROT. 31935: In ovariectomized rats, the toxicity of OMPA is considerably increased by pretreatment with natural folliculoids such as estradiol and estrone. Stilbestrol is even more effective in this respect, *cf.* Table 96, p. 283.

Selye PROT. 32307: In ovariectomized rats, the toxicity of OMPA is slightly aggravated by mestranol given as a pretreatment for four days, *cf.* Table 97, p. 283.

Selye PROT. 33905: In rats, OMPA (octamethyl pyrophosphoramide) (1 mg/100 g body weight in 0.2 ml corn oil) was administered s.c. once on the 4th day of conditioning. Dyskinesia was listed 3 hrs, mortality 24 hrs after this injection. Under these circumstances, the "Standard Conditioners" (p. VIII) caused no noteworthy change in the resulting intoxication, only estradiol exhibited an aggravating effect.

Selye PROT. 40387: Unlike most pesticides, heptachlor is comparatively insensitive to toxication or detoxication by various steroids, *cf.* Table 98, p. 283.

Selye PROT. 35804: In rats, heavy intoxication with EPN is readily prevented by the standard catatoxic steroids and by phenobarbital. Several other conditioning agents appear to have some protective effect against this pesticide whereas thyroxine aggravates its toxicity, *cf.* Table 99, p. 284.

Selye PROT. 31639, 31649: In rats (100 g ♀), pretreatment with triamterene (1 mg in 1 ml water p.o. x2/day) or amiloride (300 µg in 1 ml water p.o. x2/day) fails to protect against hexobarbital, progesterone, parathion or dioxathion.

0,0-Diethyl-0-(4-methylthio-m-tolylphosphorothioate) ← Steroids: DuBois et al. D43,878/61*, G66,247/65*

Fenthion ← Cortisone + X-irradiation(head) + Age: DuBois G77,578/67

Guthion ← Steroids: Murphy et al. D28,546/58

Morestan ← Steroids: Carlson et al. H24,653/70*

Naphthalene ← Testoids (anabolic): Booth et al. D34,656/62

Paraoxon ← Adrenalectomy + Hexamethonium: Holtz et al. C76,300/58*

Parathion ← Testosterone: DuBois et al. G66,495/49*

Phenformin ← *cf. Pancreatic Hormones*
Phenindione ← *cf. Anticoagulants*

Phenol ←

Samaras & Dietz C56,733/58: In mice, pretreatment with "swimming stress" increases sensitivity to the production of intense convulsions by phenol s.c. Cortisol does not modify phenol intoxication.

Phenol ← Prednisolone: Inscoe et al. F70,325/66

Phenoxybenzamine ←

Selye et al. G60,020/69: In the rat, pretreatment with norbolethone protects against the anesthetic effect of progesterone, desoxycorticosterone, pregnanedione, dehydroepiandrosterone, testosterone, diethylstilbestrol, pentobarbital and methyprylon. It does not significantly alter the corresponding actions of urethan, diazepam, chlorpromazine, reserpine, phenoxybenzamine, chloral hydrate, potassium bromide or magnesium chloride.

Selye et al. G60,016/69: In rats, spironolactone protects against anesthesia produced

Table 94. *Conditioning for OMPA*

Treatment[a]	Dyskinesia[b] (Positive/Total)	Mortality[b] (Dead/Total)
None	15/15	9/15
PCN	8/10 NS	6/10 NS
CS-1	10/10 NS	7/10 NS
Ethylestrenol	10/10 NS	9/10 NS
Spironolactone	10/10 NS	8/10 NS
Norbolethone	10/10 NS	10/10 *
Oxandrolone	10/10 NS	9/10 NS
Prednisolone-Ac	9/10 NS	6/10 NS
Triamcinolone	8/10 NS	4/10 NS
Progesterone	8/10 NS	1/10 *
Estradiol	10/10 NS	10/10 *
DOC-Ac	5/10 ***	2/10 NS
Hydroxydione	9/9 NS	4/9 NS
Thyroxine	4/20 ***	4/20 *
Phenobarbital	10/10 NS	8/10 NS

[a] The rats of all groups were given OMPA, octamethyl pyrophosphoramide (1.7 mg/100 g body weight in 0.2 ml corn oil, s.c., on 4th day).

[b] Dyskinesia was estimated 2 hrs after injection and mortality listed 24 hrs later ("Exact Probability Test").

For further details on technique of tabulation *cf.* p. VIII.

Table 95. *Conditioning for parathion*

Treatment[a]	Dyskinesia[b] (Positive/Total)	Mortality[b] (Dead/Total)
None	11/15	4/15
PCN	0/10 ***	0/10 NS
CS-1	0/10 ***	0/10 NS
Ethylestrenol	1/15 ***	0/15 *
Spironolactone	0/15 ***	0/15 *
Norbolethone	1/10 ***	0/10 NS
Oxandrolone	7/10 NS	3/10 NS
Prednisolone-Ac	3/10 *	7/10 *
Triamcinolone (2 mg)	11/15 NS	10/15 *
Progesterone	4/10 NS	3/10 NS
Estradiol (1 mg)	10/10 NS	10/10 ***
Estradiol (1 mg s.c.)	9/10 NS	9/10 ***
DOC-Ac	7/10 NS	4/10 NS
Hydroxydione	3/10 *	1/10 NS
Thyroxine	15/15 *	15/15 ***
Phenobarbital	1/10 ***	0/10 NS

[a] The rats of all groups were given parathion (1 mg/100 g body weight in 0.5 ml DMSO, i.p., daily, from 4th day ff.).

[b] Dyskinesia was estimated on the 5th day, 3 hrs after injection, and mortality listed on 6th day ("Exact Probability Test").

For additional pertinent data *cf. also* Table 135.

For further details on technique of tabulation *cf.* p. VIII.

Table 96. *Aggravation of OMPA toxicity by various folliculoids*

Pretreatment[a]	Prostration[b] (Positive/Total)			Mortality[b] (Dead/Total)		
	Estradiol	Estrone	Stilbestrol	Estradiol	Estrone	Stilbestrol
None	0/10	1/10	1/10	0/10	1/10	1/10
10 µg s.c.	1/10 NS	2/10 NS	2/9 NS	1/10 NS	0/10 NS	1/9 NS
10 µg p.o.	2/10 NS	0/10 NS	2/10 NS	0/10 NS	0/10 NS	0/10 NS
100 µg s.c.	2/10 NS	0/10 NS	9/10 ***	0/10 NS	0/10 NS	5/10 NS
100 µg p.o.	0/10 NS	1/10 NS	9/10 ***	0/10 NS	0/10 NS	4/10 NS
1 mg s.c.	8/10 ***	8/10 ***	10/10 ***	3/10 NS	1/10 NS	8/10 ***
1 mg p.o.	5/9 *	7/10 **	8/10 ***	2/9 NS	1/10 NS	7/10 **
10 mg s.c.	7/10 ***	7/10 **	10/10 ***	3/10 NS	0/10 NS	8/10 ***
10 mg p.o.	8/10 ***	9/10 ***	10/10 ***	8/10 ***	4/10 NS	9/10 ***

[a] All rats (100 g ♀) were ovariectomized on 1st day and then treated with the folliculoids. The doses indicated in 0.2 ml (in the case of stilbestrol in 0.4 ml) of water s.c. or in 1 ml water p.o. ,daily. They were given OMPA 1 mg/100 g body weight in 0.2 ml oil once s.c. on 4th day.

[b] The severity of the prostration was estimated 4 hrs after OMPA injection and mortality was listed 44 hrs later (Statistics Fisher & Yates).

For further details on technique of tabulation cf. p. VIII.

by progesterone, DOC, hydroxydione, pregnanedione, dehydroepiandrosterone, testosterone, diethylstilbestrol, methyprylon, pentobarbital and ethanol. It does not significantly alter the corresponding actions of morphine, codeine, urethan, diazepam, chlorpromazine, reserpine, phenoxybenzamine, chloral hydrate, potassium bromide or $MgCl_2$.

Table 97. *Doubtful aggravation of OMPA toxicity by pretreatment with mestranol*

Treatment[a]	Prostration[b] (Positive/Total)	Mortality[b] (Dead/Total)
None	1/5	0/5
Mestranol s.c.	5/5 *	2/5 NS
Mestranol p.o.	4/5 NS	2/5 NS

[a] The rats (100 g ♀) of all groups were ovariectomized on the 1st day and then received mestranol 10 mg s.c. in 0.2 ml water or p.o. in 1 ml water/day. All animals were given OMPA 1 mg per 100 g body weight in 0.2 ml oil, s.c. once, 4th day, 1 hr after mestranol administration.

[b] The severity of the prostration was estimated 3 hrs after OMPA injection and mortality was listed 48 hrs later (Fisher & Yates test).

For further details on technique of tabulation cf. p. VIII.

Table 98. *Conditioning for heptachlor*

Treatment[a]	Dyskinesia[b] (Positive/Total)	Mortality[b] (Dead/Total)
None	9/15	15/15
PCN	6/10 NS	10/10 NS
CS-1	7/10 NS	10/10 NS
Ethylestrenol	6/10 NS	10/10 NS
Spironolactone	6/10 NS	10/10 NS
Norbolethone	10/10 *	10/10 NS
Oxandrolone	6/10 NS	10/10 NS
Prednisolone-Ac	1/10 *	10/10 NS
Triamcinolone	9/10 NS	10/10 NS
Progesterone	10/10 *	10/10 NS
Estradiol	10/10 *	10/10 NS
DOC-Ac	9/10 NS	10/10 NS
Hydroxydione	4/10 NS	10/10 NS
Thyroxine	10/10 *	10/10 NS
Phenobarbital	5/10 NS	10/10 NS

[a] The rats of all groups were given heptachlor (10 mg/100 g body weight in 0.2 ml DMSO p.o., once on 4th and 5th day).

[b] Dyskinesia was estimated on 5th day, 2 hrs after the last injection. Mortality was listed on 9th day ("Exact Probability Test").

For further details on technique of tabulation cf. p. VIII.

Table 99. *Conditioning for EPN*

Treatment[a]	Dyskinesia[b] (Positive/Total)	Mortality[b] (Dead/Total)
None	14/15	9/15
PCN	1/10 ***	0/10 ***
CS-1	0/15 ***	0/15 ***
Ethylestrenol	0/15 ***	0/15 ***
Spironolactone	1/15 ***	0/15 ***
Norbolethone	0/15 ***	0/15 ***
Oxandrolone	0/15 ***	0/15 ***
Prednisolone-Ac	8/15 *	6/15 NS
Triamcinolone (2 mg)	12/15 NS	7/15 NS
Progesterone	9/15 *	4/15 NS
Estradiol (1 mg)	8/15 *	0/15 ***
DOC-Ac	12/15 NS	1/15 ***
Hydroxydione	4/15 ***	2/15 *
Cholesterol	14/15 NS	6/15 NS
Thyroxine	15/15 NS	15/15 **
Phenobarbital	0/10 ***	0/10 ***

[a] The rats of all groups were given EPN, phenylphosphonothioic acid 0-ethyl 0-p-nitrophenyl ester (0.7 mg/100 g body weight in 0.2 ml DMSO, i.p., on 4th day).

[b] Dyskinesia was estimated 1 hr after injection and mortality listed 24 hrs later ("Exact Probability Test").

For further details on technique of tabulation cf. p. VIII.

Phenylalanine ←

Reiss et al. F 81,632/66: In rabbits given large amounts of phenylalanine the blood and tissue concentration of this compound could be reduced by pretreatment with norbolethone decanoate or STH.

Phenylbutazone ← Prednisone, Man: Levi et al. F 99,523/68*

Phenytoin ← Lynestrenol, Mouse: Rümke et al. H 14,039/69*

Phenyramidol ←

Selye PROT. 42329: In rats, phenyramidol sleeping time is significantly shortened by PCN, CS-1, ethylestrenol, spironolactone, norbolethone, oxandrolone, prednisolone and phenobarbital but, somewhat unexpectedly, estradiol also shares this effect, cf. Table 100.

Table 100. *Conditioning for phenyramidol*

Treatment[a]	Sleeping Time[b] (min)
None	100 ± 8
PCN	17 ± 8 ***
CS-1	15 ± 8 ***
Ethylestrenol	15 ± 9 ***
Spironolactone	34 ± 12 ***
Norbolethone	31 ± 13 ***
Oxandrolone	45 ± 14 **
Prednisolone-Ac	55 ± 12 **
Triamcinolone	76 ± 10 NS
Progesterone	83 ± 11 NS
Estradiol	40 ± 13 ***
DOC-Ac	103 ± 19 NS
Hydroxydione	91 ± 6 NS
Thyroxine	108 ± 13 NS
Phenobarbital	30 ± 12 ***

[a] The rats of all groups were given phenyramidol (50 mg/100 g body weight in 0.2 ml water, s.c., on 4th day).

[b] Sleeping time (Student's t-test).

For further details on technique of tabulation cf. p. VIII.

Phlorhizin ←

Winter & Belanger A 36,751/41: In the rat, pretreatment with testosterone inhibits phlorhizin glycosuria and the associated renal lesions.

Phosgene ←

English F 399/64: Description of a single patient who recovered from phosgene poisoning after treatment with cortisol.

Phosphate ← cf. also Selye B 40,000/50, p. 613; C 92,918/61, p. 205.

Selye & Bois C 12,616/56: The nephrocalcinosis which develops in rats treated with DOC + NaH_2PO_4 is inhibited by cortisol.

Selye & Bois C 13,168/56: Selective corticomedullary nephrocalcinosis can be obtained in uninephrectomized rats by NaH_2PO_4 p.o. even after adrenalectomy. This effect is aggravated by DOC and virtually absent if the animals are maintained exclusively with cortisol. The action of DOC is counteracted by concurrent treatment with cortisol. "It appears that the corticoids exert an important regulating influence upon the ability of the kidney to handle an excess of phosphate."

Selye C 38,401/57: In the rat, estradiol facilitates the production of cortico-medullary nephrocalcinosis by NaH_2PO_4. A similar effect is produced by DOC. "Since oestradiol is completely devoid of mineralocorticoid, and deoxycorticosterone of folliculoid actions, the enhancement of nephrocalcinosis appears to be an 'independent steroid hormone action'."

Selye C38,768/58: The cortico-medullary nephrocalcinosis produced in rats by an excessive intake of NaH_2PO_4 is largely inhibited by ovariectomy and enhanced even in the ovariectomized animal by comparatively small doses of estradiol or stilbestrol. The nephrocalcinotic effect of estradiol is not significantly influenced under these conditions by large doses of progesterone but greatly aggravated by methyltestosterone, although luteoids and testoids counteract many of the other actions of folliculoids.

Selye C39,319/58: In rats, nephrocalcinosis produced by excess NaH_2PO_4 p.o. is aggravated by estradiol, but even the severe calcification induced by this combined treatment is prevented by hypophysectomy.

Cantin D36,815/62: In the rat, the nephrocalcinosis produced by Na_2HPO_4 is aggravated by DOC or estradiol. Parathyroidectomy prevents this change, even following combined hormone and phosphate treatment.

Cornelius D58,739/63: In sheep, large amounts of urinary calculi were regularly produced by a high phosphate diet after orchidectomy. [The author gives no evidence that the orchidectomy was essential (H.S.).]

Cantin F5,681/64: The nephrocalcinosis produced in rats by combined treatment with NaH_2PO_4 + either estradiol or DOC is prevented by parathyroidectomy or thyroparathyroidectomy, and in either case additional treatment with thyroxine prevents nephrocalcinosis.

Phosphorus ←

Berdjis F79,528/67: The hepatotoxic effect of CCl_4, phosphorus and ethionine could be diminished by cortisone and survival prolonged.

Allegri & Ferrari B53,060/49: In rats, testosterone offers moderate protection against the hepatic damage produced by phosphorus poisoning.

Selye G70,480/71: In rats, elementary yellow phosphorus (150 µg/100 g body weight in 0.4 ml corn oil) was administered p.o. once daily, from the 4th day of conditioning to the end of the experiment. Osteosclerosis and hepatic steatosis were listed on the day of death, and the mean survival was computed.

Under these circumstances, none of the "Standard Conditioners" (p. VIII) or cholesterol caused any noteworthy change in the resulting intoxication. Hydroxydione, PCN and phenobarbital were not tested.

Physostigmine ←

Selye G70,428/70: In rats, ethylestrenol powerfully inhibits the toxicity of digitoxin, nicotine, indomethacin, phenindione, dioxathion, EPN, physostigmine, hexobarbital, cyclopental, thiopental, DOC (anesthesia), meprobamate and picrotoxin. Thyroxine increases the toxicity of many among these drugs and inhibits the protective effect of ethylestrenol.

Selye G70,435/70: In rats, intoxication with physostigmine was diminished by ethylestrenol, CS-1, spironolactone, and prednisolone, but aggravated by estradiol and thyroxine. Norbolethone, oxandrolone, progesterone, triamcinolone, DOC, and hydroxydione had no significant effect.

Selye G70,480/71: In rats, the toxicity of physostigmine (unlike that of the anticholines-

Table 101. *Conditioning for physostigmine*

Treatment[a]	Dyskinesia[b] (Positive/Total)	Mortality[b] (Dead/Total)
None	6/10	2/10
PCN	1/10 *	0/10 NS
CS-1	0/10 **	0/10 NS
Ethylestrenol	0/10 **	0/10 NS
Spironolactone	1/10 *	0/10 NS
Norbolethone	3/10 NS	1/10 NS
Oxandrolone	4/10 NS	1/10 NS
Prednisolone-Ac	1/10 *	1/10 NS
Triamcinolone (2 mg)	5/10 NS	3/10 NS
Progesterone	5/10 NS	1/10 NS
Estradiol (1 mg)	10/10 *	8/10 *
Estradiol (1 mg s.c.)	10/10 *	4/10 NS
DOC-Ac	3/10 NS	2/10 NS
Hydroxydione	5/9 NS	1/9 NS
Thyroxine	10/10 *	9/10 ***
Phenobarbital	2/10 NS	0/10 NS

[a] The rats of all groups were given physostigmine sulfate (1 mg/100 g body weight in 1 ml water, p.o., once on 4th day).

[b] Dyskinesia was estimated 1 hr after injection and mortality listed 24 hrs later ("Exact Probability Test").

For further details on technique of tabulation cf. p. VIII.

Table 102. *Conditioning for picrotoxin*

Treatment[a]	Dyskinesia[b] (Positive/Total)	Mortality[b] (Dead/Total)
None	15/15	13/15
PCN	3/10 ***	0/10 ***
CS-1	2/15 ***	1/15 ***
Ethylestrenol	0/15 ***	0/15 ***
Spironolactone	4/15 ***	2/15 ***
Norbolethone	0/15 ***	0/15 ***
Oxandrolone	4/15 ***	0/15 ***
Prednisolone-Ac	2/15 ***	0/15 ***
Triamcinolone (2 mg)	13/15 NS	6/15 *
Progesterone	1/15 ***	0/15 ***
Estradiol (1 mg)	10/10 NS	5/10 NS
Estradiol (1 mg s.c.)	10/10 NS	5/10 NS
DOC-Ac	11/15 *	4/15 ***
Hydroxydione	11/15 *	6/15 *
Thyroxine	10/10 NS	10/10 NS
Phenobarbital	0/10 ***	0/10 ***
β-Sitosterol	14/15 NS	11/15 NS

[a] The rats of all groups were given picrotoxin (350 μg/100 g body weight in 0.2 ml water, s.c., on 4th day).

[b] Dyskinesia was estimated 30 min after injection and mortality listed 24 hrs later ("Exact Probability Test").

For further details on technique of tabulation cf. p. VIII.

terase pesticides) is only moderately diminished by PCN, CS-1, ethylestrenol, spironolactone and prednisolone. Estradiol and thyroxine diminish physostigmine resistance, whereas phenobarbital does not affect it significantly, cf. Table 101, p. 285.

Picrotoxin ← cf. also Selye G60,083/70, p. 385.

Clarke A36,747/41: Rats can be protected against otherwise fatal doses of picrotoxin by the administration of anesthetic doses of DOC.

Holck D28,543/49: Adult male rats are more resistant than females to toxic doses of picrotoxin. Such a sex difference is absent in one-month-old rats. Castration lowers picrotoxin resistance in rats of either sex. Testosterone raises picrotoxin resistance in normal and especially in spayed females, but not in males. Blockade of the RES abolished the sex difference but corticosterone failed to influence it.

Selye G60,070/70: In rats, picrotoxin poisoning can be prevented by ethylestrenol, CS-1, spironolactone, norbolethone, oxandrolone, prednisolone and progesterone. Triamcinolone, DOC, hydroxydione, cholesterol and β-sitosterol have no such protective effect.

Selye G60,087/70: In rats, fatal intoxication with picrotoxin is readily combated by the classic catatoxic steroids, prednisolone, progesterone and phenobarbital. To a lesser extent DOC, and hydroxydione may also be effective. β-Sitosterol (a pharmacologically inert steroid included in this series as an additional control) is quite ineffective in protecting against picrotoxin, cf. Table 102.

Selye G70,428/70: In rats, ethylestrenol powerfully inhibits the toxicity of digitoxin, nicotine, indomethacin, phenindione, dioxathion, EPN, physostigmine, hexobarbital, cyclopental, thiopental, DOC (anesthesia), meprobamate and picrotoxin. Thyroxine increases the toxicity of many among these drugs and inhibits the protective effect of ethylestrenol.

Selye PROT. 27594: In mice, pretreatment with spironolactone, ethylestrenol, triamcinolone or thyroxine had little, if any, effect upon the toxicity of picrotoxin under our experimental conditions.

Picrotoxin ← Corticosterone: Holck D28,543/49*

Picrotoxin ← Ovariectomy + Testosterone: Holck D28,543/49*

Piperidine ←

Selye G70,480/71: In rats, moderate intoxication with piperidine did not cause sufficient mortality among the controls to identify the possible protective effect of our standard conditioning agents but in any event, none of them increased susceptibility to this toxicant. On the other hand, the motor disturbances were most significantly inhibited by CS-1, ethylestrenol, norbolethone, oxandrolone, triamcinolone, progesterone, hydroxydione and phenobarbital. Even DOC and thyroxine appeared to have offered some protection. This rather nonspecific protective effect of so many among our conditioners is reminiscent of their effect upon intoxication with methyprylon (a piperidine derivative). One noteworthy difference is that methyprylon intoxication is completely prevented by PCN whereas piperidine is singularly resistant to prophylaxis by this highly potent catatoxic steroid, cf. Table 103.

Table 103. *Conditioning for piperidine*

Treatment[a]	Dyskinesia[b] (Positive/Total)	Mortality[b] (Dead/Total)
None	12/15	2/15
PCN	10/10 NS	0/10 NS
CS-1	1/10 ***	0/10 NS
Ethylestrenol	1/15 ***	0/15 NS
Spironolactone	7/15 NS	1/15 NS
Norbolethone	1/10 ***	0/10 NS
Oxandrolone	2/10 ***	0/10 NS
Prednisolone-Ac	5/10 NS	0/10 NS
Triamcinolone	2/15 ***	1/15 NS
Progesterone	1/10 ***	0/10 NS
Estradiol	8/10 NS	0/10 NS
DOC-Ac	3/10 *	1/10 NS
Hydroxydione	0/10 ***	0/10 NS
Thyroxine	5/15 *	2/15 NS
Phenobarbital	0/10 ***	0/10 NS

[a] The rats of all groups were given piperidine (50 mg/100 g body weight in 1 ml water, p.o., once on 4th day).

[b] Dyskinesia was estimated 5 hrs after injection and mortality listed on the 5th day ("Exact Probability Test"). This experiment was subsequently repeated several times and the results were too variable for reliable evaluation. Depending upon uncontrollable factors, the same conditioners, which provided good protection in certain instances, were ineffective when the experiments were repeated.

For further details on technique of tabulation *cf.* p. VIII.

Pipradol ←

Selye G 70,480/71: In rats, pipradol hydrochloride (30 mg/100 g body weight in 1 ml corn oil) was administered p.o. once on the 4th day of conditioning. Dyskinesia was listed 3 hrs, mortality 24 hrs after this injection. Under these circumstances, the "Standard Conditioners" (p. VIII) caused no noteworthy change in the resulting intoxication, only PCN exhibited an inhibitory effect. Phenobarbital was not tested.

Plant Extracts ←

Campbell C 38,327/57: In cockerels, the hepatic damage produced by the pyrrolizidine alkaloids of ragwort (Senecio jacoboea L.) disappears very slowly if at all, whereas hens recover. In both sexes, but particularly in cockerels, stilbestrol accelerates hepatic regeneration.

Plasmocid ← *cf. Selye C 50,810/58, p. 110; C 92,918/61, p. 95.*

Polyvinyl Alcohol ← *cf. Selye G 60,083/70, p. 358.*

Potassium ←

Zwemer & Truszkowski A 2,330/37: Adrenocortical extract protects intact mice and guinea pigs against otherwise fatal amounts of KCl i.p.

Lowenstein et al. A 74,481/43: In rats, pretreatment with DOC increased, whereas thyroid feeding decreased resistance to KCl i.p.

Mullins et al. 83,885/43: In rabbits, both adrenocortical extract and DOC can protect against acute potassium intoxication, but only under certain experimental conditions.

Thatcher & Radike B 4,515/47: In rats, resistance to KCl intoxication was increased by DOC or adrenocortical extract.

Robertson B 32,963/49: In mice and rats, DOC increases resistance to multiple injections of KCl, both in the absence and in the presence of the adrenals. Potassium tolerance may be used as a test for adrenocortical function.

Collins C 7,486/55: In rats, the resistance to KCl i.p. is diminished by pretreatment with glucocorticoids perhaps as a consequence of adrenal atrophy.

Collins C 12,721/56: In rats, prolonged pretreatment with cortisol decreases tolerance to the i.p. injection of KCl. This "is probably due to hypofunction of the adrenal-pituitary axis rather than to steroid-induced alterations of electrolyte balance."

Collins C 17,662/56: Survival after KCl i.p. (referred to as "potassium stress") is diminished after the induction of adrenocortical atrophy by cortisol. Concurrent administration of DOC, aldosterone, adrenocortical extract, corticosterone or ACTH counteracts this effect of cortisol upon K-tolerance.

Wallon & Browaeys C 78,322/59: Addition of KCl to the drinking water prolongs the survival of rats given large doses of cortisone.

Spremolla & Grassi G 68,941/63: Renal lesions produced in rats by a K-deficient diet can be corrected by 4-chlorotestosterone.

Grassi & Spremolla F 28,126/64: 4-Chlorotestosterone prevents the drop in K, glycogen, and nitrogen as well as the morphologic changes produced in the liver of rats kept on a K-deficient diet.

Pralidoxime ←

Selye G70,435/70: In rats, pralidoxime intoxication was counteracted by prednisolone and, to a lesser extent, by ethylestrenol and estradiol, CS-1, spironolactone, norbolethone, oxandrolone, progesterone, triamcinolone, DOC, hydroxydione, and thyroxine had no significant effect.

Selye G70,480/71: In rats, intoxication with pralidoxime (an anticholinesterase inhibitor and cholinesterase reactivator) was readily prevented by triamcinolone and prednisolone, the two glucocorticoids of our series, whereas the other conditioning agents had little if any effect upon this toxicant, *cf.* Table 104.

Table 104. *Conditioning for pralidoxime*

Treatment[a]	Dyskinesia[b] (Positive/ Total)	Mortality[b] (Dead/ Total)
None	11/13	7/13
PCN	10/10 NS	7/10 NS
CS-1	7/9 NS	5/9 NS
Ethylestrenol	3/8 *	0/8 *
Spironolactone	8/10 NS	6/10 NS
Norbolethone	6/10 NS	2/10 NS
Oxandrolone	6/10 NS	3/10 NS
Prednisolone-Ac	0/10 ***	0/10 **
Triamcinolone	0/10 ***	1/10 *
Progesterone	8/10 NS	4/10 NS
Estradiol	3/9 *	0/9 *
DOC-Ac	8/10 NS	1/10 *
Hydroxydione	8/10 NS	6/10 NS
Cholesterol	4/9 NS	2/9 NS
Thyroxine	4/9 NS	1/9 NS
Phenobarbital	3/10 *	4/10 NS

[a] The rats of all groups were given pralidoxime Cl (16 mg/100 g body weight in 0.2 ml water, s.c., on 4th and 5th day).

[b] Dyskinesia was estimated on 4th day 30 min after injection and mortality listed on 6th day ("Exact Probability Test").

For further details on technique of tabulation *cf.* p. VIII.

Primaquine ←

el-Denshary et al. G77,356/69: In rabbits, the hepatic damage produced by primaquine is most effectively prevented by choline but, to a lesser extent, also by dexamethasone.

Procaine ←

Munoz et al. G68,223/61: Male rats are more resistant than females to the convulsant action of procaine i.p. Gonadectomy decreased resistance in males but not in females. Testosterone did not significantly alter resistance in either sex.

Paeile et al. F52,633/64: Adult male rats are more resistant to procaine than adult females. Chronic CCl_4 poisoning, pretreatment with SKF 525-A and orchidectomy diminish the resistance of the males approximately to the female level. The plasma procainesterase activity is approximately the same in both sexes and not affected by orchidectomy or CCl_4 intoxication.

Brodeur et al. F99,981/67: The procainesterase activity of the liver is higher in adult male rats than in adult females or immature rats of either sex. Ovariectomy and chronic treatment with testosterone or norethandrolone increase hepatic procainesterase activity in adult females. Conversely, orchidectomy and chronic treatment with estradiol or progesterone decrease this enzyme activity in the livers of adult males. However, immature rats are more resistant to procaine in vivo than could be expected from the reduced ability of their livers to hydrolyze procaine in vitro. "Factors other than drug metabolism appear to govern the ultimate toxicity of procaine in immature rats."

Promazine ←

Rudofsky & Crawford E58,989/66: Following administration of meperidine or promazine "pregnant women, women on oral contraceptives and neonates excreted significantly more unchanged meperidine than normeperidine, whereas the reverse held for the male 'controls' and other female groups. Pregnant women, women on oral contraceptives and neonates excreted more unchanged and minimally degraded promazine than non-pregnant women. Stilbestrol and progesterone each changed the pattern of excretion by male subjects toward that associated with pregnancy." Apparently, pregnancy diminishes the capacity to metabolize meperidine and promazine, a change reflected in neonates and subjects taking oral contraceptives.

Crawford & Rudofsky G42,454/66: In women taking various oral contraceptives, as well as in pregnant women and in neonates, the urinary excretion of pethidine and promazine is increased, suggesting interference with the detoxication of these drugs.

Propionitrile ←

Gellhorn 16,839/23: In mice, resistance against acetonitrile can be increased not only by thyroid extract but, to a lesser extent, also by extracts of various other tissues. These preparations also augment resistance to KCN and propionitrile, whereas thyroidectomy and orchidectomy have an opposite effect.

Selye G70,480/71: In rats, propionitrile poisoning was aggravated by PCN, prednisolone, triamcinolone and thyroxine but not strikingly affected by the other conditioners involved in this series, although estradiol and hydroxydione may have offered barely significant protection, *cf.* Table 105.

Table 105. *Conditioning for propionitrile*

Treatment[a]	Dyskinesia[b] (Positive/Total)	Mortality[b] (Dead/Total)
None	7/15	1/15
PCN	10/10 **	9/10 ***
CS-1	4/10 NS	4/10 NS
Ethylestrenol	6/15 NS	3/15 NS
Spironolactone	3/15 NS	3/15 NS
Norbolethone	2/10 NS	4/10 NS
Oxandrolone	3/10 NS	2/10 NS
Prednisolone-Ac	10/10 **	10/10 ***
Triamcinolone	15/15 ***	14/15 ***
Progesterone	3/10 NS	3/10 NS
Estradiol	0/10 *	0/10 NS
DOC-Ac	1/10 NS	1/10 NS
Hydroxydione	0/10 *	0/10 NS
Thyroxine	15/15 ***	15/15 ***
Phenobarbital	5/10 NS	0/10 NS

[a] The rats of all groups were given propionitrile (15 mg by 100 g body weight in 0.2 ml water, s.c., once on 4th day).

[b] Dyskinesia was estimated 4 hrs after injection and mortality listed 24 hrs later ("Exact Probability Test").

For further details on technique of tabulation *cf.* p. VIII.

Puromycin Aminonucleotide (PAN) ←

Selye C38,594/57: The nephrosis and osteitis fibrosa produced by PAN in the rat is inhibited by cortisol and aggravated by DOC.

Fiegelson et al. D96,580/57: In the rat, PAN-nephrosis is adversely influenced by cortisol, whereas anti-kidney-serum nephritis is largely inhibited by it.

Wilson et al. C45,755/57: In rats, PAN nephrosis is not prevented by cortisone or ACTH.

Gupta & Giroud C73,800/59: In rats, the production of nephrosis by PAN is inhibited by spironolactone. Apparently "in aminonucleoside nephrosis the increased rate of secretion of aldosterone is one of the main factors operating in fluid retention."

Borowsky et al. D2,508/61: The course of an already-established PAN nephrosis was not altered by treatment with 0.4 mg/day of prednisolone after cessation of PAN-treatment. From this, it was concluded that "steroids do not modify this lesion."

Fisher & Gruhn D12,898/61: The histologic and electron microscopic alterations produced by PAN (6-dimethyl-aminopurine-3-amino-d-ribose) in the rat are not affected by cortisone, adrenalectomy or hypophysectomy.

Herken et al. G15,041/63: In rats, both the functional and the ultrastructural kidney lesions produced by PAN are counteracted by triamcinolone, dexamethasone and 6-methylprednisolone.

Lannigan D69,709/63: Chronic treatment with low doses of hydrocortisol (3 mg/kg in the drinking water) moderately diminished the severity of PAN-nephrosis in rats.

Pyribenzamine ←

Mayer et al. B3,674/46: Male rats are much more resistant to pyribenzamine than females. Castration of females rendered them almost as resistant as males but treatment of ovariectomized rats with "estrogen" did not give consistent results in a small series of preliminary experiments.

Pyrilamine ←

Selye G70,480/71: In rats, pyrilamine maleate (8 mg/100 g body weight in 0.2 ml water) was administered s.c. once on the 4th day of conditioning. Dyskinesia was listed 30 min, mortality 24 hrs after this injection. Under these circumstances, the "Standard Conditioners" (p. VIII) caused no noteworthy change in the resulting intoxication. PCN and phenobarbital were not tested.

Pyruvate ←

Lecoq B79,754/51: In rabbits, injection of disulfiram + ethanol or of Na-pyruvate produces essentially the same syndrome of intoxication, since pyruvic acid is the principal metabolite of ethanol after pretreatment with disulfiram. In either case, ACTH and cortisone offer little, if any, protective effect.

Lecoq et al. B66,406/51: In rats, the toxic effects of ethanol and its metabolites, pyruvate and acetaldehyde (which accumulate in the body under the influence of disulfiram) are inhibited by ACTH, cortisone, and hepatic extracts. Conversely, thyroxine, DOC, and testosterone appear to aggravate ethanol intoxication. [Statistically evaluated data are not presented (H.S.).]

Red Squill ← Gonadectomy + Testosterone: Crabtree et al. A19,999/39*

Reserpine ←

Efron D59,758/62: In rats, adrenalectomy greatly decreases resistance to reserpine, whereas hypophysectomy leaves it almost unchanged. It is assumed therefore, "that the increased toxicity of reserpine in adrenalectomized rats is related to the absolute lack of certain adrenal steroids, which in some way may condition the nervous system to the effects of the drugs, rather than to the inability of the pituitary-adrenal system to respond to so-called 'nonspecific stress' caused by the drug."

Agostini & Giagheddu G14,490/63: Reserpine catalepsy in guinea pigs is inhibited by various folliculoid, testoid and corticoid hormones as well as by epinephrine.

Räsänen & Taskinen G51,026/67: Dexamethasone protects the gastric mucosa of the rat against the production of ulcers by reserpinization. The effect is ascribed to the degranulation of the gastric mast cells induced by the glucocorticoid.

Selye et al. G60,016/69: In rats, spironolactone protects against anesthesia produced by progesterone, DOC, hydroxydione, pregnanedione, dehydroepiandrosterone, testosterone, diethylstilbestrol, methyprylon, pentobarbital and ethanol. It does not significantly alter the corresponding actions of morphine, codeine, urethan, diazepam, chlorpromazine, reserpine, phenoxybenzamine, chloral hydrate, potassium bromide or $MgCl_2$.

Selye et al. G60,020/69: In the rat, pretreatment with norbolethone protects against the anesthetic effect of progesterone, DOC pregnanedione, dehydroepiandrosterone, testosterone, diethylstilbestrol, pentobarbital and methyprylon. It does not significantly alter the corresponding actions of urethan, diazepam, chlorpromazine, reserpine, phenoxybenzamine, chloral hydrate, potassium bromide or magnesium chloride.

RES-Blocking Agents ←

Selye B39,702/49: In rats in which an arthritis was produced by intrapedal injection of formalin and India ink, phagocytosis and transport of the carbon particles to the regional lymph nodes are accelerated by ACTH. This is ascribed to glucocorticoid formation and the resulting diminution of the inflammatory barrier at the formalin injection site.

Heller et al. C40,073/57: In rats, the phagocytosis of India ink i.v. by the RES is stimulated by various folliculoids but not by testoids.

Selye et al. C70,942/59: Topical injection of cortisol acetate microcrystals into a hind paw of a rat selectively protects the surrounding region against the angiotactic sequestration of i.v. injected carbon (India ink) particles during a dextran-induced anaphylactoid edema.

Nicol et al. C92,079/60: In male mice, various diethylstilbestrol derivatives increase the blood clearance of i.v.-injected carbon owing to stimulation of the RES. There is corresponding enlargement of the spleen and liver.

Kelly et al. D32,495/62: "In livers of mice whose reticulo-endothelial system was stimulated by estradiol, it was established that the cells preparing for division and those which had recently divided were actively phagocytic."

Gabbiani et al. G19,450/65: In rats pretreated with ACTH, F-COL or restraint, a single i.v. injection of thorium dextrin (an RES-blocking agent) produces thrombohemorrhagic lesions with necrosis in the adrenals, liver and kidneys. The changes are reminiscent of the Shwartzman-Sanarelli phenomenon.

Göthe H20,084/70: In rats, cortisol p.o. does not significantly alter the accumulation of intratracheally-administered quartz dust, although it delays its transfer from the lung to the regional lymph nodes.

Göthe H20,085/70: In rats, ACTH accelerates, whereas prednisolone retards, the transport of intratracheally-administered quartz dust from the lung to the regional lymphatics.

Salicylates ←

Montuori G60,881/54: In mice, cortisone s.c. raises resistance to sodium salicylate given 6 hrs later i.p.

Barnett & Teague C56,641/58: In rats, stilbestrol antagonizes the hepatic glycogenolytic action of sodium salicylate.

Abbott & Harrisson F36,510/65: In rats, cancellous bone formation is stimulated by various salicylates. This effect is blocked by parathyroid extract and vitamin D but not influenced by cortisone.

Klingenberg & Miller F54,504/65: In rheumatic patients, prednisone given conjointly with salicylates increases the glomerular filtration and decreases the plasma concentration of the latter. "The ability of corticosteroids to increase glomerular filtration rate and diminish tubular reabsorption of water might partially explain their ability to increase the clearance of salicylate."

Selenium ←

Romeo et al. F91,552/67; H7,930/68: In the rat, the hepatic cirrhosis produced by chronic intoxication with Na_2SeO_3 is inhibited by 19-norandrostenolone and 4-chlorotestosterone.

Serine ← cf. SDH under Influence of Steroids upon Enzymes

SKF 525-A ←

Selye G70,480/71: In rats, acute and severe intoxication with SKF 525-A was significantly diminished by pretreatment with PCN, CS-1, spironolactone, oxandrolone, prednisolone, triamcinolone and progesterone. The other conditioners of our series were not or only very slightly effective, cf. Table 106.

Silicon ← cf. RES

Sodium ← cf. also Selye C50,810/58, p. 107.

Baisset et al. C84,788/58: In rats and dogs, the effects of NaCl-overdosage are ameliorated by posterior pituitary extracts and aggravated by NaCl.

Scheer et al. D3,935/61: Exposure of frogs to high concentrations of NaCl decreases Na-uptake and increases electrical resistance in the skin, as does destruction of the inter-renal bodies. These effects are reversed in both cases by aldosterone but treatment of frogs, in tap water or saline, with spironolactone has no effect on the skin. Aldosterone and spironolactone have no significant effect on either the urine or the plasma Na. "We conclude that the inter-renals of frogs are involved in control of the regulatory functions of the skin but not of the kidneys. The absence of effect of aldactone may mean that this agent is not an aldosterone antagonist in frogs, or that aldosterone is not an indispensable participant in salt regulation in these animals."

Table 106. *Conditioning for SKF 525-A*

Treatment[a]	Dyskinesia[b] (Positive/Total)	Mortality[b] (Dead/Total)
None	25/28	4/28
PCN	4/10 **	0/10 NS
CS-1	9/20 ***	0/20 NS
Ethylestrenol	12/20 *	1/20 NS
Spironolactone	9/20 ***	3/20 NS
Norbolethone	11/20 *	0/20 NS
Oxandrolone	7/20 ***	0/20 NS
Prednisolone-Ac	3/20 ***	1/20 NS
Triamcinolone (2 mg)	7/20 ***	3/20 NS
Progesterone	9/19 ***	1/19 NS
Estradiol (1 mg)	15/20 NS	0/20 NS
Estradiol (1 mg s.c.)	16/18 NS	3/18 NS
DOC-Ac	14/19 NS	1/19 NS
Hydroxydione	10/19 *	2/19 NS
Cholesterol	5/10 *	0/10 NS
Thyroxine	16/20 NS	9/20 *
Phenobarbital	5/10 *	1/10 NS

[a] The rats of all groups were given SKF 525-A, β-diethylaminoethyl diphenylpropyl-acetate (15 mg/100 g body weight in 1 ml water, i.p., once on 4th day).

[b] Dyskinesia was estimated 2 hrs after injection and mortality listed 24 hrs later ("Exact Probability Test").

For further details on technique of tabulation cf. p. VIII.

Squill ←

Crabtree et al. A19,999/39: Male rats are twice as resistant as females to the fatal action of powdered red squill (Urginea maritima). Castration has no effect in females but abolishes the increased squill resistance of the male.

Strychnine ←

Parhon & Urechia A23,732/11; 62,361/13: In dogs and rabbits, orchidectomy and thyroidectomy do not influence resistance to strychnine consistently, but thyroid feeding appears to aggravate the characteristic convulsions.

Vacek C63,230/58: DOC anesthesia protects the mouse against the convulsive and lethal effects of strychnine, pentylenetetrazol and caffeine.

Kato et al. D38,983/62: Male rats are more resistant than females to strychnine intoxication especially if the drug is given s.c. whereby its activity is delayed. The greater strychnine-metabolizing potency of hepatic microsomes from male rats than from females has also been demonstrated in vitro. SKF 525-A increases strychnine toxicity and renders both sexes equally sensitive. Castration diminishes the high strychnine resistance of the male rat but has no effect in females. Pretreatment with testosterone or 4-chlorotestosterone augments the strychnine-metabolizing ability of liver slices or isolated hepatic microsomes from both male and female castrates, whereas estradiol has no effect.

Kato et al. G64,325/62: Adult male rats are more resistant than females to pentobarbital anesthesia, carisoprodol paralysis and strychnine convulsions. Conversely, the lethal effect of OMPA is greater in the male. The sex difference is ascribed to the increased production of anabolic testoids which enhance the decomposition of these substrates, the first three of which are inactivated, the last activated in the process. The differences were also demonstrated in vitro using liver slices or microsomal fractions. The high microsomal activity of the male could be abolished by castration and restored by several anabolic testoids.

Bonta & Overbeek E5,494/65: In mice, several water-soluble esters of cortisol and prednisolone decreased sensitivity to the induction of convulsions by strychnine, but testosterone 17-glycinate offered the best protection. 16β-N-piperidino-3β-hydroxy-androst-5-en-17-one and 16β-N-piperidino-17β-hydroxy-5α-androstan-3-one actually increased strychnine sensitivity and the latter produced convulsions by itself.

Selye G70,480/71: In rats, acute fatal strychnine intoxication is readily and completely prevented by prednisolone, triamcinolone, estradiol and phenobarbital. Here, the classic catatoxic steroids have little if any prophylactic effect, cf. Table 107.

Strychnine ← Gonadectomy + Folliculoids, Testoids: Kato et al. *D38,983/62**

Strychnine ← Adrenalectomy: Kato et al. *G74,030/62*

Table 107. *Conditioning for strychnine*

Treatment[a]	Dyskinesia[b] (Positive/Total)	Mortality[b] (Dead/Total)
None	13/15	10/15
PCN	6/10 NS	2/10 *
CS-1	11/15 NS	10/15 NS
Ethylestrenol	7/15 *	5/15 NS
Spironolactone	11/15 NS	3/15 *
Norbolethone	10/15 NS	8/15 NS
Oxandrolone	8/15 NS	7/15 NS
Prednisolone-Ac	0/15 ***	0/15 ***
Triamcinolone	0/10 ***	0/10 ***
Triamcinolone (2 mg)	0/5 ***	0/5 *
Progesterone	8/15 NS	7/15 NS
Estradiol	0/10 ***	0/10 ***
Estradiol (1 mg)	0/5 ***	0/5 *
Estradiol (1 mg s.c.)	0/5 ***	0/5 *
DOC-Ac	9/15 NS	5/15 NS
Hydroxydione	10/10 NS	8/10 NS
Cholesterol	10/10 NS	5/10 NS
Thyroxine	15/15 NS	15/15 *
Phenobarbital	0/10 ***	0/10 ***

[a] The rats of all groups were given strychnine hydrochloride, 150 μg/100 g body weight in 0.2 ml water, s.c., once on 4th day.

[b] Dyskinesia was estimated 15 min after injection and mortality listed on same day p.m. ("Exact Probability Test").

For further details on technique of tabulation cf. p. VIII.

Sulfa Drugs ←

Sacra & McColl C73,654/59: Female rats are less resistant than males to chronic intoxication with hypoglycemic thiadiazoles but no such sex difference was observed in acute tests. Testosterone increased, whereas stilbestrol decreased, the resistance of female rats to these drugs.

Sulfonamide ← cf. Selye *C92,918/61, p. 219.*

Tannic Acid ←

Patrick C12,967/55: In rats and mice, cortisone or ACTH inhibited the mesenchymal reaction and delayed repair following production of hepatic damage by tannic acid or CCl_4.

Korpássy et al. B74,333/52: In rats given toxic doses of tannic acid, DOC has no protective effect.

Tannic acid ← DOC: Korpássy et al. *B74,333/52**

TEM ← cf. Carcinolytic Agents

Tetracaine ←

Zykov H 21,879/69: In mice, ACTH, cortisol and DOC failed to influence tetracaine intoxication.

Tetraethylammonium ← cf. Ganglioplegics

Tetrahydronaphthylamine ←

Borchardt 23,683/28: In cats, neither thyroparathyroidectomy nor adrenalectomy prevents the production of fever by tetrahydronaphthylamine, whereas denervation of the liver inhibits it almost completely.

Thalidomide ←

Leone & Rinaldi G 44,123/65: In pigeons, the medullary bone formation produced by estradiol is inhibited by Thalidomide.

Thallium ←

Stavinoha et al. C 94,628/59: In mice, testosterone (0.6 mg/kg) i.m. failed to protect against the lethal effect of thallium sulfate intoxication.

Selye G 70,480/71: In rats, thallium chloride (16 mg/100 g body weight in 0.5 ml corn oil) was administered s.c. once on the 4th day of conditioning. Nephrocalcinosis was estimated on day of death, and mortality listed on the 7th day. Under these circumstances, the "Standard Conditioners" (p. VIII) caused no noteworthy change in the resulting intoxication, only estradiol exhibited an inhibitory effect. Phenobarbital was not tested.

Theobromine ←

Selye PROT. 40890: In rats, severe intoxication with theobromine is well prevented by PCN, CS-1 and phenobarbital, less conspicuously by progesterone, whereas the other standard conditioning agents are ineffective, cf. Table 108.

Theophylline ←

Selye PROT. 42044: In rats, theophylline intoxication is considerably inhibited by pretreatment with PCN, CS-1, ethylestrenol, norbolethone, oxandrolone, prednisolone, progesterone and phenobarbital. Spironolactone, DOC and hydroxydione offer barely significant protection, cf. Table 109.

Table 108. *Conditioning for theobromine*

Treatment[a]	Dyskinesia[b] (Positive/Total)	Mortality[b] (Dead/Total)
None	13/15	13/15
PCN	0/15 ***	0/15 ***
CS-1	1/10 ***	1/10 ***
Ethylestrenol	12/15 NS	12/15 NS
Spironolactone	9/15 NS	9/15 NS
Norbolethone	8/10 NS	8/10 NS
Oxandrolone	9/10 NS	9/10 NS
Prednisolone-Ac	10/10 NS	10/10 NS
Triamcinolone	14/15 NS	14/15 NS
Progesterone	3/10 **	2/9 ***
Estradiol	10/10 NS	10/10 NS
DOC-Ac	6/9 NS	6/9 NS
Hydroxydione	8/10 NS	8/10 NS
Thyroxine	8/15 NS	8/15 NS
Phenobarbital	1/10 ***	1/10 ***

[a] The rats of all groups were given theobromine, 50 mg/100 g body weight in 1 ml water p.o. twice daily on the 4th and the 5th day.

[b] Dyskinesia was estimated on the 9th day and mortality listed on the same day p.m. ("Exact Probability Test").

For further details on technique of tabulation cf. p. VIII.

Table 109. *Conditioning for theophylline*

Treatment[a]	Dyskinesia[b] (Positive/Total)	Mortality[b] (Dead/Total)
None	16/20	14/20
PCN	2/15 ***	2/15 ***
CS-1	0/15 ***	0/15 ***
Ethylestrenol	2/15 ***	2/15 ***
Spironolactone	6/15 *	6/15 NS
Norbolethone	4/15 ***	4/15 *
Oxandrolone	4/15 ***	4/15 *
Prednisolone-Ac	0/15 ***	0/15 ***
Triamcinolone	13/15 NS	13/15 NS
Progesterone	2/15 ***	2/15 ***
Estradiol	12/15 NS	12/15 NS
DOC-Ac	7/15 *	7/15 NS
Hydroxydione	7/15 *	7/15 NS
Thyroxine	15/15 NS	15/15 NS
Phenobarbital	0/15 ***	0/15 ***

[a] The rats of all groups were given theophylline (20 mg/100 g body weight in 2 ml water, s.c., on 4th day).

[b] Dyskinesia was estimated on 5th day and mortality listed on the same day.

For further details on technique of tabulation cf. p. VIII.

Thiadiazoles ← *cf.* **Sulfa Drugs**

Thimerosal ←

Selye PROT. 38080: In rats, thimerosal intoxication is inhibited by all catatoxic steroids, prednisolone, and estradiol. The apparent protection by hydroxydione requires confirmation, *cf.* Table 110.

Table 110. *Conditioning for thimerosal*

Treatment[a]	Dyskinesia[b] (Positive/Total)	Mortality[b] (Dead/Total)
None	7/10	9/10
PCN	0/10 ***	10/10 NS
CS-1	1/10 **	6/10 NS
Ethylestrenol	2/10 *	3/10 **
Spironolactone	1/10 **	5/10 NS
Norbolethone	0/10 ***	4/10 *
Oxandrolone	2/10 *	6/10 NS
Prednisolone-Ac	1/10 **	7/10 NS
Triamcinolone	6/10 NS	10/10 NS
Progesterone	3/10 NS	10/10 NS
Estradiol	2/10 *	1/10 ***
DOC-Ac	6/10 NS	10/10 NS
Hydroxydione	2/10 *	10/10 NS
Thyroxine	7/10 NS	10/10 NS
Phenobarbital	7/10 NS	10/10 NS

[a] The rats of all groups were given thimerosal, 5 mg/100 g body weight in 0.2 ml water s.c. once on 4th and on 5th day.

[b] Dyskinesia was estimated on 5th day 3 hrs after injection and mortality listed on 7th day ("Exact Probability Test").

For further details on technique of tabulation *cf.* p. VIII.

Thioacetamide ←

Eger et al. E 58,108/59: In rats, prednisolone does not prevent hepatic cirrhosis induced by allyl alcohol or thioacetamide.

Arnold et al. E 27,627/63: Chemical investigations suggest that collagen formation in rats with hepatic cirrhosis induced by thioacetamide is inhibited by cortisone.

Prellwitz & Bässler E 36,762/63: Detailed biochemical studies on the effect of Δ^1-cortisone and nandrolone phenpropionate upon the hepatic cirrhosis produced by thioacetamide in the rat.

Röttger et al. D 64,427/63: In the rat, the hepatic cirrhosis produced by chronic treatment with thioacetamide is not influenced by prednisolone or testosterone, although mortality from acute intoxication with thioacetamide is diminished by prednisolone.

Becker H 22,471/68: In rats, the hepatic cirrhosis produced by chronic treatment with thioacetamide cannot be prevented by simultaneous cortisone administration.

Becker H 17,711/69: In rats, the hepatic cirrhosis produced by thioacetamide or CCl_4 is not inhibited by cortisone and damage to the parenchymal cells is actually increased.

Petzold et al. H 20,651/69: In rats, the hepatic cirrhosis produced by thioacetamide can be prevented by concurrent treatment with Turinabol (the latter is described as 4-chloro-1-dehydro-methyl-testosterone, although in the Merck Index it is listed as 4-chlorotestosterone). Turinabol administered after the induction of thioacetamide damage enhances the regeneration of the liver.

Thiophosphamide ← *cf.* **Carcinolytic Agents**

Thiourea ←

Glock B 23,056/45: In rats given normally fatal doses of thiourea, treatment with adrenocortical extract plus NaCl offers greater protection than NaCl alone. Thyroxine is a still more effective prophylactic even when given without NaCl.

DuBois et al. B 3,103/46: In dogs, adrenal cortical extract offers moderate protection against ANTU poisoning.

Threonine ← *cf.* **TDH** under **Influence of Steroids upon Enzymes**

Tolbutamide ← *cf.* **Pancreatic Hormones**

Tremorine ←

Hewett et al. D 19,834/64: Various aminosteroids possess "loss-of-righting-reflex activity" and prevent tremorine-induced tremor as well as pentylenetetrazol convulsions. Their effect is ascribed to interneuronal blockade and not to general anesthesia.

Selye G 70,480/71: In rats, tremorine dihydrochloride (5 mg/100 g body weight in 1 ml water) was administered p.o. once on the 4th day of conditioning. Dyskinesia was listed 5 hrs, mortality 24 hrs after this injection. Under these circumstances, the "Standard Conditioners" (p. VIII) caused no noteworthy change in the resulting intoxication. PCN was not tested.

Tribromoethanol ←

Eichholtz A 27,018/27: In rabbits, "destruction of the liver" by ethylene chlorhydrin does not significantly affect the length of tribromoethanol anesthesia. After bilateral nephrectomy, sleeping time is somewhat prolonged but still variable. On the other hand, bilateral adrenalectomy prolongs the sleeping time very considerably.

Eichloltz et al. B 45,516/49: Adrenalectomy greatly prolongs the tribromoethanol and thiopental sleeping time in rats. In both instances the sleeping time could be shortened again if adrenalectomized rats were treated with DOC or adrenocortical extract.

Nicol et al. F 58,460/65: In the mouse, resistance to partially decomposed solutions of tribromoethanol is increased by estradiol.

Selye PROT. 41492: In rats, β-tribromoethanol sleeping time is considerably shortened by pretreatment with PCN, CS-1, ethylestrenol, spironolactone, norbolethone and prednisolone. Progesterone and DOC tend to prolong tribromoethanol anesthesia, perhaps because these steroids possess an anesthetic effect of their own, cf. Table 111.

Tribromoethanol ← Adrenalectomy + DOC: Eichholtz et al. B45,516/49*

Trichloroethanol ←

Selye G 70,480/71: In rats, β-trichloroethanol is subject to detoxication by essentially the same conditioners as β-tribromoethanol. Its hypnotic effect is strongly counteracted by all catatoxic steroids (except oxandrolone) as well as by prednisolone and phenobarbital. Thyroxine exerts a barely significant inhibitory action whereas estradiol actually prolongs β-trichloroethanol anesthesia, cf. Table 112.

Trichloroethylene ←

de Dominicis B 3,412/42: Combined treatment with adrenocortical extracts + vitamin C raises the resistance of guinea pigs to trichloroethylene.

Triorthocresyl Phosphate ←

Glees D 7,966/61; D 14,872/61: Triorthocresyl phosphate (TOCP) is an anticholinesterase compound which induces widespread neurologic symptoms with demyelination of the central nervous system in the chick. These changes can be prevented by pretreatment with cortisone.

Table 111. *Conditioning for β-tribromoethanol*

Treatment[a]	Sleeping Time[b] (min)
None	44 ± 3
PCN	19 ± 3 ***
CS-1	25 ± 3 ***
Ethylestrenol	23 ± 5 ***
Spironolactone	20 ± 4 ***
Norbolethone	25 ± 4 ***
Oxandrolone	33 ± 6 NS
Prednisolone-Ac	23 ± 4 ***
Triamcinolone	44 ± 3 NS
Triamcinolone (2 mg)	40 ± 3 NS
Progesterone	63 ± 9 *
Estradiol	46 ± 2 NS
Estradiol (1 mg)	37 ± 3 NS
DOC-Ac	60 ± 6 *
Hydroxydione	58 ± 9 NS
Thyroxine	38 ± 3 NS
Phenobarbital	58 ± 12 NS

[a] The rats of groups were given β-tribromoethanol (25 mg/100 g body weight in 1 ml water + amylene hydrate, s.c., on 4th day).

[b] (Student's t-test.)

For further details on technique of tabulation cf. p. VIII.

Table 112. *Conditioning for β-trichloroethanol*

Treatment[a]	Sleeping time[b] (min)
None	174 ± 19
PCN	20 ± 13 ***
CS-1	63 ± 33 **
Ethylestrenol	53 ± 20 ***
Spironolactone	32 ± 14 ***
Norbolethone	86 ± 25 **
Oxandrolone	203 ± 32 NS
Prednisolone-Ac	44 ± 25 ***
Triamcinolone	107 ± 29 NS
Progesterone	123 ± 31 NS
Estradiol	261 ± 22 **
DOC-Ac	193 ± 18 NS
Hydroxydione	137 ± 17 NS
Thyroxine	99 ± 25 *
Phenobarbital	44 ± 17 ***

[a] The rats of all groups were given β-trichloroethanol (1 ml/100 g body weight of a 5% aqueous solution, p.o., once on 4th day).

[b] Student's t-test.

For further details on technique of tabulation cf. p. VIII.

Selye G70,480/71: In rats, intoxication with tri-o-cresyl phosphate could not be counteracted by any of the standard conditioners except for an inhibition of borderline significance by thyroxine. PCN, norbolethone, prednisolone, triamcinolone, and phenobarbital slightly aggravated the toxicity of this compound, whereas T_3 and propylthiouracil did not affect it, *cf.* Table 113.

Table 113. *Conditioning for tri-o-cresyl phosphate*

Treatment[a]	Dyskinesia[b] (Positive/Total)	Mortality[b] (Dead/Total)
None	5/10	5/10
PCN	10/10 *	10/10 *
CS-1	7/10 NS	7/10 NS
Ethylestrenol	9/10 NS	9/10 NS
Spironolactone	8/10 NS	8/10 NS
Norbolethone	10/10 *	9/10 NS
Oxandrolone	5/10 NS	6/10 NS
Prenisolone-Ac	9/10 NS	10/10 *
Triamcinolone	10/10 *	10/10 *
Progesterone	7/10 NS	8/10 NS
Estradiol	8/10 NS	8/10 NS
DOC-Ac	5/10 NS	5/10 NS
Hydroxydione	6/10 NS	7/10 NS
Thyroxine	0/10 *	0/10 *
Phenobarbital	10/10 *	10/10 *
T_3 50 µg s.c. x2/day	6/10 NS	8/10 NS
PTU 3 mg < 0.1 ml i.p. (DMSO) x2/day	1/10 NS	2/10 NS

[a] The rats of all groups were given tri-o-cresyl phosphate (50 mg/100 g body weight in 1 ml corn oil, p.o., daily from 4th day ff.).

[b] Dyskinesia was estimated on 7th day 3 hrs after tri-o-cresyl phosphate administration and mortality listed on 8th day ("Exact Probability Test").

For further details on technique of tabulation *cf.* p. VIII.

Trypsin ←

Bein & Jaques D41,862/60: Aldosterone protects the cat against lethal shock produced by trypsin i.v. Prednisone and prednisolone are much less effective in this respect.

Tryptophan ← *cf.* **TPO** under **Influence of Steroids upon Enzymes**

Tubocurarine Chloride ←

Selye G70,480/71: In rats, the motor disturbances produced by D-tubocurarine were completely or almost completely prevented by all typical catatoxic steroids (except oxandrolone) as well as by prednisolone, triamcinolone and progesterone. Phenobarbital provided no significant protection, *cf.* Table 114.

Table 114. *Conditioning for D-tubocurarine*

Treatment[a]	Dyskinesia[b] (Positive/Total)	Mortality[b] (Dead/Total)
None	10/15	3/15
PCN	0/10 ***	0/10 NS
CS-1	0/10 ***	0/10 NS
Ethylestrenol	1/15 ***	1/15 NS
Spironolactone	2/15 ***	0/15 NS
Norbolethone	1/10 **	1/10 NS
Oxandrolone	5/10 NS	4/10 NS
Prednisolone-Ac	0/10 ***	0/10 NS
Triamcinolone	1/15 ***	1/15 NS
Progesterone	1/10 **	1/10 NS
Estradiol	7/10 NS	1/10 NS
DOC-Ac	7/10 NS	4/10 NS
Hydroxydione	5/10 NS	4/10 NS
Thyroxine	9/15 NS	6/15 NS
Phenobarbital	5/15 NS	0/15 NS

[a] The rats of all groups were given D-tubocurarine chloride (20 µg/100 g body weight in 0.2 ml water, s.c., once on 4th day).

[b] Dyskinesia was estimated 30 min after injection and mortality listed 24 hrs later ("Exact Probability Test").

For further details on technique of tabuation *cf.* p. VIII.

Tyramine ←

Selye G70,480/71: In rats, tyramine intoxication appears to have been only slightly counteracted by ethylestrenol, spironolactone, norbolethone, prednisolone and DOC, whereas triamcinolone offered excellent protection. The other standard conditioners, including phenobarbital, were ineffective, *cf.* Table 115.

Tyramine ← Prednisolone: Inscoe et al. *F70,325/66*

Table 115. *Conditioning for tyramine*

Treatment[a]	Dyskinesia[b] (Positive/ Total)	Mortality[b] (Dead/ Total)
None	8/15	8/15
PCN	1/5 NS	1/5 NS
CS-1	2/9 NS	2/9 NS
Ethylestrenol	1/10 *	2/10 NS
Spironolactone	1/10 *	1/10 *
Norbolethone	1/10 *	1/10 *
Oxandrolone	2/10 NS	2/10 NS
Prednisolone-Ac	1/10 *	1/10 *
Triamcinolone	0/10 **	0/10 **
Progesterone	5/10 NS	5/10 NS
Estradiol	4/10 NS	4/10 NS
DOC-Ac	1/10 *	1/10 *
Hydroxydione	4/10 NS	4/10 NS
Thyroxine	4/10 NS	4/10 NS
Phenobarbital	6/9 NS	6/9 NS

[a] The rats of all groups were given tyramine (20 mg/100 g body weight in 1 ml water, i.v., on 4th day).

[b] Dyskinesia was estimated 2 hrs after injection and mortality listed on 5th day ("Exact Probability Test").

For further details on technique of tabulation *cf.* p. VIII.

Tyrosine ← *cf. also* TKT *under* Enzymes Influenced by Steroids

Alam et al. G53,636/67: In rats fed low-protein diets, excessive tyrosine intake depresses growth and causes characteristic lesions in the paws and eyes. Injections of cortisol or stress caused by infusorial earth i.p. prevented the manifestations of tyrosine intoxication, presumably as a consequence of hepatic microsomal TPO induction. The effect of infusorial earth i.p. is ascribed to the resulting stress-induced increases in corticoid secretion.

Fuller G75,131/70: In rats, exposure to cold, as well as treatment with cortisol or glucagon after adrenalectomy induced TKT activity in the liver but not in the brain. Apparently, the TKT "of brain differed from the enzyme in liver since it did not exhibit diurnal variations of activity and was not affected by hormones, drugs, or stress."

Rose & Cramp G75,215/70: In women using folliculoid-luteoid contraceptives, the plasma tyrosine level is significantly decreased. Two women treated with ethinylestradiol alone showed a similar decrease of plasma tyrosine. "It is suggested that increased levels of glucocorticoids, due to the action of oestrogen, induce elevated levels of tyrosine aminotransferase, and that as a consequence there is an enhanced rate of degradation of the amino acid in the liver."

Selye G70,468/70: In rats, dietary tyrosine intoxication results in inflammation of the eyes, pancreas, paws and snout. These changes can be prevented not only by glucocorticoids (triamcinolone, prednisolone) but also by catatoxic steroids devoid of glucocorticoid potency, such as PCN, ethylestrenol, CS-1 and, to a lesser extent, by spironolactone and norbolethone. Estradiol is likewise effective in protecting against tyrosine intoxication although it is devoid of both glucocorticoid and catatoxic potencies. Progesterone, oxandrolone, DOC, hydroxydione and cholesterol are ineffective. Thyroxine actually aggravates tyrosine intoxication, *cf.* Fig. 13, p.298

Selye G70,480/71: Rats given a great dietary excess of L-tyrosine have developed a syndrome characterized by dermatitis on the paws and around the eyes, panophthalmia, pancreatic lesions, loss of body weight and high mortality. These signs of tyrosinosis were suppressed, or at least diminished, by phenobarbital, PCN and to a lesser extent by various other catatoxic steroids. Prednisolone, triamcinolone, and thyroxine decreased the resistance to tyrosinosis. The mean food intake was actually increased by the steroids that offered protection, hence the beneficial effect of the latter could not have been the result of a diminished L-tyrosine intake consequent upon decreased food consumption, *cf.* Table 116, p. 299.

Tyrosine ← Prednisone + Methemalbumin: Marver et al. *G76,839/68*

Uranium ← *cf. also* Selye *G60,083/70*, p. 353.

Feyel 99,416/43: In mice, testosterone pretreatment does not protect either against $HgCl_2$ or uranium nitrate intoxication.

Urethan ←

Sindram 52,504/35: In rats, pretreatment with adrenocortical extract ("Cortin") increases resistance to urethan anesthesia. Adrenalectomy has an inverse effect but Cortin shortened urethan anesthesia even in the absence of the adrenals. Tribromoethanol sleeping time is likewise shortened by adrenocortical extract in intact rats.

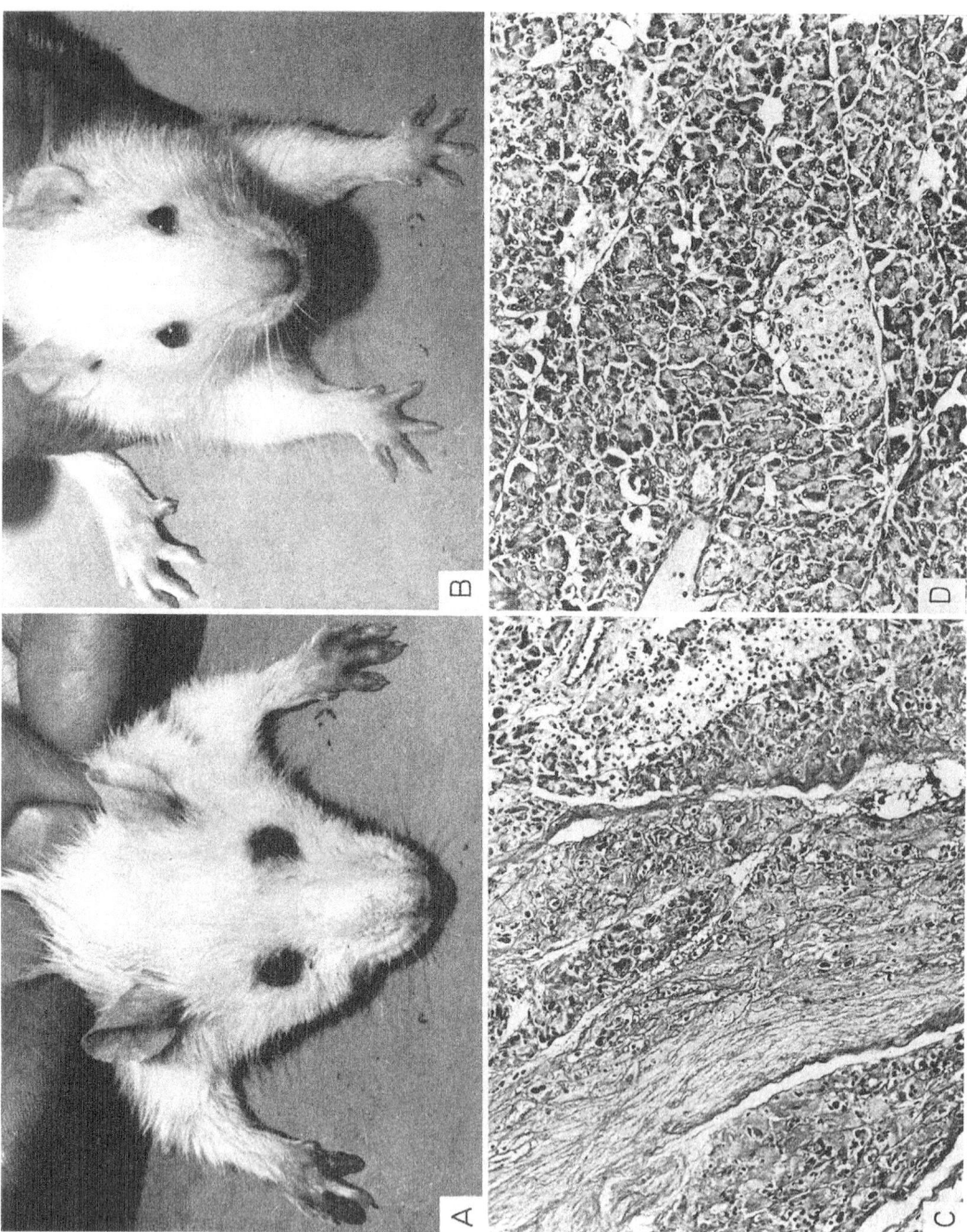

Fig. 13. **Protection by PCN against tyrosinosis.** Both rats received the same tyrosine treatment. A: Inflammatory lesions affecting the eyes, snout, and paws of the otherwise-untreated control. B: No such changes are observed in the rat pretreated with PCN. C: In the pancreas of the rat shown above, there are extensive necroses of parenchymal cells and edema in the stroma, characteristic of tyrosine intoxication. D: The pancreas of the PCN-pretreated rat shows no obvious anomaly. [Selye G 70,468/70. Courtesy of J. Nutr.]

Table 116. *Conditioning for L-tyrosine*

Treatment[a]	Eye lesions[b] (%)	Final body weight[c] (g)	Food intake per rat[c] (g)	Mortality[d] (%)
None	50	90 ± 4	10 ± 0.5	80
PCN	0 *	116 ± 3 ***	15 ± 0.6 ***	0 ***
CS-1	20 NS	88 ± 2 NS	12 ± 1.0 NS	0 ***
Ethylestrenol	10 NS	92 ± 2 NS	13 ± 0.6 **	10 ***
Spironolactone	20 NS	89 ± 2 NS	14 ± 1.0 **	20 *
Norbolethone	30 NS	87 ± 5 NS	14 ± 0.7 ***	30 *
Oxandrolone	40 NS	84 ± 2 NS	10 ± 0.9 NS	40 NS
Prednisolone-Ac	0 *	70 ± 4 **	15 ± 1.2 **	80 NS
Triamcinolone (2 mg)	0 *	74 ± 4 *	11 ± 1.7 NS	40 NS
Progesterone	0/3 NS	98 ± 16 NS	13 ± 0.5 ***	90 NS
Estradiol	0 *	70 ± 1 ***	9 ± 0.6 NS	40 NS
DOC-Ac	70 NS	86 ± 4 NS	11 ± 0.8 NS	50 NS
Hydroxydione	70 NS	76 ± 3 *	11 ± 1.0 NS	50 NS
Cholesterol	60 NS	78 ± 6 NS	10 ± 0.9 NS	60 NS
Thyroxine	80 NS	—d	10 ± 1.3 NS	100 NS
Phenobarbital	0 *	118 ± 2 ***	16 ± 0.4 ***	0 ***

[a] The rats of all groups were given a diet containing 10% L-tyrosine (from 2nd day until end of the experiment).

[b] Eye lesions were estimated from 8th day to time of death and mortality registered on 15th day ("Exact Probability Test").

[c] Student's t-test.

[d] Premature mortality.

For further details on technique of tabulation *cf.* p. VIII.

Ito et al. G42,670/66: In mice, the development of urethan-induced thymic lymphomas was enhanced by orchidectomy but not significantly affected by ovariectomy. In the early latent period, adrenalectomy accelerated the development of thymic lymphomas, especially in females.

Vesselinovitch & Mihailovich F91,584/67: In male mice, urethan induced a higher incidence of hepatomas than in females. Gonadectomy decreased the incidence in males and increased it in females, thus practically eliminating the sex difference.

Selye et al. G60,016/69: In rats, spironolactone protects against anesthesia produced by progesterone, DOC, hydroxydione, pregnanedione, dehydroepiandrosterone, testosterone, diethylstilbestrol, methyprylon, pentobarbital and ethanol. It does not significantly alter the corresponding actions of morphine, codeine, urethan, diazepam, chlorpromazine, reserpine, phenoxybenzamine, chloral hydrate, KBr or MgCl$_2$.

Selye et al. G60,020/69: In the rat, pretreatment with norbolethone protects against the anesthetic effect of progesterone, DOC, pregnanedione, dehydroepiandrosterone, testosterone, diethylstilbestrol, pentobarbital and methyprylon. It does not significantly alter the corresponding actions of urethan, diazepam, chlorpromazine, reserpine, phenoxybenzamine, chloral hydrate, potassium bromide or magnesium chloride.

Vitamin A ←

Mayer & Truant B43,456/49: Both in intact and in castrate male rats kept on a vitamin-A deficient diet, testosterone exerts its normal stimulating effect upon the seminal vesicles. The atrophy of the accessory sex organs induced by vitamin-A deficiency is presumably due to interference with the synthesis or release of testoids, not to a target organ insensitivity.

Wolbach et al. C14,796/55: The skeletal lesions produced by vitamin-A overdosage in weanling rats are aggravated by adrenalectomy but not influenced by cortisone.

Millen & Woollam C38,328/57: In rats, vitamin-A overdosage during pregnancy produces gross malformations of the brain and calvarium in the young. This teratogenic effect is considerably aggravated by cortisone.

Selye C37,276/57: Estradiol increases, whereas methyltestosterone counteracts the bone absorption and catabolism produced by hypervitaminosis A in the rat.

Selye C36,386/58: Cortisol aggravates the bone absorption produced by vitamin-A overdosage in the rat. In this respect the effect of cortisol is opposite to that of STH.

Grangaud & Conquy C71,751/58; G71,675/58: In rats kept on a vitamin-A deficient diet, progesterone induces an increase in body weight and reestablishes a normal estrus cycle.

Grangaud et al. C97,508/59; C88,406/60; C89,715/60: Progesterone s.c. protects the male rat against the manifestations of vitamin-A deficiency.

Fell & Thomas D10,358/61: In tissue culture, chick and mouse bone and cartilage implants rapidly disintegrate in the presence of excess vitamin A and this response was prevented by cortisol. Earlier observations had shown that, in vivo, cortisol sensitizes the rat for the production of skeletal lesions by vitamin A. "It is suggested that this discrepancy between the results obtained in vitro and in vivo is probably due to systemic factors that operate in the body but are eliminated in organ cultures."

Nicol & Grangaud D20,176/61: In rats, thiouracil ameliorates the manifestations of vitamin-A deficiency. Progesterone has a similar effect.

Weissmann D10,768/61: In larvae of Xenopus laevis, bone absorption and other manifestations of vitamin-A overdosage were accelerated by cortisol. "This was held to be due to liberation of vitamin A from hepatic stores by the steroid, and is in contrast to the retardation of hypervitaminosis A by hydrocortisone in vitro." Presumably an excess of vitamin A causes release of cathepsins from lysosomes.

Thomas et al. D23,234/62: In rabbits, large doses of vitamin A produce cartilage changes resulting in the collapse of the ears, and loss of basophilic and metachromatic staining of their cartilage. Pretreatment with cortisone prevents these changes.

Hulth & Westerborn D56,601/63: In rabbits, the lesions produced by cortisone in the growth cartilages are not significantly influenced by vitamin A but recovery from the papain-induced cartilaginous damage is delayed by cortisone.

Thomas et al. D57,729/63: In rabbits, acute overdosage with vitamin-A palmitate or vitamin-A acid produced loss of hair and collapse of the ear cartilage. Histologically, depletion of cartilage matrix was seen also in the articular and epiphyseal cartilages. All these changes were largely prevented by simultaneous administration of cortisone, and a local protective effect was demonstrated by intra-articular injection of cortisol in hypervitaminotic rabbits. The protective effect of cortisol may be due to lysosome stabilization. Earlier observations which showed a synergism between cortisone and vitamin A after chronic steroid treatment may have been due to excessive increases in the blood levels of vitamin A occasioned by glucocorticoids.

Weissmann et al. D64,001/63: Earlier experiments have shown that cortisone protects the cartilage of rabbits from dissolution by an excess of vitamin A. This was ascribed to the stabilizing action of cortisone upon lysosomes whose proteases may be responsible for the degradation of chondromucoprotein. Unexpectedly, the osseous and other types of lesions produced by vitamin-A alcohol overdosage in Xenopus laevis larvae is aggravated by cortisol, whereas similar hypervitaminosis induced by vitamin-A acid is prevented by this glucocorticoid. The difference is ascribed to the fact that vitamin-A acid is not stored in the liver to any degree, whereas the alcohol is stored as the ester and can then be released from the hepatic store by cortisol. The inhibitory effect of cortisol is attributed to lysosomal stabilization.

Fell F48,679/64: The degenerative changes developing in cartilaginous limb-bone rudiments of mice, when excess vitamin A is added in tissue culture, can be diminished by cortisol in vitro, perhaps owing to antagonistic effects upon lysosomal membranes.

Thomas E37,875/64: Review on the effects of papain, vitamin A and cortisone on cartilage matrix in vivo.

Goldhaber E5,596/65: Description of the optimum conditions for the inhibition of vitamin-A-induced bone resorption by cortisol on explants of murine bones.

Soriano G44,574/67: Fragments of murine esophagus cultured in vitro show inhibition of keratinization and differentiation into multistratified epithelium under the influence of vitamin A. Cortisol has the same effect and

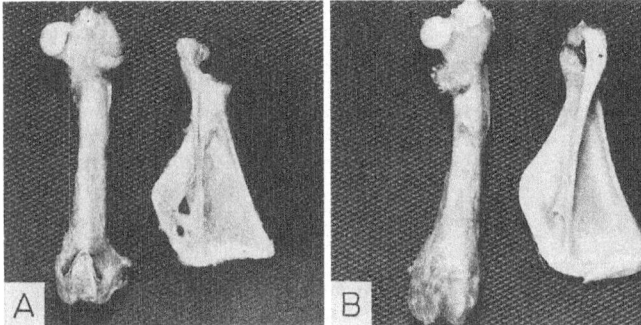

Fig. 14. **Protection by spironolactone against hypervitaminosis-A.** Both rats received the same excessive amount of vitamin A. A: In the control rat, the bones are very thin, the femur is narrow and the scapula even shows perforations. B: Spironolactone prevents these changes. [Tuchweber et al. G70,477/70. Courtesy of Int. Ztschr. Vitaminforschg.]

when given conjointly the two compounds synergize each other.

Ehrlich & Hunt G55,237/68: In rats, vitamin A has no effect upon wound healing but it overcomes the inhibitory effect of cortisone.

Janoski et al. E7,896/68 (p. 281): Review suggesting that many of the actions of glucocorticoids, particularly their inhibition of ultraviolet ray injury, vitamin-A overdosage and endotoxin shock are due to the stabilization of lysosomal membranes which prevents the escape of toxic lysosomal enzymes.

Tuchweber & Garg G70,434/70: In rats, the bone lesions characteristic of vitamin-A overdosage are inhibited by spironolactone, norbolethone and ethylestrenol; the hepatic and serum vitamin-A concentrations are simultaneously decreased.

Tuchweber et al. G70,477/70: In rats, pretreatment with spironolactone, norbolethone, ethylestrenol and oxandrolone inhibits the bone absorption and catabolism induced by hypervitaminosis A. On the other hand, estradiol, prednisolone and triamcinolone actually aggravate vitamin-A intoxication. Progesterone, DOC and thyroxine do not significantly alter this intoxication. In spironolactone and norbolethone pretreated animals, the serum clearance of vitamin A is accelerated; triamcinolone has an opposite effect, especially in chronic experiments. The hepatic vitamin-A concentration is significantly decreased by spironolactone or norbolethone, *cf.* Fig. 14.

Vitamin B ← *cf. also Aminopterin*

Hertz B18,379/48: In chickens, the responsiveness of the genital tract to folliculoids depends upon the availability of folic acid and can be suppressed by folic acid antagonists.

Weintraub et al. B49,800/50: Male mice are more sensitive than females to intoxication with the folic acid antagonist aminopterin. The low tolerance of the males was abolished by castration, but not influenced by estradiol. Testosterone failed to affect the tolerance of the female.

Meites et al. C39,753/57: Review on the effect of cortisone upon various components of the vitamin-B complex with personal observations on the guinea pig and rat.

Paroli C63,940/57: In pigeons, vitamin-B_1 deficiency is beneficially influenced by DOC.

Greengard et al. F74,421/66: Prevention by various corticoids of nicotinamide-deficiency disorders and of 6-aminonicotinamide toxicity in rats and dogs.

Greengard et al. G63,690/68: In rats, triamcinolone, dexamethasone, corticosterone and DOC protect against the syndrome of nicotinamide deficiency. "Moreover, in animals in which liver NAD and NADH had been depleted by feeding the deficient diet, the levels of these coenzymes could be restored to normal, or above normal, by steroid administration. Administration of steroids also increased the amount of NADP and NADPH. Evidence is presented that the ability of the steroids to increase the levels of the pyridine nucleotides is mediated by increasing the availability of tryptophan."

Luhby et al. H32,376/70: In women taking ethinylestradiol-containing contraceptives, there develops a derangement in tryptophan metabolism associated with "functional" vitamin-B_6 deficiency.

Vitamin C ←

Lockwood & Hartman 15,573/33: An adrenocortical extract protects guinea pigs against scurvy when given i.p., but is ineffective p.o.

Svirbely 33,140/35: In scorbutic guinea pigs, adrenocortical extract does not prolong survival.

Hyman et al. B53,374/50: "Cortisone and ACTH prolong life and reduce the hemorrhagic manifestations of scurvy in guinea pigs." [In an addendum the authors state that the large doses of ACTH and cortisone used may produce severe toxic effects which overshadow their beneficial actions (H.S.).]

Hyman et al. B57,989/51: In guinea pigs on a vitamin-C deficient diet, ACTH and cortisone ameliorate the manifestations of scurvy.

Pirani et al. B57,272/51: In guinea pigs kept on a vitamin-C deficient diet, cortisone abolishes some but not all the manifestations of scurvy.

Herrick et al. B69,259/52: In vitamin-C deficient guinea pigs, cortisone diminished the manifestations of scurvy and prolonged survival.

McGraw C68,484/59; C80,136/59: Doctor's thesis describing numerous experiments on the effect of adrenalectomy, cortisone, thyroxine, thyroidectomy, thioureas and STH upon scorbutic guinea pigs, with special emphasis upon changes in capillary resistance and cold tolerance.

Rona D26,276/62; Rona & Chappel D48, 101/63; Hajdu et al. G32,889/65; Conjugated equine estrogens (Premarin) protect the guinea pig against the production of bone lesions by vitamin-C deficiency. Estriol sodium succinate offered no such protection.

Klinger et al. F62,929/65: The normal excretion of ascorbic acid and the increase in its elimination induced by barbital are higher in male than in female rats. Orchidectomy reduced both normal excretion and its enhancement by barbital, whereas ovariectomy increased them. Thus, the sex specific differences decreased but did not disappear completely. One week's treatment of males with stilbestrol or females with testosterone diminished ascorbic acid excretion. In mice, no sex specific differences of this kind were observed. [The authors probably used hexobarbital although sometimes they speak of barbital (H.S.).]

Vitamin D, DHT ← Glucocorticoids cf.
also Selye *C50,810/58, p. 92; C92,918/61, p. 174; D15,540/62, pp. 278, 281; G60,083/70, pp. 347, 354, 385, 494.*

Polemann & Froitzheim B87,589/53: In mice, severe vitamin-D_2 intoxication could not be prevented by cortisone.

Gillman & Gilbert C31,076/56: The arterial lesions produced by heavy vitamin-D overdosage in the rat are aggravated by thyroxine or DOC, whereas cortisone and thyroidectomy offered considerable protection.

Hanssler C18,293/56: In rats on a vitamin-D deficient rachitogenic diet, cortisone decreases inorganic serum phosphorus but does not affect the calcemia or raises it slightly.

Kodicek C32,412/56: Although in patients cortisone tends to antagonize vitamin-D overdosage "cortisone treatment did not ameliorate the weight loss, clinical appearance, histological lesions or the increased urinary phosphate excretion of the hypervitaminotic rats."

Laron et al. C12,833/56: In rats first kept on a vitamin-D deficient diet, cortisone increases serum calcium and depresses alkaline phosphatase but retards the process of dental calcification during subsequent healing of the rickets induced by vitamin-D supplements.

Winberg & Zetterström C12,829/56: In a child with severe vitamin-D intoxication, cortisone brought about rapid recovery.

Harrison et al. C45,829/57: In rats kept on a vitamin-D and phosphorus deficient diet, cortisol p.o. reduced the serum citrate and prevented vitamin-D from increasing serum and bone citrate levels. On the other hand, the antirachitic effect of vitamin D (as measured by the rise in serum phosphorus and histologic evidence of rachitic cartilage and osteoid calcification) was not suppressed by cortisol. "The antirachitic action of Vit. D and its effect upon citrate metabolism can, therefore, be separated. The tibias of Vit. D deficient cortisol fed rats show evidences of increased calcification in comparison with rachitic controls which might in part be due to inhibition of bone resorption as well as retardation of cartilage growth by cortisol."

Selye & Bois C16,506/57: In rats given daily s.c. injections of ergocalciferol, which in themselves caused no pathologic calcification, calcium deposition was produced in the gastric mucosa by concurrent treatment with cortisol, whereas DOC had so such effect.

Selye C27,735/57: The cardiovascular calcification and nephrocalcinosis produced by DHT in rats are aggravated by estradiol, cortisol, DOC, ACTH and thyroxine. Conversely, methyltestosterone and STH exert a protective effect.

Wilson et al. C33,679/57: In rats, the nephrocalcinosis produced by overdosage with vitamin-D_2 could not be prevented by concurrent treatment with large doses of cortisone p.o.

Cruickshank & Kodicek C53,881/58: Cortisone did not prevent intoxication with vitamin-D_2 in rats.

Laron et al. C50,634/58: In rats kept on a vitamin-D deficient diet until rickets developed and then given dietary supplements of vitamin D, concurrent treatment with cortisone did not prevent healing, as shown by newly formed trabeculae and osteoblast proliferation although the extent of these changes was reduced. Qualitatively, the changes produced by cortisone and vitamin D are essentially different. "The findings suggest that the two steroids, vitamin D and cortisone, have different sites of action."

Thoenes & Schröter C56,987/58: In rats kept on a vitamin-D deficient diet, cortisone tends to inhibit the development of rickets, whereas ACTH does not. DOC actually aggravates vitamin-D deficiency.

Thomas & Morgan C55,688/58: In rats, chronic treatment with vitamin-D_2 or cortisone causes sclerosis of the metaphyses in long bones owing to proliferation of trabeculae. Combined administration of vitamin-D_2 and cortisone did not lessen the hypercalcemia induced by vitamin D and further intensified osteosclerosis. "These results suggest that in rats cortisone and vitamin D act independently rather than competitively on bone."

Skanse et al. C69,514/59: In a woman with vitamin-D intoxication, symptoms of psychosis and EEG manifestations developed, which disappeared together with the associated hypercalcemia under treatment with cortisone.

Bélanger & Migicovsky C95,269/60: In vitamin-D deficient chicks, norethandrolone promotes the maturation of cartilage matrix, whereas cortisone and cortisol inhibit it.

Vanha-Perttula & Näätänen C90,637/60: In rats, the calcifying mediasclerosis produced by overdosage with vitamin-D_3 is aggravated by cortisone.

Bekemeier & Leiser D76,994/61: Cortisol (unlike folliculoids) fails to cause a shift of the vitamin-D-induced nephrocalcinosis from the cortex to the cortico-medullary junction in the rat.

Kleinbaum E23,570/62: Several earlier reports and personal observations suggest that, in children heavily overdosed with vitamin-D_2, prednisone diminishes the blood calcium and in the event of interruption of vitamin-D_2 therapy may even lead to severe tetanic attacks.

Stroder et al. D36,990/62: Both in infants and in rats, the skeletal changes produced by vitamin-D deficiency are inhibited by cortisone, prednisone and prednisolone.

Schottek & Bekemeier E39,551/63: The renal calcification produced by an excess of vitamin-D_2 in the rat was not significantly influenced by DOC, cortisol, estrone, testosterone or methyltestosterone.

Strebel et al. F34,734/65: After calciphylactic sensitization with DHT, neonatal rats respond with severe thymus calcification to a challenging dose of triamcinolone.

Calandi et al. F75,662/66: Review of data suggesting that glucocorticoids counteract vitamin-D intoxication in animals and man.

← **Mineralocorticoids** *cf. also Selye C50,810/58, p. 92. Selye et al. G60,055/70:* In the rat, the calcinosis produced by a single high dose of DHT p.o. can be markedly inhibited by various testoids and antimineralocorticoids, but DOC has no protective effect.

← **Adrenalectomy.** *Bekemeier & Leiser D65,289/63:* Vitamin-D_2 overdosage produces predominantly cortical nephrocalcinosis in intact, adrenalectomized, or hypophysectomized rats. Additional treatment with dienestrol (an artificial folliculoid) shifts calcium deposition predominantly to the cortico-medullary junction, irrespective of the presence or absence of the hypophysis or adrenals.

← **Gonadectomy.** *Selye C27,682/57:* In rats, the production of cardiovascular calcification by DHT is facilitated and the loss of weight increased by orchidectomy. Presumably, "some testicular factor exerts a protective effect against this type of intoxication." *cf.* Fig. 15, p. 304.

Chury & Kasparek H29,730/69: Female rats are more sensitive than males to the production of a progeria-like syndrome by chronic treatment with DHT. Castration increases the sensitivity of the males.

Chury & Nevrtal H33,801/70: Rats, orchidectomized immediately after birth, are more sensitive to the production of the "progeria-

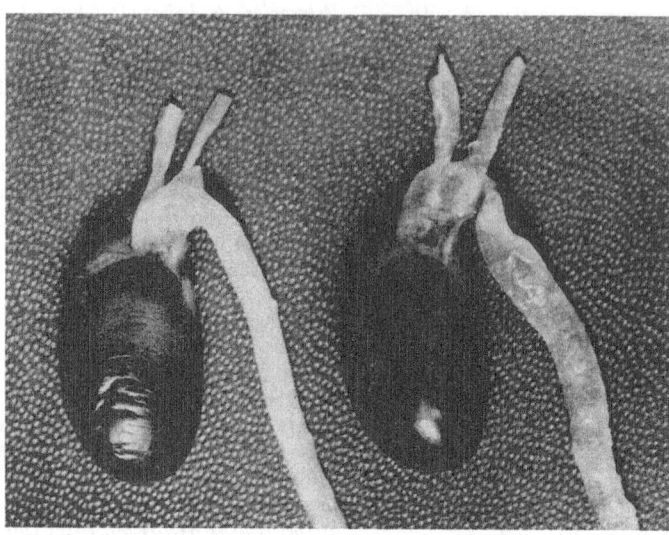

Fig. 15. **Enhancement of DHT intoxication by orchidectomy.** Both rats received the same threshold amount of DHT. In the intact male, the aorta is normal (left), whereas in the orchidectomized animal, intense calcifying arteriosclerosis has developed. [Selye C27,682/57. Courtesy of Lab. Invest.]

like syndrome" by DHT than are females or males castrated after puberty. The ECG alterations in all these groups run roughly parallel with the morphologic changes.

← **Folliculoids** *cf. also Selye D15,540/62, p. 281; G60,083/70, pp. 364, 369, 370. Korenchevsky 14,032/23:* In rats kept on a vitamin-D deficient diet, the development of rickets is not influenced by gonadectomy in either sex.

Saviano 60,155/35: Estradiol has a beneficial effect upon the vitamin-D deficiency rickets of the rat.

Norman & Mittler B18,001/48: On the basis of chemical and X-ray studies of the bones in rats kept on diets with varying vitamin-D content, the authors conclude that testosterone is "rachitogenic," whereas estradiol is "antirachitic."

Schottek & Bekemeier E39,551/63: The renal calcification produced by an excess of vitamin-D_2 in the rat was not significantly influenced by DOC, cortisol, estrone, testosterone or methyltestosterone.

Bekemeier F80,690/67: In rats, vitamin-D_2 overdosage causes predominantly cortical nephrocalcinosis which shifts to the cortico-medullary junction upon treatment with estrone. This effect is not evident in the mouse, rabbit and dog.

Chang & McGinnis F83,363/67: Male quail remain in good physical condition with vitamin-D deficient diets for at least a year, whereas females die. "Injections of testosterone and estradiol into vitamin-D deficient hens did not influence egg production, but significantly improved bone ash of tibia, sternum, and femur. Alleviation of debility caused by vitamin-D deficiency was observed in laying hens when testosterone was injected."

Pohle & Bekemeier F91,972/67: In rats overdosed with vitamin D or DHT, calcification occurs especially in the interstitial tissue of the renal cortex, whereas after simultaneous treatment with dienestrol, calcium deposition occurs intracanalicularly at the cortico-medullary junction.

Orimo et al. H20,265/70: In female Wistar-Imamichi rats, a progeria-like syndrome can be produced by chronic DHT administration, but in this strain, the emaciation, muscular weakness, kyphosis, cutaneous wrinkle formation, and nephrocalcinosis were unaccompanied by calcification of the aorta. The latter was atrophic but showed no trace of metastatic calcinosis. Also characteristic of this strain is that it reacts with osteoporosis instead of the usual osteosclerosis of DHT progeria. Treatment with "conjugated estrogens" (Premarin)

← Steroids

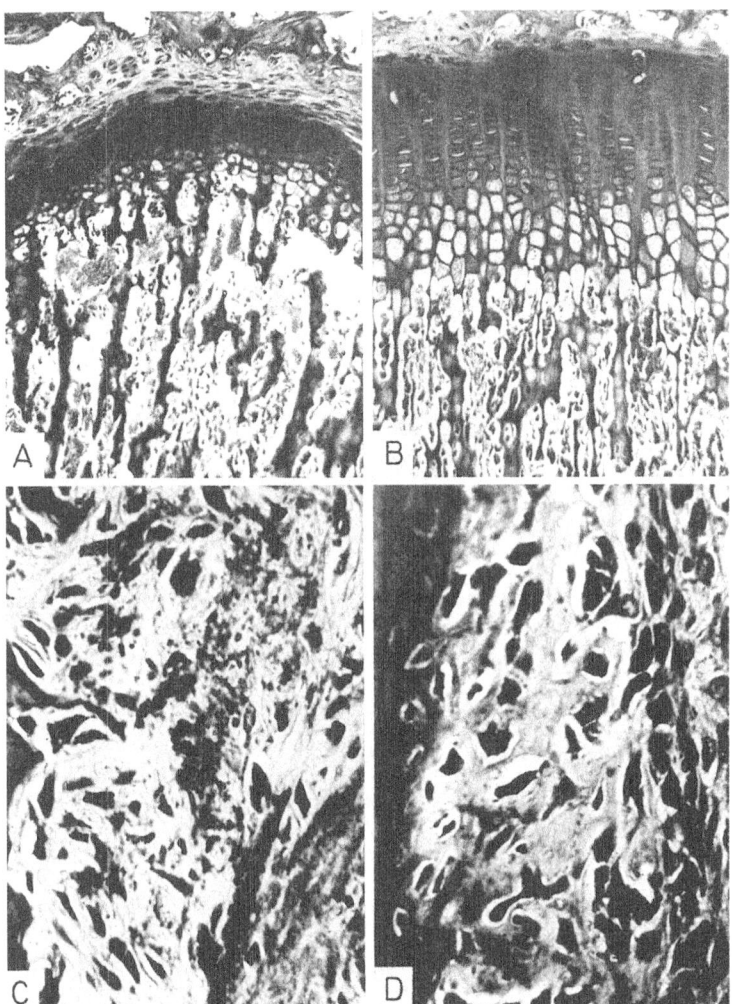

Fig. 16 (A—D). **Effect of various steroids upon DHT intoxication.** All rats were treated with the same toxic dose of DHT. A: Distal femoral growth-cartilage of otherwise-untreated controls. Atrophy of the distal layers of the cartilage plate and osteoclastic bone absorption ($\times 80$). B: Methyltestosterone protects the bone against these changes ($\times 80$). C: Periosteum of a rat simultaneously-treated with ACTH. The dark tissue near the left edge of the field is the femoral shaft. In the periosteum, numerous "basophilic bone globules" are visible, but there is no transformation of the periosteum into bone ($\times 320$). D: Treatment with DHT + STH. Here only very few "basophilic bone granules" are visible, but the periosteal connective tissue is in the process of osseous metaplasia ($\times 320$). Thus, ACTH aggravates, whereas STH slightly protects, against DHT intoxication

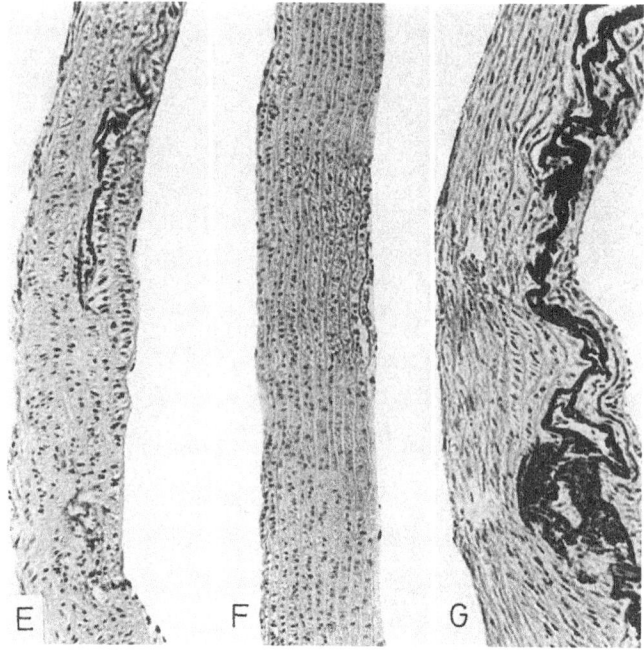

Fig. 16 (E–G). E: At the dosage used, DHT causes only mild calcification in the aorta. F: Methyltestosterone prevents this effect of DHT. G: Estradiol aggravates this effect of DHT (von Kóssa × 95)

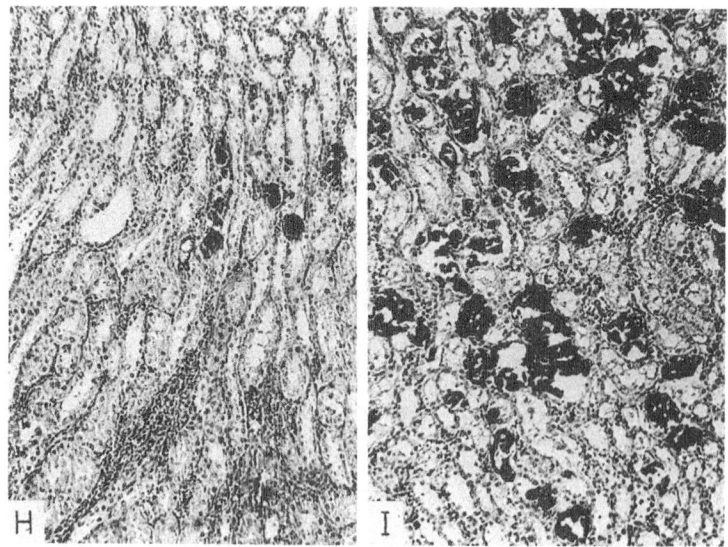

Fig. 16 (H, I). H: DHT + methyltestosterone results in the formation of only a few calcified cylinders in the cortico-medullary junction of the kidney. I: DHT + estradiol results in massive calcification of this region. The intensity of the calcification in rats treated with DHT alone was intermediate between that seen in Figs. H and I (von Kóssa × 80). [Selye C27,735/57. Courtesy of Acta endocr.]

offered virtually complete protection against all these changes.

Selye G70,467/70: In rats, the catabolism and calcinosis induced by chronic DHT intoxication is counteracted by: norbolethone > ethylestrenol > CS-1 > PCN. Spironolactone, though previously shown to antagonize acute DHT intoxication does not protect against chronic poisoning with this same compound, in fact it totally abolishes the high anti-DHT potency of norbolethone and ethylestrenol.

← **Testoids** *cf. also Selye D15,540/62, p. 281; G19,425/65, p. 142; G60,083/70, pp. 374, 376, 385. Selye C27,735/57:* The cardiovascular calcification and nephrocalcinosis produced by DHT in rats are aggravated by estradiol, cortisol, ACTH and thyroxine. Conversely, methyltestosterone and STH exert a protective effect, cf. Fig. 16, p. 305, 306.

Selye & Mishra C38,201/58: In the rat, methyltestosterone prevents the loss of body weight produced by overdosage with DHT, vitamin-D_2, partial fasting, AAN and estradiol. The catabolism elicited by IDPN or cortisol is not influenced.

Selye & Renaud C40,518/58: In the rat, norethandrolone is highly efficacious in inhibiting the cardiovascular calcinosis and catabolism produced by DHT. In these respects, it is approximately as effective as methyltestosterone.

Bélanger & Migicovsky C95,269/60: In vitamin-D deficient chicks, norethandrolone promotes the maturation of cartilage matrix, whereas cortisone and cortisol inhibit it.

Suchowsky & Junkmann D2,674/61: 1-Methyl-Δ^1-androsten-17β-ol-3-one-17β-acetate is more potent than testosterone propionate in preventing the DHT-induced catabolism and soft-tissue calcification in the rat.

Bekemeier et al. E97,156/62: In the rat, overdosage with vitamin-D_2 produces predominantly cortical nephrocalcinosis, whereas simultaneous treatment with testosterone shifts the calcium deposits to the cortico-medullary junction.

Gabbiani D32,379/62: In the rat, calciphylaxis produced by DHT + egg-white or Thorotrast is inhibited by pretreatment with methyltestosterone.

Bertolotti & Giordano D57,171/62: 19-Norandrostenolone phenylpropionate inhibits the soft-tissue calcification produced by vitamin-D overdosage in rats. [The type of vitamin-D preparation used is not indicated (H.S.).]

Mosbach & Bevans D65,362/63: In rabbits, the production of gallstones and cholecystitis by DHT is inhibited by methyltestosterone and, to a lesser extent, by testosterone. At the same time, the serum concentration of DHT falls under the influence of methyltestosterone, presumably owing to diminished intestinal absorption of the latter.

Selye et al. D28,648/63; D30,544/63: The progeria-like syndrome produced in the rat by chronic intoxication with DHT can be prevented by methyltestosterone.

Tuchweber et al. D65,261/63: Both methyltestosterone and vitamin E prevent the production of a progeria-like syndrome by DHT in the rat.

Selye et al. E24,117/64: The progeria-like syndrome produced by DHT, vitamin-D_2 or vitamin-D_3 can be prevented by ferric dextran, methyltestosterone or vitamin E in the rat.

Selye et al. G11,109/64: Methyltestosterone prevents not only the soft-tissue calcification and catabolism but also the cystic transformation of the parathyroids normally elicited by combined treatment with DHT + calcium acetate in the rat.

Baldratti E5,460/65: In rats, the catabolism and tissue calcification produced by DHT overdosage are prevented by 4-hydroxy-17α-methyltestosterone.

Bekemeier F53,774/65: In rats, folliculoids are much more active than testoids in shifting nephrocalcinosis from the cortex to the cortico-medullary junction after vitamin-D_2 intoxication.

Bekemeier G31,719/65: Ethynyltestosterone shifts calcium deposition from the renal cortex to the cortico-medullary junction in vitamin-D_2 treated rats, whereas progesterone has no such effect.

Friedrich et al. F39,223/65: Nandrolone phenpropionate does not significantly influence vitamin-D deficiency rickets in the rat, but it increases the antirachitic effect of subthreshold doses of vitamin-D_3.

Selye et al. G19,426/65: Among 36 steroids examined for their ability to protect the rat against the catabolism and soft-tissue calcification induced by DHT, the strongest anabolic steroids (e.g., norbolethone, SC-7294 and fluoxymesterone) proved to be most efficacious.

Selye et al. G60,055/70: In the rat, the calcinosis produced by a single high dose of DHT p.o. can be inhibited by pretreatment

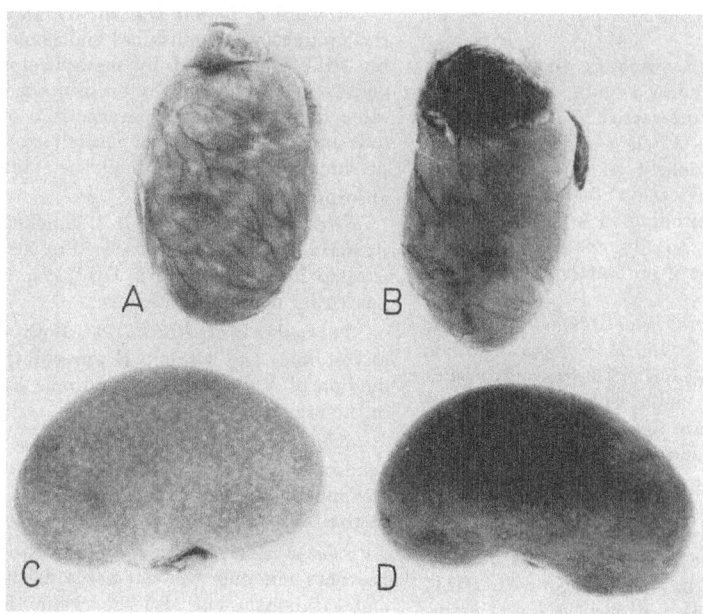

Fig. 17. **Protection by CS-1 against DHT.** Both rats received the same treatment with DHT + Na_2HPO_4. A, C: Heavy calcification of the heart and kidney in the control rat. B, D: Normal heart and kidney in the animal pretreated with CS-1 (manufacturer's code number SC-11927). [Selye *et al.* C 93,872/60. Courtesy of Lancet]

with CS-1, norbolethone, oxandrolone, ethylestrenol, methylandrostenediol (MAD), methyltestosterone, prednisone and spironolactone approximately in decreasing order of activity. A trace of inhibition was apparently also obtained with progesterone, prednisolone and triamcinolone, but with these compounds the mortality was so high that the low degree of calcification may have been caused by the premature death of the animals. DOC had no protective effect.

← **Other Steroids** *cf.* also *Selye C 92,918/61, p. 179; G 60,083/70, pp. 331, 333, 372, 373, 385.*
Selye et al. C 93,872/60: The myocarditis with calcification of the cardiac muscle and coronary arteries as well as the nephrocalcinosis produced in rats by combined treatment with DHT + Na_2HPO_4 are prevented by CS-1 s.c. It is assumed that CS-1 may act by blocking the effect of endogenous mineralocorticoids necessary for the production of lesions by DHT. However, the possibility is also considered that CS-1 may block the actions of DHT-type steroids directly as it is assumed to inhibit the actions of mineralocorticoids, *cf.* Fig. 17.

Selye C 92,918/61: Both spironolactone and CS-1 protect the rat against DHT-intoxication. Not all actions of these antagonists are due to their mineralocorticoids, blocking effect.

Selye G 60,055/70: In rats, the cardiovascular calcinosis and mortality induced by acute overdosage with DHT is inhibited by all catatoxic steroids as well as by both glucocorticoids of our standard series of conditioners and by phenobarbital, *cf.* Table 117.

Selye G 70,480/71: In rats, the fatal calcinosis induced by acute DHT intoxication is inhibited by PCN, CS-1, cyproterone, ethylestrenol, spironolactone, norbolethone, TMACN, oxandrolone, 6α-methylprednisolone, fluoxymesterone, spiroxasone, prednisolone, dexamethasone, betamethasone, MAD, emdabol, 17α-acetoxyprogesterone, testosterone, corticosterone, progesterone, 16β-methyl-16,17-epoxy-3β,11α-dihydroxy-5α-pregnan-20-one, cortisone, cortisol, and triamcinolone. It is not significantly affected by dehydroisoandrosterone, pregnanedione, 11α-hydroxyprogesterone, hydroxydione, DOC, fluorocortisol or estradiol.

← Steroids

Table 117. *Conditioning for DHT*

Treatment[a]	Cardio-vascular calcinosis[b] (Positive/Total)	Mortality[b] (Dead/Total)
None	20/30	16/20
PCN	0/15 ***	6/15 *
CS-1	5/15 ***	0/15 ***
Ethylestrenol	1/9 ***	1/10 ***
Spironolactone	4/10 ***	3/10 *
Norbolethone	0/10 ***	0/10 ***
Oxandrolone	0/10 ***	0/10 ***
Prednisolone-Ac	0/10 ***	5/10 NS
Triamcinolone	2/8 ***	9/10 NS
Triamcinolone (2 mg)	10/18 ***	14/20 NS
Progesterone	3/8 ***	4/9 NS
Estradiol	7/9 NS	5/10 NS
DOC-Ac	7/10 *	6/10 NS
Hydroxydione	8/10 NS	5/10 NS
Thyroxine	8/10 NS	6/10 NS
Phenobarbital	0/10 ***	0/10 ***

[a] The rats of all groups were given dihydrotachysterol "DHT" (3 mg per rat in 0.5 ml corn oil, p.o., once on 4th day).

[b] Cardiovascular calcinosis was estimated on day of death (but only in animals that survived at least 7 days). Mortality was listed on 9th day ("Exact Probability Test").

For further details on technique of tabulation *cf.* p. VIII.

Vitamin E ←

Aterman C35,275/57: The fatal hepatic necrosis which develops in weanling rats fed a diet deficient in sulfur-containing amino acids and vitamin E is inhibited by ACTH and cortisone, but aggravated by thyroid powder feeding. In the case of simultaneous treatment with thyroid and cortisone, the two types of hormones antagonize each other.

Vitamin K ←

Mellette D7,939/61: Female rats are more resistant to dietary vitamin-K deficiency than males. Castration increases the susceptibility of the female rat and decreases that of the male. In males, estradiol decreases, whereas testosterone increases, mortality on such diets.

W-1372 ←

W-1372

Selye G70,480/71: In rats, W-1372 is well tolerated when administered p.o. in water or mineral oil whereas, in corn oil solution, it causes severe hepatic lipidosis, sometimes with necrosis and high mortality. These toxic manifestations are very well prevented by PCN, CS-1, spironolactone and to a lesser extent by ethylestrenol, norbolethone, oxandrolone, progesterone, estradiol and phenobarbital *cf.* Table 118.

Table 118. *Conditioning for W-1372*

Treatment[a]	Hepatic lipidosis[b] (Positive/Total)	Mortality[b] (Dead/Total)
W-1372 in water	0/10	0/10
W-1372 in mineral oil	3/10	2/10
None	10/10	10/10
PCN	0/10 ***	0/10 ***
CS-1	1/10 ***	0/10 ***
Ethylestrenol	8/10 NS	2/10 ***
Spironolactone	3/10 ***	1/10 ***
Norbolethone	7/10 NS	0/10 ***
Oxandrolone	9/10 NS	4/10 **
Prednisolone-Ac	10/10 NS	10/10 NS
Triamcinolone	9/10 NS	10/10 NS
Progesterone	8/10 NS	0/10 ***
Estradiol	3/9 ***	5/10 *
DOC-Ac	9/10 NS	4/10 **
Hydroxydione	9/10 NS	5/10 *
Thyroxine	8/10 NS	9/10 NS
Phenobarbital	5/9 *	2/10 ***

[a] The rats of all groups were given W-1372 [(N-γ-phenylpropyl-N-benzyloxy acetamide), 40 mg/100 g body weight in 1 ml corn oil (except for the first two groups), p.o., twice daily, on 4th and 5th day].

[b] Hepatic lipidosis was estimated on day of death and mortality listed on the 7th day ("Exact Probability Test").

No statistics for the two first groups, but in water and mineral oil W-1372 was manifestly less toxic than in oil (compare with 3rd group).

For further details on technique of tabulation *cf.* p. VIII.

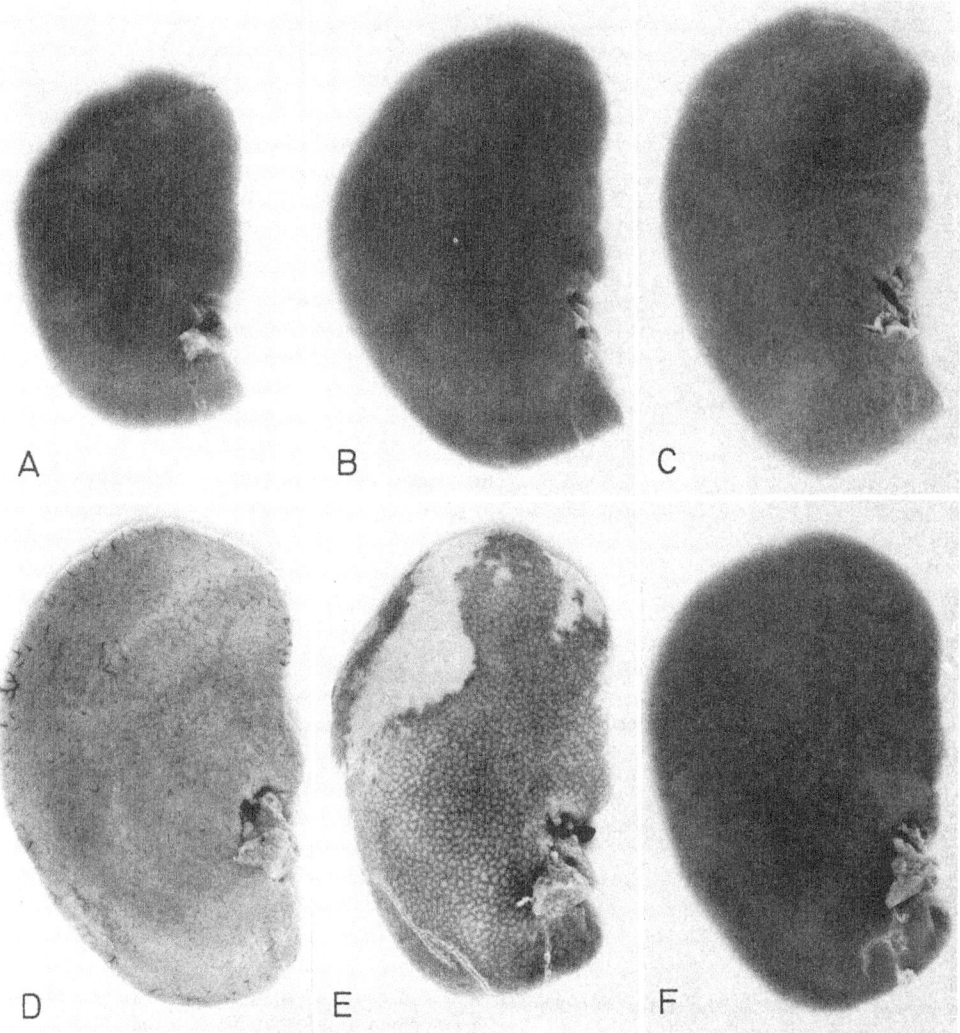

Fig. 18. **Left hepatic lobe after treatment with W-1372 (40 mg).** A: Untreated control. B: W-1372 in water. Liver hypertrophy. C: W-1372 in mineral oil. Liver hypertrophy. D: W-1372 in vegetable oil. Lipid infiltration and hypertrophy of the liver. E: W-1372 in vegetable oil + progesterone treatment. Hypertrophy, lipid infiltration and necrotic foci. F: W-1372 in vegetable oil + PCN treatment. Liver is hypertrophic but lipid infiltration and necrosis are prevented. [Selye & Lefebvre G79,005/71. Courtesy of Arch. Anat. path.]

Selye & Lefebvre G79,005/71: "Partial hepatectomy increases the intoxication produced by W-1372. Catatoxic steroids (PCN, spironolactone) inhibit, whereas glucocorticoids (prednisolone acetate, triamcinolone) aggravate, these effects." *cf.* Figs. 18 and 19.

Warfarin ← *cf. Anticoagulants*

Water ←

Gaunt A63,323/43: Large doses of adrenocortical extract or DOC protect the rat against otherwise fatal water intoxication.

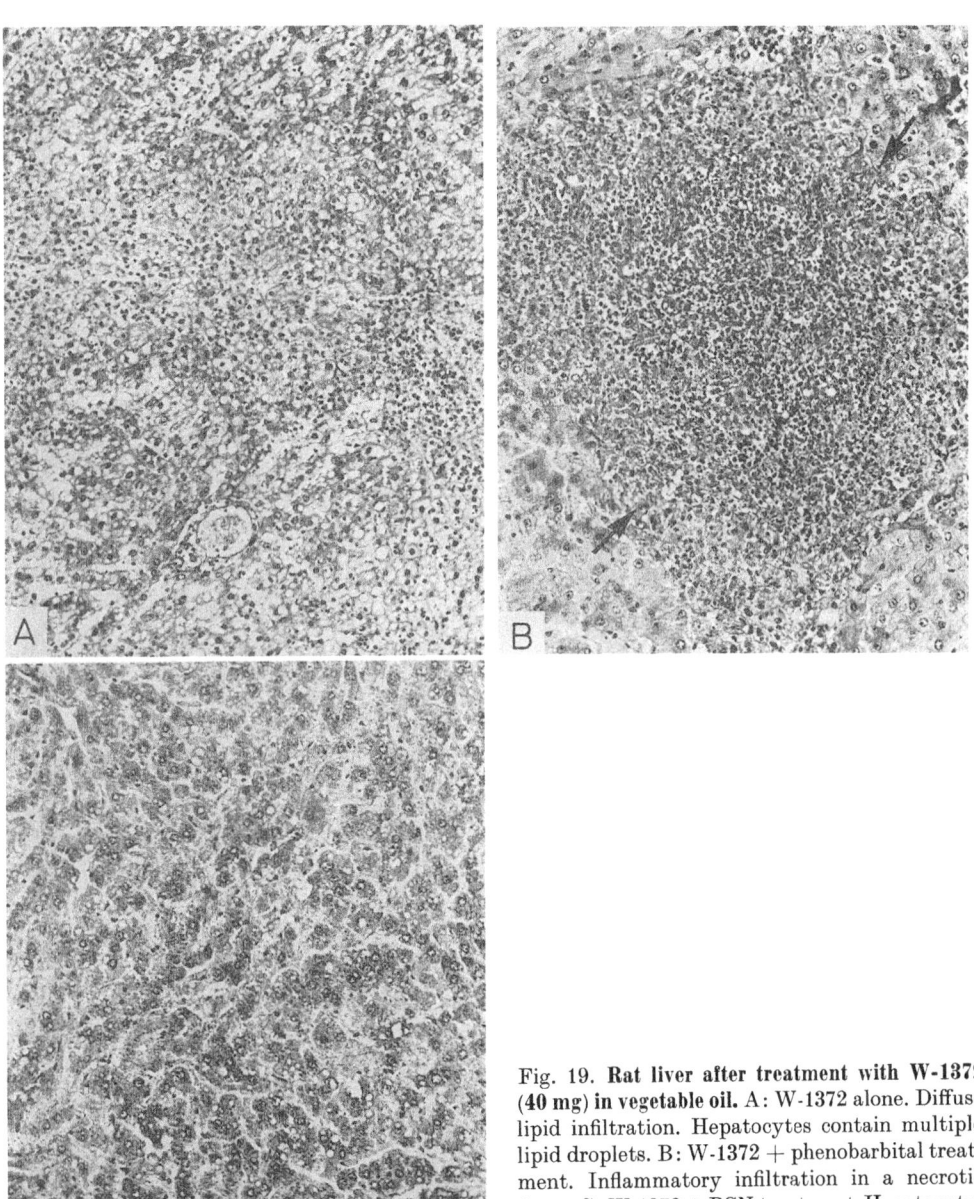

Fig. 19. **Rat liver after treatment with W-1372 (40 mg) in vegetable oil.** A: W-1372 alone. Diffuse lipid infiltration. Hepatocytes contain multiple lipid droplets. B: W-1372 + phenobarbital treatment. Inflammatory infiltration in a necrotic focus. C: W-1372 + PCN treatment. Hepatocytes are hypertrophied and show few lipid droplets (PAS×90). [Selye & Lefebvre G 79,005/71. Courtesy of Arch. Anat. path.]

Yohimbine ←

Sturtevant C 9,089/55; Sturtevant C 21,591/56: In rats with metacorticoid hypertension (produced by temporary overdosage with DOC + NaCl), the pressor effect of epinephrine, norepinephrine, vasopressin and renin was increased but the effect of histamine, 5-HT, yohimbine and TEA on the blood pressure was not consistently altered.

Zoxazolamine ←

Conney et al. D 52,543/61: Pretreatment of male rats with chlorcyclizine shortens the duration of action and increases the hepatic microsomal metabolism of hexobarbital, pentobarbital and zoxazolamine. These effects were not prevented by hypophysectomy or adrenalectomy combined with castration.

Bousquet et al. F 35,073/65: In rats with stress produced by applying a tourniquet around one hind limb for 2.5 hrs, the toxicity of hexobarbital, pentobarbital, meprobamate and zoxazolamine was significantly diminished, whereas that of barbital and phenobarbital remained unaffected. Pretreatment with ACTH or corticosterone simulated the effect of stress. After hypophysectomy or adrenalectomy, stress failed to offer the usual protection. [The barbiturates and zoxazolamine appear to have been administered immediately after release of the tourniquet, but this is not specifically stated. Allegedly a single injection of corticosterone (50 µg per animal) sufficed to offer protection (H.S.).]

Kato & Gillette F 57,816/65: The ability of rat liver microsomal enzymes to inactivate various substrates is greater in males than in females, but the sex difference varies with the substrate. There is a more than 3-fold sex difference with aminopyrine and hexobarbital but virtually none with hydroxylation of aniline and zoxazolamine. In male rats, starvation impairs sex-dependent enzymes which metabolize aminopyrine and hexobarbital but enhances those that hydroxylate aniline. On the other hand, in female rats, starvation increases the specific activity of the aminopyrine and hexobarbital-metabolizing enzymes as well as aniline hydroxylase. Starvation does not alter the metabolism of hexobarbital and enhances that of aminopyrine by microsomes of castrated rats but impairs the metabolism of these compounds by microsomes of methyltestosterone-treated castrates.

Kato & Gillette F 57,817/65: The metabolism of aminopyrine and hexobarbital by hepatic microsomes of male rats is impaired by adrenalectomy, castration, hypoxia, ACTH, formaldehyde, epinephrine, morphine, alloxan or thyroxine. The metabolism of aniline and zoxazolamine is not appreciably decreased by any of these agents; in fact, hydroxylation of aniline is enhanced by thyroxine or alloxan. Apparently, the treatments impair mainly the sex-dependent enzymes. Accordingly, the corresponding enzymic functions of the hepatic microsomes of female rats are not significantly impaired by the agents which do have an inhibitory effect in males.

Novick Jr. et al. F 63,768/66: In mice, the zoxazolamine prostration time is shortened by pretreatment with several 19-nortestosterone derivatives.

Buu-Hoi & Hien G 66,135/69: Studies on the induction of zoxazolamine-hydroxylase activity in the liver of the rat by treatment with various polycyclic aromatic hydrocarbons with the purpose of determining pharmacochemical interrelations. It is incidentally mentioned that estradiol induces this enzyme and thereby shortens zoxazolamine paralysis in the rat.

Gordon et al. H 24,106/70: In rats, medroxyprogesterone had no effect upon zoxazolamine "sleeping time." In weanling rats, medroxyprogesterone did not affect the growth-promoting action of testosterone upon the seminal vesicles but it inhibited the stimulation of the ventral prostate. In several patients the steroid accelerated the metabolic clearance of testosterone.

Selye G 70,480/71: In rats, zoxazolamine paralysis is inhibited by PCN, CS-1, cyproterone, ethylestrenol, spironolactone, TMACN, 6α-methylprednisolone, fluoxymesterone, 16β-methyl-16,17-epoxy-3β,11α-dihydroxy-5α-pregnan-20-one, MAD, cortisone, cortisol and testosterone. It is not significantly affected by norbolethone, oxandrolone, spiroxasone, prednisolone, dexamethasone, betamethasone, embadol, 17α-acetoxyprogesterone, corticosterone, dehydroisoandrosterone, pregnanedione, progesterone, triamcinolone, 11α-hydroxyprogesterone, hydroxydione, DOC, F-COL and estradiol.

Selye G 70,480/71: In rats, the duration of the muscular paralysis produced by zoxazolamine was greatly shortened by PCN, CS-1, ethylestrenol, and to a lesser extent by spironolactone, and phenobarbital. The other standard conditioners were ineffective, *cf.* Table 119.

Table 119. *Conditioning for zoxazolamine*

Treatment[a]	Paralysis time[b] min
None	225 ± 50
PCN	38 ± 7 **
CS-1	63 ± 16 **
Ethylestrenol	57 ± 20 **
Spironolactone	105 ± 23 *
Norbolethone	151 ± 34 NS
Oxandrolone	155 ± 42 NS
Prednisolone-Ac	106 ± 40 NS
Triamcinolone	201 ± 30 NS
Progesterone	144 ± 23 NS
Estradiol	342 ± 32 NS
DOC-Ac	209 ± 34 NS
Hydroxydione	247 ± 35 NS
Thyroxine	268 ± 27 NS
Phenobarbital	103 ± 25 *

[a] The rats of all groups were given zoxazolamine (10 mg/100 g body weight in 1 ml water, i.p., once on 4th day).
[b] Student's t-test.
For additional pertinent data *cf. also* Table 135.
For further details on technique of tabulation *cf.* p. VIII.

Szabo et al. G79,024/71: In rats, PCN increases resistance to indomethacin, hexobarbital, progesterone, zoxazolamine and digitoxin, both in the presence and in the absence of the pituitary. Hypophysectomy also fails to prevent the induction of SER proliferation in the hepatocytes.

Zoxazolamine ← Adrenalectomy: Kato et al. *F57,817/65*

Zoxazolamine ← Norethynodrel: Juchau et al. *G40,275/66*

Zoxazolamine ← Ovariectomy + Methyltestosterone + Phenobarbital: Kato et al. *F76,403/66*

Zoxazolamine ← Testoids: Novick et al. *F63,768/66**

DIET ←

(Chemically well-characterized factors, e.g., cholesterol, electrolytes, vitamins, choline, are listed conjointly with drugs.)

Among the complex diets to be discussed here, those containing large amounts of **yeast** are especially noteworthy because, in rats, they can produce fatal hepatic necroses. This toxic effect of the yeast is prevented by glucocorticoids and ACTH but not by progesterone, folliculoids, testoids or DOC. Aldosterone allegedly prolongs survival, but this effect cannot be ascribed to its mineralocorticoid potency since DOC is inactive in this respect. There is also some contradiction in the literature concerning the effect of folliculoids; in ovariectomized rats, the yeast-induced hepatic necroses are said to be inhibited by estradiol but aggravated by estriol.

In orchidectomized rats kept on **protein-deficient** diets, testoids still promote the growth of the levator ani muscle, although the animals lose much body weight; hence it was concluded that the hormone-induced growth of this muscle is not an appropriate index for the general "myotrophic" activity of testoid anabolics.

The hepatic necroses seen on certain high-fat low-protein diets are prevented by 4-chlorotestosterone.

In ovariectomized rats kept on low protein rations, folliculoid pellets implanted into the mesenteric circulation maintain estrus, whereas this is not the case on normal diets. Apparently, the folliculoid-inactivating system of the liver depends upon an adequate protein intake.

The weight loss and eventual death of **fasting** rats are somewhat delayed by testosterone but the effect upon the final carcass weight is minimal. On the other hand, the weight of the testicles is maintained and that of the accessory sex organs actually increased by testoids despite starvation. The renotrophic effect of testoids, though comparatively mild, continues to be demonstrable during fasting.

Among other complex dietary deficiencies the **"stiffness syndrome"** deserves special mention. It develops in guinea pigs kept on a skim milk powder diet and is said to be prevented by dietary supplements of a hitherto unidentified steroid compound isolated from cane juice.

Several investigators examined the effect of steroids upon voluntary **food consumption** but these studies are not strictly relevant to our subject. A few pertinent key references will be found in the Abstract Section.

Yeast ←

Schwartz B57,985/51: The fatal hepatic necrosis produced in rats by feeding a diet containing 30% yeast can be inhibited by cortisone.

Aterman C61,786/58: The hepatic necrosis produced in rats by feeding a diet containing yeast as the only source of protein is inhibited by cortisone, cortisol or ACTH, but not influenced by progesterone, "estrogen," testosterone or DOC. Aldosterone prolongs survival time providing 50 µg or more is administered daily. Although the author did not report any observations on the effect of aldosterone upon carbohydrate metabolism, he arrived at the conclusion that "these results, therefore, suggest that in the system examined here aldosterone has some 'glucocorticoid' activity and differs significantly from deoxycortone acetate which in doses of 0.5 and 2.5 mgm. daily has been completely ineffective."

Brenner et al. D24,411/62: In ovariectomized rats, the hepatic necrosis produced by a yeast diet is inhibited by estradiol but aggravated by estriol.

Protein Deficiency ←

Shipley & György B20,418/44: "Liver damage produced in rats by diets low in protein and high in fat was consistently reflected in the living animal by impairment in ability to inactivate estrone."

Vanderlinde & Westerfeld B51,537/50: "The estrogen draining through the liver from mesenterically implanted pellets of estrone in castrate rats was inactivated when the rats were maintained on: 1) chow ad libitum, 2) normal or 50% restricted intake of a 21% purified casein diet. The liver estrogen inactivating system was not maintained by: 1) an 8% purified casein diet ad libitum, or 2) 50% of the usual intake of chow. The results are consistent with the concept that protein intake is the critical dietary factor involved in maintaining the estrogen inactivating system in the liver."

Nimni & Geiger C31,438/57: Testosterone and norethandrolone promote the growth of the levator ani muscle in normal and castrated male rats on protein-free diets. Under these circumstances the animals lose weight despite steroid treatment. "It is, therefore, concluded that the hormone-induced growth of this muscle is not an appropriate index for the general 'myotropic,' i.e. anabolic effects of steroid compounds."

Cicchini et al. C57,934/58: In rats kept on the high-fat low-protein diet of Handler, 4-chlorotestosterone inhibits the development of hepatic steatosis.

Fasting ←

Usuelli et al. B34,756/49: The daily weight loss and eventual death of fasting rats are somewhat delayed by testosterone but the effect upon total carcass weight is minimal. Conversely, the weight of the testicles is perfectly maintained and that of the seminal vesicles actually increased by the hormone despite complete food deprivation.

Quimby B62,481/51: In rats recovering from prolonged inanition, large doses of testosterone actually delayed subsequent weight gain.

Homburger & Pettengill C8,310/55: In rats of different strains given testosterone on normal or restricted diets, "renotropism, virilization, and adrenal depressor effect occurred to almost the same degree under all experimental conditions, whether or not the animals were growing at an increased rate. Conversely, the growth stimulation of testosterone propionate in the mice on a normal diet depended on the source of the animals and did not occur either on a restricted intake nor on a high-protein diet."

Tillotson & Kochakian C14,153/56: In orchidectomized guinea pigs, testosterone was unable to prevent the loss of body and organ weight induced by fasting.

Kowalewski C68,938/59: Cortisone prolongs the survival of rats during fasting; testosterone enanthate and norethandrolone do not share this effect.

Jöchle & Langecker D22,258/62: In the rat and mouse, methenolone-enanthate counteracts the weight loss produced by cortisone or a reduction of food intake.

Rubino & Giacalone E36,677/63: In starving rats, 17α-methyl-17β-hydroxy-androsta-1,4-dien-3-one does not influence weight loss during starvation.

Selye G70,480/71: In rats, the mean survival after total fasting (with drinking water ad lib.) beginning on 4th day of conditioning was listed and the body weight measured on the 6th day. Under these circumstances none of the "Standard Conditioners" (p.VIII) or cholesterol caused any noteworthy change in the resulting intoxication. PCN, CS-1, thyroxine and phenobarbital were not tested.

Various Other Complex Dietary Deficiencies ← *cf.* also Selye C50,810/58, p. 109; G60,083/70, p. 364.

Ross et al. B37,268/49: In guinea pigs kept on a deficient regime of **skim milk powder**, the "stiffness syndrome" can be prevented by a steroid compound (probable formula $C_{28}H_{46}O$) isolated from cane juice, but not further characterized.

Larizza & Ventura B38,397/49: In rats, the hepatic steatosis produced by high **fat** diets can be partially inhibited by moderate doses of diethylstilbestrol, whereas large doses actually aggravate it.

Kalter C8,008/55: In pregnant mice, cortisone increased **food consumption** but decreased body weight.

Dewar G9,079/64: From experiments on free-fed mice bearing progesterone tablet implants "it is concluded that progesterone fundamentally affects body weight by promoting water and nitrogen retention and, at the same time, increasing energy expenditure. The increase in **food intake** usually observed is, at least in part, a secondary response to the demands created by the latter two effects and fat deposition occurs also if this response is overadjusted."

Leung et al. G60,800/68: Observations on the **food intake** and growth of rats on amino acid imbalanced diets as influenced by cortisol.

Borgman & Haselden H29,947/70: In rabbits kept on a **gallstone producing ration**, ACTH, thyroid hormones or cortisone did not inhibit the production of biliary calculi, but several of these hormones inhibited usually associated hepatic steatosis.

MICROORGANISMS AND PARASITES ←

Ever since the discovery of the nonspecific adaptive properties of glucocorticoids, numerous investigators examined the effect of these and other steroids upon the course of infections. Much of the pertinent literature has been described in our earlier monographs (Selye B40,000/50, p. 67; C92,918/61, p. 241; G60,083/70, pp. 347–354), but in view of the great importance of this topic in relation to the hormonal regulation of resistance in general, we shall have to reconsider and update these data here.

In general, the antiphlogistic effect of glucocorticoids diminishes resistance to infection, primarily because it interferes with the formation of an effective granulomatous barricade between the invader and the host, but in part also because of the immunosuppressive properties of glucocorticoids. Usually these effects are unfavorable for the host; but the glucocorticoids may also exert beneficial actions by suppressing excessive inflammatory responses to comparatively mild pathogens or their toxins. None of these actions are catatoxic, since they are not directed against the invader but merely alter the tissue reactivity of the host. The suppression of inflammatory reactions is a typical syntoxic effect in that it inhibits the development of a morbid lesion — here inflammation — without destroying the pathogen; thereby it facilitates the coexistence of host and invader.

On the other hand, certain steroids, especially testoid anabolics, have been shown to stimulate defensive reactions against some microorganisms through mechanisms which are not yet fully understood. In the final analysis, this effect may be catatoxic if it depends upon the stimulation of systematic or local immunologic and inflammatory response which facilitate the destruction of the invader.

In the following pages we shall discuss the actions of steroids upon both living and dead microorganisms and parasites in this order:

1. Bacteria and Vaccines
2. Viruses
3. Fungi and Yeasts
4. Parasites
   A. Protozoa
   B. Worms

In the immediately following pages we shall summarize only some of the most salient facts; additional detail will be found in the Abstract Section. The effects of hormones upon bacterial toxins will be discussed separately in the next section.

Bacteria and Vaccines ←

In rats, cortisone has been found to increase the pathogenicity of inherently virulent **actinomycetes**, without affecting normally avirulent strains.

The resistance of mice against **B. anthracis** does not appear to be significantly affected by testosterone, progesterone or folliculoids.

The development of Tyzzer's disease, induced in mice by inoculation with **B. piliformis** or with liver tissue from severely infected animals, is enhanced by cortisone, cortisol, and prednisolone but not by DOC or testosterone.

It is well-known that mice can be sensitized to histamine, 5-HT and anaphylaxis by pretreatment with **B. pertussis** vaccine. This hypersensitivity has been tentatively ascribed to a blockade of part of the adrenergic sympathetic nervous system. Even after adrenalectomy, cortisone and cortisol protect the pertussis-sensitized mouse against histamine, cold and anaphylaxis. This protection is dose-dependent and has been recommended as a basis for the bioassay of antiphlogistic and anti-endotoxic activity.

After injection of B. pertussis, intact mice become even more sensitive to cold than otherwise untreated adrenalectomized animals. Cortisone and cortisol protect the pertussis-treated mice from cold but not to the same extent as they protect adrenalectomized ones.

In mice, guinea pigs and rabbits, cortisone greatly aggravates the course of infection with various types of **Brucella** organisms. In cows, the progress of experimental brucellosis is allegedly inhibited by pregnancy but not by progesterone.

Neither cortisone nor DOC appears to affect the response of the mouse to tetanus toxin or to infection with tetanus spores.

In guinea pigs infected with **Cl. welchii**, survival can allegedly be prolonged by adrenocortical extract.

The resistance of mice to various types of unidentified **Corynebacteria** is diminished by cortisone and to a lesser extent by corticosterone. Furthermore, guinea pigs could not be protected by cortisone against inoculation with **diphtheriae** and cortisol activates a latent **kutscheri** infection in mice.

In rabbits, cortisone is said to inhibit the local reaction to inoculation with **pneumococci** at the same time accelerating the spread of the infection and death. DOC has no such effect.

The resistance of mice to various types of pneumococci can be raised by estrone. According to some investigators diethylstilbestrol has the same effect but others claim that this artificial folliculoid (like progesterone) is ineffective.

Cortisol increases the susceptibility of chickens to **E. rhusiopathiae**.

Various glucocorticoids reduce resistance to **E. coli** infection in different species.

In the rat, hematogenous pyelonephritis produced by i.v. inoculation of E. coli is allegedly facilitated by diethylstilbestrol.

Neither cortisone nor ACTH exerts any favorable effect upon **Leptospira** infection; no mention is made of possible detrimental effects.

In mice intracorneally inoculated with **M. lepraemurium**, cortisone inhibits both the topical and the systemic inflammatory lesions, although the liver and spleen are filled with bacilli.

In mice and rats infected with **M. paratuberculosis (johnei)**, cortisone inhibits the inflammatory lesions; yet the natural resistance of the mouse to this type of infection is diminished by pretreatment with cortisone.

Especially extensive investigations have been performed on the effect of steroids upon infection with **M. tuberculosis**. The natural resistance of rats to this infection is overcome by cortisone pretreatment, and this induced susceptibility is in turn abolished by concurrent administration of STH or norethandrolone.

In mice, cortisone greatly aggravates the course of experimental tuberculosis and overcomes the beneficial effect of vaccination. It does not impair the chemotherapeutic effect of isoniazid but reduces that of streptomycin. In this species, STH allegedly does not prevent the detrimental influence of cortisone upon tuberculosis. There is some reason to think that the decrease in tuberculosis resistance induced by glucocorticoids is not merely the consequence of an antiphlogistic action since indomethacin (which is also antiphlogistic) fails to diminish the resistance of the mouse to tuberculosis.

In guinea pigs, glucocorticoids, folliculoids and allegedly even testosterone diminish resistance to virulent strains of tuberculosis. However, cortisone does not aggravate the lesions produced by low-virulence strains (e.g., BCG). The proliferation of tubercle bacilli in macrophages isolated from cortisone-treated and control guinea pigs is virtually identical. From this it has been concluded that the increased susceptibility of cortisone-treated animals is not caused by an altered rate of intracellular multiplication of bacilli but by an enhanced susceptibility of the host cells to toxic bacterial products.

In rabbits, cortisone facilitates and estradiol retards the progress of tuberculosis. Ovariectomy and progesterone do not influence it.

In mice, infection with **Nocardia asteroides** is enhanced by cortisone, but this effect can be blocked by concurrent administration of 4-chlorotestosterone.

Cortisone allegedly protects the rabbit against the toxic effects of **typhoid** vaccine; in patients with typhoid fever, cortisol may have a beneficial effect upon the toxemia. However, these actions appear to be directed against the bacterial products, not the bacteria themselves, since in rabbits, infection by small numbers of typhoid bacilli is facilitated by cortisone.

Curiously, although cortisone aggravates the course of many infections in different species it gives definite protection against otherwise lethal infection with S. typhi in mice. It was concluded that here again, the corticoid does not attack the germs but induces resistance to their toxins.

In patients with typhoid the bactericidal effect of the blood is increased by pretreatment with certain testoid anabolics.

Resistance to **S. typhimurium** is decreased by cortisone in mice; progesterone and DOC fail to affect it.

Some of the first observations on the effect of glucocorticoids upon infections were made in connection with the so-called **"saprophytosis"** syndrome. The latter occurs in rats, mice and other species following heavy overdosage with glucocorticoids, as a consequence of the proliferation of normally saprophytic organisms (usually Corynebacteria) which in many of the earlier experiments have not been further identified. STH offers indubitable protection against this form of endogenous infection.

Data on the effect of cortisone upon **staphylococcal** infection are contradictory. Most investigators found that this and other glucocorticoids diminish resistance to various strains of staphylococci; yet, some data in the literature suggested that, under certain conditions, cortisone can protect both the rabbit and the mouse against staphylococcal infection.

Various folliculoids aggravate staphylococcal infection in mice but this effect is not directly proportional to their folliculoid potency. Progesterone is ineffective in this respect.

Streptococcal infections are likewise aggravated by glucocorticoids in rats, mice and rabbits. On the other hand, if rabbits are immunized with streptococci, prior to cortisone treatment and infection, little or no bacteremia occurs "indicating that enhancement of infection by cortisone is probably not caused by interference with the immune mechanism." Furthermore, chlortetracycline and oxytetracycline are ineffective against streptococcus infection in nonimmunized mice if these are treated with large doses of cortisone. Immunized mice similarly treated with cortisone are protected by these antibiotics. Only one team of investigators claimed that cortisone or ACTH actually increases survival following streptococcal infection in rats and further enhances the protective effect of penicillin.

"Conjugated equine estrogens" (Premarin) allegedly protect mice against streptococcal infection, perhaps owing to an increase in the acid mucopolysaccharide content of the ground substance which diminishes the spread of germs.

The spread of **Treponema pallidum** is enhanced by cortisone in the rabbit and if syphilomas are already developed they become soft and spongy. The production of Wassermann reagin is inhibited. After interruption of cortisone treatment there is a "rebound phenomenon" in that the lesions become unusually large.

Actinomycetes ←

Piantoni C 38,895/55: In rats, cortisone increases the pathogenicity of inherently virulent actinomycetes, but does not affect the activity of normally avirulent strains.

Bacillus Anthracis ←

Weinstein B 15,029/39: In mice, various anterior pituitary preparations protect against infection with B. anthracis. Parathyroid extract was also very effective, whereas thyroxine and testosterone offered little protection and progesterone, insulin, "estrin" and posterior lobe extract were virtually ineffective.

Bacillus Piliformis (Tyzzer's disease) ←

Fujiwara et al. E 34,642/63: Tyzzer's disease with hepatic necroses can be produced in various species by inoculation with liver tissue of severely infected animals, with or without cortisone treatment, although the glucocorticoid facilitates infection.

Takagaki et al. D 69,101/63: In the mouse, the production of Tyzzer's disease by infection with B. piliformis or hepatic emulsion of spontaneously-affected mice (in which the bacilli parasitize the hepatic cells), is possible only after pretreatment with cortisone or cortisol.

Fujiwara et al. F 17,247/64: In mice, Tyzzer's disease produced by inoculation of B. piliformis is enhanced by cortisone, cortisol and prednisolone, but not affected by DOC or testosterone.

Bordetella Pertussis ← cf. also Histamine + Vaccine

Kind B 81,943/53: In B. pertussis inoculated mice, cortisone inhibits the lethal effect of both histamine and B. pertussis vaccine. Cortisone also protects uninoculated mice against lethal intoxication with this vaccine.

Munoz & Schuchardt C 28,986/57: After an injection of B. pertussis cells, intact mice become even more sensitive to "cold stress" than are otherwise untreated adrenalectomized mice. Cortisone and cortisol protect pertussis-treated and, to a lesser degree, adrenalectomized mice from cold. Cortisol also increases the cold resistance of normal mice. "It is suggested that while pertussis possibly affects adrenal function, it must in addition affect other functions in the mouse which are also concerned with the protection against stress."

Munoz E 8,473/64: Cortisone and cortisol protect the pertussis-sensitized mouse against histamine, cold and anaphylaxis even after adrenalectomy.

Parfentjev F 10,707/64: Review on the use of mice hypersensitized by pertussis vaccine in testing corticoids for antiphlogistic and antiendotoxic activity.

Brucella ←

Abernathy B 57,911/51: In mice, guinea pigs and rabbits infected with Brucella abortus, Br. mellitensis or Br. suis, cortisone increased the dissemination of the lesions and the death rate. The agglutinin response was not affected.

Abernathy & Spink B 75,468/52: In mice, cortisone greatly aggravates the course of acute infection with Br. suis. Observations on the effect of cortisone upon other forms of brucellosis in various species are also reviewed.

Payne C 89,814/60: In cows, the progress of experimental brucellosis is inhibited by pregnancy but not by progesterone.

Clostridium Tetani ←

Greene et al. B 94,257/53: In mice, cortisone or DOC did not significantly affect the response to tetanus toxin or tetanus spore infection.

Clostridium Welchii ←

Kepl et al. A 56,633/43: In guinea pigs infected with Cl. welchii, treatment with adrenocortical extract prolonged survival.

Corynebacteria ← cf. also Selye C 92,918/61, p. 233.

Mason et al. C 14,288/56: Corticosterone is approximately half as active as cortisone in suppressing the resistance of mice to Corynebacterium pseudotuberculosis murium. The relative pro-infectious potency of the two steroids roughly parallels their glucocorticoid activity.

Speirs C 34,744/56: In BBF_1 mice, cortisone s.c. produces pseudotuberculosis owing to proliferation of C. pseudotuberculosis murium. Oxytetracycline p.o. reduces the incidence of these lesions.

di Nola et al. C 33,308/57: In guinea pigs, cortisone pretreatment failed to protect against inoculation of live diphtheria organisms or diphtheria toxin.

Caren & Rosenberg G41,288/66: "When mice harboring latent C. kutscheri are administered hydrocortisone, which depresses mouse serum C' levels, pseudotuberculosis is activated with equal frequency in mice of both C' types."

Diplococcus Pneumoniae ←

Magara 35,283/36: Brief description (without experimental details) stating that both "male and female hormone extracts" increase resistance of the mouse to pneumococcal infection.

von Haam & Rosenfeld A44,924/42: In mice, estrone i.p. increases resistance to experimental pneumococcus infection. Stilbestrol and progesterone are ineffective. Testosterone protects both males and females to a moderate degree.

Tobian & Strauss B28,613/48: In mice surviving from pneumococcal infection owing to penicillin treatment, no further improvement was obtained by adrenocortical extract.

Glaser et al. B57,933/51: In mice and rats with streptococcal and pneumococcal infections, cortisone depresses cellular exudation and increases mortality.

Kass et al. B69,981/51: In mice, the final mortality rate after infection with influenza virus or pneumococci is not significantly altered by ACTH or cortisone, although the course of the disease may be modified.

Robinson B57,249/51: The local lesions, bacteremia and mortality following intradermal injection of virulent Type I pneumococci were aggravated by cortisone pretreatment and larger than ordinary doses of penicillin were required to control the infection.

Germuth et al. D77,106/52: In rabbits, cortisone increases susceptibility to pneumococcal infection as manifested by greater mortality, increased bacterial growth in the locally infected sites and enhanced bacteremia. The decreased resistance is ascribed to interference with the migration of phagocytic cells to the infected sites. On the other hand, cortisone increases the resistance of the rabbit to hemolytic Staphylococcus aureus.

Kass et al. B95,353/54: In mice, resistance to pneumococcal and influenza virus infections is depressed by pretreatment with cortisone or cortisol, but not by ACTH. STH failed to overcome the effect of cortisone and did not increase resistance to infection when given alone.

Ertuganova C97,404/60: In rabbits, cortisone inhibits the local response to inoculation with pneumococci but accelerates the spread of infection and death. DOC does not influence this infection.

Nicol et al. F70,028/66: The survival time of intact or ovariectomized mice infected with Pneumococcus Type 1 is increased by pretreatment with diethylstilbestrol.

Erysipelothrix Rhusiopathiae ←

Malik D34,701/62: "Hydrocortisone increased the susceptibility of chicken to E. rhusiopathiae, shortened the course of infection, increased the percentage of deaths and resulted in septicaemia even with poorly virulent strains."

Escherichia Coli ←

Moll D38,927/56: Review of the literature on reduction of resistance by glucocorticoids against bacterial infections. Personal observations on mice showing that cortisone predisposes to the production of fatal septicemia by E. coli.

Andriole & Cohn G807/63: In the rat, hematogenous pyelonephritis produced by E. coli infection i.v. is facilitated by diethylstilbestrol.

Gonococci ← *cf. Neisseria Gonorrhoeae*

Klebsiella Pneumoniae ←

da Rocha Lagoa B49,008/47: In rabbits, an otherwise fatal infection with Klebsiella pneumoniae can be combated by adrenocortical extracts and at the same time the otherwise considerable hyperkalemia is prevented.

Leptospira ←

Derom & van Hoydonck C17,095/55: "ACTH and cortisone have not been found to have any favorable effects on the infection of guinea pigs with Leptospira ictero-haemorragiae, strain 'Afsnee'."

Mycobacterium Leprae ←

Naguib & Robson C23,199/56: In mice, intracorneally inoculated with M. lepraemurium, cortisone decreased the development of both corneal and systemic lesions; nevertheless, the liver and spleen usually contained large numbers of lepra cells filled with bacilli. Cortisone did not appreciably modify the beneficial action of isoniazid.

Mycobacterium Paratuberculosis (johnei) ←

Ford G67,455/57: Mice are normally resistant to infection by M. johnei but they become sensitive following pretreatment with cortisone.

Chandler D5,239/61: In mice infected with M. johnei, cortisone reduced the hepatic and splenic infection but had no definite effect upon the intestinal lesions.

Chandler D5,240/61: In the rat, cortisone did not enhance infection with M. johnei and may have actually reduced it.

Mycobacterium Tuberculosis ←

RAT

Michael Jr. et al. B53,378/50: Rats infected with virulent M. tuberculosis (H37Rv) do not die of tuberculosis unless they are pretreated with cortisone.

Cummings & Hudgins B66,423/51: Cortisone increases susceptibility to tuberculosis in the rat and rabbit although it diminishes the allergic manifestations of the disease.

Lemonde et al. B70,248/52; B69,349/52: The rat, which is naturally resistant to human tuberculosis, can be made sensitive to this infection by pretreatment with cortisone. This sensitivity is in turn abolished by concurrent treatment with STH. Mice which are naturally sensitive to tuberculosis can also be protected by STH.

Lemonde et al. C95,984/60: Norethandrolone inhibits the development of tuberculous lesions in the rat and counteracts the opposite effect of cortisol.

MOUSE

D'Arcy-Hart & Rees B50,249/50: Cortisone greatly aggravates the course of tuberculosis in mice following inoculation of human-type tubercle bacilli.

Solotorovsky et al. B56,305/51: "Cortisone overcame the beneficial effect of vaccination in mice infected with a highly virulent strain of M. tuberculosis, human type, but did not significantly enhance the lethality in non-vaccinated mice."

Ilavsky & Foley C7,577/54: In mice infected with massive doses of tubercle bacilli, "the chemotherapeutic effect of isoniazid was not impaired by concomitant treatment with large doses of cortisone. The effectiveness of streptomycin was reduced, and the weak effect of PAS was not significantly altered."

Youmans & Youmans B95,169/54: In mice, cortisone markedly reduced the survival time after infection with human tubercle bacilli and this effect could not be prevented by STH. Given alone, ACTH, STH and TTH likewise failed to influence the course of the infection.

Batten & McCune C53,554/57: ACTH, cortisol and cortisone greatly reduce the resistance of mice to infection with human M. tuberculosis.

Wagner & Lammers C83,426/58: The course of experimental tuberculosis is aggravated by cortisone and prednisolone in the mouse. The glucocorticoids also largely counteract the beneficial effect of streptomycin.

Robinson et al. G53,271/68: Unlike cortisol, indomethacin does not reduce the resistance of mice to virulent human strain of M. tuberculosis. A striking difference between the two drugs was also noted in respect to the high incidence of activated latent infection by cortisol, but not by indomethacin. "It would appear that indomethacin, like other nonsteroid, anti-inflammatory agents, has no influence on resistance to infection in spite of its anti-inflammatory action."

RABBIT

Lurie et al. B31,931/49; B31,932/49: In highly inbred, sexually mature rabbits, estradiol retarded the progress of tuberculosis following i.c. inoculation. In immature rabbits, estradiol was less effective. LH accelerated the progress of the disease, whereas ovariectomy or progesterone remained without effect.

Lurie et al. B31,933/49: In rabbits, estradiol retards the progress of experimental tuberculosis at the portal of entry in the skin and diminishes its dissemination to internal organs, presumably by reducing the permeability of connective tissue. Chorionic gonadotropin has an inverse effect.

Lurie et al. B55,625/51: In rabbits infected with M. tuberculosis, the number of bacilli in the pulmonary lesions as well as the number of tubercles are increased by cortisone; yet, dissemination to the tracheobronchial lymph nodes appears to be inhibited by the hormone.

Lurie et al. B68,457/52: In rabbits genetically resistant to tuberculosis, cortisone facilitated the infection.

Lepri & Fornaro D91,865/54: In rabbits rendered allergic to tuberculosis, the ocular manifestations of topical challenge by tubercle bacilli were variably influenced by ACTH and cortisone.

Bodaiji & Mori C35,586/57: In rabbits, cortisone facilitates the development of pulmonary lesions after inoculation with tubercle bacillus, H37Rv.

GUINEA PIG

Aycock & Foley B773/45: In guinea pigs, pretreatment with estradiol, diethylstilbestrol or testosterone diminishes resistance against tuberculosis.

Spain & Molomut B80,256/50; B60,878/50: Cortisone greatly aggravates the course of tuberculosis in guinea pigs and renders them very refractory to streptomycin treatment.

Spain B69,019/51: Cortisone diminishes the resistance of guinea pigs to tuberculosis.

Swedberg B59,988/51: Thyroxine diminishes the resistance of guinea pigs to tuberculosis. "Estrogen" has the same effect, whereas testosterone does not significantly change the course of the infection.

Okada et al. C18,328/55: In guinea pigs inoculated with B.C.G. or Vole bacillus, cortisone did not aggravate the lesions or increase the bacterial count.

Greuel & Schäfer E54,589/56: In guinea pigs treated with ACTH, DOC or cortisone, the progress of tuberculosis was proportional to the size of the adrenals, and least severe in animals given cortisol.

Kracht & Meissner C21,867/56: Cortisone aggravates tuberculosis in guinea pigs but infection with low virulence strains (e.g., B.C.G.) are not activated.

Tao et al. C82,168/59: Bovine type RM strain mycobacteria grew much more vigorously in the organs of rabbits and guinea pigs after treatment with cortisone; but no such enhancement of virulence was observed in hamsters and rats.

Vakilzadeh & Vandiviere E32,626/63: In guinea pigs, the beneficial effect of vaccination against tuberculosis was greatly increased by thyroxine and T3, but not by cortisone, cortisol or ACTH. None of the hormones altered natural host resistance in nonimmunized guinea pigs.

Hsu G70,576/69: The proliferation of tubercle bacilli in macrophages isolated from cortisone-treated and nontreated guinea pigs is virtually identical. Cytologic studies revealed that intracellular infection is toxic to the host cells derived from cortisone-treated animals. This toxicity is combated by serum from B.C.G.-vaccinated animals although the serum does not alter the rate of intracellular bacterial multiplication. "Hence, the increased susceptibility of cortisone-treated animals to tuberculous infection is not likely to be caused by an altered rate of intracellular multiplication of tubercle bacilli but the enhanced susceptibility of the host cells to toxic injury imposed by the intracellular multiplication of the pathogen."

VARIA

Lemonde C310/54: Doctor's thesis (186 pp., 564 refs.) on humoral factors influencing infections with special reference to the effect of STH and cortisone upon experimental tuberculosis.

Schäfer B99,955/54: Monograph (127 pp., numerous refs.) on the role of endocrine factors in tuberculosis. Special sections are devoted to the hormones of the thyroid, parathyroid, thymus, adrenals, pancreas and gonads.

Lurie C14,768/55: Review (30 pp., 128 refs.) on the effect of hormones in experimental tuberculosis. Special emphasis is placed upon the retardation of tuberculosis by folliculoids and its aggravation by cortisone.

Mycoplasma ←

Muftic & Redmann G58,918/68: In vitro tests on the effect of about 200 steroids upon cultures of Mycoplasma gallisepticum. No definite pharmaco-chemical correlations could be established.

Neisseria Gonorrhoeae ←

Rupp & Knackstedt C42,998/57: Cortisone increases the susceptibility of mice to both living and heat-killed gonococci.

Nocardia Asteroides ←

Ghione D87,868/57: 4-Chlorotestosterone enhances anaphylactic shock in guinea pigs, prolongs survival in systemic nocardiosis of mice and improves healing in cutaneous nocardiosis of rabbits.

Ghione C51,954/58: 4-Chlorotestosterone prolongs the survival time of mice infected with Nocardia asteroides or Staphylococcus aureus. Thus it counteracts the pro-infectious effect of cortisone.

Pasteurella Pestis ←

Girard C22,665/56: Infection with a comparatively avirulent strain of P. pestis is facilitated by cortisone pretreatment in the mouse.

Pasteurella Tularensis ←

Pinchot et al. B39,038/49: In rats infected with P. tularensis, survival time was not influenced by potent adrenocortical extract.

Pneumococci ← cf. Diplococcus Pneumoniae

Psittacosis — Ornithosis ←

Moritsch C15,606/56: Observations on the treatment of psittacosis by cortisone + antibiotics in the mouse.

Stewart C59,979/58: Administration of cortisone with psittacosis virus to embryonated hens' eggs prolonged the survival of the embryos.

Rickettsia ←

Jackson & Smadel E52,720/51: Intact mice pretreated with cortisone or ACTH, "were given lethal amounts of the toxins of R. tsutsugamushi, R. prowazeki, or S. typhosa. Such animals were as susceptible to the toxins as normal controls. Neither hormone had any therapeutic effect in mice infected with R. tsutsugamushi. Furthermore, treated and untreated mice in a terminal phase of infection with R. tsutsugamushi were equally susceptible to the toxin of this rickettsia when injected intravenously. In the current experiments the adrenal cortex of normal or infected animals apparently contributed as effectively as possible in the host's response to rickettsial or bacterial toxins and further stimulation was without advantage."

Salmonella Enteritidis ←

Chedid et al. B91,161/52: Infection with S. enteritidis p.o. causes an intestinal infection in intact rats but is rarely fatal. After adrenalectomy mortality is greatly increased although blood cultures are usually negative. "Death is not due to invasion by the organism but to an increase in the sensitivity to its toxic product after ablation of the adrenals."

Chedid et al. B99,547/54: In rats, pretreatment with cortisone diminishes survival following oral inoculation with S. enteritidis.

Salmonella Typhi ←

Benetato et al. 33,773/35: In rats, neither adrenocortical extract nor an adrenotrophic anterior pituitary preparation altered resistance to morphine or to typhoid-paratyphoid vaccine.

Chedid et al. B91,160/51: Although cortisone aggravates the course of various infections, it gives definite protection against otherwise lethal infections with S. typhi in mice.

Chedid et al. B91,161/52: Intact mice can be protected against otherwise fatal infections with S. typhi by a single dose of cortisone given one hour before infection. The corticoid does not appear to attack the germs but induces resistance to their toxin.

Germuth et al. D77,106/52: Rabbits are protected against the toxic effects of typhoid vaccine by cortisone pretreatment.

Mody et al. C45,962/56: Two patients with toxemia of typhoid fever resistant to chloramphenicol responded well to cortisol i.v.

Heyman & Jandl C94,285/60: In rabbits, infection by small numbers of typhoid bacilli is facilitated by cortisone.

Loschiavo G28,338/65: In patients with typhoid, the bactericidal property of the blood is increased by treatment with 19-nortestosterone-17-cyclopentylpropionate.

Salmonella Typhimurium ←

Bowen et al. C31,414/57: In mice, cortisone decreased resistance to S. typhimurium. Progesterone and DOC were without effect.

Bowen et al. C31,415/57: Cortisone reduces the survival time following infection with S. typhimurium especially in mice kept at a warm environmental temperature.

Bowen et al. C31,416/57: Cortisone given one day before infection with S. typhimurium reduces survival in various strains of mice selected for a wide range in their natural resistance to this germ.

"Saprophytosis" ←

Selye B40,000/50: Large doses of cortisone predispose the rat to the development of septicemia with abscess formation especially in the lungs (but also in other organs) as a consequence of diminished resistance against normally saprophytic organisms.

Selye B57,451/51: In rats, "saprophytosis" due to proliferation of normally nonpathogenic microorganisms, such as develops after heavy overdosage with cortisone or ACTH, can be completely prevented by concurrent administration of STH.

Ducommun & Ducommun B70,251/53: In rats, saprophytosis produced by heavy overdosage with cortisone is inhibited by concurrent administration of STH. This "anti-infectious effect of STH" is much less evident after adrenalectomy. DOC, testosterone, and estradiol alone or in combination failed to duplicate the anti-infectious action of STH in cortisone-treated rats.

von Wasielewski & Knick G68,292/58: In mice, cortisone decreases resistance to inoculation with various pathogenic, but not to saprophytic, organisms.

Staphylococcus ← cf. also Selye G60,083/70, p. 378.

Kligman et al. G64,164/51: In guinea pigs, infection with Trichophyton mentagrophytes, vaccinia virus and S. aureus is adversely influenced by cortisone.

Germuth et al. D77,106/52: In rabbits cortisone increases susceptibility to pneumococcal infection as manifested by greater mortality, increased bacterial growth in the locally infected sites and enhanced bacteremia. The decreased resistance is ascribed to interference with the migration of phagocytic cells to the infected sites. On the other hand cortisone increases the resistance of the rabbit to hemolytic S. aureus.

Debry C30,870/56: Doctor's thesis (176 pp. 578 refs.) on the influence of hormones upon infection. Personal observations on guinea pigs and rats indicate that ACTH, STH and DOC do not significantly affect the course of acute staphylococcus infection, whereas cortisone aggravates it.

Herbeuval et al. C55,674/58: Testosterone does not significantly influence staphylococcus septicemia in the rabbit. Earlier literature on the effect of testoids upon infection is reviewed.

Herbeuval et al. C55,676/58: In rabbits, DOC does not influence the development of septicemia following infection with S. aureus, whereas cortisone aggravates its course.

Smith et al. F68,892/66: Testosterone, cortisone, as well as various organ extracts, partially protect the mouse against staphylococcal infection.

Toivanen G49,847/67; G59,609/66: Staphylococcal infection in mice is enhanced by estradiol benzoate given once or several times immediately before infection. "The enhancement of the infection was also demonstrated by the use of estrone, estriol, 17α-estradiol, 17β-estradiol, estradiol sulphate, estradiol phosphate, ethynylestradiol, diethylstilbestrol, methallenestril and chlorotrianisene. The effect was not directly correlated to the estrogenic potency of the drug. Progesterone was found to be inert."

Toivanen G49,848/67: In mice, estradiol pretreatment enhanced infection with staphylococci, but the degree of this activity depended upon the time interval between infection and the initiation of hormone treatment as well as upon the magnitude of the microbial inoculum.

Streptococcus ←

Glaser et al. B58,299/50: In mice, neither ACTH nor cortisone exerted a beneficial effect upon streptococcal or pneumococcal infections; indeed they may have aggravated them.

Glaser et al. B57,933/51: In mice and rats with streptococcal and pneumococcal infections, cortisone depresses cellular exudation and increases mortality.

Glaser et al. B65,298/51: "Cortisone shortens the survival time of mice with cervical adenitis due to group A streptococci. Rats with streptococcal pneumonia were similarly affected by cortisone therapy."

Thomas et al. B57,977/51: "When the rabbits are immunized with streptococci prior to cortisone treatment and infection, bacteremia occurs briefly or not at all and the animals survive, indicating that enhancement of infection by cortisone is probably not caused by interference with the immune mechanism."

Mogabgab & Thomas B72,457/52: In rabbits, pretreatment with ACTH or cortisone greatly aggravated streptococcal septicemia. DOC had no such effect.

Foley C13,263/55: "Chlortetracycline and oxytetracycline are ineffective against streptococcus infections in nonimmunized mice which are treated with large doses of cortisone. Immunized mice similarly treated with cortisone are effectively protected by these antibiotics.'

Fazio et al. C34,111/56: In rats, cortisone or ACTH increases survival following streptococcal infection and further enhances the protective effect of penicillin.

Foley et al. C31,073/57: Prednisone, prednisolone, cortisone and cortisol aggravate streptococcus infections in mice and interfere with the efficacy of chlortetracycline.

Kuck C69,754/59: Comparative studies on the increase in tetracycline requirements for the control of streptococcal infections caused by triamcinolone, prednisolone and cortisol, in mice.

Weisskopf et al. D35,320/61: Review of the protective action of folliculoids against viruses and bacteria, with personal observations on the increase in the resistance of mice that can be induced by Premarin against virulent streptococcal infection. Females are more resistant than males, and castration increases resistance in males. The effect of folliculoids is tentatively ascribed to an increase in the acid mucopolysaccharide content of the ground substance which decreases the subcutaneous spread of germs.

Treponema Pallidum ←

Turner & Hollander B 55,488/50: In rabbits, syphilomas induced by intradermal or intratesticular injection of Treponema pallidum become soft and spongy under the influence of cortisone, and the production of Wassermann reagin is inhibited. Upon withdrawal of cortisone, there is a rebound phenomenon in which the lesions become unusually large.

Gastinel et al. D 8,309/60: In rabbits, infected with syphilis by various routes, cortisone accelerates the generalization of the lesions.

Wicher & Jakubovski G 26,810/64: In guinea pigs, cortisone prolongs the incubation period, shortens the duration and alters the character of the changes elicited by i.c. inoculation with T. pallidum. Serologic tests and the infectivity of the organisms are not affected.

Varia ←

Kass & Finland B 59,076/51: Review on the effect of ACTH and corticoids upon **various types of infections** in animals and man.

Kay et al. B 60,579/51: In dogs, cortisone offered no protection against the lethal effect of an experimental **appendical peritonitis**.

Chedid et al. B 91,161/52: Review (21 pp., 75 refs.) on the relationship between the adrenals and **infection**.

Kass & Finland C 80,582/53: Review (27 pp., 313 refs.) on the role of corticoids in **infection and immunity.**

Cavallero C 829/54: Review on the effect of STH, ACTH and cortisone upon various **infections**, especially in the rat.

Maral & Cosar C 14,760/55: Review of the literature and personal observations on the effect of cortisone upon **various types of infection** in the mouse, rabbit and rat.

Kass & Finland E 56,566/57: Review (18 pp., 181 refs.) on the effect of corticoids upon various **infections**.

Kass & Finland D 87,314/58: Review (35 pp., 151 refs.) on "Corticosteroids and **infections**."

Spink C 91,027/60: Review on the pathogenesis of shock due to **infection** and its treatment by glucocorticoid.

Ghione & Turolla G 18,525/64: Review of investigations on mice, guinea pigs and rats showing that the **infection** facilitating effect of glucocorticoids (cortisone, prednisone) is counteracted by anabolic steroids such as 4-hydroxymethyltestosterone or 4-chlorotestosterone.

Nicol et al. F 25,320/64: Review of the literature and personal observations suggest that folliculoids increase resistance against various **infections**, but the sex-stimulating and anti-infectious effects of diverse natural or synthetic folliculoids do not run parallel.

Viruses ←

The tumorigenic effect of **adenovirus-12** is greater in female than in male hamsters. Ovariectomy diminishes this effect. Estradiol increases it in males but not in females.

The susceptibility of mice to the lethal effect of various **arboviruses** is increased by cortisone but uninfluenced by DOC, testosterone, progesterone or estradiol.

Pretreatment with cortisone aggravates the course of **Coxsackie** infection in guinea pigs and mice. In mice, gonadectomy diminishes mortality from Coxsackie infection but only during the first 10 days after operation. Testosterone does not alter this beneficial effect.

In mice, cortisone increases mortality following inoculation with **Japanese encephalomyelitis** virus. Allegedly concurrent treatment with splenic extract blocks this action. DOC has no adverse effect.

In dogs, cortisone, ACTH, estradiol, stilbestrol and thyroxine all stimulate the growth of **equine encephalomyelitis** virus, whereas testosterone and progesterone do not. The hormones which aggravate the infection also counteract the prophylactic effect of mepacrine and abolish the normally greater resistance of females as compared to males.

In rats, cortisone offers partial protection against the paralysis induced by **encephalomyocarditis** virus.

Susceptibility to **virus hepatitis** is greatly increased by glucocorticoids in the mouse. The associated severe lymphoid necrosis is prevented although the hepatic lesions are aggravated. Infected animals pretreated with cortisol may show up to a 1000-fold increase in the hepatic virus concentration as compared with similarly infected but untreated animals. Suppression of immune phenomena and of RES activity may be responsible for this sensitization. STH counteracts the glucocorticoid-induced increase in virus susceptibility. In weanling mice and in rats, which are normally resistant to virus hepatitis, susceptibility can be induced by cortisone.

Pretreatment with estradiol allegedly facilitates the production of murine virus hepatitis.

In man, 4-chlorotestosterone and several other anabolic testoids allegedly protect the liver against the damaging effect of viral hepatitis.

In mice, resistance to various strains of **influenza** virus and Newcastle-disease viruses is reduced by cortisone given 24 hrs before challenge. However, under certain conditions various glucocorticoids can also increase the survival of mice infected with influenza virus and diminish the severity of the pulmonary changes.

In chick embryos, infected with influenza B., pretreatment with cortisone prolongs survival although virus proliferation is enhanced.

Various testoid anabolics have also been said to exert a protective effect against the damaging action of influenza virus upon embryonated chicken eggs; yet, in mice, testosterone allegedly accelerates the proliferation of influenza virus, presumably because of its protein anabolic effect.

Cortisone accelerates the course of **poliomyelitis** infection in mice and hamsters; DOC, progesterone and stilbestrol are ineffective. Yet, earlier investigators claimed that estradiol can protect various species against poliomyelitis, but only in the event of intranasal and not following i.p. or intracerebral inoculation.

In monkeys, cortisone did not increase susceptibility to poliomyelitis under the conditions in which the tests were performed.

Cortisone allegedly increases susceptibility of mice to **rabies** virus perhaps because of its immunosuppressive effect. Prednisolone has been claimed to protect against the paralytic complications of antirabies vaccines.

Cortisone definitely enhances **vaccinia** infection in rabbits; estradiol, estrone and pseudopregnancy have an opposite effect in this species. In guinea pigs, cortisone also exerts an adverse influence upon vaccinia infection. In mice, it depresses interferon formation but fails to inhibit the protection offered by N-ethylisatin-β-thiosemicarbazone.

Aldosterone is said to inhibit the reproduction of vaccinia virus in vitro.

Rabbits are allegedly protected against **variola** by aldosterone.

In sheep, ACTH and dexamethasone aggravate the lesions produced by the smallpox virus; STH has an opposite effect, presumably because its prophlogistic action helps to delimit the lesions.

Adenoviruses ←

Yohn et al. G57,790/68: In hamsters given adenovirus-12, strain Huie, s.c. at birth, thymectomy at one week of age increased tumor incidence in both sexes, although it remained higher in females as is usually the case. Cortisone treatment, begun at one week of age, increased tumor incidence but, again, this remained higher in females. Antibody responses to adenovirus-12 T-antigen were depressed in thymectomized and cortisone-treated animals.

Yohn & Funk G68,339/69: Adenovirus-12 produced a higher incidence of tumors in female than in male Syrian hamsters. Ovariectomy lowered tumor incidence, whereas estradiol increased it but only in males.

Arboviruses ←

Southam & Babcock B63,662/51: "Large doses of cortisone greatly increased the susceptibility of mice to lethal infection by **West Nile, Ilheus,** and **Bunyamwere** viruses. ACTH in massive dosage produced the same effect with West Nile virus. Desoxycorticosterone, testosterone, progesterone, and estradiol in massive doses had no significant effect on these virus infections in mice."

Columbia-SK Virus ←

Siegel et al. D13,002/61: "Cortisone increased the mortality and nullified the protection afforded by trypan red in mice inoculated intraperitoneally with Columbia-SK virus."

Coxsackie ←

Kilbourne & Horsfall Jr. B65,487/51: Adult mice normally resistant to Coxsackie virus can be lethally infected following pretreatment with cortisone.

Graham et al. B68,455/52: Cortisone increases the susceptibility of the mouse to Coxsackie virus infection.

Angela & di Nola C12,561/54: In guinea pigs, pretreatment with cortisone aggravates the course of the subsequent Coxsackie infection.

Berkovich & Ressel F46,105/65: In mice, mortality after Coxsackie B1 virus infection was diminished by gonadectomy in both sexes but only during the first ten days after operation. Testosterone did not significantly influence this beneficial effect.

Encephalomyelitis ←

Vollmer & Hurlbut B66,973/51: In mice, moderate doses of cortical extract or cortisone had no effect on Japanese B encephalitis virus infection, although in doses that inhibit growth, cortisone did increase the mortality rate. Testosterone had no adverse effect.

Kudo et al. C11,417/54: In mice, cortisone increases mortality following inoculation with Japanese encephalomyelitis virus, whereas DOC has no adverse effect.

Nakagawa & Kanda C9,941/55; C8,165/55: Cortisone increases the susceptibility of mice to infection with encephalomyelitis virus but concurrent administration of a splenic extract blocks this action of the glucocorticoid.

Hurst et al. C94,089/60: Cortisone, ACTH, estradiol, stilbestrol and thyroxine all stimulate the growth of the virus of equine encephalomyelitis in the dog, whereas testosterone and progesterone do not. The hormones which aggravate the infection also counteract the prophylactic effect of mepacrine and abolish the normally greater resistance of the females.

Olivier & Cheever G15,789/63: Cortisone diminishes the susceptibility of rats to the development of paralysis following inoculation of encephalomyocarditis virus.

Hepatitis ←

Melcher Jr. et al. B69,381/52: Rats normally resistant to viral hepatitis become susceptible after pretreatment with cortisone.

Starr & Pollard C60,012/58: Cortisone induced susceptibility of comparatively resistant weanling Swiss mice to infection with the Gledhill strain of mouse hepatitis virus.

Pecori et al. C89,121/59: In mice, virus hepatitis is aggravated by prednisolone and beneficially influenced by STH.

Pecori et al. C89,118/59: Prednisone, triamcinolone and dexamethasone increase sensitivity of the mouse to infection with the MHV-3 hepatitis virus. This pro-infectious effect is largely counteracted by STH.

Manso et al. C68,152/59: In mice infected with hepatitis virus, the levels of GOT, GPT, lactic dehydrogenase, and glutathione reductase increased under the influence of cortisol, whereas in intact mice the hormone did not influence these enzyme activities. It is assumed that cortisol "may exert an adverse effect on the natural course of the experimentally-induced infection."

Jones & Cohen D55,380/63: Pretreatment with estradiol valerate facilitates the production of murine virus hepatitis.

Terragna et al. G25,811/64: In man, 4-chlorotestosterone ameliorates the course of viral hepatitis.

Terragna et al. G36,590/65: In patients with viral hepatitis, various anabolic testoids protect the liver (needle biopsy) against damage.

Hirano & Ruebner G38,763/66: In mice, the severe lymphoid necrosis produced by murine hepatitis virus (MHV_3) was prevented by cortisone whereas the liver lesions were aggravated. Essentially the same results were obtained with puromycin although it failed to aggravate the hepatic lesions. Presumably suppression of protein synthesis was the common underlying mechanism. "It is concluded that multiplication of the virus alone did not produce the lymphoid necrosis but that protein synthesis induced by the infection, presumably an immune reaction, was primarily responsible for this lesion."

Ruebner et al. G48,873/67: In the mouse, cortisone not only increases the number and size of necrotic foci produced by MHV_3-virus but also alters the light-microscopic and ultrastructural appearance of the hepatocytes.

Datta & Isselbacher G68,822/69: Cortisol and methylprednisolone greatly increase the susceptibility of the mouse to virus hepatitis. "Infected animals pretreated with hydrocortisone showed from 50-fold to a more than 1.000-fold increase of virus in the liver compared with untreated infected animals."

Lavelle & Starr H18,566/69: In mice, cortisone increases susceptibility to virus hepatitis and depresses RES activity.

Nelson & Lanza G80,151/70: In nine patients with massive hepatic necrosis due to viral hepatitis, prednisone proved to be a valuable adjunct to treatment.

Influenza ←

Kalter et al. B49,656/50: In mice, the proliferation of influenza virus is accelerated by STH and testosterone, presumably because of an enhanced protein synthesis in general.

Kass et al. B69,981/51: In mice, the final mortality rate after infection with influenza virus or pneumococci is not significantly altered by ACTH or cortisone, although the course of the disease may be modified.

Kilbourne B69,376/52: Pretreatment with cortisone prolongs the survival of chick embryos infected with influenza B although virus proliferation is enhanced.

Khoobvarian & Walker C30,210/57: In mice, resistance to i.v. inoculation of PR8 influenza A, Lee influenza B, and Newcastle disease viruses was reduced by cortisone given at least 24 hrs before challenge.

Lagôa D58,191/62: Cortisol and prednisolone, unlike dexamethasone and cortisone, increase the survival of mice infected with influenza PR8 virus.

Mims G68,101/62: Glucocorticoids did not protect mice from the lethal action of ectromelia virus but increased survival and delayed death after inoculation with influenza virus.

Terragna G36,765/63: In tests on embryonated chicken eggs and in mice infected with influenza virus A-PR8, treatment with anabolic hormones (dehydroisoandrosterone, 4-chlorotestosterone) exerts a certain protective effect, but the results are variable.

Sobis G29,127/64: In mice, the pulmonary changes induced by influenza virus are diminished by cortisol.

Measles ←

Coraggio et al. D58,058/62: In rabbits immunized with measles virus, 19-norandrostenolone raises antibody formation.

Mumps ←

Kilbourne & Horsfall Jr. B55,005/51: In chicken eggs, the concentration in the allantoic fluid of Lee, PR8 or mumps virus is increased by cortisone.

Pneumonia ←

Smith et al. B64,635/51: In mice, susceptibility to pneumonia virus (PVM) is not influenced by ACTH but is enhanced by cortisone.

Poliomyelitis ←

Levaditi & Haber 33,069/35: In Macacus cynomolgus monkeys, resistance to poliomyelitis virus, acquired by prior infection, is not influenced by thyroidectomy, orchidectomy or thyroxine administration.

Foley & Aycock B764/45: Review of the literature and personal observations on the protective effect of estradiol against poliomyelitis infection in various species. In general, the folliculoids are effective against intranasal infection, but not against i.p. or intracerebral inoculation.

Shwartzman B54,248/50: "ACTH and cortisone in combination or cortisone alone produce a marked acceleration of poliomyelitis infection (strain MEF1) in mice and an extraordinary enhancement of susceptibility to this infection in hamsters giving rise to a violent and uniformly fatal disease. ACTH alone fails to produce this effect possibly due to elaboration of an unknown factor capable of reversing the enhancing effect of cortisone."

Shwartzman B66,955/51: ACTH and cortisone accelerate poliomyelitis (strain MEF) in mice and hamsters. DOC, progesterone and diethylstilbestrol are ineffective.

Findlay & Howard B81,142/52: In mice and hamsters, cortisone and ACTH increase susceptibility to poliomyelitis and other virus infections.

Shwartzman B69,778/52: Cortisone, unlike ACTH, greatly increases the susceptibility of Syrian hamsters to i.p. inoculation with strain MEF1 poliomyelitis virus.

Shwartzman & Fisher B69,580/52: In Syrian hamsters, cortisone enhances infection with MEF1 and Lansing strains of poliomyelitis virus. ACTH, DOC, progesterone and stilbestrol are without effect. Earlier literature on the influence of various hormones upon poliomyelitis is reviewed.

Shwartzman & Aronson B84,833/53: In the hamster, pretreatment with cortisone facilitates infection with poliomyelitis.

Hoosier et al. D12,216/61: "In several comparative experiments with and without cortisone, no enhancing effect of this compound on the susceptibility of monkeys to infection with poliovirus was found."

Rabies ←

Yaoi et al. C34,360/56: Cortisone increases the susceptibility of mice to rabies virus.

Finger E26,273/62: Prednisolone protects the rabbit against the paralytic complications elicited by antirabies vaccines, presumably because it depresses allergic reactions to the contaminating foreign brain tissue.

Vaccinia ←

Sprunt & McDearman A33,321/40: Treatment with estradiol or estrone, as well as pseudopregnancy, increased the resistance of the rabbit to vaccinia virus.

Kligman et al. G64,164/51: In guinea pigs, infection with Trichophyton mentagrophytes, vaccinia virus and Staphylococcus aureus is adversely influenced by cortisone.

Bugbee et al. C84,115/60: "Cortisone has a definite enhancing effect on vaccinia infection in rabbits."

Coraggio et al. D12,550/61: Aldosterone inhibits the reproduction of vaccinia virus in vitro.

Lieberman et al. F67,288/66: In mice, cortisone did not inhibit the protection offered by N-ethylisatin-β-thiosemicarbazone against neurovaccinia virus. However, it did depress interferon formation.

Variola ←

Cilli et al. D12,192/61: In sheep, STH, owing to its prophlogistic effect, delimits the lesions produced by variola virus. ACTH and dexamethasone exert an opposite effect.

Pecori et al. D12,549/61: Aldosterone protects the rabbit against inoculation with smallpox virus.

Varia ←

Altucci et al. D65,818/62: Review and personal observations on the effect of various glucocorticoids upon viral infections in vivo and in vitro.

Smart & Kilbourne G33,810/66: In chick embryos infected with various viruses, cortisol diminishes interferon formation but its effect upon survival depends upon experimental circumstances.

Poel H23,662/68: Review of the literature with personal observations on the co-carcinogenic effect of folliculoids and luteoids. Neither of these groups of steroids are truly carcinogenic in themselves but they enhance mammary cancer development under the influence of viral and chemical carcinogens. [The possible mechanism of these interactions is not discussed (H.S.).]

Fungi and Yeasts ←

Resistance to **Candida albicans** infection is decreased by cortisone in the mouse and rabbit. Testosterone allegedly enhances, whereas STH counteracts, this deleterious effect of cortisone in mice.

Cortisone also aggravates infection with **Trichophyton mentagrophytes, Histoplasma capsulatum** and various other fungi in several species of animals.

Bronchopulmonary Aspergillosis ←

Sandhu et al. G75,603/70: In mice, bronchopulmonary aspergillosis produced by inhalation of various species of these fungi was greatly enhanced by cortisone.

Candida Albicans (monilia) ←

Roth et al. C32,916/56: Pretreatment with cortisone or X-rays, singly or in combination, reduces the inherent resistance of mice to infection with Candida albicans.

Scherr C39,263/57: In mice infected with Candida albicans, the development of moniliasis may either be increased or decreased by cortisone depending upon various factors, particularly sex, pregnancy, or the severity of the infection. Testosterone enhanced and STH counteracted the deleterious effect of cortisone. Gonadotrophin (pregnant mare's serum) was without effect.

Henry & Fahlberg C81,623/60: Repeated i.p. injections of cortisol (unlike a single dose) aggravate monilial infection in mice.

Louria et al. C91,764/60: "Monilial infections in mice were enhanced to a far greater degree by cortisone than were infections due to Histoplasma capsulatum or Cryptococcus neoformans."

de Mitri et al. D64,042/63: In rabbits intrabronchially inoculated with Candida albicans, cortisone treatment causes: "1. a quicker onset of necrosis; 2. a larger extension of tissue alterations with a tendency to haematic diffusion (which could never be established in animals not treated with cortisone); 3. late occurrence of a reduced defense reaction of the mesenchyma."

Nishikawa G73,894/69: In germ-free mice, cortisone decreases host resistance so that oral inoculation with Candida albicans results in stomach ulcers in which the organisms proliferate.

Histoplasma Capsulatum ←

Vogel et al. C10,597/55: In guinea pigs, cortisone failed to cause significant aggravation of the infection following inoculation with Histoplasma capsulatum.

Grunberg & Titsworth D67,985/63: Cortisone i.m. enhances the susceptibility of mice to infection with Histoplasma capsulatum.

Trichophyton Mentagrophytes ←

Kligman et al. G64,164/51: In guinea pigs, infection with Trichophyton mentagrophytes, vaccinia virus and Staphylococcus aureus is adversely influenced by cortisone.

Varia ←

Piantoni C38,892/55: An extensive review of the literature and personal observations on rabbits and rats lead to the conclusion that cortisone does not cause normally apathogenic fungi to become virulent, but greatly enhances the virulence of normally pathogenic fungi.

Parasites ←

Protozoa ←. As judged by observations on different animal species many protozoan infections are adversely influenced by glucocorticoids. Among these are infections with various strains of **Ameba, Besnoitia, Eimeria mivati and meleagrimitis,** various forms of **Plasmodia, Trypanosomes and Toxoplasma.**

Steroids devoid of glucocorticoid activity have only rarely been noted to exert any pronounced influence on protozoan infections. Yet, it has been claimed that orchidectomy increases the severity of Trypanosoma lewisi infection in rats, although not to the same extent as adrenalectomy.

Worms ←. Glucocorticoids also diminish resistance against infestation with various worms such as **Ancylostoma caninum, Fasciola hepatica, Hymenolepis nana, Schistosoma mansoni (Bilharzia), Trichinella spiralis and Trichuris muris.** On the other hand, allegedly, under certain conditions progesterone may beneficially affect bilharziosis in the mouse, although among 30 steroids tested all folliculoids and testoids were ineffective in this respect.

Protozoa ←

Ameba ←. *Teodorovic et al. D52,087/63:* In the guinea pig, amebiasis is aggravated by cortisone or cortisol.

Besnoitia ←. *Frenkel C13,371/56:* The adrenal necrosis produced by Besnoitia jellisoni (an obligate intracellular protozoan organism) is inhibited by cortisol, corticosterone, 11-dehydrocorticosterone and possibly by DOC. This is associated with a depression of general immunity. The organisms do not proliferate around sites of corticosterone, DOC, testosterone or epinephrine injections. "It is postulated that certain glucocorticoids can so modify immunity mechanisms locally, that general immunity becomes ineffective."

Frenkel C52,043/58: Hamsters inoculated s.c. with the intracellular protozoan Besnoitia jellisoni recovered owing to sulfadiazine treatment. However, latent infection persisted and relapses could be precipitated by a subsequent treatment with cortisone, cortisol, prednisone or prednisolone. The relapse phenomenon is recommended for the assay of the immuno-depressing activity of corticoids.

Frenkel C84,036/60: Chronic latent Besnoitia infection in Golden hamsters is greatly enhanced by glucocorticoids (22 modified luteoids and corticoids have been tested). The procedure is suitable for the routine assay of pro-infectious activity.

Eimeria ←. *McLoughlin G73,149/69:* In chickens, dexamethasone permits Eimeria meleagrimitis to complete its development, whereas this is not the case in untreated chickens or in either dexamethasone treated or untreated turkeys.

Rose G73,104/70; Long & Rose G72,642/70: In partially immunized chickens, betamethasone increases oocyst production and extends the patent period of Eimeria mivati infection. In fully susceptible chickens, betamethasone had a similar but less pronounced effect, presumably because the major action of the steroid is to reduce acquired immunity to this form of coccidiosis.

Plasmodia (malaria) ←. *Bennison & Coatney B17,600/48:* Following inoculation with P. gallinaceum, the parasite counts are much higher in females than in males. This difference in parasite count was not significantly influenced by testosterone or estradiol.

Overman et al. B49,805/49: An adrenocortical extract prolongs survival of monkeys infected with P. knowlesi.

Redmond B67,882/52: Cortisone increases susceptibility to malaria in pigeons infected with P. relictum.

Jackson C11,604/55: Cortisone delays the course of Plasmodium berghei malaria in rats but increases mortality.

Cox G64,797/68: In mice, betamethasone suppresses the acquisition of immunity to infection with Plasmodium vinckei but has no effect once immunity is established.

Trypanosoma Cruzi ←. *Pizzi & Chemke C34,555/55:* In rats, cortisone aggravates the course of infection with Trypanosoma cruzi. The mechanism of this resistance and its histopathologic characteristics are extensively discussed.

Rubio C34,556/55: In mice, cortisone aggravates the course of Trypanosoma cruzi infection.

Sommer C9,937/55: The cortisone-induced increase in the susceptibility of mice to Trypanosoma cruzi infection is not abolished by STH.

Rubio C41,052/56: In mice, cortisone treatment during the first days after Trypanosoma cruzi inoculation did not significantly affect the course of the infection.

Trypanosoma Equiperdum ←. *Scott et al. 15,446/33:* The resistance of intact guinea pigs to diphtheria toxin or that of rats to **Trypanosoma equiperdum** or mice to infection with **Pneumococcus Type I** was not influenced by pretreatment with large amounts of a life-maintaining adrenocortical extract ("cortin"). It does not appear to be possible to raise resistance above normal in intact animals but there is considerable evidence to show that various types of intoxication and infection cause structural damage to the adrenal and interfere with its function.

Cantrell C64,728/59: Cortisone does not significantly influence infection with Trypanosoma equiperdum in the rat.

Trypanosoma Lewisi ←. *Perla & Marmorston-Gottesman 810/30:* In young rats, thymectomy diminishes, whereas orchidectomy increases, the severity of T. lewisi infection.

Perla & Marmorston-Gottesman 10,865/31: Intact rats infected with T. lewisi rarely succumb, whereas in adrenalectomized animals the infection is usually fatal, although the bacterial growth is not modified. The authors attributed this mortality to the toxicity of the flagellate.

Herbert & Becker G63,454/61: In rats, cortisone does not cause inhibition of the production of Taliaferro's antibody, albastin, or of its maintenance after infection with T. lewisi. Cortisone does not appear to exert a deleterious effect on antibody production or maintenance and, if anything, it diminishes the duration of the infection.

Sherman & Ruble G49,628/67: In rats, pretreatment with cortisone diminishes resistance to T. lewisi, presumably as a consequence of impaired host immune responses.

Patton & Clark G73,195/68: In rats infected with T. lewisi, dexamethasone resulted in the development of exceedingly large populations of trypanosomes which were fatal to their hosts. This effect of dexamethasone is ascribed to the inhibition of the production of ablastin and trypanocidal antibodies.

Toxoplasma ←. *Frenkel C34,875/57:* Combined treatment with cortisone and X-rays diminished the resistance of Golden hamsters with the RH strain of toxoplasma and significantly depressed acquired immunity.

Giroud et al. D68,563/62: Various strains of toxoplasma, harmless for untreated rats, become virulent following treatment of the animals with glucocorticoids.

Worms ←

Ancylostoma Caninum ←. *Sen et al. F76,261/65:* Pretreatment with cortisone increased the susceptibility of mice to infection with Ancylostoma caninum perhaps by suppression of immunity. The effect of glucocorticoids upon infestation with other worms is reviewed.

Bilharzia ← *cf.* **Schistosomiasis.**

Fasciola Hepatica ←. *Sinclair G65,622/68:* In sheep infected with Fasciola hepatica, the growth of the flukes and the development of extensive hepatic hemorrhages with severe clinical signs was aggravated by dexamethasone but the usual splenomegaly and hepatic fibrosis were prevented by this glucocorticoid.

Hymenolepis Nana ←. *Pinto D23,719/60:* Hymenolepis nana type "M" is a natural parasite of the mouse; the rat is resistant to it, unless it is pretreated with cortisone.

Schistosomiasis ←. *Nagata et al. D26,285/56:* Cortisone increases the susceptibility of the mouse to infection with S. japonicum.

Coker C42,296/57: Cortisone does not significantly alter the susceptibility to infestation with S. mansoni in the mouse, as judged by the number of worms recovered from the portal circulation.

Lagrange D57,434/62: Combined treatment with ultrasound + progesterone + estradiol protects the mouse against bilharziosis following infection with S. mansoni. None of these agents alone nor testosterone + ultrasound were effective.

Lagrange D69,093/63: In mice, a protective effect against S. mansoni has been obtained by progesterone, dexamethasone and its 16β-isomer (celestone), as well as by the hormonally inactive 21-acetoxy-nor-12-prednisone (Win 1303). Among 30 steroids tested, all folliculoids and testoids were negative, pregnan-derivatives appeared to show anti-bilharziosis activity irrespective of their steroid hormone actions. The mechanism of this protection is not known, but bilharziosis in the mouse leads to a transformation of the liver "into a veritable sponge loaded with eggs surrounded by tubercles. The circulation of the liver and intestine is greatly disturbed at the same time by the accumulation of the eggs in the mesenteric venules and the resulting phlebitis." Mortality is ordinarily 100% within 1—15 months. Even in mice killed after 6—10 months in apparently good health, adult worms are eliminated but are atrophic and sterile. It is assumed that the protective steroids act upon the parasites themselves.

Trichinella Spiralis ←. *Coker C48,693/56:* In mice immunized against Trichinella spiralis, cortisone abolishes established immunity as judged by adult worm counts in the small intestine and suppression of the characteristic cellular response following a challenging infection of immune controls.

Ritterson C78,122/59: Chinese hamsters which possess an innate resistance to Trichinella spiralis can be infected with this organism following pretreatment with cortisone.

Howard et al. D22,789/62: In rats, "the anti-inflammatory effect of cortisone appears to inhibit the cellular reaction seen in trichinous myocarditis and this may impair the destruction and removal of the migrating larvae."

Pawlowski G65,301/68: In the rat, the development of trichinella infestation is not influenced by DOC, but enhanced by norandrostenolone (Durabolin). [The brief abstract gives no experimental details (H.S.).]

Trichuris Muris ←. *Campbell & Collette D61,500/62:* Cortisone enhances infection with the whipworm Trichuris muris in the mouse. Perhaps "the normal refractoriness of albino mice to this infection may be the result of inflammation of the gut evoked by parasitic invasion or associated immunologic phenomena."

← Steroids

BACTERIAL TOXINS ←

← Corticoids

In chick embryos, hemorrhages and mortality occur after inoculation of various endotoxins into the chorio-allantoic membrane. These effects are inhibited by cortisone, cortisol, fluorocortisol and aldosterone; DOC, prednisolone and cholesterol are inactive in this respect. Thus, there does not appear to be any close relationship between this protective action and the classic, glucocorticoid and mineralocorticoid, effects of steroids.

Cats can be protected against fatal endotoxin shock by aldosterone given i.v. 30 min after endotoxin, but no such protection is observed if the aldosterone is administered 30 min before or simultaneously with the endotoxin. $3\beta,16\alpha$-Dihydroxy-allopregnan-20-one competitively antagonizes this protective action. Although cortisol and prednisolone also afford some protection against endotoxin shock, aldosterone is about 100 times more active than these glucocorticoids. When aldosterone is incubated with E. coli endotoxin, it allegedly diminishes the toxicity of the latter as judged by in vivo tests on cats. It has been suggested "that aldosterone combines with, or otherwise alters the chemical structure of the endotoxin."

In dogs, cortisone failed to modify the circulatory failure produced by meningococcus toxin. As regards E. coli endotoxin shock, the results reported are contradictory. Most investigators stated that glucocorticoids, particularly cortisol and prednisolone, do improve survival and counteract circulatory shock to some extent but the best results are obtained if glucocorticoids are given in combination with some vasoactive drugs such as metaraminol, hydralazine or isoproterenol. In 6—9 day old beagles, cortisol sodium succinate given i.v. one hour before a lethal dose of E. coli endotoxin increased the survival rate, whereas it offered no protection if given immediately after endotoxin.

According to one team of investigators, aldosterone does not prevent endotoxin shock in the dog as it does in the cat; however, since the assay technique was not the same, this difference cannot be ascribed entirely to an essentially distinct reaction form of the two species.

Early investigations on the effect of adrenocortical extracts upon diphtheria intoxication in guinea pigs have yielded contradictory results. More recently it was found that neither ACTH nor cortisone improves the resistance of the guinea pig to diphtheria toxin (or of mice to Shiga and meningococcus toxin). However, the subnormal diphtheria-toxin resistance of the hypophysectomized guinea pigs is restored to normal by cortisone.

Allegedly the bronchoconstriction induced by S. typhosa endotoxin in guinea pigs can be prevented by prednisolone, but this observation requires confirmation.

In monkeys both cortisol and aldosterone (the latter especially when given in combination with angiotensin) offer some protection against the vascular collapse of endotoxin shock.

The literature on the effect of corticoids upon endotoxin shock in mice is extremely voluminous and contradictory. Apparently the results depend not only upon the type of corticoid given but also upon numerous other technical details (e.g., dose, timing, route of administration of the toxin and corticoid, age and strain of the mice). Hence, it is virtually impossible to arrive at meaningful generalizations beyond the conclusion that under most experimental conditions, glucocorticoids offer definite protection against various endotoxins.

Curiously, pertussis vaccine abolishes the ability of cortisone to protect mice against endotoxin.

In most respects the endotoxins of various bacteria exhibit essentially similar toxic effects; yet, considerable differences appear to exist between various preparations as regards the ability of corticoids to inhibit their toxicity. It is noteworthy that mice protected by cortisone against an initial lethal challenge with Brucella endotoxin, still develop resistance to subsequent challenge by a second injection of the same endotoxin. Apparently, the manifestations of shock are not necessary for the acquisition of resistance.

Pregnancy diminishes resistance of mice to S. enteritidis endotoxin; at the same time the protective effect of cortisone is also inhibited. 5-HT is said to protect against endotoxin and to augment the prophylactic effect of cortisol at otherwise ineffective dose levels.

There appears to be some relationship between the induction of resistance and the hepatic glycogen stores; the latter are depleted by endotoxin and increased by cortisone.

The toxicity of staphylococcal α-toxin was prevented by pretreatment with either cortisol or alloxan, whereas tolbutamide increased sensitivity to α-toxin. Again the protective action of cortisol was ascribed to its gluconeogenic effect which antagonizes the hypoglycemia induced by the α-toxin.

The amyloidosis produced by chronic treatment with endotoxins is also prevented by cortisone. The hepatic glycogen-depleting effect of endotoxin is inhibited by cortisone. Aminoglutethimide (an inhibitor of corticoid biosynthesis) increases susceptibility to endotoxin as well as the associated hepatic glycogen depletion but cortisone combats even the glycogen-depleting effect of this combined treatment. Similarly, methylprednisolone increases resistance to endotoxin even if the toxicity of the latter is enhanced by concurrent treatment with certain antitumor antibiotics.

The increased endotoxin susceptibility induced by zymosan is abolished by cortisone, perhaps as a result of an antagonistic interaction at the level of the RES. On the other hand, cortisone fails to alter the clearance of radioactive endotoxin from the blood or tissues.

Reserpine inhibits the protection against endotoxin that is induced in intact mice by cortisone. (The same is true in adrenalectomized but not in hypophysectomized rats. Apparently reserpine interferes with the cortisone effect only in the presence of the pituitary.)

Stress (cold) decreases the resistance of the mouse to endotoxin (perhaps owing to a "depletion of corticoid reserves") but cortisone protects even against the combined effect of stress + endotoxin.

Aldosterone exhibited no protective value against the lethal effect of Clostridium welchii α-toxin in the mouse, perhaps because corticoids are effective only against endotoxins, not against exotoxins.

Aldosterone admixture to tetanus toxin in vitro protects the mouse against the shock.

In **rabbits**, the febrile response to diphtheria endotoxin is diminished by 48 hrs pretreatment with repeated large doses of cortisone or ACTH; pretreatment during 24 hrs with smaller doses of these hormones exerts an opposite effect. This dependence upon dosage and timing may explain the discrepancies in earlier reports on the effect of glucocorticoids upon endotoxin reactions.

Cortisone also prevents the early reaction of prostration and death produced by endotoxin i.v. but in some rabbits pretreated for three days with this hormone, a generalized Shwartzman response-like renal cortical necrosis occurred within 24 hrs after endotoxin administration. When a single injection of cortisone was given 6 hrs before the endotoxin, prostration and death were prevented without subsequent development of renal cortical necrosis.

In the rabbit, endotoxin shock is associated with a release of hepatic lysosomal acid hydrolases. This effect is likewise prevented by glucocorticoids but not by DOC, presumably because only the former stabilize lysosomal membranes.

The topical response to intradermal or intraconjunctival injection of endotoxin is also inhibited by cortisone in rabbits, but this may well be merely a manifestation of the antiphlogistic effect.

Observations on **rats** gave contradictory results; whereas some authors state that this species can be protected against endotoxin shock by glucocorticoids, others reported negative results, apparently owing to differences in timing and dosage. However, there appears to be little doubt that, under optimal experimental conditions, glucocorticoids can protect the rat against endotoxin shock. DOC is devoid of this effect.

A dose of meningococcus toxin, well tolerated by normal nonpregnant rats, produces eclampsia-like hemorrhagic lesions in the liver of pregnant or cortisone pretreated animals. On the other hand, in rats kept on hyperlipemic diets, the induction of hepatic vein thromboses by S. typhosa endotoxin is inhibited by cortisol and prednisolone.

The ability of glucocorticoids to protect against various types of endotoxin may differ but there is no definite proof of this. The great variability of the results appears to depend not upon the kind of endotoxin used but upon other hitherto unidentified factors. We found considerable variation in the prophylactic effect of glucocorticoids even in experiments in which all controllable factors (steroid, endotoxin, timing, strain, age and sex of rats) were identical. In our laboratory, the most reliable results were obtained in rats heavily overdosed by cortisol, cortisone, triamcinolone, dexamethasone, betamethasone, prednisolone or cortisol 21-sodium succinate 1—4 days before the i.v. injection of a near lethal dose of E. coli endotoxin.

In **man**, endotoxin shock appears to be particularly well prevented by combined treatment with glucocorticoids and vasoactive agents, especially metaraminol.

In **summary**, it may be said that under suitable experimental conditions glucocorticoids undoubtedly offer considerable protection against shock produced by diverse endotoxins in various species. Since the clearance of radioactive E. coli endotoxin is not significantly altered by cortisone, it was concluded that the corticoids act "by their physical presence," presumably through a syntoxic effect upon the host's tissues. The protection is not merely a "nonspecific anti-stress effect" as no similar protection is offered under identical conditions against many other stressors.

There appears to be no clear-cut relationship between the glucocorticoid and anti-endotoxic activity of steroids. For example, prednisone and prednisolone are considerably more potent antiphlogistics than cortisol, yet they exhibit essentially the same anti-endotoxic effect as the latter. However, to some extent, the two pharmacologic actions tend to run parallel. The singularly strong anti-endotoxic effect of aldosterone is exhibited only in certain species and appears to depend mainly on the immediate effect of this hormone upon the circulation.

← *Adrenalectomy*

It has been known, even before the description of the stress syndrome, that adrenalectomized rats are particularly sensitive to bacterial endotoxins. Subsequently, the important role played by the adrenal in this connection has been confirmed in various species both by the decrease in endotoxin resistance induced by adrenalectomy and by the efficacy of corticoid substitution therapy.

In adrenalectomized mice, the lethal effect of Brucella endotoxin could be inhibited by cortisone, cortisol, fluorocortisol, and aldosterone, in decreasing order of activity. Indeed, the protective effect of corticoids against the lethal action of endotoxin in adrenalectomized rats has been recommended as the basis for the bioassay of these hormones, although it was recognized that the anti-endotoxin and antiphlogistic effects do not run strictly parallel.

In mice, endotoxin resistance is greatly decreased a few hours after adrenalectomy or hypophysectomy; however, while cortisone protects normal, adrenalectomized or hypophysectomized animals against high doses of endotoxin, chlorpromazine is effective only in the presence of both the adrenals and the pituitary.

It is particularly important to note that following total sympathetic blockade (adrenal demedullation combined with blockade or depletion of catecholamines), mortality from both histamine and endotoxin is as markedly increased in rats as by complete adrenalectomy. Pretreatment with epinephrine alone suffices to counteract the lethality of endotoxin and histamine after sympathetic blockade. Cortisone alone only partially corrects the sensitization by adrenalectomy, whereas cortisone + epinephrine offers complete protection. Presumably, sympathetic stimulation is the first line of defense against the vasomotor disturbance induced by endotoxin or histamine. By contrast, the lethal effects of other stressors (formalin, tourniquet shock) though likewise increased by adrenalectomy cannot be aggravated by mere sympathetic blockade. On the other hand, cortisone alone counteracts the toxicity of these latter stressors after adrenalectomy. Apparently, "formalin and tourniquet shock is initiated by a mechanism which differs from that elicited by histamine and endotoxin and does not primarily involve the sympathetic system."

← *Luteoids*

The resistance of the mouse to S. enteritidis endotoxin is allegedly diminished by progesterone, whereas in the cat, progesterone given conjointly with, or 30 min after, endotoxin stabilizes the blood pressure and prolongs survival. These observations require confirmation.

← Testoids

Comparatively few studies have been carried out concerning the effect of testoids upon endotoxin resistance and even these yielded contradictory results. It appears, however, that 4-chlorotestosterone may increase the resistance of the guinea pig to diphtheria endotoxin under certain experimental conditions.

← Folliculoids

Even before pure folliculoids were available, it had been reported by several investigators that follicular fluid of cow's ovaries or crude folliculoid extracts can protect the mouse against tetanus toxin or the guinea pig against diphtheria toxin.

In rats, considerable protection against the lethal effect of endotoxin was allegedly obtained by conjugated estrogens given 30—60 min before endotoxin.

This protection, which lasts only a few hours, has been ascribed to the liberation of corticoids by the adrenal cortex under the influence of folliculoids. However, this interpretation must take into account that under identical conditions, the folliculoids are even more active than cortisol. Furthermore, if folliculoids are administered 24 hrs before the endotoxin they actually reduce resistance to the latter and predispose to the production of hepatic necroses.

← Other Steroids

That there is no close parallelism between glucocorticoid and anti-endotoxic activity among steroids is well illustrated by the observation that 19-oxoprogesterone and aldosterone are highly effective in preventing endotoxin shock in the cat, although they have no glucocorticoid potency. In fact, 19-oxoprogesterone is also devoid of anti-inflammatory and salt-retaining properties.

Bacterial Toxins ← *cf. also Selye B 40,000/ 50, p. 68; E 5,986/66, pp. 14, 75, 81, 82; G 60,083/ 70, pp. 347, 354.*

← Corticoids.

CHICKEN

Smith & Thomas C 5,334/55: In chick embryos, the hemorrhages and death caused by inoculation of endotoxins into the chorio-allantoic membrane, were inhibited by cortisone or cortisol administered simultaneously in the same manner.

Smith & Thomas C 97,047/56: In chick embryos, the lethal effect of various endotoxins is prevented by cortisone, cortisol and F-COL but not by DOC, prednisone or cholesterol.

Dooley & Holtman C 84,689/59: In chicks, the hypoglycemia and fever produced by Salmonella pullorum endotoxin are inhibited by cortisone. However, both endotoxin and cortisone produce similar patterns of nonprotein nitrogen excretion.

Wyler et al. D 5,696/60: In the chick embryo, dexamethasone is 1000 times more active than cortisone in preventing fatal endotoxin poisoning. Aldosterone is about as active as cortisone, whereas prednisolone is somewhat more so. DOC is inactive. "Since aldosterone, like the anti-inflammatory steroids, influences the carbohydrate metabolism, this property is discussed as an underlying common denominator for the observed effect."

CAT

Bein & Jaques D 41,862/60: Cats can be protected against fatal endotoxin shock by aldosterone i.v. However, 3β,16α-dihydroxy-allopregnan-20-one exerts a competitively antagonistic effect on this protective action of aldosterone. To a lesser extent, cortisol and prednisolone also afford protection, whereas corticosterone and DOC are inactive. Aldosterone was 100 times more active than cortisol or prednisolone, but in contrast to the latter, it also offered protection in advanced stages of endotoxin poisoning. In guinea pigs, all the corticoids tested offered protection. Furthermore, pretreatment with aldosterone "protects mice against the lethal action of E. coli or S. typhimurium toxin as well as against that of hemorrhagic snake venoms (Vipera aspis, Crotalus adamenteus), but not against the neurotoxic venom of Naja tripudians. Prednisolone, which is effective to roughly the same degree in the mouse as in the rat, has to be administered in doses some 10—30 times larger, whereas hydrocortisone and cortexone [DOC] display no protective action, even in high dosage."

Bondoc et al. D69,984/62: In cats, aldosterone given 30 min after endotoxin prolonged survival, and frequently even prevented death. No such protection was observed when aldosterone was given 30 min before, or simultaneously with, endotoxin.

Hayasaka & Howard G10,112/63: In the cat, aldosterone administered 30 min after an otherwise fatal dose of E. coli endotoxin increased survival. On the other hand, when aldosterone was incubated with diphtheria toxin it did not prevent the development of a positive Schick test when the mixture was injected into non-immunized guinea pigs. Furthermore, aldosterone given to immunized guinea pigs did not prevent the antigen-antibody reaction upon subsequent injection of diphtheria toxin.

Hayasaka & Howard D31,136/63: "d-Aldosterone, when incubated for 30 minutes at 37º C. with the lipopolysaccharide derived from E. coli, appears to reduce the resulting toxicity of the endotoxin as measured by the survival rate in cats. The possibility that aldosterone combines with, or otherwise alters, the chemical structure of the endotoxin is suggested."

Hayasaka et al. E31,522/63: Aldosterone and, to a lesser extent, cortisol given 30 min after endotoxin, protect the cat against lethal shock. Earlier literature on the prevention of endotoxin shock by various corticoids is reviewed.

DOG

Ebert et al. E56,239/55: In dogs, cortisone failed to modify the effect of meningococcus toxin on the circulation. Apparently "adrenal insufficiency was not playing an important role in the production of circulatory failure following the administration of meningococcus toxin."

Lillehei & McLean D59,725/58; D84,873/59: In dogs, cortisol treatment increased survival from endotoxin shock.

Melby et al. C65,221/59: In dogs, E. coli endotoxin i.v. raises SGOT presumably as a consequence of cellular injury and this effect can be prevented by cortisol.

Vick C84,708/60: In dogs, survival from shock due to E. coli endotoxin is prolonged by cortisol, especially if given in combination with metaraminol.

Weil & Miller D97,273/60; Weil C91,305/60: In dogs, both metaraminol and prednisolone increased survival after treatment with E. coli entotoxin. The best results were obtained by combined treatment with prednisolone and metaraminol.

Longerbeam & Lillehei D3,868/61: In dogs, pretreatment with cortisone did not appreciably alter the disturbances in intestinal hemodynamics caused by endotoxin shock. However dibenzyline did ameliorate them, and catecholamines aggravated them. Apparently "the protective action of cortisone is not mediated through a hemodynamic mechanism."

Spink & Vick C98,717/61: In the dog, endotoxin shock could not be prevented by cortisol unless metaraminol was simultaneously administered.

Vick & Spink D43,929/61: Canine endotoxin shock is effectively combated by cortisol + a pressor drug. Addition of hydralazine to this combination further augments its beneficial effect.

Smith et al. D18,862/64: Large doses of cortisol improved blood pressure, cardiac output and survival in canine endotoxin shock.

Vick F48,509/65: In the dog, cortisol and/or isoproterenol cause temporary improvement in endotoxin shock but no increase in survival time.

Vick et al. F58,531/65: In dogs, survival from endotoxin shock was not significantly altered by cortisol.

Hinshaw et al. F65,403/66: Observations on perfused organ preparations of dogs "suggest that prednisolone exerts significant vascular effects on both hepatic and forelimb vascular beds in endotoxin shock."

Thomas & Brockman F 82,789/66: In dogs, survival in lethal endotoxin shock was prolonged by pretreatment with methylprednisolone or cortisol but post treatment with the same glucocorticoids hastened death. Aldosterone was without effect. "These studies do not support the use of steroids in endotoxin shock."

Lillehei et al. G 45,335/67: Cortisol given 30—60 min after endotoxin greatly reduces mortality from shock in the dog.

Loggie et al. F 99,839/68: In 6—9 day old beagles, cortisol sodium succinate i.v. one hour before i.v. injection of lethal doses of E. coli endotoxin increased the survival rate, whereas given immediately after endotoxin, the glucocorticoid offered no protection.

Motsay et al. H 32,852/70: In dogs, massive doses of glucocorticoids (e.g., methylprednisolone) can offer protection against circulatory shock produced by overdosage with epinephrine or endotoxin. The prophylactic effect is ascribed primarily to a protection of the microcirculation.

GUINEA PIG

Scott et al. 15,446/33: The resistance of intact guinea pigs to diphtheria toxin or that of rats to Trypanosoma equiperdum or mice to infection with Pneumococcus Type I was not influenced by pretreatment with large amounts of a life-maintaining adrenocortical extract ("cortin"). It does not appear to be possible to raise resistance above normal in intact animals but there is considerable evidence to show that various types of intoxication and infection cause structural damage to the adrenal and interfere with its function.

Zwemer & Jungeblut 53,287/35: Pretreatment with an adrenocortical extract containing the "life maintaining principle" protects guinea pigs against the cutaneous necrosis elicited by i.c. injection of diphtheria toxin. The lethal effect of s.c. injected diphtheria toxin in guinea pigs is diminished upon incubation with the adrenocortical extract in vitro at room temperature.

Berger 95,075/37: Contrary to earlier claims, it has not been possible to combat diphtheria intoxication in guinea pigs by adrenocortical extracts in combination with vitamin C.

Schmidt 94,670/37: In guinea pigs, infection with diphtheria bacilli or intoxication with diphtheria toxin can be combated by adrenocortical extracts in combination with vitamin C.

de Marchi A 30,837/38: In guinea pigs, adrenocortical extract offers partial protection against diphtheria toxin.

Murray & Branham B 65,414/51: Neither ACTH nor cortisone improved the resistance of guinea pigs to diphtheria toxin or of mice to Shiga and meningococcus toxin.

Tonutti B 69,136/52: Although cortisone normalizes the low diphtheria toxin resistance of hypophysectomized guinea pigs, it does not raise the resistance of intact guinea pigs above normal.

Brainerd & Scaparone B 87,957/53: In guinea pigs, cortisone failed to influence the lethal effect of diphtheria toxin or to prevent its neutralization by diphtheria antitoxin in vivo.

Boquet et al. E 52,759/56: In guinea pigs, cortisone may either increase or decrease resistance to typhoid endotoxin, depending upon dosage.

Nola et al. C 33,308/57: In guinea pigs, cortisone pretreatment failed to protect against inoculation of live diphtheria organisms or diphtheria toxin.

Farrar & Magnani F 6,647/64: Homogenates of normal guinea pig liver rapidly detoxify endotoxins in vitro, whereas homogenates of livers damaged by CCl_4 do not. Adrenalectomized animals are notoriously sensitive to endotoxin, but pretreatment of guinea pigs with testosterone or cortisone does not influence their resistance to toxic doses of endotoxin and hence the detoxifying ability of the liver does not appear to be under steroid control.

Batliwalla & Deshpande G 43,844/66: In guinea pigs, cortisone can protect the myocardium, liver, kidney and suprarenals against damage induced by diphtheria toxin.

Kovács & Görög H 2,570/68: Salmonella typhosa endotoxin i.v. induces a bronchoconstriction in guinea pigs; this can be prevented both by antihistamine and by prednisolone.

MONKEY

Spink et al. D 61,007/63: In Mangabey monkeys, E. coli endotoxin produces hypotension, oliguria, hyperkalemia and death. These effects are counteracted by aldosterone, especially in combination with angiotensin.

Vick et al. E 20,146/63: In the dog and monkey, cortisol helped to maintain the arterial blood pressure during endotoxin shock.

MOUSE

Singer B316/40: Mice are protected against Clostridium welchii toxin i.p. by pretreatment with DOC s.c.

Beck & Voloshin B58,271/50: In mice, tolerance for Serratia marcescens tumor-necrotizing polysaccharide is increased by cortisone.

Jackson & Smadel B77,408/51: In intact mice, neither ACTH nor cortisone pretreatment raised resistance to the toxins of R. tsutsugamushi, R. prowazeki or S. typhosa.

Jackson & Smadel E52,720/51: Intact mice pretreated with cortisone or ACTH "were given lethal amounts of the toxins of R. tsutsugamushi, R. prowazeki, or S. typhosa. Such animals were as susceptible to the toxins as normal controls. Neither hormone had any therapeutic effect in mice infected with R. tsutsugamushi. Furthermore, treated and untreated mice in a terminal phase of infection with R. tsutsugamushi were equally susceptible to the toxin of this rickettsia when injected intravenously. In the current experiments the adrenal cortex of normal or infected animals apparently contributed as effectively as possible in the host's response to rickettsial or bacterial toxins and further stimulation was without advantage."

Chédid et al. B91,161/52: DOC does not alter the resistance of the intact or adrenalectomized mouse to S. enteritidis endotoxin but progesterone diminishes it considerably.

Boyer & Chédid C624/53: Cortisone protects the mouse against lipopolysaccharide antigens or infections with germs possessing such antigens, such as S. typhi, Neisseria meningitidis. Cortisone does not protect against the infection with E. coli, Shigella dysenteria, although they also possess lipopolysaccharide antigens, nor against Staphylococcus aureus, Streptococcus pyogenes, Pseudomonas aeruginosa, Klebsiella pneumoniae, which do not possess such antigens. Cortisone is also ineffective against the exotoxins of diphtheria, tetanus or dysentery organisms.

Greene et al. B94,257/53: In mice, cortisone or DOC did not significantly affect the response to tetanus toxin or tetanus spore infection.

Maral C17,604/53: Cortisone is highly effective in combating endotoxin poisoning in the mouse but comparatively less potent against tetanus toxin. It has no effect upon diphtheria intoxication in the guinea pig or Cl. histolyticum-toxin poisoning in mice. The effect of cortisone is compared with that of chlorpromazine in all these tests.

Parker et al. D77,476/53: In mice and guinea pigs, cortisone failed to alter the effect of diphtheria tetanus and botulinum toxins.

Chédid C1,930/54: Pertussis vaccine abolishes the ability of cortisone to protect the mouse against endotoxin. The protective effect of chlorpromazine is also abolished.

Chédid C622/54: Pertussis vaccine sensitizes the intact mouse both to histamine and to typhoid endotoxin. Under these conditions, both promethazine and cortisone protect the animals against fatal doses of histamine but not against endotoxin. In adrenalectomized mice, cortisone does protect against endotoxin.

Geller et al. B98,147/54: Cortisone offers definite protection in mice given otherwise lethal doses of Escherichia intermedium endotoxin. In order to be effective, cortisone must be injected simultaneously with or before the endotoxin. Complicating transient bacteremia, presumably of intestinal origin, can be suppressed by antibiotics. Interference by antibiotics with cortisone protection was demonstrable only when the antibiotics were given after cortisone.

Spink & Anderson B95,168/54: Cortisone protects mice against the lethal effect of Brucella endotoxin.

Gallut C14,519/55: Mice can be protected against fatal intoxication with cholera Vibrio endotoxin by cortisone or ACTH but the degree of protection depends upon dosage and timing.

Barbazza C13,021/55: Pretreatment with cortisol protects the mouse against fatal intoxication with typhoid endotoxin. [In the Italian text, the animals are described as "topi" which may mean rat or mouse; they are said to have weighed 20 g which would suggest mice, but in the foreign language summaries, they are consistently referred to as rats, which makes interpretation difficult (H.S.).]

Biozzi et al. E22,483/55: In mice multiple i.v. injections of killed S. typhi or of its endotoxin greatly stimulate the phagocytic activity of the RES. Cortisone inhibits this effect, "in this way it impairs the defences of the animal against invading bacteria."

Chedid & Boyer C10,098/55: In mice, resistance to S. enteritidis endotoxin is greatly diminished during pregnancy and the protective effect of cortisone is also inhibited.

Moll D38,913/56: "The resistance of weaned mice to the effects of Escherichia coli and Salmonella typhimurium endotoxins was increased during the administration of cortisone and markedly decreased subsequent to its abrupt withdrawal."

Abernathy & Spink G68,366/57: "Mice protected against an initial lethal challenge with brucella endotoxin by treatment with cortisone acetate, 9-alpha-fluorohydrocortisone acetate, or chlorpromazine develop resistance to subsequent challenge to endotoxin."

Gordon & Lipton C33,200/57: Certain strains of mice can be protected against endotoxin shock by 5-HT. While cortisol has no effect in itself, it increases the prophylactic action of 5-HT.

Tauber & Garson C51,966/58: "Cortisone significantly protected mice from the lethality of Neisseria gonorrhoeae endotoxin."

Benaceraff et al. C67,852/59: Zymosan renders mice highly susceptible to lethal effects of endotoxin at a time when the RES is greatly stimulated but this sensitization is abolished by cortisone.

Berry et al. C73,198/59: Mice of different strains were protected by cortisone against the lethal effect of various bacterial endotoxins. The effect may be related in some way to the hepatic glycogen stores which are depleted by endotoxin and increased by cortisone.

Ribble et al. C92,576/59: "Doses of cortisone that prevented death did not materially influence the rate of removal or organ distribution of lethal amounts of radioactive E. coli endotoxin in normal mice." Cortisone did not alter the resistance of mice made tolerant to E. coli endotoxin or their ability to clear radioactive endotoxin from the blood and tissue.

Gordon & Lipton C94,649/60: 5-HT reduces endotoxin mortality in mice. This effect is greater in females than in males and is potentiated by cortisol. Thyroxine aggravates the toxicity of endotoxin.

Chedid & Parant D6,761/61: The protection of intact mice against endotoxin shock by cortisone is inhibited by reserpine. The same is true in adrenalectomized rats, whereas after hypophysectomy cortisone is even more effective in offering protection against endotoxin but reserpine no longer blocks this effect. Apparently the drug interferes with the cortisone effect only in the presence of the pituitary.

Liashenko D51,368/60; D50,402/61: A single dose of cortisone can protect mice from intoxication with dysenteric endotoxin. The hormone also offers resistance against infections with Bacterium dysenteriae Flexneri and Staphylococcus aureus and increases the therapeutic efficacy of levomycetin.

Berry & Smythe E28,203/63: Review of the literature and personal observations on the protection of intact mice by cortisone against fatal endotoxin poisoning. Cortisone increases hepatic TPO activity and both nicotinamide and DPN (compounds involved in TPO induction), hence the protective effect of cortisone may be mediated through these compounds.

Previte & Berry E89,101/63: In mice, exposure to the stress of cold decreases resistance to endotoxin perhaps because of an initial "depletion of corticoid reserves." Cortisone protects even against the combined effect of endotoxin + cold.

Turner & Berry E36,911/63: In mice, various bacterial endotoxins prolong gastric emptying time while cortisone reduces this inhibition.

Berry F24,603/64: The glyconeogenetic effect of a single cortisone injection is about the same in mice whether they are kept in the cold or at room temperature. However, endotoxin causes a much more pronounced fall in hepatic glycogen in the cold and this effect cannot be readily prevented by cortisone. In cold-exposed mice, cortisone also fails to induce an increase in hepatic TPO.

Berry G68,858/64: In mice, injection of endotoxin causes a drop in TPO as well as in oxidized pyridine nucleotides in the liver, presumably DPN and TPN. (This is not unexpected since TPO catalyzes a key reaction in the conversion of tryptophan into nicotinamide, a portion of the pyridine nucleotide molecule.) Possibly, the decline in DPN and/or TPN "is one of the significant metabolic lesions avoided or corrected by the administration of corticoid to the endotoxin-poisoned animals. This suggestion is supported by the finding that either nicotinamide or DPN, when given at the same time as endotoxin, protects against lethality to about the same extent as cortisone."

Berry & Smythe D19,640/64: In mice, S. typhimurium endotoxin lowers hepatic TPO, whereas cortisone raises it; when the two are administered simultaneously a normal enzyme level is maintained and mortality greatly diminished. If cortisone injection is delayed for a few hours it fails to induce TPO or protect against the lethal effect of endotoxin. Inhibitors of enzyme protein synthesis (actinomycin D, ethionine, 2-thiouracil and 8-azaguanine) potentiate the lethal effect of endotoxin and abolish cortisone protection.

Chedid et al. E 8,476/64: In mice, moderate doses of cortisone increase resistance to endotoxin without accelerating its blood clearance and detoxication. Heavy prolonged cortisone overdosage increases susceptibility to endotoxin.

Kostrubiak & Howard G 57,804/64: In mice, aldosterone exhibited no protective value against the lethal effect of Clostridium welchi alpha-toxin. Apparently corticoids are effective only against endotoxins, not against exotoxins.

Kostrubiak & Howard F 43,646/65: Aldosterone, admixture to tetanus toxin, protects the mouse against shock.

Bóbr & Ptak G 47,053/66: Four-day pretreatment with cortisol i.p. increases the resistance of intact male or female mice to fatal doses of staphylococcal α-toxin i.v. Since alloxan had a similar effect, whereas tolbutamide increased sensitivity to α-toxin, the protective action of cortisol is ascribed to its gluconeogenic effect. "It should also be noted that α-toxin in rabbits produces disturbances in carbohydrate metabolism, leading to hypoglycaemia. Present findings of hypoglycaemia following the α-toxin inoculation in mice confirm these earlier observations."

Berry et al. H 2,124/68: Studies on the influence of hypoxia, glucocorticoids and endotoxin on hepatic enzyme induction and survival in mice. "Endotoxin inhibited the induction of tryptophan oxygenase, prevented the increase in liver glycogen, induced the transaminase, and increased the lethality of simulated altitude. Cortisone increased survival at all altitudes except the highest. These observations emphasize the importance of these metabolic adjustments for the survival of animals subjected to hypoxic stress."

Laufer et al. H 13,434/68: The amyloidosis produced in mice by tubercle bacilli in Freund's adjuvant, or by mixtures of endotoxins can be prevented by pretreatment with cortisone, but once the amyloid is deposited cortisone had no effect.

Agarwal & Berry G 65,866/69: In mice, cortisone induced liver TPO and increased liver pyridine nucleotide levels after pretreatment with zymozan or glucan. It also protected such animals against the lethal effects of endotoxin. The observations are "consistent with the view that a cause and effect relationship may exist between hormone induction of selected hepatic enzymes and survival against stress."

Jeffries H 19,361/69: In mice the liver glycogen-depleting effect of endotoxin is inhibited by cortisone. Aminoglutethimide (an inhibitor of corticosteroid synthesis) increases the susceptibility to endotoxin and the associated liver glycogen depletion but cortisone is able to combat even the glycogen depleting effect of this combination treatment to some extent.

Rose & Bradley H 19,375/69: In mice, endotoxin resistance is greatly decreased by concurrent treatment with the antitumor antibiotics, sparsomycin or pactamycin. Even this enhanced toxicity is inhibited by methylprednisolone.

Rose & Bradley G 79,576/70: In mice, endotoxin resistance is greatly decreased by simultaneous treatment with sparsomycin. Aldosterone fails to protect against the toxicity of the combined treatment.

RABBIT

Katabuchi 44,803/29: In rabbits injected with typhoid toxin, the production of an antiserum is enhanced by adrenocortical extract but to a lesser degree also by extracts of various other organs.

Duffy Jr. & Morgan B 65,399/51: In rabbits, the febrile response to Shigella dysenteriae endotoxin is diminished following pretreatment during 48 hrs with repeated large doses of ACTH or cortisone. Pretreatment during 24 hrs with smaller doses of these hormones exerts an opposite effect. "This appears to account for the discrepancies in the results previously reported."

Thomas et al. B 57,977/51: The topical response to an intradermal or intraconjunctival injection of endotoxin is inhibited by cortisone in rabbits. On the other hand, endotoxin i.v. causes bilateral cortical necroses in rabbits and hamsters pretreated with cortisone.

Bennett Jr. & Beeson B 95,351/53: In rabbits, the febrile response to a single injection of various endotoxins may be decreased, increased or unchanged by treatment with ACTH or cortisone. Acquired resistance to pyrogen fever is abolished by Thorotrast but not by cortisone although both these agents prevent the Shwartzman reaction.

Thomas B 92,009/54: In mature rabbits, the early lethal effects of endotoxin can be prevented by cortisone pretreatment, although renal necrosis does occur.

Thomas & Smith E23,202/54: In rabbits, cortisone prevented the early reaction of prostration and death produced by endotoxin i.v. but in some of the rabbits pretreated for three days bilateral renal cortical necrosis occurred within 24 hrs after endotoxin. When a single injection of cortisone was given 6 hrs before endotoxin, protection against prostration and death was demonstrable without subsequent development of renal cortical necrosis. The early lethal reaction caused by small amounts of endotoxin following colloidal iron saccharate i.v. was prevented by cortisone.

Janoff et al. D35,553/62: Studies on the hepatic lysosomal enzymes of rats and rabbits after traumatic or endotoxin shock, adrenalectomy, or treatment with cortisone suggested that "a) disruption of lysosomes and release of their contained enzymes in free, active form may occur in liver and intestine of shocked animals. b) The activation of lysosomal hydrolases within cells and their release into the circulation may play an important role in exacerbating tissue injury and accelerating the development of irreversibility during shock. c) The increased stability of lysosomes of tolerant and of cortisone-treated animals may constitute an important component of the resistance of these animals to shock."

Weissmann & Thomas D23,630/62: Following endotoxin treatment in vivo, the hepatic lysosomes of the rabbit release their enzymes readily upon ultraviolet irradiation. This increased lability is in turn prevented by pretreatment of the animals with cortisone for three days before endotoxin administration. Apparently "one action of endotoxin is to release acid hydrolases from particulate form within cells, and that glucocorticoids serve to stabilize such particles against injury by several agents."

Weissmann & Thomas D35,555/62: In rabbits, endotoxin shock is associated with the release of hepatic lysosomal acid hydrolases (β-glucuronidase, cathepsin). This effect is prevented by glucocorticoids, but not by DOC. "Thus, glucocorticoids, in a variety of experimental situations, appear to decrease the liberation of potentially harmful enzymes from lysosomes, and may in fact function physiologically to stabilize the boundaries of these subcellular particles."

Gonzalez et al. F88,028/67: In rabbits, neither corticosterone nor cortisol offered any significant protection against shock produced by E. coli endotoxin.

Dieckhoff et al. H1,991/68: Prednisolone diminished endotoxin shock and prolonged survival following production of a generalized Shwartzman-Sanarelli phenomenon in the rabbit, without significantly altering the characteristic vascular lesions.

Fine et al. G53,608/68: General review on the beneficial effect of treatment with various glucocorticoids upon hemorrhagic, endotoxin and traumatic shock in rabbits.

RAT

Ingle B42,751/47: Neither adrenocortical extract nor DOC protects the rat against diphtheria toxin.

Jasmin B80,596/53: A dose of meningococcus toxin i.v. well tolerated by nonpregnant rats produces eclampsia-like hemorrhagic lesions in the liver of pregnant or cortisone pretreated animals.

Ganley et al. C7,489/55: Rats cannot be protected against the lethal effect of Cl. perfringens toxin by ACTH, adrenocortical extract, cortisol, cortisone or DOC.

Levitin et al. C26,683/56: Cortisol, corticosterone, and cortisone, as well as ACTH protect the rat against endotoxin, whereas DOC does not.

Weil et al. F4,907/64; Weil & Allen F14,091/64: Experiments on the protection by various glucocorticoids against endotoxin shock in the mouse and rat. "The demonstration of significantly higher survival rates with prednisolone, and especially with dexamethasone in pharmacological doses indicates that a drug action rather than hormonal replacement accounts for therapeutic effectiveness."

Renaud et al. F74,449/66: In rats, kept on a hyperlipemic diet, ACTH, cortisol or prednisolone protected against the production of shock and hepatic vein thromboses by S. typhosa lipopolysaccharide. DOC increased mortality and did not protect these thromboses.

Nolan & Ali G55,490/68; Nolan et al. H5,204/68: In rats, pretreatment with cortisol, corticosterone, ACTH, Thorotrast (to block the RES) or endotoxin 24 hrs before endotoxin challenge did not increase the mortality rate.

Renaud & Latour F99,806/68: In rats kept on a hyperlipemic diet, the production of phlebothromboses by S. typhosa lipopolysaccharide is inhibited by triamcinolone.

Selye PROT. 32990: In rats, pretreatment for 4 days, or even for only one day, with large doses of cortisol, cortisone, triamcinolone, dexamethasone, betamethasone, prednisolone,

Table 120. *Protection by glucocorticoids against endotoxin poisoning*

Treatment[a]	Prostration[c] (Positive/Total) Pretreatment 1 day ff.	3 days ff.	Mortality[c] (Dead/Total) Pretreatment 1 day ff.	3 days ff.
None	5/5	2/10	5/5	9/10
Cortisol-Ac 10 mg	0/5 ***	0/10 NS	2/5 NS	2/10 ***
Cortisone-Ac 10 mg	0/5 ***	0/10 NS	2/5 NS	2/10 ***
Triamcinolone 10 mg	0/5 ***	0/10 NS	0/5 ***	1/10 ***
Dexamethasone-Ac 2 mg	0/5 ***	0/10 NS	1/5 *	0/10 ***
Betamethasone-Ac 2 mg	0/5 ***	0/10 NS	0/5 ***	0/10 ***
Prednisolone-Ac 10 mg	0/5 ***	0/10 NS	0/5 ***	0/10 ***
Prednisone-Ac 10 mg	0/5 ***	0/10 NS	1/5 *	1/10 ***
Solu-Cortef 10 mg[b]	—	0/10 NS	—	0/10 ***

[a] The rats (100 g ♀) of all groups received E. coli 026:B6 1.5 mg per 100 g body weight, in 1 ml water, i.v. once, 4th day. The glucocorticoids were given at the doses indicated in 1 ml water, p.o. x2/day, 1st day or 3rd day ff. and on the 4th day 1 hr before E.coli injection, except Solu-Cortef (cortisol-21-Na-succinate).

[b] Solu-Cortef was given in 1 ml water, i.v. once, 30 min before E.coli endotoxin administration.

[c] The severity of the prostration was estimated for the 1 day pretreated groups: 3 hrs after endotoxin injection and for the 3 days pretreated groups: 2 hrs later. Mortality was listed 24 hrs later (Fisher & Yates test).

For further details on technique of tabulation *cf.* p. VIII.

prednisone or Solu-Cortef offered considerable protection against the lethal effects of E. coli endotoxin i.v. *cf.* Table 120

Selye PROT. 41632: In rats, the inhibition of E. coli toxicity by cortisol is abolished following pretreatment with dactinomycin or cycloheximide at dose levels at which these antagonists are not demonstrably toxic by themselves. On the other hand, metyrapone, puromycin aminonucleoside (PAN) and ethionin do not block cortisol protection; indeed, metyrapone may slightly enhance it *cf.* Table 121.

SHEEP

Halmagyi et al. D68,121/63: In sheep, the cardiovascular manifestations of endotoxin shock could not be prevented by 0.2 mg/kg of d-aldosterone i.v. 30 min before the injection of E. coli endotoxin.

MAN

Abernathy & Spink C48,635/58: In man, cortisol or ACTH suppressed or ameliorated reactions to Brucella endotoxin.

Weil et al. G68,706/62: In man, endotoxin shock is very effectively prevented by combined treatment with glucocorticoids (cortisol, prednisone, dexamethasone) and vasoactive agents (especially metaraminol).

Cherry G74,846/70: Review of the use of glucocorticoids in the treatment of endotoxin shock in man.

VARIA

Chedid & Boyer C17,612/55: Review of the literature and personal observations on the effect of cortisone upon resistance to bacterial toxins in comparison with similar effects of chlorpromazine.

Weil & Spink D96,274/57: Review on the prevention of endotoxin shock by glucocorticoids in various species.

Kass D35,079/60: "In only two situations have adrenocortical hormones been shown to be protective to the host: the replacement of hormone in hypoadrenalism, and the protective action against the lethal toxicity of bacterial lipopolysaccharides." There appears to be no clear-cut relationship between the glucocorticoid and anti-endotoxic activity of steroids, as judged by Table 122.

Weil G68,214/61: Review of the literature on the prevention of endotoxin shock by glucocorticoids in the dog, mouse and rat. Personal observations on mice demonstrated the efficacy of cortisol, prednisolone, dexamethasone and methylprednisolone in increasing survival after E. coli endotoxin i.p.

Table 121. *Effect of dactinomycin, metyrapone, puromycin aminonucleoside and cycloheximide upon the prevention of endotoxin shock by cortisol*

Group	Treatment[a]	Dyskinesia[b] (Positive/Total)	Mortality[b] (Dead/Total)
1	E. coli	20/21	20/21
2	Cortisol ac. + E. coli	9/20 ***	7/20 ***
3	Dactinomycin	0/10	0/10
4	Dactinomycin + E. coli	10/10	10/10
5	Cortisol ac. + Dactinomycin + E. coli	10/10 ***	10/10 ***
6	Metyrapone	0/10	0/10
7	Metyrapone + E. coli	10/10	10/10
8	Cortisol ac. + Metyrapone + E. coli	0/10 *	0/10 *
9	PAN	0/10	0/10
10	PAN + E. coli	9/10	9/10
11	Cortisol ac. + PAN + E. coli	3/10 NS	3/10 NS
12	Cycloheximide	0/10	0/10
13	Cycloheximide + E. coli	10/10	10/10
14	Cortisol ac. + Cycloheximide + E. coli	10/10 ***	10/10 ***
15	Ethionin	0/10	0/10
16	Ethionin + E. coli	10/10	10/10
17	Cortisol ac. + Ethionin + E. coli	2/10 NS	2/10 NS

[a] The rats received E. coli 0.26: B6 (1.5 mg in 1 ml water, i.v.) at 0 hr after cortisol acetate (2 mg in 1 ml water, p.o.) was administered at −1 hr. In addition, at −30 min, certain groups received dactinomycin (70 µg in 0.2 ml water, i.v.), metyrapone (12 mg in 0.1 ml corn oil, i.p.) puromycin aminonucleoside "PAN" (10 mg in 0.2 ml water, i.p.), cycloheximide (25 µg in 0.2 ml NaCl, s.c.), or ethionin (50 mg in 2 ml 0.9% NaCl, i.p.).

[b] Dyskinesia was estimated 24 hrs after injection of E. coli, and mortality listed 24 hrs later. For statistical purposes, group 2 was compared with group 1, and groups 5, 8, 11, 14, and 17 with group 2 ("Exact Probality Test"). For further details on technique of tabulation *cf*. p. VIII.

Weil & Allen D7,883/61: A review on the protection offered by various glucocorticoids against endotoxin shock in the mouse, rat and dog. The rate of removal and organ distribution of radioactive E. coli endotoxin is unaltered by cortisone, and the steroids are assumed to protect the tissues "by their physical presence." This view is allegedly supported by the suppression of increased serum transaminase by hydrocortisone. In any event, the corticoids do not protect in a "nonspecific manner" against injuries, since prednisolone phosphate i.p. protects against the lethal effect of endotoxin but not against that of mecamylamine, chlorpromazine, metaraminol or dibenzyline as judged by experiments on intact mice. The protective effect of glucocorticoids administered i.p. at 15 min and again at 4 hrs after E. coli endotoxin i.p. decreases in the following order: cortisol sodium succinate, prednisolone phosphate, methylprednisolone sodium succinate, and dexamethasone phosphate.

Table 122. *Relative anti-inflammatory (glucocorticoid) and anti-endotoxic effects of steroids*

Steroid	Anti-inflammatory	Anti-endotoxic
Cortisol	1.0	1.0
Corticosterone	0.5	0.7
Prednisone	3.5	0.7
Prednisolone	4.0	1.3
6-α-Methylprednisone	5.0	30.0
11-Deoxycorticosterone	<0.1	0.1
11-α-OH-progesterone	<0.1	0.03

Spink D39,028/62: Review on the protective effect of glucocorticoids in endotoxin shock. "Although endotoxin shock does not appear to be associated with adrenal insufficiency except on rare occasions, this does not preclude the possibility that under severe stress physiologic amounts of adrenal hormone are inadequate, and pharmacologic doses of exogenous adrenal steroid are desirable." Protection has also been obtained with aldosterone.

Lillehei et al. E31,273/63: Review on the beneficial action of cortisol in canine endotoxin shock.

Fukui E8,467/64: Review of the literature on the increased endotoxin resistance induced by cortisone with a discussion of possible underlying mechanisms.

Janoff & Kaley E8,484/64: Review of the literature supporting the concept that endotoxins act by disruption of lysosomes with release of their contained enzymes and that cortisone protects against the resulting shock by stabilizing lysosomal membranes.

Sambhi et al. G68,985/64: Review on the action of glucocorticoids and aldosterone in traumatic and endotoxin shock in animals and men.

Weissmann & Thomas E8,482/64: Review of the literature showing that cortisone, unlike DOC, stabilizes hepatic lysosomal membranes against the permeability-increasing effect of endotoxin.

Janoski et al. E7,896/68 (p. 282): Review suggesting that many of the actions of glucocorticoids particularly the inhibition of ultraviolet ray injury, vitamin-A overdosage and endotoxin shock are due to the stabilization of lysosomal membranes which prevents the escape of toxic lysosomal enzymes.

← **Adrenalectomy.** *Belding & Wyman 3,915/26:* Adrenalectomized rats are particularly sensitive to diphtheria toxin.

Halberg et al. G68,353/56: Adrenalectomized mice are protected against the hypothermic and lethal effects of Brucella endotoxin by cortisone, cortisol, fluorocortisol and aldosterone in decreasing order of activity.

Brooke et al. D11,627/61: In adrenalectomized rats protection against the lethal effects of endotoxin can serve as the basis of an assay of corticoids. However, this effect does not parallel antiphlogistic activity.

Yokoi et al. D8,839/61: In rabbits, a biphasic fever pattern is elicited by Sh. flexneri type 6 pyrogen. The biphasic nature of the response was maintained after thyroidectomy but largely abolished by adrenal demedullation.

Higginbotham D21,395/62: In mice, resistance to 5-HT, endotoxin and anaphylactic shock is markedly decreased by adrenalectomy. Cortisol readily restored resistance to 5-HT but was less effective with regard to endotoxin and anaphylactic shock. Resistance to histamine and histamine releasers is less markedly diminished by adrenalectomy in the mouse, and large doses of cortisol are required to induce a measurable increase in resistance to histamine.

Parant D82,116/62: In mice, resistance to endotoxin is greatly decreased a few hours after adrenalectomy or hypophysectomy. Cortisone protects normal, adrenalectomized, and hypophysectomized animals against high doses of endotoxin, whereas chlorpromazine is effective only in the presence of both the adrenals and the pituitary. ACTH also protects the hypophysectomized mouse, but only if slow absorption is assured.

Krawczak & Brodie H25,296/70: In rats, complete blockade of sympathetic function can be achieved by demedullation combined with reserpine-like agents (depleting catecholamine stores), bretylium-like agents (preventing nerve impulse from releasing catecholamines) or ganglioplegics. Following such total sympathetic blockade, mortality from histamine or endotoxin is as markedly increased as by adrenalectomy. Pretreatment with epinephrine alone counteracts the increased lethality of endotoxin and histamine after sympathetic blockade. Cortisone pretreatment only partially corrects the sensitization by adrenalectomy, whereas cortisone + epinephrine offers complete protection against these agents. Presumably, sympathetic stimulation is "the first line of defense against the vasomotor disturbance elicited by endotoxin and histamine." The lethal effect of formalin or tourniquet shock is likewise greatly increased by adrenalectomy but, in contrast to that of endotoxin and histamine, it cannot be increased by sympathetic blockade. Furthermore, cortisone alone counteracts the toxicity of these stressors in adrenalectomized rats. Apparently "formalin and tourniquet shock is initiated by a mechanism which differs from that elicited by histamine and endotoxin and does not primarily involve the sympathetic system."

← **Luteoids.** *Chedid et al. B91,161/52:* DOC does not alter the resistance of the intact or adrenalectomized mouse to S. enteritidis endotoxin but progesterone diminishes it considerably.

Silk F95,477/67: In the cat, progesterone given with—or 30 min after—endotoxin stabilizes the blood pressure and markedly prolongs survival.

← **Testoids.** *Dutz et al. C 31,646/56:* In rats, gonadectomy did not significantly change the course of Masugi nephritis, whereas a folliculoid preparation (Östrasid) and testosterone ameliorated it. STH considerably aggravated the glomerular lesions and the hypertension.

Herrmann D 34,026/62: In guinea pigs, following interruption of corticoid administration, the adrenocortical hypofunction and atrophy as well as the irresponsiveness to the production of adrenocortical necrosis by diphtheria toxin reappear much more rapidly if the animals are simultaneously treated with testosterone.

Herrmann & Winkler D 20,550/62: In guinea pigs, methandrostenolone accelerates the restitution of the adrenal cortex after interruption of cortisone therapy as judged by the more rapid reappearance of sensitivity to diphtheria toxin and histologic criteria.

Farrar & Magnani F 6,647/64: Homogenates of normal guinea pig liver rapidly detoxify endotoxins in vitro, whereas homogenates of livers damaged by CCl_4 do not. Adrenalectomized animals are notoriously sensitive to endotoxin but pretreatment of guinea pigs with testosterone or cortisone does not influence their resistance to toxic doses of endotoxin and hence the detoxifying ability of the liver does not appear to be under steroid control.

Terragna et al. E 66,111/66: In guinea pigs, pretreatment with 4-chlorotestosterone increases resistance to diphtheria toxin.

Terragna et al. F 86,979/66: In the mouse, 4-chlorotestosterone administered simultaneously or soon after E. coli endotoxin protects against the lethal action of the latter but the anabolic steroid fails to protect if administered before the endotoxin. [The statistical significance of these data has not been analyzed (H.S.).]

Evangelista et al. H 16,824/69: Neither ACTH nor stanozolol gave any significant protection against endotoxin shock in dogs.

← **Folliculoids.** *Imamura 14,567/29:* In mice, resistance to tetanus toxin is increased by the injection of follicular fluid from cows' ovaries.

Crainiceanu & Copelman 67,918/35: A folliculoid extract "folliculine" prolongs the survival of guinea pigs which have received fatal doses of diphtheria toxin. [Brief abstract containing no details (H.S.).]

Herrmann & Winkler D 27,922/62: In guinea pigs, the adrenocortical atrophy and hypofunction produced by chronic cortisone treatment is prevented by simultaneous administration of estradiol. The responsiveness of the adrenal cortex to the induction of hemorrhagic necrosis by diphtheria toxin returns much more rapidly after interruption of cortisone treatment if estradiol is simultaneously administered.

Nolan F 75,232/67: In rats, a significant protection against the fatal effect of endotoxin was obtained by giving "equine estrogens" 30—60 min before the endotoxin. Protection is short-lived and does not occur when endotoxin is given 2—8 hrs after folliculoid treatment. Since earlier workers had shown that cortisol offers a similar protection, it is possible that the effect of the folliculoids is mediated through the adrenal cortex.

Nolan & Ali F 79,610/67: In rats, "conjugated estrogens administered from 0 to 2 hours before endotoxin afforded greater protection on a weight basis than hydrocortisone succinate. No protection was noted when estrogen pretreatment was 3 to 8 hours prior to challenge. In contrast, however, if conjugated estrogens or estriol was given 24 hours prior to the endotoxin, the L.D. 50 in female rats was reduced ten-fold, from 2.0 mg to 0.25 mg."

Nolan et al. H 5,204/68: In intact rats, conjugated "equine estrogens" antagonize the lethal effects of E. coli endotoxin. In this respect, the folliculoid preparation is even more active than cortisol succinate. A parallel type of blockade to the vasoconstrictive effect of endotoxin was also noted both for the folliculoid and the corticoid preparations in the isolated rat liver.

Nolan & Ali G 55,490/68: Various folliculoids administered up to one hour before an injection of E. coli endotoxin reduce the lethal effect of the latter, but when estrogens are administered 18—48 hrs before the endotoxin, the mortality rate is increased. Pretreatment with cortisol, corticosterone, ACTH, Thorotrast (to block the RES) or endotoxin 24 hrs before endotoxin challenge did not increase the mortality rate. Endotoxin doses that normally cause no hepatic damage elicited liver necrosis in rats pretreated with folliculoids.

← **Other Steroids.** *Bein D 37,982/62:* Whereas earlier work suggested that protection by steroids against endotoxin shock depends upon glucocorticoid activity, it has now been demonstrated in acute experiments on anesthetized cats that the sharp drop in blood pressure produced by endotoxin, and the lack of pressor response to epinephrine are prevented by aldosterone i.v. given just before the endotoxin. It is incidentally mentioned that 19-oxoprogesterone with the following formula:

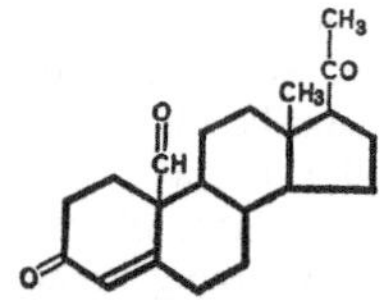

is active in this respect, although it has neither anti-inflammatory nor salt-retaining properties. It is concluded that the anti-endotoxin effect is independent of corticoid activities. [The experimental conditions of the 19-oxoprogesterone tests (experimental animal, dose, route of administration) are not given (H.S.).]

Kocsár et al. G69,983/69: In rats, incubation of tritium-labeled endotoxin with bile or Na-deoxycholate reduces its absorption when subsequently injected i.p. In rats rendered bile-deficient by cannulation of the choledochus, unlike in normal rats, endotoxin is absorbed after administration p.o. "Our experimental findings suggest that bile acids play an important role in the defense mechanism of the macroorganism against bacterial endotoxins."

Selye G70,480/71: In rats, the prostration and mortality produced by i.v. injection of E. coli endotoxin could be prevented by prednisolone, triamcinolone and cortisone. Conversely, PCN, CS-1, norbolethone, and thyroxine tended to aggravate endotoxin shock and mortality. The other members of our standard series of conditioners were ineffective, as was aldosterone even at the high dose of 1 mg p.o., twice daily, *cf.* Table 123.

Table 123. *Conditioning for E. coli endotoxin No. 08*

Treatment[a]	Dyskinesia[b] (Positive/ Total)	Mortality[b] (Dead/ Total)
None	7/12	8/13
PCN	10/10 *	10/10 *
CS-1	10/10 *	4/10 NS
Ethylestrenol	3/8 NS	4/8 NS
Spironolactone	9/10 NS	4/10 NS
Norbolethone	9/10 NS	10/10 *
Oxandrolone	7/10 NS	3/10 NS
Prednisolone-Ac	0/9 **	1/9 *
Triamcinolone (2 mg)	0/10 ***	0/10 ***
Progesterone	8/10 NS	4/10 NS
Estradiol (1 mg)	8/10 NS	9/10 NS
DOC-Ac	6/9 NS	3/9 NS
Hydroxydione	9/10 NS	6/10 NS
Cortisone-Ac	0/10 ***	4/10 NS
Cholesterol	5/5 NS	3/5 NS
Thyroxine	10/10 *	10/10 *
Phenobarbital	8/10 NS	5/10 NS
Aldosterone (1 mg)	5/5 NS	3/5 NS

[a] The rats of all groups were given E.coli endotoxin No. 08 (800 µg/100 g body weight in 0.8 ml water, i.v., once on 4th day).

[b] Dyskinesia was measured 3 hrs after injection of the endotoxin and mortality listed on 7th day ("Exact Probability Test").

For further details on technique of tabulation *cf.* p. VIII.

VENOMS AND PLANT POISONS ←

Cortisone, cortisol and other glucocorticoids have been shown to protect various mammals, including man, against venoms of snakes, spiders and wasps.

The claim that the resistance of rats against a poisonous extract of Amanita phalloides can be raised by adrenocortical extract requires confirmation. However, estradiol offers striking protection against the peliosis-like hepatic necrosis induced by pure phalloidin in the rat.

Snakes ←

Dossena B47,510/49: Female guinea pigs appear to be more sensitive than males to Cape cobra venom but pretreatment with testosterone, estradiol or progesterone failed to affect their resistance.

Maral C17,604/53: In mice, cortisone exerts a favorable influence upon intoxication with viper venom.

Schöttler C10,890/54: In mice and guinea pigs injected with the venom of Bothrops jararaca or Crotalus terrificus s.c., ACTH, cortisone and cortisol failed to offer protection.

Deichmann et al. C33,188/57: Cortisol largely protects the dog against the lethal, but not against the local, effect of Crotalus adamanteus venom i.m.

Deichmann et al. C73,854/58: In dogs, cortisol i.v. protects against the lethal but not against the local effects of rattlesnake (Crotalus adamanteus) venom i.m.

Bein & Jaques D41,862/60: Pretreatment with aldosterone "protects mice against the lethal action of E. coli or S. typhimurium toxin as well as against that of hemorrhagic snake venoms (Vipera aspis, Crotalus adamanteus), but not against the neurotoxic venom of Naja tripudians. Prednisolone, which is effective to roughly the same degree in the mouse as in the rat, has to be administered in doses some 10—30 times larger, whereas hydrocortisone and cortexone display no protective action, even in high dosage."

Russell & Emery D2,497/61: Review of the literature on the protective effect of ACTH and glucocorticoids against snake venom with personal observations on the lethality of Ancistrodon contortrix venom in mice.

Arora et al. D27,786/62: Cortisol given within an hour after s.c. injection of Echis carinatus venom protects the rat against fatal intoxication. It also greatly augments the therapeutic efficacy of the specific antivenom.

Bonta et al. F28,544/65: Estriol-16,17-disodium succinate inhibits the local hemorrhages induced by snake venom in canine heart-lung preparations.

Halmagyi et al. G31,584/65: In sheep, Crotalus venom shock was moderately counteracted by concurrent treatment with cortisol, aldosterone or β-methasone.

Ogawa F54,550/65: In adrenalectomized, as in intact rats, the toxicity of Habu snake venom is reduced by dexamethasone and F-COL, whereas DOC shortens the survival period.

Haas G38,758/66: Extensive review on the use of corticoids and ACTH in the treatment of snake bites in man and in animals.

Bonta et al. G69,044/69: Topical treatment with estriol prevents the hemorrhagic action of cobra venom placed directly upon the dog's lung. The comparable effect of Agkistrodon piscivorus venom is not prevented. The former venom does, whereas the latter does not, contain the "heparin precipitable factor."

Clark & Higginbotham G77,169/70: In mice, the lethal effect of moccasin venom i.v. is aggravated by adrenalectomy or vaccination; cortisol offers protection in both intact and adrenalectomized or vaccinated animals.

Spiders ←

Mohammed et al. C7,579/54: Rats can be protected against fatal doses of scorpion toxin by pretreatment with cortisone or ACTH.

Bettini & Cantore C21,801/55: Comparative studies on the protective effect of ACTH, cortisone and chlorpromazine against lethal poisoning with the venom of the spider Latrodectus tredecimguttatus.

Wasp ←

Jaques H13,146/69: Cortisol protects the guinea pig against lethal wasp-venom shock.

Mushrooms ←

Cheymol & Pfeiffer B54,350/49: The resistance of intact rats to intoxication with a highly poisonous extract of Amanita phalloides rises considerably following treatment with adrenocortical extract or NaCl, whereas DOC has little, if any, prophylactic potency.

Tuchweber et al. (in preparation): In rats, mortality and peliosis-like hemorrhagic necrosis of the liver induced by phalloidin i.p. are prevented by pretreatment with estradiol. PCN, ethylestrenol, spironolactone, triamcinolone, betamethasone, cortisol, progesterone and phenobarbital were ineffective in this respect.

IMMUNE REACTIONS ←

← Corticoids

The immunosuppressive effect of corticoids is so well known that it need not be discussed here in detail. Besides, this topic has been dealt with at length in our earlier monographs. Here, we shall limit ourselves to a few points of special theoretic interest.

In **guinea pigs**, allegedly neither cortisone nor ACTH can suppress passive or active anaphylaxis, or a positive Schick test. Yet, apparently, under suitable conditions, both cortisone and ACTH diminish tuberculin sensitivity. Curiously, two weeks after interruption of cortisone or ACTH administration, the hormone-treated animals become even more sensitive than the controls.

There appears to exist a singular interaction between corticoids and thyroid hormones. Thyroxine increases hypersensitivity to tuberculin in guinea pigs but, here again, 14 days after stopping the treatment the effect is reversed and the pretreated animals surpass the unpretreated controls in the degree of their tuberculin resistance. Since propylthiouracil diminishes the immunosuppressive effect of cortisone, it was postulated that thyroxine is necessary for the desensitizing action of these hormones. This assumption is not contradicted by the fact that thyroxine increases tuberculin hypersensitivity because it fails to block desensitization by ACTH or cortisone.

Much has been written about a "cabbage factor" (possibly an SH-compound) which on ingestion inhibits the desensitization to tuberculin produced by the metabolism of ascorbic acid in the tissues of allergic guinea pigs. The desensitizing action of cortisone or ACTH in cabbage-fed animals has therefore been thought to be indirect, depending upon the reversal of the cabbage effect by the hormone. Apparently, ATP prevents the desensitizing effect of cortisone upon tuberculin, whereas STH depresses tuberculin sensitivity and synergizes the action of cortisone.

Certain hypothalamic lesions can suppress anaphylactic reactivity in guinea pigs. This inhibitory effect can be partially blocked in turn by chronic treatment with thyroid hormones, adrenalectomy or adrenal inactivation by metyrapone. It has been concluded that the sharp, inhibiting effect of hypothalamic lesions may be partly due to hypothyroidism and partly to hypercorticoidism.

In hyperimmunized **rabbits**, the development of nephritis is inhibited by cortisone. Some investigators claimed that various luteoids can prolong skin homograft survival in rabbits. Curiously, combined treatment with cortisone and luteoids actually interferes with the beneficial effect of the latter.

In **mice**, pretreatment with cortisone suppresses the amyloidosis normally produced by repeated injections of killed tubercle bacilli. Also, in the mouse (unlike in the rat), triamcinolone reduces anaphylactic mortality, but various glucocorticoids act differently in this respect: betamethasone and depersolon are effective in the rat but not in the mouse; dexamethasone is active, whereas cortisol is inactive, in both species.

In **rats** hemolysin formation following i.p. injection of sheep erythrocytes is inhibited by pretreatment with cortisone, but only if the hormone is administered before the antigen. Hemolysin formation is also inhibited in rats by dexamethasone, but not by prednisolone or norandrostenolone.

Rats whose thymus is partly destroyed by calciphylaxis (DHT + triamcinolone), allegedly accept skin homografts, although the thymic medulla is usually well preserved. This finding requires confirmation.

Certain experiments on **dogs** suggest that aldosterone may prolong the life of renal homografts, but here also confirmatory evidence would be welcome.

← Adrenalectomy

For the extensive literature on the effect of adrenalectomy the reader must again be referred to our earlier monographs. Suffice it to point out here, merely for its historic interest, an observation made over 40 years ago which shows that hemolysin formation is inhibited in rats by adrenalectomy.

← Folliculoids and Luteoids

It has been claimed that medroxyprogesterone increases survival of renal allografts in dogs and of skin allografts in rabbits by immunosuppression. Melengestrol, another primarily progestational steroid with less pronounced glucocorticoid activity, is more effective than cortisol in suppressing allergic encephalomyelitis in rats. These observations have led to the supposition that both luteoid and glucocorticoid activity is somehow related to immunosuppression.

← Testoids

Several investigators presented evidence to show a regulating effect of testoids upon immune phenomena.

In rats, gonadectomy did not significantly change the course of Masugi nephritis but testosterone inhibited its development. In rats, immunized by sheep erythrocytes, various anabolic steroids enhance antibody formation. These compounds also stimulate antibody formation in infants vaccinated against diphtheria.

← Gonadectomy

In guinea pigs, allegedly gonadectomy diminishes anaphylactic shock in both sexes, whereas in rats this is not the case. Gonadectomy also fails to influence the development of allergic nephritis in the rat.

Immune Reactions ← *cf. also Selye B40, 000/ 50, p. 69; G60,083/70, pp. 347, 355.*

← **Corticoids.** *Wolfram & Zwemer 30,809/35:* In sensitized guinea pigs, anaphylactic shock caused by reinjection of crystalline ovalbumin is inhibited by "cortin."

Dworetzky et al. B52,246/50: In guinea pigs, anaphylactic shock was not significantly influenced by cortisone or ACTH.

Long & Miles D41,973/50: In guinea pigs, moderate thyrotoxicosis produced by two weeks' treatment with thyroxine increases hypersensitivity to tuberculin whereas moderate doses of propylthiouracil do not affect it. ACTH and cortisone diminish tuberculin sensitivity. Fourteen days after stopping thyroxine injections, the animals became actually less hypersensitive than the controls. A similar reversal of effect was noted two weeks after interruption of cortisone or ACTH treatment in that the animals became more hypersensitive than the controls.

Long et al. B60,189/51: In B.C.G.-infected guinea pigs, hypersensitivity to tuberculin is considerably diminished by cortisone or ACTH. This diminution is abolished by pretreatment with propylthiouracil, which alone has no effect upon hypersensitivity. Pretreatment with thyroxine increases tuberculin hypersensitivity but does not block desensitization by ACTH or cortisone. Apparently, thyroxine is necessary for the desensitizing action of ACTH and cortisone.

Long et al. D85,907/51: In guinea pigs, single injections of cortisone or ACTH diminish allergic hypersensitivity on a cabbage diet, but not on a basal diet deficient in the "cabbage factor." The authors conclude "that there is in cabbage a factor which on ingestion leads to the inhibition of the desensitisation produced by the metabolism of ascorbic acid in the tissues of the allergic guinea pig; and that the desensitising action of cortisone or of ACTH in cabbage-fed animals is indirect, depending on the reversal of the cabbage effect by the hormones. The cabbage factor may possibly be an SH-compound."

Long et al. B63,843/51: In guinea pigs, dihydroascorbic acid—unlike ascorbic acid—inhibits the tuberculin reaction after infection with B.C.G. vaccine. The desensitizing effect of dihydroascorbic acid is not inhibited by thiouracil. Alloxan, like ACTH or cortisone, does not modify desensitization by ascorbic acid on diets deprived of the "cabbage factor;" it desensitizes guinea pigs on a cabbage diet and this desensitization is inhibited by propylthiouracil.

Malkiel G71,451/51: In guinea pigs, ACTH and cortisone are without effect on the end results of histamine shock, or of passive or active anaphylaxis.

Teilum et al. B62,687/51: In hyperimmunized rabbits, the development of nephritis is inhibited by cortisone.

Cornforth & Long B77,176/53: In guinea pigs sensitized to tuberculin, single s.c. injections of ATP prevent desensitization by alloxan, cortisone and dihydroascorbic acid. Single s.c. injections of insulin do not in themselves influence sensitivity but prevent desensitization by alloxan and cortisone. Single s.c. injections of STH depress tuberculin sensitivity and synergize the action of cortisone or alloxan.

Rosenbaum & Obrinsky B85,352/53: In guinea pigs, cortisone did not affect the development of a positive Schick reaction nor did it prevent death and adrenal hemorrhage after treatment with diphtheria toxin.

Lepri & Fornaro D91,865/54: In rabbits, rendered allergic to tuberculosis, the ocular manifestations of topical challenge by tubercle bacilli were variably influenced by ACTH and cortisone.

Berglund C16,832/56: In rats, hemolysin formation following i.p. injection of sheep erythrocytes is inhibited by pretreatment with cortisone. No significant effect is obtained by cortisone administration after antigen injection.

Tolentino et al. D16,593/61: In rats, hemolysin formation against sheep erythrocytes is decreased by dexamethasone but uninfluenced by prednisolone, norandrostenolone. Under similar conditions, testosterone and dihydroisoandrosterone increase hemolysin formation.

Todd et al. G10,342/63: Experiments on dogs "suggest that in certain circumstances aldosterone is capable of prolonging the life of renal homografts in dogs."

Vakilzadeh & Vandiviere E32,626/63: In guinea pigs, the beneficial effect of vaccination against tuberculosis was greatly increased by thyroxine and T3, but not by cortisone, cortisol or ACTH. None of the hormones altered natural host resistance in nonimmunized guinea pigs.

Webster & Gentille E30,434/63: Rats "chemically thymectomized" by calciphylaxis of the thymus owing to combined treatment with triamcinolone and DHT accept skin homografts, although the thymic medulla is usually well preserved.

Hulka & Mohr G44,272/67: Although earlier observations showed that various luteoids can prolong skin-homograft survival in the rabbit, combined treatment with cortisone + medroxyprogesterone, progesterone, norethynodrel or norethindrone, actually interfered with the homograft survival-prolonging effect obtained by cortisone alone.

Laddu & Sanyal G60,298/68: Triamcinolone reduced mortality from anaphylaxis in the mouse but not in the rat. Betamethasone and depersolon were effective in the rat but not in the mouse. Dexamethasone was effective in both species and cortisol ineffective in either species.

Laufer et al. H13,434/68: Pretreatment with cortisone suppressed amyloidosis in mice injected with killed Mycobacterium tuberculosis.

Patton & Clark G73,195/68: In rats infected with Trypanosoma lewisi, dexamethasone resulted in the development of exceedingly large populations of trypanosomes which were fatal to their hosts. This effect of dexamethasone is ascribed to the inhibition of the production of ablastin and trypanocidal antibodies.

Filipp & Mess G71,129/69: In guinea pigs, suppression of anaphylactic reactivity by anterior hypothalamic lesions can be partially blocked by chronic treatment with thyroid hormones as well as by adrenalectomy or adrenal inactivation by metyrapone (Metopirone). "Combined treatment of guinea gips bearing hypothalamic lesions with Metopirone and thyroxine completely eliminated the blocking effect of the tuberal lesion on anaphylactic reactions." Apparently the shock-inhibiting effect of hypothalamic lesions is partly due to hypothyroidism and partly to hypercorticoidism.

Nyfors G76,097/70: In grass pollen-allergic patients, the skin wheal reaction was not significantly influenced by a large dose of prednisone, whereas the tuberculin test (Mantoux) was considerably diminished.

← **Adrenalectomy.** *Perla & Marmorston-Gottesman 16,042/29:* In rats, epinephrine raises the capacity for hemolysin formation after adrenalectomy.

Higginbotham D21,395/62: In mice, resistance to 5-HT, endotoxin and anaphylactic shock is markedly decreased by adrenalectomy. Cortisol readily restored resistance to 5-HT, but was less effective with regard to endotoxin and anaphylactic shock. Resistance to histamine and histamine releasers is less markedly diminished by adrenalectomy in the mouse, and large doses of cortisol are required to induce a measurable increase in resistance to histamine.

← **Folliculoids and Luteoids.** *Dutz et al. C31,646/56:* In rats, gonadectomy did not significantly change the course of Masugi nephritis, whereas a folliculoid preparation (Östrasid) and testosterone ameliorated it.

Turcotte et al. G56,529/68: Medroxyprogesterone acetate (a potent synthetic luteoid) increases survival of renal allografts in dogs and of skin allografts in rabbits by immunosuppression. Earlier literature on immunosuppression by luteoids is reviewed.

Greig et al. H24,654/70: In rats, melengestrol acetate (MGA; 6α-methyl-6-dehydro-16-methylene-17-acetoxyprogesterone) — a primarily progestational steroid with less pronounced glucocorticoid activity than that of cortisol — is more effective than the latter in suppressing allergic encephalomyelitis. Melengestrol is even effective in reversing the established disease.

← **Testoids.** *Sarre B99,950/54:* In rabbits, both the Masugi nephritis and sublimate nephrosis are inhibited by testosterone and even more actively by estradiol.

Dutz et al. C31,646/56: In rats, gonadectomy did not significantly change the course of Masugi nephritis, whereas a folliculoid preparation (Östrasid) and testosterone ameliorated it. STH considerably aggravated the glomerular lesions and the hypertension.

Ghione D87,868/57: 4-Chlorotestosterone enhances anaphylactic shock in guinea pigs, prolongs survival in systemic nocardiosis of mice and improves healing in cutaneous nocardiosis of rabbits.

Heboyan & Messeri G69,057/62: In rats vaccinated with S. typhi and maintained on the high-fat low-protein diet of Handler, the anabolic steroid 4-hydroxy-19 nortestosterone-17 cyclopentyl propionate increases the formation of agglutinins, γ-globulins, and complement.

Jannuzzi & Bassi G68,895/62: In infants vaccinated against diphtheria, serum antitoxin levels were raised by 4-chlorotestosterone and methandrostenolone.

Tolentino D34,052/62: In rats, immunized by sheep erythrocytes, various anabolic testoids enhance antibody formation. Such steroids also raise the titer of antitoxin in infants vaccinated against diphtheria.

Terragna & Jannuzzi G2,778/63: In rats, hemolysin formation following i.p. injection of sheep erythrocytes is greatly increased by various anabolic steroids such as 4-chloro-19-nortestosterone, norandrostenolone, phenylpropionate, methandrostenolone, 4-chlorotestosterone and dehydroisoandrosterone.

Ghione & Turolla G18,525/64: Review of the effect of various anabolics upon immune reactions.

Tolentino et al. G70,136/64: In rats, methandrostenolone, administered several days before or after immunization by sheep erythrocytes, failed to affect antibody formation, whereas concurrent treatment stimulated it.

Lupulescu et al. F77,999/66: In rabbits, the formation of antibodies against Brucella S_6 is stimulated by thyroxine and 4-chlorotestosterone but decreased by thiourea. The effect of 4-chlorotestosterone is evident even after destruction of the thyroid and hence is not mediated through the latter gland.

← **Gonadectomy.** *Kemény et al. B66,729/51:* In guinea pigs, both ovariectomy and orchidectomy diminish anaphylactic shock, whereas thymectomy has no effect upon it.

Dutz et al. C31,646/56: In rats, gonadectomy did not significantly change the course of Masugi nephritis, whereas a folliculoid preparation (Östrasid) and testosterone ameliorated it.

HEPATIC LESIONS ←

(*cf. also* Section on "Drugs" for lesions produced by hepatotoxic compounds and "Histology" for the effect of steroids on the normal liver).

← **Corticoids.** Probably the first definite proof of some interaction between the liver and the adrenal, in the maintenance or resistance to various damaging agents, was given by the observation that although adrenocortical extracts (rich in glucocorticoid potency) have little influence upon the resistance of intact animals to stress, they do exhibit a marked anti-shock effect in rats subjected to very extensive partial hepatectomy. In these they prevent the characteristic hypovolemia, hypochloremia, and hypoglycemia that normally develop after removal of almost the entire hepatic tissue.

The regeneration of the liver as well as the accumulation of protein and free fatty acids in hepatic tissue are enhanced by moderate doses of adrenocortical extract or ACTH. On the other hand, heavy overdosage with glucocorticoids may interfere with hepatic regeneration as part of the general catabolic effect exerted by these hormones. Allegedly, supplements of vitamin-B_{12} counteract the inhibitory action of heavy cortisone overdosage upon hepatic regeneration in partially hepatectomized rats.

After complete hepatectomy "cortin" does not prevent hypoglycemia, presumably because glucocorticoids act upon the blood sugar largely through the liver. However, after total hepatectomy or total evisceration (with intact kidneys and adrenals), rats can maintain a high blood sugar if they receive adrenocortical extract in combination with glucose and insulin. These observations show that glucocorticoids are also capable of affecting the blood sugar through extrahepatic mechanisms. On the other hand, in rats with irreversible hypovolemic shock produced by complete occlusion of the portal vein, neither cortisol nor adrenalectomy influenced the survival time significantly.

There is good reason to believe that glucocorticoids increase bile secretion; this may be of considerable importance in some of the protective effects of steroids against agents eliminated through the bile. Following complete occlusion of the choledochus, cortisol enhances the accumulation of bile in the duct stump; it also favors the formation of perforating choledochus ulcers and hepatic necroses, both in intact and in adrenalectomized rats. All these effects are counteracted by concurrent administration of STH. In dogs, with choledochus ligature, cortisone raises the level of total serum bilirubin, suggesting increased bile pigment synthesis.

← **Adrenalectomy.** In partially hepatectomized rats, adrenalectomy inhibits hepatic regeneration, and decreases the deposition of fat and protein in the liver remnant. Glucocorticoid adrenal extracts, unlike DOC, restore these responses to normal. Yet, some degree of hepatic regeneration is possible even in the absence of the adrenals.

← **Folliculoids.** In partially hepatectomized rats, stilbestrol or hexestrol does not markedly affect the mitotic proliferation of the hepatocytes. In rats with choledochus ligature, estradiol is said to shorten survival.

← **Testoids.** In the rat, testosterone prolongs survival and inhibits the body-weight loss normally observed after choledochus ligature. This steroid also inhibits hepatic steatosis during the first days following partial hepatectomy in rats, but it has no significant effect upon hepatic GPT concentration.

← Corticoids

Selye et al. A 32,768/40: Review of the earlier literature on the ability of epinephrine and "cortin" to raise resistance against various stressors. Attention is called to the fact that whereas cortin is very effective in this respect in adrenalectomized animals, it rarely increases resistance above normal in the presence of the adrenals. The slight effect that cortical extracts do possess during severe shock is presumably due to the fact that "a condition of 'relative adrenal insufficiency' exists in organisms exposed to nonspecific damage." Following extensive partial hepatectomy in rats, "suitable cortin therapy prevents the hypochloraemia, and the decrease in blood volume and in blood sugar which are usually elicited by this intervention." In rats damaged by repeated s.c. injections of formaldehyde, cortical extract prevented the hypoglycemia and hypochloremia of severe shock, whereas DOC was virtually ineffective, and in fact it aggravated the s.c. edema caused by formaldehyde. Chronic pretreatment with cortical hormones causes adrenal atrophy which counteracts their beneficial effect in protecting against stress. "These experiments should be interpreted as a warning against prolonged pretreatment with this substance in preparation for a surgical intervention." The best protective effect was obtained in rats with surgical shock produced by crushing of the intestines, if given repeated injections of cortical extract s.c. during the subsequent 24 hrs. An "Addendum" reports on similar experiments performed with corticosterone prepared for this purpose by E. C. Kendall. This compound, which differs from DOC only in that it possesses an 11β-hydroxyl group, proved to be especially effective in protecting the rat against traumatic shock caused by crushing of the intestines. [This was the first observation showing that 11-oxygenation of corticoids is required to endow them with anti-stress activity (H.S.).]

Selye & Dosne A 30,702/40: In the rat, "the decrease in blood sugar produced by complete hepatectomy is not significantly influenced even by large doses of cortin. This finding makes it probable that the cortical hormone does not inhibit the utilization of circulating sugar. It seems more likely that it prevents the hypoglycemic action of insulin or the decrease in blood sugar following the removal of a large part of the hepatic glycogen stores by stimulating gluconeogenesis in the liver."

Berman et al. 97,700/47: DOC stimulates liver regeneration in partially hepatectomized rats as judged by the weight and protein content of the liver remnant.

Ingle et al. B 2,737/47: In completely hepatectomized and eviscerated rats (with intact kidneys and adrenals) receiving continuous i.v. infusions of glucose + insulin, adrenocortical extract caused a rise in blood sugar.

Roberts B 97,023/53: In rats, the enhanced repair on the liver after treatment with ACTH or adrenocortical extract is characterized mainly by an increased protein deposition in the liver remnant. The usual decline of serum proteins occurring after partial hepatectomy was completely prevented by this treatment.

Einhorn et al. E 55,369/54: In rats, "the restoration of the weight of the liver after partial hepatectomy was not markedly affected by cortisone, the multiplication of cells was reduced to a significant degree after the first 2 days of regeneration. Liver restoration in terms of nucleic acids was similarly inhibited by cortisone."

Selye B 90,556/54: In rats with jaundice caused by bile duct ligature, minute doses of cortisone exert a strong antiphlogistic action (granuloma-pouch and topical irritation arthritis techniques), presumably because jaundice conditions for the anti-inflammatory effect of glucocorticoids.

Selye & Bois B 97,074/54: Following occlusion of the choledochus, cortisol enhances accumulation of bile in the duct stump and favors the development of perforating choledochus ulcers and hepatic necroses both in intact and in the adrenalectomized rats. All these manifestations of cortisol overdosage are inhibited by STH, *cf.* Fig. 20, p. 356.

Chandler et al. C 39,998/57: In dogs with bile duct ligature, cortisone raised the level of total serum bilirubin, indicating increased synthesis of bile pigments. At the same time, proliferation of bile ducts was inhibited.

Maros et al. D 12,784/61: In rats, inhibition of hepatic regeneration after partial hepatectomy by cortisone can be blocked by concurrent administration of vitamin-B_{12} supplements.

Miti & Memeo D 27,223/62: Aldosterone increases hepatic regeneration after partial hepatectomy in the rat. Earlier literature on this subject, including observations on hepatic regeneration after simultaneous partial hepatectomy and adrenalectomy, is reviewed.

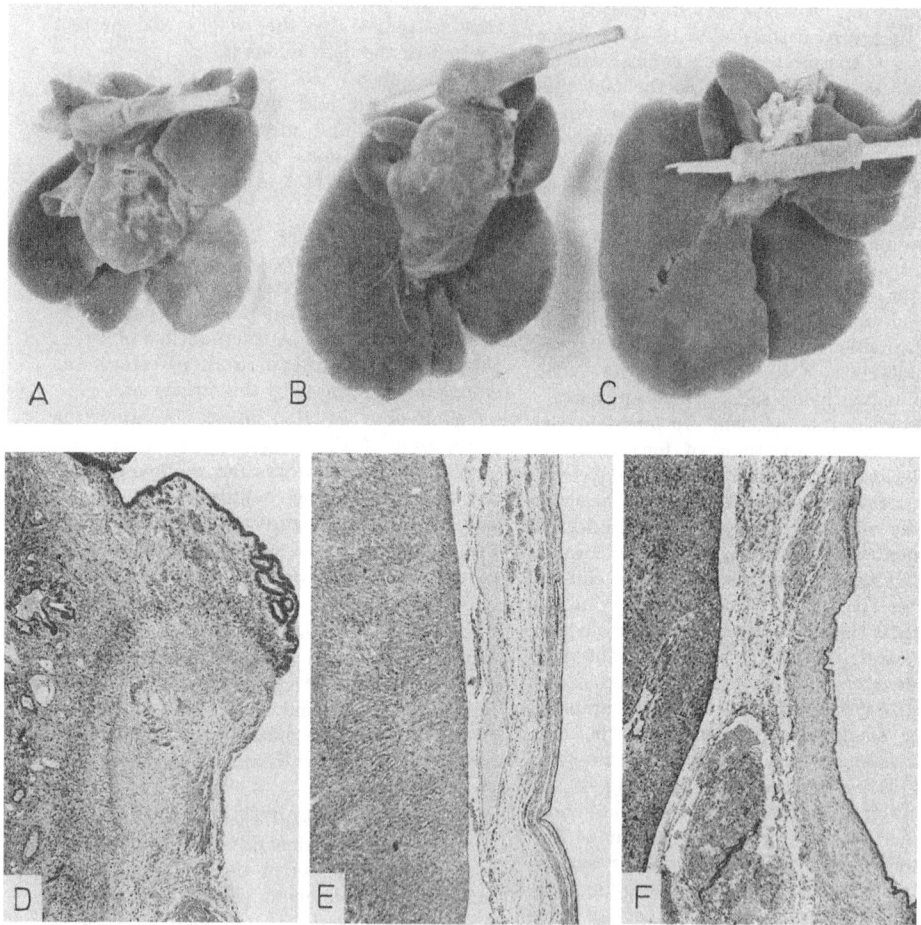

Fig. 20. **Effect of corticoids upon bile secretion and the choledochus.** In all animals, the choledochus was ligated. A: Treatment with large doses of cortisol. Macroscopic aspect of the liver (seen from its caudal aspect). To visualize the duodenum, a wooden stick is introduced into its lumen. The bile-duct, though greatly dilated, is collapsed because of a perforation near the duodenum. There are also several other very thin, ulcerated parts where perforation is imminent. B: Treatment with small doses of cortisol. Here, the bile-duct is greatly dilated and a few thin points are distinguishable, but perforation did not occur. C: Treatment with DOC. Bile-duct is only slightly dilated and of dense structure. D: Histologic section through the bile-duct shown avobe. Note the interruption of the dark epithelial lining and the large ulcer, filled with necrotic tissue (lower right quadrant). Many of the bile-duct branches within the adjacent hepatic tissue were proliferating and greatly dilated. E: Histologic section through the bile-duct shown above. Here, the wall of the choledochus is thin and the surrounding connective tissue very edematous, but actual ulceration has not occurred. The adjacent liver tissue contains several patches of focal necrosis. F: Histologic section through the bile-duct shown above. Note the dense connective tissue underneath the epithelium of the choledochus and the absence of ulcers. Though not shown here, this effect of cortisol is counteracted by concurrent administration of STH. [Selye and Bois B 97,074/54. Courtesy of Gastroenterologia (Basel)]

Souda D62,846/62: In the rat, cortisone pretreatment inhibits mitotic proliferation in the regenerating liver after partial hepatectomy.

Bucher G68,621/63: Review on the influence of adrenalectomy and corticoids upon hepatic regeneration.

Zimel & Macrineanu F35,084/64: In rats, hepatic regeneration following partial hepatectomy is moderately influenced by cytostatic derivatives of hexestrol and cortisol.

Hyde & Davis F82,461/66: Both cortisol and the diuretic drug chlorazanil depress mitotic division in the regenerating liver of the mouse, after partial hepatectomy.

Petzold & Ziegler F92,832/67: The fat and phosphatase accumulation in the liver remnant of partially hepatectomized rats is enhanced by prednisone. 4-Chlorotestosterone does not significantly affect the tissue phosphatase, but delays the removal of fats from the liver.

Deplano H23,483/68; Deplano & Fornara H23,484/68: In rats, the effect of cortisone upon hepatic regeneration following partial hepatectomy is examined with special reference to DNA and RNA synthesis and alkaline phosphatase activity.

Mejia et al. G60,637/68: In rats with irreversible hypovolemic shock produced by complete occlusion of the portal vein, neither cortisol pretreatment nor adrenalectomy influenced the survival time, whereas selective extirpation of the adrenal medulla, or continuous infusion of norepinephrine increased it. Similar infusion of epinephrine decreased survival time.

Šimek et al. G71,089/68: In intact, and even more markedly in adrenalectomized rats, the accumulation of free fatty acids in the liver is enhanced by cortisol during the early period after partial hepatectomy. ACTH has the same effect, but only in the presence of the adrenals.

Šimek et al. H13,837/68: Comparative studies on DNA synthesis, fatty acid content, and the weight of the regenerating liver in partially hepatectomized rats after treatment with cortisol, ACTH, and various stressor agents.

Bucher et al. G72,546/69: Review of the humoral factors responsible for hepatic regeneration following partial hepatectomy. Hepatic DNA synthesis is stimulated in intact rats by parabiosis or cross-circulation with partially hepatectomized partners. Furthermore, tiny liver grafts implanted outside of the portal area proliferate in response to partial ablation of the parent organ. Various stressors inhibit hepatic regeneration in partially hepatectomized rats, but this effect is not reproduced by ACTH or cortisol. On the other hand, adrenalectomy increases hepatic regeneration.

Raab & Webb H20,502/69: In rats, the biosynthesis of DNA is maximally inhibited by cortisol 17—19 hrs after partial hepatectomy.

Shigei H27,112/69: In rats, adrenalectomy changed the ultrastructure of hepatocytes by reducing the glycogen areas, increasing the number of mitochondria and lysosomes, and inducing vesicular forms of endoplasmic reticulum around the Golgi complexes. All these changes are prevented by cortisol. In partial hepatectomized rats, adrenalectomy and cortisol also exert antagonistic effects upon hepatocyte ultrastructure.

Wimberly et al. G65,769/69: In dogs and cats, methylprednisolone alone or in combination with antibiotics failed to increase survival following temporary occlusion of the portal vein and hepatic artery.

← Adrenalectomy

MacKay & Carne A14,767/38: In rats, the hepatic steatosis normally occurring during 24 hrs of fasting after partial hepatectomy is more pronounced in females than in males, and can be largely prevented by adrenalectomy.

Berman et al. 97,700/47: Adrenalectomy decreases the deposition of fat and protein as well as the increase in cell size and number normally seen in the liver remnant of rats 24 hrs after partial hepatectomy. A glucocorticoid adrenal extract unlike DOC restores these responses to normal.

Canzanelli et al. B37,729/49: In rats, hypophysectomy delays liver regeneration after partial hepatectomy but "neither adrenalectomy nor the administration of adrenal-cortex extract has any effect on the amount of liver regeneration."

Drabkin B53,844/50: In partially hepatectomized and adrenalectomized rats, active hepatic regeneration occurred despite depletion of cytochrome c.

Friedgood et al. B52,238/50: In rats, after partial hepatectomy, regeneration and protein accumulation in the liver are inhibited by adrenalectomy, but restored to a certain degree by adrenocortical extract. 11-Dehydrocorticosterone and 17-hydroxy, 11-dehydrocorticosterone share this effect, yet DOC is even more active.

Uyldert G76,358/50: In rats, the inhibition of hepatic regeneration following partial hepatectomy (about 1/3 of the liver removed) is inhibited by adrenalectomy and restored both by adrenocortical extract and by DOC.

Bucher G68,621/63: Review on the influence of adrenalectomy and corticoids upon hepatic regeneration.

Camargo et al. F72,052/66: After partial hepatectomy, lipid infiltration of the rat liver depends upon the proportion of hepatic tissue removed, and not upon surgical stress, postoperative fasting, simultaneous adrenalectomy, or hypophysectomy. The lipid infiltration reaches a maximum 6—12 hrs after the operation, and then declines.

Šimek et al. H22,183/68: In rats, the initial increase in liver triglyceride content induced by partial hepatectomy is decreased after adrenalectomy. However, within 24 hrs after the operation, this difference disappears. The effect of adrenalectomy upon the liver triglyceride changes induced by partial hepatectomy can be annulled by epinephrine or cortisone. ACTH augments the immediate rise in liver triglyceride but only in the presence of the adrenals.

Shigei H27,112/69: In rats, adrenalectomy changed the ultrastructure of hepatocytes by reducing the glucogen areas, increasing the number of mitochondria and lysosomes, and inducing vesicular forms of endoplasmic reticulum around the Golgi complexes. All these changes are prevented by cortisol. In hepatectomized rats, adrenalectomy and cortisol also exert antagonistic effects upon hepatocyte ultrastructure.

← Folliculoids

Cristensen & Jacobsen A49,204/49: In rats subjected to partial hepatectomy, neither hypophysectomy nor thyroidectomy impairs the rate of regeneration. No significant change in mitotic rate was observed after pretreatment with stilbestrol or STH.

Giuliani C15,153/55: In rats with bile duct ligature, testosterone prolongs survival and inhibits body weight loss, but its action upon the prostate is diminished. Estradiol exerts inverse effects in all these respects.

Zimel & Măcrineanu F35,084/64: In rats, hepatic regeneration following partial hepatectomy is moderately influenced by cytostatic derivatives of hexestrol and cortisol.

Kappas G43,772/67: Review (4 p., 42 refs.) on the hepatotoxic effect of folliculoids in animals and man.

Martinez-Manautou et al. H30,302/70: Women were treated for several years with oral contraceptives containing a luteoid (chlormadinone acetate) with or without folliculoids. There was "a moderate dilatation and vesiculation of the rough and smooth surfaced endoplasmic reticulum both in the women treated with microdoses of progestogens, and in those treated with a combination of progestogens and oestrogens. A more marked vesiculation of this organelle was present in those women under sequential medication. Elongation of mitochondria with crystalloid inclusions in their matrices was found in 5 to 10% of the whole population of mitochondria per cell examined in the chlormadinone treated women."

← Testoids

Giuliani C15,153/55: In rats with bile duct ligature, testosterone prolongs survival and inhibits body weight loss, but its action upon the prostate is diminished. Estradiol exerts inverse effects in all these respects.

Bengmark & Olsson D6,135/64: In rats, testosterone inhibits fatty infiltration of the liver during the first days after partial hepatectomy but has no significant effect upon liver weight or hepatic glutamic pyruvic transaminase concentration.

Petzold & Ziegler F92,832/67: The fat and phosphatase accumulation in the liver remnant of partially hepatectomized rats is enhanced by prednisone. 4-Chlorotestosterone does not significantly affect the tissue phosphatase, but delays the removal of fats from the liver.

Porto & Donato H34,703/69: In guinea pigs, hepatic regeneration after partial hepatectomy is enhanced by testosterone.

← Other Steroids

Selye G70,480/71: In rats, the bile duct was ligated on the 4th day of conditioning. Final eviscerated body weight was measured, and mortality listed on the 10th day. Under these circumstances none of the "Standard Conditioners" (p. VIII) or cortisone caused any noteworthy change in the resulting intoxication. CS-1, PCN and phenobarbital were not tested.

RENAL LESIONS ←

(*cf. also* Renal Damage Induced by Mercury and Other Toxicants *under* "Drugs")

← **Corticoids.** In mice and rats, pretreatment with DOC prolongs survival and delays the rise in blood NPN following complete nephrectomy. This effect is particularly obvious in rats maintained on high carbohydrate diets. It is possible that depletion of the potassium stores by the mineralocorticoid participates in this protective effect.

In dogs maintained on a standard high-fat diet, arterial lesions develop upon subsequent total nephrectomy. These are prevented by cortisone as well as by ACTH and pregnancy. Cortisol also prolongs survival of dogs after bilateral ligature of the ureters and in rats, the renal damage produced by obstruction of the ureters is diminished by cortisone.

On the other hand, the calcification of the kidney induced in rats by complete ligature of the renal blood vessels is increased by cortisone, whereas the cardiovascular calcification elicited by bilateral nephrectomy, especially in old rats, is not significantly influenced by glucocorticoids (e.g., prednisolone, triamcinolone) or DOC.

← **Testoids.** The most extensive studies on the effect of steroids upon the consequences of renal damage have been performed with testoids. The first pertinent observation was the demonstration that testosterone pretreatment prolongs the survival of mice after bilateral nephrectomy, and protects the kidney against atrophy following the production of hydronephrosis by unilateral ligature of the ureter. MAD also exerts a potent renotrophic effect upon the hydronephrotic mouse kidney.

Furthermore, testosterone alone or in combination with DOC delays the development of azotemia in rats, especially if they are kept on a high carbohydrate diet. However, data on the ability of testoids to maintain life after complete nephrectomy are contradictory, presumably because the diet, species, age and other factors may modify the response. It has been claimed that both MAD and nandrolone prolong the survival time of bilaterally nephrectomized rats. Similar results have been obtained with several other anabolic testoids, in various species including man, but these data have not remained unchallenged.

← **Folliculoids and Luteoids.** The arterial lesions that develop following complete nephrectomy in dogs kept on a standard high-fat diet are prevented not only by corticoids but also by diethylstilbestrol.

The cardiovascular calcification elicited by bilateral nephrectomy in aged rats is not significantly affected either by estradiol or by progesterone.

← **Gonadectomy.** Male rats are more sensitive than females to the production of hypertension by unilateral renal artery constriction. Gonadectomy does not significantly alter this change in males, although it appears to aggravate it in females.

← **Other Steroids.** Spironolactone has been claimed to protect the rat against mortality and some of the cardiovascular and renal changes normally produced by an "endocrine kidney" or by a renal encapsulation. On the other hand, the cardiovascular calcification elicited by bilateral nephrectomy in aged rats is not influenced by ethylestrenol, CS-1, spironolactone, norbolethone or oxandrolone.

← Corticoids

Selye A 34,190/40: "Experiments in mice and rats indicate that pretreatment with desoxycorticosterone acetate prolongs the survival time of animals in which acute uraemia is produced by bilateral nephrectomy."

Selye & Nielsen A 35,723/41; Dosne A 35,924/41: In the rat, pretreatment with DOC "not only prolongs the survival time and delays clinical signs of uremia, but actually inhibits the rise in the non-protein nitrogen content of the blood after complete nephrectomy."

Masson et al. B 40,204/49: DOC and testosterone, alone or in combination, delayed the development of azotemia only in rats fed a high carbohydrate diet.

Holman & Jones B 93,771/53: The arterial lesions that occur in dogs kept on a standard high fat diet upon subsequent nephrectomy are prevented by pregnancy, cortisone, ACTH, or diethylstilbestrol.

Guze & Beeson C 43,020/57: In rats with ureteral ligation, damage to the renal tissue is inhibited by cortisone.

Berman C 74,922/59: Survival in uremia, produced by bilateral ureteral ligation in dogs, is prolonged by cortisol, but not by testosterone.

Dési et al. C 69,045/59: In rats, survival after bilateral nephrectomy is prolonged by STH and DOC, alone or in combination, but the effect of STH is diminished by concurrent administration of MAD.

Laron & Laufer D 20/687/62: In rats, cortisone increases calcium deposition in the kidney following ligature of its vessels, but prevents ectopic bone formation.

Gardell et al. G 70,430/70: In rats, the cardiovascular calcification produced by bilateral nephrectomy is not significantly influenced by ethylestrenol, CS-1, spironolactone, norbolethone, oxandrolone, prednisolone, progesterone, triamcinolone, DOC, estradiol, or thyroxine.

← Testoids

Selye A 30,863/40: Testosterone pretreatment prolongs the survival of mice after bilateral nephrectomy. Cholesterol does not share this effect.

Selye & Friedman A 35,722/41: "Experiments on the mouse indicate that the renal atrophy, which usually develops subsequent to the hydronephrosis caused by unilateral ligature of the ureter, may be inhibited and delayed by testosterone administration."

Masson et al. B 40,204/49: DOC and testosterone, alone or in combination, delayed the development of azotemia only in rats fed a high carbohydrate diet.

Homburger et al. B 47,878/50: MAD exerts "a potent renotropic effect upon the experimental hydronephrotic mouse kidney."

Berman C 74,922/59: Survival in uremia produced by bilateral ureteral ligation in dogs, is prolonged by cortisol, but not by testosterone.

Dési et al. C 69,045/59: In rats, survival after bilateral nephrectomy is prolonged by STH and DOC, alone or in combination, but the effect of STH is diminished by concurrent administration of MAD.

Szold et al. C 64,498/59; C 79,889/59: Nandrolone prolongs the survival time of bilaterally nephrectomized rats.

Dési et al. D 11,138/61: 19-Norandrostenolone-decanoate (Durabolin) significantly prolongs the survival time in nephrectomized rats.

Gerber & Cottier D 12,775/61: "The 3 tested testosterone derivatives with anabolic properties (19-Nortestosteronphenylpropionate, 17-Ethyl-19-nortestosterone, 1-Dehydro-17-methyltestosterone) did not lower the daily increment of urea concentration in the blood of rats following bilateral nephrectomy, even when the hormones were given prophylactically." [The hormones were tested at a dose of 3 mg/kg body weight (H.S.).]

Köhnlein & Rehn D 44,607/62: The kidney damage produced by temporary renal artery obstruction in the rat is effectively combated by testosterone, but not by norandrostenolone phenylpropionate (Durabolin). From this, it is concluded that the nephrotrophic effect depends upon testoid and not upon anabolic activity.

Börner et al. E 85,972/66: Review and personal observations on the effect of testoids upon various clinical and experimental uremic conditions.

Schimmelpfennig et al. F 74,978/66: In castrate rats, 4-chlorotestosterone did not significantly improve the renal insufficiency caused by 30 min ligature of the left renal artery.

Tessmann H 5,695/67: Pretreatment with testosterone exerted no protective effect against the tubular damage elicited by temporary obstruction of the renal vessels in the mouse and rat.

← Folliculoids and Luteoids

Holman & Jones B93,771/53: The arterial lesions that develop in dogs kept on a standard high fat diet, upon subsequent nephrectomy are prevented by pregnancy, cortisone, ACTH, or diethylstilbestrol.

Gardell et al. G70,430/70: In rats, the cardiovascular calcification produced by bilateral nephrectomy is not significantly influenced by ethylestrenol, CS-1, spironolactone, norbolethone, oxandrolone, prednisolone, progesterone, triamcinolone, DOC, estradiol, or thyroxine.

← Gonadectomy

Bein et al. C57,714/58: In male rats, with hypertension produced by unilateral renal artery constriction, vascular lesions are more common than in females. Gonadectomy does not significantly alter these changes in males, but aggravates them in females. Parathyroidectomy has no significant effect upon them.

← Other Steroids

Fregly D15,796/61: In the rat, the antimineralocorticoid spirolactone SC-8109 diminished the hypertension produced by renal encapsulation.

Nadasdi D9,288/61: "Spironolactone significantly protects against the mortality and some of the cardiovascular-renal changes normally produced by the presence of an ischemic (or 'endocrine') kidney in rats."

Gardell et al. G70,430/70: In rats, the cardiovascular calcification produced by bilateral nephrectomy is not significantly influenced by ethylestrenol, CS-1, spironolactone, norbolethone, oxandrolone, prednisolone, progesterone, triamcinolone, DOC, estradiol, or thyroxine.

Selye G70,480/71: In rats nephrectomized on the 8th day of conditioning, none of the "Standard Conditioners" (p. VIII) or cholesterol caused any noteworthy change in mean survival. CS-1, PCN and phenobarbital were not tested.

OTHER SURGICAL PROCEDURES ←
(cf. also "Stress")

After **parathyroidectomy**, the mortality is approximately the same in male and spayed female rats, whereas intact females are said to be more resistant. In orchidectomized rats, estradiol allegedly prolongs survival after thyroparathyroidectomy, the comparatively high resistance of intact females is ascribed to folliculoids.

Extensive **partial pancreatectomy** causes diabetes more readily in male than in female rats. Postnatal orchidectomy abolishes this sex difference.

Rowinski & Manunta B64,144/51: Mortality after parathyroidectomy is equal in male and in spayed female rats, whereas intact females are more resistant.

Foglia & Penhos B79,957/52: In male rats, extensive partial pancreatectomy causes severe diabetes more frequently than in females. Postnatal orchidectomy abolishes this difference.

Manunta B73,160/52: In orchidectomized rats, estradiol prolongs survival after thyroparathyroidectomy. A comparatively high resistance of intact females to parathyroidectomy is attributed to folliculoid hormones.

IONIZING RAYS ←

← Corticoids. It has been claimed that in the **mouse**, pretreatment with DOC offers some protection against total body X-irradiation, but subsequent studies have shown that the resistance so induced, if at all significant, is very moderate. Glucocorticoids have likewise little, if any, prophylactic action against ionizing rays.

On the other hand, cortisone may enhance the protective effect of heterologous bone marrow transplants by suppressing immune reactions against the grafted cells.

Severe X-irradiation greatly increases the sensitivity of the mouse to bacterial endotoxins and this effect is counteracted by shielding the adrenals or treatment with cortisone.

In the **rat**, the recovery of hemopoietic tissue after total body X-irradiation is impaired by cortisone. Furthermore, the protection against such irradiation that may be obtained by reduction of oxygen tension is counteracted by cortisone. The renal lesion induced by topical X-irradiation of the kidneys is aggravated, whereas the pulmonary fibrosis produced by X-irradiation of the lungs is diminished by cortisone.

In **rabbits**, cortisone allegedly increases topical X-ray resistance of the skin. Betamethasone partially inhibits X-ray damage to the nervous system in rabbits.

In **guinea pigs**, cortisone is said to offer some protection against total body X-irradiation.

It has also been claimed that in **man**, radiation sickness can be prevented by DOC or by glucocorticoids, and in a few patients, prednisolone appeared to have a beneficial effect upon radiation pneumonitis. The topical X-ray resistance of the skin is allegedly also increased by cortisone.

← **Testoids.** Several investigators claimed that testosterone and other testoids offer some protection to the **mouse** against total body X-irradiation, but others found this type of treatment ineffective or even harmful. These differences may be due to variations in dosage and timing. Pretreatment with testosterone is allegedly much more efficacious in this respect than treatment after exposure.

Similarly variable protective effects have been observed in the **rat, rabbit**, and several **other species.** Various testoid anabolics are not equally potent in this respect, but none appears to have been conspicuously efficacious in counteracting the radiation syndrome.

← **Luteoids.** Virtually all the published data are in agreement stating that progesterone and other luteoids do not offer protection against X-irradiation in any animal species.

← **Adrenalectomy.** In the mouse, the polydipsia, polyuria, and hepatic steatosis seen during the first days after total body X-irradiation tend to be inhibited by adrenalectomy, but these apparent improvements are actually due to the lack of defensive adrenocortical responses. Survival after X-irradiation is undoubtedly shortened by adrenalectomy.

← **Folliculoids.** Many publications deal with the effect of various folliculoids upon X-ray resistance in the **mouse**, but the results are very contradictory. It appears that, in general, pretreatment with folliculoids increases X-ray resistance, whereas treatment after irradiation has an inverse effect; however, the outcome of such experiments depends upon too many hitherto unidentified factors to permit precise evaluation. Among these modifying influences, the type of folliculoid used, the dosage, timing, intensity of irradiation, genetic predisposition and many others may be important.

Similarly contradictory results have been obtained in the **rat** and various **other species.**

← **Gonadectomy.** Several investigators agree that male mice are less resistant than females to total body X-irradiation, although after gonadectomy, the females are even more sensitive than the males. Male, unlike female rats, fed X-irradiated beef, die of internal hemorrhages, the severity of which is aggravated by testosterone.

← **Corticoids**

MOUSE

Ellinger 93,367/46: Pretreatment with DOC lessened fatty degeneration of the liver normally induced in mice by X-irradiation but only slightly decreased mortality, and failed to protect the bone marrow and spleen.

Ellinger 93,953/47: DOC reduces mortality in mice exposed to X-rays.

Ellinger B24,015/48: DOC offers some protection against total body X-irradiation in mice. Pregnenolone is ineffective in this respect.

Ellinger B57,402/48: In mice, DOC increases resistance to X-irradiation.

Graham & Graham A49,307/49: In mice, testosterone, estradiol, stilbestrol, and DOC did not significantly alter resistance to X-radiation whereas horse serum i.p. offers considerable protection.

Straube et al. B39,082/49: Neither DOC nor adrenocortical extract altered the X-ray resistance of intact or adrenalectomized mice.

Graham & Graham B58,164/50: Review of the literature, and personal observations on the effect of folliculoids, luteoids, testoids, adrenocortical extract, and DOC upon the resistance of the mouse to total body X-irradiation.

Graham et al. B48,335/50: Survival time is increased in mice given adrenocortical extract immediately after total body X-irradiation, whereas DOC, 11-dehydrocorticosterone (Kendall's Compound A), stilbestrol, and testosterone are inactive in this respect.

Smith et al. B47,642/50: In mice, neither ACTH nor cortisone increased survival following X-irradiation.

Mirand et al. B76,197/52: In mice exposed to X-irradiation of the head, both cortisone and DOC diminish mortality.

Ellinger B95,888/54: Review (8 pp., 54 refs.) on the effect of hormones upon X-ray sensitivity. In mice, DOC increases, whereas cortisone diminishes tolerance to ionizing rays.

Kaplan et al. B98,601/54: Review (40 pp., 107 refs.) on the role of folliculoids, corticoids, luteoids, and testoids in the development of radiation-induced lymphoid tumors of mice.

Betz C13,907/55: Pretreatment with DOC enhances the resistance of the mouse to X-irradiation, but treatment after exposure is ineffective. Cortisone does not protect, even if administered before X-irradiation. There is no obvious sex difference in X-ray resistance among mice. Pretreatment with testosterone offers definite protection, especially to females, but here again, its administration after exposure is without effect. Curiously, estradiol pretreatment also offers protection, whereas given after exposure, it actually decreases resistance.

Cole et al. C14,411/55: "The administration of cortisone may enhance the protective effect of rat bone marrow in X-irradiated mice."

Brenk C57,624/58: Cortisone failed to influence acute radiation lethality in mice, but delayed the appearance of diarrhea.

Skalka C71,368/59: In mice, the hepatic steatosis induced by X-irradiation is prevented by adrenalectomy, but restored by cortisone. DOC is ineffective in this respect.

Smith et al. E21,486/63: Exposure to severe X-irradiation greatly increases the sensitivity of mice to S. typhosa endotoxin, especially on the third day after irradiation. Shielding the adrenals, or treatment with cortisone counteracted the effect of X-irradiation. Shielding the abdominal cavity, but not the adrenals, was even more effective. Possibly, the protection of the intestines plays a decisive role here. "It might be conjectured that absorption of bacterial endotoxins from the intestinal lumen influences the time of the so-called intestinal death following high doses of radiation."

Cittadini et al. G76,028/70: In X-irradiated mice, the formation of hemopoietic islets in the spleen is inhibited by dexamethasone, ACTH, or the stress of exposure to cold.

Mistry et al. H33,481/70: In certain strains of mice, cortisol inhibits the induction of leukemia by X-rays.

RAT

Thiersch et al. B76,313/52: In rats, the recovery of hemopoietic tissues following total body X-irradiation is impaired by cortisone.

Stender & Hornykiewytsch C37,079/55: In rats, the lethal effect of total body X-irradiation is diminished by a reduction in the oxygen tension of the surrounding air. This protective action is counteracted by cortisone, adrenalectomy, and thyroxine.

Berdjis & Brown C45,470/57: In rats, the pulmonary fibrosis produced by local X-irradiation is diminished by cortisone.

Haley et al. C51,851/58: In rats, adrenocortical extract did not improve the decreased muscular efficiency induced by whole body X-irradiation.

Berdjis C83,954/60: In rats, the renal lesions produced by X-irradiation of both kidneys are aggravated by cortisone. "While the control kidneys showed no alterations, the cortisone-treated animals developed glomerulosclerosis with intercapillary thickening, capillary thrombosis, hyaline masses, and cystic formations. These lesions were more marked in the irradiated groups."

Bargon et al. G78,255/70: In rats, the renal damage, particularly the sclerosis produced by topical X-irradiation, is diminished by prednisolone.

Rabbit

Lehmann et al. C46,970/56: Both in the rabbit and in man, systemic treatment with cortisone increases the topical X-ray resistance of the skin.

Giordano & Invernizzi H5,873/68: In rabbits, X-ray damage to the nervous system can be partially inhibited by betamethasone.

Guinea Pig

Cervini & Longo C9,357/55: Cortisone appears to have offered some protection against total body X-irradiation in guinea pigs.

Man

Ellinger et al. B44,439/49: In patients, radiation sickness can be prevented by DOC.

Painter & Brues B39,627/49: Discussion on the use of corticoids in combating the radiation syndrome.

Douglas C78,775/59: In a few patients with radiation pneumonitis, prednisolone had a beneficial effect.

← *Testoids*

Mouse

Graham & Graham A49,307/49: In mice, testosterone, estradiol, stilbestrol, and DOC did not significantly alter resistance to X-irradiation, whereas horse serum i.p. offers considerable protection.

Patt et al. B32,806/49: In mice, estradiol benzoate greatly enhances resistance to total body X-irradiation. Progesterone and testosterone are ineffectual. The protective action of folliculoids may be mediated through the adrenals.

Patt et al. B43,570/49: In mice, estradiol, unlike testosterone or progesterone, offers significant protection against total body X-irradiation.

Ellinger B49,654/50: Mortality following total body X-irradiation was greatly increased in mice by daily treatment with testosterone begun after exposure.

Graham et al. B48,335/50: Survival time is increased in mice given adrenocortical extract immediately after total body X-irradiation, whereas DOC, 11-dehydrocorticosterone (Kendall's Compound A), stilbestrol, and testosterone are inactive in this respect.

Langendorff & Koch B98,043/54: Male mice are more sensitive than females to X-irradiation but after gonadectomy, females are more sensitive than males. Castration increases radiosensitivity in females and decreases it in males. Estradiol causes no further increase in the radioresistance of the castrate male. Unexpectedly, after administration of testosterone, the radioresistance of females increases far beyond the norm.

Betz C13,907/55: Pretreatment with DOC enhances the resistance of the mouse to X-irradiation, but treatment after exposure is ineffective. Cortisone does not protect, even if administered before X-irradiation. There is no obvious sex difference in X-ray resistance among mice. Pretreatment with testosterone offers definite protection especially to females, but here again, its administration after exposure is without effect. Curiously, estradiol pretreatment also offers protection, whereas given after exposure it actually decreases resistance.

Loewit G23,765/64: In mice, pretreatment with decadurabolin (19-nortestosterone-decanoate) offers considerable protection against total body X-irradiation.

Ogandzhanyan et al. F7,045/64: In the mouse, survival after total body X-irradiation is diminished by pretreatment with stilbestrol, and uninfluenced by testosterone.

Rat

Darcis & Brisbois C50,953/57: In the rat, the sensitivity of the small intestine to topical X-irradiation (unlike that of the vagina) is not influenced by thyroxine or testosterone.

Oliva & Valli C50,803/58: In rats exposed to severe total body X-irradiation, the survival time was only slightly prolonged by pretreatment with estrone, stilbestrol, or testosterone. Progesterone was ineffective.

Hotterbeex & Darcis C75,318/59: In rats, the topical damage produced in the rectum or vagina by local X-irradiation is aggravated following testosterone pretreatment.

Ghys & Loiselle C83,564/60: Testosterone protects female rats against total body X-irradiation, rapid neutron rays, or radioactive phosphorus. In males, this effect is actually reversed.

Malhotra & Reber C83,177/60: A high percentage of rats fed X-irradiated meat developed a hemorrhagic syndrome with prolonged prothrombin time. Testosterone increases, whereas stilbestrol decreases the severity of the syndrome in both intact and gonadectomized males.

Szold C80,607/60: 19-Norandrostenolone offers moderate protection against X-irradiation in the rat.

Ghys D70,483/62: In hypophysectomized rats, sensitivity to cobalt irradiation is greatly increased by testosterone and estradiol.

Caprino & Gallina G10,521/63: In the rat, norandrostenolone phenylpropionate enhances anabolism and recovery after total body X-irradiation.

Ghys D54,640/63: Review of the literature on the effect of ovariectomy, orchidectomy, estradiol, and testosterone upon resistance of the rat to total body X-irradiation.

Malhotra & Reber E36,906/63: Male, unlike female rats, fed X-irradiated beef, die of internal hemorrhage, the severity and lethality of which can be aggravated by testosterone. The literature on the effect of sex, castration, and stilbestrol upon the lethality of irradiated beef feeding is discussed.

Danysz & Panek F61,858/65: Methylandrostenolone protects young rats against total body X-irradiation.

Danysz et al. G38,389/65: "A radioprotective effect in rats, resulting in an increase in the LD_{50} was found after a continuous application of methandrostenolone (1 mg/kg)."

Danysz & Panek G57,847/68: Methandrostenolone (Dianabol) protects the rat against X-irradiation.

Vodicka & Dostál G69,171/68: Nandrolone reduces the polyuria in female X-irradiated rats during the first day, but has no effect on the negative nitrogen balance or the loss of body weight.

Picha G70,118/69: In rats and mice, methenolone reduces body weight loss and increases survival following X-irradiation. These anabolics also abet the radio-protective effect in man.

RABBIT

Mairesse & Darcis D27,579/62: Testosterone increases, whereas ovariectomy decreases the resistance of the buccal mucosa to X-irradiation in rabbits.

Horváth & Horváth G55,076/68: The delay in the effect of X-irradiation upon the healing of bone fractures in rabbits is counteracted by nandrolone phenpropionate.

← *Luteoids*

Straube et al. B33,113/48: In mice, pretreatment with estradiol benzoate increases resistance to total body X-irradiation, whereas treatment on the day of irradiation has an opposite effect. Progesterone is ineffectual.

Patt et al. B32,806/49: In mice, estradiol benzoate greatly enhances resistance to total body X-irradiation. Progesterone and testosterone are ineffectual. The protective action of folliculoids may be mediated through the adrenals.

Patt et al. B43,570/49: In mice, estradiol, unlike testosterone or progesterone, offers significant protection against total body X-irradiation.

Graham & Graham B58,164/50: Review of the literature, and personal observations on the effect of folliculoids, luteoids, testoids, adrenocortical extract, and DOC upon the resistance of the mouse to total body X-irradiation.

Kaplan et al. B98,601/54: Review (40 pp., 107 refs.) on the role of folliculoids, corticoids, luteoids, and testoids in the development of radiation-induced lymphoid tumors of mice.

Rigat C10,747/55: Review (46 pp., 67 refs.) on the literature concerning the effect of hormones upon X-irradiation with special reference to ACTH, STH, vasopressin, epinephrine, cortisone, DOC, testosterone, estradiol, progesterone, and thyroxine.

Oliva & Valli C50,803/58: In rats exposed to severe total body X-irradiation, the survival time was only slightly prolonged by pretreatment with estrone, stilbestrol, or testosterone. Progesterone was ineffective.

Rooks E4,589/64: Review (10 pp., 46 refs.) on protection by hormones against X-irradiation in mammals. In general, folliculoids (particularly estradiol), and DOC exhibit a good radio-protective effect whereas glucocorticoids, testoids and luteoids, do not.

← *Adrenalectomy*

Smith & Tyree C12,045/56: In rats, the polydipsia and polyuria seen during the first days after X-irradiation tend to be inhibited by adrenalectomy or hypophysectomy.

Skalka C71,368/59: In mice, the hepatic steatosis induced by X-irradiation is prevented by adrenalectomy, but restored by cortisone. DOC is ineffective in this respect.

Etoh & Egami G11,664/63: In goldfish, resistance to X-irradiation is greatly diminished both by adrenalectomy and by hypophysectomy.

← Folliculoids

MOUSE

Treadwell et al. A56,593/43: In mice, pretreatment with estradiol diminished mortality following total body X-irradiation, whereas administration of the hormone after irradiation had a contrary result.

Straube et al. B33,113/48: In mice, pretreatment with estradiol benzoate increases resistance to total body X-irradiation, whereas treatment on the day of irradiation has an opposite effect. Progesterone is ineffectual.

Graham & Graham A49,307/49: In mice, testosterone, estradiol, stilbestrol, and DOC did not significantly alter resistance to X-radiation, whereas horse serum i.p. offers considerable protection.

Patt et al. B32,806/49: In mice, estradiol benzoate greatly enhances resistance to total body X-irradiation. Progesterone and testosterone are ineffectual. The protective action of folliculoids may be mediated through the adrenals.

Patt et al. B43,570/49: In mice, estradiol, unlike testosterone or progesterone, offers significant protection against total body X-irradiation.

Graham et al. B48,335/50: Survival time is increased in mice given adrenocortical extract immediately after total body X-irradiation, whereas DOC, 11-dehydrocorticosterone (Kendall's Compound A), stilbestrol, and testosterone are inactive in this respect.

Langendorff & Koch B98,043/54: Male mice are more sensitive than females to X-irradiation but after gonadectomy, females are more sensitive than males. Castration increases radiosensitivity in females and decreases it in males. Estradiol causes no further increase in the radioresistance of the castrate male. Unexpectedly, after administration of testosterone, the radioresistance of females increases far beyond the norm.

Betz C13,907/55: Pretreatment with DOC enhances the resistance of the mouse to X-irradiation, but treatment after exposure is ineffective. Cortisone does not protect, even if administered before X-irradiation. There is no obvious sex difference in X-ray resistance among mice. Pretreatment with testosterone offers definite protection especially to females, but here again, its administration after exposure is without effect. Curiously, estradiol pretreatment also offers protection, whereas given after exposure it actually decreases resistance.

Rugh & Wolff C19,209/56: Female mice are more resistant to total body X-irradiation than are males. Orchidectomy augments resistance, and this is further increased by treatment with estradiol. In intact males, estradiol raises X-ray resistance to the same level as in castrates.

Nuzhdin et al. D5,866/60: In mice, diethylstilbestrol offered practically no protection against the induction of gonadal atrophy by X-irradiation.

Kohn et al. D9,831/61: In the mouse, even minute doses of estradiol valerianate increase the mortality caused by total body X-irradiation.

Kohn et al. D42,858/62: Pretreatment with estradiol-17β-n-valerianate increases the mortality of mice exposed to X-irradiation.

Ogandzhanyan et al. F7,045/64: In the mouse, survival after total body X-irradiation is diminished by pretreatment with stilbestrol and uninfluenced by testosterone.

Rugh et al. F21,653/64: In ICR and CF1 mice, post-irradiation orchidectomy increased survival time, and estradiol caused a further prolongation of it; yet, the effects depended upon the time lapse between treatment and irradiation.

Flemming & Langendorff G38,381/65; Langendorff & Langendorff G42,801/66: In female mice, resistance to total body X-irradiation is greater than in males, and it can be increased in both sexes by natural and synthetic folliculoids.

Thompson et al. G44,654/67: In mice, estradiol or estriol administered two weeks after sublethal X-irradiation induced excessive mortality.

Jenkins et al. H27,688/69: In mice, treatment with estradiol during repopulation of the spleen after X-irradiation reduced the number of myelocytic colonies and increased the numbers of erythropoietic and undifferentiated colonies.

Thompson et al. G70,145/69: In mice, comparative studies were performed on the protection against total body X-irradiation offered by pretreatment with various folliculoids (esters of estradiol, estriol and estrone) in relation to their effect upon hemopoietic tissues. Earlier literature indicates a decreased X-ray resistance due to folliculoids given after X-irradiation, and an enhanced resistance induced by pretreatment with them.

RAT

Oliva & Valli C 50,803/58: In rats exposed to severe total body X-irradiation the survival time was only slightly prolonged by pretreatment with estrone, stilbestrol, or testosterone. Progesterone was ineffective.

Malhotra & Reber C 83,177/60: A high percentage of rats fed X-irradiated meat developed a hemorrhagic syndrome with prolonged prothrombin time. Testosterone increases, whereas stilbestrol decreases the severity of the syndrome, both in intact and in gonadectomized males.

Ghys D 70,483/62: In hypophysectomized rats, sensitivity to cobalt irradiation is greatly increased by testosterone and estradiol.

Shellabarger et al. D 39,218/62: In female rats, the production of mammary cancers by X-irradiation is inhibited by diethylstilbestrol in doses which in themselves are not carcinogenic. T 3 did not influence carcinogenesis under these circumstances.

Malhotra & Reber E 36,906/63: Male, unlike female rats, fed X-irradiated beef, die of internal hemorrhage, the severity and lethality of which can be aggravated by testosterone. The literature on the effect of sex, castration, and stilbestrol upon the lethality of irradiated beef feeding is discussed.

Akoev et al. F 73,202/66: Both stilbestrol and thyroid extract offered some protection against ^{60}Co γ-radiation in rats.

Mitznegg et al. G 77,075/70: In rats, pregnancy protects against X-irradiation, presumably through the increased production of endogenous folliculoids. Combined treatment with clomiphene blocks the protective effect of pregnancy perhaps because it counteracts the action of folliculoids.

Segaloff & Maxfield H 36,188/71: In rats, combined treatment with X-irradiation and diethylstilbestrol causes a higher incidence of mammary carcinoma than either of these agents alone.

← **Gonadectomy**

Langendorff & Koch B 98,043/54: Male mice are more sensitive than females to X-irradiation but after gonadectomy, females are more sensitive than males. Castration increases radiosensitivity in females and decreases it in males. Estradiol causes no further increase in the radioresistance of the castrate male. Unexpectedly, after administration of testosterone, the radioresistance of females increases far beyond the norm.

Rugh & Wolff C 19,209/56: Female mice are more resistant to total body X-irradiation than are males. Orchidectomy augments resistance, and this is further increased by treatment with estradiol. In intact males, estradiol raises X-ray resistance to the same level as in castrates.

Langendorff et al. C 36,885/57: Male mice are much more sensitive to X-irradiation than females. Orchidectomy increases resistance.

Kepp & Hofmann C 65,530/59: In rats, resistance to whole body X-irradiation is increased by ovariectomy.

Cronkite et al. C 81,609/60: In female rats, total body X-irradiation caused a high percentage of mammary carcinomas. Shielding the ovaries, or transplanting nonexposed ovaries into ovariectomized irradiated rats, did not significantly reduce the incidence of mammary neoplasms.

Mairesse & Darcis D 27,579/62: Testosterone increases, whereas ovariectomy decreases the resistance of the buccal mucosa to X-irradiation in rabbits.

Ghys D 54,640/63: Review of the literature on the effect of ovariectomy, orchidectomy, estradiol, and testosterone upon resistance of the rat to total body X-irradiation.

Hamilton et al. D 64,060/63: Male mice survived γ-irradiation somewhat longer than females. Orchidectomy has no effect upon the survival time, but ovariectomy slightly prolongs it.

Huggins & Fukunishi E 35,442/63: In rats, mammary tumors induced by DMBA or by X-irradiation regress following ovariectomy. "Tumors of this sort are, by definition, hormone-dependent."

Malhotra & Reber E 36,906/63: Male, unlike female rats, fed X-irradiated beef, die of internal hemorrhage, the severity and lethality of which can be aggravated by testosterone. The literature on the effect of sex, castration, and stilbestrol upon the lethality of irradiated beef feeding is discussed.

Rugh et al. F 21,653/64: In ICR and CF1 mice, post-irradiation orchidectomy increased survival time and estradiol caused a further prolongation of it but the effects depended upon the time lapse between treatment and irradiation.

← *Other Steroids*

Ellinger B24,015/48: DOC offers some protection against total body irradiation in mice. Pregnenolone is ineffective in this respect.

Ghys D30,012/62: Review of the literature, and personal observations on the effect of various steroid hormones on the survival of rats exposed to total body X-irradiation.

REVIEWS

Graham & Graham B58,164/50: Review of the literature, and personal observations on the effect of folliculoids, luteoids, testoids, adrenocortical extract, and DOC upon the resistance of the mouse to total body X-irradiation.

Kaplan et al. B98,601/54: Review (40 pp., 107 refs.) on the role of folliculoids, corticoids, luteoids and testoids in the development of the radiation-induced lymphoid tumors of mice.

Rigat C10,747/55: Review (46 pp., 67 refs.) on the literature concerning the effect of hormones upon X-irradiation, with special reference to ACTH, STH, vasopressin, epinephrine, cortisone, DOC, testosterone, estradiol, progesterone, and thyroxine.

Ghys & Loiselle C83,564/60: Review on the radio-protective effect of DOC.

Ghys D54,640/63: Review of the literature on the effect of ovariectomy, orchidectomy, estradiol, and testosterone upon resistance of the rat to total body X-irradiation.

Kandror E27,416/63: Review of the literature on the effect of corticoids and ACTH upon total body X-irradiation, especially in connection with the physiopathology of stress.

Davydova F23,736/64: Review and personal observations on the effect of folliculoids and testoids upon radiation injury.

Rooks E4,589/64: Review (10 pp., 46 refs.) on protection by hormones against X-irradiation in mammals. In general, folliculoids (particularly estradiol), and DOC exhibit a good radio-protective effect, whereas glucocorticoids, testoids, and luteoids, do not.

Danysz & Kocmierska-Grodzka F84,845/67: Review of the literature on the radio-protective action of folliculoids and testoids with personal observations on a prophylactic effect of methandrostenolone (Dianabol).

ULTRAVIOLET RAYS ←

The hepatic lysosomal proteases of the rat are released by ultraviolet irradiation in vitro, and this effect is diminished by glucocorticoid pretreatment of the animals in vivo.

Endotoxin treatment in vivo facilitates the subsequent release of hepatic lysosomal enzymes by ultraviolet irradiation in rabbits, and here again, cortisone exerts a stabilizing effect.

The damage caused to fetal rat skin explants by ultraviolet irradiation can be inhibited by the addition of cortisol to the culture medium. This protection has also been ascribed to the stabilization of lysosomes by the glucocorticoid.

Graham A61,343/43: In dogs, the hypotension produced by carbon arc irradiation (about 6% ultraviolet, 30% luminous and 64% infrared rays) could be prevented by DOC or adrenocortical extract, both in the presence and in the absence of the adrenals.

Weissmann & Dingle D14,268/61: The hepatic lysosomal proteases of the rat are released by ultraviolet irradiation in vitro, and this effect is greatly diminished by pretreatment of the animals with cortisol in vivo.

Weissmann & Fell D46,242/62: The damage caused to fetal rat skin explants by ultraviolet irradiation can be inhibited by the addition of cortisol to the culture medium. This protection "might be due, at least in part, to a reduced proteolytic activity in the damaged tissue through a stabilising action of the hormone on the lysosomes."

Weissmann & Thomas D23,630/62: Following endotoxin treatment in vivo, the hepatic lysosomes of the rabbit release their enzymes readily upon ultraviolet irradiation. This increased lability is in turn prevented by a three day pretreatment of the animals with cortisone before endotoxin administration. Apparently "one action of endotoxin is to release acid hydrolases from particulate form within cells, and that glucocorticoids serve to stabilize such particles against injury by several agents."

Janoski et al. E7,896/68 (p. 280): Review suggesting that many of the actions of glucocorticoids, particularly their inhibition of ultraviolet ray injury, vitamin-A overdosage, and endotoxin shock are due to the stabilization of lysosomal membranes which prevents the escape of toxic lysosomal enzymes.

HEMORRHAGE ←

In the **dog**, early experiments with adrenocortical extracts revealed no significant protection against hemorrhagic shock, but infusion of cortisol (especially in the form of its water soluble sodium hemisuccinate) 30 min after bloodletting prevented the hypotension. If aldosterone is added to the shed blood before reinfusing it, resistance to the production of hemorrhagic shock is likewise greatly increased.

In the **cat**, large doses of cortisone and dexamethasone given i.v. prior to the induction of hemorrhagic shock also prolonged survival after reinfusion of all shed blood. Aldosterone was apparently ineffective here.

In **rats** with hemorrhagic shock induced by maintaining the arterial blood pressure at 35 mm Hg for 4 hrs, large amounts of dexamethasone, cortisol, aldosterone and methylprednisolone prolonged survival, allegedly in decreasing order of activity, but since each hormone was given in different amounts, it is difficult to make comparisons between them.

Even in rats submitted to "irreversible" hemorrhagic shock followed 4 hrs later by reinfusion of the shed blood, survival time is prolonged if glucocorticoids are added to the blood transfusate.

Under special circumstances, resistance to hemorrhagic shock could also be improved by glucocorticoids in the **rabbit** and **monkey**.

Dog

Fine et al. A56,268/42: In intact dogs, adrenocortical extract is moderately effective, and DOC completely ineffective, in combating hemorrhagic shock.

Huizenga et al. A54,816/43; A59,447/43: Adrenocortical extract fails to protect intact dogs against death from hemorrhagic shock.

Connolly et al. D57,333/58; Connolly C78,861/59: In dogs, cortisol given i.v. within 30 min after induction of hemorrhagic shock is highly effective in preventing the drop of blood pressure.

Kuhn et al. C67,681/59: Exposure to cold increases the resistance of the dog to hemorrhagic shock, and this resistance is not affected by concurrent treatment with cortisone.

Hakstian et al. D10,396/61: Review of the literature, and personal observations on the control of hemorrhagic shock in dogs, by cortisol alone or in association with pressor amines.

Zapata-Ortiz & de la Mata D37,373/62: In dogs, mortality from hemorrhagic shock is greatly reduced when aldosterone is added to the reinfused blood. "Natural secretion of aldosterone probably plays an important role in the evolution of shock."

Lillehei et al. E37,842/64: Review, and personal observations on the beneficial effect of cortisol in hemorrhagic and endotoxin shock, mainly based on experiments in the dog.

Cat

Lefer & Martin H7,806/69: In cats, "pharmacologic doses of cortisol or dexamethasone given intravenously prior to induction of hemorrhagic shock prolonged survival significantly after reinfusion of all shed blood. High doses of aldosterone were ineffective in prolonging survival, as was cortisol when administered at the time of reinfusion. ... Glucocorticoids may prevent the disruption of lysosomes and/or prevent proteases from being released into the blood."

Glenn & Lefer H34,576/71: In cats subjected to hemorrhagic shock methylprednisolone increased survival time in proportion to a diminution of plasma levels of a myocardial depressant factor (MDF) and of the lysosomal enzymes, β-glucuronidase and plasma cathepsin-like activity (PCLA). Presumably, "methylprednisolone exerts a protective effect in hemorrhagic shock by preventing the release of lysosomal enzymes which may be responsible for the formation of MDF, a peptide implicated in the reduction of myocardial contractility during postoligemic shock."

RAT

Weil & Whigham F 13,600/64: Various corticoids differ in their potency to combat hemorrhagic shock in the rat. "Significantly better results were obtained with dexamethasone than with hydrocortisone in terms of early alertness and survival at the end of seven days ($p < 0.01$). Ten of 20 animals treated with methylprednisolone survived ($p < 0.001$). The largest of the three doses of d-aldosterone gave the best results with survival of six of ten rats ($p < 0.03$)."

Weil et al. F 48,510/65; F 61,024/65: In rats hemorrhagic shock was produced by maintaining the blood pressure at 30 mm Hg for 4 hrs followed by reinfusion of the withdrawn blood. Dexamethasone (8 mg/kg) given at the completion of the bleeding period kept all animals alive, whereas all untreated controls died. Cortisol and methylprednisolone were less effective, but even aldosterone offered some protection, though only over a narrow dose range.

Bouyard & Klein G 41,843/66: In rats submitted to "irreversible" hemorrhagic shock, followed 4 hrs later by reinfusion of the removed blood, the addition of various glucocorticoids (methylprednisolone, triamcinolone, dexamethasone or betamethasone) to the blood transfusate increases the survival rate.

Weil & Whigham F 52,838/65; Whigham F 75,787/67: In rats with intact adrenals, hemorrhagic shock was produced by maintaining the arterial pressure at 35 mm Hg for 4 hrs. When large amounts of corticoids were administered after blood reinfusion, survival was prolonged by dexamethasone, cortisol, d-aldosterone, and methylprednisolone in decreasing order of activity. [However, since each hormone was given in different amounts, comparisons are difficult. Aldosterone was effective only within a narrow dose range of around 0.4 mg/kg, both lower and higher doses being ineffective (H.S.).]

RABBIT

Telivuo & Louhimo G 39,506/66: In rabbits, mortality from hemorrhagic shock was only moderately diminished by concurrent treatment with cortisol i.v.

Palmerio & Fine G 66,810/69: Rabbits "that recover from an otherwise lethal degree of hemorrhagic shock with the help of special therapy (dexamethasone plus antibiotic) tolerate a subsequent exposure to the same degree of hemorrhagic shock without the need for such therapy."

MONKEY

Schumer G 64,570/69: In Rhesus monkeys, survival from hemorrhagic shock is prolonged by dexamethasone i.v.

HYPOXIA AND HYPEROXYGENATION ←

← **Corticoids.** In the **rat**, several early investigators succeeded in prolonging survival under anoxic conditions by treatment with adrenocortical extract. Death from lack of oxygen in closed vessels is accelerated by T3 and retarded by cortisone. Furthermore, the decreased altitude tolerance of thyroxine treated rats is counteracted by cortisol.

In **guinea pigs**, small doses of cortisone increase, whereas large doses decrease resistance to oxygen deficiency. The enhanced susceptibility to hypoxia induced by morphine is counteracted by pretreatment with ACTH or cortisone.

Early investigators claimed that in the **mouse**, adrenocortical extracts, unlike pure glucocorticoids or DOC, increase resistance to hypoxia, but more recent observations suggest that cortisone also improves survival at all but the very highest simulated altitudes tested.

In **man**, cortisone likewise raises resistance to various manifestations of anoxemia.

← **Adrenalectomy.** In rats, adrenalectomy greatly increases sensitivity to anoxia, and cortisol restores it towards normal. On the other hand, it has been claimed that adrenalectomy can give definite protection against the central nervous system manifestations and the lung edema characteristic of oxygen poisoning. Adrenocortical extract and cortisol — unlike cortisone and DOC — allegedly augment the susceptibility of adrenalectomized animals to hyperoxygenation.

← **Folliculoids, Testoids, Gonadectomy.** Estradiol and stilbestrol are ineffective in altering the resistance of the rat to anoxia. Females are allegedly more resistant than males, but this difference is ascribed to the larger size of the female adrenal, and not to any specific activity of the ovaries; indeed, ovariectomy is said to increase resistance to anoxia in the rat.

In hens, tolerance to acute hypoxia is allegedly enhanced by testosterone, and decreased by stilbestrol.

← *Corticoids* cf. also Selye B40,000/50, p. 67.

RAT

Dorrance et al. A38,460/42: Neither a potent adrenocortical extract nor DOC altered the work performance of intact rats under anoxic conditions.

Johnson et al. 96,626/43: The altitude tolerance is increased by adrenocortical extract in adrenalectomized, but not in intact rats.

Britton & Kline 93,980/45: Adult female rats are much more resistant to anoxia than males, perhaps because their adrenals are larger. Adrenocortical extract raises resistance to anoxia, whereas DOC does not.

Thorn et al. B335/45: Adrenocortical extract increased the survival of normal rats exposed to reduced barometric pressure.

Keminger G42,501/66: In rats, death from lack of oxygen in closed vessels is accelerated by T3, and retarded after thyroidectomy or cortisone treatment. Epinephrine further accelerates mortality in hyperthyroid animals.

Debias F69,410/66: The decreased altitude tolerance of thyroxine-treated rats is counteracted by cortisol.

GUINEA PIG

Arnould et al. C12,257/55: The resistance of guinea pigs to reduced oxygen pressure is raised by pretreatment with cortisone i.p.

Volterrani C64,384/57: In guinea pigs, tolerance to hypoxia is decreased by cortisone, but increased by ACTH pretreatment.

Volterrani C64,385/57: In guinea pigs, small doses of cortisone enhanced whereas large doses diminished, resistance to reduced oxygen tension.

Sobel et al. C90,836/60: Morphine increases the mortality of guinea pigs exposed to reduced oxygen tension. Prior administration of cortisone or ACTH protects against this combined treatment.

MOUSE

Kottke et al. B25,989/48: Resistance to hypoxia is increased in mice by adrenocortical extract, but not by DOC. The effect of the extract is not ascribed to glucocorticoids, since other investigators found cortisone to be inactive.

Berry et al. H2,124/68: Studies on the influence of hypoxia, glucocorticoids, and endotoxin on hepatic enzyme induction and survival in mice. "Endotoxin inhibited the induction of tryptophan oxygenase, prevented the increase in liver glycogen, induced the transaminase, and increased the lethality of simulated altitude. Cortisone increased survival at all altitudes except the highest. These observations emphasize the importance of these metabolic adjustments for the survival of animals subjected to hypoxic stress."

MAN

Frawley et al. B57,930/51: In man both cortisone and ACTH improve high altitude tolerance.

Tabusse et al. C10,563/54: Cortisone increases resistance to various manifestations of anoxemia (inhalation of 7.5% nitrogen in air) as seen in human volunteers, but simultaneously aggravates the characteristic EEG changes.

← *Adrenalectomy*

Taylor C47,861/58: In rats "adrenalectomy gave very definite protection against the central nervous system manifestations of oxygen poisoning, and gave some protection against lung damage." Adrenocortical extract and cortisol enhanced the susceptibility of adrenalectomized animals to oxygen poisoning, whereas cortisone, DOC, and thyroid powder had no such effect.

DeBias & Wang-Yen D22,848/62: In rats, adrenalectomy greatly increases sensitivity to hypobaric oxygenation, but cortisol treatment restores it towards normal.

← Folliculoids, Testoids, Gonadectomy

Britton & Kline 93,980/45: Adult female rats are much more resistant to anoxia than males, perhaps because their adrenals are larger. Adrenocortical extract raises resistance to anoxia, whereas DOC does not. Ovariectomy increases resistance to anoxia.

Goldsmith et al. B333/45: Thiouracil and thiourea enhance the resistance of rats to lowered barometric pressure. Estradiol and stilbestrol are ineffective in themselves and fail to influence the action of the antithyroid compounds.

Kline & Britton 85,856/45: At 16° C, female rats withstand anoxia longer than males. At higher temperatures, the difference is less pronounced. "Estrous conditions and estrogens, castration, etc., do not appear related to the different responses."

Burton et al. G67,617/69: In hens, tolerance to acute hypoxia of high altitude is increased by testosterone, and decreased by diethylstilbestrol.

TEMPERATURE VARIATIONS ←

A very large number of publications deals with the effects of steroids upon resistance to heat or cold environments, or to local burning and freezing. These findings will be discussed together.

← Corticoids

Heat ←. The earliest observations suggested that, in **rabbits**, treatment with adrenocortical extract increases resistance to high surrounding temperatures.

In **mice**, neither adrenocortical extract nor DOC offered significant protection against fatal burns, and in fact, cortisone enhanced mortality after scalding.

In the **rat**, it is likewise impossible to obtain any significant protection against burn shock by pretreatment with adrenocortical extracts or DOC, although some investigators asserted that, if applied before the burn, DOC is effective in this respect. The action of cortisone and cortisol upon the rat's ability to withstand "heat stress" has not been clearly established, some investigators claiming to have obtained positive, others negative results.

In **dogs**, adrenocortical extract offered no protection against burn shock.

In a small group of **men**, acclimatization to heat was not significantly improved by DOC.

Cold ←. In intact **rats**, neither DOC nor adrenocortical extract raised resistance to burn shock significantly. Cold tolerance was likewise not considerably altered by adrenocortical extract, cortisone or DOC, but the improvement of survival obtained by thyroxine was further ameliorated by conjoint treatment with cortisone or corticosterone.

Some increase in cold tolerance has also been obtained in rats by intermittent or prolonged pretreatment with cortisone, prednisone or prednisolone.

In the **mouse**, injection of H. pertussis enhanced sensitivity to "cold stress" even more than does adrenalectomy. Cortisone and cortisol protect the pertussis-treated mouse against cold, and to some extent, cortisol also raises the cold resistance of normal mice.

← Folliculoids, Testoids, Gonadectomy

Contrary to earlier claims, neither ovariectomy nor orchidectomy changes the heat resistance of the **rabbit** significantly.

In **rats**, orchidectomy has been said to raise resistance to cold, yet, testosterone does not alter it in either intact or castrate males. In intact or spayed rats, restrained in a cold environment, the development of gastric ulcers is allegedly reduced by ovariectomy, but not influenced by estradiol.

← Adrenalectomy

Adrenalectomy greatly diminishes the resistance of various species against cold or heat, whereas treatment with adrenocortical extract, glucocorticoids and, to a lesser extent, mineralocorticoids, restore temperature resistance towards normal.

← Other Steroids

The acquisition of adaptation to heat is allegedly inhibited by spironolactone pretreatment in the rat, but once resistance is established, the compound does not counteract it. It has been concluded that hyperaldosteronism is necessary only for the acquisition, not for the maintenance of heat resistance.

← Corticoids

Heat ←. *Maddaloni A18,244/38:* Treatment with adrenocortical extract increases the resistance of the rabbit to a high surrounding temperature.

Rosenthal B26,228/43: Neither adrenocortical extract nor DOC protected mice against fatal burns.

Bergman et al. B2,009/45: In the mouse and rat, neither adrenocortical extracts nor DOC offered protection against shock caused by a standardized skin burn.

Ingle & Kuisenga 96,155/45: In intact rats, neither DOC nor adrenocortical extract raised the resistance to burn shock.

Cope et al. B52,084/49: In dogs, adrenocortical extracts offered no protection against burn shock.

Robinson et al. B56,828/50: In four men, acclimatization to heat was not significantly improved by DOC.

You & Sellers B46,218/50: The resistance of intact rats to severe burns was increased by DOC, but not by adrenocortical extract.

Neal et al. B80,371/52: The survival time of severely burned rats is not influenced by cortisone or ACTH, whereas DOC administered before the burn offers considerable protection.

Kar & De C72,791/55: Cortisone and cortisol failed to affect the ability of rats to withstand "heat stress" upon exposure to extremely warm surrounding temperatures.

Schöttler C8,455/55: Neither ACTH nor cortisone protects the mouse against the fatal effects of severe scalding; in fact, cortisone increases mortality.

Agarkov et al. D40,496/62: In intact rats, cortisone raises resistance to heat, whereas ACTH does not.

Cold ←. *Adolph B35,581/48:* Adrenocortical extract failed to increase the resistance of rats to cold exposure.

Sellers et al. B65,310/51: The survival of clipped rats exposed to cold is considerably prolonged by combined treatment with thyroxine + cortisone. Each of these agents alone has much less protective value, and DOC is inactive.

Kirsteins C41,958/56: Short-term administration of cortisone or ACTH to rats did not significantly influence cold tolerance, whereas long-term intermittent cortisone administration prior to cold exposure definitely raised tolerance in this respect.

Dufour & Dugal C26,092/57: In rats, resistance to cold is diminished by STH or DOC given in combination with vitamin C.

Munoz & Schuchardt C28,986/57: After an injection of H. pertussis cells, intact mice become even more sensitive to "cold stress" than untreated adrenalectomized mice. Cortisone and cortisol protect pertussis-treated mice against cold, but to a lesser degree than the adrenalectomized mice. Cortisol also increases the cold resistance of normal mice. "It is suggested that while pertussis possibly affects adrenal function, it must in addition affect other functions in the mouse which are also concerned with the protection against stress."

Garrido C77,562/59: In intact rats, prednisone and ACTH enhanced resistance to cold.

Garrido D8,112/60: In rats, resistance to cold is increased by thyroxine and T3, and decreased by thyroidectomy or destruction of the thyroid with radio-iodine. Prednisolone exerted only a moderate protective effect.

Araki G11,847/63: Pretreatment with ACTH or cortisol raises the resistance of intact mice to cold exposure. Nicotinamide has a similar effect which is ascribed to the stimulation of the pituitary-adrenal system.

Bauman & Turner F81,331/67: Pretreatment of rats with thyroxine enhanced their resistance to cold. Additional administration of corticosterone greatly increases this effect although, in itself, corticosterone possesses only a slight protective action.

← *Folliculoids, Testoids, Gonadectomy*

Barella B3,397/40: In rabbits, resistance to heat stroke is diminished by orchidectomy.

Gigante & Scopinaro B67,617/46: In man, testosterone improves the circulation of skin areas affected by frostbite.

Berde & Takács B31,943/48: In rabbits, ovariectomy does not change heat resistance (in contradiction to earlier claims by others).

Berde & Takács B38,366/48: In rabbits, orchidectomy does not alter heat tolerance.

Dugal & Saucier C53,333/58: In rats, orchidectomy raises resistance to cold.

Dugal & Saucier C77,621/58: Testosterone does not alter the resistance of intact or castrate male rats to cold.

Luther et al. G70,681/69: In rats restrained in a cold environment, the development of gastric ulcers is reduced by ovariectomy. Estradiol has no effect upon the induction of these ulcers in either intact or ovariectomized rats.

← *Adrenalectomy*

Selye & Schenker A15,353/38: Adrenalectomized rats are particularly sensitive to exposure to cold but their resistance is greatly (and dose-dependently) increased by pretreatment with adrenocortical extract. This fact is used as the basis of a sensitive test for corticoid activity.

Tyslowitz & Astwood 80,678/41: In hypophysectomized rats, the decreased resistance to cold is largely corrected by ACTH and adrenocortical extract. In adrenalectomized rats, adrenocortical extract is also effective in this respect, whereas ACTH is not.

Dufour et al. C12,151/55: In adrenalectomized rats, both STH and DOC improve survival following exposure to cold.

← *Other Steroids*

Henane & Laurent F71,731/66: The acquisition of adaptation to heat (swimming in hot baths) is inhibited by spironolactone pretreatment in the rat; but once adaptation is established, the anti-aldosterone does not counteract it. It is concluded that hyperaldosteronism is necessary only for the induction, not for the maintenance of heat adaptation.

ELECTRIC STIMULI ←

← **Corticoids.** In rats, DOC (like progesterone and several testoids) increases the EST, whereas glucocorticoids (e.g., cortisone, cortisol) have an opposite effect.

In mice, progesterone, DOC, and a series of related steroids inhibit electroshock seizures (as well as pentylenetetrazol convulsions).

In cats, DOC allegedly protects against cocaine convulsions, but has no effect upon the EST. On the other hand, cortisone increases the amplitude and maintenance of muscular responses to the electrical stimulation of the corresponding nerves in the cat. From experiments in which different types of macropotentials are recorded on single nerve cell discharges of the decerebrate cats, it was concluded that prednisolone increases the excitability of each nerve cell, but the effect is potentiated by multiple neuronal connections mediated through the reticular activating system.

← **Adrenalectomy.** In rats, the EST is lowered by adrenalectomy.

← **Folliculoids, Luteoids, Testoids, Gonadectomy.** The earliest observations suggested that in **guinea pigs**, orchidectomy does not influence the convulsions produced by electric irritation of peripheral nerves.

In **rats**, progesterone (like DOC and testosterone) increases the EST, whereas gonadectomy decreases it in both sexes.

In **mice**, progesterone (like DOC and various derivatives of pregnenolone) inhibits electroshock seizures. Lynestrenol reduces the anticonvulsive effect (tested by the EST) of various drugs.

← *Corticoids*

Spiegel 83,892/43: In rats DOC, progesterone and testosterone i.p. increase the EST.

Aird B683/44: DOC i.p. protected mice against cocaine induced convulsions but had no effect upon the EST of cats.

Spiegel & Wycis 93,925/45: Among 29 steroids tested, DOC, progesterone, testosterone, acetoxypregnenolone, androstenedione, and dehydroandrosterone increased the EST significantly in the rat.

Davenport B36,663/49: Adrenalectomized rats maintained on plain water show a decreased EST, which can be restored by NaCl or DOC, but not by KCl or $MgCl_2$. From plasma electrolyte determinations "it is concluded that the electroshock seizure threshold of the adrenalectomized rat is directly correlated with the plasma sodium level."

Woodbury & Davenport B37,243/49: In rats, DOC (like NaCl or $CaCl_2$ solutions) elevates the EST.

Woodbury et al. B46,344/50: In rats, DOC elevates the EST and its effect is counteracted by ACTH or adrenocortical extracts, possibly because of some antagonism between gluco- and mineralocorticoids.

Fingl et al. D38,091/52: In rats, chronic administration of phenobarbital or diphenylhydantoin diminishes the brain hyperexcitability induced by cortisone, as judged by EST measurements.

Pozo & Negrete B68,183/52: In cats, cortisone increases the amplitude and maintenance of muscular responses to electrical stimulation of the corresponding nerves.

Minz & Domino B81,852/53: In rats, small doses of epinephrine or norepinephrine prolong the duration of electrically-induced seizures. Since glucose, ACTH, and cortisone failed to prolong seizure duration, it is unlikely that epinephrine acts by release of these substances. Histamine depresses the cortical response to electroshock.

Woodbury B98,594/54: Review (42 pp., 90 refs.) on the "Effect of Hormones on Brain Excitability and Electrolytes." In the rat, the EST is increased by DOC and decreased by cortisone and cortisol. ACTH and 11-dehydrocorticosterone, given chronically, antagonize partially the effect of cortisone.

Woodbury et al. C34,538/57: Review (33 pp., 25 refs.) on the effect of corticoids upon the EST in the rat. Cortisone and cortisol decrease it (increased excitability), whereas DOC and, to a lesser extent, aldosterone increase it. Corticosterone and other corticoids have less pronounced effects.

Vallecalle et al. C93,280/60: The EST is decreased by gonadectomy both in male and in female rats. "Folliculin" lowers the EST, whereas testosterone raises it in both sexes. The increased CNS excitability induced by ovariectomy is corrected by cortisol, but not by "folliculin."

Schulte & ten Bruggencate D32,457/62: From experiments in which different types of macropotentials are recorded on single nerve cell discharges of decerebrate cats "it is concluded that Prednisolone increases the excitability of each single nerve cell but the effect is potentiated by multiple neuronal connections from nerve centers, in our experiments for example, from the reticular activating system."

Craig F69,385/66: In mice, progesterone, DOC, a series of 3β-(aminoalkyl) esters of pregnenolone, and various other steroids proved to inhibit pentylenetetrazol convulsions and electroshock seizures.

← *Adrenalectomy*

Davenport B36,663/49: Adrenalectomized rats maintained on plain water show a decreased EST, which can be restored by NaCl or DOC, but not by KCl or $MgCl_2$. From plasma electrolyte determinations "it is concluded that the electroshock seizure threshold of the adrenalectomized rat is directly correlated with the plasma sodium level."

de Salva et al. C51,842/58: In rats, the EST was lowered by hypophysectomy and adrenalectomy, but only insignificantly by thyroidectomy. 5-HT elevated the EST.

de Salva D66,176/63: In rats, the EST is reduced in descending order of magnitude by adrenalectomy, hypophysectomy, and thyroidectomy. The effect of these endocrine deficiencies upon various depressant drugs is also described.

← Folliculoids, Luteoids, Testoids, Gonadectomy

Specht 13,475/23: In guinea pigs, neither thyroidectomy nor orchidectomy influences the course of the convulsions produced by amyl nitrate inhalation or the electric irritation of peripheral nerves.

Spiegel 83,892/43: In rats DOC, progesterone, and testosterone i.p. increase the EST.

Spiegel & Wycis 93,925/45: Among 29 steroids tested, DOC, progesterone, testosterone, acetoxypregnenolone, androstenedione, and dehydroandrosterone increased the EST significantly in the rat.

Vallecalle et al. C93,280/60: The EST is decreased by gonadectomy both in male and in female rats. "Folliculin" lowers the EST, whereas testosterone raises it in both sexes. The increased CNS excitability induced by ovariectomy is corrected by cortisol, but not by "folliculin."

Craig F69,385/66: In mice, progesterone, DOC, a series of 3β-(aminoalkyl) esters of pregnenolone and various other steroids proved to inhibit pentylenetetrazol convulsions and electroshock seizures.

Blackham & Spencer G73,813/70: In mice, lynestrenol reduced, whereas mestranol or SKF 525-A increased the anticonvulsive effect (tested with electroshock) of diphenylhydantoin, phenobarbital, chlordiazepoxide, and diazepam administered i.p. after five days of pretreatment. This may be due to an altered microsomal drug metabolism, but since mestranol and lynestrenol have opposite effects upon brain 5-HT concentrations, the latter mechanism must also be considered.

← Other Steroids

Spiegel & Wycis 93,925/45: Among 29 steroids tested, DOC, progesterone, testosterone, acetoxypregnenolone, androstenedione, and dehydroandrosterone increased the EST significantly in the rat.

Craig F69,385/66: In mice, progesterone, DOC, a series of 3β-(aminoalkyl) esters of pregnenolone, and various other steroids proved to inhibit pentylenetetrazol convulsions and electroshock seizures.

SYSTEMIC TRAUMA ←

← **Corticoids.** In the rat, adrenocortical extract (Cortin) raises resistance to various forms of systemic trauma (intestinal crushing, formaldehyde injections, extensive partial hepatectomies), but its effect is not as pronounced in the presence as in the absence of the adrenals. The increased nonspecific stress resistance characteristic of the countershock phase in the G.A.S. is largely ascribed to an enhanced corticoid production. DOC is ineffective in this respect, whereas corticosterone (which differs from DOC only in the presence of an 11β-hydroxyl group) is highly effective. Apparently, 11-oxygenation of corticoids, with the associated induction of glucocorticoid potency, is an essential prerequisite for antistress activity.

Pretreatment with DOC inhibits adrenocortical enlargement during the alarm reaction produced by various stressors. This mineralocorticoid-induced "compensatory adrenal atrophy" diminishes resistance and particularly interferes with the hyperglycemic response to cold, formalin, atropine, surgical trauma or forced muscular exercise. It is concluded that "overdosage with one of the compounds produced by an endocrine cell can interfere with the production by the same cell of other hormonal compounds (in this case corticoids, such as corticosterone, active in carbohydrate metabolism)." On the other hand, pretreatment of rats with adrenocortical extract can increase their performance during forced muscular exercise, without previous training. Here, the adrenal hypertrophy is also prevented, but since a glucocorticoid preparation is administered, the protective effect against stress is nevertheless obvious.

However, adrenocortical extract, cortisone, corticosterone, and DOC proved to be singularly ineffective in protecting the rat against tourniquet shock. Resistance to the trauma of the Noble-Collip drum is considerably increased by adrenocortical extract or DOC in adrenalectomized, but only slightly in intact rats. In fact, some investigators claimed that in the presence of the adrenals, large doses of cortisone or prednisone actually diminish resistance to the trauma of the Noble-Collip drum. The catabolic effect of bone fractures is further aggravated by betamethasone.

Under suitable conditions of dosage, the gastric ulcers produced in rats by forced muscular exercise can be prevented by pretreatment with prednisolone, but not by DOC. This is remarkable because heavy overdosage with glucocorticoids is in itself conducive to gastric ulcer formation.

In dogs, both adrenocortical extract and DOC offer only a moderate protection if any against shock produced by tourniquet or muscle trauma. On the other hand, ischemic shock elicited by temporary occlusion of the thoracic aorta appears to be favorably influenced by cortisol, methylprednisolone and methylfluorocortisol (Me-F-COL).

In the **cat**, both ACTH and cortisone have been claimed to prolong survival following traumatic shock.

In the **goat**, cortisone had no influence upon survival after trauma, nor did it counteract the sensitizing effect of thyroxine.

In the **rabbit**, combined treatment with adrenocortical extract and DOC (unlike DOC alone) allegedly reduces mortality from the shock of intestinal manipulation.

The extensive literature on the effect of corticoids on traumatic shock in **man** has been discussed in our previous monographs. Let us add here only that recent observations in patients with cardiopulmonary bypass suggest that dexamethasone pretreatment improved the clinical condition as well as diminished serum β-glucuronidase and LDH levels. It was assumed that the postoperative complications of cardiopulmonary bypass may be related in part to disruption of lysosomal membranes which can be stabilized by the glucocorticoid during "circulatory stress."

← **Adrenalectomy.** The fact that adrenalectomy diminishes stress resistance in all species and that corticoid therapy restores it towards normal is well known and has been covered extensively in our earlier monographs. However, the interactions between adrenal catecholamines and corticoids in the restoration of systemic stress resistance have been considerably clarified by recent experiments from Brodie's laboratory. Here, complete blockade of sympathetic function, with maintenance of the adrenal cortex, has been compared with complete adrenalectomy, with or without substitution therapy by catecholamines or corticoids. From these observations, it was concluded that sympathetic stimulation is the first line of defense against the vasomotor disturbance elicited by endotoxin or histamine, whereas the lethal effect of formalin or tourniquet shock, which is also increased by adrenalectomy, is not increased by mere sympathetic blockade. Cortisone alone suffices to counteract the toxicity of these stressors in adrenalectomized rats. Apparently, "formalin and tourniquet shock is initiated by a mechanism which differs from that elicited by histamine and endotoxin and does not primarily involve the sympathetic system."

The gastric ulcers produced by forced muscular exercise are not considerably modified by adrenalectomy in the rat, although they can be prevented by prednisolone.

← **Testoids.** Much work has been done in an effort to combat the catabolism of nonspecific stress by anabolic steroids. It is true that postoperative recovery of body weight may be accelerated by such steroids; for example, in cholecystectomized women, methandrostenolone enhanced the weight increase. Yet, animal experiments suggest that the anticatabolic effect of anabolics is not wholly nonspecific. Methyltestosterone is very efficient in preventing the severe catabolism produced by overdosage with DHT or vitamin-D_2, but it is much less efficacious in protecting against body-weight loss due to undernutrition, estradiol or the osteolathyrism induced by AAN. The catabolism elicited by cortisol or by the neurolathyric compound IDPN was not influenced by this testoid.

In guinea pigs, the alkaline phosphatase changes characteristic of fatigue, after exhausting exercise, are not prevented by 4-chlorotestosterone, but their return to normal is accelerated.

Anabolics also influence local stress reactions. For example, in rats, 17-ethyl-19-nortestosterone promotes, whereas cortisone inhibits, repair in bone fractures (measured by ^{35}S uptake). The regeneration of crushed murine skeletal muscle is likewise delayed by cortisone and accelerated by methandienone or methandrostenolone. Anabolics are also said to inhibit the myopathy produced in rats by ligature of the aorta and subsequent cooling of the distal part of the body.

← **Folliculoids, Luteoids, Gonadectomy.** Pretreatment with estradiol allegedly decreases the resistance of the mouse against various stressors (formalin, cold) and facilitates the development of changes characteristic of the alarm reaction. In rats, audiogenic seizures are not significantly influenced by ovariectomy. However, testosterone, progesterone, and estradiol appear to increase the seizure incidence in naturally seizure-resistant rats, whereas in seizure-prone animals, they have an opposite effect.

The development of gastric ulcers in rats restrained in a cold environment is claimed to be reduced by ovariectomy, but uninfluenced by estradiol.

← **Other Steroids.** Spironolactone diminishes the performance of rats adapted to swim in warm surroundings, allegedly because of its anti-aldosterone effect.

← *Corticoids cf. also Selye B40,000/50, pp. 64—72, 108; B58,650/51, p. 54; G60,083/70, p. 358.*

RAT

Selye et al. A32,768/40: Review of the earlier literature on the ability of epinephrine and "cortin" to raise resistance against various stressors. Attention is called to the fact that whereas cortin is very effective in this respect in adrenalectomized animals, it rarely increases resistance above normal in the presence of the adrenals. The slight effect that cortical extracts do possess during severe shock is presumably due to the fact that "a condition of 'relative adrenal insufficiency' exists in organisms exposed to nonspecific damage." Following extensive partial hepatectomy in rats, "suitable cortin therapy prevents the hypochloraemia, and the decrease in blood volume and in blood sugar which are usually elicited by this intervention." In rats damaged by repeated s.c. injections of formaldehyde, cortical extract prevented the hypoglycemia and hypochloremia of severe shock, whereas DOC was virtually ineffective, in fact it aggravated the s.c. edema caused by formaldehyde. Chronic pretreatment with cortical hormones caused adrenal atrophy which counteracted their beneficial effect in protecting against stress. "These experiments should be interpreted as a warning against prolonged pretreatment with this substance in preparation for a surgical intervention." The best protective effect was obtained in rats with surgical shock produced by crushing of the intestines, if given repeated injections of cortical extract s.c. during the subsequent 24 hrs. An "Addendum" reports on similar experiments performed with corticosterone prepared for this purpose by E. C. Kendall. This compound, which differs from DOC only in that it possesses an 11β-hydroxyl group, proved to be especially effective in protecting the rat against traumatic shock caused by crushing of the intestines. [This was the first observation showing that 11-oxygenation of corticoids is required to endow them with antistress activity (H.S.).]

Selye & Dosne A 33,299/40: "Experiments in the rat indicate that pure corticosterone administered in aqueous solution is very effective in combating shock caused by surgical trauma and other means. Desoxycorticosterone is ineffective when tested under similar conditions. From this it appears that the hydroxyl group on carbon atom 11 is important for the shock-combating action of cortical steroids."

Korényi & Hajdu A 56,945/42: In rats, adrenocortical extract increases performance during forced muscular exercise without previous training. Simultaneously, the associated adrenal hypertrophy is prevented.

Noble & Collip A 56,107/42: Adrenocortical extract and DOC greatly raise the resistance of adrenalectomized rats to the trauma of the Noble-Collip drum. In intact rats, "cortin" and DOC as well as ACTH induce only a slight increase in resistance, under similar circumstances. "From a practical viewpoint the effects of adrenal preparations on this type of shock have been disappointing."

Root & Mann A 57,542/42: Adrenocortical extract did not significantly prolong survival of rats in tourniquet shock.

Selye & Dosne A 37,249/42: Pretreatment with DOC inhibits, but does not completely prevent the adrenocortical enlargement during the alarm reaction. Under these conditions, the mineralocorticoid-induced "compensatory adrenal atrophy" diminishes the resistance and particularly the hyperglycemic response to cold, formalin, atropine, trauma or forced muscular exercise. It is concluded that "overdosage with one of the compounds produced by an endocrine cell can interfere with the production by the same cell of other hormonal compounds (in this case corticoids, such as corticosterone, active in carbohydrate metabolism). As a result of this interference symptoms of overdosage with hormones produced by a certain endocrine cell type may coexist with signs of deficiency in the hormone production of that same cell."

Ingle A 59,854/43: In intact rats, survival from tourniquet shock was not improved by adrenocortical extract, cortisone, corticosterone or DOC.

McKenna & Zweifach C 27,414/56: Large doses of cortisone or prednisone, far from increasing, actually diminish the resistance of rats to the trauma of the Noble-Collip drum. This effect is ascribed to a depression of the RES function.

Schachter et al. C 63,544/59: In rats, pretreatment with cortisone, thyroxine or both these agents shortened survival after tourniquet shock.

Kulagin D 236/60: In rats with a crush syndrome produced by clamping a thigh, survival was enhanced by ACTH, cortisone and cortisol, whereas DOC aggravated the condition by increasing edema in the injured area.

Vennet & Schneewind D 23,294/62: In rats, mortality induced by trauma in the Noble-Collip drum was significantly reduced by treatment with cortisol, prednisolone, and 6α-methylprednisolone given i.p. immediately after removal from the drum.

Campbell et al. G 9,081/64: In the rat, the catabolic effect of a bone fracture is further increased by betamethasone.

da Vanzo F 19,865/64: Pretreatment with F-COL protects the rat against tourniquet shock.

Serkes et al. F 92,105/67: Cortisol administered to tourniquet traumatized rats in infusion fluid, lowered serum β-glucuronidase but did not prolong survival time. "Serum levels of beta-glucuronidase, presumed to reflect lysosomal enzyme release, did not correlate with survival."

Robert et al. G 74,748/70: In rats, the gastric ulcers produced by forced muscular exercise can be prevented by pretreatment with prednisolone, but neither adrenalectomy nor

DOC affects their development. The ulcers were more common in females than in males, and could be totally prevented by fasting.

Dog

Shleser & Asher A 56,711/42: In dogs, both adrenocortical extract and DOC exert a mildly protective effect against shock following ligature of one common internal iliac vein.

Bourque et al. A 57,912/43: Tourniquet shock is effectively combated in dogs by combined treatment with adrenocortical extract i.v. + NaCl s.c. Neither agent alone is effective.

Swingle et al. A 61,337/43: In nonadrenalectomized dogs, shock produced by tourniquet or trauma is not alleviated either by DOC or by adrenocortical extract.

Cleghorn B 2,571/47: In dogs, shock produced by muscle trauma is not alleviated by large amounts of adrenocortical extract unless treatment is initiated at an early stage.

Pisanty & Toscano C 30,049/56: In dogs, DOC, 17-hydroxycorticosterone, and ACTH injected before surgery reduced mortality but had no effect upon the onset of shock. Corticosterone was more effective.

Levin et al. C 82,785/60: In dogs, ischemic shock produced by temporary occlusion of the thoracic aorta is favorably influenced by cortisol, methylprednisolone and Me-F-COL.

Satori & Szabo E 21,902/63: Dexamethasone administered to dogs just before application, and again before the removal of a tourniquet, increases resistance to shock.

Cat

Khrabrova D 33,557/62: Both ACTH and cortisone prolong survival following traumatic shock in the cat.

Goat

Oppenheimer et al. C 50,563/58: In goats, traumatic shock reduces the capacity of the thyroid to concentrate iodine, but recently thyroidectomized animals showed no change in survival times, although pretreatment with thyroxine greatly sensitized them to traumatic shock. Cortisone had no effect upon survival following trauma nor did it counteract the aggravating effect of thyroxine.

Rabbit

Weil et al. 78,692/40: "Adrenal cortical extract and desoxycorticosterone acetate given together both before and after trauma without other therapy reduce the mortality from experimental shock after intestinal manipulation in normal (non-adrenalectomized) rabbits." DOC alone is ineffective.

Mouse

Perla et al. A 31,863/40: In mice and rats, pretreatment with NaCl in combination with DOC or adrenocortical extract increased resistance to histamine. Favorable results have also been obtained by DOC + NaCl in a few patients suffering from surgical shock.

Man

Replogle et al. G 40,447/66: In patients with cardiopulmonary bypass, dexamethasone pretreatment appeared to improve the clinical condition, and diminished the serum β-glucuronidase and LDH levels. It is assumed that postoperative complications following cardiopulmonary bypass may be related in part to damage of lysosome membranes and that "massive doses of dexamethasone may stabilize the lysosome membrane during periods of circulatory stress."

Varia

Sambhi et al. G 68,985/64: Review on the action of glucocorticoids and aldosterone in traumatic and endotoxin shock in animals and men.

← Adrenalectomy

Krawczak & Brodie H 25,296/70: In rats, complete blockade of sympathetic function can be achieved by demedullation combined with reserpine-like agents (depleting catecholamine stores), bretylium-like agents (preventing nerve impulse from releasing catecholamines), or ganglioplegics. Following such total sympathetic blockade, mortality from histamine or endotoxin is as markedly increased as by adrenalectomy. Pretreatment with epinephrine alone counteracts the increased lethality of endotoxin and histamine after sympathetic blockade. Cortisone pretreatment only partially corrects the sensitization by adrenalectomy, whereas cortisone + epinephrine offer complete protection against these agents. Presumably, sympathetic stimulation is "the first line of defense against the vasomotor disturbance elicited by endotoxin and histamine." The lethal effect of formalin or tourniquet shock is likewise greatly enhanced by adrenalectomy but, in contrast to that of endotoxin and histamine, it cannot be increased by sympathetic blockade. Furthermore, cortisone alone counteracts the toxicity of these stressors in adrenalectomized rats. Apparently "formalin and tourniquet shock is initiated by a mechanism which differs from that elicited by histamine and endotoxin and does not primarily involve the sympathetic system."

Robert et al. G74,748/70: In rats, the gastric ulcers produced by forced muscular exercise can be prevented by pretreatment with prednisolone, but neither adrenalectomy nor DOC affects their development. The ulcers were more common in females than in males, and could be totally prevented by fasting.

← Testoids

Kowalewski C50,864/58: Experiments on rats with fractures of the humerus show "that cortisone inhibits and 17-ethyl-19-nortestosterone promotes those processes of repair which may be measured by S^{35} uptake method, and that 17-ethyl-19-nortestosterone may protect connective tissue against the catabolic effect of cortisone."

Selye & Mishra C38,201/58: In the rat, methyltestosterone prevents the loss of body weight produced by overdosage with DHT, vitamin-D_2, partial fasting, AAN and estradiol. The catabolism elicited by IDPN or cortisol is not influenced.

Gandini & Gandini-Collodel D58,657/62: In guinea pigs, the alkaline phosphatase changes characteristic of fatigue that occur following prolonged running in revolving cages are not prevented by pretreatment with 4-chlorotestosterone but the restoration to normal is greatly accelerated.

Klug G19,783/64: In cholecystectomized women postoperative weight increase was enhanced by methandrostenolone.

Werboff et al. F10,255/64: In rats, audiogenic seizures are not significantly influenced by ovariectomy. Testosterone, progesterone and estradiol significantly increased seizure incidence in naturally seizure-resistant animals, whereas they had an opposite effect in seizure-sensitive rats.

Sloper & Pegrum G49,073/67: The regeneration of crushed murine skeletal muscle is inhibited by cortisone and accelerated by methandienone (17β-hydroxy-17α-methyl-Δ^1-testosterone) or methandrostenolone.

Igic et al. H13,355/69: Methenol (an anabolic steroid possibly identical with methenolone, but here not characterized) inhibits the myopathy produced in rats by ligature of the aorta and subsequent cooling of the distal half of the animal.

← Folliculoids, Luteoids, Gonadectomy

Campbell et al. C23,145/56: Pretreatment with estradiol decreases the resistance of the mouse to various stressors (formalin, cold) and facilitates the development of organ changes characteristic of the alarm reaction.

Werboff et al. F10,255/64: In rats, audiogenic seizures are not significantly influenced by ovariectomy. Testosterone, progesterone and estradiol significantly increased seizure incidence in naturally seizure-resistant animals, whereas they had an opposite effect in seizure-sensitive rats.

Luther et al. G70,681/69: In rats restrained in a cold environment, the development of gastric ulcers is reduced by ovariectomy. Estradiol has no effect upon the induction of these ulcers either in intact or in ovariectomized rats.

← Other Steroids

Henane F52,022/65: Spironolactone diminishes the performance of rats which adapted themselves to swim in warm surroundings. The effect is ascribed to a suppression of adaptively secreted aldosterone.

LOCAL TRAUMA ←

The voluminous literature on the effect of **steroids** upon inflammation, wound healing and other forms of local trauma should be consulted in our earlier monographs on stress *(Selye B40,000/50; B58,650/51; B87,000/52; B90,100/53; C1,001/54; C9,000/55—56)*.

Even large doses of adrenocortical extract failed to increase the work capacity (swim test) of intact rats, suggesting that in this respect the **corticoids** are not very efficacious in combating the topical results of fatigue upon muscle cells.

In rats with bone fractures, 17-ethyl-19-nortestosterone promotes repair (^{35}S uptake), whereas cortisone exerts an opposite effect. Apparently, the two types of steroids antagonize each other's actions on connective tissue.

The regeneration of crushed murine skeletal muscle is inhibited by cortisone and accelerated by several anabolic testoids, the two types of steroids thus opposing each other in this respect also.

Ratsimamanga B48,447/50: Even very large doses of adrenocortical extract failed to increase the work capacity (swim test) of intact rats.

Kowalewski C50,864/58: Experiments on rats with fractures of the humerus show "that cortisone inhibits and 17-ethyl-19-nortestosterone promotes those processes of repair which may be measured by S^{35} uptake method, and that 17-ethyl-19-nortestosterone may protect connective tissue against the catabolic effect of cortisone."

Sloper & Pegrum G49,073/67: The regeneration of crushed murine skeletal muscle is inhibited by cortisone and accelerated by methandienone (17β-hydroxy-17α-methyl-Δ^1-testosterone) or methandrostenolone.

VARIA ←

In general, anabolics counteract body-weight loss and tend to prolong survival in animals with transplanted or spontaneous **neoplasms**, but this is not invariably the case.

The effect of steroids upon the toxicity of carcinogens (including their ability to induce tumors) is discussed in the section on "Drugs."

In mice with hereditary **muscular dystrophy**, survival is prolonged and catabolism lessened by various anabolic steroids.

The role of hepatic drug-metabolizing enzymes in the maintenance of the **sexual cycle** is discussed at length in the sections on "History" and "Theories." Ovarian homotransplants placed into the portal circulation fail to maintain the sexual cycle in spayed rats, whereas retransplantation of the gonads into the systemic circulation reinitiates estrus. This finding furnished one of the first proofs showing the importance of hepatic detoxifying mechanisms for the physiology of steroid hormones.

It was also of considerable importance for the development of modern ideas concerning metabolic effects of steroids, that folliculoids inhibit **somatic growth**, whereas testosterone actually enhances it.

Also to be mentioned in this connection is the production of **adrenocortical hyperplasia with sexual anomalies** by the 2α-cyano compound, TMACN, as well as the abortifacient and lactation inhibiting effect of various catatoxic steroids (ethylestrenol, spironolactone), which is now under study in our Institute.

Tumors ← cf. also Carcinogens

Beatson A50,749/1896: Ovariectomy + thyroid extract administration is recommended for the treatment of inoperable mammary carcinomas in women.

Reid B93,930/54: Review (18 pp., 181 refs.) on the effect of STH and corticoids upon carcinogen-induced and transplantable neoplasms.

Glenn et al. G70,204/60: Review (48 pp., 11 refs.) on the effect of various steroids, ACTH, GTH, ovariectomy, and adrenalectomy upon the development of C3H mammary carcinoma transplants in mice and fibroadenomas in rats.

Marmo & Miele D27,478/61: 4-Chlorotestosterone acetate and 19-nortestosterone phenpropionate prolong the survival of mice with Ehrlich ascites tumors, and of rats with Walker tumors.

Krahe & Heinen D 35,677/62: In rats, bearing Yoshida-sarcoma transplants, methandrostenolone caused a loss of body weight, whereas in those bearing Walker sarcomas, it exerted an opposite effect.

Rooks & Dorfman F 62,099/66: 2α-Methyl-17β-hydroxy-5α-androstan-3-one increases the survival time of rats bearing mammary fibroadenomas.

Bonmassar et al. F 85,891/67: Pretreatment with the anabolic steroid dimetazine increases the resistance of the rat to subsequent inoculations of Ehrlich ascites tumor. The prophylactic effect presumably depends upon the activation of immune mechanisms.

Muscular Dystrophy ←

Dowben C 79,563/59: The survival of mice with hereditary muscular dystrophy is prolonged by treatment with 17α-ethyl-19-nortestosterone and, to a lesser extent, by 17α-ethyl-Δ^4-19-norandrostenediol-3α,17β-3-propionate, but not by testosterone propionate.

Dowben & Gordon D 4,188/61: The median survival time (ST_{50}) of mice suffering from hereditary muscular dystrophy is about 17 weeks. This can be prolonged to about 40 weeks by anabolic steroids such as 17α-ethyl-19-nortestosterone, 9α-fluoro-11β-hydroxy-17α-methyltestosterone, methylandrostandiol, Δ^1-17α-methyltestosterone or 17α-methyl-19-nortestosterone. Some prolongation of the life span was also obtained by cortisone, "spirolactone" (presumably spironolactone), and SU-4885. Testosterone propionate did not prolong survival. DOC, aldosterone, and estradiol actually shortened it.

Borgman D 62,710/63: "Treatment of mice with hereditary muscular dystrophy by an anabolic steroid, methylandrostenediol dienanthoylacetate, lengthened survival time but did not otherwise alter the disease syndrome."

Dowben et al. F 10,902/64: The life span of mice with hereditary muscular dystrophy is prolonged by various anabolic-testoid compounds, but shortened by folliculoids, DOC, or aldosterone.

Dowben E 80/65: Review on the effect of anabolic steroids in experimental and clinical muscular dystrophies.

Miscellaneous Effects of Protective Steroids ←

McEuen et al. 39,157/37: First communication on the "Effect of Testosterone on Somatic Growth." Unlike folliculoids, testosterone does not inhibit **somatic growth** in the rat. Indeed, although only small amounts of the compound were available, they appeared to stimulate growth, at least in females.

Golden & Sevringhaus A 37,808/38: In ovariectomized rats, ovarian homotransplants placed into the mesenteries failed to maintain the **sexual cycle**, whereas retransplantation of the gonads into the axillary region reinitiated estrus. Apparently, folliculoids are detoxified during their passage through the liver.

Colfer A 47,355/47: In rats, **audiogenic convulsions** cause a loss of K and a gain of Na in the brain. DOC protects against audiogenic convulsions, and produces changes in the microincineration pattern of the cerebral cortex opposite to those associated with convulsive influences. A low K diet also protects against audiogenic convulsions.

Smith C 46,496/56: In brown trout, thyroxine raises, whereas thiourea and thiouracil reduce **salinity tolerance**. Anterior pituitary extracts and STH likewise raise salinity tolerance, whereas posterior lobe extracts, testosterone, gonadotrophin, TTH, and ACTH have no effect.

Aschkenasy-Lelu G 9,425/64: Review of the **various damaging agents** against which females are more resistant than males, and of the resistance-increasing effect of folliculoids.

Goldman et al. G 73,456/66: In rats given 2α-cyano-4,4,17α-trimethylandrost-5-en,17β-ol,3-one (TMACN), the fetuses at term exhibit a syndrome of **adrenocortical hyperplasia with sexual anomalies**, presumably due to persistent inhibition of fetal 3β-hydroxysteroid dehydrogenase.

ENZYMES ←

Most of the catatoxic actions of steroids, that have been adequately analyzed, were found to depend upon the stimulation of drug-metabolizing enzyme systems; hence, our selection of the data to be specifically classified under "Enzymes" is necessarily somewhat arbitrary. In the choice of pertinent facts we were guided by the principle that this section should be as concise as possible, and limited to enzymologic findings which could not be listed under any other heading. Since the purpose of this monograph is to review our knowledge on the hormonal regulation of resistance, all observations having a direct bearing upon susceptibility to morbid changes have been reserved for more detailed consideration in the section dealing with particular pathogens (*cf.* Enzymologic References).

The following pages are intended merely as a classified guide to the literature on the effect of steroids upon the enzymic activities that may play a part in resistance, although they have not been clearly related to defense against any particular pathogen. Enzyme activities totally unrelated to defense (e.g., those concerned specifically with reproduction) have been completely disregarded; however, borderline observations on enzymes which participate in the regulation of general metabolism but may assume a special role in certain intoxications are listed.

For convenient access, the data are classified according to substrates, but they have not been subjected to personal analysis and critical evaluation, since any effort to do so would have exceeded the scope of this monograph — as well as the competence of its author.

The arrangement of the material is as follows:

All enzyme activities **specifically directed against a toxic agent** are not considered here but under Drugs, together with the corresponding toxicant itself (e.g. "zoxazolaminase" with zoxazolamine).

Only enzyme activities **directed against substrates not usually administered as toxicants** [e.g., TKT (tyrosine), TPO (tryptophan), SDH (serine), DNA-polymerase] are listed here and arranged according to the pharmacologic action of the inducing steroid (e.g., corticoid, folliculoid, antimineralocorticoid).

Within the large sections "Corticoids" and "Adrenalectomy" a further subdivision is made, the first section being devoted to "TKT and TPO," the second to "Other Amino Acid Enzymes" (including GOT, TDH, GPT, SDH, OKT, methionine adenosyl transferase, etc.), and the third to "Other Enzymes." Here the material is classified according to the regulating steroid.

Separate sections deal with "All Enzymes" as influenced by steroids other than the corticoids. Here, the first criterion for classification is the steroid activity, and data on its effect upon all enzyme systems are discussed conjointly, since even so the corresponding subsections are small in comparison with the extensive accumulations of data on corticoids and adrenalectomy.

In accordance with this plan, the data in the following pages will be classified as follows:

TKT and TPO ← Corticoids	All Enzymes ← Luteoids
Other Amino Acid Enzymes[a] ← Corticoids	All Enzymes ← Testoids
Other Enzymes[b] ← Corticoids	All Enzymes ← Gonadectomy
TKT and TPO ← Adrenalectomy	All Enzymes ← Antifolliculoids
Other Amino Acid Enzymes ← Adrenalectomy	All Enzymes ← Antitestoids
Other Enzymes ← Adrenalectomy	All Enzymes ← Antimineralocorticoids
All Enzymes ← Folliculoids	All Enzymes ← Various Steroids

[a] GOT, GPT, TDH, SDH, OKT.   [b] G-6-P-ase, UDP-ase, urea-cycle enzymes, DNA- and RNA-polymerase, NAD-ase, phosphatases, etc.

← *Corticoids*

REVIEWS

Drews H 12,100/69: Review of the hepatic enzymes that can be induced by cortisol.

Hahn & Koldovský E 8,164/69: Brief summary of the effect of corticoids upon hepatic enzymes.

TKT (Tyrosine) and TPO (Tryptophan) ←.

RAT

Thomson & Mikuta B 90,975/54: Cortisol increases the hepatic TPO activity of the rat liver.

Knox & Auerbach E 76,825/55: The TPO activity of rat liver is lowered by adrenalectomy and increased in both normal and adrenalectomized animals by cortisone. The increase in TPO activity caused by histidine and other pharmacologically active amines is prevented by adrenalectomy, unless the animals receive glucocorticoids. Hormone-induced and substrate-induced enzyme adaptation must be distinguished.

Civen & Knox E 53,175/57: In rats, an increase in the hepatic TPO activity can be obtained by treatment with tryptophan, cortisone or cortisol.

Lin & Knox E 63,521/57: The hepatic TKT activity of the rat increases after injections of tyrosine or cortisol. A 4-fold increase was observed within 5 hrs. Tyrosine was an effective inducing stimulus only if the adrenal glands were present, or if cortisol was injected after adrenalectomy.

Lin & Knox C 73,824/58: In rats, the hepatic TKT activity increased after treatment with cortisone, cortisol or corticosterone and L-tyrosine. This effect was observed also following adrenalectomy. On the other hand, a comparable action of other amino acids was probably due to stress. "That a nonspecific stress-producing agent could actually increase the level of tyrosine-α-ketoglutarate transaminase was further supported by the results obtained with a compound which is unrelated to tyrosine metabolism. Injections of propylene glycol in doses of 0.5 ml. per 100 mg. of body weight caused the level of this enzyme to increase to an average of 1390 units in three intact rats." Adrenalectomized rats did not support this dose of propylene glycol.

Schor & Frieden C 57,994/58: In the rat, insulin can induce hepatic TPO activity, and this is only partly inhibited by adrenalectomy. In the intact rat, the effect of insulin and tryptophan, or insulin and cortisone, are additive. Possibly, "hormonal induction may be a form of substrate induction in that certain hormones might affect the availability of tryptophan for the enzyme-forming system."

Civen & Knox E 64,178/59: In the adrenalectomized rat, the cortisol-induced increase in hepatic TPO activity is not associated with a higher level of tryptophan in the liver of normal rats, nor with an increased tryptophan metabolite excretion by pyridoxine-deficient rats. Tryptophan induction of the enzyme is associated with a rise in hepatic tryptophan and the excretion of metabolites by the deficient rats. The inducing effect of tryptophan and cortisol given together was the sum of their separate actions. In vitro TPO is induced by addition of tryptophan, but not of cortisol, to the medium. It is concluded that cortisol is a primary inducer of enzyme and acts differently from, and independently of, the substrate.

Feigelson et al. G 67,768/59: Studies on the half-life of cortisone-induced TPO in rat liver.

Ginoulhiac G 67,780/59: Studies on the TPO-induction by various corticoids in adrenalectomized rats suggest that "the TPO test is suitable for the biological evaluation of corticoids."

Horton & Franz C 63,790/59: In the rat, the cortisone-induced increase in TPO activity is reduced by ethionine and restored again by methionine.

Lin et al. C 96,929/59: TKT activity is higher in the livers of male than of female rats. This enzyme activity is diminished by castration in males, and increased by testosterone in females. Cortisol enhances this transaminase activity in males much more than in females, both in the presence and in the absence of the adrenals.

Maickel & Brodie C 83,071/60: TPO in rat liver is increased by ACTH, cortisone, or cortisol, as well as by various stressor agents and barbiturates. Hypophysectomy prevents the effect of stressors and barbiturates, suggesting that the latter act through the pituitary-adrenal system.

Feigelson D 4,122/61: In the rat, hepatic TPO activity can be induced both by tryptophan and by cortisone.

Kenney & Flora D 12,237/61: Tryptophan and i.p. injections of diatomaceous earth (Celite) were as effective as tyrosine in inducing increases of hepatic TKT activity in intact, but not in adrealectomized rats. Cortisol was an efficacious inducer at low doses in both intact and adrenalectomized animals. In the latter, the effect of a small dose of cortisol was potentiated by simultaneous administration of tyrosine, methionine or diatomaceous earth. "It is concluded that induction of tyrosine transaminase is entirely mediated by adrenal hormone." In adrenalectomized rats, diatomaceous earth i.p. is believed to act as a stressor through adrenocortical stimulation.

Nicolis & Ginoulhiac D27,485/61: Hepatic TPO induction is so characteristic of glucocorticoid activity in the rat that it may be used as the basis of a bioassay procedure.

Feigelson et al. D25,364/62: In the rat, the induction of hepatic TPO by tryptophan or cortisone is used as a model for the study of interrelations between hormonal- and substrate-dependent enzyme induction processes. Following i.p. administration of either inducer, there is a rise in liver TPO activity, reaching a maximum after 4—5 hrs, the peak being higher for tryptophan than for cortisone. Judged by ^{14}C-glycine and ^{32}P-orthophosphate incorporation experiments, both the tryptophan and cortisone-induced stimulation of protein metabolism follow the same time course, but their effects on RNA metabolism do not coincide. Tryptophan causes no increase in RNA turnover while the enzyme level is rising. When the enzyme activity has returned to normal, precursor incorporation into RNA is stimulated. Cortisone, on the other hand, markedly stimulates RNA turnover with maximal effects at 4 hrs corresponding to peak enzyme levels. The pattern of incorporation of the purine precursor, glycine-2-^{14}C, into the RNA of various hepatic subcellular fractions showed that cortisone increases precursor incorporation into the proteins of all liver cell constituents, but much less than into RNA. On the basis of these and many other experiments concerning the mechanism of enzyme induction, a hypothesis is proposed according to which the difference between substrate and hormone induction might be explained.

Feigelson & Greengard D46,319/62: In the rat, a single i.p. injection of cortisone causes a 3-fold increase in the amount of TPO enzyme protein (immunologic assay). When assayed in the presence of saturation levels of its hematin cofactor, a proportionate rise in the catalytic activity of the enzyme is also obtained. Adrenalectomized rats react the same way. "Thus, the increase in liver tryptophan pyrrolase activity during hormonal induction and during the second phase of substrate induction are due to increased tryptophan pyrrolase protein levels."

Goldstein et al. D70,931/62: Cortisol enhanced both TKT and TPO activities in the isolated, perfused rat liver. This effect was prevented by puromycin, an inhibitor of protein synthesis. Cortisol "may exert some of its physiological effects directly on liver cells by altering the level of enzyme activities."

Greengard & Feigelson G67,329/62: Immunochemical evidence showing that an increased amount of TPO is found in the liver of adrenalectomized rats after treatment with L-tryptophan. A similar increase is obtained by cortisone. [The brief abstract does not state whether cortisone was also tested in adrenalectomized rats (H.S.).]

Kenney E89,716/62: In the rat, the induction of hepatic TKT by cortisol is associated with an equivalent increase in enzyme antigen. A cross-reactive precursor could not be detected in any of the subcellular liver fractions. Induction in the presence of ^{14}C-labeled amino acids results in extensive labeling of transaminase, with or without induction.

Knox G51,969/62: Review on the effect of stress upon hepatic TPO production. In adrenalectomized animals, only tryptophan of a series of analogues induces this enzyme, whereas, in intact rats, various stressors, ACTH, cortisone, cortisol and corticosterone (but not DOC) do so. "The recognition of the adrenal hormone-induced adaptation of the tryptophan pyrrolase has provided the unified explanation for a large number of different stressful stimuli which increase the enzyme level." Tryptophan pyrrolase is absent from the liver of newborn rabbits and in them, this enzyme cannot be induced by cortisol. Tyrosine transaminase induction is regulated in a very similar manner.

Davis D92,322/63: The decarboxylation of o-tyrosine and 5-hydroxytryptophan by livers of adrenalectomized rats, given water, was significantly lower than in controls. No significant effects on decarboxylation of these substrates were observed in adrenalectomized animals given NaCl, or in intact animals treated with DOC or exposed to cold. On the other hand, cortisone increased the inherent hepatic decarboxylating activity for both substrates, in normal as well as in pyridoxine-deficient rats.

Greengard et al. D63,145/63: In adrenalectomized rats, "the administration of puromycin inhibited the cortisone-induced elevation of tryptophan pyrrolase and tyrosine-α-ketoglutarate transaminase activity as well as the substrate-induced elevation of the latter. Actinomycin abolished the cortisone-mediated rise in the level of both enzymes but did not influence the tryptophan-mediated increase in the level of tryptophan pyrrolase." In newborn rats, the development of hepatic TKT was inhibited by actinomycin, but neither adrenalectomy nor actinomycin D interfered with the postnatal development of hepatic TPO. Apparently, accumulation of TPO (unlike that of TKT) is not under adrenal control and can proceed despite inhibited RNA synthesis.

Greengard et al. E20,258/63: In starved rats, hepatic glycogen deposition following cortisone treatment is inhibited by puromycin and actinomycin D. The former interferes with enzyme induction in general, the latter with cortisone-induced rise in hepatic enzyme, including TKT. "The regulatory effect of cortisone on carbohydrate metabolism may be brought about by its action on the cellular concentration of certain enzyme proteins."

Knox D66,995/63: In intact rats, hepatic TPO or TKT can be induced by pretreatment either with the corresponding substrates or with cortisol. However, after adrenalectomy TKT, unlike TPO, can no longer be induced by the substrate. Cortisol induces both enzymes even after adrenalectomy, and the increase is particularly pronounced if the hormone is given conjointly with these substrates.

Pitot G65,475/63: In the Morris hepatoma 5123, TPO activity is normally low and cannot be significantly altered by either tryptophan or cortisone, whereas both these substances induce the enzyme in the normal liver tissue. In adrenalectomized rats, TPO induction by tryptophan is lower than in intact animals, though cortisone induction in the host liver is actually increased. A slight enzyme induction appears to be possible even in the hepatoma when cortisone is administered to the adrenalectomized rat. Essentially similar but not quite identical results have been obtained with rats bearing Morris hepatoma 7800 or 7316. TKT, TDH and G-6-P-ase activities were either minimally or not affected by cortisone in various transplantable hepatic tumors.

Rosen et al. E32,653/63: "A period of about 48 hours is required to attain maximal activity of alanine-α-ketoglutarate transaminase in liver after subcutaneous treatment of rats with a single injection of cortisol. In contrast, tyrosine-α-ketoglutarate transaminase reaches a maximal value in liver between 4 and 5 hours after an intraperitoneal dose of cortisol." The same dose of cortisol causes even greater increases of hepatic TKT in adrenalectomized rats, but GPT or TPO induction by cortisol is not influenced by adrenalectomy.

Geller et al. G22,722/64: In rats, hepatic TKT tryptophan-α-ketoglutarate transaminase and TPO activities are increased 3.5 hrs after i.p. injection of cortisol, but no such activation was seen after stress (animals placed in a mechanical shaker) causing an increase in adrenal and plasma glucocorticoids as well as a depletion of adrenal ascorbic acid. Possibly, the amount of glucocorticoid secreted was not equivalent to that injected.

Pitot et al. G37,125/64: In intact rats bearing Reuber H-35 hepatomas, TKT activity is much greater in the tumor than in the normal hepatic tissue. Cortisone i.p. induces enzyme in the liver, but not in the tumor. In adrenalectomized hosts, however, the enzyme in the tumor is in the range of the host liver, and cortisone induces enzyme in both liver and tumor. If cortisone is added to cultures 24 hrs before the enzyme assay, a significant induction occurs in vitro, reaching a maximum in 6 hrs. Actinomycin D added to the medium delays enzyme induction without inhibiting it completely.

Schapiro et al. G21,848/64: In the rat, cortisol greatly increases hepatic TPO, TKT, and tryptophan transaminase activity, whereas stress (reciprocating shaker) stimulates corticoid secretion without any change in hepatic transaminase or pyrrolase activity. Apparently, stress not only activates the adrenal cortex, but also the mechanisms which block the induction of these enzymes by corticoids, because shaker stress inhibited the elevation of hepatic transaminase that occurred following cortisol, although it did not block the elevation of TPO in the rat.

Shiba et al. G31,114/65: The addition of cortisol to the blood perfused through a rat liver in vitro induced hepatic TPO, whereas this was not the case with livers of rats bearing large Walker tumors. The inhibitory effect upon enzyme induction is ascribed to "toxohormone" (an extract of Walker tumors), since addition of a toxohormone preparation to the perfusion fluid also prevented enzyme induction by cortisol.

Peraino et al. G40,083/66: In rats pretreated with cortisone, the dietary induction of SDH, OKT and TKT was not much affected, but carbohydrate repression was largely eliminated. Pretreatment with phenobarbital alone had little effect on the induction of SDH and OKT but, given with cortisone, it considerably enhanced the response of these enzymes to induction by casein hydrolysate feeding. Neither cortisone nor phenobarbital acted as inducers when given alone or in combination. They were active only in the presence of a dietary inducer.

Southren et al. F66,647/66: Clinical improvement has been observed in Cushing's syndrome after treatment with o,p'-DDD. This effect might have been due to a direct interference by o,p'-DDD with the biologic action of cortisol, or by its giving rise to cortisol metabolites which inhibit cortisol competitively at the effector site. In the rat, o,p'-DDD had no effect upon the induction of TPO in the liver, whereas 6β-hydroxycortisol was found to be a potent inhibitor of cortisol action in this test system. Since o,p'-DDD induces the production of 6β-hydroxycortisol, the protective effect may have been due to the latter.

Tomkins et al. G49,588/66: Glucocorticoids stimulate TKT induction in rat hepatoma cells in vitro. Inhibitor and immunochemical experiments indicate that the corticoids do not activate a precursor, but increase the number of enzyme protein molecules. Apparently, the hormones exert some control at the level of translation of the transaminase messenger by antagonizing a repressor of messenger function. "It cannot yet be determined whether the presumed increase in messenger concentration occurs as a secondary response to the stimulation of translation, or whether there is a direct effect of the hormone on gene transcription."

Gelehrter & Tomkins G51,315/67: Dexamethasone induced a 3—15-fold increase of TKT activity in a tissue culture of rat hepatoma cells, but no rise in total RNA nor its synthesis as measured by the rate of incorporation of labeled precursors. Various experiments also failed to demonstrate gross stimulation of RNA synthesis associated with enzyme induction by steroid hormones in vivo, "suggesting that these changes are not an essential part of the mechanism of enzyme induction by glucocorticoids."

Peterkofsky & Tomkins G52,839/67: TKT can be induced by dexamethasone in tissue cultures from Morris hepatoma 7288C. Cytosine arabinose completely inhibits DNA synthesis in these cells, but does not affect RNA synthesis or enzyme induction. Conversely, mitomycin C and actinomycin D preferentially inhibit RNA synthesis, and completely block induction. Kinetic experiments in which actinomycin D was added at increasing intervals after dexamethasone suggest that messenger RNA accumulates during the early phase of induction. From these and other observations, it is concluded "that messenger RNA for both tyrosine aminotransferase and general cell protein are relatively stable. After inhibition of protein synthesis by cycloheximide, tyrosine aminotransferase activity decreased exponentially with a half-life of seven hours, and this rate was not affected by either steroid or actinomycin."

Seidman et al. F88,452/67: The induction of TPO has been studied in the liver remnant of partially hepatectomized rats after treatment with cortisol, and subsequent adrenalectomy. "It seems possible, therefore that the lessened response to hydrocortisone in hepatic cells preparing to divide is related to repression of transcriptional rather than translational mechanisms and that the duplicating genome itself may be unable to participate simultaneously in other functions."

Granner et al. H11,721/68: Dexamethasone stimulates TKT synthesis when added in vitro to tissue cultures derived from a rat hepatoma.

Hager & Kenney G58,950/68: Cortisol, insulin and glucagon induced TKT in the isolated, perfused rat liver. The hormonal induction of all these enzymes was sensitive to actinomycin D, but STH (which represses TKT induction in vivo) apparently acts indirectly, since it loses this effect in vitro. Cortisol acts as long as it is present in the perfusion fluid, whereas enzyme synthesis induced by the pancreatic hormones ceases after two or three hours, regardless of the continued presence of the protein hormones. It is assumed that cortisol is a "primary inducer," whereas the pancreatic hormones probably act indirectly, as a consequence of their initial hepatic effect, and are therefore "secondary inducers." Both the primary and the secondary induction mechanisms are blocked by actinomycin D.

Schapiro H2,360/68: Stress (30 min rough agitation in a noisy laboratory shaker) had no effect upon the corticoid sensitive enzyme TKT in the liver of the intact rat, but it increased TPO activity, which is likewise corticoid inducible. Adrenalectomized rats, similarly stressed, exhibited a decreased transaminase activity with no change in TPO. This inhibitory effect was abolished by hypophysectomy. STH inhibited induction of transaminase by cortisol, but had no effect upon cortisol-induced TPO activity. The opposing actions of STH and glucocorticoids may be involved in adaptive reactions to stress.

Agarwal et al. G65,716/69: In the rat, both S. typhimurium endotoxin and Thorotrast lowered hepatic TPO activity, and prevented cortisol from inducing this enzyme in the isolated, perfused liver. Under these conditions, the TKT activity of the liver remained unaffected. Partial purification of hepatic TPO induced by endotoxin or Thorotrast indicated the presence of some inhibitory substance. "Since histological studies revealed that thorotrast is localized in Kupffer cells, it is suggested that the reticuloendothelial system contributes to the control of enzyme induction in rat liver."

Benes & Zicha G67,159/69: Exposure to 1400 R does not inhibit the TPO activity of rat liver. In fact, substrate induction of TPO is stimulated by X-irradiation applied 24 hrs earlier. Induction by cortisol is initially stimulated, and then inhibited by X-irradiation. X-irradiation before partial hepatectomy inhibits the increase in TPO normally observed 12 hrs after the operation. Similar results are obtained by actinomycin D applied one hour after partial hepatectomy. "The diminished synthesis of tryptophan oxygenase in irradiated regenerating rat liver tissue, as well as the decrease of hormonal induction after the irradiation can be explained by the inhibition of the specific messenger RNA's synthesis."

Valeriote et al. G67,621/69: Purification and properties of rat liver TKT induced by triamcinolone.

Yuwiler et al. H9,994/69: Comparative observations on fasted and cortisol-injected rats led to the conclusion that "the natural stress of fasting is accompanied by alterations in some corticoid-inducible enzymes, but that these changes are not analogous to those obtained following glucocorticoid administration."

Levitan & Webb H20,594/70: In rats, the purine analogue azaguanine does not inhibit the initial induction of hepatic TKT by cortisol. However, the continued induced synthesis of the enzyme elicited by repeated doses of cortisol is inhibited by azaguanine. "This suggests that the induction cycle involves the activation and renewal of a pool of preexisting messenger RNA."

Nakano et al. G76,247/70: "In adrenalectomized rats, hepatic TPO which can be increased in amount in intact rats by feeding either tryptophan or methionine, was activated and increased in amount by feeding tryptophan but not methionine. The feeding of tryptophan resulted in a significant increase in the level of arginase and threonine dehydratase. Methionine produced a similar increase in both threonine dehydratase and arginase activities. Administration of cortisone acetate produced a significant increase in the level of all three enzyme activities."

Mouse

Agarwal & Berry G66,479/66: In the mouse, stress produced by i.p. injection of infusorial earth or bentonite causes no significant change in hepatic TPO activity at the time when sensitization to endotoxin is already developed. The inducibility of TPO is delayed by injections of cortisone at a time when the hormone protects against endotoxin. Still, the results are considered to be "in agreement with the concept that maintenance of liver TP is necessary for continued survival of endotoxin poisoned mice. The absence of change in this enzyme seen in celite- and bentonite-injected mice sensitized to endotoxin is an apparent exception." Presumably, "suppression of TP-activity is not the only way in which mice may be sensitized to endotoxin."

Berry et al. G67,237/66: S. typhimurium endotoxin lowers liver TPO in mice and prevents the induction of the enzyme by concurrent injection of cortisone. It lowers, but does not prevent, substrate induction. Actinomycin D has a similar effect on TPO. In the intact but not adrenalectomized mouse, endotoxin induces TKT almost as well as cortisone. Actinomycin D, on the other hand, has an effect on this transaminase similar to that of TPO.

Agarwal & Berry G66,480/67: "Four hours after zymosan administration, cortisone was able to induce mouse liver tryptophan pyrrolase production almost at a normal rate and, under these conditions, protected mice against a concurrent injection of endotoxin. Administration of zymosan, at either 2 or 4 hrs after cortisone administration, resulted in little change in tryptophan pyrrolase activity while endotoxin, when similarly administered, caused a rapid decline in liver tryptophan pyrrolase activity. ... Glucan and zymosan, like endotoxin, increased tyrosine-α-ketoglutarate transaminase activity in intact but not in adrenalectomized mice. Zymosan and thorotrast, unlike endotoxin, neither lowered liver carbohydrate levels nor influenced cortisone induced neosynthesis of liver glycogen. These results suggest a cause and effect relationship between inducibility of key liver enzymes and survival against stress."

Berry et al. E7,069/67: In mice, endotoxin, zymosan, glucan and saccharated iron oxide (all RES-blocking agents) lower hepatic TPO and increase TKT in vivo, but not in vitro. Endotoxin also prevents the induction of TPO by cortisone, especially when the latter is given 2—4 hrs after endotoxin. The transaminase responds normally. Zymosan and glucan do not prevent the induction of TPO by cortisone. "Perhaps one might relate these effects to the dose of colloid used in relation to its toxicity, but even large doses of saccharated iron oxide capable of killing mice fail to prevent the induction of tryptophan pyrrolase by cortisone."

Rapoport et al. G53,334/68: Pneumococcal infection raises the hepatic TPO activity in intact, but not in adrenalectomized, mice. Cortisol increased TPO activity both in control and in pneumococcus-infected mice, but only if administered early after inoculation. Later during the course of infection, some inhibitory factor develops which counteracts the induction of TPO by cortisol.

Agarwal & Berry G65,866/69: In mice, cortisone induced liver TPO and increased liver pyridine nucleotide levels after pretreatment with zymosan or glucan. It also protected such animals against the lethal effects of endotoxin. The observations are "consistent with the view that a cause and effect relationship may exist between hormone induction of selected hepatic enzymes and survival against stress."

Finch et al. G71,208/69: In senescent mice, the induction of hepatic TKT by exposure to cold is delayed in comparison with young mice. Corticosterone and insulin are equally effective in this respect in mice of both age groups.

VARIA

Chan & Cohen D18,552/64: Vertebrates above the evolutionary level of amphibians respond to cortisol with an increased hepatic TKT activity. "Animals showing this response include the rat, guinea pig, chick, pigeon, horned toad (Phrynosoma cornatum), and painted turtle (Chrysemys picta). In contrast, vertebrates at the amphibian level or below failed to show this response. Animals failing to show this response include the bull frog (Rana catesbeiana), grass frog (Rana pipiens), marine toad (Bufo marinus), tiger salamander (Ambystoma tigrinum), mud puppy (Necturus), white bass (Roccus chrysops), and black crappie (Promoxis nigromaculatus)."

Litwack & Nemeth G26,050/65: In the rabbit, hepatic TKT activity rises 2—4-fold at birth. A similar increase is obtained precociously in the event of premature delivery by cesarian section, whereas prolonging gestation delays the rise in enzymic activity. Under all these conditions, the ability of cortisol to cause a further rise in enzymic activity coincides with delivery. In the guinea pig, TKT is absent during fetal life and increases to adult values within 24 hrs after birth. The enzyme activity in the newborn is stimulated by cortisol, though a single injection is without effect in the fetus or adult. In chickens, enzymic activity is relatively constant during the embryonic period, but rises 2—3-fold after hatching.

Other Amino Acid Enzymes: GOT (Aspartate), TDH (Threonine), GPT (Alanine), SDH (Serine), Methionine, OKT (Ornithine) ←.

Beaton et al. D83,636/57: Following STH treatment, there is a significant depression in the GPT activity of rat liver tissue, whereas cortisone has an inverse effect.

Gavosto et al. C34,243/57: In partially hepatectomized rats, cortisone does not significantly influence the rate of hepatic regeneration, but it increases the GOT and GPT activities, in both normal and regenerating liver tissue.

Rosen et al. C47,568/58: Cortisol increases the GPT activity of the rat liver. Similar results have been obtained with cortisone and prednisone. GOT activity is not similarly influenced. "These facts, added to the observation that a substantial rise in hepatic GPT occurs in rats treated with hydrocortisone, in contrast to treatment with deoxycorticosterone, strongly suggest that the control of hepatic levels of GPT by glucocorticosteroids is importantly related to the mechanism whereby these compounds exert their gluconeogenic activity."

Rosen et al. C50,741/58: In rats treated with cortisol, cortisone or prednisone for 1 week, there was an increase in hepatic GPT but not in GOT. DOC had no such effect. Hypophysectomy or adrenalectomy did not prevent this action of cortisone. STH, testosterone or insulin failed to alter GPT activity, nor did they influence its stimulation by cortisol.

Rosen et al. C71,414/59: Marked increases in GPT activity were observed in the livers of rats given cortisol, cortisone, 9α-fluorocortisol, prednisone, 6α-methylprednisolone, 9α-fluoro-21-desoxy-6α-methylprednisolone or ACTH, whereas two nonglucocorticoid cortisol derivatives, 11-epicortisol and 9α-methoxycortisol, were inactive. STH, testosterone, and insulin caused no significant change in GPT by themselves, nor did they modify the action of cortisol. On the other hand, large doses of estradiol and thyroxine caused a moderate increase in GPT activity, but when injected simultaneously with cortisol, they appeared to interfere with its action as did progesterone. Adrenalectomy slightly diminished or failed to affect the GPT inducing activity of cortisol whereas hypophysectomy caused a rise in GPT activity and augmented the effect of cortisol.

Rosen et al. G66,496/59: In the rat, cortisol, cortisone, and prednisone cause a 6—13-fold increase in hepatic GPT activity. This effect was directly related to the protein content of the ration. In alloxan diabetic rats, the rise in this enzyme activity was equivalent to that obtained by cortisol or high-protein diets, and could be inhibited by insulin. Adrenalectomy diminished but did not abolish the rise in GPT activity obtained by feeding high-protein diets. Thus, the initiation of enzyme synthesis by dietary protein is not mediated exclusively through the adrenals.

Harding et al. D14,355/61: In the rat, pretreatment with DOC depresses the hepatic GPT activity. A similar depression is obtained by adrenalectomy, but this is not further aggravated by concurrent treatment with DOC. ACTH increases GPT activity in hypophysectomized, but not in adrenalectomized, animals. In hypophysectomized rats, DOC fails to lower GPT nor does it alter the response of this enzyme to ACTH. "The inhibitory effect of DOC on alanine transaminase activity appears to be due to suppression of ACTH release by the pituitary."

Segal et al. D45,899/62: In the rat, prednisolone treatment increases the GPT activity and immunologic evidence suggests that this is due to an actual rise of enzyme protein.

Segal et al. G67,774/62: Purification and properties of hepatic GPT from normal rats or from those in which this enzyme was induced by cortisone or prednisolone.

Davis D92,322/63: The decarboxylation of o-tyrosine and 5-hydroxytryptophan by livers of adrenalectomized rats, given water, was significantly lower than in controls. No significant effects on decarboxylation of these substrates were observed in adrenalectomized animals given NaCl, or in intact animals treated with DOC, or exposed to cold. On the other hand, cortisone increased the inherent hepatic decarboxylating activity for both substrates, in normal as well as in pyridoxine-deficient rats.

Pitot G65,475/63: In the Morris hepatoma 5123, TPO activity is normally low and cannot be significantly altered by either tryptophan or cortisone, whereas both these substances induce the enzyme in the normal liver tissue. In adrenalectomized rats, TPO induction by tryptophan is lower than in intact animals, although cortisone induction in the host liver is actually increased. A slight enzyme induction appears to be possible even in the hepatoma when cortisone is administered to the adrenalectomized rat. Essentially similar but not quite identical results have been obtained with rats bearing Morris hepatoma 7800 or 7316. TKT, TDH and G-6-P-ase activities were either minimally or not affected by cortisone in various transplantable hepatic tumors.

Segal & Kim G67,769/63: Studies on the half-life of prednisolone-induced GPT in rat liver.

Freedland & Avery G67,766/64: In the rat, the TDH and SDH activity of liver homogenates was increased by high protein diets, alloxan diabetes, or cortisol. Factors affecting the activity of TDH caused a proportional change in SDH, suggesting that both of these activities may be due to a single protein. The SDH activity was decreased by adrenalectomy or hypophysectomy. Adrenalectomy had no effect upon the response of this enzyme to protein feeding, whereas after hypophysectomy, this response was diminished.

Peraino et al. G40,083/66: In rats pretreated with cortisone, the dietary induction of SDH, OKT and TKT was not much affected, but carbohydrate repression was largely eliminated. Pretreatment with phenobarbital alone had little effect on the induction of SDH and OKT, but given with cortisone, it considerably enhanced the response of these enzymes to induction by casein hydrolysate feeding. Neither cortisone nor phenobarbital acted as inducers when given alone or in combination. They were active only in the presence of a dietary inducer.

Moscona & Piddington F90,487/67: In retinal explants of 12-day chick embryos, glutamine synthetase activity can be induced by the addition of various corticoids to the culture medium. Cortisol, corticosterone, and aldosterone are particularly active in this respect, whereas pregnenolone, progesterone, DOC, 11-desoxycortisol, 17α-hydroxyprogesterone, and 11α-hydroxyprogesterone had little activity. 11β-Hydroprogesterone and 11β,17α-dihydroxyprogesterone exhibited intermediate degrees of activity. Apparently, "the 11β-position is of primary significance in the activity of these molecules in inducing retinal glutamine synthetase in this system. This conclusion is further supported by the fact that cortisone, which has a ketone group in the 11-position, had no effect under these conditions."

Schmidinger & Kröger F 92,031/67: The increase in hepatic SDH induced by protein-deficient diets and starvation in intact rats is prevented by actinomycin D, puromycin or glucose, but aggravated after adrenalectomy. Cortisone administered during the starvation period increases SDH activity, perhaps owing to utilization of inhibitors of this enzyme during gluconeogenesis.

Räihä & Kekomäki G 68,114/68: In the rat, the OKT activity of the liver is very low in the fetus, exhibits a small transient elevation around term, then drops, and eventually reaches the high adult activity level during the third postnatal week. Triamcinolone given postnatally causes a pronounced elevation of OKT, but has no such effect in fetal or adult rats. Puromycin prevents the rise in OKT activity after triamcinolone administration. In adult rats fed a protein-or arginine-free diet, OKT activity decreases and fails to rise under the influence of triamcinolone. Partial hepatectomy or STH depresses OKT-activity in the livers of adult rats.

Shou et al. H 15,277/69: In the rat, the hepatic methionine adenosyl transferase activity was not much influenced by glucagon, but during alloxan diabetes it increased considerably. Combined treatment with alloxan and triamcinolone resulted in an additive effect. The response to alloxan could be prevented and even reversed by insulin or adrenalectomy. In normal rats, insulin caused no consistent increase.

Uete H 15,157/69: Triamcinolone impairs the capacity of a special thymus microsome fraction system to incorporate amino acids into proteins in the rat. Detailed studies using labeled amino acids led to the conclusion "that both the soluble fraction and the ribosomes of thymus cells are involved in the inhibition of protein synthesis in thymus microsomes following the administration of adrenal cortical hormones."

Yuwiler et al. H 9,994/69: Comparative observations on fasted and cortisol-injected rats led to the conclusion that "the natural stress of fasting is accompanied by alterations in some corticoid-inducible enzymes, but that these changes are not analogous to those obtained following glucocorticoid administration."

Other Enzymes (G-6-P-ase, UDP-ase, Urea-Cycle Enzymes, DNA- and RNA-polymerase, Phosphatases, etc.) ←. *Weber et al. C 11,010/56:* In the liver of the rat, "cortisone caused a marked increase in the G-6-P-ase activity of the homogenate, nuclear, mitochondrial and microsomal fractions per unit weight, nitrogen and average cell."

Feigelson et al. G 68,042/62: In partially hepatectomized rats, cortisone causes a transient stimulation and subsequent depression in the incorporation of precursors into the DNA of the regenerating liver.

Willmer & Foster D 28,163/62: Studies on the effect of various diets upon carbohydrate-metabolizing hepatic enzymes in intact and adrenalectomized rats, and on the effect of substitution therapy with various corticoids after adrenalectomy.

Feigelson & Feigelson D 59,123/63: In rat liver tissue, "cortisone rapidly elevates incorporation of glycine-2-^{14}C into acid-soluble adenine nucleotides as well as into RNA. Intraperitoneal administration of a variety of L- and D-amino acids, NH_4+, and glutamine into adrenalectomized rats imitated cortisone by stimulating glycine-2-^{14}C incorporation into acid-soluble and RNA purines. Although liver adenosine triphosphate levels rise after cortisone administration, such alterations in ATP per se do not influence the rate of precursor incorporation into RNA or protein. On the basis of these findings, it is proposed that increased amino acid deamination, implicit in the gluconeogenic action of the glucocorticoids, results in the liberation of α-amino nitrogen moieties that mediate the cortisone-induced increases in hepatic purine biosynthetic rates."

Schimke D 39,880/63: Studies on the induction of urea-cycle enzymes (carbamyl phosphate synthetase, ornithine transcarbamylase, argininosuccinate synthetase, argininosuccinase, and arginase) in the liver of intact and adrenalectomized animals given cortisone or cortisol.

← Steroids

Dietrich & Yero G26,959/65: Cortisol markedly lowered the nicotinamide deamidase activity of the liver in intact, hypophysectomized, and adrenalectomized rats. Under these conditions, cortisol failed to inhibit hepatic synthesis of NAD significantly after nicotinamide challenge. Hexestrol markedly lowered hepatic deamidase activity in intact, thyroidectomized, and adrenalectomized rats. A lowering of the hepatic NAD-levels after nicotinamide challenge occurred upon hexestrol treatment in intact, but not in adrenalectomized, rats. Hypophysectomy markedly stimulated nicotinamide deamidase activity and NAD-biosynthesis after nicotinamide challenge.

Dietrich G28,103/65: In the mouse, hepatic nicotinamide deamidase, and the capacity to synthesize NAD are lowered by dienestrol, diethylstilbestrol, estradiol-17β, estrone, estriol, cortisone and cortisol. Pretreatment with large amounts of hexestrol also lowered the capacity of hepatic tissue to synthesize NAD upon nicotinamide challenge.

Franklin G32,826/65: The demethylation of morphine by rat hepatic microsomes was greatly diminished by pretreatment with cortisone, although, simultaneously, the G-6-P-ase activity of the liver increased. Pretreatment with morphine exhibited essentially similar effects upon these two enzymes.

Griffin & Cox F86,851/66: "The induction of alkaline phosphatase by prednisolone in HeLa cell cultures appears to occur at the level of protein synthesis (translation) as a result of a steroid-induced change in the conformational state of the enzyme during its synthesis."

Moses et al. G40,253/66: In a patient with glycogen storage disease, triamcinolone caused a 4-fold increase in hepatic G-6-P-ase.

Terayama & Takata F69,475/66: "Administration of cortisone had no significant effect on the N-demethylating activity of normal liver but partially prevented the decrease in enzymatic activity caused by adrenalin or partial hepatectomy."

Drews & Brawerman G52,150/67: Studies on changes in RNA-synthesis in the rat liver during regeneration and after cortisol administration. The relationship between enzyme induction and RNA-synthesis is discussed.

Wulf & Hers G53,099/67: In N.M.R.I. mice, prednisolone stimulates not only glycogen synthesis, but also the formation of glycogen synthetase in the liver.

Freedland et al. G55,808/68: Extensive studies on the effect of adrenalectomy, hypophysectomy and cortisol treatment upon a great variety of rat liver enzymes, with observations on the effect of thyroxine upon these enzymes in intact, adrenalectomized or hypophysectomized rats. The extensive data do not lend themselves to succinct presentation in the form of a summary and must be consulted in the original.

Gresham & Pover G58,354/68: In the rat, alkaline RNAse levels increase in the mucosa of the small intestine after total body or selective head X-irradiation as well as after treatment with such radiomimetic drugs as Chlorambucil or Myleran but not after treatment with ACTH, cortisol or various stressors. Still, a relationship to the G.A.S. is suspected because blockade of the normal neuroendocrine responses to stress by combined treatment with morphine + pentobarbital blocked the intestinal RNA response to X-irradiation, and the latter was also lacking in newborn rats in which hypothalamic control of anterior pituitary function has not yet developed.

← *Adrenalectomy*

TKT, TPO ←. *Knox B71,418/51:* Tryptophan induces hepatic TPO both in intact and in adrenalectomized animals. Various other compounds, including epinephrine and histamine which (to a lesser extent) have the same effect in intact animals, fail to act after adrenalectomy. "The first mechanism has been identified as that of enzyme adaptation, previously known only in microorganism, and the second has been identified as the stress reaction, acting through the adrenal glands."

Geschwind & Li B93,277/54: In the rat, the induction of the TPO enzyme system is diminished by hypophysectomy and adrenalectomy, but increased by thyroidectomy.

Thomson & Mikuta B96,579/54: In adrenalectomized rats, maintained on 1% NaCl, the activation of the hepatic TPO system is so specific for glucocorticoids (e.g., cortisone, cortisol) and so accurately dose-dependent that it is recommended as a bioassay method. DOC is ineffective.

Thomson & Mikuta B90,975/54: "Total-body X-irradiation produces within a few hours a dose-dependent increase in the tryptophan peroxidase-oxidase system of rat liver. The increase does not occur in adrenalectomized rats, and hence cannot be construed as a direct effect of X-irradiation." After hypophysectomy, enzyme induction became progressively less pronounced as adrenal atrophy developed. ACTH restored the ability of the hypophysectomized rat to respond with enzyme induction.

Knox & Auerbach E76,825/55: The TPO activity of rat liver is lowered by adrenalectomy and increased in both normal and adrenalectomized animals by cortisone. The increase in TPO activity caused by histidine and other pharmacologically active amines is prevented by adrenalectomy, unless the animals receive glucocorticoids. Hormone-induced and substrate-induced enzyme adaptation must be distinguished.

Lin & Knox E63,521/57: The hepatic TKT activity of the rat increases following injections of tyrosine or cortisol. A 10-fold increase was observed within 5 hrs. Tyrosine was an effective inducing stimulus only if the adrenal glands were present, or if cortisol was injected after adrenalectomy.

Lin & Knox C73,824/58: In rats, the hepatic TKT activity increased following treatment with cortisone, cortisol or corticosterone and L-tyrosine. This effect was observed also after adrenalectomy. On the other hand, a comparable effect of other amino acids was probably due to stress. "That a nonspecific stress-producing agent could actually increase the level of tyrosine-α-ketoglutarate transaminase was further supported by the results obtained with a compound which is unrelated to tyrosine metabolism. Injections of propylene glycol in doses of 0.5 ml per 100 gm of body weight caused the level of this enzyme to increase to an average of 1390 units in three intact rats." Adrenalectomized rats did not support this dose of propylene glycol.

Schor & Frieden C57,994/58: In the rat, insulin can induce hepatic TPO activity, and its effect is only partly inhibited by adrenalectomy. In the intact rat, the effect of insulin and tryptophan, or insulin and cortisone, are additive. Possibly, "hormonal induction may be a form of substrate induction in that certain hormones might affect the availability of tryptophan for the enzyme-forming system."

Canal & Maffei-Faccioli G66,306/59: Reserpine is a more potent inducer of TPO in the liver of adrenalectomized than in that of intact rats. Hence, the effect of reserpine is not due to stress-induced increased corticoid production; it may be due to the liberation not only of 5-HT but also of its precursor tryptophan.

Civen & Knox E64,178/59: In the adrenalectomized rat, the cortisol-induced increase in hepatic TPO activity is not associated with a higher level of tryptophan in the liver of normal rats, nor with an increased tryptophan metabolite excretion by pyridoxine-deficient rats. Tryptophan induction of the enzyme is associated with a rise in hepatic tryptophan and the excretion of metabolites by the deficient rats. The inducing effect of tryptophan and cortisol given together was the sum of their separate actions. In vitro TPO is induced by addition of tryptophan, but not of cortisol, to the medium. It is concluded that cortisol is a primary inducer of enzyme and acts differently from, and independently of, the substrate.

Ginoulhiac G67,780/59: Studies on the TPO-induction by various corticoids in adrenalectomized rats suggest that "the TPO test is suitable for the biological evaluation of corticoids."

Lin et al. C96,929/59: TKT activity is higher in the liver of male than of female rats. This enzyme activity is diminished by castration in males, and increased by testosterone in females. Cortisol increases this transaminase activity in males much more than in females, both in the presence and in the absence of the adrenals.

Sereni et al. C80,562/59: Activity of TKT is very low in the livers of fetal rats, but rapidly increases beginning 2 hrs after birth, reaching a maximum at 12 hrs. Injection of amphenone or adrenalectomy at birth delays the development of this enzyme, whereas cortisol reverses the effect of adrenalectomy.

Kenney D98,193/60: In the rat, hepatic TKT activity increases sharply after birth. This increase is prevented by adrenalectomy; tyrosine cannot substitute for cortisol in restoring transaminase development. Methionine is as active as tyrosine in increasing the response to cortisol after adrenalectomy and this process does not depend upon the specific substrate as such, but apparently upon the presence of certain amino acids. Immunochemical assays "are clearly incompatible with a mechanism of induction involving de novo synthesis of enzyme protein and suggest that adrenal steroids promote either the activation of an antigenically similar but enzymically inactive precursor protein, or the release of an inhibitor."

Kenney & Flora D12,237/61: Tryptophan and i.p. injections of diatomaceous earth (Celite) were as effective as tyrosine in inducing increases in hepatic TKT in intact, but not in adrenalectomized rats. Cortisol was an effective inducer at low doses in both intact and adrenalectomized animals. In the latter, the effect of a small dose of cortisol was potentiated by simultaneous administration of tyrosine, methionine or diatomaceous earth. "It is concluded that induction of tyrosine transaminase is entirely mediated by adrenal hormone." In adrenalectomized rats, diatomaceous earth i.p. is believed to act as a stressor through adrenocortical stimulation.

Feigelson & Greengard D46,319/62: In the rat, a single i.p. injection of cortisone causes a 3-fold increase in the amount of TPO enzyme protein (immunologic assay). When assayed in the presence of saturation levels of its hematin cofactor, a proportionate increase in the catalytic activity of the enzyme is also obtained. Adrenalectomized rats react the same way. "Thus, the increase in liver tryptophan pyrrolase activity during hormonal induction and during the second phase of substrate induction are due to increased tryptophan pyrrolase protein levels."

Greengard & Feigelson G67,329/62: Immunochemical evidence showing that an increased amount of TPO is found in the liver of adrenalectomized rats following treatment with L-tryptophan. A similar increase is obtained by cortisone. [The brief abstract does not state whether cortisone was also tested in adrenalectomized rats (H.S.).]

Kenney E98,787/62: Labeling of TKT in the livers of cortisol-pretreated and not pretreated adrenalectomized rats was followed after a single injection of L-leucine-^{14}C. The results suggest "that the rate of enzyme synthesis is increased on induction, and that alterations in the rate of enzyme degradation play little or no role in the induced increase in enzyme."

Lee & Balts D16,649/62: In rats, adrenalectomy diminishes the ability of the liver to form TPO following tryptophan injection. "Under dosage and time conditions in which hydrocortisone and the adrenocortical extract did not act as inducers, it was demonstrated that they permitted the quantitative response to substrate administration to return to normal; desoxycorticosterone was found to be ineffective. The results have been interpreted as an example of the 'permissive' action of the adrenocortical secretory products."

Rosen & Milholland D23,053/62: Administration of L-tryptophan, but not of tyrosine, stimulated hepatic TKT activity in adrenalectomized rats. No such induction was obtained by tryptophan in vitro. Adrenalectomized rats treated with tyrosine, methionine or histidine had slightly subnormal TKT levels. Tryptophan analogues (D-tryptophan, acetyl-L-tryptophan, indole, D,L-5-OH-tryptophan and 5-HT), increase both TKT and TPO activity in the livers of adrenalectomized rats. In hypophysectomized rats, tryptophan, 5-HT or 5-OH-tryptophan caused only a slight rise in the hepatic activity of TPO or TKT.

Davis D92,322/63: The decarboxylation of o-tyrosine and 5-hydroxytryptophan by livers of adrenalectomized rats, given water, was significantly lower than in controls. No significant effects on decarboxylation of these substrates were observed in adrenalectomized animals given NaCl, or in intact animals treated with DOC or exposed to cold. On the other hand, cortisone increased the inherent hepatic decarboxylating activity for both substrates, in normal as well as in pyridoxine-deficient rats.

Greengard & Gordon G15,572/63: "The tyrosine-α-ketoglutarate transaminase activity of liver extracts, assayed in the presence of excess pyridoxal phosphate, was increased by the parenteral administration of pyridoxine to adrenalectomized rats. A 3-fold rise can occur in 4 hrs. The administration of puromycin, an inhibitor of protein synthesis, prevents the pyridoxine-induced rise in the amount of tyrosine-α-ketoglutarate transaminase. The results suggest that coenzyme levels, in addition to regulating the activity of existing enzyme, may influence, in vivo, the amount of the protein moiety of appropriate enzyme systems."

Greengard et al. D63,145/63: In adrenalectomized rats, "the administration of puromycin inhibited the cortisone-induced elevation of tryptophan pyrrolase and tyrosine-α-ketoglutarate transaminase activity as well as the substrate-induced elevation of the latter. Actinomycin D abolished the cortisone-mediated rise in the level of both enzymes but did not influence the tryptophan-mediated increase in the level of tryptophan pyrrolase." In newborn rats, the development of hepatic TKT was inhibited by actinomycin D, but neither adrenalectomy nor actinomycin interfered with the postnatal development of hepatic TPO. Apparently, accumulation of TPO (unlike that of TKT) is not under adrenal control and can proceed despite inhibited RNA synthesis.

Kenney & Kull G22,373/63: In adrenalectomized rats treated with cortisol, the synthesis of nuclear RNA precedes increased cytoplasmic TKT-synthesis after about 30 min. Enzyme induction is therefore ascribed to the stimulation of messenger RNA.

Knox D66,995/63: In intact rats, TPO or TKT can be induced by pretreatment either with the corresponding substrates or with cortisol. However, after adrenalectomy, TKT, unlike TPO can no longer be induced by the substrate. Cortisol induces both enzymes even after adrenalectomy, and the increase is particularly pronounced if the hormone is given conjointly with these substrates.

Pitot G65,475/63: In the Morris hepatoma 5123, TPO activity is normally low and cannot be significantly altered either by tryptophan or by cortisone, whereas both these substances induce the enzyme in the normal liver tissue. In adrenalectomized rats, TPO induction by tryptophan is lower than in intact animals, although cortisone induction in the host liver is actually increased. A slight enzyme induction appears to be possible even in the hepatoma when cortisone is administered to the adrenalectomized rat. Essentially similar but not quite identical results have been obtained with rats bearing Morris hepatoma 7800 or 7316. TKT, TDH and G-6-P-ase activities were either minimally or not affected by cortisone in various transplantable hepatic tumors.

Rosen et al. E32,653/63: "A period of about 48 hours is required to attain maximal activity of alanine-α-ketoglutarate transaminase in liver after subcutaneous treatment of rats with a single injection of cortisol. In contrast, tyrosine-α-ketoglutarate transaminase reaches a maximal value in liver between 4 and 5 hours after an intraperitoneal dose of cortisol." The same dose of cortisol causes even greater increases in hepatic TKT in adrenalectomized rats, but GPT or TPO induction by cortisol is not influenced by adrenalectomy.

Rosen & Milholland E32,652/63: Tryptophan induced significant increases in hepatic TKT activity in intact and in adrenalectomized (NaCl-maintained) rats. Tyrosine, histidine, and methionine slightly depressed the hepatic TKT activity of the adrenalectomized rats. Analogues of tryptophan (including D-tryptophan, acetyl-L-tryptophan, indole, DL-5-hydroxytryptophan and 5-HT i.p.) increase both TKT and TPO activity by 50—300% in the livers of intact or adrenalectomized rats. 5-HT and DL-5-hydroxytryptophan were most active. After hypophysectomy, the response of each of these enzymes to tryptophan gradually diminished. After 6 months, tryptophan, 5-hydroxytryptophan and 5-HT failed to cause significant increases in the hepatic activity of these enzymes, but cortisol remained highly effective, causing increases in both enzyme activities comparable to those seen in intact or adrenalectomized rats. "Experiments with two known inhibitors of protein synthesis, DL-ethionine and puromycin, indicate that a major fraction of the induced activity of tryptophan pyrrolase seen in adrenalectomized or hypophysectomized rats treated by injection with tryptophan is due to activation rather than synthesis of new enzyme protein. The responses of tryptophan pyrrolase and tyrosine transaminase in liver following cortisol administration appear to be mainly the result of the synthesis of each of these enzymes."

Garren et al. G28,021/64: In adrenalectomized rats, a single i.p. injection of cortisol produces an increase in hepatic TPO and TKT activity. Actinomycin D did not inhibit synthesis of these enzymes, but blocked their induction when injected early after cortisol administration. Actinomycin D and fluorouracil stimulated TPO and TKT synthesis when injected 5 hrs or later after cortisol. "It is proposed that repression of the synthesis of these enzymes occurs at the level of messenger RNA translation."

Knox G65,171/64: Observations on adrenalectomized rats lead to the distinction between two types of TPO induction. One is called the "hormone type" because glucocorticoids act this way. Thus, in adrenalectomized rats, cortisol increased the amount of some limiting RNA moiety, thereby augmenting enzyme synthesis. This action is prevented by actinomycin D through the inhibition of RNA synthesis as well as by puromycin, which inhibits protein synthesis. The second form or "substrate type" of induction is obtained by tryptophan which increases the amount of TPO without stimulating RNA synthesis. This increase is not prevented by actinomycin D although it is, of course, blocked by puromycin, which inhibits protein synthesis.

Pitot et al. G37,125/64: In intact rats bearing Reuber H-35 hepatomas, TKT activity is much greater in the tumor than in the normal hepatic tissue. Cortisone i.p. induces enzyme in the liver, but not in the tumor. In adrenalectomized hosts, however, the enzyme in the tumor is in the range of the host liver and cortisone induces enzyme in both liver and tumor. If cortisone is added to cultures 24 hrs before the enzyme assay, a significant induction occurs in vitro, reaching a maximum in 6 hrs. Actinomycin D added to the medium delays enzyme induction without inhibiting it completely.

Schimke et al. G11,062/64: In adrenalectomized rats, tryptophan i.p. alone causes a linear increase in hepatic TPO reaching a level six times that of the controls within 16 hrs. Cortisol s.c. causes an exponential increase reaching a maximum of 7—8 times the control levels. Simultaneous treatment with cortisol and tryptophan produces a linear increases in TPO at a rate 7 times that produced by tryptophan alone, resulting in a 40—50-fold increase. Analysis of the enzyme kinetics led to the conclusion that "the greatest increase in TPO, then, result from both an increased rate of enzyme formation and a decreased rate of enzyme degradation."

Berlin & Schimke G37,616/65: In adrenalectomized rats, 4 days of pretreatment with cortisone increased the activity of hepatic TPO, TKT, GPT and arginase. Differences in the turnover rate of enzymes thus induced may simulate differential selective-inducing effects upon one or the other enzyme.

Kenney & Albritton G64,557/65: Review of the literature suggesting that transaminase induction in response to stressors can be due to corticoid secretion during the stress reaction. Cortisol increases enzyme synthesis following an increased rate of synthesis of ribosomal transfer and "DNA-like" RNA's. The present experiments confirm the view that repressor(s) can inhibit enzyme synthesis at the translational level because inhibition of RNA synthesis can prolong the corticoid-induced increase in enzyme synthesis under suitable conditions. "Administration of stressing agents (tyrosine, Celite) to adrenalectomized rats initiates a highly selective repression of the synthesis of hepatic TKT. The enzyme level falls with a t½ of about 2.5 hr. Immunochemical measurement of the rate of enzyme synthesis indicates that it is reduced essentially to zero in stressed, adrenalectomized rats, whereas labeling of total liver soluble proteins is unaffected. Actinomycin-D does not itself influence the enzyme level, but it blocks the stress-initiated repression of enzyme synthesis, indicating that repression acts at the translational level, whereas initiation of repression involves transcriptional processes." In hypophysectomized rats, stressors are ineffective and preliminary data suggest that STH is responsible for transaminase repression.

Nomura et al. G33,405/65: Various forms of stress (forced exercise, immobilization, cold), as well as the administration of chlorpromazine, increased the TPO activity of the liver both in intact and in adrenalectomized, but not in hypophysectomized, rats.

Schimke et al. G24,293/65: In adrenalectomized rats, both cortisol and tryptophan increase hepatic TPO, but a particularly pronounced rise is obtained by combined treatment with both these agents. An analysis of the time course of changing enzyme levels and results of isotope incorporation studies indicate that cortisol increases the rate of enzyme synthesis, whereas tryptophan decreases the rate of enzyme degradation.

Singer & Mason G66,500/65: Na-benzoate increased hepatic TKT activity both in intact and in NaCl-maintained adrenalectomized rats. Among 31 cyclic compounds tested for this inducing ability after adrenalectomy, only cortisol, its hemisuccinate and diethylstilbestrol disulfate were more effective than benzoate. Curiously, enzyme induction by cortisol was actually enhanced after adrenalectomy. "Strong inhibition of the increase by injected puromycin and actinomycin D, compounds which inhibit protein and RNA synthesis respectively, suggests that the benzoate-mediated effect occurred by a mechanism involving increases in protein and RNA synthesis. In this respect, the effect of benzoate resembles that of the glucocorticoids."

Tomkins et al. G35,353/65: Following a single injection of cortisol into adrenalectomized rats, the hepatic TPO and TKT levels rise. "Although actinomycin D blocks the initial steroid-induced increase, later administration of the antibiotic (or of 5-fluorouracil) causes an increase in the levels of these enzymes."

Berry et al. G67,237/66: S. typhimurium endotoxin lowers liver TPO in mice and prevents the induction of the enzyme by concurrent injection of cortisone. It lowers, but does not prevent, substrate induction. Actinomycin D has a similar effect on TPO. In the intact mouse, the endotoxin induces TKT almost as well as cortisone, but not in the adrenalectomized animal. Actinomycin D, on the other hand, has an effect on this transaminase similar to that on TPO.

Fiala & Fiala F65,983/66: In the rat, actidione i.p. inhibits the induction of hepatic TPO assayed 4 hrs after administration of the substrate, or of cortisol. By contrast, cycloheximide did not abolish the induction of

TKT by cortisol and, in fact, actidione increased the level of TKT even in the absence of cortisol treatment. A similar, though smaller, effect occurred in hypophysectomized or adrenalectomized rats, suggesting a direct induction of TKT by actidione. Puromycin inhibited the induction of TKT. Apparently, an inhibitor of protein synthesis, such as actidione, may also act as an inducer for the synthesis of TKT, thus simulating the action of cortisol. "This 'pseudohormonal' action of actidione may explain the toxicity of actidione in certain mammalian species and also the fact that hydrocortisone may act as an antidote in actidione poisoning. It does not explain why a similar effect of 'pseudohormonal' induction is not observed in the case of TPO, but only the inhibition of enzyme induction."

Schapiro et al. F 67,227/66: Hepatic TKT activity increased in immature, stressed (reciprocating shaker) rats, but not in the intact, stressed adults. In the stressed adrenalectomized adults, TKT activity markedly decreased, while adrenalectomized immature rats showed no change. Hypophysectomy largely abolished inhibition in the adults. TPO activity, when present, was increased by stress in old-age groups, but the increase was abolished by adrenalectomy and hypophysectomy. "The results suggest stress-activation of a pituitary mechanism that inhibits or represses activation of tyrosine transaminase and that may not function during early postnatal life."

Agarwal & Berry G 66,480/67: "Four hours after zymosan administration, cortisone was able to induce mouse liver tryptophan pyrrolase production almost at a normal rate and, under these conditions, protected mice against a concurrent injection of endotoxin. Administration of zymosan, at either 2 or 4 hours after cortisone administration, resulted in little change in tryptophan pyrrolase activity while endotoxin, when similarly administered, caused a rapid decline in liver tryptophan pyrrolase activity. ... Glucan and zymosan, like endotoxin, increased tyrosine-α-ketoglutarate transaminase activity in intact but not in adrenalectomized mice. Zymosan and thorotrast, unlike endotoxin, neither lowered liver carbohydrate levels nor influenced cortisone induced neosynthesis of liver glycogen. These results suggest a cause and effect relationship between inducibility of key liver enzymes and survival against stress."

Aitio & Hänninen G 66,417/67: Both in intact and in adrenalectomized rats, cinchophen increased the hepatic TKT activity, but had no effect upon that of GPT and GOT.

Grossmann & Mavrides G 46,206/67: Studies on the kinetics of cortisol-induced hepatic TKT activity in adrenalectomized rats. "Puromycin inhibited enzyme synthesis when it was given during the initial phase of induction. However, it unexpectedly caused a rapid reappearance of enzyme activity following its administration during the inactivation phase. This potentiated response is consistent with other observations which lead to the idea that a repressor is formed about 4 hours after hormone administration and that inhibition of repressor synthesis allows, at least temporarily, continued synthesis of enzyme." The inactivator appears to depend upon pituitary function, since adrenalectomized and hypophysectomized rats showed little or no inactivation phase following cortisol treatment.

Hänninen & Hartiala F 76,119/67: In the rat, the stress of restraint causes a linear increase in hepatic TKT to 4 times the initial level within 12 hrs. This effect was partially inhibited by actinomycin D and totally by adrenalectomy.

Kato G 54,276/67: In intact, unlike in adrenalectomized, ascites-tumor-bearing mice, the hepatic TKT activity is elevated.

Kenney G 50,810/67: In intact, hypophysectomized or adrenalectomized rats, STH inhibits the synthesis of hepatic TKT. The rate of enzyme synthesis is reduced nearly to 0 (immunochemical-isotopic analyses), whereas labeling of the bulk of the liver proteins is increased by STH. Repression is blocked when RNA synthesis is inhibited by actinomycin D. STH also appears to play a role in the repression of TKT induction by stressors. A hypophysectomized and an intact rat were united by parabiosis. When the pituitary-bearing member was stressed by tyrosine i.p., repression occurred in the livers of both treated and untreated (hypophysectomized) animals. Transaminase levels were unchanged in a single experiment where the stressing agent was administered to the hypophysectomized partner.

Kupfer & Peets F 85,854/67: Cortisol s.c. increases hepatic TKT activity in adrenalectomized male rats and this effect is further augmented by SKF 525-A which in itself has no effect. In intact rats, SKF 525-A raises hepatic TKT activity in itself but this effect is not further augmented by cortisol. Possibly, the potentiation of cortisol induction of TKT by SKF 525-A is due to an inhibition of the degradation of cortisol.

Seidman et al. F 88,452/67: The induction of TPO has been studied in the liver remnant of partially hepatectomized rats following treatment with cortisol, and after adrenalectomy. "It seems possible, therefore that the lessened response to hydrocortisone in hepatic cells preparing to divide is related to repression of transcriptional rather than translational mechanisms and that the duplicating genome itself may be unable to participate simultaneously in other functions."

Goswami et al. G 55,570/68: L-tyrosine fails to induce TKT in the liver of the adrenalectomized rats unless 8-azaguanine is administered simultaneously. Pretreatment with actinomycin D prevents this response. It is assumed that "tyrosine is a potential stimulator restrained by an inhibitor whose activity is diminished by 8-aG."

Kenney et al. H 4,503/68: When adrenalectomized rats are subjected to severe stress, or given STH, the hepatic level of TKT falls markedly. No such effect is obtained by addition of STH to the perfusion fluid of an isolated liver and, hence, the "repression response" is considered secondary to an extrahepatic factor.

Rapoport et al. G 53,334/68: Pneumococcal infection raised the hepatic TPO activity in intact, but not in adrenalectomized, mice. Cortisol increased TPO activity both in control and in pneumococcus-infected mice, but only if administered early after inoculation. Later during the course of infection, some inhibitory factor develops which counteracts the TPO induction by cortisol.

Schapiro H 2,360/68: Stress (30 min rough agitation in a noisy laboratory shaker) had no effect upon the corticoid sensitive enzyme TKT in the liver of the intact rat, but it increased TPO activity, which is likewise corticoid inducible. Adrenalectomized rats, similarly stressed, exhibited a decreased transaminase activity with no change in TPO. This inhibitory effect was abolished by hypophysectomy. STH inhibited induction of transaminase by cortisol, but had no effect upon cortisol-induced TPO activity. The opposing actions of STH and glucocorticoids may be involved in adaptive reactions to stress.

Finch et al. G 71,207/69: In mice, various stressors (cold, shaking) cause a rapid and transient increase in hepatic TKT activity during fasting. Recent feeding or adrenalectomy inhibits TKT induction by cold.

Geller et al. H 8,414/69: The stress of laparotomy increases hepatic TKT activity in the intact, but not in the adrenalectomized rat, which actually responds in an inverse manner. Hypophysectomy eliminates some, but not all of these laparotomy-induced repressions. Under these conditions, the TPO- and the TKT-responses are somewhat different.

Govier & Lovenberg G 70,841/69: In rats, the increase in hepatic TKT produced by phentolamine is almost completely abolished by adrenalectomy or hypophysectomy. If small doses of cortisol are given to adrenalectomized rats, phentolamine again increases enzyme activity. Aminoglutethimide completely eliminates both the increase in plasma corticosterone and the enzyme induction by phentolamine. "It is concluded that at least two factors are operative in the induction of tyrosine aminotransferase by phentolamine— (1) a response to an increased plasma corticosterone concentration, and (2) an additional effect which may be a direct substrate type of induction."

Kröger et al. G 66,240/69: In adrenalectomized rats, the induction of hepatic TKT and TPO is possible only if, in addition to the substrate, small amounts of cortisone are administered.

Lane & Mavrides H 12,953/69: Cortisol caused a greater increase of hepatic TKT in hypophysectomized than in adrenalectomized rats. In general, elevation of enzyme activity after cortisol was inversely proportional to the initial enzyme level, and the latter was in turn higher on protein-rich than on protein-poor diets.

Levitan & Webb G 64,051/69: Six hours after administering cortisol to adrenalectomized rats, the increased hepatic TKT level begins to fall. Upon concurrent treatment with 8-azaguanine, the increase is greater and much more prolonged. It is assumed that 8-azaguanine affects the degradation of TKT but does not significantly inhibit its synthesis.

Nicolis & Ginoulhiac H 14,045/69: In adrenalectomized rats, the hepatic TPO activity turns roughly parallel to the glucocorticoid potency of prednisone, prednisolone, 16α-methylprednisone, 16β-methylprednisone, dexamethasone and betamethasone.

Nakano et al. G 76,247/70: "In adrenalectomized rats, hepatic TPO which can be increased in amount in intact rats by feeding either tryptophan or methionine, was activated and increased in amount by feeding tryptophan but not methionine. The feeding of tryptophan resulted in a significant increase in the level of arginase and threonine dehydratase. Methionine produced a similar increase in both threonine dehydratase and arginase activities. Administration of cortisone acetate produced a significant increase in the level of all three enzyme activities."

Other Amino Acid Enzymes ←. *Brin & McKee C31,261/56:* In the rat, various stressors (total body X-irradiation, nitrogen mustard, starvation) as well as cortisone increase GOT and GPT activities in the liver. Adrenalectomy decreases the activity of these enzymes. GPT is more sensitive to stress than GOT.

Rosen et al. C50,741/58: In rats treated with cortisol, cortisone or prednisone for one week, there was an increase in hepatic GPT but not in GOT activity. DOC had no such effect. Hypophysectomy or adrenalectomy did not prevent this action of cortisone. STH, testosterone or insulin failed to alter GPT activity nor did any of them influence GPT stimulation by cortisol.

Rosen et al. C71,414/59: Marked increases in GPT activity were observed in the livers of rats given cortisol, cortisone, 9α-fluorocortisol, 6α-methylprednisolone, prednisone, 9α-fluoro-21-desoxy-6α-methylprednisolone or ACTH, whereas two nonglucocorticoid cortisol derivatives, 11-epicortisol and 9α-methoxycortisol, were inactive. STH, testosterone and insulin caused no significant change in GPT by themselves nor did they modify the action of cortisol. On the other hand, large doses of estradiol and thyroxine caused a moderate increase in GPT activity, but when injected simultaneously with cortisol they appeared to interfere with its action as did progesterone. Adrenalectomy slightly diminished or failed to affect the GPT inducing activity of cortisol, whereas hypophysectomy caused a rise in GPT activity and augmented the effect of cortisol.

Rosen et al. G66,496/59: In the rat, cortisol, cortisone and prednisone cause a 6—13 fold increase in hepatic GPT activity. This effect was directly related to the protein content of the ration. In alloxan diabetic rats, the rise in this enzyme activity was equivalent to that obtained by cortisol or high-protein diets and could be inhibited by insulin. Adrenalectomy diminished but did not abolish the rise in GPT activity obtained by feeding high-protein diets. Thus, the initiation of enzyme synthesis by dietary protein is not mediated exclusively through the adrenals.

Harding et al. D14,355/61: In the rat, pretreatment with DOC depresses the hepatic GPT activity. A similar depression is obtained by adrenalectomy, but this is not further aggravated by concurrent treatment with DOC. ACTH increases GPT activity in hypophysectomized, but not in adrenalectomized, animals. In hypophysectomized rats, DOC fails to lower GPT nor does it alter the response of this enzyme to ACTH. "The inhibitory effect of DOC on alanine transaminase activity appears to be due to suppression of ACTH release by the pituitary."

Freedland F17,044/64: In the rat, adrenalectomy considerably decreases the arginase and arginine synthetase activity of liver homogenates, but has no effect on lactic acid dehydrogenase activity. Various dietary measures, which alter the activities of arginine synthetase, arginase, and lactic acid dehydrogenase in intact rats, are also effective after adrenalectomy.

Freedland & Avery G67,766/64: In the rat, the TDH and SDH activity of liver homogenates was increased by high protein diets, alloxan diabetes, or cortisol. Factors affecting the activity of TDH caused a proportional change in SDH suggesting that both of these activities may be due to a single protein. The SDH activity was decreased by adrenalectomy or hypophysectomy. Adrenalectomy had no effect upon the response of this enzyme to protein feeding, whereas, after hypophysectomy, this response was diminished.

Ishikawa et al. F41,763/65: In alloxandiabetic rats, the SDH and TDH levels of the hepatic microsomes are greatly enhanced. SDH was readily induced by cortisol in the diabetic, but not in the normal, rat. The effects of actinomycin S, STH, and starvation upon SDH have also been studied in intact, hypophysectomized, adrenalectomized and thyroidectomized rats. It is concluded that "serine dehydratase activity in the liver plays an important role in the production of pyruvate as a starting material for gluconeogenesis."

Schmidinger & Kröger F92,031/67: The increase in hepatic SDH induced by protein-deficient diets and starvation in intact rats is prevented by actinomycin D, puromycin or glucose, but aggravated after adrenalectomy. Cortisone administered during the starvation period increases SDH activity, perhaps owing to utilization of inhibitors of this enzyme during gluconeogenesis.

Jost et al. H11,724/68: Studies on the induction and repression of SDH by rat liver microsomes. "Amino acid induction and glucose repression as well as hormonal induction by both glucagon and hydrocortisone occur in adrenalectomized animals."

Pan et al. H3,934/68: The methionine adenosyltransferase activity of hepatic homogenates is higher in female than in male rats. "Ovariectomy decreased the enzyme level, whereas the administration of 17β-estradiol or diethylstilbestrol, but not progesterone, reversed the effect of ovariectomy. Estradiol also raised the enzyme level in intact male rats to that of the female. Adrenalectomy had no effect on the response of the enzyme to estradiol. Castration of the male resulted in an increase in the activity of methionine adenosyltransferase, and the administration of androgenic-anabolic hormones brought the elevated activity down to the normal level of intact males or even lower. Adrenalectomy did not abolish the effect of castration. 17α-Ethyl-19-nortestosterone and 1-methyl-Δ^1-androstenolone were more effective in this respect than testosterone, 17α-methyl-Δ^5-androstene-3β,17β-diol and 5α-androstan-17β-ol-3-one. The effect of the steroids in decreasing methionine adenosyltransferase activity seems to be associated with their anabolic rather than their androgenic action."

Hoshino & Kröger H13,867/69: SDH was induced in the livers of adrenalectomized rats by fasting and concurrent cortisone treatment. The properties of the purified enzyme preparation are described.

Murphy & Malley G68,408/69: Studies on hepatic TKT, alkaline phosphatase (AP), GPT and TPO in relation to stress and CCl_4-intoxication in the rat. "Liver TKT elevation, but not AP elevation, was prevented by adrenalectomy prior to CCl_4. Experiments on rats subjected to simultaneous acute cold stress and CCl_4 indicated that, during the acute phase of CCl_4 hepatotoxicity, their livers had reduced capacity for induction of TKT and TPO by endogenous corticosterone. However, chronically injured livers of rats given repeated doses of CCl_4 were fully responsive to the TKT- and TPO-inducing effects of exogenous corticosterone or acute cold stress."

Shou et al. H15,277/69: In the rat, the hepatic methionine adenosyltransferase activity was not much influenced by glucagon, but during alloxan diabetes it increased considerably. Combined treatment with alloxan and triamcinolone resulted in an additive effect. The response to alloxan could be prevented and even reversed by insulin or adrenalectomy. In normal rats, insulin caused no consistent increase.

Other Enzymes ←. *Pitot G65,475/63:* In the Morris hepatoma 5123, TPO activity is normally low and cannot be significantly altered either by tryptophan or by cortisone, whereas both these substances induce the enzyme in the normal liver tissue. In adrenalectomized rats, TPO induction by tryptophan is lower than in intact animals although cortisone induction in the host liver is actually increased. A slight enzyme induction appears to be possible even in the hepatoma when cortisone is administered to the adrenalectomized rat. Essentially similar but not quite identical results have been obtained with rats bearing Morris hepatoma 7800 or 7316. TKT, TDH and G-6-P-ase activities were either minimally or not affected by cortisone in various transplantable hepatic tumors.

Garren et al. G19,151/64: Cortisol increased the rate of synthesis of nuclear RNA in the livers of adrenalectomized rats.

Dietrich & Yero G26,959/65: Cortisol markedly lowered the nicotinamide deamidase-activity of the liver in intact, hypophysectomized, and adrenalectomized rats. Under these conditions, cortisol failed to inhibit hepatic synthesis of NAD significantly after nicotinamide challenge. Hexestrol markedly lowered hepatic deamidase activity in intact, thyroidectomized, and adrenalectomized rats. A reduction of the hepatic NAD-ase-levels after nicotinamide challenge occurred upon hexestrol treatment in intact, but not in adrenalectomized, rats. Hypophysectomy markedly stimulated nicotinamide deamidase activity and NAD-biosynthesis after nicotinamide challenge.

Greenman et al. G35,063/65; Wicks et al. G35,046/65: Studies on the stimulation of hepatic ^{32}P-RNA synthesis in adrenalectomized rats treated with cortisol.

Freedland et al. G55,808/68: Extensive studies on the effect of adrenalectomy, hypophysectomy and cortisol treatment upon a great variety of rat liver enzymes, with observations on the influence of thyroxine upon these enzymes in intact, adrenalectomized or hypophysectomized rats. The extensive data do not lend themselves to succinct presentation in the form of a summary and must be consulted in the original.

Fazekas & Rengei G64,534/69: Comparative studies on the NAD and $NADH_2$ content of various tissues in intact and adrenalectomized rats treated with ethanol s.c.

Jacob et al. G64,812/69: Rat liver nucleoli were examined for RNA polymerase activity. A single injection of cortisol into adrenalectomized rats resulted in a 3-fold increase in Mg^{2+}-dependent polymerase while Mn^{2+}-dependent polymerase activity was not significantly altered.

Murphy & Malley G68,408/69: Studies on hepatic TKT, alkaline phosphatase (AP), GPT and TPO in relation to stress and CCl_4-intoxication in the rat. "Liver TKT elevation, but not AP elevation, was prevented by adrenalectomy prior to CCl_4. Experiments on rats subjected to simultaneous acute cold stress and CCl_4 indicated that, during the acute phase of CCl_4 hepatotoxicity, their livers had reduced capacity for induction of TKT and TPO by endogenous corticosterone. However, chronically injured livers of rats given repeated doses of CCl_4 were fully responsive to the TKT- and TPO-inducing effects of exogenous corticosterone or acute cold stress."

← *Folliculoids*

Rosen et al. C71,414/59: Marked increases in GPT activity were observed in the livers of rats given cortisol, cortisone, 9α-fluorocortisol, prednisone, 6α-methylprednisolone, 9α-fluoro-21-desoxy-6α-methylprednisolone or ACTH, whereas two nonglucocorticoid cortisol derivatives, 11-epicortisol and 9α-methoxycortisol, were inactive. STH, testosterone and insulin caused no significant change in GPT by themselves nor did they modify the action of cortisol. On the other hand, large doses of estradiol and thyroxine caused a moderate increase in GPT activity but when injected simultaneously with cortisol they appeared to interfere with its action as did progesterone. Adrenalectomy slightly diminished or failed to affect the GPT-inducing activity of cortisol, whereas hypophysectomy caused a rise in GPT activity and augmented the effect of cortisol.

Dietrich & Yero G26,959/65: Cortisol markedly lowered the nicotinamide deamidase-activity of the liver in intact, hypophysectomized, and adrenalectomized rats. Under these conditions, cortisol failed to inhibit hepatic synthesis of NAD significantly after nicotinamide challenge. Hexestrol markedly lowered hepatic deamidase activity in intact, thyroidectomized, and adrenalectomized rats. A lowering of the hepatic NAD-ase-levels after nicotinamide challenge occurred upon hexestrol treatment in intact, but not in adrenalectomized, rats. Hypophysectomy markedly stimulated nicotinamide deamidase activity and NAD-biosynthesis after nicotinamide challenge.

Dietrich G28,103/65: In the mouse, hepatic nicotinamide deamidase, and the capacity to synthesize NAD are lowered by dienestrol, diethylstilbestrol, estradiol-17β, estrone, estriol, cortisone and cortisol. Pretreatment with large amounts of hexestrol also lowered the capacity of hepatic tissue to synthesize NAD upon nicotinamide challenge.

Dietrich et al. H19,763/70: In mice, large amounts of hexestrol induce marked changes in the means whereby nicotinate is converted into nicotinamide within the liver.

Rose & Braidman H25,726/70: In rats, estradiol increases hepatic TPO, TKT and GPT activity. The depression which develops in some women using contraceptive pills may be due to increased metabolism of tryptophan to nicotinic acid ribonucleotide; raised aminotransferase activity may divert pyridoxal phosphate away from other metabolic functions including 5-HT synthesis.

← *Luteoids*

Rosen et al. C71,414/59: Marked increases in GPT activity were observed in the livers of rats given cortisol, cortisone, 9α-fluorocortisol, prednisone, 6α-methylprednisolone, 9α-fluoro-21-desoxy-6α-methylprednisolone or ACTH, whereas two nonglucocorticoid cortisol derivatives, 11-epicortisol and 9α-methoxycortisol were inactive. STH, testosterone and insulin caused no significant change in GPT by themselves nor did they modify the action of cortisol. On the other hand, large doses of estradiol and thyroxine caused a moderate increase in GPT activity but when injected simultaneously with cortisol they appeared to interfere with its action as did progesterone. Adrenalectomy slightly diminished or failed to affect the GPT-inducing activity of cortisol, whereas hypophysectomy caused a rise in GPT activity and augmented the effect of cortisol.

Simon et al. C84,793/59: In the rabbit and rat, progesterone, androsterone and testosterone stimulate the oxidation of galactose by surviving liver slices. The same steroids also stimulate the conversion of UDP-galactose into UDP-glucose by rabbit liver slices and extracts.

Pesch et al. C79,957/60: Earlier observations have shown that progesterone, androsterone and testosterone stimulate the oxidation of galactose by rabbit liver slices, owing to an increase in the enzymic activity of the hepatic microsomes. In vivo observations revealed that progesterone can also inhibit the formation of cataracts in rats maintained on a high galactose diet.

Galactose ← Progesterone + Galactosemia, Man: Pesch et al. C79,957/60*

Xylose ← Progesterone + Age: Pesch et al. C79,957/60*

← Testoids

Rosen et al. C50,741/58: In rats treated with cortisol, cortisone or prednisone for one week, there was an increase in hepatic GPT but not in GOT activity. DOC had no such effect. Hypophysectomy or adrenalectomy did not prevent this action of cortisone. STH, testosterone or insulin failed to alter GPT activity nor did they influence its stimulation by cortisol.

Lin et al. C96,929/59: TKT activity is higher in male than in female rat liver. This enzyme activity is diminished by castration in males, and increased by testosterone in females. Cortisol increases this transaminase activity in males much more than in females, both in the presence and in the absence of the adrenals.

Rosen et al. C71,414/59: Marked increases in GPT activity were observed in the livers of rats given cortisol, cortisone, 9α-fluorocortisol, prednisone, 6α-methylprednisolone, 9α-fluoro-21-desoxy-6α-methylprednisolone or ACTH, whereas two nonglucocorticoid cortisol derivatives, 11-epicortisol and 9α-methoxycortisol were inactive. STH, testosterone and insulin caused no significant change in GPT by themselves nor did they modify the action of cortisol. On the other hand, large doses of estradiol and thyroxine caused a moderate increase in GPT activity but when injected simultaneously with cortisol they appeared to interfere with its action as did progesterone. Adrenalectomy slightly diminished or failed to affect the GPT-inducing activity of cortisol, whereas hypophysectomy caused a rise in GPT activity and augmented the effect of cortisol.

Simon et al. C84,793/59: In the rabbit and rat, progesterone, androsterone and testosterone stimulate the oxidation of galactose by surviving liver slices. The same steroids also stimulate the conversion of UDP-galactose into UDP-glucose by rabbit liver slices and extracts.

← Gonadectomy

Lin et al. C96,929/59: TKT activity is higher in the livers of male than of female rats. This enzyme activity is diminished by castration in males, and increased by testosterone in females. Cortisol increases this transaminase activity in males much more than in females, both in the presence and in the absence of the adrenals.

Wurtman & Axelrod E36,478/63: Hepatic MAO activity is greater in male than in female rats. This difference can be reversed by estradiol in male and by testosterone in female gonadectomized rats.

Pan et al. H3,934/68: The methionine adenosyltransferase activity of hepatic homogenates is higher in female than in male rats. "Ovariectomy decreased the enzyme level, whereas the administration of 17β-estradiol or diethylstilbestrol, but not progesterone, reversed the effect of ovariectomy. Estradiol also raised the enzyme level in intact male rats to that of the female. Adrenalectomy had no effect on the response of the enzyme to estradiol. Castration of the male resulted in an increase in the activity of methionine adenosyltransferase, and the administration of androgenic-anabolic hormones brought the elevated activity down to the normal level of intact males or even lower. Adrenalectomy did not abolish the effect of castration. 17α-Ethyl-19-nortestosterone and 1-methyl-$Δ^1$-androstenolone were more effective in this respect than testosterone, 17α-methyl-$Δ^5$-androstene-3β,17β-diol and 5α-androstan-17β-ol-3-one. The effect of the steroids in decreasing methionine adenosyltransferase activity seems to be associated with their anabolic rather than their androgenic action."

Künzel & Müller-Oerlinghausen G64,178/69: In vitro glucuronide synthesis is much higher in male than female rat liver tissue because of a larger UDP-glucuronic acid supply in the male liver. Orchidectomy decreases glucuronide synthesis and this decrease can be counteracted by testosterone administration in a dose-dependent manner. However, very large doses of testosterone (more than 100 μg per day) decrease glucuronide formation. Cyproterone (an antitestoid) does not inhibit the increase in glucuronide synthesis induced by testosterone.

← Various Steroids

Thompson et al. F81,633/66: "Tyrosine α-ketoglutarate transaminase can be induced by steroid hormones in a newly established line of tissue culture cells, derived from primary culture of the ascites form of an experimental rat hepatoma." Dexamethasone, triamcinolone and cortisol were highly active, DOC and aldosterone much less potent, whereas stilbestrol, estradiol, testosterone and progesterone were virtually inactive. The induction by dexamethasone was blocked by puromycin, cycloheximide, chloramphenicol, progesterone, actinomycin D and mitomycin C. Paradoxically, after induction by the steroid had taken place, actinomycin D produced a further increase in enzyme activity.

Farese H27,025/70: In rats, TMACN inhibits cholesterol side-chain cleavage during incubation of adrenal homogenates or slices in vitro.

Leber et al. H35,676/71: In male rats, pretreatment with spironolactone stimulated the specific activity of isolated hepatic microsomes for aminopyrine demethylation and 4-methylumbelliferone glucoronidation. Microsomal cytochrome P-450 content increased about 66%. Under comparable conditions, ethacrynic acid increased the specific activity of the microsomes for the demethylation of aminopyrine and the P-450 content but, glucoronidation of 4-methylumbelliferone was not significantly altered. Another nonsteroidal diuretic, furosemid, did not influence any of these parameters.

VI. EFFECT OF OTHER HORMONES UPON RESISTANCE

← ACTH

Steroids ←

The influence of ACTH upon various actions of mineralocorticoids *(Selye C92,918/61, p. 18; G60,083/70, pp. 328–332)* and MAD *(Selye G60,083/70, pp. 328, 330)* has been discussed elsewhere. Let us add here that in rats ACTH (like adrenocortical extract) antagonizes many manifestations of overdosage with **DOC**, such as the: hypernatremia, EST-elevation, and insulin hypersensitivity, as well as the hyalinosis syndrome produced after uninephrectomy + NaCl. Conversely, the hyalinosis elicited by **MAD** is actually aggravated by ACTH. This singular "DOC-like" effect is presumably due to the inhibition by MAD of 11β-hydroxylation in the adrenals; in the presence of this enzymic defect the corticotrophic action of ACTH shifts towards an excess secretion of DOC which has no 11β-OH group.

Nonsteroidal Hormones and Hormone-Like Substances ←

ACTH shares with the glucocorticoids the property of increasing **insulin** resistance. This action is not unexpected in view of the antagonistic effect exerted by insulin and glucocorticoids upon the blood sugar.

In guinea pigs exposed to **histamine** spray, ACTH has little if any protective effect but the gastric ulcers produced in this species by conjoint treatment with histamine and antihistamines can be prevented by the concurrent administration of ACTH. In newborn rats, fatal histamine intoxication is not significantly influenced either by ACTH or by various glucocorticoids.

The production of renal infarcts by **5-HT** in the rat, though diminished by hypophysectomy, is not significantly influenced by ACTH.

Steroids ←

Woodbury et al. B47,201/50: In rats, ACTH and adrenocortical extract antagonize the following actions of DOC: 1) hypernatremia; 2) EST threshold elevation; 3) insulin hypersensitivity; 4) hyalinosis (after sensitization by uninephrectomy plus NaCl).

Molteni et al. H4,919/68: In rats, the vascular lesions produced by MAD following uninephrectomy plus NaCl are aggravated by ACTH, presumably, because MAD interferes with β-hydroxylation in the adrenals, so that under the influence of ACTH an excess of DOC is secreted.

Cortisol ← ACTH: Kuipers et al. C48,349/58*; Kumagai et al. C57,345/58; Berliner et al. G75,988/61*; Moor et al. G75,989/61*; Werk et al. F20,780/64*

Cortisone ← ACTH + Sex: Hagen et al. G77,512/60

Nonsteroidal Hormones and Hormone-Like Substances ←

Insulin ←. *Jensen & Grattan 77,887/40:* In mice, ACTH, glucocorticoids and cortical extracts increase insulin resistance, whereas other pituitary hormones and thyroxine have no such effect.

Thyroxine ← *cf. Selye G60,083/70, pp. 328, 330, 347, 355.*

Histamine and 5-HT ←. *Andreani B63,732/50:* In guinea pigs, conjoint treatment with large doses of histamine and antihistamines had previously been shown to result in gastric ulcer formation although the lethal effects of histamine are suppressed. These ulcers can be prevented by ACTH.

Friedlaender & Friedlaender B55,467/50: In guinea pigs, intoxication with histamine (aerosol) and anaphylactic shock (horse serum) were not influenced by pretreatment with ACTH.

Buttle & Squires B59,985/51: In guinea pigs exposed to histamine spray, the time required to induce convulsions is prolonged by ACTH i.p. but only during approximately an hour after the injection.

Malkiel G71,451/51: In guinea pigs, ACTH and cortisone are without effect on the end results of histamine shock, or of passive or active anaphylaxis.

Jasmin & Bois C92,099/60: Hypophysectomy partially protects the rat against the production of renal infarcts by 5-HT. ACTH does not affect this change, cortisol aggravates it, whereas DOC and testosterone offer partial protection.

Schapiro F31,856/65: In newborn rats, fatal intoxication with histamine was not significantly influenced by ACTH, cortisol, cortisone or corticosterone.

Drugs ←

The effect of ACTH upon various intoxications has been the subject of many investigations; these could hardly be condensed more than has been done in the Abstract Section to which the reader is therefore referred. Here, we shall comment only on a few particularly interesting data and on certain observations which can be clarified by correlating them with facts not mentioned by the authors of the original articles cited.

Anaphylactoid edema is essentially a special type of serous inflammation, usually studied in rats because these are particularly sensitive to this change. The edema is more or less selectively localized to the acral regions (snout, paws, ears) and is ascribed to the sudden liberation of histamine and 5-HT from the mastocytes of the affected parts. It is provoked by so-called "anaphylactoidogenic agents," such as egg-white, dextran, polymyxin and other typical dischargers of histamine and 5-HT. Like most types of inflammation, this response can be prevented by ACTH and glucocorticoids but only if very large amounts are given. It is noteworthy however, that the specific toxicity of anaphylactoidogenic agents may be uninfluenced or actually aggravated by ACTH, even when the hormone suppresses inflammation itself.

Certain **anticoagulants** such as bishydroxycoumarin (Dicoumarol) and polyanethol sulfonate (Liquoid), at doses normally well tolerated by rabbits, cause death with widespread hemorrhages when given conjointly with ACTH. Curiously bishydroxycoumarin administered with glucocorticoids (cortisol, cortisone) does not elicit this syndrome.

In mice, ACTH shortens sleeping time after treatment with various **barbiturates**, including barbital, thiopental and pentobarbital. The induction time of barbital anesthesia was not changed but its depth was diminished in mice by cortisone, cortisol or ACTH. At the same time the barbital concentration of the brain was decreased by these hormones, which presumably protect against anesthesia by inhibiting the barbital uptake of the brain. Compound "S" or DOC does not share these effects.

In the rat and in man, ACTH also shortens barbiturate sleeping time. Hexobarbital anesthesia is likewise diminished in rats by exposure to stress, presumably as a consequence of endogenous ACTH secretion.

It is highly probable that most of the barbiturates are detoxified by hepatic microsomal enzymes and some of the hormones which shorten barbital sleeping time may do so by inducing such enzymic activities. However, barbital is not significantly degraded within the body and hence, in this case the effect of ACTH is likely to be mediated through a different mechanism, perhaps a topical effect upon the cerebral barbital uptake.

In rats with tourniquet stress, the toxicity of hexobarbital, pentobarbital, meprobamate and zoxazolamine was significantly diminished, whereas that of barbital and phenobarbital remained unaffected. Pretreatment with ACTH or corticosterone simulated the effects of stress.

In rats, the organ changes produced by certain **carcinogens** are not regularly influenced by ACTH. However, hepatoma formation by N-OH-FAA is enhanced both by ACTH and by STH.

Prostatic carcinogenesis after topical 20-methylcholanthrene crystal implantation is inhibited by ACTH as well as by several thyroid and steroid hormones.

In mice, the amyloidosis produced by repeated parenteral administration of **casein** is aggravated by ACTH or glucocorticoids and it may be combined with waxy degeneration of the cardiac muscle.

The typical **cholesterol** atherosclerosis of the rabbit is diminished by ACTH as well as by several glucocorticoids. It is not clear as yet, however, whether this effect is due to increased cholesterol degradation by hepatic microsomal-enzyme systems or to some other, possibly local, effect of glucocorticoids upon the vessels.

In rats, fatal intoxication with certain **ganglioplegics** (TEA, hexamethonium, pentolinium) has been prevented by all glucocorticoids tested (triamcinolone, cortisol, prednisolone, etc.) but not by typical catatoxic steroids (ethylestrenol, CS-1, spironolactone, norbolethone, oxandrolone) or by progesterone, DOC and hydroxydione. Various stressors (bone fractures, fasting, spinal cord transection, formalin) gave excellent protection against TEA, whereas others (restraint, cold) did not. Since even large doses of ACTH failed to protect against TEA the prophylactic effect of stress cannot be ascribed exclusively to increased production of ACTH. The protective effect of glucocorticoids is not directed against ganglioplegics as such since these steroids offer no protection against trimethaphan, mecamylamine, trimethidinium or pempidine.

Although osteolathyrism produced in rats by **lathyrogens** (AAN, PNA, or the feeding of lathyrus seeds) is readily prevented by small doses of glucocorticoids, very large amounts of ACTH are required to obtain even partial protection. The dissecting aneurysms of the aorta characteristic of angiolathyrism are likewise readily suppressed by cortisone but not by ACTH.

The toxicity of **morphine** is diminished by ACTH in various species.

In guinea pigs, ACTH (like cortisone) ameliorates the manifestations of **vitamin-C** deficiency.

In rats, the generalized calcinosis produced by various **vitamin-D** and **DHT** preparations is aggravated by ACTH (as it is by glucocorticoids) but the development of rickets on vitamin-D deficient diets is not significantly affected by ACTH. These findings should be checked under varying experimental conditions of dosage and timing, since it is known that all potent catatoxic steroids prevent acute DHT intoxication in the rat, whereas only the anabolics appear to offer protection against chronic overdosage with the same compound. Indeed, catatoxic steroids with little or no anabolic potency (e.g., PCN, spironolactone) tend to aggravate DHT intoxication and to antagonize the beneficial effect of anabolic catatoxic steroids (e.g., ethylestrenol) in long lasting experiments.

Acetaldehyde ←

Lecoq et al. B66,406/51: In rats, the toxic effects of ethanol and its metabolites, pyruvate and acetaldehyde (which accumulate in the body under the influence of disulfiram) are inhibited by ACTH, cortisone, and hepatic extracts. Conversely, thyroxine, DOC, and testosterone appeared to aggravate ethanol intoxication. [Statistically evaluated data are not presented (H.S.).]

Acrylonitrile ←

Szabó & Selye G79,010/71: In rats, pretreatment with ACTH (but not with STH) prevents the production of adrenal apoplexy by acrylonitrile. Hypophysectomy protects against adrenal apoplexy, but not against mortality under similar conditions.

Allylformiate ←

Küchmeister et al. B84,244/53: In rats, ACTH offers some protection against the hepatic damage produced by allylformiate.
Allylformiate ← ACTH: Küchmeister et al. B84,244/53*

Aminocaproic Acid ←

Pataki F75,591/67: In rabbits, combined treatment with polyanetholsulfonate (Liquoid) + EACA produces thrombohemorrhagic necrosis of the adrenal cortex. Simultaneous ACTH treatment significantly reduces the number of fibrin thrombi and the extent of adrenal necrosis but enhances the cortical hemorrhages.

Aminopterin ←

Traina B72,887/51: In mice, ACTH does not influence the toxic effects of aminopterin.
Aminopterin ← ACTH, Gp., Mouse: Traina B72,887/51*

Aminopyrine ← ACTH: Kato et al. F57,817/65

Anaphylactoid Edema ← cf. also Selye B40,000/50, p. 756; G46,715/68, pp. 177, 178, 183.
Higginbotham & Dougherty C44,529/57: In mice, ACTH increased the toxicity of polymyxin B; STH and TTH had no effect upon it.

Anticoagulants ←

van Cauwenberge & Jaques C58,521/58: A dose of phenindione or bishydroxycoumarin, well tolerated by otherwise untreated rabbits, causes death with widespread hemorrhages when given together with ACTH. The hemorrhagic tendency induced by bishydroxycoumarin was not accentuated by STH, cortisone or DOC.

van Cauwenberge & Jaques C72,748/59: The "hemorrhagic death syndrome" produced by dicoumarol treatment in rats simultaneously exposed to various stressors can be reproduced by the administration of ACTH, STH or DOC, instead of stressors. Dicoumarol + cortisol or cortisone did not reproduce this syndrome.

Pataki F75,591/67: In rabbits, combined treatment with polyanetholsulfonate (Liquoid) + EACA produces thrombohemorrhagic necrosis of the adrenal cortex. Simultaneous ACTH treatment significantly reduces the number of fibrin thrombi and the extent of adrenal necrosis but enhances the cortical hemorrhages.

Arsenic ←

Beck & Voloshin B58,271/50: In mice, resistance to arsenite and other arsenicals is increased by cortisone, adrenocortical extracts and ACTH.

Beck B64,609/51: "Prior administration of beef adrenal extract increased the resistance of mice, particularly male mice, to semi-lethal doses of arsenite, oxophenarsine and clorarsen. Male mice were protected against arsenite by cortisone and ACTH, but not by desoxycorticosterone."

Barbiturates ←

Hoyrup & Vinten-Johansen B 84,197/52: In patients with acute phenobarbital or diphenylhydantoin poisoning, the use of ACTH is contraindicated as judged by impressions gained from a small series of observations.

Winter & Flataker B 73,509/52: Cortisone or ACTH, unlike DOC, shortens barbiturate anesthesia. The markedly prolonged sleeping time of mice receiving both barbiturates and diphenhydramine is also decreased by cortisone but the effect of the steroid can be fully accounted for by its antagonism to the barbiturate.

de Boer & Mukomela C 5,245/55: In rats, ACTH and cortisone shorten thiopental and pentobarbital anesthesia, especially in females whose sleeping time is normally longer than that of males.

Komiya C 8,533/55: In mice, barbital sleeping time is decreased by cortisone, cortisol and ACTH but not affected by compound S (11-desoxocortisone) or DOC.

Komiya et al. C 21,326/56: In mice, thiopental anesthesia is reduced in depth, but not in duration, by epinephrine. Barbital anesthesia was slightly reduced by norepinephrine but not by epinephrine. Unpublished experiments suggest that ACTH and glucocorticoids shorten the duration of barbital anesthesia in mice.

Komiya & Shibata C 16,708/56: In mice, the induction time of barbital anesthesia was not changed by cortisone, cortisol, 11-desoxycortisone or DOC. The duration of anesthesia was shortened, the depth of anesthesia diminished, and the barbital concentration of the brain decreased by cortisone, cortisol or ACTH, but none of these parameters was affected by 11-desoxycortisone or DOC. Apparently, the active hormones protect against anesthesia by decreasing the barbital concentration of the brain.

Kubota & Bernstein C 52,401/57: In man, ACTH ameliorates the symptoms of intoxication with various barbiturates.

Rupe et al. E 26,910/63: The sedative effect of hexobarbital and pentobarbital but not of barbital was diminished by tourniquet stress, in the intact but not in the hypophysectomized or adrenalectomized rat. In intact rats, ACTH or cortisone decreases hexobarbital sleeping time as does stress, whereas SKF 525-A completely blocks the protective action of stress. Presumably "the stress effect on the duration of drug action is mediated through increased drug metabolism."

Bousquet et al. E 39,107/64: Morphine-pretreated rats sleep longer than controls after hexobarbital or meprobamate, but not after barbital. ACTH-pretreatment overcomes the morphine inhibition of drug metabolism (verified in vitro).

Bousquet et al. F 35,073/65: In rats with stress produced by applying a tourniquet around one hind limb for 2.5 hrs, the toxicity of hexobarbital, pentobarbital, meprobamate and zoxazolamine was significantly diminished, whereas that of barbital and phenobarbital remained unaffected. Pretreatment with ACTH or corticosterone simulated the effect of stress. After hypophysectomy or adrenalectomy, stress failed to offer the usual protection. [The barbiturates and zoxazolamine appear to have been administered immediately after release of the tourniquet but this is not specifically stated. Allegedly a single injection of corticosterone (50 μg per animal) sufficed to offer protection (H.S.).]

Hexobarbital ← ACTH + Morphine: Rupe et al. E 26,910/63*; Bousquet et al. E 39,107/64*, F 35,073/65*

Pentobarbital ← ACTH + Morphine + Stress: Driever et al. G 31,872/65*

Beryllium ←

Ferris et al. B 65,475/51: In patients with beryllium granulomatosis of the lung, ACTH was found to be beneficial.

Kennedy et al. B 59,278/51: In patients, ACTH exerted beneficial effects upon beryllium granulomatosis and silicosis, presumably as a consequence of its antiphlogistic effect.

Kline et al. B 65,488/51: In patients with beryllium granulomatosis, ACTH and cortisone were found to be beneficial.

White et al. B 74,079/52: In mice, ACTH had no appreciable effect on the distribution or retention of radioberyllium or on the survival rate following acute intoxication with beryllium sulfate.

Beryllium ← ACTH, Mouse: White et al. B 74,079/52*

Bilirubin ← ACTH, Mouse: Catz et al. H 14,471/68

Carbon Tetrachloride ←

Patrick C12,967/55: In rats and mice, cortisone or ACTH inhibited the mesenchymal reaction and delayed repair following production of hepatic damage by tannic acid or CCl_4.

Carcinogens ←

Robertson et al. B88,672/53: In rats, hypophysectomy prevents the production of hepatic cirrhosis and hepatomas by 3'-Me-DAB. The susceptibility to tumorigenesis is restored by ACTH, but not by CON, DOC or testosterone. These hormones likewise failed to prevent carcinogenesis in intact rats.

Currie et al. D48,292/62: In rats, the production of adrenal necrosis by DMBA is prevented by metyrapone, but not significantly influenced by ACTH.

Morii & Huggins D45,369/62: Immature rats are refractory to the production of adrenocortical necrosis by DMBA, unless they are pretreated with ACTH. On the other hand, STH induces no DMBA sensitivity in the immature rat. "The status of susceptibility of the adrenal cortex is correlated with its content of corticosterone."

Morii & Kuwahara G33,213/63: Mice, guinea pigs, hamsters, rabbits, cats and dogs, unlike rats, are not susceptible to the production of adrenal apoplexy by DMBA, and pretreatment with ACTH did not make the adrenals of these species responsive.

Hitachi F67,866/65: In mice, ACTH inhibits the involution of the adrenal cortex produced by MC.

Huggins & Sugiama F44,582/65: In rats, DMBA produces no adrenocortical necrosis if the animals are immature or hypophysectomized. ACTH renders the adrenals of immature rats susceptible to this type of injury.

Morri G34,628/65: Pretreatment with small amounts of ACTH failed to protect the rat against DMBA-induced adrenocortical apoplexy. However, administration of ACTH to young rats or to hypophysectomized adults, which normally do not respond to the corticolytic effect of DMBA, makes them susceptible.

Shirasu et al. F76,819/67: In the rats, hepatoma formation by N-hydroxy-N-2-fluorenylacetamide (N-OH-FAA) is enhanced by ACTH and STH. Studies with ^{14}C-labeled N-OH-FAA showed "decreased dehydroxylation and deacetylation of N-OH-FAA. The radioactivity bound to liver proteins was increased, remarkably so in the animals treated with growth hormone."

Ronzoni et al. H18,409/68: In rats, prostatic carcinogenesis induced by the implantation of 20-methylcholanthrene crystals into the prostate is inhibited by ACTH, triiodothyronine and, to a lesser extent, by progesterone and 19-nortestosterone phenylpropionate. Estradiol and cortisone facilitate carcinogenesis, whereas testosterone, orchidectomy and methylthiouracil failed to influence it.

Bird et al. H30,425/70: In rats less than 30 days of age, DMBA or 7-OHM-12-MBA produces no adrenal necrosis unless animals are pretreated with ACTH. However, a single i.v. injection of 7-OHM-12-MBA on the 17th day of gestation causes adrenal necrosis in the embryos as well as in the mothers. Pretreatment with SKF 525-A protected the adrenals both of the embryos and of the mothers.

7,12-Dimethylbenz(a)anthracene ← ACTH + Age: Morii et al. D45,369/62*

9,10-Dimethyl-1,2-benzanthracene ← ACTH: Currie et al. D48,292/62*

Carcinolytics ←

Andreani et al. C14,628/55: In rats, the different organ changes produced by TEM are unequally influenced by combined treatment with ACTH + cortisone.

Casein ← cf. also Selye C92,918/61, p. 250.

Latvalahti B88,191/53: In mice, the amyloidosis produced by repeated s.c. injections of casein is aggravated by ACTH and cortisone but not by DOC or testosterone; orchidectomy facilitates its development.

Peräsalo & Latvalahti C9,661/54: The amyloidosis produced by sodium caseinate s.c. in mice is uninfluenced by DOC and testosterone but aggravated by cortisone, adrenocortical extract and ACTH.

Fanfani & Dini C48,253/57: In mice, combined parenteral administration of casein and ACTH causes necrotic lesions and waxy degeneration in the cardiac muscle but not true amyloidosis.

Cholesterol ← cf. also Selye G60,083/70, pp. 328, 329, 346.

Oppenheim & Bruger B74,288/52: In rabbits, cholesterol atheromatosis is diminished by cortisone and to a lesser extent by ACTH.

Tarantino & Natali B71,460/52: In rabbits, ACTH inhibits cholesterol atheromatosis and diminishes the associated hypercholesterolemia.

Cinchophen ←

Rodriguez-Olleros & Galindo C 17,868/56: In dogs, induction of gastric ulcers by cinchophen is not significantly affected by ACTH or cortisone.

Diphenylhydantoin ←

Hoyrup & Vinten-Johansen B 84,197/52: In patients with acute phenobarbital or diphenylhydantoin poisoning, the use of ACTH is contraindicated as judged by impressions gained from a small series of observations.

Disulfiram ← cf. Ethanol

Ethanol ←

Lecoq et al. B 66,406/51: In rats, the toxic effects of ethanol and of its metabolites pyruvate and acetaldehyde (which accumulate in the body under the influence of disulfiram) are inhibited by ACTH, cortisone, and hepatic extracts. Conversely, thyroxine, DOC, and testosterone appear to aggravate ethanol intoxication. [Statistically evaluated data are not presented (H.S.).]

Lecoq B 79,754/51: In rabbits, injection of disulfiram + ethanol or of Na-pyruvate produces essentially the same syndrome of intoxication, since pyruvic acid is the principal metabolite of ethanol after pretreatment with disulfiram. In either case, ACTH and cortisone offer little, if any, protective effect.

Ethionine ←

Farber & Segalorr D 95,996/55: In ovariectomized rats, various testoids and STH protected the liver against fatty infiltration produced by ethionine i.p., whereas cortisone and ACTH aggravated it. Estradiol, DOC and TSH had no effect.

Formaldehyde ← cf. *Selye B 40,000/50, pp. 390, 589.*

Ganglioplegics ←

Brust et al. B 57,917/51: In man, "administration of ACTH or cortisone significantly alters the blood pressure and 'TEAC floor'. The responses are independent of sodium retention and indicate that the vascular effects of these drugs are mediated by a humoral mechanism which is potentiated by autonomic blockade." Observations on both normotensive and hypertensive patients showed that "the usual depressor effects of TEAC were ultimately converted to a pressor rise, suggesting that autonomic blockade potentiates the vascular effects of ACTH and cortisone." DOC exhibited no such action.

Brust et al. B 58,739/51: In man, the "TEAC floor" rises within 24 hrs after ACTH administration and falls again after discontinuation of hormone treatment. The rise in "TEAC floor" precedes the increase in urinary 17-ketosteroid excretion and precedes or parallels eosinopenia. In patients with uncomplicated essential hypertension blood pressure alterations paralleled the "TEAC floor" changes. "The 'TEAC floor' appears to be a sensitive indicator of the adrenocortical activity produced by ACTH."

Selye G 70,448/70: In rats, intoxication with TEA, hexamethonium and pentolinium could be prevented by all of seven glucocorticoids tested. On the other hand, glucocorticoids offered no protection against trimethaphan, mecamylamine, trimethidinium or pempidine. Typical catatoxic steroids (ethylstrenol, CS-1, spironolactone, norbolethone, oxandrolone) as well as progesterone, DOC and hydroxydione failed to offer significant protection against hexamethonium or TEA. Various stressors (bone fractures, fasting, spinal cord transection and formalin) gave excellent protection against TEA, whereas others (restraint, cold) did not. "Since even large doses of ACTH are ineffective in this respect the anti-TEA effect of stressors cannot be ascribed merely to increased corticoid secretion."

Hexadimethrine ←

Tuchweber et al. D 27,884/63: In rats, hypophysectomy prevents the nephrocalcinosis, but aggravates the adrenal necrosis, produced by hexadimethrine. ACTH-treatment of the hypophysectomized rat facilitates the production of nephrocalcinosis, but protects the adrenal. Adrenalectomy prevents this form of nephrocalcinosis even in rats maintained on NaCl or DOC. On the other hand, triamcinolone- treated adrenalectomized rats react to hexadimethrine with strong nephrocalcinosis. Under similar conditions in intact rats, the corticoids did not significantly change the syndrome of hexadimethrine intoxication, except that the anaphylactoid reaction to this compound is inhibited by triamcinolone.

Isoniazid ←

Mrozikiewicz & Strzyzewski G68,152/66; H7,524/67: In the mouse, isoniazid-induced convulsions are facilitated not only by glucocorticoids (cortisol, prednisolone) and ACTH, but also by DOC.

Isoproterenol ← cf. Selye C92,918/61, p. 117.

Lathyrogens ← cf. also Selye G60,083/70, pp. 331, 357.

Selye C25,013/57: The osteolathyrism produced in rats by aminoacetonitrile (AAN) is slightly aggravated by thyroparathyroidectomy, and suppressed by large doses of thyroxine. "An amount of ACTH that more than doubles the weight of the adrenals and causes pronounced thymus atrophy also inhibits the effect of AAN, but fails to prevent it completely. This is all the more noteworthy because comparatively small doses of cortisol can totally prevent such bone lesions. Extensive partial hepatectomy greatly increases the effect of AAN upon the bones."

Selye C31,369/57: In the rat, the osteolathyrism produced by AAN is aggravated by STH, LTH and partial hepatectomy but it is inhibited by ACTH, cortisol or estradiol.

Pyörälä et al. G67,833/59: Dissecting aneurysms of the aorta developed in 40% of immature rats fed Lathyrus odoratus. The media was remarkably thickened and the ground substance showed increased metachromasia and PAS reaction. This response was suppressed by cortisone and thyroxine but not by ACTH, TSH or DOC at the doses employed.

van Cauwenberge et al. C78,726/59: In rats, osteolathyrism is inhibited by ACTH and, to a lesser extent, by salicylates and butazolidine.

Glickman et al. E24,104/63: In rats, the dental changes produced by AAN are aggravated following partial hepatectomy and thyroidectomy, reduced by ACTH and almost completely abolished by thyroxine.

Meprobamate ←

Bousquet et al. F35,073/65: In rats with stress produced by applying a tourniquet around one hind limb for 2.5 hrs, the toxicity of hexobarbital, pentobarbital, meprobamate and zoxazolamine was significantly diminished, whereas that of barbital and phenobarbital remained unaffected. Pretreatment with ACTH or corticosterone simulated the effect of stress. After hypophysectomy or adrenalectomy, stress failed to offer the usual protection.

[The barbiturates and zoxazolamine appear to have been administered immediately after release of the tourniquet but this is not specifically stated. Allegedly a single injection of corticosterone (50 µg per animal) sufficed to offer protection (H.S.).]

Mercury ←

Kádas & Zsámbéky C26,265/56; C49,522/57: The renal damage produced by $HgCl_2$ in the rat is most effectively prevented by testosterone, but, to a lesser extent, also by cortisone, particularly when the latter is given in combination with ACTH.

Morphine ←

Winter & Flataker B62,935/51: In rats, cortisone inhibits the effects of methadone and morphine upon the thermal tail-flick response. Cortisone also increases the excitatory effect of morphine in cats. On the other hand, cortisone synergizes the analgesic antagonist N-allylnormorphine. After spinal cord section, cortisone and ACTH reduce the effect of morphine on the spinal reflex activity in rats (thermal tail-flick response), whereas DOC enhances it.

Adler et al. G79,852/57: In Sprague-Dawley rats given ^{14}C-labeled morphine, the ratio of bound to free morphine is 2—3 times greater in the urine and plasma than in Long-Evans rats. The tissues of adrenalectomized rats of both strains contain higher concentrations of ^{14}-C-labeled morphine than do control rats. Plasma bound morphine levels indicate no impairment of morphine conjugation. Vasopressin increases, whereas ACTH decreases morphine sensitivity. Yet both after ACTH and after vasopressin, tissue concentrations of morphine are either reduced or unaffected in marked contrast to the increased values after adrenalectomy. Apparently, the decreased morphine sensitivity induced by ACTH is not reflected by lower brain morphine concentrations.

Sobel et al. C90,836/60: Morphine increases the mortality of guinea pigs exposed to reduced oxygen tension. Prior treatment with cortisone or ACTH protects against this combined treatment.

Markova D47,081/62: Pretreatment with ACTH or cortisone increases the morphine resistance of newborn rats although not quite to the adult level. DOC does not share this effect.

Paroli G12,543/63: In the rat, cortisol and ACTH inhibit the analgesic effect of morphine; dexamethasone and prednisolone (though more active glucocorticoids) do not share this effect.

Lecannelier & Quevedo H8,759/67: In rabbits, the analgesic effect of morphine is reduced by ACTH or cortisol.

Mustard Powder ← *cf. Selye B40,000/50, p. 390.*

Pentylenetetrazol ←

Torda & Wolff B57,149/51: In rats, the convulsions and EEG changes produced by pentylenetetrazol are inhibited by ACTH or cortisone.

Torda & Wolff B69,986/52: In rats, the convulsion-threshold of pentylenetetrazol is raised by ACTH even after hypophysectomy or adrenalectomy. Furthermore, ACTH increases the electric activity of the brain "by a mechanism that is not dependent on the presence of the adrenal cortex."

Boeri C78,610/58: In guinea pigs, cortisone, ACTH and vasopressin aggravate pentylenetetrazol convulsions.

Pentylenetetrazol ← ACTH: Torda et al. B69,986/52*

Phenyldione ← *cf. Anticoagulants*

Plasmocid ← *cf. Selye C92,918/61, p. 95.*

Polyanetholsulfonate ← *cf. Anticoagulants*

Potassium ←

Collins C17,662/56: Survival after KCl i.p. (referred to as "potassium stress") is diminished after the induction of adrenocortical atrophy by cortisol. Concurrent administration of DOC, aldosterone, adrenocortical extract, corticosterone or ACTH counteracts this effect of cortisol upon K tolerance.

Puromycin Aminonucleoside ←

Wilson et al. C45,755/57: In rats, puromycin aminonucleoside nephrosis is not prevented by cortisone or ACTH.

Pyruvate ←

Lecoq et al. B66,406/51: In rats, the toxic effects of ethanol and its metabolites pyruvate and acetaldehyde (which accumulate in the body under the influence of disulfiram) are inhibited by ACTH, cortisone, and hepatic extracts. Conversely, thyroxine, DOC, and testosterone appear to aggravate ethanol intoxication. [Statistically evaluated data are not presented (H.S.).]

Lecoq B79,754/51: In rabbits, injection of disulfiram + ethanol or of Na-pyruvate produces essentially the same syndrome of intoxication, since pyruvic acid is the principal metabolite of ethanol after pretreatment with disulfiram. In either case, ACTH and cortisone offer little, if any, protective effect.

RES-Blocking Agents ←

Selye B39,702/49: In rats in which an arthritis was produced by intrapedal injection of formalin and India ink, phagocytosis and transport of the carbon particles to the regional lymph nodes are accelerated by ACTH. This is ascribed to glucocorticoid formation and the resulting diminution of the inflammatory barrier at the formalin injection site.

Kennedy et al. B59,278/51: In patients, ACTH exerted beneficial effects upon beryllium granulomatosis and silicosis, presumably as a consequence of its antiphlogistic effect.

Michalová C56,094/58: In rabbits exposed to quartz dust, ACTH diminished the severity of silicosis, but this effect was not manifest in chronic experiments.

Gabbiani et al. G19,450/65: In rats pretreated with ACTH, fluorocortisol or restraint, a single i.v. injection of thorium dextrin (an RES-blocking agent) produces thrombohemorrhagic lesions with necrosis in the adrenals, liver and kidneys. The changes are reminiscent of the Shwartzman-Sanarelli phenomenon.

Göthe H20,085/70: In rats, ACTH accelerates, whereas prednisolone retards, the transport of intratracheally administered quartz dust from the lung to the regional lymphatics.

Silica ← *cf. RES-Blocking Agents*

Tannic Acid ←

Patrick C12,967/55: In rats and mice, cortisone or ACTH inhibited the mesenchymal reaction and delayed repair following production of hepatic damage by tannic acid or CCl_4.

Tetracaine ←

Zykov H21,879/69: In mice, ACTH, cortisol and DOC failed to influence tetracaine intoxication.

Tetraethylammonium (TEA) ← *cf. Ganglionic-Blocking Agents*

Thorium Dextrin ← *cf. RES-Blocking Agents*

Vitamin C ←

Hyman et al. B53,374/50: "Cortisone and ACTH prolong life and reduce the hemorrhagic manifestations of scurvy in guinea pigs." [In an addendum the authors state that the large doses of ACTH and cortisone used may proauce severe toxic effects which overshadow their beneficial actions (H.S.).]

Hyman et al. B57,989/51: In guinea pigs on a vitamin-C deficient diet, ACTH and cortisone ameliorate the manifestations of scurvy.

Vitamin D, DHT ← *cf. also Selye G60,083/70, pp. 329, 331.*

Selye C27,735/57: The cardiovascular calcification and nephrocalcinosis produced by DHT in rats are aggravated by estradiol, cortisol, ACTH and thyroxine. Conversely, methyltestosterone and STH exert a protective effect.

Thoenes & Schröter C56,987/58: In rats kept on a vitamin-D deficient diet, cortisone tends to inhibit the development of rickets, whereas ACTH does not. DOC actually aggravates vitamin-D deficiency.

Campeanu et al. G21,413/63: In rats, combined treatment with vitamin-D_2 and ACTH produces intense generalized calcinosis. [No mention of controls receiving vitamin-D_2 alone (H.S.).]

Zoxazolamine ←

Bousquet et al. F35,073/65: In rats with stress produced by applying a tourniquet around one hind limb for 2.5 hrs, the toxicity of hexobarbital, pentobarbital, meprobamate and zoxazolamine was significantly diminished, whereas that of barbital and phenobarbital remained unaffected. Pretreatment with ACTH or corticosterone simulated the effect of stress. After hypophysectomy or adrenalectomy, stress failed to offer the usual protection. [The barbiturates and zoxazolamine appear to have been administered immediately after release of the tourniquet but this is not specifically stated. Allegedly a single injection of corticosterone (50 μg per animal) sufficed to offer protection (H.S.).]

Selye G70,480/71: In rats, ACTH inhibited zoxazolamine paralysis and acute DHT-induced soft-tissue calcification but failed to influence poisoning with digitoxin, dioxathion, parathion, nicotine, hexobarbital, progesterone, indomethacin or the infarctoid cardiopathy produced by fluorocortisol + Na_2HPO_4 + corn oil.

Complex Diets ←

ACTH and glucocorticoids inhibit the fatal hepatic necroses which develop in young rats fed diets deficient in sulfur-containing amino acids and vitamin E, as well as in rats kept on diets containing yeast as the only source of protein.

Aterman C35,275/57: The fatal hepatic necrosis which develops in weanling rats fed a diet deficient in sulfur-containing amino acids and vitamin E is inhibited by ACTH and cortisone, but aggravated by thyroid powder feeding. In the case of simultaneous treatment with thyroid and cortisone, the two types of hormones antagonize each other.

Aterman C61,786/58: The hepatic necrosis produced in rats by feeding a diet containing yeast as the only source of protein is inhibited by cortisone, cortisol or ACTH, but not influenced by progesterone, "estrogen," testosterone or DOC. Aldosterone prolongs survival time providing 50 μg or more is administered daily. Although the author did not report any observations on the effect of aldosterone upon carbohydrate metabolism, he arrived at the conclusion that "these results, therefore, suggest that in the system examined here aldosterone has some 'glucocorticoid' activity and differs significantly from deoxycortone acetate which in doses of 0.5 and 2.5 mgm. daily has been completely ineffective."

Borgman & Haselden H29,947/70: In rabbits kept on a gallstone producing ration, ACTH, thyroid hormones, or cortisone did not inhibit the production of biliary calculi, but several of these hormones inhibited the usually associated hepatic steatosis.

Microorganisms, Parasites and Their Products ←

Bacteria and Vaccines ←. ACTH does not significantly influence the course of infection with **Clostridium tetani** in the mouse or with **Corynebacterium diphtheriae** and **leptospirosis** in the guinea pig.

Infection with **M. tuberculosis** is aggravated by ACTH in the mouse, guinea pig, rat and rabbit despite a few dissenting claims. In this respect, ACTH imitates the effects of glucocorticoids and, like the latter, it is antagonized by concurrent treatment with STH.

In rats infected with **P. pestis**, ACTH also decreased, whereas STH increased, survival.

Pneumococcal and **Rickettsial** infections are not very manifestly affected by ACTH in the mouse.

"Saprophytosis," due to proliferation of normally nonpathogenic microorganisms (usually Corynebacteria), such as occurs after severe glucocorticoid intoxication, is also induced in rats by heavy overdosage with ACTH. It can be prevented by concurrent treatment with STH.

In guinea pigs and rats, ACTH could not be shown to exert a significant influence upon infection with **staphylococci**, although cortisone decreased resistance to these organisms.

The effect of ACTH on **streptococcal infections** varies greatly depending upon experimental conditions.

Viruses ←. ACTH undoubtedly exerts an antipyretic effect in rabbits inoculated with **influenza** virus as it does in various other forms of infection. In mice and ferrets, ACTH does not significantly influence resistance to influenza. On the other hand, large doses of ACTH increase the susceptibility of mice to lethal infection with various **arboviruses**. Infection with **poliomyelitis** is likewise facilitated by ACTH in mice and hamsters, although with some strains of poliomyelitis no definite increase in susceptibility could be obtained by ACTH. In the dog, the growth of equine **encephalomyelitis** is enhanced by ACTH. This hormone also facilitates the spread of **variola** virus in sheep and it can reactivate a latent **rabies** infection in guinea pigs.

Parasites ←. In guinea pigs, ACTH did not significantly influence the course of infestation with **Trichinella spiralis**.

Bacterial Toxins ← *cf. also Selye E 5,986/66*. In **rabbits**, pretreatment during 48 hrs with large doses of ACTH or cortisone diminishes the febrile response to Shigella endotoxin, whereas 24 hrs of pretreatment with smaller doses of these hormones exerts an opposite effect.

In the **mouse**, neither ACTH nor cortisone pretreatment raised resistance against the toxins of R. tsutsugamushi, R. prowazeki or S. typhosa. However, under suitable conditions of dosage and timing, mice can allegedly be protected by ACTH or cortisone against fatal intoxication with cholera-vibrio endotoxin, diphtheria toxin and various other endotoxins. The effects of tetanus, Shiga, and meningococcus toxin are not influenced by ACTH in the mouse.

In **guinea pigs**, neither ACTH nor cortisol improved resistance to diphtheria toxin, but the production of hemorrhages and adrenal necroses by pertussis toxin was enhanced by ACTH.

Rats allegedly cannot be protected against the lethal effects of perfringens toxin by ACTH or glucocorticoids, but the resistance to many endotoxins is undoubtedly increased by these hormones. The hepatic vein thromboses produced in rats on hyperlipemic diets by S. typhosa endotoxin are prevented by ACTH, cortisol or prednisolone.

In dogs, ACTH gave no significant protection against endotoxin shock.

In man, the febrile response to killed typhoid bacilli and the reactions to Brucella endotoxin are inhibited by ACTH.

Venoms ←. ACTH has been found to protect various species against fatal doses of the venoms of scorpions, snakes and spiders.

Bacteria and Vaccines ←

Clostridium Tetani ←. *Massalski & Kulejewska C 52,338/57:* In mice, ACTH does not influence experimental tetanus, nor does it alter the actions of tetanus toxin and antitoxin.

Corynebacterium Diphtheriae ←. *di Nola et al. C 43,232/57:* In guinea pigs, ACTH offered no protection against fatal diphtheria infection.

Leptospira ←. *Derom & van Hoydonck C 17,095/55:* "ACTH and cortisone have not been found to have any favorable effects on the infection of guinea pigs with Leptospira ictero-haemorragiae, strain 'Afsnee'."

Bacillus Piliformis (Tyzzer's disease) ←. *Yamada et al. H 24,079/69:* In mice and rats inoculated with B. piliformis, pretreatment with ACTH or cortisone greatly enhances susceptibility to Tyzzer's disease.

Diplococcus Pneumoniae ←. *Kass et al. B 69,981/51:* In mice, the final mortality rate after infection with influenza virus or pneumococci is not significantly altered by ACTH or cortisone, although the course of the disease may be modified.

Kass et al. B 95,353/54: In mice, resistance to pneumococcal and influenza virus infections is depressed by pretreatment with cortisone or cortisol, but not by ACTH. STH failed to overcome the effect of cortisone and did not increase resistance to infection when given alone.

Mycobacterium Tuberculosis ←. *Reinmuth & Smith B 60,585/51:* In rabbits sensitized by tuberculosis bacilli and subsequently challenged with Old Tuberculin introduced into the trachea, the resulting pneumonia is decreased in severity by pretreatment with ACTH.

Swedberg et al. B 58,412/51: In mice, ACTH aggravates the course of experimental tuberculosis.

Lucherini et al. B 89,088/53: In guinea pigs, STH inhibits the progress of tuberculosis and counteracts the opposite effect of ACTH.

Cavallero C 829/54: Review on the effect of STH, ACTH and cortisone upon various infections, especially in the rat.

Lepri & Fornaro D 91,865/54: In rabbits rendered allergic to tuberculosis, the ocular manifestations of topical challenge by tubercle bacilli were variably influenced by ACTH and cortisone.

Youmans & Youmans B 95,169/54: In mice, cortisone markedly reduced the survival time after infection with human tubercle bacilli and this effect could not be prevented by STH. Given alone, ACTH, STH and TTH likewise failed to influence the course of the infection.

Donomae et al. C 22,935/55: In rabbits infected with human tuberculosis bacilli and reinoculated with the same germs into the lung, ACTH greatly enhances cavity formation.

Greuel & Schäfer E 54,859/56: In guinea pigs treated with ACTH, DOC or cortisone, the progress of tuberculosis was proportional to the size of the adrenals, and least severe in animals given cortisol.

Shmelev & Uvarova C 53,553/56: Contrary to earlier investigators, the authors found that in guinea pigs and rabbits, ACTH actually increases resistance to tuberculosis.

Wasz-Höckert & Backman C 30,700/56: In guinea pigs, the progress of tuberculosis can greatly be enhanced by ACTH, which is useful for the diagnosis of tuberculosis.

Wasz-Höckert & Backman C 34,801/56: In guinea pigs, ACTH aggravates the course of tuberculosis. STH in itself is without conspicuous effect, however, "the strongly deteriorating effect on tuberculosis produced by ACTH was evidently counteracted by STH when given simultaneously with ACTH."

Batten & McCune C53,554/57: ACTH, cortisol and cortisone greatly reduce the resistance of mice to infection with human tuberculosis.

Fiorentino D8,379/59: In guinea pigs, ACTH greatly accelerates the progress of tuberculosis. A test for the rapid diagnosis of tuberculosis is based upon this observation.

Renovanz C78,772/59: In guinea pigs, the course of experimental tuberculosis was not markedly influenced by ACTH, tolbutamide derivatives or antithyroid treatment with perchlorates.

Vakilzadeh & Vandiviere E32,626/63: In guinea pigs, the beneficial effect of vaccination against tuberculosis was greatly increased by thyroxine and T3, but not by cortisone, cortisol or ACTH. None of the hormones altered natural host resistance in nonimmunized guinea pigs.

Wasz-Höckert & McCune E31,145/63: In mice infected with tuberculosis, STH caused an increase in body weight but did not inhibit the development of the infection nor did it counteract the unfavorable effect of ACTH.

Kampioni G33,098/64: In tuberculous guinea pigs, ACTH inhibits the proliferation of the pleural stroma but not the thickening of the mesothelial cells.

Pasteurella Pestis ←. *Hayashida C37,366/57:* In rats infected with P. pestis, ACTH decreased, whereas STH increased, survival.

Rickettsia ←. *Jackson & Smadel E52,720/51:* Intact mice pretreated with cortisone or ACTH "were given lethal amounts of the toxins of R. tsutsugamushi, R. prowazeki, or S. typhosa. Such animals were as susceptible to the toxins as normal controls. Neither hormone had any therapeutic effect in mice infected with R. tsutsugamushi. Furthermore, treated and untreated mice in a terminal phase of infection with R. tsutsugamushi were equally susceptible to the toxin of this rickettsia when injected intravenously. In the current experiments the adrenal cortex of normal or infected animals apparently contributed as effectively as possible in the host's response to rickettsial or bacterial toxins and further stimulation was without advantage."

"Saprophytosis" ←. *Selye B57,451/51:* In rats, "saprophytosis" due to proliferation of normally nonpathogenic microorganisms, such as develop after heavy overdosage with cortisone or ACTH, can be completely prevented by concurrent administration of STH.

Staphylococcus ←. *Debry C30,870/56:* Doctor's thesis (176 pp., 578 refs.) on the influence of hormones upon infection. Personal observations on guinea pigs and rats indicate that ACTH, STH and DOC do not significantly affect the course of acute staphylococcus infection, whereas cortisone aggravates it.

Streptococcus ←. *Glaser et al. B58,299/50:* In mice, neither ACTH nor cortisone exerted a beneficial effect upon streptococcal or pneumococcal infections, indeed they may have aggravated them.

Mogabgab & Thomas B72,457/52: In rabbits, pretreatment with ACTH or cortisone greatly aggravated streptococcal septicemia. DOC had no such effect.

Fazio et al. C34,111/56: In rats, cortisone or ACTH increases survival following streptococcal infection and further enhances the protective effect of penicillin.

Viruses ←

Kass & Finland B54,130/50: In man, the febrile response to i.v. injection of killed typhoid bacilli is reduced by ACTH. A similar antipyretic effect against typhoid bacilli and influenza virus is exerted by ACTH in rabbits.

Loosli et al. B58,316/50: In mice and ferrets, ACTH did not significantly influence air-borne influenza-A infection.

Shwartzman B54,248/50: "ACTH and cortisone in combination or cortisone alone produce a marked acceleration of poliomyelitis infection (strain MEFl) in mice and an extraordinary enhancement of susceptibility to this infection in hamsters giving rise to a violent and uniformly fatal disease. ACTH alone fails to produce this effect possibly due to elaboration of an unknown factor capable of reversing the enhancing effect of cortisone."

Kass et al. B69,981/51: In mice, the final mortality rate after infection with influenza virus or pneumococci is not significantly altered by ACTH or cortisone, although the course of the disease may be modified.

Shwartzman B66,955/51: ACTH and cortisone accelerate poliomyelitis (strain MEF) in mice and hamsters. DOC, progesterone and diethylstilbestrol are ineffective.

Smith et al. B64,635/51: In mice, susceptibility to pneumonia virus (PVM) is not influenced by ACTH but is enhanced by cortisone.

Southam & Babcock B63,662/51: "Large doses of cortisone greatly increased the susceptibility of mice to lethal infection by West Nile, Ilheus, and Bunyamwere viruses. ACTH in massive dosage produced the same effect with West Nile virus. Desoxycorticosterone, testosterone, progesterone, and estradiol in massive doses had no significant effect on these virus infections in mice."

Findlay & Howard B81,142/52: In mice and hamsters, cortisone and ACTH increase susceptibility to polyomyelitis and other virus infections.

Shwartzman B69,778/52: Cortisone, unlike ACTH, greatly increases the susceptibility of Syrian hamsters to i.p. inoculation with strain MEF1 poliomyelitis virus.

Shwartzman & Fisher B69,580/52: In Syrian hamsters, cortisone enhances infection with MEF1 and Lansing strains of poliomyelitis virus. ACTH, DOC, progesterone and stilbestrol are without effect. Earlier literature on the influence of various hormones upon poliomyelitis is reviewed.

Kass et al. B95,353/54: In mice, resistance to pneumococcal and influenza virus infections is depressed by pretreatment with cortisone or cortisol, but not by ACTH. STH failed to overcome the effect of cortisone and did not increase resistance to infection when given alone.

Hurst et al. C94,089/60: Cortisone, ACTH, estradiol, stilbestrol and thyroxine all stimulate the growth of the virus of equine encephalomyelitis in the dog, whereas testosterone and progesterone do not. The hormones which aggravate the infection also counteract the prophylactic effect of mepacrine and abolish the normally greater resistance of the females.

Cilli et al. D12,192/61: In sheep, STH, owing to its prophlogistic effect, delimits the lesions produced by variola virus. ACTH and dexamethasone exert an opposite effect.

Soave D22,275/62: In guinea pigs, latent rabies virus infection can be reactivated by ACTH s.c.

Parasites ←

Luongo et al. B69,505/51: In guinea pigs, ACTH did not significantly influence the course of infestation with T. spiralis but appeared to reduce the associated toxic effects.

Sheldon & Bauer D46,962/62: Review on the role of predisposing factors, particularly alloxan diabetes and ACTH-treatment, upon various fungus infections.

Bacterial Toxins ←

RABBIT

Duffy & Morgan B65,399/51: In rabbits the febrile response to Shigella dysenteriae endotoxin is diminished following pretreatment during 48 hrs with repeated large doses of ACTH or cortisone. Pretreatment during 24 hrs with smaller doses of these hormones exerts an opposite effect. "This appears to account for the discrepancies in the results previously reported."

Bennett Jr. & Beeson B95,351/53: In rabbits, the febrile response to a single injection of various endotoxins may be decreased, increased or unchanged by treatment with ACTH or cortisone. Acquired resistance to pyrogen fever is abolished by Thorotrast but not by cortisone although both these agents prevent the Shwartzman reaction.

MOUSE

Jackson & Smadel E52,720/51; B77,408/51: Intact mice pretreated with cortisone or ACTH "were given lethal amounts of the toxins of Rickettsiae tsutsugamushi, R. prowazeki, or S. typhosa. Such animals were as susceptible to the toxins as normal controls. Neither hormone had any therapeutic effect in mice infected with R. tsutsugamushi. Furthermore, treated and untreated mice in a terminal phase of infection with R. tsutsugamushi were equally susceptible to the toxin of this rickettsia when injected intravenously. In the current experiments the adrenal cortex of normal or infected animals apparently contributed as effectively as possible in the host's response to rickettsial or bacterial toxins and further stimulation was without advantage."

Gallut C14,519/55: Mice can be protected against fatal intoxication with cholera Vibrio endotoxin by cortisone or ACTH but the degree of protection depends upon dosage and timing.

Massalski & Kulejewska C52,338/57: In mice, ACTH does not influence experimental tetanus, nor does it alter the actions of tetanus toxin and antitoxin.

Nadel et al. D12,681/61: In mice, pretreatment with ACTH offers no protection against endotoxin. Hence, the resistance induced by pretreatment with endotoxin itself cannot be due to mobilization of the pituitary-adrenal axis.

Parant D82,116/62: In mice, resistance to endotoxin is greatly decreased a few hours after adrenalectomy or hypophysectomy. Cortisone protects normal, adrenalectomized, and hypophysectomized animals against high doses of endotoxin, whereas chlorpromazine is effective only in the presence of both the adrenals and the pituitary. ACTH also protects the hypophysectomized mouse but only if slow absorption is assured.

Skuratova D 20,887/62: In mice, resistance against the fatal effect of diphtheria toxin is more markedly increased by STH than by ACTH.

GUINEA PIG

Murray & Branham B 65,414/51: Neither ACTH nor cortisone improved the resistance of guinea pigs to diphtheria toxin or of mice to Shiga and meningococcus toxin.

Okonogi et al. C 34,465/56: In guinea pigs the production by pertussis toxin of subcutaneous hemorrhages, pulmonary lesions and adrenal necrosis is enhanced by ACTH.

RAT

Ganley et al. C 7,489/55: Rats cannot be protected against the lethal effect of Cl. perfringens toxin by ACTH, adrenocortical extract, cortisol, cortisone or DOC.

Levitin et al. C 26,683/56: Cortisol, corticosterone, and cortisone, as well as ACTH protect the rat against endotoxin, whereas DOC does not.

Renaud et al. F 74,449/66: In rats kept on a hyperlipemic diet, ACTH, cortisol or prednisolone protected against the production of shock and hepatic vein thromboses by S. typhosa lipopolysaccharide. DOC increased mortality and did not protect against these thromboses.

DOG

Evangelista et al. H 16,824/69: Neither ACTH nor stanozolol gave any significant protection against endotoxin shock in dogs.

MAN

Kass & Finland B 54,130/50: In man, the febrile response to i.v. injection of killed typhoid bacilli is reduced by ACTH. A similar antipyretic effect against typhoid bacilli and influenza virus is exerted by ACTH in rabbits.

Abernathy & Spink C 48,635/58: In man, cortisol or ACTH suppressed or ameliorated reactions to brucella endotoxin.

Venoms ←

Mohammed et al. C 7,579/54: Rats can be protected against fatal doses of scorpion toxin by pretreatment with cortisone or ACTH.

Schöttler C 10,890/54: In mice and guinea pigs injected with the venom of Bothrops jararaca or Crotalus terrificus s.c., ACTH, cortisone and cortisol failed to offer protection.

Bettini & Cantore C 21,801/55: Comparative studies on the protective effect of ACTH, cortisone and chlorpromazine against lethal poisoning with the venom of the spider Latrodectus tredecimguttatus.

Haas G 38,758/66: Extensive review on the use of corticoids and ACTH in the treatment of snake bites in man and in animals.

Immune Reactions ←

The immunosuppressive effects of ACTH have been discussed in our previous monographs to which the reader is referred for a more detailed account.

In **guinea pigs**, ACTH does not strikingly influence anaphylactic shock under usual conditions, yet it may inhibit it if given during 3 days before the challenging reinjection. However, ACTH does clearly diminish tuberculine hypersensitivity although only on diets containing the "cabbage factor" (presumed to be an SH-compound).

The beneficial effect of vaccination against tuberculosis is not significantly altered by ACTH or cortisone in the guinea pig.

In **rabbits** sensitized to tuberculosis, ACTH tends to, but does not regularly, inhibit the manifestations of subsequent topical challenge.

In **rats**, ACTH decreases, whereas STH increases, antibody formation against Pasteurella pestis. The hemolytic icterus produced by appropriate agglutinin treatment, and the renal damage caused by nephrotoxic serum, can also be inhibited by ACTH.

Hepatic and Renal Lesions ←

Tolerance to temporary **hepatic** vessel ligation is increased by ACTH in the dog. In rats, ACTH (like corticoids) enhances repair and fat deposition in the liver remnant after partial hepatectomy. Various stressors inhibit hepatic regeneration under similar conditions, presumably because the stimulating effect of ACTH and corticoids is overcompensated by the stress itself.

The arterial lesions that develop after bilateral **nephrectomy** in dogs kept on a high-fat diet are prevented by ACTH and cortisone, but also by pregnancy or diethylstilbestrol.

Immune Reactions ← cf. Selye G60,083/70, pp. 328, 329, 347.

Guinea Pig

Leger et al. A 48,766/48: In sensitized guinea pigs, ACTH, given prior to a shock dose of antigen, failed to influence the course of anaphylactic shock.

Dworetzky et al. B52,246/50: In guinea pigs, anaphylactic shock was not significantly influenced by cortisone or ACTH.

Friedlaender & Friedlaender B55,467/50: In guinea pigs, intoxication with histamine (aerosol) and anaphylactic shock (horse serum) were not influenced by pretreatment with ACTH.

Long & Miles D41,973/50: In guinea pigs, moderate thyrotoxicosis produced by two week's treatment with thyroxine increases hypersensitivity to tuberculin, whereas moderate doses of propylthiouracil do not affect it. ACTH and cortisone diminished tuberculin sensitivity. Fourteen days after stopping thyroxine injections, the animals became actually less hypersensitive than the controls. A similar reversal of this effect was noted two weeks after interruption of cortisone or ACTH treatment in that the animals became more hypersensitive than the controls.

Malkiel G71,451/51: In guinea pigs, ACTH and cortisone are without effect on the end results of histamine shock, or of passive or active anaphylaxis.

Long et al. D85,907/51: In guinea pigs, single injections of cortisone or ACTH diminish allergic hypersensitivity on a cabbage diet, but not on a basal diet deficient in the "cabbage factor." The authors conclude "that there is in cabbage a factor which on ingestion leads to the inhibition of the desensitization produced by the metabolism of ascorbic acid in the tissues of the allergic guinea pig; and that the desensitizing action of cortisone or of ACTH in cabbage-fed animals is indirect, depending on the reversal of the cabbage effect by the hormones. The cabbage factor may possibly be an SH-compound."

Long et al. B60,189/51: In B.C.G.-infected guinea pigs, hypersensitivity to tuberculin is considerably diminished by cortisone or ACTH. This diminution is abolished by pretreatment with propylthiouracil, which alone has no effect upon hypersensitivity. Pretreatment with thyroxine increases tuberculin hypersensitivity but does not block desensitization by ACTH or cortisone. Apparently, thyroxine is necessary for the desensitizing action of ACTH and cortisone.

Long et al. B63,843/51: In guinea pigs, dihydro-ascorbic acid—unlike ascorbic acid—inhibits the tuberculin reaction after infection with B.C.G. vaccine. The desensitizing effect of dihydro-ascorbic acid is not inhibited by thiouracil. Alloxan, like ACTH or cortisone, does not modify desensitization by ascorbic acid on diets deprived of the "cabbage factor;" it desensitizes guinea pigs on a cabbage diet and this desensitization is inhibited by propylthiouracil.

Hoene et al. B68,152/52: In guinea pigs, ACTH given during three days before the challenging reinjection inhibits anaphylactic shock.

Vakilzadeh & Vandiviere E32,626/63: In guinea pigs, the beneficial effect of vaccination against tuberculosis was greatly increased by thyroxine and T3, but not by cortisone, cortisol or ACTH. None of the hormones altered natural host resistance in nonimmunized guinea pigs.

Rabbit

Reinmuth & Smith B60,585/51: In rabbits sensitized by M. tuberculosis and subsequently challenged with Old Tuberculin introduced into the trachea, the resulting pneumonia is decreased in severity by pretreatment with ACTH.

Lepri & Fornaro D91,865/54: In rabbits rendered allergic to tuberculosis, the ocular manifestations of topical challenge by tubercle bacilli were variably influenced by ACTH and cortisone.

RAT

Hayashida & Li C29,987/57: In rats, ACTH decreases, whereas STH increases, the formation of antibodies against a soluble protein envelope antigen extracted from P. pestis.

Vivan & Braito D22,638/62: In rats, the hemolytic icterus produced by appropriate agglutinin treatment can be prevented by concurrent administration of ACTH and glucuronic acid.

Wakim et al. D39,883/63: In rats and dogs, the renal damage produced by nephrotoxic serum can be inhibited by ACTH.

Hepatic and Renal Lesions ←

Hepatic Lesions ←. *Arrigo & Pontremoli B54,373/50:* In rats, ACTH greatly accelerates liver regeneration after partial hepatectomy but does not significantly increase hepatic steatosis.

Raffucci B83,148/53: Dogs tolerate much better repeated temporary rather than continuous occlusion of the hepatic artery and portal vein. ACTH in combination with antibiotics greatly enhances tolerance for noncontinued-occlusion of the afferent hepatic vessels.

Roberts B97,023/53: In rats, the enhanced repair of the liver following treatment with ACTH or adrenocortical extract is characterized mainly by increased protein deposition in the liver remnant. The usual decline of serum proteins occurring after partial hepatectomy was completely prevented by this treatment.

Hines & Roncoroni C40,870/57: In dogs, the hepatic damage produced by ligature of all the afferent vessels of the liver during one hour is diminished by ACTH, and survival is improved.

Šimek et al. G71,089/68: In intact and even more markedly in adrenalectomized rats, the hepatic accumulation of free fatty acids is increased by cortisol during the early period after partial hepatectomy. ACTH has the same effect but only in the presence of the adrenals.

Šimek et al. H13,837/68: Comparative studies on DNA synthesis, fatty acid content, and weight regeneration in the liver remnant of partially hepatectomized rats after treatment with cortisol, ACTH and various stressor agents.

Šimek et al. H22,183/68: In rats, the initial increase in liver triglyceride content induced by partial hepatectomy is decreased after adrenalectomy. However, within 24 hrs after the operation, this difference disappears. The effect of adrenalectomy upon the liver triglyceride changes induced by partial hepatectomy can be anulled by epinephrine or cortisone. ACTH augments the immediate rise in liver triglyceride but only in the presence of the adrenals.

Bucher et al. G72,546/69: Review of the humoral factors responsible for hepatic regeneration following partial hepatectomy. Hepatic DNA synthesis is stimulated in intact rats by parabiosis or cross-circulation with partially hepatectomized partners. Furthermore, tiny liver grafts implanted outside the portal area proliferate in response to partial ablation of the parent organ. Various stressors inhibit hepatic regeneration in partially hepatectomized rats, but this effect is not reproduced by ACTH or cortisol. On the other hand, adrenalectomy increases hepatic regeneration.

Renal Lesions ←. *Holman & Jones B93,771/53:* The arterial lesions that develop in dogs kept on a standard high-fat diet upon subsequent nephrectomy are prevented by pregnancy, cortisone, ACTH or diethylstilbestrol.

Varia ←

Ionizing Rays ←. Resistance to total body X-irradiation is not significantly influenced by ACTH in the mouse, rat or man, although some investigators claim to have obtained moderate protection by ACTH at least in rats.

Hypoxia and Hyperoxygenation ←. In mice and man, resistance to hypoxia is increased by ACTH, whereas in guinea pigs, allegedly tolerance to both hypoxia and hyperoxygenation is diminished by this hormone. It has been claimed, however, that in guinea pigs, whose resistance to hypoxia is increased by morphine, prior treatment with ACTH or cortisone protects against this combined treatment.

Temperature Variations ←. According to some investigators, the survival time of severely burned **rats** is not influenced by ACTH; others claim that the hormone prolongs survival. Cold tolerance is allegedly increased by prolonged ACTH pretreatment in this species.

In **mice**, ACTH does not protect against the fatal effects of burns, but allegedly pretreatment with ACTH increases resistance to cold.

Other Stressors ←. In rats, ACTH (like STH) and glucocorticoids decrease the **EST**.

ACTH allegedly aggravates the calcifying arteriosclerosis that tends to develop in rats exposed to the stress of **repeated breeding**.

An improvement in **muscular performance** (swimming) could be induced in rats by ACTH, but only at a critical temperature.

The resistance to **trauma** (Noble-Collip drum, tourniquet shock) is moderately enhanced by ACTH pretreatment in the rat.

In trout, **salinity tolerance** is not affected by ACTH, although it can be significantly altered by several other hormones.

Ionizing Rays ←

Smith et al. B47,642/50: In mice, neither ACTH nor cortisone increased survival following X-irradiation.

Rigat C10,747/55: Review (46 pp., 67 refs.) of the literature concerning the effect of hormones upon X-irradiation, with special reference to ACTH, STH, vasopressin, epinephrine, cortisone, DOC, testosterone, estradiol, progesterone, and thyroxine.

Taber C10,417/55: In man, ACTH increases resistance to radiation sickness.

Kedrova & Krekhova G71,665/59: In rats, ACTH offers some protection against lethal X-irradiation. Although cysteine has a similar effect by itself, it actually blocks the protective effect of ACTH.

Kandror E27,416/63: Review of the literature on the effect of corticoids and ACTH upon total body X-irradiation, especially in connection with the physiopathology of stress.

Orlova et al. G22,562/63: In rats, long-acting ACTH preparations offer protection against total body X-irradiation.

Trinci G45,713/66: In rats, resistance to X-irradiation was not markedly affected by pretreatment with ACTH.

Cittadini et al. G76,028/70: In X-irradiated mice, the formation of hemopoietic islets in the spleen is inhibited by dexamethasone, ACTH or the stress of exposure to cold.

Hypoxia and Hyperoxygenation ←

Frawley et al. B57,930/51: In man, both cortisone and ACTH improve high altitude tolerance.

Parkes B63,024/51: In mice, resistance to anoxia is increased by posterior lobe extract as well as by ACTH preparations containing posterior lobe principles.

Grognot & Senelar C41,294/57: In rats and guinea pigs, the pulmonary inflammation induced by inhalation of pure oxygen at normal barometric pressure is aggravated by ACTH or histamine.

Volterrani C64,384/57: In guinea pigs, tolerance to hypoxia is decreased by cortisone but increased by ACTH pretreatment.

Sobel et al. C90,836/60: Morphine increases the mortality of guinea pigs exposed to reduced oxygen tension. Prior treatment with cortisone or ACTH protects against this combined treatment.

Temperature Variations ←

Neal et al. B80,371/52: The survival time of severely burned rats is not influenced by cortisone or ACTH, whereas DOC administered before the burn offers considerable protection.

Schöttler C8,455/55: Neither ACTH nor cortisone protect the mouse against the fatal effects of severe scalding; in fact, cortisone increases mortality.

Kirsteins C41,958/56: Short term cortisone or ACTH administration to rats did not significantly influence cold tolerance, whereas long-term intermittent cortisone administration prior to exposure to cold definitely raised tolerance in this respect.

Koch et al. C33,922/57: In rats, ACTH, unlike STH, prolongs survival following severe burns.

Garrido C77,562/59: In intact rats, prednisone and ACTH increased resistance to cold.

Hale & Mefferd Jr. C79,669/59: In rats exposed to cold and various other stressors, pretreatment with "ACTH had a 'restraining' influence on nonspecific metabolic responses."

Yang & Lissak C77,913/59: In rats, the improvement of muscular performance (swimming) induced by ACTH is fully evident only at a critical temperature.

Knigge C97,819/60: Review on the neuroendocrine mechanisms influencing ACTH and TTH secretion, particularly during adaptation to cold.

Agarkov et al. D40,496/62: In intact rats, cortisone raises resistance to heat, whereas ACTH does not.

Araki G11,847/63: Pretreatment with ACTH or cortisol raises the resistance of intact mice to exposure to cold. Nicotinamide has a similar effect which is ascribed to stimulation of the pituitary-adrenal system.

Other Stressors ←

Electric Stimuli ←. *Minz & Domino B81,852/53:* In rats, small doses of epinephrine or norepinephrine prolong the duration of electrically-induced seizures. Since glucose, ACTH and cortisone failed to prolong seizure duration, it is unlikely that epinephrine acts by release of these substances. Histamine depressed the cortical response to electroshock.

Woodbury B98,594/54: Review (42 pp., 90 refs.) on the "Effect of Hormones on Brain Excitability and Electrolytes." In the rat, the EST is increased by DOC and decreased by cortisone and cortisol. ACTH and 11-dehydro-corticosterone, given chronically, partially antagonize the effect of cortisone.

Rosenblum C5,974/55: In rats, "ACTH and cortisone acetate in combination with vasopressin each produced a greater fall in EST than was produced by vasopressin alone. In contrast, STH in combination with vasopressin prevented the fall induced by vasopressin alone and produced its usual elevation in the EST."

Trauma ←. *Noble & Collip A56,107/42:* Adrenocortical extract and DOC greatly increase the resistance of adrenalectomized rats to the trauma of the Noble-Collip drum. In intact rats, "cortin" and DOC as well as ACTH induce only a slight increase in resistance under similar circumstances. "From a practical viewpoint the effects of adrenal preparations on this type of shock have been disappointing."

Kulagin D236/61: In rats with a crush syndrome produced by clamping a thigh, survival was increased by ACTH, cortisone and cortisol, whereas DOC aggravated the condition by increasing edema in the injured area.

Khrabrova D33,557/62: Both ACTH and cortisone prolong survival following traumatic shock in the cat.

Muscular Work ←. *Yang & Lissak C77,913/59:* In rats, the improvement of muscular performance (swimming) induced by ACTH is fully evident only at a critical temperature.

Osmosis ←. *Smith C46,496/56:* In brown trout, thyroxine raises, whereas thiourea and thiouracil reduce, salinity tolerance. Anterior pituitary extracts and STH likewise raise salinity tolerance, whereas posterior lobe extracts, testosterone, gonadotrophin, TTH and ACTH have no effect.

Tumors ←. *Glenn et al. G70,204/60:* Review (48 pp., 11 refs.) on the effect of various steroids, ACTH, GTH, ovariectomy, and adrenalectomy upon the development of C3H mammary carcinoma transplants in mice and fibroadenomas in rats.

Repeated Breeding ← cf. *Selye C50,810/58, p. 82; C92,918/61, p. 230; G60,083/70, pp. 328, 330.*

Hepatic Enzymes ←

In the rat, ACTH increases the **TPO** and **TKT** activity of the liver even without concurrent treatment with the corresponding substrates. In this respect, ACTH imitates the actions of glucocorticoids and of various stressors which cause ACTH and glucocorticoid secretion.

ACTH also increases hepatic **GPT** activity even in hypophysectomized but not in adrenalectomized rats. Presumably this effect is likewise mediated through the adrenal cortex.

Observations with the use of marked cholesterol in the rat showed that ACTH decreases the rate of **cholesterol** palmitate and oleate synthesis.

TPO, TKT ←

Geschwind & Li B95,517/53: Hypophysectomy does not abolish (and perhaps even increases) the resting TPO activity of the rat liver. However, in hypophysectomized animals, the ability to induce this enzyme by tryptophan injection is gradually diminishing during the first 14 post-operative days. Treatment with ACTH enhances the formation of this adaptive enzyme system (measured by kynurenin formation) even without treatment with tryptophan.

Knox & Auerbach E76,825/55: ACTH increases TPO activity of the liver in the rat.

Maickel & Brodie C83,071/60: TPO in rat liver is increased by ACTH, cortisone, or cortisol, as well as by various stressor agents and barbiturates. Hypophysectomy prevents the effect of stressors and barbiturates, suggesting that the latter act through the pituitary-adrenal system.

Knox G51,969/62: Review on the effect of stress upon hepatic TPO production. In adrenalectomized animals, only tryptophan of a series of analogues induces this enzyme, whereas, in intact rats, various stressors, ACTH, cortisone, cortisol and corticosterone (but not DOC) do so. "The recognition of the adrenal hormone-induced adaptation of the tryptophan pyrrolase has provided the unified explanation for a large number of different stressful stimuli which increase the enzyme level." Tryptophan pyrrolase is absent from the liver of newborn rabbits and in them, this enzyme cannot be induced by cortisol. Tyrosine transaminase induction is regulated in a very similar manner.

GPT ←

Rosen et al. C71,414/59: Marked increases in GPT activity were observed in the livers of rats given cortisol, cortisone, 9α-fluorocortisol, prednisone, 6α-methylprednisolone, 9α-fluoro-21-desoxy-6α-methylprednisolone or ACTH, whereas two nonglucocorticoid cortisol derivatives, 11-epicortisol and 9α-methoxycortisol were inactive. STH, testosterone and insulin caused no significant change in GPT by themselves nor did they modify the action of cortisol.

Harding et al. D14,355/61: In the rat, pretreatment with DOC depresses the hepatic GPT activity. A similar depression is obtained by adrenalectomy, but this is not further aggravated by concurrent treatment with DOC. ACTH increases GPT activity in hypophysectomized, but not in adrenalectomized, animals. In hypophysectomized rats, DOC fails to lower alanine transaminase, nor does it alter the response of this enzyme to ACTH. "The inhibitory effect of DOC on alanine transaminase activity appears to be due to suppression of ACTH release by the pituitary."

Cholesterolase ←

Schweppe & Jungmann H15,978/69: Observations on the metabolism of marked cholesterol added together with various hormones to hepatic microsomes of the rat led to the conclusion that "1) cholesterol palmitate and oleate were synthesized most rapidly; 2) at high concentrations, testosterone decreased the formation of all esters but at lower dose levels, testosterone increased the synthesis of cholesterol oleate and palmitate; 3) estradiol caused a two-fold increase in cholesterol oleate formation; 4) ACTH decreased the synthesis rate of cholesterol palmitate and oleate; 5) insulin had a significant inhibitory effect on cholesterol linoleate; 6) epinephrine had little significant effect at the dose level used; and 7) L-thyroxine increased the synthesis of all cholesterol esters."

← SOMATOTROPHIC HORMONE (STH)

Steroids ←

The effects of **corticoids** can be modified by STH in many respects. In rats sensitized by uninephrectomy + NaCl, STH produces a hyalinosis syndrome with malignant hypertension, similar to that elicited by mineralocorticoids. The corresponding action of DOC is aggravated by STH. Adrenalectomy or pretreatment with cortisone (in doses sufficient to produce adrenocortical atrophy) inhibits the production of hyalinosis by STH. It is assumed that STH induces malignant hypertension by increasing the production or the effect of mineralocorticoids.

Glucocorticoid overdosage symptoms (catabolism, splenic and thymic atrophy, "saprophytosis") are prevented in rats by simultaneous administration of STH. On the other hand, a synergism between STH and mineralocorticoids (DOC, aldosterone) has been demonstrated (in both intact and adrenalectomized rats) as judged by their effects upon many target organs.

The inhibition of growth by **folliculoids** (e.g., stilbestrol) can be blocked in rats by concurrent STH administration, but this conjoint treatment results in particularly severe osteosclerosis.

Corticoids ←

Selye B53,940/51: In uninephrectomized NaCl-treated rats, the hyalinosis syndrome produced by DOC is aggravated by STH; indeed, STH alone can engender malignant hypertensive disease. These effects of STH are inhibited by cortisone. Apparently STH increases mineralocorticoid production by the adrenals (unless these are rendered atrophic by cortisone) and/or sensitizes the peripheral tissue to mineralocorticoids.

Selye B65,065/52: In rats, large doses of cortisone permit the proliferation of normally saprophytic organisms which cause multiple abscesses and hepatic necroses (the "saprophytosis syndrome"). All these changes can be prevented by simultaneous treatment with STH.

Horava & Selye B70,249/53: In rats, heavy overdosage with cortisol produces intense catabolism with atrophy of the adrenals, thymus and spleen, as well as pulmonary "saprophytosis." Concurrent administration of STH inhibits the body weight loss and the saprophytosis, but not adrenal and thymus atrophy. The renal glomerular changes induced by cortisol intoxication are actually aggravated by STH.

Ducommun & Ducommun B70,251/53: In rats, saprophytosis produced by heavy overdosage with cortisone is inhibited by concurrent administration of STH. This "anti-infectious effect of STH" is much less evident after adrenalectomy. DOC, testosterone, and estradiol alone or in combination failed to duplicate the anti-infectious action of STH in cortisone-treated rats.

Selye & Bois C1,718/55: In intact and in adrenalectomized rats, a synergism between mineralocorticoids (DOC, aldosterone) and STH was evident in their effects upon many target organs.

Bavetta et al. D29,064/62: In the rat, "growth hormone, methyl testosterone or stilbestrol, when given alone or in combination were not able to counteract the inhibitory effects of 6-methyl prednisolone on body weight and collagen synthesis at the site of subcutaneously implanted polyvinyl sponges."

Folliculoids ←

Selye B70,245/53: In rats, the inhibition of growth produced by a folliculoid substance, such as stilbestrol, can be inhibited by STH, but this conjoint treatment results in severe osteosclerosis.

Drugs ←

STH conspicuously influences the toxicity of only a few drugs. For example in rats, it tends to aggravate the production of hepatic sclerosis by CCl_4 while diminishing parenchymal injury.

In rats, hepatoma formation by certain **carcinogens** is enhanced both by STH and by ACTH. Studies with ^{14}C-labeled N-OH-FAA showed decreased dehydroxylation and deacetylation of the carcinogens as well as increased binding of radioactivity to liver proteins in animals treated with STH.

Female rats are much more resistant than males to the induction of cardiovascular and renal lesions by **choline** deficient diets. However, STH sensitizes the female to the production of these changes by choline deficiency, perhaps because the increased growth rate accelerates the exhaustion of choline stores.

The bone changes produced by various **lathyrogens** are very considerably aggravated by STH. Conversely, hypophysectomy prevents these changes, and substitution with STH in doses just sufficient to maintain normal growth restores the susceptibility of the skeleton to the production of lathyrism. It was concluded that the normal STH secretion of the hypophysis decisively influences the development of this bone disease. The lathyrism-enhancing effect of STH is not mediated through the adrenals, since it is evident even after bilateral adrenalectomy.

The cardiac infarcts produced by coronary artery ligature in the rat tend to develop into rupturing cardiac aneurysms under the influence of the lathyrogen, AAN. This effect is not significantly altered by STH. Similarly, STH fails to influence the hemorrhagic tendency induced by lathyrogens such as AAN. Hence, there does not appear to be any close relationship between the effect of STH upon the skeletal and the cardiovascular manifestations of lathyrism. Furthermore, the hormones presumably act directly upon the responsiveness of individual target organs, and not by altering the metabolism of the lathyrogens.

In the rat, the catabolism produced by **nitrogen mustard** is not prevented, and even tends to be aggravated, by STH alone; yet, excellent protection is obtained by combined treatment with STH and antibiotics.

On the other hand, the growth stimulating effect of STH is greatly diminished in rats given diets deficient in **phenylalanine, tryptophan, or tyrosine.**

In rats kept on a **vitamin-A** deficient diet, STH fails to promote growth, and actually precipitates the manifestations of avitaminosis. On the other hand, the intense catabolism and bone absorption produced in rats by vitamin-A overdosage are prevented by STH.

The cardiovascular calcification engendered by **vitamin-D** derivatives, such as **DHT**, is somewhat diminished, but not prevented by STH, although the associated catabolism is markedly inhibited.

Acrylonitrile ←

Szabó & Selye G 79,010/71: In rats, pretreatment with ACTH (but not with STH) prevents the production of adrenal apoplexy by acrylonitrile. Hypophysectomy protects against adrenal apoplexy, but not against mortality under similar conditions.

Aminopyrine Barbiturates ←

Wilson H 34,926/71: In rats, implants of mammotropic tumor (which secretes STH, ACTH and LTH) decreased the hepatic metabolism of hexobarbital and aminopyrine. Similar but much less pronounced changes were observed in rats bearing very large Walker tumors.

Anaphylactoidogenic Agents ←

Higginbotham & Dougherty C 44,529/57: In mice, ACTH increased the toxicity of polymyxin B; STH and TTH had no effect upon it.

Anticoagulants ←

van Cauwenberge & Jaques C 58,521/58: A dose of bishydroxycoumarin (Dicoumarol) well tolerated by otherwise untreated rabbits, causes death with widespread hemorrhage when given together with ACTH. The hemorrhagic tendency induced by coumarol was not accentuated by STH, cortisone or DOC.

van Cauwenberge & Jaques C 72,748/59: The "hemorrhagic death syndrome" produced by Dicoumarol treatment in rats simultaneously exposed to various stressors can be reproduced by the administration of ACTH, STH, or DOC, instead of stressors. Dicoumarol + cortisol or cortisone did not reproduce this syndrome.

Carbon Tetrachloride ←

Campanacci Jr. et al. C 20,086/56: In rats, small doses of STH increase the hepatic sclerosis produced by CCl_4, whereas at high dose levels, the hormone aggravates parenchymal degeneration, but inhibits sclerosis.

Post et al. C 40,180/57: In rats, the hepatic injury produced by CCl_4 is diminished by STH.

Furukawa F 71,711/65: In rats, hepatic steatosis produced by CCl_4 is inhibited by adrenalectomy and, to some extent, also by hypophysectomy. The effect of CCl_4 after adrenalectomy is restored by corticoids, but not by epinephrine which only increases the action of the former. STH does not counteract the effect of hypophysectomy. Alloxan diabetes inhibits CCl_4-induced hepatic lipidosis.

Carcinogens ←

Reid B 93,930/54: Review (18 pp., 181 refs.) on the effect of STH and corticoids upon carcinogen-induced and transplantable neoplasms.

Shirasu et al. F 76,819/67: In the rats, hepatoma formation by N-hydroxy-N-2-Fluorenylacetamide (N-OH-FAA) is enhanced by ACTH and STH. Studies with ^{14}C-labeled N-OH-FAA showed "decreased dehydroxylation and deacetylation of N-OH-FAA. The radioactivity bound to liver proteins was increased, remarkably so in the animals treated with growth hormone."

7,12-Dimethylbenz(a)anthracene ← STH + Age: Morii et al. D 45,369/62*

Choline ←

Wilgram & Hartcroft C 14,392/55: Female rats are much more resistant than males to the production of cardiovascular lesions by choline deficiency. However, simultaneous administration of "androgens" (kind not specified) and STH sensitizes the female to the induction of these lesions by hypolipotrophic rations.

Wilgram et al. C 15,960/56: Both STH and testosterone aggravate the renal and cardiovascular lesions characteristic of choline deficiency in the rat.

Wilgram C 84,322/59: In rats, STH increases the severity of the cardiovascular lesions produced by choline deficiency.

Aterman D 15,536/61: In male weanling rats, the hepatic necrosis induced by feeding a diet containing yeast as the sole source of protein is greatly accelerated by partial hepatectomy or treatment with STH.

Chlorpromazine ←

Epple et al. F 76,569/66: In toads, the hypothermic action of chlorpromazine and ethanol is diminished by STH.

Ethanol ←

Epple et al. F 76,569/66: In toads, the hypothermic action of chlorpromazine and ethanol is diminished by STH.

Ethionine ←

Farber & Segaloff D 95,996/55: In ovariectomized rats, various testoids and STH protected the liver against fatty infiltration produced by ethionine i.p., whereas cortisone and ACTH aggravated it. Estradiol, DOC, and TSH had no effect.

Lathyrogens ← *cf. also Selye C 92,918/61, p. 137.*

Selye & Bois C 18,280/56: In rats, the osteolathyrism produced by lathyrus odoratus seeds is aggravated by STH and inhibited by cortisol. Combined treatment with DOC + uninephrectomy + NaCl resulted in dissecting aneurysms of the aorta. Very small doses of thyroxine or estradiol were without effect upon this form of lathyrism.

Dasler C 36,068/57: Brief mention of unpublished observations indicating that in rats, osteolathyrism produced by APN is not inhibited by cortisone or thyroxine, but aggravated by STH.

Selye C 25,910/57: In rats, the osteolathyrism produced by moderate doses of AAN is greatly aggravated by STH.

Selye C 31,369/57: In the rat, the osteolathyrism produced by AAN is aggravated by STH, LTH, and partial hepatectomy, but it is inhibited by ACTH, cortisol, or estradiol.

Selye C 31,790/57: In rats, osteolathyrism produced by AAN is inhibited by thyroxine, cortisol, and estradiol, but aggravated by STH even after adrenalectomy.

Selye & Bois C22,712/57: In rats, osteolathyrism (produced by AAN) is inhibited by cortisol and augmented by STH. The combination of STH and AAN enhances the development of polyarthritis in the small joints of the extremities. DOC facilitates the production of aortic aneurysms by AAN.

Selye & Bois C23,297/57: In rats, STH greatly aggravates the osteolathyrism produced by AAN.

Selye & Ventura C27,684/57: In rats, hypophysectomy greatly diminished the development of the osteolathyrism normally produced by AAN, but STH aggravated these bone lesions even more in the absence than in the presence of the pituitary. It is concluded that the normal hormonal secretion of the hypophysis exerts a decisive influence on the development of osteolathyrism.

Selye & Cantin C88,878/61: In rats, the osteolathyrism produced by AAN is inhibited by thyroxine and cortisol, but aggravated by STH. The cardiac infarcts elicited in rats by ligature of the descending branch of the left coronary artery are often transformed into rupturing cardiac aneurysms under the influence of AAN. The incidence of these cardiac ruptures is augmented by cortisol and DOC, but not significantly influenced by thyroxine and STH. Evidently, there is no direct relationship between the skeletal and the cardiac lesions under these circumstances.

Aschkenasy D30,892/62: In rats, lathyrism produced by AAN is aggravated by adrenalectomy and, in the absence of the adrenals, the usual antilathyric effect of cortisone is no longer demonstrable; in fact the glucocorticoid facilitates the production of hernias. STH aggravates the osteolathyrism, but not the induction of hemorrhages by AAN.

Nitrogen Mustard ←

Mitchell & Girerd B82,866/53: In rats, the catabolism and mortality produced by nitrogen mustard is actually aggravated by STH alone, and only slightly inhibited by antibiotics; STH + antibiotics offer excellent protection.

Phenylalanine ←

Scott & Dynes C53,564/57: In rats on a phenylalanine- and tyrosine-deficient diet, STH caused less stimulation of the epiphyseal growth plate than in pair-fed animals.

Reiss et al. F81,632/66: In rabbits given large amounts of phenylalanine, the blood and tissue concentration of this compound could be reduced by pretreatment with norbolethone decanoate or STH.

Plasmocid ← cf. Selye C92,918/61, p. 95.

Tryptophan ←

Bavetta et al. C17,656/56: In rats on a tryptophan-deficient diet, STH failed to increase body weight, but it did stimulate endochondral osteogenesis and dentin formation.

Tyrosine ←

Scott & Dynes C53,564/57: In rats on a phenylalanine- and tyrosine-deficient diet, STH caused less stimulation of the epiphyseal growth plate than in pair-fed animals.

Vitamin A ←

Ershoff & Deuel Jr. B14,516/45: In vitamin-A deficient rats, STH fails to promote growth, and actually shortens survival by the precipitation of acute vitamin-A deficiency symptoms.

Selye C36,050/57: In rats, the intense osteoclastic bone absorption produced by vitamin-A overdosage can be prevented by STH. Although the luteotrophic hormone (LTH) shares many of the actions of STH, it cannot substitute for the latter in counteracting vitamin-A intoxication, cf. Fig. 21.

Bavetta C60,277/58: In rats, STH failed to increase body weight on a vitamin-A deficient diet, but endochondral ossification was enhanced, and dentin formation stimulated. "The suggestion is made that impaired chondrogenic and osteogenic activity in vitamin A-depleted rats is due, at least in part, to an inadequate production or secretion of growth hormone."

Bottiglioni et al. C70,889/59: In rats, the atrophy of the skeletal musculature and the decreased metachromasia of the aortic wall produced by vitamin-A deficiency are aggravated by STH.

Vitamin C ←

McGraw C68,484/59; C80,136/59: Doctor's thesis describing numerous experiments on the effect of adrenalectomy, cortisone, thyroxine, thyroidectomy, thiourea, and STH upon scorbutic guinea pigs, with special emphasis upon changes in capillary resistance and cold tolerance.

Vitamin D, DHT ← cf. also Selye G60,083/70, pp. 331, 333.

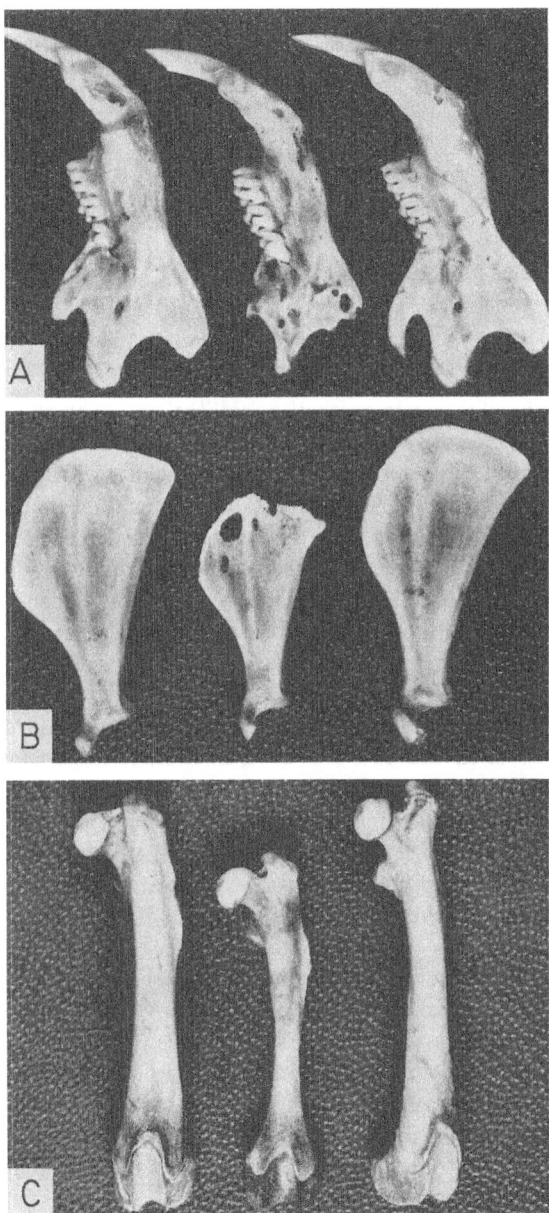

Fig. 21. **Prevention of vitamin-A induced skeletal lesions by STH.** A: Mandible of normal (left), vitamin-A treated (middle) and vitamin-A + STH-treated rats. Note that hypervitaminosis A resulted in several perforations within the flat part of the mandible and in absorption of the coronoid and condyloid processes with disappearance of the angle of the jaw. All these changes have been completely prevented by STH. B: Scapula of normal (left), vitamin-A treated (middle) and vitamin A+STH-treated rat. Again, the resorption of bone normally produced by vitamin A has been prevented by STH. C: Femur of a normal (left), a vitamin-A treated (middle) and vitamin A + STH-treated rat. The antagonism between STH and vitamin-A is clearly visible. [Selye C36,050/57. Courtesy of J. Endocrin.]

Selye C 27,735/57: The cardiovascular calcification and nephrocalcinosis produced by DHT in rats are aggravated by estradiol, cortisol, ACTH, and thyroxine. Conversely, methyltestosterone and STH exert a protective effect.

Zinc ←

Prasad et al. G 64,823/69: In rats kept on a zinc-deficient diet, STH failed to promote growth.

Varia ←

Selye G 70,480/71: In rats, STH offered some protection against progesterone anesthesia but did not alter the syndrome of intoxication with digitoxin, dioxathion parathion, nicotine, hexobarbital, zoxazolamine, indomethacin, acute DHT intoxication or the myocardial necroses produced by fluorocortisol + Na_2HPO_4 + corn oil.

Diet ← *cf. Selye G 60,083/70, pp. 331, 333.*

Microorganisms, Parasites and Their Products ←

As previously stated, STH counteracts the facilitating effect of glucocorticoids and of ACTH upon the spread of various infections. This has first been demonstrated for the "**saprophytosis**" that develops in rats as a consequence of the proliferation of normally saprophytic organisms. STH also exerts a beneficial effect upon resistance of mice to **pneumococci** and **typhoid bacilli**, and of rats to **P. pestis**. On the other hand, STH does not appear to modify the course of **staphylococcus** infection in rabbits.

The most extensive studies on the effect of STH have been conducted in connection with experimental **tuberculosis**. In the rat, there appears to exist a definite antagonism between the resistance-decreasing action of ACTH and glucocorticoids on the one hand and the protection offered by STH on the other. This has been confirmed by some investigators in guinea pigs and mice; indeed, it has been claimed that STH exerts a favorable effect even in human tuberculosis. However, many of the reports are contradictory, probably owing to genetic differences in the strains of the bacteria and hosts, as well as to variations in the potency and immunologic compatibility of the STH preparations employed.

In mice, the proliferation of influenza **virus** is accelerated by STH, perhaps as a consequence of enhanced protein synthesis in general. The detrimental effect of ACTH and cortisone upon the course of influenza virus infection in mice is not overcome by STH. However, the increase in the sensitivity of the mouse to infection with MHV-3 hepatitis virus, induced by different glucocorticoids, is largely counteracted by STH. In sheep, STH tends to delimit the lesions produced by variola virus, but in mice its effect upon vaccinia virus is not very pronounced.

In mice, STH retards the development of infection with parasites, **Plasmodium berghei**, and in frogs, it inhibits infection with **Trypanosoma inopinatum**.

The moniliasis produced by **Candida albicans** in mice is aggravated by cortisone and this deleterious effect is counteracted by STH.

STH offers no protection against **typhoid endotoxin** in the mouse, but resistance against diphtheria toxin appears to be increased.

Bacteria and Vaccines ←

Corynebacteria ← *cf. Selye C 92,918/61, p. 233.*

"Endotheliomyelosis" ← *cf. Selye C 92,918/61, p. 241.*

"Saprophytosis" ←. *Selye B 57,451/51:* In rats, "saprophytosis" due to proliferation of normally nonpathogenic microorganisms, such as develops after heavy overdosage with cortisone or ACTH, can be completely prevented by concurrent administration of STH.

Selye B65,065/52: In rats, large doses of cortisone permit the proliferation of normally saprophytic organisms which cause multiple abscesses and hepatic necroses (the "saprophytosis syndrome"). All these changes can be prevented by simultaneous treatment with STH.

Pneumococcus ←. *Kass et al. B95,353/54:* In mice, resistance to pneumococcal and influenza virus infections is depressed by pretreatment with cortisone or cortisol, but not by ACTH. STH failed to overcome the effect of cortisone and did not increase resistance to infection when given alone.

Meier & Neipp C37,215/56: In mice, the chemotherapeutic action of sulfonamides against resistant Type III pneumococci is increased by various gonadotrophic and STH preparations. However, certain bacterial polysaccharide fractions possess a similar effect, and hence, the latter is presumably not dependent upon the specific actions of the hormone preparations.

Staphylococcus ←. *Debry C30,870/56:* Doctor's thesis (176 pp. 578 refs.) on the influence of hormones upon infection. Personal observations on guinea pigs and rats indicate that ACTH, STH, and DOC do not significantly affect the course of acute staphylococcus infection, whereas cortisone aggravates it.

Herbeuval et al. C55,675/58: In rabbits, STH does not modify the course of staphylococcus infection.

Typhoid Bacilli ←. *Jude et al. C16,220/55:* In mice, STH pretreatment protects against subsequent infection with typhoid bacilli. The protection is ascribed to improved antibody formation and phagocytosis. STH offers no protection against typhoid endotoxin.

Pasteurella Pestis ←. *Hayashida C37,366/57:* In rats infected with P. pestis, ACTH decreased, whereas STH increased survival.

Mycobacterium Tuberculosis ←. *Lemonde et al. B70,248/52:* The rat which is naturally resistant to human M. tuberculosis can be made sensitive to this infection by pretreatment with cortisone. This sensitivity is in turn abolished by concurrent treatment with STH. Mice which are naturally sensitive to tuberculosis can also be protected by STH.

Lucherini et al. B89,088/53: In guinea pigs, STH inhibits the progress of tuberculosis and counteracts the opposite effect of ACTH.

Chirico et al. C5,040/54: In guinea pigs, the late pulmonary manifestations of tuberculosis are enhanced by STH and the fibrotic healing processes are improved. The effects of the hormone are ascribed to a stimulation of mesenchymal defense reactions.

Lemonde C310/54: Doctor's thesis (186 pp., 564 refs.) on humoral factors influencing infections, with special reference to the effect of STH and cortisone upon experimental tuberculosis.

Youmans & Youmans B95,169/54: In mice, cortisone markedly reduced the survival time after infection with human tubercle bacilli, and this effect could not be prevented by STH. Given alone, ACTH, STH, and TTH likewise failed to influence the course of the infection.

Carstensen et al. C12,300/55: In man, STH (Somacton) has been found useful in the treatment of tuberculosis.

Guillermand et al. C15,540/55: In man, STH [source not indicated (H.S.)] allegedly exerts a very favorable effect upon tuberculosis.

Lemonde et al. C526/55: In mice, STH is beneficial in combating chronic but not acute tuberculous infection.

Lemonde C6,400/55: In mice and rats, STH has a favorable effect upon the course of experimental tuberculosis.

Brouet et al. G72,418/56: Review (47 pp., 55 refs.) on the effect of STH upon clinical and experimental tuberculosis. Personal observations on guinea pigs showed that the hormone has a moderate protective effect.

Chirico C24,381/56: Review (32 pp., about 100 refs.) on the effects of STH, with special reference to its influence upon inflammation and tuberculosis.

Wasz-Höckert & Backman C34,801/56: In guinea pigs, ACTH aggravates the course of tuberculosis. STH in itself is without conspicuous effect, however, "the strongly deteriorating effect on tuberculosis produced by ACTH was evidently counteracted by STH when given simultaneously with ACTH."

Wasz-Höckert & McCune E31,145/63: In mice infected with tuberculosis, STH caused an increase in body weight but did not inhibit the development of the infection, nor did it counteract the unfavorable effect of ACTH.

Varia ←. *Cavallero C829/54:* Review on the effect of STH, ACTH, and cortisone upon various infections, especially in the rat.

Viruses ←

Kalter et al. B49,656/50: In mice, the proliferation of influenza virus is accelerated by STH and testosterone, presumably because of an enhanced protein synthesis in general.

Kass et al. B95,353/54: In mice, resistance to pneumococcal and influenza virus infections is depressed by pretreatment with cortisone or cortisol, but not by ACTH. STH failed to overcome the effect of cortisone and did not increase resistance to infection when given alone.

Pecori et al. C89,118/59; C89,121/59: Prednisone, triamcinolone, and dexamethasone increase the sensitivity of the mouse to infection with the MHV-3 hepatitis virus. This pro-infectious effect is largely counteracted by STH.

Cilli et al. D12,192/61: In sheep, STH, owing to its prophlogistic effect, delimits the lesions produced by variola virus. ACTH and dexamethasone exert an opposite effect.

Altucci et al. D65,819/62: In mice, STH alters the tissue reaction to infection by vaccinia virus, but has little effect upon mortality.

Parasites ←

Galliard & Lapierre E82,642/53: In mice, STH retards the development of infection with P. berghei.

Galliard et al. G70,892/53: In frogs, infection with T. inopinatum is inhibited by STH, presumably as a consequence of its phlogistic action which favors the phagocytosis of the parasites.

Galliard et al. D89,408/54: In mice, STH greatly retards infection with Plasmodium berghei. STH has no effect upon either toxoplasmosis in the mouse or infection with T. brucei in the rat or mouse.

Fungi and Yeasts ←

Scherr C39,263/57: In mice infected with Candida albicans, the development of moniliasis may be either increased or decreased by cortisone, depending upon various factors, particularly the severity of the infection, sex or pregnancy. Testosterone enhanced, and STH counteracted the deleterious effect of cortisone. Gonadotrophin (pregnant mare serum) was without effect.

Bacterial Toxins ←

Jude et al. C16,220/55: In mice, STH-pretreatment protects against subsequent infection with typhoid bacilli. The protection is ascribed to improved antibody formation and phagocytosis. STH offers no protection against typhoid endotoxin.

Skuratova D20,887/62: In mice, resistance against the fatal effect of diphtheria toxin is more markedly increased by STH than by ACTH.

Immune Reactions ←

In guinea pigs, STH has been claimed to depress tuberculin sensitivity and to synergize the desensitizing effect of cortisone.

In rats, STH aggravates the glomerular lesions characteristic of the Masugi nephritis, and increases the formation of antibodies against Pasteurella pestis. It also raises hemolysin formation following i.p. injection of sheep erythrocytes in the rat.

Hepatic and Renal Lesions ←

In partially hepatectomized rats, STH failed to further increase the high mitotic rate in the liver remnant.

In completely nephrectomized rats, STH slightly prolonged survival. The renal atrophy produced by temporary ligation of one renal pedicle is counteracted, and survival following removal of the contralateral kidney is prolonged by STH.

Various Stressors ←

In guinea pigs and rats, STH diminishes the catabolism, and to a lesser extent the mortality, induced by total body **X-irradiation.**

In the rat, STH counteracts the loss of body weight induced by chronic exposure to **cold.** Under certain circumstances it also prolongs survival in extreme cold, or after severe burns. It has been claimed that in man, STH likewise counteracts the catabolism produced by burns.

STH is said to increase the EST in the rat and the **salinity tolerance** in the trout, and to offer "moderate protection" against **various stressors** in guinea pigs.

Hepatic Enzymes ←

In rats, STH decreases hepatic arginase and GPT but not GOT activity. The TPO activity of the rat liver increases with age, as well as after STH injection.

In rats, STH inhibits the synthesis of hepatic TKT and represses TKT induction by stressors or cortisol, but it has no effect upon the cortisol-induced TPO activity.

The OKT activity of the rat liver is diminished after treatment with STH, the same as after partial hepatectomy.

In rats treated with STH during the postnatal period, the development of various drug-metabolizing hepatic microsomal enzymes is suppressed.

In mice, STH first decreases and then increases hepatic TPO activity. A similar biphasic reaction is allegedly produced by exposure to stress; this may explain some of the contradictions in the published data.

Immune Reactions ←

Cornforth & Long B77,176/53: In guinea pigs sensitized to tuberculin, single s.c. injections of ATP prevent desensitization by alloxan, cortisone, and dihydro-ascorbic acid. Single s.c. injections of insulin do not in themselves influence sensitivity but prevent desensitization by alloxan and cortisone. Single s.c. injections of STH depress tuberculin sensitivity and synergize the action of cortisone or alloxan.

Dutz et al. C31,646/56: In rats, gonadectomy did not significantly change the course of Masugi nephritis, whereas a folliculoid preparation (Östrasid) and testosterone ameliorated it. STH considerably aggravated the glomerular lesions and the hypertension.

Hayashida & Li C29,987/57: In rats, ACTH decreases whereas STH increases the formation of antibodies against a soluble protein envelope antigen extracted from P. pestis.

Ghiringhelli C90,609/60: In rabbits, the production of anti-ovalbumin antibodies is not significantly influenced by STH.

Terragna & Jannuzzi F62,290/66: Review of the literature on the influence of STH on antibody formation. Personal observations in rats show that hemolysin formation following i.p. injection of sheep erythrocytes was increased by STH, but the change was statistically not significant.

Hepatic Lesions ←

Cristensen & Jacobsen A49,204/49: In rats subjected to partial hepatectomy, neither hypophysectomy nor thyroidectomy impairs the rate of regeneration. No significant change in mitotic rate was observed after pretreatment with stilbestrol or STH.

Selye & Bois B97,074/54: In adrenalectomized rats with choledochus ligature, cortisol enhances the accumulation of bile within the bile-duct stem and furthers the development of perforating choledochus ulcers. These actions can be prevented by concurrent treatment with STH.

Moolten et al. H30,606/70: In rats, the rise in hepatic DNA synthesis after partial hepatectomy is accelerated by surgical interventions or STH. Cortisone, cortisol and ACTH were ineffective. Neither stress nor STH stimulated DNA synthesis significantly in non-hepatectomized rats.

Renal Lesions ←

Dési et al. C69,045/59: In rats, survival after bilateral nephrectomy is prolonged by STH and DOC, alone or in combination, but the effect of STH is diminished by concurrent administration of MAD.

Köhnlein et al. D38,961/62: In rats, the renal atrophy produced by temporary ligation of one renal pedicle is counteracted, and survival following subsequent removal of the healthy kidney is prolonged by STH.

Various Stressors ←

Ionizing Rays ←. *Lacassagne & Tuchmann-Duplessis E 53,832/53:* In X-irradiated guinea pigs and rats, body-weight loss and to some extent even mortality, were diminished by STH.

Hoene et al. B 92,374/54: In rats, pretreatment with STH inhibits the loss of body weight and the involution of the lymph nodes following X-irradiation, but it exerts no clear-cut effect upon the involution of the spleen and thymus or the deficient antibody formation induced by irradiation.

Rigat C 10,747/55: Review (46 pp., 67 refs.) on the literature concerning the effect of hormones upon X-irradiation, with special reference to ACTH, STH, vasopressin, epinephrine, cortisone, DOC, testosterone, estradiol, progesterone, and thyroxine.

Barlow & Sellers C 21,626/55: In rats, STH prevents body-weight loss but does not prolong survival following X-irradiation.

Bloodworth et al. C 14,328/56: In rats, weight loss and mortality following X-irradiation were diminished by STH.

Temperature Variations ←. *Dugal & Dufour C 8,603/54:* In rats, the loss of body weight produced by chronic exposure to cold is counteracted by STH.

Dufour & Dugal C 15,508/55: In rats, STH increases resistance to cold.

Dufour & Dugal C 26,092/57: In rats, resistance to cold is diminished by STH or DOC given in combination with vitamin C.

Koch et. al. C 33,922/57: In rats, ACTH, unlike STH, prolongs survival following severe burns.

Soroff et al. G 52,127/67: In man, human STH counteracts the catabolism produced by burns.

Varia ←. *Rosenblum C 5,974/55:* In rats "ACTH and cortisone acetate in combination with vasopressin each produced a greater fall in EST than was produced by vasopressin alone. In contrast, STH in combination with vasopressin prevented the fall induced by vasopressin alone and produced its usual elevation in the EST."

Smith C 46,496/56: In brown trout, thyroxine raises, whereas thiourea and thiouracil reduce **salinity tolerance**. Anterior pituitary extracts and STH likewise raise salinity tolerance, whereas posterior lobe extracts, testosterone, gonadotrophin, TTH, and ACTH have no such effect.

Amante C 62,537/58: In guinea pigs, STH "moderately protects" against the stress of burns, tourniquet, or evisceration.

Vanamee et al. H 32,254/70: In rats, the production of stress ulcers of the stomach by *restraint* is inhibited by pretreatment with STH.

Hepatic Enzymes ←

Beaton et al. B 86,367/53: In adult male rats, a single i.p. injection of STH causes a decrease in the rate of urea formation by liver slices, as well as in the hepatic arginase and GPT but not GOT activity. No such changes were noted in young male rats.

Wood Jr. & Knox D 81,779/54: In mice, STH decreases hepatic TPO activity.

Beaton et al. C 10,012/55: STH decreases the hepatic GPT and d-aminoacid oxidase activity in nonpregnant female rats. These effects are even more pronounced if the animals receive STH + "equine estrogenic substances" + progesterone. This enzyme activity also decreases during pregnancy both in intact and in hypophysectomized rats.

Wood et al. C 27,721/56: In mice bearing SC-sarcoma implants, the hepatic TPO activity was first diminished, but rose above normal as the neoplasms grew. "Changes analogous to this biphasic depression and elevation of the enzyme level in tumor-bearing animals could be produced in control mice by growth hormone and by adrenal-stimulating stress, respectively."

Beaton et al. D 83,636/57: Following STH treatment, there is a significant depression in the GPT activity of rat liver tissue, whereas cortisone has an inverse effect.

Zuchlewski & Gaebler D 91,862/57: Hepatic glutamic acid dehydrogenase activity increases after hypophysectomy in the rat, and it is not altered by STH in either hypophysectomized or sham-operated control animals. GPT and GOT activities have also been investigated under similar conditions.

Rosen et al. C 50,741/58; C 71,414/59: Marked increases in GPT activity were observed in the livers of rats given cortisol, cortisone, 9α-fluorocortisol, prednisone, 6α-methylprednisolone, 9α-fluoro-21-desoxy-6α-methylprednisolone or ACTH, whereas two nonglucocorticoid cortisol derivatives, 11-epicortisol and 9α-methoxycortisol were inactive. STH, testosterone, and insulin caused no significant change in GPT by themselves, nor did they modify the action of cortisol. On the other hand, large doses of estradiol and thyroxine caused a moderate increase in GPT activity but when injected simultaneously with cortisol, they appeared to interfere with its action as did progesterone. Adrenalectomy slightly diminished or failed to affect the GPT inducing activity of cortisol, whereas hypophysectomy caused a rise in GPT activity and augmented the effect of cortisol.

Rivlin & Knox C71,249/59: The TPO activity of rat liver increases with age and body weight, as well as after STH injection.

Kenney & Albritton G64,557/65: Review of the literature suggesting that transaminase induction in response to stressors can be due to corticoid secretion during the stress reaction. Cortisol enhances enzyme synthesis after an increased rate of synthesis of ribosomal transfer and "DNA-like" RNA's. The present experiments confirm the view that repressor(s) can inhibit enzyme synthesis at the translational level because inhibition of RNA synthesis can prolong the corticoid-induced increase in enzyme synthesis under suitable conditions. "Administration of stressing agents (tyrosine, Celite) to adrenalectomized rats initiates a highly selective repression of the synthesis of hepatic TKT. The enzyme level falls with a t½ of about 2.5 hr. Immunochemical measurement of the rate of enzyme synthesis indicates that it is reduced essentially to zero in stressed, adrenalectomized rats, whereas labeling of total liver soluble proteins is unaffected. Actinomycin does not itself influence the enzyme level, but it blocks the stress-initiated repression of enzyme synthesis, indicating that repression acts at the translational level, whereas initiation of repression involves transcriptional processes." In hypophysectomized rats, stressors are ineffective, and preliminary data suggest that STH is responsible for transaminase repression.

Rinaudo et al. F95,471/67: Studies on the induction of various hepatic enzymes by STH and LTH in toad tadpoles.

Kenney G50,810/67: In intact, hypophysectomized or adrenalectomized rats, STH inhibits the synthesis of hepatic TKT. The rate of enzyme synthesis is reduced nearly to zero (immunochemical-isotopic analyses), whereas labeling of the bulk of the liver proteins is increased by STH. Repression is blocked when RNA synthesis is inhibited by actinomycin-D. STH also appears to play a role in the repression of TKT induction by stressors. A hypophysectomized and an intact rat were united by parabiosis. When the pituitary-bearing member was stressed by tyrosine i.p., repression occurred in the livers of both treated and untreated (hypophysectomized) animals. Transaminase levels were unchanged in one single experiment, where the stressing agent was administered to the hypophysectomized partner.

Räihä & Kekomäki G68,114/68: In the rat, the OKT activity of the liver is very low in the fetus; it exhibits a small transient elevation around term, then drops, and eventually reaches the high adult activity level during the third postnatal week. Triamcinolone given postnatally causes a pronounced elevation of OKT, but has no such effect in fetal or adult rats. Puromycin prevents the rise in OKT after triamcinolone administration. In adult rats fed a protein-or arginine-free diet, OKT activity decreases and fails to rise under the influence of triamcinolone. Partial hepatectomy or STH depresses OKT-activity in the livers of adult rats.

Schapiro H2,360/68: Stress (30 min rough agitation in a noisy laboratory shaker) had no effect upon the corticoid sensitive enzyme TKT in the liver of the intact rat, but it increased TPO activity, which is likewise corticoid inducible. Adrenalectomized rats, similarly stressed, exhibited a decreased transaminase activity with no change in TPO. This inhibitory effect was abolished by hypophysectomy. STH inhibited induction of transaminase by cortisol, but had no effect upon cortisol-induced TPO activity. The opposing actions of STH and glucocorticoids may be involved in adaptive reactions to stress.

Schapiro et al. H12,411/69: Brief abstract stating (without giving experimental details) that "the severe stress of laparotomy in the intact adult rat induces a large corticoid-dependent increase in transaminase activity. STH administered simultaneously, or one hour before laparotomy will completely inhibit this enzyme increase. During the early postnatal period, however, STH will not block transaminase induction caused by cortisol or laparotomy."

Wilson G69,098/69: In the rat, in vitro studies suggest that STH depresses hexobarbital, aminopyrine and ethylmorphine metabolism. ACTH and LTH have no such effect and do not influence the corresponding action of STH. [The hormones were administered s.c. 48 hrs before removal of the liver for the metabolic studies (H.S.).]

Wilson H21,345/70: In rats, the development of various drug-metabolizing hepatic microsomal enzymes can be suppressed by postnatal treatment with STH.

← OTHER ANTERIOR PITUITARY PREPARATIONS (LTH, GTH, TTH, CRUDE EXTRACTS)

Many of the experiments concerning the protective action of LTH, GTH, TTH and other anterior pituitary extracts, were performed with more or less purified preparations in which several hormones were present; hence, we shall discuss these experiments conjointly. Most of the relevant work is concerned with the effect of anterior pituitary extract upon resistance to drugs, infections, hypoxia, and various forms of nonspecific stress.

Drugs ←

Resistance of mice to **acetonitrile** is considerably increased by thyroid preparations, and hence, it is not surprising that the thyrotrophic hormone (TTH) has a similar effect. However, gonadotrophic urinary extracts and folliculoid preparations also increase acetonitrile resistance in the mouse; hence, this phenomenon is not truly characteristic for the thyroid hormones.

Pretreatment of rats with crude lyophilized anterior pituitary preparations makes them particularly sensitive to the anesthetic effect of **pentobarbital** and **progesterone**. However, this effect is also nonspecific, since various tissue extracts and proteins, such as egg white, casein, etc., prolong pentobarbital anesthesia.

The hepatotoxic effect of CCl_4 is partially prevented by crude anterior pituitary extracts in the rat.

Among the **carcinogens**, AAF is especially active in producing neoplastic lesions in the rat liver. This effect is intensified by pregnant mare serum, gonadotrophin, but also by estradiol and testosterone. The detoxication of N-OH-FAA is inhibited in rats bearing functional pituitary-tumor transplants, which also enhance hepatic carcinogenesis.

In rabbits, **cholesterol** atheromatosis is aggravated by TTH. According to some investigators, the severity of the lesions roughly parallels the blood cholesterol level, whereas others claim that TTH decreases the hypercholesterolemia. In cockerels, neither chorionic gonadotrophin nor TTH has any clear-cut effect upon cholesterol atherosclerosis.

In rats, the production of cardiac lesions by **emetine**, as well as of vascular changes by **ergotamine**, are inhibited by various gonadotrophic preparations.

The action of **lathyrogens** upon the bones of the rat is aggravated by luteotrophic hormone (LTH) as well as by STH.

On the other hand, the osteoclastic bone absorption produced by **vitamin-A** overdosage in rats, though prevented by STH, is not influenced by LTH.

Microorganisms and Their Products ←

Various anterior pituitary preparations are said to protect mice against bacterial infection, (e.g., with B. anthracis, E. coli and Ps. pyocyaneus), but not against several other organisms.

In rabbits, the progress of tuberculosis is accelerated by LH. In mice, the tuberculosis is not significantly affected by TTH, nor is infection with **Candida albicans** demonstrably altered by gonadotrophin.

Various gonadotrophic preparations have been claimed to counteract the lethal effects of **diphtheria toxin** in guinea pigs.

Hypoxia ←

In rats and guinea pigs, pretreatment with crude anterior pituitary extracts diminishes resistance to decreased oxygen pressure, presumably as a consequence of their TTH content, since thyroidectomy abolishes this effect. Resistance to hypoxia is also decreased in guinea pigs by purified TTH, an observation which is in agreement with the well-known fact that thyroid hormones act in this manner.

Hormones ←

Masson et al. B 48,694/49: In rats sensitized by uninephrectomy + NaCl, DOC produced more severe hypertension than a crude anterior pituitary powder (APP). Combined treatment with DOC + APP had no additive effect.

Oester C 84,324/59: The calcifying arteriosclerosis produced by repeated i.v. injections of epinephrine in the rabbit is aggravated by thyroxine and T3 s.c., but not by TTH or dinitrophenol. Thyroidectomy, unlike propylthiouracil, inhibits the epinephrine arteriopathy.

Blatt et al. H 19,832/69: In frog tadpoles, prolactin antagonizes thyroxine-induced tail regression in the course of metamorphosis, but pancreatic regression and acid phosphatase development in the liver are not inhibited. Thus, prolactin does not antagonize the entire process of metamorphosis some events of which may not be directly induced by thyroxine.

Drugs ←

Acetonitrile ←. *Eufinger et al. 22,082/29:* In mice, acetonitrile resistance is increased by pretreatment with human pregnancy serum. It remains to be seen whether this is due to an increased serum level of GTH, TTH or of other metabolites.

Eufinger & Wiesbader 4,663/30: In mice, pretreatment with gonadotrophic urinary extracts or folliculoid preparations increases acetonitrile resistance and hence this phenomenon is not characteristic for thyroid hormones.

Neuweiler 43,582/32: In mice, it was not possible to increase acetonitrile resistance by a variety of gonadotrophic hormone preparations, including the serum of pregnant women.

Sommer 44,648/34: In mice, acetonitrile resistance is increased by a variety of gonadotrophic preparations, including the serum of pregnant women.

Fellinger & Hochstädt 63,744/35: In mice, the protection against acetonitrile offered by thyroxine or TTH is blocked by an extract of blood which contains the "ether soluble antithyroid substances."

Wiesbader 68,823/36: In mice, acetonitrile resistance is increased not only by thyroid extract but also by TTH and various gonadotrophic preparations.

Actinomycin ←. *Tuchmann-Duplessis & Mercier-Parot H 28,876/70:* In rats, LTH does not prevent the abortifacient and teratogenic actions of actinomycin.

Anaphylactoid Edema ←. *Higginbotham & Dougherty C 44,529/57:* In mice, ACTH increased the toxicity of polymyxin B; STH and TTH had no effect upon it.

Barbiturates ←. *Selye & Masson A 97,571/44:* Pretreatment of rats with lyophilized anterior pituitary (LAP) makes them particularly sensitive to the anesthetic effect of progesterone or pentobarbital.

Masson B 275/45: Male rats are more resistant to pentobarbital anesthesia than females. However, upon treatment with LAP s.c., resistance decreased considerably in both sexes, and eventually reached the same low level in males and females. LAP produced a similar increase in sensitivity to amobarbital, hexobarbital, cyclobarbital and inbarbital, but did not influence barbital or phenobarbital anesthesia.

Masson A 95,888/46: In rats, not only anterior pituitary preparations, but extracts of various tissues, as well as egg white, casein, and other proteins prolonged pentobarbital anesthesia. Presumably, "the assimilation of foreign proteins interferes with some important mechanism necessary for the detoxification of barbiturates."

Masson B1,217/46: In male rats, pretreatment for 6 days with crude pituitary powder s.c. "slightly prolonged the duration of anesthesia with phanodorn, thioethamyl, neonal, delvinal, nostal and amytal, and greatly prolonged (2 to 5 times) with pentothal, seconal, allyl pental, nembutal, evipal, pernoston and sigmodal." There was no difference between the pretreated and control rats as regards the anesthetic effect of phenobarbital, probarbital, barbital, aprobarbital, diallyl barbituric acid and trichloroacetaldehyde. "The action of pituitary preparations is not specific but can also be obtained with preparations from various organs and with foreign proteins." Hepatic damage is considered to be a likely cause of the prolongation of anesthesia under these conditions.

Cadmium ←. *Pařizek et al. H7,672/68:* In adult rats in which persistent estrus had been induced by a single s.c. injection of testosterone or 19-nortestosterone on the fifth day of life, cadmium s.c. elicited particularly severe ovarian changes. Pretreatment with pregnant mare serum gonadotrophin protected the ovaries of such animals.

Carbon Tetrachloride ←. *Masson 96,335/47:* The hepatotoxic action of CCl₄ is aggravated by DOC and testosterone but partially prevented by anterior-pituitary extracts in the rat.

Arrigo & Trasino C21,687/55: In rats, crude alkaline anterior-pituitary extracts (rich in STH) do, whereas acid extracts (rich in ACTH and STH) do not protect the liver and pancreas against damage by CCl₄. Cortisone protects the liver but not the pancreas.

Julius 29,127/34: In mice, the production of skin cancers by topical application of tar was not prevented by a gonadotropic extract of pregnancy urine.

Carcinogens ←. *Cantarow et al. B18,774/46:* In rats given AAF p.o., the development of cystic and neoplastic hepatic lesions was accelerated and intensified by GTH (pregnant mare serum), estradiol, and testosterone, but inhibited by thiouracil. "This phenomenon may be related on the role of the liver in the intermediary metabolism and excretion of the sex steroid." In the hyperplastic target organs of the sex hormones tumors did not occur, in contrast to the high incidence of tumors in the thyroids of rats given thiouracil simultaneously with the carcinogens.

Stasney et al. B26,653/47: In rats, 2-acetaminofluorene feeding produces mammary carcinoma only in females, and its development is not significantly accelerated by estradiol or gonadotrophin. "Malignant lesions of the liver occurred in 54.8 per cent of females and 92.3 per cent of males receiving the carcinogen alone. Administration of estradiol and PMS gonadotrophin to females and of testosterone and chorionic gonadotrophin to males intensified the cystic and neoplastic hepatic lesions induced by 2-acetaminofluorene."

Weisburger et al. D18,583/64: In rats fed a diet containing N-hydroxy-N-2-fluorenylacetamide, implantation of Furth's mammotropic tumor MtT/F4, as a source of pituitary hormones, accelerated hepatic carcinogenesis.

Shirasu et al. F65,704/66: In rats, the detoxication of N-hydroxy-N-2-fluorenylacetamide (N-OH-FAA) is inhibited by the transplantation of functional pituitary tumors which may account for their enhancing effect upon hepatic carcinogenesis.

Cholesterol ←. *Bruger & Fitz A15,324/38:* In cholesterol-fed rabbits, atheromatosis of the aorta is aggravated by chronic treatment with TTH. The severity of the lesions roughly parallels the blood cholesterol level.

Turner & De Lamater A37,602/42: In cholesterol-fed rabbits, TTH markedly reduces hypercholesterolemia even after thyroidectomy. [Vascular changes are not described (H.S.).]

Stamler et al. B91,353/53: In cholesterol-fed chicks, coronary atherosclerosis is prevented by estradiol even if the feminizing effects are eliminated by concurrent administration of testosterone. The protective effect of the folliculoid is not due to its effect upon blood cholesterol, since hypercholesterolemia remains uninfluenced by it, but estradiol elevates the plasma phospholipid levels. In itself, neither testosterone nor chorionic gonadotrophin affects coronary atherosclerosis under these conditions.

Stamler et al. C81,655/58: TTH—unlike thyroid preparations—failed to influence cholesterol atherosclerosis in cockerels.

Emetine ←. *de Gregorio & Armellini G64,277/64:* In rabbits, the production of cardiac lesions by emetine is inhibited by chorionic gonadotrophin and testosterone but not by estradiol.

Scaffidi & Arrigo G62,941/68: In rabbits, the cardiac lesions produced by emetine are inhibited by various gonadotrophic hormone preparations.

Ergotamine ←. *Bolis E 50,716/56:* In rats, various gonadotrophic preparations diminish the organ lesions produced by toxic doses of ergotamine.

Messina G 18,016/64: In rats, ergotamine produces vascular lesions conducive to tail necrosis more readily in females than in males. Hypophysectomy prevents these toxic manifestations in both sexes, whereas treatment with chorionic gonadotrophin does not affect them.

Ethionine ←. *Farber & Segaloff D 95,996/55:* In ovariectomized rats, various testoids and STH protected the liver against fatty infiltration produced by ethionine i.p., whereas cortisone and ACTH aggravated it. Estradiol, DOC, and TTH had no effect.

Glycine ←. *Hay 93,491/47:* In rats, the hepatotoxic and nephrotoxic actions of glycine-enriched diets are not significantly modified by crude anterior pituitary extracts.

Lathyrogens ←. *Selye C 31,369/57:* In the rat, the osteolathyrism produced by AAN is aggravated by STH, LTH, and partial hepatectomy, but it is inhibited by ACTH, cortisol, or estradiol.

Morphine ←. *Benetato et al. 33,773/35:* In rats, neither adrenocortical extract nor an adrenotrophic anterior pituitary preparation altered resistance to morphine or to thyphoid-parathyphoid vaccine.

p-Nitrobenzoic Acid ←. *Wilson G 63,125/68:* In young rats, transplants of a pituitary mammotropic tumor "did not prevent an increase in the liver microsomal metabolism of hexobarbital or the formation of formaldehyde from aminopyrine which followed phenobarbital pretreatment. High levels of somatotropin, corticotropin, and prolactin in blood, or possibly some other unknown factors produced by this tumor, appeared to prevent the normal development of the liver enzyme system which metabolized hexobarbital, aminopyrine, and p-nitrobenzoic acid in the rat."

Reserpine ←. *Wirtheimer D 10,158/59:* In rats, the production of gastric ulcers by reserpine is enhanced following pretreatment with various impure gonadotrophic hormone preparations.

Vitamin A ←. *Schneider & Widmann 33,725/35:* In guinea pigs, both thyroidectomy and treatment with TTH considerably alter vitamin-A metabolism.

Mayer & Goddard B 55,008/51: In rats deficient in vitamin A, the atrophy of the accessory sex organs is abolished by chorionic gonadotrophin, suggesting that the defect is not due to an inability of the gonads to secrete testoids but to inadequate pituitary gonadotrophin secretion.

Selye C 36,050/57: In rats, the intense osteoclastic bone absorption produced by vitamin-A overdosage can be prevented by STH. Although the luteotrophic hormone (LTH) shares many of the actions of STH, it cannot substitute for the latter in counteracting vitamin-A intoxication.

Vitamin C ←. *Agnoli 2,633/32:* In guinea pigs, neither crude pituitary extracts nor urinary gonadotrophins ameliorate the course of scurvy on vitamin-C deficient diets.

Varia ←. *Störtebecker 76,398/39:* Review of the early literature (1913—1937) on the effect of the pituitary upon drug resistance.

Microorganisms and Their Products ←

Bacteria ←. *Weinstein B 15,029/39:* In mice, various anterior pituitary preparations protect against infection with B. anthracis. Parathyroid extract was also very effective, whereas thyroxine and testosterone offered little protection while progesterone, insulin, "estrin" and posterior lobe extract were virtually ineffective.

Weinstein A 33,940/40: In mice, neither parathyroid extract nor a crude anterior pituitary preparation offered protection against infection with Klebsiella pneumoniae, but they did improve survival after inoculation of E. coli or Ps. pyocyaneus.

Lurie et al. B 31,933/49: In rabbits, estradiol retards the progress of experimental tuberculosis at the portal of entry in the skin and diminishes its dissemination to internal organs, presumably by reducing the permeability of connective tissue. Chorionic gonadotrophin has an inverse effect.

Lurie et al. B 31,931/49; B 31,932/49: In highly inbred, sexually mature rabbits, estradiol retarded the progress of tuberculosis following i.c. inoculation. In immature rabbits, estradiol was less effective. LH accelerated the progress of the disease, whereas ovariectomy or progesterone remained without effect.

Schäfer B 99,955/54: Monograph (127 pp., numerous refs.) on the role of endocrine factors in tuberculosis. Special sections are devoted to the hormones of the thyroid, parathyroid, thymus, adrenals, pancreas, and gonads.

Youmans & Youmans B95,169/54: In mice, cortisone markedly reduced the survival time after infection with human tubercle bacilli, and this effect could not be prevented by STH. Given alone, ACTH, STH, and TTH likewise failed to influence the course of the infection.

Meier & Neipp C37,215/56: In mice, the chemotherapeutic action of sulfonamides against resistant Type III pneumococci is increased by various gonadotrophic and STH preparations. However, certain bacterial polysaccharide fractions possess a similar effect, and hence, the latter is presumably not dependent upon the specific actions of the hormone preparations.

Scherr C39,263/57: In mice infected with Candida albicans, the development of moniliasis may be either increased or decreased by cortisone, depending upon various factors, particularly the severity of the infection, sex or pregnancy. Testosterone enhanced, and STH counteracted the deleterious effect of cortisone. Gonadotrophin (pregnant mare serum) was without effect.

Bacterial Toxins ←. *Ciulla & Razzini B50,987/39:* In guinea pigs, pretreatment with pregnancy urine gonadotrophins diminishes the lethal effect of diphtheria toxin.

Tonutti B48,892/50: In guinea pigs, diphtheria toxin produces marked hemorrhagic necrosis of the testes and ovaries only after pretreatment with gonadotrophic hormones.

Scaffidi & Fidecaro G51,129/65; G43,543/66: In guinea pigs, the cardiopathy produced by diphtheria toxin can be prevented by chorionic gonadotrophin and cocarboxylase.

Hypoxia ←

Houssay & Rietti 3,187/32; 3,283/32: In rats pretreatment with an impure pituitary extract diminishes resistance against hypoxia, but this effect is abolished by thyroidectomy, and is presumably due to TTH. In untreated rats, thyroidectomy actually increases resistance to anoxia.

Houssay & Rietti 5,793/32: In guinea pigs, resistance to decreased oxygen pressure is diminished by anterior pituitary extract, presumably through its TTH content since the effect is abolished after thyroidectomy.

Rotter A63,564/42: In guinea pigs, altitude tolerance is greatly reduced by pretreatment with TTH.

Varia ←

Henriques et al. B24,140/48: In rats sensitized by uninephrectomy, the production of hyalinosis and hypertension by crude anterior pituitary extracts is facilitated if the **diet** is rich either in protein or in aminoacids.

Smith C46,496/56: In brown trout, thyroxine raises, whereas thiourea and thiouracil reduce **salinity tolerance.** Anterior pituitary extracts and STH likewise raise salinity tolerance, whereas posterior lobe extracts, testosterone, gonadotrophin, TTH, and ACTH have no effect.

Osipovich C58,570/57: In **uninephrectomized** rats, methylthiouracil enhances compensatory hypertrophy of the remaining kidney, presumably as a consequence of increased TTH secretion. The acceleration of compensatory renal hypertrophy by exposure to cold is ascribed to a similar mechanism.

Glenn et al. G70,204/60: Review (48 pp., 11 refs.) on the effect of various steroids, ACTH, GTH, ovariectomy and adrenalectomy upon the development of C3H mammary **carcinoma transplants** in mice and fibroadenomas in rats.

Knigge C97,819/60: Review on the neuroendocrine mechanisms influencing ACTH and TTH secretion particularly during adaptation to **cold.**

Bucher G68,621/63: Review on the influence of hypophysectomy and hypophysial hormones upon **hepatic regeneration.**

Fisher & Fisher F74,176/66: In rats, the incidence of metastases from Walker **tumor transplants** is not significantly altered by thyroidectomy, propylthiouracil, thyroxine or TTH.

Preisig et al. F70,515/66: In acromegalic patients, **biliary BSP excretion** is increased. [It is not known which, if any, of the hormones secreted by the hyperactive pituitary are responsible for this effect (H.S.).]

Rinaudo et al. F95,471/67: Studies on the induction of various **hepatic enzymes** by STH and LTH in toad tadpoles.

Sakamato & Prasad F95,441/67: In mice and rats, β-MSH offers moderate protection against **X-irradiation** under certain conditions.

← *POSTERIOR PITUITARY PREPARATIONS*

In dogs and guinea pigs, vasopressor pituitary extracts offer partial protection against **histamine** intoxication. In rats, the production of renal cortical necrosis by vasopressin is greatly facilitated by **5-HT** and **folliculoids**.

It has been claimed that vasopressor posterior pituitary extracts influence the toxicity of various **drugs** through different mechanisms. They may improve resistance to hypotensive drugs because of their vasopressor effect, or aggravate the toxicity of substances normally eliminated through the kidney, because of their antidiuretic action. However, none of these effects was shown to be sufficiently striking to have deserved extensive investigation, except for the well-known aggravation of water intoxication by vasopressin.

Under certain circumstances, vasopressin has also been claimed to offer protection against various **infections, X-irradiation, hemorrhage, anoxia, electroshock** and **traumatic shock**. On the other hand, vasopressin aggravates or fails to influence the damaging effect of various **bacterial toxins, hyperoxygenation,** and exposure to **cold**.

Steroids ← *cf. Selye C50,810/58, pp. 83, 84; C92,918/61, p. 124; G60,083/70, p. 334.*

Hormones and Hormone-Like Substances ←

Best & Solandt A33,635/40: In dogs, shock produced by histamine, trauma, or hemorrhage is successfully treated by vasopressor pituitary extracts.

Kowalewski & Bain C3,897/54: In guinea pigs, a vasopressor posterior pituitary extract given s.c., 10 min before the injection of histamine, prevented the induction of gastric ulcers, presumably because of an antagonistic interaction at the level of the vascular system.

Drugs ←

Acetonitrile ←. *Paal 22,603/30:* In mice, acetonitrile resistance is not consistently influenced by posterior pituitary extract (hypophysin), a folliculoid preparation (progynon), or epinephrine.

Barbiturates ←. *Werle & Lentzen A28,007/38:* In dogs and rabbits, various vasoactive substances (epinephrine, histamine, vasopressin, kallikrein) tend to prolong the anesthetic effect of pronarcon and hexobarbital.

Rümke G69,768/63: In mice, small doses of vasopressin i.v. failed to prolong hexobarbital sleeping time.

Hexobarbital ← Vasopressin, Gp, Mouse: Lamson et al. C14,547/51*; Rümke G69,768/63*

Pentobarbital ← Vasopressin + H_2O, Mouse: Borzelleca et al. C40,953/57*

Bromoethylamine Hydrobromide ←. *Fuwa & Waugh F96,546/68:* In rats, the renal papillary necrosis produced by bromoethylamine hydrobromide is inhibited by vasopressin, presumably as a consequence of its antidiuretic effect.

Carcinolytic Agents ←. *Connors et al. G17,080/64:* In rats, Mannitol Myleran is normally excreted unchanged in the urine within 5 hrs after i.p. administration. Pretreatment with antidiuretic hormone potentiates both its lethal and antitumor action, presumably because it diminishes excretions.

Chlorpromazine ←. *Khrabrova D49,985/61:* In cats, electroshock is effectively antagonized by chlorpromazine if the hypotensive action of the latter is prevented by vasopressin.

Chloral Hydrate ←. *Fastier et al. C37,038/57:* In mice, chloral hydrate sleeping time is increased by epinephrine, norepinephrine, phenylephrine, methoxamine, 5-HT, histamine, ergotamine, yohimbine and atropine. "It is suggested that some, at least, of the drugs which prolong the effects of hypnotics do so by virtue of a hypothermic action." Vasopressin, cortisone, and DOC did not prolong chloral hydrate sleeping time at the doses tested.

Cholesterol ← *cf. also Selye G60,083/70, p. 335. Cooper & Gutstein F61,290/66:* In rabbits, calcific aortic atherosclerosis is produced by combined treatment with cholesterol and vasopressin.

Digitalis ←. *Ghedini & Ollino A 21,128/14:* Brief mention of observations on rabbits showing that pretreatment with Pituitrin modifies the hemodynamic actions of digitalis "unfavorably" and those of strophantin "favorably." [For lack of details, these findings cannot be evaluated (H.S.).]

Nash et al. G 9,641/64: In rats, the toxic cardiac effects of ouabain are antagonized by synthetic oxytocin and by reserpine.

Ethanol ←. *Baïsset & Montastruc D 34,473/62; D 37,918/62:* In dogs, the development of a polyuria and polydipsia, following administration of ethanol, as well as the gradual development of a craving for alcohol are prevented by vasopressor posterior lobe extract.

Morphine ←. *Gruber et al. 2,199/31:* In dogs, a vasopressor pituitary extract temporarily lowers the increased general tonus of the intestine produced by morphine.

Adler et al. G 79,852/57: In Sprague-Dawley rats, given ^{14}C-labeled morphine, the ratio of bound to free morphine is 2—3 times greater in the urine and plasma than in Long-Evans rats. The tissues of adrenalectomized rats of both strains contain higher concentrations of ^{14}C-labeled morphine than do control rats. Plasma bound morphine levels indicate no impairment of morphine conjugation. Vasopressin increases, whereas ACTH decreases morphine sensitivity. Yet both after ACTH and after vasopressin, tissue concentrations of morphine are either reduced or unaffected in marked contrast to the increased values after adrenalectomy. Apparently, the decreased morphine sensitivity induced by ACTH is not reflected by lower brain morphine concentrations.

Paraphenylendiamine←. *Meissner E 52,567/19:* The head and neck edema produced by paraphenylendiamine in the rabbit is not prevented by epinephrine, posterior pituitary extract of thyroid extract.

Pentylenetetrazol ←. *Boeri C 78,610/58:* In guinea pigs, cortisone, ACTH, and vasopressin aggravate pentylenetetrazol convulsions.

Phosgene ←. *Rothlin B 30,696/47:* In rats, phosgene ($COCl_2$) intoxication is effectively combated by posterior pituitary extract as well as by ergotamine, presumably as a consequence of their vasoconstrictor effect.

Potassium ← *cf. Selye C 92,918/61, pp. 83, 124, 188.*

Sodium Chloride ←. *Baïsset et al. C 55,475/57:* In the rat and dog, posterior pituitary extracts favorably influence the manifestations of chronic NaCl-overdosage and prolong survival.

Baïsset et al. C 84,788/58: In rats and dogs, the effects of NaCl-overdosage are ameliorated by posterior pituitary extracts and aggravated by NaCl.

Suxamethonium ←. *Keil D 27,254/62:* In rabbits, sheep and pigs, oxytocin did not modify resistance to suxamethonium.

Strychnine←. *Marañón & Aznar 46,926/11:* In frogs, the fatal convulsions produced by strychnine can be prevented if, prior to injection, the drug is mixed with extracts of the posterior pituitary, the thyroid, various other tissues, and particularly epinephrine. [The possibility of delayed absorption owing to local vasoconstriction has not been considered (H.S.).]

Vitamin D ← *cf. Selye C 92,918/61, pp. 124, 188; G 60,083/70, pp. 335, 336.*

Vitamin E ←. *Houchin & Smith B 6,967/44:* Rabbits deprived of vitamin E, show increased sensitivity to posterior pituitary extracts.

Water ←. *Liling & Gaunt 89,147/45:* In rats, vasopressin aggravates the manifestations of water intoxication, even if the animals are adapted by previous administration of water loads.

Waltregny & Mesdjian F 85,818/67: In cats, combined treatment with "posterior lobe extract" s.c. and large amounts of distilled water i.p. produces a condition of epilepsy with a characteristic EEG as a consequence of water intoxication.

Bacteria ← *cf. also Selye G 60,083/70, p. 335.*

Lauber 9,102/32: Observations on the effect of vasopressin, epinephrine, thyroid extract and insulin upon streptococcal and staphylococcal infections in mice.

Weinstein B 15,029/39: In mice, various anterior pituitary preparations protect against infection with B. anthracis. Parathyroid extract was also very effective, whereas thyroxine and testosterone offered little protection, while progesterone, insulin, "estrin" and posterior lobe extract were virtually ineffective.

Bacterial Toxins ← *cf. also Selye G 60,083/70, p. 335.*

Bailey A 1,154/17: In rabbits, vasopressin aggravates the vascular lesions produced by diphtheria toxin.

Altura et al. F 43,209/65: In rats, norepinephrine and angiotensin fail to prolong survival after traumatic shock, temporary ligature of the superior mesenteric artery, or endotoxin shock. However, vasopressin (PLV-2) was significantly effective in traumatic and intestinal ischemia shock, but not in endotoxinemia.

Ionizing Rays ←

Gray et al. B68,316/52: In rats, pretreatment with either epinephrine or vasopressin diminishes mortality after total body X-irradiation.

Gray et al. B69,100/52: In rats, pretreatment with vasopressin or epinephrine increases survival following exposure to lethal X-irradiation.

Hervé D78,167/54: In mice, an oxytocic posterior lobe preparation increases resistance against total body X-irradiation.

Rigat C10,747/55: Review (46 pp., 67 refs.) on the literature concerning the effect of hormones upon X-irradiation, with special reference to ACTH, STH, vasopressin, epinephrine, cortisone, DOC, testosterone, estradiol, progesterone, and thyroxine.

Bacq & Beaumariage C87,128/60: In mice, synthetic oxytocin (Syntocinon) increases resistance to total body X-irradiation.

Hemorrhage ←

Best & Solandt A33,635/40: In dogs, shock produced by histamine, trauma, or hemorrhage is successfully treated by vasopressor pituitary extracts.

Cort et al. F23,086/64: In dogs, various synthetic extended-chain analogues of vasopressin and oxytocin exert a beneficial effect upon hemorrhagic shock.

Cort et al. F96,105/68: In dogs, certain vasopressin analogues offer protection against hemorrhagic shock.

Hypoxia and Hyperoxygenation ←

Campbell A14,903/37: In rats exposed to six atmospheres of oxygen in a pressure chamber, subsequent decompression is better tolerated at low than at high external temperatures. "Using an external temperature of 24°C and white rats of about 80 g, the following substances, administered subcutaneously, are found to enhance oxygen poisoning: thyroxin (0.4 mg), dinitrophenol (1.5 mg), ac-tetrahydro-β-naphthylamine (0.5 c.c., 1 p.c.), adrenaline (0.02 mg), pituitary extract (posterior lobe, above 3.5 units), insulin (0.025 u.) and eserine (0.045 mg administered with atropine 0.075 mg). These doses in themselves are harmless."

Parkes B63,024/51: In mice, resistance to anoxia is increased by posterior lobe extract as well as by ACTH preparations containing posterior lobe principles.

Electric Stimuli ←

Rosenblum C5,974/55: In rats, "ACTH and cortisone acetate in combination with vasopressin each produced a greater fall in EST than was produced by vasopressin alone. In contrast, STH in combination with vasopressin prevented the fall induced by vasopressin alone and produced its usual elevation in the EST."

Khrabrova D49,985/61: In cats, electroshock is effectively antagonized by chlorpromazine if the hypotensive action of the latter is prevented by vasopressin.

Varia ←

Best & Solandt A33,635/40: In dogs, shock produced by histamine, **trauma** or hemorrhage is successfully treated by vasopressor pituitary extracts.

Marino et al. D58,761/63: In guinea pigs, the cardiopathy produced by vasopressin intoxication is aggravated by concurrent exposure to a **psychologic stress** situation (preconditioning followed by conflict situation).

Zilberstein C80,282/60: In rats, 5-HT, vasopressin and reserpine lower resistance to **cold** allegedly because they interfere with pituitary hormone secretion and cause a state of "temporary functional adrenalectomy."

← HYPOPHYSECTOMY AND HYPOTHALAMIC LESIONS

The effects of adrenalectomy, orchidectomy and ovariectomy are discussed with the steroids, since ablation of these glands acts upon resistance mainly by creating a lack of steroid hormones. On the other hand, hypophysectomy will be discussed here (immediately following the pituitary hormones) together with hypothalamic lesions, since both of these operations act upon resistance primarily through their effect upon pituitary hormone secretion. Yet, it must be remembered that, secondarily, several hypophyseal principles (e.g., ACTH and the gonadotrophins) do influence susceptibility to damaging agents through their regulating effect upon steroid secretion.

Steroids ←

It has long been noted that the hyalinosis, polyuria and hypertension produced by mineralocorticoids in rats (conditioned by uninephrectomy + NaCl) are prevented, or at least greatly diminished by hypophysectomy. STH, ACTH and TTH all play important roles in the pathogenesis of this syndrome (as do various steroids and thyroid hormones secreted under pituitary control); hence, it is not clear to what extent the prophylactic effect of hypophysectomy is due to the lack of one or the other hypophyseal hormone.

Phenobarbital increases the estradiol-metabolizing activity of hepatic microsomal enzymes in immature female rats. It also diminishes the uterotrophic effect of this folliculoid. Neither hypophysectomy nor adrenalectomy prevents this phenobarbital-induced estradiol resistance, indicating that the barbiturate does not act through the pituitary-adrenal axis.

In C3H mice, the females, unlike the males, regularly develop myocardial calcification following prolonged cortisol treatment; ovariectomy offers no protection but testosterone renders females more resistant. In hypophysectomized mice of this strain, neither cortisol nor ACTH produces myocardial calcification.

Nonsteroidal Hormones and Hormone-Like Substances ←

In rats, the osteosclerosis produced by small doses of **parathyroid** extract is diminished but not prevented by hypophysectomy. From this it was first concluded that STH is not necessary for all types of tissue growth.

The osteitis fibrosa and soft-tissue calcification produced by acute overdosage with parathyroid extract (like that caused by DHT) in the rat is also inhibited by hypophysectomy, although the characteristic hypercalcemia is not markedly affected. Presumably, the pituitary acts mainly by altering the calcium avidity of the organic matrix.

Hypophysectomy partially protects the rat against the production of renal necroses by **5-HT**. In hypophysectomized rats, the elevation of the EST, induced by 5-HT is preceded by hyperexcitability.

Steroids ←

Ventura & Selye C24,231/57: In rats, the hyalinosis (nephrosclerosis, myocarditis, polyuria, edema, etc.) produced by chlorocortisol following conditioning by uninephrectomy + NaCl was prevented by hypophysectomy. However, at the same time, the production of pulmonary saprophytosis by chlorocortisol was enhanced. Apparently, in the absence of the hypophysis, the mineralocorticoid activities are inhibited, whereas the glucocorticoid actions of the same steroid molecule are augmented.

Forchielli et al. D75,874/58: The rate of Δ^4 reduction of 11-desoxycortisol was 3—4-fold greater in female than in male rat liver homogenates and in microsomal fractions containing the Δ^4-5α-hydrogenase. Female rat liver contains only one Δ^4-hydrogenase (5α-microsomal), whereas the male liver contains the soluble Δ^4-5β-hydrogenase as well. Ovariectomy caused no marked change in enzyme titer, but hypophysectomy decreased it sharply. Curiously, ACTH, STH, and pregnant mare serum partially restored the enzyme level in the hypophysectomized rat. In young animals, increase in the titer of hepatic Δ^4-5α-hydrogenase occurs prior to puberty. This fact (like the negative results after ovariectomy) suggests an independence of enzyme regulation from ovarian hormones.

Lostroh C54,348/58: Female mice of the C3H strain regularly develop myocardial calcification after prolonged cortisol treatment, whereas males are comparatively resistant. Ovariectomy offers no protection, but testosterone renders females more resistant. In hypophysectomized mice, neither cortisol nor ACTH produces myocardial calcification.

Selye C39,319/58: In rats, nephrocalcinosis produced by excess NaH_2PO_4 p.o. is aggravated by estradiol, but even the severe calcification induced by this combined treatment is prevented by hypophysectomy.

Levin et al. F75,365/67: Phenobarbital increases the 17β-estradiol-metabolizing activity of hepatic microsomal enzymes in immature female rats. The in vitro activity is paralleled by in vivo blockade of the estradiol-induced uterine weight increase. The phenobarbital-induced resistance to the uterine weight-increasing effect of estradiol is not prevented by adrenalectomy or hypophysectomy, indicating that the barbiturate does not act through the pituitary-adrenal axis.

Salgado & Mulroy C84,321/59: In rats, the cardiovascular changes produced by DOC following sensitization by uninephrectomy and NaCl are inhibited by hypophysectomy or thyroidectomy, although not all the lesions are blocked to an equal extent.

Garg et al. G79,002/71: In rats, PCN p.o. induces proliferation of SER even after hypophysectomy.

Szabó et al. G79,024/71: In rats, PCN increases resistance to indomethacin, hexobarbital, progesterone, zoxazolamine and digitoxin, both in the presence and in the absence of the pituitary. Hypophysectomy also fails to prevent the induction of SER proliferation in the hepatocytes.

Adrenal Cortical Extract ← Hypophysectomy: Zauder B57,611/51*

DOC, Progesterone ← Hypophysectomy: Chamorro A57,215/42*

Estradiol ← Hypophysectomy + Phenobarbital: Levin et al. F75,365/67*

Nonsteroidal Hormones and Hormone-Like Substances ←

Parathyroid Hormone ←. *Selye et al. 30,634/34; Thomson et al. A239/34:* In rats, osteoblast proliferation and new bone formation following treatment with small doses of parathyroid extract and renal regeneration after uninephrectomy are diminished, yet not completely prevented by hypophysectomy. Apparently, STH is not necessary for all types of growth.

Selye et al. D25,666/62: In the rat, hypophysectomy greatly diminishes both soft tissue calcification and osteitis fibrosa produced by parathyroid extract or DHT. The hypercalcemia is not diminished by the absence of the hypophysis, and the latter may act by altering the metabolism of calcifiable organic matrix.

ACTH, Epinephrine ← Hypophysectomy: Zauder B57,611/51*

5-HT ←. *Jasmin & Bois C92,099/60:* Hypophysectomy partially protects the rat against the production of renal infarcts by 5-HT. ACTH does not affect this change, cortisol aggravates it, whereas DOC and testosterone offer partial protection.

de Salva D27,783/62: The "EST elevating effect of serotonin and ephedrine in intact rats was preceded by hyperexcitability in hypophysectomized rats."

Drugs ←

Much work has been done on the effect of the hypothalamus-pituitary system on **barbiturate** resistance.

In rats, thiopental sleeping time is greatly prolonged within two weeks after hypophysectomy. This increased sensitivity is restored towards normal by ACTH, DOC or testosterone. The depressant effect of phenobarbital and of several other muscle relaxants appears to be diminished after hypophysectomy.

The sedative action of hexobarbital and thiopental is diminished by tourniquet stress in intact but not in hypophysectomized or adrenalectomized rats. Various observations suggest that "the stress effect on the duration of drug action is mediated through increased drug-metabolism." The stimulation of hepatic microsomal hexobarbital and pentobarbital metabolism by the antihistamine, chlorcyclizine, is not prevented in rats by hypophysectomy or by adrenalectomy plus castration; that is, removal of both steroid hormone-producing glands.

X-irradiation of the head considerably enhances the anesthetic effect of thiopental, barbital and pentobarbital in the rat. The induction by phenobarbital of resistance to pentobarbital is not inhibited by cephalic X-irradiation. Irradiation of the head is just as effective as total body irradiation or hypophysectomy in inhibiting the rapid induction of hexobarbital-metabolizing microsomal oxidases by hexobarbital. Even X-irradiation in utero produces the same result. X-irradiation of pregnant rats results in male offspring deficient in hepatic microsomal hexobarbital-metabolizing enzymes, but still capable of responding to phenobarbital with increased enzyme activity. Apparently, "the ontogenic increase in enzyme activity is hormone-dependent, while that following phenobarbital administration is independent of hormonal regulation as evidenced by the response of hypophysectomized or sexually immature animals." Bilateral electrolytic lesions in the posterior hypothalamus inhibit hepatic hexobarbital oxidase activity in the same manner as does X-irradiation of the head or hypophysectomy.

The hepatic steatosis produced by CCl_4 in rats is less completely prevented by hypophysectomy than by adrenalectomy.

The induction of hepatic damage, and even of hepatomas, by certain **carcinogens** is inhibited by hypophysectomy in the rat. As judged by the few published observations, certain carcinogens do, whereas others do not, induce hepatic microsomal drug-metabolizing enzymes after hypophysectomy or hypothalamic lesions in the rat.

In rats, hypophysectomy greatly diminishes the skeletal changes produced by **lathyrogens**, such as AAN. STH restores the ability of the skeleton to react even after hypophysectomy. It is concluded that the normal hormonal secretion of the hypophysis exerts a decisive influence on the development of osteolathyrism.

In weanling male rats, total body X-irradiation inhibits the development of hepatic microsomal enzymes which catalyze the oxidative desulfuration of the **pesticide** Guthion. Shielding of the liver or testes does not prevent this inhibition, whereas shielding of the head area does. Irradiation did not inhibit enzyme development in hypophysectomized rats. "Thus, the pituitary is necessary for the radiation effect, but involvement of the pituitary is not the result of a radiation-induced deficiency of pituitary hormones."

The nephrocalcinosis produced in rats by oral administration of large amounts of **phosphates** (e.g., Na_2HPO_4 or NaH_2PO_4) or by $HgCl_2$ is inhibited by hypophysectomy.

The nephrosis elicited by **puromycin aminonucleoside** in the rat is not completely prevented by hypophysectomy, but the associated hypercholesterolemia and hyperlipemia are diminished.

Hypophysectomy decreases survival in rats given excessive amounts of **vitamin A** but does not significantly affect the characteristic skeletal lesions.

Hypophysectomy greatly diminishes the soft-tissue calcification and osteitis fibrosa produced by **DHT** in rats, but does not significantly affect the associated hypercalcemia. Possibly, the effect of the pituitary is mediated through metabolic changes in the calcifiable matrix. The predominantly cortical nephrocalcinosis produced by vitamin-D_2 overdosage in the rat is not altered by hypophysectomy. The calciphylaxis elicited by combined treatment with DHT and $CrCl_3$ is prevented by hypophysectomy in the rat.

Chlorcyclizine shortens the duration of action and increases the hepatic microsomal metabolism of zoxazolamine in male rats. These effects are not prevented by hypophysectomy or adrenalectomy + castration. However, the depressant action of zoxazolamine is diminished after hypophysectomy.

Acrylonitrile

Szabó & Selye G79,010/71: In rats, pretreatment with ACTH (but not with STH) prevents the production of adrenal apoplexy by acrylonitrile. Hypophysectomy protects against adrenal apoplexy, but not against mortality under similar conditions.

Aminopyrine ← Hypophysectomy + Pesticides: Hart et al. G27,102/65

Atropine ←

de Salva D27,783/62: "Atropine and diphenhydramine had no effect in intact rats but produced lowered EST in hypophysectomized rats."

Barbiturates ←

Waltz et al. C11,847/55: In rats, thiopental sleeping time is greatly prolonged within about two weeks after hypophysectomy. This increased sensitivity is restored towards normal by ACTH, DOC, or testosterone.

de Salva D27,783/62: "Drugs with skeletal muscle relaxant properties (phenobarbital, meprobamate, phenaglycodol, mephenesin, and zoxazolamine) were less effective as depressants after hypophysectomy than they were in intact rats."

Rupe et al. E26,910/63: The sedative effect of hexobarbital and thiopental, but not of barbital, was diminished by tourniquet stress, in the intact, but not in the hypophysectomized or adrenalectomized rat. In intact rats, ACTH or cortisone decreases hexobarbital sleeping time, as does stress, whereas SKF 525-A completely blocks the protective action of stress. Presumably "the stress effect on the duration of drug action is mediated through increased drug metabolism."

Conney et al. D52,543/61: Pretreatment of male rats with chlorcyclizine shortens the duration of action and increases the hepatic microsomal metabolism of hexobarbital, pentobarbital and zoxazolamine. These effects were not prevented by hypophysectomy or adrenalectomy combined with castration.

Bousquet et al. F35,073/65: In rats, stressed by application of a tourniquet to one hind leg, the duration of response to hexobarbital, pentobarbital, meprobamate and zoxazolamine is significantly reduced, but only in the presence of both the pituitary and the adrenal glands. Pretreatment with ACTH or corticosterone simulates the effects of stress in shortening hexobarbital anesthesia. "It is suggested that the pituitary-adrenal axis serves a regulatory function with respect to duration of drug responses which may be mediated by an alteration of drug metabolism."

Nair et al. F53,576/65: In the rat, X-irradiation of the head considerably enhanced the anesthetic effect of thiopental, barbital, and pentobarbital. The induction by phenobarbital of resistance to subsequent pentobarbital anesthesia was not inhibited by cephalic X-irradiation.

Nair & Bau G67,246/67: Exposure of rats to X-irradiation in utero or during early postnatal life suppresses the hexobarbital-metabolizing enzyme system in the liver. Hypophysectomy or irradiation of the head (but not of the body with the head shielded) has a similar effect in adult rats.

Yam & DuBois G58,163/67: In 23-day-old male rats, X-irradiation of the whole animal or the head only inhibited the rapid increase in hexobarbital-metabolizing hepatic microsomal oxidase normally obtained by hexobarbital treatment. Hypophysectomy produced the same result.

Nair et al. G67,245/68: X-irradiation of pregnant rats results in male offspring deficient in the hepatic microsomal enzymes which metabolize hexobarbital. However, irradiation did not suppress the increase of enzyme activity brought about by chemical inducers (phenobarbital). Actinomycin inhibited both the ontogenic and phenobarbital-induced increases in enzyme activity. "The ontogenic increase in enzyme activity is hormone-dependent, while that following phenobarbital administration is independent of hormonal regulation as evidenced by the response in hypophysectomized or sexually immature animals. It is concluded from these results that the inhibitory effect of x-irradiation on the hepatic enzyme system is mediated through an action on the hormonal regulation of enzyme activity."

Nair et al. G67,250/69: Hepatic hexobarbital oxidase activity is inhibited by head X-irradiation, hypophysectomy, or bilateral electrolytic lesions in the posterior hypothalamus. The in vitro data were verified by measurements of the hexobarbital sleeping time. "It is suggested that the microsomal enzyme system metabolizing hexobarbital is normally under the regulatory control of hypothalamo-hypophyseal hormonal activity. The light dependent circadian rhythm for this enzyme, recently reported by us, is also consistent with this interpretation."

Norton G80,572/71: Hypophysectomized rats can become dependent upon barbital and show the same withdrawal symptoms as intact animals. In barbital-dependent rats, the liver, thyroid, adrenals and secondary sex organs are enlarged but the gonads regress. The hepatic enlargement is also evident after hypophysectomy.

Szabó et al. G79,024/71: In rats, PCN increases resistance to indomethacin, hexobarbital, progesterone, zoxazolamine and digitoxin, both in the presence and in the absence of the pituitary. Hypophysectomy also fails to prevent the induction of SER proliferation in the hepatocytes.

Hexobarbital ← Hypophysectomy: Conney et al. D52,543/61; Bousquet et al. F35,073/65*; Yam et al. G58,163/67; Nair et al. H21,083/70*

Benactyzine ←

de Salva D27,783/62: In hypophysectomized rats, the EST elevating effects of reserpine, mescaline, benactyzine and phenyltoloxamine were replaced by an EST lowering action.

Bilirubin ← Hypophysectomy + Barbital, Mouse: Catz et al. H14,471/68

Cadmium ←

Pařízek D23,927/60: In rats, cadmium intoxication elicits the usual testicular lesions even if administered 3 months after hypophysectomy.

Carbon Tetrachloride ←

Furukawa F71,711/65: In rats, hepatic steatosis produced by CCl_4 is inhibited by adrenalectomy and, to some extent, also by hypophysectomy. The effect of CCl_4 after adrenalectomy is restored by corticoids but not by epinephrine which increases only the action of the former. STH does not counteract the effect of hypophysectomy. Alloxan diabetes inhibits CCl_4-induced hepatic lipidosis.

Carcinogens ←

Lacassagne & Nyka 59,016/36: Rabbits, whose pituitary was destroyed by radium, become singularly resistant to the production of papillomas by painting of the ears with benzpyrene or tar.

Korteweg & Thomas A33,075/39: In mice, hypophysectomy delays but does not prevent the growth of transplanted mammary carcinomas or the induction of cutaneous neoplasms caused by painting the skin with 3:4-benzpyrene.

Moon et al. B74,251/52: In rats hypophysectomized two weeks before s.c. implantation of methylcholanthrene pellets, the development of sarcomas was almost completely prevented.

Griffin et al. B77,163/53: In rats, hypophysectomy inhibits the induction of liver damage and hepatomas by 3-methyl-4-dimethylaminoazobenzene (3'-Me-DAB).

Richardson et al. C2,406/53: In rats, hypophysectomy interferes with the production of hepatic cancers by 3'-Me-DAB.

Robertson et al. B88,672/53: In rats, hypophysectomy prevents the production of hepatic cirrhosis and hepatomas by 3'-Me-DAB. The susceptibility to tumorigenesis is restored by ACTH, but not by CON, DOC or testosterone. These hormones likewise failed to prevent carcinogenesis in intact rats.

Richardson et al. B99,907/54: In hypophysectomized rats, 3'-Me-DAB failed to produce hepatomas. Conjoint treatment with ACTH + STH partially restored the carcinogenic activity. Other pituitary preparations, cortisone, testosterone and DOC were ineffective. Earlier literature on the effect of hypophysectomy on carcinogenesis is reviewed.

Robertson et al. E61,212/54: In rats, hypophysectomy inhibits the carcinogenic action of azo dyes. ACTH, STH and, to a lesser extent, TTH and GTH restored this activity. DOC permitted the development of cirrhosis and bile duct adenomas in carcinogen-treated hypophysectomized females, whereas testosterone and vasopressin were inactive.

Griffin et al. C 14,406/55: In rats, the hepatic carcinogenesis normally induced by 3′-Me-DAB is prevented by hypophysectomy, but may be restored by subsequent treatment with either ACTH or STH. The literature on the effect of various hormones upon the induction of neoplasms by carcinogens is reviewed.

Conney et al. D 87,867/56: Injection of 3-methylcholanthrene (3-MC) i.p. greatly increases the ability of rat liver homogenates to N-demethylate 3-methyl-4-monomethylaminoazobenzene and to reduce the azo linkage of 4-demethylaminoazobenzene. Neither of these activities was altered after adrenalectomy, but both systems were slightly depressed after hypophysectomy.

O'Neal & Griffin, C 31,971/57: In rats, hypophysectomy prevents the induction of hepatomas by 3′-methyl-4-dimethyl-aminoazobenzene. The hepatoma induction by diacetylaminofluorene (DAAF) is also reduced though not abolished by hypophysectomy, but the induction of facial tumors by DAAF is not impeded in the absence of the pituitary. "The development of hepatic neoplasms is apparently regulated by the pituitary gland, while the mechanism of face tumor carcinogenesis by the same compound is independent of this endocrine system."

Huggins et al. C 62,178/59: In rats, mammary carcinomas induced by 3-MC involute following ovariectomy or hypophysectomy and, hence, they may be regarded as "hormone-dependent." Similar regression of tumors is frequently achieved by dihydrotestosterone. Only few mammary cancers continue to grow after ovariectomy and these are considered to be "hormone-independent."

Dao & Sunderland D 79,860/59; Dao et al. E 57,368/60: In rats, the induction of mammary carcinomas by 3-MC is enhanced during pregnancy, pseudopregnancy, and progesterone treatment. Regression of neoplasms occurs after parturition. Males are virtually resistant. In fully formed tumors, regression could be induced by hypophysectomy or ovariectomy.

Kim & Furth H 31,205/60: In rats, the induction of mammary cancers by 3-MC is considerably inhibited by ovariectomy or hypophysectomy. Grafts of functional mammotropic pituitary tumors counteract the inhibitory effect of hypophysectomy in that they not only stimulate the growth of involuting preexisting cancers, but also cause the appearance of new mammary tumors.

Bielschowsky D 10,255/61: In rats, hypophysectomy, thyroidectomy and adrenalectomy inhibit the development of hepatomas by treatment with 2-acetylaminofluorene (AAF) or 2-aminofluorene (AF).

Bock & Dao D 11,892/61: In rats, 3-MC accumulation in the mammary glands is increased by hypophysectomy or ovariectomy, but diminished during pregnancy. The affinity of mammary tissue for certain carcinogens may be due to its close association with adipose tissue.

Seguy et al. D 5,238/61: In rats, high doses of folliculoids enhanced the carcinogenic action of benzpyrene. Hypophysectomy or ovariectomy did not significantly influence this type of carcinogenesis, but the number of animals used was very small.

Goodall G 77,088/62: In rats, the production of hepatomas by AF is prevented by hypophysectomy or thyroidectomy. Cortisone restores the ability of the thyroidectomized but not of the hypophysectomized rats to develop hepatomas after AF treatment. Cortisone strongly accelerates the appearance of hepatomas in intact rats.

Morii & Huggins D 45,369/62: In rats, the adrenal necrosis produced by DMBA is prevented by hypophysectomy performed three weeks earlier. ACTH (but not STH) restores the susceptibility of the adrenals in the absence of the pituitary.

Sterental et al. D 61,608/63: In rats, mammary tumors induced by DMBA regressed after adrenalectomy + ovariectomy or hypophysectomy. Folliculoid treatment reactivated tumor growth after adrenalectomy + ovariectomy but not after hypophysectomy. These tumors remained unresponsive to folliculoids after hypophysectomy even if thyroid and cortisone replacement therapy was given.

Huggins & Sugiyama F 44,582/65: In rats, DMBA produces no adrenocortical necrosis if the animals are immature or hypophysectomized. ACTH renders the adrenals of immature rats susceptible to this type of injury.

Morii G 34,628/65: Pretreatment with small amounts of ACTH failed to protect the rat against DMBA-induced adrenocortical apoplexy. However, administration of ACTH to young rats or to hypophysectomized adults, which normally do not respond to the corticolytic effect of DMBA, makes them susceptible.

Shimazu G31,110/65: 20-Methylcholanthrene increases hepatic dimethylaminoazobenzene-demethylase in the rat, even after adrenalectomy, ovariectomy, or hypophysectomy. Hypothalamic lesions decrease the basal level of the enzyme and its response to methylcholanthrene. On the other hand, glutamine synthetase (a microsomal enzyme not induced by methylcholanthrene) is unaffected by hypothalamic lesions.

Huggins & Grand F74,177/66: In rats, neither hypophysectomy nor orchidectomy causes regression of DMBA-induced mammary cancers.

Raitschew G76,731/70: In hamsters, homotransplantation of a pituitary into the kidney increases the number of melanomas produced under standardized conditions by DMBA.

Somogyi G70,416/70: In rats, spironolactone inhibits the adrenocortical necrosis, carcinogenicity and hemopoietic-tissue-damaging action of DMBA. Ethylestrenol, CS-1 and norbolethone are also effective against the DMBA-induced adrenal necrosis. Spironolactone likewise protects against the adrenocorticolytic effect of 7-OHM-MBA. Thus, the anti-DMBA action of spironolactone does not seem to be based on the blockade of the transformation of the carcinogen into this supposedly more active metabolite. The preventive action of spironolactone is abolished by ethionine, suggesting the involvement of active protein synthesis. The DMBA-induced adrenal lesions are aggravated by estradiol, testosterone, methyltestosterone, cortisol, triamcinolone, and prednisolone, as well as by the stress of muscular work or restraint. The aggravation of adrenal necrosis by estradiol is diminished but not abolished by hypophysectomy.

Somogyi & Kovacs G60,074/70: In rats, hypophysectomy does not abolish the aggravation of DMBA-induced adrenal necrosis but diminishes its intensity.

Oka & Huggins H36,569/71: In rats, 7,8,12-trimethylbenz(a)-anthracene elicits an erythroblastic leukemia which regresses considerably after hypophysectomy.

Dimethylaminoazobenzene ← Hypophysectomy: Conney et al. *D87,867/56;* Gelboin et al. *D81,074/58*;* Shimazu et al. *G76,684/59*, G31,110/65*

7,12-Dimethylbenz(a)anthracene ← Hypophysectomy: Huggins et al. *D13,007/61*;* Morii et al. *D45,369/62*;* Ford et al. *D69,790/63**

3-MC ← Hypophysectomy: Moon et al. *B74,251/52*;* Dao *G37,357/64**

Cerium ←

Snyder et al. C99,417/59: In rats, i.v. injection of cerium produced extremely high levels of liver fat in females but not in males. After castration, males reacted as strongly as females. Testosterone reduced fatty infiltration in both intact and ovariectomized females. Hypophysectomy prevented fatty liver formation in both sexes, whereas adrenalectomy did so only in males.

Chlorpromazine ← Hypophysectomy + Chlordane: Hart et al. *G27,102/65*

Cycloheximide ←

Fiala & Fiala F33,398/65: In rats, cycloheximide increases microsome-bound hepatic RNA, but this effect is prevented by hypophysectomy.

Digitalis ←

Szabó et al. G79,024/71: In rats, PCN increases resistance to indomethacin, hexobarbital, progesterone, zoxazolamine and digitoxin, both in the presence and in the absence of the pituitary. Hypophysectomy also fails to prevent the induction of SER proliferation in the hepatocytes.

Diphenhydramine ←

de Salva D27,783/62: Diphenhydramine produced lowered EST in hypophysectomized but not in intact rats.

Diphenylhydantoin ←

de Salva D66,177/63: In rats, hypophysectomy decreases the EST raising effect of diphenylhydantoin.

Ephedrine ←

de Salva D27,783/62: The "EST elevating effect of serotonin and ephedrine in intact rats was preceded by hyperexcitability in hypophysectomized rats."

Ergot ←

Messina G18,016/64: In rats, ergotamine produces vascular lesions conducive to tail necrosis more readily in females than in males. Hypophysectomy prevents these toxic manifestations in both sexes, whereas treatment with chorionic gonadotrophin does not affect them.

Hexadimethrine ←

Tuchweber et al. D27,884/63: In rats, hypophysectomy prevents the nephrocalcinosis, but aggravates the adrenal necrosis produced by hexadimethrine. ACTH-treatment of the hypophysectomized rat facilitates the production of nephrocalcinosis, but protects the adrenal. Adrenalectomy prevents this form of nephrocalcinosis even in rats maintained on NaCl or DOC. On the other hand, triamcinolone-treated adrenalectomized rats react to hexadimethrine with strong nephrocalcinosis. Under similar conditions in intact rats, the corticoids did not significantly change the syndrome of hexadimethrine intoxication, except that the anaphylactoid reaction to this compound was inhibited by triamcinolone.

Indomethacin ←

Szabó et al. G79,024/71: In rats, PCN increases resistance to indomethacin, hexobarbital, progesterone, zoxazolamine and digitoxin, both in the presence and in the absence of the pituitary. Hypophysectomy also fails to prevent the induction of SER proliferation in the hepatocytes.

Lathyrogens ←

Selye & Ventura C27,684/57: In rats, hypophysectomy greatly diminished the development of osteolathyrism normally produced by AAN but STH aggravates these bone lesions even more in the absence than in the presence of the pituitary. It is concluded that the normal hormonal secretion of the hypophysis exerts a decisive influence on the development of osteolathyrism.

Selye C31,369/57: Hypophysectomy greatly delays the development of osteolathyrism in rats treated with AAN but simultaneous administration of STH results in bone lesions even more severe than those of intact AAN-treated controls.

Bois et al. E29,177/63: In rats with lathyrism induced by AAN, the increased mitotic rate in the epiphysial cartilages is prevented by hypophysectomy and restored by subsequent STH administration. STH appears to be indispensable for the development of osteolathyrism.

Magnesium ←

Jasmin E7,631/68: In rats, certain manifestations of the magnesium-deficiency syndrome are inhibited by cortisol, hypophysectomy or thyroparathyroidectomy.

Meprobamate ←

de Salva D27,783/62: "(1) Drugs with skeletal muscle relaxant properties (phenobarbital, meprobamate, phenaglycodol, mephenesin, and zoxazolamine) were less effective as depressants after hypophysectomy than they were in intact rats; (2) threshold elevating effects in intact rats of reserpine, mescaline, benactyzine and phenyltoloxamine were replaced by a EST lowering action."

Kato & Vassanelli D40,237/62: "Rats pretreated with phenobarbital, phenaglycodol, glutethimide, nikethamide, chlorpromazine, triflupromazine, meprobamate, carisoprodol, pentobarbital, thiopental, primidone, chloretone, dyphenylhydantoin and urethane showed an accelerated metabolism of meprobamate and, at the same time, a diminished duration of sleeping time and paralysis due to meprobamate." SKF 525-A counteracted these actions of the enzyme inducers. In hypophysectomized or adrenalectomized rats, phenobarbital still increased meprobamate metabolism in vitro.

Mercury ←

Szabó & Selye G70,478/70: In rats, hypophysectomy greatly diminishes the nephrocalcinosis produced by $HgCl_2$. This effect of $HgCl_2$ is completely abolished in hypophysectomized rats treated with triamcinolone.

Morphine ←

Tanabe & Cafruny C48,625/58: "The ability of hypophysectomized rats to tolerate large doses of morphine and morphine-withdrawal stresses did not seem to be impaired."

Morphine ← Hypophysectomy: Zauder B57,611/51*

p-Nitrobenzoic Acid ← Hypophysectomy + Pesticides: Hart et al. G27,102/65

Ozone ←

Fairchild et al. E32,187/63: In rats, hypophysectomy protects against the production of pulmonary edema by ozone inhalation. This effect is not abolished by ACTH or TTH and may be dependent upon the posterior lobe.

Fairchild G71,531/63: Review (6 pp., 26 refs.) on the effect of thyroidectomy, thiourea, thyroid hormones, glucocorticoids and hypophysectomy upon the resistance of various species to inhaled irritants, especially ozone.

Pesticides ←

DuBois et al. B3,089/47: In rats, both insulin and hypophysectomy antagonize the hyperglycemic effect of ANTU, but do not prolong survival.

Hietbrink & DuBois F65,296/66: In weanling male rats, total body X-irradiation inhibits the development of hepatic microsomal-enzyme fraction that catalyzes the oxidative desulfuration of Guthion. Shielding of the liver and testes does not prevent this inhibition, whereas irradiation of the head area—while the remainder of the body is shielded—produces a degree of inhibition similar to that obtained by total body irradiation. "The same dose of irradiation did not inhibit the enzyme development in hypophysectomized weanling rats. Thus, the pituitary is necessary for the radiation effect, but involvement of the pituitary is not the result of a radiation-induced deficiency of pituitary hormones."

Szabo & Selye G70,497/70: In rats, various catatoxic steroids, and particularly PCN, offer protection against intoxication with parathion and dioxathion. This protective effect is not prevented by hypophysectomy.

Guthion ← Hypophysectomy + X-irradiation: Hietbrink et al. *F65,296/66*

Phenaglycodol, Phenyltoloxamine ←

de Salva D27,783/62: "(1) Drugs with skeletal muscle relaxant properties (phenobarbital, meprobamate, phenaglycodol, mephenesin, and zoxazolamine) were less effective as depressants after hypophysectomy than they were in intact rats; (2) threshold elevating effects in intact rats of reserpine, mescaline, benactyzine and phenyltoloxamine were replaced by a EST lowering action."

Phosphates ←

Selye et al. C16,047/56: In rats, hypophysectomy inhibits the development of nephrocalcinosis after the administration of large amounts of Na_2HPO_4 p.o. or of NaH_2PO_4 by the "granuloma-pouch" technique. However, the atrophy of the outer renal cortex, induced by repeated injections of hypertonic phosphate solutions into the granuloma pouch, is not prevented by hypophysectomy.

Selye C39,319/58: In rats, nephrocalcinosis produced by excess NaH_2PO_4 p.o. is aggravated by estradiol, but even the severe calcification induced by this combined treatment is prevented by hypophysectomy.

Puromycin Aminonucleoside ←

Oliver & Kelsch F25,772/64: In rats, the development of the nephrotic syndrome produced by puromycin aminonucleoside (PAN) is not prevented by hypophysectomy.

Hoak et al. F61,136/65: In rats with nephrosis induced by PAN the usual hypercholesterolemia and hyperlipemia are inhibited by hypophysectomy.

Reserpine ←

de Salva D27,783/62: In hypophysectomized rats, the EST-elevating effects of reserpine, mescaline, benactyzine and phenyltoloxamine were replaced by an EST-lowering action.

Efron D59,758/62: In rats, adrenalectomy greatly decreases resistance to reserpine, whereas hypophysectomy leaves it almost unchanged. It is assumed therefore, "that the increased toxicity of reserpine in adrenalectomized rats is related to the absolute lack of certain adrenal steroids, which in some way may condition the nervous system to the effects of the drugs, rather than to the inability of the pituitary-adrenal system to respond to so-called 'nonspecific stress' caused by the drug."

Strychnine ← Hypophysectomy: Kato et al. *G74,030/62*

Vitamin A ←

Wolbach & Maddock B83,297/52: In rats, hypophysectomy decreases survival during vitamin-A overdosage, but does not significantly affect the skeletal response characteristic of this type of hypervitaminosis, except that bone repair processes are inhibited.

Vitamin D, DHT ←

Selye et al. D20,710/62: In rats, hypophysectomy greatly inhibits the development of calciphylaxis following combined treatment with DHT + $CrCl_3$.

Selye et al. D25,666/62: In the rat, hypophysectomy greatly diminishes both soft tissue calcification and osteitis fibrosa produced by parathyroid extract or DHT. The hypercalcemia is not diminished by the absence of the hypophysis and the latter may act by altering the metabolism of calcifiable organic matrix.

Bekemeier & Leiser D65,289/63: Vitamin-D_2 overdosage produces predominantly cortical nephrocalcinosis in intact, adrenalectomized, or hypophysectomized rats. Additional treatment with dienestrol (an artificial folliculoid) shifts calcium deposition predominantly to the cortico-medullary junction, irrespective of the presence or absence of the hypophysis or adrenals.

Water ← Hypophysectomy, Dog: Bodo et al. 88,791/45*

Zoxazolamine ←

Conney et al. D52,543/61: Pretreatment of male rats with chlorcyclizine shortens the duration of action and increases the hepatic microsomal metabolism of hexobarbital, pentobarbital and zoxazolamine. These effects were not prevented by hypophysectomy or adrenalectomy combined with castration.

de Salva D27,783/62: "(1) Drugs with skeletal muscle relaxant properties (phenobarbital, meprobamate, phenaglycodol, mephenesin, and zoxazolamine) were less effective as depressants after hypophysectomy than they were in intact rats."

Szabó et al. G79,024/71: In rats, PCN increases resistance to indomethacin, hexobarbital, progesterone, zoxazolamine and digitoxin, both in the presence and in the absence of the pituitary. Hypophysectomy also fails to prevent the induction of SER proliferation in the hepatocytes.

Microorganisms, Bacterial Toxins and Venoms ←

Hypophysectomy greatly diminishes the resistance of the rat to **tuberculosis** and this induced susceptibility can be abolished by STH. In guinea pigs, hypophysectomy reduces resistance even to the toxic actions of killed tubercle bacilli, a defect which cannot be corrected by DOC or cortisone. After hypophysectomy, cortisone is even more effective in protecting mice against **endotoxin** shock than in the presence of the pituitary, but reserpine fails to block endotoxin shock after hypophysectomy. It has been claimed, however, that resistance to endotoxin is actually increased a few hours after hypophysectomy or adrenalectomy in the mouse. The low endotoxin resistance of hypophysectomized rats is not corrected by parabiosis with an intact partner.

The resistance of the rat to **cobra venom** is reduced by about 2/3 after hypophysectomy.

Tuberculosis ←

Steinbach et al. B7,316/44: In rats, hypophysectomy greatly diminishes resistance to experimental tuberculosis.

Tonutti & Fetzer B75,190/52: In guinea pigs, hypophysectomy greatly reduces resistance to the toxic actions of killed tubercle bacilli. This defect is uninfluenced by DOC, but abolished by cortisone, although the latter accelerates dissemination of living tubercle bacilli.

Gillissen & Busanny-Caspari C6,858/53: In guinea pigs and rabbits, hypophysectomy did not significantly influence the course of tuberculosis [Only three animals of each species were used (H.S.).]

Bisetti & Barbolini D12,624/61: Rats which are normally highly resistant to infection with tuberculosis bacilli, become sensitive after hypophysectomy. This induced susceptibility can be abolished by STH. To a much lesser extent ACTH also offers some protection.

Bacterial Toxins ←

Chedid & Parant D6,761/61: The protection of intact mice against endotoxin shock by cortisone is inhibited by reserpine. The same is true in adrenalectomized rats, whereas after hypophysectomy cortisone is even more effective in offering protection against endotoxin, but reserpine no longer blocks this effect. Apparently the drug interferes with the cortisone effect only in the presence of the pituitary.

Parant D82,116/62: In mice, resistance to endotoxin is greatly increased a few hours after adrenalectomy or hypophysectomy. Cortisone protects normal, adrenalectomized, and hypophysectomized animals against high doses of endotoxin, whereas chlorpromazine is effective only in the presence of both the adrenals and the pituitary. ACTH also protects the hypophysectomized mouse but only if slow absorption is assured.

Chedid et al. D57,924/63: The low resistance of hypophysectomized rats to endotoxin is not corrected by parabiosis with an intact partner.

Venoms ←

Ball & Samuels 7,404/32: In rats, hypophysectomy is estimated to diminish resistance to cobra venom to about 2/3 of the norm.

Immune Reactions ←

In rats, hypophysectomy does not significantly modify antibody production after treatment with various antigens. On the other hand, fatal anaphylactic shock can be produced in hypophysectomized, but not in intact, rats. In guinea pigs, anaphylactic reactivity can be suppressed by anterior hypothalamic lesions, perhaps through their effect upon adrenal and thyroid secretion.

Hepatic and Renal Lesions ←

In rats and mice, hypophysectomy does not abolish the increase in hepatic polyploidy which occurs after **partial hepatectomy**, but it diminishes mitotic regeneration of the liver. This defect is corrected by STH, but further aggravated by cortisone.

Renal regeneration after **partial nephrectomy** is inhibited, but not abolished, by hypophysectomy in the rat. This observation first called attention to the fact that STH is not necessary for all types of growth.

The compensatory hypertrophy of the remaining kidney following uninephrectomy is diminished, but not abolished, by hypophysectomy in the rat and dog. However, if hypophysectomy precedes uninephrectomy by 15 days, the inhibition of regeneration is much less evidently suppressed. Presumably by that time, involution of the kidneys is already so pronounced that even mild compensatory hypertrophy is proportionately more evident. However, if hypophysectomy is performed two weeks after uninephrectomy, it causes severe involution of the remaining kidney.

Immune Reactions ←

Molomut 76,648/39: In rats, hypophysectomy does not significantly modify antibody production after treatment with various antigens. On the other hand, fatal anaphylactic shock could be produced in hypophysectomized but not in intact rats, though both groups of animals presented a similar antibody picture.

Filipp & Mess G71,129/69: In guinea pigs, suppression of anaphylactic reactivity by anterior hypothalamic lesions can be partially blocked by chronic treatment with thyroid hormones as well as by adrenalectomy or adrenal inactivation by metyrapone (Metopirone). "Combined treatment of guinea pigs bearing hypothalamic lesions with Metopirone and thyroxine completely eliminated the blocking effect of the tuberal lesion on anaphylactic reactions." Apparently the shock-inhibiting effect of hypothalamic lesions is partly due to hypothyroidism and partly to hypoadrenalcorticoidism.

Hepatic Lesions ←

Canzanelli et al. B37,729/49: In rats, hypophysectomy delays liver regeneration after partial hepatectomy but "neither adrenalectomy nor the administration of adrenal-cortex extract has any effect on the amount of liver regeneration."

Christensen & Jacobsen A49,204/49: In rats subjected to partial hepatectomy, neither hypophysectomy nor thyroidectomy impairs the rate of regeneration. No significant change in mitotic rate was observed after pretreatment with stilbestrol or STH.

Hemingway & Cater C56,780/58: In rats subjected to hypophysectomy + partial hepatectomy, mitotic regeneration of the liver is inhibited. Cortisone further inhibits mitosis and causes nuclear degeneration. These changes can in turn be blocked by treatment with STH.

Weinbren D95,941/59: Review (11 pp., 110 refs.) and personal observations on factors influencing hepatic regeneration after partial hepatectomy in the rat, with special sections on the effects of hypophysectomy and thyroid hormones.

Bucher G68,621/63: Review on the influence of hypophysectomy and hypophysial hormones upon hepatic regeneration.

Swartz G53,670/67: Studies in rats and mice on the increase in hepatic polyploidy after partial hepatectomy. In the rat, hypophysectomy does not abolish polyploidization.

Renal Lesions ←

Selye et al. 30,634/34: In rats, osteoblast proliferation and new bone formation following treatment with small doses of parathyroid extract and renal regeneration after uninephrectomy are not prevented by hypophysectomy. Apparently, STH is not necessary for all types of growth.

Gonzalez 79,025/38; A34,057/38: In toads, hypophysectomy diminishes compensatory renal hypertrophy following uninephrectomy. This defect can be partially compensated by either anterior- or posterior-pituitary implants.

McQueen-Williams & Thompson A33,938/40: In rats, total hypophysectomy prevented the compensatory hypertrophy of the remaining kidney after uninephrectomy. Thyroidectomy did not prevent renal regeneration under identical conditions.

Winternitz & Waters A34,910/40: In dogs, hypophysectomy almost completely prevents compensatory hypertrophy of the remaining kidney after uninephrectomy.

Braun-Menendez & Houssay B45,945/49: In rats, the compensatory hypertrophy of the remaining kidney following uninephrectomy is diminished but not abolished by hypophysectomy. The earlier literature on this topic is reviewed.

Astarabadi & Essex B75,446/52: In dogs, hypophysectomy diminishes, but does not completely abolish, compensatory hypertrophy of the remaining kidney after uninephrectomy.

Astarabadi & Essex B86,411/53: In dogs, the inhibition of compensatory renal hypertrophy following uninephrectomy is largely overcome by treatment with lyophilized anterior pituitary extract. In rats, hypophysectomy is less effective in inhibiting compensatory renal hypertrophy but treatment with pituitary extract fails to restore normal renal growth after hypophysectomy and uninephrectomy.

Sandri et al. C13,150/55: In rats, compensatory hypertrophy of the remaining kidney after uninephrectomy is greatly inhibited by hypophysectomy if the two operations are performed simultaneously, but not if hypophysectomy precedes uninephrectomy by 15 days. [Presumably by that time, involution of the kidneys is already so pronounced that even mild compensatory hypertrophy is proportionately more evident (H.S.).]

Astarabadi D8,815/61: In rats, hypophysectomy performed two weeks after uninephrectomy caused involution of the remaining kidney. "The results of the experiment suggest the presence of a renotropic principle in the hypophysis which is required for the compensatory renal hypertrophy." [At the time of hypophysectomy, compensatory hypertrophy was virtually complete, hence, the experiment merely confirms that hypophysectomy causes renal involution, a fact previously established on intact rats (H.S.).]

Various Stressors ←

In rats, resistance to total body **X-irradiation** is considerably decreased after hypophysectomy, although the characteristic polyuria and polydipsia of the first few days are diminished. The tendency to develop duodenal lesions under the influence of X-irradiation is not considerably altered by hypophysectomy in the rat, and ACTH does not consistently ameliorate the irradiation syndrome in the absence of the pituitary.

In hypophysectomized rats, sensitivity to cobalt irradiation is increased by testosterone and estradiol.

Goldfish also become unusually sensitive to X-irradiation after hypophysectomy.

Resistance to increased **oxygen tension** is enhanced by hypophysectomy, presumably because the thyroid function is diminished; administration of desiccated thyroid or thyroxine restores the high oxygen resistance of the hypophysectomized rat to normal.

Resistance to **cold** is decreased after hypophysectomy in the rat, but restored towards normal by cortical extract, ACTH, or TTH.

The **EST** is lowered in rats by hypophysectomy as it is by thyroidectomy or adrenalectomy.

The growth of Walker **tumor transplants** is essentially normal in hypophysectomized rats maintained on cortisol + DOC.

Ionizing Rays ←

Tyree et al. B33,116/48; Patt et al. B33,711/48: In rats, hypophysectomy decreases resistance to total body X-irradiation.

Smith & Tyree C12,045/56: In rats, the polydipsia and polyuria seen during the first days after X-irradiation tend to be inhibited by adrenalectomy or hypophysectomy.

Baker et al. C56,998/58: In rats, hypophysectomy does not significantly alter the duodenal lesions produced by total body X-irradiation.

Ghys D70,483/62: In hypophysectomized rats, sensitivity to cobalt irradiation is greatly increased by testosterone and estradiol.

Grafov D20,890/62: In rats, the decreased resistance to total body X-irradiation induced by hypophysectomy is not consistently ameliorated by ACTH.

Etoh & Egami G11,664/63: In goldfish, resistance to X-irradiation is greatly diminished both by adrenalectomy and by hypophysectomy.

Hyperoxygenation ←

Bean & Johnson B68,165/52: In rats exposed to oxygen under high pressure, resistance was increased by hypophysectomy.

Bean & Bauer B76,951/52: In rats, desiccated thyroid augments the adverse effects of exposure to high oxygen tension. It also abolishes the protective effect of hypophysectomy.

Smith et al. C95,244/60: In rats, desiccated thyroid or thyroxine increases the noxious effects of breathing virtually pure oxygen at atmospheric pressure. Conversely, hypophysectomy increases resistance to oxygen presumably through the elimination of TTH.

Temperature Variations ←

Baird et al. 14,881/33: In rats, resistance to cold is greatly diminished after hypophysectomy but restored by cortical extract, TTH or thyroxine.

Tyslowitz & Astwood 80,678/41: In hypophysectomized rats, the decreased resistance to cold is largely corrected by ACTH and andrenocortical extract. In adrenalectomized rats, adrenocortical extract is also effective in this respect, whereas ACTH is not.

Electric Stimuli ←

de Salva D66,176/63: In rats, the EST is reduced in descending order of magnitude by adrenalectomy, hypophysectomy and thyroidectomy. The effect of these endocrine deficiencies upon various depressant drugs is also described.

de Salva et al. C51,842/58: In rats, the EST was lowered by hypophysectomy and adrenalectomy, but only insignificantly by thyroidectomy. 5-HT elevated the EST.

de Salva D66,177/63: In rats, hypophysectomy decreases the EST raising effect of diphenylhydantoin.

Gispen et al. G77,128/70: In rats exposed to unescapable electric shock the threshold for flinch, jerk, run and jump was significantly lowered by hypophysectomy. "Treatment with the ACTH analogue $ACTH_{1-10}$ did not affect threshold levels in hypophysectomized or intact rats. It is concluded that the stimulating effect of $ACTH_{1-10}$ on conditioned-avoidance acquisition in hypophysectomized rats is not caused by an influence on sensory capacities.'

Tumors ←

Korteweg & Thomas A 33,075/39: In mice, hypophysectomy delays but does not prevent the growth of transplanted mammary carcinomas or the induction of cutaneous neoplasms caused by painting the skin with 3:4-benzpyrene.

Ventura et al. C 23,299/57: In rats, the growth of transplanted Walker tumors is essentially normal after hypophysectomy and maintenance therapy with cortisol + DOC. However, the tumor cachexia is greatly increased, whereas the severe involution of the spleen and liver, as well as the development of leukemoid tissue infiltrates in the adrenals and spleen were inhibited.

Hepatic Enzymes ←

For the extensive literature concerning the effect of hypophysectomy on the basic levels of hepatic TPO, TKT, GOT, and other enzymes, as well as upon induction of such enzymes by hormones or substrates, *cf.* the Abstract Section.

TPO, TKT ←

Geschwind & Li B 95,517/53: Hypophysectomy does not abolish (and perhaps even increases) the resting TPO activity of the rat liver. However, in hypophysectomized animals, the ability to induce this enzyme by tryptophan injection is gradually diminishing during the first 14 post-operative days. Treatment with ACTH enhances the formation of this adaptive enzyme system (measured by kynurenin formation) even without treatment with tryptophan.

Geschwind & Li B 93,277/54: In the rat, the induction of the TPO enzyme system is diminished by hypophysectomy and adrenalectomy, but increased by thyroidectomy.

Thomson & Mikuta B 90,975/54: "Total-body X-irradiation produces within a few hours a dose-dependent increase in the TPO system of rat liver. The increase does not occur in adrenalectomized rats, and hence cannot be construed as a direct effect of X-irradiation." After hypophysectomy, enzyme induction became progressively less pronounced as adrenal atrophy developed. ACTH restored the ability of the hypophysectomized rat to respond with enzyme induction.

McCann et al. E 93,864/59: In rats, hypothalamic lesions interfering with ACTH-secretion, as well as hypophysectomy decrease the induction of hepatic TPO by histidine, but do not block the response completely.

Maickel & Brodie C 83,071/60: TPO in rat liver is increased by ACTH, cortisone, or cortisol, as well as by various stressor agents and barbiturates. Hypophysectomy prevents the effect of stressors and barbiturates, suggesting that the latter act through the pituitary-adrenal system.

Westermann et al. C 83,072/60: In the rat, large doses of reserpine produce an alarm reaction with an increase in the hepatic TPO activity associated with lowered brain serotonin and norepinephrine. Hypophysectomy prevents these responses.

Rosen & Milholland D 23,053/62: Administration of L-tryptophan, but not of tyrosine, stimulated hepatic TKT activity in adrenalectomized rats. No such induction was obtained by tryptophan in vitro. Adrenalectomized rats treated with tyrosine, methionine or histidine had slightly subnormal TKT levels. Tryptophan analogues (D-tryptophan, acetyl-L-tryptophan, indole, D,L-5-OH-tryptophan and 5-HT), increase both TKT and TPO activity in the livers of adrenalectomized rats. In hypophysectomized rats, trytophan, 5-HT or 5-OH-tryptophan caused only a slight rise in the hepatic activity of TPO or TKT.

Rosen & Milholland E 32,652/63: Tryptophan induced significant increases in hepatic TKT activity in intact and in adrenalectomized (NaCl-maintained) rats. Tyrosine, histidine and methionine slightly depressed the hepatic TKT activity of the adrenalectomized rats. Analogues of tryptophan (including D-tryptophan, acetyl-L-tryptophan, indole, DL-5-hydroxytryptophan and 5-HT i.p.) increase both TKT and TPO activity by 50—300% in the livers of intact or adrenalectomized rats. 5-HT and DL-5-hydroxytryptophan were most active. After hypophysectomy, the response of each of these enzymes to tryptophan gradually diminished. After 6 months, tryptophan, 5-hydroxytryptophan and 5-HT failed to cause significant increases in the hepatic activity of these enzymes, but cortisol remained highly effective, causing increases in both enzyme activities comparable to those seen in intact or adrenalectomized rats. "Experiments with two known inhibitors of protein synthesis, DL-ethionine and puromycin, indicate that a major fraction of the induced activity of tryptophan pyrrolase seen in adrenalectomized or hypophysectomized rats treated by injection with tryptophan is due to activation rather than synthesis of new enzyme protein. The responses of tryptophan pyrrolase and tyrosine transaminase in liver following cortisol administration appear to be mainly the result of the synthesis of each of these enzymes."

Nomura et al. G33,405/65: Various forms of stress (forced exercise, immobilization, cold), as well as the administration of chlorpromazine, increased the TPO-activity of the liver both in intact and in adrenalectomized, but not in hypophysectomized, rats.

Kenney & Albritton G64,557/65: Review of the literature suggesting that transaminase induction in response to stressors can be interpreted as due to corticoid secretion during the stress reaction. Cortisol increases enzyme synthesis following an increased rate of ribosomal transfer synthesis and "DNA-like" RNA's. The present experiments confirm the view that repressor(s) can inhibit enzyme synthesis at the translational level because inhibition of RNA synthesis can prolong the corticoid-induced increase in enzyme synthesis under suitable conditions. "Administration of stressing agents (tyrosine, Celite) to adrenalectomized rats initiates a highly selective repression of the synthesis of hepatic tyrosine-α-ketoglutarate transaminase. The enzyme level falls with a t½ of about 2.5 hr. Immunochemical measurement of the rate of enzyme synthesis indicates that it is reduced essentially to zero in stressed, adrenalectomized rats, whereas labeling of total liver soluble proteins is unaffected. Actinomycin does not itself influence the enzyme level, but it blocks the stress-initiated repression of enzyme synthesis, indicating that repression acts at the translational level, whereas initiation of repression involves transcriptional processes." In hypophysectomized rats, stressors are ineffective and preliminary data suggest that STH is responsible for transaminase repression.

Fiala & Fiala F65,983/66: In the rat, cycloheximide (Actidione) i.p. inhibits the synthesis of hepatic TPO assayed 4 hrs after administration of the substrate, or of cortisol. By contrast, actidione did not abolish the induction of TKT by cortisol and, in fact, actidione increased the level of TKT even in the absence of cortisol treatment. A similar, though smaller, effect occurred in hypophysectomized or adrenalectomized[1] rats, suggesting a direct induction of TKT by actidione. Puromycin inhibited the synthesis of TKT. Apparently, an inhibitor of protein synthesis such as actidione may also act as an inducer for the synthesis of TKT, thus simulating the action of cortisol. "This 'pseudohormonal' action of actidione may explain the toxicity of actidione in certain mammalian species and also the fact that hydrocortisone may act as an antidote in actidione poisoning. It does not explain why a similar effect of 'pseudohormonal' induction is not observed in the case of TPO, but only the inhibition of enzyme induction."

Schapiro et al. F67,227/66: Hepatic TKT-activity increased in immature, stressed (reciprocating shaker) rats, whereas intact stressed adults showed no change. In the stressed adrenalectomized adults, TKT activity markedly decreased, while adrenalectomized immature rats showed no change. Hypophysectomy largely abolished inhibition in the adults. TPO-activity, when present, was increased by stress in old-age groups, but the increase was abolished by adrenalectomy and hypophysectomy. "The results suggest stress-activation of a pituitary mechanism that inhibits or represses activation of tyrosine transaminase and that may not function during early postnatal life."

Grossman & Mavrides G46,206/67: Studies on the kinetics of cortisol-induced hepatic TKT activity in adrenalectomized rats. "Puromycin inhibited enzyme synthesis when it was given during the initial phase of induction. However, it unexpectedly caused a rapid reappearance of enzyme activity following its administration during the inactivation phase. This potentiated response is consistent with other observations which lead to the idea that a repressor is formed about 4 hours after hormone administration and that inhibition of repressor synthesis allows, at least temporarily, continued synthesis of enzyme." The inactivator appears to depend upon pituitary function, since adrenalectomized and hypophysectomized rats showed little or no inactivation phase following cortisol treatment.

Kenney G50,810/67: In intact, hypophysectomized or adrenalectomized rats, STH inhibits the synthesis of hepatic TKT. The rate of enzyme synthesis is reduced nearly to zero(immunochemical-isotopic analyses), whereas labeling of the bulk of the liver proteins is increased by STH. Repression is blocked when RNA synthesis is inhibited by actinomycin. STH also appears to play a role in the repression of TKT induction by stressors. A hypophysectomized and an intact rat were united by parabiosis. When the pituitary-bearing member was stressed by tyrosine i.p., repression occurred in the livers of both treated and untreated (hypophysectomized) animals. Transaminase levels were unchanged in a single experiment where the stressing agent was administered to the hypophysectomized partner.

Labrie & Korner G56,018/68: The basal level of TPO and TKT was unchanged in the liver of the hypophysectomized rat, but injected cortisol produced greater increases in these enzyme activities. STH depressed these enzyme activities only after pretreatment for four days in either hypophysectomized or adrenalectomized rats, but even shorter pretreatment counteracted the enzyme-inducing effect of cortisol. An amino-acid mixture p.o. enhanced cortisol stimulation of both enzyme activities and abolished the STH-inhibition of the cortisol effect.

Govier & Lovenberg G70,841/69: In rats, the increase in hepatic TKT produced by phentolamine is almost completely abolished by adrenalectomy or hypophysectomy. If small doses of cortisol are given to adrenalectomized rats, phentolamine again increases enzyme activity. Aminoglutethimide completely eliminates both the increase in plasma corticosterone and enzyme induction by phentolamine. "It is concluded that at least two factors are operative in the induction of TKT by phentolamine—(1) a response to an increased plasma corticosterone concentration, and (2) an additional effect which may be a direct substrate type of induction."

Lane & Mavrides H12,953/69: Cortisol caused a greater increase of hepatic TKT in hypophysectomized than in adrenalectomized rats. In general, elevation of enzyme activity after cortisol was inversely proportional to the initial enzyme level, and the latter was in turn higher on protein-rich than on protein-poor diets.

Geller et al. H8,414/69: The stress of laparotomy increases hepatic TKT activity in intact, but not in the adrenalectomized rat, which actually responds in an inverse manner. Hypophysectomy eliminates some, but not all, of this laparotomy-induced repression. Under these conditions, the TPO- and the TKT-responses are somewhat different.

GPT, GOT ←

Beaton et al. C10,012/55: STH decreases the hepatic GPT and d-amino acid oxidase activity in nonpregnant female rats. These effects are even more pronounced if the animals receive STH + "equine estrogenic substances" + progesterone. This enzyme activity also decreases during pregnancy both in intact and in hypophysectomized rats.

Rosen et al. C50,741/58: In rats treated with cortisol, cortisone or prednisone for 1 week, there was an increase in hepatic GPT but not in GOT. DOC had no such effect. Hypophysectomy or adrenalectomy did not prevent this action of cortisone. STH, testosterone or insulin failed to alter GPT activity nor did they influence its stimulation by cortisol.

Rosen et al. C71,414/59: Marked increases in GPT activity were observed in the livers of rats given cortisol, cortisone, 9α-fluorocortisol, prednisone, 6α-methylprednisolone, 9α-fluoro-21-desoxy-6α-methylprednisolone or ACTH, whereas two nonglucocorticoid cortisol derivatives, 11-epicortisol and 9α-methoxycortisol, were inactive. STH, testosterone and insulin caused no significant change in GPT by themselves nor did they modify the action of cortisol. On the other hand, large doses of estradiol and thyroxine caused a moderate increase in GPT activity but when injected simultaneously with cortisol they appeared to interfere with its action as did progesterone. Adrenalectomy slightly diminished or failed to affect the GPT inducing activity of cortisol, whereas hypophysectomy caused a rise in GPT activity and augmented the effect of cortisol.

Harding et al. D14,355/61: In the rat, pretreatment with DOC depresses the hepatic GPT activity. A similar depression is obtained by adrenalectomy, but this is not further aggravated by concurrent treatment with DOC. ACTH increases alanine transaminase activity in hypophysectomized, but not in adrenalectomized, animals. In hypophysectomized rats, DOC fails to lower alanine transaminase, nor does it alter the response of this enzyme to ACTH. "The inhibitory effect of DOC on alanine transaminase activity appears to be due to suppression of ACTH release by the pituitary."

Other Amino Acid Enzymes ←

Zuchlewski & Gaebler D91,862/57: Hepatic glutamic acid dehydrogenase activity increases after hypophysectomy in the rat, and is not altered by STH either in hypophysectomized or in sham-operated control animals. GPT and GOT activities have also been investigated under similar conditions.

Freedland & Avery G67,766/64: In the rat, the TDH and SDH activity of liver homogenates was increased by high protein diets, alloxan diabetes, or cortisol. Factors affecting the activity of TDH caused a proportional change in SDH suggesting that both of these activities may be due to a single protein. The SDH activity was decreased by adrenalectomy or hypophysectomy. Adrenalectomy had no effect upon the response of this enzyme to protein feeding, whereas, after hypophysectomy, this response was diminished.

Freedland G28,270/65: Hypophysectomy causes a marked decrease in the hepatic microsomal arginase and arginine synthetase activity in the rat, and both these urea-cycle enzyme levels are increased by cortisol and high-protein diet, even after hypophysectomy.

Ishikawa et al. F41,763/65: In alloxan-diabetic rats, the hepatic SDH and TDH activities are greatly increased. SDH was readily induced by cortisol in the diabetic, but not in the normal, rat. The effects of actinomycin S, STH, and starvation upon SDH have also been studied in intact, hypophysectomized, adrenalectomized and thyroidectomized rats. It is concluded that "serine dehydratase activity in the liver plays an important role in the production of pyruvate as a starting material for gluconeogenesis."

Shimazu G31,110/65: 20-Methylcholanthrene increases hepatic dimethylaminoazobenzene-demethylase in the rat, even after adrenalectomy, ovariectomy, or hypophysectomy. Hypothalamic lesions decrease the basal level of the enzyme and its response to methylcholanthrene. On the other hand, glutamine synthetase (a microsomal enzyme not induced by methylcholanthrene) is unaffected by hypothalamic lesions.

Various Enzymes ←

Greengard et al. D12,966/61: Hypophysectomy enormously increases the rise in hepatic DPN content induced by nicotinamide i.p. in the rat. ACTH or cortisone suppresses this increase. Many of the metabolic actions of the pituitary-adrenal system may depend upon alterations in the hepatic concentration of this coenzyme.

Abraham et al. G20,214/64: Hypophysectomy drastically reduces the citrate-cleavage enzyme activity induced in rat liver by dietary measures.

Dietrich & Yero G26,959/65: Cortisol markedly lowered the nicotinamide deamidase-activity of the liver in intact, hypophysectomized, and adrenalectomized rats. Under these conditions, cortisol failed to inhibit hepatic synthesis of NAD significantly after nicotinamide challenge. Hexestrol markedly lowered hepatic deamidase activity in intact, thyroidectomized, and adrenalectomized rats. A lowering of the hepatic NAD-levels after nicotinamide challenge occurred upon hexestrol treatment in intact, but not in adrenalectomized, rats. Hypophysectomy markedly stimulated nicotinamide deamidase activity and NAD-biosynthesis after nicotinamide challenge.

Freedland et al. G55,808/68: Extensive studies on the effect of adrenalectomy, hypophysectomy and cortisol treatment upon a great variety of rat liver enzymes, with observations on the effect of thyroxine upon these enzymes in intact, adrenalectomized or hypophysectomized rats. The extensive data do not lend themselves to succinct presentation in the form of a summary and must be consulted in the original.

← THYROID HORMONES

The role of the thyroid in resistance, and particularly in drug detoxication, is very great but poorly understood. The discovery by Reid Hunt, at the beginning of this century, that thyroid extract increases the acetonitrile resistance of the mouse was probably one of the first clear-cut demonstrations in the field of hormone-induced drug resistance. The "Hunt test" was so sensitive and reliable that it has been widely used for bioassay purposes, although the underlying mechanism remains mysterious even today.

As we shall see from the following pages, thyroid deficiency and hyperthyroidism alter reactivity to innumerable agents, including hormones, drugs, infections, stressors, and particularly exposure to temperature variations. In all these cases, it is of course tempting to hold changes in the BMR responsible for altered resistance, since a general increase or decrease in metabolism affects the activity of most chemical reactions, be they favorable or detrimental to the organism. However, recent work on the catatoxic steroids indicates that thyroid hormones can significantly influence the activity of the hepatic microsomal drug-metabolizing enzymes and through them the degradative inactivation of toxicants or, conversely, their transformation into metabolites even more toxic than the parent compounds.

Despite the voluminous literature described in the following pages, no systematic study has as yet been carried out along these lines. The exploration of the part played by the thyroid hormones in resistance appears to be particularly promising now against the background of what we have learned recently about the corresponding actions of steroids.

Steroids ←

Corticoids ←. The nephrosclerosis produced by DOC + uninephrectomy + NaCl in the rat is greatly aggravated by thyroxine. Thyroidectomy has an inverse effect, although not all the lesions are equally affected by it. The glycogenolytic action of thyroid feeding is counteracted by cortisone. Thyroxine increases the toxicity of many drugs (e.g., digitoxin, indomethacin, nicotine, phenindione, various pesticides) against which ethylestrenol offers excellent protection. The protective effect of catatoxic steroids can be counteracted by concurrent treatment with thyroid hormone.

Testoids ←. It has been claimed that in orchidectomized mice, thyroxine increases the seminal vesicle enlargement produced by testosterone. In rats, the renotrophic action of methyltestosterone is enhanced by thyroxine.

Folliculoids ←. The hypercalcemia produced in cockerels by stilbestrol is inhibited by thyroxine, and the oviduct stimulating effect of estradiol in young pullets is increased by thiouracil.

In ducks, estradiol stimulates the proliferation of fine spongy bone trabeculae. Thyroidectomy retards bone proliferation, whereas conjoint treatment with thyroxine and estradiol leads to the abundant formation of thick trabeculae.

In rats, thyroidectomy diminishes, whereas thyroid extract increases the hepatotoxicity of CCl_4.

Corticoids ← cf. also *Selye B40,000/50,* p. 552; *C92,918/61,* p. 280; *G60,083/70,* pp. 326, 401.

Selye et al. B229/45: In rats, the nephrosclerosis produced by DOC after uninephrectomy + NaCl is greatly aggravated by thyroxine.

Kusama C58,473/57: In rats, the glucogenolytic action of thyroid feeding is counteracted by cortisone.

Yates et al. C51,744/58: Studies on the Ring A reduction of cortisone by slices and homogenates of rat livers after pretreatment with thyroxine or previous thyroparathyroidectomy showed that the total hepatic activity is less in normal males than in females. "Activity was increased 37% and 45% in hyperthyroid males and females respectively, and was decreased 39% and 47% in hypothyroid animals."

Salgado & Mulroy C84,321/59: In rats, the cardiovascular changes produced by DOC following sensitization by uninephrectomy and NaCl are inhibited by hypophysectomy or thyroidectomy, although not all the lesions are blocked to an equal extent.

Selye G70,428/70: In rats, ethylestrenol powerfully inhibits the toxicity of digitoxin, nicotine, indomethacin, phenindione, dioxathion, EPN, physostigmine, hexobarbital, cyclopental, thiopental, DOC (anesthesia), meprobamate and picrotoxin. Thyroxine increases the toxicity of many among these drugs, and inhibits the protective effect of ethylestrenol.

Fluorocortisol Acetate ← *cf. also Tables 12—14*

DOC ← *cf. also Table 15*

Triamcinolone ← *cf. also Table 18*

Cortisone ← Thyroxine: McGuire et al. *E90,938/59, E91,579/59*

Testoids ← *cf. also Selye B40,000/50, p. 631; G60,083/70, p. 401.*

Caridroit & Arvy A57,397/42: In castrate mice, thyroxine increases the seminal vesicle enlargement produced by testosterone.

Selye et al. B229/45: In rats, the renotrophic action of methyltestosterone is greatly enhanced by thyroxine.

Masson 96,171/47: In orchidectomized mice, thyroxine increases the stimulation of the seminal vesicles by testosterone, but the effect is not very marked and may even be reversed depending upon the dose level at which the two hormones are given.

Bradlow et al. C27,897/56: In man, studies with radioactive testosterone suggest that T3 markedly influences the metabolism of this testoid, in that conversion into androsterone is increased with a concomitant fall in etiocholanolone.

Androst-4-ene-3,17-dione ← Thyroxine: McGuire et al. *E90,938/59, E91,579/59*

Androst-4-ene-3,17-dione ← Triiodothyronine: McGuire et al. *E90,938/59*

Folliculoids ← *cf. also Selye G60,083/70, p. 406.*

Benoit & Clavert B27,669/48: In ducks, estradiol stimulates the proliferation of spongy bone consisting of fine trabeculae. Thyroidectomy retards this bone proliferation whereas conjoint treatment with thyroxine and estradiol leads to abundant development of thick trabeculae.

von Faber C6,925/55: In cockerels, the hypercalcemia produced by stilbestrol is inhibited by concurrent administration of thyroxine.

Common et al. D12,509/61: In immature pullets, the oviduct-stimulating effect of estradiol is greatly increased by the administration of thiouracil p.o.

Kulcsar-Gergely & Kulcsar G71,532/62: In rats, thyroidectomy diminishes, whereas thyroid extract increases the hepatotoxicity of CCl_4. Correspondingly, the sexual cycle is accelerated by thyroidectomy and delayed by thyroid hormone treatment as a result of changes in hepatic folliculoid degradation.

Estradiol ← *cf. also Table 16*

Progesterone ← *cf. Table 17*

Steroidases in General (incl. Bile Acids, Cholesterol) ← *cf. also* **Cholesterol** *under* **Drugs**

Schmidt 27,511/34: In guinea pigs, gastric ulcer formation following i.p. injection of Na-glycocholate or Na-taurocholate is diminished following pretreatment with thyroxine p.o., perhaps because hyperthyroidism causes liver damage and thereby interferes with the biliary excretion of the bile acid.

McGuire Jr. & Tomkins E90,938/59: In rats, thyroxine increases the rate of reduction of Δ^4-3-ketosteroids by TPNH-dependent microsomal enzymes.

McGuire & Tomkins E91,579/59: In the rat, thyroxine causes a pronounced increase in the microsomal 5α-reductase activity of the liver, but the rate of reduction of some steroid substrates is raised more than that of others. Furthermore, when microsomes are "aged" at 0—5°C for several weeks, the decline in activity varies with different steroid substrates. "Further evidence for the substrate specificity of the 5α hydrogenases was the observation that 4-androstene-3,17-dione strongly inhibited the reduction of cortisone, while the converse was not true." These and other observations suggest that each series of 4-ene-3-ketosteroid hydrogenases, 5α and 5β, contains multiple enzymes capable of discerning small variations in the steroid molecule.

McGuire Jr. & Tomkins D5,722/60: In the microsomal fraction of rat liver, there appear to be at least 5 Δ^4-3-ketosteroid reductases (5α). When rats are treated with thyroxine, the reductase activity for cortisone, cortisol, DOC, 4-androstene-3,17-dione and 11-deoxycortisol (Cpd. S) increases, but the increment is different for each of these substrates.

Danielsson & Tchen G72,327/68 (p. 159): Brief summary of the influence of the thyroid upon cholesterol and bile acid metabolism.

Lehmann & Breuer E8,112/68: The in vitro metabolism of ^{14}C-estrone by the hepatic microsomes of the rat is markedly influenced by in vivo pretreatment with T3 or $NaClO_4$. Hyperthyroidism increases, whereas hypothyroidism and severe thyrotoxicosis diminish estrone metabolism.

Lehmann & Breuer H 15,110/69: "After incubation of oestrone with the microsomal fractions of liver of euthyroid, hyperthyroid, thyrotoxic as well as hypothyroid rats the following metabolites were identified in the ether soluble fractions: 6α-, 6β- and 7α-hydroxyoestrone, 6α-, 6β- and 7α-hydroxy-17β-oestradiol, 16α-hydroxyoestrone, oestriol and 17β-oestradiol. The amounts of metabolites formed depended upon the functional state of the thyroid."

Schweppe & Jungmann H 15,266/69: The ability of rat liver microsomes to synthesize cholesterol palmitate, oleate, and linoleate in vitro is increased by the addition of thyroxine or glucagon to the incubation medium. Testosterone increases cholesterol palmitate and oleate formation. 17β-Estradiol stimulates mainly oleate synthesis.

Schweppe & Jungmann H 15,978/69: Observations on the metabolism of marked cholesterol added together with various hormones to hepatic microsomes of the rat led to the conclusion that "1) cholesterol palmitate and oleate were synthesized most rapidly; 2) at high concentrations, testosterone decreased the formation of all esters but at lower dose levels, testosterone increased the synthesis of cholesterol oleate and palmitate; 3) estradiol caused a two-fold increase in cholesterol oleate formation; 4) ACTH decreased the synthesis rate of cholesterol palmitate and oleate; 5) insulin had a significant inhibitory effect on cholesterol linoleate; 6) epinephrine had little significant effect at the dose level used; and 7) L-thyroxine increased the synthesis of all cholesterol esters."

Pancuronium ← *cf.* Table 19

Steroids ← Thyroxine: McGuire et al. *E 90,938/59, D 5,722/60*

Nonsteroidal Hormones and Hormone-Like Substances ←

Pituitary, Thyroid and Parathyroid Hormones ←. The renotrophic action of crude anterior **pituitary extracts** is greatly enhanced by thyroxine in the rat.

Several earlier observations suggested that T2, thiourea, and thiouracil interfere with many of the characteristic effects of **thyroxine** overdosage in rats and mice.

In rats, the activity of thyroxine is greatly augmented after partial hepatectomy. However, it is only when the circulating amount of thyroxine (or T3) is above physiologic limits that the liver plays an important role in its detoxication.

The osteitis fibrosa produced by **parathyroid extract** in rats is not prevented by thyroidectomy. Apparently, parathyroid hormone does not act through the thyroid as had been claimed by earlier investigators.

On the other hand, pretreatment with thyroxine inhibits the soft tissue calcinosis, osteitis fibrosa, and hypercalcemia produced by parathyroid overdosage in the rat. This inhibition is manifested even after thyroparathyroidectomy, but not after nephrectomy, in contradistinction to calcitonin which inhibits parathyroid extract overdosage even in the absence of the kidneys.

Pancreatic Hormones ←. In rabbits and rats, thyroidectomy decreases resistance to insulin. This effect is much less evident in guinea pigs and dogs. Thyroid feeding has an opposite effect. In cats, thyroidectomy decreases resistance to insulin-induced hypoglycemia even if the parathyroids are preserved.

Thyroidectomy decreases, whereas thyroid extract increases sensitivity to the diabetogenic action of alloxan in rats. The hepatic necrosis produced by alloxan intoxication in rats is prevented by thiouracil, and aggravated by thyroid feeding.

More recent experiments suggest that in mice, sensitivity to insulin convulsions is increased by thyroxine, and that in rats, the diabetogenic effect of alloxan is antagonized by thyroid feeding.

Catecholamines ←. In most species, thyroidectomy increases, whereas thyroid hormones decrease resistance to epinephrine and, to a lesser extent, to norepinephrine. This is true not only of the acute toxicity of catecholamines but also of such chronic changes as the calcifying arteriosclerosis produced in the rabbit.

Histamine and 5-HT ←. In guinea pigs, thyroidectomy protects against otherwise fatal histamine intoxication, whereas thyroxine has an opposite effect. Rats pretreated with thyroxine become extremely sensitive to 5-HT or to anaphylactoidogenic agents which cause histamine and 5-HT liberation from mastocytes.

Thyroxine inhibits the action of 5-HT upon isolated smooth muscles in rats, whereas in the perfused hindquarter, the vasomotor effects of 5-HT are allegedly enhanced by thyroxine.

In man, wheal formation following 5-HT i.c. is reduced in myxedema and increased in thyrotoxicosis.

Hypophyseal Hormones ← cf. also Selye B40,000/50, pp. 515, 552; C92,918/61, p. 40.

Selye et al. B229/45: In rats, the renotrophic action of anterior pituitary extracts is greatly enhanced by thyroxine.

Thyroid Hormones ←

Abelin & Schönenberger 4,290/33: In rats, diiodothyronine inhibits many of the effects of thyroxine overdosage.

Dietrich & Beutner B20,412/44: In mice, thiourea and thiouracil interfere with the action of orally administered thyroid powder when the Reid Hunt test is made the basis of observations. In this test, minute amounts of whole thyroid can be detected by their protective effect against otherwise lethal doses of acetonitrile.

Kellaway et al. B14,515/45: In rats, the activity of thyroxine s.c. was estimated by an increase in pulse rate after partial hepatectomy, thyroidectomy, or bile duct ligation. "It was found (1) that thyroxine activity is greatly intensified in the absence of the liver; (2) that the liver does not play a significant role when the amount of circulating thyroxine is within physiologic limits; (3) that the liver deals with excess hormone by some process of inactivation and not by simple excretion."

3,3,5-Triiodo-L-thyronine ← cf. also Table 20
Propylthiouracil ← cf. also Tables 21, 22
Parathyroid Hormone ← cf. also Selye G60,083/70, pp. 401, 413.

Selye A36,715/42: In rats, partial hepatectomy, complete thyroidectomy, or bilateral nephrectomy do not prevent the osteitis fibrosa and soft-tissue calcification produced by large doses of parathyroid extract. Apparently, parathyroid hormone does not exert its action through either the thyroid or the kidney, as had previously been postulated by some investigators. Furthermore, hepatic detoxication does not play an important role in the metabolism of parathyroid hormone.

Côté et al. G46,713/67; Gabbiani et al. G39,934/67; G46,730/68; G46,731/68; Tuchweber et al. G46,759/68: Pretreatment with thyroxine or calcitonin inhibits the soft tissue calcification and osteitis fibrosa induced by parathyroid extract overdosage. In the event of concurrent administration, the effect of the two protective hormones is summated. Thyroxine retains its effect upon calcium metabolism in thyroparathyroidectomized or adrenalectomized but not in nephrectomized rats. The stress of restraint likewise prevents parathyroid overdosage, but the associated biochemical changes are different from those caused by thyroxine.

Pancreatic Hormones ←

Ducheneau 20,846/24: In rabbits, thyroidectomy increases sensitivity to the hypoglycemic and lethal effects of insulin.

Houssay & Busso 20,601/24: In rabbits and rats, thyroidectomy decreases resistance to the toxic effects of insulin. The phenomenon is less evident in guinea pigs and still less in dogs. Thyroid feeding has an opposite effect.

Britton & Myers 18,695/28: In cats, thyroidectomy greatly increases sensitivity to insulin-induced hypoglycemic reactions even if the parathyroids are preserved. However, about 3 weeks after operation, insulin resistance returns to normal and subsequently rises above that level.

Jensen & Grattan 77,887/40: In mice, ACTH, glucocorticoids and cortical extracts increase insulin resistance, whereas other pituitary hormones and thyroxine have no such effect.

Martinez B15,837/45; Houssay & Sara B727/45: In rats, desiccated thyroid feeding increases, whereas thyroidectomy decreases sensitivity to alloxan i.v.

Martinez B2,342/46: In rats, thiouracil diminishes the diabetic action of alloxan and of subtotal pancreatectomy.

Ershoff B24,883/48: In immature female rats fed purified rations containing both pancreas and desiccated thyroid, mortality was high. Similar diets containing only pancreas or desiccated thyroid induced no comparable mortality.

Houssay B60,812/50; Martinez B61,239/51: In rats, thyroidectomy or prolonged treatment with thiouracil or cysteine (which increase the free SH groups of tissues) markedly raises resistance to the diabetogenic action of alloxan. These procedures also diminish the incidence of diabetes after subtotal pancreatectomy in the rat, and can even produce permanent cures in a certain percentage of mild diabetic animals.

Martin B88,524/53: In rats, both chloroform and alloxan produce hepatic necrosis and their effect is increased when both agents are given in combination. Thiouracil protects against this form of hepatic necrosis, whereas thyroid feeding aggravates it.

Houssay et al. C15,702/55: In dogs, destruction of the thyroid by ^{131}I alleviates alloxan diabetes.

Hasselblatt & Bastian C59,171/58: In mice sensitivity to insulin convulsions is increased by thyroxine and even more markedly by tolbutamide.

Altieri et al. C71,565/58: In rats, the toxic and diabetogenic effects of alloxan are aggravated by thyroid feeding and inhibited by ^{131}I.

Epinephrine and Norepinephrine ← *cf. also Selye C92,918/61, pp. 112, 123, 194; G60,083/70, pp. 334, 404.*

Busso 26,684/25: In rats, thyroidectomy does not change the resistance to epinephrine or phenol. Morphine appears to be slightly more toxic to thyroidectomized than to intact rats, but the results were irregular.

Spinelli 10,086/31: In guinea pigs, thyroidectomy increases the resistance to histamine, acetonitrile, picrotoxin, aconitine, epinephrine, nicotine, and atropine but augments sensitivity to pilocarpine and guanidine.

Peltola B57,468/50: In mice, the lethal effect of epinephrine is dose-dependently increased by pretreatment with thyroid powder. This can serve as a basis for the bioassay of thyroid preparations.

Kroneberg & Hüter B69,838/51: In mice, pretreatment with thyroxine increases mortality to subsequently administered epinephrine, whereas norepinephrine sensitivity is essentially unchanged.

Thibault & Lachaze B69,990/51: In vitro, the effect of epinephrine upon the contraction of the isolated rabbit intestine, spleen and uterus is enhanced by conjoint application of thyroxamine, the "active form of thyroxine."

Kroneberg B87,448/52: In mice, the toxicity of epinephrine, unlike that of norepinephrine, is greatly increased following thyroxine pretreatment.

Brewster Jr. et al. C11,771/56: In dogs, the physiologic changes produced by thyroid extract are abolished following sympathetic blockade. The inotropic, chronotropic and calorigenic effects of epinephrine and norepinephrine are increased by thyroid feeding. "It is concluded that there is a dynamic interrelationship between the thyroid hormones and those of the adrenal medulla and sympathetic nerve endings."

Swanson C22,149/56: In rats, thyroidectomy inhibited while thyroxine potentiated the calorigenic effect of epinephrine.

Osorio C31,059/56: In rats, hypothyroidism (^{131}I, propylthiouracil, thyroidectomy) decreased, whereas hyperthyroidism (desiccated thyroid) increased vascular reactivity to epinephrine, norepinephrine, and angiotensin.

Oester C84,324/59: In rabbits, the arteriosclerosis produced by combined treatment with epinephrine + thyroxine is readily influenced by various conditioning factors.

Hoch D25,881/62: Review (68 pp., 611 refs.) on the biochemical actions of thyroid hormones with a special section on their interactions with epinephrine.

Halpern et al. G67,689/63: In mice, thyroxine greatly increases the toxicity of various sympathomimetic compounds, such as amphetamine, ephedrine, dopa, and dopamine. The toxicity of tyramine and norepinephrine is less markedly enhanced and that of mepiramine is uninfluenced.

Proulx et al. G43,289/66: In rats made hyperthyroid by feeding iodinated casein, "there was a 25% decrease in liver monoamine oxidase and this decrease does not appear to be related to a decrease in body weight. Liver catechol-0-methyl transferase activity was normal in hyperthyroid animals."

Svedmyr G39,171/66: In rabbits, thyroxine potentiates the calorigenic and hyperlactacidemic effect of epinephrine, leaving its hyperglycemic effect undiminished. Thyroidectomy decreases the calorigenic and hyperlactacidemic actions of epinephrine. The metabolic effects of norepinephrine are less strikingly affected by the thyroid.

Epinephrine ← cf. also Table 23

Histamine and 5-HT ←

Spinelli 14,294/29: In guinea pigs, thyroidectomy protects against otherwise fatal histamine intoxication.

Spinelli 10,086/31: In guinea pigs, thyroidectomy increases the resistance to histamine, acetonitrile, picrotoxin, aconitine, epinephrine, nicotine, and atropine, but augments sensibility to pilocarpine and guanidine.

Gyermek & Pataky B65,706/50: In guinea pigs, thyroxine does not influence the bronchoconstriction induced by histamine aerosol.

Sackler et al. B78,749/53: In rats, thyroparathyroidectomy increases histamine tolerance, but only in females. Intact rats show no sex difference in histamine tolerance. Gonadectomy raises histamine tolerance in both sexes.

Long C32,348/57: In guinea pigs, both anaphylactic shock (horse serum) and sensitivity to histamine are greatly increased by pretreatment with thyroxine. Thyroxine also augments the sensitivity of guinea pigs to intradermal tuberculin injection.

Jasmin & Bois C92,099/60: Rats pretreated with thyroxine become extremely sensitive to 5-HT, and readily die in a state of shock reminiscent of anaphylaxis.

Parratt & West D235/60: In rats, pretreatment with thyroxine greatly increases sensitivity to dextran, egg white, polymyxin B, compound 48/80, histamine, and 5-HT so that in addition to the anaphylactoid edema, there develops edema and hemorrhage in the intestinal tract. The effect is ascribed to inhibition of intestinal histaminase by thyroxine.

Panisset et al. F71,775/66: In vitro observations on isolated organs (duodenum, uterus, lung) of rats indicate that thyroxine inhibits the action of 5-HT upon smooth muscle. Conversely, in the perfused hindquarter, the vasomotor effect of 5-HT was enhanced by thyroxine.

Skinohø & Quaade G72,600/69: In man, wheal formation following intracutaneous injection of 5-HT is reduced in myxedema and increased in thyrotoxicosis. A control study with histamine revealed normal reactivity in myxedema and increased response in thyrotoxicosis.

Angiotensin ←

Osorio C31,059/56: In rats, hypothyroidism (^{131}I, propylthiouracil, thyroidectomy) decreased, whereas hyperthyroidism (desiccated thyroid) increased vascular reactivity to epinephrine, norepinephrine, and angiotensin.

Drugs ←

One of the earliest observations on the effect of hormones upon resistance is the great increase in **acetonitrile** tolerance induced by thyroid preparations in the mouse. During the earliest years of the present century this effect was generally used as the basis for the assay of thyroid preparations and even for the determination of thyroid hormone in blood. This so-called "Reid Hunt test" is fairly specific in that other cyanides are not detoxified by thyroid preparations, and other iodine compounds are virtually ineffective in raising acetonitrile resistance. Curiously, in many species such as the rat, thyroid preparations do not protect against acetonitrile and may even decrease resistance to it. Still, even in mice, the specificity of the acetonitrile test is far from absolute, its outcome depending among others, upon the diet, age, and genetic background of the test animals. Hence, the Reid Hunt test is no longer used for bioassay purposes, yet its underlying mechanism continues to be an intriguing problem.

In mice, thyroxine increases the toxicity of **amphetamine** (as it does that of epinephrine and norepinephrine). It has been claimed that this sensitization occurs especially when the animals are kept under crowded conditions, but the phenomenon is evident even in individually caged mice. T3 shares this effect of thyroxine. Allegedly, the mortality induced by amphetamine is actually inhibited during the first hour after thyroxine treatment. In rats, thyroidectomy does not significantly affect amphetamine tolerance, but methylthiouracil reduces it, and T3 aggravates it.

Sensitivity to **anaphylactoidogenic agents** is increased by thyroxine and decreased by thyroidectomy or methylthiouracil treatment in the rat. These observations agree with the similar effects of thyroid hormones upon 5-HT and histamine toxicity as previously discussed.

Numerous investigators dealt with the effect of thyroid hormones upon **barbiturate** intoxication. One of the first observations along these lines was made in cats in which profound phenobarbital anesthesia allegedly inhibits a rise in BMR produced by thyroxine.

In the mouse, the toxic effects of several barbiturates are aggravated, and sleeping time is prolonged by thyroid preparations. The latter also delay the removal of barbiturates from the plasma and tissues of the mouse, whereas thioureas have an inverse effect. However, thyroidectomy allegedly also increases pentobarbital sleeping time.

In rabbits, phenobarbital resistance is said to rise during the first hours following thyroxine administration, whereas the narcotic effect of chloral hydrate is not affected. In rats, thyroidectomy prolongs, while thyroxine shortens pentobarbital anesthesia. It had been claimed at first that these effects are not accompanied by changes in hepatic barbiturate detoxication in vitro upon incubation with liver slices. However, more recent observations show that the activity of hexobarbital-metabolizing enzymes in hepatic microsomes is diminished by thyroxine, which would account for the prolongation of anesthesia. It is difficult to see why both thyroidectomy and thyroid preparations prolong barbiturate sleeping time. In fact, some investigators claim that propylthiouracil shortens pentobarbital anesthesia.

Resistance to **carbon monoxide** is diminished by thyroid feeding in rats, presumably because the increased BMR augments oxygen requirements.

According to some investigators, the hepatic cirrhosis produced by **carbon tetrachloride** in the rat is aggravated both by thyroxine and by thiouracil. However, the published results are quite contradictory, presumably because of differences in dosage and timing. Extensive recent investigations suggest that thyroidectomy diminishes, whereas thyroid extract increases the hepatotoxicity of CCl_4; particularly good protection against hepatic cirrhosis is obtained in rats simultaneously thyroidectomized and ovariectomized.

The influence of the thyroid upon the actions of **carcinogens** has also been extensively investigated. The production of cystic and neoplastic hepatic lesions by 2-acetaminofluorene in rats is inhibited by thiouracil; concurrent treatment with thyroid powder and testosterone sensitizes for this carcinogen. Prostatic carcinogenesis induced by topical application of 20-methylcholanthrene is said to be inhibited by T3 without being affected by methylthiouracil.

The anesthetic effect of **chloral hydrate** is not conspicuously affected by thyroid preparations in the mouse, rat or rabbit.

The toxicity of **chlordiazepoxide** is increased by a thyroid extract or T3 in the mouse, whereas methylthiouracil appears to have an opposite effect.

The hepatotoxicity of **chloroform** is increased by a thyroid extract and diminished by thiouracil in rats and rabbits.

In rabbits, **cholesterol** atheromatosis and the associated xanthomatous lesions in the liver are inhibited by thyroxine and increased by thyroidectomy or thiouracil treatment. In chicks, various thyroid preparations diminish the hypercholesterolemia, but do not significantly suppress the coronary or aortic atherogenesis. In rats fed a high-fat, high-cholesterol diet, the increase in hepatic and plasma cholesterol is not significantly changed by thyroxine. However, both D- and L-T3 diminish the changes in plasma lipids while aggravating the hepatic lesions.

The pyrogenic effect of **cocaine** is increased to fatal levels in rabbits pretreated with thyroxine. In rats, thyroxine also aggravates cocaine intoxication.

In view of the excellent protection offered by thyroid preparations against acetonitrile in the mouse, the effects upon other **cyano-compounds** have also been investigated, but sensitivity to these is not strikingly affected by the thyroid.

Since **digitalis** compounds are extensively used in studies on protective steroids, it is of interest that thyroid preparations augment the hemodynamic effects of digitalin in the rabbit, and aggravate the cardiac lesions produced by digitalis alkaloids in cats. Sensitization to digitalis, and particularly to digitoxin, has been observed in various species using different indicators of activity. It is also noteworthy that therapeutic doses of cardiac glycosides allegedly prevent the thyroxine-induced weight loss in the guinea pig. The convulsions and mortality induced by digitoxin overdosage in the rat are not prevented by thyroidectomy or propylthiouracil, nor do these agents inhibit the antidigitoxin activity of PCN. Apparently, the mild goitrogenic effect of the latter is not involved in its protective action against digitoxin.

The toxicity of **ephedrine** (like that of amphetamine, epinephrine and norepinephrine) is increased by thyroxine, not only in "aggregated" mice as claimed previously, but also in separately caged animals.

The toxicity of **imipramine** is increased by thyroxine or T3, and decreased by thiourea in the mouse.

The catatoxic effect of ethylestrenol against **indomethacin**-induced intestinal ulceration and mortality is inhibited by thyroxine in the rat. Given by itself, thyroxine shortens survival after indomethacin intoxication.

The skeletal changes produced by **lathyrogens** in the rat are most actively prevented by various thyroid preparations and aggravated by thyroidectomy or thiouracil. Neurolathyrism produced by IDPN and other neurolathyrogens are similarly influenced, but angiolathyrism is not significantly affected by thyroid hormones. T3 is about 50 times as potent as thyroxine in preventing osteolathyrism. Since both L- and D-T3 suppress osteolathyrism in the rat, the effect is allegedly independent of the classical thyroid hormone actions.

The nephrocalcinosis characteristic of **magnesium** deficiency is prevented by thyroxine in the rat, but allegedly some manifestations of the Mg-deprivation are also inhibited by thyroparathyroidectomy.

Meprobamate intoxication is counteracted by catatoxic steroids but aggravated by thyroxine; in the case of concurrent administration of the two types of hormones, they mutually tend to antagonize each other's influence in this respect.

Morphine resistance is diminished in mice, rats, and guinea pigs by pretreatment with thyroid extracts. Thyroidectomy does not appear to have a consistent effect upon morphine intoxication or upon the development of morphine withdrawal symptoms. However, in most of these respects, the published data are contradictory.

The fatal pulmonary edema produced by **ozone** inhalation in mice and rats is prevented by thiourea and aggravated by thyroxine or T3. Thyroxine and T3 increase the sensitivity of the mouse and rat to the induction of convulsions by **pentylenetetrazol**. The influence of thyroidectomy and thiouracil is less clear-cut.

Thyroxine increases the toxicity of several **pesticides** and antagonizes the protective action of catatoxic steroids. However, this effect of the thyroid hormone is rarely very pronounced, and often absent.

The nephrocalcinosis produced in rats by dietary excess of certain **phosphates** is inhibited both by thyroparathyroidectomy and by thyroxine in the rat. However, allegedly, propylthiouracil increases this type of nephrocalcinosis.

Physostigmine intoxication is aggravated by thyroxine in the rat.

Picrotoxin poisoning is inhibited by thyroidectomy in guinea pigs. In rats, thyroxine aggravates picrotoxin poisoning and counteracts the protective effect of ethylestrenol.

In mice and rats, thyroid preparations increase the toxicity of **reserpine.**

The characteristic syndrome of **tyrosine** intoxication (keratitis, conjunctivitis, alopecia, inflammation of the paws and snout) produced under certain conditions in young rats is inhibited by thiouracil and aggravated by thyroxine.

There undoubtedly exist close interrelations between the thyroid and **vitamin-A** metabolism. Earlier observations suggested that the toxicity of thyroxine is partly inhibited by carotene (the precursor of vitamin A) in the rat. Furthermore, in goats, the milk is normally rich in vitamin A, but virtually free of carotene, whereas the reverse is true after thyroidectomy. In guinea pigs, thyroxine inhibits the hepatic storage of carotene and its transformation into vitamin A. Early investigators claimed that hypervitaminosis A can be prevented by thyroxine in the rat, but subsequent experiments failed to confirm this. The pertinent literature is very confusing. In rats kept on a vitamin-A deficient diet, thiourea blocks the protective effect of carotene, and this blockade can be in turn abolished by thyroid powder. Yet, it was claimed that thiouracil prolongs the survival of the rat on a vitamin-A deficient diet.

In rats, the hepatic storage of vitamin A is increased by thyroxine, but the total vitamin-A storage of the body is unaffected. Both L- and D-T3 aggravate hypervitaminosis A in the rat. The offspring of rats given excessive amounts of vitamin A during pregnancy often show deformities of the skull and brain, which are aggravated by methylthiouracil treatment of the pregnant mother.

In pigeons kept on **vitamin-B** deficient polished rice, wasting and death were accelerated by thyroid feeding, but this may not have been true beriberi. In vitamin-B complex deficient rats, thyroid feeding aggravates the resulting skeletal lesions. On the other hand, survival on a thiamine deficient diet is prolonged in thyroparathyroidectomized rats, but not significantly altered by desiccated thyroid. Conversely, thiamine antagonizes thyroxine overdosage in the rat.

Vitamin-B_{12} requirements are greatly augmented by thyroxine in the rat, and although vitamin-B_{12} possesses no lipotropic potency itself, it prevents the hepatic steatosis produced in thyroxine-treated rats by hypolipotropic diets.

In guinea pigs fed **vitamin-C** deficient diets, the development of scurvy is accelerated by thyroid feeding. Thyroidectomy also aggravates the scorbutic lesions but does not accelerate their onset.

The development of bone lesions on **vitamin-D** deficient diets is not very consistently influenced by thyroidectomy or thyroid administration in the rat. However, the calcinosis produced by excess of vitamin D or DHT is aggravated by thyroxine in the rat. Curiously in rabbits, the calcinosis and other manifestations of vitamin-D_2 overdosage are accentuated by methylthiouracil, whereas in the cow, the production of calcinosis by vitamin-D_3 overdosage has been said to be prevented by thyroxine.

In the chick, **vitamin-E** requirements are increased by thyroid preparations and decreased by thiourea. In rats, the muscular dystrophy produced by vitamin-E deficiency is aggravated by thyroid feeding. In rabbits, suppression of thyroid activity by radioiodine exerts a certain prophylactic effect.

Zoxazolamine paralysis is aggravated by thyroidectomy and inhibited by thyroxine or T3 in the rat owing to changes in hepatic microsomal zoxazolamine metabolism.

Acetaldehyde ←

Lecoq et al. B66,406/51: In rats, the toxic effects of ethanol and its metabolites, pyruvate and acetaldehyde (which accumulate in the body under the influence of disulfiram) are inhibited by ACTH, cortisone, and hepatic extracts. Conversely, thyroxine, DOC, and testosterone appear to aggravate ethanol intoxication. [Statistically evaluated data are not presented (H.S.).]

2-Acetaminofluorene ← cf. Carcinogens (AAF)

Acetanilide ← cf. Table 24

Acetonitrile ←

GUINEA PIG

Spinelli 10,086/31: In guinea pigs thyroidectomy increases the resistance to histamine, acetonitrile, picrotoxin, aconitine, epinephrine, nicotine, and atropine, but augments sensitivity to pilocarpine and guanidine.

MOUSE

Hunt 60,064/05: In mice, thyroid feeding greatly increases resistance to acetonitrile but not to various other cyanides, such as hydrocyanic acid or sodium ferricyanide.

Hunt 49,717/07: In mice, acetonitrile resistance is increased by injections of the blood of hyperthyroid patients.

Hunt & Seidell 46,617/10: In mice, the protective effect of thyroid extract against acetonitrile is due to the hormone itself and not to iodine. Other iodine preparations do not have a protective action. Unlike mice, rats are actually sensitized to acetonitrile by thyroid pretreatment.

Hunt 49,718/11: In mice, the resistance to acetonitrile induced by thyroid extract is subject to considerable variation depending upon the diet.

Wuth A 48,026/21: In mice, tyramine and diiodotyramine, like thyroid extract, offer protection against acetonitrile whereas histamine does not.

Miura 13,081/22: Mice are protected against acetonitrile by thyroxine and desiccated thyroid, but not by KI or T2.

Hunt 13,889/23: Pretreatment with thyroid preparations greatly increases the resistance of mice to acetonitrile, whereas the reverse is true in many other species.

Gellhorn 16,839/23: In mice, resistance against acetonitrile can be increased not only by thyroid extract, but to a lesser extent also by extracts of various other tissues. These preparations also augment resistance to KCN and propionitrile, whereas thyroidectomy and orchidectomy have an opposite effect.

von Zwehl 25,477/26: Female mice pretreated with repeated doses of T2 tolerate 2—3 lethal doses of acetonitrile, whereas in males, a significant protective effect could not be demonstrated.

Paal 22,603/30: Review of the literature, and extensive personal studies on acetonitrile test in mice, and its use for the determination of thyroid hormone in human blood. Thyroidectomy does not increase the resistance of mice to acetonitrile, but diminishes the protective effect of thyroxine. Concurrent treatment with insulin also inhibits the prevention of acetonitrile toxicity by thyroxine.

Knaab 14,828/33: Discussion of the earlier literature, and personal observations on factors influencing the effect of thyroxine upon acetonitrile resistance in the mouse.

Montgomery 18,184/33: Review of the literature on the acetonitrile test for thyroid preparations in mice. The protective effect of thyroid is confirmed, but individual variations and dietary factors alter responsiveness so much that the technique is unsuited for bioassay purposes.

Grab 44,536/33: In mice, about 50 μg of thyroxine suffices to protect with certainty against otherwise lethal acetonitrile intoxication.

Paal 18,183/33: In mice, exposure to light greatly influences sensitivity to acetonitrile. Even after thyroidectomy, daylight as well as ultraviolet irradiation increase the MLD of acetonitrile. Hence, resistance to this drug is not always influenced through variations in thyroid activity.

Santo 27,439/34: Review on the factors influencing the Reid Hunt-reaction in mice.

Fellinger & Hochstädt 63,744/35: In mice, the protection against acetonitrile offered by thyroxine or TTH is blocked by an extract of blood that contains the "ether soluble antithyroid substances."

Fleischmann & Kann 67,360/36: In mice, vitamin A antagonizes the protective effect of thyroxine against acetonitrile intoxication. Vitamin A also antagonizes the effect of thyroxine upon tadpole metamorphosis.

Dietrich & Beutner B20,412/44: In mice, thiourea and thiouracil interfere with the action of orally administered thyroid powder when the Reid Hunt test is made the basis of observations. In this test, minute amounts of whole thyroid can be detected by their protective effect against otherwise lethal doses of acetonitrile.

VARIA

Hunt 49,716/07: Comparative studies on the effect of thyroid extract upon the acetonitrile and morphine resistance of mice, rats, and guinea pigs.

Hunt & Seidell 50,346/09: Monograph (115 pp.) on the use of the acetonitrile test for thyroid function. In rats, thyroid feeding actually lowers resistance to acetonitrile.

Hunt 50,349/10: Very detailed description of the acetonitrile test for thyroid. Here, special attention is placed upon the modifying influence of the diet, seasonal variations, species, and other conditioning factors.

Oehme & Paal 62,442/32: Review (42 pp., about 200 refs.) on the technique and clinical applications of the acetonitrile test for thyroid action, with a survey of the numerous factors that can influence its outcome.

Aconitine ←

Spinelli 10,086/31: In guinea pigs thyroidectomy increases the resistance to histamine, acetonitrile, picrotoxin, aconitine, epinephrine, nicotine, and atropine, but augments sensitivity to pilocarpine and guanidine.

Acrylamide ← *cf. Table 25*
Acrylonitrile ← *cf. Table 26*

Adenosine Diphosphate ←

Chandler & Nordöy G22,017/64: In rats, the pulmonary thrombi produced by ADP i.v. are stabilized by pretreatment with propylthiouracil, perhaps because the inactivation of ADP is delayed.

Allyl Alcohol ←

Srinivasan et al. G78,977/70: In rats, pretreatment with thyroxine aggravates the hepatic damage produced by allyl alcohol (judged by hepatic histology, serum GPT and BSP).

Allylformiate ←

Spiess-Bertschinger B40,585/44: In rats, the hepatic lesions produced by allylformiate are aggravated by thyroid feeding, but regenerative phenomena are active. After thyroidectomy, the hepatic lesions are particularly severe and characterized by necrosis without regeneration.

o-Aminophenol ← 6-Propylthiouracil, Mouse: Werder et al. *G12,065/64*
Aminopyrine ← *cf. Table 27*
Aminopyrine ← Thyroxine: Kato et al. *F57,817/65*
Aminopyrine ← Thyroidectomy: Orrenius et al. *G66,249/65*

p-Aminosalicylate ←

Mehrotra & Sarna D14,287/61: In rats, the hepatic lesions and glycogen infiltration produced by p-aminosalicylate (PAS) were not prevented by thyroxine. Hence, these changes are not due to hypothyroidism.

Amphetamine ←

MOUSE

Pfeifer et al. D12,952/60: In mice, the increased motility induced by amphetamine is inhibited during the first hour after thyroxine treatment. The possible biochemical reasons for this "negative tendency" during the early phase of thyroxine action are described.

Askew G72,695/62; Halpern et al. G11,305/63: In mice, thyroxine increases the lethal effect of amphetamine.

Halpern et al. G63,588/63: In mice, thyroxine pretreatment diminishes resistance to amphetamine and DL-dopa, especially under conditions of crowding.

Gayet-Hallion & Bouvet F16,484/64: In mice kept under crowded conditions, the toxicity of amphetamine is diminished by pretreatment with the blood of thyroidectomized horses.

Halpern et al. F24,137/64: In mice, the toxicity of amphetamine and ephedrine is increased by pretreatment with thyroxine not only—as had been previously shown—when several animals are kept together in a jar, but also when they are kept in solitary cages.

Moore F36,358/65: In mice, the toxicity of d-amphetamines is greatly augmented by pretreatment with T3. Simultaneously, there develops a dose-dependent reduction in the levels of brain, heart, and spleen norepinephrine, liver glycogen and blood glucose. Similar changes are observed if amphetamine is given to mice crowded ("aggregated") in small cages.

Moore G36,616/65: In mice, pretreatment with T3 greatly increases sensitivity to the lethal effect of amphetamine. "Chlorpromazine, phenoxybenzamine, and propranolol pretreatment reduced the lethality of d-amphetamine in hyperthyroid mice while α-methyl-m-tyrosine, α-methyl-p-tyrosine, and reserpine pretreatment did not. The toxicity of α-methyl-m-tyrosine was enhanced in hyperthyroid mice."

Winter G71,836/65: In mice, the toxicity of amphetamine, imipramine, chlordiazepoxide and pentylenetetrazol is increased by T3 or thyroid powder, whereas the narcotic effect of amobarbital and morphine is decreased. Methylthiouracil has, in general, opposing effects. [The experimental conditions are not described in sufficient detail to evaluate these findings (H.S.).]

Winter F64,465/66; F98,019/68: In mice, pretreatment with thyroid extract p.o. increases the toxicity of reserpine, chlordiazepoxide, imipramine, and amphetamine.

RAT

Tormey & Lasagna C80,689/60: In rats, thyroidectomy does not significantly affect tolerance to amphetamine.

Mantegazza & Riva F47,703/65: In rats, methylthiouracil reduces various manifestations of amphetamine intoxication.

Dolfini & Kobayashi F91,611/67: In rats, amphetamine causes more pronounced hyperthermia after pretreatment with T3 than following thyroidectomy or thiouracil treatment.

Mantegazza et al. H7,676/68: In rats, pretreatment with methylthiouracil reduces the toxicity, hyperthermia, hyperglycemia, and the increase in plasma free fatty acids induced by amphetamine more than the increased spontaneous activity and anorexia. This dissociation of effects might reflect an altered metabolic pattern of amphetamine.

Amyl Nitrate ←

Specht 13,475/23: In guinea pigs, neither thyroidectomy nor orchidectomy influences the course of the convulsions produced by amyl nitrate inhalation or electric irritation of peripheral nerves.

Anaphylactoid Edema ← *cf. also Selye G46,715/68, pp. 117, 180, 184, 199.*

Parratt & West D235/60: In rats, pretreatment with thyroxine greatly increases sensitivity to dextran, egg-white, polymyxin B, compound 48/80, histamine, and 5-HT so that in addition to the anaphylactoid edema, there develops edema and hemorrhage in the intestinal tract. The effect is ascribed to inhibition of intestinal histaminase by thyroxine.

Spencer & West D32,617/62: In rats, the anaphylactoid edema produced by dextran or egg-white is diminished by thyroidectomy or methylthiouracil, and increased by thyroxine or T3.

Aniline ← Thyroxine + Orchidectomy + Methyltestosterone: Kato et al. *F57,817/65* and glutamate exert similar effects in intact but not in adrenalectomized guinea pigs.

The lengthening of barbiturate sleeping time in adrenalectomized rats can be abolished by cortisone, but not by DOC. Pretreatment of adrenalectomized mice with cortisone or cortisol reduces the high rate of barbital uptake by the brain to normal, whereas DOC has no such effect.

Adrenalectomy inhibits the degradation of hexobarbital by liver slices of male rats; this effect can be counteracted by pretreatment with cortisone.

Chlorpromazine pretreatment reduces barbiturate sleeping time even in adrenalectomized rats.

In adrenalectomized rats maintained on NaCl, pretreatment with spironolactone still induces resistance to pentobarbital and hexobarbital, but not to phenobarbital. This is so even if the anesthetics are given in doses normally causing approximately equal anesthesia.

← **Gonadectomy.** It has been known since 1933, that male rats are less sensitive to barbiturate anesthesia than females, and that castration increases sensitivity of the male but not of the female. Testosterone raises the pentobarbital resistance of intact or ovariectomized females and castrate males, but has little effect upon the barbiturate sensitivity of intact males. Upon injections of pentobarbital, repeated every 90 min, adult male rats rapidly developed resistance, whereas females did not. Castration lowered the ability of adult males to develop tolerance. In females, ovariectomy may actually increase the ability to detoxify pentobarbital once tolerance has developed.

Barbital anesthesia does not appear to be considerably affected by orchidectomy in rats, presumably because unlike other barbiturates, barbital is not metabolized in the body.

Thyroidectomy, which in itself prolongs pentobarbital anesthesia, increases even further the barbiturate sensitivity of simultaneously orchidectomized rats.

The increased hexobarbital sleeping time of females and castrate males, as compared to intact males, is associated with a delay in barbiturate metabolism as reflected by the prolonged persistence of the drug in the blood, and by the decreased rate of detoxication in vitro, by liver slices or microsomal fractions.

The hexobarbital sleeping time, which is prolonged by orchidectomy in the rat, is shortened by testosterone, whereas cyproterone (an antitestoid) fails to inhibit the anti-anesthetic effect of testosterone; indeed, it actually shares this property.

The effect of gonadectomy and sex hormone treatment depends largely upon the species under investigation. Thus, in guinea pigs, orchidectomy and ovariectomy prolong pentobarbital sleeping time while testosterone diminishes it, in agreement with the results obtained in the rat.

On the other hand, in the mouse, hexobarbital anesthesia lasts longer in males than in females and orchidectomy decreases sleeping time, whereas ovariectomy does not affect it. Testosterone prolongs hexobarbital sleeping time in orchidectomized, intact male as well as in ovariectomized mice, and in the same species, this effect is blocked by cyproterone. In vitro experiments with the 9000g liver supernatant of female mice reveals a greater hexobarbital hydroxylating activity than a similar hepatic preparation made from male mice. After orchidectomy, the in vitro metabolism of hexobarbital becomes equal to that of female mice.

← **Varia.** In rats, pretreatment with hydroxydione does not significantly influence pentobarbital sleeping time. In mice, phenobarbital given one hour before hydroxydione increases sleeping time, but when the interval is two days, single doses of phenobarbital decrease hydroxydione anesthesia.

In rats, pentobarbital sleeping time is significantly decreased by DOC, 4-chlorotestosterone, aldosterone, and stilbestrol, when given 30 min before the barbiturate. Progesterone has an inverse effect, perhaps because of its own acute anesthetic action. On the other hand, chronic pretreatment with progesterone, stilbestrol or aldosterone decreased pentobarbital sleeping time without causing any significant change in the brain pentobarbital concentration.

Typical catatoxic steroids, such as ethylestrenol, spironolactone, and norbolethone diminish the depth of hexobarbital anesthesia in rats, and increase the aliphatic hydroxylation of this barbiturate by hepatic microsomes, thereby enhancing its elimination from the blood. The effect of these catatoxic steroids upon pentobarbital anesthesia is essentially the same. On the other hand, progesterone, SC-8109, and SC-5233 failed to affect pentobarbital sleeping time in the rat.

In mice, an aza-steroid (17α-methyl-17β-hydroxy-4-aza-estran-3-one) shortened the duration of hexobarbital anesthesia. Also in the mouse, pentobarbital anesthesia is shortened by ethylestrenol, CS-1, spironolactone, and norbolethone, but not by oxandrolone, prednisolone, progesterone, triamcinolone, DOC, hydroxydione, estradiol, or thyroxine.

Bilirubin ←

In mice, α-naphthylisothiocyanate-induced hyperbilirubinemia and cholestasis are aggravated by norethandrolone and norethynodrel, but not by mestranol. This response is largely dependent upon the ambient temperature.

Carbon Tetrachloride ←

The literature on the effect of various steroids upon CCl_4 poisoning is extensive but very contradictory. Most investigators agree, however, that under suitable conditions of timing and dosage, various glucocorticoids and testoids can protect the rat and several other species against the hepatotoxic action of CCl_4, whereas DOC and various folliculoids appear to have an inverse effect.

Ovariectomy protects the liver against CCl_4 intoxication, perhaps because it removes the source of endogenous folliculoids whose hepatic degradation might compete with the defense against CCl_4. Particularly good protection is obtained if ovariectomy is combined with thyroidectomy. Even adrenalectomy and hypophysectomy inhibit the CCl_4-induced hepatic steatosis in the rat; here substitution therapy with corticoids allegedly restores normal responsiveness. Enovid (mestranol + norethynodrel) aggravates the liver damage caused by CCl_4 in rats.

The apparent contradictions in the findings of various investigators may well be due in part to differences in the actions of steroids, depending upon the criteria used (hepatic steatosis, necroses, regeneration, sclerosis), as well as the dosage and timing of the steroids and of CCl_4.

Anticoagulants ←

Lowenthal & Fisher C 40,044/57: In rats, the anticoagulant effect of warfarin is increased by thyroxine and diminished by hypothyroidism (methimazole treatment).

Owens et al. D 21,725/62: In man, dextrothyroxine potentiates the anticoagulant action of warfarin.

Solomon & Schrogie H 1,868/68: In women, thyroxine greatly potentiates the anticoagulant effect of warfarin. Analysis of the data (according to the method of Lineweaver and Burk) suggests that an increased affinity of the drug for its receptor site is responsible for the potentiation of its effect. The literature on the increase in the response to various indirect anticoagulants by thyroxine in man is briefly reviewed.

Selye G 60,094/70: In rats, the fatal hemorrhagic diathesis produced by phenindione is inhibited by ethylestrenol, CS-1, spironolactone, norbolethone, and oxandrolone. Progesterone, hydroxydione, DOC, and estradiol have a much less pronounced effect. Prednisolone, triamcinolone, and thyroxine are inactive.

Selye G 70,428/70: In rats, ethylestrenol powerfully inhibits the toxicity of digitoxin, nicotine, indomethacin, phenindione, dioxathion, EPN, physostigmine, hexobarbital, cyclopental, thiopental, DOC (anesthesia), meprobamate, and picrotoxin. Thyroxine increases the toxicity of many among these drugs and inhibits the protective effect of ethylestrenol.

Bishydroxycoumarin ← *cf. also Table 28*
Phenindione ← *cf. also Table 29*

Antimony ←

Shih-Chi et al. C 72,194/58: In mice, thyroxine decreases, whereas propylthiouracil increases resistance to the fatal effect of intoxication with ammonium antimonyl gluconate i.p. The differences are not explicable on the basis of the distribution or excretion of antimony.

Arsenic ←

Hunt & Seidell 50,346/09: In mice, pretreatment with thyroid extract does not influence resistance to sodium arsenate.

Bogdanovitch & Varagitch G 71,534/54; Bogdanovitch C 18,912/56: In rats, pretreatment with thyroid extract increases, whereas methylthiouracil decreases the toxicity of organic arsenicals such as oxophenarsine or dichlorophenarsine.

Atropine ←

Hunt & Seidell 50,346/09: In mice, pretreatment with thyroid extract does not change resistance to atropine.

Spinelli 10,086/31: In guinea pigs, thyroidectomy increases the resistance to histamine, acetonitrile, picrotoxin, aconitine, epinephrine, nicotine, and atropine, but augments sensitivity to pilocarpine and guanidine.

Barbiturates ←

CAT

von Issekutz & von Issekutz Jr. 45,261/35: In cats, profound phenobarbital anesthesia inhibits the rise in BMR normally produced by thyroxine. It is assumed that thyroxine raises oxygen consumption indirectly through an effect upon the higher nervous centers.

FROG

Richards 79,646/41: In the frog, stimulation of metabolism by thyroxine increases susceptibility to pentobarbital.

MOUSE

Prange Jr. & Lipton F 56,756/65: In mice, the toxic effects of the convulsant barbiturate 5-(1,3-dimethylbutyl)-5-ethyl barbituric acid (DMBEB) are aggravated by desiccated thyroid p.o., and diminished by propylthiouracil.

Winter G 71,836/65: In mice, the toxicity of amphetamine, imipramine, chlordiazepoxide and pentylenetetrazol is increased by T3 or thyroid powder, whereas the narcotic effect of amobarbital and morphine is decreased. Methylthiouracil has, in general, opposing effects. [The experimental conditions are not described in sufficient detail to evaluate these findings (H.S.).]

Schrogie & Solomon C 43,019/66: In mice, the metabolism of bishydroxycoumarin was markedly inhibited by both L-and D-thyroxine. The demethylation of meperidine was likewise inhibited by both isomers but particularly by D-thyroxine. L-thyroxine also increased the lethal effect of meperidine overdosage. Pentobarbital sleeping time was prolonged in mice treated with either L- or D-thyroxine, but the latter was more active in this respect.

Ellinwood F 64,417/66: In mice, dichloroisoproterenol (a β-adrenergic blocker) does not influence pentobarbital sleeping time and, far from inhibiting, actually potentiates the prolongation of anesthesia by thyroid feeding. It is unlikely therefore that thyroid would increase barbiturate hypnosis through the production of epinephrine.

Klinger F66,416/66: In mice and rats, large doses of thyroxine prolong hexobarbital sleeping time and diminish the resistance induced by barbital pretreatment. The associated changes in ascorbic acid metabolism are discussed.

Prange et al. G40,154/66: In mice, thyroid feeding increases sensitivity to various barbiturates and delays their removal from the brain, liver, and plasma. Propylthiouracil has an inverse effect. In rats, thyroxine slightly and thyroidectomy markedly increase pentobarbital sleeping time.

Spencer and Waite H30,100/70: In mice, pretreatment with thyroxine enhances the hypnotic effect of very small doses of thiopental. Earlier experimenters had shown that hyperthyroidism increases sensitivity to larger doses of barbiturates, but in the present case, metabolic studies suggest that an "enhanced rate of redistribution of thiopentone brought about by increased pheripheral and cerebral blood flow in hyperthyroid mice" was probably responsible for the diminished anesthetic effect.

Hexobarbital ← Thiouracil, Mouse: Wenzel et al. G76,357/55*

Hexobarbital ← Triiodothyronine, Mouse: Holtz et al. C76,300/58*

Pentobarbital, Thiopental ← Thyroid extract, Mouse: Ellinwood et al. E39,187/64*; Prange et al. G40,154/66*

RABBIT

Zárday & Weiner: 53,715/35: In rabbits, thyroxine s.c. does not influence the narcotic effect of chloral hydrate given a few hours later. On the other hand, the resistance to phenobarbital rises through the influence of thyroxine under similar conditions.

RAT

Scarborough 34,971/36: In rats, feeding of thyroid extract diminishes the anesthetic effect of pentobarbital.

Horinaga A36,414/41: Thyroidectomy increases barbiturate sensitivity in the rat.

Robillard et al. B66,661/51: In rats, thyroidectomy prolongs pentobarbital anesthesia and delays hepatic detoxication of the drug, whereas thyroxine pretreatment diminishes the duration and depth of this anesthesia without enhancing the hepatic detoxication of pentobarbital as determined by incubation of the drug with liver slices. After simultaneous thyroidectomy and orchidectomy, pentobarbital detoxication is more markedly delayed than after simple thyroidectomy or orchidectomy, and the anesthetic effect is correspondingly further intensified than after ablation of the thyroid or testes alone.

Holck et al. B95,270/54: In rats, thyroidectomy or propylthiouracil treatment increased the recovery time from isopropyl-β-bromallyl barbituric acid, propallylonal (Nostal), thiopental, and hexobarbital. Thyroglobulin or thyroxine caused no consistent shortening of the average recovery time from isopropyl-β-bromallyl barbituric acid; propallylonal (Nostal). Either of these effects is also largely influenced by the sex of the animals.

Robillard et al. G67,325/54: Thyroidectomy prolongs pentobarbital anesthesia in intact, and even much more in castrate adult male rats. Thyroxine decreases the anesthetic effect of pentobarbital in thyroidectomized rats even below the normal level. Liver homogenates of thyroidectomized rats metabolize pentobarbital in vitro less rapidly than those of normal rats, but pretreatment in vivo with thyroxine does not increase the pentobarbital-metabolizing activity of these homogenates above the control value.

Lanzetta C68,990/58: In rats, thyroxine or dinitrophenol given i.p. 30 min before thiopental prolongs the anesthetic effect of the latter, presumably through uncoupling of oxidative phosphorylation.

Conney & Garren D93,666/61: In the rat, thyroxine prolongs the duration of hexobarbital anesthesia by decreasing the activity of hexobarbital-metabolizing enzymes in hepatic microsomes.

Kato & Gillette F57,817/65: The metabolism of aminopyrine and hexobarbital by hepatic microsomes of male rats is impaired by adrenalectomy, castration, hypoxia, ACTH, formaldehyde, epinephrine, morphine, alloxan, or thyroxine. The metabolism of aniline and zoxazolamine is not appreciably decreased by any of these agents; in fact, the hydroxylation of aniline is enhanced by thyroxine or alloxan. Apparently, the treatments impair mainly the sex-dependent enzymes. Accordingly, the corresponding enzymic functions of the hepatic microsomes of female rats are not significantly impaired by the agents which do have an inhibitory effect in males.

Kato & Takahashi G55,715/68: Thyroxine decreased the N-demethylation of aminopyrine and hydroxylation of hexobarbital by liver microsomes of male rats. By contrast, thyroxine increased the metabolism of aminopyrine and hexobarbital in females. The hydroxylation of aniline and reduction of p-nitrobenzoic acid were increased in both sexes. The effect of thyroxine and thyroidectomy upon other microsomal enzyme systems has also been examined.

Harbison & Becker H10,917/69: Thyroidectomy greatly prolonged hexobarbital sleeping time and zoxazolamine paralysis in rats. T3 increased the response to hexobarbital but diminished the effect of zoxazolamine. The mortality rates induced by high doses of hexobarbital, thiopental, amobarbital, pentobarbital, and phenobarbital were all significantly increased in rats pretreated with T3.

Kato et al. H11,854/69: "The administration of thyroxine or starvation resulted in marked decrease in the hydroxylation of pentobarbital and hexobarbital and N-demethylation of aminopyrine in male rats, whereas the hydroxylation of aniline and zoxazolamine and N-demethylation of N-methylaniline were significantly increased."

Selye G70,428/70: In rats, ethylestrenol powerfully inhibits the toxicity of digitoxin, nicotine, indomethacin, phenindione, dioxathion, EPN, physostigmine, hexobarbital, cyclopental, thiopental, DOC (anesthesia), meprobamate, and picrotoxin. Thyroxine increases the toxicity of many among these drugs and inhibits the protective effect of ethylestrenol.

Barbiturates ← *cf. also Tables 30—34*

VARIA

Glaubach & Pick 11,431/30: In guinea pigs and rabbits, the hypothermia produced by phenobarbital is counteracted by thyroxine pretreatment.

Zárday & Weiner A52,879/34: Anesthesia with morphine in rats, and with chloral hydrate in rabbits was not significantly influenced by pretreatment with thyroxine s.c., one hour before the anesthetics. On the other hand, phenobarbital anesthesia was prolonged by thyroxine pretreatment in rabbits under identical conditions. Similar observations have been made on patients suffering from thyrotoxicosis, in that they are unusually resistant to barbiturates but not to other anesthetics. This selective antagonism is ascribed to interactions between thyroxine and barbiturates at some common receptor site in the midbrain.

Ellinwood Jr. & Prange Jr. E39,187/64: Review of earlier observations on the effect of thyroid and thiourea preparations upon pentobarbital sleeping time in mice and rats. Since thyroid hormones and epinephrine are synergistic in many respects, mice were treated with various combinations of these agents. Pentobarbital anesthesia was prolonged by desiccated thyroid and shortened by propylthiouracil pretreatment. High doses of epinephrine prolonged sleeping time in themselves and potentiated the effect of thyroid feeding. The prolongation of pentobarbital sleeping time by epinephrine may be due to depletion of hepatic glycogen which interferes with hepatic microsomal drug metabolism.

Barbital ← Thyroidectomy: Boyland et al. D47,605/62*

Hexobarbital ← Thyroxine: Conney et al. *D93,666/61**

Pentobarbital ← Thyroidectomy + Thyroxine: Robillard et al. *G67,325/54**; Prange et al. G40,154/66*

Bilirubin ← Triiodothyronine + Age, Man: Lees et al. C74,543/59*

Cadmium ← *cf. Table 35*

Caffeine ←

Hunt & Seidell 50,346/09: In mice, pretreatment with thyroid extract did not change resistance to caffeine.

Strubelt et al. G78,572/70: In rats, T3 increases, whereas thyroidectomy decreases, the calorigenic response to theophylline and caffeine, probably because the thyroid hormone activates adenyl cyclase and/or inhibits phosphodiesterase.

Caramiphen ← *cf. Table 36*

Carbon Dioxide ←

Barbour & Seevers 84,296/43: In rats, exposure to cold and an excess of CO_2 produces a state of narcosis against which considerable resistance can be induced by thyroid extract. No such effect was obtained by dinitrophenol.

Carbon Monoxide ←

Mack & Smith 45,162/34: In rats, both thyroid feeding and dinitrophenol shorten survival during CO poisoning.

Smith et al. 45,163/35: Male rats are more sensitive to the lethal action of illuminating gas than females. This difference is eliminated by gonadectomy. Thyroid feeding or dinitrophenol injections decrease survival time.

Carbon Tetrachloride ←

Lesca & Mosca B48,329/49: In rats, the hepatic cirrhosis produced by CCl_4 is aggravated both by thiouracil and by thyroxine. However, survival time is increased in the thyroxine-treated rat.

Aragona & Barone B92,455/53: In rats, thyroxine protects the liver against the damaging effect of CCl_4.

Calvert & Brody C82,829/60: In rats, brief pretreatment with thyroxine increases, whereas previous thyroidectomy diminishes the metabolic changes produced by CCl_4 intoxication. Adrenal catecholamines are strongly reduced in hyperthyroid and only slightly reduced in hypothyroid animals. "The changes are consistent with a concept of anoxia being the primary event in CCl_4 hepatotoxicity."

Calvert & Brody D61,412/61: Thyroxine pretreatment increases the susceptibility of the rat to the hepatotoxicity of CCl_4.

Kulcsár-Gergely & Kulcsár G71,532/62; E33,917/63: In rats, thyroidectomy diminishes, whereas thyroid extract increases the hepatotoxicity of CCl_4. Correspondingly, the sexual cycle is accelerated by thyroidectomy and delayed by thyroid hormone treatment as a result of changes in hepatic folliculoid degradation.

Kulcsár-Gergely et al. F32,037/64: In rats, simultaneous thyroidectomy and ovariectomy offer some protection against the induction of hepatic cirrhosis by CCl_4.

Kulcsár-Gergely & Kulcsár G1,372/64: In rats intoxicated with CCl_4, survival is increased by ovariectomy and thyroidectomy.

Berencsi et al. G33,802/65: In rats, the production of hepatic lesions by CCl_4 is diminished after thyroidectomy or methylthiouracil treatment.

Berencsi & Krompecher G43,712/66: In rats, the hepatic damage caused by CCl_4 is decreased by thyroidectomy or methylthiouracil and increased by thyroxine or T3.

Kulcsár & Kulcsár-Gergely F74,930/66: In rats, ovariectomy, thyroidectomy, or removal of both glands, offers partial protection against CCl_4 intoxication.

Srinivasan & Balwani G64,503/68: In rats, pretreatment with thyroxine increased the liver damage produced by subsequent administration of CCl_4 or thioacetamide.

Kulcsár et al. H14,649/69: In rats, thyroidectomy offers some protection against the production of hepatic damage by CCl_4; this may be due to altered mucopolysaccharide formation.

Kulcsár et al. H24,478/70: In rats, thyroxine increases, whereas thyroidectomy decreases, the hepatotoxicity of CCl_4 as judged by BSP elimination.

Carcinogens ←

Cantarow et al. B18,774/46: In rats given 2-acetaminofluorene p.o., the development of cystic and neoplastic hepatic lesions was accelerated and intensified by GTH (pregnant mare serum), estradiol, and testosterone, but inhibited by thiouracil. "This phenomenon may be related to the role of the liver in the intermediary metabolism and excretion of the sex steroid." In the hyperplastic target organs of the sex hormones, tumors did not occur, in contrast to the high incidence of tumors in the thyroids of rats given thiouracil simultaneously with the carcinogens.

Miller Jr. & Baumann G74,552/51: Rats made hyperthyroid by feeding iodinated casein + p-dimethylaminoazobenzene (DAB), exhibited a high mortality, and the incidence of tumors in the survivors was very great. Thiouracil and propylthiouracil did not alter tumor incidence remarkably. "Liver slices from hyperthyroid rats destroyed less than one-fourth as much DAB as slices from normal rats."

Bielschowsky & Hall C194/53: In rats, the production of hepatomas by AF or AAF is inhibited following thyroidectomy. The protection is manifest only if the thyroid is removed before the administration of the carcinogens and even then it is restricted to the liver. The production by AF or AAF of extrahepatic neoplasms is not prevented.

Reid B93,930/54: Review (18 pp., 181 refs.) on the effect of STH and corticoids upon carcinogen-induced and transplantable neoplasms.

Klärner & Klärner C45,812/58: In BAF_1 mice, the growth of urethan-induced pulmonary tumors is significantly inhibited by alloxan diabetes and exposure to heat, but only slightly affected by thyroxine and insulin.

Bielschowsky D10,255/61: In rats, hypophysectomy, thyroidectomy and adrenalectomy inhibit the development of hepatomas by treatment with 2-acetylaminofluorene (AAF) or 2-aminofluorene (AF).

Leathem & Oddis D2,742/61: Female rats are less responsive than males to the induction of hepatomas by AAF. Thyroid feeding increases the incidence of hepatomas in females treated with AAF. It has the same effect in mice of both sexes given DMBA.

Sherwin-Weidenreich & Herrmann D67,842/63: In mice, tumor induction by DMBA is not inhibited. and perhaps even accelerated, by T3.

Sterental et al. D61,608/63: In rats, mammary tumors induced by DMBA regressed after adrenalectomy + ovariectomy or hypophysectomy. Folliculoid treatment reactivated tumor growth after adrenalectomy + ovariectomy but not after hypophysectomy. These tumors remained unresponsive to folliculoids after hypophysectomy even if thyroid and cortisone replacement therapy was given.

Reuber F4,431/64: In rats, the production of hepatomas by N-2-fluorenyldiacetamide was prevented by orchidectomy or thyroidectomy. However, the carcinogenic effect was restored in thyroidectomized animals by thyroid feeding.

Weidenreich-Sherwin & Herrmann F16,179/64: In mice, the production of skin tumors by topical application of 3-MC is considerably enhanced by T3.

Reuber F36,234/65: Concurrent treatment with testosterone and thyroid powder sensitizes the rat for the production of hepatic cirrhosis and hepatomas by N-2-fluorenyldiacetamide.

Goodall F71,302/66: In rats, the induction of hepatic tumors by 2-aminofluorene is inhibited by thyroidectomy.

Ronzoni et al. H18,409/68: In rats, prostatic carcinogenesis induced by the introduction of 20-methylcholanthrene crystals into the prostate is inhibited by ACTH, triiodothyronine and, to a lesser extent, by progesterone and 19-nortestosterone phenylpropionate. Estradiol and cortisone facilitate carcinogenesis, whereas testosterone, orchidectomy, and methylthiouracil failed to influence it.

Davidson et al. H10,206/69: In rats made hypothyroid by ^{131}I, the incidence of mammary cancer induction by DMBA is increased. Hypothyroidism induced by iodine deficiency did not share this effect and radio-iodine may have acted by radiation injury to the breast tissue rather than the associated hypothyroidism.

3-MC ← Thyroidectomy: Boyland et al. D47,605/62*

Carisoprodol ← cf. Table 37

Carotene ← cf. **Vitamin A**

Choline ←

Tabachnick et al. C50,317/58: In mice, thyroxine increases sensitivity to decamethonium and neostigmine but not to D-tubocurarine or succinylcholine. Rabbits pretreated with thyroxine also become more sensitive to decamethonium. It is tentatively suggested that the motor disturbances associated with hyperthyroidism may be due to "a change in the muscle itself, probably at the motor endplate where these drugs act."

Chloral Hydrate ←

Hunt & Seidell 50,346/09: In mice, pretreatment with thyroid extract questionably diminishes resistance to chloral hydrate.

Zárday & Weiner A52,879/34: Anesthesia with morphine in rats, and with chloral hydrate in rabbits was not significantly influenced by pretreatment with thyroxine s.c., one hour before the anesthetics. On the other hand, phenobarbital anesthesia was prolonged by thyroxine pretreatment in rabbits under identical conditions. Similar observations have been made on patients suffering from thyrotoxicosis, in that they are unusually resistant to barbiturates but not to other anesthetics. This selective antagonism is ascribed to interactions between thyroxine and barbiturates at some common receptor site in the midbrain.

Zárday & Weiner: 53,715/35: In rabbits, thyroxine s.c. does not influence the narcotic effect of chloral hydrate given a few hours later. On the other hand, the resistance to phenobarbital rises through the influence of thyroxine under similar conditions.

Chloralose ←

Cheymol & Quinquaud 3,531/32: In dogs, thyroparathyroidectomy greatly increases sensitivity to chloralose anesthesia.

Chlordiazepoxide ← cf. also Table 38

Winter G71,836/65; F64,465/66; Winter F98,019/68: In mice, the toxicity of amphetamine, imipramine, chlordiazepoxide and pentylenetetrazol is increased by T3 or thyroid powder, whereas the narcotic effect of amobarbital and morphine is decreased. Methylthiouracil has, in general, opposing effects.

Ashford & Ross H2,686/68: In mice, pretreatment with thyroid extract increased the toxicity of imipramine, nortriptyline, chlorpromazine, perphenazine, and chlordiazepoxide, whereas the toxicity of meprobamate and reserpine was not enhanced.

Chloroform ←

Hari 40,209/21: Polemic remarks concerning the technique and interpretation of earlier data on the effect of thyroidectomy upon the resistance to cyanides, chloroform, bacterial toxins, and oxygen deficiency.

McIver A 35,431/40: In rats, susceptibility to chloroform poisoning is increased by thyroxine.

Black-Schaffer et al. B 55,142/50: In rabbits, chloroform s.c. produces midzonal necrosis of the liver following pretreatment with thyroid extract. Normal or starved rabbits respond to chloroform with centrolobular necrosis. Presumably, "the hyperthyroid state selectively affects the hepatic midzone qualitatively or quantitatively so as to amplify its sensitivity to chloroform beyond that of the periportal or central zones."

Martin B 88,524/53: In rats, both chloroform and alloxan produce hepatic necrosis and their effect is increased when both agents are given in combination. Thiouracil protects against this form of hepatic necrosis whereas thyroid feeding aggravates it.

Chlorpromazine ←

Ashford & Ross H 2,686/68: In mice, pretreatment with thyroid extract increased the toxicity of imipramine, nortriptyline, chlorpromazine, perphenazine and chlordiazepoxide, whereas the toxicity of meprobamate and reserpine was not enhanced.

Skobba & Miya G 64,738/69: In rats, the hyperthermia produced by thyroxine or dinitrophenol increases the toxicity of chlorpromazine. Cooling the animals by an air current prevents this increase in toxicity.

Cholesterol ← cf. also *Selye G 60,083/70, pp. 385, 395.*

Suzue et al. 38,509/36: In rabbits, the production of xanthomatous lesions in the liver by a high-fat high-cholesterol diet is increased by thyroidectomy and inhibited by thyroxine.

Steiner et al. B 28,166/48: In dogs, thiouracil greatly enhances the production of atheromatosis by cholesterol feeding.

Stamler et al. C 81,655/58: In cholesterol-fed chicks, desiccated thyroid, thyroxine, T3 and T2 diminished hypercholesterolemia, but a definite and consistent suppression of coronary or aortic atherogenesis was not observed.

Osumi G 34,534/65: In cholesterol-fed rabbits, combined treatment with T3 and 3,5,3'-triiodo-4-acetyl-thyroformic acid (TBF-43) inhibited fatty degeneration of the liver, adrenal and spleen, but did not noticeably influence the atheromatous changes in the arteries.

Kessler et al. F 89,469/67: In rats fed a high-fat high-cholesterol diet, the resulting increase in hepatic and plasma cholesterol and lipid is not changed by either L- or D-thyroxine but D- or L-T3 diminishes the rise of both values in the serum and increases it further in the liver.

Danielsson & Tchen G 72,327/68 (p. 159): Brief summary of the influence of the thyroid upon cholesterol and bile acid metabolism.

Hamprecht G 69,560/69: Review (7 pp., 153 refs.) on the mechanisms regulating cholesterol synthesis. A special section deals with the effect of thyroid hormones, steroids, epinephrine, norepinephrine and glucagon.

Cholesterol ← Thyroxine: Mitropoulos et al. *G 26,978/65*

Cinchophen ← cf. Table 39

Clofibrate ←

Azarnoff & Svoboda H 19,856/69: In rats, the proliferation of hepatic microbodies induced by clofibrate is not abolished by thyroidectomy nor does it occur after various other compounds which displace thyroxine from the plasma. "These observations make less tenable the hypothesis that thyroid hormone displacement is the mechanism of action of clofibrate."

Cocaine ← cf. also Table 40

Glaubach & Pick 11,431/30: In rabbits, pretreatment with thyroxine increases the fever normally produced by tetrahydro-β-naphthylamine or cocaine to fatal levels.

Glaubach & Pick 6,241/31: Studies in guinea pigs and rabbits on the increase in dibucaine, cocaine and procaine toxicity caused by thyroxine as judged by the resulting temperature variations.

Selye G 70,471/71: In rats, cocaine intoxication is inhibited by PCN, ethylestrenol, CS-1, spironolactone, norbolethone, oxandrolone, prednisolone and estradiol. Triamcinolone and DOC fail to protect and thyroxine actually aggravates cocaine intoxication.

Codeine ←

Hunt & Seidell 50,346/09: In mice, pretreatment with thyroid extract diminishes resistance to codeine.

Anan 24,228/29: In mice, thyroxine increases the toxicity of morphine and heroin but not that of other alkaloids such as ethylmorphine codeine, thebaine, papaverine and narcotine.

Colchicine ← cf. also Table 41

Vollmer & Buchholz A 48,810/30: In mice, thyroxine as well as various other "oxidizing substances" (glucose, lactate, methylene blue etc.) protect against alcohol intoxication. The same substances decrease resistance to colchicine or hydrochinone. Morphine resistance is not influenced.

Selye G60,098/70: In rats, fatal colchicine poisoning can be prevented by spironolactone, CS-1, ethylestrenol and, less constantly, by oxandrolone. Progesterone, norbolethone, prednisolone, triamcinolone, DOC, hydroxydione, estradiol and thyroxine are virtually ineffective in this respect.

Compound MO-911 ←

Carrier & Buday D 11,237/61: In rats, feeding with thyroid extracts greatly augments the lethal effect of a hydrazide (iproniazid) or of a nonhydrazide (N-methyl-N-benzyl-2-propynylamine hydrochloride; 'MO-911') enzyme inhibitor.

MO-911 ← Thyroid extract: Carrier et al. D 11,237/61*

DL-Coniine ← cf. Table 42

Curare ←

Tabachnick et al. C 50,317/58: In mice, thyroxine increases sensitivity to decamethonium and neostigmine but not to D-tubocurarine or succinylcholine. Rabbits pretreated with thyroxine also become more sensitive to decamethonium. It is tentatively suggested that the motor disturbances associated with hyperthyroidism may be due to "a change in the muscle itself, probably at the motor end-plate where these drugs act."

Croton Oil ← cf. Table 43

Cyanide ←

Hunt 60,064/05: In mice, thyroid feeding greatly increases resistance to acetonitrile but not to various other cyanides, such as hydrocyanic acid or sodium ferricyanide.

Mansfeld & Müller 35,416/11: In rabbits, thyroidectomy inhibits the protein catabolic effect of exposure to decreased oxygen tension, hydrocyanic acid intoxication or fasting.

Mansfeld 11,881/20: In rabbits and dogs, thyroidectomy diminishes the protein catabolism normally observed after intoxication with hydrocyanic acid, hemorrhage, or hypobaric oxygenation.

Hari 40,209/21: Polemic remarks concerning the technique and interpretation of earlier data on the effect of thyroidectomy upon the resistance to cyanides, chloroform, bacterial toxins and oxygen deficiency.

Gellhorn 16,839/23: In mice, resistance against acetonitrile can be increased not only by thyroid extract but, to a lesser extent, also by extracts of various other tissues. These preparations also augment resistance to potassium cyanide (KCN) and propionitrile, whereas thyroidectomy and orchidectomy have an opposite effect.

Busso 26,684/25: In rats, thyroidectomy decreases sensitivity to KCN, whereas the reverse is true in rabbits.

Tsuru 44,467/33: In rabbits, pretreatment with thyroid extract did not significantly influence resistance to hydrocyanic acid or thiocyanides.

Dietrich & Beutner B 20,412/44: In mice, thiourea and thiouracil interfere with the action of orally administered thyroid powder when the Reid Hunt test is made the basis of observations. In this test, minute amounts of whole thyroid can be detected by their protective effect against otherwise lethal doses of acetonitrile.

Cycloheximide ← cf. also Tables 44, 45

Selye G 70,403/70: In rats, cycloheximide intoxication is inhibited by ethylestrenol, CS-1 and spironolactone. Norbolethone, oxandrolone, progesterone, hydroxydione, and prednisolone offer less perfect protection. Triamcinolone, DOC, estradiol and thyroxine have no protective effect.

Cyclophosphamide ← cf. also Table 46

Selye G 70,466/70: In rats, cyclophosphamide intoxication can be prevented by PCN, CS-1 and spironolactone. Progesterone, ethylestrenol and norbolethone were slightly active; oxandrolone, DOC, hydroxydione and phenobarbital were inactive, whereas prednisolone, triamcinolone, estradiol and thyroxine actually decreased resistance to this drug, cf. Fig. 22, p. 480.

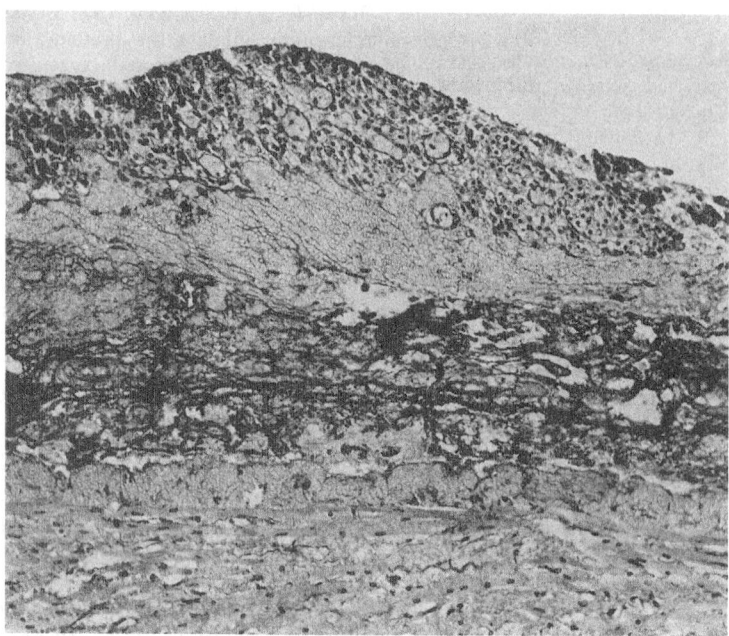

Fig. 22. **Effect of thyroxine upon cyclophosphamide intoxication.** Hemorrhagic, pericardial exudate in rat given cyclophosphamide after pretreatment with thyroxine. Leucocytes are absent because of the cyclophosphamide-induced atrophy of hemopoietic tissue. PAS X

Cystine ←

György & Goldblatt G 71,898/45: In rats kept on a hepatotoxic diet containing large amounts of cystine, the development of liver cirrhosis could be prevented by thiouracil p.o.

Decamethonium ←

Tabachnick et al. C 50,317/58: In mice, thyroxine increases sensitivity to decamethonium and neostigmine but not to D-tubocurarine or succinylcholine. Rabbits pretreated with thyroxine also become more sensitive to decamethonium. It is tentatively suggested that the motor disturbances associated with hyperthyroidism may be due to "a change in the muscle itself, probably at the motor end-plate where these drugs act."

Desipramine ← Thyroid extract, Mouse: Prange et al. F 29,162/64*

α,γ-Diaminobutyric Acid ←

Vivanco et al. G 43,566/66: In rats α,γ-diaminobutyric acid (DBA) produced a neurologic syndrome in the rat. "The animals became irritable and screamed when touched. They moved the head from side to side in the manner of a bear and leaped like kangaroos or frogs. Sometimes they got up on the rear legs with simultaneous quivering of the forearms. They showed excessive salivation. In the preagonal state they presented paresis or paralysis of the hind limbs and motor incoordination. The 'swimming test' was always negative and they did not show circling movements or backward gait as in the IDPN intoxication." Pretreatment with thyroxine prevents these changes as it does the clinically different ECC syndrome (excitation, choreiform and circling movements) elicited by β,β'-iminodipropionitrile (IDPN). DBA enters the brain substance in unpretreated but not in thyroxine-treated rats. Possibly the toxic compound is destroyed before it can enter the brain.

Dibucaine ←

Glaubach & Pick 6,241/31: Studies in guinea pigs and rabbits on the increase in dibucaine, cocaine and novocaine toxicity caused by thyroxine as judged by the resulting temperature variations.

Digitalis ← cf. also Selye G60,083/70, p. 408.

Ghedini & Ollino A21,128/14: Brief mention of observations on rabbits showing that pretreatment with thyroid extract augments the hemodynamic actions of digitalin in the rabbit.

Freund A26,153/32: Studies on the effect of thyroidectomy or pretreatment with thyroxine or insulin upon the in vitro metabolic changes induced by digitalis compounds in the cat's heart.

Kinsell et al. A37,369/42: Experiments on guinea pigs and mice suggested that "therapeutic dosage of cardiac steroid-glycosides prevents a weight loss in thyroxin-treated animals similar to that obtained with adrenal cortical hormone and desoxycorticosterone acetate. Larger dosage of these cardiac glycosides either fails to modify such weight loss or actually increased it."

Dearing et al. C41,482/43: In cats, thyroxine aggravates the myocardial lesions produced by various digitalis alkaloids.

Dearing et al. B53,571/50: In cats, various digitalis preparations produce myocardial fiber necrosis and inflammation. Pretreatment with thyroxine sensitizes the animals to these lesions.

Rosen & Moran D65,414/63: In dogs, the positive inotrophic response to ouabain was decreased by thyroxine. The arrhythmia-producing and lethal effect of large doses of this glycoside were delayed by thyroidectomy but not remarkably influenced by thyroxine. The literature on the influence of clinical hyper- and hypothyroidism upon digitalis intoxication is reviewed.

Phansalkar et al. H20,555/69: In mice, pretreatment with thyroxine greatly increases mortality from subsequent digoxin administration. Reserpine protects against this intoxication. It is suggested that digoxin toxicity is mediated through a catecholamine mechanism.

Selye G70,428/70: In rats, ethylestrenol powerfully inhibits the toxicity of digitoxin, nicotine, indomethacin, phenindione, dioxathion, EPN, physostigmine, hexobarbital, cyclopental, thiopental, DOC (anesthesia), meprobamate and picrotoxin. Thyroxine increases the toxicity of many of these drugs and inhibits the protective effect of ethylestrenol.

Selye PROT. 33541,34074: In rats, PCN is highly efficacious in preventing digitoxin poisoning, even after parathyroidectomy, thyroparathyroidectomy or concurrent treatment with propylthiouracil (PTU). No protection was obtained by thyroidectomy, parathyroidectomy or treatment with PTU, thyroxine, parathyroid extract or calcitonin. Apparently, the goitrogenic effect of PCN plays no indispensable role in its catatoxic action, cf. Table 124, p. 482.

Digitoxin ← cf. also Tables 47—50

Diisopropylfluorophosphate (DFP) ←

Schreiber C3,482/54: In mice, pretreatment with methylthiouracil increases resistance against diisopropylfluorophosphate (DFP).

"DFP" ← cf. also Table 52

Dinitrophenol ←

Glaubach & Pick 30,481/34: In rabbits, the lethal effect of dinitrophenol, and of several of its pyrogenic derivatives, is greatly aggravated by pretreatment with thyroxine.

Dihydroxyphenylalanine ←

Samiy B68,269/52: Both in rats and in rabbits, DOPA produced sustained hypertension following pretreatment with thyroxine. Presumably, thyroid hormone enhances the decarboxylation of DOPA to the pressor agent hydroxytyramine.

Halpern et al. G63,588/63: In mice, thyroxine pretreatment diminishes resistance to amphetamine and DL-dopa, especially under conditions of crowding.

Diphenylhydantoin ←cf. Table 53
Dipicrylamine ← cf. Table 54

Disulfiram ←

Lecoq et al. B66,406/51: In rats, the toxic effects of ethanol and its metabolites, pyruvate and acetaldehyde (which accumulate in the body under the influence of disulfiram) are inhibited by ACTH, cortisone, and hepatic extracts. Conversely, thyroxine, DOC, and testosterone appear to aggravate ethanol intoxication. [Statistically evaluated data are not presented (H.S.).]

Dye ←

Aterman & Howell C63,343/59: In rats, the biliary excretion of bromsulphthalein is delayed after destruction of the thyroid by ^{131}I. This defect is corrected by treatment with thyroid extract.

Table 124. *Role of the thyroparathyroid apparatus in the antidigitoxin effect of PCN*

Treatment[a]	Convulsions[b] (Positive/Total)	Mortality[b] (Dead/Total)	Mean Survival (Days)
None	14/15	15/15	4
PCN	1/10 ***	0/10 ***	∞
Thyroidectomy	12/12 NS	12/12 NS	3
Thyroidectomy + PCN	1/12 ***	0/12 ***	∞
Parathyroidectomy	9/9 NS	8/9 NS	3½
Parathyroidectomy + PCN	0/10 ***	2/10 ***	4
PTU	10/10 NS	7/10 NS	3½
PTU + PCN	0/10 ***	0/10 ***	∞
Thyroxine	10/10 NS	10/10 NS	2½
Parathyroid extract	10/10 NS	9/10 NS	3½
Calcitonin	10/10 NS	10/10 NS	3

[a] The rats of all groups were given digitoxin 2 mg in 1 ml water, p.o./day on 10th day ff. PTU 3 mg in 0.1 ml DMSO, i.p. x2/day; PCN 0.1 mg in 1 ml water, p.o. x2/day; thyroxine 100 µg in 0.2 ml water NaOH, s.c./day and surgery on the 1st day. Parathormone 20 I.U. in 0.2 ml s.c. x2/day and calcitonin 10 µg in 0.5 ml water, i.p. x3/day on the 9th day.

[b] The severity of the convulsions was estimated on the 13th day and mortality was listed on the 15th (Statistics Fisher & Yates).

For further details on technique of tabulation *cf.* p. VIII.

Dolgova & Dolgov G33,058/64: In rats, the organ distribution of parenterally administered neutral red is considerably modified by pretreatment with thyroid extract. Increased dye deposition was noted in the liver, spleen, and skeletal muscle, whereas in the brain and testes dye-uptake was reduced.

Kulcsár et al. H24,478/70: In rats, thyroxine increases, whereas thyroidectomy decreases, the hepatotoxicity of CCl_4 as judged by BSP elimination.

Emetine ← *cf.* Table 55

Ephedrine ←

Halpern et al. F24,137/64; F27,643/64: In mice, the toxicity of amphetamine and ephedrine is increased by pretreatment with thyroxine not only—as had been previously shown—when several animals are kept together in a jar, but also when they are kept in solitary cages.

EPN ← *cf. Pesticides*

Ergot ←

Griffith Jr. & Comroe A33,738/40: In rats, pretreatment with thyroxine s.c. increases mortality and the incidence of tail necrosis following s.c. injections of ergotamine tartrate.

Wells & Anderson G74,995/50: In rats, the production of tail gangrene by ergotamine is not influenced by propylthiouracil but facilitated by thyroxine. "It is assumed that thyroxin acts, not by altering the resistance of the tissues to vascular occlusion, nor by sensitizing the vascular musculature to ergotamine, but by prolonging the action of the alkaloids, possibly by interfering with their elimination or destruction."

Ethanol ←

Preusse 26,352/33: In mice, thyroxine or thyroid powder causes only a moderate increase in resistance to ethanol.

Vollmer & Buchholz A48,810/30: In mice, thyroxine as well as various other "oxidizing substances" (glucose, lactate, methylene blue etc.) protect against alcohol intoxication. The same substances decrease resistance to colchicine or hydroquinone. Morphine resistance is not influenced.

Lecoq et al. B66,406/51: In rats, the toxic effects of ethanol and its metabolites, pyruvate and acetaldehyde (which accumulate in the body under the influence of disulfiram) are inhibited by ACTH, cortisone, and hepatic extracts. Conversely, thyroxine, DOC, and testosterone appear to aggravate ethanol intoxication. [Statistically evaluated data are not presented (H.S.).]

Aragona & Barone B 92,455/53: In rats, methylthiouracil aggravates the hepatic lesions produced by ethanol intoxication.

Choisy & Potron H 28,010/68: In rabbits, pretreatment with thyroxine accelerates the oxidation of ethanol and its clearance from the blood.

Ether ←

Rutsch 7,744/33: In guinea pigs, thyroidectomy decreases, whereas thyroxine pretreatment increases, resistance to ether, paraldehyde or tribromoethanol anesthesia. These findings are ascribed to changes in the responsiveness of the brain.

Ethylene Glycol ← cf. Table 56
Ethylmorphine ← cf. Table 57
Flufenamic Acid ← cf. Table 58

Fluoride ←

Phillips et al. 34,798/35: In chicks, combined treatment with thyroid extract and NaF is particularly toxic.

Bixler et al. E 99,118/56: In rats with hypothyroidism induced by ^{131}I, the protective effect of fluorine against dental caries is diminished.

Fluphenazine ← cf. Table 59
Ganglioplegics ← cf. Tables 61, 62
Glutethimide ← cf. Table 63
Glycerol ← cf. Table 64

Guanidine ←

Hunt & Seidell 50,346/09: In mice, pretreatment with thyroid extract does not influence resistance to guanidine.

Spinelli 10,086/31; 7,409/32: In guinea pigs, thyroidectomy decreases resistance to the lethal effects of guanidine intoxication. Subsequent administration of thyroid extract restores the resistance to normal.

Parhon & Werner 34,844/35: In dogs, guinea pigs and rabbits, thyroparathyroidectomy causes only a moderate increase in sensitivity to methylguanidine.

Halothane ←

Nikki G 71,573/69: In mice, shivering and hypothermia during halothane anesthesia is diminished following pretreatment with thyroxine.

Heroin ←

Anan 24,228/29: In mice, thyroxine increases the toxicity of morphine and heroin but not that of other alkaloids such as ethylmorphine, codeine, thebaine, papaverine and narcotine.

Hydroquinone ← cf. also Table 65

Vollmer & Buchholz A 48,810/30: In mice, thyroxine as well as various other "oxidizing substances" (glucose, lactate, methylene blue etc.) protect against alcohol intoxication. The same substances decrease resistance to colchicine or hydroquinone. Morphine resistance is not influenced.

N-(p-Hydroxyphenyl) glycine ←

Li & Sos H 30,786/68: In rats, N-(p-hydroxyphenyl)glycine fails to exert its usual pressor effect after thyroidectomy.

Imipramine ← cf. also Table 66

Prange & Lipton D 42,869/62: In mice, pretreatment with thyroxine greatly increases the initial convulsive actions and the terminal mortality of imipramine intoxication.

Prange et al. D 62,707/63: In mice pretreatment with propylthiouracil increases resistance to imipramine, whereas hyperthyroidism has an opposite effect.

Winter G 71,836/65: In mice, the toxicity of amphetamine, imipramine, chlordiazepoxide and pentylenetetrazol is increased by T3 or thyroid powder, whereas the narcotic effect of amobarbital and morphine is decreased. Methylthiouracil has, in general, opposing effects. [The experimental conditions are not described in sufficient detail to evaluate these findings (H.S.).]

Winter F 64,465/66; F 98,019/68: In mice, pretreatment with thyroid extract p.o. increases the toxicity of reserpine, chlordiazepoxide, imipramine and amphetamine.

Ashford & Ross H 2,686/68: In mice, pretreatment with thyroid extract increased the toxicity of imipramine, nortriptyline, chlorpromazine, perphenazine and chlordiazepoxide, whereas the toxicity of meprobamate and reserpine was not enhanced.

Prange Jr. et al. G 76,612/70: In man, the antidepressive effect of imipramine is enhanced by TTH as well as by T3. Earlier literature is cited.

Prange et al. G69,595/69: In retarded, depressed patients, small doses of T3 enhanced the therapeutic effect of imipramine.

Prange et al. H31,796/70: In depressed patients, T3 increases the therapeutic effect of imipramine.

Imipramine ← Thyroid extract, Mouse: Prange et al. D42,869/62*

Indomethacin ← cf. also Table 67

Selye G70,428/70: In rats, ethylestrenol powerfully inhibits the toxicity of digitoxin, nicotine, indomethacin, phenindione, dioxathion, EPN, physostigmine, hexobarbital, cyclopental, thiopental, DOC (anesthesia), meprobamate and picrotoxin. Thyroxine increases the toxicity of many of these drugs and inhibits the protective effect of ethylestrenol.

Iodides ← cf. Selye G60,083/70, p. 407

Iproniazid ←

Carrier & Buday D11,237/61: In rats, feeding with thyroid extracts greatly augments the lethal effect of a hydrazide (iproniazid) or of a nonhydrazide (N-methyl-N-benzyl-2-propynylamine hydrochloride; 'MO-911') enzyme inhibitor.

Carrier & Buday E28,887/63: In rats, the toxic effects of the MAO inhibitors, pargyline and iproniazid are increased by pretreatment with desiccated thyroid.

Isoniazid ←

Hunt & Carlton F3,186/64: In Pekin ducks, combined administration of semicarbazide and isoniazid p.o. produces a neurolathyrism-like syndrome which is not significantly influenced either by thiouracil or by DL-thyroxine.

Isoproterenol ← cf. also Selye C92,918/61, pp. 117, 123; G60,083/70, pp. 405, 406.

Chappel et al. C71,409/59: In rats, thyroxine aggravates, whereas thyroidectomy or propylthiouracil treatment inhibits the development of myocardial lesions following injection of isoproterenol.

Lathyrogens ← cf. also Selye C92,918/61, p. 137; G60,083/70, p. 357.

Duck

Hunt & Carlton F3,186/64: In Pekin ducks, combined administration of semicarbazide and isoniazid p.o. produces a neurolathyrism-like syndrome which is not significantly influenced either by thiouracil or by DL-thyroxine.

Rat

Selye & Bois C18,280/56: In rats, the osteolathyrism produced by Lathyrus odoratus seeds is aggravated by STH and inhibited by cortisol. Combined treatment with DOC + uninephrectomy + NaCl resulted in dissecting aneurysms of the aorta. Very small doses of thyroxine or estradiol were without effect upon this form of lathyrism.

Dasler C36,068/57: Brief mention of unpublished observations indicating that in rats, osteolathyrism produced by APN is not inhibited by cortisone or thyroxine, but aggravated by STH.

Diaz et al. C50,497/57: Thyroxine inhibits the osteolathyrism produced in rats by methyleneaminoacetonitrile (MAAN). Estrogens allegedly have a similar, though somewhat less pronounced, effect. [The authors actually tested only estrone in combination with progesterone (H.S.).]

Ponseti E54,643/57: In rats, the osteolathyric changes produced by AAN are more readily inhibited by T3 than by thyroxine.

Selye C25,013/57: The osteolathyrism produced in rats by AAN is slightly aggravated by thyroparathyroidectomy, and suppressed by large doses of thyroxine. "An amount of ACTH that more than doubles the weight of the adrenals and causes pronounced thymus atrophy also inhibits the effect of AAN, but fails to prevent it completely. This is all the more noteworthy because comparatively small doses of cortisol can totally prevent such bone lesions. Extensive partial hepatectomy greatly increases the effect of AAN upon the bones."

Selye C31,790/57: In rats, osteolathyrism produced by AAN is inhibited by thyroxine, cortisol and estradiol but aggravated by STH even after adrenalectomy.

Selye C36,049/57: In rats, the ocular changes produced by IDPN are even more readily prevented by thyroxine than other manifestations of neurolathyrism.

Strong et al. G61,885/58: In rats, T3 or iodinated casein offered only slight protection against APN poisoning, "although skeletal changes were somewhat delayed and reduced in severity, possibly because of slower growth."

Diaz et al. D99,329/58: In rats, the osteolathyrism produced by MAAN is mildly inhibited by progesterone and estrone, completely prevented by thyroxine and aggravated by thyroidectomy.

Ponseti & Aleu C61,715/58: In rats with lathyrism produced by AAN, bone fractures produce unusually large calluses which do not ossify well. T3 diminishes the size of the callus and improves its ossification.

Selye C36,069/58: In rats, the ECC syndrome (excitement, choreiform movements, and circling) normally produced by IDPN is inhibited by thyroxine. Thyroidectomy had no effect, but since the controls were 100% positive, an aggravation could not have been noted.

Ponseti C68,050/59: In rats, the lathyric bone lesions produced by AAN were strongly suppressed by triiodothyronine and thyroxine, whereas those elicited by APN were much less evidently inhibited by these hormones. "Corticosterone and cortisone suppressed only slightly the lesions produced by aminoacetonitrile in rats."

Ponseti C78,321/59: In rats, T3 is about 50 times as potent as thyroxine in suppressing osteolathyrism after treatment with AAN.

Pyörälä et al. G67,833/59: Dissecting aneurysms of the aorta developed in 40% of immature rats fed Lathyrus odoratus. The media was remarkably thickened and the ground substance showed increased metachromasia and PAS reaction. This response was suppressed by cortisone and thyroxine but not by ACTH, TTH or DOC at the doses employed.

Gabay et al. D98,867/61: In rats, the osteolathyrism produced by MAAN is associated with a considerable increase in bone hexosamine. This change is more effectively inhibited by thyroxine than by cortisone. Both hormones are virtually ineffective in protecting against osteolathyrism produced by the feeding of Lathyrus odoratus seeds.

Khogali D10,840/61: In rats, the diminished breaking stress and stiffness of the bones, characteristic of lathyrism induced by APN, can be counteracted both by L- and by D-T3. Since both isomers are equally effective in this respect, it is considered unlikely that their antilathyric property depends upon classic thyroid hormone properties.

Selye & Cantin C88,878/61: In rats, the osteolathyrism produced by AAN is inhibited by thyroxine and cortisol but aggravated by STH. The cardiac infarcts elicited in rats by ligature of the descending branch of the left coronary artery are often transformed into rupturing cardiac aneurysms under the influence of AAN. The incidence of these cardiac ruptures is augmented by cortisol and DOC, but not significantly influenced by thyroxine and STH. Evidently there is no direct relationship between the skeletal and the cardiac lesions under these circumstances.

Vivanco et al. D10,627/61: Thyroxine prevents the osteolathyrism produced by MAAN but not that elicited by a Lathyrus odoratus diet.

Vivanco et al. D15,606/61: In rats, the neurolathyrism produced by IDPN as well as the associated histologic changes in the central nervous system are prevented by thyroxine.

Aschkenasy D30,881/62: In rats, lathyrism produced by AAN is inhibited by thyroxine and aggravated by propylthiouracil.

Glickman et al. E24,104/63: In rats, the dental changes produced by AAN are aggravated following partial hepatectomy and thyroidectomy, reduced by ACTH and almost completely abolished by thyroxine.

Lalich & Turner G44,676/67: In rats fed APN in combination with cottonseed meal, there occurred severe diarrhea, colonic dilatation and herniation in the costo-vertebral angle. These changes were uninfluenced by T3.

Morcos F80,855/67: In rats, thyroxine did not prevent the development of the ECC syndrome following injection of IDPN but only delayed its onset.

Alper & Ruegamer H17,023/69: In rats which developed lathyrism under the influence of semicarbazide, the antithyroid agent methimazole prevented the accumulation of chondroitin sulfate in the aorta.

AAN ← cf. also Table 73

Lead ←

Gabbiani et al. G46,731/68: In rats, pretreatment with thyroxine or calcitonin inhibits the soft-tissue calcification and osteitis fibrosa induced by parathyroid extract overdosage. When both hormones are given simultaneously their effects are summated. Calcitonin, but not thyroxine, inhibits the local calcergy (induced by intravenous injection of lead acetate followed by topical administration of polymyxin) and the hypercalcemia produced by a single injection of lead acetate.

LSD ← cf. Table 74

Magnesium ←

Forbes G30,402/65: In rats, thyroxine prevents the nephrocalcinosis of magnesium deficiency.

Jasmin E7,631/68: In rats, certain manifestations of the magnesium-deficiency syndrome are inhibited by cortisol, hypophysectomy or thyroparathyroidectomy.

Jacob & Forbes G69,934/69: In rats, nephrocalcinosis produced by magnesium deficiency is inhibited by approximately equal amounts of D- or L-thyroxine, but only if D-thyroxine is administered frequently enough to offset its more rapid metabolism in the tissue.

Forbes G81,277/71: In rats, the renal calcification produced by magnesium deficiency is prevented by thyroxine and aggravated by thyroid deficiency or injection of adenine. Such metabolic stimulators as Na-salicylate or 2,4-dinitrophenol are without effect.

Mechlorethamine ← *cf. Table 75*

Meperidine ←

Schrogie & Solomon C43,019/66: In mice, the metabolism of bishydroxycoumarin was markedly inhibited by both L- and D-thyroxine. The demethylation of meperidine was likewise inhibited by both isomers but particularly by D-thyroxine. L-thyroxine also increased the lethal effect of meperidine overdosage. Pentobarbital sleeping time was prolonged in mice treated with either L- or D-thyroxine but the latter was more active in this respect.

Mephenesin ← *cf. Table 76*

Meprobamate ← *cf. also Table 77*

Selye & Solymoss G70,402/70: Although in rats meprobamate intoxication is counteracted by catatoxic steroids, thyroxine actually aggravates it.

Selye G70,428/70: In rats, ethylestrenol powerfully inhibits the toxicity of digitoxin, nicotine, indomethacin, phenindione, dioxathion, EPN, physostigmine, hexobarbital, cyclopental, thiopental, DOC (anesthesia), meprobamate and picrotoxin. Thyroxine increases the toxicity of many of these drugs and inhibits the protective effect of ethylestrenol.

Mercury ← *cf. Tables 78—80*

Methadone ← *cf. also Table 82*

Sung & Way B91,323/53: Rats treated with thiouracil or methimazole showed tolerance to toxic actions of methadone (absence of general depression and body rigidity). In thyroidectomized animals, the increase in pain-threshold was also diminished. Feeding of thyroid powder exerted opposite effects. Liver slices from thiouracil and thyroid-fed rats metabolized methadone more slowly than those from controls. Tissue levels of methadone were also increased by both these agents. However, total urinary and fecal excretion of methadone was essentially the same in all groups.

n-Methylaniline ← *cf. Table 83*

Methylphenidate ←

Fregly & Black F15,674/64: In rats, pretreatment with propylthiouracil appeared to decrease the responsiveness to methylphenidate (given in the diet) as judged by the increased activity level induced by exposure to cold. However, "this difference in activity level is probably associated with differences in the food (and drug) intakes of the two groups."

Selye PROT. 27955: In rats, pretreated with thyroxine, methylphenidate produced temporary but very severe paralysis of the hind legs when given at dose levels which in nonpretreated controls caused only excitation.

α-Methyl-p-tyrosine ←

Moore G36,616/65: In mice, pretreatment with T3 greatly increases sensitivity to the lethal effect of amphetamine. "Chlorpromazine, phenoxybenzamine, and propranolol pretreatment reduced the lethality of d-amphetamine in hyperthyroid mice while α-methyl-m-tyrosine, α-methyl-p-tyrosine, and reserpine pretreatment did not. The toxicity of α-methyl-m-tyrosine was enhanced in hyperthyroid mice."

Methyprylon ← *cf. Table 84*

Morphine ←

Hunt 49,716/07: Comparative studies on the effect of thyroid extract upon the acetonitrile and morphine resistance of mice, rats and guinea pigs.

Hunt & Seidell 50,346/09: In mice, rats and guinea pigs, pretreatment with thyroid extract diminishes resistance to morphine.

Olds Jr. 34,544/10: In rats, thyroidectomy does not alter resistance to morphine.

Busso 26,684/25: In rats, thyroidectomy does not change the resistance to epinephrine or phenol. Morphine appears to be slightly more toxic to thyroidectomized than to intact rats but the results were irregular.

Anan 24,228/29: In mice, thyroxine increases the toxicity of morphine and heroin but not that of other alkaloids such as ethylmorphine, codeine, thebaine, papaverine and narcotine.

Lund & Benedict A14,206/29: In rabbits, morphine causes a more pronounced drop in the BMR in the absence than in the presence of the thyroid. Morphine does not influence the rise in BMR induced by a thyroid extract.

Glaubach & Pick 11,431/30: In guinea pigs, pretreatment with thyroxine diminishes resistance against morphine.

Vollmer & Buchholz A 48,810/30: In mice, thyroxine as well as various other "oxidizing substances" (glucose, lactate, methylene blue etc.) protect against alcohol intoxication. The same substances decrease resistance to colchicine or hydroquinone. Morphine resistance is not influenced.

Zárday & Weiner A 52,879/34: In rats, morphine, and in rabbits chloral hydrate anesthesia were not significantly influenced by pretreatment with thyroxine s.c., one hour before the anesthetics. On the other hand, phenobarbital anesthesia was prolonged by thyroxine pretreatment in rabbits under identical conditions. Similar observations have been made on patients suffering from thyrotoxicosis in that they are unusually resistant to barbiturates but not to other anesthetics. This selective antagonism is ascribed to interactions between thyroxine and barbiturates at some common receptor site in the midbrain.

Zárday & Weiner 53,715/35: In rats, pretreatment with thyroxine s.c. does not influence the narcotic action of morphine given s.c. a few hours later.

Swann 80,669/41: In rats, thyroidectomy does not alter the morphine withdrawal symptoms.

Bhagat F 9,444/64: In mice, pretreatment with thyroxine increased the analgesic action of morphine.

Cochin & Sokoloff D 29,487/60: "The effect of in vivo administration of L-thyroxin on in vitro N-demethylation of morphine by rat-liver enzyme preparations from normal and morphine-treated rats has been investigated. Thyroxin given 7 days to otherwise untreated control animals has no effect on N-demethylating activity, but after 10—14 days it significantly depresses this activity. Administration of thyroxin for 7 days prior to and during morphine withdrawal reduces further the enzyme activity already markedly depressed after chronic administration of morphine, and prevents almost completely recovery of activity which occurs some 8—10 days after morphine withdrawal."

Winter G 71,836/65: In mice, the toxicity of amphetamine, imipramine, chlordiazepoxide and pentylenetetrazol is increased by T3 or thyroid powder, whereas the narcotic effect of amobarbital and morphine is decreased. Methylthiouracil has, in general, opposing effects. [The experimental conditions are not described in sufficient detail to evaluate these findings (H.S.).]

Morphine ← Thyroxine + Morphine: Cochin et al. *D 29,487/60*

a-Naphthylisothiocyanate ← cf. Table 85

Navadel ← cf. **Dioxathion** under **Pesticides**

Neostigmine ←

Tabachnick et al. C 50,317/58: In mice, thyroxine increases sensitivity to decamethonium and neostigmine but not to D-tubocurarine or succinyl choline. Rabbits pretreated with thyroxine also become more sensitive to decamethonium. It is tentatively suggested that the motor disturbances associated with hyperthyroidism may be due to "a change in the muscle itself, probably at the motor endplate where these drugs act."

Nicotine ← cf. also Table 86

Hunt & Seidell 50,346/09: In mice, pretreatment with thyroid extract does not influence resistance to nicotine.

Spinelli 10,086/31: In guinea pigs, thyroidectomy increases the resistance to histamine, acetonitrile, picrotoxin, aconitine, epinephrine, nicotine and atropine but augments sensibility to pilocarpine and guanidine.

Gogolák et al. G 51,384/67: In hypothyroid (^{131}I, methylthiouracil, NaClO$_4$) rats, higher doses of nicotine are required to produce hippocampal-seizure discharges with the typical modifications in EEG than in intact animals. The comparable effect of pentylenetetrazol is not modified by hypothyroidism.

Selye G 70,428/70: In rats, ethylestrenol powerfully inhibits the toxicity of digitoxin, nicotine, indomethacin, phenindione, dioxathion, EPN, physostigmine, hexobarbital, cyclopental, thiopental, DOC (anesthesia), meprobamate and picrotoxin. Thyroxine increases the toxicity of many of these drugs and inhibits the protective effect of ethylestrenol.

Nikethamide ← cf. Table 87
p-Nitroanisole ← cf. Table 88

Nitrogen Dioxide ←

Fairchild & Graham D 56,574/63: In mice and rats, mortality induced by exposure to respiratory irritants such as ozone or nitrogen dioxide is inhibited by thioureas or thyroidectomy but enhanced by thyroxine or T3.

Dinitrophenol, in doses known to elevate the BMR, did not significantly affect mortality under these conditions.

Nitrogen Mustard ←

Connors & Elson G2,440/62: In rats, thioureas reduce the toxicity of certain radiomimetic alkylating agents. The same is true of other compounds containing thiol groups.

Nitrous Oxide ←

Rummel et al. D89,013/57: In guinea pigs and rabbits, thyroxine increases the threshold for N_2O anesthesia, whereas dinitrophenol has no such effect. Contrary to expectations, methylthiouracil also failed to affect the N_2O anesthesia threshold.

Rummel C79,429/59: In guinea pigs and rats, thyroxine increases, whereas thyroidectomy decreases, the threshold for N_2O anesthesia. Dinitrophenol is ineffective. DOC lowers, whereas cortisone raises, this anesthesia threshold.

Rummel & Wellensiek D96,909/68: In rats, the N_2O anesthesia threshold is diminished by thyroidectomy and restored to normal by thyroxine but not by dinitrophenol.

Nortriptyline ←

Ashford & Ross H2,686/68: In mice, pretreatment with thyroid extract increased the toxicity of imipramine, nortriptyline, chlorpromazine, perphenazine and chlordiazepoxide, whereas the toxicity of meprobamate and reserpine was not enhanced.

Novocaine ←

Glaubach & Pick 6,241/31: Studies in guinea pigs and rabbits on the increase in dibucaine, cocaine and novocaine toxicity caused by thyroxine as judged by the resulting temperature variations.

Octamethyl Pyrophosphoramide ← cf. Pesticides

Oxalate ←

Kochmann 55,946/34: In mice, fatal intoxication with Na-oxalate can be prevented by parathyroid extract in a dose-dependent manner suitable for bioassays.

Ozone ←

Fairchild & Stokinger D4,088/61; Fairchild & Graham D56,574/63: In mice and rats, mortality induced by exposure to respiratory irritants such as ozone or nitrogen dioxide is inhibited by thioureas or thyroidectomy but enhanced by thyroxine or T3. Dinitrophenol, in doses known to elevate the BMR, did not significantly affect mortality under these conditions.

Fairchild G71,531/63: Review (6 pp., 26 refs.) on the effect of thyroidectomy, thioureas, thyroid hormones, glucocorticoids and hypophysectomy upon the resistance of various species to inhaled irritants especially ozone.

Paraldehyde ←

Rutsch 7,744/33: In guinea pigs, thyroidectomy decreases, whereas thyroxine pretreatment increases, resistance to ether, paraldehyde or tribromoethanol anesthesia. These findings are ascribed to changes in the responsiveness of the brain.

Paraphenylenediamine ←

Meissner E52,567/19: The head and neck edema produced by paraphenylenediamine in the rabbit is not prevented by epinephrine, posterior pituitary extract or thyroid extract.

Pargyline ←

Carrier & Buday E28,887/63: In rats, the toxic effects of the MAO inhibitors, pargyline and iproniazid are increased by pretreatment with desiccated thyroid.

Paroxypropionine ←

Scharf et al. C91,620/60: In rats, the degenerative changes produced in the pituitary by p-hydroxypropiophenone (paroxypropionine or POP) are aggravated by methylthiouracil.

Pentachlorophenol ←

Pasley et al. G67,522/68: In cichlid fish, the toxic effect of pentachlorophenol (a herbicide, molluscacide and lumber preservative) is counteracted by thyroxine.

Pentylenetetrazol ← cf. also Table 89

Woodbury et al. B68,423/52: In rats, brain excitability (pentylenetetrazol, EST) decreases following thyroidectomy or treatment with propylthiouracil and increases after thyroxine pretreatment. There are however certain differences between thyroidectomy and propylthiouracil as regards the recovery time from electroshock seizures and their relative effect upon extensor and flexor components.

Pfeifer et al. D12,952/60: In rats, the convulsive effect of "Pentametazol" [presumably pentylenetetrazol (H.S.)] is diminished one hour after administration of thyroxine, but increased 18 hrs later. A corresponding biphasic response is also noted with regard to the EST. In mice, the increased motility induced by amphetamine is also inhibited during the first hour after thyroxine treatment. The possible biochemical reasons for this "negative tendency" during the early phase of thyroxine action are described.

Winter G71,836/65: In mice, the toxicity of amphetamine, imipramine, chlordiazepoxide and pentylenetetrazol is increased by T3 or thyroid powder, whereas the narcotic effect of amobarbital and morphine is decreased. Methylthiouracil has, in general, opposing effects. [The experimental conditions are not described in sufficient detail to evaluate these findings (H.S.).]

Gogolák et al. G51,384/67: In hypothyroid (^{131}I, methylthiouracil, NaClO$_4$) rats higher doses of nicotine are required to produce hippocampal-seizure discharges with the typical modifications in EEG than in intact animals. The comparable effect of pentylenetetrazol is not modified by hypothyroidism.

Pfeifer et al. G65,057/68: In mice, thyroxine facilitates the production of convulsions by pentylenetetrazol and electroshock. These effects are inhibited by various amphetamine derivatives.

Pentylenetetrazol ← Thiouracil, Mouse: Wenzel et al. G76,357/55*

Peptone ←

Houssay & Cisneros 26,936/25: In dogs sensitized after thyroidectomy, subsequent anaphylactic shock is diminished. Thyroidectomized dogs are also comparatively insensitive to peptone shock.

Czarnecki & Kiersz D15,579/61: In dogs, shock produced by trypan blue or peptone injection is more powerfully inhibited by thyroparathyroidectomy than by thyroidectomy.

Perchlorates ← cf. also Table 90

Bajusz & Selye C64,511/59: C57,180/59; Selye C61,814/59: The spastic muscular contractions (with positive "flick-test") produced by NaClO$_4$ in the rat can be inhibited by cortisol or triamcinolone, and aggravated by DOC or Me-Cl-COL. Thyroparathyroidectomy or parathyroidectomy exerts a sensitizing effect. Triamcinolone also protects the dog against the syndrome produced by heavy overdosage with NaClO$_4$. Methyltestosterone, estradiol and progesterone did not significantly affect the response of the rat to NaClO$_4$.

Perphenazine ←

Ashford & Ross H2,686/68: In mice, pretreatment with thyroid extract increased the toxicity of imipramine, nortriptyline, chlorpromazine, perphenazine and chlordiazepoxide, whereas the toxicity of meprobamate and reserpine was not enhanced.

Pesticides ← cf. also Tables 91—99

Byerrum B1,322/46: In rats, iodine given either as Lugol's solution or as KI protects against ANTU poisoning.

Byerrum & DuBois B3,076/47: In rats, ANTU poisoning can be prevented by KI p.o. but very little protection is offered to thyroidectomized rats by the administration of iodine. Desiccated thyroid fed for 2 days offered no protection against ANTU.

Meyer & Karel B18,102/48: Of 25 compounds tested only KI and 1-thiosorbitol were unequivocally successful in preventing lethal pulmonary edema and pleural effusion in ANTU-treated rats. Organic iodides (diiodotyrosine, cetyl iodide, n-decyl iodide, amyl iodide, and iodoacetic acid) as well as iodine were ineffective.

Carroll & Noble B32,718/49: In rats, resistance to ANTU can be produced not only by pretreatment with ANTU itself but also by previous administration of other thioureas. "Neither the anti-thyroid potency nor the acute toxicity of these substances is directly related to their ability to impart resistance." However, resistance to ANTU is also found in rats fed on certain goitrogenic diets, especially those containing seeds of the brassica species.

Wassermann et al. G74,485/69: In rats, hepatic changes induced by p,p'-DDT are aggravated following thyroidectomy and the storage of p,p'-DDT, o,p'-DDT and dieldrin is increased.

Selye G70,428/70: In rats, ethylestrenol powerfully inhibits the toxicity of digitoxin, nicotine, indomethacin, phenindione, dioxathion, EPN, physostigmine, hexobarbital, cyclopental, thiopental, DOC (anesthesia), meprobamate and picrotoxin. Thyroxine increases the toxicity of many of these drugs and inhibits the protective effect of ethylestrenol.

Selye G70,435/70: In rats, ethylestrenol, CS-1, spironolactone, and norbolethone counteract the lethal effects of ethion, dioxathion, EPN, Guthion and parathion. To a lesser extent, this is also true of oxandrolone, prednisolone and progesterone. Triamcinolone, desoxycorticosterone, hydroxydione, estradiol, and thyroxine offer no consistent protection against these pesticides. DDT is much more resistant against detoxication by even the most powerful catatoxic steroids.

Selye et al. G70,457/70: In rats, ethylestrenol, CS-1, spironolactone and norbolethone fail to alter sensitivity to OMPA, although these typical catatoxic steroids have previously been shown to induce hepatic microsomal enzymes and to detoxify numerous other pesticides. This is of interest because catatoxic barbiturates greatly increase the toxicity of OMPA, presumably by transforming it into a more toxic metabolite. On the other hand, estradiol, estrone and stilbestrol, which have no typical catatoxic actions, considerably increase OMPA toxicity in ovariectomized rats. "The protective effect of catatoxic steroids is presumably due to their structural characteristics and is independent of other pharmacologic actions. Conversely, sensitization to OMPA depends more upon the estrogenic action of compounds than upon their chemical structure, since stilbestrol, a nonsteroidal estrogen, is also highly effective in this respect." Prednisolone, triamcinolone, progesterone, DOC, hydroxydione and thyroxine fail to influence OMPA toxicity.

Selye PROT. 31612: In mice, the lethal effect of dioxathion is powerfully inhibited by ethylestrenol, norbolethone, prednisolone and estradiol, moderately by CS-1 and oxandrolone, but not influenced by spironolactone, progesterone, triamcinolone, DOC, hydroxydione and thyroxine.

DDT ← Thyroidectomy: Wassermann et al. G74,485/69*

Phenol ←

Hunt & Seidell 50,346/09: In mice, pretreatment with thyroid extract does not influence resistance to phenol.

Busso 26,684/25: In rats, thyroidectomy does not change the resistance to epinephrine or phenol. Morphine appears to be slightly more toxic to thyroidectomized than to intact rats but the results were irregular.

Phenyramidol ← *cf. Table 100*

Phosphates ←

Selye C38,627/58: In rats the nephrocalcinosis produced by a dietary excess of NaH_2PO_4 is inhibited both by thyroparathyroidectomy and by excess thyroxine administration.

Cantin F5,681/64: The nephrocalcinosis produced in rats by combined treatment with NaH_2PO_4 + either estradiol or DOC is prevented by parathyroidectomy or thyroparathyroidectomy, and in either case additional treatment with thyroxine prevents nephrocalcinosis.

Meyer & Forbes G53,688/67: In rats kept on a high-phosphate diet, nephrocalcinosis is decreased by thyroxine and increased by prophylthiouracil.

Phosphorus ←

Selye & Mishra C40,183/58: In the rat, mortality and hepatic degeneration produced by elementary yellow phosphorus is inhibited by thyroxine and aggravated by thyroidectomy. The associated osteosclerosis was not affected under the conditions of this experiment.

Physostigmine ← *cf. also Table 110*

Selye G70,435/70: In rats, intoxication with physostigmine was diminished by ethylestrenol, CS-1, spironolactone, and prednisolone, but aggravated by estradiol and thyroxine. Norbolethone, oxandrolone, progesterone, triamcinolone, DOC, and hydroxydione had no significant effect.

Selye G70,428/70: In rats, ethylestrenol powerfully inhibits the toxicity of digitoxin, nicotine, indomethacin, phenindione, dioxathion, EPN, physostigmine, hexobarbital, cyclopental, thiopental, DOC (anesthesia), meprobamate and picrotoxin. Thyroxine increases the toxicity of many of these drugs and inhibits the protective effect of ethylestrenol.

Picrotoxin ← *cf. also Table 102*

Hunt & Seidell 50,346/09: In mice, pretreatment with thyroid extract does not influence resistance to picrotoxin.

Spinelli 10,086/31: In guinea pigs, thyroidectomy increases resistance to histamine, acetonitrile, picrotoxin, aconitine, epinephrine, nicotine and atropine but augments sensibility to pilocarpine and guanidine.

Selye G70,428/70: In rats, ethylestrenol powerfully inhibits the toxicity of digitoxin, nicotine, indomethacin, phenindione, dioxathion, EPN, physostigmine, hexobarbital, cyclopental, thiopental, DOC (anesthesia), meprobamate and picrotoxin. Thyroxine increases the toxicity of many of these drugs and inhibits the protective effect of ethylestrenol.

Pilocarpine ←

Spinelli 10,086/31: In guinea pigs, thyroidectomy increases the resistance to histamine, acetonitrile, picrotoxin, aconitine, epinephrine, nicotine and atropine but augments sensibility to pilocarpine and guanidine.

Piperidine ← *cf. Table 103*
Potassium ← *cf. also Selye C92,918/61, p. 83.*
Lowenstein et al. A74,481/43: In rats, pretreatment with DOC increased, whereas thyroid feeding decreased, resistance to KCl i.p.
Pralidoxime ← *cf. also Table 104*
Selye G70,435/70: In rats, pralidoxime intoxication was counteracted by prednisolone and, to a lesser extent, by ethylestrenol and estradiol. CS-1, spironolactone, norbolethone, oxandrolone, progesterone, triamcinolone, DOC, hydroxydione, and thyroxine had no significant effect.
Propionitrile ← *cf. also Table 105*
Gellhorn 16,839/23: In mice, resistance against acetonitrile can be increased not only by thyroid extract but, to a lesser extent, also by extracts of various other tissues. These preparations also augment resistance to potassium cyanide (KCN) and propionitrile, whereas thyroidectomy and orchidectomy have an opposite effect.

Puromycin Aminonucleoside ←

Alexander & Hunt D20,284/61: In rats, pretreatment with T3 aggravates the proteinuria caused by puromycin aminonucleoside.

Pyruvate ←

Lecoq et al. B66,406/51: In rats, the toxic effects of ethanol and its metabolites pyruvate and acetaldehyde (which accumulate in the body under the influence of disulfiram) are inhibited by ACTH, cortisone, and hepatic extracts. Conversely, thyroxine, DOC, and testosterone appear to aggravate ethanol intoxication. [Statistically evaluated data are not presented (H.S.).]

Quinine ←

Karásek B52,652/37: In guinea pigs pretreated with thyroid extract or thyroxine, the isolated right auricles of the heart exhibit an accelerated pulse. In this respect quinine exerts an antagonistic effect.

Reserpine ←

Ershoff C60,006/58: In rats, reserpine and thyroid extracts, given in well-tolerated amounts, caused 100% mortality when administered concurrently.
Thier & Gravenstein C83,115/60: In isolated atria of rats, the slowing of the heart beat produced by reserpine is antagonized by thyroxine pretreatment in vivo.
Winter G71,836/65; F64,465/66; F98,019/68: In mice, pretreatment with thyroid extract p.o. increases the toxicity of reserpine, chlordiazepoxide, imipramine and amphetamine.
Ashford & Ross H2,686/68: In mice, pretreatment with thyroid extract increased the toxicity of imipramine, nortriptyline, chlorpromazine, perphenazine and chlordiazepoxide, whereas the toxicity of meprobamate and reserpine was not enhanced.

Salicylates ←

Pfeiffer 16,694/23: In guinea pigs, thyroidectomy aggravates the drop in body temperature produced by cooling or salicylate injection i.p.
Vunder & Lapshina D34,912/56: In rats, mice and chickens, the goitrogenic effect of paraamino-salycylic acid is prevented by concurrent administration of thyroid extract.

Semicarbazide ←

Hunt & Carlton F3,186/64: In Pekin ducks, combined administration of semicarbazide and isoniazid p.o. produce a neurolathyrism-like syndrome which is not significantly influenced either by thiouracil or by DL-thyroxine.
SKF 525-A ← *cf. Table 106*

Sodium Chloride ←

Fregly C77,939/59: In rats, the hypertension induced by substitution of hypertonic NaCl for drinking fluid, as well as the accompanying cardiac and renal hypertrophy, are prevented by propylthiouracil.
Strychnine ← *cf. also Table 107*

Hunt & Seidell 50,346/09: In mice, pretreatment with thyroid extract does not influence resistance to strychnine.

Bálint & Molnár 34,586/11: In guinea pigs, the fatal effect of strychnine intoxication is inhibited by epinephrine or thyroid extract i.p.

Marañón & Aznar 46,926/11: In frogs, the fatal convulsions produced by strychnine can be prevented if, prior to injection, the drug is mixed with extracts of the posterior pituitary, the thyroid, various other tissues, and particularly epinephrine. [The possibility of delayed absorption owing to local vasoconstriction has not been considered (H.S.).]

Parhon & Urechia 62,361/13: In dogs and rabbits, orchidectomy and thyroidectomy do not influence resistance to strychnine consistantly, but thyroid feeding appears to aggravate the characteristic convulsions.

Sulfa Drugs ←

Lehr & Martin C13,119/56: In rats, the production of cardiovascular lesions by "standard renal injury" (due to treatment with sulfa drugs) is prevented by thyroparathyroidectomy but not by thyroidectomy with parathyroid extract treatment. Curiously, "chemical thyroidectomy" [technique not specified (H.S.)] also inhibited, and thyroid hormone excess aggravated these lesions.

Lehr & Martin C23,011/56: In rats, the cardiovascular lesions produced by sodium acetylsulfathiazole (as a consequence of renal injury) are prevented by thyroparathyroidectomy, presumably because in the final analysis the changes observed are due to nephrogenic hyperparathyroidism.

Taurochenodeoxycholate ← Thyroxine: Voigt et al. *H25,247/70*

Tetrahydronaphthylamine ←

Borchardt 23,683/28: In cats, neither thyroparathyroidectomy nor adrenalectomy prevents the production of fever by tetrahydronaphthylamine, whereas denervation of the liver inhibits it almost completely.

Glaubach & Pick 11,431/30: In rabbits, the fever normally produced by tetrahydro-β-naphthylamine or cocaine is increased to fatal levels following pretreatment with thyroxine.

Thallium ←

Buschke 4,823/33; Buschke et al. 43,284/33: In mice, thyroxine increases, whereas thymus extract decreases, sensitivity to thallium intoxication.

Uspenskaya D34,628/39: In rabbits, thallium intoxication is aggravated by chronic pretreatment with thyroid extract but not significantly influenced by thyroidectomy.

Theobromine ← cf. Table 108

Theophylline ← cf. also Table 109

Strubelt et al. G78,572/70: In rats, T3 increases, whereas thyroidectomy decreases, the calorigenic response to theophylline and caffeine, probably because the thyroid hormone activates adenylcyclase and/or inhibits phosphodiesterase.

Thimerosal ← cf. Table 110

Thioacetamide ←

Srinivasan & Balwani G64,503/68: In rats, pretreatment with thyroxine increased the liver damage produced by subsequent administration of CCl_4 or thioacetamide.

Thiourea ←

MacKenzie & MacKenzie A49,024/43: In rats, thyroidectomy offers no protection against the production of pulmonary edema by acute thiourea-overdosage.

Glock B23,056/45: In rats given normally fatal doses of thiourea, treatment with adrenocortical extract plus NaCl offers greater protection than NaCl alone. Thyroxine is a still more effective prophylactic even when given without NaCl.

Wiberg et al. E23,265/63: The mouse anoxia test performed after thiouracil treatment permits simultaneous assessment of survival and goitre prevention. The antigoitrogenic assay is more sensitive and permits greater precision than the anoxia test in the bioassay of thyroactive materials.

Tribromoethanol ← cf. also Table 111

Pribram A47,677/29: Both in rabbits and in man, single i.v. injections of thyroxine a few hours prior to administration of tribromoethanol diminish the actions of the latter.

Rutsch 7,744/33: In guinea pigs, thyroidectomy decreases, whereas thyroxine pretreatment increases, resistance to ether, paraldehyde or tribromoethanol anesthesia. These findings are ascribed to changes in the responsiveness of the brain.

Trichlorethanol ← cf. Table 112
Tri-o-cresyl phosphate ← cf. Table 113

Triton ←

Michel & Truchot C 79,107/59: In thyroidectomized rats, the hypercholesterolemia and, to a lesser extent, perhaps also the cholesterol accumulation in the liver produced by triton WR-1339 are diminished by thyroxine.

Tryptophan ←

Bavetta et al. C 47,327/57: In rats, various manifestations of tryptophan deficiency are aggravated by thyroid feeding.

D-Tubocurarine ← cf. Table 114
Tyramine ← cf. Table 115
Tyrosine ← cf. also Table 116

Schweizer B 3,047/47: Addition of excessive amounts of L-tyrosine to the diet produces alkaptonuria, keratitis, conjunctivitis, alopecia, and inflammation of the paws in young rats. Among older animals, males are more sensitive than females. The severity of the syndrome is aggravated by thyroxine and inhibited by thiouracil.

Moore G 36,616/65: In mice, pretreatment with T3 greatly increases sensitivity to the lethal effect of amphetamine. "Chlorpromazine, phenoxybenzamine, and propranolol pretreatment reduced the lethality of d-amphetamine in hyperthyroid mice while α-methyl-m-tyrosine, α-methyl-p-tyrosine, and reserpine pretreatment did not. The toxicity of α-methyl-m-tyrosine was enhanced in hyperthyroid mice."

Boctor et al. H 22,509/70: In rats, tyrosine intoxication was aggravated by thyroxine and alleviated by thiouracil. "Plasma tyrosine concentration and liver tyrosine transaminase activity were high in rats fed a high tyrosine diet; thyroxine administration increased them further, but depressed slightly the activity of liver p-hydroxyphenylpyruvate hydroxylase."

Uranium ←

Rabboni & Milazzo B 18,975/47: In rabbits, thyroidectomy protects against the production of toxic nephritis by conjoint administration of uranium acetate and epinephrine.

Vitamin A ←

Euler & Klussmann 4,928/32: In rats, the toxicity of thyroxine is partly inhibited by carotene and the authors suggest that perhaps "thyroxine is bound to carotene and thereby inactivated." There may exist a physiologic antagonism between vitamin A and thyroxine.

Fasold & Heidemann 16,518/33: A goat normally excreted vitamin A but no carotene in its milk. After thyroidectomy, the milk of the same animal contained carotene but no vitamin A. It is assumed that thyroid hormone participates in the synthesis of vitamin A.

Abelin 57,019/33: In guinea pigs, thyroxine inhibits the hepatic storage of carotene and its transformation into vitamin A. In vitro studies suggest an actual chemical interaction between carotene and thyroxine.

Fasold & Peters A 54,337/33: In rats, hypervitaminosis A can be prevented by thyroxine. The hormone causes a resumption of growth and of carotene deposition in the liver.

Schneider & Widmann 33,725/35: In guinea pigs, both thyroidectomy and treatment with TTH considerably alter vitamin-A metabolism.

Fleischmann & Kann 67,360/36: In mice, vitamin A antagonizes the protective effect of thyroxine against acetonitrile intoxication. Vitamin A also antagonizes the effect of thyroxine upon tadpole metamorphosis. The enhancement of fatty acid oxidation by carotene in vitro is inhibited by thyroxine.

Greaves & Schmidt A 48,725/36: In rats, laparotomy and various toxic agents failed to influence vitamin-A requirements but these are increased by thyroxine or desiccated thyroid and decreased by thyroidectomy.

Sure & Buchanan A 48,611/37: In rats kept on specified diets, thiamine antagonizes the toxic actions of thyroxine but, at the same time, tends to increase vitamin-A requirements as manifested by the onset of xerophthalmia.

Logaras & Drummond A 16,392/38: Metabolic studies on rats kept on a vitamin-A-deficient diet "do not support the view that thyroxine increases the utilization or decreases storage of vitamin A."

Wohl & Feldman A 30,107/39: In patients with hyperthyroidism or hypothyroidism, dark adaptation is frequently deranged suggesting the existence of a disturbance in vitamin-A metabolism.

Baumann & Moore C 38,599/39: In rats given an excess of vitamin A, thyroxine promoted catabolism and shortened survival. Earlier literature on an alleged antagonism between thyroxine and vitamin A is reviewed.

Canadell & Valdecasas B 25,697/47: In rats kept on a vitamin-A deficient diet the characteristic trophic changes can be prevented by the administration of carotene. Thiourea blocks the protective effect of the provitamin A and the effect of the antithyroid compound is in turn blocked by thyroid powder or iodine. The action of thiouracil is ascribed to the inhibition of carotenase activity.

Wiese et al. B39,257/48: In rats, thiouracil prolongs survival on vitamin-A deficient diets.

Woollam & Millen C64,432/58: The offspring of rats given large doses of vitamin A during pregnancy often show deformities of the skull and brain. This teratogenic effect is potentiated by methylthiouracil administration to the pregnant mother.

Nicol & Grangaud D20,176/61: In rats, thiouracil ameliorates the manifestations of vitamin-A deficiency. Progesterone has a similar effect.

Anderson et al. G11,709/64: In rats kept on diets with varying vitamin-A contents, the hepatic storage of vitamin A was increased by thyroxine as compared to thiouracil-treated controls, but the total vitamin-A storage of the body remained unaffected.

Khogali F73,238/66: In rats, hypervitaminosis A is aggravated both by L- and by D-triiodothyronine.

Sundaresan et al. G50,127/67: The vitamin-A requirements of rats are greatly increased during exposure to cold; this increase is abolished by thiouracil.

Vitamin-B Complex ←

Cameron & Moore 57,815/21: In pigeons kept on polished rice, wasting and death were accelerated by thyroid feeding but it is dubious whether this was true also of the specific manifestations of polyneuritis.

Nishimura & Nitta 1,171/29: In vitamin B complex deficient rats, thyroid feeding aggravates the severity of the resulting skeletal lesions.

Templeton & Patras 9,640/33: In rats, survival on a thiamine-deficient diet is prolonged by thyroparathyroidectomy but not significantly altered by desiccated thyroid.

Perelmuter & Miletzkaja 78,650/34: In pigeons on a B-avitaminotic diet, thyroid feeding accelerates the development of polyneuritis.

Sure & Buchanan A6,259/37: In rats, the loss of weight produced by thyroxine can be combated by thiamine.

Sure & Buchanan A48,611/37: In rats kept on specified diets, thiamine antagonizes the toxic actions of thyroxine but, at the same time, tends to increase vitamin-A requirements as manifested by the onset of xerophthalmia.

Infante et al. C17,520/55: In rats, vitamin-B_{12} possesses no lipotropic potency in itself but does prevent hepatic steatosis on hypolipotropic diets supplemented with thyroxine.

Gershoff et al. C54,255/58: In rats, thyroxine greatly increases vitamin-B_{12} requirements.

Vitamin C ←

Mouriquand & Michel 12,231/21: In guinea pigs kept on a normally adequate diet, scurvy-like bone changes developed upon treatment with thyroid extract. Other manifestations of scurvy have not been noted.

Abderhalden 13,399/23: In guinea pigs on an ascorbic acid-deficient diet, thyroidectomy aggravates but does not accelerate the development of scorbutic lesions.

Svirbely 33,140/35: In guinea pigs fed a vitamin-C deficient diet, the development of scurvy is accelerated by thyroid feeding.

Ganguli et al. G71,669/56: Chlorobutanol increases ascorbic acid synthesis and this effect can be suppressed by simultaneous administration of thyroxine, ATP, or malic acid.

McGraw C68,484/59; C80,136/59: Doctor's thesis describing numerous experiments on the effect of adrenalectomy, cortisone, thyroxine, thyroidectomy, thioureas and STH upon scorbutic guinea pigs, with special emphasis upon changes in capillary resistance and cold tolerance.

Vitamin D, DHT ← *cf. also Selye G60,083/70, p. 400.*

Kunde & Williams 18,960/27: In rats thyroidectomized (without removing the parathyroids) 15—29 days after birth, even very large amounts of cod liver oil cannot prevent the development of rickets on a rachitogenic diet.

Schechet B61,419/51: In rats, addition of desiccated thyroid or iodinated casein to a rachitogenic diet assures more regular growth and thereby facilitates the bioassay of vitamin-D preparations.

Gillman & Gilbert C31,076/56: The arterial lesions produced by heavy vitamin-D overdosage in the rat are aggravated by thyroxine or DOC, whereas cortisone and thyroidectomy offer considerable protection.

Selye C27,735/57: The cardiovascular calcification and nephrocalcinosis produced by DHT in rats are aggravated by estradiol, cortisol, ACTH and thyroxine. Conversely, methyltestosterone and STH exert a protective effect.

Takens C69,439/59: In rabbits, the calcinosis and other toxic manifestations of vitamin-D_2 overdosage are accentuated by pretreatment with methylthiouracil.

Manston G69,733/69: The metastatic calcification produced by vitamin-D_3 overdosage in the cow can be prevented by thyroxine.

DHT ← cf. also Table 117

Vitamin E ←

Wheeler & Perkinson B43,572/49: In chicks, vitamin-E requirements are increased by pretreatment with thyroprotein and decreased by thiouracil.

Tentori et al. C7,904/54: In rats, thyroid feeding accelerates the development of the characteristic skeletal muscle lesions produced by vitamin-E deficiency.

Fudema et al. D23,102/62: In rabbits, the muscular dystrophy and death induced by vitamin-E deficiency are delayed following suppression of thyroid activity by ^{131}I.

Vitamins (Pantothenic Acid) ←

Haque et al. B19,204/48: In chicks fed a ration low in folic acid and pantothenic acid, thyroxine caused high mortality but the pantothenic acid-deficiency symptoms were partially counteracted. Review of the literature.

W-1372 ← cf. Table 118

Water ←

Gaunt 84,566/44: Rats are protected against water intoxication by thyroxine. This effect is largely abolished by adrenalectomy.

Zoxazolamine ← cf. also Table 119

Conney & Garren D78,956/60: In rats, pretreatment with thyroxine i.p. shortened the duration of action of zoxazolamine by increasing its metabolism in vivo. However, thyroxine unlike phenobarbital and other drugs did not accelerate zoxazolamine metabolism by increasing the activity of hepatic microsomal enzymes; the shortening of zoxazolamine action by thyroxine was correlated with increased activity of glucose-6-phosphate and 6-phosphogluconate dehydrogenases which are involved in the generation of NADPH.

Conney & Garren D93,666/61: In rats, thyroxine shortens the duration of action of zoxazolamine by accelerating its metabolism through hepatic microsomes.

Harbison & Becker H10,917/69: Thyroidectomy greatly prolonged hexobarbital sleeping time and zoxazolamine paralysis in rats. T3 increased the response to hexobarbital but decreased the effect of zoxazolamine. The mortality rates induced by high doses of hexobarbital, thiopental, amobarbital, pentobarbital and phenobarbital were all significantly increased in rats pretreated with T3.

Zoxazolamine ← Thyroxine: Conney et al. *D93,666/61**

Varia ←

Hunt & Seidell 50,346/09: Systematic studies on the effect of thyroid extract upon the resistance of mice to a great variety of toxic substances.

Störtebecker 76,398/39: Review of the early literature on the effect of thyroid hormone upon resistance to various drugs.

Selye G70,480/71: In rats, pretreatment with thyroxine diminished resistance to intoxication with dioxathion and parathion. It failed to affect poisoning with digitoxin, nicotine, hexobarbital, progesterone (anesthesia), zoxazolamine, indomethacin, acute DHT induced tissue calcinosis or the infarctoid myocardial necroses produced by fluorocortisol + Na_2HPO_4 + corn oil.

Complex Diets ←

In rabbits, thyroidectomy moderately decreases the catabolic effect of fasting. Thyroid feeding accelerates catabolism in rats kept on vitamin-free diets.

Nutritional hepatic cirrhosis (such as is seen on various hypolipotropic diets) is prevented by propylthiouracil and other thioureas in proportion to their goitrogenic effect, whereas thyroid feeding has an opposite action.

In hamsters, gallstone formation on a diet containing 24% rice starch is increased by concurrent treatment with thyroxine.

Blum 38,401/00; 38,405/06: Studies on the effect of thyroidectomy upon the resistance of dogs, rabbits, and sheep to feeding various diets led to the conclusion that the thyroid is not an organ of internal secretion but acts by accumulating and destroying endogenous toxic substances especially those derived from meat diets.

Mansfeld & Müller 35,416/11: In rabbits, thyroidectomy inhibits the protein catabolic effect of exposure to decreased oxygen tension, hydrocyanic acid intoxication or fasting.

Hari 51,049/19: Contrary to earlier claims, even thyroidectomized rabbits show intense protein catabolism during fasting.

Cameron & Moore 57,815/21: In rats kept on a vitamin-free diet (oatmeal and water), thyroid feeding produced a particularly rapid loss of weight.

György et al. G71,701/48: In rats, hepatic cirrhosis produced by a complex hepatotoxic diet is prevented by propylthiouracil and other thioureas in proportion to their goitrogenic effect.

Sellers & You B68,641/51: In rats kept on a choline-deficient diet, propylthiouracil retards the development of hepatic cirrhosis and fatty cyst formation; thyroid feeding has an opposite effect.

Dryden & Hartman C66,416/59: In rats kept on various complex diets during treatment with thyroprotein, no single nutrient could be found which would antagonize the manifestations of hyperthyroidism.

Bergman & van der Linden G30,642/65: In hamsters, gallstone formation on a diet containing 24% rice starch, is increased by concurrent treatment with D-thyroxine. At the same time, the animals develop fatty livers. On a diet containing 72.3% rice starch, the gallstone-forming action of D-thyroxine is blocked although hepatic steatosis still occurs.

Bergman & van der Linden G43,913/66; G39,200/66: In hamsters kept on certain diets, thyroxine promotes gallstone formation. Cholestyramine prevents this effect.

Borgman & Haselden H29,947/70: In rabbits kept on a gallstone producing ration, ACTH, thyroid hormones or cortisone did not inhibit the production of biliary calculi, but several of these hormones inhibited the usually associated hepatic steatosis.

Microorganisms, Parasites and Their Products ←

Bacteria and Vaccines ←. Numerous investigations dealt with the effect of thyroid hormones upon the course of various bacterial infections but special attention was given in this connection to tuberculosis. In guinea pigs, thyroidectomy and thiouracil diminish, whereas thyroxine and T3 increase, resistance to tuberculosis. Essentially similar observations were made in rabbits and in mice. However, in the latter species, pretreatment with thyroxine or dinitrophenol in doses sufficient to limit the weight gain of noninfected controls, diminished resistance to infection with tuberculosis.

Heavy overdosage with thyroxine also diminishes resistance to various other bacterial infections (e.g., plague bacilli, S. typhi, staphylococcus, streptococcus) although it increases resistance to some infections (e.g., chicken cholera); we have no valid explanation for this dual effect although it may be due to incidental conditioning factors (dosage, timing, diet, etc.) as much as to the type of microbe used.

Viruses ←. In monkeys, resistance to poliomyelitis virus is allegedly not affected either by thyroidectomy or by thyroxine, but in mice, it is increased by thyroid extract and decreased by thiouracil.

In rats, sensitivity to various strains of encephalitis virus is augmented by thyroxine and the same appears to be the case in mice vaccinated and subsequently infected with influenza.

Parasites ←. Thyroid feeding has an adverse effect upon mice infected with Hymenolepis tapeworms, whereas thiouracil increases resistance to these parasites.

In chickens, thiouracil did not appear to alter resistance to cecal coccidiosis (Eimeria tenella) significantly but mild hyperthyroidism, induced by thyroactive iodocasein, increased the ability of chicks to overcome infection with Ascaridia galli or Heterakis gallinae.

Allegedly thyroidectomy or pretreatment with thioureas also slightly decreases resistance to toxoplasma and to Trichinella spiralis in the mouse.

Bacterial Toxins ←. In guinea pigs and rabbits, thyroidectomy or treatment with thyroid preparations produced only minor and variable changes in resistance to various endotoxins. Allegedly, in mice, the lethal action of endotoxins is enhanced by T3 or thyroxine, whereas in guinea pigs thyroxine diminishes the lethal effect of tetanus toxin.

Bacteria and Vaccines ←

Bacillus Anthracis ←. *Weinstein B15,029/39:* In mice, various anterior pituitary preparations protect against infection with B. anthracis. Parathyroid extract was also very effective, whereas thyroxine and testosterone offered little protection and progesterone, insulin, "estrin" and posterior lobe extract were virtually ineffective.

Brucella Melitensis ←. *Bradley & Spink C76,042/59:* In mice, infected with small numbers of B. melitensis, hepatic granulomas occurred without necrosis. Severe necrosis developed after pretreatment with T3 without multiplication of brucellae and with minimum inflammatory lesions. Necrosis was not induced by T3 in mice given brucella endotoxin after T3 treatment.

Klebsiella Pneumoniae ←. *Martin & Bullard H15,263/69:* In mice, resistance to infection by K. pneumoniae is increased by propylthiouracil and decreased by thyroxine.

Mycobacterium Tuberculosis ←.

GUINEA PIG

Kepinow & Metalnikow 40,285/22: Thyroidectomized guinea pigs infected with tubercle bacilli do not respond with fever to a subsequent tuberculin injection although their survival rate is not altered.

Izzo & Cicardo B23,261/47; B67,482/47: In guinea pigs, thyroidectomy diminishes, whereas thyroxine increases, resistance to infection with tubercle bacilli. The clinical literature on the effect of hyperthyroidism upon tuberculosis is reviewed.

Swedberg B59,988/51: Thyroxine diminishes the resistance of guinea pigs to tuberculosis. "Estrogen" has the same effect, whereas testosterone does not significantly change the course of the infection.

Wasz-Höckert et al. C30,699/56: In guinea pigs, methylthiouracil aggravated, whereas thyroid extract ameliorated, the course of experimental tuberculosis.

Renovanz C78,772/59: In guinea pigs, the course of experimental tuberculosis was not markedly influenced by ACTH, tolbutamide derivatives or antithyroid treatment with perchlorates.

Solanki & Junnarkar D21,370/61: In guinea pigs, pretreatment with thyroxine increases the resistance to tuberculosis by augmenting the phagocytic capacity of mononuclear leukocytes.

Bloch D61,174/63: In guinea pigs, resistance to tuberculosis is increased by T3.

Vakilzadeh & Vandiviere E32,626/63: In guinea pigs, the beneficial effect of vaccination against tuberculosis was greatly increased by thyroxine and T3, but not by cortisone, cortisol or ACTH. None of the hormones altered natural host resistance in nonimmunized guinea pigs.

RABBIT

Lurie & Ninos C14,387/56: In rabbits pretreatment with T3 inhibits, whereas thiouracil aggravates, the course of experimental tuberculosis.

Lurie et al. C14,963/56; C52,055/58: In rabbits, the course of pulmonary tuberculosis is ameliorated by treatment with T3 or thyroxine and aggravated by propylthiouracil or thyroidectomy. Dinitrophenol exerts no conspicuous effect.

Lurie et al. C64,295/59: In rabbits, thyroidectomy or propylthiouracil reduced the native resistance to human tubercle bacilli. T3 exerted no consistent effect upon tuberculin sensitivity but greatly inhibited the growth of bacilli and enhanced resistance to infection.

Lurie et al. C65,610/59: Various strains of inbred rabbits were infected with tuberculosis bacilli. "Hyperthyroidism induced by L-triiodothyronine or L-thyroxine suppressed to a greater or lesser degree the inception and progress of the pulmonary tuberculosis produced by the quantitative inhalation of human tubercle bacilli in four races, AD, III, IIIC, CaC, and IIIA, with low or intermediate genetic resistance to the disease. L-Triiodothyronine also exerted a definite suppressive influence on the development of an already existing tuberculosis when the hormone was administered three weeks after the infection."

Dzyubinskaya C97,348/60: Pretreatment with methylthiouracil aggravates the course of experimental tuberculosis in rabbits.

Mouse

Dubos D93,317/55; G71,484/55: In mice, resistance to tuberculosis is decreased by pretreatment with thyroxine or dinitrophenol p.o. in amounts sufficient to limit the weight gain of noninfected controls. These findings, as well as observations on dietary factors influencing resistance to tuberculosis, led to "the hypothesis that a decrease in resistance to infection can be brought about by metabolic disturbances which cause either a depletion of the glycogen reserves of the body, or a reduction in the glycolytic activity of inflammatory cells, or an increase in the concentration of certain polycarboxylic acids and ketones in the tissues."

Maśliński C50,519/56: In mice, the histologic reaction to infection with tuberculosis is somewhat altered by pretreatment with "thyroid hormone" or methylthiouracil, but survival is not significantly changed.

Maśliński C50,520/56: In mice, severe overdosage with methylthiouracil or desiccated thyroid aggravates the course of tuberculosis. There is, however, an optimum state of hyperthyroidism in which the intensity of the tuberculous changes is the lowest.

Chirico et al. C67,012/59: In mice, small doses of thyroxine diminish mortality and prolong the mean survival time following infection with tubercle bacilli.

Backman C94,674/60: In mice, both methylthiouracil and desiccated thyroid aggravate the course of experimental tuberculosis.

Rat

Steinbach 92,528/32: In rats, parathyroidectomy lowers resistance to infection with bovine but not with human tuberculosis. Thyroparathyroidectomy makes rats susceptible to both human and bovine tubercle bacilli.

Varia

Schäfer B99,955/54: Monograph (127 pp., numerous refs.) on the role of endocrine factors in tuberculosis. Special sections are devoted to the hormones of the thyroid, parathyroid, thymus, adrenals, pancreas and gonads.

Maśliński C48,845/57: Review (55 pp., 114 refs.) on the relationship between tuberculosis and the thyroid. Personal observations on mice revealed that following infection with tuberculosis mortality was increased by methylthiouracil in comparison with controls receiving thyroid preparations or no hormone treatment.

Debry et al. D34,828/62: Review (14 pp., 64 refs.) on the relationship between tuberculosis and thyroid activity.

Mycoplasma ←. *Tripi et al. B12,732/49:* In rats, the production of polyarthritis by PPLO organisms was enhanced and the mortality increased following chronic pretreatment with thiouracil. Thyroidectomy (inducing a similar or greater drop in BMR) did not change this form of polyarthritis. Presumably, thiouracil acts "through some peculiar intrinsic action" rather than by merely diminishing thyroid activity.

Pasteurella ←. *Marbé 34,321/10:* In guinea pigs, pretreatment with thyroid extract diminishes resistance to infection with plague bacilli and counteracts the protective effect of antiplague serum.

Parhon & Parhon 36,340/14: During a chicken cholera epidemic, a small number of thyroid extract-treated chickens survived better than controls.

Salmonella Typhi ←. *Marbé 34,320/10; A23,018/10:* In guinea pigs, resistance to infection with typhoid bacilli is diminished by pretreatment with thyroid extract.

Marbé A23,015/12: Addition of thyroid extract to cultures of typhimurium bacilli in vitro increases their virulence.

Shigella ←. *Melnik 26,134/25:* In rabbits, thyroidectomy offers some protection against infection with Shiga bacilli.

Staphylococcus ←. *Lauber 9,102/32:* Observations on the effect of vasopressin, epinephrine, thyroid extract and insulin upon streptococcal and staphylococcal infections in mice.

Sealy A56,716/42: In rabbits, desiccated thyroid does not produce liver necrosis in itself but facilitates its production after infection by S. aureus. A review of the literature also suggests that uncomplicated hyperthyroidism does not result in liver necrosis either in experimental animals or in man unless there is a complicating infection.

Dubos et al. C 21,520/55; Dubos G 71,484/55: In mice, thyroxine pretreatment diminishes resistance to infection with S. aureus. The resistance-diminishing effect of thyroxine and dinitrophenol against other infections is briefly mentioned.

Smith & Dubos C 12,130/56: In mice, pretreatment with thyroid extract or dinitrophenol decreases resistance to staphylococcal infection.

Hedwall & Heeg D 14,804/61: In rats, an experimental staphylococcus pyelonephritis is aggravated by pretreatment with thyroxine.

Streptococcus ←. *Lauber 9,102/32:* Observations on the effect of vasopressin, epinephrine, thyroid extract and insulin upon streptococcal and staphylococcal infections in mice.

Schultz 99,001/38: In guinea pigs and rabbits, pretreatment with thyroxine increases susceptibility to the development of purulent myocarditis after s.c. inoculation with hemolytic streptococci.

Varia ←. *Marbé A 4,623/08; A 4,624/08; A 4,625/08; A 4,626/09; A 4,627/09; A 23,010/09; A 23,011/09; A 23,012/09; A 23,013/09; A 23,016/10; 34, 561/10:* Studies on the effect of thyroidectomy and thyroid extract upon opsonin formation and phagocytosis of bacteria in guinea pigs and rabbits.

Murphy et al. C 60,008/58: In mice, resistance to infection with C. albicans or S. pyrogens is increased by pretreatment with T3 but this hormone does not significantly alter resistance to transplanted leukemia.

Nutter et al. C 65,285/59: In mice, T3 decreases survival time after infection with tubercle bacilli or pneumococci.

Viruses ←

Levaditi & Haber 33,069/35: In Macacus cynomolgus monkeys, resistance to poliomyelitis virus, acquired by prior infection, is not influenced by thyroidectomy, orchidectomy or thyroxine administration.

Holtman B 1,287/46: In mice, resistance to infection with polio virus is increased by thyroid extract and decreased by thiouracil. The comparative polio resistance of mice kept in a cool environment may be secondary to increased thyroid hormone production.

Hurst et al. C 94,089/60: Cortisone, ACTH, estradiol, stilbestrol and thyroxine all stimulate the growth of the virus of equine encephalomyelitis in the dog whereas testosterone and progesterone do not. The hormones which aggravate the infection also counteract the prophylactic effect of mepacrine and abolish the normally greater resistance of the females.

Jandásek C 88,870/60: In suckling rats infected with tick encephalitis survival was greatly shortened by thyroxine. Neither antibody production nor the number of virus carriers was influenced by the hormone.

Jandásek C 92,117/60: Mice become particularly sensitive to infection by encephalitis virus (strain Hypr) following pretreatment with thyroxine.

Lungu et al. F 84,406/67: In mice vaccinated against influenza, subsequent infection with the virus causes an increased mortality following treatment with thyroxine or thiouracil.

Jannuzzi et al. H 27,335/70: In patients with viral hepatitis, various anabolics, including stanozolol and 4-chlorotestosterone, exert a beneficial effect.

Parasites ←

Larsh Jr. A 47,571/47: In old mice, thyroid feeding has an adverse effect on infestation with Hymenolepis tapeworms, whereas thiouracil increases resistance to the parasites. In young mice, the infestation was much less dependent upon the thyroid status.

Wheeler et al. A 48,602/48: In chickens, a preliminary study suggests that thiouracil-induced hypothyroidism does not significantly affect resistance to cecal coccidiosis induced by infection with Eimeria tenella.

Todd G 71,890/48: In chickens infected with Ascardia galli or Heterakis gallinae, mild hyperthyroidism induced by feeding thyroactive iodocasein (Protamone) increased the ability of the birds to overcome the worm infestation. Thiouracil had a detrimental effect.

Todd B 40,185/49: In chickens infected with Ascardia galli or Heterakis gallinae, treatment with thyroactive iodocasein or thiouracil caused no significant difference in the development of either worm; however, "specimens of H. gallinae attained significantly greater lengths in mildly hypothyroid birds."

Hirschlerowa C 35,235/56: Thyroidectomy or pretreatment with methylthiouracil decreases resistance to infection with toxoplasma unless the animals are given substitution therapy with thyroid extract.

Krupa et al. G 45,694/67: In mice, propylthiouracil slightly decreased resistance to infestation with Trichinella spiralis larvae but the results were not consistent.

Bacterial Toxins ←

Marbé 35,374/11: In guinea pigs, thyroid feeding increases sensitivity to diphtheria toxin.

Hari 40,209/21: Polemic remarks concerning the technique and interpretation of earlier data on the effect of thyroidectomy upon the resistance to cyanides, chloroform, bacterial toxins and oxygen deficiency.

Houssay & Sordelli A 48,113/21: In rabbits, thyroidectomy does not change sensitivity to diphtheria toxin. In guinea pigs, sensitivity to diphtheria toxin, tetanus toxin and to cobra venom is likewise not modified by removal of the thyroid.

Locatelli 28,678/34: In dogs, thyroidectomy diminishes the wave of mitosis in hepatocytes normally produced by small doses of diphtheria toxin.

Sealy & Lyons B 46,719/49: In rabbits, sterile inflammation produced by staphylococcus toxin s.c. causes hepatic necrosis if the animals are pretreated with thyroid extract.

Kroneberg & Pötzsch E 54,858/52: In mice, thyroxine pretreatment increases sensitivity to endotoxin.

Melby et al. C 86,232/58: In mice, T3 increases the lethal effect of Br. melitensis endotoxin. In mice infected with Br. melitensis, unique hepatic lesions develop under the influence of T3 pretreatment which are not seen in unpretreated controls.

Bradley & Spink C 76,042/59: In mice, infected with small numbers of Brucella melitensis, hepatic granulomas occurred without necrosis. Severe necrosis developed after pretreatment with T3 without multiplication of brucellae and with minimum inflammatory lesions. Necrosis was not induced by T3 in mice given Brucella endotoxin after T3 treatment.

Melby & Spink C 72,440/59: In mice, the lethal action of various endotoxins is enhanced by pretreatment with T3.

Gordon & Lipton C 94,649/60: 5-HT reduces endotoxin mortality in mice. This effect is greater in females than in males and is potentiated by cortisol. Thyroxine aggravates the toxicity of endotoxin.

Yokoi et al. D 8,839/61: In rabbits, a biphasic fever pattern is elicited by Sh. flexneri type 6 pyrogen. The biphasic nature of the response was maintained after thyroidectomy but largely abolished by adrenal demedullation.

Schoen & Voss D 11,906/61: In guinea pigs, the lethal effect of tetanus toxin is inhibited by pretreatment with thyroxine.

E-coli Endotoxin ← *cf. also Table 123*

Venoms ←

Houssay & Sordelli A 48,113/21: In rabbits, thyroidectomy does not change sensitivity to diphtheria toxin. In guinea pigs, sensitivity to diphtheria toxin, tetanus toxin and cobra venom is likewise not modified by removal of the thyroid.

Immune Reactions ←

Most of the studies on the effect of thyroid hormones upon immune reactions have been performed on guinea pigs which are notoriously sensitive to anaphylaxis.

The formation of various antibodies has been claimed to be inhibited by thyroidectomy and stimulated by thyroid extract. In sensitized guinea pigs, thyroid extract, administered a few days before a challenging dose of horse serum, protects against fatal anaphylactic shock. However, thyroidectomy prior to sensitization allegedly has the same effect, whereas this is not the case if the thyroid is removed after sensitization. Indeed, it has been claimed that, in guinea pigs, thyroidectomy blocks anaphylaxis unless the animals are treated with thyroid. Suppression of anaphylactic reactivity by anterior hypothalamic lesions can be partially overcome by thyroid hormones in guinea pigs.

Particularly extensive studies have been performed in guinea pigs concerning the role of the thyroid apparatus in the reaction to tuberculin. Moderate thyrotoxicosis produced by two weeks' pretreatment with thyroxine increases tuberculin hypersensitivity. Propylthiouracil does not affect it, but the suppression of hypersensitivity by cortisone or ACTH is allegedly abolished by pretreatment with this goitrogen.

The beneficial effect of vaccination against tuberculosis is also increased in guinea pigs by thyroxine or T3.

If dogs are sensitized after thyroidectomy, subsequent anaphylactic shock is mild. Thyroidectomized dogs are also relatively insensitive to peptone shock. In rabbits, Masugi nephritis is considerably aggravated by pretreatment with thioureas.

Marbé A4,623/08; A4,624/08; A4,625/08; A4,627/09; A4,626/09; A23,010/09; A23,011/09; A23,012/09; A23,013/09; A23,016/10; 34,561/10: Studies on the effect of thyroidectomy and thyroid extract upon opsonin formation and phagocytosis of bacteria in guinea pigs and rabbits.

Müller A47,855/11: In guinea pigs, the formation of various antibodies is inhibited by thyroidectomy as well as by surgical interference with hepatic circulation. Treatment with thyroid extract has an opposite effect. The latter is not due to shock, since removal of all abdominal organs except the liver is ineffective. Furthermore, the blood loses its "alexic power" when perfused through an isolated liver preparation.

Savini & Savini A24,559/15: In sensitized guinea pigs, pretreatment with thyroid extracts a few days before administration of a challenging dose of horse serum protects against fatal anaphylactic shock.

Képinow 13,298/22: In guinea pigs, thyroidectomy blocks anaphylaxis unless they are treated with thyroid extract.

Képinow & Lanzenberg 13,258/22: Preliminary studies on the effect of thyroidectomy upon anaphylaxis and antibody formation in guinea pigs.

Lanzenberg & Képinow 13,117/22: In guinea pigs, thyroidectomy prior to sensitization prevents subsequent anaphylactic shock, whereas this is not the case if the thyroid is removed after sensitization.

Appelmans 14,085/23: Anaphylactic shock develops normally in thyroidectomized guinea pigs even if both the sensitizing and the challenging dose of antigen are administered after the operation.

Houssay & Sordelli 13,430/23: Comparative studies on the influence of thyroidectomy upon anaphylaxis in the guinea pig, rabbit and dog.

Képinow 13,941/23: Discussion of the optimal conditions for the prevention of anaphylaxis by thyroidectomy in guinea pigs.

Parhon & Ballif 13,548/23; 17,302/23: In guinea pigs, anaphylaxis is diminished after thyroidectomy but not significantly influenced by thymectomy.

Houssay & Cisneros 26,936/25: In dogs sensitized after thyroidectomy, subsequent anaphylactic shock is diminished. Thyroidectomized dogs are also comparatively insensitive to peptone shock.

Fleisher & Wilhelmj 23,337/27: In guinea pigs, thyroidectomy before sensitization diminishes the severity of subsequent anaphylactic shock. In rabbits, this inhibition is not clear-cut although there does appear to occur some change in the reaction of thyroidectomized rabbits following the second injection of antigens. Immunological studies suggest that thyroidectomy does not prevent the formation of antibodies but merely alters the reaction during shock.

Spinelli 7,369/32: In guinea pigs, thyroidectomy increases resistance to anaphylactic shock.

Long & Miles D41,973/50: In guinea pigs, moderate thyrotoxicosis produced by two weeks' treatment with thyroxine increases hypersensitivity to tuberculin, whereas moderate doses of propylthiouracil do not affect it. ACTH and cortisone diminish tuberculin sensitivity. Fourteen days after stopping thyroxine injections, the animals became actually less hypersensitive than the controls. A similar reversal of effect was noted two weeks after interruption of cortisone or ACTH treatment in that the animals became more hypersensitive than the controls.

Strehler & Sollberger B54,646/50: In rabbits, Masugi nephritis is greatly aggravated by pretreatment with tetramethylthiourea.

Long et al. B60,189/51: In B.C.G.-infected guinea pigs, hypersensitivity to tuberculin is considerably diminished by cortisone or ACTH. This diminution is abolished by pretreatment with propylthiouracil, which alone has no effect upon hypersensitivity. Pretreatment with thyroxine increases tuberculin hypersensitivity but does not block the sensitization by ACTH or cortisone. Apparently, thyroxine is necessary for the desensitizing action of ACTH and cortisone.

Long et al. B63,843/51: In guinea pigs, dihydroascorbic acid—unlike ascorbic acid—inhibits the tuberculin reaction after infection with B.C.G. vaccine. The desensitizing effect of dihydroascorbic acid is not inhibited by thiouracil. Alloxan, like ACTH or cortisone, does not modify desensitization by ascorbic acid on diets deprived of the "cabbage factor;" it desensitizes guinea pigs on a cabbage diet and this desensitization is inhibited by propylthiouracil.

Long & Shewell G71,833/54: In guinea pigs, allergic hypersensitivity to B.C.G. is increased by thyroxine or insulin. Partial pancreatectomy has no effect on sensitivity by itself but prevents the action of thyroxine, although not that of insulin.

Long & Shewell G71,832/55: In guinea pigs, thyroxine increases immunity as judged by the local response to diphtheria toxin injected intradermally and of circulating antitoxin after immunization with diphtheria toxoid. Partial pancreatectomy prevents this effect of thyroxine.

Long C32,348/57: In guinea pigs, both anaphylactic shock (horse serum) and sensitivity to histamine are greatly increased by pretreatment with thyroxine. Thyroxine also augments the sensitivity of guinea pigs to intradermal tuberculin injection.

Vakilzadeh & Vandiviere E32,626/63: In guinea pigs, the beneficial effect of vaccination against tuberculosis was greatly increased by thyroxine and T3, but not by cortisone, cortisol or ACTH. None of the hormones altered natural host resistance in nonimmunized guinea pigs.

Lupulescu et al. F77,999/66: In rabbits, the formation of antibodies against brucella S_6 is stimulated by thyroxine and 4-chlorotestosterone but decreased by thiourea. The effect of 4-chlorotestosterone is evident even after destruction of the thyroid and hence is not mediated through the latter gland.

Filipp & Mess G71,129/69: In guinea pigs, suppression of anaphylactic reactivity by anterior hypothalamic lesions can be partially blocked by chronic treatment with thyroid hormones as well as by adrenalectomy or adrenal inactivation by metyrapone (Metopirone). "Combined treatment of guinea pigs bearing hypothalamic lesions with Metopirone and thyroxine completely eliminated the blocking effect of the tuberal lesion on anaphylactic reactions." Apparently the shock-inhibiting effect of hypothalamic lesions is partly due to hypothyroidism and partly to hyperadrenalcorticoidism.

Special Surgical Interventions ←

Hepatic Lesions ←. In rats, desiccated thyroid feeding increases the weight of the liver under normal conditions and the rate of regeneration after partial hepatectomy. Curiously, thiouracil has also been claimed to accelerate liver regeneration under similar conditions but this was denied by several investigators, who found that even thyroidectomy had no significant effect upon the regeneration of hepatic tissue in the rat.

In dogs, the manifestations of shock produced by constriction of the hepatic veins were aggravated by thyroid feeding and constriction of the portal vein caused ascites only after pretreatment with methylthiouracil.

Ascites produced by subdiaphragmatic constriction of the inferior vena cava was inhibited by thyroidectomy and restored by a thyroid extract in one series of experiments. However, other investigators pointed out that subdiaphragmatic constriction of the inferior vena cava causes ascites in itself and that this can be ameliorated by thyroidectomy, though only if the operation is performed after the caval constriction.

Renal Lesions ←. In uninephrectomized rats, compensatory hypertrophy of the remaining kidney is diminished, but not prevented, by thyroidectomy. Regeneration is inhibited by thiouracil and enhanced by thyroxine under these conditions.

The pressor effect of renal encapsulation is diminished by methylthiouracil and increased by thyroxine in the rat. However, thyroidectomy performed after the kidneys had been encapsulated for 9-19 weeks has only a slight effect upon the blood pressure.

The metastatic calcification produced by complete nephrectomy in rats is uninfluenced by thyroxine although it can be prevented by calcitonin. Presumably, the previously described protective effect of thyroxine against exogenous parathyroid hormone depends upon the presence of the kidney.

In dogs and rats, destruction of the thyroid by radio-iodine increases survival after bilateral nephrectomy perhaps merely because general metabolism is greatly diminished.

Hepatic Lesions ←

Higgins 9,809/33: In rats, desiccated thyroid feeding increases the weight of the liver under normal conditions, and the rate of regeneration after partial hepatectomy.

Hepler & Simonds A15,174/38: In dogs, the manifestations of shock produced by constriction of the hepatic veins are aggravated following thyroid feeding.

Fogelman & Ivy B23,357/48: In rats, thiouracil accelerates liver regeneration after partial hepatectomy.

Drabkin B17,795/48: In rats, thyroidectomy moderately diminishes liver regeneration after partial hepatectomy and reduces cytochrome c in skeletal muscle, heart, liver and kidney.

Spigolon B52,689/49: In dogs, gradual constriction of the portal vein caused ascites only if the animals were pretreated with methylthiouracil.

Christensen & Jacobsen A49,204/49: In rats subjected to partial hepatectomy, neither hypophysectomy nor thyroidectomy impairs the rate of regeneration. No significant change in mitotic rate was observed after pretreatment with stilbestrol or STH.

Drabkin D18,388/50: In rats, thyroidectomy or thiouracil treatment does not significantly impair liver regeneration after partial hepatectomy, whereas thyroxine markedly inhibits it.

Giberti et al. B82,948/53: In rats, propylthiouracil does not inhibit liver regeneration after partial hepatectomy but prevents hepatic steatosis.

Weinbren D95,941/59: Review (11 pp., 110 refs.) and personal observations on factors influencing hepatic regeneration after partial hepatectomy in the rat, with special sections on the effects of hypophysectomy and thyroid hormones.

Canter et al. C67,855/59; Baronofsky & Canter C85,341/60: In dogs, the production of ascites by subdiaphragmatic constriction of the inferior vena cava is inhibited by thyroidectomy and restored by subsequent treatment with thyroid extract.

Poll et al. D4,775/61: In dogs, ascites produced by supradiaphragmatic constriction of the vena cava inferior is usually ameliorated by thyroidectomy, but only if the operation is performed after caval constriction.

Girkin & Kampschmidt C99,934/61: In rats, the hepatic enlargement induced by Walker tumor transplants or by partial hepatectomy is inhibited by thiouracil and largely restored by subsequent thyroxine treatment.

Renal Lesions ←

McQueen-Williams & Thompson A33,938/40: In rats, total hypophysectomy prevented the compensatory hypertrophy of the remaining kidney after uninephrectomy. Thyroidectomy did not prevent renal regeneration under identical conditions.

Zeckwer 84,592/44: In rats, thyroidectomy does not significantly alter renal regeneration following unilateral nephrectomy.

Herlant B30,957/47: In uninephrectomized rats, regeneration in the remaining kidney is inhibited by thiouracil.

Herlant B30,956/48: In uninephrectomized rats, thyroxine greatly increases the number of mitoses in the proximal tubules of the remaining kidney.

Valori B46,667/48: In rats, thyroidectomy diminishes but does not abolish compensatory hypertrophy of the remaining kidney after uninephrectomy.

Kleinsorg & Loeser B41,137/49: In rats, compensatory hypertrophy of the remaining kidney following uninephrectomy is enhanced by thyroxine and inhibited by methylthiouracil.

Bächtold B60,463/50: In rats, the pressor effect of renal encapsulation is diminished by pretreatment with methylthiouracil and increased by thyroxine.

Marshall & Freeman B68,239/52; B96,575/54: In dogs and rats, destruction of the thyroid by ^{131}I increases survival time after bilateral nephrectomy.

Braun-Menéndez C4,927/54: In rats, the hypertension produced by figure-of-8 ligature is diminished by thyroidectomy or thiouracil and increased by thyroid powder p.o.

Osipovich C58,570/57: In uninephrectomized rats, methylthiouracil enhances compensatory hypertrophy of the remaining kidney, presumably as a consequence of increased TTH secretion. The acceleration of compensatory renal hypertrophy by exposure to cold is ascribed to a similar mechanism.

Fregly et al. C66,042/59: In rats, the hypertension produced by bilateral renal encapsulation is prevented by thyroidectomy or propylthiouracil.

Fregly et al. C80,398/60: In rats, after renal encapsulation, propylthiouracil reduced the systolic blood pressure even more than did complete thyroidectomy. However, the cardiac hypertrophy of renal hypertension was not prevented by propylthiouracil, suggesting that the diastolic pressure remained unaffected. Thyroidectomy performed after the kidneys had been encapsulated for 9—19 weeks had only a slight effect on blood pressure.

Fregly & Cook C88,371/60: In rats, various thioureas inhibit the development of hypertension and cardiac hypertrophy following bilateral renal encapsulation. This effect is counteracted by feeding desiccated thyroid.

Mandel et al. D6,027/60: In rats, the compensatory renal hypertrophy and RNA synthesis in the remaining kidney, which normally occur after uninephrectomy, are inhibited by propylthiouracil.

Eades Jr. et al. F89,204/67: In rats with renal hypertension (uninephrectomy + figure-of-8 ligature), propylthiouracil inhibits hypertension and coronary atherosclerosis but not the hypercholesterolemia.

Lefort et al. G46,725/67: In rats, metastatic calcification produced by bilateral nephrectomy is largely inhibited by calcitonin but uninfluenced by thyroxine pretreatment. Presumably the previously demonstrated protective effect of thyroxine against exogenous parathyroid hormone depends upon the presence of the kidney.

Côté et al. G46,741/68: In rats, calcitonin inhibits the metastatic calcification and bone lesions induced by bilateral nephrectomy. In nephrectomized animals, thyroxine does not modify the changes induced by endogenous hyperparathyroidism consequent to bilateral nephrectomy. "Presumably, to be effective against soft-tissue calcification and bone resorption induced by parathyroid extract overdosage, thyroxine requires the presence of the kidney."

Eades Jr. et al. H9,590/69: In rats with renal hypertension produced by uninephrectomy and a meat diet, thiouracil or sulfadiazine diminishes the blood pressure and protects the remaining kidney from damage.

Gardell et al. G70,430/70: In rats, the cardiovascular calcification produced by bilateral nephrectomy is not significantly influenced by ethylestrenol, CS-1, spironolactone, norbolethone, oxandrolone, prednisolone, progesterone, triamcinolone, DOC, estradiol or thyroxine.

Blood-Vessel Ligatures ←

Dau & Weber G20,433/63: Contrary to earlier claims, the recovery of the spinal cord (disappearance of motor disturbances) after temporary aorta ligature is not significantly influenced by "blockade of the thyroid" through pretreatment with iodine or $KClO_4$ in rabbits.

Ionizing Rays ←

In the mouse, according to most investigators, resistance to X-irradiation is decreased by thyroid hormones and increased by thioureas. However, some workers claim that neither thioureas nor thyroidectomy influences X-ray resistance significantly in this species. The timing and dosage of the thyroid treatment also appears to be important since in one series of observations, pretreatment with thyroid extract until five days before X-irradiation diminished the resulting mortality induced by X-irradiation.

In **rats** also, pretreatment with thyroid hormones generally diminishes X-ray resistance, whereas thiouracil offers little if any protection. Indeed, it has been stated that conjoint treatment with thyroxine and thiourea induces the greatest drop in X-ray resistance.

In **rabbits**, both systemic damage following total body irradiation, and the renal changes induced by topical X-irradiation of the kidney, are aggravated by thyroxine and T3.

The thyroxine-induced differentiation of limb-buds in **toad** tadpoles is only insignificantly retarded by X-irradiation.

In the **goldfish**, as in mammals, thyroxine diminishes X-ray resistance.

MOUSE

Blount & Smith B30,000/49: In mice exposed to total X-irradiation, mortality was greatly increased by feeding desiccated thyroid and insignificantly diminished by thiouracil.

Haley et al. B49,990/50: Contrary to earlier claims, no protection against X-irradiation could be obtained in mice given large doses of thiouracil, propylthiouracil or methylthiouracil.

Limperos & Mosher B49,737/50: In mice, pretreatment with thiourea increases resistance to X-irradiation.

Mole et al. D96,011/50: In mice, thiourea reduces mortality following whole body X-irradiation.

Haley et al. B58,913/51: In rats, thyroparathyroidectomy offers no protection against X-irradiation. The small degree of protection noted by previous investigators after thiouracil may have been due to its sulfhydryl group. On the other hand, thyroxine causes a significant increase in mortality rate, though not in total mortality.

Smith B66,170/51: In mice, thyroid feeding increases the mitotic index of the epidermis, but does not influence the effect of X-irradiation upon epidermal mitotic proliferation.

Pospíšil & Novák C67,534/58: Mice pretreated with thyroid extract until 5 days before X-irradiation were more resistant than unpretreated mice against mortality induced by ionizing rays. These findings are in sharp contrast with those of earlier authors who have found an increased mortality in animals given thyroid both before and during, or even continuing after X-irradiation.

Léonard & Maisin E26,654/63: In mice, β-aminoethylisothiourea offers moderate protection against the toxic effects of X-irradiation.

Maisin et al. E36,751/63: In mice, the protection against X-irradiation offered by 2-β-aminoethylisothiourea (AET) is only slightly improved by concurrent administration of 5-HT.

RAT

Haley et al. B60,616/51: In rats, pretreatment with thiourea or thyroxine did not significantly alter mortality after X-irradiation. However, an increase in mortality rate was observed in animals which had received both thyroxine and thiourea.

Smith & Smith B60,347/51; B60,348/51: In rats, desiccated thyroid or dinitrophenol increased radiation lethality, but thiouracil and propylthiouracil exerted no significant protective effect.

Haley et al. G71,834/52: In rats, mortality after X-irradiation is increased both by propylthiouracil and by thyroxine.

Stender & Hornykiewytsch C37,079/55; C37,086/55: In rats the lethal effect of total body X-irradiation is diminished by a reduction in the oxygen tension of the surrounding air. This protective effect is counteracted by cortisone, adrenalectomy, and thyroxine.

Darcis & Brisbois C50,953/57: In the rat, the sensitivity of the small intestine to topical X-irradiation (unlike that of the vagina) is not influenced by thyroxine or testosterone.

Krahe & Künkel C77,236/58: In rats, pretreatment with thyroxine decreases resistance to X-irradiation.

Shellabarger et al. D39,218/62: In female rats, the production of mammary cancers by X-irradiation is inhibited by diethylstilbestrol in doses which in themselves are not carcinogenic. T3 did not influence carcinogenesis under these circumstances.

Caprino & Gallina G13,680/63: Contrary to earlier claims, propylthiouracil does not offer significant protection against total body X-irradiation in rats.

Greig et al. E60,304/65: In rats, irradiation of the thyroid inhibits its capacity to undergo hyperplasia under the influence of a goitrogen. Pretreatment with methylthiouracil before irradiation reduces the degree of this inhibition.

Akoev et al. F73,202/66: Both stilbestrol and thyroid extract offered some protection against ^{60}C γ-radiation in rats.

Srebo et al. H32,848/70: In rats, thyroxine decreases, whereas propylthiouracil increases, resistance to subsequent X-irradiation.

Slebdodzinski and Srebro H29,972/71: In rats, thyroxine pretreatment aggravates the syndrome of total body irradiation, whereas propylthiouracil offers considerable protection.

RABBIT

Vittorio et al. C76,156/59: Rabbits treated with a mixture of thyroxine and T3 became unusually sensitive to the lethal effect of X-irradiation. Neither untreated nor methimazole treated rabbits succumbed after the dose of irradiation used.

Caldwell et al. D54,096/63: In rabbits, renal damage produced by topical X-irradiation of the kidney is aggravated by T3.

FISH, TOAD

Allen & Ewell C92,110/59: In tadpoles of Bufo boreas halophilus, thyroxine-induced differentiation of limb-buds is only insignificantly retarded by X-irradiation.

Srivastava et al. G23,764/64: In the goldfish (Carassius auratus L.), resistance to X-irradiation is diminished by thyroxine the same as in mammals.

VARIA

Rigat C10,747/55: Review (46 pp., 67 refs.) on the literature concerning the effect of hormones upon X-irradiation, with special reference to ACTH, STH, vasopressin, epinephrine, cortisone, DOC, testosterone, estradiol, progesterone, and thyroxine.

Hypoxia ←

In the **rat**, thyroid hormones increase whereas thyroidectomy and thioureas decrease sensitivity to hypoxia. This phenomenon became the basis of what was known as "Asher's method" for testing thyroid function. Pretreatment with thyroxine also predisposes the liver and the brain of the rat to the production of degenerative changes by hypoxia.

Similar observations have subsequently been confirmed by numerous investigators in the **mouse** in which the sensitization by thyroxine is so consistent and evident that it was made the basis of the Emmens and Parkes "closed vessel technique" for the bioassay of thyroid preparations. If mice are placed in closed vessels, the speed of their mortality during the developing anoxia is proportional to the amount of thyroid hormone with which they have been pretreated. T3 is about five times as active as thyroxine in this respect. The sodium salt of L-thyroxine is about seven times more potent than that of D-thyroxine. Among a series of T2 compounds only 3:5-diiodo-L-thyronine was effective, but even this was much less active than T3.

In **rabbits** and **dogs**, thyroidectomy diminishes the protein catabolic effect of hypobaric oxygenation and of several other stressors.

In **guinea pigs**, thyroidectomy is said not to affect resistance to lack of oxygen, whereas T3 has been claimed actually to increase it.

Fish and various other species are made unusually resistant to asphyxia by thioureas.

RAT

Klinger 51,094/18: Contrary to earlier claims, thyroparathyroidectomized rats do not tolerate hypoxia better than normals; in fact, they become hypersensitive to it.

Streuli 32,220/18: In rats, thyroidectomy increases resistance to hypoxia. Splenectomy has an opposite effect, and rats simultaneously thyroidectomized and splenectomized exhibit a normal resistance to hypoxia.

Duran A 10,045/20: In rats, thyroid extract increases, whereas thyroidectomy decreases sensitivity to hypobaric oxygenation.

Cameron & Carmichael 42,188/26: In young rats, thyroid feeding produces a predisposition for tetany; in animals so treated, diminished oxygen tension rapidly induces tetanic convulsions.

Rydin 22,940/28: In rats, thyroxine pretreatment increases sensitivity to hypobaric oxygenation.

Asher & Wagner 23,903/29: Both rats and guinea pigs become highly sensitive to anoxia after pretreatment with thyroid extract. This phenomenon is the basis of what the authors describe as "Asher's method for the testing of thyroid function by lack of oxygen."

Houssay & Rietti 3,187/32: In rats, pretreatment with an impure pituitary extract diminishes resistance against hypoxia, but this effect is abolished by thyroidectomy and is presumably due to TTH. In untreated rats, thyroidectomy actually increases resistance to anoxia.

McIver & Winter B 33,399/43: In rats pretreated with thyroxine, exposure to diminished atmospheric oxygen tension causes hepatic injury.

Goldsmith et al. B 333/45: Thiouracil and thiourea increase the resistance of rats to lowered barometric pressure. Estradiol and stilbestrol are ineffective in themselves and fail to influence the action of the antithyroid compounds.

Gordon et al. B 761/45: Review of the literature, and personal observations on the raised resistance to lowered barometric pressures induced in rats by thiourea, para-aminobenzoic acid (PABA), and other agents interfering with the thyroid function.

Blood et al. B 48,970/49: As judged by observations in rats pretreated with thyroxine or thiouracil "oxygen availability becomes a limiting factor in oxygen consumption only at altitudes approaching 40,000 feet in normal rats, but at much lower altitudes in animals whose metabolism has been stimulated by cold or by thyroxin."

Bargeton et al. B 50,869/49: In rats, pretreatment with thiouracil increases resistance against reduced barometric pressure.

Zarrow et al. B 63,316/51: In rats exposed to hypobaric oxygenation, thyroxine diminished survival time, whereas in mice it caused an initial increase followed by a decrease. Thiouracil enhanced survival time in rats and, to a much lesser extent, in mice also.

Flückiger & Verzár B 86,489/52: In rats, thyroidectomy does not markedly influence the development of hypothermia upon exposure to decreased oxygen pressure.

DeBias D 41,419/62: The survival of rats exposed to reduced oxygen tension was not significantly altered by thyroidectomy.

Riedel F 22,473/64: In rats and rabbits, chronic thyroxine overdosage produces morphologic changes in the brain, which are aggravated by hypoxia.

Keminger G 42,501/66: In rats, death from lack of oxygen in closed vessels is accelerated by T3, and retarded after thyroidectomy or cortisone treatment. Epinephrine further accelerates mortality in hyperthyroid animals.

Trojanová G 42,905/66: In newborn rats, the survival of the respiratory centre (gasping) during anoxia is greatly reduced by thyroparathyroidectomy.

Smoake & Mulvey Jr. H 23,262/70: In rats, thyroidectomy and propylthiouracil increase, whereas feeding of desiccated thyroid decreases resistance to hypobaric hypoxia.

Mouse

Emmens & Parkes B 4,928/47: Male mice are considerably more sensitive than females to anoxia (closed vessel technique). Various thyroid preparations increase sensitivity to anoxia.

Smith B 4,939/47: In mice, thyroxine shortens, whereas thiourea prolongs, survival in closed vessels. L-thyroxine is considerably more active than d-thyroxine. T2 is even less active, whereas thyroxamine, diiodothyronamine, tetrachlorothyronine, tetrabromothyronine, and T2 are inactive.

Reisfield & Leathem B 46,491/50: In mice, survival in closed vessels is reduced by thyroid globulin p.o., but unaffected by propylthiouracil.

Basil et al. B 53,039/50: The mouse anoxia test has been found useful in assaying the biologic activity of various thyroxine derivatives.

Smith & Smith B 60,348/51: In mice, desiccated thyroid or thyroxine pretreatment decreases resistance to progressive hypoxia or forced muscular exercise. Death may have been due to cardiac failure. "Irradiated mice, whether given thyroid or not, lived longer in the closed vessel and were still alive at lower O_2 concentrations than their corresponding controls."

Gemmill B 85,291/53: In mice, T3 is only slightly more potent than thyroxine as judged by the anoxia test.

Anderson B94,669/54: In mice, T3 is about 5 times as active as thyroxine in increasing sensitivity to anoxia.

Tabachnick et al. C22,161/56: "Using the mouse anoxia assay, Na L-thyroxine was found to be seven times more potent than Na D-thyroxine."

Tomich et al. C83,307/60: Six iodo-L-thyronines, viz. 3:3':5'-triiodo-, 3:5-diiodo-, 3:3'-diiodo-, 3':5'-diiodo, 3-monoiodo-, and 3'-monoiodo-L-thyronine, have been compared with 3:5:3'-triiodo-L-thyronine, in mice by the anoxia method. The only compound with any significant activity was 3:5-diiodo-L-thyronine but even this was much less active than 3:5:3'-triiodo-L-thyronine.

Wiberg et al. E23,265/63: The mouse anoxia test performed after thiouracil treatment permits simultaneous assessment of survival and goitre prevention. The antigoitrogenic assay is more sensitive and permits greater precision than the anoxia test in the bioassay of thyroactive materials.

RABBIT

Mansfeld & Müller 35,416/11: In rabbits, thyroidectomy inhibits the protein catabolic effect of exposure to decreased oxygen tension, hydrocyanic acid intoxication, or fasting.

GUINEA PIG

Stämpfli 931/27: In guinea pigs, thyroidectomy does not significantly alter resistance to lack of oxygen.

Lamarche & Pluche F68,410/66: In guinea pigs, resistance to hypobaric oxygenation is increased by T3 but not by triiodothyroacetic acid.

FISH

Tinacci B28,546/47: Fish (Mustelus laevis) pretreated with various thioureas become unusually resistant to asphyxia.

VARIA

Mansfeld 11,881/20: In rabbits and dogs, thyroidectomy diminishes the protein catabolism normally observed after intoxication with hydrocyanic acid, hemorrhage, or hypobaric oxygenation.

Hári 40,209/21: Polemic remarks concerning the technique and interpretation of earlier data on the effect of thyroidectomy upon the resistance to cyanides, chloroform, bacterial toxins, and oxygen deficiency.

Hyperoxygenation ←

In rats exposed to six atmospheres of oxygen in a pressure chamber, resistance is diminished by thyroxine. Similar diminutions of tolerance for hyperoxygenation have been noted with various other thyroid preparations, whereas thioureas have an opposite effect.

In the cat also, thyroid extract increases, whereas thyroidectomy decreases sensitivity to oxygen poisoning.

Campbell A14,903/37: In rats exposed to six atmospheres of oxygen in a pressure chamber, subsequent decompression is better tolerated at low than at high external temperatures. "Using an external temperature of 24°C and white rats of about 80 g., the following substances, administered subcutaneously, are found to enhance oxygen poisoning: thyroxin (0.4 mg), dinitrophenol (1.5 mg), ac-tetrahydro-β-naphthylamine (0.5 c.c., 1 p.c.), adrenaline (0.02 mg), pituitary extract (posterior lobe, above 3.5 units), insulin (0.025 u.) and eserine (0.045 mg administered with atropine 0.075 mg). These doses in themselves are harmless."

Gersh & Wagner B1,140/45: In cats, thyroid extract increases, whereas thyroidectomy decreases sensitivity to the convulsive effect of oxygen poisoning.

Grossman & Penrod B36,303/49: In rats exposed to high oxygen tension, the mortality is increased by pretreatment with desiccated thyroid, and decreased by propylthiouracil.

Bean & Bauer B76,951/52: In rats, desiccated thyroid augments the adverse effects of exposure to high-oxygen tension. It also abolishes the protective effect of hypophysectomy.

Taylor C47,861/58: In rats "adrenalectomy gave very definite protection against the central nervous system manifestations of oxygen poisoning, and gave some protection against lung damage." Adrenocortical extract and cortisol increased susceptibility of adrenalectomized animals to oxygen poisoning, whereas cortisone, DOC, and thyroid powder had no such effect.

Smith et al. C95,244/60: In rats, desiccated thyroid or thyroxine increases the noxious effects of breathing virtually pure oxygen at atmospheric pressure. Conversely, hypophysectomy increases resistance to oxygen, presumably through the elimination of TTH.

Szilagyi et al. G68,248/69: In rats and rabbits, mortality from hyperbaric oxygenation is increased by pretreatment with thyroid extract, but uninfluenced by thyroidectomy.

Temperature Variations ←

In **rabbits**, thyroid hormones increase resistance to cold, and conversely, tolerance to desiccated thyroid is augmented in a cold environment. Thyroparathyroidectomy and thioureas diminish cold resistance. Tolerance to a warm environment is decreased by desiccated thyroid.

In **rats**, sensitivity to warm surroundings also rises after pretreatment with thyroid preparations, whereas resistance to cold is increased. Thyroidectomy and thioureas diminish cold resistance. In rats fed thyroid, exposure to cold causes marked pentosuria, whereas thiouracil has an opposite effect. The decreased ability of old rats to adapt themselves to cold is also improved by T3. In thyroidectomized rats, resistance to cold is restored towards normal by intraocular thyroid transplants. The vitamin-A requirements of rats are greatly increased during exposure to cold unless they are pretreated with thiouracil.

In **mice**, thyroid feeding increases sensitivity to heat stroke and predisposes to the production of hepatic lesions during exposure to high temperature.

In **hamsters**, thyroidectomy diminishes cold resistance much less than in rats. However, radiothyroidectomy renders them sensitive to cold. Hamsters presumably possess ectopic thyroids which are not eliminated by ordinary thyroidectomy.

Thyroidectomized **goats** are also very resistant to cold, but this has been ascribed to increased epinephrine secretion.

In various strains of **fish**, heat tolerance is increased by thiourea. Immature salmon can be completely radiothyroidectomized and yet continue to grow, but their heat tolerance is impaired.

RABBIT

Cori 17,210/22: In rabbits, thyroidectomy diminishes resistance to cold and increases its hypothermic effect.

Draize & Tatum 3,901/31: The resistance of rabbits to survival at a temperature of 33°C is recommended as a basis for the bioassay of desiccated thyroid preparations.

Draize & Tatum 3,657/32: In rabbits, the tolerance for desiccated thyroid is increased in a cold and decreased in a warm environment.

Sanfilippo & Ricca 31,704/35: In rabbits, pretreatment with thyroxine increases resistance to cold.

di Macco 34,121/35: In rabbits, the hyperthermia induced by exposure to heat is aggravated by thyroxine.

Capitolo A1,730/36: In rabbits, thyroparathyroidectomy decreases the resistance to heat stroke, and death occurs at a lower body temperature level than in controls.

Martinengo & Beghelli B3,426/39: In rabbits, pretreatment with T2 diminishes resistance to heat.

Lange et al. B23,962/48: In rabbits, resistance to cold is increased by pretreatment with thyroid extract and diminished following partial suppression of thyroid function by thiouracil.

Medvedeva F96,027/68: Biochemical studies on the decreased cold resistance of thiourea-treated rabbits.

RAT

Abderhalden & Wertheimer 19,292/28: Rats pretreated with thyroxine are unusually sensitive to warm surrounding temperature.

Genitis et al. 68,723/35: In young thyroparathyroidectomized rats, exposure to heat 24 hrs after the operation greatly increased the mortality rate, whereas cold surrounding temperature diminished it. The number of tetanic convulsions was greatest at an intermediate temperature. [From the brief abstract, it is difficult to differentiate between the role of parathyroid and of thyroid deficiency (H.S.).]

Barbour & Seevers 84,296/43: In rats, exposure to cold and an excess of CO_2 produce a state of narcosis against which considerable resistance can be induced by thyroid extract. No such effect was obtained by dinitrophenol.

Zarrow & Money B27,880/49: In rats, pretreatment with thiouracil diminishes the resistance to cold, a phenomenon which is ascribed to the adrenal cortical involution elicited by thiourea.

Blood et al. B48,970/49: As judged by observations in rats pretreated with thyroxine or thiouracil "oxygen availability becomes a limiting factor in oxygen consumption only at altitudes approaching 40.000 feet in normal rats, but at much lower altitudes in animals whose metabolism has been stimulated by cold or by thyroxine."

Roe & Coover B54,246/51: In rats, thyroid feeding or exposure to cold markedly increases urinary pentose excretion, whereas thiouracil reduces the output of urinary pentose and decreases resistance to cold. Apparently "the thyroid gland has a dominating role in the production of urinary pentose and that adjustment of animals to cold takes place, at least in part, through activity of the thyroid gland."

Sellers et al. B65,310/51: The survival of clipped rats exposed to cold is considerably prolonged by combined treatment with thyroxine + cortisone. Each of these agents alone has much less protective value, and DOC is inactive.

Money C5,393/54: Female rats lose their ability to resist a cold environment if they are pretreated with thiouracil.

Weiss C34,561/57: Studies on tissue metabolism in rats exposed to cold after thyroidectomy by ^{131}I. "The hypothesis is advanced the thyroid gland exerts its effects by way of a few selected tissues only, in which it regulates the level of metabolism so as to provide adequate heat production for suitable adaptation to cold of the entire animal."

Weiss C66,153/59: The decreased ability of old rats to adapt themselves to cold is greatly improved by T3.

Garrido D8,112/60: In rats, resistance to cold is increased by thyroxine and T3, and decreased by thyroidectomy or destruction of the thyroid with radio-iodine. Prednisolone exerted only a moderate protective effect.

Fregly D5,800/61: In rats, propylthiouracil does not reduce spontaneous running activity in itself, but when exposed to cold, rats thus treated do not increase their activity as much as controls.

Hsieh D20,969/62: Rats fed propylthiouracil for four weeks before exposure to cold died in about 17 days, while those fed an iodine-deficient diet and propylthiouracil, for the same period before exposure, died in less than one day. Rats maintained for four weeks in the cold and on T3 died when the dose levels of the thyroid hormone were reduced. "Thus cold adaptation does not reduce the requirement for thyroid hormone."

Beaton D55,998/63: Review of the literature, and personal observations on the effect of thyroid feeding or thyroidectomy upon the cold resistance of rats given diets of varying protein content.

Pavlovic-Hournac & Andjus E33,972/63: In rats, the decreased resistance to cold induced by thyroidectomy is restored towards normal by intraocular thyroid transplants.

Weiss G21,456/63: In rats, resistance to cold can be increased with T3 acetate as it can with T3 or thyroxine.

Hamburgh & Lynn G21,782/64: In rats raised at 20°C, the delay in skeletal maturation induced by propylthiouracil is more severe than in controls raised at 30°C.

Hsieh F71,817/66: Systematic studies on the thyroid hormone (thyroxine, T3) requirements of thyroidectomized curarised rats for resistance to cold in the absence of shivering.

Weihe F69,421/66: In rats, thyroxine impedes acclimatization to high altitude.

Bauman & Turner F81,331/67: Pretreatment of rats with thyroxine raises their resistance to cold. Additional administration of corticosterone greatly increases this effect, although in itself, corticosterone possesses only a slight protective action.

Sundaresan et al. G 50,127/67: The vitamin-A requirements of rats are greatly increased during exposure to cold, this increase is abolished by thiouracil.

MOUSE

Lübke C 12,952/56: In mice, thyroid feeding increases sensitivity to heat stroke and causes particularly severe hepatic lesions upon exposure to high temperature.

GUINEA PIG

Pfeiffer 16,694/23: In guinea pigs, thyroidectomy aggravates the drop in body temperature produced by cooling or salicylate injection i.p.

Amante & Mancini C 21,222/56: In guinea pigs, pretreatment with methylthiouracil prolongs survival following severe burns. The data are discussed primarily in connection with the role of the thyroid in the alarm reaction.

HAMSTER

Chaffee et al. G 71,307/63: In hamsters, thyroidectomy does not diminish cold resistance nearly as much as in the rat.

Yousef et al. F 86,757/67: Hamsters, unlike rats, are very resistant to cold even after complete surgical thyroidectomy. In order to determine whether this difference is due to the existence of ectopic thyroids, radio-iodine was administered; since this caused an even more severe drop in plasma PBI than thyroidectomy, it was concluded that hamsters may possess accessory thyroid tissue. However, upon exposure to cold, the BMR rose significantly in both groups and yet, the surgically thyroidectomized hamsters survived, whereas most of the radio-thyroidectomized animals succumbed. Apparently, "increased thyroid activity in cold exposure has no significant effect upon survival" in this species.

Yousef et al. F 98,470/68: Hamsters are resistant to cold even after surgical thyroidectomy, but not after treatment with ^{131}I. The plasma PBI is lowered by thyroidectomy, but not as much as by ^{131}I. Presumably the hamsters have ectopic thyroid tissue which permits survival after surgical thyroidectomy.

GOAT

Andersson et al. G 45,246/67: Thyroidectomized goats maintain body temperature during exposure to acute cold ($-3°C$) and also react to cooling of the hypothalamic thermoregulatory "centre" by a rise in body temperature. However, under these conditions, shivering and urinary catecholamine excretion were greatly increased. "It is concluded that to maintain thermal homeostasis in the cold markedly hypothyroid goats have to compensate the lack of thyroid hormone by a conspicuous increase in adrenaline secretion."

CAT

Boatman C 68,449/59: In cats "thyroidectomy prior to cold exposure makes heat conservation responses less efficient than in the normal animal and the intact thyroid plays a role in maintaining body fluids in an efficient equilibrium for rapid adjustment to a cold environment."

FISH

Evropeitzeva A 49,151/49: Larvae of the fish Coregonus lavaretus ludoga withstand exposure to $29°C$ for five min after treatment with thiourea, whereas untreated animals die.

La Roche & Leblond C 434/54: Immature salmon can be completely "thyroidectomized" by radio-iodine; yet, they continue to grow, although their resistance to a rise in water temperature is greatly impaired.

Suhrmann D 76,901/55: Immersion into a solution of thiourea increases the upper lethal temperature tolerated by goldfish (Carassius auratus).

Fortune C 17,485/55; C 21,670/56: In the minnow (Phoxinus phoxinus L.), the thermal death point is raised considerably by treatment with thiourea.

Cheverie & Lynn D 68,411/63: In the fish (Tanichthys albonubes), inactivation of the thyroid by immersion into a thiourea solution slightly reduces tolerance to high temperatures. The literature on opposite results in other species of fish is reviewed.

Dodd & Dent E 21,585/63: In minnows (Phoxinus phoxinus L.), neither thiourea nor thyroxine pretreatment induced any significant change of heat tolerance.

Electric Stimuli ←

In **guinea pigs**, the EST is diminished within two days after initiation of thyroid feeding, and augmented after thyroidectomy.

In rats, the EST is only insignificantly lowered by thyroidectomy. It is allegedly also diminished one hour after thyroxine administration but increased 18 hrs later. This biphasic response may explain some of the contradictions in the literature.

In mice, thyroxine facilitates the production of convulsions by electroshock, and in dogs, it increases irritability of the sympathetic nervous system.

Specht 13,475/23: In guinea pigs, neither thyroidectomy nor orchidectomy influences the course of the convulsions produced by amylnitrate inhalation or electric irritation of peripheral nerves.

Gerlich B49,124/49: In guinea pigs, the EST is diminished within two days after initiation of thyroid feeding. Thyroidectomy has an opposite effect.

Woodbury et al. B68,423/52: In rats, brain excitability (pentylenetetrazol, EST) decreases following thyroidectomy or treatment with propylthiouracil and increases after thyroxine pretreatment. There are however certain differences between thyroidectomy and propylthiouracil as regards the recovery time from electroshock seizures and their relative effect upon extensor and flexor components.

Thiéblot et al. C18,452/56: In dogs, thyroxine pretreatment increases the electric irritability of the sympathetic nervous system.

de Salva et al. C51,842/58: In rats, the EST was lowered by hypophysectomy and adrenalectomy, but only insignificantly by thyroidectomy. 5-HT elevated the EST.

Pfeifer et al. D12,952/60: In rats, the convulsive effect of "Pentametazol" [presumably pentylenetetrazol (H.S.)] is diminished one hour after administration of thyroxine, but increased 18 hrs later. A corresponding biphasic response is also noted with regard to the EST. In mice, the increased motility induced by amphetamine is also inhibited during the first hour after thyroxine treatment. The possible biochemical reasons for this "negative tendency" during the early phase of thyroxine action are described.

de Salva D66,176/63: In rats, the EST is reduced in descending order of magnitude by adrenalectomy, hypophysectomy, and thyroidectomy. The effect of these endocrine deficiencies upon various depressant drugs is also described.

Pfeifer et al. G65,057/68: In mice, thyroxine facilitates the production of convulsions by pentylenetetrazol and electroshock. These effects are inhibited by various amphetamine derivatives.

Various Stressors ←

Dogs fed desiccated thyroid are particularly susceptible to **traumatic shock**, whereas methylthiouracil offers some protection against it. Similar observations have been made in rats. The formation of peritoneal adhesions in response to local injury is diminished by methylthiouracil.

In mice, thyroid preparations diminish resistance to forced **muscular exercise**.

In rabbits and dogs, thyroidectomy diminishes the protein catabolism that follows **hemorrhage**.

Following pretreatment with T3, the **audiogenic seizures** produced in susceptible mice by strong sound are accelerated in onset, but their pattern remains unchanged. T3 does not induce audiogenic seizure-proneness in nonsusceptible strains.

Trauma ←

Schachter & Huntington A32,970/40: Dogs fed desiccated thyroid are particularly susceptible to the production of traumatic shock by manipulation of their intestines.

D'Aste & Ardau B56,421/49: In dogs, methylthiouracil offers some protection against various forms of traumatic shock, but this effect is ascribed to the antihistaminic property of the drug.

Takács et al. C29,459/54: In rats, traumatic shock (produced by freezing the hind limbs) is diminished by methylthiouracil, but aggravated by thyroxine, thyroid extract, or dinitrophenol.

Dobrokhotova C55,431/57: In rats, survival following hemorrhagic shock with trauma is prolonged by methylthiouracil.

Kovách et al. C50,699/57: In rats, survival from shock (produced by freezing a hind leg with liquid air) is shortened by thyroid feeding, thyroxine, dinitrophenol or epinephrine, all of which accelerate the metabolic rate. Conversely, methylthiouracil increases survival time.

Oppenheimer et al. C50,563/58: In goats, traumatic shock reduces the capacity of the thyroid to concentrate iodine, but recently thyroidectomized animals showed no change in survival times, although pretreatment with thyroxine greatly sensitized to traumatic shock. Cortisone had no effect upon survival following trauma nor did it counteract the aggravating effect of thyroxine.

Schachter et al. C63,544/59: In rats, pretreatment with cortisone, thyroxine, or both these agents shortened survival after tourniquet shock.

Németh & Vigaš F98,055/68: In rats, resistance to trauma in the Noble-Collip drum is reduced by pretreatment with thyroxine or dinitrophenol but increased by thyroidectomy.

Rusakov & Chernov H9,072/69: In rabbits, the formation of adhesions by removal of the serosa of peritoneal organs is considerably diminished by pretreatment with methylthiouracil.

Muscular Work ←

Smith & Smith B60,348/51: In mice, desiccated thyroid or thyroxine pretreatment decreases resistance to progressive hypoxia or forced muscular exercise. Death may have been due to cardiac failure. "Irradiated mice, whether given thyroid or not, lived longer in the closed vessel and were still alive at lower O_2 concentrations than their corresponding controls."

Valtin & Tenney C66,148/59: In rats, resistance to forced muscular exercise is diminished following pretreatment with T3.

Hemorrhage ←

Mansfeld 11,881/20: In rabbits and dogs, thyroidectomy diminishes the protein catabolism normally observed after intoxication with hydrocyanic acid, hemorrhage, or hypobaric oxygenation.

Sound ←

Hamburgh & Vicari C71,704/58; D11,010/60: In mice susceptible to audiogenic seizures, T3 does not change the seizure pattern nor does it induce seizures in nonsusceptible strains. It merely accelerates the onset of the period during which susceptible animals respond by convulsions to audiogenic stimulation.

Tumors ←

In rats, the production of cystic and neoplastic hepatic lesions by 2-acetaminofluorene is inhibited by thiouracil. The hepatic enlargement induced by Walker tumor transplants is also diminished by this goitrogen and restored by a subsequent thyroxine treatment.

The growth of transplanted fibrosarcomas is increased by thyroid extract or T3, and decreased by propylthiouracil. The lifespan of rats bearing transplantable leukemia is prolonged by thyroidectomy, but in mice this does not seem to be the case.

Cantarow et al. B18,774/46: In rats given 2-acetaminofluorene p.o., the development of cystic and neoplastic hepatic lesions was accelerated and intensified by GTH (pregnant mare serum), estradiol, and testosterone, but inhibited by thiouracil. "This phenomenon may be related to the role of the liver in the intermediary metabolism and excretion of the sex steroid." In the hyperplastic target organs of the sex hormones, tumors did not occur, in contrast to the high incidence of tumors in the thyroids of rats given thiouracil simultaneously with the carcinogens.

Murphy et al. C60,008/58: In mice, resistance to infection with Candida albicans or Streptococcus pyogenes is increased by pretreatment with T3, but this hormone does not significantly alter resistance to transplanted leukemia.

Girkin & Kampschmidt C 99,934/61: In rats, the hepatic enlargement induced by Walker tumor transplants or by partial hepatectomy is inhibited by thiouracil, and largely restored by subsequent thyroxine treatment.

Claus et al. D 29,754/62: In rats, the growth of transplanted fibrosarcomas was increased by thyroid extracts or T3 and decreased by propylthiouracil or an iodine-deficient diet.

Morris & Mokal D 65,803/63: In rats bearing transplantable leukemia, survival is prolonged by thyroidectomy.

Fisher & Fisher F 74,176/66: In rats, the incidence of metastases from Walker tumor transplants is not significantly altered by thyroidectomy, propylthiouracil, thyroxine or TTH.

Varia ←

Smith C 46,496/56: In brown trout, thyroxine raises, whereas thiourea and thiouracil reduce salinity tolerance. Anterior pituitary extracts and STH likewise raise **salinity tolerance**, whereas posterior lobe extracts, testosterone, gonadotrophin, TTH, and ACTH have no such effect.

Czarnecki & Kiersz D 15,579/61: In dogs, shock produced by **trypan blue or peptone** injection is more powerfully inhibited by thyroparathyroidectomy than by thyroidectomy.

Hepatic Enzymes ←

TPO activity is allegedly increased by thyroidectomy in the rat, and substrate-induced TPO synthesis is inhibited by thyroxine.

Hepatic GPT activity is moderately increased by thyroxine. α-GPDH activity is raised by T3 or thyroxine, but diminished by thyroidectomy or radiothyroidectomy.

TPO, TKT ←

Geschwind & Li B 93,277/54: In the rat, the induction of the TPO enzyme system is diminished by hypophysectomy and adrenalectomy, but increased by thyroidectomy.

Kulcsar et al. G 72,002/69: In rats, the substrate-induced synthesis of TPO was inhibited by hepatic injury (CCl_4) as well as by thyroxine. Thyroidectomy was without effect, and actually inhibited the influence of CCl_4.

GPT ←

Rosen et al. C 71,414/59: Marked increases in GPT activity were observed in the livers of rats given cortisol, cortisone, 9α-fluorocortisol, prednisone, 6α-methylprednisolone, 9α-fluoro-21-desoxy-6α-methylprednisolone or ACTH, whereas two nonglucocorticoid cortisol derivatives, 11-epicortisol and 9α-methoxycortisol were inactive. STH, testosterone, and insulin caused no significant change in GPT by themselves nor did they modify the action of cortisol. On the other hand, large doses of estradiol and thyroxine caused a moderate increase in GPT activity, but when injected simultaneously with cortisol, they appeared to interfere with its action as did progesterone. Adrenalectomy slightly diminished or failed to affect the GPT inducing activity of cortisol, whereas hypophysectomy caused a rise in GPT activity and augmented the effect of cortisol.

SDH ←

Ishikawa et al. F 41,763/65: In alloxan-diabetic rats, SDH and TDH levels of the hepatic microsomes are greatly enhanced. SDH was readily induced by cortisol in the diabetic, but not in the normal, rat. The effects of actinomycin S, STH, and starvation upon serine dehydratase have also been studied in intact, hypophysectomized, adrenalectomized, and thyroidectomized rats. It is concluded that "serine dehydratase activity in the liver plays an important role in the production of pyruvate as a starting material for gluconeogenesis."

α-GDPH ←

Rivlin & Wolf H 13,055/69: In rats, the hepatic α-GPDH activity is greatly increased by T3 or thyroxine, but diminished by thyroidectomy or ^{131}I treatment. Both the basal

a-GPDH activity and the maximal increment induced by triiodothyronine are dependent upon adequate intake of riboflavin.

Other Enzymes ←

Spinks & Burn B72,891/52: Thyroid feeding diminishes the amine oxydase activity of the liver in rabbits, whereas thyroidectomy increases it both in rabbits and in rats.

Metzenberg et al. D86,024/61: Thyroxine induces carbamyl phosphate synthetase in hepatic microsomes of the liver in tadpoles.

Freedland F46,702/65: In hepatic homogenates of rats pretreated with thyroxine "there was a marked increase in glucose-6-phosphatase, a decrease in phosphorylase, and relatively smaller changes in other glycolytic enzyme activities after treatment. The enzymes of the pentose phosphate pathway increased as did malic enzyme activity, although a fourth TPN-linked dehydrogenase, isocitric, decreased. L-a-Glycerolphosphate dehydrogenase decreased in the hyperthyroid animals. All 3 of the tricarboxylic acid cycle enzymes measured increased in activity after thyroxine injection."

Kato & Takahashi H11,853/69: "The magnitude of increase in the activities of microsomal drug-metabolizing enzymes and NADPH-linked electron transport system in the alloxan diabetic rats was greater than in normal rats, in contrast, the magnitude of increase in the thyroxine-treated rats was smaller than in normal rats."

Kato et al. H11,851/69: Studies on the effects of thyroxine upon hepatic microsomal enzyme induction by various drugs in diverse species.

← PARATHYROIDS

Comparatively few investigators have examined the effect of the parathyroids on resistance in general.

Steroids ← cf. Selye *C50,810/58, p. 89; C92,918/61, pp. 77, 164, 280; G60,083/70, pp. 410, 412.*

Hormones and Hormone-Like Substances ←

The effect of the parathyroids on the action of **steroids** has been discussed elsewhere. (For references *cf.* Abstract Section.) Parathyroidectomized dogs are allegedly much less resistant against **histamine** than intact controls, and in rabbits, parathyroid extract protects against histamine, **insulin**, and a number of other toxicants. However, these early experiments require confirmation.

Histamine ←

Dragstedt et al. 17,561/23: "Parathyroidectomized dogs are much less resistant to guanidine, methyl-guanidine, trimethylamine, histamine, and the various intestinal poisons than are normal dogs."

McDonagh 19,285/28: In rabbits, parathyroid extract protects against the toxic effects of histamine, insulin, guanidine, coniine and "somnifaine" [superficial description of observations which do not inspire confidence (H.S.)].

Insulin ←

McDonagh 19,285/28: In rabbits, parathyroid extract protects against the toxic effects of insulin [superficial description of observations which do not inspire confidence (H.S.)].

Epinephrine ← cf. Selye *C92,918/61, p. 194; G60,083/70, pp. 410, 413.*

Drugs ←

The parathyroids play an important role in resistance only against very few drugs. Even the effects of such compounds as **copper** or **beryllium** salts which cause definite bone changes are not markedly influenced by parathyroid extract.

It has been claimed that in mice, parathyroid extract can protect against fatal **fluoride** intoxication, but this has been denied by subsequent investigators.

During the early part of this century, it was assumed that parathyroidectomy causes tetany because it interferes with the detoxication of **guanidine**, but this could not be confirmed.

On the other hand, the topical calcification produced by **indium chloride** in the rat is prevented by parathyroidectomy, although the associated hepatic necrosis and icterus remain unaffected. Pretreatment with parathyroid extract (or DHT) prevents the hepatic necrosis, but augments the topical calcergy.

Resistance to $MgSO_4$ i.v. is increased by parathyroid extract in the dog, presumably because of the well-known antagonism between Ca- and Mg-ions. In mice, parathyroid extract inhibits the development of Mg-anesthesia in a dose-dependent manner.

The nephrocalcinosis induced by a dietary excess of **phosphate** (NaH_2PO_4) in the rat is inhibited by thyroparathyroidectomy as well as by excessive thyroxine administration.

The production of cardiovascular lesions by "standard renal injury" following treatment with **sulfa drugs** is prevented by thyroparathyroidectomy in the rat — as is the osteitis fibrosa produced by **uranium** intoxication — probably because these toxicants elicit renal damage with secondary hyperparathyroidism. The latter is presumed to be responsible for the disturbances in skeletal metabolism.

The calcinosis elicited by **vitamin-D** compounds, including **DHT**, is not prevented by parathyroidectomy; hence it cannot be ascribed to a secondary hypersecretion of parathyroid hormone as had been originally thought.

Anaphylactoidogens ← cf. Selye G46,715/68, pp. 179, 199.

Antibiotics ← cf. Selye C92,918/61, p. 91; G60,083/70, pp. 410, 413.

Barbiturates ←

McDonagh 19,285/28: In rabbits, parathyroid extract protects against the toxic effects of histamine, insulin, guanidine, coniine and "somnifaine" [superficial description of observations which do not inspire confidence (H.S.)].

Copper ←

Ulmansky & Sela G70,273/69: In mice, copper administration causes thickening, and fluoride treatment thinning, of the epiphyseal plates. Neither of these responses is influenced by parathyroid extract, which in itself causes some thickening of epiphyseal plates.

Beryllium ←

Jones 33,139/35: In dogs with beryllium rickets, parathyroid extract failed to raise the blood calcium.

Coniine ←

McDonagh 19,285/28: In rabbits, parathyroid extract protects against the toxic effects of histamine, insulin, guanidine, coniine and "somnifaine" [superficial description of observations which do not inspire confidence (H.S.)].

Digitoxin ←

Selye PROT. 33541, 34074: In rats, PCN is highly efficacious in preventing digitoxin poisoning, even after parathyroidectomy, thyroparathyroidectomy, or concurrent treatment with propylthiouracil (PTU). No protection was obtained by thyroidectomy, parathyroidectomy, or treatment with PTU, thyroxine, parathyroid extract or calcitonin. Apparently, the goitrogenic effect of PCN plays no indispensable role in its catatoxic action.

Fluoride ←

Kochmann 55,947/34: In mice, fatal intoxication with NaF or oxalic acid can be prevented by pretreatment with parathyroid extract. These inhibitions are dose-dependent and may serve for the assay of parathyroid preparations.

Muñoz 67,126/36: In rats, parathyroid extract fails to prevent the manifestations of fluorosis.

Ulmansky & Sela G70,273/69: In mice, copper administration causes thickening, and fluoride treatment thinning, of the epiphyseal plates. Neither of these responses is influenced by parathyroid extract, which in itself causes some thickening of epiphyseal plates.

Guanidine ←

Dragstedt et al. 17,561/23: "Parathyroidectomized dogs are much less resistant to guanidine, methyl-guanidine, trimethylamine, histamine, and the various intestinal poisons than are normal dogs."

Süssmann 24,462/27: In mice, very impure parathyroid extracts protect against guanidine and picrotoxin but not against strychnine.

McDonagh 19,285/28: In rabbits, parathyroid extract protects against the toxic effects of histamine, insulin, guanidine, coniine and "somnifaine" [superficial description of observations which do not inspire confidence (H.S.)].

Indium ←

Selye et al. D25,667/62: In rats, $InCl_3$ s.c. produces topical calcification and severe hepatic necrosis with icterus. Parathyroidectomy prevents the topical (calcergic) calcification at the injection site, but not the hepatic necrosis. Pretreatment with parathyroid extract (or with DHT) prevents the hepatic necrosis, although it augments the local tissue calcification at the injection site.

Magnesium ←

Matthews & Austin 21,067/27: In dogs, resistance to $MgSO_4$ i.v. is increased by parathyroid extract, and decreased by parathyroidectomy, presumably because of the well-known antagonism between Ca- and Mg-ions.

Simon 31,369/35: In mice, parathyroid extract inhibits the development of magnesium narcosis in a dose-dependent manner. This phenomenon can be used for the standardization of parathyroid preparations.

Perchlorate ← *cf. Selye C92,918/61, p. 280.*
Permanganate ← *cf. Selye D15,540/62, p. 303.*

Oxalate ←

Kochmann 55,947/34: In mice, fatal intoxication with NaF or oxalic acid can be prevented by pretreatment with parathyroid extract. These inhibitions are dose-dependent and may serve for the assay of parathyroid preparations.

Peptone ←

Czarnecki & Kiersz D15,579/61: In dogs, shock produced by trypan blue or peptone injection is more powerfully inhibited by thyroparathyroidectomy than by thyroidectomy.

Phosphate ← *cf. also Selye G60,083/70, p. 410.*

Selye C38,627/58: In rats, the nephrocalcinosis produced by a dietary excess of NaH_2PO_4 is inhibited both by thyroparathyroidectomy and by excess thyroxine administration.

Picrotoxin ←

Süssmann 24,462/27: In mice, very impure parathyroid extracts protect against guanidine and picrotoxin, but not against strychnine.

Potassium ←

Thatcher & Radike B4,515/47: In rats, resistance to KCl intoxication was increased by DOC or adrenocortical extract. Parathyroid extract decreased potassium resistance.

Puromycin Aminonucleoside ←

Johnston & Follis Jr. D12,799/61: In rats, the osteitis fibrosa-like changes produced by puromycin aminonucleoside (PAN) are not prevented by parathyroidectomy.

Salicylates ←

Abbott & Harrisson F36,510/65: In rats, cancellous bone formation is stimulated by various salicylates. This effect is blocked by parathyroid extract and vitamin D, but not influenced by cortisone.

Strychnine ←

Süssmann 24,462/27: In mice, very impure parathyroid extracts protect against guanidine and picrotoxin, but not against strychnine.

Sulfa Drugs ← *cf. also Selye C92,918/61, p. 194; G60,083/70, pp. 413, 414.*

Lehr & Martin C13,119/56: In rats, the production of cardiovascular lesions by "standard renal injury" (due to treatment with sulfa drugs) is prevented by thyroparathyroidectomy, but not by thyroidectomy with parathyroid extract treatment. Curiously, "chemical thyroidectomy" [technique not specified (H.S.)] also inhibited, and thyroid hormone excess aggravated these lesions.

Lehr & Martin C23,011/56: In rats, the cardiovascular lesions produced by sodium acetyl sulfathiazole (as a consequence of renal injury) are prevented by thyroparathyroidectomy, presumably because in the final analysis, the changes observed are due to nephrogenic hyperparathyroidism.

Lehr C84,326/59: In rats, the role of parathyroid hormone in the production of cardiovascular lesions by renal damage (Na-acetylsulfathiazole, surgery) was subjected to systematic analysis.

Okano et al. H25,894/70: In rats, the calcification and necrosis of the aortic media induced by the "obstructive nephropathy" developing after injection of sodium sulfaacetylthiazole (SAT) can be prevented by parathyroidectomy, and to a lesser extent by calcitonin.

Uranium ←

Eger B35,694/42: In rats, the osteodystrophia fibrosa produced by uranium intoxication can be prevented by parathyroidectomy, presumably because the renal damage induced by the heavy metal acts on the bones only through the intermediary of the parathyroids.

Vitamin A ← *cf. Selye G60,083/70, pp. 410, 413.*

Vitamin C ←

Kalnins & Ledina B19,372/47: In guinea pigs, parathyroid extract accelerates the development of scorbutic changes on a vitamin-C deficient diet.

Vitamin D, DHT ← *cf. Selye C92,918/61, p. 176; D15,540/62, p. 281; G60,083/70, pp. 408, 410.*

Diet ← *cf. also Selye G60,083/70, pp. 410, 413.*

Dragstedt & Peacock 17,556/23: In dogs, parathyroid tetany is highly subject to modification by certain diets. It is concluded that "the parathyroid glands do not furnish a hormone necessary for life, and dogs may be kept alive indefinitely after their removal if treatment directed to the prevention of this toxemia of intestinal origin is carried out."

Bacteria ←

In guinea pigs, parathyroid extract allegedly delays the course of experimental tuberculosis, whereas in rats removal of the parathyroids has been claimed to lower resistance to this infection. In mice, parathyroid extract offers some protection against infection with P. anthracis, E. coli or Ps. pyocyaneus but not against Klebsiella pneumoniae.

Bacterial Toxins ←

In dogs and rabbits, tetanus intoxication is not significantly affected by parathyroid extract, but the spread of this toxin is allegedly delayed by parathyroid preparations in the mouse.

Renal Lesions ←

Hypertension produced by unilateral renal artery constriction in rats is not significantly affected by parathyroidectomy. However, the cardiovascular calcification produced by nephrectomy and by certain renal lesions in the rat can be prevented by parathyroidectomy presumably because here the calcinosis is a secondary result of increased parathyroid hormone secretion.

In rats, calciphylaxis produced by bilateral nephrectomy + ferric dextrin is prevented by parathyroidectomy. From this it was concluded that endogenous parathyroid hormone in amounts secreted by the gland can act as a calciphylactic sensitizer.

Stressors ←

Several investigators claimed that the parathyroids play an important part in resistance to cold, X-irradiation and other forms of stress, but all these findings require confirmation.

Bacteria ←

Pelouze & Rosenberger 62,508/24: In guinea pigs, parathyroid extract or calcium feeding delays the course of experimental tuberculosis.

Steinbach 92,528/32: In rats, parathyroidectomy lowers resistance to infection with bovine but not with human tuberculosis. Thyroparathyroidectomy makes rats susceptible to both human and bovine tubercle bacilli.

Weinstein B15,029/39: In mice, various anterior pituitary preparations protect against infection with B. anthracis. Parathyroid extract was also very effective, whereas thyroxine and testosterone offered little protection, and progesterone, insulin, "estrin" and posterior lobe extract were virtually ineffective.

Weinstein A33,940/40: In mice, neither parathyroid extract nor a crude anterior pituitary preparation offered protection against infection with Klebsiella pneumoniae, but they did improve survival after inoculation of E. coli or Ps. pyocyaneus.

Schäfer B99,955/54; G58,597/54: Monograph (127 pp., numerous refs.) on the role of endocrine factors in tuberculosis. Special sections are devoted to the hormones of the thyroid, parathyroid, thymus, adrenals, pancreas, and gonads.

Bacterial Toxins ←

Lissák 29,256/34: In dogs and rabbits, tetanus intoxication is not significantly modified by parathyroid extract.

Weinstein A33,940/40: In mice, parathyroid extract prevents the spread of tetanus toxin from the site of inoculation and delays death.

Quattrocchi & Foresti G43,535/66: Anaphylactic shock in guinea pigs and the Shwartzman-Sanarelli phenomenon in rabbits are inhibited by pretreatment with parathyroid extract. [The statistical significance of the apparent differences has not been appraised (H.S.).]

Immune Reactions ←

Quattrocchi & Foresti G43,535/66: Anaphylactic shock in guinea pigs and the Shwartzman-Sanarelli phenomenon in rabbits are inhibited by pretreatment with parathyroid extract. [The statistical significance of the apparent differences has not been appraised (H.S.).]

Renal Lesions ←

Quadri 45,920/06: In rabbits, i.v. injection of a parathyroid extract ("Paratiroidina") prolongs survival following bilateral ureter ligature. This fact is ascribed to an antitoxic action of the parathyroid hormone, although the hormonal activity of the extract has not been ascertained.

Bein et al. C57,714/58: In male rats with hypertension produced by unilateral renal artery constriction, vascular lesions are more common than in females. Gonadectomy does not significantly alter these changes in males, but aggravates them in females. Parathyroidectomy has no significant effect upon them.

Lehr C84,326/59: In rats, the role of parathyroid hormone in the production of cardiovascular lesions by renal damage (Na-acetylsulfathiazole, surgery) was subjected to systematic analysis.

Selye et al. D32,610/63: In rats, calciphylaxis produced by bilateral nephrectomy + ferric dextrin can be prevented by parathyroidectomy. Hence, it may be concluded that autologous parathyroid hormones in amounts secreted by the glands can act as calciphylactic sensitizers.

Stressors ←

Genitis et al. 68,723/35: In young thyroparathyroidectomized rats, exposure to heat 24 hrs following the operation greatly increased the mortality rate, whereas **cold** surrounding temperature diminished it. The number of tetanic convulsions was greatest at an intermediate temperature. [From the brief abstract it is difficult to differentiate between the role of parathyroid and of thyroid deficiency (H.S.).]

Sanfilippo 56,085/35: In rabbits, parathyroid extract increases resistance to **cold**.

Rixon et al. C61,789/58: In rats, parathyroid extract prolongs survival after **X-irradiation**.

Czarnecki & Kiersz D15,579/61: In dogs, **shock produced by trypan blue or peptone** injection is more powerfully inhibited by thyroparathyroidectomy than by thyroidectomy.

← CALCITONIN

Parathyroid Hormone ←. Calcitonin inhibits the production of soft tissue calcification by parathyroid extract in the rat. Thyroxine has a similar effect, and combined treatment with the two hormones leads to a summation of their actions.

Drugs ←. In rats, the organ lesions produced by intoxication with **holmium** or **indium** chlorides, unlike the nephrocalcinosis produced by **mercury**, are completely prevented by calcitonin. The calcergy, induced by **lead** acetate i.v. + topical administration of polymyxin, is inhibited by calcitonin in the rat simultaneously with the hypercalcemia resulting from lead acetate administration.

The myocardial lesion, produced in rats as a consequence of the obstructive nephropathy caused by **sulfa compounds** is also inhibited by calcitonin.

The bone lesions characteristic of **vitamin-A** overdosage in the rat are prevented by calcitonin, although those elicited by various other techniques are not influenced by this hormone.

Renal Lesions ←. Calcitonin inhibits the metastatic calcification and the osteitis fibrosa induced by bilateral nephrectomy in the rat.

Parathyroid Hormone ← cf. also Selye *G60,083/70, p. 413.*

Tuchweber et al. G46,759/68; Gabbiani et al. G46,731/68; G46,730/68: Pretreatment with thyroxine or calcitonin inhibits the soft tissue calcification and osteitis fibrosa induced by parathyroid extract overdosage. In the event of concurrent administration, the effect of the two protective hormones is summated. Thyroxine retains its effect upon calcium metabolism in thyroparathyroidectomized or adrenalectomized but not in nephrectomized rats. The stress of restraint likewise prevents parathyroid overdosage, but the associated biochemical changes are different from those caused by thyroxine.

Drugs ←

Digitoxin ←. *Selye PROT. 33541, 34074:* In rats, PCN is highly efficacious in preventing digitoxin poisoning, even after parathyroidectomy, thyroparathyroidectomy, or concurrent treatment with propylthiouracil (PTU). No protection was obtained by thyroidectomy, parathyroidectomy or treatment with PTU, thyroxine, parathyroid extract or calcitonin. Apparently, the goitrogenic effect of PCN plays no indispensable role in its catatoxic action.

Holmium, Indium ←. *Gabbiani & Tuchweber G70,453/70:* In rats, the organ lesions produced by toxic doses of holmium and indium chlorides—unlike the nephrocalcinosis elicited by $HgCl_2$—are completely prevented by calcitonin.

Lead ←. *Gabbiani et al. G46,731/68:* In rats, calcitonin (but not thyroxine) inhibits the local calcergy induced by intravenous injection of lead acetate followed by topical administration of polymyxin and the hypercalcemia produced by a single injection of lead acetate.

Mercury ←. *Gabbiani & Tuchweber G70,453/70:* In rats, the organ lesions produced by toxic doses of holmium and indium chlorides—unlike the nephrocalcinosis elicited by $HgCl_2$—are completely prevented by calcitonin.

Sulfa Drugs ←. *Fujita et al. H2,733/68:* In rats, calcitonin inhibits the myocardial lesions that occur as a consequence of the obstructive nephropathy after the administration of Na-sulfacetylthiazole (SAT).

Okano et al. H25,894/70: In rats, the calcification and necrosis of the aortic media induced by the "obstructive nephropathy" developing after injection of sodium sulfacetylthiazole (SAT) can be prevented by parathyroidectomy, and to a lesser extent by calcitonin.

Vitamin A ←. *Clark et al. H5,009/68:* In rats, the bone lesions produced by vitamin-A overdosage were prevented by calcitonin, but those induced by various other techniques were not influenced, or actually aggravated.

Renal Lesions ←

Lefort et al. G46,725/67; Côté et al. G46,741/68: In rats, calcitonin inhibits the metastatic calcification and bone lesions induced by bilateral nephrectomy. In nephrectomized animals, thyroxine does not modify the changes induced by endogenous hyperparathyroidism consequent to bilateral nephrectomy. "Presumably, to be effective against soft-tissue calcification and bone resorption induced by parathyroid extract overdosage, thyroxine requires the presence of the kidney."

← PANCREATIC HORMONES

The pancreatic hormones affect resistance to various agents, mainly through their influence upon carbohydrate metabolism. It is interesting, however, that while the effect of insulin and surgically or drug-induced diabetes have been studied in connection with many toxicants, virtually no attention has been given to the possible corresponding effects of glucagon.

Steroids ←

Progesterone anesthesia is aggravated by insulin and prevented by epinephrine, presumably by virtue of the blood sugar changes produced by these hormones.

Nonsteroidal Hormones and Hormone-Like Substances ←

Thyroid feeding greatly increases mortality in rats on a diet containing desiccated pancreas. However, there is no proof that here pancreatic hormones play a role.

The toxicity of **histamine, 5-HT**, and of the **anaphylactoidogenic** agents that liberate these amines from mastocytes, is greatly influenced by pancreatic hormones. The anaphylactoid edema produced by dextran or egg-white in the rat is inhibited by alloxan diabetes and aggravated by insulin. The response to Cpd. 48/80 is less consistently influenced by these agents. In mice, sensitized with pertussis vaccine, alloxan also inhibits the response to 5-HT, histamine or anaphylaxis.

Steroids ← *cf. also Selye G60,083/70, pp. 414—419.*

Winter & Selye A35,658/41; Winter A36,333/41: Epinephrine increases, whereas insulin decreases, the resistance of the rat to the anesthetic action of progesterone.

Hydroxydione ← Carbutamide, Mouse: Rümke G69,768/63*

Nonsteroidal Hormones and Hormone-Like Substances ←

Thyroid Hormones ←. *Ershoff B24,883/48:* In immature female rats fed purified rations containing both pancreas and desiccated thyroid, mortality was high. Similar diets containing only pancreas or desiccated thyroid induced no comparable mortality.

Histamine and 5-HT ←. *Goth et al. C43,836/57:* In rats, alloxan diabetes inhibits the anaphylactoid edema produced by dextran or egg white; insulin aggravates it. Cpd. 48/80 is not influenced by these agents. "These results suggest a hitherto unrecognized role of insulin in certain types of inflammation and histamine release."

Adamkiewicz & Adamkiewicz C73,760/59: In rats, alloxan diabetes prevents the anaphylactoid reaction caused by dextran; insulin restores this reactivity.

Ganley & Robinson C66,305/59: In mice, sensitized with B. pertussis vaccine, alloxan inhibits the response to 5-HT and somewhat less to histamine and anaphylaxis.

Sanyal et al. C79,555/59: In rats, anaphylactoid edema produced by egg white is aggravated by insulin pretreatment.

Ganley D31,168/62: In mice, alloxan diabetes inhibits the sensitizing properties of Bordetella pertussis vaccine as measured by challenge with histamine, 5-HT or anaphylaxis. This effect is reversed by insulin.

Insulin ←. *Hasselblatt & Bastian C59,171/58:* In mice, sensitivity to insulin convulsions is increased by thyroxine and even more markedly by tolbutamide.

Tolbutamide ← Tolbutamide, Dog: Charbon G76,685/61*; Remmer et al. D19,894/64*

Drugs ←

Among the drug actions subject to regulation by pancreatic hormones, one of the most interesting is the previously mentioned response to **anaphylactoidogens**. Various antigen-antibody reactions are influenced in a similar way and since overdosage with sugars, cortisol or epinephrine also inhibit the anaphylactoid edema, it is assumed that the latter agents, like insulin and alloxan, act through their effect upon the blood sugar. Since these interrelations have been discussed at length in a previous monograph *(Selye G19,425/65)* they need not be discussed here in detail.

Barbiturate anesthesia can be markedly influenced by insulin but in a somewhat unpredictable manner. In mice, hexobarbital sleeping time is allegedly prolonged both by epinephrine and by insulin, whereas in rabbits, pentobarbital sleeping time is shortened by the same two hormones. In guinea pigs, hexobarbital sleeping time is also reduced by insulin and it has been postulated that here a direct effect upon both the CNS and upon hepatic detoxication may be involved. In mice, thiopental anesthesia is prolonged by alloxan diabetes, perhaps as a consequence of a deranged metabolic degradation of the barbiturate, but insulin fails to correct this effect.

Pancreatic hormones also appear to affect the toxicity of **digitalis** alkaloids. In dogs, pancreatectomy offers moderate protection against lethal doses of k-strophanthin; in rats, insulin enhances the cardiac action of this compound but not of its aglycon, strophanthidin.

The beriberi produced in pigeons by **vitamin-B$_1$** deficiency is aggravated by insulin, but only under certain circumstances. In rats, moderate alloxan diabetes does not significantly affect thiamine deficiency.

In rats pretreated with **vitamin D**, alloxan produces selective calcification of the Langerhans islets as a consequence of calciphylaxis.

Acetone ←

Hirschfelder & Maxwell 26,930/24: In rabbits, insulin fails to antagonize the toxic effects of ethanol or acetone.

Acetonitrile ←

Paal 22,603/30: Review of the literature and extensive personal studies on the acetonitrile test in mice and its use for the determination of thyroid hormone in human blood. Thyroidectomy does not increase the resistance of the mice to acetonitrile but diminishes the protective effect of thyroxine. Concurrent treatment with insulin also inhibits the prevention of acetonitrile toxicity by thyroxine.

Aminopyrine ← Alloxan + Insulin: Dixon et al. E35,705/63; Kato et al. F57,817/65

Anaphylactoidogens ← cf. also Selye *G 46,715/68, pp. 104, 108, 177, 179, 184, 197*.

Adamkiewicz & Langlois C 31,853/57: In rats, insulin sensitizes to the production of anaphylactoid edema by the systemic or intrapedal injection of small doses of dextran. The sensitization manifests itself even despite cortisone treatment.

Adamkiewicz D 61,626/63: Review showing that "hyperglycemias resulting from overdosage with sugars, cortisol, adrenaline, or from diabetes inhibit the anaphylactoid reactions; anaphylaxis, and the tuberculin reaction, but potentiate infections. Hypoglycemias resulting from fasting, insulin and adrenalectomy potentiate the anaphylactoid reactions, anaphylaxis, and the tuberculin reaction; but inhibit infections. The hypothesis is proposed that hyperglycemia inhibits certain antigen-antibody combinations; this results in an inhibition of hypersensitivity, but an aggravation of infection."

Sacra & Adamkiewicz F 49,352/65: In rats, the toxicity of Cpd. 48/80 is increased by insulin and diminished by glucose.

Aniline ← Alloxan + Insulin: Dixon et al. *E 35,705/63*

Aniline ← Alloxan + Orchidectomy + Methyltestosterone: Kato et al. *F 57,817/65*

Anticoagulants ← Tolbutamide, Rb, Man: Chaplin et al. *D 99,463/58**

Anticoagulants ← Glucagon, Man: Koch-Weser *G 73,494/70**

Barbiturates ←

Reinhard B 283/45: In mice, the hexobarbital sleeping time is prolonged by epinephrine or insulin.

Westfall B 31,306/46: In rabibts, pentobarbital sleeping time is shortened by epinephrine and insulin despite their opposite effect upon blood sugar.[This contradicts Reinhard B 283/45 (H.S.).]

Holck B 42,745/48: In mice, neither epinephrine nor insulin altered significantly the fatal dose of hexobarbital given 20 min later.

Dixon et al. D 9,331/61: In alloxan diabetic rats, the ability of the hepatic microsomal fractions to inactivate hexobarbital, chlorpromazine or codeine in vitro is diminished and the sleeping time following hexobarbital injection in vivo prolonged. These effects can be reversed by insulin and roughly parallel the glycogen content of the liver. "Factors leading to severe depletion of hepatic glycogen will probably affect the rate at which drugs are metabolized by the microsomes."

Shrotri et al. D 27,239/62: In guinea pigs, hexobarbital sleeping time is reduced by insulin. "A direct effect on the CNS as well as a role in the detoxification in liver are postulated."

Dixon et al. E 35,705/63: In alloxan-diabetic rats, "a depressed metabolism of hexobarbital and aminopyrine in vitro, an increased in vitro hydroxylation of aniline, and a prolonged in vivo effect of hexobarbital were evident. The O-dealkylation of codeine was unaffected by the chronic diabetic state. Insulin treatment returned the rate of metabolism of hexobarbital to normal levels but had no effect on aminopyrine metabolism. Metabolism of aniline was decreased below the normal rate after insulin treatment. Phenobarbital treatment of diabetic animals resulted in a stimulation of most of the drug-metabolizing enzyme systems studied. However, the hydroxylation of aniline by livers from diabetic rats treated with phenobarbital was decreased." A relationship between hepatic glycogen and drug-metabolizing enzyme activity is suspected.

Kato & Gillette F 57,817/65: The metabolism of aminopyrine and hexobarbital by hepatic microsomes of male rats is impaired by adrenalectomy, castration, hypoxia, ACTH, formaldehyde, epinephrine, morphine, alloxan or thyroxine. The metabolism of aniline and zoxazolamine is not appreciably decreased by any of these agents; in fact, hydroxylation of aniline is enhanced by thyroxine or alloxan. Apparently, the treatments impair mainly the sex-dependent enzymes. Accordingly, the corresponding enzymic functions of the hepatic microsomes of female rats are not significantly impaired by the agents which do have an inhibitory effect in males.

Vincent & Motin G 51,414/67: Description of a patient who recovered from severe combined intoxication with barbiturates and insulin.

Quevauviller & Podevin G 57,209/68: In mice, alloxan diabetes prolongs thiopental anesthesia by interfering with the metabolic degradation of the barbiturate. Insulin fails to correct this effect.

Weiner et al. H 24,942/70: In rats, glucagon, alloxan and starvation all increased hexobarbital sleeping time. This effect was markedly antagonized by insulin. Perhaps, cyclic AMP may be involved since theophylline greatly increases the action of glucagon. This synergism also occurred in isolated, perfused rat livers and, hence, "inhibition of hexobarbital metabolism by cyclic AMP would appear to be mediated in the liver."

Amobarbital ← Insulin + Glucose, Rb: Maloney et al. 61,235/31*

Hexobarbital ← Insulin, Mouse: Reinhard B283/45*; Holck B42,745/48*, D28,543/49*

Hexobarbital ← Alloxan + Insulin: Dixon et al. D9,331/61*; Fouts G77,514/62; Dixon et al. E35,705/63

Hexobarbital ← Tolbutamide: Remmer G66,542/62*; Rümke et al. G74,669/60*; Kato et al. E47,494/64; Remmer et al. D19,894/64*, G66,868/65*; Remmer F90,864/67*

Bilirubin ←

Müller-Oerlinghausen & Schinke G79,199/70: In rats, the maximal transport capacity of the liver (Tm) for bilirubin is reduced in diabetes caused by alloxan or anti-insulin serum. "It is suggested that the reduced synthesis of UDP-glucuronic acid which has been found in former experiments in vitro is responsible for the impaired bilirubin excretion." The excretion of indocyanine green is likewise inhibited in experimental diabetes.

Bilirubin ← Tolbutamide, Dog: Singh et al. D6,799/61*

Caffeine ←

Labbé & Théodoresco 17,831/24: In dogs and rabbits, resistance to caffeine is somewhat increased by insulin but the results are not impressive.

Carbon Tetrachloride ←

Furukawa F71,711/65: In rats, hepatic steatosis produced by CCl_4 is inhibited by adrenalectomy and, to some extent, also by hypophysectomy. Corticoids restore the effect of CCl_4 after adrenalectomy; epinephrine does not, but it increases the effect of corticoids. STH does not counteract the effect of hypophysectomy. Alloxan diabetes inhibits CCl_4-induced hepatic lipidosis.

Carcinogens ←

Dunning et al. A48,770/48: In rats, "the diabetic condition induced by alloxan shortened the life span of the affected individuals, thereby reducing both the percentage of rats surviving long enough to develop benzpyrene sarcomas and the average latent period of those which did, but did not prevent or delay the malignant process in the rats surviving to the average time of occurrence for these neoplasms."

Salzberg & Griffin B68,802/52: In rats, hepatic carcinogenesis following treatment with 3'-Me-DAB is inhibited by alloxan diabetes.

Klärner & Klärner C45,812/58: In BAF_1 mice, the growth of urethan-induced pulmonary tumors is significantly inhibited by alloxan diabetes and exposure to heat, but only slightly affected by thyroxine and insulin.

Tinozzi & Pannella D54,092/61: In rats, alloxan diabetes largely prevents the induction of tumors by 20-methylcholanthrene.

Lacassagne & Hurst G78,530/69: In rats, tolbutamide (a hypoglycemic sulfonamide) accelerates, whereas diazoxide (a hyperglycemic sulfonamide) retards hepatoma formation after treatment with AAF. When the two compounds are given together, they nullify each other's actions.

Heuson G78,138/70: In rats, DMBA-induced mammary tumors appear to be influenced by insulin, both in vivo and in vitro. DNA synthesis in organ cultures of these carcinomas is stimulated by insulin. Large doses have a strong, probably direct stimulating effect on DMBA-induced neoplasms in vivo, whereas regression is noted in alloxan-diabetic rats.

Carisoprodol ← Tolbutamide: Kato et al. E47,494/64

Chlorpromazine ←

Wisniewski & Danysz G40,054/66: In rats, insulin administered simultaneously with chlorpromazine increases the potency and the brain concentration of the latter. "It can be supposed that insulin increases the velocity of the penetration of chlorpromazine across cell membranes in both directions. Hypoglycemia does not show any influence on this effect of insulin and it may be concluded that insulin acts directly on cell membranes."

Wisniewsky & Buczko G51,489/67: In rats, the depressive effect of chlorpromazine is decreased by alloxan and restored to normal by concurrent treatment with insulin.

Chlorpromazine ← Alloxan + Insulin: Dixon et al. D9,331/61*

Cholesterol ← *cf. also Selye B40,000/50, p. 551; G60,083/70, pp. 414—419, 430.*

Cholesterol ←

McGill et al. B32,954/49: In rabbits, cholesterol atherosclerosis is inhibited by alloxan diabetes contrary to the author's expectations.

Hamprecht G69,560/69: Review (7 pp., 153 refs.) on the mechanisms regulating cholesterol synthesis. A special section deals with the effect of thyroid hormones, steroids, epinephrine, norepinephrine and glucagon.

Wellmann et al. H9,536/69: In cholesterol-fed rabbits, alloxan aggravates the characteristic renal lesions.

Chromium ←

Zondek 36,326/14: In rabbits, the hypertension produced by uranium and mercury nephritis, unlike that of chromium nephritis, is counteracted by i.v. injection of a beef pancreas extract.

Cobalt ←

Avezzu C46,134/57: In rabbits, cobalt destroys the alpha cells, alloxan the beta cells, of the Langerhans islets, and hence, there exists a mutual antagonism between these two substances as regards the consequent metabolic effects also.

Codeine ← Alloxan + Insulin: Dixon et al. *D9,331/61, E35,705/63*

Digitalis ←

Freund A26,153/32: Studies on the effect of thyroidectomy or pretreatment with thyroxine or insulin upon the in vitro metabolic changes induced by digitalis compounds in the cat's heart.

Travis et al. C18,863/56: In dogs, pancreatectomy offers a slight but significant degree of protection against lethal doses of k-strophanthin. "This would appear to be related to the absence of insulin since hyperglycemia per se, does not afford any protection. Thus these results are in harmony with the concept that insulin facilitates the transport of glycosides having d-glucose as a terminal sugar in somewhat the same manner as it facilitates the transport of the simple sugar."

Adamkiewicz C97,998/61: In rats, insulin enhances the cardiac action of k-strophanthin but not of the aglycon strophanthidin.

Cohn et al. H26,723/70: In dogs, glucagon abolishes ouabain-induced arrhythmias. The mechanism of this anti-arrhythmic action could not be clarified but glucagon causes an immediate rise, followed by a fall in serum potassium and this may have been involved.

Dyes ←

Müller-Oerlinghausen & Schinke G79,199/70: In rats, the maximal transport capacity of the liver (Tm) for bilirubin is reduced in diabetes caused by alloxan or anti-insulin serum. "It is suggested that the reduced synthesis of UDP-glucuronic acid which has been found in former experiments in vitro is responsible for the impaired bilirubin excretion." The excretion of indocyanine green is likewise inhibited in experimental diabetes.

Dye (BSP) ← Tolbutamide, Rb: Hasselblatt et al. *G77,523/62**

Dye (BSP) ← Tolbutamide + Ethionine, Mouse: Fujimoto et al. *G30,289/65**

Ethanol ←

Hirschfelder & Maxwell 26,930/24: In rabbits, insulin fails to antagonize the toxic effects of ethanol or acetone.

Hiestand et al. B78,576/53: In mice, alloxan diabetes and epinephrine increase, whereas insulin decreases, sensitivity to lethal doses of ethanol.

Hirvonen et al. G59,966/68: In rats, moderate chronic ethanol intoxication causes hypertrophy of the adrenal glomerulosa. This effect is inhibited by insulin. On the other hand, the ethanol-induced activation of the fasciculata is actually enhanced by insulin.

Ethanol ← Alloxan, Mouse: Hiestand et al. *B78,576/53**

Ethanol ← Insulin + Glucose, Dog: Greenberg *A48,342/42**; Sammalisto *G76,362/62**

Hexadimethrine ←

Kovács & Szijj F96,892/68: In rats, insulin increases sensitivity to hexadimethrine-induced pituitary necrosis; alloxan fails to affect it.

Lathyrogens ←

Franchimont et al. D13,136/61: In rats, osteolathyrism produced by AAN is aggravated by 5-HT, whereas glucagon does not modify it significantly.

van Cauwenberge & Lefebvre G58,189/64: In rats, osteolathyrism produced by AAN is not influenced by glucagon.

Meprobamate ← Tolbutamide: Kato et al. *E47,494/64*

Mercury ←

Zondek *36,326/14:* In rabbits, the hypertension produced by uranium and mercury nephritis, unlike that of chromium nephritis, is counteracted by i.v. injection of a beef pancreas extract.

Methampyrone ← Tolbutamide: Remmer *F90,864/67*

Methylaminoantipyrine ← Tolbutamide: Remmer *G6,542/62*

Monomethylaminoantipyrine ← Tolbutamide: Remmer et al. *D19,894/64*

Morphine ←

Wiśniewski *E32,005/63:* In rabbits, insulin increases the analgesic action of morphine and dolantin.

Pentylenetetrazol ←

Waltregny & Mesdjian *F78,025/66:* In cats, insulin hypoglycemia raises sensitivity to pentylenetetrazol convulsions.

Peptone ←

Barral et al. *8,860/32:* In guinea pigs, anaphylactic and peptone shocks are aggravated by insulin and diminished by glucose.

Pesticides ←

DuBois et al. *B3,089/47:* In rats, both insulin and hypophysectomy antagonize the hyperglycemic effect of ANTU but do not prolong survival.

Dieldrin ← Tolbutamide: Matsumura et al. *G74,472/68*

Picrotoxin ← Insulin: Holck *D28,543/49**

Salicylates ←

Wiśniewski & Zarebski *F85,977/67; F96,973/68:* In mice, insulin greatly increases the analgesic effect of Na-salicylate and its concentration in the brain, heart and skeletal muscle. Alloxan has an opposite effect.

Strychnine ← Tolbutamide: Kato et al. *E47,494/64*

Thiouracil ←

Pyatnitskaya *C43,809/56:* In rats, the fatty degeneration of the liver produced by thiouracil is prevented by conjoint administration of insulin and glucose.

Thioacetamide ←

Georgii et al. *C69,388/59:* In rats, the hepatic lesions produced by chronic treatment with thioacetamide are at first inhibited and later aggravated by concurrent administration of an antidiabetic sulfanil urea preparation (D 860, artosin, tolbutamide).

Toluene Diisocyanate ←

Thompson & Scheel *G55,229/68:* In rats, the toxicity of toluene diisocyanate is diminished by alloxan and increased by insulin or pertussis vaccine. Yet, other evidence suggests that the pulmonary changes produced by this drug are not due to an allergic reaction but to direct chemical damage.

Uranium ←

Zondek *36,326/14:* In rabbits, the hypertension produced by uranium and mercury nephritis, unlike that of chromium nephritis, is counteracted by i.v. injection of a beef pancreas extract.

Vitamin-B Complex ← cf. also Selye *C92,918/61, p. 231.*

Chahovitch *26,462/25:* In pigeons, insulin aggravates the already manifest symptoms of incipient thiamine deficiency.

Chahovitch *26,685/25:* In pigeons, insulin pretreatment retards the development of beriberi on a thiamine-deficient diet.

Baglioni & Console *45,284/34:* In pigeons on a thiamine-deficient diet, the development of beriberi is delayed by daily treatment with insulin, but only under certain experimental circumstances. The extensive literature on the effect of insulin upon beriberi is reviewed.

Janes & Brady *98,541/47; B23,359/48:* In rats, alloxan diabetes does not significantly alter the thiamine-deficiency syndrome.

Vitamin D ←

Kodousková et al. *D69,797/63:* In rats pretreated with vitamin D, alloxan causes calcification of the Langerhans islets as a manifestation of calciphylaxis.

Zinc ←

Kamikubo *D7,362/59:* In rats, alloxan decreased the comparatively high zinc content of Yoshida's ascites tumor.

Varia ←

Störtebecker *76,398/39:* Review of the early literature (1924—1937) on the effect of the pancreas upon resistance to various drugs.

Selye *G70,480/71:* In rats, tolbutamide protects against intoxication with dioxathion, parathion, hexobarbital, progesterone (anesthesia), indomethacin but not against digitoxin, nicotine, zoxazolamine, DHT or the infarctoid cardiopathy produced by fluorocortisol + Na_2HPO_4 + corn oil.

Microorganisms, Vaccines and Parasites ←

It is a well-known fact that both pancreatic and alloxan diabetes increase sensitivity to a great variety of **bacteria**, including Mycobacterium tuberculosis, pneumococcus, staphylococcus, streptococcus, perfringens and many others.

Alloxan diabetes also aggravates the course of infestation with various **parasites**, especially, fungus infections.

In mice, insulin decreases resistance to **endotoxins** allegedly because the hypoglycemic state interferes with defense against the stressor effect of these lipopolysaccharides.

Bacteria and Vaccines ←

Bordetella Pertussis ←. Ganley & Robinson *C66,305/59:* In mice, sensitized with B. pertussis vaccine, alloxan inhibits the response to 5-HT and somewhat less to histamine and anaphylaxis.

Ganley *D31,168/62:* In mice, alloxan diabetes inhibits the sensitizing properties of B. pertussis vaccine as measured by challenge with histamine, 5-HT or anaphylaxis. This effect is reversed by insulin.

Clostridium Welchii ←. Wishart & Pritchett *12,285/20:* In dogs, partial pancreatectomy, conducive to severe glycosuria, fails to diminish resistance to infection with Cl. welchii.

Escherichia Coli ←. Krizek & Davis *F14,734/64:* In rats given alloxan and maintained with insulin, the proliferation of E. coli injected s.c. was not greatly altered.

Mycobacterium Tuberculosis ←. Schäfer *B99,955/54:* Monograph (127 pp., numerous refs.) on the role of endocrine factors in tuberculosis. Special sections are devoted to the hormones of the thyroid, parathyroid, thymus, adrenals, pancreas and gonads.

Renovanz *C78,772/59:* In guinea pigs, the course of experimental tuberculosis was not markedly influenced by ACTH, tolbutamide derivatives or antithyroid treatment with perchlorates.

Schäfer & Greuel *D54,900/62:* In guinea pigs, the oral antidiabetic, tolbutamide has a deleterious effect upon the development of experimental tuberculosis.

Dobrev *G23,362/64:* In rabbits, alloxan diabetes aggravates the course of experimental tuberculosis and diminishes the allergic response to tuberculin.

Pneumococcus ←. Drachman et al. *F81,617/66:* In rats, alloxan diabetes increases susceptibility to experimental Type 25 pneumococcal pneumonia presumably through a depression in phagocytosis.

Staphylococcus, Streptococcus ← *cf. also* Selye *G60,083/70, p. 418.* Lauber *9,102/32:* Observations on the effect of insulin upon streptococcal and staphylococcal infections in mice.

Schultz & Rose *B31,347/39:* "Guinea pigs treated with maximum tolerated doses of protamine insulin and subjected to chronic, hemolytic streptococcus, focal infection develop nonpurulent carditis. This susceptibility to cardiac damage during infection is probably associated with the altered metabolic activity incident to insulin treatment."

Bóbr *G30,418/65:* In mice, alloxan diabetes raises susceptibility to Staphylococcus pyogenes.

Welchia Perfringens ←. Adamkiewicz et al. *F99,983/67:* Mice rendered diabetic by alloxan are sensitive to doses of washed Welchia perfringens which are innocuous for normal controls.

Parasites ←

Mucormycosis ←. Elder & Baker *C12,831/56:* In rabbits, alloxan diabetes aggravates the course of pulmonary mucormycosis following intratracheal inoculation of Rhizopus spores.

Trypanosoma Equiperdum ←. *Ewing et al. B50,244/50:* In mice infected with T. equiperdum, severe hypoglycemia develops and both alloxan and glucose exert an immediate analeptic effect.

Varia ←. *Sheldon & Bauer D46,962/62:* Review on the role of predisposing factors, particularly alloxan diabetes and ACTH-treatment, upon various fungus infections.

Bacterial Toxins ← *cf. also Selye E5,986/66, p. 82.*

Pieroni & Levine G68,105/69: In mice, insulin increases mortality produced by endotoxin. "This result is consistent with the thesis that there is a reciprocal relationship between the glycemic state of a host and its susceptibility to a wide variety of stressor agents."

Immune Reactions ←

We have already mentioned that insulin increases, whereas alloxan diabetes decreases, the anaphylactoid reaction as well as various antigen-antibody responses in different species. Similar effects have been noted in connection with the response to histamine and 5-HT in normal or pertussis sensitized animals. Let us add here that in guinea pigs, anaphylactic and peptone shock are aggravated by insulin and diminished by glucose. Alloxan also desensitizes the guinea pig to tuberculin and this effect is inhibited by insulin.

Barral et al. 8,860/32; 8,858/32: In guinea pigs, anaphylactic and peptone shocks are aggravated by insulin and diminished by glucose.

Cornforth & Long B77,176/53: In guinea pigs sensitized to tuberculin, single s.c. injections of ATP prevent desensitization by alloxan, cortisone and dihydroascorbic acid. Single s.c. injections of insulin do not in themselves influence sensitivity but prevent desensitization by alloxan and cortisone. Single s.c. injections of STH depress tuberculin sensitivity and synergize the action of cortisone or alloxan.

Long & Shewell G71,833/54: In guinea pigs, allergic hypersensitivity to BCG is increased by thyroxine or insulin. Partial pancreatectomy has no effect on sensitivity by itself but prevents the action of thyroxine, although not that of insulin.

Long & Shewell G71,832/55: In guinea pigs, thyroxine increases immunity as judged by the local response to diphtheria toxin injected intradermally and of circulating antitoxin after immunization with diphtheria toxoid. Partial pancreatectomy prevents this effect of thyroxine.

Ganley & Robinson C66,305/59; Ganley D31,168/62: In mice, alloxan diabetes inhibits the sensitizing properties of Bordetella pertussis vaccine as measured by challenge with histamine, 5-HT or anaphylaxis. This effect is reversed by insulin.

Stressors ←

There is no conclusive evidence to suggest that resistance to **ionizing rays** can be significantly affected by pancreatic preparations. However, in rats, both insulin and carbutamide diminish resistance to **hypoxia**.

In cats, dogs and chickens, insulin delays the appearance of the shivering reflex upon exposure to **cold**, whereas glucose reinstalls it. Combined treatment with cold and insulin elicits a state simulating hibernation. Both insulin and alloxan diminish resistance to cold in various species; however, in guinea pigs, insulin allegedly increases resistance to heat stroke.

Combined treatment with insulin + glucose increases the resistance of the rat to trauma in the Noble-Collip drum.

Ionizing Rays

Cavallot & Einaudi C 30,084/56: In guinea pigs, resistance to whole body X-irradiation is increased by treatment with an insulin-free pancreatic extract.

Gordeyeva C 97,407/60: In rats, resistance to total body X-irradiation is increased by glucose but additional administration of insulin is of no further advantage.

Hypoxia and Hyperoxygenation

Campbell A 14,903/37: In rats exposed to six atmospheres of oxygen in a pressure chamber, subsequent decompression is better tolerated at low than at high external temperatures. At 24°C, the following substances, administered s.c., enhance oxygen poisoning: thyroxine, dinitrophenol, ac-tetrahydro-β-naphthylamine, epinephrine, pituitary extract (posterior lobe), insulin, and eserine + atropine. These doses in themselves are harmless.

Fister C 97,077/59: In the rat, both insulin and carbutamide lower resistance to hypoxia.

Kawashima & Ueda F 68,970/66: In rats, insulin sensitizes to hypoxia. This effect is inhibited by urethan.

Cold

Cassidy et al. 24,604/25: In cats and dogs, insulin hyperglycemia abolishes the shivering reflex elicited by exposure to cold. Glucose causes its reappearance. Combined treatment with cold and insulin elicits a state simulating hibernation in cats and dogs.

Cassidy et al. 26,459/26: In chickens, insulin delays the appearance of shivering upon exposure to cold until the blood sugar rises.

Tullio 22,671/30: In rabbits, exposure to cold decreases the blood sugar, and insulin hypoglycemia decreases resistance to cold.

Poe & Davis D 27,155/62: In rats, alloxan diabetes diminishes resistance to cold.

Poe et al. E 21,412/63: In rats, alloxan diabetes diminishes resistance to cold but some adaptation to low temperature is possible even during the diabetic stage.

Heat

Grazia & Sardo 27,853/34: In guinea pigs, insulin increases resistance to heat stroke.

Trauma

Triner et al. D 65,801/63: In rats, treatment with insulin + glucose increases resistance to trauma in the Noble-Collip drum.

Varia

Ouzelatz C 36,618/57: In rats, insulin aggravates the production of gastric ulcers by pylorus ligature.

Hepatic Changes

In rats, alloxan and various antidiabetics can produce severe, often necrotizing, hepatic lesions.

Scharf et al. F 69,957/66: In rats, chronic treatment with methylthiouracil or paroxypropion produces essentially similar hepatic lesions. T2 reduces liver glycogen and the size of the hepatocytes. Single large doses of alloxan cause severe necrotizing lesions followed by cell proliferation. Concurrent treatment with methylthiouracil inhibits the alloxan-induced hepatic lesions and diminishes mortality.

Klatskin G 65,221/69: Review (103 pp., 809 refs.) on toxic and drug-induced hepatitis with special sections on the hepatotoxic effect of testoids, corticoids, thioureas, luteoids, folliculoids and oral antidiabetics.

Hepatic Enzymes

For the literature concerning the effect of pancreatic hormones upon the basic levels of hepatic TPO, TKT, GOT, GPT, SDH, TDH *cf.* Abstracts.

TPO, TKT

Schor & Frieden C57,994/58: In the rat, insulin can induce TPO activity, and its effect is only partly inhibited by adrenalectomy. In the intact rat, the effect of insulin and tryptophan, or insulin and cortisone, are additive. Possibly, "hormonal induction may be a form of substrate induction in that certain hormones might affect the availability of typtophan for the enzyme-forming system."

Finch et al. G71,208/69: In senescent mice, the induction of hepatic TKT by exposure to cold is delayed in comparison with young mice. Corticosterone and insulin are equally effective in this respect in mice of both age groups.

SDH, TDH

Freedland & Avery G67,766/64: In the rat, the TDH and SDH activity of liver homogenates was increased by high-protein diets, alloxan diabetes, or cortisol. Factors affecting the activity of TDH caused a proportional change in SDH suggesting that both of these activities may be due to a single protein. The SDH activity was decreased by adrenalectomy or hypophysectomy. Adrenalectomy had no effect upon the response of this enzyme to protein feeding, whereas, after hypophysectomy, this response was diminished.

Ishikawa et al. F41,763/65: In alloxan-diabetic rats, the SDH and TDH levels of the hepatic microsomes are greatly enhanced. SDH was readily induced by cortisol in the diabetic, but not in the normal rat. The effects of actinomycin S, STH, and starvation upon SDH have also been studied in intact, hypophysectomized, adrenalectomized and thyroidectomized rats. It is concluded that "serine dehydratase activity in the liver plays an important role in the production of pyruvate as a starting material for gluconeogenesis."

GPT, GOT

Rosen et al. C50,741/58: In rats treated with cortisol, cortisone or prednisone for 1 week, there was an increase in hepatic GPT but not in GDT. DOC had no such effect. Hypophysectomy or adrenalectomy did not prevent this action of cortisone. STH, testosterone or insulin failed to alter GPT activity nor did they influence its stimulation by cortisol.

Rosen et al. C71,414/59: Marked increases in GPT activity were observed in the livers of rats given cortisol, cortisone, 9α-fluorocortisol, prednisone, 6α-methylprednisolone, 9α-fluoro-21-desoxy-6α-methylprednisolone or ACTH, whereas two nonglucocorticoid cortisol derivatives, 11-epicortisol and 9a-methoxycortisol were inactive. STH, testosterone and insulin caused no significant change in GPT by themselves nor did they modify the action of cortisol. On the other hand, large doses of estradiol and thyroxine caused a moderate increase in GPT activity but when injected simultaneously with cortisol, they appeared to interfere with its action as did progesterone. Adrenalectomy slightly diminished or failed to affect the GPT-inducing activity of cortisol, whereas hypophysectomy caused a rise in GPT activity and augmented the effect of cortisol.

Rosen et al. G66,496/59: In the rat, cortisol, cortisone and prednisone cause a 6—13 fold increase in hepatic GPT activity. This effect was directly related to the protein content of the ration. In alloxan diabetic rats, the rise in this enzyme activity was equivalent to that obtained by cortisol or high-protein diets and could be inhibited by insulin. Adrenalectomy diminished but did not abolish the rise in GPT activity obtained by feeding high-protein diets. Thus, the initiation of enzyme synthesis by dietary protein is not mediated exclusively through the adrenals.

Other Enzymes

Schweppe & Jungmann H15,266/69: The ability of rat liver microsomes to **synthesize cholesterol palmitate**, oleate and linoleate in vitro is increased by the addition of thyroxine or glucagon to the incubation medium. Testosterone increases cholesterol palmitate and oleate formation. 17β-Estradiol stimulates mainly oleate synthesis.

Harada et al. H15,156/69: The **acetyl-CoA-synthetase** activity of the rat liver increases 2—3-fold during alloxan diabetes, fasting, or high-fat diet feeding.

Kato & Takahashi H11,853/69: "The magnitude of increase in the activities of microsomal drug-metabolizing enzymes and **NADPH**-linked electron transport system in the alloxan diabetic rats was greater than in normal rats, in contrast, the magnitude of increase in the thyroxine-treated rats was smaller than in normal rats."

Müller-Oerlinghausen et al. G64,175/69: Hepatic tissue of mice which had been injected with tolbutamide, synthesizes an increased amount of glucuronide when incubated in vitro with o-aminophenol. Insulin given at a dose causing a similar degree of hypoglycemia is much less effective in enhancing **glucuronide synthesis**. Adrenalectomy diminishes the formation of o-aminophenol glucuronide, despite hypoglycemia. However, adrenalectomized mice given cortisone again respond with increased glucuronide synthesis following tolbutamide.

Shou et al. H15,277/69: In the rat, the hepatic **methionine adenosyl transferase** activity was not much influenced by glucagon, but during alloxan diabetes it increased considerably. Combined treatment with alloxan and triamcinolone resulted in an additive effect. The response to alloxan could be prevented and even reversed by insulin or adrenalectomy. In normal rats, insulin caused no consistent increase.

← EPINEPHRINE AND NOREPINEPHRINE

Even before Walter Cannon put forth his classic concept of the "emergency reaction," it had been realized that the adrenal medulla plays an important part in defense, especially through its effect upon the cardiovascular system. In a sense, the secretion of vasopressor catecholamines into the blood stream complements the protective and adaptive effects of the sympathetic nervous system. On the other hand, we know very little about the possible direct effects of these hormones upon detoxication mechanisms apart from the fact that they may influence these by altering the liver glycogen and blood sugar concentrations.

Steroids ←

In the rat, epinephrine increases, whereas insulin decreases the anesthetic effect of progesterone. Also in rats, epinephrine and norepinephrine produce eclampsia-like manifestations following pretreatment with DOC + NaCl.

Nonsteroidal Hormones and Hormone-Like Substances ←

In mice, pretreatment with **epinephrine** increases resistance to this catecholamine in a rather specific manner.

The diabetogenic action of **alloxan** is diminished by epinephrine in the rabbit.

In dogs, many of the changes produced by **thyroid preparations** are abolished by sympathetic blockade and increased by epinephrine and norepinephrine.

The toxicity of **histamine** is as markedly increased by complete sympathetic blockade as it is by total adrenalectomy in the rat. Epinephrine counteracts the increased susceptibility to histamine, but not to several other stressor agents. It appears that the adrenergic system is the first line of defense against certain stressors (e.g., histamine, endotoxin), whereas resistance to others (e.g., formalin, tourniquet shock) is more dependent upon glucocorticoids.

Steroids ← *cf. also Selye G60,083/70, pp. 331, 358, 360.*

Winter & Selye A35,658/41; Winter A36,333/41: Epinephrine increases, whereas insulin decreases, the resistance of the rat to the anesthetic action of progesterone.

Pellanda C7,961/55: In rats pretreated with DOC and NaCl, epinephrine or norepinephrine produces an eclampsia-like syndrome.

Cortisol ← Epinephrine: Kumagai et al. *C57,345/58*

Steroids ← Norepinephrine, Cattle: Cooper et al. *D20,337/62*

17α-Hydroxyprogesterone ← Epinephrine, Cattle: Cooper et al. *D20,338/62*

Nonsteroidal Hormones and Hormone-Like Substances ← *cf. also Selye C92,918/61, pp. 112, 121; G60,083/70, pp. 358—362.*

Brewster Jr. et al. C11,771/56: In dogs, the physiologic changes produced by **thyroid** extract are abolished following sympathetic blockade. The inotrophic, chronotrophic and calorigenic effects of epinephrine and norepinephrine are increased by thyroid feeding. "It is concluded that there is a dynamic interrelationship between the thyroid hormones and those of the adrenal medulla and sympathetic nerve endings."

Carrasco-Formiguera & Escobar B19,877/48: In rabbits, epinephrine i.m. inhibits the diabetogenic action of **alloxan**.

Gasic B17,561/47: In mice, pretreatment with **epinephrine** increased resistance to this catecholamine but not to formalin. Apparently, at least under these conditions, cross-resistance does not occur.

Krawczak & Brodie H25,296/70: In rats, complete blockade of sympathetic function can be achieved by demedullation combined with reserpine-like agents (depleting catecholamine stores), bretylium-like agents (preventing nerve impulse from releasing catecholamines) or ganglioplegics. Following such total sympathetic blockade, mortality from histamine or endotoxin is as markedly increased as by adrenalectomy. Pretreatment with epinephrine alone counteracts the increased lethality of endotoxin and **histamine** after sympathetic blockade. Cortisone pretreatment only partially corrects the sensitization by adrenalectomy, whereas cortisone + epinephrine offers complete protection against these agents. Presumably, sympathetic stimulation is "the first line of defense against the vasomotor disturbance elicited by endotoxin and histamine." The lethal effect of formalin or tourniquet shock is likewise greatly increased by adrenalectomy but, in contrast to that of endotoxin and histamine, it cannot be increased by sympathetic blockade. Furthermore, cortisone alone counteracts the toxicity of these stressors in adrenalectomized rats. Apparently "formalin and tourniquet shock is initiated by a mechanism which differs from that elicited by histamine and endotoxin and does not primarily involve the sympathetic system."

Drugs ←

The **anaphylactoid** edema produced in rats by egg-white can be prevented by epinephrine or norepinephrine, but not by isoproterenol. The gastric hemorrhages elicited by polymyxin (another anaphylactoidogen) are even more effectively prevented by epinephrine than by various antihistamines.

In guinea pigs, epinephrine injected on awakening from **barbiturate** anesthesia produced a return of sleep. This effect could be duplicated by glucose, lactate or glutamate in intact animals but after adrenalectomy only epinephrine was effective. In mice, epinephrine also prolongs the hypnotic effect of various barbiturates, although allegedly thiopental and barbital anesthesia is mildly reduced by it, under certain circumstances, perhaps because epinephrine (unlike norepinephrine) enhances the penetration of barbital into the brain. In any event barbital and epinephrine (but not norepinephrine) may cause very peculiar neurologic manifestations — associated with ataxia, incoordination and loss of righting reflex — at doses at which barbital alone has no such effect.

In rabbits, pentobarbital sleeping time is shortened by epinephrine, but if administered just after awakening from thiopental anesthesia, epinephrine reinduces sleep; yet, epinephrine (unlike norepinephrine) causes rapid awakening if given to rabbits during thiopental anesthesia.

Carbon tetrachloride given simultaneously with epinephrine to the dog often leads to fatal ventricular fibrillation. In rats, epinephrine or norepinephrine fails to potentiate the hepatotoxic effect of CCl_4 and, in isolated perfused rat livers, the hemodynamic effects of norepinephrine are increased by CCl_4. On the other hand, in mice the hepatotoxicity of CCl_4 has been claimed to be considerably increased by concurrent administration of either epinephrine or norepinephrine.

In dogs, epinephrine injected during **chloroform** anesthesia readily produces collapse and death. Pretreatment with epinephrine has no such effect, indeed it may protect the dog against subsequent combined treatment with chloroform and epinephrine. The chloroform-epinephrine collapse can be prevented in dogs by lithium carmine or induced hypothermia.

The muscular paralysis produced by **curare** derivatives can be inhibited by epinephrine in several species.

Various observations suggest that at least under certain circumstances norepinephrine may increase the effect of **digitalis** derivatives.

The toxicity of **ganglioplegics** (e.g., hexamethonium) is counteracted by epinephrine in the guinea pig. On the other hand, tetraethylammonium may considerably sensitize the dog to the pressor effect of epinephrine and other vasopressor agents. In rabbits, combined treatment with epinephrine and tetraethylammonium may also result in dangerous intoxication.

There is some evidence that in rats and dogs, epinephrine offers some protection against **mescaline** intoxication.

The head and neck edema induced by **paraphenylenediamine** is moderately inhibited by epinephrine.

In mice, **pentylenetetrazol** convulsions can be inhibited by combined administration of norepinephrine and 5-HT into certain regions of the brain. In one-day old chicks in which the blood-brain barrier is still incompletely formed, epinephrine (as well as 5-HT or histamine) prevent pentylenetetrazol convulsions and produce sleep.

Picrotoxin convulsions are also inhibited by intracerebral administration of epinephrine or 5-HT in mice.

In various species, **reserpine** intoxication is counteracted by epinephrine.

In rabbits, concurrent treatment with **sparteine** and epinephrine causes cardiac and hepatic lesions which are not obtained at comparable dose levels by either agent alone.

Epinephrine offers considerable protection against **strychnine** convulsions in frogs, guinea pigs and mice.

In cholesterol-fed rabbits, the anti-atheromatous action of **Tween 80** is inhibited by norepinephrine.

It has been claimed that, in **vitamin-D** deficient rats, the healing of rickets can be initiated by epinephrine, but these observations require confirmation. On the other hand, the production of cardiovascular calcification by DHT is enhanced by norepinephrine in the rat. The progeria-like syndrome produced by chronic treatment with small doses of DHT in rats is not influenced by epinephrine. However, a single large dose of this catecholamine often causes calcifying mural ball valve thrombi in the left atrium of rats pretreated with large doses of DHT (or parathyroid extract).

Acetonitrile ←

Paal 22,603/30: In mice, acetonitrile resistance is not consistently influenced by posterior pituitary extract (hypophysin), a folliculoid preparation (progynon), or epinephrine.

Dessau 34,845/35: In rats, adrenalectomy decreases resistance to acetonitrile. Resistance can be slightly restored by adrenocortical transplants, but not by the adrenocortical extract tested or by epinephrine.

Allyl Alcohol ←

Strubel et al. G80,282/70: In rats, norepinephrine did not augment the hepatotoxicity of CCl_4 or allyl alcohol at doses of 0.25 mg/kg or less. However, at the dose of 1 mg/kg, at which norepinephrine itself causes liver damage, it potentiates the hepatotoxicity of these agents. Earlier claims that CCl_4 causes liver damage only through the massive liberation of endogenous catecholamines could not be confirmed.

Aminopyrine ← Norepinephrine + Phenoxybenzamine: Dixon et al. G11,757/64

Amitriptyline ←

Nymark & Rasmussen G42,054/66: In rabbits, norepinephrine offered no considerable protection against the ECG changes produced by amitriptyline.

Anaphylactoidogens ← cf. also Selye B40,000/50, p. 758; G46,715/68, pp. 177, 178, 181, 187.

Clark & MacKay B36,925/49: In rats, the anaphylactoid edema produced by egg white i.p. is prevented by epinephrine or norepinephrine s.c.; isoproterenol is ineffective.

Moreno & Brodie D20,261/62: In rats, the gastric hemorrhages that occur 2 hrs after polymyxin s.c. are more effectively prevented by epinephrine than by various antihistamines (cyproheptadine, chlorpheniramine, pyrilamine). At very high doses, chlorpromazine and dibenzyline were also effective but anticholinergic drugs and antacids were not. Presumably, lesions were due to gastric vascular changes without involvement of the secretory mechanism.

Adamkiewicz D61,626/63: Review showing that "hyperglycemias resulting from overdosage with sugars, cortisol, adrenaline, or from diabetes inhibit the anaphylactoid reactions; anaphylaxis, and the tuberculin reaction; but potentiate infections. Hypoglycemias resulting from fasting, insulin and adrenalectomy, potentiate the anaphylactoid reactions, anaphylaxis, and the tuberculin reaction; but inhibit infections. The hypothesis is proposed that hyperglycemia inhibits certain antigen-antibody combinations; this results in an inhibition of hypersensitivity, but an aggravation of infection."

Aniline ← Norepinephrine + Phenoxybenzamine: Dixon et al. G11,757/64

Antibiotics ← cf. Selye G60,083/70, pp. 358, 361.

Anticoagulants ←

Jaques G70,979/68: Review (30 pp., 13 refs.) on the "hemorrhagic stress syndrome" that is produced in various mammals treated with indirect anticoagulants (e.g., phenindione, dicoumarol) and then exposed to stress or treated with DOC, ACTH, or STH. Conversely, cortisone, epinephrine, ephedrine and adrenochrome inhibit this syndrome.

Arsenic ←

Hanzlink & Karsner 10,286/20: In guinea pigs, epinephrine can prevent true anaphylactic shock but not the anaphylactoid shock produced by peptone, dextrin or agar. The arsphenamine-induced disturbances (which have been regarded by some as anaphylactoid) are diminished by epinephrine, presumably as a consequence of its circulatory action.

Barbiturates ←

Dog

Werle & Lentzen A28,007/38: In dogs and rabbits, various vasoactive substances (epinephrine, histamine, vasopressin, kallikrein) tend to prolong the anesthetic effect of pronarcon and hexobarbital.

Rolf & Campbell H18,467/69: In dogs, anesthesia by various thiobarbiturates sensitizes for the production of cardiac arrhythmias by epinephrine.

Hexobarbital ← Epinephrine, Dog: Dallemagne A47,748/41*

Guinea Pig

Lamson et al. B89,712/52: In guinea pigs, epinephrine injected i.p. on awakening from barbiturate anesthesia produced a return to sleep. A similar effect was caused by glucose, lactate, or glutamate. However, in adrenalectomized animals, only epinephrine was effective.

Hexobarbital ← Epinephrine, Gp: Lamson et al. C14,547/51*

Mouse

Reinhard B283/45: In mice, the hexobarbital sleeping time is prolonged by epinephrine or insulin.

Holck B42,745/48: In mice, neither epinephrine nor insulin altered significantly the fatal dose of hexobarbital given 20 min later.

Fastier D95,950/56: In mice, 5-HT considerably potentiates the hypnotic effect of cyclobarbital and chloral hydrate. However, this property is not very specific, since bufotenine, tryptamine, histamine, and epinephrine likewise prolong cyclobarbital hypnosis. Literature on numerous other drugs which prolong barbiturate anesthesia is cited. "It therefore seems possible that the ability of 5-HT to prolong hypnosis may be due to a relatively unspecific, vascular effect."

Pradhan et al. C13,632/56: In 3 strains of mice, urethan sleeping time was greatly increased by epinephrine and norepinephrine. Phenobarbital sleeping time was only mildly increased by epinephrine.

Komiya et al. C21,326/56: In mice, thiopental anesthesia is reduced in severity, but not in duration, by epinephrine. Barbital anesthesia was slightly reduced by norepinephrine but not by epinephrine. Unpublished experiments suggest that ACTH and glucocorticoids shorten the duration of barbital anesthesia in mice.

Holtz et al. C76,300/58: In mice just awakening from hexobarbital anesthesia, sleep is reinduced by norepinephrine but not by epinephrine.

Kato C78,047/59: In mice, the prolongation of pentobarbital or hexobarbital sleeping time by 5-HT (administered in the form of its precursor 5-HTP which penetrates the brain barrier more readily) is inhibited by DOPA; the latter presumably acts as a precursor of norepinephrine.

Mazel & Bush D4,194/61: In mice, the penetration of barbital into the brain and the resulting anesthesia are enhanced by epinephrine but not by norepinephrine.

Fouts D43,347/62: Repeated injections of epinephrine i.p. increase the hexobarbital- and chlorpromazine-destroying effect of hepatic microsomal fractions in the rat.

Ellinwood & Prange E39,187/64: In mice, high doses of epinephrine prolonged sleeping time in themselves and potentiated the effect of thyroid feeding. The prolongation of pentobarbital sleeping time by epinephrine may be due to depletion of hepatic glycogen which interferes with hepatic microsomal-drug metabolism.

Kato & Gillette F57,817/65: The metabolism of aminopyrine and hexobarbital by hepatic microsomes of male rats is impaired by adrenalectomy, castration, hypoxia, ACTH, formaldehyde, epinephrine, morphine, alloxan or thyroxine. The metabolism of aniline and zoxazolamine is not appreciably decreased by any of these agents; in fact, hydroxylation of aniline is enhanced by thyroxine or alloxan. Apparently, the treatments impair mainly the sex-dependent enzymes. Accordingly, the corresponding enzymic functions of the hepatic microsomes of female rats are not significantly impaired by the agents which do have an inhibitory effect in males.

Vizet F77,760/67: In mice, combined treatment with barbital and epinephrine causes "spectacular neurologic modifications," with ataxia, muscular incoordination and loss of righting reflex, at dose levels at which barbital alone has no such effect. Norepinephrine does not markedly influence barbital intoxication. There is a parallel increase in the cerebral concentration of the barbiturate when epinephrine is added to barbital, but an augmentation of the blood-brain barrier permeability does not completely account for the increase in toxicity.

Mazel & Bush G65,299/69: In mice, epinephrine increases the anesthetic effect and brain concentration of barbital. "The epinephrine effect, however, cannot be attributed to increased brain barbital levels alone, because at 10 min the controls showed no signs of depression with the same brain barbital levels as the 'anesthetized' epinephrine-treated animals."

Hexobarbital ← Epinephrine, Mouse: Reinhard B283/45*; Holck B42,745/48*; Holtz et al. C76,300/58*; Mathies et al. D84,334/61*

Pentobarbital ← Epinephrine + Thyroid extract, Mouse: Ellinwood et al. E39,187/64*

RABBIT

Westfall B31,306/46: In rabbits, pentobarbital sleeping time is shortened by epinephrine and insulin despite their opposite effect upon blood sugar.

Fenu C17,650/54: In rabbits just awakening from thiopental anesthesia, epinephrine i.v. reinduces sleep. A smaller dose of epinephrine injected intracysternally, though equivalent as regards its stressor effects, does not reinduce sleep under these conditions. Since other stressors likewise failed to share this effect of epinephrine, the latter cannot be merely due to an activation of the pituitary-adrenocortical axis.

Cahn et al. G 71,537/56: In rabbits, the prolongation of barbiturate (Kemithal, Mebubarbital) anesthesia by 5-HT is further prolonged by phentolamine, neostigmine and several other drugs, whereas epinephrine and pantheline have an opposite effect.

Savoldi et al. C 92,984/60: In rabbits, epinephrine, unlike norepinephrine, causes rapid awakening from thiopental anesthesia.

RAT

Milošević C 39,053/56: In rats, epinephrine i.p. administered almost simultaneously with thialbarbital i.v. prolongs anesthesia. The effect of several other anesthetics (chloral hydrate, paraldehyde, tribromoethanol, chlorobutanol, chloralose and ethanol) is likewise significantly prolonged by epinephrine pretreatment. Norepinephrine, cobefrine, synephrine, suprifen and ephedrine also prolong thialbarbital anesthesia, whereas amphetamine and methamphetamine exert an inverse effect. The somewhat contradictory earlier literature on the effect of catecholamines upon anesthesia is briefly reviewed.

Slocombe C 14,144/56: In rats under thiopental anesthesia, epinephrine, norepinephrine, adrenochrome, and 5-HT cause a flattening of the electrical activity both at cortical and at subcortical sites.

MAN

von Reis C 76,244/59: In patients with barbiturate intoxication, norepinephrine i.v. is beneficial presumably because it prevents anuria by inhibiting the hypotension.

  Hexobarbital ← Epinephrine: Fouts D 43,347/62, G 76,304/63

  Hexobarbital ← Norepinephrine + Phenoxybenzamine: Dixon et al. G 11,757/64

Benzol ←

Dautrebande 8,083/32: In dogs, benzol inhalation during epinephrine treatment tends to produce fatal collapse.

Caffeine ←

Johnson & Siebert C 91,021/28; C 91,037/28: In rabbits, the cardiac lesions produced by caffeine are greatly aggravated by concurrent treatment with epinephrine.

Carbon Tetrachloride ←

Hermann et al. 10,215/31; Hermann & Vial 32,885/35: In dogs, fatal ventricular fibrillation is elicited by epinephrine not only when the hormone is given in combination with chloroform but also when administered with CCl_4 or CH_2Cl_2.

Furukawa F 71,711/65: In rats, hepatic steatosis produced by CCl_4 is inhibited by adrenalectomy and, to some extent, also by hypophysectomy. Corticoids restore the effect of CCl_4 after adrenalectomy; epinephrine does not but it increases the effect of corticoids. STH does not counteract the effect of hypophysectomy. Alloxan diabetes inhibits CCl_4-induced hepatic lipidosis.

Larson & Plaa F 29,496/65: In rats, infusion of large amounts of epinephrine or norepinephrine did not potentiate the hepatotoxic effect of CCl_4 nor did it induce CCl_4-like hepatic lesions after transection of the spinal cord. These and other observations suggest that protection of the liver against CCl_4-induced lesions by cervical cordotomy is not due to blockade of adrenergic mechanisms but to reduced hepatic metabolism consequent to hypothermia.

Rice et al. G 55,767/67: In isolated perfused rat livers, the hemodynamic effects of norepinephrine are increased by CCl_4.

Schwetz & Plaa G 67,000/69: In mice, the hepatotoxicity of CCl_4 i.p. is greatly increased by simultaneous treatment with epinephrine or norepinephrine s.c. "Epinephrine and norepinephrine may play a secondary potentiating role in CCl_4-induced hepatotoxicity."

Strubelt et al. G 80,282/70: In rats, norepinephrine did not augment the hepatotoxicity of CCl_4 or allyl alcohol at doses of 0.25 mg/kg or less. However, at the dose of 1 mg/kg, at which norepinephrine itself causes liver damage, it potentiates the hepatotoxicity of these agents. Earlier claims that CCl_4 causes liver damage only through the massive liberation of endogenous catecholamines could not be confirmed.

Chloral Hydrate ←

Fastier et al. C 37,038/57: In mice, chloral hydrate sleeping time is increased by epinephrine, norepinephrine, phenylephrine, methoxamine, 5-HT, histamine, ergotamine, yohimbine and atropine. "It is suggested that some, at least, of the drugs which prolong the effects of hypnotics do so by virtue of a hypothermic action." Vasopressin, cortisone and DOC did not prolong chloral hydrate sleeping time at the doses tested.

Chloroform ←

Davis & Whipple 58,731/19: In dogs, pretreatment with epinephrine protects against the production of hepatic necrosis produced by chloroform anesthesia. This resistance requires several days of pretreatment and cannot be obtained by a single epinephrine injection just before chloroform administration.

Bardier & Stillmunkès 25,803/26: The collapse produced by epinephrine + chloroform is inhibited by scorpion and vipera venom [species is not stated but presumably dog (H.S.).] In dogs, epinephrine injected during chloroform anesthesia readily produces collapse and death. Injected before chloroform, epinephrine is harmless at similar dose levels. Indeed, pretreatment with epinephrine can protect the dog against subsequent combined administration of chloroform plus epinephrine.

Hermann et al. 10,215/31; Hermann & Vial 32,885/35: In dogs, fatal ventricular fibrillation is elicited by epinephrine not only when the hormone is given in combination with chloroform but also when administered with CCl_4 or CH_2Cl_2.

Tournade & Raymond-Hamet 7,436/32: In dogs, norepinephrine i.v. produces fatal collapse during chloroform anesthesia.

Velluda & Russu 38,782/36: In dogs, chloroform-epinephrine collapse can be prevented by lithium carmine.

Szilágyi et al. D21,498/61: In dogs, the epinephrine-chloroform syncope is inhibited by hypothermia.

Chlorpromazine ← Epinephrine: Fouts *D43,347/62, G76,304/63*

Cholesterol ← cf. also Selye *G60,083/70, pp. 358, 359.*

Trentini et al. G71,152/68: In rabbits, the cholesterol-atherosclerosis-inhibiting effect of Tween 80 is diminished both by 5-HT and by norepinephrine.

Hamprecht G69,560/69: Review (7 pp., 153 refs.) on the mechanisms regulating cholesterol synthesis. A special section deals with the effect of thyroid hormones, steroids, epinephrine, norepinephrine and glucagon.

Cocaine ←

Avant & Weatherby C81,325/60: Review on the inhibition of the systemic toxicity of various local anesthetics by admixture of epinephrine which delays their absorption. Personal observations on mice showed that among five cocaine derivatives, only one (tetracaine) exhibited considerably decreased systemic toxicity upon addition of epinephrine to the s.c. injected anesthetic.

Curare ←

Bremer & Titeca 23,673/28: In decerebrate cats, the abolition of rigidity by curare is counteracted by epinephrine i.v.

Maddock et al. B18,670/48: In dogs, intra-arterial injection of epinephrine blocks the effect of i.v.-administered curare upon the musculature. This blockade is abolished by Dibenamine.

Constantin & Bouyard H15,750/69: In rabbits, the muscular paralysis produced by alcuronium is inhibited by epinephrine presumably through an α-adrenergic mechanism.

Cyclohexylamine ← cf. Selye *G60,083/70, pp. 358, 363.*

Digitalis ←

Ghedini & Ollino A21,128/14: Brief mention of observations on rabbits showing that epinephrine i.v. "favorably influences" the hemodynamic actions of digitalin, whereas pancreatic powder influences them "unfavorably."

Lage & Spratt F86,237/67: In mice, norepinephrine does not influence the toxicity of digitoxigenin. However, the protection by reserpine against digitoxigenin poisoning is inhibited by large doses of norepinephrine which "would suggest that the depletion of catecholamines by reserpine may be responsible for the protection."

Morrow G47,272/67: In dogs under pentobarbital anesthesia, ouabain tolerance was diminished by large doses of norepinephrine. "The studies suggest that a therapeutic level of digitalis may become toxic during the administration of large doses of norepinephrine."

Ergotamine ←

Tinel & Ungar 14,897/33: In guinea pigs, epileptoid convulsions are produced by epinephrine given conjointly with ergotamine, peptone or yohimbine.

Ethanol ←

Hiestand et al. B78,576/53: In mice, alloxan diabetes and epinephrine increase, whereas insulin decreases, sensitivity to lethal doses of ethanol.

Ethanol ← Epinephrine, Mouse: Hiestand et al. B78,576/53*

Formalin ←

Gasic B17,561/47: In mice, pretreatment with epinephrine increased resistance to this catecholamine but not to formalin. Apparently, at least under these conditions, cross-resistance does not occur.

Ganglioplegics ←

Page & Taylor B24,841/47: In earlier publications, epinephrine "has been recommended as the antidote of choice after excessive doses of tetraethyl ammonium chloride." In the present experiments on dogs, it is shown that under certain circumstances, especially during pentobarbital anesthesia, TEA may considerably sensitize to the pressor effect of epinephrine, renin and angiotensin.

Byrne C46,341/56: In rabbits, the effect of various drugs upon pulmonary embolisms produced by graphite particles has been investigated. "The combination of epinephrine and tetraethyl-ammonium was dangerous, since epinephrine is a ganglion blocking agent and enhances the effect of tetraethyl-ammonium."

Orione C37,851/56: Guinea pigs are protected by epinephrine against the hypothermia and mortality of hexamethonium intoxication.

Halothane ←

Nikki & Rosenberg G71,574/69: In mice, shivering and hypothermia are prevented by norepinephrine and 5-HT but not by dopamine. "The results suggest that brain catecholamines participate in the control of shivering and return of normothermia after halothane anesthesia in mice."

Hexamethonium ← cf. Ganglioplegics

Lathyrogens ← cf. also Selye G60,083/70, pp. 358, 361.

Kohn & Rivera-Velez F73,678/65: In rats made lathyric by APN fumarate, the vasopressor effect of norepinephrine is diminished.

Lead Acetate ← cf. Selye C19,425/65, p. 137.

Meperidine ←

Radouco-Thomas et al. E60,201/57: In guinea pigs, the analgesic effect of meperidine is diminished by reserpine and counteracted by concurrent administration of norepinephrine.

Meprobamate ←

Belaval & Widen C76,528/58: In a few patients, some of the effects of meprobamate intoxication were antagonized by norepinephrine.

Mescaline ←

Speck C31,193/57: In rats, epinephrine inhibits the bradycardia and hypoglycemia but not the mortality induced by mescaline.

Schopp et al. E92,442/61: In the dog, epinephrine (like KCl and neostigmine) can oppose the paralyzing action of mescaline.

Methanol ←

Severin & Bashkurov G49,801/67: In patients with acute methanol poisoning, combined treatment with norepinephrine, cortisone and various other agents facilitated recovery. [In view of the complex treatment given, it is impossible to ascertain the relative value of each component of the therapeutic regimen (H.S.).]

Methoxyflurane ←

Catton G71,124/69: In rabbits given epinephrine i.v., methoxyflurane anesthesia depends largely upon CO_2 and O_2 tensions.

Methyltropolone ←

Murnaghan & Mazurkiewicz D68,260/63: In mice, the toxicity of 4-methyltropolone is greatly increased by epinephrine. "The results suggest that the in vivo effects of methyltropolone are not only due to inhibition of O-methyltransferase but are also due to a blockade at both alpha and beta receptor sites. Blockade of alpha receptors by methyltropolone suggests that attachment of the ring hydroxyls of the adrenergic amine is a prerequisite for excitation at this receptor."

Morphine ←

Miller et al. G73,877/55: Review of earlier literature suggesting that morphine analgesia is mediated through the release of epinephrine from the adrenal medulla. It had been claimed that adrenalectomy decreases the pain reaction threshold to morphine and that morphine itself has an analgesic effect. However, in the authors' experiments on rats these observations could not be confirmed and TEA failed to reverse the effect of morphine on pain. In mice, near lethal doses of epinephrine or norepinephrine were required to raise the pain threshold.

Heller et al. H 2,707/68: In mice, epinephrine, norepinephrine, and isoproterenol possess a certain analgesic effect of their own and enhance analgesia produced by morphine.

Heller et al. H 13,896/68: In mice and rats, the analgesic effect of morphine is increased by epinephrine or norepinephrine i.v.

Nicotine ←

Hueper 91,722/43: In rats, the cardiovascular lesions produced by chronic nicotine intoxication are aggravated both by epinephrine and by DOC.

Papain ← *cf. also Selye C 50,810/58, p. 106; C 92,918/61, p. 110; G 60,083/70, pp. 358, 361.*

Zacco & Pratesi B 37,559/47: In guinea pigs, papain shock can be prevented by pretreatment with epinephrine.

Paraoxon ←

de Candole C 25,237/56: In rabbits, resistance to the anticholinesterase paraoxon is increased, under certain conditions, by norepinephrine.

Paraphenylenediamine ←

Meissner E 52,567/19: The head and neck edema produced by paraphenylenediamine in the rabbit is not prevented by epinephrine, posterior pituitary extract or thyroid extract.

Tainter 25,429/26; 23,737/28: In rabbits, the head and neck edema produced by paraphenylenediamine is inhibited by epinephrine and related catecholamines.

Cohen et al. 92,880/33: In rabbits, paraphenylenediamine-induced head and neck edema is delayed but not completely abolished by epinephrine.

Pentylenetetrazol ←

Schmidt & Matthies D 34,219/62: In mice, 5-HT or norepinephrine injected into certain regions of the brain is without effect upon pentylenetetrazol injections in itself, but counteracts the inhibitory effect of intracerebrally-injected reserpine.

Schmidt E 32,188/63: In mice, pentylenetetrazol convulsions are inhibited by combined administration of 5-HT and norepinephrine into certain regions of the brain.

Kobrin & Seifter F 74,422/66: In one day old chicks, in which the blood-brain barrier is still incompletely formed, various ω-amino acids as well as 5-HT, histamine and epinephrine, produce sleep and prevent pentylenetetrazol convulsions.

Jones & Roberts G 60,654/68: In mice, the convulsive effect of pentylenetetrazol is inhibited by norepinephrine administered intracerebroventricularly.

Schlesinger et al. G 69,565/69: In mice, intracranial injections of 5-HT or norepinephrine protect against pentylenetetrazol convulsions.

Peptone ←

Hanzlink & Karsner 10,286/20: In guinea pigs, epinephrine can prevent true anaphylactic shock but not the anaphylactoid shock produced by peptone, dextrin or agar. The arsphenamine-induced disturbances (which have been regarded by some as anaphylactoid) are diminished by epinephrine, presumably as a consequence of its circulatory action.

Tinel & Ungar 14,897/33: In guinea pigs, epileptoid convulsions are produced by epinephrine given conjointly with ergotamine, peptone or yohimbine.

Pesticides ←

Cueto Jr. G 72,544/70: In dogs, o,p'-DDD produces a selective glucocorticoid deficiency due to its damaging effect upon the fasciculata and reticularis of the adrenal. Epinephrine and norepinephrine produce hypotensive failure in DDD-treated dogs presumably as the consequence of their stressor action. Prednisolone largely restores the resistance of the DDD-treated animals.

Phenylethylamine ←

Fischer et al. G 48,517/67: In mice pretreated with iproniazid (as a MAO-inhibitor), phenylethylamine produces amphetamine-like motor effects which are inhibited by epinephrine.

Picrotoxin ←

Saito et al. E 27,616/63: In mice, picrotoxin convulsions are inhibited by the intracerebral administration of epinephrine or 5-HT.

Picrotoxin ← Epinephrine: Holck D 28,543/49*

Plasmocid ← *cf. Selye C 50,810/58, p. 110; C 92,918/61, p. 83; C 92,918/61, pp. 96, 110; G 60,083/70, pp. 358, 361.*

Potassium ←

Lum H 22,940/70: In anesthetized dogs, epinephrine i.v. protected against the lethal effects of potassium i.v.

Procaine ←

Cole & Hulpieu B32,910/49; B57,578/50: In dogs the toxicity of procaine is not consistently counteracted by epinephrine.

Reserpine ←

Schmidt & Matthies D34,219/62: In mice, 5-HT or norepinephrine injected into certain regions of the brain is without effect upon pentylenetetrazol injections in itself, but counteracts the inhibitory effect of intracerebrally injected reserpine.

Agostini & Giagheddu G14,490/63: Reserpine catalepsy in guinea pigs is inhibited by various folliculoid, testoid and corticoid hormones as well as by epinephrine.

Simionovici et al. F43,099/65: In mice, epinephrine and norepinephrine, as well as histamine, offer partial protection against reserpine intoxication (sedation blepharoptosis, hypothermia). 5-HT has no such effect.

Sparteine ←

Christian D1,675/11; Christian et al. C81,653/11: In rabbits given concurrent treatment with sparteine and epinephrine, cardiac and hepatic lesions develop which are not seen if either of these agents is given alone.

Strychnine ←

Falta & Jvcovic A1,273/09: In frogs and guinea pigs, epinephrine protects against strychnine-induced convulsions, even if the two compounds are injected in different points of the body.

Januschke 50,228/10: In frogs, epinephrine i.v. does not protect against strychnine intoxication. Protection following treatment with mixtures of the two compounds by routes other than i.v. is ascribed to a delay in strychnine absorption.

Bálint & Molnár 34,586/11: In guinea pigs, the fatal effect of strychnine intoxication is inhibited by epinephrine or thyroid extract i.p.

Marañón & Aznar 46,926/15: In frogs, the fatal convulsions produced by strychnine can be prevented if, prior to injection, the drug is mixed with extracts of the posterior pituitary, the thyroid, various other tissues, and particularly epinephrine. [The possibility of delayed absorption owing to local vasoconstriction has not been considered (H.S.).]

Amici C5,836/54: In mice, mortality from acute strychnine intoxication can be diminished by epinephrine and norepinephrine as well as by some of their derivatives.

Tetraethylammonium (TEA) ← cf. Ganglioplegics

Tremorine ←

Falutz F85,463/67: In cats, tremorine-induced tremor is uninfluenced by norepinephrine and epinephrine but inhibited by L-dopa.

Tween 80 ←

Scilabra & Pugliese G68,796/68; Trentini et al. G71,152/68: In cholesterol-fed rabbits, norepinephrine inhibits the anti-atheromatous action of Tween 80.

Urethan ←

Pradhan et al. C13,632/56: In 3 strains of mice, urethan sleeping time was greatly increased by epinephrine and norepinephrine. Phenobarbital sleeping time was only mildly increased by epinephrine.

Vitamin D, DHT ← *cf. also Selye C92,918/61, pp. 183, 188; G19,425/65, p. 137; G60,083/70, pp. 358, 361.*

de Bosányi 367/25: In rats kept on a vitamin-D deficient diet, the healing of rickets can be initiated by epinephrine.

Yohimbine ←

Tinel & Ungar 14,897/33: In guinea pigs, epileptoid convulsions are produced by epinephrine given conjointly with ergotamine, peptone or yohimbine.

Varia ←

Schou E92,436/61: Review (23 pp., 147 refs.) on factors influencing the absorption of drugs from subcutaneous connective tissue. Special sections deal with the effect of epinephrine, folliculoids and glucocorticoids which can alter the actions of various drugs by modifying their absorption rate.

Microorganisms, Vaccines and Venoms ←

Comparatively few investigators dealt with the effect of catecholamines upon **bacterial** infections. In guinea pigs, infection with Clostridium welchii is enhanced by the addition of epinephrine to the inoculum and, in rats, acute hypertension produced by epinephrine (or angiotensin) facilitates the production of pyelonephritis by E. coli. Topical resistance to inoculation with various pathogenic microbes is diminished by the injection of epinephrine into the site of inoculation.

Injection of epinephrine conjointly with various **viruses** enhances their infectivity in mice. In rabbits, herpes simplex infection followed by norepinephrine treatment may cause plaques of demyelination in the central nervous system.

At the beginning of this century, it has been claimed that epinephrine can inactivate **bacterial toxins**, e.g., diphtheria or tetanus toxin in guinea pigs, mice and rabbits, both in vivo and in vitro. It has subsequently been shown, however, that neutralization only occurs if epinephrine and the toxin, are mixed before injection, presumably because the vasopressor hormone delays absorption. In rabbits, combined administration of typhoid toxin and norepinephrine produces cardiac necroses. Data on the effectiveness of catecholamines in preventing endotoxin shock in various species are rather conflicting. Under certain circumstances, combined treatment with endotoxin and epinephrine produces a generalized Shwartzman-Sanarelli phenomenon in the rabbit.

In rats, complete blockade of the sympathetic function greatly diminishes resistance to endotoxins and this effect can be counteracted by epinephrine.

In guinea pigs, intoxication with cobra **venom** applied to skin erosions can be inhibited by the delay of absorption that results from topical treatment with epinephrine.

Bacteria ←

Lauber 9,102/32: Observations on the effect of vasopressin, epinephrine, thyroid extract and insulin upon streptococcal and staphylococcal infections in mice.

Evans et al. B65,652/48: In guinea pigs and rabbits, epinephrine diminishes local resistance to a large series of pathogenic microbes.

Bishop & Marshall C95,338/60: In guinea pigs, infection with Clostridium welchii is greatly enhanced by addition of epinephrine in oil or water to the inoculum.

Jones & Shapiro D55,793/63: In rats, an acute episode of hypertension produced by epinephrine or angiotensin i.v. facilitates the production of pyelonephritis following infection with E. coli.

Viruses ←

Sellers H10,893/69: In mice, epinephrine or 5-HT injected simultaneously with various viruses i.v. enhances their infectivity and their penetration into the brain.

Connor H23,400/70: In rabbits, infection with herpes simplex followed by treatment with norepinephrine may cause plaques of demyelination in the subcortical white matter and brain-stem. Possibly, in man, disseminated sclerosis is "multifactorial in origin" resulting from an apparently innocuous infection with herpes simplex in childhood followed later by challenge through physical or mental stress resulting in norepinephrine liberation. [A largely speculative "Letter to the Editor" (H.S.).]

Bacterial Toxins ← *cf. also Selye E5,986/66, pp. 14, 72; G60,083/70, p. 362.*

Marie 37,085/13: In guinea pigs, the lethal effect of diphtheria or tetanus toxin s.c. is diminished by previous incubation with epinephrine.

Marie 32,348/18; 37,087/19: In mice and rabbits, tetanus toxin is largely inactivated by epinephrine in vivo or in vitro.

Tawara 12,478/21: In mice, the lethal effect of tetanus toxin is not significantly influenced by epinephrine unless the two compounds are mixed before injection. This neutralizing effect may be due to the acidity of the epinephrine solution employed, since various acids are equally effective.

Mezzano & Peluffo D9,328/60: In rabbits, combined administration of typhoid toxin and norepinephrine produces cardiac necrosis not observed following treatment with either of these agents alone.

Altura et al. F43,209/65: In rats, norepinephrine and angiotensin fail to prolong survival after traumatic shock, temporary ligature of the superior mesenteric artery or endotoxin shock. However, vasopressin (PLV-2) was significantly effective in traumatic and intestinal ischemia shock but not in endotoxinemia.

Patel & Rao G36,076/65: In mice, epinephrine offers virtually no protection against tetanus toxin.

Vick F48,509/65: In the dog, cortisol and/or isoproterenol cause temporary improvement in endotoxin shock but no increase in survival time.

Bruce & Brunson F79,682/67: In dogs, mortality from endotoxin shock is diminished after pretreatment with norepinephrine. Survival is further improved by concurrent administration of the tranquilizer propiomazine.

Kutner et al. G46,379/67: In dogs, norepinephrine considerably decreases thoracic-duct lymph-flow both under normal conditions and during endotoxin shock.

Zeller et al. F92,117/67: In rats, simultaneous treatment with endotoxin and large amounts of 5% glucose solution i.v. produces a generalized "Shwartzman reaction" which can be blocked by phenoxybenzamine but is not modified by norepinephrine.

Brown et al. H456/68: In dogs, survival from endotoxin shock was improved by combined treatment with norepinephrine and adrenergic blockade.

Hruza & Stetson Jr. H455/68: Pretreatment with depot epinephrine or norepinephrine increased resistance to trauma in the Noble-Collip drum and to endotoxin.

Anas et al. G64,139/69: In dogs, norepinephrine, isoproterenol and phenoxybenzamine increase oxygen consumption during endotoxin shock. In this respect, norepinephrine is most active, but its effect is transient.

Boler et al. G65,722/69: "Treatment of endotoxin-shocked dogs with propiomazine and levarterenol promoted their survival and prevented or reduced the severity of most of the previously described ultrastructural alterations of the liver."

Barksdale et al. H21,684/70: In rabbits prepared and challenged for the generalized Shwartzman reaction by two i.v. injections of endotoxin spaced at an interval of 24 hrs, "epinephrine treatment was shown to increase the mortality when the normal optimum dose of endotoxin was used, ie, 100 µg per injection, but did not increase the incidence of the generalized Shwartzman reaction. When sublethal doses of endotoxin were used, ie, 25 µg or 10 µg, epinephrine treatment profoundly increased the mortality and incidence of the generalized reaction."

Krawczak & Brodie H25,296/70: In rats, complete blockade of sympathetic function can be achieved by demedullation combined with reserpine-like agents (depleting catecholamine stores), bretylium-like agents (preventing nerve impulse from releasing catecholamines) or ganglioplegics. Following such total sympathetic blockade, mortality from histamine or endotoxin is as markedly increased as by adrenalectomy. Pretreatment with epinephrine alone counteracts the increased lethality of endotoxin and histamine after sympathetic blockade. Cortisone pretreatment only partially corrects the sensitization by adrenalectomy, whereas cortisone + epinephrine offers complete protection against these agents. Presumably, sympathetic stimulation is "the first line of defense against the vasomotor disturbance elicited by endotoxin and histamine." The lethal effect of formalin or tourniquet shock is likewise greatly increased by adrenalectomy but, in contrast to that of endotoxin and histamine, it cannot be increased by sympathetic blockade. Furthermore, cortisone alone counteracts the toxicity of these stressors in adrenalectomized rats. Apparently "formalin and tourniquet shock is initiated by a mechanism which differs from that elicited by histamine and endotoxin and does not primarily involve the sympathetic system."

Venoms ←

Bardier & Stillmunkès 13,522/23: In dogs and rabbits, scorpion venom exerts cardiovascular actions similar to those of epinephrine but does not produce collapse during chloroform anesthesia. The pharmacologic interactions between the venom and epinephrine are briefly discussed.

Douglas 21,321/24: In guinea pigs, intoxication with cobra venom applied to skin erosions can be inhibited by the delay of absorption that results from topical treatment with epinephrine.

Stahnke F57,253/65: In rats treated with various scorpion and snake venoms, resistance was decreased by pretreatment with heat, cold or epinephrine. In all three cases, the change in resistance is ascribed to stress as such.

Immune Reactions ←

In guinea pigs and dogs, anaphylactic shock can be inhibited by epinephrine and norepinephrine. In rats, allegedly large amounts of epinephrine depress antibody formation against sheep serum. In rabbits, massive doses of epinephrine + norepinephrine decrease the incidence of chicken anti-rabbit-kidney nephritis.

Hanzlik & Karsner 10,286/20: In guinea pigs, epinephrine can prevent true anaphylactic shock but not the anaphylactoid shock produced by peptone, dextrin or agar. The arsphenamine-induced disturbances (which have been regarded by some as anaphylactoid) are diminished by epinephrine, presumably as a consequence of its circulatory action.

Marmorston-Gottesman & Perla 23,446/28: In rats, large amounts of epinephrine, injected repeatedly before and after injection of an antigen (sheep serum), depress antibody formation.

Cirstea & Suhaciu G2,471/63: In dogs, anaphylactic shock is diminished by epinephrine and norepinephrine.

Hinton et al. G21,390/64: In rabbits, large doses of epinephrine + norepinephrine decrease the incidence of chicken anti-rabbit-kidney nephritis. Fluorescent antibody studies "suggest the final antigen-antibody reaction may be of lesser magnitude in the treated animals."

Ionizing Rays ←

In mice, cutaneous purpura produced by heavy X-irradiation is allegedly inhibited by adrenochrome. Resistance to total body X-irradiation is increased by numerous amines including norepinephrine, epinephrine, histamine and 5-HT, allegedly because these compounds reduce the oxygen tension in tissues. Even topical treatment with norepinephrine is said to protect the hair follicles against radiation injury.

In rats, mortality after total body X-irradiation is likewise diminished by epinephrine; similar observations with epinephrine and its derivatives have been made in guinea pigs, hamsters and chicks.

Hervé & Lecomte B46,855/49: In mice, the cutaneous purpura produced by heavy X-irradiation is inhibited by adrenochrome semicarbazone.

Gray et al. B68,316/52: In rats, pretreatment with either epinephrine or vasopressin diminishes mortality after total body X-irradiation.

Gray et al. B69,100/52: In rats, pretreatment with Pitressin or epinephrine increases survival following exposure to lethal X-irradiation.

Bacq D77,006/54: In mice, resistance to whole body X-irradiation is increased by numerous amines, particularly cysteamine (β-mercaptoethylamine), norepinephrine, 5-HT and histamine.

Stearner et al. B92,163/54: In chicks, both epinephrine and decreased oxygen tension protect against mortality from X-irradiation. Presumably both agents act by decreasing oxygen supply to tissues during an early phase of the events initiated by ionizing rays.

Rigat C10,747/55: Review (46 pp., 67 refs.) on the literature concerning the effect of hormones upon X-irradiation with special reference to ACTH, STH, vasopressin, epinephrine, cortisone, DOC, testosterone, estradiol, progesterone, and thyroxine.

van der Meer & van Bekkum G71,673/59: In mice, the radioprotective effect of histamine, epinephrine and other biologic amines is related to their pharmacologic activity and can be blocked by their pharmacologic antagonists. "It is concluded that histamine, epinephrine and a number of other biological amines protect against irradiation by reducing the oxygen tension in the spleen and possibly in other blood forming organs."

Semenov D7,087/60: In mice, 5-HT offers better protection against radiation sickness than epinephrine although the latter is also effective, especially when given in combination with acetylcholine.

Gabler G40,828/66: In guinea pigs and rats, mortality from whole body X-irradiation is diminished by epinephrine and metaproterenol.

Letov H19,253/68: In mice, topical treatment with norepinephrine protects the hair follicles against radiation-induced injury.

Prewitt & Musacchia H16,155/69: In hamsters exposed to ^{60}Co radiation, survival was improved by pretreatment with norepinephrine > epinephrine and > isoproterenol. It is dubious whether these agents act simply through tissue hypoxia.

Cold ←

In rats, in which gastrointestinal ulcers were produced as part of an alarm reaction elicited by cold or other stressors, epinephrine p.o. produces lung edema, presumably because the hormone is well absorbed from the wound surfaces of the stress ulcers. Also in rats, epinephrine "appears to improve survival during exposure to cold, and adaptation to low temperatures increases the calorigenic effect of norepinephrine." However, depending upon circumstances, the catecholamines may also have an adverse effect upon survival during exposure to cold. In cold adapted guinea pigs, nonshivering thermogenesis is induced by cold or norepinephrine. It is suggested that nonshivering thermogenesis is essentially a catecholamine-mediated mechanism.

In **dogs**, norepinephrine infusions during cooling reduce the incidence of ventricular fibrillation, whereas epinephrine has an opposite effect.

In **minipigs**, nonshivering thermogenesis plays a major role in adaptation to cold only during neonatal life, if at all. Epinephrine and norepinephrine fail to stimulate nonshivering thermogenesis in minipigs, whereas they do have this effect in cold adapted rats.

In the **ground squirrel**, norepinephrine produces nonshivering thermogenesis after curarization.

De Gaetani 33,111/35: In dogs, the cardiovascular changes produced by epinephrine are greatly altered by exposure to cold.

Selye A8,052/38: Rats and guinea pigs normally tolerate very large doses of epinephrine or histamine p.o. but these substances cause toxic manifestations (lung edema, emphysema) if administered following the production of an alarm reaction by cold, forced muscular exercise or other stressors. Presumably the gastrointestinal lesions characteristic of the alarm reaction facilitate the absorption of substances which normally do not traverse the intestinal epithelium in active form.

DesMarais & Dugal B51,093/50; B64,359/51: In rats exposed to cold, epinephrine "appears to improve survival." [Brief abstract without details (H.S.).]

Hannon & Larson D4,112/61: In rats, the effect of norepinephrine upon calorigenesis and the mobilization of nonesterified fatty acids is considerably modified by cold.

Evonuk & Hannon E21,027/63: In rats, adaptation to cold increases the calorigenic effect of norepinephrine.

Schönbaum et al. E21,028/63: In rats, norepinephrine (like epinephrine) has an adverse effect upon survival during exposure to cold. This effect is less pronounced following adaptation to cold. Adrenal-demedullated animals (whether receiving guanethidine or not) showed evidence of acclimation to cold. "These observations suggest that increased amounts of adrenaline and noradrenaline in tissues or circulation are not essential for acclimation."

Leblanc & Pouliot F4,622/64: In rats, norepinephrine facilitates adaptation to cold.

Pohl & Hart F62,568/66: In the ground squirrel (Citellus tridecemlineatus), exposure to cold or injection of norepinephrine produced nonshivering thermogenesis after curarization.

Zeisberger & Brück F89,184/67; Zeisberger et al. F89,185/67: In cold-adapted guinea pigs, nonshivering thermogenesis is induced by exposure to cold or by injection of norepinephrine. Several observations suggest "that the nonshivering thermogenesis in the guinea pig is essentially due to a catecholamine-mediated mechanism."

Angelakos & Daniels G64,739/69: In dogs, infusion of norepinephrine during cooling reduced the incidence of ventricular fibrillation, whereas epinephrine had an opposite effect.

Brück et al. H13,180/69: In minipigs, as in most species other than the rat, nonshivering thermogenesis plays a major role in adaptation to cold only during neonatal life if at all. Epinephrine and norepinephrine, which stimulate considerable nonshivering thermogenesis in cold-adapted adult rats, failed to do so in minipigs.

Other Stressors ←

In rats, various adrenergic blocking agents inhibit, whereas epinephrine increases mortality during traumatic shock in the **Noble-Collip** drum. However, some investigators failed to observe any effect of epinephrine or norepinephrine upon this type of shock; indeed, occasionally they noted an increase in resistance when the catecholamines were administered in the form of depots.

In rabbits, survival following trauma in the Noble-Collip drum has been said to be moderately improved by epinephrine and other vasopressor amines. On the other hand, rabbits, made tolerant to normally lethal doses of epinephrine, showed an increased susceptibility to "rotational shock," whereas drum-tolerant animals were less susceptible to the lethal effect of epinephrine.

Death from **hypoxia** in rats kept in closed vessels is accelerated by epinephrine. Mortality from **hyperoxygenation** (exposure to 6 atmospheres of oxygen) is increased in rats by pretreatment with epinephrine, whereas survival from **hemorrhagic shock** is improved by long-lasting infusions of norepinephrine.

Small doses of epinephrine or norepinephrine prolong the duration of **electrically-induced seizures** in the rat.

In rats, irreversible hypovolemic shock, produced by complete **occlusion of the portal vein**, is effectively combated by continuous infusions of norepinephrine, whereas epinephrine has an inverse effect.

In rats, with complete **blockade of the sympathetic nervous system**, epinephrine considerably increases resistance to certain stressors (endotoxin, histamine) but not to others (formalin, tourniquet shock). Apparently, the adrenergic system is of special importance only in combating certain types of stress.

Trauma ←

Levy et al. C10,848/54: In rats, various adrenergic-blocking agents increase resistance to traumatic shock (Noble-Collip drum), whereas epinephrine has an opposite effect.

Noble C10,541/55: In rats, mortality from trauma in the Noble-Collip drum is strikingly increased by pretreatment with epinephrine but not diminished by various adrenergic-blocking agents.

Brunson et al. C78,005/59: In rabbits, survival following trauma in the Noble-Collip drum is moderately improved by epinephrine and other vasopressor amines.

Walden & Brunson G5,968/63: Studies on rabbits gradually adapted to trauma in the Noble-Collip drum led to the conclusion that "animals tolerant to normally lethal doses of epinephrine showed an increased susceptibility to rotational shock, but drum tolerant animals were less susceptible to lethal doses of epinephrine."

Altura et al. F 36,124/65; F 43,209/65: In rats, survival following temporary ligation of the superior mesenteric artery was improved by PLV-2 but not by epinephrine or angiotensin. The associated changes in the microcirculation of the meso-appendix are described.

Cronin & Tan F 29,408/65: In dogs, the inotropic effect of norepinephrine is increased during cardiogenic shock elicited by closed-chest coronary embolization.

Hruza & Stetson Jr. H 455/68: In rats, pretreatment with depot epinephrine or norepinephrine increased resistance to trauma in the Noble-Collip drum and to endotoxin.

Calof & Smith H 10,412/69: In rats, mortality from traumatic shock (Noble-Collip drum) is not modified by epinephrine or norepinephrine but considerably reduced by various β-adrenergic agents.

Hruza & Zweifach G 77,195/70: Rats adapted to trauma in a Noble-Collip drum show an increased catecholamine content in their fat tissue and an increased resistance to epinephrine. Conversely, rats rendered resistant to epinephrine or norepinephrine become more resistant to trauma in the Noble-Collip drum. [This may be one of the mechanisms involved in the induction of cross resistance (H.S.).]

Hypoxia and Hyperoxygenation ←

Campbell A 14,903/37: In rats exposed to six atmospheres of oxygen in a pressure chamber, subsequent decompression is better tolerated at low than at high external temperatures. "Using an external temperature of 24°C and white rats of about 80 g, the following substances, administered subcutaneously, are found to enhance oxygen poisoning: thyroxin (0.4 mg), dinitrophenol (1.5 mg), ac-tetrahydro-β-naphthylamine (0.5 c.c., 1 p.c.), adrenaline (0.02 mg), pituitary extract (posterior lobe, above 3.5 units), insulin (0.025 u.) and eserine (0.045 mg administered with atropine 0.075 mg). These doses in themselves are harmless."

Keminger G 42,501/66: In rats, death from lack of oxygen in closed vessels is accelerated by T3 and retarded after thyroidectomy or cortisone treatment. Epinephrine further accelerates mortality in hyperthyroid animals.

Hemorrhage ←

Lansing et al. C 30,227/57: In rats, survival from hemorrhagic shock is improved by long-lasting infusions of norepinephrine.

Electric Stimuli ←

Minz & Domino B 81,852/53: In rats, small doses of epinephrine or norepinephrine prolong the duration of electrically-induced seizures. Since glucose, ACTH and cortisone failed to prolong seizure duration, it is unlikely that epinephrine acts by release of these substances. Histamine depressed the cortical response to electroshock.

Varia ← *cf. also Selye B 40,000/50, p. 64; B 58,650/51, p. 53; G 60,083/70, pp. 358, 361.*

Mejia et al. G 60,637/68: In rats with irreversible hypovolemic shock produced by complete occlusion of the portal vein, neither cortisol pretreatment nor adrenalectomy influenced the survival time, whereas selective extirpation of the adrenal medulla or continuous infusion of norepinephrine increased it. Similar infusion of epinephrine decreased survival time.

Krawczak & Brodie H 25,296/70: In rats, complete blockade of sympathetic function can be achieved by demedullation combined with reserpine-like agents (depleting catecholamine stores), bretylium-like agents (preventing nerve impulse from releasing catecholamines) or ganglioplegics. Following such total sympathetic blockade, mortality from histamine or endotoxin is as markedly increased as by adrenalectomy. Pretreatment with epinephrine alone counteracts the increased lethality of endotoxin and histamine after sympathetic blockade. Cortisone pretreatment only partially corrects the sensitization by adrenalectomy, whereas cortisone + epinephrine offers complete protection against these agents. Presumably, sympathetic stimulation is "the first line of defense against the vasomotor disturbance elicited by endotoxin and histamine." The lethal effect of formalin or tourniquet shock is likewise greatly increased by adrenalectomy but, in contrast to that of endotoxin and histamine, it cannot be increased by sympathetic blockade. Furthermore, cortisone alone counteracts the toxicity of these stressors in adrenalectomized rats. Apparently "formalin and tourniquet shock is initiated by a mechanism which differs from that elicited by histamine and endotoxin and does not primarily involve the sympathetic system."

Hepatic Enzymes ←

For the effect of adrenergic agents upon hepatic enzyme induction *cf.* the Abstract Section as well as the individual toxicants, whose metabolism is affected (*cf.* "Drugs").

Dixon et al. G11,757/64: In the rat, both norepinephrine and adrenergic blocking agents inhibit the hepatic drug-metabolizing enzyme activity as judged by tests in vitro.

Terayama & Takata F69,475/66: Epinephrine markedly reduces the N-demethylating activity of rat liver.

← SPECIAL SURGICAL PROCEDURES

← Thymectomy

Hormones and Hormone-Like Substances ←. During the early part of this century, a great deal of work has been done on the influence of thymus extract upon the toxicity of **thyroid** preparations. In tadpoles, thyroid extract inhibits growth, and concurrent administration of thymus extract neutralizes this effect. In mice, the toxic manifestations of thyroid feeding are allegedly inhibited also by feeding thymus tissue.

In pigeons, the loss of weight elicited by thyroid extract or thyroid feeding is inhibited by dietary administration of thymus tissue. This effect could not be duplicated by equivalent amounts of nucleic acid preparations, but the specificity of an antithyroid thymus principle remains in doubt.

In rats, the hypercalcemia and osteitis fibrosa produced by **parathyroid extract** overdosage are said to be inhibited by concurrent treatment with a thymus extract and thymectomy is claimed to raise **histamine** resistance, but all these findings require confirmation.

Cameron & Carmichael 27,015/25: In young rats, feeding of desiccated **thyroid** frequently produces tetany, perhaps as a consequence of the decreased blood supply to the entire thyroparathyroid apparatus. This tetany cannot be influenced by simultaneous feeding of thymus.

Kříženecký & Podhradský 4,186/26: In frog tadpoles, feeding of thyroid extract inhibits growth; concurrent administration of thymus extract neutralizes this effect.

Sklower 25,299/27: In mice, the toxic manifestations of thyroid feeding can be inhibited by concurrent thymus feeding. Earlier literature on antagonistic interactions between thyroid and thymus is reviewed.

Kříženecký 4,176/28; 23,688/28; 277/30: In pigeons, the loss of weight produced by desiccated thyroid is greatly diminished by concurrent administration of a thymus extract. Equivalent amounts of nucleic acid preparations do not have this effect. "The thymus appears to be a regulator of the thyroid gland."

Scholtz 4,272/32: In rats, the hypercalcemia and osteofibrosis produced by excess **parathyroid extract** are inhibited by concurrent treatment with thymus extract.

Weltman & Sackler D14,302/61: In adult rats, thymectomy raises resistance to **histamine** and to swimming in cold water. The effect is ascribed to a raised resistance to nonspecific stress. [The results are not statistically significant (H.S.).]

Drugs ←. The thymus involution of the alarm reaction is one of the most sensitive indicators of exposure to the stress of any toxicant, yet, we have very little evidence to show that the thymus could influence resistance to drugs. Except for the well-known immunologic disturbances produced by neonatal thymectomy, neither removal of the organ nor treatment with extracts of its tissue succeeded in altering general resistance in a significant and reproducible manner.

It has been stated that the hepatic changes caused in rats by such **carcinogens** as dimethylaminoazobenzol are diminished by treatment with thymus extract, and that in newborn mice, the induction of pulmonary tumors by DMBA is facilitated by the injection of neonatal thymus tissue. Furthermore, in neonatal mice, the otherwise permanent immunosuppression induced by DMBA can be reversed by syngenic thymus, bone marrow, or spleen cell transplants.

Probably, one of the first observations on the effects of neonatal thymectomy was that removal of the thymus during the first days of life increases the sensitivity of the rabbit to **morphine, heroin,** and **codeine**. However, the change in resistance was not very pronounced and was presumably due to the general debilitation of neonatally thymectomized animals.

At about the same time, it had been claimed that thymus extract decreases the sensitivity to **thallium** intoxication in mice, but this observation has never been confirmed.

Resistance to **vitamin A** or **vitamin D** is not significantly affected in rats thymectomized at 2-3 weeks of age. The claim that thymectomy partially protects the adult rabbit against overdosage with irradiated ergosterol remained unconfirmed. In vitamin-D deficient rats, the development of rickets could not be significantly altered by lipid soluble thymus extracts.

Anaphylactoidogens ← cf. Selye G46,715/68, pp. 180, 184, 200.

Carcinogens ←

Fumarola & Giordano D33,779/62: In rats, the production of tumors by benzpyrene is allegedly somewhat inhibited after thymectomy and accelerated by treatment with thymus extract.

Potop et al. E39,894/62: In rats, the hepatic changes produced by dimethylaminoazobenzol are diminished by treatment with a thymus extract.

Simpson et al. F2,965/64: In rats, neonatal thymectomy did not significantly influence the induction of tumors by DMBA.

Balner & Dersjant G37,980/66: In mice, neonatal thymectomy does not significantly influence the induction of cutaneous tumors by intradermal 3-MC administration. Surprisingly, tumor incidence in mice with depressed homograft reactivity was, if anything, lower than in the immunologically competent animals.

Grant et al. F66,117/66: In mice, the induction of cutaneous papillomas and carcinomas by 3,4-benzopyrene is accelerated by neonatal thymectomy. "It may be that some tumours initiated by benzopyrene do not differ sufficiently from the host to evoke a homograft reaction against them even when the immunological competence is unimpaired. It may be that factors such as the growth-rate of the tumour allow it to progress in spite of a reaction against it, or it may be that under some conditions an animal may become specifically tolerant to a tumour which it bears."

Allison & Taylor F83,300/67: From experiments on mice treated with DMBA and various viruses, "it is concluded that neonatal thymectomy does not consistently increase the incidence of chemically induced tumors but does increase the incidence of tumors after exposure to polyoma and SV40 viruses and adenovirus type 12."

Flaks F95,414/67: In mice, the induction of pulmonary tumors by DMBA, soon after birth, is intensified by injections of neonatal thymus tissue.

Smiecinski & Górski H20,765/68: In 2—3 week old female mice, topical tumorigenesis by intravaginal application of 20-methylcholanthrene is "slightly retarded" by thymectomy. This effect has been tentatively ascribed to the removal of "promine," an allegedly tumor growth-stimulating substance of thymic origin. [The results do not lend themselves to statistical evaluation (H.S.).]

Ball & Dawson G67,723/69: In neonatal mice "the permanent immunosuppression induced by DMBA could be reversed by the injection of normal syngeneic bone marrow and spleen cells but not with thymic implants."

Kobayashi H 27,113/69; H 27,114/69: In mice, thymectomy inhibits the production of cutaneous papillomas by DMBA, whereas transfusion of thymus cells has an opposite effect.

Schneiberg & Gorski G 68,745/69: In mice, thymectomy followed by whole-body X-irradiation increases the incidence of skin cancers after serial spraying with methylcholanthrene. In itself, neither thymectomy nor X-irradiation was effective in this respect.

Cholesterol ← *cf. Selye G 60,083/70, p. 442.*

Chloroform ←

Bomskov et al. A 56,954/42: In rats and guinea pigs, sensitivity to chloroform can be diminished by a thymus extract.

Curare ←

Blaw et al. F 65,571/66: In mice, neonatal thymectomy increases the sensitivity of the myoneural junction to blockade by tubocurarine.

Morphine ←

Arima 60,156/35: In rabbits thymectomized during the first few days of life, sensitivity to morphine, heroin, and codeine is slightly diminished. Treatment with thymus extract has an opposite effect.

Sulfa Drugs ← *cf. Selye G 60,083/70, p. 442.*

Thallium Acetate ←

Buschke et al. 43,284/33; 4,823/33: In mice, thyroxine increases, whereas thymus extract decreases sensitivity to intoxication with thallium acetate.

Vitamin A ←

Vogt et al. B 36,750/48: In rats thymectomized at 2—3 weeks of age, resistance to vitamin-A or vitamin-D deficiency was not significantly affected.

Vitamin C ←

Lopez-Lomba 17,165/23: In guinea pigs, thymectomy prolonged survival on a vitamin-C deficient diet. [The difference was not impressive (H.S.).]

Vitamin D ←

Coppo 3642/32: In rabbits, thymectomy does not characteristically influence the syndrome of overdosage with irradiated ergosterol.

Messini & Coppo 31,827/35: In rabbits, thymectomy partially protects against intoxication with irradiated ergosterol.

Vogt et al. B 36,750/48: In rats thymectomized at 2—3 weeks of age, resistance to vitamin-A or vitamin-D deficiency was not significantly affected.

Nassi G 1,107/62; G 1,108/62: In vitamin-D deficient rats, treatment with a lipid soluble thymus extract did not significantly affect the development of rickets.

Microorganisms, Parasites and Their Products ←. Despite several claims to the contrary, there does not seem to be any convincing evidence that thymectomy or thymus extracts have any specific effect upon **bacterial infections**.

Mice thymectomized at birth become extremely resistant to the **virus of lymphocytic choriomeningitis**, but this infection may aggravate the course of the wasting syndrome produced by neonatal thymectomy. The susceptibility of neonatally thymectomized mice against this virus is restored by implants of Millipore diffusion chambers containing newborn thymic tissue. It is assumed that the neurologic symptoms in mice and man result from an antigen-antibody reaction in the brain which can be prevented by neonatal thymectomy.

In newborn mice infected with **polyoma virus**, neonatal thymectomy delays mortality of certain strains only. Inoculation of polyoma virus into neonatally thymectomized weanling hamsters resulted in tumor formation, whereas sham operated litter mates developed no neoplasms. Apparently, "neonatal thymectomy may render some resistant animals susceptible to the effects of an oncogenic virus."

In inbred BALB/c mice, inoculated with **Rauscher virus,** thymectomy did not influence the erythroblastic reaction, but thymectomy did alter the response to a variety of other viruses in various species.

In neonatally thymectomized mice, susceptibility to infection with **C. albicans** is increased.

In chickens from embryos inoculated in ovo with testosterone, after about one week of incubation, the bursa of Fabricius spleen and thymus are permanently atrophic and the antibody formation against repeated infection with **Eimeria tenella** fails to develop antibodies. Surgical thymectomy 90 min after hatching was rarely complete and did not constantly block immunization against Eimeria tenella.

Neonatally thymectomized rats infected with **P. berghei** are highly subject to parasitemia, whereas neonatally thymectomized hamsters are comparatively resistant and develop the disease slowly. It is postulated that the thymectomized hamsters failed to develop an antibody that normally causes microembolization of the cerebral capillaries with agglutinated parasites.

In neonatally thymectomized mice, susceptibility to the toxic effects of E. coli or S. typhosa **endotoxins** is increased.

Bacteria and Vaccines ←

Cody & Code G4,417/63: In rats sensitized with Bordetella pertussis vaccine, the anaphylaxis produced by challenge with horse serum is inhibited by concurrent thymectomy and splenectomy but not by thymectomy alone.

Schäfer B99,955/54: Monograph (127 pp., numerous refs.) on the role of endocrine factors in tuberculosis. Special sections are devoted to the hormones of the thyroid, parathyroid, thymus, adrenals, pancreas, and gonads.

Kratter & Martelli B60,263/49: In adult rabbits, thymectomy increases susceptibility to staphylococcus infection.

Viruses ←

Lymphocytic Choriomeningitis ←. *Levey et al. E30,471/63:* In mice, neonatal thymectomy protects against the virus of lymphocytic choriomeningitis, but susceptibility is restored by implants of Millipore diffusion chambers containing newborn thymic tissue. "A humoral mechanism of action of the tissue in the chamber is proposed."

Rowe et al. E29,673/63; East et al. E38,279/64; Földes et al. G29,263/65: Mice thymectomized at birth become resistant to lymphocytic choriomeningitis virus infection.

Szeri et al. G56,565/66: In mice, infection with lymphocytic choriomeningitis virus accelerates and aggravates the course of the wasting syndrome produced by neonatal thymectomy.

Schmuñis et al. G55,003/67: In mice, neonatal thymectomy protects against lymphocytic choriomeningitis produced by Junin virus. Presumably, the "neurological symptoms in mice and human patients result from an antigen-antibody reaction in the brain and that this reaction between the virus and its antibody is prevented by thymectomy."

Polyoma ←. *Kodama & Moore D56,877/63:* In newborn mice infected with polyoma virus, thymectomy (performed two weeks later) delayed mortality in the AKR but not in the C3H strain. The incidence and latency of parotid tumors were not affected by thymectomy in either strain.

Lang G55,002/68: "Inoculation of polyoma virus into weanling hamsters, thymectomized as neonates, has resulted in the production of tumors. In contrast, the sham operated litter mates developed no demonstrable neoplasms over a 12—18 month period of observation. Thus, it has been confirmed in these studies that neonatal thymectomy may render some resistant animals susceptible to the effects of an oncogenic virus."

Rauscher ←. *Dunn & Green G40,311/66:* In inbred BALB/c mice inoculated with Rauscher virus "thymectomy had no apparent effect on the erythroblastic reaction, while splenectomy intensified the process in the liver and erythroblastic foci appeared in the lymph nodes. Granulocytopoiesis was also stimulated in some mice."

Varia ←. *Dunn E 29,253/63:* "When BALB/c mice given the **Moloney virus** were thymectomized, splenectomized or subjected to both procedures, the incidence of lymphocytic leukemia was reduced." *Li et al. E 33,523/63:* Various types of calf thymus extracts exhibit antiviral and antibacterial activity **in vitro**.

Crispens & Rey F 87,332/67: In mice, neonatal thymectomy increases sensitivity to **lactate dehydrogenase virus**.

van Hoosier Jr. et al. F 78,860/67: In hamsters, thymectomy facilitates tumor formation by weakly oncogenic **adenoviruses**.

Jahkola et al. G 47,813/67: In mice, the infection by **cytomegalic inclusion** virus is aggravated by thymectomy.

Yohn et al. G 57,790/68: In hamsters given **adenovirus-12**, strain Huie, s.c. at birth, thymectomy at one week of age increased tumor incidence in both sexes, although it remained higher in females as is usually the case. Cortisone treatment, begun at one week of age, increased tumor incidence but, again, this remained higher in females. Antibody responses to adenovirus-12 T-antigen were depressed in thymectomized and cortisone-treated animals.

Fungi and Yeasts, Parasites ←

Candida Albicans ←. *Salvin et al. G 30,533/65; F 35,876/65:* In mice thymectomy diminishes resistance to infection with C. albicans as well as to the endotoxins of E. coli and S. typhosa but not to C. albicans endotoxin.

Eimeria ←. *Pierce & Long G 36,006/65:* Chickens from embryos inoculated in ovo with testosterone hatched between the 6th and 9th day of incubation without a detectable bursa of Fabricius; their spleen and thymus weights were also significantly reduced. These fowls failed to develop antibodies as a result of repeated infection with Eimeria tenella. Surgical thymectomy 90 min after hatching was rarely complete and did not consistently lead to a failure of immunization against E. tenella.

Rose & Long G 74,020/70: Review of the literature with personal observations on the effect of thymectomy and removal of the bursa of Fabricius upon Eimeria infections in the chicken.

Plasmodium Berghei ←. *Stechschulte H 15,256/69:* "Neonatally thymectomized rats infected with P. berghei develop higher percentage parasitemias and have a higher percentage mortality than sham-operated animals."

Brown et al. H 1,304/68: In rats, neonatal thymectomy decreases resistance to infection with P. berghei. [Although throughout the paper the authors speak of rats, in their conclusion they refer to mice (H.S.).]

Wright H 1,836/68: In hamsters, neonatal thymectomy delays death from infection with P. berghei. "It is postulated that the non-thymectomized animals develop an agglutinin, in response to the malarial infection, that causes microembolisation of the cerebral capillaries with agglutinated parasitised RBC, and that neonatal thymectomy inhibits or delays the production of this agglutinin."

Trypanosoma Lewisi ←. *Perla & Marmorston-Gottesman 810/30:* In young rats, thymectomy diminishes, whereas orchidectomy increases the severity of T. lewisi infection.

Bacterial Toxins ←

Salvin et al. G 30,533/65; F 35,876/65: In mice, thymectomy diminishes resistance to infection with C. albicans as well as to the endotoxins of E. coli and S. typhosa, but not to C. albicans endotoxin.

Immune Reactions ←. The extensive literature on neonatal thymectomy upon immune reactions is beyond the scope of this monograph and should be consulted in the reviews cited in the Abstract Section which are specifically devoted to this topic. Let us point out merely that in rats sensitized with Bordetella pertussis vaccine, anaphylaxis to horse serum is inhibited by concurrent thymectomy and splenectomy, but not by thymectomy alone. In adult rats which had been neonatally thymectomized, the production of nephrotoxic serum nephritis remains possible.

Kemény et al. B 66,729/51: In guinea pigs, both ovariectomy and orchidectomy diminish anaphylactic shock, whereas thymectomy has no effect upon it.

Miller E 37,260/63: Review on the role of the thymus in immunity.

Cody & Code G 4,417/63: In rats sensitized with B. pertussis vaccine, the anaphylaxis produced by challenge with horse serum is inhibited by concurrent thymectomy and splenectomy, but not by thymectomy alone.

Fisher & Fisher F690/64: In adult rats which had been neonatally thymectomized, the production of nephrotoxic serum nephritis remains possible. This "indicates that progression of the disease is not necessarily dependent upon those immunologic functions related to thymic function, at least during the time interval studied."

Hepatic Lesions ←. In partially hepatectomized adult rats, thymectomy inhibits mitotic proliferation of the hepatocytes, but does not significantly affect the associated enzymic changes.

Forabosco & Narducci G70,746/69; Forabosco & Toni G70,747/69; Forabosco & Guli G70,748/69; Forabosco et al. G70,749/69: In adult rats, thymectomy inhibits mitotic proliferation in hepatocytes after partial hepatectomy. Earlier literature is reviewed.

Ionizing Rays ←. In mice, thymectomy increases the incidence of epithelial tumor formation after X-irradiation. Thymus transplants do not significantly influence the incidence of leukemia.

In neonatally thymectomized mice, both thymus implants and cystamine tend to correct the comparatively low X-ray resistance. The intercapillary glomerulosclerosis produced by neonatal X-irradiation is potentiated by neonatal thymectomy, but reduced by splenectomy in mice. In adult, unlike in neonatal mice, thymectomy does not reduce resistance to total body X-irradiation. X-ray resistance is restored in neonatally thymectomized mice by the i.p. implantation of thymus-bearing diffusion chambers.

O'Gara & Ards D12,341/61: In mice, thymectomy appears to increase the incidence of epithelial tumors following X-irradiation. In thymectomized mice bearing intrasplenic thymus transplants, the incidence of leukemia was not significantly altered in comparison to thymectomized controls.

Méwissen & Lagneau G14,713/64: In mice thymectomized at 40 days of age, cystamine retains its protective action, and implantation of a thymus lobe likewise increases resistance.

Goedbloed & Vos G33,427/65: In mice, neonatal thymectomy had little if any effect on the incidence of secondary disease in radiation chimeras.

Méwissen et al. F45,017/65: Mice thymectomized during the first days of life show a very low resistance to total body X-irradiation, but this can be improved by thymus transplants.

Guttman G45,255/67: In mice, the intercapillary glomerulosclerosis produced by neonatal X-irradiation is potentiated by neonatal thymectomy but reduced by splenectomy.

Schneiberg et al. G56,009/67; G58,580/67: In three-week old mice, thymectomy reduces natural resistance to whole body X-irradiation, but this is not the case in rats thymectomized at a later age.

Schneiberg et al. G69,791/68: In mice, sensitization to X-irradiation produced by thymectomy is restored by i.p. implantation of thymus-bearing diffusion chambers, presumably owing to the production of a humoral lymphopoietic factor by the thymus implant.

Schneiberg et al. G58,579/68: In mice, thymectomy does not significantly affect the blood protein changes produced by acute X-irradiation, although it does increase mortality.

Varia ←. In germ-free mice, the lethality of **parabiotic** intoxication is aggravated by neonatal thymectomy, presumably because here the thymus-dependent immune reactions are actually beneficial. Adaptive **enzyme formation** does not appear to be significantly affected by neonatal thymectomy in the rat.

Cold ←

Weltman & Sackler D14,302/61: In adult rats, thymectomy raises resistance to histamine and to swimming in cold water. The effect is ascribed to a raised resistance to nonspecific stress. [The results are not statistically significant (H.S.).]

Tumors ←

Potop et al. F38,309/65: In the mouse and rat as well as in chick embryos, the growth of various experimental tumors is stimulated by a lipoprotein extract of the thymus.

Parabiosis ←

Anderson et al. H11,186/69: In germ-free mice, the lethality of parabiotic intoxication is aggravated by neonatal thymectomy. "It is concluded that with respect to parabiotic union of germ-free mice, the primary consequence of neonatal thymectomy is a dampening of the characteristic anemia-polycythemia which is not associated with an enhanced survival, and that thymic dependent immune reactions may actually promote survival."

Hepatic Enzymes ←

Bonetti et al. G48,030/67: Induction of hepatic TPO-activity by tryptophan i.p. is not prevented by postnatal thymectomy in the rat. These observations do not confirm the view that adaptive enzyme formation depends upon a mechanism similar to that of immunologic defense.

← Splenectomy

Splenectomy does not appear to have any conspicuous effects upon detoxicating mechanisms.

It has been claimed that immunosuppression induced by neonatal administration of **DMBA** in mice could be reversed by syngenic spleen, bone marrow, or thymus cell implants. In rats sensitized with B. pertussis vaccine, the anaphylaxis produced by challenge with horse serum is inhibited by concurrent splenectomy and thymectomy, but not by thymectomy alone. In certain inbred strains of mice inoculated with **Rauscher virus**, splenectomy intensified the erythroblastic reaction in the liver, whereas thymectomy had no such effect. In rats, splenectomy does not significantly alter the regeneration of the liver after **partial hepatectomy**, although some investigators claimed that splenectomy accelerates it. This acceleration does not occur if the spleen is reimplanted into either the portal or the systemic circulation. However, all these claims have been challenged by some investigators.

The intercapillary glomerular sclerosis produced by neonatal **X-irradiation** in mice is said to be reduced by splenectomy.

Drugs ←

Ball & Dawson G67,723/69: In neonatal mice "the permanent immunosuppression induced by **DMBA** could be reversed by the injection of normal syngenic bone marrow and spleen cells but not with thymic implants."

Brodeur & Marchand H37,030/71: In rats, splenectomy significantly decreases cytochrome P-450 during the first few days after the operation but not at seven days. **Parathion, p-nitroanisole** and **zoxazolamine** metabolism is also decreased, whereas that of **hexobarbital** is unchanged during the first four days after splenectomy. Apparently, splenectomy inhibits certain hepatic microsomal enzymes, perhaps by influencing the blood supply of the liver.

Microorganisms and Vaccines ←

Cody & Code G4,417/63: In rats sensitized with **B. pertussis vaccine**, the anaphylaxis produced by challenge with horse serum is inhibited by concurrent thymectomy and splenectomy, but not by thymectomy alone.

Dunn E29,253/63: "When BALB/c mice given the **Moloney virus** were thymectomized, splenectomized or subjected to both procedures, the incidence of lymphocytic leukemia was reduced."

Dunn & Green G40,311/66: In inbred BALB/c mice inoculated with **Rauscher virus** "thymectomy had no apparent effect on the erythroblastic reaction, while splenectomy intensified the process in the liver and erythroblastic foci appeared in the lymph nodes. Granulocytopoiesis was also stimulated in some mice."

Hepatectomy Partial ←

Pontremoli & Arrigo D63,528/50: In rats partially hepatectomized and splenectomized simultaneously, hepatic regeneration is just as rapid, and sometimes even accelerated, in the absence of the spleen.

Trasino B56,794/50: In rats, splenectomy does not significantly alter the regeneration of the liver remnant after partial hepatectomy.

Zaltzman D92,764/56: Splenectomy enhances regeneration of the liver after partial hepatectomy in the rat.

Pérez-Tamayo & Romero D38,897/58: In rats, splenectomy stimulates hepatic regeneration after partial hepatectomy. This acceleration does not occur if the spleen is reimplanted either into the portal circulation or s.c. Apparently, a humoral factor is involved.

Molimard & Benozio G75,048/70: In rats, splenectomy does not influence hepatic regeneration after partial hepatectomy, but the latter operation causes an increase in splenic weight.

Ionizing Rays ←

Guttman G45,255/67: In mice, the intercapillary glomerulosclerosis produced by neonatal X-irradiation is potentiated by neonatal thymectomy but reduced by splenectomy.

← Other Surgical Interventions

← Pinealectomy. In rats, pinealectomy inhibits the induction of hepatic cancers by some but not by all **carcinogens.**

← Sympathectomy. The extensive literature on the effect of sympathectomy with or without adrenal demedullation has been discussed in many earlier review articles to which the reader must be referred. Suffice it here to summarize certain recent investigations which show that in rats, complete blockade of the sympathetic function by demedullation combined with reserpine-like, bretylium-like or gangliopleic agents, increases mortality from **histamine** or **endotoxin** as much as does complete adrenalectomy. Pretreatment with epinephrine alone counteracts this diminished resistance. On the other hand, the lethal effect of other stressors such as **formalin** or **tourniquet shock** is greatly increased by adrenalectomy, but not by a sympathetic blockade. In this event cortisone is especially effective in restoring resistance. Apparently "formalin and tourniquet shock is initiated by a mechanism which differs from that elicited by histamine and endotoxin and does not primarily involve the sympathetic system."

← Pinealectomy

Jelínek & Křeček H2,778/68: In young, unlike in adult rats, pinealectomy inhibits the adrenal regeneration hypertension that results from an excessive mineralocorticoid production by the regenerating adrenal cortex.

Lacassagne et al. G74,931/69: In rats, removal of the pineal inhibits the induction of hepatic cancers by 4-dimethylaminoazobenzene, but does not influence the carcinogenic effect of 2-acetylaminofluorene and diethylnitrosamine.

Aubert & Bohuon G77,483/70: In hamsters, certain carcinogens (DMBA, urethan) induce melanomas, preceded by depigmentation. Epiphysectomy does not alter this result.

← Sympathectomy

Krawczak & Brodie H25,296/70: In rats, complete blockade of sympathetic function can be achieved by demedullation combined with reserpine-like agents (depleting catecholamine stores), bretylium-like agents (preventing nerve impulse from releasing catecholamines) or gangliopleics. Following such total sympathetic blockade, mortality from histamine or endotoxin is as markedly increased as by adrenalectomy. Pretreatment with epinephrine alone counteracts the increased lethality of endotoxin and histamine after sympathetic blockade. Cortisone pretreatment only partially corrects the sensitization by adrenalectomy, whereas cortisone + epinephrine offers complete protection against these agents. Presumably, sympathetic stimulation is "the first line of defense against the vasomotor disturbance elicited by endotoxin and histamine." The lethal effect of formalin or tourniquet shock is likewise greatly increased by adrenalectomy but, in contrast to that of endotoxin and histamine, it cannot be increased by sympathetic blockade. Furthermore, cortisone alone counteracts the toxicity of these stressors in adrenalectomized rats. Apparently "formalin and tourniquet shock is initiated by a mechanism which differs from that elicited by histamine and endotoxin and does not primarily involve the sympathetic system."

← HISTAMINE

Drugs ←. Histamine does not considerably influence drug-resistance in general, but it does tend to increase the anesthetic effect of **barbiturates, chloral hydrate** and several other hypnotics.

In rats given **lead acetate** i.v., subcutaneous injection of histamine causes topical calcergy, and if the dose of histamine is large, this may be associated with widespread calcification in the autonomic nervous system ("neurocalcergy").

Varia ←. Sensitivity to histamine is greatly increased in mice by pretreatment with B. pertussis **vaccine**, but resistance to botulinum **toxin** and nereis toxin is not affected.

Several investigators reported that histamine offers protection against total body **X-irradiation** in mice. It has also been claimed that histamine aggravates the pulmonary lesions produced by **hyperoxygenation** and depresses the cortical response to **electroshock**. On the other hand, an alarm reaction produced by exposure to **cold** increases the toxicity of orally administered histamine in rats, presumably because the amine is readily absorbed from the exulcerated gastrointestinal mucosa.

Drugs ←

Acetonitrile ←. *Wuth A 48,026/21:* In mice, tyramine and diiodotyramine—like thyroid extract—offer protection against acetonitrile, histamine does not.

Barbiturates ←. *Werle & Lentzen A 28,007/38:* In dogs and rabbits, various vasoactive substances (epinephrine, histamine, vasopressin, kallikrein) tend to prolong the anesthetic effect of pronarcon and hexobarbital.

Fastier D 95,950/56: In mice, 5-HT considerably potentiates the hypnotic effect of cyclobarbital and chloral hydrate. However, this property is not very specific, since bufotenine, tryptamine, histamine, and epinephrine likewise prolong cyclobarbital hypnosis. Literature on numerous other drugs which prolong barbiturate anesthesia is cited. "It therefore seems possible that the ability of 5-HT to prolong hypnosis may be due to a relatively unspecific, vascular effect."

Hexobarbital ← Histamine, Mouse: Ambrus et al. C 16,607/52*; Bousquet et al. F 35,073/65*

Chloral Hydrate←. *Fastier et al. C 37,038/57:* In mice, chloral hydrate sleeping time is increased by epinephrine, norepinephrine, phenylephrine, methoxamine, 5-HT, histamine, ergotamine, yohimbine, and atropine. "It is suggested that some, at least, of the drugs which prolong the effects of hypnotics do so by virtue of a hypothermic action." Vasopressin, cortisone, and DOC did not prolong chloral hydrate sleeping time at the doses tested.

Lead ←. *Selye et al. G 11,123/64:* "In rats simultaneously given an intravenous injection of lead acetate and a subcutaneous injection of histamine, extensive calcium deposition occurs in various parts of the autonomic nervous system. This neurotropic form of mastocalcergy can be inhibited by pretreatment with various mast-cell dischargers (compound 48/80, polymyxin, chlorpromazine), mast-cell components (histamine, 5-HT) or drugs known to inhibit the pharmacologic actions of such mast-cell components (cyproheptadine, neo-antergan). This prophylactic effect appears to be largely specific to compounds related to mast-cell activity since it was not shared by various other drugs and stressors tested."

Pentylenetetrazol ←. *Kobrin & Seifter F74,422/66:* In one day old chicks, in which the blood-brain barrier is still incompletely formed, various ω-amino acids as well as 5-HT, histamine, and epinephrine, produce sleep and prevent pentylenetetrazol convulsions.

Reserpine ←. *Simionovici et al. F43,099/65:* In mice, epinephrine and norepinephrine, as well as histamine, offer partial protection against reserpine intoxication (sedation blepharoptosis, hypothermia). 5-HT has no such effect.

Varia ←

Microorganisms, Vaccines, and Bacterial Toxins ←. *Kind E67,787/58:* Review (9 pp., 80 refs.) on increased sensitivity to 5-HT, histamine, and anaphylaxis induced in mice by **B. pertussis vaccine**.

Fishel et al. E8,474/64: Review (8 pp., 26 refs.) on the mechanism of sensitization by **B. pertussis vaccine** to histamine and 5-HT. The published data "indicate that the basis of this hypersensitivity is a blockade of a part of adrenergic division of the sympathetic nervous system. Preliminary experiments are also described, which suggest that a similar mechanism may also be operative in the local Shwartzman reaction."

Simpson H5,300/68: In mice, 5-HT increases, whereas pargyline decreases resistance to both **botulinum toxin** and **nereis toxin**. Histamine has no effect on either intoxication.

Ionizing Rays ←. *Bacq D77,006/54:* In mice, resistance to whole body X-irradiation is increased by numerous amines, particularly cysteamine (β-mercaptoethylamine), norepinephrine, 5-HT, and histamine.

van der Meer & van Bekkum G71,673/59: In mice, the radioprotective effect of histamine, epinephrine, and other biologic amines is related to their pharmacologic activity and can be blocked by their pharmacologic antagonists. "It is concluded that histamine, epinephrine and a number of other biological amines protect against irradiation by reducing the oxygen tension in the spleen and possibly in other blood forming organs."

Langendorff et al. G34,793/65: In mice, incorporation of ^{59}Fe in the erythrocytes can be used as a test for the radioprotective effect of 5-HT, histamine, and other chemicals.

Langendorff et al. G38,385/65: In mice, an open skin wound considerably increases mortality following total body X-irradiation. After this combined treatment, 5-HT has no protective effect, whereas histamine diminishes mortality.

Langendorff & Messerschmidt G45,424/66: In mice, the effect of 5-HT and histamine upon whole body irradiation combined with standard skin wounds is examined.

Koch G51,862/67: Theoretical considerations on the protective effect of 5-HT and histamine against X-irradiation.

Hyperoxygenation ←. *Grognot & Senelar C41,294/57:* In rats and guinea pigs, the pulmonary inflammation induced by inhalation of pure oxygen at barometric pressure is aggravated by ACTH or histamine.

Electric Stimuli ←. *Minz & Domino B81,852/53:* In rats, small doses of epinephrine or norepinephrine prolong the duration of electrically-induced seizures. Since glucose, ACTH, and cortisone failed to prolong seizure duration, it is unlikely that epinephrine should act by release of these substances. Histamine depressed the cortical response to electroshock.

Cold ←. *Selye A8,052/38:* Rats and guinea pigs normally tolerate very large doses of epinephrine or histamine p.o., but these substances cause toxic manifestations (lung edema, emphysema) if administered following the production of an alarm reaction by cold, forced muscular exercise, or other stressors. Presumably the gastrointestinal lesions characteristic of the alarm reaction facilitate the absorption of substances which normally do not traverse the intestinal epithelium in active form.

← *5-HT*

Nonsteroidal Hormones and Hormone-Like Substances ←. Comparatively little is known about the protective effect of 5-HT against overdosage with hormones and related compounds. The duration of hydroxydione anesthesia is prolonged by 5-HT in rats and mice. The toxicity of epinephrine is allegedly unaffected by 5-HT in the mouse, but it is diminished in the rabbit.

Drugs ←. 5-HT greatly potentiates the action of various **barbiturates** in the mouse, rabbit, and rat.

5-HT is also said to augment the antitumor actions of various chemical **carcinogens** diminishing at the same time their damaging effect upon the hemopoietic system.

The toxicity of **carbon tetrachloride** upon rat liver is decreased by 5-HT.

5-HT also prolongs **chloral hydrate, ethanol, ether, halothane** and **chloroform anesthesia** and tends to protect rabbits and dogs against **curare**.

The toxic effects of **harmine** in chickens are inhibited by 5-HT, whereas the bone lesions caused by **lathyrogens** in rats are aggravated.

In mice, the depression of spontaneous activity produced by **LSD** is converted into stimulation by 5-HT, but the prolonging effect of this amine upon hexobarbital narcosis is augmented by LSD.

5-HT potentiates the effects of **mephenesin** and **meprobamate** in the mouse. In rabbits, it increases the analgesic effect of **morphine**.

In rats, 5-HT increases the effects of **nitrogen mustard** but diminishes the myotoxic action of **paraphenylenediamine**.

Pentylenetetrazol convulsions are inhibited by combined treatment with 5-HT and norepinephrine in the mouse. 5-HT also antagonizes pentylenetetrazol in newly hatched chicks in which the blood-brain barrier is still incomplete; here the amine has an anesthetic effect. In mice, intracranial injection of 5-HT protects against pentylenetetrazol convulsions. In strains susceptible to audiogenic and pentylenetetrazol-induced seizures, 5-HTP presumably protects because it raises the 5-HT concentration in the brain.

Picrotoxin convulsions are also inhibited by intracerebral administration of 5-HT in mice. On the other hand, the inhibition of pentylenetetrazol convulsions by intracerebrally injected **reserpine** is counteracted by 5-HT injected into certain regions of the brain.

In dogs, 5-HT inhibits the epilepsy provoked by direct application of **strychnine** or of an electric current to the brain.

In **DHT**-sensitized rats, calcification of the submaxillary glands can be obtained by 5-HT given s.c.

Microorganisms and Their Products ←. 5-HT (like histamine) is especially toxic to mice sensitized with Bordetella pertussis vaccine. If injected simultaneously with various viruses i.v., 5-HT tends to enhance their infectivity and their penetration into the brain.

In mice, resistance to **botulinum toxin** is increased by 5-HT given 30-60 min earlier. 5-HT also increases resistance to various endotoxins in the mouse. This effect, which is greater in females than in males, is potentiated by cortisol and aggravated by thyroxine.

Ionizing Rays ←. In mice, resistance to total body X-irradiation is increased by numerous amines including 5-HT, histamine, norepinephrine, and cystamine. 5-HTP offers similar protection, and the beneficial effect of 5-HT can be enhanced by concurrent administration of other radioprotective substances such as MAO-inhibitors and sulfhydryl-containing compounds. The radioprotective effect of 5-HT has also been confirmed in rats.

Various Stressors ←. 5-HT also increases the resistance of mice against **hyperoxygenation**. In rats it is said to decrease resistance to **cold**. In dogs it inhibits the epilepsy produced by direct **electric** stimulation of the brain, and in rats it elevates the EST. The characteristic response of rats treated with **methionine sulfoximine** is reduced by 5-HT. Finally, in susceptible strains of mice, **audiogenic seizures** are prevented by 5-HTP, presumably because of the resulting increase in brain 5-HT.

Steroids ← cf. also Selye G60,083/70, p.429.

Bianchi & de Maio C54,169/58: In rats, anesthesia produced by hydroxydione i.p. is aggravated by 5-HT, reserpine or hexamethonium.

Vacek D10,919/61: In mice, 5-HT prolongs the duration of hydroxydione anesthesia, whereas LSD shortens it.

Estradiol ← 5-HT: Inscoe et al. F70,325/66

Nonsteroidal Hormones and Hormone-Like Substances ←

Milošević C41,594/57: In mice, reserpine potentiates the toxicity of epinephrine, but this effect should not be ascribed to depletion of 5-HT, since the latter given i.v. does not significantly modify the lethal effect of epinephrine.

Sanyal G55,044/68: In rabbits, 5-HT prevents production of pulmonary edema by epinephrine.

5-HT(N-acetyl) ← 5-HT: Inscoe et al. F70,325/66

Drugs ←

N-Acetyl-p-aminophenol ← 5-HT: Inscoe et al. F70,325/66

N-Acetyltyramine ← 5-HT: Inscoe et al. F70,325/66

Anaphylactoid Edema ← cf. Selye G46,715/68, p. 201.

Barbiturates ←.

MAN

Poloni D95,333/55; D99,472/55: Studies on the effect of 5-HT upon barbiturate or LSD intoxication in man (especially in schizophrenics) and in leeches.

MOUSE

Shore et al. C18,383/55: In mice, 5-HT markedly potentiates the hypnotic action of hexobarbital. In addition, 5-HT i.v. given to mice which have just recovered from hexobarbital hypnosis, immediately causes them to fall asleep again. Thus, it acts like chlorpromazine or reserpine by increasing the sensitivity of the brain to barbiturates, rather than like SKF 525-A which inhibits drug detoxication.

Fastier D95,950/56: In mice, 5-HT considerably potentiates the hypnotic effect of cyclobarbital and chloral hydrate. However, this property is not very specific, since bufotenine, tryptamine, histamine, and epinephrine likewise prolong cyclobarbital hypnosis. Literature on numerous other drugs which prolong barbiturate anesthesia is cited. "It therefore seems possible that the ability of 5-HT to prolong hypnosis may be due to a relatively unspecific, vascular effect."

Zanowiak & Rodman C85,018/59: In mice, 5-HT potentiates the effects of various barbiturates, mephenesin, and meprobamate. This potentiation is counteracted by LSD.

Kato C78,047/59: In mice, the prolongation of pentobarbital or hexobarbital sleeping time by 5-HT (administered in the form of its precursor 5-HTP which penetrates the brain barrier more readily) is inhibited by DOPA; the latter presumably acts as a precursor of norepinephrine.

Rümke G76,693/62: In the mouse, hexobarbital anesthesia is prolonged by an immediately preceding i.p. or s.c. injection of 5-HT.

Hexobarbital ← 5-HT, Mouse: Shore et al. C18,383/55*; Sturtevant D87,568/56*; Brown C31,328/57*; Holtz et al. C76,300/58*; Matthies et al. D84,334/61*; Rümke G76,693/62*, G69,768/63*

RABBIT

Antona C11,379/55: In rabbits, large doses of 5-HT increase the duration and depth of thiopental anesthesia.

Cahn et al. G71,537/56: In rabbits, the prolongation of barbiturate (Kemithal, Mebubarbital) anesthesia by 5-HT is further prolonged by phentolamine, neostigmine, and several other drugs, whereas epinephrine, and pantheline have an opposite effect.

Mantegazzini C33,637/56: In rabbits, the potentiation of pentobarbital anesthesia by 5-HT does not depend upon the hypotensive action of large doses of the latter.

Cahn et al. C64,625/58: In rabbits, thiopental anesthesia is prolonged by pretreatment with 5-HT i.v. This is associated with characteristic changes in the carbohydrate metabolism of the brain.

Lauria & Sharma F67,259/66: In mice, pentobarbital sleeping time is prolonged by 5-HT and several other indole derivatives.

Kadzielawa & Widy-Tyszkiewicz H18,469/69: In mice, p-chlorophenylalanine decreases the duration of hexobarbital sleeping time. This effect is counteracted by 5-HTP, presumably as a consequence of increased 5-HT formation.

RAT

Correll et al. E57,669/52: In rats, anesthesia with various barbiturates or ether diminishes resistance to the lethal effect of 5-HT.

Pierre & Cahn C24,570/55: In rats, 5-HT prolongs thiopental anesthesia, but has no definite effect upon pentobarbital, urethan, or ether narcosis. In rabbits, 5-HT prolongs pentobarbital anesthesia, but has no definite effect upon thiopental and urethan narcosis.

Cahn et al. C19,722/56: In rats thiopental anesthesia is prolonged by 5-HT and this effect can be inhibited by a variety of 5-HT antagonists; further prolongation of sleep is obtained in decreasing order by chlorpromazine, Hydergine, acetylcholine, neostigmine, and phentolamine.

Slocombe C14,144/56: In rats under thiopental anesthesia, epinephrine, norepinephrine, adrenochrome, and 5-HT cause a flattening of the electrical activity both at cortical and at subcortical sites.

Gaddum C25,117/56: Brief review on the synergism between barbiturates and 5-HT.

Garattini & Valzelli G71,229/56: In rats, the prolongation of pentobarbital anesthesia by 5-HT is influenced by numerous drugs.

Salmoiraghi et al. C21,596/56: 5-HT prolongs the hypnotic action of hexobarbital both in mice and in rats.

Fornaroli C47,728/57: In rats, 5-HT prolongs anesthesia produced by various barbiturates or ether. Earlier literature is reviewed.

Bose et al. D58,773/63: In rats, hexobarbital sleeping time is prolonged by 5-HT. This prolongation is inhibited by Cannabis resin.

Phenobarbital ← 5-HT(N-acetyl): Inscoe et al. *F70,325/66*

Bemegride ← 5-HT, Mouse: Rümke *G76,692/62**

Carcinolytic Agent ←. *Man'ko F74,715/66; F82,459/66:* In mice and rats, 5-HT increases the carcinolytic action of dopan, chlorambucil and cyclophosphamide upon certain transplantable tumors, and simultaneously decreases their damaging effect upon the hemopoietic system.

Carbon Tetrachloride ←. *Fiore-Donati et al. C62,200/58; C78,953/59:* In rats, 5-HT offers partial protection against the hepatic lesions produced by CCl_4.

Erspamer E5,915/66: A monograph on 5-HT and related indolealkylamines, with a special section on their protective effect against radiation injury, hepatic cirrhosis produced by CCl_4 or allyl alcohol, and cardiovascular calcifications produced by DHT.

Cholesterol ←. *Trentini et al. G71,152/68:* In rabbits, the cholesterol-atherosclerosis-inhibiting effect of Tween 80 is diminished both by 5-HT and by norepinephrine.

Chloral Hydrate ←. *Fastier D95,950/56:* In mice, 5-HT considerably potentiates the hypnotic effect of cyclobarbital and chloral hydrate. However, this property is not very specific, since bufotenine, tryptamine, histamine and epinephrine likewise prolong cyclobarbital hypnosis. Literature on numerous other drugs which prolong barbiturate anesthesia is cited. "It therefore seems possible that the ability of 5-HT to prolong hypnosis may be due to a relatively unspecific, vascular effect."

Fastier et al. C37,038/57: In mice, chloral hydrate sleeping time is increased by epinephrine, norepinephrine, phenylephrine, methoxamine, 5-HT, histamine, ergotamine, yohimbine, and atropine. "It is suggested that some, at least, of the drugs which prolong the effects of hypnotics do so by virtue of a hypothermic action." Vasopressin, cortisone, and DOC did not prolong chloral hydrate sleeping time at the doses tested.

Chloroform ←. *Wulfsohn & Politzer D22,421/61:* In mice, 5-HT greatly prolongs chloroform anesthesia but has little or no effect upon ether or halothane narcosis.

Curare ←. *Sala & Perris C78,420/58:* In rabbits treated with D-tubocurarine, 5-HT causes a rapid but transient restoration of neuromuscular transmission.

Schopp & Rife E24,636/63: In dogs, 5-HT exerts a mild anticurare action upon the indirectly stimulated peroneal-tibialis-anticus nerve-muscle preparation.

Ethanol ←. *Rosenfeld G72,151/60:* In mice, ethanol anesthesia is prolonged by 5-HT, tryptamine, and dopamine. "Analytical data provided experimental proof that the potentiating effect of the aromatic amines was not attributable either to an increase in the brain alcohol content or to an interference with the over-all rate of alcohol destruction in the body."

Ethanol ← 5-HT + Iproniazid, Mouse: Besendorf et al. C31,623/56*

Ether ←. *Fornaroli C47,728/57:* In rats, 5-HT prolongs anesthesia produced by various barbiturates or ether. Earlier literature is reviewed.

Wulfsohn & Politzer D22,421/61: In mice, 5-HT greatly prolongs chloroform anesthesia, but has little or no effect upon ether or halothane narcosis.

Halothane ←. *Wulfsohn & Politzer D22,421/61:* In mice, 5-HT greatly prolongs chloroform anesthesia, but has little or no effect upon ether or halothane narcosis.

Nikki & Rosenberg G71,574/69: In mice, shivering and hypothermia are prevented by norepinephrine and 5-HT, but not by dopamine. "The results suggest that brain catecholamines participate in the control of shivering and return of normothermia after halothane anaesthesia in mice."

Harmine ←. *Bowman & Osuide F98,712/68:* In chickens, the toxic effects of tremorine and harmine are inhibited by 5-HT and numerous other drugs.

Lathyrogens ←. *Franchimont et al. D13,136/61:* In rats, osteolathyrism produced by AAN is aggravated by 5-HT, whereas glucagon does not modify it significantly.

Lead ←. *Selye et al. G11,123/64:* "In rats simultaneously given an intravenous injection of lead acetate and a subcutaneous injection of histamine, extensive calcium deposition occurs in various parts of the autonomic nervous system. This neurotropic form of mastocalcergy can be inhibited by pretreatment with various mast-cell dischargers (compound 48/80, polymyxin, chlorpromazine), mast-cell components (histamine, 5-HT) or drugs known to inhibit the pharmacologic actions of such mast-cell components (cyproheptadine, neo-antergan). This prophylactic effect appears to be largely specific to compounds related to mast-cell activity since it was not shared by various other drugs and stressors tested."

LSD ←. *Poloni D95,333/55; D99,472/55:* Studies on the effect of 5-HT upon barbiturate or LSD intoxication in man (especially in schizophrenics) and in leeches.

Brown C31,328/57: In mice, the depression of spontaneous activity induced by LSD is converted into stimulation by 5-HT.

Salmoiraghi & Page C38,518/57: In mice, LSD and various other hallucinogens (bufotenine, mescaline, ibogaine) augment the prolonging effect of 5-HT upon hexobarbital narcosis.

Mephenesin, Meprobamate ←. *Zanowiak & Rodman C85,018/59:* In mice, 5-HT potentiates the effects of various barbiturates, mephenesin, and meprobamate. This potentiation is counteracted by LSD.

Mercury ←. *Erspamer B84,587/53:* In rats given large doses of $HgCl_2$ survival is prolonged and mortality decreased by repeated s.c. injections of 5-HT, perhaps because the latter diminishes renal blood flow.

Menthionine Sulfoximine ←. *Wada et al. G48,380/67:* Rats treated with methionine sulfoximine show a characteristic response to audiogenic stimuli, which is reduced by 5-HT and increased by DOPA.

Morphine ←. *Nicák F47,918/65:* In rats and mice, the analgesic effect of small doses of morphine is potentiated by 5-HT.

Saarnivaara H2,855/68; G71,565/69: In rabbits, 5-HT increases morphine analgesia.

Nitrogen Mustard ←. *Uroić et al. E37,637/64:* In rats, 5-HT increases the toxicity of mustine hydrochloride (nitrogen mustard), a typical radiomimetic poison.

Ballerini & Bosi G31,956/65: In rats, 5-HT increases the lethality of intoxication with uracil mustard. Antiserotonins have an opposite effect.

Paraphenylenediamine ←. *Jasmin & Bois C73,640/59; C83,058/60:* In rats, the myotoxic action of paraphenylenediamine can be partially prevented by 5-HT, but also by KCl, methylene blue, and vitamin C. The mechanism of protection is not understood.

Pentylenetetrazol ←. *Bonnycastle et al. C37,036/57:* In rats, anticonvulsants increase the 5-HT concentration of the brain, but administration of 5-HT, iproniazid, or 5-hydroxytryptophan, in doses which elevate the brain levels of 5-HT, did not protect against the convulsant or lethal action of pentylenetetrazol.

Schmidt & Matthies D34,219/62: In mice, 5-HT or norepinephrine injected into certain regions of the brain is without effect upon pentylenetetrazol injection in itself, but counteracts the inhibitory effect of intracerebrally injected reserpine.

Schmidt E32,188/63: In mice, pentylenetetrazol convulsions are inhibited by combined administration of 5-HT and norepinephrine into certain regions of the brain.

Seifter et al. G71,087/63: In chicks, pentylenetetrazol convulsions can be inhibited by 5-HT and some of its analogues.

Kobrin & Seifter F74,422/66: In one day old chicks, in which the blood-brain barrier is still incompletely formed, various ω-amino acids as well as 5-HT, histamine, and epinephrine, produce sleep and prevent pentylenetetrazol convulsions.

Schlesinger et al. G61,802/68: In susceptible mice, audiogenic and pentylenetetrazol-induced seizures are prevented by 5-HTP, presumably because of the resulting increase in brain 5-HT concentration.

Schlesinger et al. G69,565/69: In mice, intracranial injections of 5-HT or norepinephrine protect against pentylenetetrazol convulsions.

Pentylenetetrazol ← 5-HTP + Genetics, Mouse: Schlesinger et al. G61,802/68*

Picrotoxin ←. *Saito et al. E27,616/63:* In mice, picrotoxin convulsions are inhibited by the intracerebral administration of epinephrine or 5-HT.

Plasmocid ← *cf. Selye G60,083/70, p. 429.*

Reserpine ←. *Schmidt & Matthies D34,219/62:* In mice, 5-HT or norepinephrine injected into certain regions of the brain is without effect upon pentylenetetrazol injection in itself, but counteracts the inhibitory effect of intracerebrally injected reserpine.

Simionovici et al. F43,099/65: In mice, epinephrine and norepinephrine, as well as histamine, offer partial protection against reserpine intoxication (sedation blepharoptosis, hypothermia). 5-HT has no such effect.

Strychnine ←. *Scarinci G66,316/55:* In dogs, 5-HT inhibits the epilepsy produced by direct application of strychnine to, or direct electric stimulation of the brain.

Tremorine ←. *Bowman & Osuide F98,712/68:* In chickens, the toxic effects of tremorine and harmine are inhibited by 5-HT and numerous other drugs.

Tween 80 ←. *Trentini et al. G71,152/68:* In rabbits, the cholesterol-atherosclerosis-inhibiting effect of Tween 80 is diminished both by 5-HT and by norepinephrine.

Tyramine ← 5-HT: Inscoe et al. F70,325/66

Urethan ←. *Pierre & Cahn C24,570/55:* In rats, 5-HT prolongs thiopental anesthesia, but has no definite effect upon pentobarbital, urethan, or ether narcosis. In rabbits, 5-HT prolongs pentobarbital anesthesia but has no definite effect upon thiopental and urethan narcosis.

Vitamin D, DHT ← *cf. also Selye G60,083/70, p. 429. Selye & Gentile D6,950/61:* In rats pretreated with DHT p.o., selective calcification of the submaxillary glands can be obtained by 5-HT s.c. as a manifestation of calciphylaxis.

Erspamer E5,915/66: A monograph on 5-HT and related indolealkylamines, with a special section on their protective effect against radiation injury, hepatic cirrhosis produced by CCl_4 or allyl alcohol, and cardiovascular calcifications produced by DHT.

Microorganisms ←

Fishel et al. E8,474/64: Review (8 pp., 26 refs.) on the mechanism of sensitization by B. pertussis vaccine to histamine and 5-HT. The published data "indicate that the basis of this hypersensitivity is a blockade of a part of adrenergic division of the sympathetic nervous system. Preliminary experiments are also described, which suggest that a similar mechanism may also be operative in the local Shwartzman reaction."

Sellers H10,893/69: In mice, epinephrine or 5-HT injected simultaneously with various viruses i.v. enhances their infectivity and their penetration into the brain.

Bacterial Toxins ← *cf. also Selye E5,986/66, p. 85.*

Boroff C75,371/59: In mice, both the toxicity and ultraviolet fluorescence of Cl. botulinum toxin are inhibited by 5-HT and tryptophan, as well as by substances releasing 5-HT into the circulation (e.g. reserpine, chlorpromazine).

Gordon & Lipton C94,649/60: 5-HT reduces endotoxin mortality in mice. This effect is greater in females than in males and is potentiated by cortisol. Thyroxine aggravates the toxicity of endotoxin.

Boroff & Fleck F87,254/67: In mice, 5-HT increases resistance to botulinum toxin given 30—60 min later.

Simpson G60,451/68; H5,300/68: In mice, botulinal poisoning is prevented by 5-HT. Although both 5-HT and the toxin act upon mechanisms of cholinergic synaptic transmission, work with isolated nerve-muscle preparations showed that the synaptic junction is not the site of 5-HT and toxin interaction, suggesting "that it is the circulatory system rather than the nervous system at which the two drugs interact."

Ionizing Rays ←

MOUSE

Bacq D77,006/54: In mice, resistance to whole body X-irradiation is increased by numerous amines, particularly cysteamine (β-mercaptoethylamine), norepinephrine, 5-HT, and histamine.

Langendorff & Koch C36,881/57: In mice, both tryptamine and 5-HT offered protection against X-irradiation, whereas amphetamine and d,l-ephedrine were ineffective.

Melching et al. C76,527/58: In mice, 5-HT i.p. increases resistance against whole body X-irradiation, but only under certain conditions of dosage and timing.

Langendorff et al. C69,396/59: In mice, 5-HT exerts a prophylactic effect against total body X-irradiation.

Semenov D7,087/60: In mice, 5-HT offers better protection against radiation sickness than epinephrine, although the latter is also effective, especially when given in combination with acetylcholine.

Doull & Tricou D4,271/61: In mice, pretreatment with 5-HT increases resistance to whole body X-irradiation.

Feinstein & Seaholm E29,638/63: In mice, both 5-HT and the 5-HT antagonist KB-95 exhibit some radioprotective activity. Conjoint administration of both compounds is somewhat less effective than treatment with either drug alone.

Maisin et al. E36,751/63: In mice, the protection against X-irradiation offered by 2-β-aminoethylisothiourea (AET) is only slightly improved by concurrent administration of 5-HT.

Vittorio et al. D56,243/63: Review of the literature and personal observations in mice on the radio protective effect of 5-HT.

Abe & Langendorff G23,763/64: In mice, 5-HT protects the testes against damage caused by X-irradiation. The histologic manifestations of the damage and protection have been studied under varying circumstances.

Langendorff et al. G34,793/65: In mice incorporation of ^{59}Fe in the erythrocytes can be used as a test for the radioprotective effect of 5-HT, histamine, and other chemicals.

Langendorff et al. G38,385/65: In mice, an open skin wound considerably increases mortality following total body X-irradiation. After this combined treatment, 5-HT has no protective effect, whereas histamine diminishes mortality.

Kobayashi et al. G73,566/66: In mice, under suitable experimental conditions, 5-HTP offers as good, or even better, protection against whole body X-irradiation as does 5-HT.

Langendorff & Langendorff G38,396/66: In mice, the protective effect of 5-HT against X-irradiation largely depends upon the age of the animals.

Langendorff & Messerschmidt G45,424/66: In mice, the effect of 5-HT and histamine upon whole body irradiation combined with standard skin wounds is examined.

Maisin & Mattelin F78,796/67: In mice, the radioprotective effect of 5-HT can be enhanced by conjoint administration of other radioprotectors.

Cier et al. F85,815/67: In mice, the protection against total body X-irradiation given by 5-HT is considerably increased by concurrent treatment with thiosulfate. Various other radioprotective compounds offer likewise better protection and are less toxic if administered conjointly than if given singly.

Graul & Rüther G66,718/67: In mice and rabbits, 5-HT, cysteamine, and AET (β-animoethylisothiuronium) have proved to be particularly effective as radioprotective substances against ^{60}CO-γ and X-irradiation.

Hasegawa & Landahl G48,428/67: In mice, the radioprotective effect of 5-HT depends upon the oxygen content of the air.

Maisin & Mattelin H719/67: In mice, the radioprotective effect of 5-HT is enhanced by concurrent treatment with one or more sulfhydryl compounds.

Westphal & Hagen G45,683/67: In mice, the chromosome aberrations in the thymus induced by X-irradiation are reduced by 5-HT and cysteamine.

Barnes & Lowman G63,518/68: In mice, the radioprotective effect of 5-HT can be augmented by simultaneous administration of phenelzine, a MAO-inhibitor.

Maisin et al. G59,894/68: In mice, the radioprotective effect of 5-HT can be increased by simultaneous treatment with other radioprotectors.

Streffer et al. G55,078/68: In mice, the protective effect of 5-HT against X-irradiation was compared under different experimental conditions.

Barnes & Lowman G64,917/69: In mice, 5-HT gave better protection against total body X-irradiation than did 5-HTP. Earlier claims to the contrary are not confirmed.

Léonard et al. G71,644/69: In mice, the radio-protective effect of various chemicals given conjointly is increased by the addition of 5-HT to the mixture.

RAT

Gray et al. B92,332/52: In rats, 5-HT greatly increases survival following total body X-irradiation. The production of methemoglobinemia by para-aminopropiophenone has a similar effect; hence, the protection is ascribed to temporary tissue anoxia.

van den Brenk & Elliott C76,268/58: In rats, the protective effect of 5-HT against whole body X-irradiation is compared with that of tryptamine and other agents.

van den Brenk & Moore C71,353/59: In rats, the protective effect of 5-HT upon total body X-irradiation is reversed by breathing oxygen under high pressure.

Ladner et al. G31,673/65: In rats, 5-HT protects against whole body X-irradiation especially when combined with tryptophan.

Frölén G43,045/66: In rats "the genetic radio-protective effects of cysteamine, AET, cystamine, glutathion and serotonin have been studied. Only cysteamine showed a clear mutation-reducing effect on spermatids and spermatozoa."

Rixon & Baird G55,192/68: In rats, studies on the radioprotective effect of 5-HT suggest that intense vasoconstriction and hypoxia-induced reduction in cellular respiration may have a beneficial effect.

VARIA

Maisin & Doherty C91,781/60: A review on chemical protection against X-irradiation, with special emphasis upon the protective effect of 5-HT alone or given in combination with MEA [bis(2-aminoethyl)disulfide (cystamine)] or AET (2-aminoethylisothiourea).

Erspamer E5,915/66: A monograph on 5-HT and related indolealkylamines with a special section on their protective effect against radiation injury, hepatic cirrhosis produced by CCl_4 or allyl alcohol, and cardiovascular calcifications produced by DHT.

Koch G51,862/67: Theoretical considerations on the protective effect of 5-HT and histamine against X-irradiation.

Various Stressors ←

Hyperoxygenation ←. *Laborit et al. C48,371/57; C52,731/58; C77,964/59:* In mice, 5-HT protects against the convulsions produced by exposure to oxygen under high pressure.

Cold ←. *Zilberstein C80,282/60:* In rats, 5-HT, vasopressin, and reserpine lower resistance to cold, allegedly because they interfere with pituitary hormone secretion and cause a state of "temporary functional adrenalectomy."

Electric Stimuli ←. *Scarinci G66,316/55:* In dogs, 5-HT inhibits the epilepsy produced by direct application of strychnine to, or direct electrical stimulation of the brain.

de Salva et al. C51,842/58: In rats, the EST was lowered by hypophysectomy and adrenalectomy, but only insignificantly by thyroidectomy. 5-HT elevated the EST.

Sound ←. *Wada et al. G48,380/67:* Rats treated with methionine sulfoximine show a characteristic response to audiogenic stimuli, which is reduced by 5-HT and increased by DOPA.

Schlesinger et al. G61,802/68: In susceptible mice, audiogenic and pentylenetetrazol-induced seizures are prevented by 5-HTP, presumably because of the resulting increase in brain 5-HT concentration.

← VARIOUS OTHER HORMONE-LIKE SUBSTANCES

Prostaglandin E_1 partially protects mice against strychnine-induced convulsions.

Erythropoietin increases the resistance of mice against X-irradiation.

In dogs and rabbits, **kallikrein** (like other vasoactive substances) prolongs the anesthetic effect of barbiturates.

"Toxohormone" (a Walker tumor extract) allegedly causes pronounced changes in the microsomal steroidases of the rat liver.

Drugs (Var) ← cf. *Selye B87,000/52, pp. 59—66, 210—216, 250, 256, 264, 269, 277, 278; B90,100/53, pp. 86—93, 267—277, 321, 322, 335, 336; C1,001/54, pp. 294—301, 451—460, 465—468, 478, 490, 491; C9,000/56, pp. 233—241, 348—352, 449—460, 470—476, 485, 486; D15,540/62, p. 275; G46,715/68, p. 176, 202.*

Bacterial Toxins ← cf. *Selye E5,986/66, pp. 71, 85, 86.*

Stress ← cf. *Selye B58,650/51, p. 50; B87,000/52; B90,100/53; C1,001/54; C9,000/56.*

Varia ←

Werle & Lentzen A 28,007/38: In dogs and rabbits, various vasoactive substances (epinephrine, histamine, vasopressin, **kallikrein**) tend to prolong the anesthetic effect of pronarcon and hexobarbital.

Čapek D 54,290/62: In mice, **bradykinin** decreases the seizure threshold to strychnine, pentylenetetrazol, and electroshock. Substance P has the opposite effect.

Jones & Shapiro D 55,793/63: In rats, an acute episode of hypertension produced by epinephrine or **angiotensin** i.v. facilitates the production of pyelonephritis following infection with E. coli.

Altura et al. F 36,124/65: In rats, survival following temporary ligation of the superior mesenteric artery was improved by PLV-2, but not by epinephrine or **angiotensin**. The associated changes in the microcirculation of the mesoappendix are described.

Altura et al. F 43,209/65: In rats, norepinephrine and **angiotensin** fail to prolong survival after traumatic shock, temporary ligature of the superior mesenteric artery, or endotoxin shock. However, vasopressin (PLV-2) was significantly effective in traumatic and intestinal ischemia shock, but not in endotoxinemia.

Naidu & Reddi F 80,336/67: In mice, resistance to X-irradiation is increased by **erythropoietin** preparations.

Duru & Türker H 10,307/69: In mice, **prostaglandin** E_1 partially protects against strychnine-induced convulsions.

Takahashi & Kato H 15,250/69: Studies on changes in hepatic microsomal steroidases induced in rats by treatment with **"toxohormone"** (a Walker tumor extract).

Vittorio et al. H 7,759/69: In mice, polycythemia induced by transfusion, increases resistance to X-irradiation. A similar result can be obtained by stimulation of stem cell activity by **erythropoietin.**

← TISSUE EXTRACTS

← **Hepatic Extracts.** In view of the important role played by the liver in detoxicating mechanisms, many investigations have been performed to determine whether drug resistance could be conferred by pretreatment with hepatic extracts. In rats, a certain hepatic preparation ("Yakriton") has been claimed to offer protection against a variety of toxicants. Hepatic extracts have also been said to protect the rat against methanol and its metabolites, pyruvate and acetaldehyde. Finally, rats have been protected against thyroxine intoxication by feeding hepatic extracts containing an "antitoxic factor."

← **Other Tissue Extracts.** In order to test the specificity of the acetonitrile test, mice have been pretreated with a great variety of tissue extracts; it has been found that these offer also some protection against acetonitrile, KCN and propionitrile, although they are much less efficacious than thyroid preparations. Resistance to pentobarbital anesthesia is decreased in male rats by a variety of tissue extracts (anterior pituitary, thymus, pancreas, liver, kidneys, spleen, testis, brain). On the other hand "among eight damaging agents given in doses sufficient to elicit an alarm reaction, only colchicine and atropine prolong the duration of anesthesia because of their high degree of toxicity." It remains questionable, however, whether the increase in barbiturate sleeping time produced by tissue extracts is solely due to their stressor action.

Vitamin-D_3 intoxication is largely inhibited by placenta extracts in the rat.

In frogs, fatal strychnine convulsions can be prevented if the drug is mixed with various tissue extracts prior to injection, but this may well be due to delayed absorption as a consequence of local inflammatory phenomena.

← Hepatic Extracts

Ravdin et al. B25,566/39: In rats, xanthine, allantoin, caffeine, sodium ricinoleate and suspensions of colloidal carbon injected s.c. protect the liver against injury from chloroform, presumably as a consequence of the resulting inflammatory reaction which is associated with the absorption of protein split-products. This would also explain the protective effect of various hepatic extracts (including Yakriton) and of high protein diets.

Lecoq et al. B66,406/51: In rats, the toxic effects of ethanol and its metabolites, pyruvate and acetaldehyde (which accumulate in the body under the influence of disulfiram), are inhibited by ACTH, cortisone, and hepatic extracts. Conversely, thyroxine, DOC, and testosterone appear to aggravate ethanol intoxication. [Statistically evaluated data are not presented (H.S.).]

Ershoff D5,818/61: Review of the literature, and personal observations on the protection of rats against toxic doses of thyroxine by feeding hepatic extracts containing the "antitoxic factor of liver."

Grandpierre & Robert H22,252/69: In rats, i.p. administration of a lyophilized liver extract detoxifies estradiol as judged by a diminished sex hormone activity in prepubertal animals.

← Other Tissue Extracts

Marañón & Aznar 46,926/15: In frogs, the fatal convulsions produced by strychnine can be prevented if, prior to injection, the drug is mixed with extracts of the posterior pituitary, the thyroid, various other tissues, and particularly epinephrine. [The possibility of delayed absorption owing to local vasoconstriction has not been considered (H.S.).]

Gellhorn 16,839/23: In mice, resistance against acetonitrile can be increased not only by thyroid extract, but to a lesser extent, also by extracts of various other tissues. These preparations likewise augment resistance to KCN and propionitrile, whereas thyroidectomy and orchidectomy have an opposite effect.

Masson 94,205/47: Various tissue extracts (anterior pituitary, thymus, pancreas, liver, kidney, spleen, testis, brain) as well as casein s.c. decrease resistance to pentobarbital anesthesia in male rats. On the other hand, "among eight damaging agents given in doses sufficient to elicit an alarm reaction, only colchicine and atropine prolonged the duration of anesthesia, because of their high degree of toxicity." Yet, the prolongation of barbiturate anesthesia by pituitary extracts must be ascribed to a nonspecific stressor effect.

Wietek & Taupitz C40,028/57: In rats, the syndrome of vitamin-D_3 intoxication is largely inhibited by placenta extract i.m.

VII. EFFECT OF NONHORMONAL FACTORS UPON RESISTANCE

← DRUGS

There exists a very extensive literature on the effect of various drugs upon resistance to toxicants. In fact, as regards the induction of defensive hepatic microsomal enzymes, much more has been published in this connection about drugs than about hormones (particularly steroids) as inducers. However, this book deals primarily with the role of hormones in resistance, hence the defensive action of drugs will be considered only in as far as it sheds some light upon our principal subject.

We shall deal here mainly with such classic hepatic microsomal-enzyme inducers as the barbiturates, pesticides and carcinogens whose actions are closely related to those of steroids. However, we shall also consider the protective effects of other drugs against certain substrates (e.g., anesthetics and hypnotics, digitalis alkaloids, indomethacin, steroids) that are highly subject to detoxication through hormones and often help to illustrate the actions of the latter. On the other hand, specific pharmacologic antagonisms (e.g., between histamine and antihistamines, 5-HT and antiserotonins, vasopressor and vasodilator substances) will not be considered. The so-called phenomena of nonspecific cross-resistance, that are related to stress, will be mentioned only in passing.

In the Abstract Section, the resistance-modifying drugs will be considered in alphabetic order, always together with all the toxicants that they affect. Here, we shall comment only on a few particularly interesting data, and on observations which can be clarified by correlating them with facts not mentioned by the authors of the original articles cited.

As with hormones, we may distinguish **syntoxic** and **catatoxic** drugs. The syntoxic effect is due to the suppression of excessive tissue reactions to an irritant, without destroying the latter; the catatoxic effect is the consequence of the destruction of the aggressor, e.g., through the induction of hepatic microsomal drug-metabolizing enzymes.

Weight for weight **amiloride** is even more active than spironolactone in protecting the rat against various forms of infarctoid cardiopathies produced by gluco-mineralocorticoids plus Na-salts and other conditioning factors. However, this effect is apparently quite unrelated to steroid-metabolizing enzyme induction, it depends upon the potassium-sparing action of amiloride. Accordingly, this drug is ineffective in protecting the rat against hexobarbital, progesterone, parathion or dioxathion, all of which are readily detoxified by spironolactone and other steroidal or nonsteroidal hepatic microsomal-enzyme inducers.

Perhaps the most carefully studied class of nonhormonal drug-metabolizing enzyme inducers are the **barbiturates**. Several investigators found that phenobarbital counteracts the uterotrophic effect of estradiol in immature intact or ovariectomized rats.

It also enhances the estradiol-metabolizing activity of isolated hepatic microsomal fractions in rats treated in vivo with phenobarbital. This action of the barbiturate remains obvious after adrenalectomy or hypophysectomy. The uterine weight-increasing effect of synthetic luteoids, such as norethindrone and norethynodrel, is likewise inhibited by phenobarbital, as is that of synthetic folliculoids. When isotope-marked folliculoids are used, e.g., tritiated diethylstilbestrol, this inhibition is paralleled by decreased radioactivity in the uterus and increased diethylstilbestrol degradation by hepatic microsomes.

In mice, the uterotrophic effect of estrone, estradiol and stilbestrol is also reduced by phenobarbital pretreatment. Endogenous folliculoid production is presumably likewise inhibited by this drug, since phenobarbital interferes with the maintenance of normal uterine weight in intact mice.

There is some evidence that in immature or gonadectomized male rats, phenobarbital diminishes the effect of testosterone upon the accessory sex organs.

Finally, in rats the half-life of i.v.-injected cortisol is decreased by pretreatment with phenobarbital; in man, this barbiturate accelerates the plasma clearance of cortisol.

Experiments with radioactive thyroxine indicate that phenobarbital increases the turnover of thyroid hormone and stimulates the function of the thyroid after enhancing the hepatocellular binding of thyroxine. Furthermore, the hepatic microsomes of phenobarbital-pretreated rats exhibit an increased ability to de-iodinate thyroxine and T3 in vitro.

There is good experimental evidence that phenobarbital and other barbiturates also enhance the metabolism of certain anticoagulants (bishydroxycoumarin, coumarin, warfarin) in various species, including man. They even promote the enzymic biotransformation of many barbiturates, bilirubin, carbon disulfide, cholesterol (at the same time inhibiting the atheromatosis produced by cholesterol feeding), diphenylhydantoin, antipyrine, ethanol, various pesticides, phenylbutazone, picrotoxin, quinine, strychnine, etc. The elimination of ascorbic acid is enhanced by phenobarbital in the rat. On the other hand, unlike various catatoxic steroids, phenobarbital does not appear to protect against cyclophosphamide, digitoxin, D-tubocurarine, tribromoethanol, mephenesin etc. *(cf. also* Tables 137, 138).

The effect of barbiturates upon hepatic enzymes has already been mentioned, especially in connection with the increase in various steroidases; for additional data, the reader is referred to the Abstract Section.

The extensive literature on the effect of **carbon tetrachloride** on hepatic microsomal-enzyme induction is discussed, with that of other hepatotoxic blockers, in the section on "General Pharmacology."

Next to the barbiturates, probably the most intensively studied class of microsomal-enzyme inducers is that of the **carcinogens.** The relationship, if any, between carcinogenic and enzyme-inducing potency is not clear but empirical observations show that many carcinogens enhance the activity of thiophosphate-oxidizing enzymes, steroidases and several other enzyme systems, including those that accelerate the biotransformation of other carcinogens. Thus, it has been possible in some instances to protect animals against the tumorigenic action of a strong carcinogen by pretreating it with a weaker one. The spectrum of enzyme induction exhibited by carcinogens does not correspond to that of the barbiturates or of steroids.

It is of special interest that some factors naturally occurring in **cedar chips** can induce various hepatic enzymes and diminish hexobarbital sleeping time. This is of practical importance in that mice and rats kept on soft wood bedding may develop a great resistance to certain toxicants.

Desipramine (an antidepressant) reduces the activity of modaline by inhibiting its biotransformation into a more active compound in the hepatic microsomes of the rat. Furthermore, desipramine potentiates the uterotrophic action of estrone in immature rats by delaying its degradation in the hepatic microsomes.

Diphenylhydantoin (an anticonvulsant and anti-epileptic drug) alters corticoid metabolism in man, but this effect will be discussed under "Clinical Implications."

In our most recent experiments on rats, we found that diphenylhydantoin offers excellent protection against digitoxin dioxathion, parathion, nicotine, hexobarbital, progesterone, zoxazolamine and indomethacin, but only at the very high dose of 100 mg, twice daily, per 100 g body weight. At lower dose levels, the protective effect decreases rapidly (*cf.* Table 137).

Curiously, in dogs or guinea pigs just awakening from barbiturate anesthesia, i.v. injection of **glucose** produces a return of sleep, perhaps because it increases barbiturate penetration into the brain.

In view of the important role played by thyroid hormones in the regulation of drug-metabolizing enzyme induction, it is of interest that in rabbits inhibition of thyroid function by **iodine** accelerates the recovery of the spinal cord following anoxia induced by temporary compression of the abdominal aorta. Destruction of the thyroid with radio-iodine has essentially the same effect as surgical thyroidectomy.

Iproniazid is discussed with the other MAO-inhibitors, under inhibitors of microsomal-enzyme induction in the section on "General Pharmacology" (p. 68).

In rats, the adrenal necrosis produced by DMBA or 7-OH-MBA is prevented by **metyrapone** and related inhibitors of corticoid synthesis. This drug delays the blood clearance of exogenous cortisol presumably because it "inhibits the liver enzyme system(s) responsible for inactivation of adrenal steroids." Addition of metyrapone to liver microsomes of mice does not interfere with electron transport; hence, the point of attack of the inhibitor on the hydroxylation of substrate appears to be on cytochrome P-450.

The well-known adrenal-stimulating effect of metyrapone and of related compounds is ascribed to a compensatory ACTH secretion, resulting from a diminished feed-back because of the inhibition of steroid 11β-hydroxylase activity in the adrenals. However, the compound also acts on hepatic enzyme induction since it prolongs hexobarbital sleeping time and inhibits the oxidative metabolism of hexobarbital, aminopyrine and acetanilide by hepatic microsomes in vitro.

In rats, metyrapone inhibits the catatoxic effect of spironolactone against digitoxin and indomethacin poisoning; it also prolongs the anesthetic action of progesterone, DOC and hydroxydione.

Pesticides were among the first compounds shown to possess hepatic microsomal drug-metabolizing enzyme-inducing capacity. They stimulate the SER of the hepatocytes, diminish hexobarbital sleeping time, inhibit the effect of various carcinogens and interfere with the metabolism of steroids (including corticoids, folliculoids and testoids). This latter action has caused some concern with regard to the probable effect of pesticides, as pollutants of the atmosphere, upon fertility, particularly among birds.

The stimulation by pesticides of the metabolism of bilirubin and of excess corticoids in Cushing's syndrome, cardiovascular diseases, etc. will be discussed at length in the section on "Clinical Implications."

Several **phenothiazines** appear to have microsomal enzyme-blocking actions similar to those of SKF 525-A. Thus they prolong hexobarbital anesthesia, potentiate the effect of various spasmolytic compounds, and inhibit DMBA-induced adrenal necrosis in the rat.

Phenylbutazone as a typical anti-inflammatory (and hence syntoxic) drug, deserves special attention as regards its effect upon hepatic microsomal enzyme induction. In vitro, when added to pig liver homogenates, it inhibits the enzymic inactivation of cortisone. However, treatment of immature rats with phenylbutazone increases several-fold the hepatic microsomal enzymes that hydroxylate testosterone and 4-androstene-3,17-dione.

In man, phenylbutazone increases the urinary excretion of 6β-hydroxycortisol. In rabbits, cholesterol atherosclerosis is diminished by phenylbutazone and oxyphenylbutazone, although to a lesser extent than by glucocorticoids.

Phenylbutazone also increases its own metabolism. That is allegedly why rats treated for short periods develop gastric ulcers which disappear upon more prolonged treatment.

Unlike salicylic acid, phenylbutazone does not significantly affect the plasma concentration or biliary and fecal excretion of ^{14}C-indomethacin.

RES-blocking agents allegedly abolish the sex difference in the picrotoxin sensitivity of rats, a species in which males are normally more resistant to this drug than females.

On theoretic grounds, it has been postulated that the anti-endotoxic activity of corticoids "in some way involves the reticuloendothelial system." However, up to now this possibility has remained purely speculative.

On the other hand, several RES-stimulants prolong pentobarbital sleeping time in the mouse. Furthermore, in this species, endotoxin, zymosan, glucan and saccharated iron oxide (all RES-blocking agents) lower TPO and increase TKT in vivo but not in vitro. "These results suggest a cause and effect relationship between inducibility of key liver enzymes and survival against stress."

In rats, pretreated with India ink i.v., phenobarbital elimination is delayed.

Salicylic acid decreases the plasma concentration of ^{14}C-indomethacin and increases its urinary and biliary excretion in the rat. Probenecid raises the plasma concentration of indomethacin. These interrelations are tentatively ascribed to the similarity in the chemical structure of the three compounds.

In rabbits, salicylic acid causes dilatation of the endoplasmic reticulum and its spaces become filled with electron-dense material.

Sucrose feeding, like starvation, interferes with the detoxication of zoxazolamine, barbiturates, strychnine, carisoprodol and OMPA in the rat, presumably through the depression of the synthesis of hepatic microsomal enzymes.

The detoxifying action of **sulfur** compounds has been known since time immemorial. Thiosulfates and various other sulfur compounds inhibit methemoglobin formation following treatment with aniline or sodium nitrite; they also counteract intoxication with iodine, arsenic, cyanides, thallium and many other toxicants.

It has been claimed that thiosulfate protects against anaphylactic shock and other immune reactions, but these observations require confirmation. On the other hand, it appears definitely established that various sulfur compounds — especially those containing SH- and SS-groups — offer protection against total body X-irradiation. In this respect, cysteamine and cysteine are particularly efficacious.

High doses of **vitamin C** offer some protection against mercurial intoxication and large doses of **vitamin E** combat the progeria-like syndrome produced by DHT in the rat.

← *Actidione cf.* **Cycloheximide**

Actinomycin *cf.* Blockers *under* Pharmacology (p. 73).

← *Adrenochrome*

Hervé B61,654/51: In mice, adrenoxyl (adrenochrome) is as active p.o. as i.p. in preventing the purpura induced by X-irradiation, but it does not prolong survival.

← *Allyl Alcohol*

Varga & Fischer G76,189/69: In rats, hepatic damage produced by bromobenzene, CCl_4, allyl alcohol and thioacetamide is associated with prolonged hexobarbital sleeping time owing to interference with the hepatic microsomal metabolism of the barbiturate. However, the degree of hepatic injury does not run strictly parallel with the prolongation of the hexobarbital sleeping time; hence, the latter cannot serve as an accurate hepatic function test.

← *Amiloride*

Selye PROT. 31639,31649: In rats (100 g ♀), pretreatment with triamterene (1 mg in 1 ml water p.o. x2/day) or amiloride (300 µg in 1 ml water p.o. x2/day) fails to protect against hexobarbital, progesterone, parathion or dioxathion.

← *Amphenone*

Gaunt et al. G63,202/68: A review on the metabolic effects of metyrapone- and amphenone-derivatives.

← *Antibiotics cf. also* **Clinical Implications**

Common et al. B59,914/50: In pullets given chlortetracycline, the changes in blood calcium and serum riboflavin following folliculoid treatment are enhanced. "It seems possible from this experiment that the addition of antibiotics to a reasonably adequate diet may modify its nutritional effects in such a way that the responsiveness of the pullet to parenteral oestrogen is enhanced."

Geller et al. B98,147/54: Cortisone offers definite protection in mice given otherwise lethal doses of Escherichia intermedium endotoxin. In order to be effective, cortisone must be injected simultaneously with, or before, the endotoxin. Complicating transient bacteremia, presumably of intestinal origin, can be suppressed by antibiotics. Interference by antibiotics with cortisone protection was demonstrable only when the antibiotics were given after cortisone.

← *Anticoagulants cf. also* **Clinical Implications**

Aggeler & O'Reilly G68,730/69: In man, pretreatment with heptabarbital diminished the reduction in prothrombin level, the amount of bishydroxycoumarin in plasma and half-life of bishydroxycoumarin more markedly after p.o. than after i.v. administration of the anticoagulant. Unchanged bishydroxycoumarin was found in the stool only after p.o. administration. Presumably, part of the response to heptabarbital was caused by increased hepatic enzymic destruction of bishydroxycoumarin although, in the event of p.o. administration, decreased absorption from the gastrointestinal tract also played a role.

← *Antihistamines*

Holten & Larsen G74,395/56: In mice, hexobarbital anesthesia is considerably prolonged by benactyzine (a compound used for the treatment of psychoneuroses). The effect resembles that of SKF 525-A and when given together, the two compounds synergize each other. Extensive review of the literature and of numerous personal observations concerning the barbiturate potentiating effect of various antihistamines and spasmolytic compounds.

McColl et al. H 24,915/70: In rats, dimenhydrinate (an antihistamine) increases the abortifacient effect of various folliculoids when given conjointly with the latter on the second day of gestation. In itself, dimenhydrinate has no such effect.

Salvador et al. G 74,397/70: In cholesterol-fed rabbits, phenobarbital inhibits the increase in serum cholesterol and phospholipids as well as the development of aortic atheroma. At the same time, "the protein concentration of liver microsomes increased significantly in cholesterol-fed rabbits given phenobarbital, and phenobarbital stimulated the activity of liver microsomal enzymes that hydroxylate testosterone in the 6β-, 7α- and 16α-positions." Chlorcyclizine was ineffective in this respect.

Salvador et al. G 75,529/70: In mice, chlorcyclizine (an antihistamine) and phenobarbital reduced serum cholesterol, triglycerides and phospholipids more markedly than phenobarbital. In rats, chlorcyclizine had little or no effect on the serum concentration of cholesterol and phospholipids but the serum triglycerides were markedly reduced. These changes were not clearly related to any increase in hepatic fat content.

← Atropine

Selye A 35,659/41: "Pretreatment with atropine prevents, while vagotomy actually intensifies the anesthetic action of progesterone."

Selye A 36,210/41: "Short pretreatment with atropine increases and chronic pretreatment with this drug decreases resistance to the anesthetic action of progesterone."

← Barbiturates

Corticoids ←. *Burstein & Klaiber F 31,533/65:* Phenobarbital increases the urinary 6β-hydroxycortisol excretion in otherwise untreated, as well as in cortisol-treated, patients possibly through enzyme induction.

Conney et al. G 29,083/65: Treatment of guinea pigs with diphenylhydantoin or phenobarbital increases the 6β-hydroxylase-activity of the liver as shown by incubation of hepatic homogenates with ^{14}C-cortisol.

Birchall et al. F 76,581/66: In Cebus albifrons monkeys, phenobarbital pretreatment increases the urinary elimination of 6β-hydroxycortisol.

Hagino et al. F 69,360/66: Pentobarbital can inhibit the estradiol-induced precocious ovulation in the rat, presumably as a consequence of hepatic microsomal enzyme induction.

Burstein & Bhavnani F 77,040/67: In guinea pigs, pretreatment with phenobarbital stimulated the hepatic microsomal metabolism of cortisol, 2α- and 6β-hydrocortisol but not to the same extent. In rats, phenobarbital pretreatment enhanced hepatic microsomal 6β-hydroxylation of cortisol without causing a significant change in the overall metabolism of substrate or product. 2α-Hydroxylation of cortisol was not observed with rat liver microsomes.

Burstein F 95,565/68: Pretreatment with phenobarbital increased hepatic microsomal 2α-hydroxylation of cortisol in two strains of guinea pigs, distinguished by high and low production of hydroxylated cortisol derivatives. Under the same conditions, phenobarbital caused no significant change in the hepatic 6β-hydroxylation activity of either strain.

Marc & Morselli G 71,617/69: In rats, the half-life of i.v.-injected cortisol is greatly decreased by pretreatment with phenobarbital. Preliminary data suggest that in man the disappearance rate of exogenous cortisol is also enhanced by phenobarbital.

Morselli et al. G 76,129/70: In man, phenobarbital accelerates the plasma clearance of cortisol injected i.v.

Fluorocortisol Acetate ← *cf. also Tables 12—14*

DOC ← *cf. also Table 15*

Triamcinolone ← *cf. also Table 18*

Testoids ←. *Garren et al. G 66,660/61:* Pretreatment of rats with phenobarbital increases the metabolism of androsterone to a more polar compound by hepatic microsomes.

Conney & Klutch D 65,813/63: "Treatment of rats with phenobarbital or chlorcyclizine stimulates several fold the activity of triphosphopyridine nucleotide-dependent enzyme systems in liver microsomes that hydroxylate testosterone and Δ^4-androstene-3,17-dione."

King et al. H 16,446/68: In orchidectomized rats, phenobarbital pretreatment diminishes the effect of testosterone upon the seminal vesicles and prostate presumably as a consequence of increased hepatic microsomal enzyme production. These findings may "offer a therapeutic modality for gynecologic syndromes that are associated with overproduction of androgens."

Heinrichs & Colás H 11,717/68: Studies on the hepatic microsomal hydroxylations of 3β-hydroxyandrost-5-en-17-one (DHA) by microsomes of rats treated in vivo with phenobarbital. The effect upon such hydroxylations of aminopyrine, and SU-9055 additions to the incubation medium are also described.

Levin et al. G 64,184/69: "Treatment of immature male rats with phenobarbital or chlordane for several days prior to an injection of testosterone or testosterone propionate inhibits the growth-promoting effect of these androgens on the seminal vesicles. It is suggested that phenobarbital and chlordane decrease the action of the androgens by enhancing their metabolism."

Orrenius et al. E 8,231/69: In rats, pretreatment with phenobarbital increases the in vitro hydroxylation of testosterone by hepatic microsomal enzymes in the 2β-, 6β-, 7α-, and 16α positions.

Conney et al. E 8,232/69: The microsomal enzymes required for the 6β-, 7α- and 16α-hydroxylation of testosterone are selectively influenced, as shown by the speed of their development with age or after treatment with phenobarbital or 3-methylcholanthrene. Addition of Chlorthion in vitro to hepatic microsomes markedly inhibits the 16α-hydroxylation of testosterone, has a lesser effect on 16β-hydroxylation and no effect on 7α-hydroxylation.

Fahim et al. G 77,345/70: In rats, phenobarbital accelerates testoid metabolism as reflected by significant reductions in the weight and RNA content of male accessory sex organs.

Folliculoids ←. *Levin & Conney F 64,557/66:* In immature, intact or adrenalectomized rats, the uterine weight increase produced by small doses of estradiol i.p. is markedly inhibited by pretreatment of animals with phenobarbital. At the same time, the estradiol-metabolizing activity of hepatic microsomal enzymes is augmented. In order to demonstrate the inhibition of uterine growth, very small doses of estradiol must be used (less than 0.5 μg) and phenobarbital must be administered for several days prior to the test.

Levin et al. F 75,365/67: Phenobarbital increases the 17β-estradiol-metabolizing activity of hepatic microsomal enzymes in immature female rats. The in vitro activity is paralleled by in vivo blockade of the estradiol-induced uterine weight increase. The phenobarbital-induced resistance to the uterine weight-increasing effect of estradiol is not prevented by adrenalectomy or hypophysectomy, indicating that the barbiturate does not act through the pituitary-adrenal axis.

Conney G 69,760/67: "Pretreatment of immature female rats with phenobarbital for several days inhibits the uterotropic effect of tritiated estradiol and decreases the concentration of the labeled steroid in the uterus."

Singhal et al. G 67,770/67: Phenobarbital pretreatment inhibits the uterotrophic effect of estradiol as well as the induction of phosphofructokinase in the uterus of the ovariectomized rat. The most marked results were obtained with threshold doses of estradiol.

Levin et al. F 94,711/68: The uterotrophic action of estrone and estradiol is inhibited in phenobarbital-pretreated rats. Furthermore, "the metabolism of estradiol by liver microsomes in vitro is enhanced when the microsomes are harvested from animals pretreated with several unrelated microsomal enzyme inducers such as phenobarbital, chlordane, orphenadrine, chlorcyclizine, norchlorcyclizine and phenylbutazone. Pretreatment of rats with these chemicals also inhibits the action of estradiol on the uterus and decreases the concentration of estradiol in this organ."

Levin et al. H 894/68: Pretreatment of immature female rats with phenobarbital inhibits the uterotrophic action of synthetic folliculoids such as ethynylestradiol, ethynylestradiol-3-methyl ether (mestranol), and diethylstilbestrol. The inhibitory effect of phenobarbital upon the action of diethylstilbestrol-³H is paralleled by decreased radioactivity in the uterus, and increased diethylstilbestrol-metabolizing activity in hepatic microsomes. The uterine weight-increasing effect of synthetic luteoids such as norethindrone and norethynodrel is likewise inhibited by phenobarbital pretreatment.

Fahim et al. G 67,772/68: Phenobarbital reduces the uterotrophic action of both exogenous estradiol and endogenous folliculoids. This effect is somewhat lessened by ovariectomy. The authors consider the possibility that the barbiturate may induce steroidases not only in the hepatic microsomes, but also in the ovary. Enzyme determinations in the liver were not performed, but phenobarbital significantly increased hepatic weight and total nitrogen content.

Welch et al. F96,172/68: Pretreatment with phenobarbital accelerates the disappearance from the whole carcass of the rat of tritium-labeled estrone more markedly than that of tritium-labeled estradiol.

Fahim et al. G65,075/69: In mice, the uterotrophic action of estrone, estradiol, and stilbestrol was significantly reduced following phenobarbital pretreatment. This effect, which was accompanied by an increase in hepatic weight, is ascribed to hepatic microsomal enzyme induction. Endogenous folliculoid production is presumably likewise inhibited by phenobarbital, since the drug interferes with the maintenance of normal uterine weight in intact mice. It is suggested "that the biologic activity observed for estrogens is dependent upon the level of activity of hepatic microsomal enzymes." [The possibility that prolonged phenobarbital pretreatment may have caused uterine atrophy through the well-known stress-induced inhibition of gonadotropin secretion has not been controlled by the use of stressors which do not share the enzyme-inducing action of phenobarbital (H.S.).]

Estradiol ← *cf. also Table 16*

Various Steroids ←. *Kuntzman et al. F27,893/64:* The rat liver contains a steroid hydroxylase system which metabolizes testosterone and estradiol to more polar compounds (incubation of microsomal fraction). The steroid hydroxylase and hexobarbital oxydase systems are similar as regards the following points:

"1. Localized in liver microsomes and require TPNH and oxygen for activity.
2. Present in mammalian liver but absent in fish liver.
3. Higher activity in male Sprague-Dawley rats than in male CF1 mice.
4. Higher activity in adult male rats than in adult female rats.
5. Little or no sex difference in enzyme activity in mice.
6. Activity is higher in adult male rats than in immature rats.
7. Inhibition by the in vitro addition of SKF 525-A.
8. Activity is increased after treatment of rats with phenobarbital or chlordane.
9. Activity not increased after treatment of rats with 3-methylcholanthrene."

Conney & Schneidman F35,870/65: Pretreatment of male rats with phenobarbital stimulates the hepatic microsomal metabolism of progesterone, testosterone, Δ^4-androstene-3,17-dione, androsterone and DOC.

Conney et al. G65,135/65: In the rat, phenobarbital stimulates the hepatic microsomal metabolism of testosterone, Δ^4-androstene-3,17-dione, androsterone and estradiol, but not of corticosterone, cortisone or cortisol. Similar effects were obtained with chlorcyclizine and phenylbutazone. Administration of "the carcinogenic hydrocarbon 3-methylcholanthrene to rats caused a several-fold increase in the oxidative metabolism of certain drugs such as zoxazolamine and acetophenetidin but had little or no effect on the oxidation of hexobarbital or the hydroxylation of testosterone and Δ^4-androstene-3,17-dione." In female rats, chlordane stimulates the metabolism of estradiol to more polar metabolites. Similar observations have also been made in the mouse and dog.

Remmer & Merker G66,868/65: The hepatic Δ_{4-3}-ketoreductase activity is much higher in female than in male rats, but cannot be further increased by phenobarbital, although the barbiturate does induce two similar TPHN-dependent microsomal reductases involved in the metabolism of p-aminoazobenzol and of chloramphenicol.

Kuntzman et al. G57,741/68: The nonhypnotic barbiturate n-phenylbarbital (phetharbital) increases the formation of polar metabolites from estradiol, testosterone and DOC added in vitro to the hepatic microsomal fraction. The effect is essentially the same as that of phenobarbital. Hepatic microsomes of n-phenylbarbital-treated guinea pigs exhibit an increased capacity to introduce a 6β-hydroxyl into cortisol added in vitro. In man, chronic treatment with phetharbital greatly increases urinary excretion of 6β-hydroxycortisol but not that of 17-OHCS, suggesting that an increased adrenal output of cortisol is not responsible for the observed rise in 6β-hydroxycortisol elimination. In the guinea pig, this nonhypnotic barbiturate increases the 6β-hydroxycortisol-forming ability of the hepatic microsomes.

Ying & Meyer H13,672/69: In immature rats, the induction of ovulation by a single injection of PMS is inhibited by phenobarbital. This block was prevented by progesterone and other ovarian steroids administered 3.5 hrs after phenobarbital. The effect of the barbiturate may have been due to the induction of hepatic microsomal steroidases.

Progesterone ← *cf. also Table 17*

Pancuronium ← *cf. also Table 19*

Nonsteroidal Hormones and Hormone-Like Substances ←. *Brown & Wells F 57,759/65:* In mice, pretreatment with barbital diminishes the ovulatory response to gonadotrophic hormone preparations. It is uncertain however whether this is due to accelerated biotransformation of the pituitary factors.

Oppenheimer et al. F 99,583/68: In rats, phenobarbital increases thyroxine turnover and thyroidal function after stimulation of hepatocellular binding of thyroxine as judged by studies with radioactive thyroxine.

Schwartz et al. H 9,326/69: In rats treated with phenobarbital, the hepatic microsomes exhibit an increased ability to de-iodinate L-thyroxine and L-T3 in vitro.

Schwartz et al. H 26,012/70: In rats, the inhibition of somatic growth induced by thyroxine was enhanced by phenobarbital. At the same time, oxygen consumption was reduced and mitochondrial α-glycerophosphate dehydrogenase (GPD) activity in the liver, kidney and heart was lowered.

3,3,5-Triiodo-L-thyronine ← *cf. also Table 20*
Propylthiouracil ← *cf. also Tables 21, 22*
Epinephrine ← *cf. also Table 23*
Acetanilide ← *cf. Table 24*
Acrylamide ← *cf. Table 25*
Acrylonitrile ← *cf. Table 26*
Aminopyrine ← *cf. Table 27*
Anticoagulants ← *cf. also Tables 28, 29.*
Dayton et al. D 42,366/61: In the guinea pig, dog and man pretreatment with barbiturates antagonizes the hypoprothrombinemic effect of coumarin anticoagulants. At the same time the plasma level of the coumarin is depressed.

Cucinell et al. G 66,286/65: In the rat, dog and man, phenobarbital accelerates the metabolism of bishydroxycoumarin, diphenylhydantoin and antipyrine.

Goss & Dickhaus F 53,987/65: Phenobarbital increases the daily maintenance dose of bishydroxycoumarin in man.

Corn H 33,065/66: In man, phenobarbital or gluthethimide treatment decreases the life span of warfarin.

Robinson & MacDonald F 69,377/66: Phenobarbital antagonizes the anticoagulant effect of warfarin in man.

Barbiturates ← *cf. also Tables 30—34*
Buchel & Levy G 74,850/70: In mice, pretreatment with phenobarbital decreases pentobarbital sleeping time; this phenomenon is detectable within 24 hrs and reaches a maximum 48 hrs after phenobarbital administration. The resistance is no longer detectable in males after 96, in females after 120 hrs.

Klinger H 25,517/70: In rats, hexobarbital sleeping time is shortened following pretreatment with barbital.

Bile Pigments ← *cf. also* **Clinical Implications.** *Catz & Yaffe G 71,888/62:* In mice, pretreatment with sodium barbital i.p. increased the hepatic bilirubin-conjugating activity.

Schmid et al. G 68,199/66: Study on enhanced formation of rapidly-labeled bilirubin by phenobarbital through the stimulation of hepatic microsomal cytochromes. In the rat, the amount of bilirubin formed from non-hemoglobin sources in the liver may equal that produced on sequestration of senescent erythrocytes.

Lüders H 34,593/70: In Gunn rats, biliary bilirubin excretion is normally minimal, presumably because of a deficiency in bilirubin glucuronyltransferase activity. Phenobarbital decreases the serum bilirubin level owing to the formation of water soluble metabolites as shown by ^{14}C-bilirubin determinations.

Bromobenzene ←. *Brodie et al. G 80,473/71:* In rats, pretreatment with phenobarbital greatly facilitates the production of hepatic necrosis by bromobenzene and other chemically inert halogenated hydrocarbons. Radioautographic and other studies suggest that "a number of aromatic halogenated hydrocarbons are converted by microsomes in vitro to active intermediates which form covalent complexes with glutathione (GSH)."

Cadmium ← *cf. Table 35*
Caramiphen ← *cf. Table 36*
Carbon Disulfide ←. *Bond et al. H 18,559/69:* In rats, pretreatment with phenobarbital does not change the LD_{50} of CS_2 p.o. but results in the production of central lobular hepatic necrosis. After pretreatment with SKF 525-A these hepatic lesions no longer occur in rats pretreated with phenobarbital and then given CS_2. SKF 525-A may inhibit the production of toxic CS_2 metabolites by hepatic microsomal enzymes.

Carbon Tetrachloride ←. *Stenger et al. G 78,940/70:* In rats, pretreatment with phenobarbital in doses which cause proliferation of the SER and a decrease in hexobarbital sleeping time greatly diminished resistance to the fatal effects of CCl_4. Phenobarbital pretreatment delayed the onset of CCl_4-induced hepatic necrosis, but greatly aggravated its eventual severity. "This altered hepatotoxic response might be related either to the increase of smooth-surfaced membranes or to the augmentation of drug-metabolizing enzyme systems in the livers of the phenobarbital-pretreated animals."

Carisoprodol ← *cf. Table 37*
Chlordiazepoxide ← *cf. Table 38*
Cholesterol ←. *Jones & Armstrong F51,262/65:* In the hamster, the hepatic SER undergoes hypertrophy following treatment with phenobarbital and, at the same time, cholesterol biosynthesis is increased.

Wada et al. G67,771/67: In rats pretreated with phenobarbital, cholesterol synthesis from either acetate or mevalonate by hepatic microsomes is increased in vitro.

Wada et al. H15,247/69: In rats, cholesterol synthesis from various precursors is inhibited by CO and accelerated by phenobarbital as shown by incubation with hepatic microsomes in vitro. Cholesterol synthesis requires NADPH, molecular oxygen, and cytochrome P-450.

Salvador et al. G74,397/70: In cholesterol-fed rabbits, phenobarbital inhibits the increase in serum cholesterol and phospholipids as well as the development of aortic atheroma. At the same time, "the protein concentration of liver microsomes increased significantly in cholesterol-fed rabbits given phenobarbital, and phenobarbital stimulated the activity of liver microsomal enzymes that hydroxylate testosterone in the 6β-, 7α- and 16α-positions." Chlorcyclizine was ineffective in this respect.

Salvador et al. G75,529/70: In mice, chlorcyclizine (an antihistamine) and phenobarbital reduced serum cholesterol, triglycerides and phospholipids more markedly than phenobarbital. In rats, chlorcyclizine had little or no effect on the serum concentration of cholesterol and phospholipids but the serum triglycerides were markedly reduced. These changes were not clearly related to any increase in hepatic fat content.

Cinchophen ← *cf. Table 39*
Cocaine ← *cf. Table 40*
Colchicine ← *cf. Table 41*
DL-Coniine ← *cf. Table 42*
Croton Oil ← *cf. Table 43*
Cycloheximide ← *cf. Tables 44, 45*
Cyclophosphamide ← *cf. also Table 46.*

Cohen & Jao H27,933/70: In rats, pretreatment with phenobarbital increases the cyclophosphamide-activating enzyme system in the liver as demonstrated in vitro and, at the same time, augments mortality following treatment with cyclophosphamide in vivo. A number of observations confirmed "the thesis that the activation of cyclophosphamide by liver is mediated through the mixed function oxidase system involved in the metabolism of drugs, steroids and carcinogens."

Selye G70,466/70: In rats, cyclophosphamide intoxication can be prevented by PCN, CS-1 and spironolactone. Progesterone, ethylestrenol and norbolethone were slightly active; oxandrolone, DOC, hydroxydione and phenobarbital were inactive, whereas prednisolone, triamcinolone, estradiol and thyroxine actually decreased resistance to this drug.

Digitalis ← *cf. Clinical Implications*
Diisopropyl Fluorophosphate ← *cf. Table 52*
Diphenylhydantoin ← *cf. also Table 53.*
Cucinell et al. G66,286/65: In the rat, dog and man, phenobarbital accelerates the metabolism of bishydroxycoumarin, diphenylhydantoin and antipyrine.

Dyes ←. *Klaassen & Plaa F99,395/68:* In rats, pretreatment with phenobarbital accelerated the plasma clearance of BSP. There was no change in hepatic storage but significant increases of in vitro metabolism, biliary transport maximum and bile flow were observed. With a dibrominated analog of BSP and with indocyanine green, which are apparently not biotransformed before excretion; enhanced plasma clearance was also elicited by phenobarbital. It is assumed "that the enhanced biliary excretion of these dyes is an important factor after phenobarbital treatment and that the role of increased biotransformation is not as important for the enhanced plasma disappearance of these dyes as might be expected from the effect of phenobarbital on the biologic half-life of other substances."

Reyes et al G71,233/69: In rats, phenobarbital "enhanced hepatic uptake of an organic anion, bromsulphalein, in vivo and simultaneously increased the amount of Y, a hepatic cytoplasmic organic anion-binding protein. This study supports the postulate that Y is a major determinant in the selective hepatic uptake of certain organic anions from plasma." Induction of Y may enhance hepatic uptake and metabolism of various substrates following treatment with phenobarbital and other inducers.

Dipicrylamine ← *cf. Table 54*
Emetine ← *cf. Table 55*
Ethanol ←. *Koff et al. G76,179/70:* In rats, pretreatment with phenobarbital reduces the hepatic steatosis produced by a single dose of ethanol. The inhibition is associated with a striking elevation of blood ethanol and no increase in blood lactate. In phenobarbital pretreated animals, the enhanced incorporation of fatty acids into triglyceride by micro-

somal preparations, after in vivo ethanol treatment, also failed to occur. Furthermore, liver slices and supernatant fractions of phenobarbital-pretreated rats exhibit a diminished capacity to oxidize ethanol. "It is suggested that the inhibitory effect of phenobarbital pretreatment on the ethanol-induced fatty liver is due to inhibition of the alcohol dehydrogenase-mediated oxidation of ethanol."

Ethylene Glycol ← cf. Table 56
Ethylmorphine ← cf. Table 57
Flufenamic Acid ← cf. Table 58
Fluphenazine ← cf. Table 59
Ganglioplegics ← cf. Tables 61, 62
Glutethimide ← cf. Table 63
Glycerol ← cf. Table 64
Hydroquinone ← cf. Table 65
Imipramine ← cf. Table 66
Indomethacin ← cf. Table 67
Lidocaine ←. *Heinonen et al. G80,898/70:* In epileptic patients, phenobarbital decreases the plasma lidocaine level only very slightly.
LSD ← cf. Table 74
Mechlorethamine ← cf. Table 75
Mephenesin ← cf. Table 76
Meprobamate ← cf. Table 77
Mercury ← cf. Tables 78—80
Methadone ← cf. Table 82
n-Methylaniline ← cf. Table 83
Methyprylon ← cf. Table 84
α-Naphthylisothiocyanate ← cf. Table 85
Nicotine ← cf. also Table 86. *Stålhandske G80,388/70:* In mice, phenobarbital increases the metabolism of ^{14}C-labelled nicotine and accelerates its disappearance from blood and tissues. Tolerance to the fatal effect of nicotine overdosage is also increased by nicotine.
Nikethamide ← cf. Table 87
p-Nitroanisole ← cf. Table 88
Pentylenetetrazol ← cf. Table 89
Perchlorate ← cf. Table 90
Pesticides ← cf. also Tables 91—99. *DuBois & Kinoshita G66,349/68:* In mice and rats, pretreatment with phenobarbital either decreased or failed to affect the toxicity of 15 anticholinesterase organic phosphates. The only exception was OMPA whose toxicity was actually increased after phenobarbital pretreatment, but only in rats.

Carlson & DuBois H24,653/70: Male rats are much more susceptible to the insecticide 6-methyl-2,3-quinoxalinedithiol cyclic carbonate (Morestan) than females. "The toxicity to rats could not be altered by castration, administration of testosterone to females and estradiol to males. Pretreatment with phenobarbital decreased the toxicity to adult males and increased the toxicity to adult females." Chronic Morestan feeding caused hepatic enlargement and inhibition of microsomal enzymes.

Phenylbutazone ←. *Zbinden G66,033/66:* Following pretreatment with phenylbutazone or phenobarbital p.o., rats become resistant to the production of peritoneal adhesions by phenylbutazone i.p. "Since the peritoneal reaction appears to be related to a direct injury of the peritoneal cells which occurred before the drug had been absorbed into the blood stream and before it had a chance to be metabolized by the liver, it is most unlikely that the differences in local toxicity could be due to a faster removal of phenylbutazone from the general circulation."

Phenyramidol ← cf. Table 100
Physostigmine ← cf. Table 101
Picrotoxin ← cf. also Table 102. *Cole A 30,204/43:* In rats, pentobarbital and phenobarbital antagonizes strychnine or picrotoxin convulsions even if the convulsives are given long after the narcotic effect of the barbiturates has disappeared. Indeed, phenobarbital was more effective against death from strychnine when given 22 hrs than when given 20 min before strychnine. Phenobarbital was equally effective against death from picrotoxin whether given 20 min or 22 hrs before picrotoxin. It is considered unlikely that active amounts of the barbiturates would persist in the body for such a long time but their decomposition products may still possess anticonvulsant activity. [Enzyme induction is not considered (H.S.).]

Piperidine ← cf. Table 103
Pralidoxime ← cf. Table 104
Propionitrile ← cf. Table 105
Quinine ←. *Saggers et al. G73,683/70:* In rat liver microsomes, quinine is metabolized by enzymes requiring NADPH; this metabolism is increased by phenobarbital.

SKF 525-A ← cf. Table 106
Strychnine ← cf. also Table 107. *Cole A 30,204/43:* In rats, pentobarbital and phenobarbital antagonizes strychnine or picrotoxin convulsions even if the convulsives are given long after the narcotic effect of the barbiturates has disappeared. Indeed, phenobarbital was more effective against death from strychnine when given 22 hrs than when given 20 min before strychnine. Phenobarbital was equally effective against death from picrotoxin whether given 20 min or 22 hrs before picrotoxin. It is considered unlikely that active amounts of the barbiturates would persist in the body

for such a long time but their decomposition products may still possess anticonvulsant activity. [Enzyme induction is not considered (H.S.).]

Kato D46,405/61: Following pretreatment with phenaglycodol or thiopental resistance to strychnine is increased, whereas resistance to OMPA is considerably diminished in the rat.

Chiesara et al. G75,314/70: In rats, a single injection of phenobarbital suffices to stimulate the SER and to increase the hexobarbital and strychnine-metabolizing enzyme activity of the hepatic microsomes. The effect of partial hepatectomy, performed either immediately before or at various times after the administration of the inducer drug, was investigated in relation to these phenomena.

Theobromine ← *cf. Table 108*
Theophylline ← *cf. Table 109*
Thimerosal ← *cf. Table 110*
Tribromoethanol ← *cf. Table 111*
Trichloroethanol ← *cf. Table 112*
Tri-o-cresyl Phosphate ← *cf. Table 113*
D-Tubocurarine ← *cf. Table 114*
Tyramine ← *cf. Table 115*
L-Tyrosine ← *cf. Table 116*
Vitamin C ←. *Klinger et al. F62,929/65:* The normal excretion of ascorbic acid and the increase in its elimination induced by barbital are higher in male than in female rats. Orchidectomy reduced both normal excretion and its enhancement by barbital, whereas ovariectomy increased them. Thus, the sex-specific differences decreased but did not disappear completely. One week's treatment of males with stilbestrol or females with testosterone diminished ascorbic acid excretion. In mice, no sex-specific differences of this kind were observed. [The authors probably used hexobarbital although sometimes they speak of barbital (H.S.).]

Vitamin D, DHT ← *cf. also Table 117.* *Dent et al. H30,946/70; Richens & Rowe H30,947/70:* In four epileptic patients, osteomalacia developed during long-term treatment with diphenylhydantoin and barbiturates. Vitamin D exerted a curative effect. "It is suggested that drug-mediated enzyme induction may be the mechanism responsible by causing a greatly increased inactivation of vitamin D in these patients."

Hahn et al. H34,347/71: In patients on phenobarbital, osteomalacia is allegedly common, perhaps because of accelerated biotransformation of vitamin D. The hepatic microsomes of phenobarbital pretreated rats readily convert tritiated vitamin D_3 to metabolites other than 25-hydroxy-cholecalciferol, the biologically active metabolite. Presumably, "the increased incidence of osteomalacia in individuals on anticonvulsant therapy can be attributed to accelerated in vivo inactivation of vitamin D by liver microsomes."

W-1372 ← *cf. Table 118*
Zoxazolamine ← *cf. Table 119*
Various Drugs ←. *Selye G70,480/70:* In rats, phenobarbital and phetharbital inhibit intoxication with dioxathion, parathion, nicotine, hexobarbital, progesterone (anesthesia), zoxazolamine (paralysis), indomethacin (intestinal ulcers) and acute DHT-induced calcinosis. Phenobarbital does, while phetharbital does not, inhibit the toxicity of digitoxin. On the other hand, both barbiturates fail to affect the production of infarctoid cardiac necroses by fluorocortisol + Na_2HPO_4 + corn oil.

E. coli endotoxin No. 08 ← *cf. Table 123*

Pregnancy ←. *Fahim et al. G77,383/70:* In pregnant rats, phenobarbital given throughout gestation "results in a significant increase in embryonic death and a 28 per cent incidence of fetal subcutaneous hemorrhage. Placentas of treated animals weighed less than controls and exhibited a significant increase in demethylation activity."

Hepatic Enzymes ←. *Cucinell et al. G66,286/65:* In the rat, dog and man, phenobarbital accelerates the metabolism of bishydroxycoumarin, diphenylhydantoin and antipyrine.

Zbinden G66,033/66: Following pretreatment with phenylbutazone or phenobarbital p.o., rats become resistant to the production of peritoneal adhesions by phenylbutazone i.p. "Since the peritoneal reaction appears to be related to a direct injury of the peritoneal cells which occurred before the drug had been absorbed into the blood stream and before it had a chance to be metabolized by the liver, it is most unlikely that the differences in local toxicity could be due to a faster removal of phenylbutazone from the general circulation."

← *Benactyzine cf.* **Phenothiazines**

← ***Benzydamine***

Burberi et al. G80,224/70: Benzydamine, although a potent anti-inflammatory agent, does not produce gastric ulcers in the rat but prevents the production of gastric ulcers such as occur 18 hrs after s.c. administration of indomethacin. [No mention of intestinal ulcers (H.S.).]

← *Bradykinin cf. Hormone-Like Substances*

← **Bromobenzene**

Varga & Fischer G76,189/69: In rats, hepatic damage produced by bromobenzene, CCl_4, allyl alcohol and thioacetamide is associated with prolonged hexobarbital sleeping time owing to interference with the hepatic microsomal metabolism of the barbiturate. However, the degree of hepatic injury does not run strictly parallel with the prolongation of the hexobarbital sleeping time; hence, the latter cannot serve as an accurate hepatic function test.

← **Carbon Tetrachloride** *cf.* **Blockers** under **General Pharmacology** (p. 79).

← **Carcinogens**

Richardson et al. B70,382/52: Review of the literature and personal observations on the inhibition of tumor formation by one carcinogen through concurrent treatment with another.

Murphy & DuBois D28,546/58: The activity of the microsomal enzyme system which oxidizes thiophosphates to potent anticholinesterase agents is considerably higher in male than in female rats (incubation of liver homogenates with Guthion or ethyl p-nitrophenyl thionobenzenephosphonate or "EPN"). Yet, in vivo, adult males are more resistant to EPN than females perhaps because the accelerated formation of toxic oxidation products is overcompensated by a more efficient detoxication of the latter. The low enzyme activity of female livers is enhanced by pretreatment with testosterone in vivo, whereas the high activity of male livers is diminished by previous castration, partial hepatectomy or treatment with progesterone or diethylstilbestrol. SKF 525-A inhibits, whereas pretreatment with carcinogens or a protein-deficient diet enhances, the activity of the thiophosphate-oxidizing enzyme.

Conney & Burns G66,473/63: Review (25 pp., 73 refs.) on the induced synthesis of oxidative enzymes in hepatic microsomes by polycyclic hydrocarbons and drugs.

Conney & Schneidman F24,913/64: "Treatment of immature rats and dogs with phenylbutazone increased several-fold the activity of enzymes in liver microsomes that hydroxylate testosterone and Δ^4-androstene-3,17-dione. Treatment of rats with phenylbutazone or phenobarbital stimulated a minor pathway of corticosteroid metabolism to polar metabolites chromatographically similar to hydroxylated substrate. Administration of the carcinogenic hydrocarbon 3-methylcholanthrene to rats did not stimulate polar metabolite formation but markedly inhibited the microsomal metabolism of corticosteroids to metabolites chromatographically less polar than the substrate."

Conney et al. E8,232/69: The microsomal enzymes required for the 6β-, 7α- and 16α-hydroxylation of testosterone are selectively influenced, as shown by the speed of their development with age or after treatment with phenobarbital or 3-methylcholanthrene. Addition of Chlorthion in vitro to hepatic microsomes markedly inhibits the 16α-hydroxylation of testosterone, has a lesser effect on 16β-hydroxylation and no effect on 7α-hydroxylation.

Chivers et al. H25,819/70: In mice, the peak of mitotic index induced by partial hepatectomy occurs after 48 hrs. DMBA given 34—38 hrs after partial hepatectomy inhibits mitosis, whereas given after 48 hrs it increases the mitotic index.

Dewhurst & Kitchen G73,848/70: In mice, zoxazolamine paralysis is greatly shortened soon after a single dose of the carcinogen, whereas upon prolonged treatment, an inverse response is obtained. It is speculated that "an active metabolite formed in relatively small amounts may gradually accumulate or the stimulation of microsomal enzymes by the first dose might lead to enhanced conversion of a subsequent dose into an active metabolite."

Soyka et al H33,315/70: Partial hepatectomy sensitized only slightly to the anesthetic effect of 5β-pregnane-3α-ol-20-one, whereas it greatly prolonged sleeping time following treatment with progesterone and many other steroids. Neither inhibition of hepatic mixed function oxydase activity by SKF 525-A nor its stimulation by 3-MC affected the duration of pregnanolone narcosis and even phenobarbital reduced its length only slightly. These findings, and distribution studies, "suggest that termination of hypnosis is due mainly to redistribution with hepatic metabolism playing a relatively minor role." [Species not mentioned; probably rat (H.S.).]

← **Cedar Chips**

Vesell F88,031/67: In mice and rats kept on softwood bedding of either red cedar, white pine, or ponderosa pine, three drug-metabolizing hepatic enzymes (morphine N-demethylase, aniline hydroxylase, and hexobarbital oxidase) were induced. Hexobarbital sleeping time was reduced. Apparently, the drug-metabolizing enzyme mechanism of an animal can be significantly altered by changes in its natural habitat.

Hart & Adamson G69,481/69: In mice, "SKF 525-A and Lilly 18947 reduced the lethality of cyclophosphamide over a 28 day observation period, while pretreatment with phenobarbital did not change the 28 day lethality. Neither SKF 525-A nor phenobarbital had an effect on the antitumor efficacy of cyclophosphamide. Mice housed on cedar chip bedding were less susceptible to the lethal effects of cyclophosphamide, but tumor-bearing mice on this bedding showed greater antitumor response to the drug than those on hardwood bedding."

← *Chloramphenicol cf.* **Inhibitors** *under* **General Pharmacology** (p. 67).

← *Chlorcyclizine cf.* **Antihistamines**

← *Chlordane cf.* **Pesticides**

← **Chlorpromazine**

Parant D82,116/62: In mice, resistance to endotoxin is greatly decreased a few hours after adrenalectomy or hypophysectomy. Cortisone protects normal, adrenalectomized, and hypophysectomized animals against high doses of endotoxin, whereas chlorpromazine is effective only in the presence of both the adrenals and the pituitary. ACTH also protects the hypophysectomized mouse but only if slow absorption is assured.

Wurtman et al. F99,396/68: In rats, pretreatment with chlorpromazine or other phenothiazines increases the level of i.v. administered ^{3}H-melatonin in brain and blood. Chlorpromazine has no effect on the level of ^{3}H-melatonin when the latter is injected into the lateral cerebral ventricle. Since chlorpromazine inhibits the in vitro metabolism of ^{3}H-melatonin by liver slices, the drug presumably alters the tissue levels of the indole by slowing its metabolism.

← **Cholesterol**

Farson et al. A49,680/47: In dogs and rabbits, cholesterol i.v. or i.p. intensifies thiopental anesthesia. The anesthesia induced by ether inhalation was not affected but that caused by ether s.c. was prolonged. "It is reasonable to assume that any compound which elicits a depression of the central nervous system would exert an additive effect or potentiation of the action of a general anesthetic. The mechanism of action of cholesterol in these studies may be explained on such a basis."

← **Cinchophen**

Aitio & Hänninen G66,417/67: Both in intact and in adrenalectomized rats, cinchophen increased the hepatic TKT activity, but had no effect upon that of alanine and aspartate aminotransferase.

← **Cobaltous Chloride**

Tephly & Hibbeln G81,868/71: In rats, CoCl$_2$ inhibits the synthesis of P-450 and the N-dealkylation of ethylmorphine by hepatic microsomes. The induction by phenobarbital of P-450 and ethylmorphine N-demethylation are likewise prevented by CoCl$_2$, but cobalt does not influence NADPH-cytochrome c reductase either under normal conditions or after stimulation by phenobarbital.

← **Cycloheximide** *cf. also* **Blockers** *under* **Pharmacology** (p. 77).

Verbin et al. G70,538/69: In rats, single i.p. injections of cycloheximide during, following or prior to DNA synthesis induced by partial hepatectomy completely abolished the first wave of mitosis seen in regenerating liver. Presumably, "this interference with cell division can be attributed to a block in the S phase as indicated by a 98 per cent inhibition of incorporation of thymidine-C^{14} into DNA, and to a block in G-2 as evidenced by a 95 per cent inhibition of incorporation of leucine-C^{14} into protein."

Alonso G81,092/70: In rats, hepatic carcinogenesis induced by diethylnitrosamine is not prevented by cycloheximide. The associated electron microscopic changes in the liver are described.

← **Desipramine**

Jori & Pugliatti G70,112/67: In rats, in vivo and in vitro experiments suggest that desipramine reduces the activity of modaline by inhibiting its biotransformation into an active compound in the hepatic microsomes. The in vivo tests were gaged by the "tryptamine symptomatology" (hunching of the back, backward locomotion, Straub tail, salivation and clonic convulsions of the anterior paws) induced by modaline.

Levin et at. H26,593/70: In rats, CCl₄ given to immature females 24 hrs before sacrifice inhibited the activity of hepatic microsomal enzymes that hydroxylate estradiol-17β and estrone. This inhibition was reflected in vivo by an altered metabolism of estradiol-17β and estrone, by a potentiation of the uterotrophic action of folliculoids and by an increased concentration of these steroids in the uterus. By contrast, tetrachloroethylene did not influence the action of estrone. SKF 525-A and desipramine, which are also inhibitors of drug metabolism, likewise potentiate the uterotrophic action of estrone in immature rats.

← Digitalis

Pines et al. C87,661/59: Intracardiac or i.v. injections of prednisolone produce premature ventricular beats and ventricular bigeminy (ECG) in the dog. These changes can be prevented or suppressed by digitalis, chlorothiazide or chloroquine.

Selye G70,480/71: In rats, pretreatment with digitoxin offered no protection against intoxication with digitoxin, dioxathion, parathion, nicotine, hexobarbital, progesterone (anesthesia), zoxazolamine, indomethacin, acute DHT-induced calcinosis or the infarctoid cardiopathy produced by fluorocortisol + Na₂HPO₄ + corn oil.

← Dimenhydrinate cf. Antihistamines

← Dimethyl Sulfoxide (DMSO)

Highman et al. H19,382/69: In rats exposed to X-irradiation or hypoxia, i.v. injections of Streptococcus mitis produce severe bacterial endocarditis. "The radioprotective compound, DMSO, did not affect the lesions in nonirradiated animals but reduced the incidence and severity of lesions in irradiated rats."

← Diphenylhydantoin cf. also Clinical Implications and Table 136

Tyler et al. G79,955/69: In epileptic patients on diphenylhydantoin, a negative metyrapone test for pituitary insufficiency may result from increased glucuronic acid conjugation of metyrapone by the liver.

Dent et al. H30,946/70; Richens & Rowe H30,947/70: In four epileptic patients, osteomalacia developed during long-term treatment with diphenylhydantoin and barbiturates. Vitamin D exerted a curative effect. "It is suggested that drug-mediated enzyme induction may be the mechanism responsible by causing a greatly increased inactivation of vitamin D in these patients."

← Disulfiram

Scholler G75,794/70: In rats, disulfiram inhibits whereas phenobarbital aggravates, the toxic effects of chloroform anesthesia, as manifested by hepatic necroses and plasma enzyme GOT and GPT determinations.

← Ethanol

Waltman et al. H19,551/69: In women, i.v. injection of ethanol just before delivery, reduces serum bilirubin levels in their infants on the 3—5th day of life. "The findings suggest a simple, safe, and expedient agent which may be used to prevent raised levels of bilirubin in the newborn—levels which may affect mental and motor development in the first year of the infant's life."

← Ethionine cf. Blockers under General Pharmacology (p. 78).

← Ferric Dextran

Selye et al. E24,117/64: The progeria-like syndrome produced by DHT, vitamin-D₂ or vitamin-D₃ can be prevented by ferric dextran, methyltestosterone or vitamin E in the rat.

← Glucose

Lamson et al. C14,547/51: In dogs, awakening from anesthesia induced by various barbiturates, glucose i.v. (as well as certain intermediates of the tricarboxylic-acid cycle) reinitiates sleep and increases barbiturate penetration into the brain. The effect is presumably due to interference with the brain barrier.

Lamson et al. B89,712/52: In guinea pigs, epinephrine when injected i.p. on awakening from barbiturate anesthesia, produced a return to sleep. A similar effect was produced by glucose, lactate or glutamate. However, in adrenalectomized animals, only epinephrine was effective.

← Glutethimide cf. Clinical Implications

← Hydrazine

Kato et al. H15,638/69: The inhibitory action of various hydrazine derivatives on the oxidation of pentobarbital and carisoprodol, and the N-demethylation of aminopyrine, closely parallel their lipid solubility.

← Indomethacin

Jeremy & Towson G77,324/70: In patients with rheumatoid arthritis, ^{14}C-2-indomethacin plasma clearance is accelerated, and urinary excretion decreased, by acetylsalicylic acid. "The study showed interference between aspirin and indomethacin, the mechanism possibly being due to decreased gastro-intestinal absorption. This could account for clinical reports that the combination of the two drugs was no better than aspirin alone."

Selye G70,480/71: In rats, pretreatment with indomethacin offered no significant protection against indomethacin itself, digitoxin, dioxathion, parathion, nicotine, hexobarbital, progesterone (anesthesia), zoxazolamine, DHT or the infarctoid cardiopathy produced by fluorocortisol + Na_2HPO_4 + corn oil.

Iodine

Voss & Walther E53,093/60; Walther & Voss G71,664/60: In rabbits, inhibition of thyroid function by iodine accelerates the recovery time of the spinal cord following anoxia induced by temporary compression of the abdominal aorta.

← Iproniazid cf. Inhibitors under General Pharmacology (p. 68).

← Isoproterenol

Zwadyk & Harrison H19,753/70: Soterenol is considerably more potent than the structurally related isoproterenol in reducing endotoxin lethality in chick embryos and mice.

← Lactone

Cosmides et al. G45,832/56: "Tetrahydrofurfuryl alcohol and butyrolactone protected chicken embryos from digitoxin toxicity. They also prolonged the time for A-V blockade to appear when perfused simultaneously with digitoxin in the frog heart. Tetrahydrofurfuryl alcohol abolished cardiac arrhythmias in the dog and permitted the failing heart to return to relative regularity. The results appear to support the theory that the unsaturated lactone of digitoxin is essential for cardiotonic activity and that a chemically related structure may compete for the same receptor to antagonize its action on the myocardium."

← Methoxyflurane

Berman & Bochantin G75,502/70: In rats, subanesthetic concentrations or methoxyflurane decreased hexobarbital sleeping time, increased aminopyrine demethylase activity in the hepatic microsomal fraction and raised resistance to otherwise fatal doses of methoxyflurane.

← Methylenedioxyphenyl Compounds

Fujii et al. G77,242/70: In mice, 61 methylenedioxyphenyl compounds (including synthetic insecticide synergists, natural products, and related open-ring analogs) showed approximately parallel potency as regards hepatic microsomal-enzyme inhibition manifested by prolongation of hexobarbital narcosis and zoxazolamine paralysis.

←Metyrapone

Currie et al. D48,292/62: In rats, the production of adrenal necrosis by DMBA is prevented by metyrapone, but not significantly influenced by ACTH.

Jull F74,180/66: In rats, the induction of mammary carcinomas by DMBA is inhibited by progesterone, DOC and metyrapone.

Gaunt et al. G63,202/68: Metyrapone has been compared to other inhibitors of adrenal steroidogenesis, mostly acting at different sites. Some of these comparisons are shown on p. 583.

Jellinck et al. F96,053/68: In rats, the DMBA-induced adrenocortical necrosis is prevented both by metyrapone (which inhibits 11β-hydroxylation and the synthesis of corticosterone) and by Su-9055 (which inhibits 17α-hydroxylation of steroids). Since the rat adrenal normally does not synthesize 17α-hydroxylated corticoids it is suggested that "competition for specific receptor sites in the adrenals occurs between the metabolites of DMBA, Metopirone and Su-9055 rather than the original compounds."

Wheatley F98,919/68: In rats, adrenal cortical necrosis produced by DMBA or 7-OH-MBA is prevented by metyrapone and related inhibitors of corticoid synthesis (Su 9055, Su 10603) but not by Ay 9944 or aminoglutethimide (Elipten). No correlation was found between the influence of these drugs on corticoidogenesis and their ability to protect against adrenal necrosis. Pretreatment with ethionine abolished the protective action of metyrapone, Su 9055 and Su 10603. It is concluded that these drugs protect by virtue of

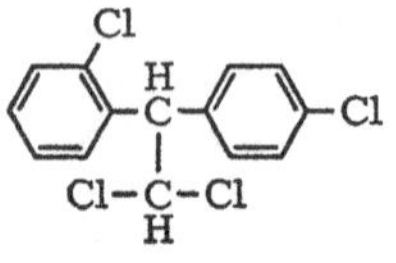

o,p'-DDD

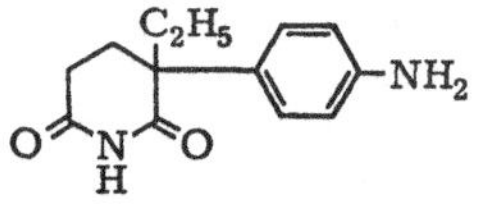

Aminoglutethimide

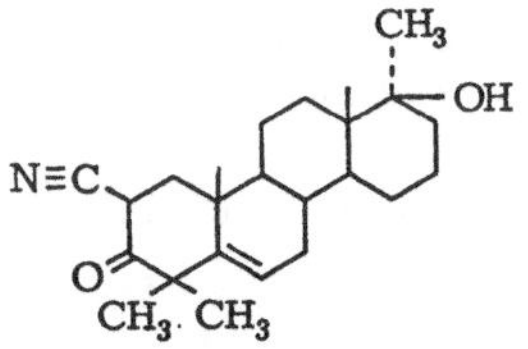

Cyanotrimethylandrostenolone

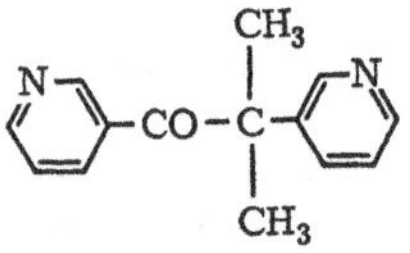

Metyrapone

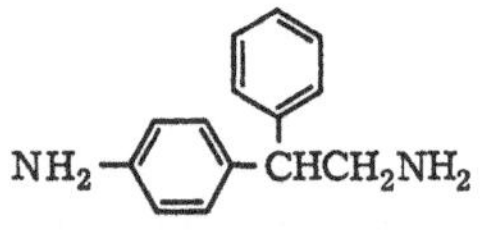

2-(p-aminophenyl)-2-phenylethylamine (SKF-12185)

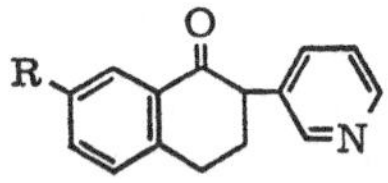

Su-9055 - R=H
Su-10603 - R-Cl

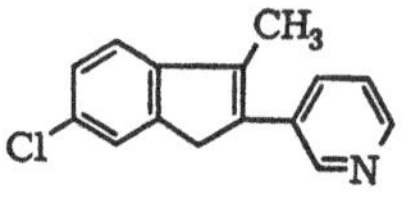

Su-8000

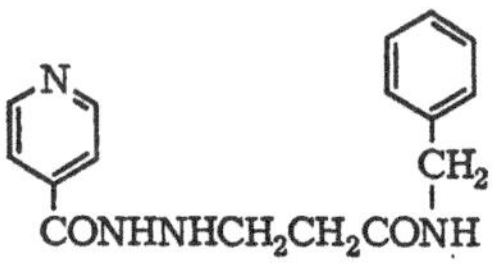

Nialamide

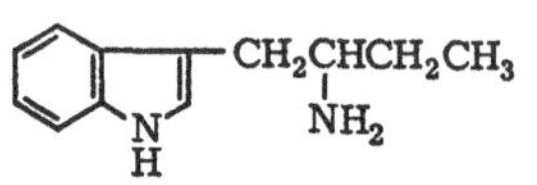

α-Ethyltryptamine

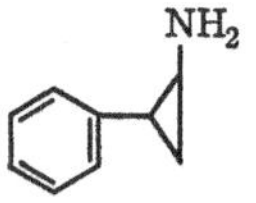

Tranylcypromine

their hepatic drug-metabolizing enzyme inducing ability, not by direct effect upon corticoidogenesis. Brief reference is made to the observation "that pretreatment of rats with Su 4885 (Metyrapone), while initially potentiating the action of Nembutal, subsequently led to a considerably enhanced rate of detoxification and a shorter duration of narcosis."

Kahl G69,105/69: Addition of metyrapone to liver microsomes of mice does not interfere with electron transport. The point of attack of the inhibitor on the hydroxylation of substrate appears to be on cytochrome P-450.

Leibman G66,210/69: Metyrapone [SU-4885, 2-methyl-1,2-bis(3-pyridyl)-1-propanone] is a potent inhibitor of adrenal steroid 11β-hydroxylase which also blocks hydroxylation of steroids at other points during their biogenesis in the adrenal gland. The 11β-hydroxylase system of the adrenal cortex is dependent upon NADPH oxygen and cytochrome P-450 thus resembling hepatic microsomal enzymes. It is of interest therefore that metyrapone prolongs hexobarbital sleeping time in rats and inhibits the oxidative metabolism of hexobarbital, aminopyrine and acetanilide by hepatic microsomes in vitro.

Netter et al. G71,785/69: In mouse liver microsomes, the inhibition by metyrapone of p-nitroanisole and N-monomethyl-p-nitroaniline was shown to be competitive. The degree of inhibition was correlated to the amount of metyrapone bound to cytochrome P-450. On the other hand, metyrapone does not seem to displace naphthalene from its binding to P-450. Possibly, simultaneous binding of substrate and inhibitor may occur at different binding sites of the same enzyme.

Szeberényi & Garattini G66,140/69: In rats, pretreatment with metyrapone delays the disappearance from the blood of i.v.-injected cortisol presumably because the compound "inhibits the liver enzyme system(s) responsible for inactivation of adrenal steroids." This effect must be taken into consideration in evaluating the metyrapone test for pituitary function.

Selye & Mécs G60,095/70: In rats, metyrapone inhibits the catatoxic effect of spironolactone against digitoxin and indomethacin poisoning.

Magalhães & Magalhães G76,648/70: In rats, metyrapone causes hypertrophy of the hepatic SER and almost complete glycogen depletion. The relative volume of the SER (calculated by stereological methods) is also increased. These changes may be related to the increase by metyrapone of non-11β-hydroxylated corticoids.

Dardachti et al. G79,006/71: In rats, metyrapone stimulates the proliferation of SER, even after adrenalectomy.

Selye PROT. 26163: In rats, metyrapone (at dose levels which produce no obvious signs of toxicity) prolongs the anesthetic effect of progesterone, DOC and hydroxydione.

Table 125. *Effect of metyrapone upon progesterone, DOC and hydroxydione anesthesia*

Treatment[a]	Anesthesia[b] (Positive/Total)		Mortality[b] (Dead/Total)	
	Control	Metyrapone	Control	Metyrapone
None	—	0/10	—	0/10
Progesterone	0/10	6/10 **	0/10	1/10
DOC	0/10	6/10 **	0/10	1/10
Hydroxydione	0/10	6/9 ***	0/10	0/9

[a] Progesterone, DOC acetate and hydroxydione sodium hemisuccinate 5 mg in 1 ml oil, i.p. were administered once to each of the two groups respectively designated. The controls received no other treatment, whereas the experimental animals were given metyrapone 8 mg in 0.1 ml oil, i.p., once, 30 min before the steroid anesthetic.

[b] The severity of anesthesia was read after 3 hrs for progesterone and DOC, after 1 hr for the more rapidly acting hydroxydione. Mortality was listed 24 hrs after metyrapone administration "Exact Probability Test."

For further details on technique of tabulation cf. p. VIII.

DOC ← Metyrapone: Netter et al. *G53,255/67;* Colby et al. *G75,695/70*

17α-Hydroxyprogesterone ← Metyrapone: Netter et al. *G53,255/67*

Acetanilide, Aminopyrine ← Metyrapone + Phenobarbital, Mouse: Netter et al. *G53,255/67*

Carcinogens ← Metyrapone: Currie et al. *D48,292/62*;* Dao et al. *D67,132/63*;* Helfenstein et al. *G76,331/63*;* Dao et al. *F21,633/64;* Wheatley *F98,919/68**

N-Monomethyl-p-nitroaniline, p-Nitroanisole ← Metyrapone + Phenobarbital: Netter et al. *G53,255/67*

← **Nicotine**

Beckett & Triggs G70,154/67: In man, nicotine excretion in the urine following intravenous injection of nicotine, inhalation of nicotine vapor or smoking is greater among nonsmokers than among smokers. The difference is ascribed to the induction of drug-metabolizing enzymes by nicotine. Following discontinuation of smoking, the accelerated nicotine metabolism persists for many months.

Welch et al. G65,788/69: No detectable benzpyrene hydroxylase or aminoazo dye N-demethylase activity was observed in the placentas of women who did not smoke but these enzymes were found in the placentas of smokers. In rats, treatment with 3,4-benzpyrene, 1,2-benzanthracene, 1,2,5,6-dibenzanthracene, chrysene, 3,4-benzofluorene, anthracene, pyrene, fluoranthene, perylene, or phenanthrene during pregnancy increased benzpyrene hydroxylase activity in the placenta.

Stålhandske & Slanina G73,544/70: In mice, repeated i.p. injections of nicotine impaired nicotine metabolism in vitro, whereas nicotine p.o. slightly increased its own metabolism. "However, the increase was not significant and the stimulating effects of nicotine on hepatic metabolism under the experimental conditions used, must be considered to be limited."

Selye G70,480/71: In rats, pretreatment with nicotine offered some protection against intoxication with digitoxin and indomethacin but not against any of the other toxicants tested.

← **Nikethamide**

Brazda & Baucum D48,613/61: In rats, five days' pretreatment with nikethamide decreases pentobarbital sleeping time and increases the pentobarbital-destroying potency of hepatic microsomes in vitro.

← *Nitrogen Mustard*

Brin & McKee C31,261/56: In the rat, various stressors (total body X-irradiation, nitrogen mustard, starvation) as well as cortisone increase glutamic-aspartic and glutamic-alanine transaminase activities in the liver. Adrenalectomy decreases the activity of these enzymes. The glutamic-alanine enzyme is more sensitive to stress than the glutamic-aspartic enzyme.

← *Pentylenetetrazol*

Dille & Seeberg 84,277/41: In cats, the acute toxicity of pentylenetetrazol is not influenced by bilateral nephrectomy, whereas liver damage induced by yellow phosphorus greatly increases sensitivity to pentylenetetrazol.

Selye A 36,443/42: In rats, the anesthesia produced by progesterone or DOC can be interrupted by pentylenetetrazol. Conversely, these anesthetic steroids protect the rat against otherwise fatal doses of pentylenetetrazol.

Kerman A 43,330/47: In the rat, DOC anesthesia is sometimes preceded by a state of catalepsy which can be interrupted by pentylenetetrazol.

← *Pesticides cf. also Clinical Implications*

Nichols & Hinnigar C 48,736/57: In dogs, DDD tends to produce abortion and increases the toxicity of barbiturates.

Welch & Conney F 36,508/65: Observations on the hydroxylation of testosterone by microsomes of the rat liver showed that different types of hydroxylation are selectively inhibited by various organophosphate insecticides. Treatment of immature male rats with phenobarbital revealed a selective increase in the various hydroxylase activities. "These results suggest that the 16α-hydroxylation of testosterone is catalysed by a different enzyme system than that required for the 6β- and 7α-hydroxylation of testosterone."

Conney et al. G 65,135/65: In the rat, phenobarbital stimulates the hepatic microsomal metabolism of testosterone, Δ^4-androstene-3,17-dione, androsterone and estradiol, but not of corticosterone, cortisone or cortisol. Similar effects were obtained with chlorcyclizine and phenylbutazone. Administration of "the carcinogenic hydrocarbon 3-methylcholanthrene to rats caused a several-fold increase in the oxidative metabolism of certain drugs such as zoxazolamine and acetophenetidin but had little or no effect on the oxidation of hexobarbital or the hydroxylation of testosterone and Δ^4-androstene-3,17-dione." In female rats, chlordane stimulates the metabolism of estradiol to more polar metabolites. Similar observations have also been made in the mouse and dog.

Azarnoff et al. G 42,999/66: In the rat, pretreatment with DDD markedly shortens anesthesia produced by various steroids and barbiturates. Simultaneously, there is proliferation of the SER and a rise in the level of hepatic hexobarbital-metabolizing enzyme. In dogs, DDD decreases hexobarbital sleeping time, but prolongs pentobarbital anesthesia. Cortisone prevents the prolongation of pentobarbital sleep.

Conney et al. F 73,731/66: In rats, pretreatment with phenobarbital, chlorcyclizine, phenylbutazone, chlordane or DDT stimulates in vitro hydroxylation of various anesthetic steroids and decreases their anesthetic effect in vivo. "The ability of liver microsomal-enzyme stimulators to decrease the central depressant effects of progesterone raises the possibility that liver microsomal-enzyme stimulators may also alter physiologic actions of endogenous steroids in the body."

Kupfer & Peets G 40,053/66: In the rat, o,p'-DDD stimulates the cortisol- and hexobarbital-metabolizing ability of the hepatic microsomal fraction.

Peakall F 90,310/67: In pigeons pretreated with DDT or dieldrin, incubation of the hepatic microsomal fraction with progesterone and testosterone revealed increased rates of steroid metabolism.

Welch et al. F 76,642/67: "The in vitro addition of organic phosphorothionate insecticides, such as parathion, malathion and chlorthion, or halogenated hydrocarbon insecticides, such as chlordane and DDT, inhibited the liver microsomal hydroxylation of testosterone. Treatment of rats with chlorthion for 10 days inhibited the liver microsomal hydroxylation of testosterone, estradiol-17β, progesterone and deoxycorticosterone, whereas chronic treatment of rats with chlordane or DDT stimulated the hydroxylation of these steroids." Chlorthion had a more marked inhibitory effect upon the 16α-hydroxylation than on the 6β- or 7α-hydroxylation. Chlordane or DDT-pretreatment stimulated 6β-, 7α- and 16α-hydroxylation of testosterone, but particularly the latter reaction. Apparently, the microsomal enzyme system responsible for 16α-hydroxylation of testosterone differs from the systems regulating 6β- and 7α-hydroxylation.

Conney et al. G43,018/67: Review of the literature and personal observations on the induction of steroid hydroxylases in hepatic microsomes by various pesticides. "In contrast to the stimulatory effect of halogenated hydrocarbon insecticides on hepatic steroid hydroxylases, treatment of rats with organophosphate insecticides, such as chlorthion, inhibits the liver microsomal metabolism of several steroid hormones. Chlorthion has a greater inhibitory effect on the 16α-hydroxylation of testosterone than on the 6β- or 7α-hydroxylation of this steroid, suggesting that separate enzyme systems are required for the various hydroxylation reactions."

Good & Ware G76,670/69: In mice, feeding of the insecticides endrin or dieldrin did not significantly affect fertility, fecundity or the number of young produced per day.

Lacassagne et al. G74,932/69: In rats, production of hepatic cancers by DAB is powerfully inhibited by Δ⁵-pregnenolone, DOC or DDD. Various other steroids give less clear-cut results.

Levin et al. G64,184/69: "Treatment of immature male rats with phenobarbital or chlordane for several days prior to an injection of testosterone or testosterone propionate inhibits the growth-promoting effect of these androgens on the seminal vesicles. It is suggested that phenobarbital and chlordane decrease the action of the androgens by enhancing their metabolism."

Fahim et al. G81,358/70: In rats, "DDT administered to cycling females or estrogen-maintained castrated animals causes decreased uterine weight and alkaline phosphatase."

Greim G76,366/70: In patients with constitutional hyperbilirubinemia (Gilbert- or Meulengracht syndrome) as well as in Cushing's disease, the stimulation of hepatic microsomal-enzyme induction by DDT or DDD is followed by remissions. Because of its corticolytic effect in the dog, it is assumed that DDD acts by blocking corticoid production, but in vitro experiments with rat liver microsomes, show that DDD and DDT increase the metabolism of corticoids and hence their therapeutic effect is ascribed to this action.

Kimbrough et al. G81,969/71: In rats, DDT and dieldrin reduce hexobarbital sleeping time, increase liver weight and cause proliferation of the SER with the formation of a typical mitochondria which often contain numerous longitudinally arranged parallel cristae.

← *Phenaglycodol*

Kato D46,405/61: In the rat, following pretreatment with phenaglycodol or thiopental, resistance to strychnine is increased, whereas resistance to OMPA is considerably diminished.

← *Phentolamine*

Selye G70,480/71: In rats, pretreatment with phentolamine protected against intoxication with digitoxin and dioxathion but not against any of the other nonadrenergic drugs tested.

← *Phenothiazines*

Holten & Larsen G74,395/56: In mice, hexobarbital anesthesia is considerably prolonged by benactyzine (a compound used for the treatment of psychoneuroses). The effect resembles that of SKF 525-A and when given together, the two compounds synergize each other. Extensive review of the literature and numerous personal observations concerning the barbiturate-potentiating effect of various antihistamines and spasmolytic compounds.

Wattenberg & Leong F38,140/65: In rats, the production of adrenal necrosis by DMBA is inhibited by phenothiazine and several of its derivatives which increase benzpyrene hydroxylase activity.

← *Phenylbutazone*

Kersten & Staudinger G67,796/56: Addition of phenylbutazone to pig liver homogenates inhibits the enzymic inactivation of cortisone in vitro.

Conney & Schneidman F24,913/64: "Treatment of immature rats and dogs with phenylbutazone increased several-fold the activity of enzymes in liver microsomes that hydroxylate testosterone and Δ⁴-androstene-3,17-dione. Treatment of rats with phenylbutazone or phenobarbital stimulated a minor pathway of corticosteroid metabolism to polar metabolites chromatographically similar to hydroxylated substrate. Administration of the carcinogenic hydrocarbon 3-methylcholanthrene to rats did not stimulate polar metabolite formation but markedly inhibited the microsomal metabolism of corticosteroids to metabolites chromatographically less polar than the substrate."

Kuntzman et al. G67,761/66: In man, phenylbutazone increases the urinary excretion of 6β-hydroxycortisol, and simultaneously decreases the nonpolar 17-OHCS. These findings are in agreement with earlier in vitro observations showing that the hydroxylation of cortisol to 6β-hydroxycortisol by guinea pig liver microsomes is increased following pretreatment with phenylbutazone in vivo.

Welch et al. G47,232/67: "When rats received 75 mg/kg of phenylbutazone twice a day for 1 day, a high incidence of gastric ulcers was observed 24 hours later. However, when rats received the same dose daily for 14 days, the metabolism of the drug was markedly stimulated and no ulcers were observed."

Bailey et al. H450/68: In rabbits, cholesterol atherosclerosis is inhibited by cortisone, prednisone, triamcinolone, methylprednisolone, dexamethasone and 9α-fluorocortisol, although hyperlipemia is aggravated. Phenylbutazone and oxyphenylbutazone also diminished cholesterol atherosclerosis, although to a lesser extent and without augmenting hyperlipemia.

Klinger et al. H28,896/70: In rats, phenylbutazone reduces hexobarbital sleeping time and increases the fresh weight of the liver as well as the ability of the hepatic 9000 g supernatant to enhance aminophenazone-N-demethylation. An increase in the ascorbic acid concentration of the liver was noted only in young animals, but the urinary excretion of ascorbic acid was as pronounced as after barbital treatment. Phenylbutazone administration to the pregnant mother failed to elicit an induction effect in the fetuses as judged by hepatic ascorbic acid determinations and by ultrastructural studies of the fetal livers. Proliferation of the SER was obtained by phenylbutazone in 10-day-old or older rats, often in association with an increase in the number of lysosomes and mitochondrial changes, as well as by evidence of intrahepatic cholestasis.

Yesair et al. G75,388/70: In rats, salicylic acid i.v. decreases the plasma concentration of indomethacin. Simultaneously, the urinary excretion of ^{14}C-indomethacin is decreased, whereas biliary and fecal excretions are increased. Phenylbutazone, chlorogenic acid and acetic acid had no effect on plasma radioactivity. Probenecid increased plasma concentration of indomethacin. "The specificity of salicylic acid in decreasing concentrations of indomethacin in plasma of rats and of probenecid in increasing indomethacin concentrations in plasma of both rat and man may arise from the similarity in structure of the benzoyl group of the three compounds."

Selye G70,480/71: In rats, phenylbutazone pretreatment protects against intoxication with dioxathion, parathion, nicotine, hexobarbital, progesterone and indomethacin but not against poisoning with digitoxin, zoxazolamine, DHT or the infarctoid cardiopathy produced by fluorocortisol + Na_2HPO_4 + corn oil.

← *Probenecid*

Yesair et al. G75,388/70: In rats, probenecid increased the plasma concentration of indomethacin.

← *Puromycin cf. Inhibitors under General Pharmacology* (p. 75).

← *Pyridinolcarbamate*

Shimamoto G70,917/69: In cholesterol-fed rabbits, pyridinolcarbamate induced the regression of the atheromatous lesions and their replacement by regenerating smooth muscle fibers.

← *RES-Blockers*

Holck D28,543/49: Adult male rats are more resistant than females to toxic doses of picrotoxin. Such a sex difference is absent in one-month-old rats. Castration lowers picrotoxin resistance in rats of either sex. Testosterone raises picrotoxin resistance in normal and especially in spayed females, but not in males. Blockade of the RES abolished the sex difference but corticosterone failed to influence it.

Kass D35,079/60: "The antiendotoxic activity of corticosteroids seems to be sufficiently different from the anti-inflammatory activity to offer the possibility that these two activities may be structurally separable. The anti-inflammatory action of corticosteroids is apparently related largely to an effect on vascular permeability, whereas the antiendotoxic activity in some way involves the reticuloendothelial system."

DiCarlo et al. F74,536/65: Several RES stimulants prolong pentobarbital sleeping time in the mouse. There is no evidence of this effect being due to induction of pentobarbital-metabolizing enzymes. "An alternative hypothesis is that the stimulants induce the biological inactivation of corticosterone, which may regulate barbiturate hydroxylase as well as tryptophan pyrrolase and certain transaminases of liver microsomes."

Wooles & Borzelleca F93,374/66: Repeated administration of zymosan i.v. prolongs hexobarbital, pentobarbital and barbital sleeping time in the mouse. This effect is ascribed to stimulation of the RES.

Agarwal & Berry G66,480/67: "Four hours after zymosan administration, cortisone was able to induce mouse liver tryptophan pyrrolase production almost at a normal rate and, under these conditions, protected mice against a concurrent injection of endotoxin. Administration of zymosan, at either 2 or 4 hours after cortisone administration, resulted in little change in tryptophan pyrrolase activity while endotoxin, when similarly administered, caused a rapid decline in liver tryptophan pyrrolase activity. ... Glucan and zymosan, like endotoxin, increased tyrosine-α-ketoglutarate transaminase activity in intact but not in adrenalectomized mice. Zymosan and thorotrast, unlike endotoxin, neither lowered liver carbohydrate levels nor influenced cortisone induced neosynthesis of liver glycogen. These results suggest a cause and effect relationship between inducibility of key liver enzymes and survival against stress."

Berry et al. E 7,069/67: In mice, endotoxin, zymosan, glucan, and saccharated iron oxide (all RES-blocking agents) lower hepatic TPO and increase TKT in vivo, but not in vitro. Endotoxin also prevents the induction of TPO by cortisone, especially when the latter is given 2—4 hrs after endotoxin. The transaminase responds normally. Zymosan and glucan do not prevent the induction of TPO by cortisone. "Perhaps one might relate these effects to the dose of colloid used in relation to its toxicity, but even large doses of saccharated iron oxide capable of killing mice fail to prevent the induction of tryptophan pyrrolase by cortisone."

Timar et al. F 82,696/67: In rats pretreated with India ink i.v., phenobarbital elimination is delayed.

← Reserpine

Radouco-Thomas et al. E 60,201/57: In guinea pigs, the analgesic effect of meperidine is diminished by reserpine and counteracted by concurrent administration of norepinephrine.

Westermann et al. C 83,072/60: In the rat, large doses of reserpine produce an alarm reaction with an increase in the hepatic tryptophan peroxydase activity associated with lowered brain serotonin and norepinephrine. Hypophysectomy prevents these responses.

← Salicylic Acid

Jeremy & Towson G 77,324/70: In patients with rheumatoid arthritis, ^{14}C-2-indomethacin plasma clearance is accelerated, and urinary excretion decreased, by acetylsalicylic acid. "The study showed interference between aspirin and indomethacin, the mechanism possibly being due to decreased gastro-intestinal absorption. This could account for clinical reports that the combination of the two drugs was no better than aspirin alone."

Katczak et al. G 75,716/70: In rabbits chronically treated with acetylsalicylic acid, the liver shows considerable dilatation of the endoplasmic reticulum whose spaces are filled with electron dense material. At the same time, various enzyme activities of the liver are changed and the glycogen content of the hepatocytes is diminished.

Yesair et al. G 75,388/70: In rats, salicylic acid i.v. decreases the plasma concentration of indomethacin. Simultaneously, the urinary excretion of ^{14}C-indomethacin is decreased, whereas biliary and fecal excretions are increased. Phenylbutazone, chlorogenic acid and acetic acid had no effect on plasma radioactivity. Probenecid increased plasma concentration of indomethacin. "The specificity of salicylic acid in decreasing concentrations of indomethacin in plasma of rats and of probenecid in increasing indomethacin concentrations in plasma of both rat and man may arise from the similarity in structure of the benzoyl group of the three compounds."

Selye G 70,480/71: In rats, acetylsalicylic acid or sodium salicylate protected against progesterone anesthesia and indomethacin-induced intestinal ulcers. Acetylsalicylic acid, unlike sodium salicylate, also offered some protection against zoxazolamine paralysis and sodium salicylate against parathion intoxication but neither of these salicylates protected against poisoning with digitoxin, dioxathion, nicotine, hexobarbital or DHT, nor did they prevent the infarctoid necroses produced by fluorocortisol + Na_2HPO_4 + corn oil.

← Soterenol

Zwadyk & Harrison H 19,753/70: Soterenol is considerably more potent than the structurally-related isoproterenol in reducing endotoxin lethality in chick embryos and mice.

← Sucrose

Kato & Takanaka F 88,660/67: Observations on the in vivo and in vitro detoxification of zoxazolamine, hexobarbital, pentobarbital, strychnine, carisoprodol, and OMPA show that sucrose feeding or starvation for 48 hrs before the tests markedly decreases the hepatic microsomal detoxication of those substrates, which are less toxic for male than for female rats. It is assumed that sucrose depresses the synthesis of hepatic microsomal enzymes.

← Sulfur

Sakurai E67,662/25: In cats, unlike in rabbits, thiosulfate inhibits methemoglobin formation following treatment with aniline or sodium nitrite.

Myers & Ferguson A48,023/28: In rabbits, intoxication with tincture of iodine s.c. is counteracted by sodium thiosulfate i.v. or p.o.

Young & Taylor A48,227/30; A48,535/31: In rabbits, sodium thiosulfate does not appreciably decrease the toxicity of mercury compounds.

Kabelik 9,032/32: In guinea pigs, sodium or magnesium thiosulfate i.p. offers considerable protection against otherwise lethal anaphylactic shock. This "anti-anaphylaxis" persists several days. Even better results are obtained with the serum of horses which have received sodium thiosulfate i.v. 4 hrs before bleeding. The serum of unpretreated horses is ineffective. The protective action of "thiosulfate serum" cannot be due to the presence of thiosulfate, since activity persists after no more thiosulfate can be detected by chemical means in the serum. The protective factor can be extracted from the serum by ethanol.

Schreiber A48,020/33: Review on the detoxifying action of sulfur compounds (particularly SH- and SS-groups) upon various drugs.

Vandestrate A48,036/33: Contrary to earlier claims, sodium thiosulfate does not protect the guinea pig against tuberculin.

Chambon & Bouvet A48,279/33: In dogs returned to an atmosphere of pure air after CO-intoxication, treatment with sodium thiosulfate does not improve detoxication as had been previously suggested.

Hochwald 36,114/36: In guinea pigs, anaphylactic shock is diminished by pretreatment with cysteine or sodium thiosulfate.

Wendt A48,250/38: Review (19 pp., 264 refs.) on the use of sodium thiosulfate in the treatment of various intoxications and diseases with special reference to the detoxication of arsenic and cyanides.

Vauthey & Vauthey A48,670/47: In guinea pigs, acute intoxication with mercuric cyanide (excitation, paralysis, death) is partially combated by 20 days' pretreatment with 100 mg of ascorbic acid per day s.c. A similar moderate protection is obtained by sodium thiosulfate and, to a much lesser extent, by glucose. [The very preliminary experiments suggest that none of the protective actions was very evident (H.S.).]

Patt et al. B54,521/49: In rats, resistance to total body X-irradiation is increased by pretreatment, 5 min before exposure, with cysteine (but not with cystine) i.v. Injection of cysteine immediately after exposure is ineffective.

Patt et al. B54,522/50: In rats and mice, cysteine-pretreatment increases resistance to whole body X-irradiation. Cysteine, methionine, sodium sulfide, and ascorbic acid are ineffective under similar conditions. When administered after X-irradiation, cysteine also fails to protect.

Bacq et al. E91,032/51: In mice, cysteamine i.p. protects against total body X-irradiation.

Stavinoha et al. C94,628/59: Review and personal observations on protection by various sulfur compounds against thallium intoxication.

Cahn & Herold G72,124/60: Review (9 pp., 58 refs.) on the importance of sulfhydryl groups in the detoxication of various agents.

Passow et al. G38,172/61: Review (39 pp., 130 refs.) on the general pharmacology of heavy metals with special reference to their detoxication by sulfur compounds.

Langendorff F42,481/65: Review on radioprotective agents with special reference to sulfur containing compounds.

Lumper & Zahn G72,128/65: Review (38 pp., 187 refs.) on the biochemistry of disulfide exchange reactions with special reference to their detoxicating value.

Cier et al. F85,815/67: In mice, the protection against total body X-irradiation given by 5-HT is considerably increased by concurrent treatment with thiosulfate. Various other radioprotective compounds likewise offer better protection, and are less toxic if administered conjointly than if given singly.

Varga & Fischer G76,189/69: In rats, hepatic damage produced by bromobenzene, CCl_4, allyl alcohol and thioacetamide is associated with prolonged hexobarbital sleeping time owing to interference with the hepatic microsomal metabolism of the barbiturate. However, the degree of hepatic injury does not run strictly parallel with the prolongation of the hexobarbital sleeping time; hence, the latter cannot serve as an accurate hepatic function test.

← Tetrachloroethylene

Levin et al. *H 26,593/70:* In rats, CCl_4 given to immature females 24 hrs before sacrifice inhibited the activity of hepatic microsomal enzymes that hydroxylate estradiol-17β and estrone. This inhibition was reflected in vivo by an altered metabolism of estradiol-17β and estrone, by a potentiation of the uterotrophic action of folliculoids and by an increased concentration of these steroids in the uterus. By contrast, tetrachloroethylene did not influence the action of estrone. SKF 525-A and desipramine, which are also inhibitors of drug metabolism, likewise potentiate the uterotrophic action of estrone in immature rats.

← Thiadiazoles cf. Sulfa Drugs

← Threonine

Sidransky et al. *G 65,724/69:* In rats, forcefed a threonine-devoid diet for 3—7 days, hepatic protein synthesis is enhanced as shown by various techniques. This increase is further augmented by cortisone, and causes a shift in hepatic polyribosomes toward heavier aggregates.

← Tolbutamide cf. Pancreatic Hormones

← Tryptamine

Langendorff & Koch *C 36,881/57:* In mice, both tryptamine and 5-HT offered protection against X-irradiation, whereas benzedrine and d,l-ephedrine were ineffective.

← Triamterene

Selye *PROT. 31649:* In rats (100 g ♀), pretreatment with triamterene (1 mg in 1 ml water p.o. x2/day) or amiloride (300 μg in 1 ml water p.o. x2/day) fails to protect against hexobarbital, progesterone, parathion or dioxathion.

← Vitamin A

Ehrlich & Hunt *G 55,237/68:* In rats, vitamin A has no effect upon wound healing but it overcomes the inhibitory effect of cortisone.

Selye *G 70,480/71:* In rats, pretreatment with vitamin A offered no significant protection against digitoxin, dioxathion, parathion, nicotine, hexobarbital, progesterone, zoxazolamine, indomethacin, DHT or the infarctoid cardiopathy produced by fluorocortisol + Na_2HPO_4 + corn oil.

← Vitamin-B_{12}

Bengmark & Olsson *E 34,736/63:* Review and personal observations on the effect of vitamin-B_{12} upon hepatic regeneration following partial hepatectomy in the rat.

← Vitamin C

Vauthey & Vauthey *A 48,670/47:* In guinea pigs, acute intoxication with mercuric cyanide (excitation, paralysis, death) is partially combated by 20 days pretreatment with 100 mg of ascorbic acid per day s.c. A similar moderate protection is obtained by sodium thiosulfate and, to a much lesser extent, by glucose. [The very preliminary experiments suggest that none of the protective actions was very evident (H.S.).]

Selye *G 70,480/71:* In rats, pretreatment with large doses of vitamin C offered no significant protection against digitoxin, dioxathion, parathion, nicotine, hexobarbital, progesterone (anesthesia), indomethacin, acute DHT intoxication or the infarctoid cardiopathy produced by fluorocortisol + Na_2HPO_4 + corn oil. Ascorbic acid actually aggravated zoxazolamine intoxication.

← Vitamin D

Selye *G 70,480/71:* In rats, pretreatment with vitamin D_2 offered no significant protection against intoxication with digitoxin, dioxathion, parathion, nicotine, hexobarbital, progesterone (anesthesia), zoxazolamine, indomethacin, acute DHT poisoning or the infarctoid cardiac necroses produced by fluorocortisol + Na_2HPO_4 + corn oil.

← Vitamin E

Tuchweber et al. *D 65,261/63:* Both methyltestosterone and vitamin E prevent the production of a progeria-like syndrome by DHT in the rat.

Selye et al. *E 24,117/64:* The progeria-like syndrome produced by DHT, vitamin-D_2 or vitamin-D_3 can be prevented by ferric dextran, methyltestosterone or vitamin E in the rat.

Cawthorne et al. *H 26,441/70:* In rats, the acute toxicity of CCl_4 p.o. is greater in males than in females. Vitamin E and various antioxidants exert a protective effect. It is suggested that the protection may be partly dependent upon the induction of hepatic microsomal enzymes.

Selye G70,480/71: In rats, pretreatment with vitamin E offered some protection against dioxathion intoxication, hexobarbital and progesterone anesthesia, and acute DHT intoxication, but not against any of the other toxicants tested.

← W-1372

Selye G70,480/71: In rats, W-1372 protects against intoxication with dioxathion, parathion, hexobarbital, progesterone (anesthesia), zoxazolamine and indomethacin but not against digitoxin, nicotine, acute DHT intoxication or the infarctoid cardiopathy produced by fluorocortisol $+$ Na_2HPO_4 $+$ corn oil.

← Xanthine

Ravdin et al. B25,566/39: In rats, xanthine, allantoin, caffeine, sodium ricinoleate and suspensions of colloidal carbon injected s.c. protect the liver against injury from chloroform, presumably as a consequence of the resulting inflammatory reaction which is associated with the absorption of protein split products. This would also explain the protective effect of various hepatic extracts (including Yakriton) and of high-protein diets.

← Varia

Fastier et al. C37,038/57: In mice, chloral hydrate sleeping time is increased by **epinephrine, norepinephrine, phenylephrine, methoxamine, 5-HT, histamine, ergotamine, yohimbine and atropine.** "It is suggested that some, at least, of the drugs which prolong the effects of hypnotics do so by virtue of a hypothermic action." **Vasopressin, cortisone and DOC** did not prolong chloral hydrate sleeping time at the doses tested.

Kato & Vassanelli D40,237/62: "Rats pretreated with **phenobarbital, phenaglycodol, glutethimide, nikethamide, chlorpromazine, triflupromazine, meprobamate, carisoprodol, pentobarbital, thiopental, primidone, chloretone, diphenylhydantoine and urethane** showed an accelerated metabolism of meprobamate and, at the same time, a diminished duration of sleeping time and paralysis due to meprobamate." SKF 525-A accelerated meprobamate metabolism and counteracted the action of the enzyme inducers. In hypophysectomized or adrenalectomized rats, phenobarbital still increased meprobamate metabolism in vitro.

Conney & Schneidman F35,870/65: Treatment of young male rats with phenobarbital stimulated the liver microsomal metabolism of progesterone, testosterone, Δ^4-androstene-3,17-dione, androsterone, and DOC to polar metabolites identified in most cases as hydroxylated derivatives of the substrates. These in vitro effects were associated with a decreased hypnotic action of high doses of these steroids. Similar effects in vitro and in vivo were obtained with **chlorcyclizine, phenylbutazone or chlordane.**

Kuntzman et al. F55,537/65: In the rats, anesthesia produced by progesterone, DOC, androsterone, or Δ^4-androstene-3,17-dione is inhibited by phenobarbital. Progesterone anesthesia is also inhibited by **chlorcyclizine-, phenylbutazone-, chlordane-** and **DDT-**pretreatment. These effects are tentatively ascribed to a stimulation of hepatic drug-metabolizing enzyme synthesis.

Burns et al. G66,103/67: **Review** (8 pp., 22 refs.) on "Drug Effects on Enzymes" with special reference to chronic toxicity tests.

Groppetti & Costa H31,959/69: In adult male rats, the disappearance of amphetamine is faster than in adult females. Estradiol retards the rate of **amphetamine** disappearance in adult males. Such potent hepatic microsomal enzyme inducers as **phenobarbital, 3-MC,** or **diphenylhydantoin** do not change the tissue levels of amphetamine.

Pérez E8,836/69: A **review** (270 pp., numerous refs.) on the role of the liver in drug detoxication and the hepatotoxic activity of certain drugs (Spanish).

Jori et al. G81,674/70: In the rat, there is linear correlation between sleeping time and brain pentobarbital concentration. This correlation was abolished or modified by various drugs, suggesting that **SKF 525-A, DDT** and low doses of **chlorpromazine** act only by modifying barbiturate metabolism, whereas **amphetamine,** high doses of chlorpromazine and **diazepam** affect pentobarbital sleeping time without altering its metabolism.

Shafer & Adicoff G80,179/70: In dogs, **tetrahydrofurfuryl alcohol** (THFA), despite its resemblance to the **lactone** moiety of **digoxin** offers no protection against the latter compound in vivo. The authors emphasize that despite these "negative results, the development of a specific nontoxic pharmacological antagonist to digitalis would be of major clinical importance." [These investigators appear to be unaware of the inhibition of digitalis toxicity by spironolactone (H.S.).]

Calhoun et al. H34,806/71: In immature rats, the uterotrophic effect of **mestranol** or **norethynodrel** was affected by numerous drugs.

"Pretreatment with phenobarbital or SKF 525 A was found to decrease and increase, respectively, the uterine wet weight in controls as well as in mestranol-treated groups. Of the other drugs tested, only tolbutamide increased uterine wet weights in both control and mestranol-treated groups. In addition, the response to mestranol was increased following pretreatment with p-aminosalicylic acid, chlorpromazine, and imipramine and decreased following diphenylhydantoin, phenylbutazone, or scopolamine pretreatment. The response to norethynodrel was decreased after pretreatment with phenobarbital or diphenylhydantoin and increased following SKF 525 A pretreatment."

← DIET

Dietary factors undoubtedly exert an important influence upon defensive reactions in general and upon the induction of microsomal enzymes in particular. For example, the protein intake is a critical factor involved in maintaining the **folliculoid**-inactivating system of the liver.

A good deal of work has been done on the influence of dietary factors on the detoxication of **barbiturates**. In mice, starvation prolongs hexobarbital sleeping time and diminishes the ability of isolated hepatic microsomes to metabolize this drug. Following repeated periods of fasting (as after other types of stress), hexobarbital hypnosis is also prolonged in male rats. Allegedly, hexobarbital detoxication by hepatic microsomes of rats is optimal if the diet contains about 3% of the calories in the form of corn oil (or equivalent amounts of linoleate). Both higher and lower essential fatty acid concentrations are detrimental.

The toxicity of **carcinogens** and **chloroform** is also considerably influenced by the diet.

In rats, 24 hrs fasting after a single injection of **indomethacin** can prevent intestinal ulcer formation, whereas earlier or later fasting had no such effect. The intestinal ulcers could also be prevented by ligature of the common bile duct; consequently it is possible that fasting acts through its influence upon bile secretion.

Pesticide detoxication is likewise modified by nutritional factors. In rats kept on a protein-deficient diet, the activity of the thiophosphate-oxidizing system is enhanced. The detoxication of heptachlor (as that of hexobarbital) proceeds most favorably if the diet contains about 3% of the calories in the form of corn oil or of equivalent amounts of linoleate.

Much attention has been given also to the action of nutritional factors upon the detoxication of **other drugs** and on the activity of various **hepatic enzyme systems** as well as on liver regeneration after **partial hepatectomy** but for corresponding data the reader is referred to the Abstract Section.

Steroids ←

György E 86,573/45: Review of the literature and personal observations on the influence of the diet upon the hepatic detoxication of estrone in the rat.

Vanderlinde & Westerfeld B 51,537/50: "The estrogen draining through the liver from mesenterically implanted pellets of estrone in castrate rats was inactivated when the rats were maintained on: 1) chow ad libitum, 2) normal or 50% restricted intake of a 21% purified casein diet. The liver estrogen inactivating system was not maintained by: 1) an 8% purified casein diet ad libitum, or 2) 50% of the usual intake of chow. The results are consistent with the concept that protein intake is the critical dietary factor involved in maintaining the estrogen inactivating system in the liver."

Drugs ←

Barbiturates ←. *Dixon et al. G 65,886/60:* In mice, starvation prolongs sleeping time after hexobarbital i.p. and simultaneously diminishes the ability of isolated hepatic microsomes to metabolize the drug.

Kalyanpur et al. F99,270/68: Review of the literature and personal observations on the effect of dietary factors upon barbital sleeping time in rats.

Hässler et al. H23,853/69: Male rats are more resistant than females to the anesthetic effect of hexobarbital. In rats raised under extreme conditions of stress (cold or repeated periods of fasting) hexobarbital sleeping time is prolonged.

Caster et al. G73,426/70: In rats, hexobarbital and heptachlor detoxication by hepatic microsomes in vitro, is optimal if the diet contains about 3% of the calories in the form of corn oil (or equivalent amounts of linoleate). Both higher and lower levels of fatty acids are detrimental for the detoxication of these substrates and this was confirmed by determinations of hexobarbital sleeping time in vivo. The results are interpreted as indicating that an optimum amount of essential fatty acid is required for the most efficient functioning of the hepatic microsomal drug-metabolizing system.

Weiner et al. H24,942/70: In rats, glucagon, alloxan and starvation all increased hexobarbital sleeping time. This effect was markedly antagonized by insulin. Perhaps, cyclic AMP may be involved since theophylline greatly increases the action of glucagon. This synergism also occurred in isolated, perfused rat livers and, hence, "inhibition of hexobarbital metabolism by cyclic AMP would appear to be mediated in the liver."

Carbon Tetrachloride ←. *Nayak et al. G80,728/70:* In rats, a protein-free diet or starvation caused deterioration of the ER and diminution of drug-metabolizing enzymes, but failed to make the hepatocytes less susceptible to the effects of CCl_4.

Carcinogens ←. *Brown et al. G57,030/54:* "The activity of an enzyme system in mouse and rat liver which N-demethylates 3-methyl-4-monomethylaminoazobenzene has been found to depend on the nature of the diet. The lowest activity occurred when a grain or purified diet was fed. The activity of mouse liver approximately doubled when any of several commercial chows was fed; the activity of rat liver increased about 30 per cent. The factor was also contained in a number of aged or otherwise treated animal products, such as an old cholesterol preparation, liver extracts, and peptones. A variety of pure sterols were inactive, but could be made active by peroxidation."

Chloroform ←. *Ravdin et al. B25,566/39:* In rats, xanthine, allantoin, caffeine, sodium ricinoleate and suspensions of colloidal carbon injected s.c. protect the liver against injury from chloroform, presumably as a consequence of the resulting inflammatory reaction which is associated with the absorption of protein-split products. This would also explain the protective effect of various hepatic extracts (including Yakriton) and of high-protein diets.

Digitoxin ←. *Selye PROT. 24423:* In rats (100 g ♀) fasting 24 hrs before or after administering 2 mg of digitoxin p.o. failed to prevent the development of convulsions and actually seemed to aggravate the resulting mortality.

Indomethacin ←. *Brodie et al. G67,797/69:* In rats given a single injection of indomethacin s.c., starvation during the following 24 hrs completely prevented intestinal ulcer formation, whereas starvation for 24 hrs on the second, third, or second + third day had no such effect. Intestinal ulcers could also be prevented by ligature of the common bile duct. When segments of small intestine were isolated by Thiry-Vella loops, ulceration was prevented in the loops but not in the adjacent anastomosed intestine.

Selye PROT. 24733,25025,24423: In rats (100 g ♀) complete fasting during a 24 hrs period before or after the injection of 3 mg of indomethacin s.c., or even 24 hrs before and continuing until 24 hrs after this injection, failed to prevent the development of perforating intestinal ulcers.

Pesticides ←. *Murphy & DuBois D28,546/58:* The activity of the microsomal enzyme system which oxidizes thiophosphates to potent anticholinesterase agents is considerably higher in male than in female rats (incubation of liver homogenates with Guthion or ethyl p-nitrophenyl thionobenzenephosphonate or "EPN"). SKF 525-A inhibits, whereas pretreatment with carcinogens or a protein-deficient diet enhances, the activity of the thiophosphate-oxidizing enzyme.

Caster et al. C73,426/70: In rats, hexobarbital and heptachlor detoxication by hepatic microsomes in vitro, is optimal if the diet contains about 3% of the calories in the form of corn oil (or equivalent amounts of linoleate). Both higher and lower levels of fatty acids are detrimental for the detoxication of these substrates and this was confirmed by determinations of hexobarbital sleeping time in vivo. The results are interpreted as indicating that an optimum amount of essential fatty acid is required for the most efficient functioning of the hepatic microsomal drug-metabolizing system.

Varia ←. *Conney & Burns G67,166/62:* Review on the effect of starvation on drug metabolism with special reference to microsomal enzymes.

Kato & Gillette F 5,638/64: In female rats, 3 days starvation "increases the activity of TPNH-dependent enzymes that catalyze the metabolism of TPNH, aniline, aminopyrine, p-nitrobenzoate, neotetrazolium, and neoprontosil, but does not alter the activity of TPNH-cytochrome c reductase. In contrast, starvation of male rats decreases the activity of aminopyrine demethylase, although it increases the activity of aniline hydroxylase and does not alter the activity of nitroreductase, TPNH-cytochrome c reductase or TPNH oxidase." Sucrose fed to rats of either sex for 3 days lowers the activity of all these enzymes, but does not interfere with their induction by phenobarbital.

Kato & Gillette F 57,816/65: The ability of rat liver microsomal enzymes to inactivate various substrates is greater in males than in females but the sex difference varies with the substrate. There is a more than 3-fold sex difference with aminopyrine and hexobarbital but virtually none with hydroxylation of aniline and zoxazolamine. In male rats, starvation impairs sex-dependent enzymes which metabolize aminopyrine and hexobarbital but enhances those that hydroxylate aniline. On the other hand, in female rats, starvation increases the specific activity of the aminopyrine and hexobarbital-metabolizing enzymes as well as aniline hydroxylase. Starvation does not alter the metabolism of hexobarbital and enhances that of aminopyrine by microsomes of castrated rats but impairs the metabolism of these compounds by microsomes of methyltestosterone-treated castrates.

Kato G66,471/67: "The metabolism of hexobarbital, aminopyrine and aniline by liver microsomes were increased in rats fasted for 72 hrs and they were drastically decreased by refeeding on a standard diet as well as on sucrose. ... The relationship between the activities of drug metabolisms and NADPH dehydrogenase and content of P-450 was discussed."

Kato & Takanaka F 88,660/67: Observations on the in vivo and in vitro detoxication of zoxazolamine, hexobarbital, pentobarbital, strychnine, carisoprodol, and OMPA showed that starvation for 48 hrs before the tests markedly decreases the hepatic microsomal detoxication of those substrates, which are less toxic for male than for female rats. Sucrose feeding had an effect similar to that of starvation and it is assumed that sucrose depresses the synthesis of hepatic microsomal enzymes.

Kato et al. H 11,854/69: "The administration of thyroxine or starvation resulted in marked decrease in the hydroxylation of pentobarbital and hexobarbital and N-demethylation of aminopyrine in male rats, whereas the hydroxylation of aniline and zoxazolamine and N-demethylation of N-methylaniline were significantly increased."

Partial Hepatectomy ← cf. also Effect of Partial Hepatectomy Upon Nutritional Disorders

Brues et al. A 45,962/36: In rats submitted to partial hepatectomy, "the number of cells in the residual fragment shows no significant increase in the first 24 hours" although the mass of the liver remnant increases about 50%. After the first day, cell number and liver mass increase approximately at the same rate. The effect of various dietary constituents upon hepatic regeneration is described.

Hepatic Enzymes ←

Brin & McKee C 31,261/56: In the rat, various stressors (total body X-irradiation, nitrogen mustard, starvation) as well as cortisone increase glutamic-aspartic and glutamic-alanine transaminase activities in the liver. Adrenalectomy decreases the activity of these enzymes. The glutamic-alanine enzyme is more sensitive to stress than the glutamic-aspartic enzyme.

Freedland et al. G 66,662/62: The phenylalanine hydroxylase activity of rat liver increases with age from embryonic life to 50—60 days and then declines to stabilize at a lower level in females than in males after maturity. Fasting and diets deficient in phenylalanine cause a rapid decrease in this enzymic activity.

Gillette G 67,333/67: Brief review on the effect of dietary factors upon hepatic microsomal-enzyme induction.

Freedland et al. H 2,949/68: Review (5 pp., 33 refs.) on the relationship of nutritional and hormonal influences in hepatic enzyme activity.

Harada et al. H15,156/69: The acyl-CoA synthetase activity of the rat liver increases 2—3-fold during alloxan diabetes, fasting, or high-fat diet feeding.

Lane & Mavrides H12,953/69: Cortisol caused a greater increase of hepatic tyrosine aminotransferase in hypophysectomized than in adrenalectomized rats. In general, elevation of enzyme activity after cortisol was inversely proportional to the initial enzyme level, and the latter was in turn higher on protein-rich than on protein-poor diets.

Yuwiler et al. H9,994/69: Comparative observations on fasted and cortisol-injected rats led to the conclusion that "the natural stress of fasting is accompanied by alterations in some corticoid-inducible enzymes, but that these changes are not analogous to those obtained following glucocorticoid administration."

← MICROORGANISMS, VACCINES AND PARASITES

Pneumococcal infection raises the hepatic TPO in intact but not in adrenalectomized mice. In rats infected with **malaria** (P. berghei), the hepatic microsomal metabolism of ethylmorphine, aniline, p-nitroanisole and hexobarbital progressively decrease and correspondingly hexobarbital sleeping time is prolonged. However, the malarial infection does not prevent the induction of microsomal enzymes by phenobarbital.

Endotoxin shock is associated in rabbits with a release of hepatic lysosomal acid hydrolases. This effect is prevented by glucocorticoids but not by DOC. It is assumed that the glucocorticoids may protect against endotoxin shock by decreasing the liberation of potentially harmful lysosomal enzymes.

In mice, hepatic TPO is lowered by S. typhimurium endotoxin, which also prevents the induction of the enzyme by concurrent injection of cortisone. In the intact unlike in the adrenalectomized mouse, the endotoxin induces TKT almost as well as does cortisone.

← Bacteria

Rapoport et al. G53,334/68: Pneumococcal infection raised the hepatic TPO-activity in intact, but not in adrenalectomized, mice. Cortisol increased TPO-activity both in control and in pneumococcus-infected mice, but only if administered early after inoculation. Later during the course of infection, some inhibitory factor develops which counteracts the induction of TPO by cortisol.

Einheber et al. G75,665/70: In mice infected with P. berghei, hexobarbital sleeping time is prolonged. "This may be due to a disturbance in function of hepatocellular smooth endoplasmic reticulum and its associated drug-metabolizing enzymes because phenobarbital treatment, which ordinarily stimulates an increase of the latter, corrects the 'defect' in hexobarbital sleeping time."

McCarthy et al. G75,511/70: In rats infected with malaria (P. berghei) "the hepatic microsomal metabolism of ethylmorphine, aniline, p-nitroanisole and hexobarbital showed progressive decreases in rates over the 8-day period. The decreases in metabolism were accompanied by progressive increases in hexobarbital sleeping time." The malarial infectoin did not prevent the induction of microsomal enzymes by phenobarbital.

← Bacterial Toxins

Weissmann & Thomas D35,555/62: In rabbits, endotoxin shock is associated with the release of hepatic lysosomal acid hydrolases (β-glucuronidase, cathepsin). This effect is prevented by glucocorticoids, but not by DOC. "Thus, glucocorticoids, in a variety of experimental situations, appear to decrease the liberation of potentially harmful enzymes from lysosomes, and may in fact function physiologically to stabilize the boundaries of these subcellular particles."

Berry et al. G67,237/66: S. typhimurium endotoxin lowers liver TPO in mice and prevents the induction of the enzyme by concurrent injection of cortisone. It lowers, but does not prevent, substrate induction. Actinomycin D has a similar effect on TPO. In the intact mouse, the endotoxin induces TKT almost as well as does cortisone, but not in the adrenalectomized animal. Actinomycin D, on the other hand, has an effect on this transaminase similar to that on TPO.

← IMMUNE REACTIONS

Comparatively little work has been done on the influence of immune reactions upon resistance to nonimmunologic pathogens. In rats with adjuvant arthritis, the hepatic microsomal N-demethylase and $NADPH_2$-oxidase enzyme activity, as well as the levels of P-450, are reduced. This implies a diminished capacity for the oxidative metabolism of steroids and drugs.

Morton & Chatfield G73,681/70: In rats with adjuvant arthritis, "the liver microsomal N-demethylase and $NADPH_2$-oxidase enzyme activity and levels of cytochrome P-450 are greatly reduced. This implies a diminished capacity for the oxidative metabolism of steroids and foreign compounds in adjuvant arthritic rats which should influence the toxicity and half-life of any administered compound. The ability of the liver to form β-glucuronide conjugates is also reduced."

← HEPATIC LESIONS

Steroids ←

The role of the liver in the detoxication of steroids is now well established. The first observations along these lines gave somewhat variable results but in ovariectomized rats, hepatic damage induced by CCl_4 appeared to increase sensitivity to threshold amounts of estrone.

More conclusive results were obtained in rats by the demonstration that partial hepatectomy greatly increases their sensitivity to the anesthetic effect of DOC, whereas nephrectomy is virtually ineffective in this respect. It was subsequently demonstrated that such partial hepatectomy also increases the anesthetic effect of many other steroids, including progesterone, pregnanedione, pregnanediol, testosterone, estradiol and even the nonsteroidal folliculoid, stilbestrol. Since this operation does not increase sensitivity to many other anesthetics (e.g., ether, $MgCl_2$), it was concluded "that the liver is the site at which all the above mentioned (steroid and stilbene) compounds are normally detoxified."

In immature rabbits, estradiol and progesterone given s.c., are much more effective in causing uterine changes than if administered p.o., presumably because an important portion of the injected steroids is inactivated during its passage through the liver.

In ovariectomized rats, the uterotrophic effect of estradiol is reduced 12 hrs after partial hepatectomy; it increases only later, as hepatic regeneration progresses. Hence, contrary to virtually every other report, it was concluded that the presence of hepatic tissue is essential for the folliculoid effect and that the liver actually activates estradiol. This view has not received confirmation by subsequent investigators.

In orchidectomized rats poisoned with CCl_4, implantation of testosterone into the spleen fails to increase prostatic weight, presumably because even the severely-damaged liver can detoxicate this steroid.

In rats, an ^{14}C-marked androstene derivative was eliminated mainly in the feces and to a much lesser extent in the urine. In rats bearing bile-duct fistulas, the major fraction of the isotopic carbon is excreted in the bile, but after choledochus ligature the ^{14}C is almost quantitatively recovered from the urine. In rats with bile-duct ligature, testosterone prolongs survival and inhibits the body weight loss, but its effect upon the prostate is diminished. Curiously, estradiol has been claimed to exert inverse effects in all these respects.

In rats, progesterone given i.v. was extensively metabolized within one hour, even after total evisceration (including liver, kidneys and adrenals). Among the recovered metabolic products of progesterone, there were no polar metabolites, similar to the conjugates of glucuronic or sulfuric acid. Some steroids such as desoxycortisone (Cpd. S) produce convulsions instead of the usual anesthesia, when given in large amounts to rats; allegedly partial hepatectomy does not sensitize to this convulsive effect of desoxycortisone. These observations have not yet been confirmed, but it is difficult to interpret them on the basis of the generally accepted view that hepatic insufficiency augments the effects of steroids by diminishing their degradation. Of course it is conceivable that lack of hepatic tissue also interferes with metabolic processes necessary for muscular contraction and thereby compensates for the delay in steroid degradation with respect to the convulsive effect.

In hepatectomized cats, the elimination of endogenous cortisol and corticosterone is greatly delayed, and in totally eviscerated animals it is completely abolished. Perhaps part of the extrahepatic steroid elimination occurs in the intestine.

In rats, spironolactone shortens the half-life of its main metabolite (the dethioacetylated 4,6-dienone) and partial hepatectomy delays the blood clearance of this metabolite. Apparently, spironolactone accelerates its own hepatic metabolism.

In rats, the activity of the hepatic enzymes metabolizing progesterone is decreased within 16 hrs following partial hepatectomy and reaches a minimum on the 4—5th post-operative day.

Pincus & Martin A 34,939/40: Following liver damage induced by CCl_4, threshold doses of estrone become more efficacious in producing vaginal estrus in ovariectomized rats. Although the results are inconstant and not very pronounced, they suggest "that liver damage by CCl_4 results in a decreased inactivation of administered estrone."

Selye A 35,003/41: First description of the anesthetic effect of steroids. Among those tested in rats, DOC and progesterone were most potent, several testoids and folliculoids showed mild hypnotic activity (often complicated by convulsions), whereas cholesterol, stigmasterol and Δ^4-cholestenone were inactive. Partial hepatectomy greatly increased sensitivity to anesthesia induced by DOC, whereas bilateral nephrectomy caused only a slight prolongation of the sleeping time, which may have been due to nonspecific stress.

Selye A 35,150/41: Partial hepatectomy sensitizes the rat to the production of anesthesia by DOC, progesterone, testosterone, estradiol, and stilbestrol. "Since this operation does not increase sensitivity to other anesthetics such as ether and magnesium chloride, but is known to sensitize animals to the action of anesthetics which are detoxified in the liver (e.g., tribromethanol), it appears most probable that the liver is the site at which all the above mentioned compounds are normally detoxified."

Leblond 82,066/42: Even 20 mg of pregnanediol i.p. produced only little or no anesthesia in intact young female rats, whereas in partially hepatectomized animals it elicited profound narcosis. "It is concluded, therefore, that pregnanediol is at least partly detoxified by the liver and is probably not the last link of the various compounds that may result from progesterone degradation in the rat."

Leblond A 55,928/42: In partially hepatectomized rats, pregnanediol and pregnanedione produce a much more pronounced anesthetic effect than in intact controls. The "detoxification of these substances by the liver is not essentially dependent upon the path of absorption; it is not due to storage in the liver or to excretion in the bile, but is the result of an inactivation by the liver cells."

Selye A 36,447/42: The partially hepatectomized immature female rat is particularly sensitive to the anesthetic effect of various steroids and represents a suitable test object for the detection of this activity.

György E 86,573/45: Review of the literature and personal observations on the influence of the diet upon the hepatic detoxication of estrone in the rat.

Masson & Hoffman B 513/45: In immature rabbits pretreated with estradiol, progesterone s.c. is much more effective in causing progestational changes in the uterus than if administered p.o. In the partially hepatectomized rabbit, even comparatively small doses of progesterone are active in this respect, "indicating that the liver plays an important role in the inactivation of progesterone in the rabbit." Earlier data on the role of the liver in the inactivation of progesterone are reviewed.

Roberts & Szego A 49,254/47: In ovariectomized rats, the uterotrophic effect of estradiol was markedly reduced 12 hrs after partial hepatectomy and thereafter increased to or even above the normal level in proportion to the ensuing liver regeneration. Contrary to earlier reports, it is concluded that the liver is essential for the folliculoid effect, and that hepatic tissue activates rather than inactivates estradiol.

Grayhack & Scott B 58,923/51: In orchidectomized rats poisoned with CCl_4, implantation of testosterone propionate into the spleen fails to increase prostatic weight, whereas under identical conditions, testosterone propionate implanted s.c. does stimulate the prostate. Apparently, even the severely damaged liver can detoxicate testoids.

Szego & Roberts B 73,573/53: In rats, partial hepatectomy diminishes the "estrogenic effect" of estradiol as judged by increased uterine water imbibition. Since various stressors exert a similar effect, this imbibition might have been due to stress but neither hypophysectomy nor adrenalectomy prevent it. "It seems evident that a major portion of this inhibition must be referable to the removal of functional hepatic tissue, which appears to be necessary for estrogen activity."

Hyde et al. D 99,140/54: In rats, 17α-methyl-C^{14}-Δ^5-androstene-3β,17β-diol administered by gavage was mostly eliminated in the feces and, to a lesser extent, in the urine. "Rats with two types of bile fistula excreted the major fraction of administered isotopic carbon in the bile. Almost quantitative recovery of the administered C^{14} was obtained in the urine of rats after ligation of the bile ducts."

Giuliani C 15,153/55: In rats with bile duct ligature, testosterone prolongs survival and inhibits body weight loss, but its effect upon the prostate is diminished. Estradiol exerts inverse effects in all these respects.

Berliner & Wiest C 22,807/56: Progesterone given i.v. is extensively metabolized in one hour by totally eviscerated rats, even if the kidneys and adrenals are also removed. After one hour, 7 compounds could be isolated from the tissues of these animals, although there were no polar metabolites similar to the conjugates with glucuronic or sulfuric acid, and the 7 isolated compounds retained their Δ^4-3-ketone configuration.

Heuser C 54,451/58: Desoxycortisone (Cpd. S)—like dehydroisoandrosterone—given in large amounts i.p. or p.o. produces no anesthesia but intense convulsions in the rat. Allegedly, "neither adrenalectomy nor partial hepatectomy sensitized the rat to the convulsive actions of Cpd. S."

Yates et al. C 56,413/58: In rats, passive venous congestion of the liver, induced surgically, impairs the enzymic reduction of ring A of DOC, cortisol, cortisone, and aldosterone.

Witzel C 68,395/59: Review (29 pp., 113 refs.) on steroid anesthesia including chapters on adaptation to steroids, the effect of partial hepatectomy, and the influence of steroid anesthetics upon various types of convulsions.

Bojesen & Egense G 75,996/60: In adrenalectomized cats, the elimination of endogenous corticoids (cortisol and corticosterone) is greatly delayed by hepatectomy and totally abolished by evisceration. "A few experiments suggested that the intestine is responsible for the main part of the extrahepatic elimination. In experiments with the perfused isolated hindquarter preparation it was impossible to demonstrate any elimination of corticosteroids in spite of electrical stimulation or the administration of large amounts of insulin."

Kulcsár-Gergely & Kulcsár C 99,083/60: In ovariectomized rats, estrone aggravates the hepatic damage produced by CCl_4. The activity of endogenous folliculoids (estrus) is increased by hepatic damage, which again shows that these hormones are inactivated by the liver. Presumably, this process of inactivation diminishes the resistance of hepatic tissue to damage.

Balabanski & Dachev F 68,584/66: Hepatic cirrhosis produced in rats by CCl_4 greatly increases the folliculoid effect of an "estrogenic preparation vitestrol." This effect is ascribed to interference with hepatic detoxication.

Crane et al. H 25,068/70: In rats, the activity of the hepatic enzymes metabolizing progesterone is decreased within 16 hrs following partial hepatectomy, and becomes minimal on the 4—5th postoperative day. "The fraction of the radioactivity present in the several metabolites from incubations of progesterone with liver tissue 7 days following hepatectomy suggests that the ring A reductases appear earlier than the 20α-steroid reductase."

Hellman et al. H 21,323/70: In patients with extrahepatic bile duct obstruction owing to compression by carcinoma tissue, the metabolism of ³H-estradiol is characteristically altered. "The similarity of these changes to those reported in cirrhosis suggests a major role for cholestasis in the causation of the altered estrogen metabolism of cirrhosis."

Solymoss et al. G 70,464/70: In rats, spironolactone shortens the half-life of its main metabolite, the dethioacetylated 4,6-dienone (metabolite A), which is interconvertible with the 17-hydroxy carboxylic acid derivative (metabolite B). This alteration is only slightly accentuated if the steroid is given chronically, and it wears off within eight days after spironolactone treatment is interrupted. After a test dose of spironolactone or of its metabolites A and B, partial hepatectomy delays the blood clearance of metabolite A. Cycloheximide and SKF 525-A also suppress the blood clearance of metabolite A under these conditions. Presumably "spironolactone influences its own biotransformation and the steroid is also a substrate of the hepatic drug-metabolizing enzymes which are induced by spironolactone itself."

Soyka et al. H 33,315/70: Partial hepatectomy sensitized only slightly to the anesthetic effect of 5β-pregnane-3α-ol-20-one, whereas it greatly prolonged sleeping time following treatment with progesterone and many other steroids. Neither inhibition of hepatic mixed function oxidase activity by SKF 525-A nor its stimulation by 3-MC affected the duration of pregnanolone narcosis and even phenobarbital reduced its length only slightly. These findings, and distribution studies, "suggest that termination of hypnosis is due mainly to redistribution with hepatic metabolism playing a relatively minor role." [Species not mentioned; probably rat (H.S.).]

Selye PROT. 42214: In rats, choledochus ligature offered considerable protection against the toxicity of indomethacin and dioxathion, slightly prolonged hexobarbital sleeping time, and failed to affect digitoxin poisoning. Partial hepatectomy had little, if any, effect upon indomethacin, dioxathion and digitoxin poisoning under the prevailing experimental conditions, but considerably prolonged hexobarbital sleeping time. Partial nephrectomy (removal of 80% of the kidney tissue) likewise prolonged hexobarbital sleeping time without significantly influencing indomethacin, dioxathion and digitoxin overdosage. The protective effect of spironolactone against indomethacin, dioxathion and digitoxin remained manifest after most of these surgical interventions. But the protection against indomethacin offered by choledochus ligature could not be further improved by spironolactone, nor was the considerable prolongation by hepatectomy of hexobarbital sleeping time markedly reduced by spironolactone. It must be kept in mind, however, that in these experiments only a single dose of spironolactone was given 5 min after the surgical interventions and 24 hrs before a single dose of the toxicants. These observations can be summarized as shown in Table 126, p. 600.

Nonsteroidal Hormones and Hormone-Like Substances ←

There is some evidence that **catecholamines** are detoxified in the liver. In the rat, the amount of radioactive norepinephrine accumulating in hepatic tissue is sufficiently large to decrease the total amount of circulating hormone considerably.

In rats, partial hepatectomy facilitates the production of gastric ulcers by **insulin**. Here probably, excessive hypoglycemia with the resulting strong stress response is the cause of the enhanced effect; other observations suggest, however, that hepatic tissue is involved in the degradation of insulin.

After partial hepatectomy or bile duct ligation, rats become unusually sensitive to the tachycardia and the increase in metabolism produced by excessive amounts of **thyroxine**. It is assumed that the liver both metabolizes the hormone and eliminates it in the bile, but hepatic inactivation does not appear to play an important role when circulating thyroxine is within physiologic limits.

Table 126. *Influence of various hepatic and renal interventions upon resistance to certain toxicants and upon the catatoxic effect of spironolactone*[a]

Treatment	1 None		2 Choledochus ligature	
	Readings	Mortality	Readings	Mortality
A. Indomethacin	10/10	10/10	3/10 ***	2/10 ***
B. Indomethacin + Spironolactone	8/10 NS	2/10 ***	0/8 NS	3/10 NS
A. Dioxathion	15/15	12/15	10/10 NS	0/10 ***
B. Dioxathion + Spironolactone	1/15 ***	0/15 ***	0/10 ***	0/10 NS
A. Hexobarbital	58 ± 5	0/15	78 ± 7 *	0/10 NS
B. Hexobarbital + Spironolactone	28 ± 2 ***	0/16 NS	80 ± 14 NS	1/11 NS
A. Digitoxin	6/10	2/10	5/10 NS	3/10 NS
B. Digitoxin + Spironolactone	0/10 **	0/10 NS	0/10 *	0/10 NS

Treatment	3 Hepatectomy (70%)		4 Nephrectomy (80%)	
	Readings	Mortality	Readings	Mortality
A. Indomethacin	8/9 NS	6/10 *	4/4 NS	10/10 NS
B. Indomethacin + Spironolactone	0/10 ***	1/10 *	1/9 **	3/9 ***
A. Dioxathion	10/10 NS	10/10 NS	10/10 NS	10/10 NS
B. Dioxathion + Spironolactone	3/10 ***	3/10 ***	5/10 *	5/10 *
A. Hexobarbital	168±25 ***	0/10 NS	99±13 **	1/10 NS
B. Hexobarbital + Spironolactone	177±30 NS	0/11 NS	62±7 *	1/10 NS
A. Digitoxin	8/10 NS	3/10 NS	7/10 NS	5/10 NS
B. Digitoxin + Spironolactone	1/10 ***	1/10 NS	0/10 ***	0/10 *

[a] All surgical interventions were performed under light ether anesthesia 24 hrs before treatment with the toxicants. The latter were given as follows: indomethacin 5 mg in 0.2 ml water, s.c.; dioxathion 4 mg in 1 ml corn oil, p.o.; hexobarbital 7.5 mg in 1 ml water, i.p.; digitoxin 2 mg in 1 ml water, p.o. Spironolactone (10 mg in 1 ml water, p.o.) was administered once 5 min after surgery. For statistical purposes, the results obtained after choledochus ligature, partial hepatectomy and partial nephrectomy (Series 2—4) were compared with the corresponding readings in intact animals (Series 1) given the same toxicant (without spironolactone). The results obtained with a toxicant alone (A), or following pretreatment with spironolactone (B), were compared with each other, separately in the intact animals and in those subjected to each of the three types of surgical interventions. That is Series 2,3 and 4 were compared with 1, and Series A with B for the corresponding readings obtained with each toxicant. The readings and mortality were listed as follows: indomethacin — intestinal ulcers on day of death, mortality on 6th day; dioxathion — dyskinesia and mortality on 3rd day; hexobarbital — sleeping time immediately after injection of the anesthetic; digitoxin — convulsions and mortality on 4th day. For further details on the technique of tabulation *cf.* p. VIII.

Partial hepatectomy does not appear to have a striking effect upon the toxicity of **5-HT** in the rat, and treatment with 5-HTP brings about an increase in the 5-HT content of the brain which is essentially the same in intact and in completely hepatectomized dogs. Yet, both the 5-HT and the 5-hydroxyindole acetic acid (5-HIAA) content of the brain increases in dogs after complete hepatectomy. Thus, the role of the liver in 5-HT metabolism is still not clear.

Hepatic detoxication does not appear to play an important role in the metabolism of **parathyroid hormone**, at least partial hepatectomy fails to affect the soft tissue calcification elicited in rats by **parathyroid extract**.

The pressor effect of **vasopressin** injected into a peripheral vein is greater than if the same amount is injected into the spleen. Hence, it was concluded that vasopressin is detoxified during its passage through the liver.

Catecholamines ←

Caskey 20,936/27: In dogs, ligation of the hepatic artery and portal vein inhibits the rise in muscle temperature normally produced by epinephrine.

Guerra & Siccardi D69,656/62: Studies on the catecholamine content of the hepatic residue following partial hepatectomy in the rat confirm earlier literature showing that epinephrine and norepinephrine are detoxified in the liver.

Eckhardt F36,030/65: It has been suggested that the liver is implicated in limiting pressor responses to norepinephrine i.v. In the rat, the amount of radioactive norepinephrine accumulating in the liver is sufficiently large to decrease considerably the total amount of circulating norepinephrine. Methylphenidate slows the rate of norepinephrine disappearance in intact but much less in partially hepatectomized rats.

Insulin ←

Selye et al. 58,020/36: Removal of the median and left lateral lobes of the rat liver produces gastric ulcers only occasionally but these are severe if the animals are treated with small doses of insulin, or if the hepatectomy is combined with adrenalectomy or hypophysectomy. Similarly severe gastric ulcers are produced when the median, left lateral, and right lateral lobes (about 85% of the hepatic tissue) are removed. In all these instances, hypoglycemia is regarded as the cause of gastric erosion.

Elgee & Williams C430/54: Review of earlier data, and personal observations on the degradation of insulin by hepatic tissue in vivo and in vitro.

Thyroid Hormones ←

Kellaway et al. B14,515/45: In rats, the activity of thyroxine s.c. was estimated by an increase in pulse rate after partial hepatectomy, thyroidectomy, or bile duct ligation. "It was found (1) that thyroxine activity is greatly intensified in the absence of the liver; (2) that the liver does not play a significant role when the amount of circulating thyroxine is within physiologic limits; (3) that the liver deals with excess hormone by some process of inactivation and not by simple excretion."

Grad & Leblond B23,328/48; B49,686/50: In rats, the increase in oxygen consumption and heart rate induced by thyroxine is raised by partial hepatectomy, bile duct ligation, and especially by the conjoint effect of both interventions. "These results are taken to indicate that the liver excretes and inactivates excess amounts of thyroid hormone."

5-HT ←

Garattini et al. D4,913/61: In rats, partial hepatectomy has no effect upon the toxicity of 5-HT.

Tyce et al. D23,092/62: Treatment with 5-HTP brought about an increase in the 5-HT content of the brain, which was essentially the same in intact and in completely hepatectomized dogs.

Tyce et al. G47,432/67: The 5-HT and 5-hydroxyindole acetic acid (5-HIAA) content of the brain increases in dogs and rats after complete hepatectomy. The literature on the role of the liver in 5-HT metabolism is reviewed.

Varia ←

Selye A36,715/42: In rats, partial hepatectomy, complete thyroidectomy or bilateral nephrectomy does not prevent the osteitis fibrosa and soft-tissue calcification produced by large doses of **parathyroid extract**. Apparently, the parathyroid hormone does not exert its action through either the thyroid or the kidney, as had previously been postulated by some investigators. Furthermore, hepatic detoxication does not play an important role in the metabolism of parathyroid hormone.

Møller-Christensen B56,243/51: In rabbits and cats, a greater increase in blood pressure is obtained by **vasopressin** injected into a peripheral vein than if the same amount is injected into the spleen. It is hence concluded that vasopressin is detoxified by the liver.

Drugs and Individual Dietary Constituents ←

In dogs, complete hepatectomy resulted in an increased urinary excretion of 18 amino acids but, to a lesser extent, glucose infusion produced a similar result. Indeed, glycine excretion was more markedly stimulated by glucose than by complete hepatectomy.

The role of hepatic lesions upon **barbiturate** detoxication has been extensively investigated. In dogs, liver damage produced by prolonged chloroform anesthesia enhances the anesthetic effect of pentobarbital, suggesting inadequate detoxication. Hepatectomy with evisceration prolongs the narcotic effect of hexobarbital in dogs, but after administration of threshold doses recovery is possible. This suggests that extrahepatic tissues also participate in barbiturate clearance. On the other hand, in dogs with an Eck fistula and ligature of both the portal vein and the hepatic artery, thiopental anesthesia was prolonged to such an extent that here extrahepatic detoxication was considered to play a very minor role. This view received further confirmation from the observation that heart-lung-liver preparations of dogs clear thiopental from the blood much more rapidly than heart-lung or heart-lung-kidney preparations.

In mice, CCl_4-induced liver damage prolongs thiopental sleeping time.

In rats bearing an Eck fistula, thiopental anesthesia is prolonged, and this barbiturate is degraded in vitro by rat liver slices and mince. Rats with liver cirrhosis produced by CCl_4 are particularly sensitive to pentobarbital anesthesia. An increase in pentobarbital sleeping time also occurs after partial hepatectomy in the rat, but the effect of thiopental is allegedly not influenced by this operation. A systematic study of 25 barbiturates revealed that in the rat, some are mainly detoxified in the liver (e.g., phenobarbital), others in the kidney (e.g., barbital), still others are about equally detoxified in the liver and kidney (e.g., cyclobarbital) and finally certain barbiturates (e.g., thiopental) appear to be detoxified in other tissues but not to any great extent in liver or kidney.

In rabbits, pentobarbital anesthesia is also prolonged following induction of liver damage by CCl_4 or elementary yellow phosphorus.

Carbon tetrachloride does not markedly interfere with the regeneration of the liver following partial hepatectomy in rats.

Certain **carcinogens** accelerate hepatic regeneration after partial hepatectomy in the rat. The induction of adrenal necrosis by DMBA is greatly increased by dietary production of fatty livers but not by CCl_4.

Hepatic lipidosis induced by a **choline**-deficient diet in the rat is not significantly altered by partial hepatectomy, although regeneration of the liver remnant is moderately delayed.

Digitalis compounds are also largely detoxified in the liver. Thus, in rats, hepatectomy or poisoning with elementary phosphorus or CCl_4 increases the lethal effect of acute g-strophanthin overdosage. No more than 10% of a given dose of digitoxin is excreted in the bile of the rat, rabbit, and dog and virtually none is excreted in that of man. Partial hepatectomy greatly increases the digitoxin concentration in the blood and tissues of rats, but has little effect upon it in rabbits and dogs.

Partial hepatectomy reduces digitoxin clearance in the rat approximately in proportion to its aggravating effect upon digitoxin convulsions.

In dogs with an Eck fistula and ligature of the hepatic artery, the clearance of certain **dyes**, such as BSP, is diminished. After partial hepatectomy, the plasma clearance of BSP, rose bengal, and colloidal radio-gold is immediately decreased, but the excretory and phagocytic capacity of the liver returns to normal within about two months. In rats, a liver bypass — established by ligature of the hepatic artery and deviation of the portal blood into the femoral vein — interferes with BSP clearance much more than does partial hepatectomy or CCl_4 intoxication.

In rats, partial hepatectomy increases sensitivity to indomethacin, but even after this operation spironalactone has a good protective effect, presumably because its detoxication is also impeded by hepatic insufficiency. The induction of intestinal ulcers by indomethacin can also be prevented by ligature of the common bile duct and, depending upon circumstances (e. g., timing, dosage), the protective effect of diminished biliary secretion or the sensitizing effect of partial hepatectomy may prevail.

The effect of **lathyrogens** (e.g., AAN) upon the skeleton of the rat is greatly enhanced by partial hepatectomy.

The nephrocalcinosis and acute mortality induced by **mercury** intoxication in the rat are inhibited by choledochus ligature.

It had been claimed that **pentylenetetrazol** given p.o. is highly active in guinea pigs, rats and rabbits, although it must pass through the liver before reaching its target organs, and that after bilateral renal hilus ligature, rats become extremely sensitive to the convulsive effect of this drug. Furthermore, perfusion of pentylenetetrazol through the liver of the frog or cat did not alter its activity. It was concluded that the principal detoxicating organ for pentylenetetrazol is the kidney, not the liver.

However, later observations were diametrically opposed to these findings. It was noted that in cats, the acute toxicity of pentylenetetrazol is not influenced by bilateral nephrectomy, but it is greatly increased following liver damage by yellow phosphorus. In rabbits, the disappearance rate of pentylenetetrazol from the blood and tissues was not influenced by bilateral nephrectomy, but greatly delayed after CCl_4 poisoning. Still more recent observations suggest that neither partial hepatectomy nor complete nephrectomy increases the resistance of the rat to the convulsive or fatal action of pentylenetetrazol. Hence, it was concluded that neither the liver nor the kidney plays an important role in the detoxication of this drug, although it is readily detoxified by catatoxic steroids.

The **pesticide**, OMPA, is well tolerated by completely hepatectomized rats in doses which kill sham operated controls. Apparently, in the liver this compound normally undergoes biotransformation into a more toxic metabolite. Yet, the comparative resistance of male rats to anticholinesterase phosphorothioates is diminished by partial hepatectomy.

The resistance of the rat to dioxathion is greatly increased by choledochus ligature.

The toxicity of **strychnine** is greatly increased by partial hepatectomy and other interventions which damage the liver. At the same time, the blood clearance of strychnine is delayed. Incubation of strychnine with liver pulp results in the destruction of strychnine as shown by observations made as early as 1931.

In rabbits in which the liver was "destroyed" by ethylene chlorohydrin, no prolongation of **tribromoethanol** anesthesia was noted. This finding was taken to mean that the liver plays no important part in the detoxication of this compound. However, in mice and rats, partial hepatectomy greatly prolongs tribromoethanol sleeping time.

The detoxication of **vitamin D** and **DHT** is also dependent upon hepatic factors. Following ligature of the common bile duct, the production of soft tissue calcinosis by DHT is inhibited in the rat. This may be due to insufficient intestinal DHT absorption in the absence of bile, or to an interruption of the enterohepatic circulation. On the other hand, the production of topical calciphylaxis (by vitamin-D_2 p.o. and Fe-Cl_3 s.c.), as well as the associated generalized calcinosis are aggravated by partial hepatectomy in the rat. This aggravation was ascribed to a decrease in the hepatic storage of iron or of vitamin D, but the possible role of deficient hepatic vitamin-D degradation should also be considered. The calcifying arteriosclerosis and atheromatosis produced in rabbits by combined treatment with cholesterol and vitamin-D_2 is aggravated by hepatotoxic amounts of CCl_4. On the other hand, "hepatectomy" (technique not further characterized) prevents the conversion of vitamin-D_3 to 25-hydroxycholecalciferol. Furthermore perfused liver can hydroxylate vitamin-D_3 through an enzyme which has been identified in liver homogenates. In rats, isolation of the liver from the circulation, almost completely abolishes the conversion of vitamin-D_3 into its biologically active metabolite, 25-hydroxycholecalciferol. It was concluded that the liver is the major if not the only physiologic site of vitamin-D_3 activation. It is noteworthy however that the technique used for the exclusion of the liver from the circulation includes bile duct ligation which — as we have said before — suffices in itself to protect against such vitamin-D derivatives as DHT.

Allylformiate ←

Rabes & Tuczek H30,729/68: In rats, the hepatic necroses produced by allylformiate elicit regenerative phenomena mainly near the periphery of the lobules, whereas after partial hepatectomy the maximum of cell proliferation shifts towards the intermediary and central portions of the liver lobules.

Amino Acid ←

Freeman & Svec B64,175/51: In dogs, the plasma concentration of 18 free amino acids was followed after complete hepatectomy. "a) An increase occurred in the concentration of glycine, histidine, glutamic acid and lysine. b) A decrease occurred in the plasma concentration of methionine, tryptophane, leucine, arginine, and valine. c) There were variable or inconclusive results on the other amino acids studied." Glucose infusion increased the urinary excretion of all 18 amino acids, but a considerable further increase was obtained by complete hepatectomy except for glycine as illustrated on p. 605.

ANIT (α-Naphthylisothiocyanate) ←

Bar-Maor & Ungar D41,800/61: ANIT stimulates mitotic proliferation in the liver of the rat, and this effect is further enhanced by partial hepatectomy.

Barbiturates ←

Dog

Pratt et al. G72,105/32: In dogs with an Eck fistula and ligature of the hepatic artery, bromsulphalein's clearance is inhibited, suggesting "that the bromsulphalein injected into the blood is eliminated, specifically, by the liver." Following hepatic damage caused by protracted chloroform anesthesia, the narcotic effect of pentobarbital is greatly prolonged, indicating that the barbiturate is inadequately detoxified when the liver is damaged.

Martin et al. A48,575/40: In dogs, hepatectomy with evisceration greatly prolongs the narcotic effect of hexobarbital, but the fact that after administration of threshold doses recovery is possible suggests that extrahepatic tissues also participate in the detoxication of this barbiturate.

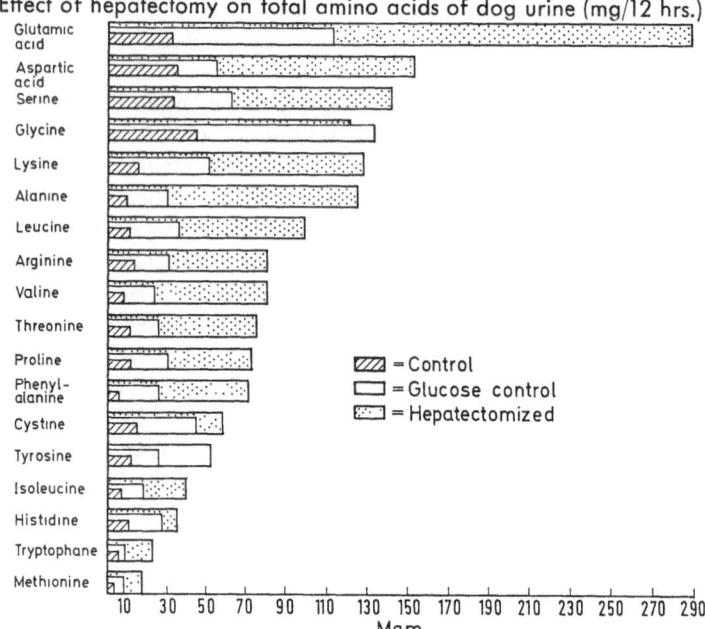

Average urinary excretion of amino acids in normal dogs, glucose-infused dogs prior to hepatectomy, and hepatectomized dogs infused with glucose (Freeman & Svec B64,175/51).

Kelly & Shideman A49,706/49: In dogs with Eck fistula, thiopental anesthesia is greatly prolonged. In heart-lung-liver preparations, the plasma levels of thiopental decline much more rapidly than in heart-lung or heart-lung-kidney preparations. The liver is primarily responsible for the detoxication of this barbiturate.

Meyers & Peoples G70,570/54: In dogs, thiopental anesthesia is greatly prolonged following establishment of an Eck fistula with ligature of the portal vein and hepatic artery. "It is believed that tissues other than the liver are quantitatively unimportant in the rapid detoxification of thiopental in the dog."

MOUSE

Shideman et al. E60,046/47: In mice, CCl_4-induced liver damage prolongs the effect of thiopental. The same is true after subtotal hepatectomy (85—90%) in rats. Diminished blood flow through the liver (Eck fistula) likewise increases the duration of thiopental anesthesia in rats. Thiopental is degraded in vitro by rat liver slices and mince.

RAT

Cameron & Saram G72,101/39: Rats with liver cirrhosis produced by CCl_4 are particularly sensitive to pentobarbital anesthesia.

Scheifley & Higgins A48,663/40: In rats, anesthesia produced by ethyl-o-ethylphenyl-urea or pentobarbital was markedly prolonged by partial hepatectomy. The effect of thiopental was not influenced by this operation.

Masson & Beland A72,286/44; B344/45: The site of barbiturate detoxication was investigated by comparative studies in bilaterally nephrectomized or partially hepatectomized rats as judged by the prolongation of sleeping time. "From the data obtained with twenty-five compounds, barbiturates can be classified into four groups. Group I: Those mainly detoxified in the kidney (e.g. barbital). Group II: Those mainly detoxified in the liver (e.g., ipral, amytal, nembutal, ortal, phenobarbital, alurate, nostal, seconal, allyl-pental, evipal, thioethamyl, sec. hexyl-ethyl, 1-methyl-allyl-isobutyl, 1-methyl-propylcrotyl and n-allyl-1-methyl-butyl-ethyl barbiturates. Group III: Those approximately equally detoxified in the liver and kidney (e.g., neonal, delvinal, phanodorn, dial). Group IV: Those possibly detoxified in other tissues of the body, but not to any great extent in liver or kidney (pentothal, 1-methyl-allyl-propyl and 1-methyl-allyl-allyl thiobarbiturates)."

Scheifley A48,124/46: In rats, the anesthetic effect of pentobarbital, unlike that of thiopental, was greatly prolonged by partial hepatectomy. "These data suggest that the liver is instrumental in protecting against the action of pentobarbital sodium but does not play a significant part in the detoxication of pentothal sodium" (thiopental). Uninephrectomy had no effect upon the production of anesthesia by either of these barbiturates.

Masson B1,217/46: In male rats, pretreatment for 6 days with crude pituitary powder s.c. "slightly prolonged the duration of anesthesia with phanodorn, thioethamyl, neonal, delvinal, nostal and amytal, and greatly prolonged (2 to 5 times) with pentothal, seconal, allyl pental, nembutal, evipal, pernoston and sigmodal." There was no difference between the pretreated and control rats as regards the anesthetic effect of phenobarbital, probarbital, barbital, aprobarbital, allobarbital and trichloroacetaldehyde. "The action of pituitary preparations is not specific but can also be obtained with preparations from various organs and with foreign proteins." Hepatic damage is considered to be a likely cause of the prolongation of anesthesia under these conditions.

Walker & Parry B46,639/49: In rats, partial hepatectomy increases the anesthetic effect of chloral hydrate, tribromoethanol, phenobarbital, and thiopental. Tests at various time intervals after the operation lead to the conclusion that "there is no apparent correlation between the regeneration of the liver by weight and its power to detoxicate these drugs."

Butler et al. G76,364/52: In rats, "partial hepatectomy has such a large effect on the rate of disappearance of mephobarbital and on the rate of production of phenobarbital from mephobarbital as to suggest that the liver is the principal, if not the only, site of the demethylation of mephobarbital."

Sandberg G71,886/53: Studies on partially hepatectomized or completely nephrectomized rats suggest that "for 5,5-diallyl-barbituric acid and its 1-(N,N-diethylcarbamylmethyl) derivative the kidneys participate as much as the liver in the detoxication. 1-benzyl-5, 5-diallyl-barbituric acid is destroyed mainly in the liver. 1-carbethoxymethyl-5,5-dialkyl-barbiturates are probably hydrolyzed to the corresponding carbonic acid, 1-carboxymethyl-5,5-dialkyl-barbituric acid."

Robillard et al. G67,325/54: Adult males are more resistant than females to pentobarbital anesthesia. Castration decreases the resistance in males. Testosterone raises pentobarbital resistance to the normal male level in both male and female castrates, whereas estradiol and progesterone prolong anesthesia in castrates of both sexes. [The hormones were administered as pellets 15 days before the test, but the amounts are not stated (H.S.).] Partial hepatectomy prolongs pentobarbital anesthesia and accentuates the differences induced by the various interventions just mentioned, without causing qualitative changes in the outcome.

Fouts et al. G68,041/61: Partially hepatectomized rats are deficient in the ability to oxidize the side-chain of hexobarbital or the ring-sulfur of chlorpromazine, and to reduce the nitro-group of p-nitrobenzoic acid. Full recovery of these activities occurs only after complete regeneration of the hepatic mass (about ten days after operation). O-dealkylation of codeine is impeded only during the first few days when the regeneration is most active. Sham-hepatectomy (with exteriorization of the liver) has a similar, though much less, pronounced effect.

Dingell & Heimberg G72,112/68: In rats, pretreatment with CCl_4 prolongs hexobarbital sleeping time and interferes with the metabolism of the barbiturate by hepatic microsomes in vivo and in vitro.

Selye PROT. 42214: In rats, choledochus ligature offered considerable protection against the toxicity of indomethacin and dioxathion, slightly prolonged hexobarbital sleeping time, and failed to affect digitoxin poisoning. Partial hepatectomy had little, if any, effect upon indomethacin, dioxathion and digitoxin poisoning under the prevailing experimental conditions, but considerably prolonged hexobarbital sleeping time. Partial nephrectomy (removal of 80% of the kidney tissue) likewise prolonged hexobarbital sleeping time without significantly influencing indomethacin, dioxathion and digitoxin overdosage. The protective effect of spironolactone against indomethacin, dioxathion and digitoxin remained manifest after most of these surgical interventions. But the protection against indomethacin offered by choledochus ligature could not be further improved by spironolactone, nor was the considerable prolongation by hepatectomy of hexobarbital sleeping time markedly reduced by spironolactone. It must be kept in mind, however, that in these experiments only a single dose of spironolactone was given 5 min after the surgical interventions and 24 hrs before a single dose of the toxicants, *cf.* Table 126, p, 600.

RABBIT

Pratt G71,897/33: In rabbits, pentobarbital anesthesia is prolonged following the induction of liver damage by CCl$_4$ or elementary phosphorus.

McLuen & Fouts E99,285/61: In rabbits, obstructive jaundice affects the hepatic microsomal metabolism of hexobarbital in rough proportion to the degree of histologically observable cell damage.

VARIA

Richards & Appel A48,718/41: Review (13 pp., 44 refs.) on "The Barbiturates and the Liver." Special attention is given to observations on the effect of hypolipotropic diets, CCl$_4$ and partial hepatectomy upon barbiturate detoxication.

Richards & Taylor H19,235/56: Review on barbiturates with a special section on the role of the liver in their detoxication. (Effect of hepatectomy, hepatotoxic drugs, liver disease).

Bilirubin ←

Weinbren & Billing G76,309/56: In rats, 24 hrs after partial hepatectomy, the bilirubin excretory capacity does not increase as rapidly as the relative weight of the regenerating liver, but thereafter the excretory capacity tends to increase with the weight rise.

n-Butylamine ←

Merli & Gandini F32,684/64: n-Butylamine produces a mixture of neuro and osteolathyrism in the rat. Hepatectomy, performed 7 days before initiation of the n-butylamine treatment, actually delayed the onset of the lathyric manifestations, perhaps as a consequence of overcompensating hepatic regenerative phenomena. [These findings are contrasted with our observation of an increase in the severity of APN-induced lathyrism by partial hepatectomy, without commenting upon the fact that, in our experiments, the operation was performed concurrently with the initiation of APN-treatment, that is, before significant hepatic regeneration could have occurred (H.S.).]

Carbon Tetrachloride ←

Costa & Smorlesi E34,570/51: In rats, hepatic cirrhosis induced by CCl$_4$ is favorably influenced by partial hepatectomy.

Kaufmann E60,536/53: In rats, liver regeneration following partial hepatectomy occurs normally after hepatic damage induced by CCl$_4$. Earlier claims that, under these conditions, partial hepatectomy actually causes remission in the CCl$_4$-induced sclerosis could not be fully confirmed.

Novelli & Mor D36,206/62: In rats, the regeneration of mitochondria in hepatocytes after partial hepatectomy is disturbed by treatment with small doses of CCl$_4$.

McLean et al. H18,569/69: In rats, simultaneous treatment with phenobarbital accelerates and aggravates the production of hepatic cirrhosis by CCl$_4$. This aggravation may depend upon an activation of CCl$_4$ toxicity by the induction of hepatic microsomal enzymes but the hepatic growth stimulating effect of phenobarbital could also be involved.

Carcinogens ←

Gershbein G71,667/58: In rats, liver regeneration following partial hepatectomy was greatly accelerated by treatment with various carcinogens.

Brody G71,680/60: In rats, the immediate and prolonged effect of p-dimethylaminoazobenzene (DAB) on the regeneration of the liver after partial hepatectomy has been studied.

von der Decken & Hultin G68,039/60: Observations on the induction of microsomal enzymes by 3-methylcholanthrene in the liver of the rat as affected by partial hepatectomy.

Tanaka & Dao G34,593/65: In rats, the induction of adrenal necrosis by DMBA is greatly increased by the dietary production of fatty livers but not by CCl$_4$.

Hughes C74,311/70: In rats subjected to a first or a second partial hepatectomy, the mitotic responses are essentially similar in magnitude and time with a mitotic peak 28 hrs postoperatively. In rats fed 3'-methyl-4-dimethylaminoazobenzene (3'-MeDAB) or 2-methyl-4-dimethylaminoazobenzene (2-MeDAB), partial hepatectomy elicits a similar mitotic response if the pretreatment is of short duration. However, following more prolonged feeding with the above agents, the mitotic peak may be delayed up to 60 hrs postoperatively. This delayed mitotic responsiveness may play a part in pre-neoplasia.

Chloral Hydrate ←

Walker & Parry B46,639/49: In rats, partial hepatectomy increases the anesthetic effect of chloral hydrate, tribromoethanol, phenobarbital and thiopental. Tests at various time intervals after the operation lead to the conclusion that "there is no apparent correlation between the regeneration of the liver by weight and its power to detoxicate these drugs."

Chloramphenicol ←

Firkin & Linnane H 31,607/70: In rats, the toxicity of chloramphenicol is greatly augmented by partial hepatectomy.

Cholesterol ←

Olivecrona & Fex G74,083/70: In rats, the disappearance from the circulation of fatty acid labeled chylomicra is retarded by partial hepatectomy. When chylomicra labeled in vitro with cholesteryl palmitate were injected, about 80% of the radioactivity was in the liver within an hour in both intact and partially hepatectomized rats.

Choline ←

Saint Omer & Mincione D53,460/60: In rats, partial hepatectomy does not significantly change hepatic lipidosis on a choline deficient diet but regeneration of the liver remnant is inhibited during the first 72 hrs after the operation.

Cyclophosphamide ←

Brock & Hohorst G71,533/62: Cyclophosphamide has no cytotoxic effect upon Yoshida sarcoma cells in vitro, but is rapidly transformed into an active compound in mice, rats and dogs in vivo. The active form is demonstrable in the blood and urine by bioassay if added to tumor cells in vitro. In completely hepatectomized rats, only a little fraction of cyclophosphamide is thus activated. However, activation can be demonstrated in vitro by incubation with liver slices. Pretreatment of rats with SKF 525-A inhibits in vivo activation which presumably takes place in hepatic microsomes.

Digitalis ←

Farah & Smuskowicz A49,134/49: In rats, total hepatectomy with evisceration or poisoning with elementary phosphorus or CCl_4 increases the lethal effect of acute g-strophanthin-overdosage. "This reduction is due to the reduced excretion of g-strophanthin by the liver and to an increase in the sensitivity of the rat heart to g-strophanthin."

St. George et al. G71,843/52: No more than 10% of a given dose of digitoxin is excreted in the bile of the rat, rabbit and dog, whereas none could be detected in the bile of two humans. Partial hepatectomy greatly increases the digitoxin concentration in the blood and tissues of rats, but has comparatively little effect upon digitoxin clearance in rabbits, and virtually none in dogs.

Gibson & Becker E65,709/67: In mice, "hypoexcretory states" were produced by penile ligation, bile duct ligature or drugs (phenylisothiocyanate, α-naphthylisothiocyanate) which reduce bile flow. "Intraperitoneal administration of ouabain to mice with no or diminished bile flow resulted in enhanced mortality rates. Digoxin and digitoxin effected enhanced lethality in anuric mice. Lanatoside-C was not more toxic to hypoexcretory mice. The use of hypoexcretory mice in toxicologic evaluations of pharmacologic agents is suggested."

Greenberger et al. H13,503/69: In rats and guinea pigs, the absorption of six tritium-labeled cardiac glycosides was studied, using isolated intestinal loops in vivo and everted duodenal and jejunal gut sacs in vitro. The nonpolar glycosides (digitoxin, digoxin and proscillaridin) were more readily absorbed than the polar glycosides (ouabain, dihydroouabain and convallatoxol). Bile duct ligation did not affect the absorption of digitoxin from isolated intestinal loops in rats. Furthermore, " the transport of digitoxin was not inhibited by another cardiac glycoside, digoxin, suggesting that there are no specific transport sites that allow for competition between glycosides. These observations indicate that digitoxin is absorbed by a passive (nonsaturable) transport process."

Solymoss et al. G70,463/70; G70,461/70: In rats, pretreatment with spironolactone, norbolethone, or ethylestrenol accelerated the plasma clearance of digitoxin, in proportion to the in vivo protective effect of these catatoxic steroids. Partial hepatectomy reduces digitoxin clearance. The effect of spironolactone is suppressed by SKF 525-A and cycloheximide.

Solymoss G70,484/70: In rats, the plasma clearance of digitoxin is accelerated by spironolactone, norbolethone, and ethylestrenol in doses that protect against the toxicity of the alkaloid in vivo. On the other hand, partial hepatectomy reduces digitoxin plasma clearance and increases the severity of the convulsions. The protective action of the steroids is suppressed by SKF 525-A and cycloheximide.

Selye PROT. 42214: In rats, choledochus ligature offered considerable protection against the toxicity of indomethacin and dioxathion, slightly prolonged hexobarbital sleeping time, and failed to affect digitoxin poisoning. Partial hepatectomy had little, if any, effect upon indomethacin, dioxathion and digitoxin poisoning under the prevailing experimental conditions, but considerably prolonged hexobarbital sleeping time. Partial nephrectomy (removal of 80% of the kidney tissue) likewise prolonged hexobarbital sleeping time without significantly influencing indomethacin, dioxathion and digitoxin overdosage. The protective effect of spironolactone against indomethacin, dioxathion and digitoxin remained manifest after most of these surgical interventions. But the protection against indomethacin offered by choledochus ligature could not be further improved by spironolactone, nor was the considerable prolongation by hepatectomy of hexobarbital sleeping time markedly reduced by spironolactone. It must be kept in mind, however, that in these experiments only a single dose of spironolactone was given 5 min after the surgical interventions and 24 hrs before a single dose of the toxicants, *cf.* Table 126, p. 600.

Dyes ←

Pratt et al. G72,105/32: In dogs with an Eck fistula and ligature of the hepatic artery, bromsulphalein clearance is inhibited, suggesting "that the bromsulphalein injected into the blood is eliminated, specifically, by the liver."

Cherrick et al. E98,251/60: Indocyanine green is rapidly and completely bound to plasma protein and excreted in the bile in unconjugated form. It is not cleared by extrahepatic mechanisms in detectable amounts. Its plasma clearance is similar to that of BSP in controls and patients with liver lesions.

Eckhardt & Armstrong F79,670/67: In rats, a liver bypass can be established by ligature of the hepatic artery combined with a deviation of the portal vein into the femoral vein through a cannula. Under these conditions, bromsulphalein (BSP) disappears much more slowly from the plasma than after partial hepatectomy or intoxication with CCl_4.

Aronsen et al. H22,143/69: In dogs, immediately after partial hepatectomy, the plasma clearance of bromsulphalein ^{131}I, rose bengal, and colloidal radio-gold is decreased. The excretory and phagocytic capacity of the liver returned to normal within 6—8 weeks.

Ethyl-o-Ethylphenylurea ←

Scheifley & Higgins A48,663/40: In rats, anesthesia produced by ethyl-o-ethylphenylurea or pentobarbital was markedly prolonged by partial hepatectomy. The effect of thiopental was not influenced by this operation.

Hexadimethrine ←

Selye et al. D25,745/63: Partial hepatectomy does not significantly influence the nephrocalcinosis produced by hexadimethrine in the rat.

Indomethacin ←

Selye G60,058/69: In the rat, partial hepatectomy increases sensitivity to toxic doses of indomethacin. Comparatively small doses of spironolactone readily inhibit this form of indomethacin intoxication even in the presence of surgically induced hepatic insufficiency. "These results are compatible with the assumption that both indomethacin and spironolactone are subject to hepatic detoxification, and hence, their respective pathogenic and prophylactic actions are enhanced after extensive resection of liver tissue."

Brodie et al. G67,797/71: In rats given a single injection of indomethacin s.c., starvation during the following 24 hrs completely prevented intestinal ulcer formation, whereas starvation for 24 hrs on the second, third or second + third day had no such effect. Intestinal ulcers could also be prevented by ligature of the common bile duct. When segments of small intestine were isolated by Thiry-Vella loops, ulceration was prevented in the loops but not in the adjacent anastomosed intestine.

Selye PROT. 42214: In rats, choledochus ligature offered considerable protection against the toxicity of indomethacin and dioxathion, slightly prolonged hexobarbital sleeping time, and failed to affect digitoxin poisoning. Partial hepatectomy had little, if any, effect upon indomethacin, dioxathion and digitoxin poisoning under the prevailing experimental conditions, but considerably prolonged hexobarbital sleeping time. Partial nephrectomy (removal of 80% of the kidney tissue) likewise prolonged hexobarbital sleeping time without significantly influencing indomethacin, dioxathion and digitoxin overdosage. The protective effect of spironolactone against indomethacin, dioxathion and digitoxin remained manifest after most of these surgical interventions. But the protection against indomethacin offered by choledochus ligature could not be further improved by spironolactone, nor was the considerable prolongation by hepatectomy of hexobarbital sleeping time markedly reduced by spironolactone. It must be kept in mind, however, that in these experiments only a single dose of spironolactone was given 5 min after the surgical interventions and 24 hrs before a single dose of the toxicants, cf. Table 126, p. 600.

Lathyrogens ←

Selye C25,013/57; C31,369/57: In rats, extensive partial hepatectomy greatly increases the effect of AAN upon the bones.

Glickman et al. E24,104/63: In rats, the dental changes produced by AAN are aggravated following partial hepatectomy and thyroidectomy, whereas they are reduced by ACTH or almost completely abolished by thyroxine.

Lead ←

Selye et al. D25,657/63: Topical calcergy produced by local trauma after i.v. injection of lead acetate in the rat is uninfluenced by partial hepatectomy, but inhibited by hypophysectomy or bilateral nephrectomy. Splenectomy itself does not influence this response, but when combined with partial hepatectomy, the animals die within a few hours after the lead-acetate injection, before calcification could develop.

Lidocaine ←

Aldrete et al. G78,399/70: In dogs, the disappearance of i.v. injected lidocaine from the blood was retarded by hepatectomy. Similar observations were made in hepatectomized patients with liver transplants in the stage of rejection.

Mercury ←

Selye PROT. 30550: In rats in which the bile duct had been ligated prior to the injection of $HgCl_2$ i.v., the usual nephrocalcinosis and mortality failed to occur. The mechanism of this protective effect is not clear but it may be related to the interruption of the enterohepatic circulation, cf. Fig. 23.

Nicotine ←

Biebl et al. 44,898/32: Hepatectomy sensitizes the dog to the pressor effect of nicotine. Perfusal of nicotine through a canine heart-lung preparation inactivates the compound rapidly. In frogs, both complete and partial hepatectomy diminish the maximum tolerable amount of nicotine. It is concluded that nicotine is destroyed by the liver.

Octamethyl Pyrophosphamide (OMPA) ← cf. Pesticides

Pentylenetetrazol ←

Voss A47,860/26: In guinea pigs, rats and rabbits, pentylenetetrazol p.o. is highly active, although it must pass through the liver before reaching its target organs. On the other hand, following bilateral ligation of the renal hilus rats become extremely sensitive to the production of convulsions by pentylenetetrazol. It is concluded that the principal detoxicating organ for pentylenetetrazol is the kidney, whereas the liver plays no important role in this respect.

Ridder A47,894/27: Perfusion of pentylenetetrazol through the liver of the frog or cat does not alter its activity. "The surviving liver of cold- or warm-blooded animals is hence unable to destroy Cardiazol."

Dille & Seeberg 84,277/41: In cats, the acute toxicity of pentylenetetrazol is not influenced by bilateral nephrectomy, whereas liver damage induced by yellow phosphorus greatly increases sensitivity to pentylenetetrazol.

Tatum & Kozelka 81,376/41: In rabbits, the disappearance rate of pentylenetetrazol from blood, liver and muscle was not influenced by bilateral nephrectomy, but it was greatly delayed by CCl_4 poisoning which caused a 50% decrease in the functional capacity of the liver as judged by the bromsulphalein test. It is concluded that, contrary to earlier reports, the liver plays an important part in the detoxication of pentylenetetrazol whereas the kidney does not.

Fournier & Selye 81,980/42: In the rat, partial hepatectomy does not alter sensitivity to pentylenetetrazol. Apparently, hepatic detoxication does not significantly alter resistance to this compound.

Fournier 84,151/43: Partial hepatectomy or complete nephrectomy does not increase the resistance of the rat to the convulsive or fatal effect of pentylenetetrazol. It is concluded that neither the liver nor the kidney plays an important role in the detoxication of this drug.

Peptone ←

deNicola 43,101/30: Review of the literature, and personal observations on the prevention of peptone shock (with the characteristic leuko-

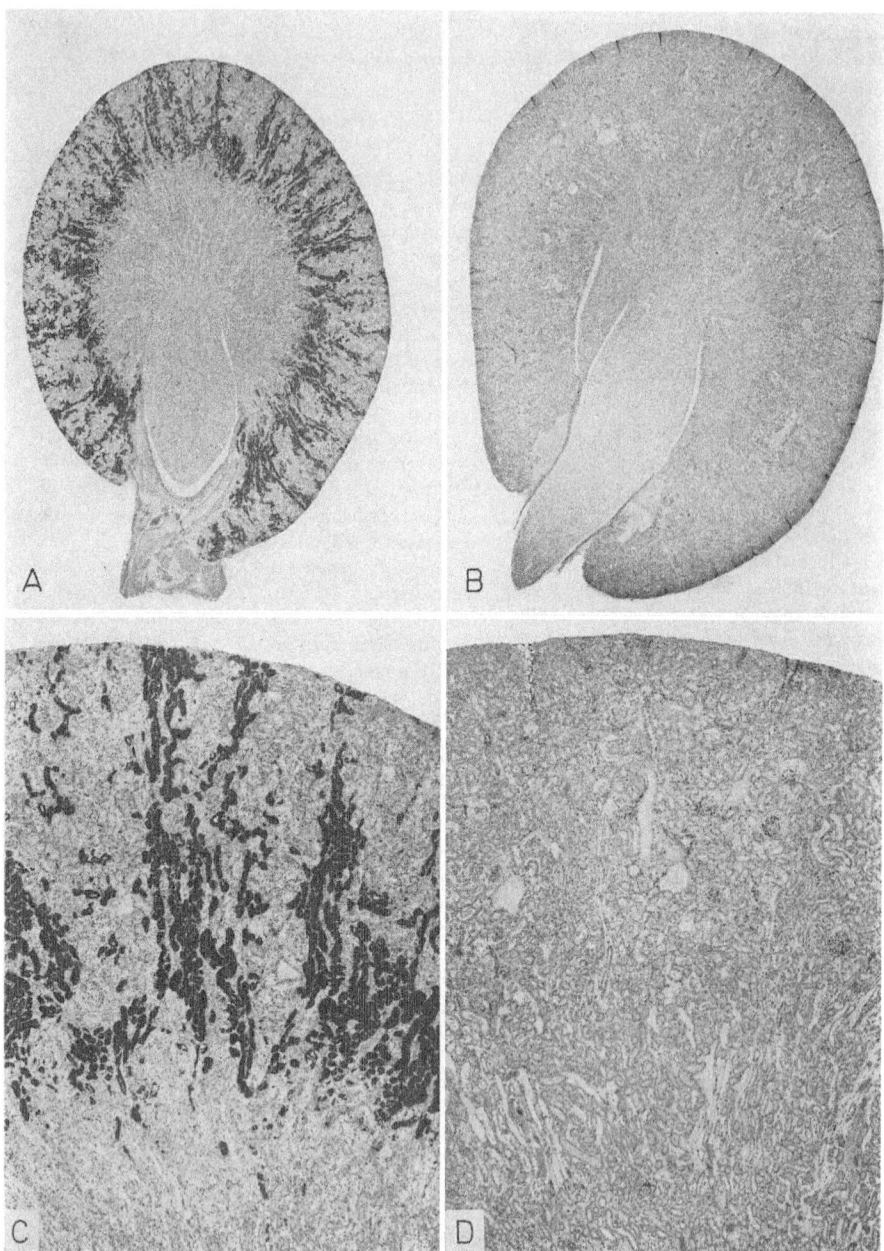

Fig. 23. **Prevention of mercury poisoning by choledochus ligature.** A + C: Kidney of rat given $HgCl_2$ shows heavy cortical calcification. B + D: Similarly-treated rat in which the choledochus had been ligated. Here, calcification is prevented (von Kóssa: A and B, X 9; C and D, X 32)

Pesticides ←

Cheng G71,450/51: Completely hepatectomized rats survived the injection of a dose of OMPA which killed sham-operated controls.

Murphy & DuBois D28,546/58: The activity of the microsomal enzyme system which oxidizes thiophosphates to potent anticholinesterase agents is considerably higher in male than in female rats (incubation of liver homogenates with Guthion, or ethyl p-nitrophenyl thionobenzenephosphonate or "EPN"). Yet, in vivo, adult males are more resistant to EPN than females, perhaps because the accelerated formation of toxic oxidation products is overcompensated by a more efficient detoxication of the latter. The low enzyme activity of female liver is enhanced by pretreatment with testosterone in vivo, whereas the high activity of male liver is diminished by previous castration, partial hepatectomy, or treatment with progesterone or diethylstilbestrol. SKF 525-A inhibits, whereas pretreatment with carcinogens or a protein-deficient diet enhances the activity of the thiophosphate-oxidizing enzyme.

DuBois & Puchala D43,878/61: Male rats are much more resistant than females to various anticholinesterase phosphorothioates. Male mice and guinea pigs are not particularly resistant to DMP. Partial hepatectomy and/or castration abolishes the comparative resistance of the male rat, whereas testosterone restores resistance in hepatectomized or orchidectomized rats. It is concluded "that androgens govern the development of this system."

Selye PROT. 42214: In rats, choledochus ligature offered considerable protection against the toxicity of dioxathion. Partial hepatectomy or partial nephrectomy (removal of 80% of the kidney tissue) had little, if any, effect upon experimental conditions. The protective effect of spironolactone against dioxathion remained manifest after these surgical interventions, *cf.* Table 126, p. 600.

Phalloidin ←

Tuchweber et al. (in preparation): In rats, mortality and peliosis-like hemorrhagic necrosis of the liver induced by phalloidin i.p. are prevented by partial hepatectomy performed 1 to 5 days prior to this treatment.

Phosphorothioates ← *cf.* Pesticides

Phlogogens ←

Novelli & Zinnari H8,990/68: In rats, collagen formation in carrageenin granulomas is inhibited by partial hepatectomy.

RES-Blockers ←

Aronsen et al. H22,143/69: In dogs, immediately after partial hepatectomy, the plasma clearance of bromsulphalein ^{131}I, rose bengal, and colloidal radio-gold is decreased. The excretory and phagocytic capacity of the liver returned to normal within 6—8 weeks.

Gans et al. G71,042/69: Thrombin rapidly disappears from the blood of intact, but not of completely hepatectomized heparinized dogs. Thrombin clearance appears to depend mainly upon phagocytosis by the Kupffer cells.

Silica ←

Novelli et al. H24,185/69: In rats, collagen formation in pulmonary silicotic granulomas is inhibited by partial hepatectomy during liver regeneration, perhaps as a consequence of diminished collagen synthesis.

Strychnine ←

Priestley et al. 9,158/31: The following six methods have been tested for the study of hepatic detoxication using strychnine as a substrate.

1. Comparison of dogs with Eck fistula and normal dogs.
2. Comparison of the effectiveness of strychnine injected into the peripheral vascular system, and injection into the portal vein.
3. The ability of incubated pulp of liver to destroy strychnine.
4. Estimation of strychnine introduced into the circulation of a heart-lung-liver perfusion, compared with that introduced into a heart-lung-limb preparation.
5. Susceptibility of normal and dehepatized dogs to strychnine.
6. Rate of disappearance of strychnine from the blood stream of normal and dehepatized dogs.

Among these six methods "the study of the dehepatized dog and the perfused liver appears to have yielded the most conclusive and accurate data. The exclusive use of any single method is not recommended. However, by the combined use of the analytic and the synthetic methods (organism without a liver and surviving liver without the organism), respectively, definite evidence concerning the liver as a detoxicating organ can be obtained." The canine liver possesses a highly specialized ability to immediately arrest and subsequently destroy strychnine.

Tetrahydronaphthylamine ←

Borchardt 23,683/28: In cats, neither thyroparathyroidectomy nor adrenalectomy prevents the production of fever by tetrahydronaphthylamine, whereas denervation of the liver inhibits it almost completely.

Tribromoethanol ←

Eichholtz A 27,018/27: In rabbits, "destruction of the liver" by ethylene chlorohydrin does not significantly affect the length of tribromoethanol anesthesia. After bilateral nephrectomy, sleeping time is somewhat prolonged but still variable. On the other hand, bilateral adrenalectomy prolongs the sleeping time very considerably.

Waelsch & Selye 3,972/31: First description of a technique for the removal of about 70% of the liver in mice which lends itself for the detection of drugs that are detoxified in the liver. Thus, in such partial hepatectomized mice, tribromoethanol (Avertin) causes much more prolonged anesthesia than in intact controls, whereas magnesium anesthesia is not significantly affected by this hepatic insufficiency; presumably because tribromoethanol is, whereas $MgCl_2$ is not detoxified by the liver.

Walker & Parry B 46,639/49: In rats, partial hepatectomy increases the anesthetic effect of chloral hydrate, tribromoethanol, phenobarbital, and thiopental. Tests at various time intervals after the operation lead to the conclusion that "there is no apparent correlation between the regeneration of the liver by weight and its power to detoxicate these drugs."

Urethan ←

Chernozemski & Warwick H 33,929/70: In female mice, hepatic tumors are much more rarely induced by urethan than in males. Partial hepatectomy greatly increases the hepatocarcinogenic effect of urethan.

Vitamin D, DHT ←

Selye C 27,736/57: In rats pretreated with DHT, the pressure building up in the renal pelvis after ureter ligature causes calcification of the renal papilla; after choledochus ligature, hepatic calcification is not observed, although small necrotic islets are formed in the liver parenchyme. "Apparently, necrotic tissue does not necessarily calcify even in the DHT overdosed animal." [The effect of bile duct ligature upon DHT-induced extrahepatic calcinosis is not described (H.S.).]

Rosenfeld et al. G 55,854/67; G 67,785/67: Partially hepatectomized rats given vitamin-D_2 (Calciferol) p.o. and $FeCl_3$ s.c. developed calciphylaxis at the iron injection site, as well as generalized calcinosis, of greater intensity than intact animals given the same combined treatment, or than hepatectomized rats given Calciferol without iron. The aggravating effect of partial hepatectomy is ascribed to a decrease in the storage of iron which, consequently, floods the organism and challenges for calciphylaxis. [The possible role of hepatic vitamin-D detoxication has not been considered (H.S.).]

Rosenfeldová et al. G 55,855/67: In rats given vitamin-D_2 (Calciferol) at the dose of 7.5 mg in 0.5 ml oil [route of administration not stated (H.S.)], 48 hrs after partial hepatectomy, mortality was significantly greater than in sham-operated rats given the same amount of vitamin-D_2. Additional treatment with $FeCl_3$ s.c., in order to produce calciphylaxis, caused a further increase of the mortality rate, particularly after partial hepatectomy. It is concluded that "the liver by storing calciferol, protects the organism against its toxic effects."

Hass et al. H 19,697/69: Under standard conditions, rabbits develop particularly severe calcifying arteriosclerosis and atheromatosis when given combined treatment with cholesterol + vitamin-D_2 p.o. The vascular damage is further aggravated by the production of hepatic damage with CCl_4.

DeLuca H 17,327/69: Brief mention of unpublished experiments indicating that "hepatectomy" prevents the conversion of vitamin-D_3 to 25-hydroxycholecalciferol. In addition, perfused liver can hydroxylate vitamin-D_3. The enzyme for the 25 hydroxylation has been identified in liver homogenates.

Ponchon et al. H 18,243/69: In rats, isolation of the liver from the circulation (portocaval shunt + hepatic artery ligation and bile duct ligation) "eliminates almost completely their ability to convert [1,2]-H_3 vitamin D_3 into its biologically active metabolite, 25-hydroxycholecalciferol, as well as certain other metabolites. It is concluded that the liver is the major if not the only physiologic site of hydroxylation of vitamin D_3 (cholecalciferol) into 25-hydroxycholecalciferol."

W-1372 ←

Selye & Lefebvre G 79,005/71: "Partial hepatectomy increases the intoxication (hepa-

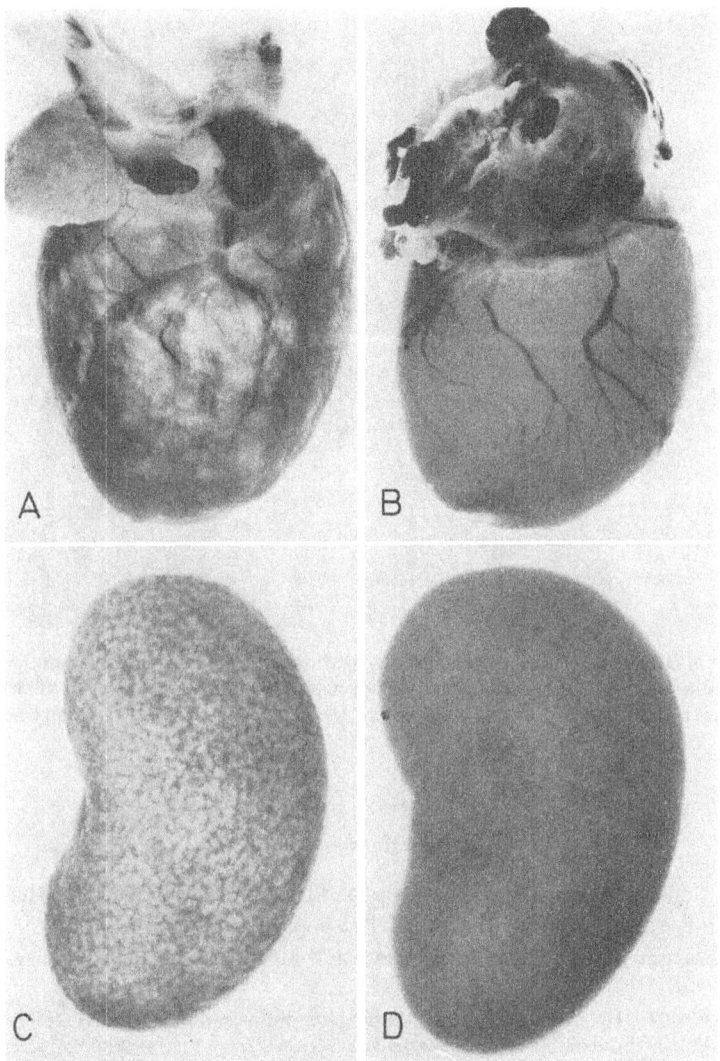

Fig. 24. **Protection against DHT intoxication by choledochus ligature.** A + C: Heavily calcified heart and kidney of rat treated with HgCl$_2$. B + D: Corresponding organs of similarly-treated rat in which the choledochus had been ligated

tic steatosis and necrosis) produced by W-1372. Catatoxic steroids (PCN, spironolactone) inhibit, whereas glucocorticoids (prednisolone acetate, triamcinolone) aggravate, these effects."

Varia ←

Selye G70,480/71: In rats, complete occlusion of the choledochus diminished resistance to hexobarbital, progesterone and zoxazolamine but offered considerable protection against intoxication with indomethacin and the acute tissue calcinosis elicited by DHT. The infarctoid cardiopathy produced by fluorocortisol + Na$_2$HPO$_4$ + corn oil was also prevented but in view of the high mortality this latter finding is difficult to interpret.

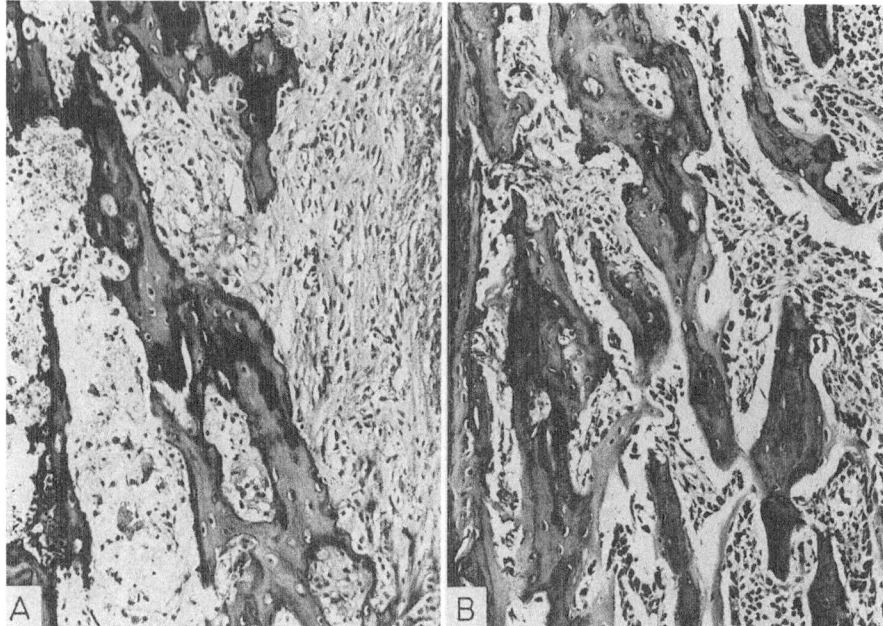

Fig. 25. **Prevention of DHT intoxication by choledochus ligature.** A: Femur of rat given toxic doses of DHT. Intense fibrosis, bone absorption and partial necrosis of bone marrow. B: Similarly-treated rat in which the choledochus was ligated before DHT administration. Essentially normal bone structure

Complex Diets ←

In rats, the hepatic necrosis produced by a diet containing yeast as the sole source of protein is greatly accelerated by partial hepatectomy.

In mice, starvation inhibits hepatic regeneration after partial hepatectomy.

Aterman D15,536/61: In male weanling rats, the hepatic necrosis induced by feeding a diet containing yeast as the sole source of protein is greatly accelerated by partial hepatectomy or treatment with STH.

Vilchez et al. H15,524/68: In mice, a first mitotic wave occurs in the liver 40—48 hrs after partial hepatectomy. Mitotic counts and DNA content indicate that starvation produces a significant decrease in the number of cells undergoing mitosis, and a parallel reduction in DNA.

Olivecrona & Fex G74,083/70: In rats, the disappearance from the circulation of fatty acid labeled chylomicra is retarded by partial hepatectomy. When chylomicra labeled in vitro with cholesteryl palmitate were injected, about 80% of the radioactivity was in the liver within an hour, in both intact and partially hepatectomized rats.

Hepatic Changes ←

A considerable amount of work has been done upon hepatic regeneration and other changes in the liver remnant after partial hepatectomy. It is not within the scope of this volume to discuss the pertinent literature in detail. Suffice it to say that during the first 24 hrs after operation, hepatic steatosis occurs and its intensity is increased by hemorrhage, withdrawal of drinking water, intravenous injection of NaCl, and other stressor agents. The fat content tends to return to normal within 3 to 4 days. Mitotic proliferation in the liver remnant does not begin immediately after partial hepatectomy but only after a latency period of several hours and it tends to reach a maximum after 48 hrs. In the regenerating rat liver there is a marked proliferation of the endoplasmic reticulum. The capacity of the liver to regenerate is maintained in rats even after 12 successive partial hepatectomies performed within one year. In rats subjected to a first or a second partial hepatectomy, the mitotic responses are essentially similar in magnitude and time, with a mitotic peak at about 28 hrs postoperatively.

In rats, choledochus ligature inhibits the growth of liver cells in autotransplanted hepatic segments, but hepatic regeneration after partial hepatectomy is not diminished by simultaneous choledochus ligature. The claim that in rats, liver regeneration after partial hepatectomy is accelerated by hepatic extracts requires confirmation.

Mann et al. 712/31: In dogs with an Eck fistula, partial hepatectomy failed to stimulate regeneration in the remnant. Such regenerative phenomena were also inhibited by CCl_4, or by ligation of the common bile duct.

Cameron A 48,168/35: In rats, choledochus ligature inhibits the growth of liver cells in autotransplanted small hepatic segments, but leaves the bile ducts unaffected.

Selye et al. 32,783/35: Following partial hepatectomy, fatty degeneration of the liver developed within the first 24 hrs after the operation. The reaction was increased by hemorrhage, withdrawal of drinking water, or intravenous injection of NaCl.

Collip et al. 36,231/35: Following partial hepatectomy, the remnant undergoes fatty metamorphosis within the first 2 days in the rat, rabbit and dog. Experiments on rats show that the fat content returns to normal within 3 to 4 days, and that neither hypophysectomy nor adrenalectomy can completely abolish this response.

Brues et al. A 45,962/36: In rats submitted to partial hepatectomy, "the number of cells in the residual fragment shows no significant increase in the first 24 hours," although the mass of the liver remnant increases about 50%. After the first day, cell number and liver mass increase approximately at the same rate. The effect of various dietary constituents upon hepatic regeneration is described.

Brues & Marble A 47,729/37: Following partial hepatectomy, rats evince a latent period of one day during which the rapidly growing organ shows no increase in cell number. Mitosis then begins and reaches a rate of 2.13% but rapidly diminishes again.

Ludewig 74,865/39: In rats, the fatty acid, phospholipid, and cholesterol concentrations in the liver at first increased and then decreased after partial hepatectomy.

Christensen & Jacobsen A 49,204/49: In rats, the mitotic rate in the liver remnant reaches a maximum 48 hrs after partial hepatectomy. If two rats are united by parabiosis, one being partially hepatectomized, some increase in mitotic proliferation occurs also in the nonhepatectomized partner, suggesting the formation of cell division stimulating substances.

Harkness E 80,279/52: Studies on the biochemical changes in the liver remnant after partial hepatectomy in the rat.

Weinbren B 90,949/53: In rats, hepatic regeneration is not diminished when bile duct ligature is performed simultaneously or 18—21 days before partial hepatectomy.

Jaffe G 77,570/54: Studies on the diurnal mitotic periodicity of regenerating rat liver.

Harkness E 57,419/57: Extensive review on the structural biochemical and functional changes induced by partial hepatectomy in the rat.

Ingle & Baker C 40,980/57: "The capacity of liver to regenerate was maintained in rats which were subjected to partial hepatectomy 12 times within a period of one year. At the end of the experiment, only minor cytological changes were observed in the regenerated liver and there was no neoplasia."

Pérez-Tamayo & Romero D 38,897/58: Review of various factors which influence regeneration of liver tissue after partial hepatectomy in the rat.

Weinbren D 95,941/59: Review (11 pp., 110 refs.) and personal observations on factors influencing hepatic regeneration after partial hepatectomy in the rat, with special sections on the effects of hypophysectomy and thyroid hormones.

Kahlson G 52,949/60: The rate of histamine formation in the regenerating liver of the rat is particularly rapid during the first week after partial hepatectomy. When radioactive histidine is injected at this time, decarboxylation is particularly rapid.

Rogers et al. E 93,548/61: In rats, liver regeneration following partial hepatectomy was studied in parabiotic pairs and triplets. The results "do not support the conclusion that the blood in parabiotic rats carries stimulating or inhibitory 'humoral factors' directly governing hepatic regeneration."

Dagradi & de Candia D 56,609/62: Comparative studies on hepatic regeneration in the dog, mouse, rat and man after partial hepatectomy.

Dagradi & Galanti D 62,332/62: In rats, a technique for the successive removal of several hepatic lobes has been employed to study the regenerative phenomena in the remnant.

MacDonald et al. D 41,743/62: In newts (Triturus viridescens), hepatic regeneration was studied by means of autoradiographs to quantitate DNA synthesis.

Marsilii & de Simone G 1,552/62: In rats, liver regeneration following partial hepatectomy leads to marked proliferation of the endoplasmic reticulum.

Oehlert et al. D 36,669/62: In rats, DNA synthesis after partial hepatectomy is studied with autoradiographic techniques.

Bucher G 68,621/63: Review (55 pp., about 400 refs.) on factors influencing the regeneration of mammalian liver.

Scheffler & Westphal D 56,080/63: In rats, hepatic regeneration after partial hepatectomy can be accelerated by feeding a mixture of adenosine, xanthine, hypoxanthine, and orotic acid.

Leduc G 79,104/64: Review (26 pp., about 130 refs.) on "Regeneration of the Liver" after various types of surgical or chemical injuries. Special attention is given to regeneration after superficial wounds, lobectomies and bile-duct obstruction.

Trotter G 71,660/64: Electron-microscopic studies on liver regeneration following partial hepatectomy in the mouse.

Rizzo and Webb H 21,587/68: In rats, during liver regeneration after partial hepatectomy, the correspondence between the rate of transport of newly-synthesized ribosome to the cytoplasm and the size of the nonfunctional monomer pool, suggests that the two parameters are directly, or indirectly coupled.

Stöcker G 76,916/68: Autoradiographic and isotopic studies on cellular proliferation in the liver of the rat following an injection of ^{3}H-thymidine and partial hepatectomy with special reference to intracellular RNA and protein synthesis.

Ronzoni et al. H 18,986/68: In rats, the hydroxyproline content of the liver furnishes a better quantitative index of sclerosis than histologic studies. The technique is recommended for the evaluation of sclerosis and its regression after various types of liver damage, e.g., partial hepatectomy or CCl_4 poisoning.

Rosene Jr. G 71,661/68: In mice, partial hepatectomy greatly elevates mitotic proliferation in the liver, which reaches a peak on the third day after the operation and returns to near normal by the fifth day. Injections of Ehrlich ascites tumor homogenates moderately accelerated the rate of hepatic mitosis. Partial hepatectomy accelerated tumor cell proliferation.

Bader G 70,347/69: Detailed description of the ultrastructural changes induced by partial hepatectomy in the rat.

Bengmark et al. G 71,689/69: In rats, ligature of the hepatic artery does not markedly alter regeneration of the liver after partial hepatectomy.

Bengmark G 74,917/69: Review (25 pp., about 375 refs.) on the chemical and structural changes in the regenerating hepatic tissue based mainly upon the effects of partial hepatectomy in the rat.

Günther et al. H 18,480/69: Correlative study of weight increase and mitotic index in the liver of partially hepatectomized rats.

Bucher and Swaffield H 21,579/69: In rats, the rate of RNA synthesis during early stages of regeneration after partial hepatectomy has been evaluated with a radioactive precursor technique.

Zelioli-Lanzini H 19,493/69: In rats, small doses of X-rays as well as hepatic extracts improve liver regeneration following partial hepatectomy.

Ove et al. H 23,725/69: In rats, following partial hepatectomy, liver polymerase had a preference for native DNA primer, whereas the deoxyribonuclease in the same preparation acted preferentially on denatured DNA.

Parks H 28,647/69: In mice, electron-microscopic studies showed the source and direction of movement of lipid granules appearing in the hepatic perisinusoidal space following partial hepatectomy.

Simmons & Boyle H 22,141/69: In partially hepatectomized rats, heterologous serum albumin or saline i.p. is followed by the same increase in the mitotic rate of the hepatocytes. The results do not support the hypothesis that lowered extra-cellular albumin plays an important role in controlling hepatic regeneration.

Johnson H 18,571/69: In mice "after partial hepatectomy the regenerating liver shows a mitotic response characterized by a lag phase during the first postoperative day, a rather sudden burst of mitotic activity at 24—48 hr, and a decline to normal levels within a week. This unexplained pattern of hyperplasia, characteristic of compensatory growth in other tissues as well as in liver, can be accounted for by the 'critical mass' hypothesis, which proposes that cell division is triggered when the growing cell reaches a certain critical mass or size."

Sugihara H 18,030/69; Kimura G 75,331/69: Detailed description of the ultrastructural changes in the hepatic remnant after partial hepatectomy in the rat.

Ungváry et al. G 72,366/69: In rats, hepatic regeneration was carefully investigated with special reference to changes in the vascular structure. Attention is called to the work of Cruveilhier (A 73,454/1829—35) who "was the first to describe hepatic regeneration in 1833. He found that removal of 75% of the liver was followed by complete regeneration of the organ in eight weeks in dogs and in three weeks in rats." [A careful search of Cruveilhier's works failed to confirm that he ever made this statement (H.S.).]

Hughes C 74,311/70: In rats subjected to a first or a second partial hepatectomy, the mitotic responses are essentially similar in magnitude and time, with a mitotic peak 28 hrs postoperatively.

Orlova & Rodionov G 73,079/70: In rats, following partial hepatectomy "the amount of histones in the nuclei of regenerating liver cells and the incorporation of ^{3}H-leucine in them started to increase and reached the maximum earlier than the respective onset and peak of the DNA content and uptake of ^{14}C-thymidine."

Lancker H 28,381/70: Summary of literature, and personal observations on DNA synthesis in regenerating rat liver.

Rabes & Tuczek H 33,839/70: In rats, quantitative autoradiographic studies revealed a great heterogeneity of liver cell proliferation after partial hepatectomy.

Tavassoli & Crosby G 73,038/70: In rats, liver fragments implanted into ectopic sites do not survive even if the regenerative stimulus is activated by partial hepatectomy.

Varia ←

In eviscerated rats, survival is shortened by simultaneous **nephrectomy** and vice versa.

Partial hepatectomy diminishes resistance to **cold** in guinea pigs and spontaneous **muscular activity** is reduced by this operation in rats. However, these effects are probably due to the stress of the operation rather than to any specific hepatic deficiency.

In rats, the growth of some transplantable **tumors** is increased, whereas that of others is not influenced by partial hepatectomy. Intraportal injection of Walker tumor suspensions, immediately followed by partial hepatectomy, increases the incidence of hepatic metastases in the rat. Several observers claimed that under certain circumstances, partial hepatectomy can accelerate the growth of transplantable tumors in rats and mice, or that the tumor transplants enhance hepatic regeneration after partial hepatectomy. These effects were ascribed to the production of some humoral growth factors, by the regenerating liver or the proliferating neoplasm but such substances have not yet been identified with certainty.

Comparatively little work has been done about the importance of the liver for resistance to **bacterial toxins** and to damaging **immune reactions**. In adrenalectomized mice, E. coli endotoxin injected i.v. or into the spleen is about equally toxic. "Thus, the liver does not appear to play an immediate role in the detoxication of this antigen."

Surgical **interference with the hepatic circulation** impedes the formation of various antibodies in the guinea pig, but a detailed discussion of hepatic influences upon immune reactions would be beyond the scope of this monograph.

In **pregnant** rats, partial hepatectomy often causes fetal absorption but liver regeneration is essentially normal.

Renal Lesions ←

Ingle et al. B42,752/47: In eviscerated rats, survival is shortened by simultaneous nephrectomy and vice versa.

Cold ←

Calcagno & Quercio G46,022/65: Partial hepatectomy as well as various other surgical operations diminish the resistance of the guinea pig to cold, presumably as an expression of an increased sensitivity to stress in general.

Muscular Contraction ←

Dugal & Ross 84,992/43: In rats, spontaneous running activity stops after partial hepatectomy as well as after a sham-operation. However, motor activity becomes normal within 72 hrs after a sham-operation, and within only seven days following partial hepatectomy.

Smith & Dugal F65,692/66: In rats, partial hepatectomy does not influence spontaneous running activity more than does a sham-operation.

Tumors ←

Paschkis et al. C8,982/55: In rats, the growth of Walker tumors and of transplantable hepatomas—unlike that of Jensen sarcomas and Murphy lymphosarcomas—was increased after partial hepatectomy. Perhaps "the regenerating liver may release a humoral agent causing increased growth of some tumors." Hepatic regeneration was enhanced by the presence of a growing tumor regardless of whether the latter was influenced or not by partial hepatectomy.

Fisher & Fisher G72,106/59: In rats, intraportal injection of Walker tumor suspensions immediately followed by partial hepatectomy increases the incidence of hepatic metastases. No such increase was observed if partial hepatectomy was performed 48 hrs prior to or after partial hepatectomy.

Llanos & Saffe G71,663/61: In C3H/mza mice, the development of spontaneous hepatomas is accelerated by partial hepatectomy.

Peyster et al. G71,671/61: In rats, partial hepatectomy enhances the growth of s.c. injected Walker tumor cells. When two rats are joined in parabiosis and one is partially hepatectomized, tumor growth is accelerated in both partners. Presumably "a humoral growth accelerator induced by liver regeneration is a major factor influencing distant tumor takes and growth."

Trotter E90,324/61: In mice, partial hepatectomy increases mitotic proliferation in some s.c.-transplanted hepatomas, but not in others.

Gershbein E71,030/63: In rats, s.c. transplantation of Walker or Flexner-Jobling tumors did not significantly alter the extent of hepatic regeneration. However, under certain circumstances, partial hepatectomy accelerated tumor growth.

Gershbein F71,304/66: Studies on the effect of various agents upon liver regeneration and Walker tumor growth in partially hepatectomized rats.

Rosene Jr. G71,661/68: In mice, partial hepatectomy greatly elevates mitotic proliferation in the liver, which reaches a peak on the third day after the operation, and returns to nearly normal by the fifth day. Injections of Ehrlich ascites tumor homogenates moderately accelerated the rate of hepatic mitosis. Partial hepatectomy increased tumor cell proliferation.

Bacterial Toxins ←

Chedid et al. B99,547/54: In mice rendered particularly sensitive by adrenalectomy, E. coli endotoxin injected i.v. or into the spleen is equally toxic. Similar results have been obtained in intact rats. "Thus the liver does not appear to play an immediate role in the detoxification of this antigen." In partially hepatectomized rats "which become more sensitive to any toxic substance" cortisone continues to exert its protective effect against endotoxin.

The same is true of the splenectomy or thymectomy.

Kocsár et al. G69,983/69: In rats, incubation of tritium-labeled endotoxin with bile or Na-deoxycholate reduces its absorption when subsequently injected i.p. In rats rendered bile-deficient by cannulation of the choledochus, unlike in normal rats, endotoxin is absorbed after administration p.o. "Our experimental findings suggest that bile acids play an important role in the defense mechanism of the macroorganism against bacterial endotoxins."

Wardle & Wright H32,903/70: In rats, a single dose of endotoxin i.v., given after choledochus ligature, causes death from intravascular coagulation (generalized Sanarelli Shwartzman phenomenon) owing to delayed clearance of endotoxin from the circulation. [Earlier pertinent data of Bertók and Kocsár are not discussed (H.S.).]

Immune Reactions ←

Müller A47,855/11: In guinea pigs, the formation of various antibodies is inhibited by thyroidectomy as well as by surgical interference with hepatic circulation. Treatment with thyroid extract has an opposite effect. The latter is not due to shock, since removal of all abdominal organs except the liver is ineffective. Furthermore, the blood loses its "alexic power" when perfused through an isolated liver preparation.

Pregnancy ←

Paschkis et al. C14,122/56: In pregnant rats partial hepatectomy causes absorption of many fetuses, but liver regeneration is not affected by pregnancy.

Varia ←

Selye & Dosne A30,702/40: "Experiments on partially hepatectomized rats indicate that the decrease in the blood volume, blood chlorides and blood sugar caused by ablation of 85 per cent of the liver tissue in fasted rats is inhibited by administration of an adrenal cortical extract, rich in the life-preserving principle. ... The decrease in blood sugar produced by complete hepatectomy is not significantly influenced even by large doses of cortin. This finding makes it probable that the cortical hormone does not inhibit the utilization of circulating sugar."

Heim & Kerrigan G68,369/63: The serum concentration of slow a_2-globulin increases in rats after partial hepatectomy or CCl_4 intoxication.

Menguy & Masters F61,098/65: The increase in serum glycoproteins, and the changes in serum glycoprotein fractions produced by parathyroid extract in intact rats are abolished by partial hepatectomy, whereas the hypercalcemia and nephrocalcinosis are not influenced by it.

Heim & Ellenson F77,887/67: A slow a_2-globulin appears among the serum proteins of the rat after partial hepatectomy or treatment with Salmonella endotoxin, s.c. as well as postpartum or after implantation of Walker tumors. Adrenalectomy prevents the appearance of the a_2-globulin in all these situations, unless substitution therapy with corticosterone is administered.

Hepatic Enzymes ←

The induction by hepatic lesions of enzyme changes specifically related to certain toxicants is discussed with the latter under "Drugs." For other hepatic enzyme alterations consult the Abstract Section.

TPO, TKT ←

Cabibbe et al. G52,346/67: Hepatic TPO-activity is increased by partial hepatectomy in the rat, allegedly as a mere consequence of the resulting "surgical stress."

Seidman et al. F88,452/67: The induction of TPO has been studied in the liver remnant of partially hepatectomized rats following treatment with cortisol, and after adrenalectomy. "It seems possible, therefore that the lessened response to hydrocortisone in hepatic cells preparing to divide is related to repression of transcriptional rather than translational mechanisms and that the duplicating genome itself may be unable to participate simultaneously in other functions."

Terawaki et al. G50,735/67: Studies on the phenylalanine hydroxylase activity of normal and regenerating rat liver after tyrosine and tryptophan injection.

Benes & Zicha G67,159/69: Exposure to

1400 R does not inhibit the tryptophan oxygenase activity of rat liver. In fact, substrate induction of tryptophan oxygenase is stimulated by X-irradiation applied 24 hrs earlier. Induction by cortisol is initially stimulated, and then inhibited by X-irradiation. X-irradiation before partial hepatectomy inhibits the increase in tryptophan oxygenase normally observed 12 hrs after the operation. Similar results are obtained by actinomycin D applied one hour after partial hepatectomy. "The diminished synthesis of tryptophan oxygenase in irradiated regenerating rat liver tissue, as well as the decrease of hormonal induction after the irradiation can be explained by the inhibition of the specific messenger RNA's synthesis."

Kulcsár et al. G72,002/69: In rats, the substrate-induced synthesis of TPO was inhibited by hepatic injury (CCl_4) as well as by thyroxine. Thyroidectomy was without effect, and actually inhibited the influence of CCl_4.

OKT ←

Räihä & Kekomäki G68,114/68: In the rat, the OKT activity of the liver is very low in the fetus, exhibiting a small transient elevation around term; it then drops, and eventually reaches the high adult activity level during the third postnatal week. Triamcinolone given postnatally causes a pronounced elevation of OKT, but has no such effect in fetal or adult rats. Puromycin prevents the rise in OKT after triamcinolone administration. In adult rats fed a protein- or arginine-free diet, OKT activity decreases and fails to rise under the influence of triamcinolone. Partial hepatectomy or STH depresses OKT activity in the livers of adult rats.

GOT, GPT ←

Cohen & Hekhuits 93,220/41: GOT activity was subnormal in six types of mouse tumors, regenerating rat liver, and fetal kitten (compared with adult cat) tissues. Apparently, an inverse relationship exists between transaminase activity and protein synthesis.

Bengmark & Olsson E34,627/63: Studies on the GPT content of the hepatic remnant after partial hepatectomy in the rat.

DNA-Polymerase ←

Feigelson et al. G68,042/62: In partially hepatectomized rats, cortisone causes a transient stimulation and subsequent depression in the incorporation of precursors into the DNA of the regenerating liver.

Hayasaki & Tsukada G73,554/70: In rats, partial hepatectomy increases the serum DNA inhibitor concentration. This inhibitor may control the activity of DNA and is therefore of considerable importance.

Glucuronidase ←

Yano & Nobunaga E21,714/63: Studies on the serum transaminase and β-glucuronidase activity following partial hepatectomy in the guinea pig and rat.

Phosphatase ←

Brachet & Jeener B23,118/46: In rats, partial hepatectomy increases alkaline phosphatase activity in the nuclei but decreases it in the cytoplasm of hepatocytes. It is assumed that alkaline phosphatase in chromatin facilitates the renewal of phosphorus in thymonucleic acid.

Oppenheimer & Flock B4,738/47: Alkaline phosphatase activity is elevated in the plasma and liver after partial hepatectomy in the rat. Since the initial elevation is greater in the liver, it is assumed that plasma alkaline phosphatase originates in hepatocytes.

Thrombin ←

Gans et al. G71,042/69: Thrombin rapidly disappears from the blood of intact, but not of completely hepatectomized heparinized dogs. Thrombin clearance appears to depend mainly upon phagocytosis by the Kupffer cells.

Other Enzymes ←

von der Decken & Hultin G37,124/60: Studies on the enzymic composition of rat liver microsomes during hepatic regeneration after partial hepatectomy.

Myers et al. D48,663/61: Studies on the deoxycytidylate deaminase content of regenerating liver tissue after partial hepatectomy in the rat.

Bucher G68,621/63 (p. 255): Review on hepatic regeneration, with a special section on enzyme changes, in the liver remnant.

Terayama & Takata F69,475/66: The N-demethylating activity of rat liver is considerably reduced during regeneration after partial hepatectomy but, for a much shorter period, also after sham-operations.

Gram et al. G62,231/68: In rats, "the regenerating liver, like the fetal or newborn liver and certain rodent hepatomas, although exhibiting low levels of microsomal enzymes, has the capacity to respond to the enzyme inducers, phenobarbital and 3-MC."

Bengmark G74,917/69: Review on hepatic regeneration with a special chapter on enzymic changes in the liver remnant.

Barker et al. H13,059/69: In the rat, CCl_4-induced liver injury decreases the P-450 level in hepatic microsomes and diminishes both steps in the oxidative N-demethylation of dimethylalanine (N-oxide accumulation and formaldehyde release). Cytochrome b_5 was rapidly restored to control levels. Partial hepatectomy decreased the cytochromes and formaldehyde production but increased N-oxide accumulation. These results are unaffected by adrenalectomy.

Henderson & Kersten G77,181/70: In partially hepatectomized rats, "the *p*-hydroxylating and N-demethylating activities decreased during the period of rapid cellular proliferation and subsequently rose to about 100 and 80 per cent respectively of their initial values within 7 days postoperatively. The UDPglucuronyltransferase activity, measured in ultrasonicated homogenates, however was not reduced during the regeneration process. Pretreatment of the rats with phenobarbital resulted in a considerable increase of the drug-oxidizing enzymes even during the period of rapid growth."

Hutterer et al. G75,925/70: In rats, 4 days after bile duct ligation, the activity of aminopyrine demethylase was greatly decreased, while the content of cytochrome P-450 and the activities of aniline hydroxylase, NADPH-cytochrome c reductase, and cytochrome P-450 reductase were only slightly decreased in the hepatic microsomes. Binding of type II substrate to cytochrome P-450 was unimpaired, and its modifier effect on P-450 reductase was intact. The binding of type I substrate was greatly decreased, and its stimulating effect on P-450 reductase was abolished. Presumably cholestasis alters the type I binding sites of the hepatic SER, which is responsible for the hypoactivity of the biotransformation system.

Kaltiala G79,608/70: In male rats in which 50% of the liver was removed, "hexobarbital, chlorpromazine and pethidine were metabolized significantly less well by the microsomal enzymes of the regenerating livers than by those of the controls (sham-operated)."

← RENAL LESIONS

Next to the liver, the kidney appears to be the most important organ of detoxication. Thus, in various species, **pentylenetetrazol** is highly active when given p.o. although it has to traverse the portal circulation, whereas after bilateral ligature of the renal hilus, rats become extremely sensitive to the convulsive effect of this drug. It had been concluded from these observations that the principal detoxicating organ for pentylenetetrazol is the kidney. However, subsequent investigations showed that the disappearance rate of pentylenetretrazol from the blood and tissues of rabbits is not significantly influenced by bilateral nephrectomy; conversely, it is greatly delayed by CCl_4-poisoning, presumably owing to the resulting hepatic damage. Essentially similar observations have been made in comparing nephrectomy with other types of chemically or surgically-induced hepatic damage. In the case of very acutely acting drugs, detoxication or excretion may not be rapid enough to induce a detectable change; hence it is not surprising that certain investigators found no effect of either partial hepatectomy or complete nephrectomy upon pentylenetretrazol poisoning.

The effect of the kidney upon **barbiturate** intoxication has also been extensively examined, but here the relative importance of the liver and the kidney appears to differ depending on the type of compound examined. Allegedly, some barbiturates are detoxified mainly in the kidney, others in the liver, yet, others in both organs or in extrahepatic and extrarenal tissues. It is important to retain, however, that for the detoxication of certain barbituric acid derivatives, the kidney can be even more important than the liver.

The renal damage produced in rats and rabbits by systemic intoxication with **mercury** is prevented by previous ureter ligature. This may be related to the disappearance of alkaline phosphatase from the proximal convoluted tubules and a diminished accumulation of Hg in the nonexcreting organ. Following temporary ligature of one ureter, the production of nephrocalcinosis and sclerosis is prevented on this side, whereas the contralateral kidney undergoes severe damage resulting in atrophy and loss of function. If after several weeks, the protected kidney is removed, the contralateral organ undergoes ragid and pronounced hypertrophy so that, at least in many instances, it can maintain life by itself.

It has been stated that in rabbits, **tribromoethanol** anesthesia is not markedly affected if the liver is "destroyed" by ethylene chlorhydrin but prolonged after bilateral nephrectomy.

The osteitis fibrosa and soft tissue calcification produced by large doses of **parathyroid extract** are not prevented by bilateral nephrectomy in the rat. From this it was concluded that, contrary to earlier views, parathyroid hormone does not exert its action exclusively through its effect upon the renal elimination of electrolytes.

Finally, it might be mentioned in this connection that the mitotic index in the **regenerating rat liver** rises after one hour of renal ischemia but not after bilateral nephrectomy.

Voss A 47,860/26: In guinea pigs, rats and rabbits, **pentylenetetrazol** p.o. is highly active although it must pass through the liver before reaching its target organs. On the other hand, following bilateral ligation of the renal hilus, rats become extremely sensitive to the production of convulsions by pentylenetetrazol. It is concluded that the principal detoxicating organ for pentylenetetrazol is the kidney, whereas the liver plays no important role in this respect.

Eichholtz A 27,018/27: In rabbits, "destruction of the liver" by ethylene chlorhydrin does not significantly affect the length of **tribromoethanol** anesthesia. After bilateral nephrectomy, sleeping time is somewhat prolonged but still variable. On the other hand, bilateral adrenalectomy prolongs the sleeping time very considerably.

Holck et al. A 8,011/37: In rats, bilateral nephrectomy does not alter the sex difference in **hexobarbital** sleeping time.

Dille & Seeberg 84,277/41: In cats, the acute toxicity of **pentylenetetrazol** is not influenced by bilateral nephrectomy, whereas liver damage induced by yellow phosphorus greatly increases sensitivity to pentylenetetrazol.

Tatum & Kozelka 81,376/41: In rabbits the disappearance rate of **pentylenetetrazol** from blood, liver and muscle was not influenced by bilateral nephrectomy but greatly delayed by CCl$_4$ poisoning causing a 50% decrease in the functional capacity of the liver as judged by the bromsulphalein test. It is concluded that, contrary to earlier reports, the liver plays an important part in the detoxication of pentylenetetrazol, whereas the kidney does not.

Selye A 36,715/42: In rats, partial hepatectomy, complete thyroidectomy or bilateral nephrectomy do not prevent the osteitis fibrosa and soft-tissue calcification produced by large doses of **parathyroid extract**. Presumably, parathyroid hormone does not exert its action either through the thyroid or through the kidney, as had previously been postulated by some investigators. Furthermore, hepatic detoxication does not play an important role in the metabolism of parathyroid hormone.

Fournier 84,151/43: Neither partial hepatectomy nor complete nephrectomy decreases the resistance of the rat to the convulsive or fatal effect of **pentylenetetrazol**. It is concluded that neither the liver nor the kidney plays an important role in the detoxication of this drug.

Wilmer A 48,603/43: In rabbits, unilateral permanent ureter ligature protects the corresponding kidney against **HgCl$_2$** and many other nephrotoxic substances, whereas the contralateral kidney shows severe damage. The protection offered by hydronephrosis is associated with a disappearance of alkaline phosphatase from the convoluted tubules which may reflect lack of elimination and concentration of the nephrotoxic substances in the renal tissue.

Masson & Beland B344/45: Review of the literature on the effect of partial hepatectomy and other forms of liver damage upon **barbiturate** anesthesia. Personal observations on a series of 29 barbiturates tested on partially hepatectomized or completely nephrectomized rats led to the conclusion that the compounds can be classified into four groups: "Group I, those detoxified mainly in the kidney; Group II, those detoxified mainly in the liver; Group III, those detoxified approximately equally in both liver and kidney; Group IV, those possibly detoxified in other tissues of the body, but not to any great extent in the liver and the kidney."

Scheifley A48,124/46: In rats, the anesthetic effect of **pentobarbital** unlike that of thiopental, was greatly prolonged by partial hepatectomy. "These data suggest that the liver is instrumental in protecting against the action of pentobarbital sodium but does not play a significant part in the detoxication of pentothal sodium" (thiopental). Uninephrectomy had no effect upon the production of anesthesia by either of these barbiturates.

Sandberg G71,886/53: Studies on **barbiturate** intoxication in partially hepatectomized or completely nephrectomized rats suggest that, "for 5,5-diallyl-barbituric acid and its 1-(N,N-diethylcarbamylmethyl) derivative the kidneys participate as much as the liver in the detoxication. 1-benzyl-5,5-diallyl-barbituric acid is destroyed mainly in the liver. 1-carbethoxymethyl-5,5-dialkyl-barbiturates are probably hydrolyzed to the corresponding carbonic acid, 1-carboxymethyl-5,5-dialkyl-barbituric acid."

Richards & Taylor H19,235/56: Review on **barbiturates** with a special section on the role of the kidney in their detoxication. (Nephrectomy, nephrotoxic drugs, patients with liver disease).

Gibson & Becker E65,709/67: In mice, "hypoexcretory states" were produced by pe-

Table 127. *Protection of the kidney against mercury by temporary ureter ligature*

Group	Treatment[a]	Renal weight (mg)		Nephrocalcinosis (Positive/Total)		Mortality (Dead/Total)
		Left	Right	Left	Right	
1	None		648	0/15	0/15	0/15
2	HgCl$_2$	—	—	18/18 a	18/18 f	18/18 b
3	Nephrectomy (right)	945 ± 17 d	557 ± 14 d:d'***	0/15	—	0/15
4	HgCl$_2$+ureter ligature (left)	1183 ± 76 c	277 ± 44 c':c:c'*** e	0/6 a':a:a'***	6/6 f':f:f' NS	0/6 b':b:b'***
5	HgCl$_2$+ureter ligature (left) + nephrectomy (left)	799	977 ± 43 e':e:e'***	0/17	11/16 f'':f:f''*	6/17 b'':b:b''***

[a] In groups 4 and 5, the left ureter was ligated on the 1st day. In groups 2, 4 and 5, HgCl$_2$ (400 µg in 1 ml water) was given i.v. on 2nd day in groups 4 and 5, the ureter ligature was removed 4 hrs. after this injection. In group 3 the right, and in group 5 the left kidney was removed and examined for calcinosis (by loupe inspection and by staining with the von Kóssa technique) on 34th day. All rats of group 2 died by the 3rd day. In the other groups, mortality was registered on the 54th day the experiment was terminated and the presence of nephrocalcinosis appraised in all survivors. The surgically removed kidneys in groups 3 and 5 were weighed immediately after nephrectomy on the 34th day, the others upon termination of the experiment 20 days later. The statistical significance of the apparent differences between the readings in groups indicated by the same letter (a—f) was determined by the "Exact Probability Test" for nephrocalcinosis and mortality, by Student's t-test for renal weight.

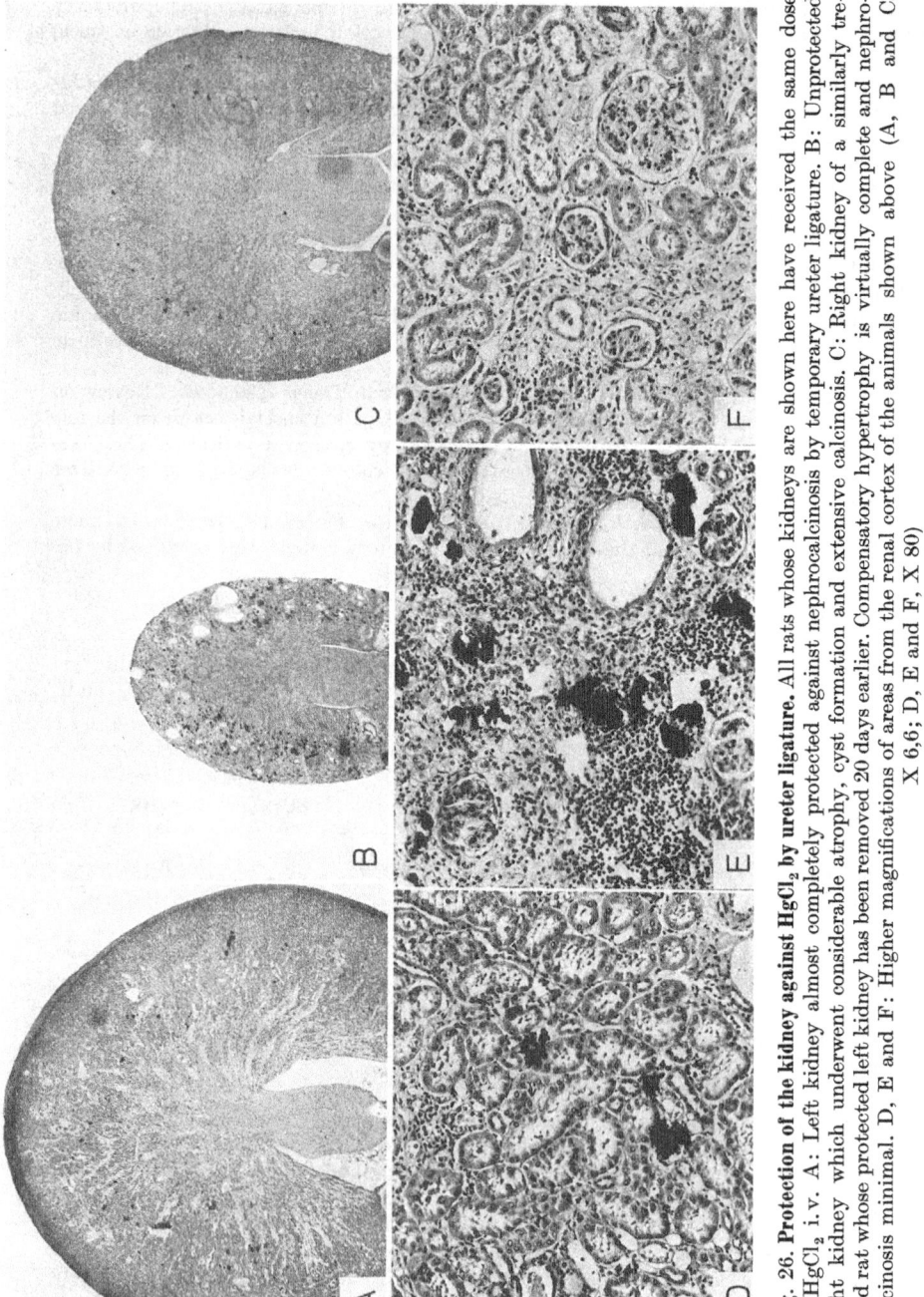

Fig. 26. **Protection of the kidney against HgCl$_2$ by ureter ligature.** All rats whose kidneys are shown here have received the same dose of HgCl$_2$ i.v. A: Left kidney almost completely protected against nephrocalcinosis by temporary ureter ligature. B: Unprotected right kidney which underwent considerable atrophy, cyst formation and extensive calcinosis. C: Right kidney of a similarly treated rat whose protected left kidney has been removed 20 days earlier. Compensatory hypertrophy is virtually complete and nephrocalcinosis minimal. D, E and F: Higher magnifications of areas from the renal cortex of the animals shown above (A, B and C, X 6,6; D, E and F, X 80)

nile ligation, bile duct ligature or drugs (phenylisothiocyanate, α-naphthylisothiocyanate) which reduce bile flow. "Intraperitoneal administration of ouabain to mice with no or diminished bile flow resulted in enhanced mortality rates. **Digoxin** and **digitoxin** affected enhanced lethality in anuric mice. Lanatoside-C was not more toxic to hypoexcretory mice. The use of hypoexcretory mice in toxicologic evaluations of pharmacologic agents is suggested."

Hyde H 15,523/69: In rats, the mitotic index in **regenerating liver** rises after one hour of renal ischemia but not after bilateral nephrectomy.

Selye & Szabo PROT. 35492: In rats, comparatively small doses of **HgCl$_2$** regularly produce fatal bilateral nephrocalcinosis (*cf.* Table 127, p. 624 in which values to be compared are identified by the same letter). Nephrocalcinosis (a : a') and mortality (b : b') are completely prevented if one of the ureters (here left) is temporarily obstructed by a ligature, from 24 hrs before to 4 hrs after the injection of the HgCl$_2$ *cf.* Fig. 26.

In order to occlude the ureter, its middle section was placed into a cranio-caudal slit of the psoas muscle and constricted by a thick silk ligature placed around the ureter-containing segment. Correspondingly, the unprotected kidney becomes sclerotic and atrophic, whereas the contralateral organ undergoes compensatory hypertrophy (c : c') such as is also seen in otherwise untreated unilaterally nephrectomized rats (d : d'). In the present experiment, this physiologic compensatory hypertrophy (d : d') was less evident than that noted in the kidney protected by temporary ligature following calcinotic destruction of the contralateral kidney (c : c'), because in the latter group, the protected kidney was weighed on the 54th day after destruction of the right kidney by mercury, whereas normal compensatory hypertrophy of the left kidney was determined 20 days after ablation of the right kidney.

Survival in group 4 was possible only because the kidney protected by ureter ligature suffices to maintain life as did the normal kidney after right nephrectomy in group 3. In group 5, removal of the protected left kidney on the 34th day resulted in hypertrophy of the nephrocalcinotic and atrophic right kidney (e : e') which also lost most of its pathological calcium deposits (f : f' and f''). This regenerative impulse also has a life-maintaining effect in that the previously atrophic calcinotic right kidney suffices by itself to maintain the life of more than half of the rats which had received the dose of mercury ordinarily sufficient to produce nephrocalcinosis resulting in a 100% mortality (*cf.* b'' with b'). Apparently, under such conditions, the increased demand occasioned by contralateral nephrectomy promotes the functional and structural rehabilitation of a kidney severely damaged by a normally fatal mercurial intoxication.

Selye PROT. 42214: In rats, choledochus ligature offered considerable protection against the toxicity of **indomethacin** and **dioxathion**, slightly prolonged **hexobarbital** sleeping time, and failed to affect **digitoxin** poisoning. Partial hepatectomy had little, if any, effect upon indomethacin, dioxathion and digitoxin poisoning under the prevailing experimental conditions, but considerably prolonged hexobarbital sleeping time. Partial nephrectomy (removal of 80% of the kidney tissue) likewise prolonged hexobarbital sleeping time without significantly influencing indomethacin, dioxathion and digitoxin overdosage. The protective effect of spironolactone against indomethacin, dioxathion and digitoxin remained manifest after most of these surgical interventions. But the protection against indomethacin offered by choledochus ligature could not be further improved by spironolactone, nor was the considerable prolongation by hepatectomy of hexobarbital sleeping time markedly reduced by spironolactone. It must be kept in mind, however, that in these experiments only a single dose of spironolactone was given 5 min after the surgical interventions and 24 hrs before a single dose of the toxicants' *cf.* Table 126, p 600.

← SEX

Resistance to many agents is sex-dependent. In some species, the female, in others, the male is more resistant to a given toxicant.

Thus, female rats are generally much more sensitive than males to the production of anesthesia by steroids and by most barbiturates; indeed even in vitro, their hepatic microsomes are less active in metabolizing these anesthetics than those of males. On the other hand, the catatoxic action of spironolactone against indomethacin, digitoxin and pentobarbital is evident both in male and in female rats. However, allegedly, hexobarbital sleeping time is greatly shortened by spironolactone in female but not in male rats.

Epinephrine arteriosclerosis is more readily produced in female than in male rabbits, and male rats are more resistant than females to the toxic actions of thyroxine.

The tumorigenic effect of certain carcinogens is also sex-dependent, but in this respect, it is difficult to generalize since some of these compounds are more effective in females, others in males.

In certain strains of mice, males are unusually sensitive to the production of renal tubular necrosis by chloroform vapor, and treatment with testoids renders females as susceptible as males.

Many additional examples of such sex differences in sensitivity will be discussed in the following pages and we shall see that in most instances, castration tends to abolish and treatment with the appropriate sex hormones to reestablish them. Since, furthermore, these differences usually appear only after puberty, it may be assumed that in many cases, they depend upon the continued presence within the body of the corresponding sex hormones. Yet, in a few instances, sex-dependent resistance phenomena have been observed even after gonadectomy.

Steroids ←

The first publication on the anesthetic effect of steroids emphasized already that male **rats** are less sensitive than females. This observation has repeatedly been confirmed with a great variety of anesthetic steroids, including progesterone, DOC, and many others that do not exhibit obvious hormonal actions.

There is also a sex difference in the metabolism of ^{14}C-marked androstane derivatives during perfusion through the isolated rat liver. The protection by spironolactone against indomethacin, digitoxin, and pentobarbital is obvious in both sexes, but quantitative studies concerning the comparative efficacy of catatoxic steroids in males and females have not been performed.

In the **mouse**, females are more resistant than males to toxic doses of estradiol and stilbestrol. Female C3H mice regularly develop myocardial calcification after prolonged cortisol treatment, whereas males are comparatively resistant.

Although some investigators claimed that female mice are more sensitive than males to hydroxydione anesthesia, this has not been confirmed, so that in this respect the mouse appears to differ essentially from the rat.

In mature female dogs, the production of hypertension and vascular changes by DOC is more difficult than in males.

Steroids ← *cf. also Selye G60,083/70, pp. 475, 477.*

RAT

Selye A35,003/41: First description of the anesthetic effect of steroids. Male rats are less sensitive than females of equal size.

Selye A35,150/41: Female rats are more sensitive to anesthesia produced by various steroids than are males, and young animals of either sex are more sensitive than adults.

Winter & Selye A35,658/41; Winter A36,333/41: Female rats are more sensitive than males to the anesthetic action of progesterone but this sex difference is obvious only after maturity. "The normal endocrine activity of the testis is largely, if not entirely, responsible for this comparative resistance of the males since castration increases sensitivity in males but is without effect in female rats. Conversely the resistance of castrate males and females may be raised by methyl testosterone administration."

Selye & Pentz A 59,789/43: Female rats are much more sensitive than males to the production of hyalinosis and hypertension by DOC + uninephrectomy + NaCl.

Emmens A 46,574/46: In immature rats of both sexes, pentobarbital has an approximately equal anesthetic effect, whereas DOC and progesterone are twice as potent in females as in males.

Allardyce et al. B 29,416/48: Following a single i.m. injection of DOC, male rats exhibit a greater rise in blood pressure than do females.

Fonts et al. B 54,459/50: Female rats are about ten times more sensitive to progesterone and DOC anesthesia than are males.

Forchielli et al. D 75,874/58: The rate of Δ^4 reduction of 11-desoxycortisol was 3—4 fold greater in female than in male rat liver homogenates and in microsomal fractions containing the Δ^4-5α-hydrogenase. Female rat liver contains only one Δ^4-hydrogenase (5α-microsomal), whereas the male liver contains the soluble Δ^4-5β-hydrogenase as well. Ovariectomy caused no marked change in enzyme titer, but hypophysectomy decreased it sharply. Curiously, ACTH, STH and pregnant mare serum partially restored the enzyme level in the hypophysectomized rat. In young animals, increase in the titer of hepatic Δ^4-5α-hydrogenase occurs prior to puberty. This fact (like the negative results after ovariectomy) suggests an independence of enzyme regulation from ovarian hormones.

Yates et al. C 61,952/58: "Homogenates of livers from adult female rats reduce Ring A of Δ^4-3-keto-steroids at rates 3 to 10 times greater than those from males. This large sex difference has been observed for all substrates so far tested: aldosterone, desoxycorticosterone, hydrocortisone, cortisone, corticosterone, testosterone and progesterone. ... Castration increases and testosterone decreases Δ^4-steroid hydrogenase activity in males. In females, neither castration nor estrogen administration had appreciable effect."

Leybold & Staudinger C 77,908/59: Description of sex differences in the ability of the hepatic microsomes of the rat to metabolize various steroid hormones.

Rummel et al. C 80,035/59: Male rats are more resistant than females to the anesthetic effect of DOC.

Colás D 20,925/62: The livers of male rats contain more dehydroepiandrosterone 16α-hydroxylase than that of males. Castration reduces the enzyme activity but not quite to the low level of the female.

Kuntzman et al. F 27,893/64: The steroid hydroxylase of the microsomal fraction of rat liver is more active in males than in females.

Schriefers & Wassmuth G 23,742/64: "The Δ^4-5α-hydrogenase activity in liver microsomes of female rats is 8.5 times that of males; but liver slices from females reduce cortisone at only twice the rate of slices from males." Comparative kinetic analysis showed that, in the female, the rate of diffusion, whereas, in the male, the low enzyme activity, is the limiting factor.

Kuntzmann & Jacobson F 35,869/65: "Incubation of progesterone-4-C^{14} with liver microsomes from adult male rats resulted in oxidation of the steroid to a more polar fraction made up of 6β- and 16β-hydroxyprogesterone and an unidentified U.V. absorbing product. In contrast, female rats metabolized progesterone primarily by reduction of the A ring followed by subsequent metabolism to polar compounds. Unlike the female rat, female rabbits and guinea pigs metabolized progesterone by hydroxylation. With microsomes from immature male rats, both hydroxylation and reduction occurred. Chronic administration of phenobarbital, chlorcycline or chlordane to female rats caused an increased formation of polar metabolites but had little effect on the disappearance of progesterone, since the main pathway in the female rat is A-ring reduction. In contrast, chronic phenobarbital administration to female rabbits increased markedly the metabolism of progesterone to hydroxylated derivatives when measured either by formation of polar metabolites or by progesterone disappearance."

Conney et al. G 65,135/65: In the male rat, the oxidative metabolism of hexobarbital, testosterone and estradiol by hepatic microsomes is more pronounced than in the female. The mouse shows no comparable sex difference.

Remmer & Merker G 66,868/65: The hepatic Δ^4-3-ketoreductase activity is much higher in female than in male rats, but cannot be further increased by phenobarbital, although the barbiturate does induce two similar TPHN-dependent microsomal reductases involved in the metabolism of p-amino-azobenzol and of chloramphenicol.

Denef & de Moor H15,811/69: The sexual differentiation of steroid-metabolizing enzymes appears in the rat liver from the 30th day of life on. From experiments on neonatally-gonadectomized or intact rats treated with folliculoid or testoid compounds, "it is concluded that, as far as the differentiation of cortisol metabolizing enzymes is concerned, estradiol is able to counteract the organizing action of testosterone at birth as well as the expression of these neonatal testosterone effects after the 30th day of life."

Grossman et al. H18,545/69: In male rats, adrenalectomy decreases the protein content and the number of zymogen granules in the pancreas. "The female rat does not demonstrate these changes following adrenalectomy. However, if the ovaries are removed in addition to the adrenal glands, alterations similar to those observed in the adrenalectomized rat with triamcinolone acetonide reverts the pancreas to normal. In contrast to the male, the female rat apparently had dual control of the pancreas through estrogenic as well as adrenal cortical hormones."

Schriefers et al. H21,007/70: Demonstration of sex differences in the metabolism of ^{14}C-marked androstane derivatives during perfusion through the isolated rat liver.

Kato et al. H34,571/71: Male rats are more resistant to the anesthetic effect of progesterone than females. Correspondingly the formation of hydroxylated metabolites of this steroid is greater with hepatic microsomes from males, whereas the formation of Δ^4-reduced metabolites is greater with female microsomes. In mice, there was no such difference either in the anesthetic action or in the in vitro metabolism of progesterone. In rats, the blood and tissue level of polar metabolites of tritiated progesterone was higher in males, whereas that of nonpolar metabolites was higher in females. "These results suggest that the stronger anesthetic action of progesterone in female rats is associated with higher tissue levels of progesterone and Δ^4-reduced metabolites, possessing the anesthetic action."

Selye PROT. 29733: In rats weighing 100—200 g, the catatoxic action of spironolactone against indomethacin, digitoxin and pentobarbital is evident in both sexes.

Selye PROT. 42911: In male rats, the protective effect of PCN, spironolactone, ethylestrenol, betamethasone, phenobarbital and phenylbutazone against intoxication with digitoxin, indomethacin, dioxathion, parathion, nicotine, progesterone, hexobarbital and zoxazolamine has been systematically examined (*cf.* Table 128, p. 630). Hexobarbital sleeping time was not shortened by PCN, spironolactone or betamethasone. For betamethasone, this is not remarkable since this compound failed to affect hexobarbital sleeping time in females also (*cf.* Table 136), but PCN and spironolactone were effective in this respect in females. In order to evaluate these data, the effect of each conditioner against each toxicant should be compared with similar experiments on females (Table 136).

Testosterone ← Sex, Rat: Kuntzman et al. *F27,893/64;* Conney et al. *G65,135/65*

Mouse

Selye & Stevenson 77,177/40: In Strong's C3H strain mice, females are more resistant than males to toxic doses of estradiol or stilbestrol. This sex difference is even more pronounced in the case of combined administration of folliculoids and progesterone, which increases the toxicity of folliculoids. The gonads of both sexes show considerable atrophy under the influence of folliculoids but this is inhibited by progesterone.

Koller C19,288/56: Mice of both sexes are approximately equally sensitive to hydroxydione anesthesia. Gonadectomy increases sensitivity to this form of narcosis especially in females but to a lesser extent also in males.

Lostroh C54,348/58: Female mice of the C3H strain regularly develop myocardial calcification following prolonged cortisol treatment, whereas males are comparatively resistant. Ovariectomy offers no protection but testosterone renders females more resistant. In hypophysectomized mice neither cortisol nor ACTH produces myocardial calcification.

Atkinson et al. D33,188/62: Female mice are more sensitive than males to hydroxydione anesthesia but allegedly there is no such sex difference to the anesthesia produced by 3α-hydroxy-5β-pregnane-11,20-dione 3-phosphate disodium.

Rümke G68,532/66: The anesthetic effect of hydroxydione is greater in female than in male mice.

Jelinek H1,518/68: There was no difference in the duration of hydroxydione anesthesia in male and female intact or gonadectomized mice. Pretreatment with methyltestosterone p.o. prolonged hydroxydione anesthesia in males but not in females or castrate males.

Neither thiopental nor pentobarbital anesthesia was influenced by methyltestosterone. Pretreatment with methandrostenolone or 17α-methyl-androst-2-ene-17β-ol failed to influence hydroxydione anesthesia in mice.

Cortisone ← Sex + Adrenalectomy, Mouse: Wragg et al. B74,080/52*; Kato et al. H31,735/70

Estradiol ← Sex, Mouse, Rat: Kuntzman et al. F27,893/64; Conney et al. G65,135/65

DOG
Rowinski et al. B64,142/51; de Muro & Rowinski B66,413/51: The production of hypertension and vascular changes by DOC is more difficult in mature female than in male dogs.

FROG
Rybová & Janáček G78,569/70: In frog bladders, aldosterone exerts a sex dependent effect in that the water and ion contents are reduced in males and increased in females.

Table 128. *Catatoxic action of various conditioners in male rats*[a]

Toxicants / Conditioners	Digitoxin (2 mg in 1 ml water p.o. x2)		Indomethacin (1mg in 0.2 ml water s.c. x5)		Dioxathion (5.3 mg in 1 ml corn oil p.o. x1)		Parathion (1.3 mg in 0.5 ml DMSO i.p. x3)	
	Convulsions +4th day	Mortality +6th day	Intestinal Ulcers	Mortality +6th day	Dyskinesia +6 hrs	Mortality +48 hrs	Dyskinesia +3rd day +4 hrs.	Mortality +4th day
None	17/30	9/30	29/29	28/30	29/30	19/30	30/30	30/30
PCN	0/10 ***	0/10 NS	0/10 ***	0/10 ***	0/10 ***	0/10 ***	1/10 ***	0/10 ***
Spironolactone	0/10 ***	0/10 NS	0/10 ***	0/10 ***	8/10 NS	4/10 NS	4/10 ***	3/10 ***
Ethylestrenol	0/10 ***	0/10 NS	0/10 ***	0/10 ***	2/10 ***	0/10 ***	0/10 ***	0/10 ***
Betamethasone-Ac	0/10 ***	0/10 NS	5/9 **	9/10 NS	7/10 NS	6/10 NS	10/10 NS	10/10 NS
Phenobarbital	9/10 NS	2/10 NS	0/10 ***	0/10 ***	0/10 ***	0/10 ***	0/10 ***	0/10 ***
Phenylbutazone	7/10 NS	4/10 NS	4/9 ***	1/10 ***	4/10 ***	1/10 *	0/10 ***	0/10 ***

[a] The conditioners were administedred as follows: PCN, spironolcatone, ethylestrenol and phenylbutazone 10 mg, phenobarbital 6 mg and betamethasone 1 mg, all in 1 ml water, p.o., twice daily from the −4th day (counting the day of toxicant administration as the first day) until the end of the experiment. Only the groups treated with digitoxin received the conditioners until the second day a.m., and those given dioxathion until the first day a.m.

MAN

Southren & Gordon G77,117/70: Review and personal observations on the application of radioisotopes to the in vivo study of the kinetics of testoid metabolism in man, with special reference to sex differences, adrenalectomy, orchidectomy, and various diseases upon the plasma clearance of testosterone.

Corticoids ← Sex: Hübener et al. B91,352/53; Forchielli et al. D75,874/58; Yates et al. C56,413/58; Leybold et al. C77,908/59; Hagen et al. G77,512/60; Leybold et al. C88,830/60; Sholiton F23,871/64

Testoids ← Sex: Rubin G76,315/57; Forchielli et al. D75,874/58; Leybold et al. C77,908/59; C88,830/60; Colas D20,925/62; Kuntzman et al. G66,245/66; Kato et al. H31,734/70, H31,735/70

Folliculoids ← Sex: Kuntzman et al. G66,245/66; Zumoff et al. H1,151/68*; Jellinck et al. H32,603/70

Luteoids ← Sex: Forchielli et al. D75,874/58; Leybold et al. C77,908/59; C88,830/60; Kuntzman et al. G66,245/66; Kato et al. H30,605/70

Steroids (Var) ← Sex: Yates et al. C61,952/58; Heinrichs et al. F72,860/66

Nonsteroidal Hormones and Hormone-Like Substances ←

Female rats are allegedly more resistant than males to the acute effects of **epinephrine** i.v., and, in female rabbits, it is more difficult to produce arteriosclerosis by chronic treatment with epinephrine than in males.

The **insulin** resistance of male rabbits is greater than that of females, and alloxan produces diabetes more readily in female than in male rats.

Male rats are more sensitive than females to overdosage with **thyroxine**.

Table 128 (continued)

Toxicants / Conditioners	Nicotine (1 ml of 1.3% aqueous solution p.o. x5)		Progesterone (15 mg in 1 ml corn oil i.p. x1)	Hexobarbital (10 mg in 1 ml water i.p. x1)	Zoxazolamine (15 mg in 1 ml water i.p. x1)
	Dyskinesia +3rd day +30 min	Mortality +6th day	Sleeping time	Sleeping time	Paralysis time
None	25/25	25/25	251 ± 29	40 ± 3	292 ± 19
PCN	8/10 NS	7/10 NS	0 ***	36 ± 3 NS	77 ± 17 ***
Spironolactone	10/10 NS	10/10 NS	0 ***	34 ± 3 NS	248 ± 23 NS
Ethylestrenol	0/10 ***	0/10 ***	0 ***	3 ± 2 ***	143 ± 27 ***
Betamethasone-Ac	10/10 NS	10/10 NS	51 ± 34 ***	46 ± 5 NS	186 ± 7 ***
Phenobarbital	0/10 ***	0/10 ***	0 ***	1 ± 1 ***	128 ± 20 ***
Phenylbutazone	2/10 ***	2/10 ***	0 ***	7 ± 2 ***	230 ± 24 NS

Resistance to **histamine** shows no distinct sex specificity in normal rats, but thyroparathyroidectomy allegedly increases histamine tolerance in females only. After sensitization with pertussis vaccine, female mice become more sensitive to histamine than males. In rats, in which acetic acid was administered by aerosol, subsequent inhalation of vaporized histamine produces an asthmatic attack among females only.

Catecholamines ← cf. also Selye G60,083/70, p. 478.

Astarabadi & Essex B75,437/52: Female rats are more resistant to epinephrine i.v. than males. Gonadectomy was without effect on the resistance of males but caused females to become as susceptible as males.

Plotka et al. C51,239/57: In rabbits, the production of aortic lesions by epinephrine i.v. is partly inhibited by adrenosterone; yet, normally males are more sensitive than females to epinephrine arteriosclerosis.

ACTH ← cf. Selye G60,083/70, pp. 476, 479.

Pancreatic Hormones ←

Dotti 34,994/36: Female rabbits are more sensitive to insulin than males.

Beach et al. B61,498/51: The diabetogenic effect of alloxan is greater in female than in male rats.

Foglia & Penhos B79,957/52: In male rats, extensive partial pancreatectomy causes severe diabetes more frequently than in females. Postnatal orchidectomy abolishes this difference.

Thyroid Hormones ←

Garvin et al. D21,160/62: Male rats are more sensitive than females to the production of hyperthyroidism by thyroxine.

Fonzo et al. G77,635/70: In rats, the hepatic storage of ^{125}I-thyroxine is greater and its subsequent deiodation smaller among females than among males. "It may be concluded that the female liver has a greater affinity for thyroxin and that a stronger binding of the hormone with the proteins of hepatocytes accounts for the decreased deiodation among females."

Parathyroid Hormone ←

Rowinski & Manunta B64,144/51: Mortality after parathyroidectomy is equal in male and in spayed female rats, whereas intact females are more resistant.

Histamine ← Sex: Sackler et al. B78,749/53*

Histamine ←

Sackler et al. B78,749/53: In rats, thyroparathyroidectomy increases histamine tolerance, but only in females. Intact rats show no sex difference in histamine tolerance. Gonadectomy raises histamine tolerance in both sexes.

Chedid C1,930/54: After sensitization with pertussis vaccine, female mice become more sensitive to histamine than males.

Gross C30,649/55: In rats, administration of histamine by aerosol or of egg-white i.p. elicits an asthmatic attack if the lung was previously irritated by inhalation of acetic acid given by a spray. This response is obtained in females, castrate males or males treated with folliculoids but not in normal males. Testosterone and progesterone abolish this effect in females and castrate males.

Drugs ←

The toxicity of innumerable drugs is sex-dependent to some extent. Here, we shall deal mainly with those toxicants which are of particular interest in connection with the problem of hormonal regulation of resistance. A more complete enumeration of pertinent observations will be found in the Abstract Section.

It is difficult to make any generalizations concerning the sex difference in the sensitivity to **barbiturates** since this differs depending upon the particular compound and animal species used. In the mouse, susceptibility to hexobarbital anesthesia does not appear to be sex-dependent, but females are more sensitive to amobarbital and pentobarbital than males. There are strains of mice, however, in which hexobarbital produces longer lasting anesthesia in males than in females and the 9000 g liver supernatant of the latter hydroxylates hexobarbital faster than that of males. The resistance to pentobarbital anesthesia induced by pretreatment with phenobarbital lasts longer in female than in male mice.

Most of the investigations concerning the sex dependence of barbiturate anesthesia have been performed in **rats**. It has been noted as early as 1932, that in this species, males are more resistant to amobarbital anesthesia than females. Similar observations have subsequently been made with numerous other barbiturates. This sex difference appears only after puberty and is abolished by castration. On the other hand, testosterone treatment raises the barbiturate resistance both in females and in castrate males to approximately the normal male level. Upon repeated pentobarbital injections, rats of both sexes become comparatively tolerant to this barbiturate, but when treatment is interrupted, susceptibility rises more rapidly in females and male castrates than in intact males.

Sexual activity as such does not significantly influence ectylurea sleeping time in rats of either sex; however, females are comparatively resistant during and shortly after pregnancy.

Unlike most other barbiturates, thiopental is about equally effective in male and in female rats.

Liver slices of male rats detoxify hexobarbital in vitro more actively than similar preparations of female rats, but no such sex difference could be demonstrated for thiopental. Certain microsomal enzyme-inhibitors, such as Sch 5712, prolong hexobarbital sleeping time about 12-fold in female and only 3-fold in male rats in vivo. Yet, this difference is absent when Sch 5712 is added to unfortified liver homogenate from rats of either sex.

The D-enantiomer of hexobarbital has a much greater anesthetic effect in female than in male rats, whereas no such sex difference in sleeping time is observed for the L-enantiomer. This is unexpected, since the metabolism of both enantiomers is more rapid in males.

In general, it may be said that the sex differences in sensitivity to barbiturate anesthesia appear only after puberty, being virtually abolished by gonadectomy in both sexes, and that they can be raised to the male level by the administration of testoids to females or gonadectomized males. The sex differences are attributed to an increased microsomal enzyme activity in the livers of males, since even in vitro liver slices or microsomal fractions of males are more potent in detoxifying most barbiturates than those of females. Yet, not all barbiturates are subject to such sex differences of their detoxication in rats, and no clear-cut and constant sex dependence of hexobarbital anesthesia could be demonstrated in **mice, guinea pigs, rabbits** and **dogs**.

Under identical dietary conditions, male rats are more susceptible than females to the hepatotoxic and nephrotoxic actions of CCl_4. However, some investigators obtained opposite results, presumably because this sex difference appears to be highly dependent upon incidental circumstances, such as dosage, duration of exposure and the strain of rat used.

A definite sex difference has also been noted with regard to the tumorigenic effects of various **carcinogens**. In certain strains of mice, o-aminoazotoluene produces hepatomas much more frequently in females than in males. Furthermore, intact females are more susceptible than spayed females; castrate males approach intact females in the degree of their susceptibility. The incidence of pulmonary tumors produced by this carcinogen is not dependent upon any of the factors just mentioned.

AAF induces hepatomas only in male mice. Male rats develop hepatomas on various azo-dyes more readily than females: they are also more sensitive than females to aflatoxin and to various other carcinogens.

On the other hand, diacetamidofluorene allegedly produces more hepatic tumors in female than in male mice.

The fact that carcinogens which elicit mammary tumors easily in females fail to do so in males is too well-known to deserve detailed discussion.

The adrenal necrosis produced by DMBA in the rat does not appear to be sex dependent.

A sex difference in susceptibility to **carcinolytic agents** has also been described. In the mouse, rat and man, females are more sensitive than males to the toxic effects of numerous antineoplastic compounds. Thus cycloheximide is more toxic to female than to male rats or mice, but no such sex difference is noted in dogs. On the other hand, in rats, females are more resistant than males to vinblastine, and cyclophosphamide produces less extensive and less lasting bladder lesions in female than in male rats.

In adult male mice of various strains, exposure to **chloroform** vapor produced necrosis of the renal tubules, whereas females showed no such change. Testoids rendered females susceptible, whereas folliculoids decreased the sensitivity of males.

Female rats are much more resistant than males to the production of cardiovascular lesions by **choline** deficiency. Mature intact or ovariectomized females — but not intact males — develop fatty infiltration of the liver when fed a choline-containing but methionine-deficient diet, for three days. Castrate males are as susceptible as females, and testosterone raises resistance both in females and in castrate males.

Sensitivity to certain **digitalis** compounds is also sex-dependent, at least in some species. Female mice are more resistant to ouabain than males, but resistance to strophanthin-k is the same in both cases. Adult female rats are also more resistant to ouabain than males, but the sex difference does not become evident before 2-4 months of age. The lethal dose of ouabain for the isolated heart of female rats is considerably higher than that for the heart of male rats. Male and castrate female dogs are more sensitive than intact females to intoxication with digoxin.

The tail necrosis produced in rats by large doses of **ergotamine** does not appear to be conspicuously sex-dependent. However, males are allegedly more sensitive than females to the production of neurofibromas and renal calcification by chronic ergot intoxication.

Male rats are more resistant than females to the production of fatty livers by **ethionine**. Orchidectomy abolishes this resistance, and testosterone protects both females and castrate males.

Ethylene glycol intoxication elicits oxalate and calcium precipitation in the kidneys more readily in male than in female rats.

Lathyrogens produce aortic aneurysms more readily in young males than in females. On the other hand, in male rats — unlike in females or orchidectomized males — the osteolathyrism produced by AAN is inhibited by rich casein diets.

Data on the sex-dependence of **nicotine** intoxication are so contradictory that they cannot be profitably discussed.

Periportal fatty degeneration of the liver is produced by chronic **orotic acid** feeding more readily in female than in male rats. Orchidectomy abolishes this resistance unless testosterone treatment is administered.

There is also a definite sex difference in the response of animals to various **pesticides**. Data concerning DDT sensitivity are somewhat contradictory, but male rats are more resistant than females to various cholinergic phosphorothioates, and particularly to parathion. On the other hand, the toxicity of OMPA is about the same in rats of either sex. In an extensive series in which 98 pesticides and two metabolites of DDT were tested in the rat, most compounds proved to be more toxic to females; yet, nine pesticides were more toxic to males. Morestan, which belongs to the exceptional pesticides that are more toxic to males, appears to be equally damaging after orchidectomy or estradiol treatment of males, and after testosterone treatment of females.

Female rats are more sensitive than males to intoxication with **strychnine**. This difference is abolished by SKF 525-A.

Excessive **tyrosine feeding** causes more pronounced manifestations of tyrosinosis (conjunctivitis, alopecia, pancreatic lesions, inflammation of the paws) in male than in female rats.

Male rats are much more resistant than females to intoxication with **vitamin D** or **DHT**. Earlier claims that female mice are more resistant than males to irradiated ergosterol intoxication require confirmation.

Acetophenetidin ← Sex, Man, Rat: Kuntzman et al. H30,992/66

Acetylcholine ←

Bonino C30,089/56: Female guinea pigs are more sensitive to lethal acetylcholine intoxication than males. Earlier literature is reviewed.

Aminopterin ←

Goldin et al. D76,907/50: There is no sex difference in the toxicity of aminopterin in immature mice, but among adults, males are more resistant than females. Estradiol increases aminopterin tolerance in immature and mature males, whereas testosterone does not influence it.

Aminopterin ← Sex + Steroids, Mouse: Goldin et al. D76,907/50*

Aminopyrine ←

Soyka G66,626/69: In rat liver, the aminopyrine demethylase activity of the microsomal fraction increased considerably during the first 30 days after birth. Evidence of an inhibitor was not found during this newborn period. After puberty, the activity in male rats was about twice as high as in females. Testosterone produced only an insignificant rise in females.

Aminopyrine ← Sex: Herken et al. G74,662/58; Siegert et al. G71,866/64*; Kato et al. F57,817/65, F76,403/66, G68,411/66, G80,897/68; Kato G74,104/66; Kinoshita et al. G71,863/66; Schenkman et al. G67,777/67

Amphetamine ←

Groppetti & Costa H31,959/69: In adult male rats, the disappearance of amphetamine is faster than in adult females. Estradiol retards the rate of amphetamine disappearance in adult males. Such potent hepatic microsomal enzyme inducers as phenobarbital, 3-MC, or diphenylhydantoin do not change the tissue levels of amphetamine.

Anaphylactoidogens ← *cf.* Selye G46,715/68, p. 209.

Aniline ← Sex: Quinn et al. E89,993/58*; Kato G74,104/66; Kato et al. F76,403/66, G68,411/66; Schenkman et al. G67,777/67

Antibiotics ←

Hurst D33,743/58: Female mice are much more susceptible than males to the therapeutic action of streptomycin on streptococcal infection.

Anticoagulants ← Sex: Feuer et al. G76,853/67

Antipyrine ← Sex, Dog, Gp, Man, Mouse, Rat, Rb: Quinn et al. E89,993/58*

Arsenic ←

Durham et al. A49,445/29: Female mice weighing over 18 g are more sensitive to novarsenobenzene (Neosalvarsan) than males, whereas mice weighing less than 15 g show no such sex difference.

Agduhr A51,257/37: In mice and rats of both sexes, sexual intercourse increases resistance against As_2O_3 and vitamin D.

Agduhr E70,688/41: Repeated mating increases the resistance of both male and female mice to arsenic. Pregnancy further augments this protective effect in females.

Skanse A72,698/41: Review on the effect of sex, sexual intercourse and gonadectomy upon the storage of arsenic in the tissues of mice.

Barbiturates ←
MOUSE

Kennedy A43,060/34: The susceptibility of mice and rats to hexobarbital anesthesia does not appear to be sex dependent. These findings are contrasted with those obtained with amobarbital to which females are more sensitive.

Buchel & Liblau E89,233/63: In Swiss mice, there is no sex difference in hexobarbital sleeping time or in the disappearance rate of this drug from the brain.

Westfall et al. F2,504/64: Pentobarbital anesthesia is more prolonged in male than in female mice. Sleeping time in males is shortened by stilbestrol and, in females, prolonged by testosterone. Apparently, the mechanism for barbiturate detoxication is different in mice and rats.

Rümke G71,098/68: In mice of the CPB-N strain, hexobarbital anesthesia lasts longer in males than in females, but only after puberty. Following gonadectomy of mature animals, the sex difference persists for about 2 weeks but then disappears.

Rümke & Noordhoek H21,659/69: Among mice of many strains, hexobarbital produces longer anesthesia in males than in females. This difference is evident only after sexual maturation. If 10 week old males are castrated, the difference persists for at least 2 weeks, but it disappears after a month. Ovariectomy has no effect upon sleeping time; testosterone increases it in females but not in males.

Noordhoek & Rümke H21,660/69: In mice, the 9000 g liver supernatant of females hydroxylates hexobarbital faster than that of males. After orchidectomy, the in vitro metabolism of hexobarbital becomes equal to that of females but ovariectomy has no effect upon it. Testosterone decreases the rate of in vitro hexobarbital hydroxylation in females but not in males. Female livers contain more cytochrome P-450 and testosterone lowers its concentration in female but not in male livers.

Buchel & Levy G74,850/70: In mice, pretreatment with phenobarbital decreases pentobarbital sleeping time; this phenomenon is detectable within 24 hrs and reaches a maximum 48 hrs after phenobarbital administration. The resistance is no longer detectable in males after 96, in females after 120 hrs.

Gerald & Feller G74,396/70: In mice, spironolactone and its Δ^6-dethioacetylated metabolite reduce hexobarbital sleeping time and cause nearly identical increases in liver weight, microsomal protein content, NADPH-cytochrome c reductase, cytochrome P-450 content and the N-demethylation of ethylmorphine. Preliminary observations suggest that these actions of spironolactone and of its metabolite are evident in both sexes.

Amobarbital, Butallylonal, Hexobarbital ← Sex, Mouse: Holck et al. A8,011/37*

Barbital, Hexobarbital, Pentobarbital ← Sex, Mouse: Blackham et al. G69,913/69*

Hexobarbital ← Sex + Testosterone, Mouse: Holck et al. A55,755/42*

Hexobarbital ← Sex + Genetics, Mouse: Fujii et al. H28,618/68*

Pentobarbital ← Sex + Testosterone, Mouse: Westfall et al. F2,504/64*

Secobarbital ← Sex + Disulfiram, Mouse: Gruber et al. D41,363/54

RAT

Nicholas & Barron 62,223/32: Male rats are more resistant than females to amobarbital anesthesia.

Barron A42,858/33: Male rats are more resistant than females to amobarbital anesthesia. Castration increases the sensitivity of the male but not quite to the female level. Castration before puberty does not diminish resistance. Ancillary experiments suggest that the effect of castration is due to changes in water metabolism.

Holck & Kanan 31,302/35: Female rats are more sensitive than males to various barbiturate anesthetics. No such sex difference could be detected in the dog, cat, rabbit, guinea pig, mouse, turtle or frog.

Holck et al. 68,297/37: Female rats are much more sensitive to anesthesia by various barbiturates than are males. Orchidectomy diminished barbiturate sensitivity, but not quite to the low level of normal females. Barbital anesthesia was not influenced by sex. Testosterone increased barbiturate resistance in normal or ovariectomized females, but not quite to the level of normal males.

Holck et al. A8,011/37: "Using duration of hypnosis and incidence of mortality as criteria, no sex-difference was found in the white or hybrid rat to barbiturates with two short side-chains, or one such with an iso-aliphatic or a phenyl group (barbital, ipral, alurate, diallyl barbiturate, nostal, dichlor allyl barbiturate, phenobarbital). No sex-difference was found to chloral hydrate. A slight to moderately higher male resistance was seen with barbiturates having one short and one longer straight aliphatic chain (neonal, ortal; also to ethyl 2-methyl-amyl barbiturate). Much higher male resistance was present with barbiturates having one short and one long, forked chain (not of the iso type) or a cyclohexenyl group (amytal, pentobarbital, seconal, pernoston and its chlorine homologue, rectidon (sigmodal), phanodorn and evipal), or those with a methylated nitrogen (eunarcon, evipal). These are the short acting ones, but nostal is also short acting and the rat exhibits no sex-difference to it. No sex-difference was found to evipal in certain other species of animals (dog, cat, rabbit, guinea pig, mouse, frog). In mice sex-difference was also absent to amytal, but was present in case of pernoston to a slight extent."

Moir E54,544/37: Very young female rats are more resistant to pentobarbital than males, whereas the reverse was true in mature rats. Both males and females developed tolerance to pentobarbital upon repeated injections, but when treatment was interrupted and then resumed, susceptibility was greatly increased in females and castrate males but not in intact males. "Inasmuch as the castrated males still remained more resistant than females, the superior resistance of the males was held to be due at least in part to some factor or factors other than the male gonads."

Carmichael D68,076/38: The LD 50 of pentobarbital increases with age but "there does not seem to be a definite sex difference in reaction to the median lethal dose of nembutal of either young or old rats." In earlier observations in which males were found to be more resistant to barbiturates, the anesthetic action and not the lethal effect was determined.

Holck & Fink A35,663/40: Sexual activity or the absence of it failed to influence ectylurea (Nostal, isopropyl bromallyl barbituric acid) anesthesia in male or female rats. However, resistance to this barbiturate was markedly raised during pregnancy and in females which recently had been pregnant although, even in these, it was not brought up to the male level.

Kinsey A39,742/40: Female rats sleep about twice as long as males when given either single or repeated injections of pentobarbital. Testosterone increases pentobarbital resistance in females. Ovariectomy diminishes the sleeping time.

Holck & Mathieson 80,435/41: Male rats are more resistant than females to the lethal effect of pentobarbital. Castration reduced the tendency to develop tolerance following repeated pentobarbital injections in males but increased it in females. Testosterone pretreatment increased resistance in castrate males and intact females, but not in intact males.

Horinaga A36,414/41: Male rats are more resistant to barbiturate anesthesia than females. Orchidectomy and treatment with folliculoids increase sensitivity, whereas ovariectomy does not affect it.

Holck et al. 84,766/43: Adult male rats are more resistant than females to sodium vinbarbital and calcium 5-ethyl 5-(2-butyl) N-methyl barbituric acid.

Holck & Mathieson B644/44: In rats, the development of tolerance to pentobarbital was determined by injecting increasing doses every 90 min day and night for periods up to 5 days. 1–2 Month-old rats practically all developed tolerance as did adult males in contrast to females. Castration lowered the ability of adult males to develop tolerance, but did do so in 2 month-old males. Ovariectomy of 2 month-old females increased their ability to detoxify pentobarbital, once tolerance had developed.

Masson B275/45: Male rats are more resistant to pentobarbital anesthesia than females. However, upon treatment with LAP (lyophilized anterior pituitary) s.c., resistance decreased considerably in both sexes and eventually reached the same low level in males and females. LAP produced a similar increase in sensitivity to amobarbital, hexobarbital, cyclobarbital and vinbarbital, but did not influence barbital or phenobarbital anesthesia.

Emmens A46,574/46: In immature rats of both sexes, pentobarbital has an approximately equal anesthetic effect, whereas DOC and progesterone are twice as potent in females as in males.

Homburger et al. E61,371/47: Female rats are more sensitive than males to pentobarbital but not to thiopental anesthesia. Age and strain differences in barbiturate resistance have also been noted in the rat.

Crevier et al. B54,151/50: Pentobarbital anesthesia lasts longer in female than in male rats as judged by the linguo-maxillary reflex. Castration abolishes the high resistance of the male, but testosterone restores it again to the normal level. In ovariectomized rats, estradiol has virtually no effect but testosterone raises resistance to the male level. These in vivo effects run parallel to the in vitro pentobarbital detoxifying power of the liver.

Jarcho et al. B59,706/50: Adult male rats require larger amounts of pentobarbital than do females for the prolonged maintenance of deep surgical anesthesia.

Maloney et al. E48,771/52: The pentobarbital sleeping time is greatly increased after adrenalectomy in rats of both sexes, males being more resistant than females. Vitamin C lengthened the sleeping time in both intact and adrenalectomized animals. Cortisone shortened the sleeping time of adrenalectomized, but lengthened that of intact animals. DOC diminished sleeping time more markedly in females than in males. [This brief abstract gives, as the authors themselves are careful to point out, "somewhat of a confused picture" (H.S.).]

Grewe D35,140/53: Male rats are more resistant than females to barbiturate (eunarcon, hexobarbital) anesthesia. After gonadectomy both sexes exhibit the longer sleeping time characteristic of females. Twenty-eight days following orchidectomy, the sleeping time is reduced to the level seen in intact males. Testosterone shortens the sleeping time of females.

Buchel D59,654/53: Extensive investigations on the influence of sex upon the sensitivity of the rat to numerous barbiturates, chloral hydrate and ethyl urethan.

Buchel D73,669/54: Review on the literature and personal observations on the increased sleeping time of female as compared to male rats after treatment with certain barbiturates particularly hexobarbital. The increased sleeping time is associated with a prolonged persistence of the concentration of the drug in the blood. Gonadectomy prolongs the sleeping time of males but does not influence that of females. In immature rats no such sex difference is observed.

Quinn et al. G67,327/54: The biologic half-life of hexobarbital was found to be 15 min for mice, 60 min for rabbits, 140 min for rats, and 260 min for dogs and man. There was an inverse relationship between the rate of biotransformation of hexobarbital to ketohexobarbital and the duration of its hypnotic effect. Male rats are more resistant to hexobarbital anesthesia than females but in the latter, resistance as well as the enzyme activity of the microsomes was increased by testosterone.

Robillard et al. G67,325/54: Adult males are more resistant than females to pentobarbital anesthesia. Castration decreases the resistance in males. Testosterone raises pentobarbital resistance to the normal male level in both male and female castrates, whereas estradiol and progesterone prolong anesthesia in castrates of both sexes. [The hormones were administered as pellets 15 days before the test, but the amounts are not stated (H.S.).] Partial hepatectomy prolongs pentobarbital anesthesia and accentuates the differences induced by the various interventions just mentioned, without causing qualitative changes in the outcome. Liver homogenates of adult male rats destroy pentobarbital in vitro (spectrophotocolorimetric determination) more rapidly than those of castrate males. Pretreatment of the castrates in vivo with testosterone increases the detoxication process, whereas estradiol pretreatment has an opposite effect.

de Boer & Mukomela C5,245/55: In rats, ACTH and cortisone shorten thiopental and pentobarbital sleeping times, especially in females whose sleeping time is normally longer than that of males.

Streicher & Garbus G76,681/55: Hexobarbital sleeping time is much longer in females than in male rats. This sex difference is evident also if the hexobarbital effect is augmented by concurrent treatment with SKF 525-A or chlorpromazine.

Brodie C12,157/56: The hexobarbital sleeping time of female rats is about four times that of males; correspondingly, the plasma levels of hexobarbital drop much more rapidly in males, whose hepatic microsomes also inactivate the drug more actively in vitro than those of females. Male rats, pretreated with estradiol, sleep as long as females and their hepatic microsomes lose much of their activity to metabolize hexobarbital. Females, pretreated with testosterone, assume the characteristics of males in all these respects. No sex differences were seen in mice, guinea pigs, rabbits, and dogs, and their ability to handle hexobarbital is not influenced by estradiol or testosterone.

Edgren C45,010/57: Female rats are more sensitive than males to the anesthetic effect of hexobarbital. Gonadectomy prolongs hexobarbital sleeping time in males and shortens it in females. Estrone prolongs hexobarbital sleeping time in ovariectomized females, whereas testosterone is ineffective. In orchidectomized rats, testosterone shortens hexobarbital sleeping time, whereas estrone is ineffective.

Remmer G79,941/57: In female rats, cortisone and prednisolone are much more efficacious than testosterone in shortening hexobarbital anesthesia and increasing microsomal hexobarbital metabolism. Adrenalectomy diminishes the capacity of hepatic microsomes of male rats to metabolize hexobarbital unless the animals are pretreated with cortisone or prednisolone.

Remmer D86,916/58: The anesthetic effect of hexobarbital is greater in female than in male rats and liver slices of males detoxify the compound more actively in vitro. No such sex difference could be demonstrated for thiopental.

Quinn et al. E89,993/58: In rats, hexobarbital sleeping time is considerably longer in females than in males; it can be reduced in females by testosterone and in males by estradiol. The plasma levels of hexobarbital run parallel with the sleeping time and the hepatic microsomal-enzyme activity inversely. The guinea pig and mouse show no such sex differences in hexobarbital metabolism.

Remmer C 73,857/58: The oxidation of hexobarbital and the demethylation of methylaminoantipyrine by liver slices in vitro are inhibited by adrenalectomy performed 10—12 days before the experiment, unless the animals are given prednisolone substitution therapy. Addition of prednisolone to the incubation medium has no effect. The drug-metabolizing activity is contained in the microsomal fraction and, in this respect, the microsomes of males are more active than those of females.

Kramer & Arrigoni-Martelli G 74,673/59: The hexobarbital metabolism by hepatic microsomal-enzyme systems is inhibited, whereas hexobarbital sleeping time is prolonged by certain malonic and succinic acid derivatives, such as Sch 5712. The latter compound prolongs hexobarbital sleeping time about 12-fold in female and only 3-fold in male rats, yet it inhibits hexobarbital metabolism in vitro about equally when tested with the unfortified liver homogenate from rats of either sex. Furthermore, Sch 5712 is singularly ineffective in prolonging hexobarbital sleeping time in rats pretreated with phenobarbital.

King & Becker E 38,612/60: Male rats are more resistant than females to anesthesia produced by pentobarbital.

Buchel & Liblau E 87,108/62: In rats, the prolonged hexobarbital sleeping time of females, compared to males, is associated with a delayed disappearance of the drug from the blood and brain; yet, at the time of awakening, the blood and brain concentration of hexobarbital is the same in both sexes.

King & Becker G 78,964/63: In rats, pregnancy prolongs pentobarbital sleeping time, and males are even less susceptible than non-pregnant females.

Backus & Cohn D 92,313/66: The hexobarbital sleeping time of female mice is shorter than that of males, and varies also according to strain. In general, the length of the sleeping time is inversely proportional to the hexobarbital-metabolizing potency of liver homogenates.

Nair & Zeitlin G 65,099/67: The hexobarbital-metabolizing activity of the rat liver is extremely low after birth and rises gradually up to the age of 80 days to levels much higher in males than in females. Prenatal X-irradiation suppresses this normal development of enzyme activities in the male so that it only reaches the normal female level. Irradiation at 21 days (total body or head alone) also suppresses the developmental increase of enzyme activity, but to a lesser extent. Adults are still more resistant.

Schenkman et al. G 67,777/67: Sex differences in the drug-oxidizing ability of liver microsomes appear to be related to substrate affinity for mixed function oxidases, and not to a difference in the content of cytochrome P-450. "These results, as well as spectral studies of substrate interaction with microsomal cytochrome, showed that microsomes isolated from livers of male rats had over twice the magnitude of substrate (hexobarbital and aminopyrine) binding than did microsomes isolated from the livers of female rats."

Bardin et al. H 12,120/69: In pseudohermaphrodite rats [not otherwise characterized (H.S.)], unlike in castrates, testosterone fails to increase hexobarbital metabolism and other hepatic microsomal-enzyme activities. The weight of the preputial glands is not increased by testosterone in pseudohermaphrodite rats and the rate of dihydrotestosterone formation from testosterone is diminished in these preputial glands in vitro. It is concluded that the pseudohermaphrodite rat has an end-organ insensitivity to testosterone.

Ganesan H 12,504/69: Male rats are more resistant than females to pentobarbital anesthesia. Orchidectomy or treatment with estradiol decreases the pentobarbital resistance of male rats.

Furner et al. H 17,931/69: In rats of both sexes, L-hexobarbital has a longer latency, a longer half-life and achieves higher blood concentrations after equivalent doses of the two enantiomers. The L-enantiomer has a much greater anesthetic effect for females than for males, whereas no such sex difference in sleeping time was observed for the L-enantiomer. This is unexpected since the metabolism of both enantiomers is more rapid in males. Pretreatment with phenobarbital always accelerated the metabolism of both enantiomers. D-hexobarbital is about twice as susceptible to inhibition by SKF 525-A as the L-enantiomer.

Hässler et al. H 23,853/69: Male rats are more resistant than females to the anesthetic effect of hexobarbital. In rats raised under extreme conditions of stress (cold or repeated periods of fasting) hexobarbital sleeping time is prolonged.

Stripp et al. H 22,743/70: In rats, spironolactone pretreatment shortened hexobarbital sleeping time. "Moreover, treatment of female rats with spironolactone doubled the rate of the in vitro metabolism of hexobarbital and benzpyrene by liver microsomes and quadrupled that of ethylmorphine. The inducing effects of spironolactone were very different from those of phenobarbital and 3-methylcholanthrene. The amount of cytochrome P-450 was either unaltered or decreased, but the NADPH cytochrome c reductase activity was increased 2-fold. Although the endogenous rate of cytochrome P-450 reduction by NADPH was not altered, the stimulatory effects of ethylmorphine or hexobarbital on the rate of cytochrome P-450 reduction were significantly greater with microsomes from spironolactone-treated animals. By contrast, treatment of male rats with spironolactone caused no change in hexobarbital sleeping time and no change or a slight decrease in hexobarbital and benzpyrene metabolism by liver microsomes."

Gillette H 34,126/71: In male rats, spironolactone caused a relatively small increase in ethylmorphine N-demethylation and decreased the oxidation of hexobarbital and 3,4-benzpyrene. However, like in females, spironolactone did not affect the type I spectral changes induced in males by ethylmorphine and hexobarbital but caused a small decrease in cytochrome P-450 content and increased NADPH-cytochrome c reductase. Moreover, in males, spironolactone increased the substrate-dependent cytochrome P-450 reduction but not its endogenous reduction. The sex difference in the effect of spironolactone upon hepatic microsomal drug metabolism is illustrated by the tabulation of data concerning ethylmorphine and hexobarbital biotransformation.

Stripp et al. G 79,538/71: In rats, the induction of hepatic microsomal enzymes by spironolactone "differed from the phenobarbital or methylcholanthrene induction in that it did not increase cytochrome P-450 content or microsomal protein. Furthermore the induction seemed to be sex dependent."

Selye PROT. 42911: In male rats, the protective effect of PCN, spironolactone, ethylestrenol, betamethasone, phenobarbital and phenylbutazone against intoxication with digitoxin, indomethacin, dioxathion, parathion, nicotine, progesterone, hexobarbital and zoxazolamine has been systematically examined (*cf.* Table 128). Hexobarbital sleeping time was not shortened by PCN, spironolactone or betamethasone. For betamethasone, this is not remarkable since this compound failed to affect hexobarbital sleeping time in females also (*cf.* Table 136), but PCN and spironolactone were effective in this respect in females. In order to evaluate these data, the effect of each conditioner against each toxicant should be compared with similar experiments on females (Table 136).

VARIA

Holck & Kanân A 43,097/34: No definite sex difference could be established in the amobarbital sensitivity of dogs and rabbits, but, on the whole, females appeared to be more resistant.

Donatelli B 38,172/47: Extensive investigations on the sex difference in barbiturate sensitivity of guinea pigs, mice, rabbits and man.

Barbiturates ← Sex, Cat, Dog, Frog, Gp, Mouse, Rat, Rb, Turtle: Holck et al. 31,302/35*

Hexobarbital ← Sex, Mouse, Rat: Kennedy A 43,060/34*

Hexobarbital ← Sex, Cat, Dog, Frog, Gp, Rb: Holck et al. A 8,011/37*

Hexobarbital ← Sex, Dog, Gp, Man, Mouse, Rat, Rb: Quinn et al. E 89,993/58*

Hexobarbital ← Sex, Mouse, Rat: Kramer et al. G 74,673/59*; Kuntzman et al. F 27,893/64; Conney et al. G 65,135/65

Pentobarbital ← Sex, Man, Rat: Weisburger et al. G 78,956/65*; Kuntzman et al. H 30,992/66

Amobarbital ← Sex: Nicholas et al. 62,223/32*; Barron A 42,858/33*

Barbiturates ← Sex: Homburger E 61,371/47*; Herken et al. G 74,662/58*; Remmer E 47,874/63*

Hexobarbital ← Sex: Holck et al. A 55,755/42*; Buchel G 67,326/54*; Streicher et al. G 76,681/55*; Brodie et al. E 92,716/58*; Herken et al. G 74,662/58*; Remmer C 73,857/58, D 86,728/58*; Remmer et al. G 67,790/58; Remmer E 52,112/59*, G 66,542/62*, F 31,499/64*; Kato et al. F 57,817/65, G 68,411/66; Kuntzman et al. G 66,245/66; Schenkman et al. G 67,777/67; Yam et al. G 58,163/67

Pentobarbital ← Sex: Moir E 54,544/37*; Holck et al. A 35,663/40*, A 55,755/42*, B 644/44*; Shaw et al. A 52,203/48*; Crevier et al. B 54,151/50*; Jarcho et al. B 59,706/50*; Robillard et al. G 67,325/54*; Brazda et al. D 48,613/61*; Kato et al. F 76,403/66, F 88,660/67*; Soyka H 30,981/68

Phenobarbital ← Sex: Kato et al. G 64,325/62*; Remmer et al. G 74,636/62*

Thiopental ← Sex: Remmer *D86, 916/58**

Pronarcon ← Sex + Genetics: Siegert et al. *G71,866/64**

BCP ←

Tanabe F92,176/67: BCP (5-n-butyl-1-cyclohexyl-2,4,6-trioxoperhydropyrimidine) is more toxic for female than for male rats, and pregnant females are more sensitive than nonpregnant controls.

Benzene ←

Hirokawa G71,106/55: Female rabbits are more sensitive to chronic benzene poisoning than males. Gonadectomized estradiol-treated males respond like females.

Ito E44,788/62: There is very little sex difference in the resistance to daily benzene inhalation in mice and rats, but the characteristic anemia occurred somewhat later in males than in females.

Bilirubin ← Sex + Barbital, Mouse: Catz et al. *H14,471/68;* Halac et al. *G77,576/69*

Bilirubin ← Sex + Steroids: Lathe et al. *C55,335/58*

Butylated Hydroxyanisole ← Sex: Brown et al. *G69,691/59**

Butylated Hydroxytoluene ← Sex: Johnson et al. *E51,900/61**; Daniel et al. *G72,354/65**

Butynamine ← Sex + Phenobarbital: Kato et al. *F76,403/66*

Cadmium ←

Ishizaki et al. F94,533/66: Female rats are more sensitive than males to the production of bone decalcification by cadmium on a calcium-deficient diet.

Tanabe G72,457/68: Female rats are more sensitive to cadmium intoxication than males.

Caffeine ←

Peters & Boyd F77,819/67: Male rats are more sensitive to caffeine intoxication than females.

Carbon Monoxide ←

Smith et al. 45,163/35: Male rats are more sensitive to the lethal action of illuminating gas than females. This difference is eliminated by gonadectomy. Thyroid feeding or dinitrophenol injections decrease survival time.

Carbon Tetrachloride ←

György et al. E86,574/46: Under identical dietary conditions, male rats are more susceptible than females to the hepatotoxic and nephrotoxic effects of CCl_4.

Bengmark & Olsson D48,932/62: Female rats are more susceptible to the hepatotoxic action of CCl_4 than males. Testosterone raised the resistance of females to this form of liver damage.

Glover & Reuber F77,043/67: In inbred buffalo strain rats, chronic thyroiditis is produced by CCl_4 more commonly among females than among males. There was no clear-cut relationship between the occurrence of thyroiditis and hepatic sclerosis.

Chaturvedi G69,350/69: Female rats are less susceptible than males to the hepatotoxic effect of CCl_4 and other hepatotoxic agents.

Cawthorne et al. H26,441/70: In rats, the acute toxicity of CCl_4 p.o. is greater in males than in females. Vitamin E and various antioxidants exert a protective effect. It is suggested that the protection may be partly dependent upon the induction of hepatic microsomal enzymes.

CCl_4 ← Sex + Diet: György et al. *E86,574/46**

CCl_4 ← Sex + CFT 1201: Maibauer et al. *G74,663/58**

CCl_4 ← Sex + 3-MC + Age: Reuber *G73,605/70**; Reuber et al. *H26,492/70**

Carcinogens ←

Andervont et al. A94,080/42; Andervont & Dunn A96,182/47: Among strain C mice, o-aminoazotoluene produced hepatomas more frequently in females than in males. Furthermore, "intact females were more susceptible than castrate females; castrate males approached intact females in their degree of susceptibility; castrate females and castrate males bearing testosterone propionate-cholesterol pellets approached intact males in their degree of susceptibility." The incidence of pulmonary tumors produced by this carcinogen, was not dependent upon any of the factors just mentioned.

Kirby B30,101/47: Female rats are less susceptible than males to the production of hepatomas and hepatic cirrhosis by AAF. Rats simultaneousy treated with pellets of estradiol or testosterone and AAF showed no carcinoma formation in the target organs of the sex hormones.

Stasney et al. B26,653/47: In rats, 2-acetaminofluorene feeding produces mammary carcinoma only in females, and its development is not significantly accelerated by estradiol or gonadotrophin. "Malignant lesions of the liver occurred in 54.8 per cent of females and 92.3 per cent of males receiving the carcinogen alone. Administration of estradiol and PMS gonadotrophin to females and of testosterone and chorionic gonadotrophin to males intensified the cystic and neoplastic hepatic lesions induced by 2-acetaminofluorene."

Shay et al. H26,763/49: In intact female rats, 3-MC p.o. produces a high incidence of mammary adenocarcinomas, whereas this is exceptional in intact or castrate males as well as in spayed females.

Bielschowski & Hall G71,797/51: In intact female rats joined in parabiosis with gonadectomized litter-mates, AAF induced a 50% incidence of malignant tumors, mostly of the granulosa. The gonadectomized partners were free of neoplastic lesions.

Leathem G74,736/51: In male mice, 2-acetylaminofluorene induced hepatomas only on certain semi-synthetic diets and only in males. In rats receiving this carcinogen in fox chow diet, hepatomas likewise developed exclusively in males [hepatic cyst formation was observed in one female only (H.S.).]

Rumsfeld et al. G73,677/51: Male rats fed 3'-methyl-4-dimethylaminoazobenzene or 4'-fluoro-4-dimethylaminoazobenzene develop hepatomas more readily than females. "The ability of liver slices or homogenates to destroy DAB, 3'-Me-DAB, or 4'-F-DAB in vitro did not vary with sex unless a carcinogen had been fed for a long period of time."

Shay et al. H31,719/52: In rats, chronic administration of 3-MC p.o. produces glandular tumors of the breast (predominantly in females and estradiol-treated males), spindle-cell and collagenous tumors of the breast and mesenteric sarcomas (predominantly in males and testosterone-treated females), and fibroadenomas of the breast (predominantly in ovariectomized and orchidectomized animals "in which the sex hormone effects were experimentally counterbalanced").

Dao & Sunderland D79,860/59; Dao et al. E57,368/60: In rats, the induction of mammary carcinomas by 3-methylcholanthrene is enhanced during pregnancy, pseudopregnancy, and progesterone treatment. Regression of neoplasms occurs after parturition. Males are virtually resistant. In fully formed tumors, regression could be induced by hypophysectomy or ovariectomy.

Dao & Greiner D91,850/61: In male rats, unlike in females or castrate males, 3-MC rarely produces mammary tumors. Ovarian transplants placed into castrate males induce predisposition for mammary carcinogenesis under these conditions.

Leathem & Oddis D2,742/61: Female rats are less responsive than males to the induction of hepatomas by AAF. Thyroid feeding increases the incidence of hepatomas in females treated with AAF. It has the same effect in mice of both sexes given DMBA.

Sidransky et al. C99,347/61: In rats fed N-2-fluorenylacetamide hepatic tumors developed in all males but only in 5 of 14 females. "Although castrated males had liver changes similar to those seen in females, these males receiving testosterone had the same changes as were found in the intact males. Intact females receiving testosterone developed earlier and more extensive changes regularly found only in the livers of males." Testosterone may accelerate hepatic tumorigenesis by this carcinogen.

Dao D36,011/62: In male, unlike in female rats, 3-MCA fails to induce mammary cancer irrespective of the dose given. In gonadectomized males or females, ovarian grafts enable the production of mammary cancers by 3-MCA.

Morii G34,628/65: Male rats are less susceptible to DMBA-induced adrenal necrosis than females.

Colafranceschi & Tosi G59,115/67: The adrenal necrosis produced by DMBA in the rat is of equal severity in males and females and cannot be influenced by ovariectomy, orchidectomy, testosterone or estradiol.

Weisburger et al. F78,862/67: Male rats are more prone to liver cancer induction by N-hydroxy-N-2-fluorenylacetamide (N-OH-FAA) than females. In newborn males treated with estradiol and placed on a diet containing N-OH-FAA, the incidence of hepatic carcinomas was decreased, whereas testosterone did not change it. In females, estradiol had a "mixed effect," and testosterone enhanced hepatoma induction.

Bates H13,409/68: Male Swiss mice are more sensitive than females to the induction of cutaneous carcinomas by DMBA + croton oil. This is especially true of females in which the initiator was applied during diestrus. Gonadectomy before application of DMBA increased tumor incidence in females but decreased it in males.

Glover et al. H 12,898/68: In Buffalo strain rats, single s.c. injections of 3-methylcholanthrene produce thyroiditis more often among females than among males.

Reuber & Glover H 5,582/68: In female Buffalo strain rats, a single s.c. injection of 3-methylcholanthrene produces thyroiditis more constantly than in males.

Newberne & Williams G 69,601/69: In rats, hepatic carcinogenesis produced by aflatoxin is inhibited by diethylstilbestrol. Male rats are less resistant to aflatoxin than females.

Svoboda et al. G 64,564/69: Hepatocytes of male rats given CPIB (ethyl-α-p-chlorophenoxyisobutyrate) show a pronounced increase in microbodies and in catalase activity while those of intact females do not. In castrate males given estradiol and CPIB, the increase in catalase activity and microbody proliferation is abolished, whereas in ovariectomized rats given testosterone and CPIB, there is an increase in microbodies and catalase activity.

Dehnen et al. G 74,165/70: In rats, the ability of hepatic microsomal enzymes to metabolize benzo(a)pyrene is not influenced by sex. The highest breakdown values were found at about 20 days of age in both sexes. After 50 days, hydroxylase activity decreased slowly but inducibility remained constant throughout life.

Kozuka H 27,469/70: "Repeated injection of reserpine and simultaneous administration of 2,7-diacetamidofluorene in SMA/Ms strain mice prevented the development of liver tumors but failed to induce gastric cancer. Female mice developed more hepatic tumors than males both in the carcinogen groups and in the reserpine-treated group. Castration increased the formation of hepatic cancer in male mice but not in females. In castrated female mice, estradiol benzoate had little effect and testosterone propionate reduced liver tumor incidence somewhat."

Levine H 31,806/70: In rats, 3,4-benzpyrene is rapidly excreted through the bile in the form of its metabolic products. Pretreatment with microsomal drug-metabolizing enzyme inducers (e.g., phenobarbital, methylcholanthrene, 3,4-benzpyrene) greatly enhances the rate of biliary excretion of this compound. Both the rate of metabolism and of biliary excretion are enhanced to a similar extent throughout the induction period. Male rats both metabolize 3,4-benzpyrene and excrete its metabolites in the bile at rates approximately 2.5 times that of females. The induction by methylcholanthrene of both the metabolism and the biliary excretion of 3,4-benzpyrene can be partially blocked by ethionine. It has been concluded that conversion to its metabolites is the rate-limiting step in the biliary excretion of 3,4-benzpyrene.

Stripp et al. H 22,743/70: In rats, spironolactone pretreatment shortened hexobarbital sleeping time. "Moreover, treatment of female rats with spironolactone doubled the rate of the in vitro metabolism of hexobarbital and benzpyrene by liver microsomes and quadrupled that of ethylmorphine. The inducing effects of spironolactone were very different from those of phenobarbital and 3-methylcholanthrene. The amount of cytochrome P-450 was either unaltered or decreased, but the NADPH cytochrome c reductase activity was increased 2-fold. Although the endogenous rate of cytochrome P-450 reduction by NADPH was not altered, the stimulatory effects of ethylmorphine or hexobarbital on the rate of cytochrome P-450 reduction were significantly greater with microsomes from spironolactone treated animals. By contrast, treatment of male rats with spironolactone caused no change in hexobarbital sleeping time and no change or a slight decrease in hexobarbital and benzpyrene metabolism by liver microsomes."

Stromberg & Reuber G 75,306/70: Males are more sensitive than females to the production of hepatic carcinomas by N-4-(4'-fluorodiphenyl)acetamide.

Young et al. G 77,809/70: In rats given single oral doses of DMBA during diestrous, the mean number of tumors per animal was significantly greater than when the carcinogen was given during other stages of the estrous cycle.

Gillette H 34,126/71: In male rats, spironolactone caused a relatively small increase in ethylmorphine N-demethylation and decreased the oxidation of hexobarbital and 3,4-benzpyrene. However (like in females), spironolactone did not affect the type I spectral changes induced in males by ethylmorphine and hexobarbital but caused a small decrease in cytochrome P-450 content and increased NADPH-cytochrome c reductase. Moreover, in males, spironolactone increased the substrate-dependent cytochrome P-450 reduction but not its endogenous reduction. The sex difference in the effect of spironolactone upon hepatic microsomal drug metabolism is illustrated by the tabulation of data concerning ethylmorphine and hexobarbital biotransformation.

Benzo(α)pyrene ← Sex + Genetics, Mouse: Kodama et al. H 28,307/70

7,12-Dimethylbenz(α)anthracene ← Sex: Huggins et al. D 13,007/61*

N-2-Fluorenylacetamide ← Sex: Kirby B 30,101/47*; Stasney et al. B 26,653/47*; Miyaji et al. D 24,881/53*

3-MC ← Sex, Mouse: Klein G 76,354/59*; Kelly et al. E 26,075/63*

3-Methyl-4-methylaminoazobenzene ← Sex: Kuntzman et al. H 30,992/66; Bresnick et al. H 215/68; Sladek et al. G 66,220/69

Carcinolytic Agents ←

Bennette D 77,417/52: Male mice are much more sensitive than females to the toxic and tumor growth-inhibiting effects of methotrexate.

Pallotta et al. D 26,380/62: "Acetoxycycloheximide, an antibiotic with anti-tumor activity, was much more toxic to female rats than to males. It was also more toxic to female mice than to males, but no such difference occurred in dogs." Two closely related cycloheximide derivatives showed no such sex difference.

Rall G 72,239/64: In the mouse, rat and man, females are more sensitive than males to the toxic effects of various antineoplastic agents such as methotrexate, cyclophosphamide, nitrogen mustard and 6-mercaptopurine. Rats also show a similar sex difference in their sensitivity to acetoxycycloheximide, but no such difference is noted in mice with regard to this compound.

Cutts H 22,100/68: In rats, diethylstilbestrol protects against lethal doses of vinblastine. Among otherwise untreated rats, females are more resistant to vinblastine than males.

Koss & Lavin G 75,309/70: In rats, the production of bladder lesions by cyclophosphamide is sex dependent. "In the female, the initial epithelial necrosis was less extensive, epithelial regeneration was more rapid, and subsequent hyperplasia and atypia were less pronounced and of shorter duration. One week after injection, the histology of the bladder epithelium was close to normal in the female, whereas in the male the epithelium was still markedly hyperplastic and atypical."

Methotrexate ← Sex, Mouse: Bennette D 77,417/52*

Carisoprodol ←

Kato et al. G 66,023/61: Adult (but not immature) male rats are less sensitive to carisoprodol-induced muscular paralysis than females. Castration or treatment with SKF 525-A abolishes the increased resistance of the adult male rat. Incubation of liver slices with carisoprodol shows that the resistance of the male is due to accelerated substrate inactivation. No sex difference is noted in adult mice or guinea pigs.

Carisoprodol ← Sex + SKF 525-A + Age: Kato et al. G 66,023/61*

Carisoprodol ← Sex + Testosterone: Kato et al. G 64,325/62*

Carisoprodol ← Sex + Phenobarbital: Kato et al. F 76,403/66

Carisoprodol ← Sex + Starvation: Kato et al. F 88,660/67*

Cerium ←

Snyder et al. C 99,417/59: In rats, i.v. injection of cerium produced extremely high levels of liver fat in females but not in males. After castration males reacted as strongly as females. Testosterone reduced fatty infiltration in both intact and ovariectomized females. Hypophysectomy prevented fatty liver formation in both sexes, whereas adrenalectomy did so only in males.

Chloral Hydrate ←

Buchel D 59,654/53: Extensive investigations on the influence of sex upon the sensitivity of the rat to numerous barbiturates, chloral hydrate and ethyl urethan.

Buchel D 73,669/54: Male rats are only questionably more resistant than females to chloral hydrate anesthesia.

Chloral Hydrate ← Sex: Holck et al. A 8,011/37*

Chloramphenicol ← Sex: Remmer et al. G 66,868/65

Chlorcyclizine ← Sex: Kuntzman et al. F 45,464/65*

Chloroform ←

Eschenbrenner 93,202/45: Chloroform induces renal necrosis in male but not in female strain A mice.

Eschenbrenner & Miller 94,309/45: Following administration of large amounts of chloroform p.o., "there was extensive necrosis of portions of the proximal and distal convoluted tubules in normal male and in testosterone-treated castrated male mice and no necrosis in female and in castrated male mice."

Deringer et al. G64,723/53: Chloroform inhalation produced renal damage in male but not in female C3H mice.

Shubik & Ritchie D67,964/53: Small doses of chloroform produce fatal tubular necrosis in the kidneys of male but not of female DBA mice.

Hewitt C41,385/56: Exposure to chloroform vapor produces renal tubular necrosis in male, but not in female mice.

Culliford & Hewitt C28,738/57: In adult male mice of two strains, exposure to chloroform vapor produced necrosis of the renal tubules, whereas females showed no such change. Testoids rendered females fully susceptible, whereas folliculoids decreased the sensitivity of the males. Orchidectomy abolished susceptibility in one strain of mice but only diminished it in another, although the residual sensitivity could be annulled by adrenalectomy. In gonadectomized mice, methyltestosterone, testosterone propionate, dehydroepiandrosterone, progesterone and very large doses of cortisone induced susceptibility.

Cholesterol ← cf. *Selye G60,083/70*, pp. 474, 476.

Cholesterol ← Sex: Kritchevsky et al. G16,024/63

Choline ←

Wilgram & Hartcroft C14,392/55: Female rats are much more resistant than males to the production of cardiovascular lesions by choline deficiency. However, simultaneous administration of "androgens" [kind not specified (H.S.)] and STH sensitizes the female to the induction of these lesions by hypolipotropic rations.

Nakamura et al. C41,067/57: Among rats about 30 days of age, males are more sensitive than females to the production of renal lesions by choline-deficient diets.

Sidransky & Farber C55,020/58: "Force-feeding of purified choline-containing diets devoid of methionine for 3 to 6 days induces fatty liver in adult female rats, but not in adult male rats. Excess lipid accumulates in the periportal region of liver lobule." Force-feeding of threonine-devoid diet also induces periportal fatty infiltration but without sex difference. Since choline does not protect against hepatic steatosis induced by methionine deficiency, the latter amino acid must play some role in the regulation of fatty liver formation other than the contribution of methyl groups for the synthesis of choline.

Sidransky et al. G48,110/67: In rats, mature intact or ovariectomized females, but not intact males, develop fatty infiltration of the liver when first fed a choline containing methionine-deficient diet for three days. Castrated males are as susceptible as females and testosterone raises the resistance in females as well as in castrated males. Presumably, testosterone is responsible for the natural resistance of male rats to this type of hepatic steatosis. Earlier literature on sex differences in susceptibility to fatty liver formation is reviewed.

Reuber H29,035/69: In male Buffalo strain rats, the liver cirrhosis produced by a choline-deficient diet is more severe than in females.

Griffith A33,347/70: Among young rats, females are more resistant than males to the production of hepatic steatosis and hemorrhagic renal lesions by choline deficiency.

Wilson et al. G79,508/70: In mice on hypolipotropic diets, the development of atrial thrombosis was independent of sex and not markedly influenced by gonadectomy. The same was true of castrated males given testosterone. Only gonadectomized females on estrone showed an unusually low incidence of thromboses.

Cocaine ←

Downs & Eddy 58,426/32: Female rats are more resistant than males to the lethal action of cocaine i.p.

Guerrero et al. F70,995/65: Resistance to cocaine is significantly lower in male than in female rats, but no such sex difference is observed in castrates. Testosterone diminished the cocaine-resistance of castrates in either sex, whereas estradiol did not influence it. At the time of death, the plasma cocaine concentration was the same in both sexes, and hence it was concluded that testosterone interferes with the enzymic inactivation of cocaine.

Paeile et al. G75,994/65: Male rats are significantly more resistant than females to lidocaine and dibucaine, whereas females are more resistant than males to cocaine.

Cyanide ← Sex, Mouse: Störtebecker 76,398/39*

Cyclural ← Sex: Graham et al. G77,527/51*

Dibucaine ←

Paeile et al. G75,994/65: Male rats are significantly more resistant than females to lidocaine and dibucaine, whereas females are more resistant than males to cocaine.

Digitalis ←

Holck & Kimura 84,604/44: Female mice are more resistant to ouabain than males. Resistance to strophanthin-K is the same in both sexes. Ovariectomy, orchidectomy and treatment with "estrogenic hormones" produced inconsistent changes in ouabain resistance.

Holck & Kimura D99,625/51: One month old rats of both sexes are equally sensitive to ouabain. Adult female rats are more resistant to ouabain than males but the difference does not become evident before 2—4 months of age. Rats rapidly become resistant to ouabain, and upon repeated injections, the sex difference tends to disappear. Castration does not alter the sex difference in ouabain resistance significantly in either sex. "However, in case of pentobarbitalized rats the usual higher female resistance was plainly seen and spaying definitely decreased the number of injections required to cause death."

Wollenberger & Karsh D95,331/51: The lethal dose of ouabain for the isolated heart of female rats is considerably higher than that for the heart of male rats.

Grinnell & Smith C31,428/57: On the basis of studies in dogs treated with estrone, estradiol or diethylstilbestrol, it is concluded that folliculoids protect the rat against the induction of cardiac arrhythmia by digoxin. "Male dogs and castrate female dogs have been found to be highly sensitive to toxic manifestations of a cardiac glycoside on cardiac rhythm, in comparison with normal females in anestrus, or castrate females treated with estrogenic substance. A high degree of resistance to toxicity of digoxin was exhibited by the 3 normal females in natural estrus which were available."

Selye PROT. 42911: In male rats, the protective effect of PCN, spironolactone, ethylestrenol, betamethasone, phenobarbital, and phenylbutazone against intoxication with digitoxin, indomethacin, dioxathion, parathion, nicotine, progesterone, hexobarbital and zoxazolamine has been systematically examined (*cf.* Table 128). Hexobarbital sleeping time was not shortened by PCN, spironolactone or betamethasone. For betamethasone, this is not remarkable since this compound failed to affect hexobarbital sleeping time in females also (*cf.* Table 136), but PCN and spironolactone were effective in this respect in females. In order to evaluate these data, the effect of each conditioner against each toxicant should be compared with similar experiments on females (Table 136).

N,N-Dimethylaniline ← Sex: Kato et al. *F76,403/66*; Ziegler et al. *G79,382/66*; Machinist et al. *H15,503/68*

N,N-Dimethylnaphthylamine ← Sex + Methylcholanthrene: Kato et al. *F76,403/66*

N-Nitrosodimethylamine ← Sex + 3-MC + Age: Venkatesan et al. *H31,273/70*

Dinitrophenol ←

Chamberlin & Hall 66,611/36: Male cats are more resistant than females to the fatal action of dinitrophenol.

Diphenhydramine ← Sex + Phenobarbital: Kato et al. *F76,403/66*

Dye ←

Reuber G64,737/69: In Buffalo strain rats, chronic treatment with trypan blue s.c. causes thyroiditis more often among females than among males.

Reuber G77,295/70: Among rats chronically treated with trypan blue, females develop chronic thyroiditis more often than males.

Ergot ← *cf.* also Selye *G60,083/70, pp. 476, 479.*

McGrath A29,208/35: In rats of both sexes, tail necrosis is produced by large amounts of ergotamine. Estrone prevents this change in females but not in males.

Loewe & Lenke A43,451/38: In the rat, the tail-necrosis produced by ergotamine s.c. is essentially the same in both sexes. Contrary to earlier claims, it cannot be prevented by folliculoid hormones and/or orchidectomy.

Suzman et al. A44,452/38: Repeated administration of estrone completely protects female rats against the tail-necrosis produced by ergotamine; males are only partially protected. Orchidectomy has no effect in itself, but enhances the protective effect of estrone in the male. Otherwise untreated rats showed no marked sex difference in their sensitivity to ergotamine.

Fitzhugh et al. A46,537/44: In rats, chronic intoxication with ergot leads to the formation of neurofibromas and renal calcification. Males are more sensitive than females.

Messina G18,016/64: In rats, ergotamine produces vascular lesions conducive to tail necrosis more readily in females than in males. Hypophysectomy prevents these toxic manifestations in both sexes, whereas treatment with chorionic gonadotrophin does not affect them.

Contreras et al. F81,599/67: In intact male rats, unlike in females or castrate males, ergonovine induced an analgesic effect (electrical stimulation of the genital papilla) unless the latter were treated with testosterone.

Ether ←

Störtebecker A1,993/37: Rabbits pretreated with "folliculin" tolerate normally anesthesia-producing doses of butallylonal (Pernocton). Subsequent experiments were conducted to determine the blood ether level during ether anesthesia at the time the corneal reflex is lost in intact and gonadectomized rabbits and mice. Similar observations were made during pregnancy and in relation to the estrous cycle. [Several conclusions were drawn suggesting an influence of sex hormones upon anesthesia but the number of animals per group was small and hence statistical evaluation impossible (H.S.).]

Ethionine ←

Farber et al. B47,283/50; D24,923/51: Male rats are more resistant than females to the production of fatty livers by ethionine. Orchidectomy abolished this resistance, whereas ovariectomy did not influence the lesions. Testosterone protected both females and castrate males.

Jensen et al. D83,567/51: DL- or L-ethionine i.p. causes hepatic steatosis in fasted female but not in fasted male rats.

Ethionine ← Sex + CFT 1201: Herken et al. G74,662/58*; Maibauer et al. G74,663/58*

Ethyl Alcohol ←

Abderhalden & Wertheimer A49,424/27: Female mice are more resistant than males to chronic ethanol poisoning.

Mallov C47,222/58: Ethanol p.o. produces more severe fatty infiltration of the liver in female than in male rats. Ovariectomy or administration of estradiol to males did not influence fatty infiltration but testosterone reduced hepatic steatosis in females, whereas castration increased it in males.

Ethyl-O-Ethylphenylurea ←

Hjort et al. A32,832/40: Male rats are more resistant than females to the anesthetic effect of unsymmetrical ethyl-O-ethylphenylurea.

Ethylene Glycol ←

Tanret et al. G68,367/61: Female rats are much more resistant than males to the production of renal oxalate deposits by ethylene glycol.

Tanret et al. D44,140/62: Prolonged oral administration of ethylene glycol produces calcium oxalate precipitation in the kidney of male, but not of female, rats. Estradiol abolishes the susceptibility of intact or castrated males, but orchidectomy does not. Intact, unlike ovariectomized, females cannot be made susceptible by treatment with testosterone.

Richardson D88,284/65: In rats, dietary supplements of glycolic acid or ethylene glycol produce oxaluria and kidney oxalate deposition in males but not in females.

Ethyl Ether ←

Störtebecker 76,398/39: Review of the literature (up to 1935) on the effect of sex and sex hormones upon ether anesthesia.

Ethylmorphine ←

Gerald & Feller G74,396/70: In mice, spironolactone and its Δ^6-dethioacetylated metabolite reduce hexobarbital sleeping time and cause nearly identical increases in liver weight, microsomal protein content, NADPH-cytochrome c reductase, cytochrome P-450 content and the N-demethylation of ethylmorphine. Preliminary observations suggest that these actions of spironolactone and its metabolite are evident in both sexes.

Stripp et al. G79,538/71: In rats, the induction of hepatic microsomal enzymes by spironolactone "differed from the phenobarbital or methylcholanthrene induction in that it did not increase cytochrome P-450 content or microsomal protein. Furthermore the induction seemed to be sex dependent. Thus ethylmorphine N-demethylation, hexobarbital oxidation and 3,4-benzpyrene hydroxylation were increased 2—4 fold in female rats, but of these activities only ethylmorphine N-demethylase was increased in male rats."

Ethylmorphine ← Sex: Castro et al. G77,558/67; Davies et al. H22,054/68; Gigon et al. G76,365/68; Sasame et al. G72,114/68; Davies et al. G76,865/69; Gigon et al. G66,216/69; Sladek et al. G66,220/69

Ethyl Urethan ←

Buchel *D 59,654/53:* Extensive investigations on the influence of sex upon the sensitivity of the rat to numerous barbiturates, chloral hydrate and ethyl urethan.

Fluoride ←

Ramseyer et al. *C 29,608/57:* Following chronic administration of NaF p.o., female rats store more fluoride in their bones than males.

Glycolic Acid ←

Richardson *D 88,284/65:* In rats, dietary supplements of glycolic acid or ethylene glycol produce oxaluria and kidney oxalate deposition in males but not in females.

Griseofulvin ← Sex: Busfield et al. *D 10,983/60, G 74,680/64*;* Epstein et al. *H 30,997/67**

Heliotrine ← *cf. Plant Extracts*

Hexachlorobenzene ←

Viale et al. *G 74,147/70:* Female rats are more sensitive than males to the production of porphyria by hexachlorobenzene.

Hexaethyl Tetraphosphate ←

Hagan & Woodard *A 48,819/47:* The insecticide hexaethyl tetraphosphate is more toxic to female than to male rats.

Hexamethonium ←

Bonino *C 30,099/56:* Female guinea pigs are more sensitive than males to hexamethonium intoxication.

Indomethacin ←

Selye *PROT. 42911:* In male rats, the protective effect of PCN, spironolactone, ethylestrenol, betamethasone, phenobarbital, and phenylbutazone against intoxication with digitoxin, indomethacin, dioxathion, parathion, nicotine, progesterone, hexobarbital and zoxazolamine has been systematically examined (*cf.* Table 128). Hexobarbital sleeping time was not shortened by PCN, spironolactone or betamethasone. For betamethasone, this is not remarkable since this compound failed to affect hexobarbital sleeping time in females also (*cf.* Table 136), but PCN and spironolactone were effective in this respect in females. In order to evaluate these data, the effect of each conditioner against each toxicant should be compared with similar experiments on females (Table 136).

Isoniazid ← Sex + Age, Man: Murray *G 77,553/62**

Isoproterenol ← *cf. Selye G 60,083/70, pp. 475, 478.*

Lasiocarpine ← *cf. Plant Extracts*

Lathyrogens ← *cf. also Selye G 60,083/70, pp. 475, 478.*

Wajda et al. *C 33,241/57:* Among weanling rats fed Lathyrus odoratus seeds, males developed aortic aneurysms more frequently than females. "Androgens" [kind not stated (H.S.)] considerably increased the incidence and severity of aortic medionecrosis on this diet.

McCallum *C 61,614/58:* In mice, Lathyrus odoratus feeding, initiated at the age of two weeks or later, causes aortic damage predominantly among males.

Aschkenasy *C 91,685/60; C 90,362/60:* In male rats, the osteolathyrism produced by AAN is inhibited by a diet containing 18—30% casein. This protective effect is not seen in females or in orchidectomized males.

Lidocaine ←

Paeile et al. *G 75,994/65:* Male rats are significantly more resistant than females to lidocaine and dibucaine, whereas females are more resistant than males to cocaine.

Lithium ←

Schmidt & Bernauer *D 65,293/63:* Female rats are more resistant than males to chronic lithium citrate intoxication.

Magnesium ←

Störtebecker *A 1,993/37:* In rabbits and mice, the depth of $MgSO_4$ anesthesia is influenced by sex hormones as judged by observations in different phases of the estrous cycle as well as after injection of folliculin or androsterone. [In view of the wide individual variations and the small number of animals, the significance of the data is in doubt (H.S.).]

$MgSO_4$ ← Sex, Mouse: Störtebecker 76,398/39*

MAO-Inhibitors ←

Wurtman & Axelrod *E 36,478/63:* Hepatic MAO activity is greater in male than in female rats. This difference can be reversed by estradiol in male and by testosterone in female gonadectomized rats.

Mepacrine ←

Hurst D33,743/58: Female mice are much more sensitive than males to the curative action of mepacrine following infection with equine encephalomyelitis.

Meperidine ← Sex: Axelrod *D28,544/56;* Remmer et al. *G67,790/58;* Timmler *E48,422/60;* Remmer *G66,542/62;* Clouet et al. *F14,837/64*;* Siegert et al. *G71,866/64*;* Kato et al. *F76,403/66*

Mercury ←

Donatelli B38,554/47: Women are much more sensitive to $HgCl_2$ intoxication than men. Testosterone pretreatment gives appreciable protection against $HgCl_2$ poisoning in mice and guinea pigs.

Heimburg & Schmidt C69,587/59: Female rats are more resistant than males to chronic intoxication with $HgCl_2$. Ovariectomy abolishes this difference. Neither estradiol nor progesterone caused any significant change in resistance to mercurial intoxication.

Spode G72,979/60: In mice, the renal storage of ^{203}Hg acetate given s.c. or i.p. reaches higher values in males than in females.

Haber & Jennings G10,684/64: Female rats are more resistant than males to the production of renal tubular necroses by $HgCl_2$.

Tessman G65,320/68: In mice and rats, there was no sex difference in the speed of regeneration of the renal epithelium following $HgCl_2$-intoxication.

Methionine ← cf. **Choline**
Methotrexate ← cf. **Carcinolytic Agents**
Methylaminoantipyrine ← Sex: Remmer *C73,857/58, G66,542/62*

N-Methylaniline ← Sex + Phenobarbital: Kato et al. *F76,403/66*

Monocrotaline ←

Ratnoff & Mirick B48,154/49: Monocrotaline i.p. produces necrosis of the liver and of the renal tubules, as well as pulmonary edema in rats. Males are somewhat more susceptible than females, especially if kept on protein-deficient diets. Testosterone increases monocrotaline susceptibility in both sexes, but neither castration nor estradiol influences survival time.

Goldenthal et al. G18,384/64: "The oral and intravenous LD_{50}'s were determined for monocrotaline. The LD_{50} was essentially the same for males and females and for oral and intravenous administration for a 90-day observation period. There was a marked sex difference with respect to the median survival time, females living significantly longer than males. Castration of either male or female rats had no significant effect on the median survival time. Pretreatment of males with estradiol cyclopentyl propionate caused the median survival time to correspond to that of females. Pretreatment of females with testosterone propionate caused the median survival time to approximate that of male animals. Pretreatment of female rats with methandrostenolone (Dianabol), an anabolic agent, caused the median survival time to correspond to that of males."

Monocrotaline ← Sex + Testosterone + Diet: Ratnoff et al. *B48,154/49**

Morphine ←

MacKay & MacKay 56,167/36: Female rats are more resistant to morphine than males, a difference ascribed to their larger adrenals.

Yeh & Woods H17,933/69: Twenty-four hours after s.c. injection of ^{14}C-DHM the recovery (as expired $^{14}CO_2$) in nontolerant female and male rats was 0.5 and 3.7%, respectively.

Stripp et al. H22,743/70: In rats, spironolactone pretreatment shortened hexobarbital sleeping time. "Moreover, treatment of female rats with spironolactone doubled the rate of the in vitro metabolism of hexobarbital and benzpyrene by liver microsomes and quadrupled that of ethylmorphine. The inducing effects of spironolactone were very different from those of phenobarbital and 3-methylcholanthrene. The amount of cytochrome P-450 was either unaltered or decreased, but the NADPH cytochrome c reductase activity was increased 2-fold. Although the endogenous rate of cytochrome P-450 reduction by NADPH was not altered, the stimulatory effects of ethylmorphine or hexobarbital on the rate of cytochrome P-450 reduction were significantly greater with microsomes from spironolactone treated animals. By contrast, treatment of male rats with spironolactone caused no change in hexobarbital sleeping time and no change or a slight decrease in hexobarbital and benzpyrene metabolism by liver microsomes."

Hayes Jr. E53,090/71: Female rats store more DDT in their fat than males when fed this insecticide at the same dose level.

Selye PROT. 42911: In male rats, the protective effect of PCN, spironolactone, ethylestrenol, betamethasone, phenobarbital, and phenylbutazone against intoxication with digitoxin, indomethacin, dioxathion, parathion, nicotine, progesterone, hexobarbital and zoxazolamine has been systematically examined (*cf.* Table 128). Hexobarbital sleeping time was not shortened by PCN, spironolactone or betamethasone. For betamethasone, this is not remarkable since this compound failed to affect hexobarbital sleeping time in females also (*cf.* Table 136), but PCN and spironolactone were effective in this respect in females. In order to evaluate these data, the effect of each conditioner against each toxicant should be compared with similar experiments on females (Table 136).

Aldrin, Heptachlor, Isodrin ← Sex: Wong et al. G77,538/65

Benzene Hexachloride ← Sex: Davidow et al. H27,655/51*

Chlorthion ← Sex, Gp, Mouse, Rat: Neal et al. F40,198/65

Dieldrin ← Sex, Pig, Sheep: Street et al. G75,678/66*

0,0-Diethyl 0-(4-methylthio-m-tolyl) phosphorothioate ← Sex, Gp, Mouse, Rat: DuBois et al. D43,878/61*

EPN ← Sex: Murphy et al. *D28,546/58;* Neal et al. *F40,198/65;* DuBois et al. H24,226/66*; Kinoshita et al. G71,863/66

Guthion ← Sex + Age: Murphy et al. *D28,546/58*

Methylparathion ← Sex, Gp, Mouse, Rat: Neal et al. *F40,198/65*

OMPA ← Sex: DuBois et al. D92,992/50*; Kato et al. G64,325/62*, F88,660/67*, H34,342/67*

Parathion ← Sex: DuBois et al. G66,495/49*; Neal et al. *F40,198/65*

Phenylbutazone ←

Selye PROT. 42911: In male rats, the protective effect of PCN, spironolactone, ethylestrenol, betamethasone, phenobarbital, and phenylbutazone against intoxication with digitoxin, indomethacin, dioxathion, parathion, nicotine, progesterone, hexobarbital and zoxazolamine has been systematically examined (*cf.* Table 128).

Phosphorus ← Sex + CFT 1201: Maibauer et al. G74,663/58*

Picrotoxin ←

Holck D28,543/49: Adult male rats are more resistant than females to toxic doses of picrotoxin. Such a sex difference is absent in one-month-old rats. Castration lowers picrotoxin resistance in rats of either sex. Testosterone raises picrotoxin resistance in normal and especially in spayed females, but not in males. Blockade of the RES abolished the sex difference but corticosterone failed to influence it.

Picrotoxin ← Sex + Testosterone: Holck D28,543/49*

Piperonyl Butoxide ← Sex + Age, Mouse: Epstein et al. H29,385/67*

Plant Extract ←

Campbell C38,327/57: In cockerels, the hepatic damage produced by the pyrrolizidine alkaloids of ragwort (Senecio jacobaea L.) disappears very slowly if at all, whereas hens recover. In both sexes, but particularly in cockerels, stilbestrol accelerates hepatic regeneration.

Bull et al. C49,278/58: Personal observations on rats and review of the entire literature on the pronounced sex differences in resistance against heliotrine, lasiocarpine and other plant alkaloids of Senecio species.

Propyl Gallate ← Sex: Johnson et al. E51,900/61*

Potassium ←

Robertson B70,810/52: Female rats are more tolerant than males to i.p. injection of KCl. No such sex difference was observed in mice.

Procaine ←

Muñoz et al. G68,223/61: Male rats are more resistant than females to the convulsant action of procaine i.p. Gonadectomy decreased resistance in males but not in females. Testosterone did not significantly alter resistance in either sex.

Paeile et al. F52,633/64: Adult male rats are more resistant to procaine than adult females. Chronic CCl_4 poisoning, pretreatment with SKF 525-A and orchidectomy diminish the resistance of the males approximately to the female level. The plasma procainesterase activity is approximately the same in both sexes and not affected by orchidectomy or CCl_4 intoxication.

Brodeur et al. F99,981/67: The procainesterase activity of the liver is higher in adult male rats than in adult females or immature rats of either sex. Ovariectomy and chronic treatment with testosterone or norethandrolone increase hepatic procainesterase activity in adult females. Conversely, orchidectomy and chronic treatment with estradiol or progesterone decrease this enzyme activity in the livers of adult males. However, immature rats are more resistant to procaine in vivo than could be expected from the reduced ability of their livers to hydrolyze procaine in vitro. "Factors other than drug metabolism appear to govern the ultimate toxicity of procaine in immature rats."

Pyribenzamine ←

Mayer et al. B3,674/46: Male rats are much more resistant to pyribenzamine than females. Castration of females rendered them almost as resistant as males but treatment of ovariectomized rats with "estrogen" did not give consistent results in a small series of preliminary experiments.

RES-Blocking Agents ←

Bernick et al. C39,526/56: The Kupffer cells of male rabbits take up more i.v. injected Thorotrast, Evans blue and colloidal carbon than those of females.

Hartveit & Andersen G67,345/69: I.v.-injected carbon particles are cleared more rapidly from the blood by female than by male mice. The difference is ascribed to the phagocytosis stimulating effect of folliculoids.

Safrole ←

Homburger et al. E94,913/62: In male rats, safrole (4-allyl-1,2-methylene dioxybenzene), a flavoring agent, is less active in causing hepatic fibrosis and ceroid deposition than in females.

Salicylates ←

Hanzlik A49,483/13: "For females the toxic dose of salicylates is approximately 80% of that for males. Individuals show idiosyncrasy towards toxic doses of the synthetic salicylate, but no connection was found between these idiosyncrasies and the factors of age, sex, race, and diseased condition. The idiosyncrasy generally varies in the same patient, and is not influenced by previous salicylate medication."

Scilliroside ← Sex: Rothlin et al. G75,565/52*

Selenium ←

Fitzhugh et al. A45,940/44: Female rats are more sensitive than males to the toxic actions of selenium p.o., especially to the production of hepatic cirrhosis.

Sodium Chloride ← cf. Selye G60,083/70, p. 477.

Squill ←

Winton A42,964/27: "Female rats succumb to doses of red squills, only one-half as great as those needed to kill males."

Crabtree et al. A19,999/39: Male rats are twice as resistant as females to the fatal action of powdered red squill (Urginea maritima). Castration has no effect in females but abolishes the increased squill resistance of the male.

Red Squill ← Sex: Winton A42,964/27*; Crabtree et al. A19,999/39*

Strychnine ←

Poe et al. A45,388/36: Female rats are more susceptible to strychnine than males and, in both sexes, toxicity decreases with age.

Ward & Crabtree A29,199/42: Female rats are more sensitive than males to strychnine i.p. or p.o.

Poe & Suchy D75,977/51: Female rats are more sensitive than males to strychnine poisoning.

Kato & Chiesara G68,581/60: Male rats are more resistant than females to the toxic action of strychnine. This difference is abolished by SKF 525-A.

Kato et al. D38,983/62: Male rats are more resistant than females to strychnine intoxication especially if the drug is given s.c. whereby its activity is delayed. The greater strychnine-metabolizing potency of microsomes from male rats than from females has also been demonstrated in vitro. SKF 525-A increases strychnine toxicity and renders both sexes equally sensitive. Castration diminishes the high strychnine resistance of the male rat but has no effect in females. Pretreatment with testosterone or 4-chlortestosterone augments the strychnine-metabolizing ability of liver slices or isolated hepatic microsomes from both male and female castrates, whereas estradiol has no effect.

Strychnine ← Sex: Poe et al. A45,388/36*; Ward et al. A29,199/42*; Kato et al. D38,983/62*, G64,325/62*, F88,660/67*

Sulfa Drugs ←

Krems et al. A46,116/41: Female rats are more susceptible than males to sulfanilamide i.p.

Sacra & McColl C73,654/59: Female rats are less resistant than males to chronic intoxication with hypoglycemic thiadiazoles but no such sex difference was observed in acute tests. Testosterone increased, whereas stilbestrol decreased, the resistance of female rats to these drugs.

Sulfanilamide ← Sex: Krems et al. A46,116/41*

Tannic Acid ←

Korpássy et al. B74,333/52: Male rats are more sensitive than females to the acute lethal effects of tannic acid.

Tannic Acid ← Sex: Korpássy et al. B74,333/52*

Tyrosine ←

Schweizer B3,047/47: Addition of excessive amounts of l-tyrosine to the diet produces alkaptonuria, keratitis, conjunctivitis, alopecia, and inflammation of the paws in young rats. Among older animals, males are more sensitive than females. The severity of the syndrome is aggravated by thyroxine and inhibited by thiouracil.

Urethan ←

Vesselinovitch & Mihailovich F91,584/67: In male mice, urethan induced a higher incidence of hepatomas than in females. Gonadectomy decreased the incidence in males and increased it in females, thus practically eliminating the sex difference.

Chernozemski & Warwick H33,929/70: In female mice, hepatic tumors are much more rarely induced by urethan than in males. Partial hepatectomy greatly increases the hepatocarcinogenic effect of urethan.

Urethan ← Sex + Hepatectomy, partial, Mouse: Lane et al. H28,306/70*

Vitamin-B Complex ←

Taylor & Carmichael A49,002/49: Male mice are much more resistant than females to fatal overdosage with folic acid.

Vitamin C ←

Klinger et al. F62,929/65: The normal excretion of ascorbic acid and the increase in its elimination induced by barbital are higher in male than in female rats. Orchidectomy reduced both normal excretion and its enhancement by barbital, whereas ovariectomy increased them. Thus, the sex specific differences decreased but did not disappear completely. One week's treatment of males with stilbestrol or females with testosterone diminished ascorbic acid excretion. In mice, no sex specific differences of this kind were observed. [The authors probably used hexobarbital although sometimes they speak of barbital (H.S.).]

Vitamin D, DHT ← *cf. also Selye D15,540/62, p. 291; G60,083/70, pp. 476, 479.*

Agduhr 52,908/34; 70,849/35: Female mice are more resistant than males to overdosage with irradiated ergosterol. Repeated mating increases ergosterol resistance in both sexes.

Agduhr A51,257/37: In mice and rats of both sexes, sexual intercourse increases resistance against As_2O_3 and vitamin D.

Strebel et al. F25,229/64: Male rats are much more resistant than females to the production by DHT of the progeria-like syndrome (with soft-tissue calcification and osteosclerosis).

Fiumara et al. H34,170/68: Male rats are more resistant than females to the production of the progeria-like syndrome by DHT.

Chury & Kasparek H29,730/69: Female rats are more sensitive than males to the production of a progeria-like syndrome by chronic treatment with DHT. Castration increases the sensitivity of the males.

Chury & Nevrtal H33,801/70: Rats, orchidectomized immediately after birth, are more sensitive to the production of the "progeria-like syndrome" by DHT than are females or males castrated after puberty. The ECG alterations in all these groups run roughly parallel with the morphologic changes.

Vitamin D_2 ← Sex + Age, Mouse: Agduhr A51,257/37*

Vitamin K ←

Mellette D7,939/61: Female rats are more resistant to dietary vitamin-K deficiency than males. Castration increases the susceptibility of the female rat and decreases that of the male. In males, estradiol decreases, whereas testosterone increases, mortality on such diets.

Zoxazolamine ←

Selye PROT. 42911: In male rats, the protective effect of PCN, spironolactone, ethylestrenol, betamethasone, phenobarbital, and phenylbutazone against intoxication with digitoxin, indomethacin, dioxathion, parathion, nicotine, progesterone, hexobarbital and zoxazolamine has been systematically examined (*cf.* Table 128). Hexobarbital sleeping time was not shortened by PCN, spironolactone or betamethasone. For betamethasone, this is not remarkable since this compound failed to affect hexobarbital sleeping time in females also (*cf.* Table 136), but PCN and spironolactone were effective in this respect in females. In order to evaluate these data, the effect of each conditioner against each toxicant should be compared with similar experiments on females (Table 136).

Zoxazolamine ← Sex: Kato et al. *F 57,817/65, F 76,403/66,* F 88,660/67*

Varia ←

Holck et al. A 8,011/37: Female rats are more sensitive than males to various **barbiturates** and **nicotine**. Orchidectomy abolishes this increased resistance to barbiturates. Pretreatment with an androgenic urinary extract shortens the anesthesia produced by hexobarbital in intact or spayed females. Androsterone is ineffective.

Agduhr 75,856/39: **Review** of the effect of sex and sexual intercourse upon the resistance of various species to diverse toxic substances.

Agduhr A 39,060/41: **Review** of the author's investigations on the effect of sex and mating upon drug resistance in animals.

Hurst D 33,743/58: **Review** (25 pp. 87 refs.) on sex differences in the toxicity of various drugs.

Booth & Gillette D 34,656/62: **Review** of sex differences in drug resistance.

Kato et al. G 64,325/62: Adult male rats are more resistant than females to **pentobarbital** anesthesia, **carisoprodol** paralysis and **strychnine** convulsions. Conversely, the lethal effect of **OMPA** is greater in the male. The sex difference is ascribed to the increased production of anabolic testoids which enhance the decomposition of these substrates, the first three of which are inactivated, the last activated in the process. The differences were also demonstrated in vitro using liver slices or microsomal fractions. The high microsomal activity of the male could be abolished by castration and restored by several anabolic testoids.

Conney & Burns G 67,166/62: **Review** on sex differences in drug metabolism.

Meier E 690/63: **Monograph** on "Experimental Pharmacogenetics" (213 pp., about 400 refs.) with special sections on the influence of sex and genetic factors, including species variations, upon drug sensitivity.

Kato & Gillette F 5,638/64: In female rats, 3 days' starvation "increases the activity of TPNH-dependent enzymes that catalyze the metabolism of **TPNH, aniline, aminopyrine, p-nitrobenzoate, neotetrazolium,** and **neoprontosil,** but does not alter the activity of TPNH-cytochrome c reductase. In contrast, starvation of male rats decreases the activity of aminopyrine demethylase, although it increases the activity of aniline hydroxylase and does not alter the activity of nitroreductase, TPNH-cytochrome c reductase or TPNH oxidase." Sucrose fed to rats of either sex for 3 days lowers the activity of all these enzymes, but does not interfere with their induction by phenobarbital.

Kato & Gillette F 57,816/65: The ability of rat liver microsomal enzymes to inactivate various substrates is greater in males than in females but the sex difference varies with the substrate. There is a more than 3-fold sex difference with **aminopyrine** and **hexobarbital** but virtually none with hydroxylation of **aniline** and **zoxazolamine**. In male rats, starvation impairs sex-dependent enzymes which metabolize aminopyrine and hexobarbital but enhances those that hydroxylate aniline. On the other hand, in female rats, starvation increases the specific activity of the aminopyrine and hexobarbital-metabolizing enzymes as well as aniline hydroxylase. Starvation does not alter the metabolism of hexobarbital and enhances that of aminopyrine by microsomes of castrated rats, but impairs the metabolism of these compounds by microsomes of methyltestosterone-treated castrates.

Gillette G 67,333/67: Brief **review** on the effect of sex on hepatic microsomal-enzyme induction.

Kato et al. H 11,854/69: "There was marked sex difference in the hydroxylation of **pentobarbital** and **hexobarbital**, in contrast only slight or negligible sex difference was observed in the hydroxylation of **aniline** and **zoxazolamine**. Similarly, there are marked sex differences in the N-demethylation of **aminopyrine**, while only slight sex difference was observed in the N-demethylation of **N-methylaniline**. The administration of methylcholanthrene to female and male rats resulted in marked increase in the hydroxylation of aniline and zoxazolamine and N-demethylation of N-methylaniline, whereas the hydroxylation of pentobarbital and hexobarbital and N-demethylation of aminopyrine were not significantly altered in female rats and they were markedly decreased in male rats."

Microorganisms and Their Products, Venoms ←

Allegedly, female rats and mice are more resistant than males to various types of infections with **plasmodia** and **bacteria**. Variable observations have been reported with regard to **viruses**. In the mouse, but not in the guinea pig, males are more susceptible than females to infection with equine encephalomyelitis. Female hamsters are more sensitive than males to inoculation with adenovirus-12, and also show a greater incidence of tumors. Among mice infected with Coxsackie virus B_1, a much higher percentage of males than of females developed hepatic necrosis.

Sex difference to various **bacterial toxins** was not found to be very pronounced.

Female guinea pigs are more sensitive than males to **Cape cobra venom**, but this difference does not appear to be subject to modification by testosterone, estradiol, or progesterone.

Bacteria, Plasmodia ←

Bennison & Coatney B17,600/47: Following inoculation with P. gallinaceum, the parasite counts are much higher in females than in males. This difference in parasite count was not significantly influenced by testosterone or estradiol.

Greenberg et al. G70,739/53: Female mice of various strains survive longer than males after infection with Plasmodium berghei.

Weisskopf et al. D35,320/61: Review of the protective action of folliculoids against viruses and bacteria, with personal observations on the increase in the resistance of mice that can be induced by Premarin against virulent streptococcal infection. Females are more resistant than males, and castration increases resistance in males. The effect of folliculoids is tentatively ascribed to an increase in the acid mucopolysaccharide content of the ground substance which decreases the subcutaneous spread of germs.

Viruses ←

Hurst et al. C94,088/60: In the mouse, but not in the guinea pig, males are more susceptible than females to infection with equine encephalomyelitis.

McFarlane & Embil H18,880/68: Female hamsters (Mesocricetus auratus) are much more sensitive (90%) than males (15%) to the inoculation of adenovirus-12. After gonadectomies, 42% of the female and 38% of the male hamsters developed tumors. The somewhat contradictory earlier literature on this sex difference is reviewed.

Yohn et al. G57,790/68: In hamsters given adenovirus-12, strain Huie, s.c. at birth, thymectomy at one week of age increased tumor incidence in both sexes, although it remained higher in females as is usually the case. Cortisone treatment, begun at one week of age, increased tumor incidence but, again, this remained higher in females. Antibody responses to adenovirus-12 T-antigen were depressed in thymectomized and cortisone-treated animals.

Yohn & Funk G68,339/69: Adenovirus-12 produced a higher incidence of tumors in female than in male Syrian hamsters. Ovariectomy lowered tumor incidence, whereas estradiol increased it but only in males.

Minkowitz & Berkovich H23,844/70: Among mice infected with Coxsackie virus Bl, 73% of the males and only 9% of the females showed extensive hepatic necrosis.

Bacterial Toxins ←

Lamanna et al. G60,750/55: The resistance of mice to type A botulinus toxin shows no sex difference, but females are more resistant than males to type B and type C toxin even if the animals have the same body weight.

Gordon & Lipton C94,649/60: 5-HT reduces endotoxin mortality in mice. This effect is greater in females than in males and is potentiated by cortisol. Thyroxine aggravates the toxicity of endotoxin.

Venoms ←

Dossena B47,510/49: Female guinea pigs appear to be more sensitive than males to

Cape cobra venom but pretreatment with testosterone, estradiol or progesterone failed to affect their resistance.

Immune Reactions ←

Lippman et al. B68,238/52: Female rats are much more sensitive than males to the production of nephrotoxic nephritis by anti-rat kidney gamma globulin.

Varia ←

According to some investigators, the hepatic steatosis produced by fasting, plus partial hepatectomy, is more pronounced in female than in male rats. Other authors maintain the opposite.

Hypertension caused by unilateral **renal artery constriction** is more readily produced in male than in female rats.

Several investigators claimed that female mice and rats are more resistant to total body **X-irradiation** than males. However, this difference is not particularly pronounced and may not be obvious under extreme experimental conditions. Male rats (unlike females), fed X-irradiated beef, die of internal hemorrhages, the severity of which is aggravated by testosterone.

Female rats and mice are more resistant to **anoxia** than males.

In rats, resistance to **burns** or exposure to **cold** is not clearly related to sex.

Rats in proestrus and estrus show a subnormal **EST**.

Male rats are allegedly less resistant than females to **trauma** in the Noble-Collip drum.

Gastric ulcer formation under the stressor effect of forced **muscular exercise** is more common in female than in male rats.

Tumor formation following inoculation with adenovirus-12 is more common in female than in male hamsters.

Certain investigators also reported sex-dependent differences in hepatic **enzyme activities**; these will be described in greater detail in the Abstract Section.

Hepatic Lesions ←

MacKay & Carne A14,767/38: In rats, the hepatic steatosis normally occurring during 24 hrs of fasting after partial hepatectomy is more pronounced in females than in males and can be largely prevented by adrenalectomy.

Berman A46,758/46: Contrary to earlier claims less hepatic fat deposition has been found following partial hepatectomy in female than in male rats.

Chambon et al. F80,788/66: In the rat, hepatic regeneration following partial hepatectomy is more rapid in females than in males. However, castration stimulates hepatic regeneration in both sexes.

Gershbein H31,893/70: In intact male rats, unlike in females, DDT caused liver enlargement. This and other insecticides also enhance liver regeneration after partial hepatectomy in males but not in females.

Renal Lesions ←

Bein et al. C57,714/58: In male rats with hypertension produced by unilateral renal artery constriction, vascular lesions are more common than in females. Gonadectomy does not significantly alter these changes in males but aggravates them in females. Parathyroidectomy has no significant effect upon them.

Ionizing Rays ←

Dobrolvolskaïa-Zavadskaïa et al. 86,799/41: Female rats are much more resistant than males to total body X-irradiation.

Abrams B58,956/51: "In general, sex appears to exert no significant influence on the capacity of mice to withstand whole body irradiation."

Ingbar & Freinkel B68,221/52: Post-pubertal male mice are more sensitive to total body X-irradiation than females.

Langendorff & Koch B98,043/54: Male mice are more sensitive than females to X-irradiation but after gonadectomy females are more sensitive than males. Testosterone increases the radioresistance of the female far beyond the norm. Estradiol causes no further increase in the radioresistance of the castrated male.

Betz C13,907/55: There is no obvious sex difference in X-ray resistance among mice. Pretreatment with testosterone offers definite protection especially to females, but here again, treatment after exposure is without effect. Curiously, estradiol pretreatment also offers protection, whereas given after exposure it actually decreases resistance.

Rugh & Clugston C11,209/55: Male CF_1 mice are more X-ray sensitive than females regardless of the phase of the estrous cycle in the latter. Females are most resistant during estrus.

Kohn & Kallman C25,371/56: Female mice are only very slightly more resistant to total body X-irradiation than males.

Rugh & Wolff C19,209/56: Female mice are more resistant to total body X-irradiation than are males. Orchidectomy raises resistance, and this is further increased by treatment with estradiol. In intact males, estradiol raises X-ray resistance to the same level as in castrates.

Langendorff et al. C36,885/57: Male mice are much more sensitive to X-irradiation than females. Orchidectomy increases resistance.

Hamilton et al. D64,060/63: Male mice survived γ-irradiation somewhat longer than females. Orchidectomy has no effect upon the survival time, but ovariectomy slightly prolongs it.

Malhotra & Reber E36,906/63: Male, unlike female, rats fed X-irradiated beef die of internal hemorrhage with severity and lethality which can be aggravated by testosterone. The literature on the effect of sex, castration and stilbestrol upon the lethality of irradiated beef feeding is discussed.

Flemming & Langendorff G38,381/65; Langendorff & Langendorff G42,801/66: Females are more resistant than males to total body X-irradiation, and resistance can be increased in both sexes by natural and synthetic folliculoids.

Hypoxia ←

Britton & Kline 93,980/45: Adult female rats are much more resistant to anoxia than males perhaps because their adrenals are larger. Adrenocortical extract raises resistance to anoxia, whereas DOC does not.

Kline & Britton 85,856/45: At 16°C female rats withstand anoxia longer than males. At higher temperatures the difference is less pronounced. "Estrous conditions and estrogens, castration, etc., do not appear related to the different responses."

Emmens & Parkes B4,928/47: Male mice are considerably more sensitive than females to anoxia (closed vessel technique). Various thyroid preparations increase sensitivity to anoxia.

Temperature Variations ←

Denison & Zarrow B77,713/52: Female rats are more resistant than males to chronic exposure to cold.

Einheber et al. B68,195/52: Male rats are more resistant to burn shock than females.

Munan & Einheber B74,511/52: Female rats are more resistant than males when exposed to the combined stressor effect of scalding and starvation.

Munan & Einheber B82,207/53: In rats, mortality from burn shock is not influenced by sex.

Electric Stimuli ←

Woolley et al. D4,062/61: "Rats in proestrus and estrus showed a greater excitability, as evidenced by a significantly lower EST (-6%), than rats in postestrus and diestrus."

Stressors ← cf. also Selye B40,000/50, p. 81.

Hruza & Poupa C44,659/57; Hruza C74, 576/59; D5,993/61: Male rats are less resistant than females to trauma in the Noble-Collip drum.

Aschkenasy-Lelu G9,425/64: Review of the various damaging agents against which females are more resistant than males, and of the resistance-increasing effect of folliculoids.

Kato & Gillette F57,817/65: The metabolism of aminopyrine and hexobarbital by hepatic microsomes of male rats is impaired by adrenalectomy, castration, hypoxia, ACTH, formaldehyde, epinephrine, morphine, alloxan or thyroxine. The metabolism of aniline and zoxazolamine is not appreciably decreased by any of these agents; in fact, hydroxylation of aniline is enhanced by thyroxine or alloxan. Apparently, the treatments impair mainly the sex-dependent enzymes. Accordingly, the corresponding enzymic functions of the hepatic microsomes of female rats are not significantly impaired by the agents which do have an inhibitory effect in males.

Robert et al. G74,748/70: In rats, the gastric ulcers produced by forced muscular exercise were more common in females than in males and could be totally prevented by fasting.

Diet ←

Silberberg & Silberberg B48,364/50: "Under the influence of a high fat diet, female C57 mice showed less acceleration of epiphyseal development and articular aging than males."

Tumors ←

McFarlane & Embil H18,880/68: Female hamsters (Mesocricetus auratus) are much more sensitive (90%) than males (15%) to the inoculation of adenovirus-12. After gonadectomies, 42% of the female and 38% of the male hamsters developed tumors. The somewhat contradictory earlier literature on this sex difference is reviewed.

Hepatic Enzymes ←

TKT ←. *Lin et al. C96,929/59:* TKT activity is higher in the liver of male than of female rats. This enzyme activity is diminished by castration in males, and increased by testosterone in females. Cortisol increases this transaminase activity in males much more than in females, both in the presence and in the absence of the adrenals.

Glucuronidase ←. *Inscoe & Axelrod D1,700/60:* The ability of microsomes from liver of male rats to form o-aminophenol glucuronide in vitro is four times as great as in females. Estradiol diminishes this enzyme activity in males, whereas testosterone increases it in females.

Künzel & Müller-Oerlinghausen G64,178/69: In vitro glucuronide synthesis is much higher in male than female rat liver tissue because of a larger UDP-glucuronic acid supply in the male liver. Orchidectomy decreases glucuronide synthesis and this decrease can be counteracted by testosterone administration in a dose-dependent manner. However, very large doses of testosterone (more than 100 µg per day) decrease glucuronide formation. Cyproterone (an antitestoid) does not inhibit the increase in glucuronide synthesis induced by testosterone.

Other Enzymes ←. *Knox et al. E83,471/56:* Review (90 pp., 752 refs.) on "Enzymatic and Metabolic Adaptations in Animals" with special reference to hormonal, sex-dependent and diet-induced adaptive enzymic changes, but without special reference to hepatic microsomes.

Freedland et al. G66,662/62: The phenylalanine hydroxylase activity of rat liver increases with age from embryonic life to 50—60 days and then declines to stabilize at a lower level in females than in males after maturity. Fasting and diets deficient in phenylalanine cause a rapid decrease in this enzymic activity.

Pan et al. H3,934/68: The methionine adenosyltransferase activity of hepatic homogenates is higher in female than in male rats. "Ovariectomy decreased the enzyme level, whereas the administration of 17β-estradiol or diethylstilbestrol, but not progesterone, reversed the effect of ovariectomy. Estradiol also raised the enzyme level in intact male rats to that of the female. Adrenalectomy had no effect on the response of the enzyme to estradiol. Castration of the male resulted in an increase in the activity of methionine adenosyltransferase, and the administration of androgenic-anabolic hormones brought the elevated activity down to the normal level of intact males or even lower. Adrenalectomy did not abolish the effect of castration. 17α-Ethyl-19-nortestosterone and 1-methyl-Δ^1-androstenolone were more effective in this respect than testosterone, 17α-methyl-Δ^5-androstene-$3\beta,17\beta$-diol and 5α-androstan-17β-ol-3-one. The effect of the steroids in decreasing methionine adenosyltransferase activity seems to be associated with their anabolic rather than their androgenic action."

← PREGNANCY

Pregnancy greatly changes the resistance of mammals to many agents. This altered tolerance may carry over into the postpartum period or it may terminate sharply at the time of delivery.

The altered tolerance during gestation can be primarily due to activities of the embryo, the placenta, the ovaries or other organs. In some cases, the underlying mechanism has been, at least partially, clarified. For example, some types of resistance persist in pregnant animals whose embryos have been removed as long as the placentas remain intact. In other cases, when resistance to a toxicant continues during lactation, there is good reason to suspect that excretion of the poisons through the milk or the characteristic hormone-secretion pattern necessary for the maintenance of milk secretion are responsible.

In most cases, the reasons for altered tolerance are not known, but they will be discussed in the following pages because of their possible dependence upon protective hormone secretion and drug-metabolizing enzyme induction.

Steroids ←

Pregnant rats are unusually resistant to various actions of glucocorticoids, such as glycogen deposition in the liver, adrenocortical atrophy, catabolism, and decreased resistance to infection. This tolerance persists, as long as the placenta remains intact, even if the fetuses are removed.

Pregnant rats are also very resistant to the production of various cardiopathies in which corticoids act as conditioning factors, for example, against the infarctoid necroses elicited by methylchlorocortisol + NaH_2PO_4.

Glucocorticoids ←

Chedid et al. *C621/54:* Pregnancy interferes with various actions of cortisone in the rat, e.g., decreased resistance to infection by S. enteritidis, glycogen deposition in the liver and adrenocortical atrophy.

Beaton & Curry *C42,333/57:* Pregnant rats are unusually resistant to intoxication with cortisone even after removal of the fetuses, as long as the placentas remain intact.

Curry & Beaton *C56,647/58:* Although pregnant rats are particularly resistant towards the toxic effects of cortisone, their sensitivity to glucagon is not diminished.

Cortisone ← Pregnancy: Hagen et al. *G77,512/60*

Gluco-Mineralocorticoids ← cf. also
Selye *C50,810/58, p. 140; G60,083/70, pp. 480, 483, 484.*

Selye *C44,470/58:* In rats, the infarctoid cardiac necrosis and the nephrocalcinosis produced by Me-Cl-COL + NaH_2PO_4 are largely inhibited by pregnancy.

Mineralocorticoids ← cf. Selye *G60,083/ 70, pp. 480, 482.*

Progesterone ← cf. Selye *E5,986/66, pp. 43, 46; G60,083/70, pp. 480, 483.*

Progesterone ← Pregnancy, Rb: Chatterton et al. *H31,456/70**

Nonsteroidal Hormones and Hormone-Like Substances ←

Pregnant rats are unusually resistant to overdosage with **thyroxine** and **parathyroid hormone**; however, their sensitivity to **glucagon** is not diminished. On the other hand, the production of intracapillary glomerular thrombi and hepatic necroses by **5-HT** is facilitated by pregnancy in rats.

Thyroid Hormones ←

Bodansky & Duff *63,084/36:* Pregnant rats are extraordinarily resistant to the catabolic effect of heavy overdosage with thyroxine.

Parathyroid Hormone ← cf. also Selye *G60,083/70, pp. 479, 482.*

Lehr & Krukowski *D81,044/61; D22,446/ 61:* In rats, late pregnancy (third week) offers considerable protection against the nephrocalcinosis, myocardial injury, hypercalcemia, and hyperphosphatemia normally produced by heavy parathyroid extract overdosage.

This protective effect does not extend to the immediate postpartum period.

Lehr & Krukowski *E21,312/63:* Pregnancy protects against soft-tissue calcification produced by parathyroid extract, even in adrenalectomized rats.

Pancreatic Hormones ←

Curry & Beaton *C56,647/58:* Although pregnant rats are particularly resistant towards the toxic effects of cortisone, their sensitivity to glucagon is not diminished.

← Pregnancy

Catecholamines ← cf. Selye *C* 92,918/61, p. 114; *G* 60,083/70, pp. 480, 483, 484.
Vasopressin ← cf. Selye *G* 60,083/70, p. 484.
5-HT ← cf. also Selye *E* 5,986/66, pp. 44, 47; *G* 60,083/70, pp. 480, 483.

Waugh & Pearl C 83,389/60: In rats, intracapillary glomerular thrombi and hepatic necroses are produced by 5-HT only during pregnancy.

Drugs ←

The **barbiturate** resistance of the rat increases during pregnancy, and allegedly remains high during lactation. A shortening of barbiturate anesthesia has also been reported during gestation in guinea pigs. However the relevant literature is somewhat contradictory. For example, certain investigators found that though sleeping times are shorter, mortality and respiratory depression are significantly greater in pentobarbital-treated virgin rats than in pregnant rats. Indeed, pregnancy may increase sleeping time, although it diminishes mortality after pentobarbital treatment.

The resistance of the rat to the production of bone lesions by **lathyrogens** is likewise increased during gestation; this has been ascribed mainly to a rise in glucocorticoid secretion.

During pregnancy, the detoxication of **meperidine, pethidine,** and **promazine** is impeded as judged by the fact that increased amounts of these drugs are eliminated in the urine.

There is a considerable rise in resistance to overdosage with **vitamin-D derivatives** and **DHT** during pregnancy in the rat, but apparently not in the cow.

o-Aminophenol ← Pregnancy + o-Aminobenzoic acid: Schmid et al. *G* 76, 338/59; Feuer et al. *H* 14,579/69*

Aminopyrine ← Pregnancy: Eriksson *H* 30,468/70

Anaphylactoidogens ← cf. Selye *G* 46,715/68, p. 209.

Aniline ← Pregnancy: Guarino et al. *H* 15,843/69

Anticoagulants ←

Feuer & Liscio H 14,579/69: Review of the literature and personal observations on the unusually low drug-metabolizing enzyme activity of the liver in newborn rats. In pregnant rats, the pentobarbital sleeping time is prolonged, and there is a reduction in the activities of 4-methylcoumarin-3-hydroxylase and uridine diphosphoglucuronic acid: o-aminophenol transglucuronylase in the liver. The low activities of these and other enzymes can be raised to or even above those of nonpregnant animals by giving inducers in vivo, such as 4-methylcoumarin, 3-methylcholanthrene, or phenobarbital. Among newborn rats, those weaned early had a shorter pentobarbital sleeping time than nonweaned controls. The reversible reduction of enzyme activity during pregnancy is ascribed to an excess of folliculoids.

4-Methylcoumarin ← Pregnancy + Phenobarbital: Feuer et al. *H* 14,579/69

Arsenic ←

Agduhr E 70,688/41: Repeated mating increases the resistance of mice to arsenic. Pregnancy further augments this protective effect in females.

Agduhr G 37,252/41: In the mouse, sexual intercourse as well as some sex hormone preparations increase the storage of arsenic in the ground substance of various organs, especially the skin, whereas repeated pregnancies have an opposite effect and at the same time augment resistance against intoxication with As_2O_3.

Barbiturates ←

Holck & Fink A 35,663/40: Sexual activity or the absence of it failed to influence ectylurea (Nostal) (isopropyl bromallyl barbituric acid) anesthesia in rats. However, resistance to this barbiturate was markedly raised in females which were or recently had been pregnant although, even in these, it was not brought up to the male level.

Holck & Mathieson B644/44: In the rat, pregnancy increases the ability to develop tolerance against pentobarbital injected every 90 min over several days and nights. This increase in tolerance persisted during lactation, but disappeared 8 weeks after parturition.

Giotti & Donatelli B39,580/48: In guinea pigs, barbiturate (Enallylpropymal) anesthesia is considerably shortened during the later part of pregnancy but returns to its normal length after parturition.

King & Becker E38,612/60: Although sleeping times are shorter, mortality and the degree of respiratory depression are significantly greater in pentobarbital-treated virgin rats than in pregnant rats.

King & Becker D5,106/61: Pregnancy increases sleeping time, but diminishes the mortality following pentobarbital treatment.

King & Becker G78,964/63: In rats, pregnancy prolongs pentobarbital sleeping time, and males are even less susceptible than nonpregnant females.

King G78,963/64: Review of earlier reports and personal observations showing that, in the rat, pentobarbital anesthesia is prolonged, but lessened in depth during pregnancy. Correspondingly, pentobarbital disappears more rapidly from the blood and tissues of nonpregnant than of pregnant rats.

Neale & Parke G67,965/69: In rats, during pregnancy, the hepatic microsomal enzymes responsible for the hydroxylation of diphenyl, reduction of p-nitrobenzoic acid, microsomal protein, and cytochrome P-450, are all increased when expressed as a function of total liver weight. However, when calculated per g liver weight, the 4-hydroxylation of diphenyl and cytochrome P-450 content are both significantly decreased. Since, during pregnancy, the animal increases in body weight, these findings may explain why the hexobarbital sleeping time is increased in full-term pregnant rats.

Barbital(sodium) ← Pregnancy: Franke et al. H31,874/66*

Pentobarbital, Propallylonal ← Pregnancy: Holck et al. A35,663/40*; Holck et al. B644/44*; Feuer et al. H14,579/69*

BCP ←

Tanabe F92,176/67: BCP (5-n-butyl-l-cyclohexyl-2,4,6-trioxoperhydropyrimidine) is more toxic for female than for male rats, and pregnant females are more sensitive than nonpregnant controls.

Bile Pigments ←

Soffer 7,166/33: The excretion of injected bilirubin is almost invariably delayed in pregnant women, suggesting impairment of the hepatic function.

Shibata et al. G80,058/66: In rats, hepatic glucuronyl transferase activity is greatly increased during the last third of gestation, whereas enzymic activity is virtually absent in the fetal liver. These divergent changes "raise doubt as to whether low enzymic activity in the fetus and increased activity after birth are the consequence, respectively, of high hormone levels in pregnancy, and falling hormone concentrations in the postpartum period. The maximal rate of bilirubin excretion into bile, the bilirubin T_m, remained unchanged in pregnancy despite the potential for increased bilirubin conjugation. When coupled with other observations, this suggests that the rate of delivery of conjugated bilirubin into bile is the rate-limiting step involved in the maximal transfer rate of bilirubin from blood to bile, and that the excretory step for bilirubin remains unaffected during pregnancy in the rat."

Song & Kappas G89,521/70: Brief review of the literature on the effect of various hormones and of pregnancy upon the activity of hepatic UDP-glucuronyltransferase.

Bilirubin ← Pregnancy: Halac et al. G77,576/69

Cadmium ←

Pařízek F31,959/65: In rats, pregnancy increases susceptibility to the fatal effect of cadmium intoxication. At autopsy, the kidneys are found to be swollen, hyperemic and hemorrhagic, especially in the medulla, and there is a high incidence of adrenal hemorrhages and thrombi in the pulmonary vessels.

Carbon Tetrachloride ←

Douglas & Clower H20,791/68: In rats, pregnancy offers some protection against the hepatotoxic effect of CCl_4.

Carcinogens ←

Dao & Sunderland D79,860/59; Dao et al. E57,368/60: In rats, the induction of mammary carcinomas by 3-MC is enhanced during pregnancy, pseudopregnancy, and progesterone treatment. Regression of neoplasms occurs after parturition. Males are virtually resistant. In fully formed tumors, regression could be induced by hypophysectomy or ovariectomy.

Bock & Dao D11,892/61: In rats, 3-MC accumulation in the mammary glands is increased by hypophysectomy or ovariectomy, but diminished during pregnancy. The affinity of mammary tissue for certain carcinogens may be due to its close association with adipose tissue.

Huggins et al. C99,772/61: In rats, the production of mammary cancers by DMBA or 3-MC is inhibited by pregnancy, estradiol, progesterone, or combined treatment of estradiol + progesterone.

Bird et al. H30,425/70: In rats less than 30 days of age, DMBA or 7-OHM-12-MBA produces no adrenal necrosis unless animals are pretreated with ACTH. However, a single i.v. injection of 7-OHM-12-MBA on the 17th day of gestation causes adrenal necrosis in the embryos as well as in the mothers. Pretreatment with SKF 525-A protected the adrenals both of the embryos and of the mothers.

3-MC ← Pregnancy: Huggins et al. C99,772/61*; Bresnick et al. H215/68*

Chlorcyclizine ← Pregnancy + SKF 525-A: Posner et al. H31,661/67*

3-Methyl-4-monomethylaminoazo-benzene ← Pregnancy: Bresnick et al. H215/68

Cholesterol ← *cf. Selye G60,083/70, pp. 479, 480.*

Choline ← *cf. also Selye G60,083/70, pp. 480, 483.*

Calabro B48,121/49; Bozzo B50,296/49: In rats the production of hepatic steatosis by hypolipotropic high-fat diets is greatly facilitated by pregnancy.

Colchicine ← *cf. Selye E5,986/66, pp. 44, 46.*

Dyes ←

Mueller & Kappas G81,288/64: Review and personal observations on the impairment of hepatic BSP excretion following treatment with natural folliculoids and during pregnancy in women.

Tindall & Beazley G34,865/65: Review of the literature and personal observations on women indicate that "during pregnancy the essential changes in liver cellular function are: (i) a slight increase in the uptake of BSP from the plasma; (ii) a twofold increase in the return of dye to the plasma; (iii) a reduction by one half to two-thirds in the elimination of dye into the bile, and (iv) an alteration in the proportion of dye lost from the liver cells per minute to the plasma and bile respectively." These changes are tentatively ascribed to excess folliculoid production.

Dye (BSP) ← Pregnancy, Man: Combes et al. E26,415/63*

Lathyrogens ←

Walker & Wirtschafter C29,985/56: In rats, a Lathyrus odoratus diet does not produce osteolathyrism during pregnancy, although fetal absorption ensues.

Dasler C36,068/57: In rats, pregnancy offers protection against osteolathyrism produced by APN.

Schuurmans D23,829/62: Theoretical considerations concerning the influence of pregnancy upon the formation of dissecting aneurysms, based upon experimental observations of others showing that corticoids greatly influence angiolathyrism.

Meperidine ←

Rudofsky & Crawford E58,989/66: After administration of meperidine or promazine "pregnant women, women on oral contraceptives and neonates excreted significantly more unchanged meperidine than normeperidine, whereas the reverse held for the male 'controls' and other female groups. Pregnant women, women on oral contraceptives and neonates excreted more unchanged and minimally degraded promazine than non-pregnant women. Stilbestrol and progesterone each changed the pattern of excretion by male subjects towards that associated with pregnancy." Apparently, pregnancy diminishes the capacity to metabolize meperidine and promazine, —a change reflected in neonates and subjects taking oral contraceptives.

Morphine ←

Bonino C64,366/57: In rats, pregnancy shortens the duration of the morphine-induced contraction of the tail muscles.

Ethylmorphine ← Pregnancy: Guarino et al. H15,843/69

p-Nitrophenol ← Pregnancy: Halac et al. G77,576/69

Papain ← *cf. Selye C92,918/61, p. 105; G60,083/70, p. 484*

Pesticides ← Pregnancy, Man: Polishuk et al. G72,380/70*

Pethidine ←

Crawford & Rudofsky G42,454/66: In women taking various oral contraceptives, as well as in pregnant women and in neonates, the urinary excretion of pethidine and promazine

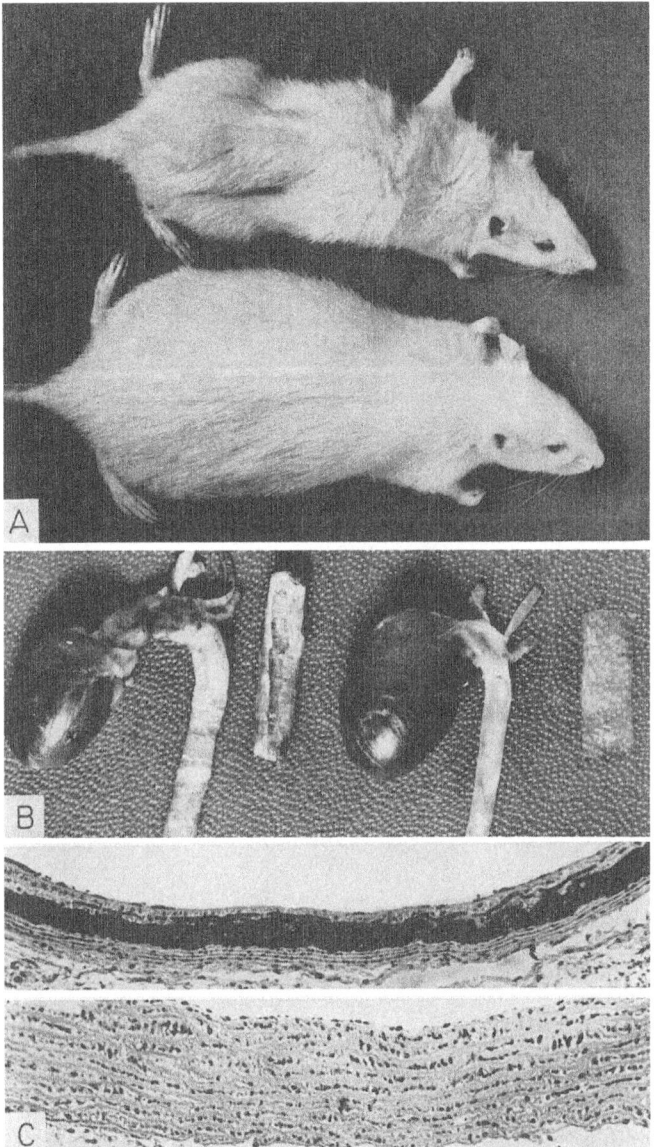

Fig. 27. **Protection by pregnancy against DHT.** All rats received the same dose of DHT. A: Considerable emaciation and shaggy fur of the control rat (top) in comparison with the normal appearance of the animal protected against DHT by pregnancy. B: Heart and thoracic aorta, with a separate opened piece of the abdominal aorta, of a nonpregnant rat (left) and of one which was pregnant during the experiment. White calcified spots in the heart and "gooseneck" appearance of the thoracic aorta due to intensely calcified cross bands. The portion of abdominal aorta (incised lengthwise) is stiff and its edges do not readily separate. The heart and aorta of the animal protected by pregnancy retain their normal appearance. The opened piece of abdominal aorta is so supple that it flattens out, and so transparent that the background pattern shines through its wall. C: In the nonpregnant rat (top), DHT caused intense calcification (demonstrated by von Kóssa stain) and dilatation (thinning) of the aorta. In the pregnant animal the aorta remained normal. [Selye C25,011/57. Courtesy of Amer. J. Obstet. Gynec.]

is increased, suggesting interference with the detoxication of these drugs.

Picrotoxin ← Pregnancy: Holck D28, 543/49*

Plasmocid ← cf. Selye C92,918/61, p. 96.

Promazine ←

Crawford & Rudofsky G42,454/66: In women taking various oral contraceptives, as well as in pregnant women and in neonates, the urinary excretion of pethidine and promazine is increased, suggesting interference with the detoxication of these drugs.

Rudofsky & Crawford E58,989/66: After administration of meperidine or promazine "pregnant women, women on oral contraceptives and neonates excreted significantly more unchanged meperidine than normeperidine, whereas the reverse held for the male 'controls' and other female groups. Pregnant women, women on oral contraceptives and neonates excreted more unchanged and minimally degraded promazine than non-pregnant women. Stilbestrol and progesterone each changed the pattern of excretion by male subjects toward that associated with pregnancy." Apparently, pregnancy diminishes the capacity to metabolize meperidine and promazine — a change reflected in neonates and subjects taking oral contraceptives.

Promazine ← Pregnancy, Man: Crawford et al. G78,958/65*

Tetraethylammonium (TEA) ←

Brust et al. B18,590/48: Observations on women revealed that "in normal term pregnancy the TEAC blood pressure floor is strikingly low and rises to normal levels after delivery. In toxemia the TEAC floor is higher than normal and consistently falls to normal levels after recovery." The TEA (or TEAC) floor is defined as the lowest point to which the blood pressure descends in the first 5 min following injection.

Vitamin D, DHT ← cf. also Selye C50,810/58, p. 140; G60,083/70, pp. 479, 480

Selye C25,011/57: The generalized calcinosis produced by heavy DHT overdosage in the rat is inhibited by pregnancy, cf. Fig. 27.

Potvliege E98,323/62: Pregnancy affords considerable protection against vitamin-D intoxication in the rat.

Greig G68,415/63: In cows given vitamin-D_3 i.v., intense metastatic calcification occurred in the subendocardium and the subintima of the aorta. "These lesions occurred whether or not the cows were pregnant at the time of injection and whether or not lactation followed."

Strebel et al. F35,901/65: Cardiovascular calcification produced by DHT in the rat is inhibited by pregnancy.

Vitamin E ← cf. Selye G60,083/70, pp. 480, 483

Diet ← cf. Selye E5,986/66, pp. 43, 45.

Microorganisms ←

The progress of **brucellosis** is inhibited in the cow by pregnancy, but not by injections of progesterone.

Pregnancy increases the susceptibility of mice to poliomyelitis **virus** and makes the otherwise resistant rat sensitive to the virus of ovine enzootic abortion. Even pseudopregnancy increases resistance of the rabbit to vaccine virus.

On the other hand, resistance of pregnant rats and mice to various types of **endotoxins** is considerably increased during gestation.

Varia ←

The arterial lesions that develop in dogs kept on a high fat diet upon subsequent **nephrectomy** are prevented by pregnancy.

Regeneration of the liver following **partial hepatectomy** is accelerated during pregnancy in the rat.

In rats exposed to strong auditory and visual stimuli, pregnancy did not prevent the usual manifestations of **stress**.

Microorganisms ←

Bacteria ←. *Payne C 89,814/60:* In cows, the progress of experimental brucellosis is inhibited by pregnancy but not by progesterone.

Viruses ←. *Sprunt & McDearman A 33, 321/40:* Treatment with estradiol or estrone, as well as pseudopregnancy, increased the resistance of the rabbit to vaccine virus.

Knox B 47,631/50: Pregnancy enhances the susceptibility of mice to inoculation with Col. SK-strain murine poliomyelitis virus p.o. This increased susceptibility does not appear to depend wholly on a greater permeability of the intestinal mucosa, since in a small series, essentially similar results were obtained by i.v. inoculation.

Payne & Belyavin C 95,892/60: Pregnancy renders the otherwise resistant rat susceptible to infection with the virus of enzootic abortion of sheep (E.A. virus). This resistance is probably "due to the presence of placental tissue, which allows the virus to establish itself."

Bacterial Toxins ← *cf. also Selye E 5,986/66, pp. 43, 44.*

Jasmin B 80,596/53: A dose of meningococcus toxin i.v. well tolerated by nonpregnant rats produces eclampsia-like hemorrhagic lesions in the liver of pregnant or cortisone pretreated animals.

Chedid & Boyer C 10,098/55: In mice, resistance to S. enteritidis endotoxin is greatly diminished and the protective effect of cortisone is also inhibited during pregnancy.

Tarján et al. G 54,411/67: Review of the literature, and personal observations on the sensitization to endotoxin shock by pregnancy.

Varia ←

Ionizing Rays ←. *Mitznegg et al. G 77,075/70:* In rats, pregnancy protects against X-irradiation, presumably through the increased production of endogenous folliculoids. Combined treatment with clomiphene blocks the protective effect of pregnancy perhaps because it counteracts the action of folliculoids.

Renal Lesions ←. *Holman & Jones B 93, 771/53:* The arterial lesions that develop in dogs kept on a standard high-fat diet upon subsequent nephrectomy, are prevented by pregnancy, cortisone, ACTH, or diethylstilbestrol.

Hepatic Lesions ←. *Gershbein G 71,666/58:* Pregnancy greatly accelerates regeneration of rat liver after partial hepatectomy.

Gonzáles-Angulo et al. H 30,301/70: In normal pregnant women, liver biopsies revealed elongation, gigantism and lamellar osmiophilic material in hepatocytes during the last trimester of gestation. In women with hydatidiform mole or choriocarcinoma, mild focal dilatation and vesiculation of both RER and SER were noted.

Stressors ←. *Soiva et al. C 97,218/60:* In rats exposed to strong auditory and visual stimuli, "pregnancy could not protect the organism from the consequences of stress."

Hepatic Enzymes ←. *Beaton et al. A 49,354/54:* In rats, on about the fifteenth day of gestation, there is a marked increase in protein anabolism accompanied by a decrease in hepatic GPT and in the rate of urea formation in liver slices.

Beaton et al. C 10,012/55: STH decreases the GPT and d-amino acid oxidase activity in nonpregnant female rats. These effects are even more pronounced if the animals receive STH + "equine estrogenic substances" + progesterone. This enzyme activity also decreases during pregnancy both in intact and in hypophysectomized rats.

← AGE

Steroids ←

There appear to be considerable differences in the biotransformation of steroids, which depend upon age or, at least, upon changes (e.g., sexual maturation, senile involution of the gonads) that are, in themselves, age-dependent.

Female rats are more sensitive to steroid anesthesia than males, but this sex difference is obvious only after maturity, and young animals of either sex are more sensitive than adults.

The effect of age upon the metabolites formed from various steroid hormones has been studied in detail. (cf. Abstract Section.)

Drugs ←

In general, the metabolizing ability of the liver for a variety of substrates is low in newborn rats.

The **aminopyrine** demethylase activity of the microsomal fraction, though low at birth, rises during the first 30 days, and after puberty, particularly in males.

Much work has been done on the age-dependence of **barbiturate** detoxication. Pentobarbital resistance increases with age up to puberty, particularly in male rats. Among 2-month-old rats, practically all developed tolerance to the injection of pentobarbital (given at 90 min intervals, day and night, for periods up to five days). The same was true of adult males in contrast to females. Orchidectomy decreased the ability to develop tolerance in adults, but not in 2-month-old males. There is good evidence to suggest that the lack of a clear-cut sex difference in the barbiturate-detoxifying ability of immature rats is due to the comparatively low level of catatoxic testoid secretions.

Among newborn rats, those weaned early exhibit a shorter pentobarbital sleeping time than nonweaned controls.

According to recent observations, the LD_{50} of hexobarbital rises considerably between the 12th and 130th day of life; however, the blood concentration of the barbiturate at waking time is not age-dependent.

The hexobarbital-metabolizing activity of the rat liver is extremely low during the neonatal period and rises gradually, up to the 80th day of life, to a level which is much higher in males than in females. X-irradiation of pregnant rats results in a deficiency of hexobarbital-metabolizing enzymes in their male offspring. However, such irradiation does not suppress the subsequent induction of this enzyme activity by phenobarbital. Actinomycin D inhibits both ontogenic and phenobarbital-induced increases in enzyme activity. Apparently, the X-ray-induced inhibition of hepatic enzymes is mediated through an effect upon the hormonal regulation of enzyme-induction, whereas the substrate-induced enzyme synthesis is independent of such endocrine controls.

In young and old rats, the anti-**indomethacin** effect of PCN is essentially the same if the dose levels are adjusted to body weight.

In pregnant women and in their neonates, the capacity to metabolize meperidine, pethidine and promazine is low as judged by the increased urinary excretion of these drugs.

Immature rats are especially sensitive to certain **pesticides** (e.g., Malathion), and their livers detoxify such compounds at a slow rate.

Female rats are more sensitive to **strychnine** intoxication than males, but resistance increases with age in both sexes.

Hepatic Enzymes ←

The **TPO and TKT** activity of rat liver is very low during fetal life but begins to rise a few hours after birth. This increase in TKT activity is prevented by adrenalectomy, and tyrosine cannot substitute for cortisol in restoring it towards normal. Premature delivery by cesarean section is also rapidly followed by increased TKT activity. Under all these conditions, the possibility to induce enzymic activity by cortisol coincides with delivery.

In guinea pigs, TKT activity is also absent during fetal life and increases to adult values within 24 hrs after birth.

In chickens, enzymic activity is relatively constant during the embryonic period, but rises after hatching.

Hepatic TKT activity increases in immature stressed (reciprocating shaker) rats, whereas intact stressed adults show no change. In stressed adrenalectomized adults, TKT activity dropped precipitously, whereas this was not the case in immature adrenalectomized rats.

TPO activity, when present, was increased by stress in old rats, but this increase was abolished by adrenalectomy or hypophysectomy. From these and other observations, it was concluded that "stress-activation of a pituitary mechanism that inhibits or represses activation of tyrosine transaminase may not function during early postnatal life."

Several **other enzyme mechanisms** (e.g., GOT, phenylalanine hydroxylase, OKT) have been found to be largely age-dependent.

Steroids ←

Selye A 35,150/41: Female rats are more sensitive to anesthesia produced by various steroids than are males, and young animals of either sex are more sensitive than adults.

Winter & Selye A 35,658/41; Winter A 36, 333/41: Female rats are more sensitive than males to the anesthetic action of progesterone, but this sex difference is obvious only after maturity. "The normal endocrine activity of the testis is largely, if not entirely, responsible for this comparative resistance of the males since castration increases sensitivity in males but is without effect in female rats. Conversely the resistance of castrate males and females may be raised by methyl testosterone administration."

Karnofsky et al. B 69,772/52: Newborn mice are extremely sensitive to the anesthetic and lethal effect of progesterone, but within 2—3 days resistance develops, and by the 7th day the mouse can tolerate about 100 times as much progesterone as on the day of birth. "The rapid development of resistance to progesterone within a few days after birth suggests that a system or mechanism has appeared which is capable of detoxifying, catabolizing, counterbalancing or accelerating the excretion of progesterone."

Forchielli et al. D 75,874/58: The rate of Δ^4 reduction of 11-desoxycortisol was 3-4-fold greater in female than in male rat liver homogenates and in microsomal fractions containing the Δ^4-5α-hydrogenase. Female rat liver contains only one Δ^4-hydrogenase (5α-microsomal), whereas the male liver contains the soluble Δ^4-5β-hydrogenase as well. Ovariectomy caused no marked change in enzyme titer, but hypophysectomy decreased it sharply. Curiously, ACTH, STH, and pregnant mare serum partially restored the enzyme level in the hypophysectomized rat. In young animals, an increase in the titer of hepatic Δ^4-5α-hydrogenase occurs prior to puberty. This fact (like the negative results after ovariectomy) suggests an independence of enzyme regulation from ovarian hormones.

Lehmann & Schütz H 14,215/69: The microsomal fraction of the liver of the mature human fetus metabolizes 4-^{14}C-estrone twice as fast as that of the 12-week-old fetus. The highest rate of metabolism was found in the microsomal fraction of the liver of an adult man. "By paperchromatography, microchemical reactions and crystallization to constant specific activity, the following metabolites were identified: 6α-, 6β-, 7α-, 15α- and 16α-hydroxyoestrone, 6α-, 6β- and 7α-hydroxyoestradiol-17β and oestriol."

Conney et al. E 8,232/69: The microsomal enzymes required for the 6β-, 7α- and 16α-hydroxylation of testosterone are selectively influenced, as shown by the speed of their development with age or after treatment with phenobarbital or 3-methylcholanthrene. Addition of chlorthion, in vitro, to hepatic microsomes markedly inhibits the 16α-hydroxylation of testosterone, whereas it has a lesser effect on 16β-hydroxylation and no effect on 7α-hydroxylation.

Cortisol ← Age: Houck et al. E 21,446/63*

Cortisone ← Age: Hagen et al. G 77, 512/60

Dehydroepiandrosterone ← Age, Man, Mky, Rat: Heinrichs et al. *F72,860/66*

Dehydroepiandrosterone ← Age, Gp, Man, Rat: Pulkkinen *G39,295/66*

Estradiol ← Age: Kuntzman et al. *F27,893/64;* Conney et al. *G65,135/65;* Kuntzman et al. *G66,245/66;* Nobuyoshi et al. *F69,360/66*;* Hertogh et al. *H31,447/70**

Estrone ← Age, Gp, Man, Rat: Pulkkinen *G39,295/66*

Pregnanolone ← Age: Soyka et al. *H31,803/70**

Progesterone ← Age: McCormack et al. *F9,493/64*;* Kuntzman et al. *G66,245/66*

Synthetic Estrogens ← Age: Noble *A30,160/39**

Testosterone ← Age: Kuntzman et al. *F27,893/64;* Conney et al. *G65,135/65;* Kuntzman et al. *G66,245/66, G71,857/68*

Drugs ←

Acetaminophen ← Age, Dog: Baader et al. *D43,960/64**

Acetanilide ← Age, Rb: Fouts et al. *H24,325/59;* Fouts *G77,514/62*

Acetazolamide ← Age, Mouse, Rat: Petty et al. *F58,540/65**

Acetophenetidin ← Age, Gp: Jondorf et al. *E90,586/58;* Baader et al. *D43,960/64**

p-Aminobenzoic Acid ← Age, Gp: Dutton *G70,064/59*

o-Aminophenol ← Age: Brown *H28,215/57;* Dutton *G70,064/59;* Schmid et al. *G76,338/59;* Gartner et al. *E28,857/63;* Baader et al. *D43,960/64*;* Flint et al. *G78,603/64;* Dutton *G78,598/66*

Aminopyrine ←. *Soyka G66,626/69:* In rat liver, the aminopyrine demethylase activity of the microsomal fraction increased considerably during the first 30 days after birth. Evidence of an inhibitor was not found during this newborn period. After puberty, the activity in male rats was about twice as high as in females. Testosterone produced only an insignificant rise in females.

Aminopyrine ← Age: Jondorf et al. *E90,586/58;* Fouts et al. *H24,325/59;* Fouts *G77,514/62;* Hart et al. *D27,689/62, G69,761/63;* Dallner et al. *G74,691/65, G74,693/65, G78,599/66;* Kato *G74,104/66;* Kato et al. *H15,796/68;* Klinger et al. *H30,598/68;* Tardiff et al. *H11,752/69;* Mitoma et al. *H31,720/70*

Amphetamine ← Age, Rb: Fouts *G77,514/62;* Fouts et al. *H24,325/59*

Aniline ← Age: Kato et al. *H15,796/68;* Gram et al. *G68,711/69;* Eling et al. *H27,047/70*

Anticoagulants ← Age: Saidi et al. *F32,236/65*;* Feuer et al. *H14,579/69*

Barbiturates ←. *Carmichael D68,076/38:* The LD_{50} of pentobarbital (Nembutal) increases with age but "there does not seem to be a definite sex difference in reaction to the median lethal dose of Nembutal of either young or old rats." In earlier observations in which males were found to be more resistant to barbiturates, the anesthetic action and not the lethal effect was determined.

Holck & Mathieson B644/44: In rats, the development of tolerance to pentobarbital was determined by injecting increasing doses every 90 min, day and night, for periods up to 5 days. Practically all 1—2-month-old rats developed tolerance as did adult males in contrast to females. Castration lowered the ability of adult males to develop tolerance, but did not do so in 2 month-old males. Ovariectomy of 2 month-old females increased their ability to detoxify pentobarbital, once tolerance had developed.

Homburger et al. E61,371/47: Female rats are more sensitive than males to pentobarbital but not to thiopental anesthesia. Age and strain differences in barbiturate resistance have also been noted in the rat.

Buchel D73,669/54: Review on the literature, and personal observations on the increased sleeping time of female as compared to male rats, after treatment with certain barbiturates, particularly hexobarbital. The increased sleeping time is associated with a prolonged persistence of the concentration of the drug in the blood. Gonadectomy prolongs the sleeping time of males but does not influence that of females. In immature rats no such sex difference is observed.

Kato E87,340/60: Chlorpromazine pretreatment reduces barbiturate sleeping time even in adrenalectomized or immature rats.

Nair & Zeitlin G65,099/67: The hexobarbital-metabolizing activity of the rat liver is extremely low after birth and rises gradually, up to the 80th day of life, to levels much higher in males than in females. Prenatal X-irradiation suppresses this normal development of enzyme activities in the male so that it only reaches the normal female level. Irradiation at 21 days (total body or head alone) also suppresses the developmental increase of enzyme activity, but to a lesser extent. Adults are still more resistant.

Nair et al. G67,245/68: X-irradiation of pregnant rats results in male offspring deficient in hepatic microsomal enzymes which metabolize hexobarbital. However, irradiation did not suppress the increase of enzyme activity brought about by chemical inducers (phenobarbital). Actinomycin inhibited both the ontogenic and phenobarbital-induced increases in enzyme activity. "The ontogenic increase in enzyme activity is hormone-dependent, while that following phenobarbital administration is independent of hormonal regulation as evidenced by the response in hypophysectomized or sexually immature animals. It is concluded from these results that the inhibitory effect of x-irradiation on the hepatic enzyme system is mediated through an action on the hormonal regulation of enzyme activity."

Feuer & Liscio H14,579/69: Review of the literature and personal observations on the unusually low drug-metabolizing enzyme activity of the liver in newborn rats. Among newborn rats, those weaned early had a shorter pentobarbital sleeping time than nonweaned controls.

Klinger H25,517/70: In male rats, the LD_{50} of hexobarbital in mg/kg rises from 160 to 343, between 12—130 days after birth; however, the blood concentration of hexobarbital at waking time is not age-dependent. The sleeping time is directly correlated with the speed of biotransformation by hepatic microsomes in vitro. CCl_4-prolongs sleeping time. Following acute habituation in CCl_4-treated rats, the hexobarbital concentration of the plasma at waking time is comparatively high.

Barbital(sodium) ← Age(Embryo): Franke et al. H31,874/66*; Kuhlmann et al. G74,362/70*

Hexobarbital ← Age: Jondorf et al. E90,586/58; Fouts et al. H24,325/59; Fouts G77,514/62; Hart et al. D27,689/62, G69,761/63; Kato et al. G17,077/64; Kuntzman et al. F27,893/64; Conney et al. G65,135/65; Kuntzman et al. G66,245/66; Kupfer et al. G40,053/66; Yam et al. G58,163/67*; Fujii et al. H28,618/68*; Kato et al. H15,796/68; Klinger et al. H30,598/68*; Dixon et al. H30,692/68; Traeger et al. H23,856/69*; Kuhlmann et al. G74,362/70*

Mephobarbital ← Age, Fowl: Strittmatter et al. G66,629/69

Pentobarbital ← Age: Boer A52,450/47*, A48,817/48*; Kato E87,340/60*; Weatherall G76,306/60*; Kato et al. G17,077/64*; Kato G74,104/66; Soyka H30,981/68; Feuer et al. H14,579/69*

Phenobarbital ← Age, Mouse, Rat: Petty et al. F58,540/65*; Mitoma et al. H31,720/70

Thiopental ← Age+Sex, Dog: Boer A52,450/47*

Bilirubin ← Age: Brown H28,215/57; Schmid et al. G76,338/59*; Sutherland et al. G78,607/61*; Catz et al. G71,888/62*; Hargreaves et al. H30,986/62*; Flint et al. G78, 603/64; Brown et al. G78,957/65*; Tomlinson et al. G76,303/66; Jacobsen et al. H30,765/67*; DeLeon et al. G71,826/67*; Halac et al. G77, 576/69

Carcinogens ←. *Bird et al. H30,425/70:* In rats less than 30 days of age, DMBA or 7-OHM-12-MBA produces no adrenal necrosis unless animals are pretreated with ACTH. However, a single i.v. injection of 7-OHM-12-MBA on the 17th day of gestation causes adrenal necrosis in the embryos as well as in the mothers. Pretreatment with SKF 525-A protected the adrenals both of the embryos and of the mothers.

Benzo(a)pyrene ← Age, Mouse: Epstein et al. G77,545/67*

Carcinogens ← Age: Noble A30,160/39*; Schoental H27,417/70*

7,12-Dimethylbenz(a)anthracene ← Age: Ford et al. D69,790/63*; Huggins et al. E35,442/63*, G14,366/64*

3-MC ← Age, Mouse: Klein G76,354/59*

3-Methyl-4-monomethylaminoazobenzene ← Age: Bresnick et al. H215/68

N-Nitrosodimethylamine ← Age + Sex + Methyltestosterone: Venkatesan et al. H31,273/70

2-Naphtylamine ← Age: Dewhurst G76,687/63*

Carisoprodol ← Age: Kato et al. G74,632/61, G17,077/64*

CCl_4 ← Age(newborn): Dawkins G78,605/63*; Reuber G73,605/70*

CO_2 ← Age, Mouse, Rat: Petty et al. F58,540/65*

Chloramphenicol ← Age(newborn), Man: Weiss et al. H33,308/60*

Chlorcyclizine ← Age (Embryo+ SKF 525-A: Posner et al. H31,661/67*

Chlorpromazine ← Age, Rb: Fouts et al. H24,325/59; Fouts G77,514/62

Codeine ← Age, Rb: Eddy A50,050/39* Fouts G77,514/62

Dimethylaniline ← Age, Bullfrog: Machinist et al. H15,503/68

Diphenyl ← Age, Hamster, Mouse, Rat, Rb: Creaven et al. G77,565/64

Diphenylhydantoin ← Age, Mouse, Rat: Petty et al. F58,540/65*

Dyes (BSP), Phenolphthalein ← Age: Brown H28,215/57; Jondorf et al. E90,586/58; Dutton G78,598/66

Ethyl Ether ← Age, Rat, Rb: Weatherall G76,306/60*

Freons (112, 113) ← Age (infant), Mouse: Epstein et al. G77,545/67*

Gonadotrophins ← Age: Zarrow et al. E20,351/63*

Griseofulvin ← Age, Mouse: Epstein et al. G77,545/67*; H30,997/67*

Indomethacin ←. *Selye PROT. 34038, 34405:* In rats of different age groups, the anti-indomethacin effect of PCN is essentially the same if administered at dose levels adjusted to body weight.

Menthol ← Age, Gp: Dutton *G70,064/59*

Meperidine, Pethidine, Promazine ←. *Rudofsky & Crawford E58,989/66:* Apparently, pregnancy diminishes the capacity of women to metabolize meperidine and promazine, a change reflected in their neonates.

Crawford & Rudofsky G42,454/66: In women taking various oral contraceptives, as well as in pregnant women and in neonates, the urinary excretion of pethidine and promazine is increased, suggesting interference with the detoxication of these drugs.

Meprobamate ← Age: Kato et al. H27, 665/61*; *G17,077/64*

Monomethyl-4-aminoantipyrine ← Age, Gp: Jondorf et al. *E90,586/58*

N-Monomethyl-p-nitroaniline ← Age (Embryo) + Phenobarbital (to mother), Man, Mouse: Pomp et al. *H14,237/69*

Morphine ← Age: Chesler et al. A52, 010/42*

Morphine Derivatives ← Age, Rb: Eddy A50,050/39*; Kupferberg et al. E21,867/63*

Ethylmorphine ← Age: Davies et al. *H22,054/68;* Sasame et al. *G72,114/68;* Gram et al. *G68,711/69*

Neoprontosil ← Age, Rb: Fouts *G77,514/62*

Nikethamide ← Age: Brazda et al. *B32,015/48;* Wilson et al. E43,062/50*

p-Nitroanisole ← Age: Pomp et al. *H14,237/69;* Strittmatter et al. *G66,629/69;* Tardiff et al. *H11,752/69;* Mitoma et al. *H31,720/70*

p-Nitrobenzoic Acid ← Age: Fouts et al. *H24,325/59;* Fouts *G77,514/62;* Hart et al. *D27,689/62;* Kato et al. *H15,796/68*

p-Nitrophenol ← Age: Dutton *G78,598/66;* Neubaur et al. *H30,996/66;* Pulkkinen *G39,295/66;* Halac et al. G77,576/69

p-Nitrophenyl ← Age, Rb: Tomlinson et al. *G76,303/66*

Norchlorcyclizine ← Age (Embryo) +SKF 525-A: Posner et al. H31,661/67*

Pesticides ←. *Brodeur & DuBois F40,590/65:* Immature rats are more sensitive to malathion than adults, and their livers detoxify the insecticide at a slow rate. Orchidectomy decreases, whereas testosterone increases, malathion detoxication. All of this suggests that testoids play an important role in the maintenance of the malathion-hydroxylating enzyme system.

Aldrin ← Age: Gillett *G74,480/69*

Chlorthion ← Age, Gp, Mouse, Rat: Neal et al. *F40,198/65*

DDT ← Age: Neal et at. 17,438/45*; Laug et al. A94,356/50*

EPN ← Age, Gp, Mouse, Rat: Neal et al. *F40,198/65;* Tardiff et al. *H11,752/69*

Fenthion ← Age: DuBois G77,578/67*

Guthion ← Age: Hietbrink et al. G26,464/64*; Du Bois G77,578/67

Methylparathion ← Age, Gp, Mouse, Rat: Neal et al. *F40,198/65*

OMPA ← Age: Kato et al. G17,077/64*

Organochlorine ← Age(newborn), Man: Polishuk et al. G72,380/70*

Parathion ← Age, Gp, Mouse, Rat: Neal et al. *F40,198/65*

Pesticides ← Age: Brodeur et al. E33, 487/63*

Picrotoxin ← Age: Holck D28,543/49*

Phenylbutazone ←. *Klinger et al. H28,896/70:* In rats, phenylbutazone reduces hexobarbital sleeping time and increases the fresh weight of the liver as well as the ability of the hepatic 9000 g supernatant to enhance aminophenazone-N-demethylation. An increase in the ascorbic acid concentration of the liver was noted only in young animals, but the urinary excretion of ascorbic acid was as pronounced as after barbital treatment. Phenylbutazone administration to the pregnant mother failed to elicit an induction effect in the fetuses as jugded by hepatic ascorbic acid determinations and by ultrastructural studies of the fetal livers. Proliferation of the SER was obtained by phenylbutazone in 10-day-old or older rats, often in association with an increase in the number of lysosomes and mitochondrial changes, as well as by evidence of intrahepatic cholestasis.

Promazine ← Age(Embryo, newborn), Man: Crawford et al. G78,958/65*

Strychnine ←. *Poe et al. A45,388/36:* Female rats are more susceptible to strychnine than males and, in both sexes, toxicity decreases with age.

Strychnine ← Age: Kato et al. *G17, 077/64**
Sulfanilamide ← Age: Krems et al. *A46,116/41**; Petty et al. *F58,540/65**
Urethan ← Age, Rat, Rb: Weatherall *G76,306/60**
Zoxazolamine ← Age: Fujii et al. *H28,618/68**; Dixon et al. *H30,692/68*

Varia ←. *Done G81,518/64:* Review (47 pp., 417 refs.) on differences in the drug sensitivity of immature and adult animals.

Done G81,512/66: Review (20 pp., 143 refs.) on "perinatal pharmacology" with a special section on drug-enzyme interactions.

Goldenthal G81,411/71: Extensive tabulation of LD_{50} values for newborn and adult mammals (rat, mouse, dog) from the literature and the files of the U.S. Food and Drug Administration.

Hepatic Lesions ←

Bucher G68,621/63: Review on the influence of age upon hepatic regeneration.

Hepatic Enzymes ←

TPO, TKT ←. *Rivlin & Knox C71,249/59:* The TPO activity of rat liver increases with age and body weight, as well as after STH-injection.

Sereni et al. C80,562/59: TKT activity is very low in the livers of fetal rats, but rapidly increases 2 hrs after birth, reaching a maximum (at least twice the usual adult level) at 12 hrs. Adrenalectomy or injection of amphenone at birth delays the development of this enzyme, whereas cortisol reverses the effect of adrenalectomy.

Kenney D98,193/60: In the rat, hepatic TKT activity increases sharply after birth. This increase is prevented by adrenalectomy, and tyrosine cannot substitute for cortisol in restoring transaminase development. Methionine is as active as tyrosine in increasing the response to cortisol after adrenalectomy, and this process does not depend upon the specific substrate as such, but apparently upon the presence of certain amino acids. Immunochemical assays "are clearly incompatible with a mechanism of induction involving de novo synthesis of enzyme protein and suggest that adrenal steroids promote either the activation of an antigenically similar but enzymically inactive precursor protein, or the release of an inhibitor."

Greengard et al. D63,145/63: In adrenalectomized rats, "the administration of puromycin inhibited the cortisone-induced elevation of tryptophan pyrrolase and tyrosine-α-ketoglutarate transaminase activity as well as the substrate-induced elevation of the latter. Actinomycin D abolished the cortisone-mediated rise in the level of both enzymes but did not influence the tryptophan-mediated increase in the level of tryptophan pyrrolase." In newborn rats, the development of hepatic TKT was inhibited by actinomycin, but neither adrenalectomy nor actinomycin interfered with the postnatal development of hepatic TPO. Apparently, accumulation of TPO (unlike that of TKT) is not under adrenal control and can proceed despite inhibited RNA synthesis.

Litwack & Nemeth G26,050/65: Hepatic TKT activity increases in the rabbit 2-4-fold at birth. A similar increase is obtained precociously in the event of premature delivery by cesarian section, whereas prolonging gestation delays the rise in enzymic activity. Under all these conditions, the ability of cortisol to cause a further rise in enzymic activity coincides with delivery. In the guinea pig, TKT is absent during fetal life, and increases to adult values within 24 hrs after birth. The enzyme activity in the newborn is stimulated by cortisol, though a single injection is without effect in the fetus or adult. In chickens, enzymic activity is relatively constant during the embryonic period, but rises 2-3-fold after hatching.

Schapiro et al. F65,746/65—66: "Infant rats, four and eight days after birth, respond to the stress of 30 minutes on a noisy reciprocating shaker with a large increase in liver aromatic amino acid transaminase activities. Adult rats exposed to the same stress do not exhibit this change. In the adult rat the inducing effects of cortisol on transaminase activities are blocked by this stress. These results suggest the activation of a mechanism(s) in the adult rat which opposes the enzyme inducing effects of cortisol."

Schapiro et al. F67,227/66: Hepatic TKT activity increased in immature, stressed (reciprocating shaker) rats, whereas intact stressed adults showed no change. In the stressed adrenalectomized adults, TKT activity markedly decreased, while in adrenalectomized immature rats it showed no change. Hypophysectomy largely abolished inhibition in the adults. TPO activity, when present, was increased by stress in old-age groups, but the increase was abolished by adrenalectomy and hypophysectomy. "The results suggest stress-activation of a pituitary mechanism that inhibits or represses activation of tyrosine transaminase and that may not function during early postnatal life."

Adelman H 32,850/70: Brief review on age-dependent enzyme induction with personal observations on ACTH-induced hepatic TKT in the rat.

Other Enzymes ←. *Cohen & Hekhuis 93, 220/41:* GOT activity was subnormal in six types of mouse tumors, regenerating rat liver, and fetal kitten (compared with adult cat) tissues. Apparently, an inverse relationship exists between transaminase activity and protein synthesis.

Knox et al. E 83,471/56: Review on metabolic and particularly enzymic adaptations, with a special section on the effect of age.

Conney & Burns G 67,166/62: Review on drug metabolism in the newborn.

Freedland et al. G 66,662/62: The phenylalanine hydroxylase activity of rat liver increases with age, from embryonic life to 50—60 days, and then declines to stabilize after maturity at a lower level in females than in males. Fasting and diets deficient in phenylalanine cause a rapid decrease in this enzymic activity.

Conney F 88,649/67 (p. 338): A review of the literature on enzyme induction in animals of different species, strains and age.

Gillette G 67,333/67: Brief review of the effect of age upon hepatic microsomal enzyme induction.

Goldstein et al. E 165/68 (p. 274): Review on the age factor in the induction of microsomal drug-metabolizing enzymes.

Nair & DuBois G 67,244/68: Review on hepatic microsomal enzyme induction in prenatal and early postnatal life.

Räihä & Kekomäki G 68,114/68: In the rat, the OKT activity of the liver is very low in the fetus, exhibiting a small transient elevation around term; it then drops, and eventually reaches the high adult activity level during the third postnatal week. Triamcinolone given postnatally causes a pronounced elevation of OKT, but has no such effect in fetal or adult rats. Puromycin prevents the rise in OKT after triamcinolone administration. In adult rats fed a protein- or arginine-free diet, OKT activity decreases and fails to rise under the influence of triamcinolone. Partial hepatectomy or STH depresses OKT activity in the livers of adult rats.

Vest et al. H 14,687/68: Brief review on changes in hepatic enzyme production during the perinatal period.

← GENETIC AND SPECIES-DEPENDENT FACTORS
(For Data on Man *cf. also* "Clinical Implications")

Steroids ←

There are considerable differences in the influence of hormones upon resistance in various species. The chemical basis of this genetic variation has not yet been adequately studied, but a few facts are known especially as regards the activation of enzymes by sex hormones.

The steroid hydroxylase activity of hepatic microsomes is higher in male than in female rats, but no such sex difference exists in mice. Fish liver does not contain this enzyme. Incubation of radio-marked progesterone with hepatic microsomes of male rats results in the oxidation of the steroid to a more polar fraction containing 6β- and 16β-hydroxyprogesterone, whereas microsomes of female rats metabolize progesterone mainly by reduction of the A ring, and its subsequent transformation into more polar compounds. By contrast, female rabbits and guinea pigs metabolize progesterone by hydroxylation. There is also a species difference in the type of steroid metabolism induced by phenobarbital and chlordane in rats and rabbits of both sexes. In monkeys, phenobarbital increases the urinary elimination of 6β-hydroxycortisol. In two strains of guinea pigs, distinguished by high and low production of hydroxylated cortisol derivatives, phenobarbital increased hepatic microsomal 2α-hydroxylation of cortisol, but caused no significant change in the 6β-hydroxylation activity in either strain.

There is some controversy in the literature concerning the existence of a sex difference in the susceptibility of the mouse to hydroxydione anesthesia (perhaps owing to the use of different strains), but in rats, the males are definitely more resistant.

It has been claimed that neither thiopental nor pentobarbital anesthesia can be influenced by catatoxic steroids in the mouse. Our own observations failed to confirm this; we have obtained a significant shortening of pentobarbital sleeping time in female mice by pretreatment with ethylestrenol, CS-1, spironolactone, and norbolethone.

Kuntzman et al. F 27,893/64: The steroid hydroxylase present in the microsome fraction of rat liver exhibits higher activity in male than in female rats, but no such sex difference is seen in mice. Fish liver does not contain this enzyme.

Kuntzman & Jacobson F 35,869/65: "Incubation of progesterone-4-C^{14} with liver microsomes from adult male rats resulted in oxidation of the steroid to a more polar fraction made up of 6β- and 16β-hydroxyprogesterone and an unidentified U.V. absorbing product. In contrast, female rats metabolized progesterone primarily by reduction of the A ring followed by subsequent metabolism to polar compounds. Unlike the female rat, female rabbits and guinea pigs metabolized progesterone by hydroxylation. With microsomes from immature male rats, both hydroxylation and reduction occurred. Chronic administration of phenobarbital, chlorcycline or chlordane to female rats caused an increased formation of polar metabolites but had little effect on the disappearance of progesterone, since the main pathway in the female rat is A-ring reduction. In contrast, chronic phenobarbital administration to female rabbits increased markedly the metabolism of progesterone to hydroxylated derivatives when measured either by formation of polar metabolites or by progesterone disappearance."

Birchall et al. F 76,581/66: In Cebus albifrons monkeys, phenobarbital pretreatment increases the urinary elimination of 6β-hydroxycortisol.

Rümke G 68,532/66: The anesthetic effect of hydroxydione is greater in female than in male mice.

Burstein & Bhavnani F 77,040/67: In guinea pigs, pretreatment with phenobarbital stimulated the hepatic microsomal metabolism of cortisol, 2α- and 6β-hydrocortisol, but not to the same extent. In rats, phenobarbital pretreatment enhanced hepatic microsomal 6β-hydroxylation of cortisol without causing a significant change in the overall metabolism of substrate or product. 2α-Hydroxylation of cortisol was not observed with rat liver microsomes.

Burstein F 95,565/68: Pretreatment with phenobarbital increased hepatic microsomal 2α-hydroxylation of cortisol in two strains of guinea pigs distinguished by high and low production of hydroxylated cortisol derivatives. Under the same conditions, phenobarbital caused no significant change in the hepatic 6β-hydroxylation activity of either strain.

Jelinek H 1,518/68: There was no difference in the duration of hydroxydione anesthesia in male and female intact or gonadectomized mice. Pretreatment with methyltestosterone p.o. prolonged hydroxydione anesthesia in males but not in females or castrate males. Neither thiopental nor pentobarbital anesthesia was influenced by methyltestosterone. Pretreatment with methandrostenolone or 17α-methylandrost-2-ene-17β-ol failed to influence hydroxydione anesthesia in mice.

Kato et al. H 34,571/71: Male rats are more resistant to the anesthetic effect of progesterone than females. Correspondingly the formation of hydroxylated metabolites of this steroid is greater with hepatic microsomes from males, whereas the formation of Δ^4-reduced metabolites is greater with female microsomes. In mice, there was no such difference either in the anesthetic action or in the in vitro metabolism of progesterone. In rats, the blood and tissue level of polar metabolites of tritiated progesterone was higher in males, whereas that of nonpolar metabolites was higher in females. "These results suggest that the stronger anesthetic action of progesterone in female rats is associated with higher tissue levels of progesterone and Δ^4-reduced metabolites, possessing the anesthetic action."

Epinephrine ← Genet, Rat, Rb: Inscoe et al. *F 70,325/66*

Drugs ←

Pretreatment with various thyroid preparations greatly increases the **acetonitrile** resistance of mice, whereas this is not so in most other species.

Female rats are more sensitive than males to various **barbiturates** but no such sex difference could be observed by most investigators in the dog, cat, rabbit, guinea pig, mouse, turtle or frog. However, strain differences in barbiturate resistance have been noted by some workers in the rat and mouse also. In Swiss mice, there is allegedly no sex difference in hexobarbital sleeping time. Rats can be separated into "long-sleepers" and "short-sleepers" on the basis of their response to hexobarbital. Hepatic "post-mitochondrial supernatant fraction" from long-sleepers possesses correspondingly less drug-metabolizing activity than that from short-sleepers not only with respect to hexobarbital but also as regards several other substrates. Rats that show a particularly long hexobarbital sleeping time are also especially sensitive to zoxazolamine, strychnine and methyprylon. Repeated administration of phenobarbital causes resistance in the rat but not in the guinea pig.

Male rats are more sensitive to **carisoprodol** paralysis than females but no such sex difference exists in mice or guinea pigs.

Small doses of **chloroform** produce fatal tubular necrosis in the kidneys of DBA mice, but no comparable renal lesion is elicited by chloroform in other species.

In mice, **digitoxin** poisoning is inhibited by CS-1, spironolactone, norbolethone, oxandrolone, prednisolone, progesterone, and thyroxine. Hence, contrary to earlier claims, mice are sensitive to catatoxic steroid actions, although in some respects their responsiveness differs from that of the rat.

Indomethacin intoxication is prevented in mice by ethylestrenol, CS-1, spironolactone, norbolethone, and to a lesser extent perhaps, by prednisolone, and estradiol.

Certain strains of rats which are particularly sensitive to **methyprylon** also have a low resistance to **zoxazolamine, strychnine,** and **hexobarbital**.

Male rats are more resistant than females to various anticholinesterase **pesticides**, whereas no such sex difference is noted in mice and guinea pigs. In mice, the lethal effect of dioxathion (Navadel) is strongly inhibited by ethylestrenol, norbolethone, prednisolone, and estradiol, but not significantly influenced by spironolactone, although the latter is effective in this respect in the rat.

Picrotoxin poisoning is not significantly influenced in mice by spironolactone, ethylestrenol, triamcinolone, or thyroxine, whereas in rats, this intoxication is readily prevented by pretreatment with various catatoxic steroids.

Acetonitrile ←

Hunt 13,889/23: Pretreatment with thyroid preparations greatly increases the resistance of mice to acetonitrile, whereas the reverse is true in many other species.

Anticoagulants ←

Dayton et al. D42,366/61: In the guinea pig, dog and man, pretreatment with barbiturates antagonizes the hypoprothrombinemic effect of coumarin anticoagulants. At the same time, the plasma level of the coumarin is depressed.

Goss & Dickhaus F53,987/65: Phenobarbital increases the daily maintenance dose of bishydroxycoumarin in man.

Robinson & MacDonald F69,377/66: Phenobarbital antagonizes the anticoagulant effect of warfarin in man.

Barbiturates ←

Holck & Kanan 31,302/35: Female rats are more sensitive than males to various barbiturate anesthetics. No such sex difference could be detected in the dog, cat, rabbit, guinea pig, mouse, turtle or frog.

Holck et al. A8,011/37: In the dog, cat, rabbit, guinea pig, mouse and frog (unlike in the rat), males are no more sensitive to hexobarbital anesthesia than females. In mice, the sex difference was also absent to amobarbital, but the butallylonal sleeping time was slightly longer in females.

Homburger et al. E 61,371/47: Female rats are more sensitive than males to pentobarbital but not to thiopental anesthesia. Age and strain differences in barbiturate resistance have also been noted in the rat.

Quinn et al. G 67,327/54: The biologic half-life of hexobarbital was found to be 15 min for mice, 60 min for rabbits, 140 min for rats, and 260 min for dogs and man. There was an inverse relationship between the rate of biotransformation of hexobarbital to keto-hexobarbital and the duration of its hypnotic effect. Male rats are more resistant to hexobarbital anesthesia than females but in the latter, resistance as well as the enzyme activity of the microsomes were increased by testosterone.

Jay G 71,140/55: Various strains of mice show considerable differences in their responsiveness to hexobarbital anesthesia.

Quinn et al. E 89,993/58: Guinea pigs and mice, unlike rats, show no sex difference in the metabolism of hexobarbital. In the rat, the sex difference is also manifest with regard to antipyrine and amidopyrine. The difference is largely dependent upon the effect of sex hormones upon microsomal drug metabolism, although variations in the inherent sensitivity of the central nervous system may also play a part.

Catz & Yaffe G 37,059/61: Description of striking differences in hexobarbital sensitivity among various strains of mice. Curiously, mortality and sleeping time do not run parallel, perhaps because toxicity is due to a metabolite of the drug.

Brodie G 55,013/62: Review on species differences in the duration of action and in the metabolism of hexobarbital in the mouse, rat, guinea pig, rabbit, dog and man. Fish, aquatic species of frogs and aquatic salamanders do not oxidize drugs in vivo, nor do their liver microsomes carry out the oxidative mechanisms of N- or O-dealkylation, hydroxylation, deamination and sulfoxidation, common to mammals. Presumably, fish can dispose of foreign compounds by diffusion through the gills, whereas aquatic frogs and salamanders eliminate them unchanged through their skins which behave as lipid membranes. Terrestrial arthropods which must conserve water, e.g., crickets (Acheta domestica) and grasshoppers (Romlea microptera) metabolize hexobarbital, amphetamine, chlorpromazine and amidopyrine very rapidly. Surprisingly, aquatic athropods such as crayfish and lobsters also metabolize these substances although at a much slower rate. However, these animals lead a partly terrestrial existence and possess rigid gills which are impermeable to lipid-soluble drugs.

Buchel & Liblau E 89,233/63: In Swiss mice, there is no sex difference in hexobarbital sleeping time or in the disappearance rate of this drug from the brain.

Backus & Cohn D 92,313/66: The hexobarbital sleeping time of female mice is shorter than that of males, and varies also according to strain. In general, the length of the sleeping time is inversely proportional to the hexobarbital-metabolizing potency of liver homogenates.

Gessner et al. F 77,776/67: In mice, "testosterone pretreatment produces a biphasic effect on the duration of action of hexobarbital, prolonging the action initially and shortening the action in 4—8 days after the pretreatment. The early action of testosterone appears to be associated with an effect on the hypnotic property of a drug, since both hexobarbital and barbital sleep times are prolonged while the duration of action of the muscle relaxant chlorzoxasone remains unaffected. The long-term pretreatment with testosterone leads to a shorter duration of action of drugs that are deactivated by detoxification, notably hexobarbital and chlorzoxasone, but has no effect on the duration of hypnosis produced by barbital, a drug which is predominantly eliminated unchanged." Folliculoids (ethinylestradiol, diethylstilbestrol) prolong the actions of both drugs.

Mitoma et al. G 69,268/67: Rats were separated into "long-sleepers" and "short-sleepers" on the basis of their response to hexobarbital. "The drug-metabolizing activities of the hepatic postmitochondrial supernatant fraction from long-sleepers were less than those from short-sleepers with respect to hexobarbital, acetanilide, aminopyrine, and o-nitroanisole, each of which represents a different drug-metabolism pathway. This trend was observed in all 5 strains of rats examined."

Timar et al. F 82,696/67: Repeated administration of phenobarbital causes resistance in the rat but not in the guinea pig.

Selye PROT. 31380: In the mouse, the duration of pentobarbital anesthesia is shortened by ethylestrenol, CS-1 spironolactone, and norbolethone, but not significantly by oxandrolone, prednisolone, progesterone, triamcinolone, DOC, hydroxydione, estradiol, or thyroxine, *cf.* Table 129.

Table 129. *Conditioning for pentobarbital anesthesia in mice*

Group	Treatment[a]	Anesthesia time (min)[b]	Mortality (dead/total)
1	None	52 ± 7	0/12
2	Ethylestrenol	4 ± 3***	0/14
3	CS-1	15 ± 5***	0/13
4	Spironolactone	19 ± 5**	0/13
5	Norbolethone	1 ± 1***	0/12
6	Oxandrolone	37 ± 9 NS	0/13
7	Prednisolone acetate	37 ± 6 NS	0/13
8	Progesterone	43 ± 6 NS	0/13
9	Triamcinolone	89 ± 15 NS	0/13
10	Desoxycorticosterone acetate	68 ± 14 NS	0/12
11	Hydroxydione sodium hemisuccinate	97 ± 20 NS	1/14
12	Estradiol	32 ± 7 NS	0/13
13	Thyroxine	91 ± 17 NS	0/13

[a] In 20 g ♀ mice all steroids (Groups 2—12) were administered (at the dose of 10 mg in 0.2 ml water p.o. x2/day, 1st day ff.), and thyroxine as Na salt (at the dose of 200 µg in 0.2 ml water/100 g body weight s.c., once daily, 1st day ff.). In addition, the mice of all groups were given pentobarbital (6 mg in 0.2 ml oil/100 g body weight i.p. once on the 4th day).

[b] Statistics: Student's t-test.

For further details on technique of tabulation *cf.* p. VIII.

Feller & Gerald H 22,744/70: In male mice, pretreatment with spironolactone shortened pentobarbital and "testosterone-potentiated" pentobarbital sleeping times. It also increased liver microsomal protein, liver weight, aniline hydroxylation and ethylmorphine N-demethylation.

Gerald & Feller G 74,092/70: In mice, pretreatment with spironolactone shortens pentobarbital sleeping time as well as "testosterone-potentiated pentobarbital sleeping time." Furthermore, spironolactone enhances the microsomal metabolism of aniline and ethylmorphine, and increases hepatic weight. It is concluded that the in vivo protective effect of spironolactone is due to the induction of hepatic microsomal enzymes.

Gerald & Feller G 78,804/70: In mice, pretreatment with spironolactone reduces pentobarbital sleeping time and accelerates the hepatic microsomal metabolism of hexobarbital in vivo and in vitro.

Mitoma H 25,522/70: Rats that show a long hexobarbital sleeping time are also particularly sensitive to zoxazolamine, strychnine and methyprylon.

Bilirubin ←

Lüders G 81,789/70: In Gunn rats which have a high serum bilirubin level, Na-dehydrocholate i.v. decreased the serum and increased the brain bilirubin content. This effect was also seen when the initial serum bilirubin level was raised by infusion of bilirubin. The decrease in serum bilirubin induced by Na-dehydrocholate did not coincide with an increased biliary excretion of the pigment. Indeed, Gunn rats with

Table 130. *Conditioning for digitoxin intoxication in mice*

Treatment[a]	Convulsions[b] (positive/total)	Mortality[b] (dead/total)
None	14/20	9/20
Ethylestrenol	6/16 NS	3/16 NS
CS-1	0/14***	0/14***
Spironolactone	0/14***	2/14 NS
Norbolethone	1/14***	2/14 NS
Oxandrolone	2/14***	1/14*
Prednisolone-Ac	3/14**	4/14 NS
Progesterone	4/14*	0/14***
Triamcinolone (2 mg)	13/15 NS	14/15***
DOC-Ac	5/14 NS	4/14 NS
Hydroxydione	6/14 NS	1/14*
Estradiol	7/14 NS	4/14 NS
Thyroxine (200 µg)	3/16***	10/16 NS

[a] The mice (20 g ♀) of all groups were given digitoxin (1 mg/100 g body weight in 0.2 ml water, p.o./day, daily from 4th day ff.). In addition, certain groups received thyroxine (200 µg/100 g body weight in 0.2 ml water + NaOH + Tween, s.c./day, on 1st day ff.), triamcinolone (2 mg/100 g body weight) and other steroids (10 mg/100 g body weight in 0.2 ml water, p.o. x2/day, on 1st day ff.).

[b] Convulsions were estimated on 7th day, and mortality listed on 9th day ("Exact Probability Test").

For further details on technique of tabulation *cf.* p. VIII.

→ Sex 651

and rats, with a rapid procedure for the measurement of brain, plasma and erythrocyte cholinesterase. "The oral LD_{50}'s for these compounds for male and female rats are DFP, 13.5 and 7.7 mgm/kgm; Parathion 30 and 3 mgm/kgm; TEPP 2 and 1.2 mgm/kgm; EPN 91 and 14.5 mgm/kgm; OMPA 13.5 and 35.5 mgm/kgm; and E-838 42 and 19 mgm/kgm. The administration of oral LD_{75} doses of these compounds caused brain cholinesterase inhibition varying with each compound: DFP > Parathion > E-838 > EPN > TEPP > OMPA."

Durham et al. C14,264/55: Diethylstilbestrol increased DDT and DDE storage in the fat of male rats, whereas testosterone decreased the storage of these compounds in the female.

Durham et al. C27,425/55: In rats, DDT increased the liver weight/body weight ratio. Diethylstilbestrol increased the storage of DDT and of its metabolite DDE in the fat of male rats, whereas testosterone propionate decreased these values in females. "An endocrine mechanism may account for the sex differences in this regard."

Ortega et al. E40,218/56: When repeatedly exposed to moderate levels of DDT, male rats show much more frequent and extensive histologic changes in the liver than females.

Swann et al. C73,379/58: Male rats are more resistant than females to parathion poisoning. Testosterone increases the resistance of females, whereas estrone diminishes that of the males. Curiously, testosterone decreases the resistance of intact males although it increases that of castrated males. After orchidectomy, estrone slightly decreases resistance over that of untreated male castrates.

Murphy & DuBois D28,546/58: The activity of the microsomal-enzyme system which oxidizes thiophosphates to potent anticholinesterase agents is considerably higher in male than in female rats (incubation of liver homogenates with Guthion or ethyl p-nitrophenyl thionobenzenephosphonate or "EPN"). Yet, in vivo, adult males are more resistant to EPN than females, perhaps because the accelerated formation of toxic oxidation products is overcompensated by a more efficient detoxication of the latter. The low enzyme activity of female livers is enhanced by pretreatment with testosterone in vivo, whereas the high activity of male livers is diminished by previous castration, partial hepatectomy or treatment with progesterone or diethylstilbestrol. SKF 525-A inhibits, whereas pretreatment

with carcinogens or a protein-deficient diet enhances the activity of the thiophosphate-oxidizing enzyme.

DuBois & Puchala D43,878/61: Male rats are much more resistant than females to various cholinergic phosphorothioates. Male mice and guinea pigs are not particularly resistant to DMP. Partial hepatectomy and/or castration abolishes the comparative resistance of the male rat, whereas testosterone restores resistance in hepatectomized or orchidectomized rats. It is concluded "that androgens govern the development of this system."

DuBois & Kinoshita G66,247/65: Female rats are much more sensitive than males to several phosphorothioates.

Gaines G67,102/69: LD_{50} values have been determined for 98 pesticides, and 2 metabolites of DDT in the rat. Most compounds were more toxic to females than to males, but 9 of 85 compounds were more toxic in males. In chickens, several of the pesticides produced paralysis.

Carlson & DuBois H24,653/70: Male rats are much more susceptible to the insecticide 6-methyl-2,3-quinoxalinedithiol cyclic carbonate (Morestan) than females. "The toxicity to rats could not be altered by castration, administration of testosterone to females and estradiol to males. Pretreatment with phenobarbital decreased the toxicity to adult males and increased the toxicity to adult females." Chronic Morestan feeding caused hepatic enlargement and inhibition of microsomal enzymes.

Gershbein H31,893/70: In intact male rats, unlike in females, DDT caused liver enlargement. This and other insecticides also enhance liver regeneration after partial hepatectomy in males but not in females.

Gish & Chura G80,046/70: In Japanese quails, sensitivity to DDT is increased by starvation and during the breeding season. Males are more sensitive than females.

Kinoshita & Du Bois G78,681/70: Male rats are more susceptible than females to the induction of hepatic microsomal enzymes by substituted urea herbicides (diuron, Herban).

Kleavy G80,049/70: Radiolabelled dieldrin added to perfusates of rat liver appears in the bile of male donors much more rapidly than in that of females. "These findings are consonant with both the lesser toxicity of dieldrin for male rats and the greater storage of dieldrin in adipose tissue by female rats reported by other investigators."

Morphine → Sex + Testosterone: Axelrod D28,544/56
Morphine → Sex: Timmler E48,422/60*; Kato et al. G68,411/66
Morphine → Sex + Phenobarbital: Kato et al. F76,403/66
Neopontosil → Sex + Phenobarbital: Kato et al. F76,403/66

Nickel Sulfide →

Jasmin et al. D68,263/63: In rats a single i.m. injection of nickel sulfide produces metastatic rhabdomyosarcomas whose incidence is increased by methylandrostenolone but is uninfluenced by sex, ovariectomy or orchidectomy.

Nicotine → *cf. also Selye G60,083/70, pp. 476, 478.*

Kosoboda A39,432/29—30: Male rabbits are much more resistant than females to the production of cardiovascular lesions by chronic nicotine intoxication.

Lee 32,854/35: No pronounced sex difference to nicotine intoxication could be observed in the mouse or rabbit.

Holck et al. A8,011/37: Male rats are more resistant to fatal nicotine intoxication than females.

Yun & Lee 34,178/35: Female mice and rabbits are more resistant to nicotine than males. Ovariectomy diminishes nicotine resistance, whereas orchidectomy does not change it. Treatment with "luteohormone" increases nicotine resistance, whereas "follicular hormone" has no effect.

Hueper 91,722/43: Female rats are much more sensitive than males to chronic nicotine intoxication.

Selye PROT. 42911: In male rats, the protective effect of PCN, spironolactone, ethylestrenol, betamethasone, phenobarbital, and phenylbutazone against intoxication with digitoxin, indomethacin, dioxathion, parathion, nicotine, progesterone, hexobarbital and zoxazolamine has been systematically examined (cf. Table 128). Hexobarbital sleeping time was not shortened by PCN, spironolactone or betamethasone. For betamethasone, this is not remarkable since this compound failed to affect hexobarbital sleeping time in females also (cf. Table 136), but PCN and spironolactone were effective in this respect in females. In order to evaluate these data, the effect of each conditioner against each toxicant should be compared with similar experiments on females (Table 136).

p-Nitroanisole → Sex + Phenobarbital: Kato et al. F76,403/66
p-Nitroanisole → Sex + Pesticides: Kinoshita et al. G71,863/66
Nitrobenzoic Acid → Sex: Kato et al. F76,403/66; Kinoshita et al. G71,863/66
p-Nitrophenol → Sex: Halac et al. G77,576/69
Norchlorocyclizine → Sex: Kuntzman et al. F45,464/65
Nortriptyline ← Sex, Man: Hammer et al. G79,581/67*

Octamethyl Pyrophosphamide ← cf. Pesticides

Orotic Acid →

Sidransky D64,556/63: The periportal fatty degeneration of the liver produced by chronic orotic acid feeding is more pronounced in female than in male rats. Orchidectomized males developed more severe fatty changes than intact males, or castrate males treated with testosterone. Ovariectomized females developed marked fatty liver changes similar to those of intact females, but this response was diminished by testosterone or estradiol.

Sidransky et al. G4,354/63: The production of fatty livers by orotic acid supplements to the diet is more pronounced in female than in male rats. Orchidectomized males develop more severe fatty livers than intact controls unless they are treated with testosterone propionate.

Pesticides →

Fitzhugh & Nelson A47,885/47: Among rats given DDT in the diet, females showed a greater mortality than males. The difference was attributed to an increased DDT intake by the females.

Deichmann et al. D98,307/50: In rats, the acute toxicity of DDT in oil p.o. appears to be essentially the same in both sexes.

DuBois et al. D92,992/50: In rats, there is no sex or age difference in the toxicity of OMPA.

Aldridge & Barnes G41,307/52: Several organophosphorus insecticides are more toxic for female than for male rats. However, the reverse is true of octamethyl pyrophosphoramide and bis-dimethylaminofluorophosphine oxide.

Frawley et al. G69,644/52: Comparative toxicologic studies on organic phosphate-anticholinesterase compounds in guinea pigs, mice bile fistulas showed that Na-dehydrocholate interferes with the biliary excretion of diazopositive substances.

Carisoprodol ←

Kato et al. G66,023/61: Adult (but not immature) male rats are more sensitive to carisoprodol-induced muscular paralysis than females. Castration or treatment with SKF 525-A abolishes the increased resistance of the adult male rat. Incubation of liver slices with carisoprodol shows that the resistance of the male is due to accelerated substrate inactivation. No sex difference is noted in adult mice or guinea pigs.

Chloroform ←

Shubik & Ritchie D67,964/53: Small doses of chloroform produce fatal tubular necrosis in the kidneys of male but not of female DBA mice.

Digitalis ←

Szabo et al. G79,013/71: In hamsters, spironolactone and ethylestrenol pretreatment prevents digitoxin convulsions and indomethacin-induced intestinal ulcers. Curiously, hamsters are resistant to as much as 100 mg of digitoxin p.o. given repeatedly, whereas 1 mg i.v. produces strong convulsions. Apparently, in this species, the absorption of digitoxin from the gastrointestinal tract is deficient. Indomethacin intoxication is also different in rats and hamsters since in the latter, unlike the former, the drug produces predominantly pyloric ulcers which often perforate.

Selye PROT. 27594, 28284, 29742, 29751: In mice, digitoxin poisoning is inhibited by CS-1 spironolactone, norbolethone, oxandrolone, prednisolone, progesterone and thyroxine. Ethylestrenol, triamcinolone, DOC, hydroxydione and estradial are ineffective, cf. Table 130, p. 677.

Ethanol ←

Jabbari & Leevy G45,526/67: Various anabolics (norethandrolone, testosterone, oxandrolone) protect the liver of the rat against ethanol-induced fatty degeneration and various functional disturbances. They are also useful in the management of alcoholic patients.

Table 131. *Conditioning for indomethacin intoxication in mice*

Treatment[a]	Intestinal ulcers (Positive/Total)[b]			Mortality (Dead/Total)[b]		
	Subcutaneous	Intraperitoneal	Oral	Subcutaneous	Intraperitoneal	Oral
None	4/9	8/11	10/13	6/10	8/11	12/14
Ethylestrenol	0/5 NS	1/5 NS	0/13 ***	1/5 NS	2/5 NS	0/13 ***
	0/5 NS	0/5 *	0/12 ***	0/5 *	0/5 *	2/12 ***
Spironolactone	0/5 NS	0/5 *	0/12 ***	1/5 NS	1/5 NS	3/12 ***
Norbolethone	0/3 NS	0/5 *	2/11 **	5/5 NS	0/5 *	0/11 ***
Oxandrolone	2/4 NS	0/5 *	4/9 NS	4/5 NS	1/5 NS	6/10 NS
Prednisolone-Ac	0/3 NS	0/4 *	0/5 **	5/5 NS	5/5 NS	4/8 NS
Progesterone	0/4 NS	2/4 NS	3/9 NS	5/5 NS	4/5 NS	6/12 NS
Triamcinolone 2 mg	—	—	4/12 *	—	—	14/14 NS
Triamcinolone 10 mg	0/3 NS	0/2 NS	—	5/5 NS	5/5 NS	—
DOC-Ac	0/3 NS	3/5 NS	4/7 NS	2/5 NS	4/5 NS	6/12 NS
Hydroxydione	0/4 NS	1/4 NS	5/10 NS	5/5 NS	5/5 NS	8/11 NS
Estradiol	0/4 NS	1/3 NS	1/8 **	4/5 NS	3/5 NS	9/9 NS
Thyroxine 200 μg	2/7 NS	—	—	15/15 *	—	—

[a] The mice (25 g ♀) of all groups received indomethacin s.c. 1 mg/day, from the 4th day to the 7th day, and 2 mg/day on the 8th day ff. Thyroxine 200 μg/day, triamcinolone 2 or 10 mg as indicated, and other catatoxic steroids 10 mg x2/day, subcutaneous, intraperitoneal or oral, as described in the table, on the 1st day ff. Every substance was given per 100 g body weight in 0.2 ml water.

[b] Intestinal ulcers and mortality listed on the 12th day (Statistics Fisher & Yates). For further details on technique of tabulation cf. p. VIII.

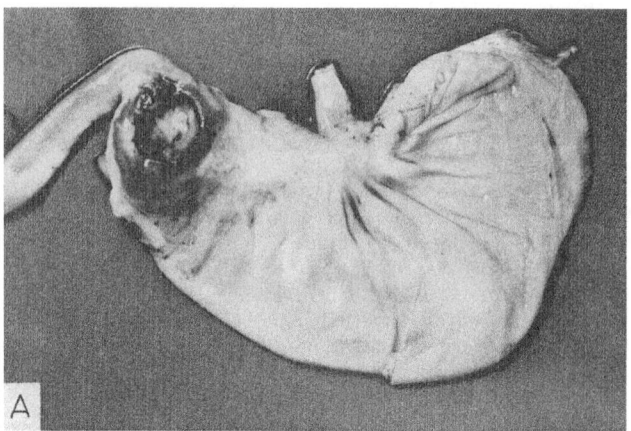
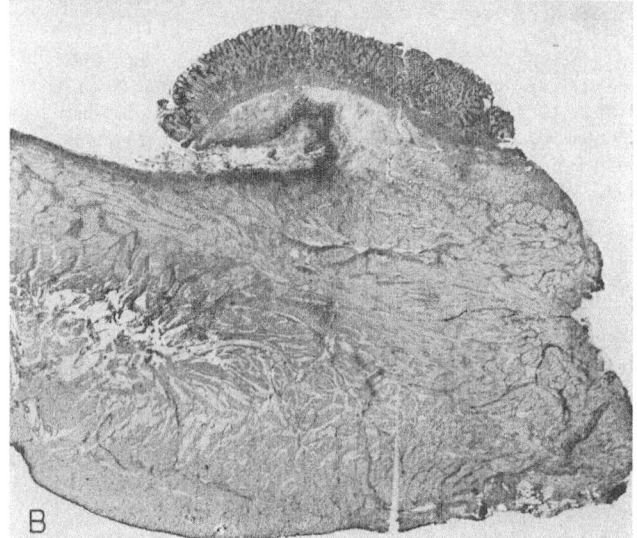

Fig. 28. **Typical perforating pyloric ulcer produced by indomethacin in the rabbit.** A: Naked eye view from anterior surface. B: Histologic appearance of the ulcer which undermines the still well-preserved portion of the stomach which is covered by an intact mucosa (PAS X 29)

Indomethacin ←

Szabo et al. G79,013/71: In hamsters, spironolactone and ethylestrenol pretreatment prevents digitoxin convulsions and indomethacin induced intestinal ulcers. Curiously, hamsters are resistant to as much as 100 mg of digitoxin p.o. given repeatedly, whereas 1 mg i.v. produces strong convulsions. Apparently, in this species, the absorption of digitoxin from the gastrointestinal tract is deficient. Indomethacin intoxication is also different in rats and hamsters since in the latter, unlike the former, the drug produces predominantly pyloric ulcers which often perforate.

Selye PROT. 28397: In mice, indomethacin intoxication can be prevented by ethylestrenol, CS-1, spironolactone, norbolethone and to a lesser extent, perhaps also by prednisolone, and estradiol administered by various routes. Thyroxine appears to have an opposite effect. Progesterone, triamcinolone, DOC, and hydroxydione had little if any effect, *cf.* Table 131, p. 678.

Methyprylon ←

Mitoma H 25,522/70: Rats that show a long hexobarbital sleeping time are also particularly sensitive to zoxazolamine, strychnine, and methyprylon.

Morphine ←

Adler et al. G79,852/57: In Sprague-Dawley rats, given ^{14}C-labeled morphine, the ratio of bound to free morphine is 2—3 times greater in the urine and plasma than in Long-Evans rats. The tissue of adrenalectomized rats of both strains contains higher concentrations of ^{14}C-labeled morphine than do control rats. Plasma bound morphine levels indicate no impairment of morphine conjugation. Vasopressin increases, whereas ACTH decreases morphine sensitivity. Yet both after ACTH and after vasopressin, tissue concentrations of morphine are either reduced or unaffected in marked contrast to the increased values after adrenalectomy. Apparently, the decreased morphine sensitivity induced by ACTH is not reflected by lower brain morphine concentrations.

Table 132. *Conditioning for dioxathion intoxication in mice*

Group	Treatment[a]	Prostration[b] (Positive/Total)	Mortality[b] (Dead/Total)
1	None	8/11	8/11
2	Ethylestrenol	0/11***	0/11***
3	CS-1	3/11*	2/11*
4	Spironolactone	6/11 NS	6/11 NS
5	Norbolethone	0/11***	0/11***
6	Oxandrolone	5/11 NS	3/11*
7	Prednisolone-Ac	1/11***	1/11***
8	Progesterone	8/11 NS	8/11 NS
9	Triamcinolone	10/11 NS	7/11 NS
10	DOC-Ac	7/11 NS	7/11 NS
11	Hydroxydione	8/11 NS	8/11 NS
12	Estradiol	0/11***	0/11***
13	Thyroxine	11/11 NS	11/11 NS

[a] In 20 g ♀ mice all steroids (Groups 2—12) were administered at the dose of 10 mg in 0.1 ml water, p.o., x2/day on the 1st day ff.; thyroxine as Na salt at the dose of 200 µg in 0.2 ml water, s.c., once daily on the 1st day ff. All drugs/100 g body weight. In addition, the mice of all groups received dioxathion 15 mg in 0.2 ml oil/100 g body weight, p.o., once on the 4th day.

[b] Mortality was listed 24 hrs after dioxathion. (Statistics: Fisher & Yates.)
For further details on technique of tabulation cf. p. VIII.

Pesticides ←

DuBois & Puchala D43,878/61: Male rats are much more resistant than females to various cholinergic phosphorothioates. Male mice and guinea pigs are not particularly resistant to dimethyl phthalate (DMP). Partial hepatectomy and/or castration abolishes the comparative resistance of the male rat, whereas testosterone restores resistance in hepatectomized or orchidectomized rats. It is concluded "that androgens govern the development of this system."

Selye PROT. 31563, 31612: In mice, the lethal effect of dioxathion is powerfully inhibited by ethylestrenol, norbolethone, prednisolone, and estradiol, and only moderately by CS-1 and oxandrolone, but it is not influenced by spironolactone, progesterone, triamcinolone, DOC, hydroxydione, or thyroxine, cf. Table 132.

Picrotoxin ←

Selye PROT. 27594: In mice, pretreatment with spironolactone, ethylestrenol, triamcinolone or thyroxine had little if any effect upon the toxicity of picrotoxin under our experimental conditions, cf. Table 133.

Table 133. *Conditioning for picrotoxin intoxication in mice*

Treatment[a]	Convulsions[b] (Positive/Total)	Mortality[b] (Dead/Total)
None	6/6	3/6
Spironolactone	4/6 NS	2/6 NS
Ethylestrenol	4/6 NS	2/6 NS
Triamcinolone	6/6 NS	5/6 NS
Thyroxine	6/6 NS	4/6 NS

[a] The mice (20 g ♀) of all groups were given picrotoxin 0.6 mg/100 g body weight in 0.4 ml water, s.c., once on the 4th day. Thyroxine 200 µg/100 g body weight in 0.2 ml water + NaOH + Tween, s.c./day, on the 1st day ff.; triamcinolone 2 mg/100 g body weight, spironolactone and ethylestrenol 10 mg/100 g body weight in 0.2 ml water, p.o. x2/day, on the 1st day ff.

Strychnine, Zoxazolamine ←

Mitoma H 25,522/70: Rats that show a long hexobarbital sleeping time, are also particularly sensitive to zoxazolamine, strychnine, and methyprylon.

Varia ←

Kalow E 695/62: A monograph on "Pharmacogenetics, Heredity and the Response to Drugs" containing special sections on human hereditary defects with altered drug response and racial differences in drug sensitivity.

Meier E 690/63: Monograph on "Experimental Pharmacogenetics" (213 pp., about 400 refs.) with special sections on the influence of sex and genetic factors, including species variations, upon drug sensitivity.

Brodie et al. F 42,949/65: Considerations on species variations in drug sensitivity. Unlike most other drugs, antitumor agents (usually antimetabolites of alkylating compounds) interact with pathways of metabolism common to normal and neoplastic tissues. These drugs exert an antitumor action because, in being metabolized, they become enmeshed in mechanisms essential to the normal economy of the body and are usually toxic for the same reason. Their toxicity in various animal species agrees well with the maximum tolerated doses in man when expressed on the basis of weight to the 0.7 power. Species variations are also of lesser importance as regards tolerance of poorly liposoluble compounds, such as tubocurarine or ganglionic blocking agents. If a drug affects the target organ equally in various species, dependable predictions might be made from experimental animals to man, even with regard to agents that are unequally metabolized, provided that the effects are expressed in terms of plasma or tissue concentrations, rather than dosage per body weight. Thus, despite a 20- to 50-fold variation in the duration of narcosis produced by hexobarbital and other barbiturates in various animal species and man, the plasma concentration of the drugs at waking time is essentially the same in various species.

Varia ←

Guinea pigs, unlike rats and rabbits, are not protected against **endotoxin** by cortisone. Correspondingly, cortisone increases TPO in rats and rabbits but not in guinea pigs. Actinomycin D and ethionine augment the lethal effect of endotoxin and abolish the protective action of cortisone, presumably because both endogenous and exogenous glucocorticoids exert their prophylactic effect through the induction of hepatic enzymes whose synthesis can be inhibited by actinomycin D and ethionine.

Vertebrates above the evolutionary level of amphibians respond to cortisol with an increased hepatic **TKT** activity, but lower vertebrates do not respond in this manner. The appearance of TKT in the course of ontogenesis, as well as the possibility of inducing this enzyme by glucocorticoids, is subject to considerable species variation.

It is generally assumed that aquatic animals, especially fish, which can excrete **nonpolar toxicants** through the gills or skin are less dependent upon the induction of microsomal drug-metabolizing enzymes than are mammals, which must depend mainly upon renal excretion of polar compounds and polar metabolites of lipid soluble toxicants.

Bacterial Toxins ←

Berry G 68,858/64: Both actinomycin D and ethionine increase the lethal effect of endotoxin in the mouse and abolish the protection offered by cortisone. Presumably, both endogenous and exogenous glucocorticoids protect through the induction of hepatic enzymes whose synthesis can be inhibited by actinomycin D and ethionine. Cortisone increases TPO in rats and rabbits, but not in guinea pigs. Correspondingly, guinea pigs cannot be protected against endotoxin by cortisone.

---

b The severity of the convulsions was estimated 30 min after picrotoxin injection. Mortality was listed 24 hrs later. (Statistics: Fisher & Yates.)

For further details on technique of tabulation cf. p. VIII.

Hepatic Lesions ←

Bucher G68,621/63: Review on the influence of species and strain differences upon hepatic regeneration.

Hepatic Enzymes ←

TPO, TKT ←. *Chan & Cohen D18,552/64:* Vertebrates above the evolutionary level of amphibians respond to cortisol with an increased hepatic TKT activity. "Animals showing this response include the rat, guinea pig, chick, pigeon, horned toad (Phrynosoma cornatum), and painted turtle (Chrysemys picta). In contrast, vertebrates at the amphibian level or below failed to show this response. Animals failing to show this response include the bull frog (Rana catesbeiana), grass frog (Rana pipiens), marine toad (Bufo marinus), tiger salamander (Ambystoma trigrinum), mud puppy (Necturus), white bass (Roccus chrysops), and black crappie (Promoxis nigromaculatus)."

Litwack & Nemeth G26,050/65: In the rabbit hepatic TKT activity increases 2-4-fold at birth in the rabbit. A similar increase is obtained precociously in the event of premature delivery by cesarian section, whereas prolonging gestation delays the rise in enzymic activity. Under all these conditions, the ability of cortisol to cause a further rise in enzymic activity coincides with delivery. In the guinea pig, TKT is absent during fetal life and increases to adult values within 24 hrs after birth. The enzyme activity in the newborn is stimulated by cortisol, though a single injection is without effect in the fetus or adult. In chickens, enzymic activity is relatively constant during the embryonic period, but rises 2-3-fold after hatching.

Other Enzymes ←. *Brodie & Maickel G67,800/62:* Review (25 pp., no refs.) on the authors' work on microsomal drug-metabolizing enzymes in fish, amphibia, reptiles, birds and mammals.

Conney & Burns G67,166/62: Review on species differences in drug metabolism with special emphasis upon microsomal enzyme induction.

Conney F88,649/67 (p. 338): A review of the literature on enzyme induction in animals of different species, strains and age.

Goldstein et al. E165/68 (p. 266): Review on species and strain differences as factors influencing the induction of drug-metabolizing microsomal enzymes.

Kato et al. H11,851/69: Studies on the effect of thyroxine upon hepatic microsomal enzyme induction by various drugs in diverse species.

Dewaide G80,406/70: Comparative studies on the effect of adaptation to cold or heat upon hepatic drug oxidation in various species. Contrary to earlier claims, drug metabolizing enzymes do play a decisive role in the resistance of fishes to changes in their environment. "The effect of a change of ambient temperature on the liver of the hamster, rat, roach, and trout becomes manifest in an almost equal way for the different species."

← IONIZING RAYS

Drugs ←

In the rat, X-irradiation of the head increases the anesthetic effect of such barbiturates as thiopental, barbital and pentobarbital. However, the induction by phenobarbital of resistance to pentobarbital is not inhibited. X-irradiation of entire 23-day-old male rats, or of the head only, inhibited the rapid increase in hexobarbital-metabolizing microsomal oxidases following hexobarbital pretreatment in the same manner as did hypophysectomy. Normally, the hexobarbital metabolizing activity of rat liver is extremely low after birth, but rises rapidly up to the age of 80 days, to levels much higher in males than in females. Prenatal X-irradiation suppresses this normal development of enzyme activities in the male so that it reaches only the normal female level. The effect of the irradiation decreases as the animals mature. In adult rats, selective irradiation of the head does not inhibit microsomal enzyme induction by phenobarbital but does, nevertheless, increase the anesthetic effect, presumably by raising the permeability of the blood-brain barrier.

In summary, it may be said that whereas the ontogenic increase in enzyme activity is hormone dependent, the phenobarbital-induced induction is not, since it is evident even in hypophysectomized or sexually immature animals. Presumably, the inhibitory effect of X-irradiation is due to interference with the hormonal regulation of enzyme activity.

In weanling male rats, total body X-irradiation or irradiation of the head only inhibits the development of microsomal enzymes which metabolize the **pesticide** Guthion.

Barbiturates ←

Nair et al. F53,576/65: In the rat, X-irradiation of the head considerably enhanced the anesthetic effect of thiopental, barbital, and pentobarbital. The induction by phenobarbital of resistance to subsequent pentobarbital anesthesia was not inhibited by cephalic X-irradiation.

Nair G67,247/67: In adult male rats, selective irradiation of the head did not inhibit hepatic microsomal enzyme induction by phenobarbital. In such experiments, the increased anesthetic effect of the barbiturate is ascribed to enhanced permeability of the blood-brain barrier.

Nair & Bau G67,246/67: Exposure of rats to X-irradiation in utero or during early postnatal life suppresses the hexobarbital-metabolizing enzyme system in the liver. Hypophysectomy or irradiation of the head (but not of the body with the head shielded) has a similar effect in adult rats.

Nair & Zeitlin G65,099/67: The hexobarbital-metabolizing activity of the rat liver is extremely low after birth and rises gradually up to the age of 80 days to levels much higher in males than in females. Prenatal X-irradiation suppresses this normal development of enzyme activities in the male so that it only reaches the normal female level. Irradiation at 21 days (total body or head alone) also suppresses the developmental increase of enzyme activity, but to a lesser extent. Adults were still more resistant.

Yam & DuBois G58,163/67: In 23-day-old male rats, X-irradiation of the whole animal, or the head only, inhibited the rapid increase in hexobarbital-metabolizing hepatic microsomal oxidase normally obtained by hexobarbital treatment. Hypophysectomy produced the same result.

Nair et al. G67,245/68: X-irradiation of pregnant rats results in male offspring deficient in the hepatic microsomal enzymes which metabolize hexobarbital. However, irradiation did not suppress the increase of enzyme activity brought about by chemical inducers (phenobarbital). Actinomycin inhibited both the ontogenic and phenobarbital-induced increases in enzyme activity. "The ontogenic increase in enzyme activity is hormone-dependent, while that following phenobarbital administration is independent of hormonal regulation as evidenced by the response in hypophysectomized or sexually immature animals. It is concluded from these results that the inhibitory effect of x-irradiation on the hepatic enzyme system is mediated through an action on the hormonal regulation of enzyme activity."

Nair et al. G67,304/68: Comparative studies suggest that the induction of drug-metabolizing enzymes by phenobarbital in the rat can be inhibited by both X-irradiation and actinomycin, but through different mechanisms.

Carcinogens ←

Terayama & Takata F69,475/66: "Whole body irradiation of rats with Co^{60}-γ rays did not affect either the aminoazo dye N-demethylating activity or the hydroxylating activity of rat-liver. It also had no significant effect on the induction of the enzymatic activities by methylcholanthrene. The ionizing irradiation, however, appeared to increase the reduction of enzymatic activity following partial hepatectomy."

Pesticides ←

Hietbrink & DuBois F65,296/66: In weanling male rats, total body X-irradiation inhibits the development of the hepatic microsomal enzyme fraction that catalyzes the oxydative desulfuration of Guthion. Shielding of the liver and testes does not prevent this inhibition, whereas irradiation of the head area (while the remainder of the body is shielded) produces a degree of inhibition similar to that obtained by total body irradiation. "The same dose of irradiation did not inhibit the enzyme development in hypophysectomized weanling rats. Thus, the pituitary is necessary for the radiation effect, but involvement of the pituitary is not the result of a radiation-induced deficiency of pituitary hormones."

Varia ←

Studies on the effect of X-irradiation upon **microbial** infection, **endotoxin** poisoning and **hepatic regeneration** are not particularly instructive in connection with the hormonal regulation of resistance.

Among the **enzymic** changes induced by total body X-irradiation in the rat, a dose-dependent increase in TPO activity is noteworthy in that it occurs within a few hours, but only in the presence of the adrenals. The substrate induction of TPO is stimulated by X-irradiation applied 24 hrs earlier. Induction by cortisol is initially stimulated but later inhibited by X-irradiation.

Microorganisms and Their Toxins ←

Cremer & Watson C 37,986/57: Deposition of endotoxin of S. typhosa was followed in normal and stressed rabbits by the fluorescein tagging technique."Pretreatment with cortisone and x-irradiation did not affect initial phagocytosis of toxin but inhibited degradation and elimination of toxin by the RES."

Vick F 79,609/67: X-irradiation prolongs the survival of dogs following subsequent endotoxin treatment.

Highman et al. H 19,382/69: In rats exposed to X-irradiation or hypoxia, i.v. injection of Streptococcus mitis produces severe bacterial endocarditis. "The radioprotective compound, dimethyl sulfoxide (DMSO), did not affect the lesions in nonirradiated animals but reduced the incidence and severity of lesions in irradiated rats."

Hepatic Lesions ←

Fabrikant H 8,091/68: In mice, X-irradiation interferes with hepatic regeneration after partial hepatectomy. A radiation free interval prior to partial hepatectomy improves the regenerative capacity of the liver.

Zelioli-Lanzini H 19,493/69: In rats, small doses of X-rays as well as hepatic extracts improve liver regeneration following partial hepatectomy.

Hepatic Enzymes ←

TPO, TKT ←. *Thomson & Mikuta B 90,975/54:* "Total-body x-irradiation produces within a few hours a dose-dependent increase in the tryptophan peroxydase-oxydase system of rat liver. The increase does not occur in adrenalectomized rats, and hence cannot be construed as a direct effect of X-irradiation." After hypophysectomy, enzyme induction became progressively less pronounced as adrenal atrophy developed. ACTH restored the ability of the hypophysectomized rat to respond with enzyme induction.

Benes & Zicha G 67,159/69: Exposure to 1400 R does not inhibit the TPO activity of rat liver. In fact, substrate induction of TPO is stimulated by X-irradiation applied 24 hrs earlier. Induction by cortisol is initially stimulated and then, inhibited by X-irradiation. X-irradiation before partial hepatectomy inhibits the increase in TPO normally observed 12 hrs after the operation. Similar results are obtained by actinomycin D applied 1 hr after partial hepatectomy. "The diminished synthesis of tryptophan oxygenase in irradiated regenerating rat liver tissue, as well as the decrease of hormonal induction after the irradiation can be explained by the inhibition of the specific messenger RNA's synthesis."

Other Enzmyes ←. *Brin & McKee C 31,261/56:* In the rat, various stressors (total body X-irradiation, nitrogen mustard, starvation) as well as cortisone increase glutamic-aspartic and glutamic-alanine transaminase activities in the liver. Adrenalectomy decreases the activity of these enzymes. The glutamic-alanine enzyme is more sensitive to stress than the glutamic-aspartic enzyme.

Gresham & Pover G 58,354/68: In the rat, alkaline RNAse levels increase in the mucosa of the small intestine after total body or selective head X-irradiation, as well as after treatment with such radiomimetic drugs as chlorambucil or busulfan but not after treatment with ACTH, cortisol or various stressors. Still, a relationship to the G.A.S. is suspected because blockade of the normal neuroendocrine responses to stress by combined treatment with morphine + pentobarbital blocked the intestinal RNAse response to X-irradiation. The latter was also lacking in newborn rats in which hypothalamic control of anterior pituitary function has not yet developed.

← ULTRAVIOLET RAYS

In mice, daylight or ultraviolet irradiation increases acetonitrile resistance even after thyroidectomy; hence, this effect of the rays is not necessarily mediated through the thyroid.

Paal 18,183/33: In mice, exposure to light greatly influences sensitivity to acetonitrile. Even after thyroidectomy, daylight as well as ultraviolet irradiation increase the MLD of acetonitrile. Hence, resistance to this drug is not always influenced through variations in thyroid activity.

Ellinger 78,163/38: In mice, ultraviolet irradiation increases resistance against acetonitrile, presumably through activation of the thyroid.

← HYPOXIA

In mice, reduced oxygen tension does not necessarily diminish and may even increase resistance to X-rays.

Barbiturates ←

DeFeo et al. H 32,863/70: "Mice under acute hypobaric conditions exhibited lower levels of pentobarbital in the body at the time of awakening than did control mice at room atmosphere. The fact that the hypoxic animals remain asleep at otherwise inadequate concentration of drug suggests enhanced sensitivity to barbiturates." The pentobarbital concentration of the body declined at a subnormal rate in mice exposed to hypobaric hypoxia. In isolated mice (1 per cage), the duration of hexobarbital, pentobarbital, barbital or chloral hydrate sleeping time was markedly reduced in comparison with controls kept in a more normal social environment (10 per cage). The magnitude of the reduction of sleeping time was greatest with hexobarbital, and least with barbital. Furthermore, "in vitro studies showed that the hepatic microsomal fractions isolated from socially deprived mice metabolized hexobarbital at a rate higher than the hepatic fractions isolated from control mice." In male mice, in which aggressive behavior develops following prolongend deprivation of social interaction (isolation), hexobarbital sleeping time was also reduced. In females which did not develop fighting behavior, the reduction in hexobarbital sleeping time was likewise evident which "would suggest that development of aggressive behavior during isolation has a different biological basis and is not related to the alteration in pharmacological activity."

Medina & Merritt G 81,699/70: In mice, the in vivo effect and hepatic metabolism of various barbiturates, zoxazolamine and other drugs are significantly altered by a reduced barometric pressure, but the action of this stressor largely depends on the length of exposure.

Bacteria ← cf. also Selye *G 60,083/70, pp. 455, 456.*

Highman et al. H 19,382/69: In rats exposed to X-irradiation or hypoxia, i.v. injection of Streptococcus mitis produces severe bacterial endocarditis. "The radioprotective compound, dimethyl sulfoxide (DMSO), did not affect the lesions in nonirradiated animals but reduced the incidence and severity of lesions in irradiated rats."

Ionizing Rays ←

Smith et al. B 48,252/48: In mice, reduced oxygen tension did not adversely influence survival following X-irradiation.

Limperos B 50,944/50: In X-irradiated mice, "low oxygen atmosphere exerts a protective effect possibly because it decreases the concentration of OH and HO_2 radicals and of H_2O_2."

Hepatic Enzymes ←

Kato & Gillette F 57,817/65: The metabolism of aminopyrine and hexobarbital by hepatic microsomes of male rats is impaired by adrenalectomy, castration, hypoxia, ACTH, formaldehyde, epinephrine, morphine, alloxan or thyroxine. The metabolism of aniline and zoxazolamine is not appreciably decreased by any of these agents; in fact, hydroxylation of aniline is enhanced by thyroxine or alloxan. Apparently, the treatments impair mainly the sex-dependent enzymes. Accordingly, the corresponding enzymic functions of the hepatic microsomes of female rats are not significantly impaired by the agents which do have an inhibitory effect in males.

Agarwal & Berry G66,480/67: Brief mention of unpublished experiments showing that mice "exposed to hypoxic stress clearly establish that enzyme induction occurs in the absence of exogenous hormone, and hence from stress alone, and that this induction is also subject to inhibition by endotoxin."

← TEMPERATURE VARIATIONS

Variations in atmospheric temperature may greatly influence **barbiturate** toxicity. Rats kept in the cold for several weeks show an increased hexobarbital sleeping time which does not correspond to an increased hexobarbital metabolism of the liver in vitro.

Lynestrenol reduced, whereas mestranol prolonged the duration of pentobarbital and hexobarbital anesthesia in mice. The effect of the luteoid was inhibited, whereas that of the folliculoid was increased when pentobarbital was prevented from inducing hypothermia.

During the acute phase of CCl_4 intoxication, the induction of TKT and TPO activity in the livers of rats is diminished by the stress of exposure to cold and the associated decrease in corticosterone production. However, after chronic hepatic injury is induced by repeated doses of CCl_4, TKT and TPO induction by cold or exogenous corticosterone may be virtually normal.

In mice, exposure to the stress of cold decreases resistance to endotoxin, possibly because of an initial "depletion of corticoid reserves." Cortisone protects even against the combined effect of endotoxin + cold. After one week of acclimatization to low temperatures, endotoxin resistance is increased, perhaps owing to the induction of excess TPO. In senescent mice, the induction of TKT by cold is delayed.

Drugs ←

Barbiturates ←. *Richards 79,646/41:* The toxicity of thiopental to frogs is higher at 10 than at 20° C, but this does not hold true of paraldehyde.

Blackham & Spencer G69,913/69: Mestranol (a folliculoid) prolonged, while lynestrenol (a luteoid) reduced the duration of pentobarbital and hexobarbital sleep in mice. Barbital was not affected. The effects of lynestrenol were abolished by SKF 525-A, while those of mestranol were markedly potentiated. Lynestrenol increased, whereas mestranol and SKF 525-A reduced the rate of clearance of barbiturate from the plasma. The effect of lynestrenol disappeared and that of mestranol was increased when pentobarbital was prevented from inducing hypothermia.

Hässler et al. H23,853/69: Male rats are more resistant than females to the anesthetic effect of hexobarbital. In rats raised under extreme conditions of stress (cold or repeated periods of fasting) hexobarbital sleeping time is prolonged.

Kalser & Kunig G65,211/69: "Rats exposed to 5° for at least 3 days and for as long as 7 weeks sleep longer than their age-matched 25° controls when given hexobarbital. This increase in sleep time does not correspond with a diminished metabolism in vitro, since the rate of metabolism by the liver of the cold-exposed rats remains essentially constant for the entire 7 weeks."

Carbon Tetrachloride ←. *Murphy & Malley G68,408/69:* Studies on hepatic TKT, alkaline phosphatase (AP), and tryptophan pyrrolase (TP) in relation to stress and CCl_4-intoxication in the rat. "Liver TKT elevation, but not AP elevation, was prevented by adrenalectomy prior to CCl_4. Experiments on rats subjected to simultaneous acute cold stress and CCl_4 indicated that, during the acute phase of CCl_4 hepatotoxicity, their livers had reduced capacity for induction of TKT and TP by endogenous corticosterone. However, chronically injured livers of rats given repeated doses of CCl_4 were fully responsive to the TKT- and TP-inducing effects of exogenous corticosterone or acute cold stress."

Chloral Hydrate ←. *Fastier et al. C 37,038/57:* In mice, chloral hydrate sleeping time is increased by epinephrine, norepinephrine, phenylephrine, methoxamine, 5-HT, histamine, ergotamine, yohimbine, and atropine. "It is suggested that some, at least, of the drugs which prolong the effects of hypnotics do so by virtue of a hypothermic action." Vasopressin, cortisone and DOC did not prolong chloral hydrate sleeping time at the doses tested.

Cholesterol ←. *cf. Selye G 60,083/70, p. 453.*

Dinitrophenol ←. *Haydu & Wolfson C 77, 942/59:* In mice, the toxicity of DPN is increased by exposure to either cold or heat; the effect of temperature extremes is further aggravated by cortisone.

Magnesium ←. *cf. Selye G 60,083/70, pp. 453, 455.*

Tyrosine ←. *Fuller G 75,131/70:* In rats, exposure to cold, as well as treatment with cortisol or glucagon after adrenalectomy, induced TKT activity in the liver but not in the brain. Apparently, the TKT "of brain differed from the enzyme in liver since it did not exhibit diurnal variations of activity and was not affected by hormones, drugs, or stress."

Varia ←. *Keplinger et al. G 70,208/59:* In rats, the acute i.p. toxicity of 58 drugs was compared at 8°, 26°, and 36° C. "Except for strychnine, chlorpromazine, and promazine, all compounds were most toxic at 36° C. Strychnine was equally toxic at 8° and 36° C, while promazine and chlorpromazine were most toxic at 8° C."

Furner & Stitzel G 54,558/68: The hepatic microsomal metabolism of ethylmorphine, aniline, and hexobarbital is diminished in vitro by previous adrenalectomy in the rat. Phenobarbital pretreatment of adrenalectomized rats raised the metabolism of all three substrates above the level characteristic of otherwise untreated, adrenalectomized controls. Exposure of adrenalectomized rats to cold stress, or treatment with cortisol, increased the metabolism of aniline and ethylmorphine, but further depressed that of hexobarbital. In intact rats, cold stress diminished hexobarbital metabolism in vitro. Apparently, both stress and phenobarbital can bring about changes in hepatic drug metabolism independent of the presence of the adrenals, and the two agents act through different mechanisms, since phenobarbital invariably stimulates, whereas stress either increases or decreases microsomal enzyme activity, depending upon the drug pathway examined.

Bacterial Toxins ←

Previte & Berry E 89,101/63: In mice, exposure to the stress of cold decreases resistance to endotoxin, perhaps because of an initial "depletion of corticoid reserves." Cortisone protects even against the combined effect of endotoxin + cold.

Berry F 69,416/66: When exposed to extremes of temperature, the resistance of mice to the lethal effect of endotoxin is greatly reduced. "It is believed that endotoxin sensitizes mice to heat and cold rather than these temperatures sensitizing to endotoxin. After 1 week of acclimatization at 5°C of 37°C, the LD_{50} of endotoxin increased, respectively, to 790 µg and 260 µg. Inducibility of the liver enzyme tryptophan pyrrolase, believed to play a role in an animal's response to endotoxin, was evaluated at each invironmental temperature. Only at the extremes was it suppressed."

Venoms ←

Stahnke F 57,253/65: In rats treated with various scorpion and snake venoms, resistance was decreased by pretreatment with heat, cold or epinephrine. In all three cases, the change in resistance is ascribed to stress as such.

Cittadini et al. G 76,028/70: In X-irradiated mice, the formation of hemopoietic islets in the spleen is inhibited by dexamethasone, ACTH or the stress of exposure to cold.

Immune Reactions ← *cf. Selye G 60,083/70, pp. 453, 455, 456.*

Hepatic Enzymes ←

Metzenberg et al. D 86,024/61: Thyroxine induces carbamyl phosphate synthetase in hepatic microsomes of the liver in tadpoles.

Davis D 92,322/63: The decarboxylation of o-tyrosine and 5-hydroxytryptophan by livers of adrenalectomized rats, given water, was significantly lower than in controls. No significant effects on decarboxylation of these substrates were observed in adrenalectomized animals given NaCl, or in intact animals treated with DOC or exposed to cold. On the other hand, cortisone increased the inherent hepatic decarboxylating activity for both substrates, in normal as well as in pyridoxine-deficient rats.

Finch et al. G 71,208/69: In senescent mice, the induction of hepatic TKT by exposure to cold is delayed in comparison with young mice. Corticosterone and insulin are equally effective in this respect in mice of both age groups.

Klain & Hannon H 13,174/69: In rats, exposure to cold induces an increase in the hepatic glucose-6-phosphatase, fructose-1,6-diphosphatase, phosphoenolpyruvate carboxykinase and glutamic-pyruvic transaminase, presumably as a consequence of increased corticoid and thyroid hormone production.

Dewaide G 80,406/70: Comparative studies on the effect of adaptation to cold or heat upon hepatic drug oxidation in various species. Contrary to earlier claims, drug metabolizing enzymes do play a decisive role in the resistance of fishes to changes in their environment. "The effect of a change of ambient temperature on the liver of the hamster, rat, roach, and trout becomes manifest in an almost equal way for the different species."

← STRESSORS

The effect of stress on the action of various pathogens is of special importance in connection with our topic, since stress can influence resistance through its effect upon the secretion of hormones as well as through nonhormonal mechanisms. It can also both diminish susceptibility to disease through "cross-resistance" and increase it by the activation of various "conditioning" mechanisms.

Steroids ←

The effect of stressors upon the biogenesis, metabolism and especially the hydroxylation of steroids by hepatic microsomes has been the subject of extensive studies. In connection with our topic, it is of special interest that the infarctoid cardiopathies produced by various corticoids + sodium salts are very regularly aggravated by diverse stressors, including even the noise made by a loud bell.

Rats pretreated with various stressors are particularly sensitive to progesterone anesthesia.

Selye A 36,210/41: Rats pretreated with various stressors become particularly sensitive to progesterone anesthesia.

Mäkinen et al. E 20,847/63: Conjoint treatment with cortisone + NaCl produces myocardial necroses in orchidectomized but not in normal male rats. Testosterone restores the resistance of the male castrates to normal, whereas concomitant exposure to the stress of a loud bell aggravates the cardiopathy.

Kuntzman et al. G 66,245/66: Review (11 pp., 19 refs.) on factors influencing steroid hydroxylases in hepatic microsomes.

Corticoids ← *cf. Selye C 50,810/58, pp. 88, 114—122, 143; C 92,918/61, pp. 58, 75, 254; G 60,083/70, pp. 446, 449, 452, 457, 459, 462.*

Corticosterone ← Stress (Cold): Maikkel et al. G 41,515/66*

Cortisol ← Stress (Tourniquet shock): Firschein et al. C 30,553/57*

Cortisone ← Stress + Genetics, Mouse: Wragg et al. B 74,080/52*

Estradiol ← Stress (Cold): Inscoe et al. F 70,325/66

Nonsteroidal Hormones and Hormone-Like Substances ←

In rabbits, epinephrine arteriosclerosis can be prevented by concurrent exposure to electroshock. There is very little evidence to suggest that sublethal amounts of **catecholamines** can be detoxicated by catatoxic steroids that increase hepatic drug metabolism; acute epinephrine or norepinephrine poisoning is actually aggravated by the syntoxic glucocorticoids.

In rabbits, the organ changes produced by heavy **thiouracil** intoxication can be prevented by electroshock.

In rats, the stress of restraint tends to prevent **parathyroid hormone** overdosage.

In mice sensitized with pertussis vaccine, the increased sensitivity to **histamine** and **5-HT** is inhibited by various stressors. In rats, the renal necroses elicited by acute 5-HT intoxication are also inhibited by forced restraint. This protection occurs even after adrenalectomy and is not shared by cortisol, hence here the action of stress is presumably not mediated through glucocorticoid secretion.

Epinephrine ← cf. also Selye B40,000/50, p. 55; B58,650/51, pp. 322, 373; G60,083/70, pp. 446, 450, 457.

Delfini B52,659/50: In rabbits, epinephrine arteriosclerosis can be prevented by concurrent exposure to electroshock.

Epinephrine ← Stress (Cold): Inscoe et al. F70,325/66

Hypophyseal Hormones ← cf. Selye B40,000/50, p. 616.

STH ← cf. also Selye G60,083/70, p. 457.

Wakabayashi et al. H27,784/70: In rats, exposure to stressors [kind not stated (H.S.)] or administration of dexamethasone suppresses plasma STH (radio-immunoassay) both in the presence and in the absence of the adrenals. Adrenalectomy increases plasma STH. [These findings support the view that during stress — perhaps owing to increased ACTH and/or glucocorticoid secretion, the "shift in pituitary hormone production" results in a diminished STH secretion (H.S.).]

Thyroid Hormones ← cf. also Selye C50, 810/58, p. 88; C92,918/61, p. 121.

Baraldi B52,651/50: In rabbits, the organ changes produced by heavy methylthiouracil intoxication can be prevented by electroshock.

Parathyroid Hormone ← cf. also Selye G60,083/70, pp. 446, 451.

Tuchweber et al. G46,759/68: Pretreatment with thyroxine or calcitonin inhibits the soft tissue calcification and osteitis fibrosa induced by parathyroid extract overdosage. In the event of concurrent administration, the effect of the two protective hormones is summated. Thyroxine retains its effect upon calcium metabolism in thyroparathyroidectomized or adrenalectomized but not in nephrectomized rats. The stress of restraint likewise prevents parathyroid overdosage, but the associated biochemical changes are different from those caused by thyroxine.

Histamine, 5-HT ← cf. also Selye B40,000/50, p. 55.

Munoz E8,473/64: In mice sensitized with B. pertussis, the development of increased sensitivity to histamine or 5-HT is inhibited by various stressors.

Selye et al. E24,146/64: The renal necroses normally produced by acute intoxication with 5-HT, can be inhibited by forced restraint both in intact and in adrenalectomized rats. Cortisol has no such inhibitory effect; hence, the action of stress is not mediated through glucocorticoid secretion.

5-HT ← Stress (Cold): Inscoe et al. F70,325/66

Drugs ←

The effect of numerous drugs can be either increased or decreased by pretreatment or concurrent treatment with stressors. Such interactions are important in the pathogenesis of the so-called "pluricausal diseases," in which stress plays a decisive but not an exclusive role.

In particular, stress can greatly alter the toxicity of **agar** (thrombohemorrhagic syndromes), **amphetamine, anaphylactoidogens** and **antibiotics**. In combination with several indirect **anticoagulants**, stress can elicit the "hemorrhagic syndrome of Jaques."

The anesthetic effect of various **barbiturates** is prolonged in rats pretreated with various toxic organ extracts, casein or colchicine, presumably as a consequence of their stressor effect. A similar prolongation of barbiturate sleeping time has been noted following treatment with toxic drugs, electroshock, etc.

On the other hand, the sedative effect of hexobarbital and pentobarbital (unlike that of barbital) was diminished by tourniquet stress in intact but not in hypophysectomized or adrenalectomized rats. In intact rats, ACTH or cortisone decreases hexobarbital sleeping time, whereas SKF 525-A blocks the protective action of stress; hence, protection by stressors has been ascribed to the liberation of glucocorticoids. The blood levels of hexobarbital, pentobarbital and meprobamate (but not of phenobarbital) were diminished by tourniquet stress in intact but not in hypophysectomized or adrenalectomized rats. However, many of these experiments gave inconsistent results, presumably because stress has a dual action in general, inhibiting barbiturate anesthesia through the liberation of glucocorticoids but aggravating it perhaps through some extra-adrenal mechanism.

For the effect of stressors upon the toxicity of other drugs, consult the Abstract Section. However, in evaluating all these data, we must keep in mind that timing is particularly important here, since pretreatment or concurrent treatment with stressors may affect potential pathogens in opposite ways.

N-Acetyl-p-aminophenol ← Stress (Cold): Inscoe et al. *F70,325/66*

N-Acetyltyramine ← Stress (Cold): Inscoe et al. *F70,325/66*

Agar ← cf. Selye *E5,986/66*, p. 150.

Aminopyrine ←

Nakanishi et al. *G79,299/70:* "Cold exposure or immobilization of intact or adrenalectomized rats significantly impaired side-chain oxidation of hexobarbital and N-demethylation of aminopyrine in vitro. In contrast, p-hydroxylation of aniline in vitro was not affected under stress conditions." The pertinent literature is somewhat contradictory but, possibly, the effect of stress on drug-metabolizing enzyme induction may vary with the substrate employed.

Amphetamine ←

Clark et al. *F92,621/67:* Crowding increases the toxicity of amphetamine in the mouse. "The administration of either dexamethasone, ethanol, glucose, 2-deoxy-d-glucose or diphenylhydantoin reduced the excitement, hyperactivity and morality in aggregated mice given d-amphetamine. The reduction in mortality was proportional to the decrease in excitement and hyperactivity."

Amphetamine ← Stress, Mouse: Hardinge et al. *E26,072/63**

Anaphylactoidogens ← cf. Selye *B40,000/50*, pp. 56, 754; *G46,715/68*, pp. 209, 212.

Aniline ←

Stitzel & Furner *G48,920/67:* In rats, stress (cold) increases the rate of p-hydroxylation of aniline and N-dealkylation of ethylmorphine simultaneously with an increase in adrenal ascorbic acid content. The stress-induced stimulation of microsomal metabolism and adrenal ascorbic acid levels are additive with those produced by phenobarbital. "It is tentatively concluded that stress and phenobarbital appear to act through different mechanisms in inducing increases in enzyme activity, although each treatment may have a common final step, namely an increased net synthesis of enzyme protein."

Nakanishi et al. *G79,299/70:* "Cold exposure or immobilization of intact or adrenalectomized rats significantly impaired side-chain oxidation of hexobarbitel and N-demethylation of aminopyrine in vitro. In contrast, p-hydroxylation of aniline in vitro was not affected under stress conditions." The pertinent literature is somewhat contradictory but, possibly, the effect of stress on drug-metabolizing enzyme induction may vary with the substrate employed.

Antibiotics ← cf. Selye *G60,083/70*, pp. 460, 464, 465.

Anticoagulants ←

Jaques *G70,979/68:* Review (30 pp., 13 refs.) on the "hemorrhagic stress syndrome" that is produced in various mammals treated with indirect anticoagulants (e.g., phenindione, dicoumarol) and then exposed to stress or treated with DOC, ACTH, or STH. Conversely, cortisone, epinephrine, ephedrine and adrenochrome inhibit this syndrome.

Barbiturates ←

Masson *B1,217/46:* In male rats, pretreatment for 6 days with crude pituitary powder s.c. "slightly prolonged the duration of anesthesia with phanodorn, thioethamyl, neonal, delvinal, nostal and amytal, and greatly prolonged (2 to 5 times) with pentothal, seconal, allyl pental, nembutal, evipal, pernoston and sigmodal." There was no difference between the pretreated and control rats as regards the anesthetic effect of phenobarbital, probarbital, barbital, aprobarbital, allobarbital and chloral. "The action of pituitary preparations is not specific but can also be obtained with preparations from various organs and with foreign proteins." Hepatic damage is considered to be a likely cause of the prolongation of anesthesia under these conditions.

Masson 94,205/47: Various tissue extracts (anterior pituitary, thymus, pancreas, liver, kidney, spleen, testis, brain) as well as casein s.c. decrease resistance to pentobarbital anesthesia in male rats. On the other hand, "among eight damaging agents given in doses sufficient to elicit an alarm reaction, only colchicine and atropine prolonged the duration of anesthesia, because of their high degree of toxicity." Yet, the prolongation of barbiturate anesthesia by pituitary extracts must be ascribed to a nonspecific stressor effect.

Cook et al. D23,923/54: A review of the literature shows that barbiturate anesthesia can be prolonged by alcohol, cholesterol, antihistaminics, histamine, certain nitrates, thiamine, ascorbic acid, cystine, disulfiram, glycerin and many other agents.

Kato E87,340/60: Mention of unpublished experiments which show "that, in rats pretreated with electroshock, the sleeping-time induced by barbiturates (48—72 h later) is much longer than in normal animals."

Rupe et al. E26,910/63: The sedative effect of hexobarbital and pentobarbital, but not of barbital, was diminished by tourniquet stress, in the intact but not in the hypophysectomized or adrenalectomized rat. In intact rats, ACTH or cortisone decreases hexobarbital sleeping time, the same as stress does, whereas SKF 525-A completely blocks the protective action of the latter. Presumably "the stress effect on the duration of drug action is mediated through increased drug metabolism."

Driever & Bousquet G31,872/65; Driever et al. F73,812/66: In rats with tourniquet stress, the blood levels of hexobarbital, pentobarbital and meprobamate, but not of phenobarbital, were diminished after injection of these drugs. These effects are prevented by hypophysectomy or adrenalectomy. Pentobarbital blood levels are lowered in adrenalectomized rats by corticosterone, but not by ACTH, whereas in hypophysectomized rats, both these hormones are active. "The ability of stress situations to stimulate drug metabolism and its dependence upon an intact pituitary-adrenal axis is suggestive of a regulatory function of the endocrine system in mediating a rapid induction of liver microsomal enzymes responsible for drug metabolism." [An addendum states that the experiments could not be repeated in the summer (H.S.).]

Wooles & Borzelleca F93,374/66: Repeated administration of zymosan i.v. prolongs hexobarbital, pentobarbital, and barbital sleeping time in the mouse. This effect is ascribed to stimulation of the RES.

Dairman & Balazs G78,636/70: Individually caged rats tend to become aggressive; they show enlarged adrenals and thyroids, but atrophic spleens and thymus glands as compared with community-caged controls. This has been referred to as "isolation stress." Individually caged rats also exhibit diminished barbiturate sleeping times, possibly as a consequence of microsomal enzyme induction.

DeFeo et al. H32,863/70: "Mice under acute hypobaric conditions exhibited lower levels of pentobarbital in the body at the time of awakening than did control mice at room atmosphere. The fact that the hypoxic animals remain asleep at otherwise inadequate concentration of drug suggests enhanced sensitivity to barbiturates." The pentobarbital concentration of the body declined at a subnormal rate in mice exposed to hypobaric hypoxia. In isolated mice (1 per cage), the duration of hexobarbital, pentobarbital, barbital or chloral hydrate sleeping time was markedly reduced in comparison with controls kept in a more normal social environment (10 per cage). The magnitude of the reduction of sleeping time was greatest with hexobarbital, and least with barbital. Furthermore, "in vitro studies showed that the hepatic microsomal fractions isolated from socially deprived mice metabolized hexobarbital at a rate higher than the hepatic fractions isolated from control mice." In male mice, in which aggressive behavior develops following prolonged deprivation of social interaction (isolation), hexobarbital sleeping time was also reduced. In females which did not develop fighting behavior, the reduction in hexobarbital sleeping time was likewise evident which "would suggest that development of aggressive behavior during isolation has a different biological basis and is not related to the alteration in pharmacological activity."

Nakanishi et al. G79,299/70: "Cold exposure or immobilization of intact or adrenalectomized rats significantly impaired side-chain oxidation of hexobarbital and N-demethylation of aminopyrine in vitro. In contrast, p-hydroxylation of aniline in vitro was not affected under stress conditions." The pertinent literature is somewhat contradictory but, possibly, the effect of stress on drug-metabolizing enzyme induction may vary with the substrate employed.

Sethy et al. G77,511/70: In rats, pentobarbital sleeping time is reduced immediately after stress (centrifugation), but returns to normal eight hours later. In adrenalectomized animals, this effect of stress is abolished.

Weiner et al. H24,942/70: In rats, glucagon, alloxan and starvation all increased hexobarbital sleeping time. This effect was markedly antagonized by insulin. Perhaps, cyclic AMP may be involved since theophylline greatly increases the action of glucagon. This synergism also occurrred in isolated, perfused rat livers and, hence, "inhibition of hexobarbital metabolism by cyclic AMP would appear to be mediated in the liver."

Barbiturates ← Stress: Rupe et al. E26,910/63*; Bosquet et al. F35,073/65*; Driever et al. G31,872/65*, F73,812/66*

Hexobarbital ← Stress: Rupe et al. E26,910/63*; Bosquet et al. F35,073/65*

Pentobarbital ← Stress: Driever et al. G31,872/65*, F73,812/66*

Brombenzene ←

Schultz B18,183/46: In rabbits, the detoxication of brombenzene as mercapturic acid is enhanced by the presence of a sterile abscess. Presumably, "a specific metabolic reaction can utilize the tissue breakdown products resulting from the formation of a sterile abscess."

Bromides ←

Prioreschi C68,485/59: In the rat, exposure to stress intensifies NaBr anesthesia.

Calcium ← *cf. Selye G60,083/70, pp. 446, 452, 453.*

Carbon Tetrachloride ←

Calvert & Brody C82,653/60: "A hypothesis is proposed which states that the characteristic hepatic changes seen after the administration of carbontetrachloride are the result of stimulation of central sympathetic areas which produce a massive discharge of the peripheral sympathetic nervous system." This hypothesis is based mainly upon the observation that in rats, adrenergic blocking agents, reserpine, adrenalectomy, and section of the spinal cord are all effective in preventing the changes characteristic of CCl_4 intoxication. [The possibility that the protection might be due to stress or the associated hypothermia has not been considered. (H.S.).]

Carcinogens ←

Wheatley et al. F68,548/66: Partial hepatectomy protects the adrenals of the rat against the hemorrhagic necrosis produced by DMBA. On the other hand, "operative stress," as in sham-hepatectomy or nephrectomy, actually increases the susceptibility of the adrenals to DMBA. Other factors influencing DMBA-induced adrenal necrosis are reviewed.

Somogyi G70,416/70: In rats, spironolactone inhibits the adrenocortical necrosis, carcinogenicity and hemopoietic-tissue-damaging action of DMBA. Ethylestrenol, SC-1, and norbolethone are also effective against the DMBA-induced adrenal necrosis. Spironolactone likewise protects against the adrenocorticolytic effect of 7-OHM-MBA. Thus, the anti-DMBA action of spironolactone does not seem to be based on the blockade of the transformation of the carcinogen into this supposedly more active metabolite. The preventive action of spironolactone is abolished by ethionine, suggesting the involvement of active protein synthesis. The DMBA-induced adrenal lesions are aggravated by estradiol, testosterone, methyltestosterone, cortisol, triamcinolone, and prednisolone, as well as by the stress of muscular work or restraint. The aggravation of adrenal necrosis by estradiol is diminished but not abolished by hypophysectomy.

Somogyi & Kovács G70,482/70: In rats, the stress of restraint or of forced muscular exercise significantly increases the adrenocorticolytic effect of DMBA. Spironolactone can abolish this stress-induced aggravation. The mammary carcinogenicity of DMBA is not influenced by stress.

Carrageenin ← *cf. Selye E5,986/66, p. 150.*

Chloral Hydrate ←

DeFeo et al. H32,863/70: "Mice under acute hypobaric conditions exhibited lower levels of pentobarbital in the body at the time of awakening than did control mice at room atmosphere. The fact that the hypoxic animals remain asleep at otherwise inadequate concentration of drug suggests enhanced sensitivity to barbiturates." The pentobarbital concentration of the body declined at a subnormal rate in mice exposed to hypobaric hypoxia. In isolated mice (1 per cage), the duration of hexobarbital,

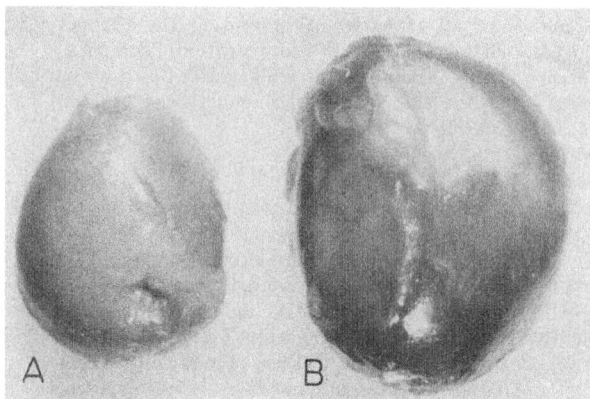

Fig. 29. **Aggravation by stress of DMBA-induced adrenocortical necrosis.** Adrenals of rat given threshold amounts of DMBA. A: Without exposure to stress, this amount of the carcinogen causes no obvious adrenal change. B: Following exposure to stress of restraint increases sensitivity to the carcinogen and results in severe adrenocortical necrosis and hemorrhage. [Courtesy of Somogyi & Kovacs.]

pentobarbital, barbital or chloral hydrate sleeping time was markedly reduced in comparison with controls kept in a more normal social environment (10 per cage). The reduction of sleeping time was greatest with hexobarbital, and least with barbital. Furthermore, "in vitro studies showed that the hepatic microsomal fractions isolated from socially deprived mice metabolized hexobarbital at a rate higher than the hepatic fractions isolated from control mice." In male mice, in which aggressive behavior develops following prolonged deprivation of social interaction (isolation), hexobarbital sleeping time was also reduced. In females which did not develop fighting behavior, the reduction in hexobarbital sleeping time was likewise evident which "would suggest that development of aggressive behavior during isolation has a different biological basis and is not related to the alteration in pharmacological activity."

Chlorides ← cf. Selye C92,918/61, p. 88; G60,083/70, pp. 460, 464.

Chloroform ←

Ravdin et al. B25,566/39: In rats, xanthine, allantoin, caffeine, sodium ricinoleate and suspensions of colloidal carbon injected s.c. protect the liver against injury from chloroform, presumably as a consequence of the resulting inflammatory reaction which is associated with the absorption of protein split products. This would also explain the protective effect of various hepatic extracts (including Yakriton) and of high protein diets.

Cholesterol ← cf. also Selye C92,918/61, p. 229; G60,083/70, pp. 445, 447, 457, 458, 459, 464, 486, 487.

Conney & Kuntzman G70,540/70: Review on the metabolism of cholesterol as influenced by the induction of hepatic drug-metabolizing enzymes.

Ethanol ←

Fazekas & Rengei G58,271/68: In rats, not pretreated with ethanol, the alcohol-dehydrogenase (ADH) activity of the liver, heart, and kidneys is diminished by adrenalectomy. Upon s.c. administration of ethanol, the ADH-activity of the liver increases both in intact and in adrenalectomized rats. The authors speculate that ADH-activity may result not only in the microsomes but also in other cellular fraction, and that part of the enzyme induction may be due to the stressor effect of ethanol.

Formaldehyde ← cf. Selye B40,000/50, p. 387; B58,650/51, p. 248.

Ganglioplegics ←

Selye G70,448/70: In rats, intoxication with TEA, hexamethonium and pentolinium could be prevented by all of the seven glucocorticoids tested. On the other hand, glucocorticoids offered no protection against trimethaphan, mecamylamine, trimethidinium or pempidine. Typical catatoxic steroids (ethylestrenol, CS-1, spironolactone, norbolethone, oxandrolone) as well as progesterone, DOC, and hydroxydione failed to offer significant protection against hexamethonium or TEA. Various stressors (bone fractures, fasting, spinal cord transection and formalin) gave excellent protection against TEA, whereas others (restraint, cold) did not. "Since even large doses of ACTH are ineffective in this respect the anti-TEA effect of stressors cannot be ascribed merely to increased corticoid secretion."

Indomethacin ←

Selye PROT. 22977,22161: In rats (100 g ♀) various severe stressors (restraint, spinal cord transection, intestinal traumas, bone fractures, formalin injections) did not significantly modify the development of perforating intestinal ulcers.

Isoproterenol ← cf. *Selye G60,083/70, pp. 453, 455.*

Lipids, Fatty Acids ←

Conney & Kuntzman G70,540/70: Review on the metabolism of fatty acids as influenced by the induction of hepatic drug-metabolizing enzymes.

Magnesium ← cf. *Selye C92,918/61, p. 88; G60,083/70, pp. 460, 464.*

Meprobamate ← Stress: Rupe et al. E26,910/63*; Bousquet et al. F35,073/65*; Driever et al. F73,812/66*

α-Methyltyrosine ←

Smookler & Buckley H32,862/70: In rats, exposure to a combination of stressors (noise, flashing lights, oscillation of the cage) causes pronounced hypertension and increased sensitivity to salicylate (gastric ulcers) and reserpine (mortality) intoxication. α-Methyltyrosine prevents the stress-induced hypertension, perhaps because it reduces the level of catecholamines by inhibiting their synthesis but leaving the catecholamine binding system intact. "The combination of a reduced amount of liberated transmitter plus rapid inactivation by an intact binding system may serve to dampen the stress-induced activation of central sympathetic centers." Whereas both reserpine and α-methyltyrosine prevent the stress-induced hypertension, the former does, whereas the latter does not cause mortality.

Morphine ←

Stitzel & Furner G48,920/67: In rats, stress (cold) increases the rate of p-hydroxylation of aniline and N-dealkylation of ethylmorphine simultaneously with an increase in adrenal ascorbic acid content. The stress-induced stimulation of microsomal metabolism and adrenal ascorbic acid levels are additive with those produced by phenobarbital. "It is tentatively concluded that stress and phenobarbital appear to act through different mechanisms in inducing increases in enzyme activity, although each treatment may have a common final step, namely an increased net synthesis of enzyme protein."

Nicotine ←

Beckett & Triggs G70,154/67: In man, nicotine excretion in the urine following intravenous injection of nicotine, smoking or inhalation of nicotine vapor is greater among nonsmokers than among smokers. The difference is ascribed to the induction of drug-metabolizing enzymes by nicotine. Following discontinuation of smoking, the accelerated nicotine metabolism persists for many months.

p-Octopamine ← Stress (Cold): Inscoe et al. F70,325/66

Papain ← cf. *Selye C50,810/58, p. 106; C92,918/61, pp. 102, 266; G60,083/70, pp. 446, 450, 459, 460.*

Perchlorates ←

Selye & Bajusz C55,656/59: A great variety of stressors sensitizes the rat to the production of spastic muscular contractions by $NaClO_4$.

Permanganates ← cf. *Selye D15,540/62, p 302.*

Pesticides ←

Brown G78,684/70: In rats, various forms of stress (exercise, starvation, temperature variations) decrease the blood and tissue clearance of DDT and of its metabolites.

Gish & Chura G80,046/70: In Japanese quails, sensitivity to DDT is increased by starvation and during the breeding season. Males are more sensitive than females.

Phenol ←

Samaras & Dietz C56,733/58: In mice, pretreatment with "swimming stress" increases sensitivity to the production of intense convulsions by phenol s.c. Cortisol does not modify phenol intoxication.

Phenol ← Stress (Cold): Inscoe et al. F70,325/66

Plasmocid ← cf. *Selye C92,918/61, pp. 95, 96, 266; G60,083/70, pp. 459, 460.*

Potassium ← cf. *Selye C92,918/61, pp. 82, 257; G60,083/70, pp. 447, 452, 460, 464.*

Reserpine ←

Smookler & Buckley H32,862/70: In rats, exposure to a combination of stressors (noise, flashing lights, oscillation of the cage) causes

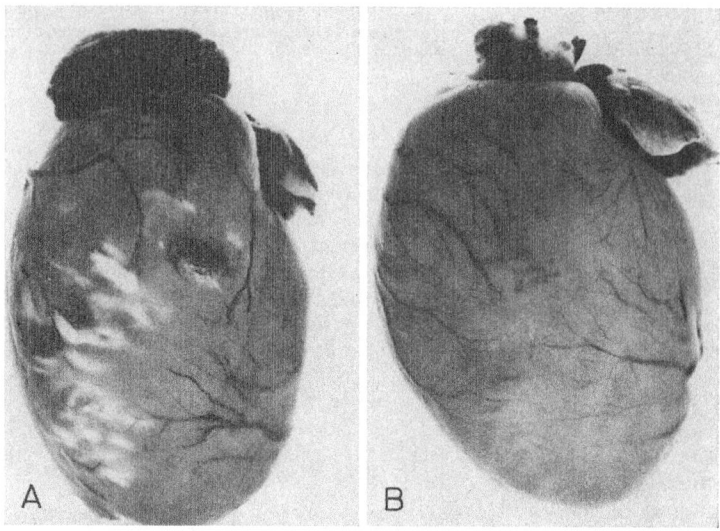

Fig. 30. **Protection by restraint against papain.** Both rats received the same dose of papain i.p. A: Many "tigroid necroses" in the otherwise untreated control. All rats of this group died within 48 hrs. B: No lesion in rat restrained (8 hrs) on day preceding papain injection. All animals of this group survived. [Selye C92,918/61. Courtesy of Charles C Thomas.]

pronounced hypertension and increased sensitivity to salicylate (gastric ulcers) and reserpine (mortality) intoxication. α-Methyltyrosine prevents the stress-induced hypertension, perhaps because it reduces the level of catecholamines by inhibiting their synthesis but leaving the catecholamine binding system intact. "The combination of a reduced amount of liberated transmitter plus rapid inactivation by an intact binding system may serve to dampen the stress-induced activation of central sympathetic centers." Whereas both reserpine and α-methyltyrosine prevent the stress-induced hypertension, the former does, whereas the latter does not cause mortality.

Salicylates ←

Smookler & Buckley H 32,862/70: In rats, exposure to a combination of stressors (noise, flashing lights, oscillation of the cage) causes pronounced hypertension and increased sensitivity to salicylate (gastric ulcers) and reserpine (mortality) intoxication. α-Methyltyrosine prevents the stress-induced hypertension, perhaps because it reduces the level of catecholamines by inhibiting their synthesis but leaving the catecholamine binding system intact. "The combination of a reduced amount of liberated transmitter plus rapid inactivation by an intact binding system may serve to dampen the stress-induced activation of central sympathetic centers." Whereas both reserpine and α-methyltyrosine prevent the stress-induced hypertension, the former does, whereas the latter does not cause mortality.

Salicylic Acid ← Stress (immobilization) + Pregnancy: Goldman et al. E 35,710/63*

Synephrine ← Stress (Cold): Inscoe et al. *F 70,325/66*

Tyramine ← Stress (Cold): Inscoe et al. *F 70,325/66*

Tyrosine ←

Alam et al. G 53,636/67: In rats fed low-protein diets, excessive tyrosine intake depresses growth and causes characteristic lesions in the paws and eyes. Injections of cortisol or stress produced by infusorial earth i.p. prevented the manifestations of tyrosine intoxication, presumably as a consequence of hepatic microsomal TPO induction. The effect of infusorial earth i.p. is ascribed to the resulting stress-induced increase in corticoid secretion.

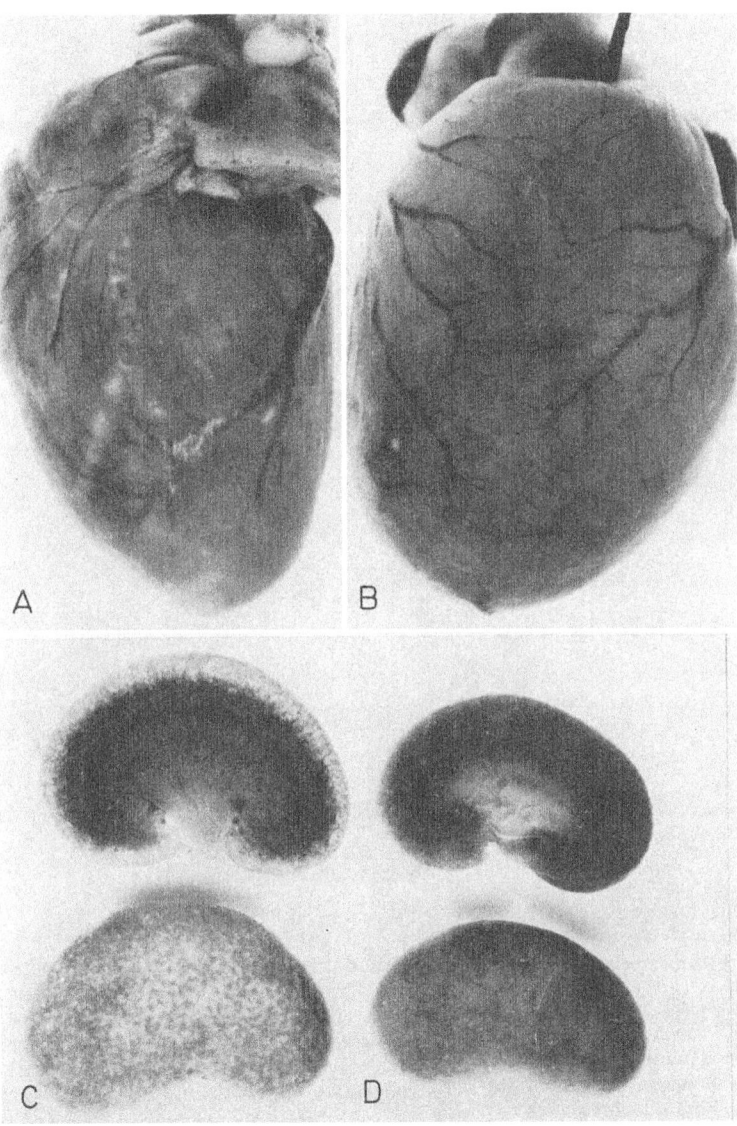

Fig. 31. **Protection by restraint against DHT.** Both rats received the same DHT-treatment during 4 days. In addition, one (A, C), was restrained on the first (3 hrs), third (5 hrs) and fifth (7 hrs) day. A, C: DHT alone produced the usual predominantly vascular calcification (white calcareous rings along the course of the major coronary branches) and, almost exclusively cortical, nephrocalcinosis with renal hypertrophy. B, D: The stress of restraint prevented this effect. [Selye C 92,918/61. Courtesy of Charles C Thomas.]

Fig. 32. **Protection by restraint against DHT.** Both rats received the same DHT-treatment. A + B: Intense "tigroid" and vascular calcification of the myocardium (visible on the cut surface of the heart) and calcification of the aorta, shown by blackening upon treatment with silver nitrate. C + D: Prevention of this calcification by repeated pretreatment with short periods of restraint. [Selye et al. C91,680/61. Path.-Biol.]

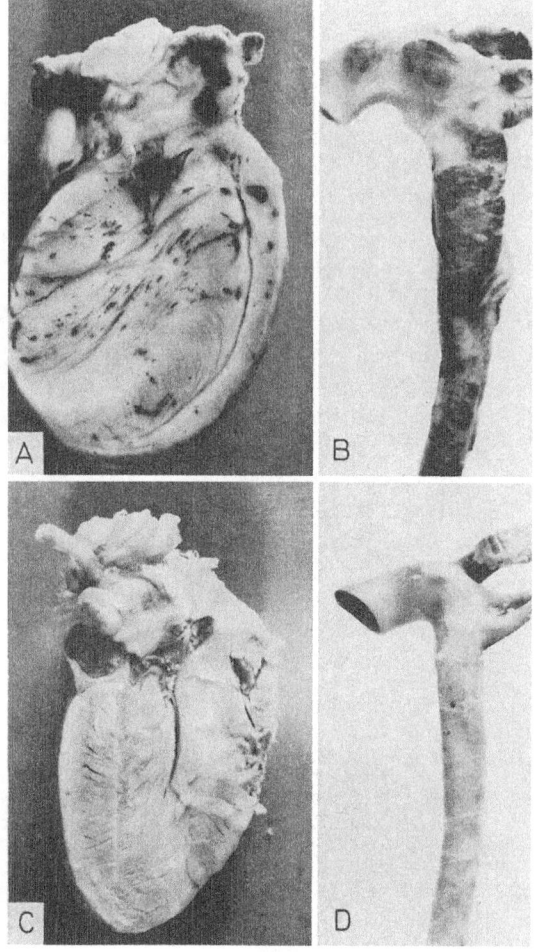

Vitamin A ←

Greaves & Schmidt A48,725/36: In rats, laparotomy and various toxic agents failed to influence vitamin-A requirements, but these are increased by thyroxine or desiccated thyroid, and decreased by thyroidectomy.

Vitamin D, DHT ←*cf. Selye C50,810/58, pp. 90, 115; C92,918/61, pp. 179, 181, 260, 266; D15,540/62, pp. 261, 282; G60,083/70, pp. 446, 451, 459, 461.*

Zoxazolamine ← Stress: Bousquet et al. F35,073/65*

Varia ←

Fouts et al. G68,041/61: Partially hepatectomized rats are deficient in the ability to oxidize the side-chain of **hexobarbital** or the ring-sulfur of **chlorpromazine**, and to reduce the nitro-group of **p-nitrobenzoic acid**. Full recovery of these activities occurs only after complete regeneration of the hepatic mass (about ten days after operation). O-dealkylation of **codeine** is impeded only during the first few days, when the regeneration is most active. Sham-hepatectomy (with exteriorization of the liver) has a similar, though much less pronounced effect.

Bousquet et al. F35,073/65: In rats with stress produced by applying a tourniquet around one hind limb for 2.5 hrs, the toxicity of **hexobarbital, pentobarbital, meprobamate** and **zoxazolamine** was significantly diminished, whereas that of barbital and phenobarbital remained unaffected. Pretreatment with ACTH or corticosterone stimulated the effect of stress. After hypophysectomy or adrenalectomy, stress failed to offer the usual protection. [The barbiturates and zoxazolamine appear to have been administered immediately after release of the tourniquet, but this is not specifically stated. Allegedly, a single injection of 50 µg per animal sufficed to offer protection (H.S.).]

Diet (Complex) ← *cf. Selye G60,083/70, p. 452.*

Parasites ←

Noble G81,736/71: In hamsters, various stressors as well as glucocorticoids aggravate infection with Leishmania braziliensis.

Varia ←

Innumerable publications deal with the effect of stressors upon **microbial infections** and the stressor effect of the infections themselves.

Rats, in which tolerance to **bacterial endotoxins** is induced by repeated daily injections, become highly resistant also to traumatic and hemorrhagic shock, but rats adapted to traumatic shock do not develop any significant degree of endotoxin tolerance. In general, exposure to stress increases mortality from endotoxin shock in various species of animals.

In rats, resistance to the **venoms** of scorpions and snakes is decreased by pretreatment with various stressors (heat, cold, epinephrine.)

It has been claimed that in mice, moderate sensitivity to various stressors is associated with the highest **X-ray** tolerance, whereas individuals especially sensitive or insensitive to stress have a low X-ray tolerance. In rats, repeated exhaustive muscular exercise after X-irradiation increases the ensuing mortality.

For the extensive literature on the effect of stressors upon the response to subsequent exposure to the same or other **stressors** (that is "nonspecific cross-resistance"), the reader must be referred to our earlier monographs quoted in the Abstract Section.

Among the first studies on the mechanism through which stress-induced hormone secretion could affect resistance are those dealing with **defensive enzyme** induction. Tryptophan induces hepatic **TPO** both in intact and in adrenalectomized rats, but various stressors which are equally effective in intact animals are ineffective in the absence of the adrenals. These findings called attention to the fact that in addition to substrate-induced hepatic enzyme activity, there is a second corticoid-mediated response which produces essentially the same results and is presumably responsible for much of the stress-induced nonspecific resistance. In agreement with this interpretation, hypophysectomy also prevents stress-induced TPO induction in rat liver. In intact rats, an i.p. injection of diatomaceous earth acts as a strong stressor and increases hepatic **TKT** activity. This effect is abolished by adrenalectomy, whereas cortisol is a good inducer of TKT both in intact and in adrenalectomized rats. In the latter, the effect of small doses of cortisol is potentiated by a simultaneous administration of either tyrosine or diatomaceous earth. Presumably, the glucocorticoid not only induces TKT but also acts as a conditioning agent for TKT activation both by its substrate and by nonspecific stress. The induction of TPO is regulated essentially in the same manner.

There is some evidence that at least certain stressors (reciprocating shaker) can stimulate corticoid secretion without any change in hepatic TKT or TPO activity. This was ascribed to the activation of mechanisms which specifically inhibit the induction of enzymes by glucocorticoids. However, the possibility must also be considered that certain types of stressors do not produce a sufficient quantity of glucocorticoids for effective enzyme induction. Extensive investigations have shown that cortisol enhances enzyme synthesis following an increased rate of synthesis of ribosomal transfer and "DNA-like" RNA. A repressor can inhibit enzyme synthesis at the translational level because inhibition of RNA synthesis prolongs corticoid-induced increases in enzyme synthesis.

Addition of cortisol to the blood perfused through a normal rat liver in vitro induces TPO, whereas this is not the case with livers of rats bearing large Walker tumors. The inhibition of induction is ascribed to a "toxohormone" which arises in the tumor tissue. This finding again suggests that stress may be associated not only with enzyme-inducing but also with induction-inhibiting mechanisms.

During the first days of life, rats exposed to the stress of a noisy reciprocating shaker respond with a large increase in TPO and TKT, whereas adult rats do not exhibit this change. Presumably, an induction-opposing mechanism is more developed in the adult than in the infant rat. In stressed adrenalectomized adults, TKT activity decreased markedly, whereas this was not the case in adrenalectomized immature rats. Hypophysectomy essentially abolished the inhibition in adults.

There is some evidence that STH may play a role in the repression of TKT induction by stressors. In any event, STH inhibits the synthesis of hepatic TKT in intact, hypophysectomized or adrenalectomized rats. Stress (reciprocating shaker) had no effect on hepatic TKT of intact rats, but increased TPO activity, although both these enzymes are corticoid inducible. Similarly stressed adrenalectomized rats exhibited a decreased TKT activity with no change in TPO. This inhibition was abolished by hypophysectomy. STH inhibited induction of TKT by cortisol, but had no effect upon cortisol-induced TPO activity.

The claim that the stress of forced muscular work, immobilization or cold can increase hepatic TPO activity even in adrenalectomized (though not in hypophysectomized) rats, requires confirmation.

Extensive studies on rats and rabbits exposed to various types of stress suggest that **lysosomal hydrolases** are released from the liver and intestine under the influence of various stressors and that this process may play a decisive role in the development of irreversible shock. The increase in lysosomal stability produced by glucocorticoids may constitute an important defensive response.

For the effect of stress upon **GOT, GPT, DNA-** and **RNA-polymerase** and other enzyme activities influenced by stress cf. the Abstract Section.

Microorganisms and Venoms ←

Bacteria ←. cf. also Selye G60,083/70, pp. 447, 453. Schäfer B99,955/54: Monograph (127 pp., numerous refs.) on the role of endocrine factors in tuberculosis. Special sections are devoted to the hormones of the thyroid, parathyroid, thymus, adrenals, pancreas and gonads. The hormonal defense reaction is viewed especially as a manifestation of the G.A.S.

Munoz E8,473/64: In mice sensitized with B. pertussis, the development of increased sensitivity to histamine or 5-HT is inhibited by various stressors.

Bacterial Toxins ← cf. also Selye E5,986/66, p. 119; G60,083/70, pp. 464, 465. Zweifach & Thomas D91,826/57: "Rats in which tolerance to bacterial endotoxin is induced, by repeated doses given daily, become highly resistant to the lethal effects of both drum trauma and hemorrhagic shock. However, rats in which the adaptation to traumatic shock is produced by repeated exposure to drum trauma, do not develop a significant degree of tolerance to lethal doses of endotoxin."

Renaud C 77,620/63: Review of the literature showing that exposure to stress greatly increases mortality in rats, rabbits and guinea pigs given E. coli endotoxin.

Venoms ←. *Stahnke F 57,253/65:* In rats treated with various scorpion and snake venoms, resistance was decreased by pretreatment with heat, cold or epinephrine. In all three cases, the change in resistance is ascribed to stress as such.

Immune Reactions ← *cf. Selye B 40,000/ 50, p. 752.*

Ionizing Rays ← *cf. also Selye B 87,000/ 52, p. 58; B 90,100/53, p. 83; C 1,001/54, p. 293.*

Kimeldorf et al. B 49,240/50: In rats, repeated exhaustive muscular exercice (swimming) after X-irradiation increases the resulting mortality.

Vácha & Pospíšil H 17,170/69: In mice, moderate sensitivity to various stressors is associated with the highest X-ray tolerance. Individuals exhibiting a specially mild or severe stress reaction are comparatively intolerant to X-irradiation.

Hypoxia and Hyperoxygenation ←

Campbell A 14,903/37: In rats exposed to six atmospheres of oxygen in a pressure chamber, subsequent decompression is better tolerated at low than at high external temperatures. "Using an external temperature of 24° C and white rats of about 80 g, the following substances, administered subcutaneously, are found to enhance oxygen poisoning: thyroxin (0.4 mg), dinitrophenol (1.5 mg), ac-tetrahydro- β-naphthylamine (0.5 c.c., 1 p.c.), adrenaline (0.02 mg), pituitary extract (posterior lobe, above 3.5 units), insulin (0.025 u.) and eserine (0.045 mg administered with atropine 0.075 mg). These doses in themselves are harmless."

Berry et al. H 2,124/68: Studies on the influence of hypoxia, glucocorticoids and endotoxin on hepatic enzyme induction and survival in mice. "Endotoxin inhibited the induction of tryptophan oxygenase, prevented the increase in liver glycogen, induced the transaminase, and increased the lethality of simulated altitude. Cortisone increased survival at all altitudes except the highest. These observations emphasize the importance of these metabolic adjustments for the survival of animals subjected to hypoxic stress.

Hepatic Lesions ← *cf. also "Hepatic Lesions" as Agents*

Bucher et al. G 72,546/69: Review of the humoral factors responsible for hepatic regeneration following partial hepatectomy. Hepatic DNA synthesis is stimulated in intact rats by parabiosis or cross-circulation with partially hepatectomized partners. Furthermore, tiny liver grafts implanted outside the portal area proliferate in response to partial ablation of the parent organ. Various stressors inhibit hepatic regeneration in partially hepatectomized rats, but this effect is not reproduced by ATCH or cortisol. On the other hand, adrenalectomy increases hepatic regeneration.

Moolten et al. H 30,606/70: In rats, the rise in hepatic DNA synthesis after partial hepatectomy is accelerated by surgical interventions or STH. Cortisone, cortisol and ACTH were ineffective. Neither stress nor STH stimulated DNA synthesis significantly in nonhepatectomized rats.

Hepatic Enzymes ←

TPO, TKT ←. *Knox B 71,418/51:* Tryptophan induces hepatic TPO both in intact and in adrenalectomized animals. Various other compounds (including epinephrine and histamine) which, to a lesser extent, have the same effect in intact animals, fail to act after adrenalectomy. "The first mechanism has been identified as that of enzyme adaptation, previously known only in micro-organism, and the second has been identified as the stress reaction, acting through the adrenal glands."

Wood et al. C 27,721/56: In mice, bearing sarcoma implants, the hepatic TPO activity was first diminished, but rose above normal as the neoplasms grew. "Changes analogous to this biphasic depression and elevation of the enzyme level in tumor-bearing animals could be produced in control mice by growth hormone and by adrenal-stimulating stress, respectively."

Lin & Knox C 73,824/58: In rats, the hepatic TKT activity increased after treatment with cortisone, cortisol, or corticosterone, and L-tyrosine. This effect was observed also following adrenalectomy. On the other hand, a comparable effect of other amino acids was probably due to stress. "That a nonspecific stress-producing agent could actually increase the level of tyrosine-α-ketoglutarate transaminase was further supported by the results obtained with a compound which is unrelated to tyrosine metabolism. Injections of propylene glycol in doses of 0.5 ml per 100 gm of body weight caused the level of this enzyme to increase to an average of 1390 units in three intact rats." Adrenalectomized rats did not support this dose of propylene glycol.

Knox G67,799/58: Review of the literature and personal observations lead to the conclusion that hepatic microsomal TPO activity plays an important role in metabolic adaptation to stress. Stressors act through the pituitary and adrenal axis upon hepatic TPO, whereas tryptophan, STH and cortisol may act upon the liver directly.

Maickel & Brodie C83,071/60: TPO in rat liver is increased by ACTH, cortisone, or cortisol, as well as by various stressor agents and barbiturates. Hypophysectomy prevents the effect of stressors and of barbiturates, suggesting that the latter act through the pituitary-adrenal system.

Kenney & Flora D12,237/61: Tryptophan and i.p. injections of diatomaceous earth (Celite) were as effective as tyrosine in inducing increases in hepatic TKT in intact, but not in adrenalectomized rats. Cortisol was an effective inducer at low doses in both intact and adrenalectomized animals. In the latter, the effect of a small dose of cortisol was potentiated by simultaneous administration of tyrosine, methionine or diatomaceous earth. "It is concluded that induction of tyrosine transaminase is entirely mediated by adrenal hormone." In not adrenalectomized rats, diatomaceous earth i.p. is believed to act as a stressor through adrenocortical stimulation.

Knox G51,969/62: Review on the effect of stress upon hepatic TPO production. In adrenalectomized animals, only tryptophan of a series of analogues induces this enzyme, whereas, in intact rats, various stressors, ACTH, cortisone, cortisol and corticosterone (but not DOC) do so. "The recognition of the adrenal hormone-induced adaptation of the tryptophan pyrrolase has provided the unified explanation for a large number of different stressful stimuli which increase the enzyme level."

Geller et al. G22,722/64: In rats, hepatic TPO and TKT activities are increased 3.5 hrs after i.p. injection of cortisol, but no such activation was seen after stress (animals placed in a mechanical shaker) which causes an increase in adrenal and plasma glucocorticoids, as well as a depletion of adrenal ascorbic acid. Possibly, the amount of glucocorticoid secreted was not equivalent to that injected.

Schapiro et al. G21,848/64: In the rat, cortisol greatly increases hepatic TPO, TKT and tryptophan transaminase activity, whereas stress (reciprocating shaker) stimulates corticoid secretion without any change in hepatic transaminase or pyrrolase activity. Apparently, stress activates not only the adrenal cortex, but also the mechanisms which block the induction of these enzymes by corticoids, because shaker stress inhibited the elevation of hepatic transaminase that occurred following cortisol, although it did not block the elevation of tryptophan pyrrolase in the rat.

Kenney & Albritton G64,557/65: Review of the literature suggesting that transaminase induction in response to stressors can be due to corticoid secretion during the stress reaction. Cortisol enhances enzyme synthesis following an increased rate of synthesis of ribosomal transfer and "DNA-like" RNAs. The present experiments confirm the view that repressor(s) can inhibit enzyme synthesis at the translational level because inhibition of RNA synthesis can prolong the corticoid-induced increase in enzyme synthesis under suitable conditions. "Administration of stressing agents (tyrosine, Celite) to adrenalectomized rats initiates a highly selective repression of the synthesis of hepatic tyrosine-α-ketoglutarate transaminase. The enzyme level falls with a $t^1/_2$ of about 2.5 hr. Immunochemical measurement of the rate of enzyme synthesis indicates that it is reduced essentially to zero in stressed, adrenalectomized rats, whereas labeling of total liver soluble proteins is unaffected. Actinomycin does not itself influence the enzyme level, but it blocks the stress-initiated repression of enzyme synthesis, indicating that repression acts at the translational level, whereas initiation of repression involves transcriptional processes." In hypophysectomized rats stressors are ineffective and preliminary data suggest that STH is responsible for transaminase repression.

Nomura et al. G33,405/65: Various forms of stress (forced exercise, immobilization, cold), as well as the administration of chlorpromazine, increased the TPO activity of the liver in both intact and adrenalectomized, but not in hypophysectomized, rats.

Shiba et al. G31,114/65: The addition of cortisol to the blood perfused through a normal rat liver in vitro induced hepatic TPO, whereas this was not the case with livers of rats bearing large Walker tumors. The inhibitory effect upon enzyme induction is ascribed to "toxohormone" (an extract of Walker tumors), since addition of a toxohormone preparation to the perfusion fluid also prevented enzyme induction by cortisol.

Schapiro et al. F65,746/65—66: "Infant rats, four and eight days after birth, respond to the stress of 30 minutes on a noisy reciprocating shaker with a large increase in liver aromatic amino acid transaminase activities. Adult rats exposed to the same stress do not exhibit this change. In the adult rat the inducing effects of cortisol on transaminase activities are blocked by this stress. These results suggest the activation of a mechanism(s) in the adult rat which opposes the enzyme inducing effects of cortisol."

Schapiro et al. F67,227/66: Hepatic TKT-activity increased in immature, stressed (reciprocating shaker) rats, but not in intact stressed adults. In the stressed adrenalectomized adults, TKT activity markedly decreased, while adrenalectomized immature rats showed no change. Hypophysectomy largely abolished inhibition in the adults. TPO activity, when present, was increased by stress in old-age groups, but the increase was abolished by adrenalectomy and hypophysectomy. "The results suggest stress-activation of a pituitary mechanism that inhibits or represses activation of tyrosine transaminase and that may not function during early postnatal life."

Agarwal & Berry G66,479/66: In the mouse, stress produced by i.p. injection of celite or bentonite causes no significant change in hepatic TPO activity at the time when sensitization to endotoxin is already developed. The inducibility of TPO is delayed by injections of cortisone at a time when the hormone protects against endotoxin. Still, the results are considered to be "in agreement with the concept that maintenance of liver (TPO) is necessary for continued survival of endotoxin poisoned mice. The absence of change in this enzyme seen in celite- and bentonite-injected mice sensitized to endotoxin is an apparent exception." Presumably, "suppression of TP-activity is not the only way in which mice may be sensitized to endotoxin."

Kenney G50,810/67: In intact, hypophysectomized or adrenalectomized rats, STH inhibits the synthesis of hepatic TKT. The rate of enzyme synthesis is reduced nearly to 0 (immunochemical-isotopic analyses), whereas labeling of the bulk of the liver proteins is increased by STH. Repression is blocked when RNA synthesis is inhibited by actinomycin. STH also appears to play a role in the repression of TKT induction by stressors. A hypophysectomized and an intact rat were united by parabiosis. When the pituitary-bearing member was stressed by tyrosine i.p., repression occurred in the livers of both treated and untreated (hypophysectomized) animals. Transaminase levels were unchanged in a single experiment, where the stressing agent was administered to the hypophysectomized partner.

Schapiro H2,360/68: Stress (30 min rough agitation in a noisy laboratory shaker) had no effect upon the corticoid sensitive enzyme TKT in the liver of the intact rat, but it increased TPO activity, which is likewise corticoid inducible. Adrenalectomized rats similarly stressed exhibited a decreased TKT activity with no change in TPO. This inhibitory effect was abolished by hypophysectomy. STH inhibited induction of TKT by cortisol but had no effect upon cortisol-induced TPO activity. The opposing actions of STH and glucocorticoids may be involved in adaptive reactions to stress.

Finch et al. G71,207/69: In mice, various stressors (cold, shaking) cause a rapid and transient increase in hepatic TKT activity during fasting. Recent feeding or adrenalectomy inhibits TKT induction by cold.

Geller et al. H8,414/69: The stress of laparotomy increases hepatic TKT activity in intact, but not in the adrenalectomized rat, which actually responds in an inverse manner. Hypophysectomy eliminates some, but not all of this laparotomy-induced repression. Under these conditions, the TPO- and the TKT-responses are somewhat different.

Schapiro et al. H12,411/69: Brief abstract stating (without giving experimental details) that "the servere stress of laparotomy in the intact adult rat induces a large corticoid-dependent increase in transaminase activity. STH administered simultaneously, or one hour before laparotomy will completely inhibit this enzyme increase. During the early postnatal period, however, STH will not block transaminase induction caused by cortisol or laparotomy."

Lysosomal Hydrolases ←. *Janoff et al. D35,553/62:* Studies on the hepatic lysosomal enzymes of rats and rabbits after traumatic or endotoxin shock, adrenalectomy, or treatment with cortisone suggested that "a) disruption of lysosomes and release of their contained enzymes in free, active form may occur in liver and intestine of shocked animals. b) The activation of lysosomal hydrolases within cells and their release into the circulation may play an important role in exacerbating tissue injury and accelerating the development of irreversibility during shock. c) The increased stability of lysosomes of tolerant and of cortisone-treated animals may constitute an important component of the resistance of these animals to shock."

GOT, GPT ←. *Brin & McKee C 31,261/56:* In the rat, various stressors (total body X-irradiation, nitrogen mustard, starvation) as well as cortisone increase GOT and GPT activities in the liver. Adrenalectomy decreases the activity of these enzymes. The glutamic-alanine enzyme is more sensitive to stress than the glutamic-aspartic enzyme.

Hänninen & Hartiala F 76,119/67: In the rat, the stress of restraint causes within 12 hrs a linear increase in hepatic GOT to 4 times the initial level. This effect was partially inhibited by actinomycin D and totally by adrenalectomy.

DNA-, RNA-Polymerase ←. *Gresham & Pover G 58,354/68:* In the rat, alkaline RNAse levels increase in the mucosa of the small intestine after total body or selective head X-irradiation, as well as after treatment with such radiomimetic drugs as chlorambucil or busulfan but not after treatment with ACTH, cortisol or various stressors. Still, a relationship to the G.A.S. is suspected because blockade of the normal neuroendocrine responses to stress by combined treatment with morphine + pentobarbital blocked the intestinal RNAse response to X-irradiation, and the latter was also lacking in newborn rats in which hypothalamic control of anterior pituitary function has not yet developed.

Šimek et al. H 13,837/68: Comparative studies on DNA synthesis, fatty acid content, and weight regeneration in the liver remnant of partially hepatectomized rats after treatment with cortisol, ACTH and various stressor agents.

Trypsin ← cf. *Selye C 92,918/61, p. 106.*

Other Enzymes ←. *Remmer C 73,857/58:* Drug-metabolizing enzyme formation in hepatic microsomes of adrenalectomized rats is inhibited unless the rats receive glucocorticoid treatment. The decreased general resistance of adrenalectomized animals may depend upon an interference with defensive enzyme formation.

Terayama & Takata F 69,475/66: The N-demethylating activity of rat liver is considerably reduced during regeneration after partial hepatectomy but, for a much shorter period, also after sham-operations.

Morton & Chatfield G 73,681/70: In rats with adjuvant arthritis, "the liver microsomal N-demethylase and NADPH$_2$-oxidase enzyme activity and levels of cytochrome P-450 are greatly reduced. This implies a reduced capacity for the oxidative metabolism of steroids and foreign compounds in adjuvant arthritic rats which should influence the toxicity and half-life of any administered compound. The ability of the liver to form β-glucuronide conjugates is also reduced."

← VARIA

Here, we shall briefly discuss the effect upon resistance and particularly upon hepatic detoxication, of a few additional agents which are only indirectly, related to hormonal mechanisms, if at all.

← *Parabiosis*

The factors regulating the intense mitotic proliferation induced by **partial hepatectomy** in the regenerating liver remnant have aroused the interest of many investigators. If two rats are joined in parabiosis, one being partially hepatectomized, mitotic proliferation is stimulated to some extent even in the intact partner. It was concluded that some blood-borne humoral factor is involved in this type of growth stimulation. Although this claim has been contradicted, negative data have been ascribed to the inadequate establishment of a cross-circulation, especially since even tiny liver grafts implanted outside of the portal area proliferate in response to partial ablation of the parent organ.

In another experiment, a hypophysectomized and an intact rat were united by parabiosis. When the pituitary-bearing member was stressed, hepatic TKT induction was repressed in both partners. Since repression can also be obtained by STH, this hormone was held responsible for the stress-induced repression.

← Diurnal Variations

In rats, the incorporation of radioactive acetate into **cholesterol** reaches a maximum at about midnight, and a minimum at about noon.

Hepatic **hexobarbital oxidase** induction is likewise subject to a light-dependent circadian rhythm. **TKT** activity in rat liver undergoes also considerable diurnal change.

← Nervous Lesions

In rats, the anesthetic effect of progesterone is prevented by pretreatment with atropine, and intensified by vagotomy, but it remains to be seen whether these actions are specific.

← Tumors

In young rats transplants of a pituitary mammotrophic tumor did not prevent the induction by phenobarbital of hepatic microsomal **hexobarbital-** and **aminopyrine-metabolizing enzymes**. However, the normal development of these enzyme systems was inhibited, presumably by the STH, ACTH, LTH or other hormones secreted by the hypophysial neoplasms.

Tumor transplants and tumor extracts have also been shown to affect microsomal **steroidases** in the rat liver.

In mice, small subcutaneous sarcoma implants depress the hepatic **TPO** activity, whereas large tumors have an opposite effect. In intact (unlike in adrenalectomized, ascites-tumor-bearing) mice, hepatic **TKT** activity is elevated.

The growth of Walker tumors and transplantable hepatomas, unlike that of Jensen sarcomas and Murphy lymphosarcomas, is increased by **partial hepatectomy** in the rat. It has been postulated that the regenerating liver may release humoral agents which stimulate the growth of some neoplasms. Conversely, both in rats and in mice, hepatic regeneration was enhanced by the presence of growing tumor tissue irrespective of whether the latter was affected by partial hepatectomy.

← Parabiosis

Christensen & Jacobsen A 49,204/49; Bucher et al. D 42,066/51: In rats, the mitotic rate in the liver remnant reaches a maximum 48 hrs after partial hepatectomy. If two rats are united by parabiosis, one being partially hepatectomized, some increase in mitotic proliferation occurs also in the nonhepatectomized partner, suggesting the formation of cell division stimulating substances.

Bielschowsky & Hall G 71,797/51: In intact female rats joined in parabiosis with gonadectomized litter-mates, AAF induced a 50% incidence of malignant tumors, mostly of the granulosa. The gonadectomized partners were free of neoplastic lesions.

Bucher G 68,621/63 (p. 281): Review of the conflicting data on the stimulation of hepatic regeneration in the intact partner of a pair of parabiotic rats in which the other partner is partially hepatectomized. Apparent contradictions may be due to differences in the efficiency of the cross-circulation.

Kenney G 50,810/67: In intact, hypophysectomized or adrenalectomized rats, STH inhibits the synthesis of hepatic TKT. The rate of enzyme synthesis is reduced nearly to 0 (immunochemical-isotopic analysis), whereas labeling of the bulk of the liver proteins is increased by STH. Represssion is blocked when RNA synthesis is inhibited by actinomycin. STH also appears to play a role in the repression of TKT induction by stressors. A hypophysectomized and an intact rat were united by parabiosis. When the pituitary-bearing member was stressed by tyrosine i.p., repression occurred in the livers of both treated and untreated (hypophysectomized) animals. TKT levels were unchanged in a single experiment where the stressing agent was administered to the hypophysectomized partner.

Bucher et al. G72,546/69: Review of the humoral factors responsible for hepatic regeneration following partial hepatectomy. Hepatic DNA synthesis is stimulated in intact rats by parabiosis or cross-circulation with partially hepatectomized partners. Furthermore, tiny liver grafts implanted outside the portal area, proliferate in response to partial ablation of the parent organ. Various stressors inhibit hepatic regeneration in partially hepatectomized rats, but this effect is not reproduced by ACTH or cortisol. On the other hand, adrenalectomy increases hepatic regeneration.

← *Diurnal Variations*

Barbiturates ←. *Roberts et al. H31,840/70:* In rats, the degradation of marked barbiturates by hepatic microsomal enzymes in vitro reached a maximum at 8.00 A.M. and a minimum at 8.00 P.M. The diurnal rhythm in vivo was much less pronounced. "A variation in the sensitivity of the central nervous system to barbiturate has also been observed, rats being least sensitive at a time when they were normally highly active." The literature on diurnal variations in drug metabolism is briefly reviewed.

Cholesterol ←. *Hamprecht G69,560/69:* In rats, the incorporation of radioactive acetate into cholesterol is subject to pronounced diurnal variations with a minimum at about noon, and a maximum at midnight.

Hepatic Enzymes ←. *Nair et al. G67,250/69:* Hepatic hexobarbital oxidase induction is inhibited by head X-irradiation, hypophysectomy or bilateral electrolytic lesions in the posterior hypothalamus. The in vitro data were verified by measurements of the hexobarbital sleeping time. "It is suggested that the microsomal enzyme system metabolizing hexobarbital is normally under the regulatory control of hypothalamo-hypophyseal hormonal activity. The light dependent circadian rhythm for this enzyme, recently reported by us, is also consistent with this interpretation."

Civen et al. H12,169/69: TKT activity in rat liver undergoes a 4-fold diurnal change, which is independent of steroid secretion, although the enzyme is inducible by glucocorticoids.

← *Nervous Lesions*

Selye A35,659/41: "In rats, pretreatment with atropin prevents, while vagotomy actually intensifies the anesthetic action of progesterone."

← *Tumors (in Animals) cf. also Carcinogens under Drugs*

Wilson G63,125/68: In young rats, transplants of a pituitary mammotrophic tumor "did not prevent an increase in the liver microsomal metabolism of hexobarbital or the formation of formaldehyde from aminopyrine which followed phenobarbital pretreatment. High levels of somatotropin, corticotropin, and prolactin in blood, or possibly some other unknown factors produced by this tumor, appeared to prevent the normal development of the liver enzyme system which metabolized hexobarbital, aminopyrine, and p-nitrobenzoic acid in the rat."

Wood Jr. & Knox D81,779/54: In mice bearing small subcutaneous sarcoma implants, the hepatic TPO activity was depressed, whereas animals with large tumor transplants showed a marked increase in the activity of this enzyme.

Paschkis et al. C8,982/55: In rats, the growth of Walker tumors and of transplantable hepatomas, unlike that of Jensen sarcomas and Murphy lymphosarcomas, was increased after partial hepatectomy. Perhaps "the regenerating liver may release a humoral agent causing increased growth of some tumors." Hepatic regeneration was enhanced by the presence of a growing tumor regardless of whether the latter was influenced by partial hepatectomy or not.

Gershbein E71,030/63: In rats, s.c. transplantation of Walker or Flexner-Jobling tumors did not significantly alter the extent of hepatic regeneration. However, under certain circumstances, partial hepatectomy accelerated tumor growth.

Kato G54,276/67: In intact, unlike in adrenalectomized, ascites-tumor-bearing mice, the hepatic TKT activity is elevated.

Rosene Jr. G71,661/68: In mice, partial hepatectomy greatly elevates mitotic proliferation in the liver, which reaches a peak on the third day after the operation and returns to near normal by the fifth day. Injections of Ehrlich ascites tumor homogenates moderately accelerated the rate of hepatic mitosis. Partial hepatectomy accelerated tumor cell proliferation.

Saint-Omer et al. G71,148/68: In mice bearing ascites tumors, mitotic proliferation and regeneration of the liver after partial hepatectomy is delayed.

Konishi H14,720/69: Changes in Δ^4-steroid hydrogenase activity in rat liver after tumor implantation.

Takahashi & Kato H15,250/69: Studies on changes in hepatic microsomal steroidases induced in rats by treatment with toxohormone (a Walker tumor extract).

Theologides & Zaki H19,577/69: In C3H mice bearing transplanted mammary carcinomas s.c., increased mitotic activity in the liver remnant after partial hepatectomy began earlier than in controls.

Wilson H34,926/71: In rats, implants of mammotropic tumor (which secretes STH, ACTH and LTH) decreased the hepatic metabolism of hexobarbital and aminopyrine. Similar but much less pronounced changes were observed in rats bearing very large Walker tumors.

VIII. CLINICAL IMPLICATIONS

To evaluate the clinical applicability of the hormonal regulation of resistance, a few introductory words may be in order.

We need say little here about the major applications of **syntoxic** hormones, particularly glucocorticoids (e.g., in inflammatory diseases or as immunosuppressants), since these have been extensively discussed in our earlier monographs on stress, and are by now generally known. Suffice it to call attention to the possible future clinical applicability of a few new syntoxic hormones which, in animals, have proven their value as antagonists of systemic intoxications with various drugs (e.g., ganglionic blocking agents, lathyrogens, endotoxins, certain barbiturates). These effects are manifest even in the presence of normally functioning adrenals. They suggest that glucocorticoids do not merely act against the excessive stress-sensitivity of hypocorticoid organisms or as anti-inflammatory compounds, but possess certain rather specific protective effects against some toxicants. It remains to be seen to what extent these prophylactic actions are due to so-called "physiologic antagonisms" between certain effects of glucocorticoids and toxicants which happen to be opposed (e.g., the glyconeogenic effect which prevents insulin hypoglycemia; the potassium loss which counteracts potassium intoxication.)

Here we shall try to survey primarily the possible clinical uses of **catatoxic** hormones under the following headings:

1. Hepatic microsomal drug metabolism in man
    Contraceptives
    Other steroids
    Barbiturates
    Diphenylhydantoin
    Other drugs (glutethimide, griseofulvin, salicylates, etc.)
2. Diseases
    Hyperbilirubinemia
    Adrenal tumors and Cushing's syndrome
    Other diseases (cardiac diseases, hepatic lesions, osteoporosis, galactosemia, v. Gierke's disease, endotoxin shock)
3. Pregnancy (abortifacient action of microsomal enzyme inducers)

1. HEPATIC MICROSOMAL DRUG METABOLISM IN MAN

There is ample evidence that many of the drugs which have been shown to induce drug-metabolizing enzymes in animals exert the same effect in man. Of these inducers, contraceptives, barbiturates, diphenylhydantoin, glutethimide, meprobamate, phenylbutazone and griseofulvin have received the greatest attention. Among the substrates whose metabolism is accelerated by these inducers are various steroids, anticonvulsants, anticoagulants, bilirubin, meprobamate, aminopyrine, salicylamide and many others. Chlorinated insecticides are particularly effective enzyme inducers in man, but their use is limited by their toxicity. Smoking during pregnancy may induce benzpyrene hydroxylase in the placenta.

The widespread use of **contraceptives** poses an especially important problem, in that some of them may induce microsomal enzymes which interfere with the action of various drugs, and in turn, other microsomal enzyme inducers may inactivate the contraceptives. In addition, these pills may interfere with hepatic function in general (as reflected by demonstrable increases in GOT, GPT, bilirubin or prolonged BSP retention) and thereby enhance the action of drugs. Liver biopsies have repeatedly revealed signs of hepatocellular damage, proliferation of the SER, and intrahepatic cholestasis. The commonly used oral contraceptives contain folliculoids and luteoids in combination; hence, it is often difficult to verify which of the two components is responsible for an observed change. Some authors claimed that hepatotoxicity is primarily referrable to the folliculoid component, whereas stimulation of drug metabolism is predominantly due to the luteoid element, but this view has been challenged.

Following administration of meperidine, pethidine or promazine, women on oral contraceptives, like pregnant women, excreted a larger than normal amount of these drugs unchanged in the urine. Similar effects were observed in neonates as well as in males given stilbestrol or progesterone. Apparently, pregnancy diminishes the capacity to metabolize meperidine, pethidine and promazine, a change also seen in neonates and subjects taking oral contraceptives.

The plasma tyrosine level is sometimes significantly decreased in women taking contraceptives, presumably because the folliculoid component stimulates the production of glucocorticoids which elevate the TPO activity. This view is supported by observations in rats, in which estradiol increases hepatic TPO, TKT and GPT.

In man, **barbiturates** (e.g., phenobarbital) increase tolerance to digitoxin by enhancing its conversion and urinary excretion as digoxin. Because of its almost negligible hypnotic effect, phetharbital has been used by some clinicians and was shown to increase urinary excretion of 6β-hydroxycortisol in man. Phenobarbital also accelerates the plasma clearance of i.v. injected cortisol. Heptabarbital and several other barbiturates increase the hepatic destruction of bishydroxycoumarin as well as of related anticoagulants. This fact is of considerable practical importance, since in patients receiving both types of drugs simultaneously, the dosage of the anticoagulant must be raised in order to obtain the usual action. Furthermore, when barbiturate administration is suddenly stopped, the effect of the anticoagulant may rise sufficiently to cause severe hemorrhagic complications.

A farmer from an area of heavy pesticide usage was given phenobarbital and diphenylhydantoin for the treatment of epilepsy. His blood levels of DDT, DDE, dieldrin and hepatachlor were far below those of other farmers living in the same area.

In man, **diphenylhydantoin** increases 6-hydroxycortisol excretion and simultaneously decreases the elimination of conjugated tetrahydro derivatives. As previously stated, diphenylhydantoin diminishes the blood level of various pesticides in man.

Following prolonged treatment with diphenylhydantoin, usually in combination with barbiturates, osteomalacia-like changes have been observed to develop in epileptic patients. These skeletal lesions respond well to vitamin-D compounds, and have been attributed to the acceleration of vitamin-D metabolism by enhanced microsomal enzyme activity.

In cases of **glutethimide** abuse, the gradual development of tolerance is apparently due to a transient acceleration of its own metabolic inactivation.

The anticoagulant activity of warfarin is sometimes markedly depressed in patients treated with **griseofulvin**. This has been ascribed to an accelerated metabolic degradation of the anticoagulant.

In patients with rheumatoid arthritis, the plasma clearance of radiomarked indomethacin is accelerated, and its urinary excretion diminished by **acetylsalicylic acid**. However, this effect has been ascribed to diminished gastrointestinal absorption rather than to accelerated metabolic degradation of indomethacin.

In patients given **phenylbutazone**, the urinary excretion of 6β-hydroxycortisol is increased, whereas the elimination of 17-OHCS is decreased. It will be recalled that 6β-hydroxycortisol formation from cortisol is enhanced by hepatic microsomes of guinea pigs in vitro, following pretreatment of the animals with phenylbutazone in vivo.

Reviews

Williams G77,567/63: Review (21 pp., 84 refs.) on drug detoxication mechanisms in man.

Burns & Conney G71,448/64: Review (25 pp., 57 refs.) on the therapeutic implications of drug-metabolism in man.

Conney F88,649/67 (p. 348): Review of the literature on enzyme induction in man.

Mannering G71,818/68 (pp. 74, 90): Review on species differences in susceptibility to the induction of hepatic microsomal drug-metabolizing enzymes. Special attention is given to the induction of drug-metabolizing enzymes in man.

Mannering G75,979/69: Review (4 pp., 32 refs.) briefly summarizing the salient facts about stimulation and inhibition of drug metabolism. Observations of drug-induced stimulation of drug metabolism in man are tabulated as follows:

Inducing agent	Substrate	Reference
Phenobarbital	Diphenylhydantoin	Cucinell et al., 1965
	Digitoxin	Jelliffee and Blankenhorn, 1966
	Griseofulvin	Busfield et al., 1963
	Coumadin	Robinson and MacDonald, 1966
	Bishydroxycoumarin	Cucinell et al., 1965; Corn and Rockett, 1965; Goss and Dickhaus, 1965
	Salicylamide	Crigler and Gold, 1966
	Bilirubin	Yaffe et al., 1966; Crigler and Gold, 1966
Barbital	Dipyrone	Remmer, 1962
Heptobarbital	Acenocoumarin	Catalano and Cullen, 1966
	Biscoumacetate	Catalano and Cullen, 1966
	Bishydroxycoumarin	Catalano and Cullen, 1966
Diphenylhydantoin	Cortisol	Werk et al., 1964
Glutethimide	Glutethimide	Schmid et al., 1964
Meprobamate	Meprobamate	Douglas et al., 1963
Phenylbutazone	Aminopyrine	Chen et al., 1962
Griseofulvin	Coumadin	Catalano and Cullen, 1966

Mannering G74,881/71: Review of the literature concerning drugs known to influence metabolism of other drugs in man. The following drugs have been shown to induce increased rates of metabolism of coumarins in man: barbiturates, chloral hydrate, griseofulvin and meprobamate. Phenobarbital stimulates the metabolism of diphenylhydantoin, griseofulvin, digitoxin, and the glucuronidation of salicylamide in man. Phenylbutazone increases the metabolism of aminopyrine, whereas meprobamate and glutethimide enhance their own rates of metabolism in man. Chlorinated insecticides are particularly effective in this respect. For example, DDT shortens the plasma half-lives of antipyrine in man.

Clinical Implications

Prescott H19,333/69: Review (5 pp., 89 refs.) on pharmacokinetic drug interactions with special reference to clinical problems.

Tuohy G66,351/69: Brief review (3 pp., 26 refs.) on microsomal drug-metabolizing enzyme induction as it affects clinical medicine.

← Contraceptives

Eisalo et al. F18,828/64: In postmenopausal women treated during 28 days with contraceptive pills containing various folliculoids and luteoids, hepatic impairment was regularly demonstrable by increased serum GOT and GPT levels associated with BSP retention. The luteoid component in itself was inactive, but the folliculoid showed essentially the same hepatotoxic activity as the whole drug.

Palva & Mustala F21,067/64: In women taking contraceptive pills, hepatotoxic damage is clearly demonstrable by increased BSP retention associated with a rise in serum bilirubin and GOT.

Borglin F40,990/65: Among 36 patients treated with oral contraceptives "in only a few instances did the values obtained deviate from normal — namely, an increase of the transaminase activity and a slight increase of the BSP retention. The serum alkaline phosphatase values, the serum bilirubin level, and the thymol turbidity tests were invariably normal. In those cases where abnormal laboratory values were noted, the S.G.P.T. proved the most sensitive value."

Cullberg et al. F34,942/65: "A case of jaundice which appeared during treatment with the oral contraceptive Lyndiol is reported. It is probable that the jaundice was caused by the drug. Laboratory data of the case include elevated levels of bilirubin, alkaline phosphatases, and transaminases. Biopsy of the liver showed intrahepatic cholestasis and hepatocellular damage." The relevant literature is reviewed.

Swyer & Little F42,188/65: Review of the literature, and personal observations on the rarity of hepatic damage among women who have used various oral contraceptives for long periods.

Crawford & Rudofsky G42,454/66: In women taking various oral contraceptives, as well as in pregnant women and in neonates, the urinary excretion of meperidine and promazine is increased, suggesting interference with the detoxication of these drugs.

Rudofsky & Crawford E58,989/66: Following administration of meperidine or promazine "pregnant women, women on oral contraceptives and neonates excreted significantly more unchanged meperidine than normeperidine, whereas the reverse held for the male 'controls' and other female groups. Pregnant women, women on oral contraceptives and neonates excreted more unchanged and minimally degraded promazine than nonpregnant women. Stilbestrol and progesterone each changed the pattern of excretion by male subjects toward that associated with pregnancy." Apparently, pregnancy diminishes the capacity to metabolize meperidine and promazine, a change reflected in neonates and subjects taking oral contraceptives.

Conti & Neglia H30,753/68: In 18 women kept on contraceptive pills (norethinodrel + mestranol) up to six months, no derangement in hepatic function tests (GOT, GPT, serum-proteins, cholesterol, bilirubin) was noted. Yet, the authors recommend caution in the use of such contraceptives in women with hepatic disease.

Larsson-Cohn G74,875/69: In women continuously taking norethindrone (NET) or chlormadinone acetate (CMA), no significant changes were observed in serum alanine aminotransferase activity or BSP clearance. Apparently "low doses of NET and CMA have a lower tendency to influence liver function than combined oral contraceptive agents."

Mowat & Arias G74,246/69: "Oral contraceptive agents cause a predictable and reversible fall in hepatic excretory function in all subjects appropriately tested." At the same time, there is induction of hepatic drug-metabolizing enzymes which may alter the responsiveness of women to various drugs, and conversely, others have shown that the uterotrophic effect of oral contraceptives is reduced by phenobarbital, at least in rats. "We can only speculate as to what this may mean for the insomniac on phenobarbitone who relies on the pill for contraception."

Perez et al. H 14,794/69: In women on oral contraceptives (chlormadinone + mestranol or noretisterone + ethinylestradiol) for 1—6 months, liver biopsies showed proliferation of the SER, whereas after 12—30 months, there were also often striking changes in the shape and size of the mitochondria, with the development of paracrystalline inclusions. Liver function tests were unaltered.

Eisalo H 29,326/70: In women on various types of contraceptive pills containing luteoids and folliculoids, the most common anomalies of hepatic functions are elevation of SGOT and SGPT with increased BSP-retention.

Kreek & Sleisenger G 77,590/70: "Classification of patients developing abnormal liver function tests or clinical jaundice while receiving oral contraceptive agents is proposed. The results of a recent study concerning the effects on liver function of low dose estrogen-progestin replacement therapy in menopausal and post-menopausal females are discussed."

Luhby et al. H 32,376/70: In women taking ethinylestradiol-containing contraceptives, there develops a derangement in tryptophan metabolism associated with "functional" vitamin-B_6 deficiency.

Martinez-Manautou et al. H 30,302/70: In women treated for several years with oral contraceptives containing a luteoid (chlormadinone acetate) with or without folliculoids "a moderate dilatation and vesiculation of the rough and smooth surfaced endoplasmic reticulum both in the women treated with microdoses of progestogens, and in those treated with a combination of progestogens and oestrogens. A more marked vesiculation of this organelle was present in those women under sequential medication. Elongation of mitochondria with crystalloid inclusions in their matrices was found in 5 to 10% of the whole population of mitochondria per cell examined in the chlormadinone treated women."

Rose & Braidman H 25,726/70: In rats, estradiol increases hepatic TPO, TKT and GPT. The depression which develops in some women using contraceptive pills may be due to an increased metabolism of tryptophan to nicotinic acid ribonucleotide, and to a raised aminotransferase activity which may divert pyridoxal phosphate away from other metabolic functions, including 5-HT synthesis.

Rose & Cramp G 75,215/70: In women using folliculoid-luteoid contraceptives, the plasma tyrosine level is significantly decreased. Two women treated with ethinylestradiol alone showed a similar decrease of plasma tyrosine. "It is suggested that increased levels of glucocorticoids, due to the action of oestrogen, induce elevated levels of tyrosine aminotransferase, and that as a consequence there is an enhanced rate of degradation of the amino acid in the liver."

← *Other Steroids*

Kory et al G 75,742/59: In patients given norethandrolone to induce weight gain, abnormal BSP retention is frequently noted but other evidence of hepatic damage is exceptional.

Marquardt et al. D 82,860/61: In man, 6 anabolic testoids increased BSP retention, creatine and creatinine excretion in the following order of decreasing potency: norethandrolone, SC-7294, methandrostenolone, fluoxymesterone, methyltestosterone and SC-6507.

Kleiner et al. F 47,209/65: In women on oral contraceptives (norethynodrel and mestranol), BSP-excretion through the bile was impaired. The effect is ascribed to the luteoid component since estradiol does not cause BSP-retention.

Aspinall H 32,269/70: In rats, spironolactone can inhibit the ulcerogenic effect of indomethacin without blocking its antiphlogistic property (adjuvant arthritis test). This dissociation may be due to 1. a direct protective action of spironolactone upon the intestinal tract, 2. the formation of indomethacin metabolites which retain antiphlogistic but loose ulcerogenic properties or 3. a mere diminution of indomethacin activity to a level sufficient to inhibit inflammation without causing intestinal ulceration.

Linèt G 79,963/70: Detailed review of the literature and personal observations on the effect of anabolic testoids upon glucocorticoid overdosage in animals and man. Special attention is given to the effect of anabolic testoids upon glucocorticoid-induced loss of body weight and other metabolic changes, adrenal atrophy, osteoporosis, wound healing, inflammation and gastric ulcer formation. Antiglucocorticoids devoid of anabolic properties are also surveyed. In clinical medicine, various forms of hyperglucocorticoidism are not, or only moderately, improved by treatment with anabolic testoids. [Excellent source of pertinent references (H. S.).]

Nelson & Lanza G80,151/70: In nine patients with massive hepatic necrosis due to viral hepatitis, prednisone proved to be a valuable adjunct to treatment.

Shafer & Adicoff G80,179/70: In dogs, tetrahydrofurfuryl alcohol (THFA), despite its resemblance to the lactone moiety of digoxin, offers no protection against the latter compound in vivo. The authors emphasize that despite these "negative results, the development of a specific nontoxic pharmacological antagonist to digitalis would be of major clinical importance." [These investigators appear to be unaware of the inhibition of digitalis toxicity by spironolactone (H.S.).]

Tolckmitt G77,793/70: In man, prednisolone increases the turnover of tryptophan with a shortening of its biologic half-life. Methandrostenolone exerts an inverse effect.

←Barbiturates

Burstein & Klaiber F31,533/65: In man, phenobarbital increases urinary excretion of 6-hydroxycortisol. This effect is tentatively ascribed to "enhancement of cortisol 6β-hydroxylase activity by enzyme induction."

Jelliffe & Blankenhorn E65,188/66: In man, pretreatment with phenobarbital increases tolerance to digitoxin by enhancing its conversion to, and urinary excretion as, digoxin. "These findings show that phenobarbital stimulates the metabolic conversion of digitoxin to digoxin, possibly by its marked effect upon smooth endoplasmic reticulum (ER) of mammalian hepatic cells."

Kuntzman et al. G57,741/68: In man, chronic treatment with phetharbital greatly increases urinary excretion of 6β-hydroxycortisol, but not that of 17-OHCS, suggesting that an enhanced adrenal output of cortisol is not responsible for the observed rise in 6β-hydroxycortisol elimination. In the guinea pig, this nonhypnotic barbiturate increases the 6β-hydroxycortisol-forming ability of the hepatic microsomes.

Aggeler & O'Reilly G68,730/69: In man, pretreatment with heptabarbital diminished the reduction in prothrombin level, the amount of bishydroxycoumarin in plasma, and the half-life of bishydroxycoumarin more markedly after p.o. than after i.v. administration of the anticoagulant. Unchanged bishydroxycoumarin was found in the stool only after p.o. administration. Presumably, part of the response to heptabarbital was caused by increased hepatic enzymic destruction of bishydroxycoumarin although, in the event of p.o. administration, decreased absorption from the gastrointestinal tract also played a role.

Davies et al. G77,532/69: In patients exposed to DDT, treatment with diphenylhydantoin or (to a lesser extent) with phenobarbital resulted in a decrease in the plasma level of DDE, the principle metabolite of DDT.

Glogner & Ermert H27,073/70: In man, the de-ethylation of phenacetin cannot be accelerated by methylphenobarbital, a good hepatic microsomal enzyme inducer. It is assumed that, under ordinary conditions, in man, the transformation of phenacetin into its metabolite N-acetyl-p-aminophenol (NA-PAP) is optimal, and hence not subject to acceleration. [The possibility has not been considered that certain inducers are substrate specific, and that methylphenobarbital may not be a potent inducer of phenacetin-metabolizing enzymes (H.S.).]

Morselli et al. G76,129/70: In man, phenobarbital accelerates the plasma clearance of cortisol injected i.v.

Riegelman et al. H27,268/70: In healthy men, phenobarbital failed to influence the metabolism of griseofulvin. However, the absorption of the orally administered antibiotic was considerably diminished. The barbiturate may increase the secretion of bile which in turn would stimulate peristalsis. There is some evidence of increased bile secretion and enhanced biliary elimination of dyes following barbiturate treatment in animals.

Schoor H28,965/70: A farmer from an area of heavy pesticide usage, was given phenobarbital and diphenylhydantoin for the treatment of epilepsy. His blood levels of DDT, DDE, diledrin and heptachlor were far below those of other farmers living in the same area. It is assumed that either the drugs activated, microsomal enzymes which destroy the pesticides or "that the pesticides are bound by serumproteins, and are consequently relatively inert. The action of the drugs on the pesticides depends on the competition of both for the same binding sites on the proteins."

Sotaniemi et al. G78,917/70: In epileptic patients treated simultaneously with phenobarbital and diphenylhydantoin, the serum levels of both drugs were significantly lower than in those given one of these drugs only. Presumably, the two drugs accelerate each other's metabolism.

← *DDD cf. "Cushing's Disease"*

← *Diphenylhydantoin*

Werk et al. F 20,780/64: In man, diphenylhydantoin increases the 6-hydroxycortisol excretion and decreases the elimination of conjugated tetrahydro derivatives. These effects were accentuated by ACTH.

Werk et al. G 67,762/66: In man, "diphenylhydantoin alters cortisol catabolism by increasing 6-hydroxylation and decreasing A-ring reduction; it may also inhibit ACTH release." In two women with nontumorous Cushing's syndrome, diphenylhydantoin diminished the urinary output of 17-OHCS and increased that of 6-OH cortisol.

Choi et al. H 12,299/69: Brief abstract on the enhancement of tissue uptake and turnover of cortisol by diphenylhydantoin in man.

Davies et al. G 77,532/69: In patients exposed to DDT, treatment with diphenylhydantoin or (to a lesser extent) with phenobarbital resulted in a decrease in the plasma level of DDE, the principle metabolite of DDT.

Tyler et al. G 79,955/69: In epileptic patients on diphenylhydantoin, a negative metyrapone test for pituitary insufficiency may result from increased glucuronic acid conjugation of metyrapone by the liver.

Schoor H 28,965/70: A farmer, from an area of heavy pesticide usage was given phenobarbital and diphenylhydantoin for the treatment of epilepsy. His blood levels of DDT, DDE, dieldrin and heptachlor were far below those of other farmers living in the same area. It is assumed that either the drugs activated the microsomal enzymes which destroy the pesticides or "that the pesticides are bound by serumproteins, and are consequently relatively inert. The action of the drugs on the pesticides depends on the competition of both for the same binding sites on the proteins."

Sotaniemi et al. G 78,917/70: In epileptic patients treated simultaneously with phenobarbital and diphenylhydantoin, the serum levels of both drugs were significantly lower than in those given one of these drugs only. Presumably, the two drugs accelerate each other's metabolism.

Westmoreland & Bass G 80,590/71: Pregnant rats are unusually sensitive to the toxic effects of diphenylhydantoin, and show a more prolonged and intense rise in the blood level of the drug than do nonpregnant controls. The drug is readily transported across the placenta and may damage the fetus. Presumably, "inhibition of hydroxylation in maternal liver by high concentrations of female sex hormones is a probable mechanism for the accumulation of toxic concentrations of the drug in the tissues of the pregnant rat and fetus."

← *Glutethimide*

Schmid et al. G 34,008/64: "In two cases of glutethimide abuse, it was demonstrated that tolerance to glutethimide is due to marked acceleration of its metabolic inactivation. After a 20-day withdrawal cure, the metabolism of glutethimide was found to have reverted to normal."

Corn H 33,065/66: In man, phenobarbital or glutethimide treatment decreases the life span of warfarin.

← *Griseofulvin*

Cullen & Catalano G 68,707/67: In three out of four patients, the anticoagulant activity of warfarin was significantly depressed by concurrent treatment with griseofulvin, but it returned to the initial level after discontinuation of the latter drug. Possibly, griseofulvin induces enzymes which metabolize warfarin.

← *Salicylates*

Jeremy & Towson G 77,324/70: In patients with rheumatoid arthritis, ^{14}C-2-indomethacin plasma clearance is accelerated and urinary excretion decreased by acetylsalicylic acid. "The study showed interference between aspirin and indomethacin, the mechanism possibly being due to decreased gastro-intestinal absorption. This could account for clinical reports that the combination of the two drugs was no better than aspirin alone."

← *Phenylbutazone*

Kuntzman et al. G 67,761/66: In men given cortisol, the urinary excretion of 6β-hydroxycortisol is increased by phenylbutazone. At the same time, the urinary excretion of a nonpolar 17-hydroxycorticosteroid is diminished. Similar changes in the pattern of endogenous urinary corticoids were observed in man treated with phenylbutazone without exogenous cortisol administration.

Poland et al. G 78,061/70: In men who work in DDT factories, the serum DDT level was

20—30 times that in a control population. The serum half-life of phenylbutazone was 19% lower and the urinary excretion of 6β-cortisol 57% higher in the DDT factory workers.

← *Thyroxine*

Owens et al. *D 21,725/62*: In man, D-thyroxine potentiates the anticoagulant action of warfarin.

Solomon & Schrogie *H 1,868/68:* In women, thyroxine greatly potentiates the anticoagulant effect of warfarin. Analysis of the data (according to the method of Lineweaver and Burk) suggests that an increased affinity of the drug for its receptor site is responsible for the potentiation of its effect. The literature on the increase in the response to various indirect anticoagulants by thyroxine in man is briefly reviewed.

2. DISEASES

Hyperbilirubinemia ←

The various types of hyperbilirubinemia may be considered here conjointly, especially since some of them are closely related to each other, and since in many instances the clinical descriptions do not permit exact classification. According to an extensive study on 23,000 infants observed during the first eight months of life, there seems to exist a positive relationship between increasing neonatal hyperbilirubinemia and the incidence of low motor and/or mental scores. It appears therefore, that the development of the central nervous system may be inhibited by jaundice even in the absence of severe kernicterus; hence, prophylactic and therapeutic measures designed to diminish neonatal hyperbilirubinemia may have far-reaching effects upon the intellectual development of mankind, and deserve most serious consideration.

In newborn infants, **barbiturates** (e.g., phenobarbital) may induce a glucuronide conjugating enzyme system and considerably lower the serum bilirubin concentration in congenital, unconjugated hyperbilirubinemia, kernicterus and various other types of jaundice. The effect is not due entirely to bilirubin conjugation, but in part also to the proven effect of barbiturates upon biliary excretion. There is also some evidence that barbiturates induce an acceptor protein "Y", which takes up bilirubin as well as BSP and may play a crucial part in hepatic detoxication. The most important contraindication to this form of treatment is that at effective dose levels, phenobarbital causes drowsiness. In adult epileptic patients, the total bilirubin level is considerably reduced by phenobarbital. In Chinese babies, among whom neonatal jaundice is very common (as a consequence of ABO incompatibility, glucose-6-phosphatase dehydrogenase deficiency, cephalhematoma and other causes), phenobarbital likewise proved to be effective.

In 10 out of 13 patients with Gilbert's syndrome, phenobarbital induced a rapid fall in plasma bilirubin. A beneficial result was also noted in a patient with hepatitis followed by chronic unconjugated hyperbilirubinemia. In the Crigler-Najjar-syndrome, favorable effects have been obtained with phenobarbital only if the glucuronyltransferase activity was not completely absent to start with.

Unlike phenobarbital, **DDT** causes no drowsiness when administered for the treatment of neonatal hyperbilirubinemia, yet it appears to be equally effective. In patients with constitutional hyperbilirubinemia (Gilbert or Meulengracht syndrome), induction of hepatic microsomal enzymes by DDT or BDT is followed by remissions. DDT appears to have the same efficacy in "physiological" as in familial unconjugated hyperbilirubinemia with nonhemolytic jaundice.

Certain studies suggest that human **milk** contains **steroids** which may cause unconjugated hyperbilirubinemia. Early observations implied that the responsible factor may be pregnane-3α,20α-diol, since this steroid allegedly does induce hyperbilirubinemia when fed to normal full term infants, in amounts corresponding to those isolated from human milk. However, subsequent investigations failed to confirm this claim. In fact, neither pregnane-3α,20β-diol nor pregnane-3α,20α-diol inhibited bilirubin conjugation by human liver slices or by solubilized human liver microsomes. On the other hand, estradiol was effective in this respect. In newborn infants, progesterone increased folliculoid excretion and serum bilirubin concentrations. Hence, sex steroids in mother's milk may influence the course of neonatal jaundice.

The common association of congenital myxedema with prolonged icterus neonatorum suggested a relationship between the **thyroid** and jaundice of the newborn. In support of this assumption, T3 decreased peak bilirubin levels in both mature and premature infants but significantly only in the latter.

Adrenal Tumors and Cushing's Syndrome

Since hepatic microsomal enzyme inducers have been shown to accelerate the metabolic degradation of steroids, including corticoids, it was natural to test their possible efficacy in the treatment of hypercorticoidism.

In patients with Cushing's disease, a **barbiturate** (N-phenylbarbital, or phenetharbital) caused a moderate decrease in the metabolic clearance and production rates of testosterone, associated with an appreciable decrease in urinary excretion of androsterone, etiocholanolone, and 11-oxyketosteroids. However, the clinical usefulness of this form of therapy remains to be demonstrated.

DDD was tested as a possible treatment for hypercorticoidism because, in dogs, it causes adrenocortical necrosis and involution. However, its effects, like those of DDT, may be due in part to the powerful microsomal enzyme-inducing properties of these pesticides. Allegedly, o,p'-DDD can cause regression of metastatic adrenal cancer in man, at the same time inhibiting its hormone secretion. The compound is said to suppress even the normal hormonal secretion of the human adrenal cortex. On the other hand, patients given large amounts of exogenous cortisol, like those with Cushing's disease, respond to o,p'-DDD with a prompt decrease of urinary 17-OHCS excretion and plasma 17-OHCS levels. From these and other metabolic studies it was concluded that o,p'-DDD altered the extra-adrenal metabolism of cortisol so as to decrease the proportion of cortisol excreted as tetrahydrocortisol and tetrahydrocortisone, whereas 6β-hydroxycortisol elimination was increased. In the rat, 6β-hydroxycortisol is a potent inhibitor of the induction of hepatic TPO by cortisol. Hence the induction by o,p'-DDD of 6β-hydroxycortisol, the direct adrenal damaging effect of the pesticide, as well as the induction of steroid inactivating hepatic microsomal enzymes may all participate in the production of clinical improvement.

The cortisol-binding capacity of the plasma does not seem to be significantly affected by o,p'-DDD in patients with Cushing's disease.

Other Diseases ←

It was reasonable to suspect that the use of microsomal enzyme inducers might be of value in the prophylaxis and treatment of various additional diseases in whose pathogenesis, endogenous or exogenous toxicants play an important role. This was to be expected especially in maladies related to an excess of steroid hormones, cholesterol and other known substrates of microsomal enzymes. This therapeutic approach was primarily based upon animal experiments.

For example, the use of spironolactone in **mineralocorticoid hypertension** was introduced because of the potent antimineralocorticoid effect of this steroid, but later investigations have shown that it also possesses catatoxic activities against many other substrates, and hence, part of its beneficial action may be due to the accelerated detoxication of endogenous steroids and other compounds.

In cholesterol-fed rabbits, phenobarbital diminishes **atherosclerosis** and hypercholesterolemia. It remains to be seen whether this effect of folliculoids and thyroid hormones in experimental atherosclerosis, as well as in certain clinical cardiovascular diseases, is related to a catatoxic activity.

Anabolic agents have been claimed to be beneficial in the treatment of certain **hepatic lesions**, such as virus hepatitis, in man. On the other hand, several steroids in common clinical use — especially testoids and the folliculoids contained in contraceptive pills — can cause hepatic lesions of possible practical significance. Only extensive clinical tests will be able to reveal whether the typical catatoxic steroids, such as PCN or CS-1 can be used therapeutically in liver diseases, which damage the hepatic parenchyme and thereby interfere with detoxication processes. However, animal experiments suggest that after partial hepatectomy such steroids do improve resistance to many drugs in that they compensate for the loss of liver tissue by increased drug-metabolizing enzyme induction in the remnant. Furthermore, mitotic regeneration of healthy hepatic tissue is enhanced by catatoxic steroids after partial hepatectomy.

Since **prostatic hypertrophy** and certain types of **hormone-dependent cancers** (prostatic, mammary) are beneficially influenced by gonadectomy, it is conceivable that the induction of steroidases by hormonally inactive catatoxic steroids may be beneficial here also. The same considerations apply to various endogenous intoxications by **hormone-producing neoplasms, porphyria**, etc. Indeed, there may even exist specific diseases of the endoplasmic reticulum with defects in microsomal enzyme production, but meanwhile we have no evidence for this.

It is unlikely that the beneficial effect of anabolics in **osteoporosis**, or of progesterone in congenital **galactosemia**, are related to hepatic enzyme induction, but this possibility should be more seriously considered in relation to the favorable effects exerted by glucocorticoids in **v. Gierke's glycogen storage disease** and in **endotoxin shock**.

Hyperbilirubinemia ← cf. also Bilirubin under Drugs

Boggs et al. G71,887/67: Data on 23,000 infants who have been observed from birth to eight months of age "appear to indicate a positive relationship between increasing neonatal hyperbilirubinemia and the incidence of low motor and/or mental scores attained at 8 months."

Koivisto et al. G78,915/70: The serum bilirubin level of neonates whose mothers had been given estradiol for induction of labor was considerably higher than normal.

← **Barbiturates.** *Yaffe et al. G67,125/66:* In a female infant with congenital unconjugated hyperbilirubinemia, phenobarbital lowered the serum bilirubin concentration. "This constitutes the first indication of the apparent induction of a glucuronide-conjugating enzyme system by phenobarbital in man and therefore may also represent the first therapeutic application of enzyme induction."

Crigler Jr & Gold G68,552/66; G68,705/67: Phenobarbital lowers the serum bilirubin concentration in infants with congenital nonhemolytic jaundice and marked kernicterus.

Thompson & Williams G71,813/67; Kreek & Sleisenger G71,811/68; Maurer et al. G71,810/68; Trolle G71,807/68; G71,809/68: In various forms of icterus, serum bilirubin can be depressed by treatment with phenobarbital.

McMullin G77,713/68: Neonates with comparatively high serum bilirubin levels showed a decrease in bilirubinemia following treatment with phenobarbital.

Trolle G77,159/68: In low-birth-weight infants treated with phenobarbital during the first 3 days of life, the first week mortality rate was 34/1000, whereas in controls it was 101/1000. This improvement may have been due to suppression of hyperbilirubinemia, but this point was not checked in the present investigation.

Anonymous H19,246/69: Editorial on the beneficial effects of immediate postnatal barbital treatment upon neonatal hyperbilirubinemia, and its secondary consequences. The beneficial effect of phenobarbital may not be due entirely to increasing bilirubin conjugation, but in part also to its proven enhancing effect upon biliary excretion. There is also some evidence that barbiturates induce an acceptor protein "Y" which takes up bilirubin as well as BSP and may play an important role in hepatic detoxication. The necessary dose of phenobarbital may cause drowsiness, but DDT is equally effective, both in "physiological" and in congenital unconjugated hyperbilirubinemia, at well tolerated dose levels.

Arias et al. G72,103/69: In patients with chronic nonhemolytic unconjugated hyperbilirubinemia and glucuronyl transferase deficiency, phenobarbital exerted a dramatic therapeutic effect.

Crigler Jr. G72,545/69: Historical remarks on the use of phenobarbital in infants with nonhemolytic hyperbilirubinemia.

Crigler & Gold H7,119/69: In a male infant with congenital nonhemolytic, unconjugated hyperbilirubinemia and severe kernicterus, phenobarbital decreased serum bilirubin, whereas T3, STH and testosterone had little or no effect. During phenobarbital treatment, liver specimens obtained by biopsy showed proliferation of the SER and an increased in vitro capacity to conjugate p-nitrophenol.

Cunningham et al. G77,715/69: In healthy full-term neonates, phenobarbital given daily from the time icterus neonatorum first appeared about 24 hrs after birth, serum bilirubin levels did not differ significantly from those of untreated controls. "Once unconjugated hyperbilirubinaemia exists in the neonate, it is unresponsive to phenobarbitone." Apparently, treatment has to start prior to or immediately after birth.

Ertel & Newton Jr. G68,390/69: "These studies suggest that phenobarbital is the agent of choice for therapy of congenital hyperbilirubinemia. The medical indications for therapy are the prevention of kernicterus and the psychological advantage of rendering these children anicteric."

Powell et al. H17,195/69: It was noted previously that pre-eclamptic toxemia is associated with a reduction in the incidence and severity of nonhemolytic jaundice in the neonate. Reexamination of these data have now shown "that for nontoxaemic mothers receiving any barbiturate at any time there was a slight but statistically insignificant reduction (11.3%) in incidence of jaundice in their infants. Toxaemic mothers not receiving barbiturate had a similar insignificant reduction (10.4%). When both P.E.T. and barbiturate were present together, however, the reduction was 30.7% and this was statistically significant ($P < 0.01$)."

Ramboer et al. H12,643/69: Controlled trials of phenobarbital therapy in neonatal jaundice.

Thompson et al. G71,801/69: In a boy with familial unconjugated, nonhemolytic jaundice who had previously shown a good response to phenobarbital, DDT (dicophane) also rapidly reduced the plasma bilirubin.

Thompson et al. G71,802/69: In epileptic patients, the plasma-total-bilirubin level is considerably reduced by phenobarbital, presumably "by the persistent induction of glucuronyl transferase or by increased excretion of bilirubin from the hepatic cell."

Walker et al. G77,714/69: Earlier studies suggested that neonatal jaundice is comparatively rare in the infants of mothers who were treated with barbiturate for preeclampsia. In reexamining the question, "no significant difference between the infants of mothers receiving or not receiving barbiturate could be demonstrated. It is confirmed that hyperbilirubinaemia is less common in infants or women with pre-eclamptic toxiaemia. The apparent effect of toxaemia could not be explained as a feature secondary to the administration of barbiturate in these patients."

Yeung & Field G73,821/69: In Chinese babies, among whom neonatal jaundice is very common, phenobarbital therapy reduced bilirubin levels when these were high as a consequence of ABO incompatibility, glucose-6-phosphate dehydrogenase deficiency, cephalhematoma and other causes. The relevant literature is discussed in detail.

Behrman & Fisher G75,312/70: Review (4 pp., 16 refs.) on the use of phenobarbital for neonatal jaundice in man.

Black & Sherlock H26,290/70: In 13 patients with Gilbert's syndrome, phenobarbital induced a rapid fall in plasma bilirubin, and in 3 of the 10 symptomatic patients the symptoms improved. The reduction in plasma bilirubin was associated with, and thought to be the results of, an increased hepatic bilirubin UDP-glucuronyl transferase activity.

Christoforov et al. G77,086/70: The heterozygous Gunn rat has a lower capacity for bilirubin excretion than the Wistar rat. However, this defect can be corrected by phenobarbital.

Jouppila & Suonio G78,916/70: In neonates of toxemic mothers who were treated with phenobarbital during the last two weeks of pregnancy, the serum bilirubin content dropped below the control level.

Kobayashi et al. H28,794/70: In a 30-year-old male with Gilbert's syndrome, phenobarbital restored the serum bilirubin level to normal, and at the same time caused pronounced proliferation of the SER. Less pronounced but qualitatively similar changes were observed in a patient with Dubin-Johnson's syndrome.

Levin et al. G73,664/70: From a study on 24 babies given phenobarbital for three days after the first appearance of jaundice, "it is concluded that phenobarbitone has no place in the management of established neonatal jaundice."

Lüders H24,062/70: Review (8 pp., 117 refs.) on the use of barbiturates, particularly phenobarbital, in the treatment of neonatal hyperbilirubinemias. In the Crigler-Najjar-syndrome, beneficial effects can be expected only if the glucuronyltransferase is not completely absent to start with. Among the major dangers of prolonged barbiturate treatment, the following are mentioned (mainly on the basis of animal experiments): depression of the central nervous system, increased perinatal mortality (in animals pretreated during gestation), derangement of steroid hormone and cholesterol metabolism, inhibition of thyroid hormone production, intrahepatic cholestasis, barbiturate withdrawal or hypersensitivity symptoms, and hepatic enlargement.

Maurer H29,765/70: Review (8 pp., 9 refs.) on the reduction in serum bilirubin of neonates after barbital treatment of the mother. Essentially similar results are obtained by exposure of premature infants to artificial light. Possibly, "photodecomposition is a normal alternate route of excretion of bilirubin and is increased or activated in newborn infants by the use of light." Hence possibly combined barbiturate and phototherapy may prove especially efficacious.

McMullin et al. H31,772/70: In infants affected by Rhesus hemolytic disease, phenobarbital, given from the first few hours of life, is of considerable value.

Oya et al. H28,966/70: In a patient with hepatitis, followed by chronic unconjugated hyperbilirubinemia, phenobarbital corrected the jaundice and caused a considerable drop in plasma bilirubin.

Specchia H27,907/70: In an adult patient with nonhemolytic indirect hyperbilirubinemia, treatment with phenobarbital was followed by a marked decrease in blood bilirubin and icterus.

Stern et al. G76,135/70: In full-term newborns, phenobarbital, given during the first four days of life, significantly lowered the serum concentration of indirect bilirubin. In vivo glucuronidation of salicylamide was similarly increased "suggesting that the effect of phenobarbital in reducing serum bilirubin levels is mediated, at least in part, by enhanced glucuronide formation."

Thaler et al. H23,990/70: In patients suffering from various forms of jaundice, microsomal enzyme induction was studied in biopsy material, simultaneously with a quantitative analysis of the biliary excretion of i.v.-administered ^{131}I-Rose-Bengal, a cholephil whose excretion does not require biotransformation. The results indicate that phenobarbital (PB) "induces an enzyme essential to drug and steroid metabolism in human liver. PB also stimulates hepatic excretion of inert dyes and endogenous cholephils, e.g., Rose Bengal and conjugated bilirubin, respectively. Enzyme induction and excretory stimulation can occur independently. These effects are greatest in patients with relatively well preserved hepatic functions, suggesting diagnostic and therapeutic applications of PB in several cholestatic conditions."

Theile & Reich G73,421/70: In premature infants, 5 mg of phenobarbital/kg i.m., daily, decreased the serum bilirubin level; the effect was more pronounced with higher dosages; however these caused marked sedation.

Vest et al. H32,456/70: Description of beneficial results in phenobarbital treated babies with neonatal hyperbilirubinemia.

Windorfer H28,824/70: Review and personal observations on the treatment of neonatal icterus with phenobarbital.

Felsher et al. H34,479/71: In patients with hepatic cirrhosis and elevated unconjugated serum bilirubin values, phenobarbital inhibited the previously demonstrated acute rise in serum bilirubin during fasting.

Felsher et al. H34,480/71: In patients with acute icteric viral hepatitis, the hepatic glucuronyl transferase activity is enhanced by phenobarbital.

Hunter et al. H36,993/71: In epileptic patients, the urinary excretion of D-glucaric (a metabolite of glucuronic acid) is considerably increased during phenobarbital treatment. Similar observations have been made in patients with Gilbert's syndrome after administration of various drugs known to induce hepatic enzymes. Because of its simplicity and sensitivity, the D-glucaric acid excretion test is recommended for the clinical assessment of drug-metabolizing enzyme induction. It is noteworthy, however, that except in primates and guinea pigs, glucuronolactone is converted to ascorbic acid and, in the rat, inducers of drug metabolizing enzymes increase the excretion of ascorbic acid rather than of D-glucaric acid.

← **DDD, DDT.** *Anonymous H19,246/69:* Editorial on the beneficial effects of immediate postnatal barbital treatment upon neonatal hyperbilirubinemia and its secondary consequences. The necessary dose of phenobarbital may cause drowsiness, but DDT is equally effective, both in "physiological" and in congenital, unconjugated hyperbilirubinemia, at well-tolerated dose levels.

Thompson et al. G71,801/69: In a boy with familial unconjugated, nonhemolytic jaundice who had previously shown a good response to phenobarbital, DDT (dicophane) also rapidly reduced the plasma bilirubin.

Greim G76,366/70: In patients with constitutional hyperbilirubinemia (Gilbert- or Meulengracht syndrome) as well as in Cushing's disease, the stimulation of hepatic microsomal enzyme induction by DDT or DDD is followed by remissions. Because of its corticolytic effect in the dog, it had been assumed that DDD acts by blocking corticoid production, but in vitro experiments with rat liver microsomes show that DDD and DDT increase the metabolism of corticoids, and hence, their therapeutic effect is ascribed to this action.

← **Steroids.** *Arias et al. G76,756/63:* In neonates, unconjugated hyperbilirubinemia is often associated with breast feeding. The milk contains a factor that inhibits glucuronide formation in vitro by rat, guinea pig and rabbit liver microsomes.

Arias & Gartner F21,711/64: "Unconjugated hyperbilirubinaemia can be produced in very young, full-term infants by feeding pregnane-3(α), 20(β)-diol in amounts equivalent to that isolated from inhibitory human milk."

Ramos et al. G38,868/66: Newborn infants fed pregnane-3α, 20α-diol or pregnane-3α, 20β-diol from the fifth to the tenth day of life showed no anomaly in serum bilirubin levels or in the rate of the physiologic decline of the bilirubin values. "In the doses used these two pregnanediol isomers are not responsible for the conjugation inhibition effect seen in the breast milk of infants with 'physiologic' jaundice."

Kreek et al. F92,343/67: Review of the literature and personal observations suggesting that idiopathic cholestatic jaundice during pregnancy may result from increased folliculoid production and is aggravated by challenge with ethinylestradiol.

Kreek et al. G51,605/67: In one patient, cholestatic jaundice recurred during each of eight pregnancies, and during periods of menorrhagia. Liver biopsies revealed intrahepatic cholestasis during pregnancy with a return to normal after delivery. An identical picture with jaundice and abnormal liver function was obtained upon treatment of the patient with ethinylestradiol.

Crigler & Gold H7,119/69: In a male infact with congenital nonhemolytic, unconjugated hyperbilirubinemia and severe kernicterus, phenobarbital decreased serum bilirubin, whereas T3, STH and testosterone had little or no effect. During phenobarbital treatment, liver specimens obtained by biopsy showed proliferation of the SER and an increased in vitro capacity to conjugate p-nitrophenol.

Adlard & Lathe G74,759/70: In newborn infants, jaundice develops more frequently on breast feeding than on cow's milk, and earlier investigators assumed that $3\alpha, 20\beta$-pregnanediol present in human milk may competitively inhibit glucuronyl transferase, thereby interfering with bilirubin clearance. The present observations suggest that "neither $3\alpha, 20\beta$-pregnanediol nor $3\alpha, 20\alpha$-pregnanediol inhibited conjugation by human liver slices or by solubilized human liver microsomes. $3\alpha, 20\beta$-pregnanediol is unlikely to be the inhibitor causing breast milk jaundice." However, estriol inhibited conjugation by human liver slices.

Rosta et al. G77,094/70: In 4 cases of neonatal jaundice, an increased pregnanediol content was observed in the mother's milk, but on the whole, "clinical trials failed to support the role of steroid inhibition in our cases of protracted neonatal jaundice."

Sas & Herczeg G77,093/70: In newborn infants, progesterone increases folliculoid excretion and serum bilirubin concentrations. Sex steroids in mother's milk may influence the course of neonatal jaundice.

← **Thyroid Hormones.** *Akerrén G76,866/54:* Compilation of 10 cases of congenital myxedema with prolonged icterus neonatorum. A relationship between the thyroid and jaundice of the newborn is suspected.

Less & Ruthven C74,543/59: "In a trial of L-triiodothyronine by mouth in the treatment of neonatal hyperbilirubinaemia, mean peak bilirubin levels were decreased in both mature and premature-treated infants compared with controls, but this difference was statistically significant in the premature group only. ... Triiodothyronine may act by stimulating the maturation of glucuronyl transferase and other enzyme systems which are responsible for conjugating bilirubin."

MacGillivray et al. G48,968/67: In a newborn with congenital myxedema and hyperbilirubinemia, T_3 treatment caused a prompt fall in bilirubin and improvement of hypothyroidism. Accidental withdrawal of treatment was followed by an early recurrence of both jaundice and myxedema. Earlier reports of an association between intense neonatal jaundice and congenital myxedema are reviewed.

← **Pregnancy.** *Kreek et al. F92,343/67:* Review of the literature and personal observations suggesting that idiopathic cholestatic jaundice during pregnancy may result from increased folliculoid production and is aggravated by challenge with ethinylestradiol.

Kreek et al. G51,605/67: In one patient, cholestatic jaundice recurred during each of eight pregnancies, and during periods of menorrhagia. Liver biopsies revealed intrahepatic cholestasis during pregnancy with a return to normal after delivery. An identical picture with jaundice and abnormal liver function was obtained upon treatment of the patient with ethinylestradiol.

← **Light.** *Giunta & Rath H35,532/69; Lucey H35,539/69:* In the newborn and especially in premature babies, exposure to light diminishes the risk of hyperbilirubinemia.

Adrenal Tumors and Cushing's Syndrome ←

← **Aminoglutethimide.** *Bochner et al. H31,656/69:* In a patient with metastatic adrenocortical carcinoma and Cushing's syndrome, DDD caused gradual diminution in the size of metastases and some fall in 17-hydroxycorticoid excretion. Aminoglutethimide caused clinical evidence of hypocorticoidism despite an increase in the size of the metastases.

← **Barbiturates.** *Southren et al. H8,265/69:* In patients with Cushing's disease, N-phenylbarbital (phenetharbital) caused "a moderate decrease in the metabolic clearance and plasma production rates of testosterone. In addition, there occurred an appreciable decrease in the urinary excretions of androsterone, etiocholanolone and the 11-oxyketosteroids, associated with an increased excretion of polar metabolites of testosterone."

← **DDD.** *Sheehan et al. B77,668/53:* In a woman with Cushing's syndrome, no beneficial results could be obtained by DDD, suggesting that the human adrenal may be resistant to this compound.

Bergenstal et al. G74,073/59: "Preliminary observations with the use of o,p'-DDD have shown it capable of producing regression of metastatic adrenal cancer in man and inhibition of its hormonal secretion. At the present time this appears to be reversible. o,p'DDD has likewise suppressed the function of the normal human adrenal."

Bergenstal et al. C94,436/60: o,p'-DDD causes regression of adrenocortical carcinoma metastases in some, but not in all, patients.

Wallace et al. E89,875/61: In two cases of Cushing's syndrome due to adrenocortical hyperplasia, clinical improvement and dimished excretion of 17-hydroxycorticosteroids and 17-ketosteroids were obtained by o,p'-DDD.

Geyer D27,915/62: In a patient with Cushing's syndrome o,p'-DDD caused remission of the disease manifestations.

Geyer & Schüller D38,170/62: Both in normal man and in patients suffering from various forms of adrenocortical hyperactivity, o,p'-DDD was found to be beneficial.

Bar-Hay et al. G1,283/64: A 10-year-old girl with nontumorous Cushing's syndrome showed dramatic improvement following treatment with o,p'-DDD.

Bledsoe et al. E20,690/64: In patients with Cushing's disease or given large amounts of exogenous cortisol, treatment with o,p'-DDD resulted in "a prompt 50—80% decrease in urinary 17-OHCS, regardless of whether the patient's source of cortisol was endogenous or exogenous. Plasma 17-OHCS levels and cortisol secretion rates, however, did not fall. Evaluation of the pattern of cortisol metabolites excreted in the urine of these patients revealed that o,p'DDD altered the extra-adrenal metabolism of cortisol so as to decrease the proportion of cortisol excreted as tetrahydrocortisol and tetrahydrocortisone and to increase the proportion excreted as 6β-hydroxycortisol."

Pichler G43,794/66: In a young girl with adrenal hyperplasia and Cushing's syndrome "complete remission" was obtained after 7 months of DDD treatment. Pigmentation and decreased steroid excretion were noted at this time. However, 9 months after discontinuation of treatment, urinary steroid secretion increased again. The effect is ascribed to a blockade of corticoid production by the adrenals.

Southren et al. F63,163/66: In two patients with Cushing's syndrome, a remission with a reduction of urinary and plasma 17-OH-CS levels has been obtained by treatment with o,p'-DDD.

Southren et al. F73,262/66: o,p'-DDD accelerates the metabolism of infused cortisol-7-^{3}H in a patient with Cushing's disease, as well as in an adrenalectomized castrated subject.

Southren et al. F66,647/66: Clinical improvement has been observed in Cushing's syndrome after treatment with o,p'-DDD. This effect might have been due to a direct interference by o,p'-DDD with the biologic action of cortisol or by giving rise to cortisol metabolites which inhibit cortisol competitively at the effector site. In the rat, o,p'-DDD had no effect upon the induction of TPO in the liver, whereas 6β-hydroxycortisol was found to be a potent inhibitor of cortisol action in this test system. Since o,p'-DDD induces 6β-hydroxycortisol, the protective effect may have been due to the latter.

Bochner et al. H31,656/69: In a patient with metastatic adrenocortical carcinoma and Cushing's syndrome, DDD caused gradual diminution in the size of metastases and some fall in 17-hydroxycorticoid excretion. Aminoglutethimide caused clinical evidence of hypocorticoidism despite an increase in the size of the metastases.

Temple Jr. et al. H17,091/69: In patients with Cushing's disease, o,p'-DDD diminished cortisol secretion. Since adrenal responsiveness to ACTH infusion was reduced and the adrenals showed electron-microscopic changes in the mitochondria of the fasciculata, the effect was ascribed to the adrenolytic action of the drug.

Burger et al. H28,702/70: In patients with Cushing's disease, the cortisol-binding capacity (CBC) of the plasma was not significantly altered by o,p'-DDD.

Greim G76,366/70: In patients with constitutional hyperbilirubinemia (Gilbert- or Meulengracht syndrome) as well as in Cushing's disease, the stimulation of hepatic microsomal enzyme induction by DDT or DDD is followed by remissions. Because of its corticolytic effect in the dog, it had been assumed that DDD acts by blocking corticoid production, but in vitro experiments with rat liver microsomes show that DDD and DDT increase the metabolism of corticoids, and hence, their therapeutic effect is ascribed to this action.

Hellman et al. H28,347/70: In a patient with Cushing's syndrome, treatment with o,p'-DDD "converted the cortisol secretory pattern from a well-defined series of peaks and valleys to an almost level pattern fluctuating about the lowest plasma concentration measured in the untreated state." The changes in plasma cortisol pattern are ascribed to direct adrenal damage.

Other Diseases ←

Cardiac Diseases ← *cf. also Selye G60,083/70. Salvador et al. G68,113/67:* Pretreatment with phenobarbital diminished hypercholesterolemia and atherosclerosis in cholesterol-fed rabbits. The cholesterol content of the aorta was likewise diminished.

Orrenius et al. E 8,231/69: Review of the literature, and personal observations on the increase in the synthesis of cholesterol from ^{14}C-acetate obtained by phenobarbital pretreatment in rats and hamsters.

Tourniaire et al. G 66,481/69: "Spironolactone is now the drug of choice in severe heart failure complicated by increased myocardial sensitivity. It enables one to stop other drugs such as digitalis and salt diuretics which are liable to increase the arrhythmia and lead to fibrillation. ... This action on myocardial excitability in heart failure may probably be explained by the antagonism between spironolactone and aldosterone in the kidney and its effects on potassium metabolism."

Hepatic Lesions ←. *Krüskemper & Noell G 48,300/66:* Methyltrienolone (17α-methyl-4, 9, 11-estratriene-17β-ol-3-one), though a strong anabolic agent, is definitely hepatotoxic as judged by various function tests in man.

Caviles H 30,761/68: In patients receiving massive doses of stanozolol for the treatment of aplastic anemia, indications of significant hepatic disturbances were not observed.

Adlercreutz H 21,321/70: Review (34 pp., about 240 refs.) on folliculoid metabolism in liver disease.

Jannuzzi et al. H 27,335/70: In patients with viral hepatitis, various anabolics, including stanozolol and 4-chlorotestosterone, exert a beneficial effect.

Osteomalacia ←. *Dent et al. H 30,946/70; Richens & Rowe H 30,947/70:* In four epileptic patients, osteomalacia developed during long-term treatment with diphenylhydantoin and barbiturates. Vitamin D exerted a curative effect. "It is suggested that drug-mediated enzyme induction may be the mechanism responsible by causing a greatly increased inactivation of vitamin D in these patients."

Osteoporosis ←. *Heather G 67,332/63:* SKF-6612 is recommended for the treatment of osteoporosis in man, owing to its anabolic effect.

Galactosemia ←. *Pesch et al. C 79,957/60:* "Administration of progesterone to three prepubertal patients with congenital galactosemia resulted in a significant increase in ability to oxidize a tracer dose of galactose-1-C^{14} to $C^{14}O_2$."

v. Gierke's Disease ←. *Moses et al. G 40,253/66:* In a patient with glycogen storage disease, triamcinolone caused a 4-fold increase in hepatic glucose-6-phosphatase activity.

Endotoxin Shock ←. *Weil et al. G 68,706/62:* In man, combined treatment with glucocorticoids (cortisol, prednisone, dexamethasone) and vasoactive agents (especially metaraminol) is particularly efficacious in preventing endotoxin shock.

3. PREGNANCY (ABORTIFACIENT ACTION OF HEPATIC MICROSOMAL ENZYME INDUCERS)

It has been noted some time ago that in dogs, DDD tends to produce abortion, and in rats, phenobarbital increases embryonic death causing subcutaneous hemorrhages in the fetuses. The placentas of the rats so treated were small and showed an increased demethylation activity. Our own hitherto unpublished observations suggest that various catatoxic steroids such as ethylestrenol, spironolactone and CS-1 interrupt pregnancy in the rat and, if administered after delivery, interfere with lactation. It is tempting to assume that these effects result from the induction by catatoxic steroids of microsomal enzymes that metabolize the hormones necessary for the maintenance of gestation and milk production; yet, in our experience, highly catatoxic amounts of PCN and phenobarbital failed to interrupt pregnancy in the rat.

Dille 45,154/34: In cats, guinea pigs and rabbits, a single anesthetic dose of barbital or amital does not interrupt pregnancy, but "in no case where barbiturates were administered over a major part of pregnancy was a successful delivery obtained."

Courrier 86,924/45: Monograph (396 pp., about 1250 refs.) on the endocrinology of gestation, with a special section (70 pp.) on hormonal interventions which interrupt pregnancy. An excellent survey of the literature up to 1945.

Nichols & Hennigar C 48,736/57: In dogs, DDD tends to produce abortion.

Pincus E 689/65: Monograph (360 pp., 1459 refs.) on the control of fertility. Special attention is given to the abortifacient action of drugs and hormones.

Badarau et al. G69,247/68: In rats, various adrenal and ovarian steroids can produce necrosis of the trophoblast during the early stages of gestation. In certain steroid combinations, a mutual antagonism has been noted. [The cursory descriptions in this brief abstract do not permit evaluation of the data (H.S.).]

Einer-Jensen G75,787/68: Review of the literature on the abortifacient action of natural and artificial folliculoids. Personal observations show that in the dog, mouse, rat and rabbit, early pregnancy can be interrupted with comparatively small doses of "F6066" [Bis(p-acetoxyphenyl)-cyclohexylidene-methane] and "F6103" [Bis-(p-acetoxyphenyl)-2-methyl-cyclohexylidene-methane.]

Jacob & Morris G73,856/69: In rabbits, norethindrone, testosterone, dehydrotestosterone and certain so-called "nonsteroidal antifolliculoids" inhibited implantation when given during the first three days after copulation. With the exception of chlormadinone, all these compounds showed some degree of folliculoid (uterotrophic) activity which parallels the antifertility potency. Progesterone and chlormadinone failed to inhibit implantation under similar conditions.

Morrison & Kilpatrick G69,282/69: Observation of a personal case and report of several others from the literature, showing that in women taking glucocorticoids during pregnancy, estriol excretion is diminished. "The effect could be the result of direct depression of the placental enzymic systems."

Szontagh & Kovacs G73,899/69: Brief postcoital treatment with dienestrol prevents pregnancy in women.

Adams & Wagner G80,309/70: In cattle, dexamethasone i.m. readily induces parturition during late pregnancy. In ewes, it is much less effective. The plasma corticoid level spontaneously rises just prepartum in cattle and ewes. "This abrupt elevation in maternal plasma corticoids may result from increased synthesis by the fetal adrenals and provide the signal for termination of the pregnancy." Early literature on the effect of corticoids, ACTH and hypophysectomy upon pregnancy is reviewed.

Bačić et al. G75,837/70: In women, the administration of large doses of ethinylestradiol during early pregnancy failed to cause abortion or bleeding. It is concluded that, unlike in several other species, folliculoids are not reliable abortifacients in man.

Bačić et al. H28,711/70: In women, the artificial folliculoid F-6103 (Bis-(p-acetoxyphenyl)-2-methyl-cyclohexylidene-methane) has no abortifacient effect, although earlier studies showed that it does interrupt early pregnancy in rats and mice.

Fahim et al. G77,383/70: In pregnant rats, phenobarbital given throughout gestation "results in a significant increase in embryonic death and a 28 per cent incidence of fetal subcutaneous hemorrhage. Placentas of treated animals weighed less than controls and exhibited a significant increase in demethylation activity."

Jean H33,486/70: In mice and rats, estradiol dipropionate injected on the 14th day of gestation failed to interrupt gestation but moderately diminished the subsequent growth of the offspring.

Jean & Jean H33,485/70: In rats and mice, estradiol injected during the second third of gestation interferes with parturition and causes considerable fetal and perinatal mortality. The earlier literature on postcoital contraception by folliculoids and testoids is reviewed.

O'Leary et al. G80,260/70: In women living in areas where DDT and DDE are extensively used for pest control, spontaneous abortions are not correlated with the blood pesticide levels. There is no reason to believe that the pesticides have a significant abortifacient action.

Nocke et al. H29,580/70: Brief abstract indicating that in pregnant women, spironolactone decreases the urinary elimination of folliculoids, 17-hydroxycorticoids and 17-oxosteroids. It is concluded that spironolactone "may have an influence on the biogenesis and/or metabolism of steroid hormones."

Meyers G77,432/70: In rats, stimulation of the sterile uterine horn of the 1—4th day of pregnancy does not lead to the usual deciduoma formation whether the animals are intact or ovariectomized and maintained on progesterone + esterone. However, the deciduoma response (DR) produced by trauma with a needle or intra-uterine instillation of oil was not equally influenced by the antifolliculoids I.C.I. 46474, CN-55945-27, U-11100A, and U-11555A. "The oil-induced, but not the trauma-induced DR, in intact pregnant rats was completely inhibited by all the antiestrogenic compounds when they were given on Day 4, while administration of the same drugs on Day 1 prevented both the oil-induced and the trauma-induced DR. Implantation was uniformly prevented by these compounds after administration on either Day 1 or Day 4. It was concluded that, in the rat, oil installation is preferable to the use of trauma for deciduoma induction, since it more closely resembles the conditions under which implantation takes place."

Sananès & Psychoyos G78,230/70: In rats, deciduoma formation is inhibited by actinomycin D presumably by interfering with RNA formation.

Bloch et al. H34,907/71: In mice, unlike in rats, TMACN administered during gestation often causes fetal absorption but no gross malformations in the reproductive tract.

SUMMARY

In the preceding pages we have surveyed evidence suggesting that catatoxic steroids may be of use in patients suffering from the most varied forms of endogenous or exogenous intoxications with bilirubin, steroids, digitalis compounds, pesticides, carcinogens, etc. In addition, knowledge of the catatoxic mechanism is indispensable in evaluating the possible effect that enzyme-inducing hormones or drugs (e.g., contraceptive pills, antimineralocorticoids, barbiturates, anticonvulsants) may exert upon the efficacy of simultaneously administered pharmaceuticals and vice versa, since many inducers are also substrates for inducible microsomal enzymes.

Furthermore, attention is called to the fact that catatoxic steroids are comparatively ineffective in attacking near physiologic levels of hormones and other normal body constituents. Yet they may interfere with pregnancy and lactation, through the enhanced metabolic degradation of the excess steroids necessary for the maintenance of these states, or through other mechanisms.

Finally, catatoxic steroids may be useful when only topical drug or hormone actions are required. Here these steroids would selectively prevent undesirable systemic side effects through the induction of hepatic microsomal enzymes which could degrade only the blood-borne fraction of the topical medications.

IX. MORPHOLOGY ←

HEPATIC TISSUE ←
Cf. also Hepatic Lesions ← Steroids p. 354

← *Steroids*

In general it may be said that glucocorticoids decrease, whereas catatoxic steroids increase, the weight of the liver in various species. However, these effects largely depend upon a variety of conditioning factors such as the dosage of the hormones, as well as the age, diet and species of the animals under investigation. Here we shall deal only with those changes which have been shown or at least suspected to be related to adaptive enzyme formation.

← **Corticoids.** In the fowl, DOC causes hypertrophy and hyperplasia of the liver. This is all the more remarkable since after adrenalectomy, DOC is singularly ineffective in promoting hepatic regeneration induced by partial hepatectomy. Conversely, heavy overdosage with cortisone causes involution and sometimes even focal necrosis of hepatic tissue in the rat and mouse. Unilateral nephrectomy which sensitizes the rat to many of the toxic actions of DOC, very markedly increases its ability to enlarge the liver.

On the other hand, in the rabbit, cortisone causes pronounced increase in liver weight with glycogen deposition and cellular hypertrophy, whereas DOC is ineffective in this respect. Small doses of cortisone may even cause hepatic enlargement in rats when liver weight is expressed as a percentage of body weight. However, at high dose levels the general catabolic action of the hormone predominates.

Flumedroxone and its unsaturated analogue cause hepatic enlargement and SER proliferation in mice and rats. Furthermore in mice, the mean mitochondrial volume increased 4-fold after cortisone treatment, possibly as a result of mitochondrial fusion.

← **Adrenalectomy.** In adrenalectomized mice, cortisone increases protein synthesis in the liver with the formation of heavy polysomes during the first hour. After 3 hrs cortisone represses protein synthesis under otherwise comparable conditions.

In adrenalectomized rats, the number of hepatic mitochondria and lysosomes increases and vesicular forms of endoplasmic reticulum arise around the Golgi complexes. All these changes are prevented by cortisol.

← **Folliculoids.** In C3H mice, chronic treatment with estradiol or diethylstilbestrol increases hepatic weight. A similar increase is obtained in pullets by estradiol. In the mouse, stilbestrol derivatives induce mitochondrial swelling and dilatation of the RER with considerable changes in the activity of various enzymes but no obvious proliferation of SER.

Heavy overdosage with natural and artificial folliculoids may cause enlargement of the liver hepatitis, hepatic necroses, and even death with severe icterus in certain strains of mice. In immature pullets, thyroxine antagonizes the hepatic changes produced by estradiol.

The hepatotoxic effects of folliculoids in man have been discussed in the section on "Clinical Implications," especially in connection with oral contraceptives.

← **Luteoids.** In hamsters, progesterone increases hepatic weight and causes proliferation of the SER accompanied by chemically demonstrable augmentation of microsomal phospholipid content. The changes are similar to those produced by barbiturates. In rats, lynestrenol causes increased vacuole formation in the Golgi apparatus without any alterations in the endoplasmic reticulum.

← **Testoids.** In mice, large doses of testosterone failed to produce significant changes in hepatic weight, although in rats it does elicit moderate hepatic hypertrophy. The capacity to excrete conjugated bilirubin is impaired in rats by norethandrolone and even more strikingly by icterogenin. Simultaneously, ultrastructural changes appear in the hepatocytes and bile canaliculi.

Methyltrienolone, a strong anabolic agent, is definitely hepatotoxic as judged by various function tests in man. In partially hepatectomized rats, the fat and phosphatase accumulation in the liver remnant is enhanced by prednisolone but not significantly affected by 4-chlorotestosterone.

Norbolethone produces pronounced proliferation of the SER in the hepatocytes of the rat presumably reflecting increased microsomal-enzyme induction.

← **Antitestoids.** In rats, cyproterone stimulates the proliferation of the SER in hepatocytes presumably again as a manifestation of microsomal enzyme induction.

← **Catatoxic Steroids in General.** Both in intact and in partially hepatectomized rats, spironolactone increases hepatic weight and the mitotic activity of hepatocytes. Several of the most active catatoxic steroids (spironolactone, norbolethone, CS-1, ethylestrenol) stimulate the SER of the hepatocytes in the rat. Progesterone and testosterone are much less effective. However, alterations in the endoplasmic reticulum are also produced by noncatatoxic steroids (estradiol) and nonsteroidal folliculoids (stilbestrol). "Thus it can be concluded that there is no close correlation between the catatoxic potency and the proliferation of the SER although all the catatoxic compounds tested lead to a marked transformation of the endoplasmic reticulum in the hepatocytes."

PCN, one of the most active catatoxic steroids, induces intense proliferation of the SER in the hepatocytes of the rat. This is accompanied by swelling of the mitochondria and a moderate increase in the lipid content of hepatocytes as well as by some hypertrophy of the microvilli in the bile canaliculi.

← **Other Steroids.** We have already mentioned the great capacity of icterogenin to reduce the elimination of conjugated bilirubin, without producing any obvious light microscopic changes in the liver. Electron microscopic lesions are noted however in hepatocytes and bile canaliculi.

For an extensive study concerning the effect of various steroids, thyroxine and phenobarbital upon body and organ weights in rats, *cf.* Table 140, p. 860.

← *Nonsteroidal Hormones and Hormone-Like Substances*

← **Anterior Pituitary Hormones.** It had long been noted that in rats, treatment with crude anterior lobe extract causes a disproportionate increase in hepatic weight. From this it has been concluded that certain anterior pituitary extracts selectively stimulate hepatic growth and that the hepatotrophic effect is not merely due to their STH content. The anterior pituitary extracts not only increase hepatic size but produce extreme polymorphism of hepatocyte nuclei and an outburst of mitotic divisions some of which are abnormal and conducive to the formation of large polymorphonuclear giant cells. In addition, crude lyophilized anterior pituitary may cause infiltration of the hepatic stroma with hemopoietic cells and megakaryo cytes. It remains to be seen however whether these latter effects are due to a specific hormone or to impurities in the crude hypophyseal extracts. Curiously in intact (unlike in hypophysectomized) rats, purified STH also causes disproportionate hepatic enlargement possibly by stimulating the secretion of a hypophyseal hepatotrophic principle.

ACTH causes hepatic steatosis in rats especially if they are maintained on high-carbohydrate diets or force-fed. Particularly pronounced hepatotrophic effects have been obtained in rats upon combined treatment with ACTH + STH. The production of fatty livers by purified ACTH is prevented by adrenalectomy in the rat.

← **Thyroid Hormones.** High doses of thyroxine may cause functional and occasionally even structural hepatic damage in various species and even in man (Selye 94,572/49).

In rats, thyroid feeding increases hepatic weight and produces diffuse basophilia with palisade-like basophilic rods in the cytoplasm of the hepatocytes, but similar changes have been described previously using a variety of stressor agents (epinephrine, bleeding). Thiourea also stimulates mitotic proliferation in the rat liver. The ESR shows no important changes in rats overdosed with thyroxine or in thyrotoxic patients.

← **Pancreatic Hormones.** In mice, insulin causes some increase in the mean mitochondrial volume of hepatocytes.

← *Drugs*

In the rat, hepatic microsomal-enzyme induction by **barbiturates** (e.g. phenobarbital) is regularly associated with a pronounced proliferation of the hepatic SER, apparently at the expense of the RER. Essentially similar changes are produced by barbiturates in the rabbit and hamster. These morphologic abnormalities are usually first seen around the central parts of the lobule gradually spreading to the periphery. Concurrent treatment with SKF 525-A further aggravates these changes but in itself SKF 525-A produces no detectable anomalies in the hepatocytes. In rats, a single injection of phenobarbital suffices to stimulate the SER. Enzyme histochemical studies on rats treated with phenobarbital suggested that NADPH tetrazolium red is directly involved in the hydroxylation chain, whereas G6PD and ICD are more indirectly affected.

CCl_4 greatly increases the proliferation of the SER in hepatocytes but apparently it stimulates only the synthesis of abnormal microsomal membranes, since protein synthesis is greatly impaired, whereas incorporation of ^{35}P into the membrane phospholipids is enhanced.

Chlorazanil, a diuretic drug, depresses mitotic division in the regenerating liver of the mouse after partial hepatectomy.

In rats, **clofibrate** first causes deformation of hepatic mitochondria and depletion of succinic oxidase and after 12 hrs proliferation of the SER.

Sublethal doses of **digitoxin** cause proliferation of the hepatic SER in the rat with enzyme changes which have been interpreted as suitable for the enhancement of glycoside metabolism. However, our in vivo experiments showed no increase in digitoxin resistance following pretreatment with the same compound.

In rats treated with **metyrapone**, the SER of the hepatocytes becomes hypertrophic concurrently with a loss of glycogen. This effect is not obtained in vitro when liver slices are incubated with metyrapone.

Various **pesticides**, which act as microsomal enzyme inducers, stimulate the proliferation of the SER in the hepatocytes of the rat. DDT is particularly effective in this respect and in addition produces inclusion bodies with myelin-like capsules.

In the hepatocytes of the rat, dieldrin (a chlorinated hydrocarbon pesticide) produces characteristic lesions which develop in three stages: 1. Increase in liver weight and microsomal protein, with SER proliferation, associated with increased activity of aniline hydroxylase and p-nitroreductase as well as a rise in the concentration of P-450 hemoprotein. 2. A "steady state" in which the elevated levels are maintained and tolerance to otherwise fatal doses of dieldrin develops. 3. A "stage of decompensation" elevation of liver weight, microsomal proteins, and P-450 persists, and the SER is abundant but drug-handling enzyme ability is diminished. The authors speak of a hypoactive hypertrophic SER which reflects a stage of exhaustion. [It is interesting to speculate upon the similarity between these three stages and those of the G.A.S. (H.S.).]

In rats, large parenteral doses of **salicylates** increase a number of peroxisomes in multivesicular bodies around the Golgi zone of the hepatocytes but the endoplasmic reticulum remains normal.

In addition to those mentioned above, a large variety of **other drugs** are capable of stimulating the SER of hepatocytes. However, not all of these are effective enzyme inducers.

← Steroids

← **Corticoids.** *Selye A 56,607/43:* In chickens, chronic treatment with DOC or methyltestosterone produces hepatic enlargement.

Selye and Pentz A 59,789/43: In the rat, many of the toxic manifestations of DOC overdosage are considerably increased by uninephrectomy + NaCl administration. Under these conditions, DOC also produces an unusually pronounced hepatic enlargement.

Antopol B 47,052/50: In mice, heavy cortisone overdosage produces considerable atrophy of the liver associated with other manifestations of the alarm reaction.

Selye B 40,000/50: Early observations on the induction of hepatic hypertrophy by DOC in the fowl and rat. Cortisone causes involution and sometimes focal necrosis in the rat liver. Unilateral nephrectomy which sensitizes the rat to many toxic actions of DOC, markedly increases its ability to enlarge the liver.

Timiras & Koch B 53,947/51; B 54,551/52: In the rabbit, cortisone causes a pronounced increase in liver weight with glycogen deposition and cellular hypertrophy; DOC has no such effect.

Clark Jr. & Pesch C 18,864/56: In female rats kept on an adequate diet, cortisone increases hepatic weight and protein content, although it arrests somatic growth. On a protein-deficient diet, cortisone increases the relative weight of the liver and maintains its protein content.

Korenchevsky C 18,714/56: In male rats, testosterone and to a lesser extent cortisone increased hepatic weight.

Klatskin G 65,221/63: Review (103 pp., 809 refs.) on toxic and drug-induced hepatitis with special sections on the hepatotoxic effect of testoids, corticoids, thioureas, luteoids, folliculoids and oral antidiabetics.

Koike et al. H 15,766/68: In adrenalectomized mice, cortisone increases protein synthesis in the liver with the formation of heavy polysomes within about 30—60 min. However, after 3 hrs, cortisone represses protein synthesis in the mouse liver, and the repressive factor is present in the polysomal fraction and the S-105 fluid. The early and late effects of cortisone are similar in intact mice. The "cytoplasmic repression" factor of the S-105 fluid is larger than that of the polysomal fraction.

Birchmeier G69,512/69: In mice, hepatic ultrastructure studies were performed after temporary treatment with cortisone or insulin. "The mean mitochondrial volume increased up to fourfold in the cortisone-treated series and to a much lesser extent in the insulin-treated series. The increase in mean mitochondrial volume was balanced by a decrease in the number of mitochondria per cell such that the total cell mitochondrial volume remained relatively constant. It is suggested that the changes in mitochondrial volume and number were a result of mitochondrial fusion. These changes were temporary. Ten days after the hormone treatment the cells were only slightly different from the control cells."

Hines G68,829/69: Flumedroxone and its unsaturated analogue cause liver enlargement and proliferation of the SER in hepatocytes of mice and rats. This change may be related to the induction by these steroids of certain esterases as previously reported.

Garg et al. G79,011/71: In rats, betamethasone and dexamethasone cause mild dilatation and irregularities of the RER in hepatocytes. There is a marked increase in the amount of glycogen granules, and the mitochondria show slight swelling and partial loss of cristae.

← **Adrenalectomy.** *Koike et al. H15,766/68:* In adrenalectomized mice, cortisone increases protein synthesis in the liver (with the formation of heavy polysomes) within about 30—60 min. However, after 3 hrs, cortisone represses protein synthesis in the mouse liver, and the repressive factor is present in the polysomal fraction and the S-105 fluid. The early and late effects of cortisone are similar in intact mice. The "cytoplasmic repression" factor of the S-105 fluid is larger than that of the polysomal fraction.

Shigei H27,112/69: In rats, adrenalectomy, changed the ultrastructure of hepatocytes by reducing the glycogen areas, increasing the number of mitochondria and lysosomes, and inducing vesicular forms of endoplasmic reticulum around the Golgi complexes. All these changes are prevented by cortisol. In partially hepatectomized rats, adrenalectomy and cortisol also exert antagonistic effects upon hepatocyte ultrastructure.

Dardachti et al. G79,006/71: In rats, metyrapone stimulates the proliferation of SER, even after adrenalectomy.

← **Folliculoids.** *Selye A18,206/39:* In certain strains of mice, heavy overdosage with estradiol or diethylstilbestrol produces considerable increase in the weight of the liver often associated with hepatitis, hepatic necrosis, severe icterus and even death. Estrone and estradiol are somewhat less toxic than diethylstilbestrol.

Selye & Stevenson 77,177/40: In Strong's C3H strain mice, the liver shows a transitory increase in weight under the influence of chronic treatment with estradiol or diethylstilbestrol.

Common et al. B23,003/48: In immature pullets, estradiol increases the weight, as well as the fat and protein content of the liver. Concurrent treatment with testosterone does not modify these changes but thyroxine i.v. antagonizes them.

Kottra & Kappas F79,911/67: Review (7 pp., 40 refs.) on the hepatotoxic action of various steroids (particularly folliculoids) especially in man.

Kemmer & Müller F89,190/67: In the mouse, "oestrastilben D" induces mitochondrial swelling and a dilatation of the RER associated with a considerable change in activity of various enzymes, but no obvious proliferation of the SER.

Klatskin G65,221/69: Review (103 pp., 809 refs.) on toxic and drug-induced hepatitis with special sections on the hepatotoxic effect of testoids, corticoids, thioureas, luteoids, folliculoids and oral antidiabetics.

← **Luteoids.** *Emans & Jones H20,754/68:* In hamsters, progesterone increases liver weight and the proliferation of the SER accompanied by chemically demonstrable augmentation of microsomal phospholipid content. The changes are similar to those produced by phenobarbital. Presumably "stimulation by steroids may be responsible in part for the maintenance of microsomal hydroxylases and smooth reticulum in the normal hepatic cell."

Klatskin G65,221/69: Review (103 pp., 809 refs.) on toxic and drug-induced hepatitis with special sections on the hepatotoxic effect of testoids, corticoids, thioureas, luteoids, folliculoids and oral antidiabetics.

Bartók et al. G74,513/70: In rats, six day treatment with lynestrenol caused no light

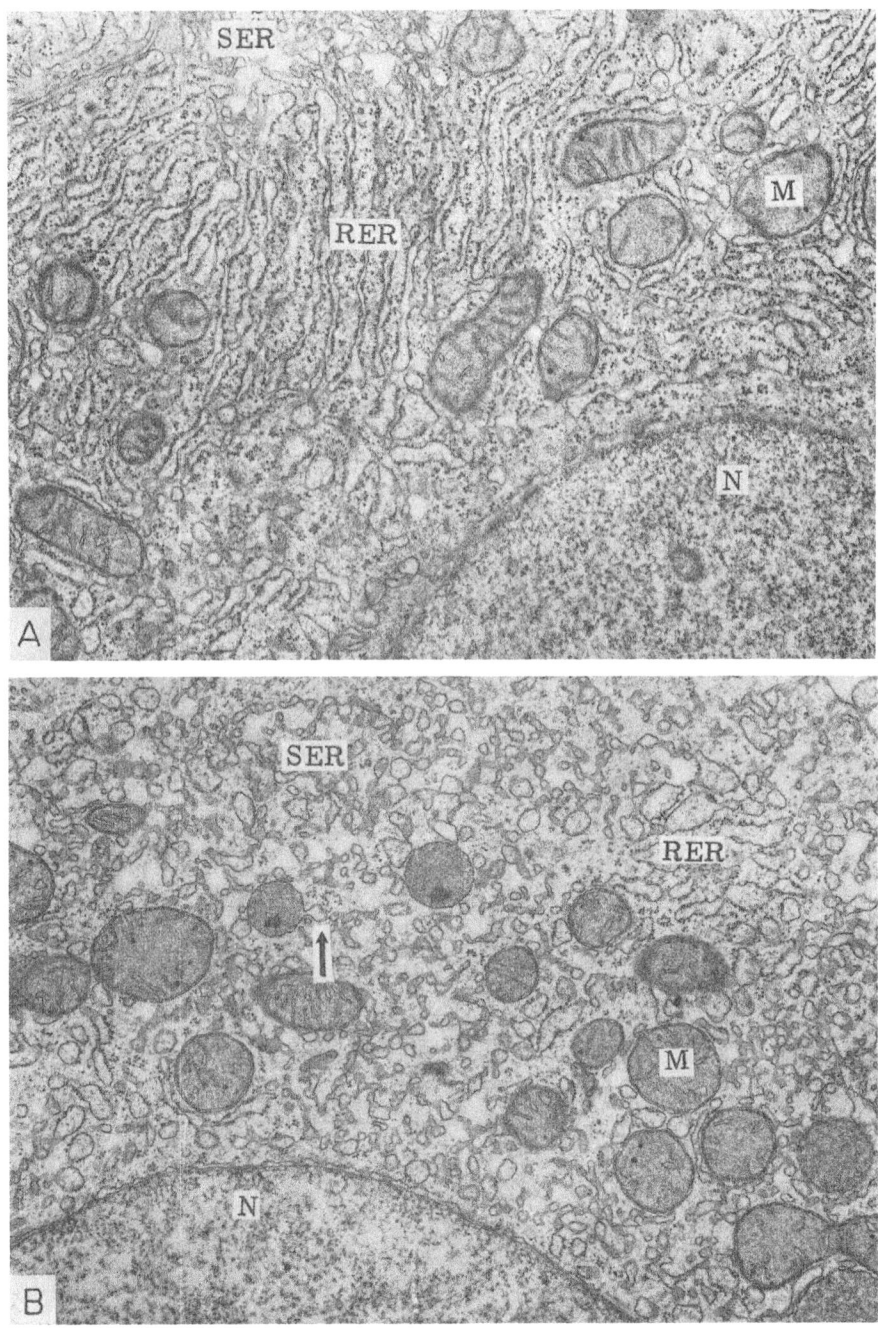

Fig. 33. **Effect of norbolethone upon the SER in the hepatocytes.** A: Normal hepatocyte of a rat. Nucleus (N), mitochondrion (M), rough endoplasmic reticulum (RER), smooth endoplasmic reticulum (SER). × 16,400. B: Hepatocyte after 5 days of norbolethone treatment. Marked proliferation of the SER with comparative scarcity of RER. One vesicle of the SER is continuous with a microbody (arrow). × 16,800. [Gardell et al. G 60,062/70. Courtesy of J. Micr.]

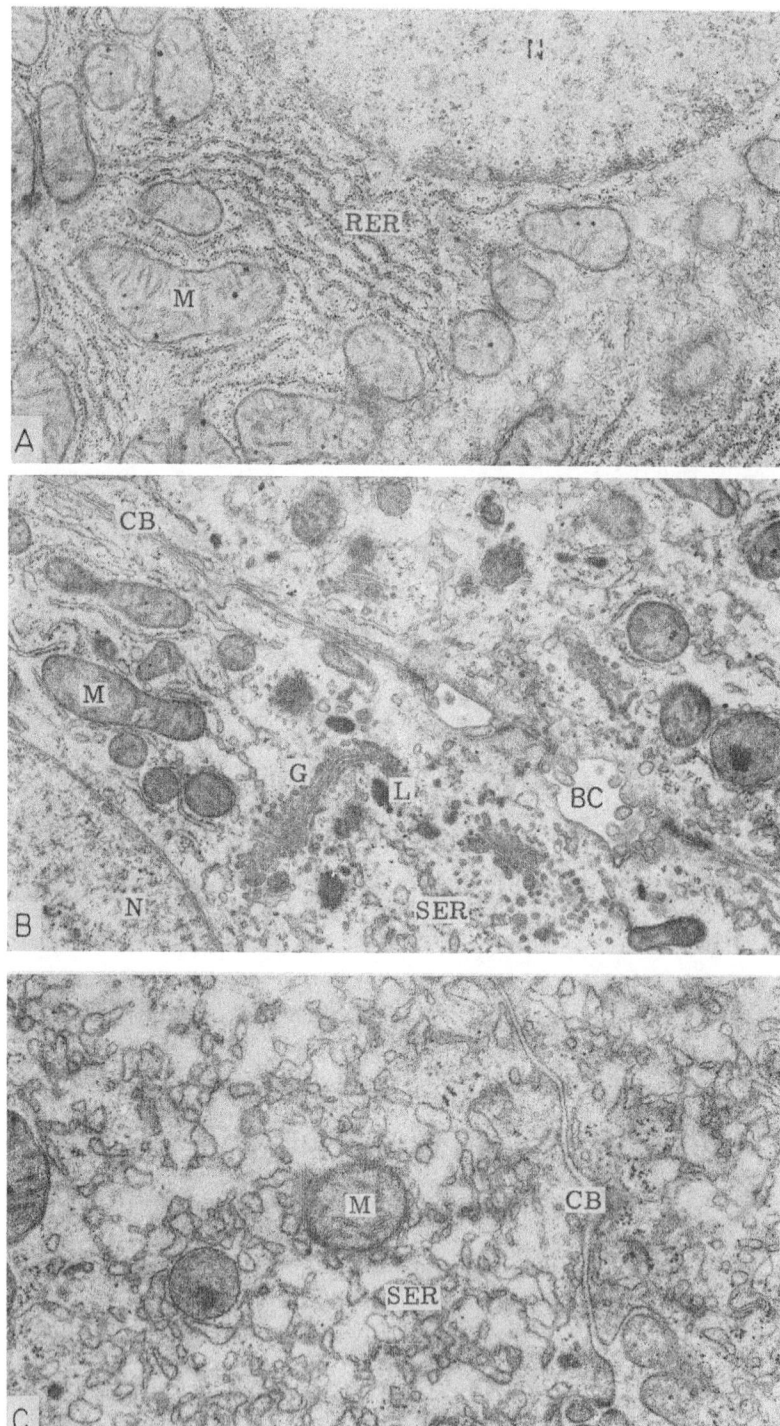

Fig. 34. **Effect of spironolactone upon the SER of hepatocytes.** A: Untreated rat. Portion of hepatocyte showing the normal nucleus (N), RER and mitochondria (M). × 13,400. B: Spironolactone-treated rat. Portions of two hepatocytes. The SER is increased, the mitochondria are essentially normal. Parts of the Golgi complex (G) are visible, as well as lysosomes (L), biliary canaliculi (BC) and the cell border (CB). × 10,600. C: Portions of two other hepatocytes in a spironolactone-treated rat. There is again proliferation of the SER. Note also mitochondrion and cell border. × 19,500. [Kovacs et al. G 60,045/70. Courtesy of Z. ges. exp. Med.]

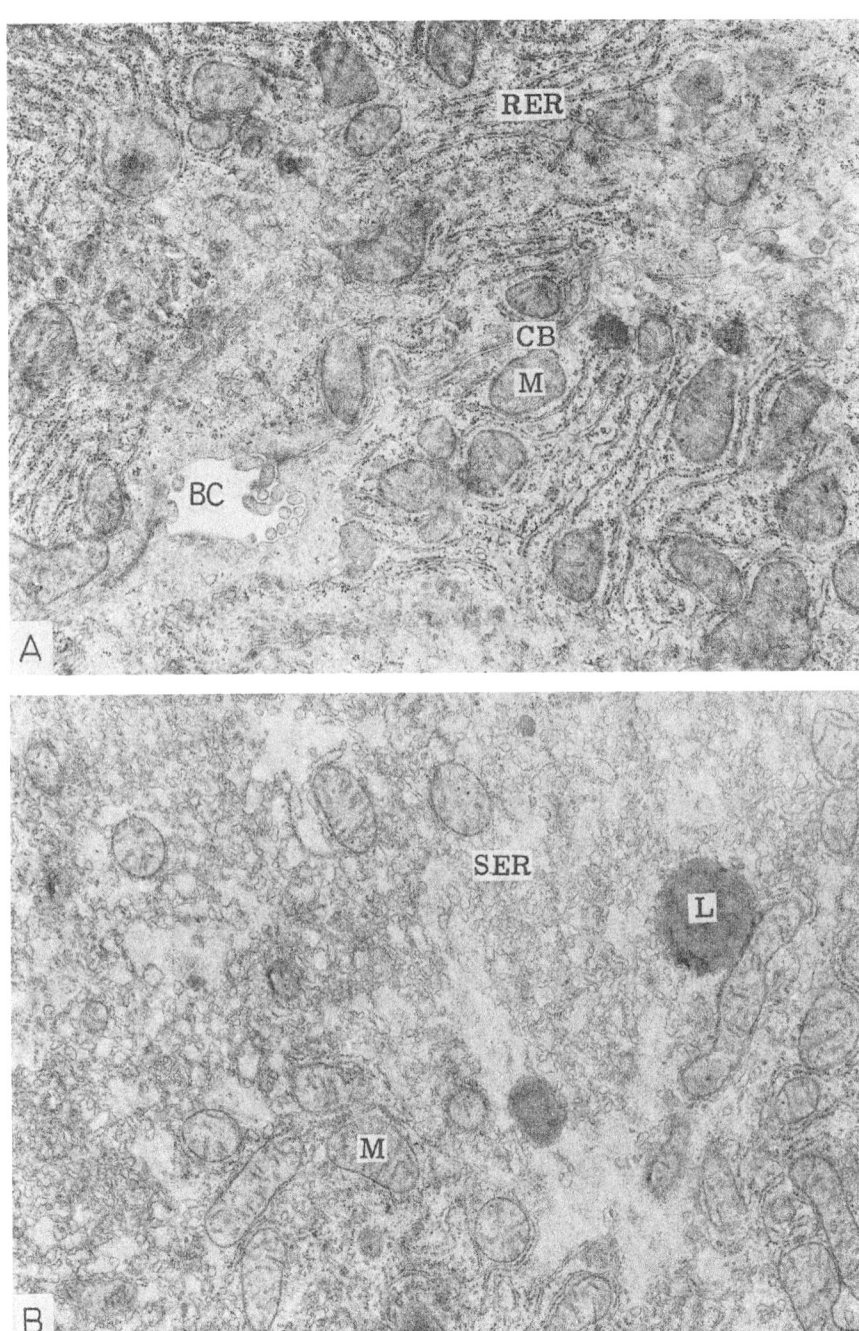

Fig. 35. **Ultrastructural changes induced by PCN in the hepatocytes.** A: Untreated control rat. Portions of two hepatocytes showing characteristic features of rough endoplasmic reticulum (RER), mitochondria (M), biliary canaliculus (BC) and of the cell border (CB) between the two hepatocytes. × 12,000. B: PCN-treated rat. Accumulation of smooth endoplasmic reticulum (SER) in a portion of the hepatocyte in small lipid granules (L). × 11,000. [Garg et al. G 70,474/70. Courtesy of J. Pharm. Pharmacol.]

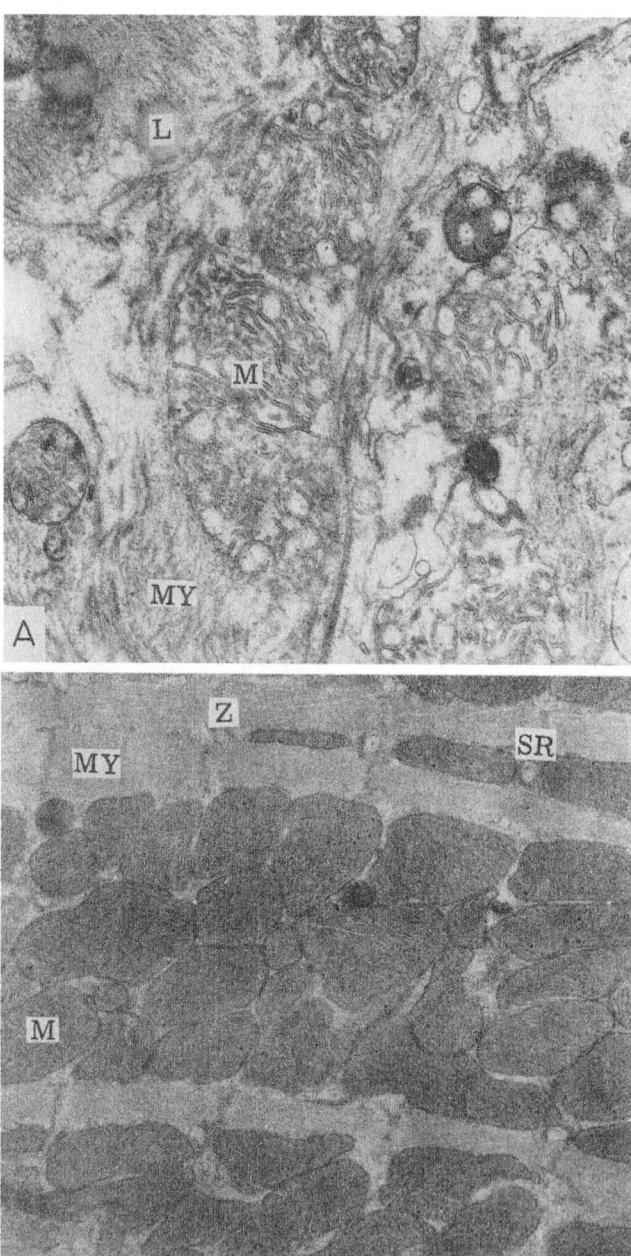

Fig. 36. **Protection by spironolactone against cardiopathy produced by digitoxin + Na_2HPO_4 + oil.** A: Apex of myocardium in the rat after 72 hrs of cardiotoxic treatment. There is an advanced stage of necrosis, the myofibrils (MY) are almost completely destroyed and the glycogen granules have virtually disappeared. The mitochondria (M) show vacuoles with destruction of their internal structure. Occasional lipid (L) granules are visible. × 20,000. B: Region from the cardiac apex of a rat which in addition to the cardiotoxic treatment has received spironolactone. The ultrastructure is virtually normal. Z-band (Z), sarcoplasmic reticulum (SR). × 14,000. [Gardell et al. G 60,065/70. Courtesy of Path. Biol.]

microscopically visible hepatic changes but the electron microscope revealed increased vacuole formation in the Golgi apparatus without any alterations of the endoplasmic reticulum.

← **Testoids.** *Selye A 18,308/39:* In mice, large doses of testosterone sufficient to cause ovarian and adrenal atrophy as well as renal hypertrophy did not significantly alter the weight of the liver.

Common et al. B 23,003/48: In immature pullets, estradiol increases the weight, as well as the fat and protein content of the liver. Concurrent treatment with testosterone does not modify these changes but thyroxine i.v. antagonizes them.

Korenchevsky C 18,714/56: In male rats, testosterone and, to a lesser extent, cortisone increased hepatic weight.

Goldfischer et al. D 20,605/62: In rats treated with norethandrolone, and even more strikingly in those given icterogenin, the capacity to excrete conjugated bilirubin is impaired although light microscopically no obvious hepatic change is noted. There are, however, histochemical and electron microscopic lesions in hepatocytes and bile canaliculi.

Krüskemper & Noell G 48,300/66: Methyltrienolone (17α-methyl-4,9,11-estratriene- 17β-ol-3-one), though a strong anabolic agent, is definitely hepatotoxic as judged by various function tests in man.

Petzold & Ziegler F 92,832/67: The fat and phosphatase accumulation in the liver remnant of partially hepatectomized rats is enhanced by prednisone. 4-Chlorotestosterone does not significantly affect the tissue phosphatase but delays the removal of fats from the liver.

Klatskin G 65,221/69: Review (103 pp., 809 refs.) on toxic and drug-induced hepatitis special sections on the hepatotoxic effect of testoids, corticoids, thioureas, luteoids, folliculoids and oral antidiabetics.

Gardell et al. G 60,062/70: In the rat, norbolethone an active catatoxic steroid produces pronounced proliferation of the SER in hepatocytes, presumably a morphologic reflection of increased microsomal enzyme production.

Mikuni et al. H 28,797/70: In rats, norethandrolone decreased iodipamide (Biligrafin) excretion into the bile. In electron micrographs, the pinocytic vesicles and lysosomes of Kupffer cells and hepatocytes contained a homogenous material interpreted to be deposits of the injected X-ray contrast medium.

← **Antitestoids.** *Kovács et al. G 70,476/71:* In rats, cyproterone acetate p.o. causes marked proliferation of the SER in hepatocytes, perhaps reflecting microsomal-enzyme induction.

← **Catatoxic Steroids.** *Horvath et al. G 70, 405/70:* Both in intact and in partially hepatectomized rats, spironolactone increases the weight of the liver and the mitotic activity of hepatocytes.

Horvath et al. G 70,408/70: In rats "treatment with the most active catatoxic steroids (spironolactone, norbolethone, SC-11927, ethylestrenol) invariably induced marked proliferation of the SER. Progesterone and testosterone had a less pronounced effect. However, alterations of the endoplasmic reticulum can also be produced by some non-catatoxic steroids (estradiol) or non-steroidal compounds (stilbestrol). Thus it can be concluded that there is no close correlation between the catatoxic potency and the proliferation of the SER although all the catatoxic compounds tested lead to a marked transformation of the endoplasmic reticulum in the hepatocytes."

Kovács et al. G 60,045/70: In the rat, spironolactone given in amounts suitable to produce a catatoxic effect causes marked proliferation of smooth-surfaced endoplasmic reticulum in hepatocytes. This change presumably reflects and induction of drug-metabolizing microsomal enzymes and may explain why spironolactone protects against the injurious effects of different compounds.

Garg et al. G 70,474/70: In rats, PCN causes proliferation of the SER in the hepatocytes, with some swelling of the mitochondria and a moderate increase in the lipid content of hepatocytes, as well as some hypertrophy of the microvilli in the bile canaliculi.

Garg et al. G 60,031/71: In rats, PCN p.o. induced proliferation of the SER in hepatocytes. At the high dosage used, it also caused disorganization of the RER, a slight increase in ribosome granules and lipid droplets with mitochondrial injury and myelin figure formation.

Garg et al. G 79,002/71: In rats, PCN p.o. induces proliferation of SER even after hypophysectomy.

Garg et al. G 70,495/71: In rats, phenobarbital, 3-MC, spironolactone, cyproterone and PCN cause proliferation of the SER in hepatocytes without producing marked changes in other cell organelles. In comparing electron microscopic with biochemical and toxicity studies "it seems that there is no obligatory parallelism between SER proliferation and catatoxic potency. However, it is clear that all catatoxic substances tested so far, lead to SER accumulation."

Garg et al. G79,008/71: In rats, hypophysectomy causes a decrease of SER and glycogen granules as well as disorganization of the RER. PCN induces SER proliferation in the hepatocytes even after hypophysectomy.

Garg et al. G79,030/71: In rats, neither spironolactone nor PCN prevents the dilatation, disorganization and breakdown of the RER induced by dactinomycin.

Horvath et al. G70,490/71: In rats, the SER of the hepatocytes proliferates under the influence of CS-1. Ethylestrenol, oxandrolone, and hydroxydione are less effective; progesterone, testosterone, estradiol, stilbestrol, prednisolone, triamcinolone, and DOC are virtually inactive in this respect.

Khandekar et al. G79,014/71: In rats, cycloheximide elicited nucleolar alterations in hepatocytes with disruption, dilatation, degranulation and ballooning of the RER. Accumulation of SER also occurred when spironolactone or PCN was administered one hour before cycloheximide. It is concluded "that the steroids enhance the metabolic degradation of cycloheximide and thus SER proliferation is not inhibited; that this morphologic change does not always denote enzyme induction and the two can therefore be dissociated; or that SER accumulation is a nonspecific response to cellular injury."

Khandekar et al. G79,026/71: In rats, the hepatic SER proliferation induced by spironolactone or PCN is not prevented by concurrent administration of cycloheximide. Either the catatoxic steroids enhance the metabolic degradation of cycloheximide (thereby blocking its effect upon the SER) or this morphologic change does not necessarily indicate active enzyme induction.

Solymoss et al. G79,015/71: In rats, PCN (unlike the naturally-occurring pregnenolone) enhances the plasma clearance of pentobarbital and the production of ^{14}C-pentobarbital metabolites. It also increases liver weight, microsomal protein concentration, NADPH-cytochrome c-reductase activity and cytochrome P-450 content. It is concluded "that microsomal enzyme-induction accounts for the remarkable resistance-increasing effect of this steroid against many toxicants."

Szabo et al. G79,024/71: In rats, PCN increases resistance to indomethacin, hexobarbital, progesterone, zoxazolamine and digitoxin, both in the presence and in the absence of the pituitary. Hypophysectomy also fails to prevent the induction of SER proliferation in the hepatocytes.

Tuchweber et al. G79,020/71: In rats, PCN causes liver hypertrophy with SER proliferation, even if administered during pregnancy.

Tuchweber et al. G79,031/71: In pregnant rats, PCN produces the usual characteristic SER accumulation associated with the formation of intramitochondrial lamellae whose significance is not clear.

← **Other Steroids.** *Goldfischer et al. D20,605/62:* In rats treated with norethandrolone, and even more strikingly in those given icterogenin, the capacity to excrete conjugated bilirubin is impaired although light microscopically no obvious hepatic change is noted. There are, however, histochemical and electron microscopic lesions in hepatocytes and bile canaliculi.

Kottra & Kappas F79,911/67: Review (7 pp., 40 refs.) on the hepatotoxic action of various steroids (particularly folliculoids) especially in man.

Song & Kappas G68,413/68: Review (48 pp., numerous refs.) on the influence of folliculoids, luteoids and pregnancy upon the structure and chemical composition of the liver.

Song et al. G70,575/69: Review (34 pp., 390 refs.) on the effect of various steroid hormones and pregnancy upon hepatic function in animals and man.

← *Nonsteroidal Hormones and Hormone-Like Substances*

← **Anterior Pituitary Hormones.** *Selye A75, 044/44:* In rats, crude lyophilized anterior pituitary extracts cause not only hepatic enlargement, but also infiltration of the liver with hemopoietic cells and megakaryocytes. However, this response may not be entirely specific since various impure protein extracts (especially if they are infected) can cause ectopic hemopoiesis in rodents.

Selye and Nielsen 84,644/44: In rats, crude anterior pituitary extracts cause disproportionate hepatic weight increase, hence the effect cannot be merely considered to be one aspect of the general growth-promoting effect of pituitary STH.

Baker et al. B26,490/48: In rats maintained on a high-carbohydrate diet, ACTH produced a specially pronounced hepatic steatosis.

Li and Evans B29,320/48: In intact (unlike in hypophysectomized) rats, purified STH causes disproportionate hepatic enlargement, possibly by stimulating the secretion of a hypophyseal "hepatotrophic principle."

Payne B32,809/49: In rats (especially if they are maintained on high carbohydrate diets or force-fed) ACTH causes fatty degeneration of the liver. This effect can be prevented by adrenalectomy. Particularly pronounced hepatotrophic effects are obtained in rats upon combined treatment with ACTH + STH.

Selye 94,572/49: In rats, treatment with crude anterior pituitary extracts causes a disproportionate increase in hepatic weight. Particularly pronounced hepatotrophic effects have been obtained in rats upon combined treatment with ACTH + STH.

Garg et al. G79,008/71: In rats, hypophysectomy causes a decrease of SER and glycogen granules as well as disorganization of the RER. PCN induces SER proliferation in hepatocytes even after hypophysectomy.

← **Thyroid Hormones.** *Common et al. B23, 003/48:* In immature pullets, estradiol increases the weight, as well as the fat and protein content of the liver. Concurrent treatment with testosterone does not modify these changes but thyroxine i.v. antagonizes them.

Selye 94,572/49: High doses of thyroxine may cause functional or even structural hepatic damage in various species including man.

Stenram B69,173/52: In rats, thyroid feeding increases hepatic weight and produces diffuse basophilia and palisade-like basophilic rods in the cytoplasm of the hepatocytes. Similar structures had been described previously, by others, after epinephrine treatment or acute bleeding.

Fautrez et al. C23,124/55: In rats, thiourea stimulates mitotic proliferation in hepatocytes.

Scharf et al. F69,957/66: In rats, chronic treatment with methylthiouracil of paroxypropion (POP) produces essentially similar hepatic lesions. T2 reduces liver glycogen and the size of the hepatocytes. Single large doses of alloxan cause severe necrotizing lesions followed by cell proliferation. Concurrent treatment with methylthiouracil inhibits the alloxan-induced hepatic lesions and diminishes mortality.

Funahashi F98,400/67: In rats overdosed with thyroxine, as well as in thyrotoxic patients, the hepatic SER shows no important changes.

Klatskin G65,221/69: Review (103 pp., 809 refs.) on toxic and drug-induced hepatitis with special sections on the hepatotoxic effect of testoids, corticoids, thioureas, luteoids, folliculoids and oral antidiabetics.

Stenram G70,339/69: The literature on the effects of thyroid hormone upon the ultrastructure of hepatocytes is reviewed. Personal observations on the rat, show disappearance of cytoplasmic glycogen. "Mitochondria, endoplasmic reticulum, and free ribosomes and polysomes are evenly distributed all over the cytoplasm. There seems to be an increase in the ratio of free to membrane-bound ribosomes and polysomes in the thyroid-fed. rats."

← **Pancreatic Hormones.** *Birchmeier G69, 512/69:* In mice, hepatic ultrastructure studies were performed after temporary treatment with cortisone or insulin. "The mean mitochondrial volume increased up to fourfold in the cortisone-treated series and to a much lesser extent in the insulin-treated series. The increase in mean mitochondrial volume was balanced by a decrease in the number of mitochondria per cell such that the total cell mitochondrial volume remained relatively constant. It is suggested that the changes in mitochondrial volume and number were a result of mitochondrial fusion. These changes were temporary. Ten days after the hormone treatment the cells were only slightly different from the control cells."

← *Drugs*

← **Barbiturates.** *Remmer & Merker D61, 064/63:* In the rat, hepatic microsomal-enzyme induction by phenobarbital is associated with a proliferation of the hepatic SER.

Remmer & Merker E36,389/63: In the rabbit, "repeated administration of phenobarbital and several other drugs results in a quantitative increase of the smooth endoplasmic reticulum of the liver cell. The marked increase in drug-metabolizing enzymes is found to occur in this enlarged smooth membrane fraction of the endoplasmic reticulum."

Jones & Armstrong F51,262/65: In the hamster, the hepatic SER undergoes hypertrophy following treatment with phenobarbital and, at the same time, cholesterol biosynthesis is increased.

Orrenius et al. G66,249/65: Ultrastructural studies on the hepatic endoplasmic reticulum in relation to phenobarbital-induced synthesis of microsomal drug-metabolizing enzyme systems in the rat.

Burger & Herdson G66,499/66: In the rat, phenobarbital causes liver enlargement and ultrastructural changes characterized by "proliferation of smooth endoplasmic reticulum with concomitant shortening and dispersion of rough endoplasmic cisternae, mitochondrial abnormalities, and the development of myelin figures. The morphologic abnormalities at first affect only central cells, but progressively involve cells further out in the lobule so that after medication for 10 days most of the lobule is involved. Nevertheless, a peripheral zone of normal-looking cells is always present." Concurrent treatment with SKF 525-A further aggravates these changes, but SKF 525-A itself causes no detectable abnormalities in the liver.

Koudstaal & Hardonk G69,482/69: In male rats given phenobarbital i.p., "enzymhistochemically an increase in activity was noted for NADPH tetr. red., G6PD, ICD, and Naftol AS-D-esterase; a decrease was seen in G6Pase and glycogen, but no difference was found in NADH tetr. red. From these results it has been suggested that NADPH tetr. red. is directly involved in the hydroxylation chain, while G6PH and ICD are more indirectly involved."

Chiesara et al. G75,314/70: In rats, a single injection of phenobarbital suffices to stimulate the SER and to increase the hexobarbital and strychnine-metabolizing enzyme activity of the hepatic microsomes. The effect of partial hepatectomy, performed either immediately before or at various times after the administration of the inducer drug, was investigated in relation to these phenomena.

Franken & Hagelskamp H28,823/70: Review (4 pp., 58 refs.) on hepatic lesions produced by barbiturates.

Brodie et al. G80,473/71: In rats, pretreatment with phenobarbital greatly facilitates the production of hepatic necrosis by bromobenzene and other chemically inert halogenated hydrocarbons. Radioautographic and other studies suggest that "a number of aromatic halogenated hydrocarbons are converted by microsomes in vitro to active intermediates which form covalent complexes with glutathione (GSH)."

← **Carbon Tetrachloride.** *Meldolesi et al. G69,793/68:* In rats, CCl_4 greatly increases the proliferation of the SER in hepatocytes and the incorporation of ^{32}P in structural membrane phospholipids. Concurrently, protein synthesis is greatly impaired. Presumably, CCl_4 stimulates the rate of synthesis only of abnormal microsomal membranes.

Smuckler G80,996/68: Brief report on the structural and functional alterations of the endoplasmic reticulum in the hepatocytes of rats intoxicated with CCl_4. "The morphological alterations that have been observed include a dilation and vesiculation of the cisternae of the endoplasmic reticulum, a loss of ordered array of free ribosomes in the cytoplasm and on the endoplasmic reticulum, a dispersal of ribosomes from the membrane surface, and the formation of dense smooth-membrane aggregates." The associated changes in protein synthesis, microsomal electron transport, etc., are briefly noted.

← **Chlorazanil.** *Hyde & Davis F82,461/66:* Both cortisol and the diuretic drug chlorazanil depress mitotic division in the regenerating liver of the mouse, following partial hepatectomy.

← **Clofibrate.** *Kaneko et al. H19,398/69:* In rats, clofibrate at first causes deformation of hepatic mitochondria and depletion of succinic oxidase but these changes disappear within 24 hrs. At 12 hrs after administration of the drug, the SER proliferates, reaching maximal development on the 4th day conjointly with an increase in drug-metabolizing enzyme activity. After 24 hrs there begins an increased formation of microbodies without nucleoides.

← **Dieldrin** *cf.* **Pesticides**

← **Digitalis.** *Arcasoy & Smuckler C63,705/69:* In the rat, a single sublethal dose of digitoxin causes proliferation of the hepatic SER and, concomitantly, an increase in aromatic ring hydroxylation and microsomal cytochrome P-450. Presumably, "digitoxin may induce in the liver enzyme systems capable of glycoside metabolism."

← **Ethanol.** *Leevy & Paumgartner G72,234/68:* In three volunteers who developed alcoholic hepatitis on an ethanol + low-protein regimen, jaundice appeared only in advanced stages of liver necrosis and inflammation. In earlier stages, there was proliferation of SER which was further increased by norethandrolone and yet, this anabolic reduced serum bilirubin.

Mincis H30,210/70: In patients, hepatic biopsies taken after ingestion of large amounts of ethanol show various ultrastructural lesions including the proliferation of SER lamellae which take on a vesicular form.

← **Metyrapone.** *Magalhães & Magalhães G76,648/70:* In rats treated with metyrapone, the SER of the hepatocytes becomes hypertrophic currently with glycogen depletion. Hepatic slices incubated with metyrapone show no ultrastructural changes. The effect of metyrapone is ascribed to increased production of 11β-hydroxylated corticoids.

Dardachti et al. G79,006/71: In rats, metyrapone stimulates the proliferation of SER, even after adrenalectomy.

← **Pesticides.** *Ortega G76,671/66:* Detailed description of the electron microscopic changes in the livers of rats treated with DDT. There was marked proliferation of the SER, inclusion bodies appeared to represent specialization of this system with myelin-like capsules. These changes were compatible with protein synthesis, glycogen storage and normal weight gain. Necrosis, cirrhosis or bile-duct proliferation were not observed.

Ortega H 15,674/69: In rats pretreated with DDT for four months, partial hepatectomy was followed by an essentially normal liver regeneration, yet it developed much more rapidly than after DDT or partial hepatectomy alone.

Hutterer et al. G66,323/69: In rats given daily injection of dieldrin (a chlorinated hydrocarbon pesticide) i.p. hepatic changes developed in three stages. "The first stage, that of induction, is characterized by an increase in liver weight, microsomal protein, smooth endoplasmic reticulum, the activity of aniline hydroxylase and p-nitroreductase, and the concentration of P-450 hemoprotein. During the second stage, a 'steady state,' the elevated levels are maintained and tolerance to otherwise fatal doses of dieldrin prevails. In the third stage, that of decompensation, elevation of liver weight, microsomal proteins, and P-450 hemoproteins persists, and the smooth endoplasmic reticulum appears as abundant as in the previous stages, but the activity of the drug-handling enzymes decreases. The smooth endoplasmic reticulum, however, in this last stage consisted of packed tubules. This hypoactive, hypertrophic, smooth endoplasmic reticulum is accompanied by biochemical and morphologic alterations of mitochondria." 3'-Methyl-4-dimethylaminoazobenzene (butter yellow) produces an essentially similar but accelerated three-stage response.

Kimbrough et al. G81,969/71: In rats, DDT and dieldrin reduce hexobarbital sleeping time, increase liver weight and cause proliferation of the SER with the formation of a typical mitochondria which often contain numerous longitudinally arranged parallel cristae.

← **Phenylbutazone.** *Klinger et al. H28,896/70:* In rats, phenylbutazone reduces hexobarbital sleeping time and increases the fresh weight of the liver as well as the ability of the hepatic 9000 g supernatant to enhance aminophenazone-N-demethylation. An increase in the ascorbic acid concentration of the liver was noted only in young animals but urinary excretion of ascorbic acid was as pronounced as after barbital treatment. Phenylbutazone administration to the pregnant mother failed to elicit an induction effect in the fetuses as judged by hepatic ascorbic acid determinations and by ultrastructural studies of the fetal livers. Proliferation of the SER was obtained by phenylbutazone in 10-day-old or older rats, often in association with an increase in the number of lysosomes and mitochondrial changes as well as by evidence of intrahepatic cholestasis.

← **Salicylates.** *Bullock et al. G73,358/70:* In rats, given large parenteral doses of Na-salicylate, there was an electronmicroscopically detectable "early increase in the number of peroxisomes, and multivesicular bodies were in evidence around the Golgi zone. The endoplasmic reticulum and attached ribosomes exhibited a normal appearance." The corresponding changes in plasma and hepatic enzyme activity are described.

← **W-1372.** *Khandekar et al. G79,016/71:* In rats, W-1372 in oil p.o. causes hepatic steatosis with liposome accumulation, dilatation disorganization, ballooning and degranulation of the RER.

Kovacs et al. G79,003/71: In rats, W-1372 causes electron microscopic changes in the liver characterized by "accumulation of lipid droplets and liposomes, progressive dilatation, disorganization and degranulation of the RER, injury to mitochondria and distension of the sacs of the Golgi apparatus." [This is of interest in view of earlier findings showing that depending upon dosage, W-1372 can produce hepatic necrosis and death or induce resistance to many of the drugs amenable to detoxication by catatoxic steroids (H.S.).]

Selye & Lefebvre G79,005/71: In rats, W-1372 causes hepatic enlargement and fatty degeneration, often with necrosis, if the compound is administered in vegetable oil. W-1372 is much less toxic when given in propylene glycol, mineral oil or DMSO, and virtually nontoxic in water.

← *Hepatic Lesions*

Rigatuso et al. G80,722/70: In rats, partial hepatectomy enhances microbody formation in the liver remnant. "It is suggested that the formation of new microbodies from pre-existing microbodies may be an important general method of microbody proliferation."

Rohr et al. H30,433/70: In rats, an ultrastructural morphometric study of liver cells has been performed during the early regenerative phase after partial hepatectomy.

Stenram et al. H 30,015/70: In rats fed low- or high-protein diets, liver ultrastructure and RNA-labelling was studied after partial hepatectomy. "The results suggest that the protein-deprived rats have a good ability to regenerate liver cell structures after partial hepatectomy, that their enlarged liver cell nucleoli have a high synthesis of RNA, and that the processing and delivering of nucleolar RNA to the cytoplasm proceeds in a normal way."

← Bile Duct Ligation

Hutterer et al. G75,925/70: In rats, 4 days after bile duct ligation the activity of aminopyrine demethylase was greatly decreased, while the content of cytochrome P-450 and the activities of aniline hydroxylase, NADPH-cytochrome c reductase, and cytochrome P-450 reductase were only slightly decreased in the hepatic microsomes. Binding of type II substrate to cytochrome P-450 was unimpaired and its modifier effect on P-450 reductase was intact. The binding of type I substrate was greatly decreased, and its stimulating effect on P-450 reductase was abolished. Presumably cholestasis alters the type I binding sites of the hepatic SER, which is responsible for the hypoactivity of the biotransformation system.

← Sex

Koudstaal and Hardonk G78,115/70: Enzyme histochemical studies suggest that "the difference in hydroxylating capacity between male and female rats may be caused by the fact that the number of cells with hydroxylating activity in the liver lobule, as judged by the NADPH-nitro-BT reductase and Naphthol-AS-D esterase activity, is higher in male than in female rats."

←Tumors

Theologides & Zaki H 19,577/69: In C3H mice bearing transplanted mammary carcinomas s.c., increased mitotic activity in the liver remnant after partial hepatectomy began earlier than in controls.

Kovacs et al. G46,737/71: In rats bearing Walker tumor transplants, the RER is dilated, disorganized and degranulated, whereas the SER proliferates.

← Varia

Fouts D43,347/62: A **review** of evidence suggesting that the SER of the liver is responsible for the induction of drug-metabolizing enzymes.

Remmer G67,786/64: **Review** (20 pp., 55 refs.) on the relationship between hepatic microsomal-enzyme induction and the development of the SER.

Fouts & Rogers F29,497/65: In the rat, "**phenobarbital and chlordane** stimulate a variety of microsomal drug metabolisms and also appear to cause a marked proliferation of smooth-surfaced endoplasmic reticulum (SER) in the hepatic cell. **Benzpyrene and methylcholanthrene** stimulate only a few microsomal drug metabolizing enzymes **and do not appear** to cause any pronounced increase in hepatic cell SER."

Conney F88,649/67 (p. 334): **Review** of the literature on the participation of the SER in the induction of drug-metabolizing hepatic enzymes.

Meldolesi G66,053/67: A **review** of the literature shows that the following drugs are capable of producing hypertrophy of the SER: ethionine, dimethyl-, and diethylnitrosamine, 2-aminofluorene, flurenyldiacetamide, thioacetamide, p-dimethylaminoazobenzene, 3-4-benzopyrene, p-dimethylcholanthrene, α-naphthylisothiocyanate, SKF 525-A, carbon tetrachloride, chlordane, DDT, ethanol, phosphorus, phenobarbital, Bax 422 Z (a thiohydantoin derivative), cysteine, 2-methyldiazobenzene, nikethamide, tolbutamide. In some cases, this hypertrophy is associated with an increased, in others with a decreased microsomal enzyme activity. Possibly, "SER hypertrophy may be produced by one and the same mechanism and all substances capable of producing SER hypertrophy may act as inducers of microsomal enzymes, thus stimulating hepatic cell to produce both endoplasmic reticulum membranes and enzymes. However, some of these substances, or their metabolites, are inhibitors of protein synthesis. In this case synthesis of new enzyme molecules is impossible and the response of the hepatic cell to the pharmacological stimulus is limited to the formation of the SER membranes."

Gran G80,994/68: **Monograph** (101 pp., numerous refs.) representing the proceedings of a symposium on the "Structure and Function of the Endoplasmic Reticulum in Animal Cells."

Mannering G71,818/68 (p. 78): Review of the literature on the production of mitosis in the enlarged livers of rats treated with **phenobarbital, nikethamide, chlorcyclizine** and **hexachlorocyclohexane.**

Claude E8,217/69: **Review** on "Microsomes, Endoplasmic Reticulum and Interactions of Cytoplasmic Membranes."

EXTRAHEPATIC TISSUES

Endocrine Glands

Partial hepatectomy protects the rat against the production of **adrenal** necrosis by DMBA. A similar inhibition is obtained by CCl_4 pretreatment.

In patients treated with spironolactone, concentric lamellar formations ("spironolactone bodies") develop in the adrenal cortical cells. Electronmicroscopically, these phospholipid-containing structures correspond to concentric whorls of SER which may reflect a compensatory increase in mineralocorticoid secretion.

In rats, phenobarbital and PCN produce **thyroid** hypertrophy and hyperplasia which are inhibited by hypophysectomy or thyroxine. These changes may correspond to an increased TTH secretion evoked by interference with the biosynthesis of thyroid hormones or an increase in their metabolic degradation.

Other Tissues

In rats treated with DDT or some of its analogues, a folliculoid effect upon the **uterus** occurs even after ovariectomy. The effect is inhibited by CCl_4 and may depend upon the conversion of DDT into folliculoids.

Spironolactone pretreatment inhibits the ultrastructural changes characteristic of the **myocardial necroses** produced in rats by digitoxin + Na_2HPO_4 + oil.

An entirely unexpected side effect of one of the steroids tested for catatoxic activity was its anticoagulant property, which resulted in **multiple hemorrhages** affecting primarily the facial connective tissue and the thymus of the rat. Such changes had been seen exceptionally in our earliest work with PCN, and even than only with huge doses (25 mg twice daily p.o.). Little attention was attached to this side effect since as much as $30-50$ µg of PCN possesses sufficient catatoxic potency to protect the rat against otherwise fatal doses of indomethacin or digitoxin. However, recently we noted that very small doses of androstanolone-5β-carbonitrile (ACN) occasionally produce a similar hemorrhagic syndrome within a few days, although the compound appears to be totally devoid of catatoxic activity. These findings suggest that the anticoagulant effect of steroids can be separated from their catatoxic potency; indeed, it may represent another independent pharmacologic action, since ACN is not known to possess any of the classical hormonal properties either. Yet, further work will be required to prove this point with certainty, since death from multiple hemorrhages interferes with the bioassay of ACN at high dose levels. In any event the production of hemorrhages is so inconstant that it may depend on variable amounts of some contaminant.

Endocrine Glands

Wheatley et al. F68,548/66: Partial hepatectomy protects the adrenals of the rat against the hemorrhagic necrosis produced by DMBA. On the other hand, "operative stress," as in sham-hepatectomy or nephrectomy, actually increases the susceptibility of the adrenals to DMBA. Other factors influencing DMBA-induced adrenal necrosis are reviewed.

Colafranceschi & Tosi G61,860/67: The induction of adrenal necrosis by DMAB is inhibited in the rat by pretreatment with CCl_4 or partial hepatectomy. The results confirm the view that DMBA becomes toxic only after it is metabolized in the liver.

Japundzic G74,862/69: In rats, phenobarbital produces thyroid enlargement with hypertrophy and hyperplasia of the follicular cells. This effect is inhibited by hypophysecto-

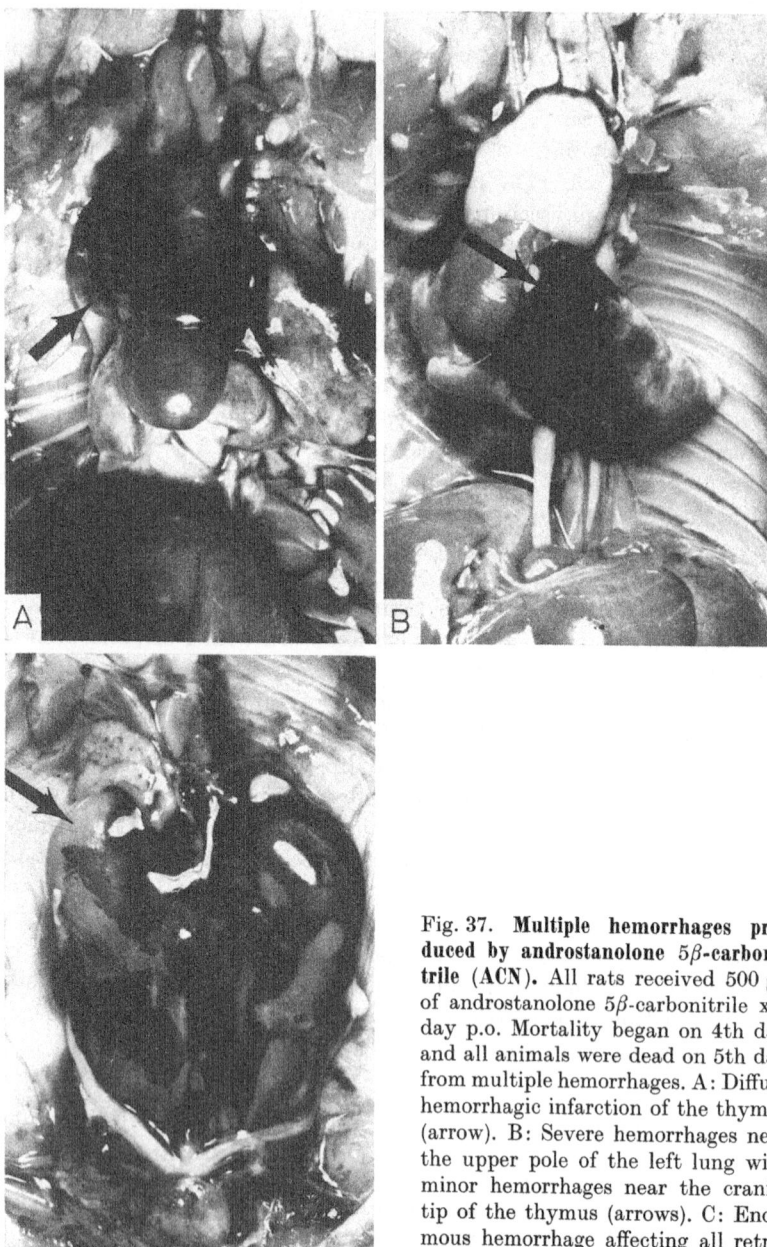

Fig. 37. **Multiple hemorrhages produced by androstanolone 5β-carbonitrile (ACN).** All rats received 500 μg of androstanolone 5β-carbonitrile x2/day p.o. Mortality began on 4th day and all animals were dead on 5th day from multiple hemorrhages. A: Diffuse hemorrhagic infarction of the thymus (arrow). B: Severe hemorrhages near the upper pole of the left lung with minor hemorrhages near the cranial tip of the thymus (arrows). C: Enormous hemorrhage affecting all retroperitoneal organs except part of the right kidney (arrow)

my or thyroxine and may therefore be ascribed to increased TSH secretion. Earlier data on the effect of thiopental and other barbiturates upon the thyroid are reviewed. Possibly barbiturates interfere with the biosynthesis of thyroid hormones, increase their metabolic degradation or their storage in the liver.

Davis & Medline G76,611/70: Description of concentric lamellar formations, the so-called "spironolactone bodies," in the adrenal cortical cells of patients treated with spironolactone. Earlier literature is described. "These phospholipid-containing bodies, as disclosed by electron microscopy, are concentric whorls of smooth membranes arranged in a pattern similar to that in many organs under experimental conditions . . . the authors believe that these structures represent a compensatory attempt on the part of the cell to produce increased mineralocorticoid."

Selye G70,480/71: In rats, unusually large doses of PCN produce thyroid hyperplasia and hypertrophy.

Other Tissues ←

Welch et al. G65,737/69: In rats, DDT and some of its analogs exhibit a folliculoid effect upon the uterus, even after castration. Since this action is inhibited by CCl_4, it may depend on the conversion of DDT analogs into folliculoids.

Gardell et al. G60,065/70: In rats, spironolactone pretreatment inhibits the ultrastructural changes characteristic of the myocardial necroses induced by digitoxin + Na_2HPO_4 + corn oil.

Selye PROT. 35304: In rats 500 μg of androstanolone-5β-carbonitrile (ACN) x2/day p.o. occasionally causes multiple, eventually fatal, hemorrhages affecting most frequently the thymus and the retroperitoneal organs, but sometimes also the lung, the facial connective tissue and other sites. The blood remains incoagulable even many hours after being shed. Subsequent experiments have shown that almost the same effect is produced at a dose level of 100 μg x2/day or even less. When given at enormous dose levels (e.g., 25 mg x2/day p.o.), PCN can produce similar manifestations, but ACN is the only steroid known to possess a high degree of anticoagulant potency. It remains to be seen whether any of the naturally occurring steroids can exert similar effects under appropriate conditions.

X. THEORIES

In this last section, we shall survey the theories concerning the role of hormones in the maintenance of resistance in general, as well as current concepts concerning certain links in the mechanism of individual, hormonally controlled resistance phenomena. This chapter is based upon what we have learned from the entire literature on the subject as listed in all the other sections of this monograph. Hence, the abstracts supporting our discussion will often be found elsewhere in this book; only those of the most pertinent original publications are reproduced here. In agreement with the general principles that have guided us throughout this treatise, major emphasis will be placed upon the newly discovered catatoxic actions of steroids, particularly on their effect upon general resistance through the induction of hepatic enzymes. However, for comparative purposes, some resistance effects of syntoxic hormones and a few extrahepatic defense mechanisms will also be considered.

The main theoretic problems shall be classified as follows:

1. Hepatic participation in general;
2. The role of hepatic enzymes;
3. SER and microsomes;
4. RNA and DNA;
5. Lysosomes;
6. Reticulo-endothelial system (RES);
7. Hepatic glycogen;
8. Vitamin C;
9. Defense against "natural" vs. "foreign" compounds;
10. Stressors;
11. Homeostasis and the nonspecificity of steroid-induced resistance.

1. HEPATIC PARTICIPATION IN GENERAL

cf. also Abstract Sections *under* "History," "General Pharmacology," "← Hepatic Lesions"

It has been demonstrated beyond any possible doubt that most of the known protective effects of steroids against exogenous or endogenous toxicants depend upon the stimulation of defensive responses in hepatic tissue. Perhaps, most important among these defensive reactions is the induction of the so-called drug-metabolizing microsomal enzymes. However, undoubtedly other phenomena are also involved in many cases: activation of enzymes which regulate intermediate metabolism in general provides building blocks for structural or enzymic proteins; stimulation of the Kupffer cells or increased storage in hepatocytes can offer temporary protection against acute flooding of the blood with poisons until they are gradually excreted or inactivated through other mechanisms.

Yet, the liver is rarely the only organ involved in detoxication. Usually, toxicants are first subjected to biotransformation — for example in the SER — into compounds especially suitable for elimination through the urine or bile. In this respect, the transformation of a nonpolar toxicant into a more polar metabolite offers the advantage of making it unsuitable for reabsorption by the renal tubules after its filtration through the glomerulus; normally the ready reabsorption of lipid soluble compounds prevents their elimination. However, even the hormonal control of biliary excretion depends not only upon a cholagogue effect; it is also modified by biotransformations which render compounds more or less suitable for excretion into the bile.

Evidence showing the relative importance of these hepatic activities has been obtained by many techniques, e.g.: the increase in sensitivity to toxicants induced by partial or complete hepatectomy and hepatotoxic agents, or the decrease in the in vivo activities of many agents when they are forced to traverse the liver before getting into the general circulation. The latter can be accomplished in many ways, for example by administration per os or through the portal vein, injection of drugs and hormones (or implantation of hormone-producing glands) into the spleen or other parts of the portal area.

Additional evidence of hepatic detoxication has been obtained by the demonstration that certain toxicants are inactivated by incubation with liver slices, liver homogenates and various liver fractions (e.g., those rich in microsomes). Biliary excretion has been followed by the chemical determination of toxicants or their metabolites in bile obtained through a fistula. The importance of the enterohepatic circulation could frequently be demonstrated by the observation that the effects of a drug are diminished or abolished following ligature of the choledochus. As has been shown by the literature cited in the sections referred to, virtually all these forms of hepatic participation in detoxication mechanisms are influenced by one or the other hormonal principle.

In connection with the action of catatoxic steroids, the most important mechanisms involved in hepatic detoxication are the induction of enzymes in the membrane systems of the endoplasmic reticulum which become smooth (SER) and break up into small vesicles, the microsomes.

Zondek 30,531/34: Estrone injected into a mouse rapidly disappears and can no longer be extracted from its tissues. On theoretic grounds, it is assumed that hepatic enzymes are responsible for this inactivation.

Weiner et al. H 24,942/70: In rats, glucagon, alloxan and starvation all increased hexobarbital sleeping time. This effect was markedly antagonized by insulin. Perhaps, cyclic AMP may be involved since theophylline greatly increases the action of glucagon. This synergism also occurred in isolated, perfused rat livers and, hence, "inhibition of hexobarbital metabolism by cyclic AMP would appear to be mediated in the liver."

2. THE ROLE OF HEPATIC ENZYMES

It has been demonstrated in various ways that synthesis of new enzyme protein, rather than mere enzyme activation, is involved in the increased biotransformation of various substrates by hormonal and nonhormonal catatoxic substances. For example in the rat, the induction of hepatic TKT by cortisol is associated with an equivalent increase in enzyme antigen. Tryptophan also induces significant increases in hepatic TKT activity. Isotope incorporation studies, combined with the analysis of the time course of changing enzyme levels, indicate that cortisol accelerates the rate of enzyme synthesis, whereas tryptophan acts predominantly by decreasing the rate of enzyme degradation. Certain additional studies suggest, however, that some enzyme activation may also play a role in connection with the augmentation of TPO and TKT.

The defensive role of TPO induction has by no means been demonstrated. It is true that in mice, endotoxin lowers TPO, whereas glucocorticoids which increase endotoxin resistance augment TPO activity. However, a-methyltryptophan maintains TPO activity without increasing survival and 5-hydroxytryptophan lowers TPO activity without sensitizing to endotoxin.

The so-called nonspecific drug-metabolizing hepatic enzymes are presumably subject to similar regulatory mechanisms. It is difficult to understand why these systems are so largely nonspecific. It has been assumed that either a multitude of specific oxidases or an oxidase of remarkable nonspecificity is at work. There are arguments in favor of both these possibilities. It must not be forgotten however that the degree of the nonspecificity of protection (and hence presumably of enzyme induction) is subject to great variations. Probably none of the microsomal enzyme inducers is completely specific, but some act only against few, others against many toxicants, and the particular combination of substrates inactivated by any one inducer is quite unpredictable. It is also impossible to determine from in vitro data alone whether inhibitors of cytochrome P-450 enzymes will significantly block the metabolism of drugs in vivo. In view of the innumerable factors which can influence the synthesis, degradation, activation and inactivation of the microsomal enzymes (as well as of the inducers, the toxicants and their metabolites) in the living organism, our approach to these problems must meanwhile depend almost entirely on empiricism.

Work on catatoxic steroids has brought out with particular clarity one additional complication, namely that the enzyme inducers may or may not enhance their own metabolic degradation. Thus, spironolactone enhances not only the inactivation of digitoxin and indomethacin but also its own metabolism as judged by blood clearance rates. However, the capacity of the catatoxic steroids to inactivate themselves is limited, and hence, they continue to detoxify drugs in chronic experiments for many weeks or months as long as the toxicant is administered in combination with an appropriate inducer. As soon as administration of the latter ceases, the toxicant again exhibits its usual effects indicating that whatever the mechanism of enzymic defense, its persistence depends upon continued stimulation by the inducer.

TPO, TKT

Kenney E 89,716/62: In the rat, the induction of hepatic TKT by cortisol is associated with an equivalent increase in enzyme antigen. A cross-reactive precursor could not be detected in any of the subcellular liver fractions. Induction in the presence of ^{14}C-labeled amino acids results in extensive labeling of transaminase, with or without induction.

Rosen & Milholland E 32,652/63: Tryptophan induced significant increases in hepatic TKT activity in intact and in adrenalectomized (NaCl-maintained) rats. Tyrosine, histidine and methionine slightly depressed the hepatic TKT activity of the adrenalectomized rats. Analogues of tryptophan (including D-tryptophan, acetyl-L-tryptophan, indole, DL-5-hydroxytryptophan and 5-HT i.p.) increase both TKT and TPO activity by 50—300% in the livers of intact or adrenalectomized rats. 5-HT and DL-5-hydroxytryptophan were most active. After hypophysectomy, the response of each of these enzymes to tryptophan gradually diminished. After 6 months, tryptophan, 5-hydroxytryptophan and 5-HT failed to cause significant increases in the hepatic activity of these enzymes, but cortisol remained highly effective, causing increases in both enzyme activities comparable to those seen in intact or adrenalectomized rats. "Experiments with two known inhibitors of protein synthesis, DL-ethionine and puromycin, indicate that a major fraction or the induced activity of tryptophan pyrrolase seen in adrenalectomized or hypophysectomized rats treated by injection with tryptophan is due to activation rather than synthesis of new enzyme protein. The responses of tryptophan pyrrolase and tyrosine transaminase in liver following cortisol administration appear to be mainly the result of the synthesis of each of these enzymes."

Schimke et al. G24,293/65: In adrenalectomized rats, both cortisol and tryptophan increase hepatic TPO, but a particularly pronounced rise is obtained by combined treatment with both these agents. An analysis of the time course of changing enzyme levels, and the results of isotope incorporation studies indicate that cortisol increases the rate of enzyme synthesis, whereas tryptophan decreases the rate of enzyme degradation.

Moon & Berry G57,245/68: "Using substrate induction as a tool, we attempted to determine the role of tryptophan pyrrolase in the response to endotoxin in mice. Previous results have shown that the administration of the LD_{50} of endotoxin lowers tryptophan pyrrolase activity. α-Methyltryptophan was found to maintain tryptophan pyrrolase activity above control levels in endotoxin-poisoned mice without increasing survival. 5-Hydroxytryptophan, by contrast, lowered tryptophan pyrrolase activity but did not sensitize mice to endotoxin. These results suggest that tryptophan pyrrolase per se does not play a unique role in survival of mice poisoned with endotoxin."

Microsomal Enzymes

Karlson & Sekeris F73,338/66: Review of the literature and personal observations on the biochemical mechanisms of hormone actions. It is postulated "that hormones may act as gene activators ... Gene activation would lead to production of messenger-RNA and induced enzyme synthesis."

Conney F88,649/67 (p. 330): Review on the role of enzyme synthesis and degradation in the induction of drug-metabolizing activity.

Mannering G71,818/68 (pp. 57, 84): The comparative nonspecificity of detoxication by microsomal enzymes suggests "that a multitude of oxidases of remarkable substrate specificity exists or, at the other extreme, that an oxidase of remarkable nonspecificity exists." The arguments for and against each of these possibilities are carefully reviewed.

Mannering G71,818/68 (p. 79): Review of the data suggesting that inducers actually increase the synthesis of new hepatic microsomal drug-metabolizing enzyme proteins.

Selye et al. G60,020/69: The antianesthetic and antidigitoxin activities of spironolactone and norbolethone may depend upon competitive inhibition or induction of hepatic microsomal enzymes.

Various authors G68,203/69: Review (27 pp., 42 refs.) on "Application of metabolic data to the evaluation of drugs. A report prepared by the Committee on Problems of Drug Safety of the Drug Research Board, National Academy of Sciences—National Research Council." A large section of this report is devoted to the inactivation of drugs by microsomal enzymes. It is emphasized that "it is difficult to predict from in vitro data alone whether inhibitors of the cytochrome P-450 enzymes will significantly block the metabolism of drugs in laboratory animals and in patients." Furthermore, "phenobarbital administration leads to an increase in virtually all known enzymatic pathways by causing an increase in both NADPH cytochrome C reductase and cytochrome P-450. Although phenobarbital is known to act by increasing the synthesis of enzyme protein, it may also act by slowing the turnover of the various components of the endoplasmic reticulum."

Solymoss & Selye G70,409/70: Rats given daily treatment with normally fatal amounts of indomethacin or digitoxin can survive for an apparently indefinite period if they are concurrently treated with spironolactone or oxandrolone. Upon interruption of catatoxic steroid administration, death ensues within a few days. "Spironolactone enhances not only the degradation of digitoxin and indomethacin but also its own metabolism as judged by their disappearance rate from the blood. However, the capacity of the steroids to inactivate themselves is limited and, hence, they continue to detoxify both drugs, even in chronic experiments."

3. SER and MICROSOMES
cf. also Electron Microscopic Data *under* "Morphology"

It appears to be well established that the induction of microsomal enzymes takes place within the endoplasmic reticulum. The electron microscopic expression of such enzyme induction is the gradual transformation of the rough into the smooth ER whose membrane systems eventually are broken up into vesicles which may become very large and give the cytoplasm a spongy appearance. It is assumed that the substrates enter these vesicles and are therein destroyed by the induced enzymes. For several of the enzyme activities, both the microsomes and soluble cell constituents are necessary as shown by the fact that pure microsomes isolated by ultracentrifugation are active only if supernatant cytosol is added.

There is some doubt about the relative participation in detoxication of the highly substrate specific amino acid deaminating (TPO, TKT) enzymes and the relatively nonspecific microsomal enzymes. Glucocorticoids, which are good inducers of TPO and TKT, shorten barbiturate and meperidine sleeping time and combat endotoxin shock. However, these latter effects may be unrelated to the activation of TPO and TKT; they have been tentatively ascribed to the induction of microsomal enzymes by glucocorticoids.

Several review articles list the many drugs and hormones capable of transforming the RER into an SER, simultaneously activating microsomal enzymes. Among these there are even typical hepatotoxic substances such as CCl_4 which increase the SER in hepatocytes and enhance the incorporation of ^{32}P in structural membrane phospholipids. Yet, concurrently, protein synthesis is impaired presumably because CCl_4 stimulates the rate of synthesis only in abnormal microsomal membranes.

Recent studies suggest that cortisol, which is a substrate for microsomal enzymes, is bound rapidly in the SER of hepatocytes, poorly in the RER, and virtually not at all in ribosomes.

Microsomal mixed function oxidases and cytochrome P-450 are relatively more concentrated in the SER than in the RER. Curiously, benzpyrene does not affect the SER or microsomal protein although it stimulates the biotransformation of many substrates. Apparently, this carcinogen acts through a mechanism different from that of the barbiturates and of most other drug-metabolizing enzyme inducers.

Certain herbicides inhibit the induction by phenobarbital of cytochrome P-450 and of drug hydroxylase activity, yet, they do not prevent the proliferation of the SER. Presumably, induced increases in cytochrome P-450 and proliferation of the SER are controlled by separate mechanisms.

Review of the entire pertinent literature suggests that most, if not all, typical catatoxic steroids do induce proliferation of the SER but not all steroids that produce this latter effect are also potent inducers of resistance in vivo. It is possible that following excessive or abnormal stimulation of the SER, its enzyme-producing activity declines without there being any morphologically detectable manifestations of its functional exhaustion.

Bucher & McGarrahan G67,470/56: For the biosynthesis of cholesterol from acetate in vitro, both microsomes and soluble cell constituents of the rat liver are required. In vivo, over 90% of newly formed cholesterol, obtained shortly after the injection of labeled acetate, is in the microsomal fraction.

Remmer D86,728/58: In the rat, cortisone and prednisolone shorten the meperidine and hexobarbital sleeping time as well as the detoxication of these sedatives by liver slices. This effect is tentatively ascribed to an activation of hepatic microsomal enzymes, since the known effect of glucocorticoids upon the deamination of amino acids depends upon highly substrate-specific enzymes.

Fouts G 79,654/61: When SER and RER particles of rabbit liver are separated by ultracentrifugation in various sucrose gradients, the NADPH oxidase and drug-metabolizing enzyme activity can be shown to be higher in the SER than in the RER.

Remmer & Merker E 36,389/63: In the rabbit, "repeated administration of phenobarbital and several other drugs results in a quantitative increase of the smooth endoplasmic reticulum of the liver cell. The marked increase in drug-metabolizing enzymes is found to occur in this enlarged smooth membrane fraction of the endoplasmic reticulum."

Fouts & Rogers F 29,497/65: Benzpyrene and methylcholanthrene which stimulate only few microsomal drug-metabolizing enzymes do not cause any pronounced increase in the SER of hepatocytes.

Conney F 88,649/67 (p. 336): Review on the effect of drugs on electron transport systems in liver microsomes.

Meldolesi G 66,053/67: A review of the literature shows that the following drugs are capable of producing hypertrophy of the SER: ethionine, dimethyl-, and diethylnitrosamine, 2-aminoflourene, flurenyl diacetamide, thioacetamide, p-dimethylaminoazobenzene, 3-4-benzopyrene, p-dimethylcholanthrene, α-naphthylisothiocyanate, SKF 525-A, carbon tetrachloride, chlordane, DDT, ethanol, phosphorus, phenobarbital, Bax 422 Z (a thiohydantoin derivative), cysteine, 2-methyldiazobenzene, nikethamide, tolbutamide. In some cases, this hypertrophy is associated with an increased, in others with a decreased, microsomal enzyme activity. Possibly, "SER hypertrophy may be produced by one and the same mechanism and all substances capable of producing SER hypertrophy may act as inducers of microsomal enzymes, thus stimulating hepatic cell to produce both endoplasmic reticulum membranes and enzymes. However, some of these substances, or their metabolites, are inhibitors of protein synthesis. In this case synthesis of new enzyme molecules is impossible and the response of the hepatic cell to the pharmacological stimulus is limited to the formation of the SER membranes."

Meldolesi et al. G 69,793/68: In rats, CCl_4 greatly increases the proliferation of the SER in hepatocytes and the incorporation of ^{32}P in structural membrane phospholipids. Concurrently, protein synthesis is greatly impaired. Presumably CCl_4 stimulates the rate of synthesis only of abnormal microsomal membranes.

Mannering G 71,818/68 (pp. 52, 78): Review on the participation of the SER in drug metabolism.

Hutterer et al. G 66,323/69: In rats, treated with dieldrin, serial ultrastructural studies of the liver showed a three-stage response. "The first stage, that of induction, is characterized by an increase in liver weight, microsomal protein, smooth endoplasmic reticulum, the activity of aniline hydroxylase and p-nitroreductase, and the concentration of P-450 hemoprotein. During the second stage, a 'steady state,' the elevated levels are maintained and tolerance to otherwise fatal doses of dieldrin prevails. In the third stage, that of decompensation, elevation of liver weight, microsomal proteins, and P-450 hemoprotein persists, and the smooth endoplasmic reticulum appears as abundant as in the previous stages, but the activity of the drug-handling enzymes decreases. The smooth endoplasmic reticulum, however, in this last stage consisted of packed tubules. This hypoactive, hypertrophic, smooth endoplasmic reticulum is accompanied by biochemical and morphologic alterations of mitochondria." 3-Methyl-4-dimethylaminoazobenzene caused a rapid decompensation without significant steady state. Literature concerning other observations on hypoactive hypertrophic SER is summarized.

Mayewski & Litwack G 70,720/69: In adrenalectomized rats, radioactive cortisol is bound rapidly to the SER of hepatocytes, poorly to the RER and virtually not at all to the ribosomes.

Williams & Rabin G 77,164/69: In rats, the effect of aflatoxin B_1 and steroid hormones on polysome binding to microsomal membranes has been measured by the activity of an enzyme-catalyzing disulfide interchange. Corticosterone and, to a much lesser extent cortisol, antagonizes the effect of aflatoxin, presumably by competition at a site on microsomal membranes responsible for polysome binding. The authors postulate the "simple hypothesis that a steroid hormone, related to corticosterone, can occupy specific sites on the membrane and that, when these sites are occupied, polysome binding can occur. The difference between 'rough' and 'smooth' endoplasmic reticulum would then be that the specific sites of the former are occupied by hormone, whereas those of the latter are not."

Fouts G76,868/70: Review of the literature showing that in rats and rabbits, microsomal mixed-function oxidases and cytochrome P-450 are relatively more concentrated in the SER than in the RER. It is noteworthy, furthermore, that benzpyrene treatment does not affect hepatic weight, microsomal protein or the appearance of the SER in the rat liver, indicating that this carcinogen acts through a mechanism different from that of barbiturates and of most other microsomal drug-metabolizing enzyme inducers.

Raisfeld et al. G75,045/70: In rats, the herbicide 3-amino-1,2,4,-triazole inhibits the induction by phenobarbital of cytochrome P-450 and drug hydroxylase activity, but does not prevent the proliferation of the SER in hepatocytes. Presumably "induced increases of cytochrome P-450 and of the membranes of endoplasmic reticulum may be controlled by separate mechanisms."

Stenger G74,578/70: Review (21 pp., 177 refs.) with special reference to the alterations in RER and SER produced by various agents and the relationship of these changes to glycogen and drug metabolism.

Stenger et al. G78,940/70: In rats, pretreatment with phenobarbital in doses which cause proliferation of the SER and a decrease in hexobarbital sleeping time greatly diminished resistance to the fatal effects of CCl_4. Phenobarbital pretreatment delayed the onset of CCl_4-induced hepatic necrosis, but greatly aggravated its eventual severity. "This altered hepatotoxic response might be related either to the increase of smooth-surfaced membranes or to the augmentation of drug-metabolizing enzyme systems in the livers of the phenobarbital-pretreated animals."

Garg et al. G79,002/71: In rats, PCN p.o. induces proliferation of SER even after hypophysectomy.

Garg et al. G70,495/71: In rats, phenobarbital, 3-MC, spironolactone, cyproterone, and PCN cause proliferation of the SER in hepatocytes without producing marked changes in other cell organelles. In comparing electron-microscopic with biochemical and toxicity studies "it seems that there is no obligatory parallelism between SER proliferation and catatoxic potency. However, it is clear that all catatoxic substances tested so far, lead to SER accumulation."

Khandekar et al. G79,026/71: In rats, the hepatic SER proliferation induced by spironolactone or PCN is not prevented by concurrent administration of cycloheximide. Either the catatoxic steroids enhance the metabolic degradation of cycloheximide (thereby blocking its effect upon the SER) or this morphologic change does not necessarily indicate active enzyme induction.

Kovacs et al. G46,737/71: In rats bearing Walker tumor transplants, the RER is dilated, disorganized and degranulated, whereas the SER proliferates.

4. RNA and DNA

The many and often conflicting concepts concerning the manner in which RNA and DNA participate in the induction of microsomal enzymes will be described in the following Abstract Section. However, it would by far exceed the scope of this monograph and the competence of its author to attempt a critical integration of all pertinent data.

Feigelson et al. D25,364/62: The induction of hepatic TPO by tryptophan or cortisone in the rat is used as a model for the study of interrelations between hormonal- and substrate-dependent enzyme induction processes. Following i.p. administration of either inducer, there is a rise in liver TPO activity, reaching a maximum after 4—5 hrs, the peak being higher for tryptophan than for cortisone. Judged by ^{14}C-glycine and ^{32}P-orthophosphate incorporation experiments, both tryptophan- and cortisone-induced stimulation of protein metabolism follow the same time course, but their effects on RNA metabolism do not coincide. Tryptophan causes no increase in RNA turnover, while the enzyme level is rising. When enzyme activity has returned to normal, precursor incorporation into RNA is stimulated. Cortisone, on the other hand, markedly stimulates RNA turnover with a peak at 4 hrs corresponding to peak enzyme levels. The pattern of incorporation of the purine precursor, glycine-2-^{14}C, into the RNA of various hepatic subcellular fractions showed that cortisone increases precursor incorporation into the proteins of all liver cell constituents, but much less than into RNA. On the basis of these and many other experiments concerning the mechanism of enzyme induction, a hypothesis is proposed according to which the difference between enzyme and hormone induction might be explained. "This hypothesis rests on the assumption that the increase in enzyme activity, in excess of that due to hematin activation, is due to the presence of increased levels of enzyme protein derived from an increased rate either of enzyme protein synthesis or of release. It is herein proposed that apotryptophan pyrrolase is synthesized at a specific vacant enzyme-forming site. Furthermore, it is postulated that apoenzyme molecules (E) on the enzyme-forming site or template are in dynamic equilibrium with the apoenzyme molecules of the cytoplasm. Holoenzyme molecules (EH), however, are incapable of binding at this site. It follows that saturation of apotryptophan pyrrolase with hematin, promoted by tryptophan, would render many enzyme-forming sites vacant, thus shifting the equilibrium toward further enzyme protein synthesis. With the fall in intracellular tryptophan concentration, EH combination would be retarded, apotryptophan pyrrolase would accumulate, occupying the enzyme-forming site, and inhibit its own synthesis; a gradual return to basal enzyme levels would then take place. In this manner, a tryptophan-regulated saturation of the enzyme with hematin cofactor would control the synthetic rate and the level of this enzyme in liver. Cortisone clearly influences the level of tryptophan pyrrolase by a different mechanism. As indicated by the arrow, it is proposed that cortisone may stimulate enzyme protein synthesis by interfering with the equilibrium between the template-bound and soluble apotryptophan pyrrolase in such a way as to prevent the accumulated apotryptophan pyrrolase from binding to the template and inhibiting its own synthesis. This interference might be envisaged as a cortisone-induced alteration of the structure of the apotryptophan pyrrolase, or as a change in the ribosome itself."

Feigelson & Feigelson D59,123/63: In rat liver tissue, "cortisone rapidly elevates incorporation of glycine-2-C^{14} into acid-soluble adenine nucleotides as well as into RNA. Intraperitoneal administration of a variety of L- and D-amino acids, NH_4+, and glutamine into adrenalectomized rats imitated cortisone by stimulating glycine-2-C^{14} incorporation into acid-soluble and RNA purines. Although liver adenosine triphosphate levels rise after cortisone administration, such alterations in ATP per se do not influence the rate of precursor incorporation into RNA or protein. On the basis of these findings, it is proposed that increased amino acid deamination, implicit in the gluconeogenic action of the glucocorticoids, results in the liberation of α-amino nitrogen moieties that mediate the cortisone-induced increases in hepatic purine biosynthetic rates."

Knox D66,995/63: The "push-pull theory" of enzyme induction is formulated on the basis of experiments concerning the production of TPO and TKT by cortisol or by the respective substrates in intact and adrenalectomized rats. As illustrated by the diagram on p. 751, the substrate-type induction "pulls protein synthesis through the existing templates and, by depleting the species of marked enzyme, slows the rate of enzyme degradation. The hormone-type induction acts by causing the production of more of the limited, essential species of RNA that is necessary for making the tryptophan pyrrolase. Thus hormonal induction pushes additional enzyme synthesis through the provision of additional RNA templates."

Lindergren G66,494/63: Discussion of the receptor-hypothesis of induction of gene-controlled adaptive enzymes.

Garren et al. G28,021/64: In adrenalectomized rats, a single i.p. injection of cortisol produces an increase in hepatic TPO and TKT activity. Actinomycin D did not inhibit synthesis of these enzymes, but blocked their induction when injected early after cortisol administration. Actinomycin D and fluorouracil stimulated TPO and TKT synthesis when injected 5 hrs or later after cortisol. "It is proposed that repression of the synthesis of these enzymes occurs at the level of messenger RNA translation."

Knox G65,171/64: Observations on adrenalectomized rats lead to the distinction between two types of TPO induction, one called the "hormone type" because glucocorticoids act this way. Thus, in adrenalectomized rats,

Model of the two known mechanisms of enzymic adaptation in animal tissues: substrate-type induction, which accumulates more total enzyme by combining with the free enzyme in effective equilibrium with its precursors, and hormone-type induction, which provides more of the limiting RNA species for the specific enzyme synthesis.

cortisol increased the amount of some limiting RNA moiety, thereby augmenting enzyme synthesis. This action is prevented by actinomycin through the inhibition of RNA synthesis as well as by puromycin, which inhibits protein synthesis. The second form or "substrate type" of induction is obtained by tryptophan which increases the amount of TPO without simulating RNA synthesis. This increase is not prevented by actinomycin although it is, of course, blocked by puromycin, which inhibits protein synthesis. These and other observations led to the formulation of the "push-pull" theory of enzyme induction which is illustrated on p. 752.

Gelboin F62,759/65: Review of the literature on the role played by RNA in the induction of hepatic microsomal enzymes.

Greenman et al. G35,063/65; Wicks et al. G35,046/65: Studies on the stimulation of hepatic ^{32}P-RNA synthesis in adrenalectomized rats treated with cortisol.

Singer & Mason G66,500/65: Na-benzoate increased hepatic TKT activity both in intact and in NaCl-maintained adrenalectomized rats. Among 31 cyclic compounds tested for this inducing ability after adrenalectomy, only cortisol, its hemisuccinate and diethylstilbestrol disulfate were more effective than benzoate. Curiously, enzyme induction by cortisol was actually enhanced after adrenalectomy. "Strong inhibition of the increase by injected puromycin and actinomycin D, compounds which inhibit protein and RNA synthesis respectively, suggests that the benzoate-mediated effect occurred by a mechanism involving increases in protein and RNA synthesis. In this respect, the effect of benzoate resembles that of the glucocorticoids."

Tomkins et al. G35,353/65: Following a single injection of cortisol into adrenalectomized rats, the hepatic TPO and TKT levels rise. "Although actinomycin D blocks the initial steroid-induced increase, later administration of the antibiotic (or of 5-fluorouracil) causes an increase in the levels of these enzymes. A mechanism is proposed to account for the late response to inhibitors of RNA synthesis in which a 'cytoplasmic repressor' can inhibit the translation of the messenger RNA's corresponding to tryptophan pyrrolase and tyrosine transaminase. Cytoplasmic repression is postulated to depend on continued RNA and protein synthesis, and the 'repressor' is thought to have a rapid rate of turnover."

Griffin & Cox F86,851/66: "The induction of alkaline phosphatase by prednisolone in HeLa cell cultures appears to occur at the level of protein synthesis (translation) as a result of a steroid-induced change in the conformational state of the enzyme during its synthesis."

Tomkins et al. G49,588/66: Glucocorticoids stimulate TKT induction in rat hepatoma cells in vitro. Inhibitor and immunochemical experiments indicate that the corticoids do not activate a precursor but increase the number of enzyme protein molecules. Apparently, the hormones exert some control at the level of translation of the transaminase messenger by antagonizing a repressor of messenger function. "It cannot yet be determined whether the presumed increase in messenger concentration occurs as a secondary response to the stimulation of translation, or whether there is a direct effect of the hormone on gene transcription."

Conney F88,649/67 (pp. 330, 333, 334): Review on the role of enzyme synthesis and

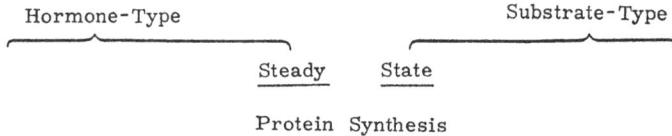

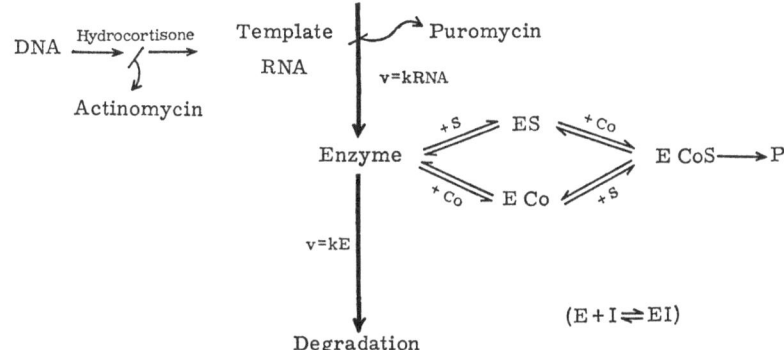

The "push-pull" model of enzyme inductions in animal tissues. In the steady state of enzyme synthesis and degradation, accumulations of total enzyme are "pushed" by temporarily increased synthesis of nascent enzyme (E) through the extra RNA templates produced by hydrocortisone (hormone-type induction), or "pulled" by the temporary specific combination of substrates, coenzymes, and inhibitors with the nascent enzyme (substrate-type induction). Sites of action are indicated for actinomycin, which distinguishes between the two mechanisms, and of puromycin.

degradation in the induction of drug-metabolizing activity.

Drews & Brawerman G52,150/67: Studies on changes in RNA-synthesis in the rat liver during regeneration and after cortisol administration. The relationship between enzyme induction and RNA-synthesis is discussed.

Gelboin G53,802/67: Review (81 pp., about 90 refs.) on enzyme induction in connection with carcinogenesis and gene action.

Gelehrter & Tomkins G51,315/67: Dexamethasone induced a 3-15-fold increase in TKT activity in hepatoma cells of the rat (in tissue culture) but no increase in total RNA nor its synthesis as measured by the rate of incorporation of labeled precursors. Various experiments also failed to demonstrate gross stimulation of RNA synthesis associated with enzyme induction by steroid hormones in vivo, "suggesting that these changes are not an essential part of the mechanism of enzyme induction by glucocorticoids."

Grossman & Mavrides G46,206/67: Studies on the kinetics of cortisol-induced hepatic TKT activity in adrenalectomized rats. "Puromycin inhibited enzyme synthesis when it was given during the initial phase of induction. However, it unexpectedly caused a rapid reappearance of enzyme activity following its administration during the inactivation phase. This potentiated response is consistent with other observations which lead to the idea that a repressor is formed about 4 hours after hormone administration and that inhibition of repressor synthesis allows, at least temporarily, continued synthesis of enzyme." The inactivator appears to depend upon pituitary function, since adrenalectomized and hypophysectomized rats showed little or no inactivation phase following cortisol treatment.

Peterkofsky & Tomkins G52,839/67: TKT can be induced by dexamethasone in tissue cultures from Morris hepatoma 7288C. Cytosine arabinose completely inhibits DNA synthesis in these cells, but does not affect RNA synthesis or enzyme induction. Conversely, mitomycin C and actinomycin D preferentially inhibit RNA synthesis and completely block induction. Kinetic experiments in which actinomycin D was added at increasing intervals after dexamethasone suggest that messenger RNA accumulates during the early phase of induction. From these and other observations, it is concluded "that messenger RNA for both tyrosine aminotransferase and general cell protein are relatively stable. After inhibition of protein synthesis by cycloheximide, tyrosine aminotransferase activity decreased exponentially with a half-life of seven hours, and this rate was not affected by either steroid or actinomycin."

Benes & Zicha G67,159/69: Exposure to 1400 R does not inhibit the TPO activity of rat liver. In fact, substrate induction of TPO is stimulated by X-irradiation applied 24 hrs earlier. Induction by cortisol is initially stimulated and then, inhibited by X-irradiation. X-irradiation before partial hepatectomy inhibits the increase in tryptophan oxygenase normally observed 12 hrs after the operation. Similar results are obtained by actinomycin D applied one hour after partial hepatectomy. "The diminished synthesis of tryptophan oxygenase in irradiated regenerating rat liver tissue, as well as the decrease of hormonal induction after the irradiation can be explained by the inhibition of the specific messenger RNA's synthesis."

Lindegren E8,182/69: Review of the receptor hypothesis of gene action.

Tomkins et al. H19,499/69: Review of the evidence in favor of the following theory of enzyme induction by steroids.

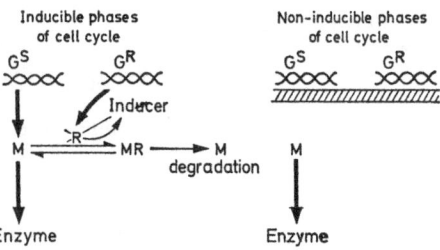

Theory of enzyme induction in mammalian cells. The configuration shown on the left is assumed to exist during the inducible phases of the cell cycle, while that on the right, during the noninducible phases. The G^S refers to the structural gene for the inducible enzyme, while G^R refers to the regulatory gene. During the inducible periods, G^S is transcribed and the resulting messenger, M, can be translated to form the enzyme. The G^R is likewise transcribed and its messenger translated to produce the protein R. The R combines reversibly with M to produce the inactive complex MR which leads to M degradation. The R itself is labile, as shown by the thin arrow leading away from R. The inducer is indicated to inactivate R by an unknown mechanism. During the noninducible phases of the cycle, neither G^S nor G^R is transcribed, but M can be translated. Although for the case of tyrosine aminotransferase the degradation of the enzyme might also be depicted, we have not done so because its concentration is not regulated by changing the rate of its inactivation under constant cultural conditions.

5. LYSOSOMES

According to certain investigators an excess of vitamin A or ultraviolet irradiation may liberate lysosomal proteases; this effect is counteracted by glucocorticoids, such as cortisol, allegedly through the stabilization of lysosomal membranes. A similar mechanism has been invoked to explain the protective action of glucocorticoids against endotoxins which are also thought to cause damage by the release of lysosomal enzymes. The interactions between glucocorticoids and other toxicants may likewise act by preventing a kind of autointoxication with lysosomal proteases. This concept appears to have been confirmed using many model systems, yet, it is not uniformly agreed to play a decisive role in glucocorticoid-induced resistance phenomena in vivo. In particular, serum levels of β-glucuronidase (presumed to reflect lysosomal enzyme release) do not correlate with survival in rats given cortisol during tourniquet shock. In fact, even in vitro studies suggest that neither glucocorticoids nor nonsteroidal anti-inflammatory drugs stabilize lysosomes with respect to the release of enzymes, when the lysosomes are thermally labilized.

Weissmann D10,768/61: In larvae of Xenopus laevis, bone absorption and other manifestations of vitamin-A overdosage were accelerated by cortisol. "This was held to be due to liberation of vitamin A from hepatic stores by the steroid, and is in contrast to the retardation of hypervitaminosis A by hydrocortisone in vitro." Presumably an excess of vitamin A causes release of cathepsins from intracellular lysosomes.

Weissmann & Dingle D14,268/61: The hepatic lysosomal proteases of the rat are released by ultraviolet irradiation in vitro and this effect is greatly diminished by pretreatment of the animals with cortisol in vivo.

Weissmann & Fell D46,242/62: The damage caused to fetal rat skin explants by ultraviolet irradiation can be inhibited by the addition of cortisol to the culture medium. This protection "might be due, at least in part, to a reduced proteolytic activity in the damaged tissue through a stabilising action of the hormone on the lysosomes."

Weissmann & Thomas D23,630/62: Following endotoxin treatment in vivo, the hepatic lysosomes of the rabbit release their enzymes readily upon ultraviolet irradiation. This increased lability is in turn prevented by pretreatment of the animals with cortisone for three days before endotoxin administration. Apparently, "one action of endotoxin is to release acid hydrolases from particulate form within cells, and that glucocorticoids serve to stabilize such particles against injury by several agents."

Weissmann & Thomas D65,709/63: Various in vivo and in vitro experiments "are compatible with the hypothesis that excess vitamin A releases acid hydrolases from liver and cartilage lysosomes in vivo and in vitro, and that cortisone antagonizes this action." This interaction may explain earlier observations on the protective effect of glucocorticoids against intoxication with vitamin-A.

Janoff G68,991/64: A review of the literature and personal observations. It is concluded that "(1) disruption of lysosomes and release of their contained enzymes in free, active form occurs in the liver of shocked animals; (2) the activation of lysosomal hydrolases within cells and their release into the circulation may play an important role in exacerbating tissue injury and accelerating the development of irreversibility at the cellular level during shock; (3) rendering animals tolerant or pretreating them with cortisone selectively stabilizes lysosomes and this effect may constitute an important component of the resistance of such animals to shock; (4) the exacerbating effect of reticuloendothelial-blocking colloids on the lethality of shock procedures may be due, in part, to a direct action of these agents on lysosomes."

Janoff & Kaley E8,484/64: Review of the literature supporting the concept that endotoxins act by disruption of lysosomes with release of their contained enzymes and that cortisone protects against the resulting shock by stabilizing lysosomal membranes.

Weissmann & Thomas E4,216/64: Review (30 pp., 81 refs.) on the stabilizing action of glucocorticoids upon lysosome membranes.

Weissmann & Thomas E8,482/64: Review of the literature showing that cortisone, unlike DOC, stabilizes hepatic microsomal membranes against the permeability-increasing effect of endotoxin.

Replogle et al. G40,447/66: In patients with cardiopulmonary bypass, dexamethasone pretreatment appeared to improve the clinical condition and diminished the serum beta-glucuronidase and LDH levels. It is assumed that postoperative complications following cardiopulmonary bypass may be related in part to damage of lysosome membranes and that "massive doses of dexamethasone may stabilize the lysosome membrane during periods of circulatory stress."

Serkes et al. F92,105/67: Cortisol administered to tourniquet-traumatized rats in infusion fluid lowered serum β-glucuronidase but did not prolong survival time. "Serum levels of beta-glucuronidase presumed to reflect lysosomal enzyme release, did not correlate with survival."

Janoski et al. E7,896/68 (p. 280): Review suggesting that many of the actions of glucocorticoids—particularly their inhibition of ultraviolet ray injury, vitamin-A overdosage and endotoxin shock—are due to the stabilization of lysosomal membranes which prevents the escape of toxic lysosomal enzymes.

Lefer & Martin H7,806/69: In cats, "pharmacologic doses of cortisol or dexamethasone given intravenously prior to induction of hemorrhagic shock prolonged survival significantly after reinfusion of all shed blood. High doses of aldosterone were ineffective in prolonging survival, as was cortisol when administered at the time of reinfusion. ... Glucocorticoids may prevent the disruption of lysosomes and/or prevent proteases from being released into the blood."

Brown & Schwartz H 14,096/69: In vitro studies on the hepatic lysosomes of the rat suggest that "neither steroidal nor non-steroidal anti-inflammatory drugs, in general, stabilized lysosomes with respect to release of enzymes when the lysosomes were labilized thermally.... That anti-inflammatory drugs exert their prime pharmacologic action at the level of the lysosome is thus very doubtful."

Curreri et al. H 11,525/69: In rabbits with cholesterol atherosclerosis various hydrolytic enzymes present in lysosomes (β-glucuronidase, acid phosphatase, cathepsin and aryl sulfatase) showed a marked increase in activity. Cortisone inhibited this atherosclerosis and the increased enzyme activity despite very high levels of serum cholesterol.

Weissmann G 79,855/69: Review (20 pp., 105 refs.) on "The Effects of Steroids and Drugs on Lysosomes." Special attention is given to the effect of lysosome stabilization by glucocorticoids which may be responsible for the prevention by these steroids of endotoxin shock, etiocholanolone fever, hypervitaminosis E and other conditions.

Lewis et al. G 80,342/70: In general, glucocorticoids stabilize rabbit liver lysosomes in vitro, although at very high concentrations they have an inverse effect. Etiocholanolone, a pyrogenic steroid, has a lytic action on lysosomes, even at comparatively low concentrations.

Polliack et al. H 32,366/70: In hamsters, tumor formation by topical application of DMBA to the cheek pouch is partially suppressed by concurrent application of cortisone, perhaps owing to depression of DNA synthesis and of mitotic activity be the hormone. "Cortisone stabilizes biological membranes; its action on cell multiplication may be related to decreased membrane permeability with consequent inhibition of release of lysosomal enzymes which play a part in early stages of cell division. Decreased membrane permeability may also have resulted in less effective penetration of carcinogen into cells. Results are in accordance with those of previous studies, which demonstrated promotion of tumor formation by labilizers of biological membranes such as vitamin A and estrogen."

Symons et al. G 80,345/70: Rabbit hepatic lysosomes take up ^{3}H-labeled cortisol and cortisone from the surrounding medium in vitro. It may be that the lytic effect exerted by high doses of glucocorticoids upon lysosomes is due to structural changes produced in the membrane.

Glenn & Lefer H 34,576/71: In cats subjected to hemorrhagic shock, methylprednisolone increased survival time in proportion to a diminution of plasma levels of a myocardial depressant factor (MDF) and of the lysosomal enzymes, β-glucuronidase and plasma cathepsin-like activity (PCLA). Presumably, "methylprednisolone exerts a protective effect in hemorrhagic shock by preventing the release of lysosomal enzymes which may be responsible for the formation of MDF, a peptide implicated in the reduction of myocardial contractility during postologemic shock."

6. RETICULO-ENDOTHELIAL SYSTEM (RES)

It is generally agreed that the RES helps to prevent sudden flooding of the circulation with blood-borne particulate substances. It is more questionable whether some particles engulfed by the RES cells are topically digested; certainly most of them are gradually released (through shedding and decomposition of the phagocytes) for subsequent degradation in other tissues and/or eventual excretion. It has been suggested that RES cells also participate in the enzymic degradation of soluble toxicants. In isolated RES cells, acetylation of foreign compounds has allegedly been demonstrated. Furthermore, such RES active agents as Thorotrast or endotoxin lower the hepatic TPO (but not TKT) activity and prevent cortisol from inducing these enzymes in the isolated perfused liver. It has been assumed that the RES cells can produce some "inhibitory substances."

The interpretation of pertinent data is somewhat complicated by the fact that the same particulate substances can both inhibit and stimulate RES cells depending upon dosage and other factors. Still, it is of considerable interest that there exists some relationship between the functional status of the RES and drug detoxication.

Thus, in mice, various compounds which decrease the blood clearance of colloidal carbon, prolong hexobarbital anesthesia; however, the same is true of zymosan, endotoxin and stilbestrol, which enhance RES activity. On the other hand, typical catatoxic drugs (e.g., phenobarbital) and inhibitors of drug-metabolizing enzymes (e.g., SKF 525-A) do not appreciably alter RES activity.

These and many other observations suggest that the RES may participate in drug metabolism but its role remains to be elucidated and it certainly does not appear to be as important as that of the hepatic parenchyme.

Govier F 57,820/65: In rabbits, acetylation of sulfanilamide and p-aminobenzoic acid (one of the major routes of metabolism of acrylamines) has been examined utilizing isolated intact hepatic and RES cells of various other tissues. "The acetylation of these compounds, usually attributed to the liver, was found to occur in cells of the reticulo-endothelial system. No acetylation could be demonstrated in the hepatic parenchymal cells. Lung and spleen, organs known to contain a high percentage of reticuloendothelial cells, were also found to acetylate these compounds."

Agarwal et al. G 65,716/69: In the rat, both S. typhimurium endotoxin and Thorotrast lowered hepatic TPO activity, and prevented cortisol from inducing this enzyme in the isolated, perfused liver. Under these conditions, the TKT activity of the liver remained unaffected. Partial purification of hepatic TPO induced by endotoxin or Thorotrast indicated the presence of some inhibitory substance. "Since histological studies revealed that thorotrast is localized in Kupffer cells, it is suggested that the reticuloendothelial system contributes to the control of enzyme induction in rat liver."

Benveniste et al. G 80,804/70: In axenic mice, the phagocytic function of the RES is regularly depressed by prednisolone. Holoxenic mice are more resistant to this effect. Various observations suggest "that depression of the immune response by cortisone, obtained under septic conditions, is more probably related to a lymphoid atrophy than to a depression of the RES."

Greisman & Woodward G 80,339/70: In rabbits, extensive studies (RES blockade, liver perfusion, etc.) "fully support the concept that tolerance to the pyrogenic activity of bacterial endotoxin is based upon increased uptake of the toxin by hepatic Kupffer cells which have become refractory to further release of endogenous pyrogen."

Munson et al. H 22,843/70: "Drugs which alter the phagocytic activity of the RES have been shown to prolong barbiturate anesthesia. In this study, these observations were extended to include agents which decrease RES activity. Methyl palmitate, thorium dioxide and pyran copolymer (PCP) markedly decreased the intravascular clearance of colloidal carbon and prolonged hexobarbital anesthesia. Zymosan, endotoxin, diethylstilbestrol and PCP enhance RES activity and also prolong hexobarbital narcosis. Conversely, chlorcyclizine, SKF 525 A and phenobarbital, which markedly alter drug metabolism, did not alter RES activity. PCP and zymosan prolonged the half life of hexobarbital in brain, liver and serum. Hexobarbital metabolism was markedly depressed in 9000x g liver supernatant fractions from PCP and zymosan-treated mice. Further studies demonstrated that the inhibition of barbiturate metabolism was non-competitive. PCP and SKF 525A were additive in microsomal inhibitory ability whereas chlorcyclizine, given in a protocol which stimulates microsomal enzyme activity, reverses the inhibitory effect of zymosan. The toxicity of cyclophosphamide, which requires hepatic microsomal enzyme activity for cytotoxicity, was markedly enhanced by PCP suggesting the enzymes necessary for the activation of cyclophosphamide are stimulated by PCP."

Song & Kappas G 80,521/70: Review (21 pp., 215 refs.) on the "Influence of Hormones on Hepatic Function" with special sections on their effect upon phagocytosis, drug metabolism and biliary excretion. Folliculoids stimulate whereas glucocorticoids inhibit the RES, whereby they may influence drug resistance.

Wooles & Munson G 78,975/71: Review of the literature and personal observations on mice suggest that there is a relationship between the functional activity of the RES and the duration of hexobarbital anesthesia. It is suggested that the RES plays an important role in drug detoxication.

7. HEPATIC GLYCOGEN

Glucocorticoids which protect mice against bacterial endotoxins also increase hepatic glycogen stores, whereas the noxious endotoxins deplete the liver of its glycogen content. In alloxan diabetic rats, hexobarbital and aminopyrine metabolism is depressed in vitro. These and several studies on the effect of insulin upon such enzyme activities raised the suspicion of some relationship between hepatic glycogen and drug-metabolizing enzyme activity.

This view appeared to receive further support from the observation that SKF 525-A and other inhibitors of enzyme activities share the property of reducing liver glycogen. However, it must be kept in mind that virtually all stressors, if sufficiently severe, reduce liver glycogen and hence a causal relationship between this change and responsiveness to enzyme inducers is difficult to prove. Besides, PAS, which increases heptic glycogen, also prolongs hexobarbital sleeping time and it has been assumed that, here, the glycogen infiltration of the liver is responsible for the enzyme inhibitory effect.

Berry et al. C73,198/59: Mice of different strains were protected by cortisone against the lethal effect of various bacterial endotoxins. The effect may be related in some way to the hepatic glycogen stores which are depleted by endotoxin and increased by cortisone.

Dixon et al. E35,705/63: In alloxan-diabetic rats, "a depressed metabolism of hexobarbital and aminopyrine in vitro, an increased in vitro hydroxylation of aniline, and a prolonged in vivo effect of hexobarbital were evident. The O-dealkylation of codeine was unaffected by the chronic diabetic state. Insulin treatment returned the rate of metabolism of hexobarbital to normal levels but had no effect on aminopyrine metabolism. Metabolism of aniline was decreased below the normal rate after insulin treatment. Phenobarbital treatment of diabetic animals resulted in a stimulation of most of the drug metabolizing enzyme systems studied. However, the hydroxylation of aniline by livers from diabetic rats treated with phenobarbital was decreased." A relationship between hepatic glycogen and drug-metabolizing enzyme activity is suspected.

Rogers et al. E31,897/63: In rats, PAS feeding induces glycogen infiltration of the liver and prolongation of hexobarbital sleeping time. This is apparently due to its diminished ability to excrete the barbiturate. The in vitro metabolism of hexobarbital and aminopyrine, by the microsomes of rats pretreated with PAS, is diminished. Acute administration of PAS had no effect on hexobarbital sleeping time, nor did addition of PAS in vitro inhibit drug-metabolizing enzymes. There may exist some relationship between hepatic glycogen deposition and changes in the SER. This might account for the inhibitory effect of PAS which is definitely different from that of chloramphenicol and SKF 525-A.

Rogers & Fouts F27,894/64: In studies with SKF 525-A and other inhibitors, a relationship has been noted between reduced glycogen content of hepatocytes and low enzymic activities.

Stenger G74,578/70: Review (21 pp., 177 refs.) with special reference to the alterations in RER and SER produced by various agents and the relationship of these changes to glycogen and drug metabolism.

8. VITAMIN C

Induction of hepatic microsomal drug-metabolizing enzymes is usually associated with increased ascorbic acid synthesis and a rise in the urinary elimination of vitamin C. However, a loss of urinary ascorbic acid is characteristic of stressors, and incidentally, shared not only by microsomal enzyme inducers but also by SKF 525-A and other inhibitors of induction.

Longenecker et al. A 47,520/40: In rats, various barbiturates, paraldehyde, chlorobutanol, aminopyrine, antipyrine, phenols, salicylates, sulfanilamide, sulfapyridine, and several other compounds increased ascorbic acid excretion. Earlier work had shown that vitamin C helps in the detoxication of such compounds as elementary phosphorus, phenol, phenylquinolinecarboxylic acid, benzene, lead and arsenicals. "No evidence was obtained to indicate that the urinary ascorbic acid was conjugated with any of the toxic substances fed, but its endogenous production appeared to be related to the animal's detoxication processes."

Kato et al. D 27,768/62: In rats, urinary vitamin-C excretion was enhanced by pretreatment with inhibitors of microsomal drug metabolism such as SKF 525-A, Lilly 18947, Lilly 32391 and MG 3062. Apparently in this respect the inducers and inhibitors of microsomal enzymes exert similar effects. [The possibility that the increase in ascorbic acid excretion may have been due to the stressor effect of the drugs should also be considered (H.S.).]

Stitzel & Furner G 48,920/67: In rats, stress (cold) increases the rate of p-hydroxylation of aniline and N-dealkylation of ethylmorphine simultaneously with an increase in adrenal ascorbic acid content. The stress-induced stimulation of microsomal metabolism and adrenal ascorbic acid levels are additive with those produced by phenobarbital. "It is tentatively concluded that stress and phenobarbital appear to act through different mechanisms in inducing increases in enzyme activity, although each treatment may have a common final step, namely an increased net synthesis of enzyme protein."

Mannering G 71,818/68 (pp. 61, 97): Review of data showing that induction of hepatic microsomal drug-metabolizing enzymes is usually associated with increased ascorbic acid synthesis.

Klinger et al. H 28,896/70: In rats, phenylbutazone reduces hexobarbital sleeping time and increases the fresh weight of the liver as well as the ability of the hepatic 9000 g supernatant to enhance aminophenazone-N-demethylation. An increase in the ascorbic acid concentration of the liver was noted only in young animals, but urinary excretion of ascorbic acid was as pronounced as after barbital treatment. Phenylbutazone administration to the pregnant mother failed to elicit an induction effect in the fetuses as judged by hepatic ascorbic acid determinations and by ultrastructural studies of the fetal livers. Proliferation of the SER was obtained by phenylbutazone in 10-day-old or older rats, often in association with an increase in the number of lysosomes and mitochondrial changes as well as by evidence of intrahepatic cholestasis.

Hunter et al. H 36,993/71: In epileptic patients, the urinary excretion of D-glucaric (a metabolite of glucuronic acid) is considerably increased during phenobarbital treatment. Similar observations have been made in patients with Gilbert's syndrome after administration of various drugs known to induce hepatic enzymes. Because of its simplicity and sensitivity, the D-glucaric acid excretion test is recommended for the clinical assessment of drug-metabolizing enzyme induction. It is noteworthy, however, that except in primates and guinea pigs, glucuronolactone is converted to ascorbic acid and, in the rat, inducers of drug metabolizing enzymes increase the excretion of ascorbic acid rather than of D-glucaric acid.

9. DEFENSE AGAINST "NATURAL" VS. "FOREIGN" COMPOUNDS

It had been thought initially that the microsomal enzyme systems in the liver may be there just to detoxicate foreign compounds. It seemed tempting to "speculate that these systems are not essential to the normal economy of the body, but operate primarily against the toxic influences of foreign compounds that gain access to the body from the alimentary tract." It has been assumed, furthermore, that perhaps the SER membranes are ordinarily permeable only to nonpolar compounds, which would present "a plausible picture of the way the body protects its essential substrates from wasteful metabolism due to the non-specific microsomal enzyme." Indeed, the view that the microsomal enzyme system exists merely to attack foreign material has led to the suggestion that the substrates of microsomal mixed-function oxygenases should be designated as "xenobiotics" (from the Greek "xenos" and "bios" for "stranger to life"). However, in many cases it is difficult to draw a sharp line of demarcation between "natural" and "foreign" compounds. In mice and rats kept on soft wood bedding of either cedar, white pine, or ponderosa pine, several drug-metabolizing hepatic enzymes were induced and hexobarbital sleeping-time was reduced. Apparently, the microsomal enzyme mechanism of an animal can be significantly altered by changes in its natural habitat.

Finally, numerous recent observations, especially with catatoxic steroids, but also with many nonsteroidal enzyme inducers, have amply demonstrated that these can stimulate the microsomal enzyme systems to metabolize such natural compounds as tyrosine, hormones, cholesterol, bilirubin, and many others. For reasons explained in the Introduction, we prefer to think of the catatoxic compounds as especially suited for the detoxication of abnormally high blood concentrations of substrates, be they "natural" or "foreign"; their metabolizing activities are much less evident at near physiologic concentrations of the substrates. In this sense, the catatoxic substances are primarily guardians of homeostasis (*cf. also* p. 763.).

Brodie et al. G66,772/55: Although SKF 525-A inhibits various hepatic microsomal-enzyme activities in the rabbit's liver it is relatively nontoxic and, hence, "one can speculate that these systems are not essential to the normal economy of the body, but operate primarily against the toxic influences of foreign compounds that gain access to the body from the alimentary tract."

Brodie C12,157/56: "The microsomal enzyme systems in liver may be there just to 'detoxicate' foreign compounds. ... We have found no normal substrate which is metabolized by the drug enzyme systems in microsomes. ... If we think of the microsomes as particles with a membrane which will, ordinarily, pass non-polar compounds but not polar compounds, we have a plausible picture of the way the body protects its essential substrates from wasteful metabolism due to the non-specific microsomal enzymes."

Williams G73,007/62: In connection with the theory that drug detoxication depends upon a special class of microsomal enzymes, it is noteworthy that several toxic compounds foreign to the body, can be metabolized by "normal enzymes" which perform a physiologic role in ordinary metabolism. This is well illustrated by the following table:

Franklin G32,826/65: When incubated under appropriate conditions with hepatic microsomes of male rats, "morphine, atropine, aminopyrine, lysergic acid, streptomycin, eserine, caffeine, N-methyl urethan, and 6-amino-N-methyl nicotinamide were N-demethylated at various rates. Those compounds not demethylated were N-methyl nicotinamide, N-methyl glycine, betaine, N-methyl guanidine, creatine, and methylamine. None of the compounds tested which occur naturally in mammalian tissues were demethylated, whereas those from exogenous sources were demethylated." Of the tested foreign compounds, only ephedrine was not demethylated.

Table 134. Some foreign compounds metabolized by "normal enzymes"

Foreign compound	"Normal" enzyme acting on foreign compound
p-Nitrobenzyl alcohol (and some other foreign alcohols)	alcohol dehydrogenase
p-Nitrobenzaldehyde (and other foreign aldehydes)	aldehyde dehydrogenase
Benzylamine	monoamine oxidase
Procaine Succinylcholine	non-specific plasma cholinesterase
8-Azaguanine	guanase, purine nucleotide phosphorylase
Azuridine	nucleosidase
2:6-Diaminopurine 6-Mercaptopurine 6-Thioxanthine 4-Aminopyrazolopyrimidine	xanthine oxidase

Mason et al. F51,528/65: The authors recommend the term "xenobiotics" (from the Greek "xenos" and "bios" for "stranger to life") for compounds which "are foreign to the metabolic network of the organism." It is clearly recognized that the mixed-function oxidases responsible for the degradation of many xenobiotic compounds are also participating in the metabolism of steroids, lipids and other normal components of the body and food.

Vesell F88,031/67: In mice and rats kept on softwood bedding of either red cedar, white pine, or ponderosa pine, three drug-metabolizing hepatic enzymes (morphine N-demethylase, aniline hydroxylase, and hexobarbital oxidase) were induced. Hexobarbital sleeping time was reduced. Apparently, the drug-metabolizing enzyme mechanism of an animal can be significantly altered by changes in its natural habitat.

Gillette et al. E8,216/69: The term "xenobiotics" is used (in the preface of a symposium on "Microsomes and Drug Oxidations") to denote the substrates which "are metabolized by mixed-function oxidases localized in the endoplasmic reticulum of the liver."

Calhoun et al. H34,806/71: In immature rats, the uterotrophic effect of mestranol or norethynodrel was affected by numerous drugs. "Pretreatment with phenobarbital or SKF 525A was found to decrease and increase, respectively, the uterine wet weight in controls as well as in mestranol-treated groups. Of the other drugs tested, only tolbutamide increased uterine wet weights in both control and mestranol-treated groups. In addition, the response to mestranol was increased following pretreatment with p-aminosalicylic acid, chlorpromazine, and imipramine and decreased following diphenylhydantoin, phenylbutazone, or scopolamine pretreatment. The response to norethynodrel was decreased after pretreatment with phenobarbital or diphenylhydantoin and increased following SKF 525A pretreatment."

10. STRESSORS

The very first indication of an improvement of nonspecific resistance by steroids was based on the observation that adrenalectomized animals are extraordinarily sensitive to virtually every kind of damage and that their resistance can be restored by treatment with glucocorticoids. It was difficult to imagine an antidote that could impart such a wide spectrum of protection unless the glucocorticoids would act by antagonizing a common endogenous endproduct of exposure to any type of stressor or would induce a similarly nonspecific protective enzyme mechanism. In fact, conceivably both types of defense against stressors may be of importance: glucocorticoids might help to increase resistance to some such common metabolites as histamine, or to some byproduct of energy liberation, which would be produced under the influence of the most diverse stressors. In addition, a stress-induced increase in some endogenous substances (e.g., catatoxic steroids) might evoke nonspecific multipurpose oxygenases which could inactivate a great variety of toxicants.

In support of the view that many stimuli may induce enzyme systems which act through common pathways, it has been emphasized that an increase in TPO—produced by histidine, epinephrine or histamine and other compounds — occurs as a consequence of stress with the resulting increase in glucocorticoid secretion. Even X-irradiation, starvation or terminal tumor growth can enhance TPO activity through this mechanism. Accordingly, adrenalectomy prevents this form of stress-induced enzyme synthesis, whereas the glucocorticoid or substrate-induced TPO synthesis proceeds unimpeded.

These and other observations led to the conclusion that hepatic TPO activity plays an important role in metabolic adaptation to stress. The stressors are thought to act upon hepatic TPO induction through the pituitary-adrenal axis, whereas STH and cortisol may act directly. There is some evidence that STH actually inhibits certain hepatic enzyme induction mechanisms and it is conceivable that stress exerts a corresponding action either directly or through the intermediary of the pituitary. If so, exposure to stress would have a dual effect in that the inhibitory actions just mentioned could be compensated, or even overcompensated, by enhanced glucocorticoid production.

The fact that adrenalectomized rats are extraordinarily sensitive to endotoxin and that cortisone antagonizes this effect both in the absence and in the presence of the adrenals appeared to support the concept of a close relationship between stress and enzymic defense. Curiously, the adrenals of mice given endotoxin failed to respond sufficiently to exogenous ACTH. It must be kept in mind however, that enormous doses of glucocorticoids are required to antagonize the fatal effect of endotoxin and it is unlikely that the glands could produce equivalent amounts under the influence of either exogenous or endogenous ACTH.

Hypoxia produces enzymic changes reminiscent of those elicited by endotoxin, and cortisone increases survival at high altitudes. These and other observations led to the conclusion that hypoxia also acts upon enzyme induction as a stressor and is correspondingly subject to the protective effect of cortisone.

Perhaps the most interesting recent observations in this connection are those showing that complete blockade of sympathetic function achieved by various means increases mortality from endotoxin or histamine as markedly as does adrenalectomy. This decrease in resistance is counteracted by treatment with epinephrine alone, whereas cortisone offers only partial protection. Presumably sympathetic stimulation is "the first line of defense against vasomotor disturbances elicited by endotoxin and histamine." On the other hand, the lethal effect of formalin or tourniquet shock, which is also greatly increased by adrenalectomy, is not increased by sympathetic blockade. Furthermore, cortisone counteracts the toxicity of these latter stressors in adrenalectomized rats suggesting that "formalin and tourniquet shock is initiated by a mechanism which differs from that elicited by histamine and endotoxin."

Knox et al. E83,471/56: Review of the literature suggesting that many stimuli which induce specific enzyme systems may act through common pathways. This is especially true of adaptive reactions to stress. "Thus increases in the tryptophan peroxidase produced by the administration of histidine, of epinephrine, of histamine, and of certain other compounds were found to occur by the common mechanism of adrenal cortical stimulation. Other stressing conditions such as X-irradiation, starvation, and terminal tumor growth have also been recognized to increase this enzyme by the same mechanism. These effects can all be eliminated by adrenalectomy, and thus can be distinguished as a group from the increase in tryptophan peroxidase induced by substrate administration. Further investigation along these lines of changes in other specific proteins which occur with X-irradiation, starvation, stress, or other agents causing adrenal cortical stimulation (e.g. colchicine) may be expected to identify still more adrenal hormone-induced adaptations."

Knox G67,799/58: Review of the literature and personal observations lead to the conclusion that hepatic microsomal TPO activity plays an important role in metabolic adaptations to stress. Stressors act through the pituitary-adrenal axis upon hepatic TPO whereas tryptophan, STH and cortisol may act upon the liver directly.

Berry et al. C73,199/59: The observation that adrenalectomized rats are extraordinarily sensitive to endotoxin strengthens the stress concept and would "place injections of endotoxin in the category of 'stressful situation'. Completely contradictory to this notion is the total loss in the ability of the adrenals of mice given endotoxin to respond to exogenous ACTH... These results might be explained by a destruction or inactivation of ACTH in vivo.

One is still at a loss, however, to understand why adrenalectomized animals should be more susceptible to endotoxin poisoning unless it is assumed that adrenal hormones other than glycocorticoids act beneficially against endotoxin." [Here, the antagonism between glucocorticoids and endotoxin was tested mainly by changes in glyconeogenesis (liver and muscle glycogen, total carbohydrate of carcass, urinary nitrogen). Hence, the alternative hypothesis should also be considered that these effects of endotoxin could be antagonized by the large dose of cortisone (5 mg p.o.), whereas the glucocorticoids secreted under the influence of ACTH did not, suffice to block these biochemical consequences of endotoxin poisoning (H.S.).]

Inscoe & Axelrod D1,700/60: In rats, exposure to stress (cold) depressed the ability of the liver to produce o-aminophenol glucuronide. However, this was due only to a diminution of microsomal protein per gram liver. The ability of microsomes to hydroxylate acetanilide was stimulated by exposure to cold, whereas N-demethylation of meperidine and methadon was depressed. Apparently, the effect of stress upon drug-detoxication depends upon the substrate used.

Rupe et al. E26,910/63: In rats, stress produced by placing a tourniquet on one hind leg decreases the pharmacologic response to hexobarbital, meprobamate and pentobarbital. This effect is prevented by hypophysectomy or adrenalectomy, but simulated by ACTH or corticosterone. No such effect on stress was noted with barbital, a compound not metabolized by hepatic microsomal enzymes. Furthermore, the protective effect of stress is counteracted by SKF 525-A. Apparently, the "pituitary-adrenal activity exerts a regulating influence on drug responses."

Bousquet et al. F35,073/65: In rats, stressed by application of a tourniquet to one hind leg, the duration of response to hexobarbital, pentobarbital, meprobamate and zoxazolamine is significantly reduced, but only in the presence of both the pituitary and the adrenal glands. Pretreatment with ACTH or corticosterone simulates the effects of stress in shortening hexobarbital anesthesia. "It is suggested that the pituitary-adrenal axis serves a regulatory function with respect to duration of drug responses which may be mediated by an alteration of drug metabolism."

Juchau et al. E50,728/65: In rats, benzpyrene hydroxylase activity can be induced even in the perfused liver in which systemic stress and the actions of the pituitary-adrenal axis cannot intervene.

Stitzel & Furner G48,920/67: In rats, stress (cold) increases the rate of p-hydroxylation of aniline and N-dealkylation of ethylmorphine simultaneously with an increase in adrenal ascorbic acid content. The stress-induced stimulation of microsomal metabolism and adrenal ascorbic acid levels are additive with those produced by phenobarbital. "It is tentatively concluded that stress and phenobarbital appear to act through different mechanisms in inducing increases in enzyme activity, although each treatment may have a common final step, namely an increased net synthesis of enzyme protein."

Berry et al. H2,124/68: Studies on the influence of hypoxia, glucocorticoids and endotoxin on hepatic enzyme induction and survival in mice. "Endotoxin inhibited the induction of tryptophan oxygenase, prevented the increase in liver glycogen, induced the transaminase, and increased the lethality of simulated altitude. Cortisone increased survival at all altitudes except the highest. These observations emphasize the importance of these metabolic adjustments for the survival of animals subjected to hypoxic stress."

Furner & Stitzel G54,558/68: In rats, adrenalectomy reduces the rate of metabolism of ethylmorphine, aniline and hexobarbital. Cortisol or stress (cold) stimulates ethylmorphine and aniline metabolism, even in adrenalectomized animals, whereas phenobarbital enhances the metabolism of all three compounds. Apparently, "both stress and phenobarbital can bring about changes in drug metabolism independent of the presence of an intact adrenal."

Krawczak & Brodie H25,296/70: In rats, complete blockade of sympathetic function can be achieved by demedullation combined with reserpine-like agents (depleting catecholamine stores), bretylium-like agents (preventing nerve impulse from releasing catecholamines) or gangioplegics. Following such total sympathetic blockade, mortality from histamine or endotoxin is as markedly increased as by adrenalectomy. Pretreatment with epinephrine alone counteracts the increased lethality of endotoxin and histamine after sympathetic blockade. Cortisone pretreatment only partially corrects the sensitization by adrenalectomy, whereas cortisone + epinephrine offers complete protection against these agents. Presumably, sympathetic stimulation is "the first line of defense against the vasomotor disturbance elicited by endotoxin and histamine." The lethal effect of formalin or tourniquet shock is likewise greatly increased by adrenalectomy but, in contrast to that of endotoxin and histamine, it cannot be increased by sympathetic blockade. Furthermore, cortisone alone counteracts the toxicity of these stressors in adrenalectomized rats. Apparently "formalin and tourniquet shock is initiated by a mechanism which differs from that elicited by histamine and endotoxin and does not primarily involve the sympathetic system."

11. HOMEOSTASIS AND THE NONSPECIFICITY OF STEROID-INDUCED RESISTANCE

Two of the most intriguing problems in connection with the hormonal regulation of resistance are that:

1. The actions of the adaptive hormones are primarily homeostatic; they readily correct severe deviations from the norm but have little or no effect upon near normal blood and tissue concentrations of most chemical compounds.

2. The defensive actions of protective hormones are largely nonspecific; they raise the resistance of the body against the damaging actions of many toxicants upon the most diverse organs.

We have already touched upon the first problem in the previous sections in connection with the old debate about whether catatoxic compounds act only against "foreign compounds" and came to the conclusion that this is not the case, at least not in the original formulation of this concept. These compounds do act against numerous natural constituents of the body, but mainly if the latter are present in abnormally large amounts. This postulate is, of course, most readily fulfilled with "foreign compounds" (e.g., barbiturates) which are "present in abnormally large amounts" whatever their blood concentration.

One must also consider the possibility that the magnitude of a detoxifying reaction may depend primarily on the amount of substrate present. If an enzyme system is more than sufficient to cope with near physiologic amounts of substrates, induction of further enzymic activity can be beneficial only when abnormally high demands are imposed by considerable increase in substrate concentration. In other words, under near-physiologic circumstances, the available enzyme concentration is not the rate-limiting factor in detoxication.

We also saw that the glucocorticoids are most effective in **raising resistance to stress towards normal, but not above a near-physiologic level.** This was probably one of the first pertinent observations. It seemed odd that small doses of the earliest impure cortical extracts should be so eminently effective in restoring the subnormal resistance of adrenalectomized rats to a stressor such as cold, whereas even large amounts of the same preparations (or of the subsequently discovered highly potent synthetic glucocorticoids) failed to make intact rats more than normally resistant to cold. Yet, selectively homeostatic actions of drugs are not unprecedented: antipyretics are highly active in decreasing fever but cause no hypothermia; antiphlogistics combat inflammatory edema but do not diminish the hydration of normal tissues.

It remains to be seen why this type of homeostatic arrangement is effective against so many potential pathogens. We have no definite information about this point but, for example in the case of glucocorticoids, it is conceivable that their effect upon capillary permeability, or membrane permeability in general, endows them with the properties of "tissue tranquilizers" in that, by diminishing fluid transport and metabolic turnover, they paralyze topical reactivity in general. This would explain why they are "syntoxic" and facilitate tolerance of potential irritants even without attacking the latter. This hypothesis is also compatible with the observation that the defensive effect of syntoxic compounds is so largely nonspecific, since innumerable agents cause damage not by directly destroying or attacking tissues, but by evoking excessive reactions through their irritating effect.

But how could we explain the almost equally great nonspecificity of the protective effect of catatoxic steroids which act against different toxicants and through a different mechanism? These hormones (or at least the great majority of those among them that have been adequately studied) act by destroying pathogens, not by rendering tissues insensitive to them. Furthermore, catatoxic steroids are most effective in raising resistance far above normal whereas syntoxic steroids are especially efficacious in restoring the subnormal stress-resistance of the hypocorticoid organism to the normal level. In other words, here again, the actions of catatoxic compounds are virtually the opposite of those elicited by syntoxic steroids.

In both these instances it is difficult to imagine through what chemical mechanisms the same steroid could offer nonspecific resistance against so many kinds of damaging agents, especially since this nonspecificity, though considerable, is not absolute. Both syntoxic and catatoxic steroids protect against numerous potential pathogens, quite unrelated in their chemical structure or toxicologic activities; yet both types of hormones offer considerable protection against some, but little or none against other forms of damage. In the case of the catatoxic steroids it is highly unlikely that Nature would have foreseen a specific enzyme for the destruction of each of the many substrates which they detoxify, including even newly synthesized toxicants to which no defense mechanism could have been developed during evolution of the species or the individual. On the other hand, if the body would manufacture a single enzyme (or a small set of enzymes) with an enormous range of detoxifying power, how could this protection nevertheless be specific to some extent in that certain catatoxic compounds are more selectively effective or ineffective against individual toxicants.

In reviewing all our data concerning the effect of hormones upon resistance, and particularly the Synoptic Tables 138 and 139 it appears that, at least in theory, we should distinguish between the following actions:

I. Nonspecific detoxication. The power of many steroids to protect against a large number of apparently unrelated toxicants.

II. Nonspecific toxication. The property of decreasing resistance to many toxicants.

III. Specific detoxication. The ability of increasing resistance selectively to one, or only a few, of the toxicants tested.

IV. Specific toxication. The selective diminution of resistance to one or few toxicants.

It is remarkable that most catatoxic steroids exhibit the "Type I" action in that they increase nonspecific resistance to many agents. Only very few, if any, catatoxic steroids show a "Type II" effect, although to some extent this may be true of estradiol and of the only nonsteroidal hormone in our series, thyroxine. These do impair resistance to numerous toxicants; yet, their effect is by no means as pronounced or general as that of actinomycin, puromycin, ethionine or SKF 525-A, which interfere with various steps in enzyme-protein synthesis or function. Finally, among the intoxications included in our series, only few are specifically prevented or aggravated by steroids, thyroxine or phenobarbital.

We cannot explain the great predominance of "Type I" activity among the catatoxic steroids nor do we understand through what mechanism a single compound could provide resistance against so many toxicants. However, as a tentative working hypothesis, it is tempting to assume the existence of some nonspecific "common prerequisites" which might participate, and even be rate-limiting, in numerous chemical reactions that influence resistance. This could be achieved by general regulators of enzyme synthesis and degradation, as well as by factors influencing the availability of common co-enzymes or of substrates which provide the energy necessary for the most diverse chemical reactions. Similarly, very different types of defensive responses could be modified by factors affecting membrane permeability (e.g., fat solubility), or the binding of toxicants to blood proteins.

To take the most common "Type I" effect as an example, it may be postulated that some common prerequisites of defense reactions are used up in the fight against stress or for the development of resistance to substrates of catatoxic steroids. If so, the need for such adjuvant substances would be a nonspecific prerequisite for the activation of many specific defense reactions. The syntoxic and catatoxic steroids may produce such common adjuvants and thereby exert a highly nonspecific protective effect. Understandably, supplements of the common prerequisites (provided through appropriate steroid treatment) would have little effect under near-physiologic circumstances when they are in ample supply to start with. Conversely, at times of excessive demands, an appropriate increase in the availability of the common adjuvants may be the decisive rate-limiting factor in the development of resistance to many agents.

In summary, we might assume as a tentative working hypothesis that the protective steroids (both syntoxic and catatoxic) activate a limited number of comparatively nonspecific enzyme systems which can attack diverse substrates by facilitating prototypes of biotransformation reactions (e.g., oxidation, reduction, conjugation) and by providing "common adjuvants" (cofactors, energy yielding substances) which enhance many types of enzymic responses.

On the other hand, certain protective steroids are selectively effective against certain toxicants or, conversely (despite a very general protective effect), selectively fail to induce resistance against certain drugs. This fact might be ascribed to specific characteristics of either the substrates or the protective steroids which happen to block the degradation of individual toxicants or interfere with their effect by fortuitous pharmacologic synergisms or antagonisms. Such interactions could occur either at the site of enzyme induction or even in the peripheral target organs. Furthermore, a certain type of enzymic reaction (e.g., S-demethylation, aliphatic oxidation or aromatic hydroxylation) may abolish the damaging effects of many toxicants and yet have no effect or actually aggravate those of others, depending upon the pharmacologic properties of the resulting metabolites. It is not unexpected therefore that the enzyme induced by very "broad spectrum" catatoxic steroids may selectively be without avail in offering protection against a given substrate and conversely that the substrate easily detoxified by numerous steroids may be resistant to one of them.

The following schematic drawing may help to remember what we consider to be the principal facts concerning the observations just mentioned. At least in theory, we assume the existence of four basic types of hormonal influences upon resistance.

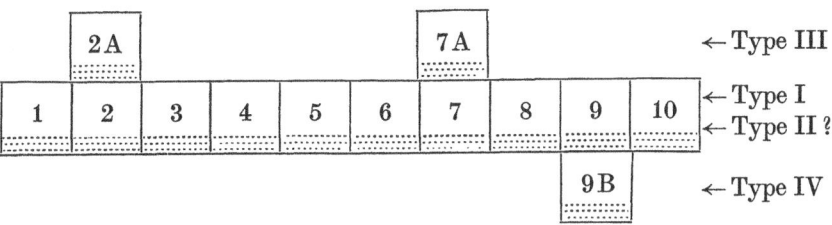

Here, the horizontal bar represents a series of ten intoxications (the consecutively numbered squares). The numbers themselves indicate the amenability of these intoxications to various types of hormonal regulations. In this theoretical series, every toxicant (1—10) is shown as amenable to the nonspecific detoxication of "Type I". The narrow shaded lower part of this series would correspond to nonspecific toxication of the "Type II" variety, but it is questionable whether any hormone actually possesses sufficiently nonspecific toxifying actions to fulfill the requirements for this hypothetic category. Among those tested, several (thyroxine, folliculoids) tend to enhance the toxicity of many agents, but no hormone or hormone derivative possesses as broad a spectrum of toxicant actions as the detoxicant effects of "Type I" steroids or the resistance aggravating actions of such antagonist drugs, as SKF 525-A, puromycin or actinomycin.

"Type III," specific detoxication, is indicated by the squares 2A and 7A, whereas "Type IV," specific toxication, is represented by 9B. The same intoxication is not necessarily amenable to modification by specific (Type III & IV) and nonspecific (Type I & II) conditioning agents; in fact these positive and negative conditioning effects (detoxication and toxication) obviously cannot occur at the same time as might be implied by the drawing, which only attempts to illustrate all possibilities. Spironolactone definitely possesses considerable "Type I" activity, but its protective effect upon mercury intoxication is specific (Type III). On the other hand, triamcinolone and other glucocorticoids may exert specific protective actions (Type III) against various ganglionic blocking agents, lathyrogens or inflammation without possessing nonspecific catatoxic properties of "Type I."

It remains to be shown whether this attempt at a classification will prove to be of heuristic value, but it is clear that any attempt to explain the relative nonspecificity of catatoxic steroids must be compatible with the fact that none of them has an identical protective spectrum; the type and degree of protection they offer against different toxicants is as individualistic as the fingerprints or the genetic code of a man.

Solymoss et al. G79,023/71: In rats, pretreatment with PCN or spironolactone increases liver weight, glutathione S-aryltransferase activity and bile flow. At the same time, the plasma clearance and biliary excretion of BSP and its conjugated metabolites are enhanced. Ethylestrenol likewise increases liver weight but does not alter the other parameters mentioned above. Spiroxasone, SC-9376 and CS-1 (antimineralocorticoids), unlike norbolethone and oxandrolone (anabolics), also enhance plasma clearance of BSP, probably through the same mechanism. In contrast to these effects of pretreatment, administration of spironolactone, ethylestrenol or estradiol immediately before BSP delays plasma clearance of the dye, probably through competitive inhibition of biliary excretion. SKF 525-A does not suppress the enhanced BSP clearance induced either by spironolactone or by phenobarbital. [Although the authors did not evaluate their data from this point of view, these observations clearly show that the catatoxic activity of steroids is not merely the result of hepatic microsomal drug metabolizing enzyme induction. It may also be mediated through extramicrosomal enzyme mechanisms or even through enhanced biliary excretion (H.S.).]

XI. SYNOPSIS OF PHARMACO-CHEMICAL AND PHARMACO-PHARMACOLOGIC INTERRELATIONS

In analyzing the mechanisms through which hormones can influence resistance, we must consider first the various forms of drug interactions in general and second the structural prerequisites for the protective actions of hormones. It is obvious that drugs and hormones may interact by influencing each other's absorption, excretion, distribution within the organism, metabolism, as well as by direct chemical or pharmacologic interactions that occur between drugs in vivo. However, these mechanisms are the subject of general pharmacology and hence they will only receive cursory attention here.

The principal objective of this section is to correlate the many experiments which we performed to obtain material for a glimpse into the structural (chemical) or pharmacologic prerequisites for the ability of steroids to protect the body against toxicants.

VARIOUS FORMS OF DRUG INTERACTIONS

In discussing the various forms of interactions between drugs (including hormones), several mechanisms must be considered, for example:

1. The gastrointestinal **absorption** of one drug can be affected by another which alters the pH of the alimentary tract, the permeability of its epithelium or peristalsis.

2. Drugs may affect the renal, biliary, or intestinal **excretion** of other drugs.

3. One drug may alter the **distribution** of another drug within the organism, e.g.:

a) by altering the permeability of the hemato-encephalic barrier;

b) by competing for shared protein-binding sites in the plasma, thus augmenting the biologic activity of the displaced drug;

c) by competing for receptor sites in tissues, thus diminishing the activity of the displaced drug.

4. Drugs may affect the synthesis, degradation or activity of microsomal and extramicrosomal **drug-metabolizing enzymes.**

5. Direct **chemical interactions between drugs** (e.g., chelation) may lead to their inactivation in vivo. Addition of a pharmacologically inert radical to a potent drug may also alter the susceptibility of the latter to microsomal enzyme activity (e.g., morphine and barbital are resistant, whereas ethylmorphine and phenobarbital are highly susceptible to degradation by microsomal enzymes). Such an "opsonization" by addition of a radical may increase the liposolubility of a drug and hence, its capacity to penetrate through membranes. This type of synthesis has not been definitely proven to occur in vivo, but it may play a role in drug interactions.

6. Direct **pharmacologic interactions between drugs** (e.g., between a vasoconstrictor and a vasodilator, or between two vasodilators) may lead to an increase or a decrease in their activity.

Drug Interactions in General

Fouts G77,566/64: Review (5 pp., 18 refs.) on the effect of drugs upon drug metabolism.

McIver G78,391/65: Review (4 pp., 43 refs.) on drug incompatibilities.

Remmer G78,385/65: Review (24 pp., 156 refs.) on the mechanism of drug interactions.

Gillette G78,390/67: Review (19 pp., 96 refs.) on theoretical aspects of drug interaction.

McIver G77,708/67: Review (6 pp., 41 refs.) on drug incompatibilities.

Block & Lamy G81,054/68: Review (6 pp., 82 refs.) on therapeutic incompatibilities of importance to pharmacists.

Hartshorn G78,178/68: Greatly simplified but excellent revue (8 pp., about 35 refs.) enumerating various ways in which drugs can interact and illustrating each type with a few examples.

Hartshorn G81,056/68: Review (4 pp., 17 refs.) with practical hints on drug interactions useful to the pharmacist.

Hartshorn G81,057/68: Review (7 pp., 3 refs.) consisting mainly of tables concerning drug interactions.

Hussar G81,059/68: Review (11 pp., 82 refs.) on drug incompatibilities.

Pelissier & Burgee, Jr. G79,655/68: A brief guide to drug incompatibilities irrespective of the underlying mechanism.

Block & Lamy G81,052/69: Review (5 pp., 27 refs.) on drug interactions with tabular summaries on changes in metabolism, binding to plasma and urinary pH changes produced by one substance which may alter the activity of another compound.

Dunphy G77,712/69: Review (11 pp., about 30 refs.) on drug interactions with an outline of an extremely simplified index listing a few examples of these.

Hartshorn G81,055/69: Review (7 pp., 33 refs.) on interactions among anti-infective agents.

Hussar G81,053/69: Practical hints concerning drug interactions of interest to the pharmacist.

Visconti G77,709/69: Review (10 pp., no refs.) on how drug interaction information may be used preventively.

Ariëns G79,943/70: Review (48 pp., about 160 refs.) on drug interactions with special reference to antagonisms, metabolic inactivation and metabolic activation. [Excellent summary, but the poor English is difficult to follow (H.S.).]

Neumann G80,018/70; G80,550/70: Review (5 pp., no refs.) on drug interactions in the style of a postgraduate lecture.

Mannering G74,881/71: Review of the literature on drug interactions in general leads to the conclusion that "a drug may alter the action of another drug in several ways: a) by producing one or more effects similar or opposite to those of the drug in question, b) by direct chemical or physical interaction of drugs, c) by displacement of drugs bound to plasma or other proteins, d) by altered renal clearance of drugs, e) through conditioning by previous drug effects, f) by interaction of drugs with receptor sites, and g) by inhibition or stimulation of the metabolic site. Examples of all of these interactions are given ..."

Lipid Solubility

Brodie G55,013/62: "Metabolism of the microsomal enzymes seems to be governed by lipid solubility, for only substances that are highly lipid soluble are metabolized by microsomes."

Mannering G71,818/68 (p. 74): A survey of the literature shows that compounds with low lipid solubility are poor inducers of drug-metabolizing microsomal enzymes, whereas potent inducers are, in general, highly soluble in organic solvents. [Yet all steroids are lipid soluble but are not good inducers (H.S.).]

Carriers

Baird & Reid G51,827/67: Pancuronium bromide produces neuromuscular blockade in man.

Lewis et al. F95,691/67: In various test procedures, steroidal monoquaternary ammonium salts exhibited non-depolarizing neuromuscular blocking activity.

Bonta & Goorissen G75,052/68; Buckett G75, 531/68: Pharmacologic studies on the neuromuscular-blocking effect of pancuronium.

Buckett et al. G56,175/68: "Pancuronium possesses up to ten times the potency of tubocurarine according to the species used for testing, while possessing similar duration of action."

Reyes et al. G71,233/69: In rats phenobarbital "enhanced hepatic uptake of an organic anion, bromsulphalein, in vivo and simultaneously increased the amount of Y, a hepatic cytoplasmic organic anion-binding protein. This study supports the postulate that Y is a major determinant in the selective hepatic uptake of certain organic anions from plasma." Induction of Y may enhance hepatic uptake and metabolism of various substrates following treatment with phenobarbital and other inducers.

Wall et al. G69,969/69: A series of steroid esters of p-[N,N-bis(2-chloroethyl)amino] phenylacetic acid (BCAPAA), steroidal sulfides of p-(N,N-bis-2-chloroethylamino)thiophenol, and a variety of steroidal ethylenimine derivatives were synthesized and tested for antitumor activity. "Activity was found only in those instances in which the steroid and potential oncolytic agent were connected by ester or heterocyclic ether linkages. The steroidal BCAPAA esters were of particular interest showing excellent inhibition of a DMBA-induced and transplantable mammary adenocarcinoma, and marked increase in survival when tested on a variety of rat leukemias. . . . The steroidal BCAPAA esters were judged to be less toxic than some of the well-known nitrogen mustards in general use."

Chaouki et al. G77,223/70: In 50 patients, pancuronium bromide was found to be an active non-depolarizing neuromuscular blocking agent, about 5 times as active as curare and 25 times more potent than gallamine triethiodide. Its advantages are rapid onset of action, no release of histamine and little disturbance in blood pressure, because of a weak ganglioplegic action.

Dick et al. G77,777/70: Favorable clinical experiences with pancuronium as a muscle relaxant in anesthetized patients.

Feldman & Tyrrell G76,666/70: Dacuronium bromide (2β, 16β-dipiperidino-5x-androstane-17β-diol-3x-acetate dimethobromide) is closely related to pancuronium bromide but the acetoxy group at C_{17} is replaced by a hydroxyl group. It has proven its usefulness as a non-depolarizing muscle relaxant in man. Its effect is fully reversible by edrophonium or neostigmine.

PREREQUISITES FOR THE PROTECTIVE ACTIONS OF HORMONES

Looking back upon research on hormones and resistance, as outlined in this monograph, it may be instructive to reexamine the justification of the path followed and to summarize the main points.

It is not without hesitation that we embarked upon this project some 35 years ago; we realized, to start with, that this would be a life-long undertaking with virtually no background data for logical planning. On the basis of what we had learned in 1936 about the role of the adrenal cortex in defense against stress, no other course seemed to be open to us but that of a purely empirical, large-scale screening of many steroids (more or less closely related to the corticoids) for possible protective effects against many toxicants.

However, the possibility of finding highly potent and comparatively nontoxic protective steroids appeared to hold considerable promise of practical applicability and the screening did not have to rely on chance alone. To some extent, we could be guided by the pharmacologic and chemical characteristics of compounds previously shown to have protective potency against certain substrates. We used the same guide lines for the identification of toxicants amenable to prophylaxis by steroids. It is on the basis of this kind of empirical research that we are now beginning to see outlines of a classification which permits us to predict, with some degree of probability, what compounds are likely to possess protective effects against what types of toxicants.

Because of the large number of experiments required to explore the many possible combinations of such interactions, we had to rely on simple in vivo observations in which directly visible (functional or structural) changes and mortality rates were our principal indices of activity. Yet, in the early days we were encouraged by the knowledge that similar screening efforts did prove to be eminently successful in many other fields. The classification of bacteria on the basis of their ability to grow on certain media or to take up the Gram stain, the screening of antibiotics on plates inoculated with various bacteria, the blind testing of 606 chemotherapeutic agents that finally led Ehrlich to the discovery of "Salvarsan," are but a few examples to illustrate this point.

In our own work we could demonstrate the nonspecificity of the pituitary-adrenal response only by countless in vivo tests with many stressors; only the screening of numerous calciphylactic sensitizers and challengers permitted us eventually to induce localized tissue calcification in a predictable and highly specific manner.

Naturally, as soon as any new protective phenomenon was discovered, in vitro studies in depth became necessary to clarify the underlying mechanisms; for example, after we noted the prevention by spironolactone of digitoxin and mercurial intoxication, or the extraordinary degree and spectrum of protective effects that can be induced in steroids by the introduction of a nitrile group. Much of this work is still to be done, but before we could even think about elucidating the manner in which a protective phenomenon works, we had to know first that the phenomenon exists.

So much for self-justification.

To begin with, we had to develop an economic procedure which permitted large scale experimentation with a minimum waste of steroids, many of which are difficult to synthesize. Then we had to design a technique for the correlative evaluation of the many individual observations made.

Our assay procedure consisted of the following three steps:

1. Establishment of possible protective potency against two standard toxicants: digitoxin and indomethacin.

2. Determination of the "protective spectrum" of the steroids found to be active in step 1.

3. Identification of damaging agents amenable to prophylaxis by steroids which have revealed interesting activities in step 2.

Before describing these steps in detail, we shall have to say a few words about the evaluation of the data obtained. The results of the **first screening** have been tabulated in the conventional way (Table 135) by listing the mean severity of the actual changes as previously described for comparable studies on the effect of 304 steroids upon indomethacin and digitoxin poisoning (*Selye G70,421/70*).

In addition, we constructed **Synoptic Tables** (Tables 136, 137, 138) in which these and many additional results are summarized on the basis of the degree of the significance ratings (*cf.* "Statistical Evaluation," p. IX) according to a system developed by Mrs. I. Mécs of this Institute. The figures indicate the means of the statistical significance grades of the changes (functional or structural) used as indicators, plus that of the mortality rates divided by 2. Thus, in an experiment in which the protection against intestinal ulcers had a significance rating of "0" (no protection), and the significance of the protection against mortality was 3 "***" (perfect protection), the figure given in the tables would be 1.5. Only in the case of compounds which normally cause no mortality (e.g., anesthetics, muscle relaxants) do the grades correspond to structural or functional lesions alone.

The Synoptic Tables (136, 137, 138) also list the **"Mean Overall Protective Index"** computed according to a procedure closely related to the "Simplified Activity Grading" system previously described (*Selye G70,421/70*). This index represents the allgebraic sum of all the individual activity gradings for a certain protective substance divided by the number of toxicants against which it was tested.

In addition, we computed the **"Total Overall Protective Index"** which represents the arithmetic sum of all the individual activity gradings (disregarding negative grades).

Furthermore, we computed the **"Protective Spectrum Index"** which is the percentage of those toxicants tested against which significant protection is obtained (irrespective of the degree of significance). Thus, if a steroid offers significant protection against 6 out of 10 toxicants examined, its "Protective Spectrum Index" is 60%.

In the Synoptic Tables, these Indexes have also been computed for the amenability to protection of the various toxicants (three bottom horizontal lines). In other words, here the figures indicate the mean degree or the percentile frequency of protection offered by the entire series of conditioners against any one toxicant.

Finally, to further facilitate the overview of this complex field we constructed a **"Diagram Table"** (Table 139) which graphically summarizes the highlights of Table 138, except that the results are registered only for one dose level of the toxicants and are expressed in a scale in which intermediates between the four grades are not recognized (for details cf. footnote on Table 139). Furthermore, in Table 138, the toxicants are listed in alphabetical order for easy identification, whereas in Table 139, they are enumerated according to decreasing "Total Overall-Protective Index" values.

Since the large number of experiments to be reported here was performed over a considerable period of time, in each case, a group of unpretreated controls received the same toxicant, simultaneously with the rats that had been pretreated with potentially protective substances. The statistical significance of the resulting changes in the pretreated animals was always calculated in comparison with the corresponding group of unpretreated controls handled under identical circumstances, at the same time and by the same technician.

Using these procedures for the evaluation of our data, we examined the steroids available for this work according to the above mentioned three-step procedure.

First Step: Protection Against Digitoxin and Indomethacin

The first systematic investigations designed to identify protective steroids consisted of a series of bioassays in which 304 natural and synthetic steroidal compounds were tested for their ability to protect the rat against digitoxin and indomethacin, under the experimental conditions outlined in the preceding section. Since these results have been the subject of an extensive review *(Selye G70,421/70)*, we shall limit ourselves here to a brief description of the principal conclusions derived from them.

Protective activity was widespread among the steroids of this first series; it was demonstrable among gonanes, estranes, androstanes, androstenes, 5β- and 5α-pregnanes as well as among pregnenes, with one or more double bonds, and with or without halogen substitution in the ring system. On the other hand, cholanes, cholestanes and genins were uniformly inactive, with the sole exception of methylnordeoxycholanate ($3\alpha,12\alpha$-dihydroxy-24-nor-5β-cholan-23-oic acid methyl ester).

Because of this widespread distribution of anti-indomethacin and antidigitoxin activity throughout various classes of steroids, it was difficult to formulate any clear-cut rules about pharmaco-chemical correlations in this field. It does appear, however, that although catatoxic activity is not strictly dependent upon any single structural prerequisite, in general the 17α-propionic acid-γ-lactone side-chain is advantageous for both antidigitoxin and anti-indomethacin activity. It is perhaps also not purely coincidental that a very large number of active catatoxic steroids is found among the 1,4-androstadienes as well as among halogenated androstene and pregnene derivatives. It is likewise noteworthy that several of the most active catatoxic steroids are 19-nor compounds, hence the angular methyl group at C_{10} is not only dispensable but often advantageous. The most striking observation in this series of tests was that among all 304 steroids tested the most active against both substrates proved to be a cyano-compound, namely PCN.

This first systematic screening series also revealed that the catatoxic activity is not strictly dependent upon any other known pharmacologic property, although most of the highly potent antidigitoxin and anti-indomethacin steroids also exhibit antimineralocorticoid or anabolic properties.

Because of the comparatively small number of animals that could be used for the bioassay of the many, not readily available, steroids, only the lowest and the highest activity grades were given serious consideration. However, even on this rigid basis of appraisal, we found that at a 10 mg dose level, among 304 steroids tested, there were:

>Active only against indomethacin: 42
>Active only against digitoxin: 32
>Active against both substrates: 24
>the remainder being inactive or of doubtful activity.

At the 0.5 mg dose level, we found:

>Active only against indomethacin: 1
>(Cpd. 277 and betamethasone acetate)
>Active only against digitoxin: 1
>(CS-1)
>Active against both substrates: 1
>(PCN)

These compounds correspond to the following structures:

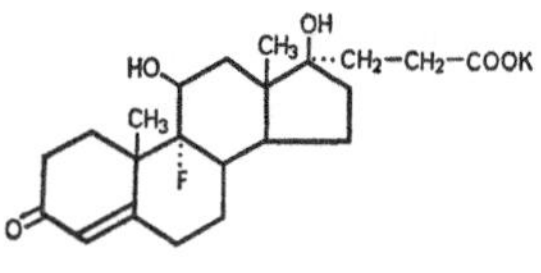

CS-1
9α-Fluoro-11β-,17-dihydroxy-
3-oxo-4-androstene-17α-propionic
acid potassium salt (SC-11927)

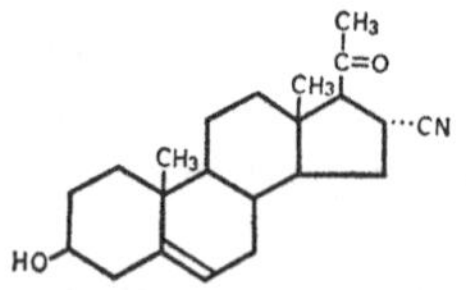

PCN
3β-Hydroxy-2-oxo-5-pregnene-
16α-carbonitrile (SC-4674)

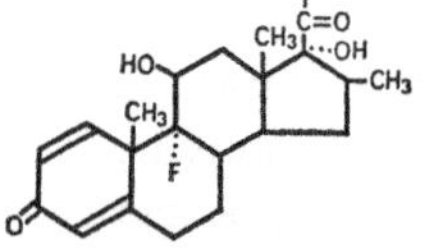

Betamethasone acetate
9α-Fluoro-16β-methyl-11β,17,21-
trihydroxy-1,4-pregnadiene-3,20-
dione 21-acetate

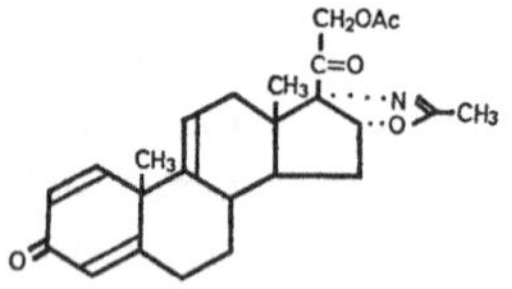

"Cpd. 277"
21-Hydroxy-3-oxo-1,4,9(11)-
pregnatrieno-[17α,16α-d]-
2'-methyl-oxazoline acetate

It is especially noteworthy that several of the active catatoxic steroids are naturally occurring hormones, hormone precursors or hormone metabolites such as: progesterone, 17α-hydroxyprogesterone, 5-pregnenolone, dehydroisoandrosterone.

Encouraged by these first observations, we then proceeded to repeat some of the key observations at lower dose levels. We also performed similar tests on many additional steroids, especially carbonitriles and other compounds related to the most active members in the preliminary series. This work (Selye G 70,480/71) was done under experimental conditions exactly corresponding to those of the first screening tests, and the results are summarized in Table 135.

However, before describing these most recent experiments, we must say a few words about the SSS steroid terminology. Up to now, in discussing the literature, we used essentially the same terms as did the authors quoted. This was far from satisfactory, but unfortunately unavoidable, because we could not have taken the responsibility of translating into any accepted steroid nomenclature the often ambiguous mixtures of trivial and systematic designations that are sometimes employed even by the most reputable pharmacologists and clinicians. However, in the following description of our own experiments with fully characterized compounds, these will be identified not only by their structure formulas and the official designations accepted by the International Union for Pure and Applied Chemistry (IUPAC Commission G82,068/69), but also by the much more easily understandable and simpler SSS terms. The SSS (Symbolic Shorthand System of steroid terminology) (Selye et al. G79,034/71) can be briefly summarized as follows:

Basic Principles

The main advantages of the SSS nomenclature are: **shortness** of code terms, **logical consistency**, and **simplicity**. The principles which guided its design are:

Rigid observance of left-to-right precedence order in the coining of symbols. The parent hydrocarbon comes first, then its substituents in a strictly determined sequence. Each substituent is named by a symbol followed by a positional number according to the principle of: "first what, then where" (e.g., 17β-Hydroxyandrostan-3-one = $Aol_{17\beta}on_3$).

We deviate from this rule only in the case of "secondary parent hydrocarbons" in which the main parent hydrocarbons (e.g., estrane, androstane) are provided with side-chains attached by C—C linkages (e.g., methylandrostane or cyanopregnane). In such cases, substituents of the side-chains are mentioned immediately after the latter. E.g., an androstane with a hydroxylated (ol) methyl group (I) attached at 16β is written $\underline{AIol_{16\beta}}$ and the whole expression is underlined (or boldface) to distinguish it from substituents on the main parent hydrocarbon itself which follow according to the order of precedence described below. For example, if the methylandrostane just mentioned also contains a ketone group at 3 and a fluorine in the 9α-position, we write $\underline{AIol_{16\beta}}on_3F_{9\alpha}$.

No signs to indicate two or more identical characteristics (e.g., diene, triol, dione). The sign Δ and the suffix "-ene" are also omitted since appropriate position numbers make them superfluous. After the symbol of the parent hydrocarbon (e.g., A = Androstane) superscript numerals suffice to designate the degree of unsaturation, while subscripts qualify the position and number of functional groups (e.g.: $A^{4,6}ol_{11\beta,17\alpha}on_3$ = 11β,17α-Dihydroxy-4,6-androstadien-3-one).

No silent "e" (e.g., in "one"). This is always omitted, not only when the next syllable begins with a vowel. The final "e" does not change either the meaning or the pronunciation of the syllable and, in many languages, it is not used in any case. Besides, SSS (like IUPAC) is not meant for oral communication.

Since esters are always formed with alcohols, the **esterified OH groups are not separately indicated**. E.g., instead of 5α-Androstane-3β,17α-diol 3-acetate 17-propionic acid ester, we merely write $A5\alpha*II''_{3\beta}*III''_{17\alpha}$ (* = ester; '' = acid), since the 3β-acetate or 17α-propionate can only be formed with the corresponding alcohols (*cf. also* p. 775 and 776). Furthermore, we employ short symbols instead of writing out the full names of the esterified acids and, instead of the usual "-", we separate ester functions from the parent hydrocarbon by an asterisk which uses no more space than the dash and yet further characterizes the following symbols as an ester.

No prefixes. It is superfluous to burden a codifier with a complex dictionary of rules according to which he must write a given symbol as a prefix or suffix. In SSS, the parent hydrocarbon is the first part of any designation; all other symbols are added as suffixes.

No synonyms. Every structural feature receives one name or symbol. This procedure is greatly facilitated by the omission of prefixes which complicate other systems. For example in IUPAC:

Carboxylic acids are named "Carboxy-" as prefix, and "-oic", "-ic" or "carboxylic acid" as suffix.

Alcohols are "Hydroxy-" as prefix and "-ol" as suffix.

Aldehydes are "Oxo-" as prefix and "-al" as suffix.

Most confusingly, ketones are also "Oxo-" as prefix, but "-one" as suffix.

Typesetting and punctuation are used to specify chemical characteristics without lengthening names. Instead of separating all parts of a term by dashes (-), SSS uses no separating sign or (where there may be ambiguity) the shorter comma (,). The latter is replaced by an asterisk (*) to indicate ester function. Commas also separate the position numerals of identical functions (e.g., ol$_{3\beta,9\beta,17\alpha}$). No punctuation is used to separate the constituents of a single functional group. E.g., *III"$_{3\beta}$, fully characterizes the location on C_3 and the steric position of an alcohol group esterified with propionic acid; the three ingredients (3, β, III") need not be separated by dashes or any other sign which would only tend to break up what is actually one unit of expression.

The simplest symbolic code terms are used for the most common expressions. Thus, the main parent hydrocarbons have symbols consisting only of the first letter of their full name (e.g., **G** = Gonane, **E** = Estrane, **A** = Androstane) although, in some instances, one or two additional letters are added to avoid ambiguity (e.g., **CH** = Cholane, **CHT** = Cholestane, etc.). For emphasis, the symbols of the main and secondary parent hydrocarbons — including signs of intrinsic modifications such as: isomerism, unsaturation, nor, homo, abeo — are underlined and always capitalized (in printing, italicized or set in boldface).

Whenever possible, simple, selfexplanatory **mnemonic abbreviations** are used for all substituent radicals, e.g., for normal alkyls roman numerals, indicating the number of carbon atoms contained:

I = Methyl II = Ethyl III = Propyl
IV = Butyl V = Pentyl.

Longer and more complex radicals are represented by letter symbols, usually contractions of the IUPAC names (*cf.* below).

When **alkyls appear as side chains** (secondary parent hydrocarbons), they follow the name of the parent hydrocarbon (on the same line) and, like the latter, are boldface (e.g., **AI** = methylandrostane).

Whenever the chemical formula characterizing a substituent is shorter than a meaningful corresponding word or abbreviation could be, we use the former (e.g., =CH_2, =NH, -CN, K, F respectively for methylene, imino, carbonitrile, potassium or fluorine). In order to avoid three-line symbols, the positional numbers of such formulas as =CH_2 are appended to a bracketed symbol e.g. $(CH_2)_{16\beta}$.

The Main Parent Hydrocarbons
(in order of precedence)

Gonane	= **G**	Ergostane	= **ER**
Estrane	= **E**	Stigmastan	= **ST**
Androstane	= **A**	Cardanolide	= **CAR**
Pregnane	= **P**	Bufanolide	= **BUF**
Cholane	= **CH**	Spirostane	= **SP**
Cholestane	= **CHT**	Other nuclei	

All ring modifications, other than those recognized above as parent hydrocarbons, are listed as derivatives at the end of each main category in this order:

Heterocyclic steroids, *cf.* p. 777
Nor-ring steroids = **n** (e.g., **AnA** = A-nor-androstane, **PnB** = B-nor-pregnane).
Homo = **ho** (e.g., PhoD=D-homo-pregnane)
Abeo = **ab**
Cyclo = **cyc**
Retro = **ret**
Seco = **sec**

Derivatives (in order of precedence)

With each parent hydrocarbon, its immediate derivatives are classified in the following order:

Isomerism: Isomerism at C_5 is indicated by 5α or 5β following the symbol of the parent hydrocarbon (e.g., **A**5α = 5α-androstane). Isomers are listed next to each other, α before β. For ring-isomers, *cf.* below.

Unsaturation: -C-C- (an), e.g., **A** (for Androstane),

—C=C— (en), e.g., Δ^4 (for Androst-4-ene), $\Delta^{4,6}$ (for Androsta-4,6-diene).

The number of unsaturations is not indicated as it is evident from the positional number(s) in the superscript. Thus, $\Delta^{4,6}$ suffices to indicate that we are dealing with a diene. [Not $\Delta^{1,2,etc.}$]. Cyclosteroids are also identified by superscripts, e.g., $\Delta^{3(5)}$. The superscript numbers of triple bonds (-yn) are repeated (e.g., P^{20-20}).

Alcohols: —OH (ol), e.g., $Aol_{17\alpha}$ (for Androstan-17α-ol), $Aol_{3\beta,17\alpha}$ (for Androstane-3β,17α-diol). [Not hydroxy, dihydroxy, etc.]

Esters: —CO$\boxed{OHH}$OC— (*), e.g., $P*Bz''_{3\alpha}*II''_{17\beta}$ (for 3α,17β-Dihydroxypregnane 3-benzoate 17-acetate).

Esters are identified by an asterisk preceding the symbol of the acid, with which the steroid hydroxy group is esterified; they are listed immediately following the corresponding free alcohols. Since ester formation is possible only with alcohol groups, it is redundant to identify the position of each (the alcohol and acid) separately (*cf. also* below). [Not oxy (e.g., acetoxy) or "acid ester" (e.g., acetic acid ester)]. Esters of steroid acids are distinguished by placing the symbol for acid (″) immediately after that of the steroid, before the asterisk (e.g., $P''*IIol_{21}$ for 21-pregnanoic acid esterified with ethanol).

Ketones: C=O (-on), e.g., $E^{1,3,5(10)}ol_3on_{17\beta}$ (for 3-Hydroxy-1,3,5(10)-estratrien-17-one or estrone). [Not oxo, keto, one (with terminal "e") and the redundant indication of the number of ketone groups by dione, trione, etc.]

Carboxylic acids: —COOH (″), e.g., P''_{21} (for Pregnan-21-oic acid). Here the carboxyl group itself is considered to be part of the steroid skeleton, not an oxidized methyl side-chain on 21-norpregnane. However, a carboxyl which is not part of a recognized main parent hydrocarbon, but is attached to it by a C—C linkage, is written as an oxidized methyl side-chain (e.g., $AI''_{16\alpha}$ for androstane 16α-carboxylic acid). Carboxylic acids not attached to the steroid skeleton by C—C linkages, e.g., those of esters, are similarly identified (by ″), e.g., I'' = formic, III'' = propionic, V'' = pentanoic. Bz'' = benzoic acid (*cf.* p. 778) for alkane symbols). [Not carboxylic acid or -oic acid.]

Steroid acid esterified (e.g., $P''*IIIol_{16\alpha}$).

Steroid alcohol esterified (e.g., $P*III''_{16\alpha}$).

Ethers: —CO$\boxed{HHO}$C— (θ), e.g., θI, θII, θPIII (for methyl, ethyl or propyl ethers). [Not methoxy or methyl ether.]

Lactones: $\overset{O}{\overset{\|}{-C-O-}}$ (-lac, -γlac), e.g., $\Delta^4III''\gamma lac_{17\alpha}ol_{11\beta,17}on_3F_{9\alpha}$ (for 9α-Fluoro-11β,17-dihydroxy-3-oxo-4-androstene-17α-propionic acid γ-lactone).

Aldehydes: —CHO (-al), e.g., $P^4ol_{11\beta,21}on_{3,20}al_{18}$ (for 11β,21-Dihydroxy-3,20-dioxo-4-pregnen-18-al or aldosterone). As with the carboxylic acids, here the carbon bearing the aldehyde function is considered part of the parent hydrocarbon and is not derived from a methyl side chain. Otherwise, we would have the grotesque situation of deriving aldosterone from an 18nor, but 18 methylated pregnane.

Hemiacetals, acetals, hemiketals and ketals: The symbols used for hydroxy and other groups (e.g., ol, θI) will be applied.

Hemiacetals: $R-\underset{\underset{OR^1}{|}}{\overset{\overset{H}{|}}{C}}-OH$ (½acetal) reaction product of an aldehyde with one alcohol group.

Acetals: $R-\underset{\underset{OR^2}{|}}{\overset{\overset{H}{|}}{C}}-OR^1$ (acetal, not abbreviated) reaction product of an aldehyde with two alcohol groups.

Hemiketals: $R-\underset{\underset{OR^2}{|}}{\overset{\overset{R^1}{|}}{C}}-OH$ (½ketal) combination of a ketone with one alcohol group.

Ketals: $R-\underset{\underset{OR^3}{|}}{\overset{\overset{R^1}{|}}{C}}-OR^2$ (ketal, not abbreviated) combination of a ketone with two alcohol groups.

Epoxy: $\overset{\overset{O}{\diagup\diagdown}}{C-C}$ (regarded as ethers). An oxygen attached to two vicinal carbons, e.g., $A\theta_{1\alpha-2}$ (for 1,2α-epoxy-androstane).

Halo compounds: Br, Cl, F, i (-bromo, -chloro, -fluoro, -iodo), e.g., $P^4Cl_{9\alpha}$ (for 9α-Chloro-4-pregnene). Instead of "I" for iodine write "i" (e.g., $P^4i_{9\alpha}$) to avoid confusion with methyl, whose symbol is roman one.

Nitrogen containing steroids: NH_2 (for amino), NH (for imino), CN (for carbonitrile or cyano). These symbols are used as such in SSS terms. However, symbols with subscript numbers (NH_2) are bracketed.

e.g., ANH_{17} (for 17-imino-androstane),

$P^5CN_{16\alpha}ol_{3\beta}on_{20}$ (for 3β-Hydroxy-20-oxo-5-pregnene-16α-carbonitrile or PCN). All other N-containing steroids, including the alkaloids, belong to this group. The aza-steroids are listed last, in the heterocyclic category (cf. below).

Sulfosteroids: All thio compounds, e.g., —SH (-thiol), C—C epithio, (θS), thioether.

Heterocyclic steroids: These are listed separately for each element replacing carbon in the ring structure. They are indicated by the chemical symbol of the substituent in brackets, followed by a subscript number identifying the position of the replaced ring carbon after the symbol of the parent hydrocarbon (e.g., $A(O_2)$ for 2-Oxa-androstane, $P(N_3)$ for 3-Aza-pregnane).

Ring modifications: (cf. p. 775).

Other non alkyl-substituted compounds: Here, we list all those non alkyl-substituted compounds for which no category has been foreseen above.

Secondary Parent Hydrocarbons

All radicals attached to the parent hydrocarbon by a **carbon-to-carbon linkage** are considered to form "secondary parent hydrocarbons." They are written by attaching the symbol for the substituent following that of the parent hydrocarbon, both being underlined (e.g., $A5\alpha I_{17\alpha}$ = 17α-methyl-5α-androstane).

All alkyl derivatives, except those listed themselves as main parent hydrocarbons (e.g., 17β-ethyl-androstane = pregnane), are regarded as alkyl derivatives of the latter. This includes even 17α-ethyl-androstane whose essential difference from pregnane is further emphasized by attaching the side chain to the structure formula of androstane, not only by an alpha (...) bond, but horizontally.

The alkyl side-chains are enumerated:
1. according to the increasing numbers of the carbon atoms to which they are attached on the skeleton of the main parent hydrocarbon and 2. according to increasing numbers of the carbon atoms they contain (methyl, ethyl, propyl, butyl, etc.). Saturated radicals are mentioned first, and those with double bonds in the order of increasing unsaturation. Triple bonds (superscript position numbers boldface e.g.: P^{20}) are mentioned after all multiple double bonds. Branched and ring-substituents are listed in the order of increasing complexity. (For corresponding symbols, cf. p. 778.)

Among the aliphatic 17-alkyl-androstanes, only pregnanes, cholanes, cholestanes, ergostane and stigmastan are regarded as special parent hydrocarbons because of their common occurrence.

Order of Precedence in General

The order of precedence for the above mentioned substituents is rigidly observed except in the first (underlined or boldface) portion of the SSS terms of secondary parent hydrocarbons. As previously stated, here all substituents attached to a side-chain are listed immediately after the positional number of the latter, to avoid subsequent repetition of the locant, e.g., $A5I''_{16\beta}III_{17\alpha/on//1}ol_{3\beta}$.

When two or more identical substituents appear in the same molecule, all these must be enumerated before considering compounds possessing additional substituents mentioned later in the above list (e.g., all -enes before -dienes, before -trienes, etc.; all -ols before -diols, before -triols, etc.). Only after this do we proceed to compounds having an additional type of substituent (e.g., only after all mono- and polyols do we proceed to -ones).

All unsaturations (double, triple and cyclizing bonds) and substitution products are listed according to the **ascending order of the affected carbons** (e.g., in pregnanes 1—21). Ring modifications, such as contractions (nor), expansions (homo), openings (sec), etc. are listed in the **order of the ring lettering (A—D)**.

Computerization

Subscript and superscript notations are unsuitable for computerization but SSS names can be written in a single line without loss of precision. E.g., normally we write dehydro-epiandrosterone thus: $A^5ol_{17\beta}on_3$ and the corresponding 5α saturated compound thus: $A5\alpha ol_{17\beta}on_3$. For computer use, these two steroids can be written respectively A5 ol 17β on 3 and A5α ol 17β on 3.

The superscript position of a number following the symbol for the parent hydrocarbon (e.g., A^5) merely facilitates its immediate recognition as a double bond. Similarly the subscript position of numbers helps to identify them as locants. But actually, this style is not indispensable if the constituent symbols are properly separated. The rule of "first what, then where" makes it obvious that the "5" belongs to the "A", the "17β" to the "ol", and the "3" to the "on". The number 5 could only indicate a double bond; it would have to be followed by α, β, or ξ if it were to denote the steric position of the 5-hydrogen. Even the omission of underlining (or boldface printing) of the parent hydrocarbon would not introduce any ambiguity. Greek letters such as α, β, or ξ, can be written out as alpha, beta or xi, and the roman numerals can be composed by capitals on computers, just as on typewriters that do not have corresponding signs. The use of capital and small letters is likewise not necessary, but it helps rapid reading and is recommended for those who have the appropriate modern computer equipment.

Chemical Symbols

, = sign of separation. To be used at discretion of codifier, wherever two adjacent symbols might be read as one (e.g., on$_{4,6}$).

* = ester (precedes symbol of acid. E.g.: *III = propyl ester).

θ = ether (precedes symbol of alkyl. E.g.: θI = methoxy or methyl ether).

A = androstan (for symbols of other parent hydrocarbons, cf. p. 775). Only parent hydrocarbons and all alkyls attached to them by carbon-to-carbon linkages are bold face (E.g.: **AIII**$_{17β}$**I**$_{2α}$ol$_{4β}$on$_{11}$ = 17β-propyl-2α-methyl androstane with 4β-alcohol and 11-keto groups.)

/,// = successive levels (subdivisions) in a code, obviating the need for more than one subscript line (e.g., 2-methylbutane = IV$_{I/2}$). The successive levels of more complex branchings coded according to the general formula: R$_{R'/2//R''///3}$ (e.g., 2(3-methylbutyl)-heptane = VII$_{IV/2//I///3}$.)

( ) = brackets are used to enclose symbols with subscript numbers which might be confused with locants, e.g., (NH$_2$), (CH$_2$).

Substituents	Methyl Formic	Ethyl Acetic	Propyl Propionic	Butyl	
Alkanes, normal	I	II	III	IV	
Alkanes, branched	—	—	III$_{1/2}$ (2-methyl-propane)	IV$_{1/2,3}$ (2,3-dimethyl-butane)	
Alcohols	I ol	II ol	III ol	IV ol	Symbols of side chains bound to ring by carbon-to-carbon linkages, follow roman numerals.
Acids	I''	II''	III''	IV''	
Aldehydes	Ial	IIal	IIIal	IVal	
Esters	*I	*II	*III	*IV	Symbols of groups bound to ring by oxygen, precede roman numerals.
Ethers	θI	θII	θIII	θIV	

The 92 carbonitriles of Table 135 have been arranged according to the increasing number of the skeletal carbon atoms to which the —CN groups or —CN-bearing side-chains are attached. A few additional steroids, other than nitriles (Cpds. 93—99) are listed in arbitrary order.

The most potent catatoxic steroids against both substrates of this test were those bearing a 2α- or 16α-carbonitrile group. Among these, several showed potency against one or both substrates at individual dose levels as low as 100 µg or even 30 µg. In general, protection against indomethacin was more readily obtained than against digitoxin.

Table 135. *First step: Screening of steroids against digitoxin and indomethacin intoxication*

Group	Steroids	Dose (mg)	Digitoxin[a]	Indomethacin[a]
CN1,2,3 Steroid Carbonitriles				
1 IM 433[b]	17β-Hydroxy-3-oxo-5α-androstane-1α-carbonitrile acetate (SC-16027) A5αCN$_{1\alpha}$*II''$_{17\beta}$on$_3$	0.5	0	0
2 IM 427	17β-Hydroxy-3-oxo-5α-androstane-1α-carbonitrile (SC-16026) A5αCN$_{1\alpha}$ol$_{17\beta}$on$_3$	0.5	0	0
3 IM 364	17β-Hydroxy-4,4,17-trimethyl-3-oxo-5-androstene-2α-carbonitrile. *Trimethylandrostenolone carbonitrile,* "TMACN" (Winthrop) A^{5}I$_{4,4,17\alpha}$CN$_{2\alpha}$ol$_{17}$on$_3$	10 0.5 0.1 0.03	3 2.5 2 0	3 3 2 0
4 IM 568	17β-Hydroxy-4,4-dimethyl-3-oxo-5-pregnene-2α-carbonitrile (U-26854) A^{5}I$_{4,4}$CN$_{2\alpha}$ol$_{17\beta}$on$_3$	0.5 0.03	2 0	0.5 —
5 IM 368	17β-Hydroxy-5α-androst-2-ene-3-carbonitrile (Lepetit) A5$\ddot{\alpha}^2$CN$_3$ol$_{17\beta}$	10 0.5	0.5 0	2 0
6 IM 365	17-Oxo-5α-androst-2-ene-3-carbonitrile (Lepetit) A5α^2CN$_3$on$_{17}$	10 0.5	2 0	2 0
7 IM 367	20,20-(Ethylenedioxy)-5β-pregn-2-ene-3-carbonitrile (Lepetit) P5β^2CN$_3\theta\theta$II$_{20}$	10	0	0

[a] For details, see Digitoxin and Indomethacin in the list of techniques used to produce and appraise various types of damage.

[b] Underneath the serial number of the compounds, the "IM" numbers (for Institut de Médecine et de Chirurgie expérimentales) are mentioned. These identify steroids in our collection and remain the same in all Tables as well as in other publications from this Institute.

Table 135 (continued)

Group	Steroids	Dose (mg)	Digi-toxin[a]	Indo-methacin[a]
8 IM 366	20,20-(Ethylenedioxy)-5α-pregn-2-ene-3-carbonitrile (Lepetit) $P5α^2CN3θ,θII_{20}$	10 0.5 0.03	0.5 0 —	2 2 0
9 IM 424	17β-Hydroxy-3ξ-amino-5α-androstane-3-carbonitrile (SC-13265) $A5αCN_{3ξ}ol_{17β}(NH_2)_3$	0.5	0	0
CN$_5$				
10 IM 420	17β-Hydroxy-3-oxo-5β-androstane-5-carbonitrile (SC-13389) $A5βCN_5ol_{17β}on_3$	10 0.03 0.015 0.005 0.001	0 0 0 0 0	0 0 0 0 0
11 IM 434	17β-Hydroxy-3-oxo-5α-androstane-5-carbonitrile (SC-13269) $A5αCN_5ol_{17β}on_3$	0.5	0	0
12 IM 432	3α,17-Dihydroxy-5α,17α-pregn-20-yne-5-carbonitrile (SC-13675) $A5αCN_5II^{1-1}{}_{17α}ol_{3α,17}$	0.5	0	0
13 IM 431	17-Hydroxy-3,20-dioxo-5α-pregnane-5-carbonitrile acetate (SC-13795) $P5αCN_5*II''_{17}on_{3,20}$	0.5	0	0
14 IM 430	5ξ-Cyano-17-hydroxy-17α-(2-methylallyl)-estran-3-one (SC-13969) $E5ξCN_5III^2{}_{17α/I//2}ol_{17}on_3$	0.5	0	0

Table 135 (continued)

Group	Steroids	Dose (mg)	Digi-toxin[a]	Indo-methacin[a]
15 IM 428 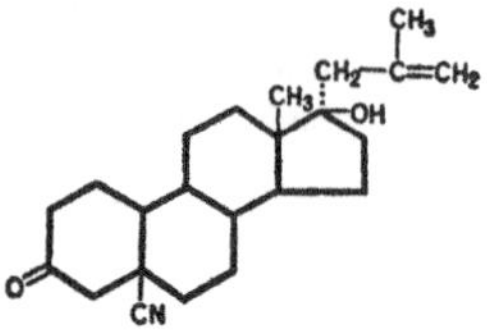	5β-Cyano-17-hydroxy-17α-(2-methyl-allyl)-estran-3-one (SC-14373) E5βCN$_5$III^2$_{17α/1//2}$ol$_{17}$on$_3$	0.5	0	0
16 IM 435	17-Hydroxy-3-oxo-19-nor-5β,17α-pregn-20-yne-5-carbonitrile (SC-13823) E5βCN$_5$II$^{1-1}$$_{17α}ol_{17}on_3$	0.5	0	0
17 IM 426 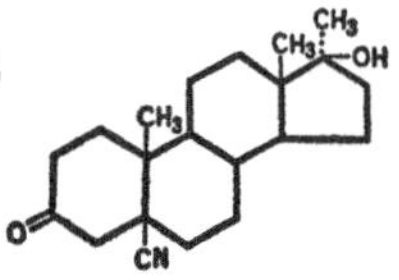	17β-Hydroxy-17-methyl-3-oxo-5β-androstane-5-carbonitrile (SC-13754) A5βI$_{17α}$CN$_5$ol$_{17}$on$_3$	0.5	0	0
18 IM 425 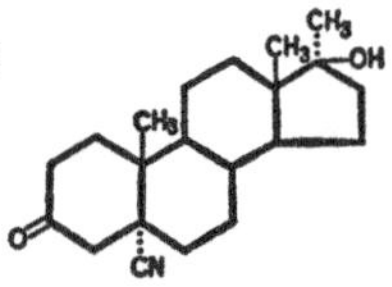	17β-Hydroxy-17-methyl-3-oxo-5α-androstane-5-carbonitrile (SC-13503) A5αI$_{17α}$CN$_5$ol$_{17}$on$_3$	0.5	0	0
19 IM 422 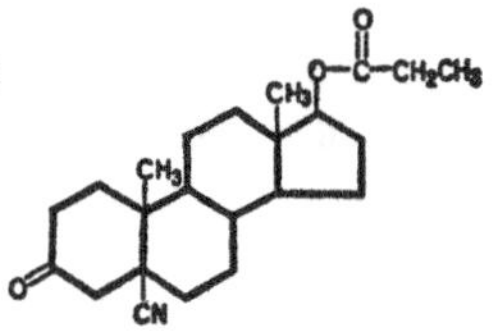	17β-Hydroxy-3-oxo-5β-androstane-5-carbonitrile propionate (SC-14175) A5βCN$_5$*III''$_{17β}$on$_3$	0.5	0	0
20 IM 421 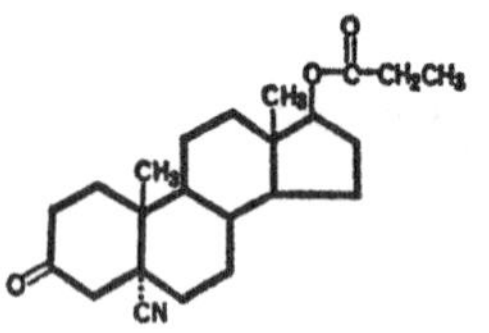	17β-Hydroxy-3-oxo-5α-androstane-5-carbonitrile propionate (SC-14174) A5αCN$_5$*III''$_{17β}$on$_3$	0.5	0	0

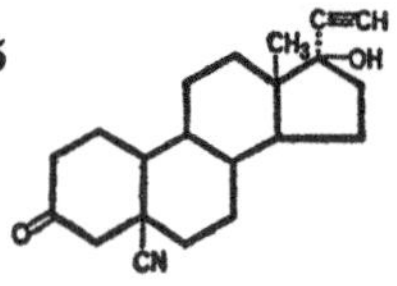

CN$_6$

Group	Steroids	Dose (mg)	Digi-toxin[a]	Indo-methacin[a]
21 IM 449 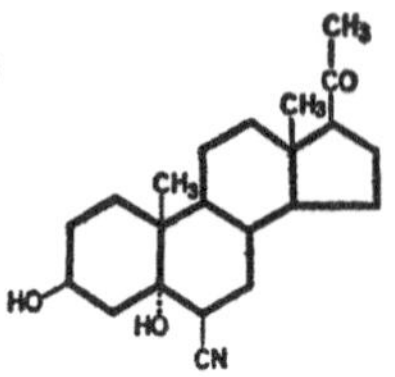	3β,5α-Dihydroxy-20-oxopregnane-6β-carbonitrile (Syntex) P5αCN$_{6β}$ol$_{3β,5}$on$_{20}$	0.5	0	0

Table 135 (continued)

Group	Steroids	Dose (mg)	Digi-toxin[a]	Indo-methacin[a]
22 IM 455	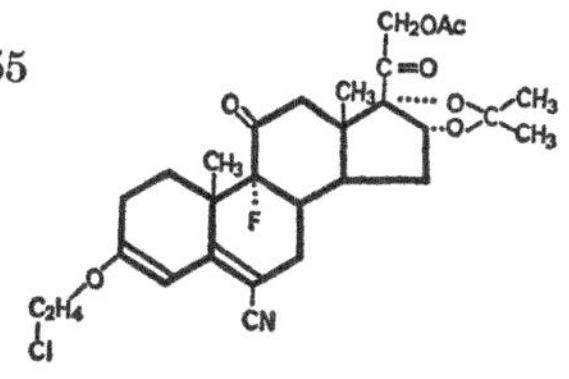 3-(2'-Chloroethoxy)-6-cyano-9α-fluoro-3,5-pregnadiene-16α,17α,21-triol-11,20-dion-21-acetate-16,17-acetonide (Farmitalia) $P^{3,5}CN_6*II''_{21}on_{11,20}\theta II_{3\beta/Cl//2}\theta\theta I_{16\alpha-17/I,I}F_{9\alpha}$	0.5	0	1
23 IM 456	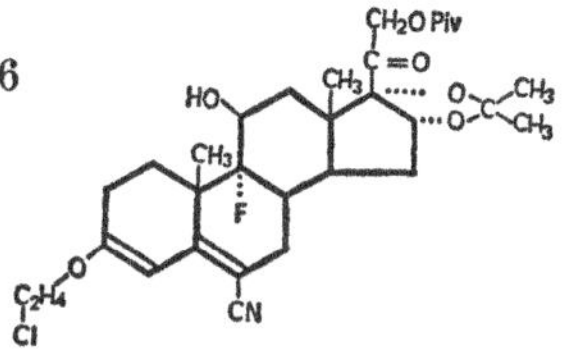 3-(2'-Chloroethoxy)-6-cyano-9α-fluoro-3,5-pregnadiene-11β,16α,17α,21-tetrol-20-one-21-pivalat-16,17-acetonide (Farmitalia) $P^{3,5}CN_6ol_{11\beta}*III''_{21/I//2,20}on_{20}\theta II_{3/Cl//2}\theta\theta I_{16\alpha-17/I,I}F_{9\alpha}$	0.5	0	
24 IM 457	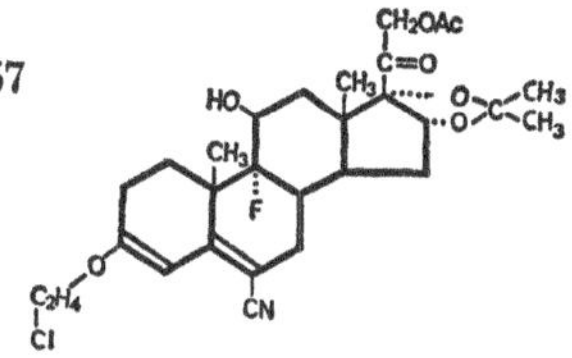 3-(2'-Chloroethoxy)-6-cyano-9α-fluoro-3,5-pregnadiene-11β,16α,17α,21-tetrol-20-one-21-acetate-16,17-acetonide (Farmitalia) $P^{3,5}CN_6ol_{11\beta}*II''_{21}on_{20}\theta II_{3/Cl//2}\theta\theta I_{16\alpha-17/I,I}F_{9\alpha}$	0.5	0	0
25 IM 458	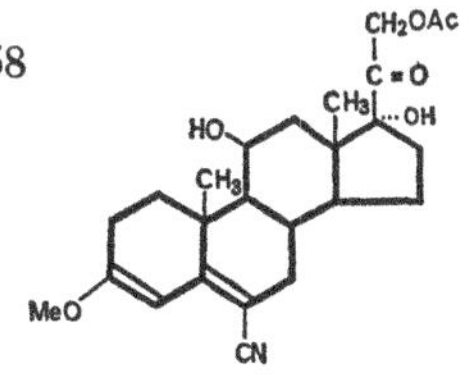 3β,11β,17α,21-Tetrahydroxy-20-oxo-3,5-pregnadiene-6-carbonitrile 3-methyl ether, 21-acetate (BDH) $P^{3,5}CN_6ol_{11\beta,17\alpha}*II''_{21}on_{20}\theta I_3$	0.5	0	0
26 IM 459	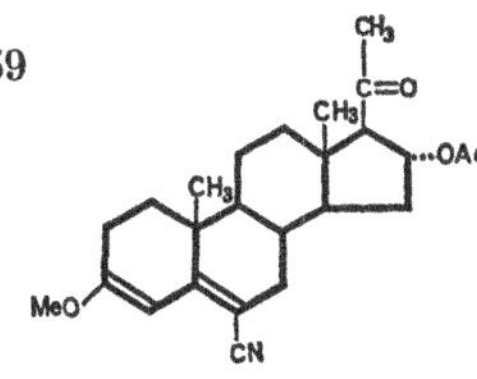 3,16α-Dihydroxy-20-oxo-3,5-pregnadiene-6-carbonitrile 3-methyl ether, 16-acetate (Glaxo Canada Ltd.) $P^{3,5}CN_6*II''_{16\alpha}on_{20}\theta I_3$	0.5	0	0

CN_{16}

Group	Steroids	Dose (mg)	Digi-toxin[a]	Indo-methacin[a]
27 IM 346	3β-Hydroxy-20-oxo-5-pregnene-16α-carbonitrile (SC-4674), (U-14975) *Pregnenolone carbonitrile "PCN"* $P^5CN_{16\alpha}ol_{3\beta}on_{20}$	10 1 0.5 0.2 0.1 0.03 0.015	3 3 3 3 3 2 0	3 3 3 3 3 3 0

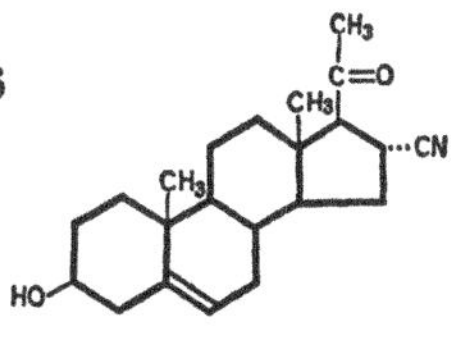

Table 135 (continued)

Group	Steroids	Dose (mg)	Digi-toxin[a]	Indo-metha-cin[a]
28 IM 413	3β-Hydroxy-20-oxo-5-pregnene-16α-carbonitrile acetate (U-34889, Syntex) Pregnenolone carbonitrile acetate "PCN-ac" P5CN$_{16α}$*II''$_{3β}$on$_{20}$	0.5 0.1 0.03 0.015	2.5 0.5 1 0	2 2 1.5 0
29 IM 483	3β-Hydroxy-20-oxo-5-pregnene-16α-carbonitrile 3-sulfate ammonium salt (U-37863C) "PCN-ammonium sulfate" P5CN$_{16α}$*(S''NH$_4$)$_{3β}$on$_{20}$	0.5 0.03 0.015	3 3 1	3 3 0.5
30 IM 478	3β-Hydroxy-20-oxo-5-pregnene-16α-carbonitrile 3(1'adamantoate) (U-36789) "PCN-adamantoate" P5CN$_{16α}$*adamantoate$_{3β}$ on$_{20}$	0.5 0.03	0.5 —	3 0
31 IM 476	3β-Hydroxy-20-oxo-5-pregnene-16α-carbonitrile 3-hemisuccinate sodium salt (U-36278A) "PCN-hemisuccinate sodium" P5CN$_{16α}$*1/2suc''Na$_{3β}$on$_{20}$	0.5 0.03 0.015 0.005	3 2.5 2 0	3 3 1.5 2
32 IM 479	3β-Hydroxy-20-oxo-5-pregnene-16α-carbonitrile 3-heptanoate (U-37001) "PCN-heptanoate" P5CN$_{16α}$*VII''$_{3β}$on$_{20}$	0.5 0.03 0.015	3 1 0	3 1.5 0
33 IM 444	3β,20-Dihydroxy-5-pregnene-16α-carbonitrile (Syntex) P5CN$_{16α}$ol$_{3β,20}$	0.5 0.1 0.03	1.5 1 0	3 1.5 0
34 IM 423	3β-Hydroxy-7,20-dioxo-5-pregnene-16α-carbonitrile (SC-6813) P5CN$_{16α}$ol$_{3β}$on$_{7,20}$	0.5 0.03	3 0	1.5 0.5

Table 135 (continued)

Group	Steroids	Dose (mg)	Digi-toxin[a]	Indo-methacin[a]
35 IM 429	3β-Hydroxy-7,20-dioxo-5-pregnene-16α-carbonitrile acetate (SC-6703) P5CN$_{16\alpha}$*II''$_{3\beta}$on$_{7,20}$	0.5 0.03	3 0	2 1.5
36 IM 474	4,4-Dimethyl-3,20-dioxo-5-pregnene-16α-carbonitrile (U-35641) P5I$_{4,4}$CN$_{16\alpha}$on$_{3,20}$	0.5 0.03	0.5 —	3 0
37 IM 411	3,3-(Ethylenedioxy)-11,20-dioxo-5-pregnene-16α-carbonitrile (U-35006) P5CN$_{16\alpha}$on$_{11,20}\theta\theta$II$_{3,3}$	0.5 0.1 0.03 0.015	2.5 2.5 0 0	2 2 1.5 1.5
38 IM 418	3β-Hydroxy-11,20-dioxo-5β-pregnane-16α-carbonitrile acetate (U-34575) P5βCN$_{16\alpha}$*II''$_{3\beta}$on$_{11,20}$	0.5 0.1 0.03 0.015	2.5 2.5 0 0	2 2 1.5 1.5
39 IM 464	16α-Cyano-5-pregnene-3β,20β-diol diacetate (SC-5482) P5CN$_{16\alpha}$*II''$_{3\beta,20\beta}$	0.1 0.03	0 —	2 0
40 IM 462	3β-Hydroxy-20-oxo-5-pregnene-16α-carbonitrile,20-oxime (U-37722) P5CN$_{16\alpha}$ol$_{3\beta}$NOH$_{20}$	0.5 0.03 0.015 0.010	3 2.5 0.5 —	3 3 1 0
41 IM 482	3β-Hydroxy-20-oxo-5-pregnene-16α-carbonitrile,20-methyloxime (U-37694) P5CN$_{16\alpha}$ol$_{3\beta}$(NOCH$_3$)$_{20}$	0.5 0.03 0.015	1 1.5 0	1.5 0 —

Table 135 (continued)

Group	Steroids	Dose (mg)	Digi-toxin[a]	Indo-metha-cin[a]
42 IM 414	20,20-(Ethylenedioxy)-3β-hydroxy-5-pregnene-16α-carbonitrile (U-19553)	0.5 0.1 0.03 0.015	2.5 2 0.5 0	2 2 1.5 0
	$P^5CN_{16\alpha}ol_{3\beta}\theta\theta II_{20}$			
43 IM 445	3β-Hydroxy-20,20-ethylene-dioxy-5-pregnene-16α-carbonitrile acetate (Syntex)	0.5 0.1 0.03	1.5 0 0	3 1.5 0
	$P^5CN_{16\alpha}*II''_{3\beta}\theta\theta II_{20}$			
44 IM 412	3,3,20,20-Bis-ethylenedioxy-11-oxo-5-pregnene-16α-carbonitrile (U-35910)	0.5 0.1 0.03 0.015	2.5 0 0 0	2 2 1.5 0
	$P^5CN_{16\alpha}on_{11}\theta\theta II_{3,20}$			
45 IM 475	3,20-Dioxo-4-pregnene-16α-carbonitrile,20-cyclic(2',2'-dimethyltrimethylene acetal) (U-35655)	0.5 0.03	1.5 0.5	3 0
	$P^4CN_{16\alpha}on_3\theta\theta III_{20/I//2,2}$			
46 IM$_a^1$461	3β-Hydroxy-20-oxo-5-pregnene-16α-carbonitrile, cyclic(2,2-dimethyltrimethylene acetal) (U-36961)	0.5 0.03 0.015	2 2 0	3 0 —
	$P^5CN_{16\alpha}ol_{3\beta}\theta\theta III_{20/I//2,2}$			
47 IM 481	4,4-Dimethyl-3,20-dioxo-5-pregnene-16α-carbonitrile,20-cyclic(2'2'-dimethyltrimethylene acetal) (U-37542)	0.5	0	0
	$P^5I_{4,4}CN_{16\alpha}on_3\theta\theta III_{20/I//2,2}$			
48 IM 480	6β-Hydroxy-20-oxo-3α,5α-cyclo-pregnane-16α-carbonitrile, cyclic(2',2'-dimethyltrimethylene acetal) (U-37483)	0.5 0.03	1 0	3 0
	$P^{3\alpha(5)}5\alpha CN_{16\alpha}ol_{6\beta}\theta\theta III_{20/I//2,2}$			

Table 135 (continued)

Group	Steroids	Dose (mg)	Digi-toxin[a]	Indo-methacin[a]
49 IM 477	6β-Hydroxy-20-oxo-3α,5α-cyclo-pregnane-16α-carbonitrile (U-36710)	0.5 0.03	2 0	3 0
	P3α(5)5αCN$_{16α}$ol$_{6β}$on$_{20}$			
50 IM 466	16α-Cyano-4-pregnene-3,20-dione (SC-4688)	0.1 0.015	3 0	0 0
	P4CN$_{16α}$on$_{3,20}$			
51 IM 471	16α-Cyano-3-hydroxy-3,5-pregnadiene-7,20-dione (SC-6963)	0.1	0	—
	P^{3,5}CN$_{16α}$ol$_3$on$_{7,20}$			
52 IM 470	16α-Cyano-3,5-pregnadiene-7,20-dione (SC-6786)	0.1	0	0
	P^{3,5}CN$_{16α}$on$_{7,20}$			
53 IM 395	3-Methoxy-16-methyl-17-oxo-estra-1,3,5(10)-triene-16ξ-carbonitrile (Roussel)	0.5	0	0
	E$^{1,3,5(10)}$I$_{16ξ}$CN$_{16}$on$_{17}$θI$_3$			
54 IM 392	17β-Hydroxy-3-methoxy-16-methylestra-1,3,5(10)-triene-16β-carbonitrile acetate (Roussel)	0.5	0	0
	E$^{1,3,5(10)}$I$_{16α}$CN$_{16}$*II″$_{17β}$θI$_3$			
CN$_{17}$ 55 IM 386	3α-Hydroxy-5β-androstane-17β-carbonitrile acetate (Roussel)	0.5	0	0
	A5βCN$_{17β}$*II″$_{3α}$			
56 IM 377	3α,17-Dihydroxy-5β-androstane-17ξ-carbonitrile 3-acetate (Roussel)	0.5	0	0
	A5βCN$_{17}$ol$_{17ξ}$*II″$_{3α}$			

Table 135 (continued)

Group	Steroids	Dose (mg)	Digitoxin[a]	Indomethacin[a]
57 IM 369	17-Cyano-3α-hydroxy-11-oxo-5β-androstane-17β-malononitrile (Roussel) $A\,5\,\beta I_{17\beta/CN//1,1}\,CN_{17}ol_{3\alpha}on_{11}$	0.5	0	0
58 IM 382	3β,17-Dihydroxy-16β-methyl-5α-androstane-17ξ-carbonitrile (Roussel) $A\,5\,\alpha I_{16\beta}CN_{17}ol_{3\beta,17\xi}$	0.5	0	0
59 IM 374	17-Hydroxy-3,11-dioxo-4-androstene-17ξ-carbonitrile (Roussel) $A^4 CN_{17}ol_{17\xi}on_{3,11}$	0.5	0	0
60 IM 378	3α-Hydroxy-5β-androst-16-ene-17-carbonitrile acetate (Roussel) $A\,5\,\beta^{16}CN_{17}*II''_{3\alpha}$	0.5	0	0
61 IM 389	3-Oxo-4,16-androstadiene-17-carbonitrile (Roussel) $A^{4,16}CN_{17}on_3$	0.5	0	0
62 IM 396	3β-Hydroxy-5,16-androstadiene-17-carbonitrile acetate (Roussel) $A^{5,16}CN_{17}*II''_{3\beta}$	0.5	0	0
63 IM 390	3,3-(Ethylenedioxy)-17-hydroxy-5-pregnene-17β-carbonitrile (Roussel) $A^5 CN_{17\alpha}ol_{17}\vartheta\vartheta II_3$	0.5	0	0
64 IM 380	3-Hydroxy-1,3,5(10),16-estratetraene-17-carbonitrile acetate (Roussel) $E^{1,3,5(10)16}CN_{17}*II''_3$	0.5	0	0

Table 135 (continued)

Group	Steroids	Dose (mg)	Digitoxin[a]	Indomethacin[a]
65 IM 400	3-Methoxy-1,3,5(10),16-estratetraene-17-carbonitrile (Roussel) $E^{1,3,5(10)16}CN_{17}\theta I_3$	0.5	0	0
66 IM 417	17-Cyano-3β-hydroxy-5-androstene-17β-malononitrile (U-28406) $A^5I_{17\beta/CN//1,1}CN_{17}ol_{3\beta}$	0.5	0	0
67 IM 391	17-Hydroxy-3-oxo-4-androstene-17ξ-carbonitrile acetate (Roussel) $A^4CN_{17}*II''_{17\xi}on_3$	0.5	0	0
68 IM 375	17-Hydroxy-3,11-dioxo-4-androstene 17ξ-carbonitrile acetate (Roussel) $A^4CN_{17}*II''_{17\xi}on_{3,11}$	0.5	0	0
16-Side chain CN				
69 IM 469	16α-Cyanomethyl-3β-hydroxy-5-pregnen-20-one (SC-6939) $P^5ICN_{16\alpha}ol_{3\beta}on_{20}$	0.5	0	0
70 IM 472	16α-Cyanomethyl-4-pregnene-3,20-dione (SC-7097) $P^4ICN_{16\alpha}on_{3,20}$	0.5	0	0
71 IM 409	α-Cyano-3β-hydroxy-20-oxo-5-pregnen-16α-acetic acid ethyl ester (SK & F) $P^5II''_{16\alpha/CN//2}*IIol_{///1}ol_{3\beta}on_{20}$	10	0	0
17-Side chain CN				
72 IM 381	3α-Hydroxy-5β-androstan-17β-acetonitrile (Roussel) $A5\beta ICN_{17\beta}ol_{3\alpha}$	0.5	0	0

Table 135 (continued)

Group	Steroids	Dose (mg)	Digi-toxin[a]	Indo-methacin[a]
73 IM 383	3α,20-Dihydroxy-5β-pregnane-20ξ-carbonitrile 3-acetate (Roussel) P 5 β CN$_{20}$ol$_{20\xi}$*II''$_{3\alpha}$	0.5	0	0
74 IM 371	20-Cyano-3α-hydroxy-5β-pregn-17(20)-en-21-oic acid acetate ethyl ester (Roussel) P 5 β$^{17(20)''}$CN$_{20}$*II''$_{3\beta}$*IIol$_{21}$	0.5	0	0
75 IM 376	20-Cyano-3α-hydroxy-11-oxo-24-nor-5β-cholan-21-oic acid amide (Roussel) CHn(24) 5 β CN$_{20}$ol$_{3\alpha}$on$_{11}$(CONH$_2$)$_{20}$	0.5	0	0
76 IM 388	3β,20,21-Trihydroxy-5β-pregnane-20ξ-carbonitrile 3,21-diacetate (Roussel) P 5 β CN$_{20}$ol$_{20\xi}$*II''$_{3\beta,21}$	0.5	0	0
77 IM 403	3α,20ξ-Dihydroxy-11-oxo-5β-pregnane-20ξ-carbonitrile 3-acetate (Roussel) P 5 β CN$_{20}$ol$_{20\xi}$*II''$_{3\alpha}$on$_{11}$	0.5	0	0
78 IM 401	20-Cyano-3α-acetoxy-11-oxo-24-norcholan-21-oic acid ethyl ester (Roussel) CHn(24) 5 β''CN$_{20}$*II''$_{3\alpha}$*IIol$_{21}$on$_{11}$	0.5	0	0
79 IM 398	20-Cyano-3α-hydroxy-5β-pregnan-21-oic acid (Roussel) P 5 β''$_{21}$CN$_{20}$ol$_{3\alpha}$	0.5	0	0

Table 135 (continued)

Group	Steroids	Dose (mg)	Digi-toxin[a]	Indo-methacin[a]
80 IM 385	3α-Hydroxy-11-oxo-5β-androstan-17β-acetonitrile acetate (Roussel) A 5 β ICN$_{17\beta}$*II''$_{3\alpha}$on$_{11}$	0.5	0	0
81 IM 384	3β-(Tetrahydropyran-2-yloxy)-5β-androstan-17β-acetonitrile (Roussel) A 5 β ICN$_{17\beta}\theta$tetrahydropyranyl$_{3\beta}$ol$_{//2}$	0.5	0	0
82 IM 406	3α-Hydroxy-11-oxo-5β-androstane-Δ^{17}-malononitrile (Roussel) A 5 β$^{17(20)}$I$_{17/CN//1,1}$ol$_{3\alpha}$on$_{11}$	0.5	0	0
83 IM 393	3α-Hydroxy-11-oxo-5β-androstan-Δ^{17}-acetonitrile acetate (Roussel) A 5 β$^{17(20)}$ICN$_{17\alpha}$*II''$_{3\alpha}$on$_{11}$	0.5	0	1.5
84 IM 408	20-Cyano-3α-hydroxy-11-oxo-5β-pregn-17(20)-en-21-oic acid acetate ethyl ester (Roussel) P 5 β$^{17(20)}$''CN$_{20}$*II$_{3\alpha}$*IIol$_{21}$on$_{11}$	0.5	0	0
85 IM 405	20-Cyano-3α-hydroxy-11-oxo-5β-pregn-17(20)-en-21-oic acid (Roussel) P 5 β$^{17(20)''}{}_{21}$CN$_{20}$ol$_{3\alpha}$on$_{11}$	0.5	0	0
86 IM 394	3α-Hydroxy-11-oxo-5β-pregn-17(20)-ene-20-carbonitrile acetate (Roussel) P5 β$^{17(20)}$ CN$_{20}$*II''$_{3\alpha}$on$_{11}$	0.5	0.5	1.5

Table 135 (continued)

Group	Steroids	Dose (mg)	Digi-toxin[a]	Indo-methacin[a]
87 IM 404	20-Cyano-3β-hydroxy-5-pregnen-21-oic acid acetate ethyl ester (Roussel) $P5''CN_{20}*IIol_{21}*II''_{3\beta}$	0.5	0	0
88 IM 373	20-Cyano-3β-hydroxy-5,17(20)-pregnadien-21-oic acid 3-acetate ethyl ester (Roussel) $P5,17(20)''CN_{20}*IIol_{21}*II''_{3\beta}$	0.5	0	0
89 IM 407	20-Hydroxy-3-oxo-19-norpregna-4,9,11-triene-20ξ-carbonitrile (Roussel) $Pn19^{4,9,11}CN_{20\xi}ol_{20}on_3$	0.5	0	0
90 IM 399	3α-Hydroxy-5β-androstan-17β-glutaronitrile acetate (Roussel) $P5\beta CN_{21}ICN_{20}*II''_{3\alpha}$	0.5	0	0
91 IM 402	21-Cyano-3β-hydroxy-5α-pregn-20-ene-21-carboxylic acid ethyl ester (Roussel) $P5\alpha^{20}I''_{21/}*_{IIoI}CN_{21}ol_{3\beta}$	0.5	0	0
92 IM 370	21-Cyano-3α-hydroxy-5β-pregn-20-ene-21-carboxylic acid ethyl ester (Roussel) $P5\beta^{20}I''_{21/}*_{IIoI}CN_{21}ol_{3\alpha}$	0.5	0	0

Table 135 (continued)

Group	Steroids	Dose (mg)	Digi-toxin[a]	Indo-methacin[a]
Other Active Steroids				
93 IM 448	$3\beta,20$-Dihydroxy-17α-pregn-5-ene-16β-carboxylic acid (Syntex) $A^5I''_{16\beta}II_{17\alpha/ol//1}ol_{3\beta}$	0.5 0.1 0.03	1.5 0.5 0	3 0 0
94 IM 446	3β-Hydroxy-20-oxo-17α-pregn-5-ene-16β-carboxamide (Syntex) $A^5II_{17\alpha/on//1}(CONH_2)_{16\alpha}ol_{3\beta}$	0.5 0.1	0 0	1.5 0
95 IM 304	3-Methoxy-19-nor-17α-pregna-1,3,5(10)-trien-20-yn-17-ol (Lilly) *Mestranol* $E^{1,3,5(10)}II^{1-1}{}_{17\alpha}ol_{17}\theta I_3$	10 0.5	0 —	3 0
96 IM 410	17-Hydroxy-4-aza-17α-pregnan-3-one (Organon) $A(N_4)II_{17\alpha}ol_{17}on_3$	10 0.5	1.5 0	3 0
97 IM 454	$16\alpha,17$-Dihydro-3'H-cyclopropa(16,17)-5α-androstane-$3\beta,17\beta$-diol diacetate (SC-21940) $A5\alpha I_{16\alpha-17}*II''_{3\beta,17}$	10 0.5	3 0	— 0
98 IM 489	3α-Hydroxy-11-oxo-5β-androstane-17β-malonic acid (Roussel) $A5\beta I_{17\beta/I''//1,1}ol_{3\alpha}on_{11}$	0.5 0.03	0 —	1.5 0
99 IM 527	9α-Fluoro-16α-methyl-$11\beta,17,21$-trihydroxy-1,4-pregnadiene-3,20-dione 21-sodium m-sulfobenzoate *Dexamethasone sodium m-sulfobenzoate* (B.R.L.) $P^{1,4}I_{16\alpha}ol_{11\beta,17}$m-sulfobenzoate $Na_{21}on_{3,20}F_{9\alpha}$	0.5 0.03	0 —	1.5 0

Cpd. 54, the only 16β-carbonitrile of our series, as well as Cpd. 53 in which the steric position of the 16-carbonitrile is unknown, were inactive in protecting against either substrate, even at the dose level of 500 μg. Cpds. 69—71 in which the —CN group is attached to a 16α-side-chain (rather than to the C_{16} carbon of the steroid skeleton itself) showed no protective activity, even at the dose of 10 mg. On the other hand, it is hardly coincidental that among 28 16α-carbonitriles tested (Cpds. 27—54) all but three (Cpds. 47, 51, 52) were active, and most of them even at very low dose levels. This suggests that the attachment of a —CN group in the 16α-position directly to the steroid skeleton is very favorable for this type of protective effect; the configuration of the rest of the steroid molecule, though capable of influencing the degree of activity, is of much lesser importance.

It is known from our previous work that a carbonitrile group in position 2α (e.g., Cpd. 3, TMACN) is also compatible with high catatoxic activity against a variety of substrates; additional evidence justifying this conclusion is given in Tables 135, 136.

Carbonitrile groups in position 3, may or may not convey some potency (Cpds. 5—9), but steroids with carbonitriles attached to C_1 (Cpds. 1, 2), C_5 (Cpds. 10—20) or C_6 (Cpds. 21—26) were uniformly inactive at all dose levels tested.

Carbonitrile substitution at C_{17}, C_{20}, C_{21} or in side-chains resulted in no remarkable catatoxic potency at the dose levels tested, with the exception of Cpds. 83 and 86 which were moderately effective in this respect at the dose level of 500 μg.

Among the steroids of Table 135 other than carbonitriles (Cpds. 93—99), special interest is attached to Cpd. 96 (an aza-steroid), Cpd. 95 (mestranol), a strong folliculoid used in anticonceptional pills, and Cpd. 93 (a 16β-carboxylic acid) all of which showed some catatoxic activity at comparatively high dose levels. This degree of activity is of little practical significance, but it is interesting that a heterocyclic aza-compound, a 16β-carboxylic acid and a folliculoid can possess some catatoxic potency.

Finally, it is noteworthy that (except for the moderate potency of Cpd. 93) all 16-carboxylic acids (Cpds. 66, 67 and 69 in Table 135 A) are devoid of catatoxic potency against both substrates. A priori, the possibility could not have been excluded that nitriles are metabolized in vivo into the corresponding carboxylic acids and that the latter would be responsible for catatoxic activity, but this does not appear to be the case.

Additional inactive steroids are listed in Table 135 A *cf.*, p. 794.

First Step: Synopsis of all 500 Steroids Tested for Their Ability to Prevent Digitoxin and Indomethacin Intoxication

The preceding tables summarize our hitherto unpublished data on the protection by steroids, and particularly by carbonitriles, against digitoxin and indomethacin intoxication. However, in order to obtain a proper overview of this field, the following list summarizes the results obtained with *all 500 steroids tested up to now, cf.* Table 135 B, p. 807. It will be kept in mind that all these experiments were performed under essentially identical conditions as outlined on p. VIII and in earlier publications (Selye G 70,421/70, G 70,480/71). Since no other laboratory has published comparable data on the detoxication of digitoxin and indomethacin by steroids, the list is assumed to be a reasonably complete inventory of all steroids tested for this effect and

Table 135A. *First step (Ctd.): Other inactive steroids.* (Tested at 0.5 mg dose level unless otherwise stated)

#			
1 IM 522[a]		17β-Hydroxy-4-estren-3-one 17-trichloroacetate *19-Nortestosterone trichloroacetate* (Bio. Research Lab.) (B.R.L.)	
		E^4 *$II''_{17\beta/Cl//2,2,2}$ on$_3$	
2 IM 505		3,17β-Dihydroxy-1,3,5(10)-estratriene 17-tribromoacetate (B.R.L.)	
		$E^{1,3,5(10)}$ ol$_3$ *$II''_{17\beta/Br//2,2,2}$	
3 IM 504		3,17β-Dihydroxy-1,3,5(10)-estratriene 17-trichloroacetate (B.R.L.)	
		$E^{1,3,5(10)}$ ol$_3$ *$II''_{17\beta/Cl//2,2,2}$	
4 IM 506		3,17β-Dihydroxy-1,3,5(10)-estratriene 17-trifluoroacetate (B.R.L.)	
		$E^{1,3,5(10)}$ ol$_3$ *$II''_{17\beta/F//2,2,2}$	
5 IM 513		3,17β-Dihydroxy-1,3,5(10)-estratriene 17-[2'-hydroxy]propionate (B.R.L.)	
		$E^{1,3,5(10)}$ ol$_3$ *$III''_{17\beta/ol//2}$	
6 IM 507		3,17β-Dihydroxy-1,3,5(10)-estratriene 17-[2'-hydroxy-2'-methyl]propionate (B.R.L.)	
		$E^{1,3,5(10)}$ ol$_3$ *$III''_{17\beta/Iol//2}$	
7 IM 509		3,17β-Dihydroxy-1,3,5(10)-estratriene 17-pentanoate (B.R.L.)	
		$E^{1,3,5(10)}$ ol$_3$ *$V''_{17\beta}$	
8 IM 510		3,17β-Dihydroxy-1,3,5(10)-estratriene 17-heptanoate (B.R.L.)	
		$E^{1,3,5(10)}$ ol$_3$ *$VII''_{17\beta}$	

[a] Underneath the serial number of the compounds, the "IM" numbers (for Institut de Médecine et de Chirurgie expérimentales) are mentioned. These identify steroids in our collection and remain the same in all Tables as well as in other publications from this Institute.

Table 135 A (continued)

#	ID		Name	Code
9	IM 511		3,17β-Dihydroxy-1,3,5(10)-estratriene 17-palmitate (B.R.L.)	$E^{1,3,5(10)}$ ol$_3$ *XVI''$_{17\beta}$
10	IM 512		3,17β-Dihydroxy-1,3,5(10)-estratriene 17-benzoate (B.R.L.)	$E^{1,3,5(10)}$ ol$_3$ *Bz''$_{17\beta}$
11	IM 508		3,17β-Dihydroxy-1,3,5(10)-estratriene 17-adamantoate (B.R.L.)	$E^{1,3,5(10)}$ ol$_3$ *adamantoate$_{17\beta}$
12	IM 519	(0.1mg)	3,17β-Dihydroxy-1,3,5(10)-estratriene 3-[2'-bromo-2'-methyl]propionate (B.R.L.)	$E^{1,3,5(10)}$ ol$_{17\beta}$ *III''$_{3/I, Br//2}$
13	IM 518		3,17β-Dihydroxy-1,3,5(10)-estratriene 3-trimethylacetate (B.R.L.)	$E^{1,3,5(10)}$ ol$_{17\beta}$ *II''$_{3/I//2,2,2}$
14	IM 514		3,17β-Dihydroxy-1,3,5(10)-estratriene 17-trichloroacetate 3-trimethylacetate (B.R.L.)	$E^{1,3,5(10)}$ *II''$_{3/I//2,2,2}$ *II''$_{17\beta/Cl//2,2,2}$
15	IM 516	(0.1mg)	3,17β-Dihydroxy-1,3,5(10)-estratriene 3-trimethylacetate 17-methyltartrate (B.R.L.)	$E^{1,3,5(10)}$ *II''$_{3/I//2,2,2}$ *methyltartrate$_{17\beta}$
16	IM 515		3,17β-Dihydroxy-1,3,5(10)-estratriene 3-propargyl ether 17-trichloroacetate (B.R.L.)	$E^{1,3,5(10)}$ *II''$_{17\beta/Cl//2,2,2}$ θIII$^2_3$
17	IM 517	(0.1mg)	3,17β-Dihydroxy-1,3,5(10)-estratriene 3,17-difuroate (B.R.L.)	$E^{1,3,5(10)}$ *furoate$_{3,17\beta}$

Table 135 A (continued)

#		Name
18 IM 191		3α-Hydroxy-5α-androstan-17-one 3-sodium sulphate (Organon) A 5 α *S''Na$_{3α}$ on$_{17}$
19 IM 313		2β-Hydroxy-3α-methylamino- 5α-androstan-17-one hydrochloride hydrate (Organon) A 5 α ol$_{2β}$on$_{17}$NHI$_{3α}$ · HCl 15 H$_2$O
20 IM 140		3α-Dimethylamino-2β-hydroxy- 5α-androstan-17-one hydrochloride monohydrate (Organon) A 5 α ol$_{2β}$on$_{17}$N$_{3α/I//1,1}$ · HCl H$_2$O
21 IM 284		2β-Diethylamino-3α-hydroxy-5α-androstan -17-one methobromide 3-acetate (Organon) [A 5 α *II''$_{3α}$ on$_{17}$N$_{2β/I,II,II}$] · Br$^-$
22 IM 260		2β-Dipropylamino-3α-hydroxy-5α-androstan- 17-one methobromide 3-acetate (Organon) [A 5 α *II''$_{3α}$ on$_{17}$N$_{2β/I,III,III}$] · Br$^-$
23 IM 453		2β,16β-Dipiperidino-5α-androstane-3α, 17β-diol diacetate dihydrochloride (Organon) A 5 α *II''$_{3α,17β}$ piperidino$_{2β,16β}$ · 2 HCl 15 H$_2$O
24 IM 185		2β, 16β-Dipiperidino-3α-hydroxy-5α-androstan- 17-one dimethobromide (Organon) [A 5 α ol$_{3α}$ on$_{17}$ piperidino$_{2β,16β/I//1,1}$] · 2 Br$^-$
25 IM 419		Thiocyanic acid 3α, 17β-dihydroxy-17-methyl-5α- androstan-2-yl-ester (SC-12697) A 5 α I$_{17α}$ ol$_{3α,17}$SCN$_{2β}$
26 IM 442		17α-Methyl-3β, 17-dihydroxy-5α-androstane-2α- hydroxymethyl (Syntex) A 5 α I$_{17α}$Iol$_{2α}$ ol$_{3β,17}$

Table 135 A (continued)

27 IM 451		17β-Hydroxy-3-oxo-5α-androstane-2-hydroxy-methylene (Syntex) A5αCHOH2ol17βon3
28 IM 443		17α-Methyl-17-hydroxy-3-oxo-5α-androstan-2-aminomethylene (Syntex) A5αI17α(CH NH2)2ol17on3
29 IM 441		3β-Hydroxy-20-oxo-5α,17α-pregnane-16β-carboxylic acid (Syntex) A5αI″16βII17α/on//1ol3
30 IM 495		3α-Hydroxy-11-oxo-5β-androstane-17β[α-benzyloxymethyl]-dimethyl-malonate (Roussel) **A5β benzyloxy methyl-dimethyl malonate** 17βol3αon11
31 IM 150		17β-Hydroxy-17-methyl-5α-androstan-[2,3-d]isoxazol (Sterling Winthrop) A5α²I17αisoxazolyl2-3/3,4ol17
32 IM 563		11α-Hydroxy-4-androstene-3,17-dione (U-1680) A⁴ol11αon3,17
33 IM 199		17β-Hydroxy-4-androsten-3-one 17-sodium sulphate (Organon) A⁴ *S″Na17βon3
34 IM 502		3-Oxo-4-androstene-17β-carboxylic acid (Roussel) A⁴I″17βon3
35 IM 450		17β-Hydroxy-3-oxo-4-androstene-7β-carboxamide (Syntex) A⁴(CONH2)7βol17βon3

Table 135 A (continued)

#			
36 IM 362		3β-Hydroxy-5-androsten-17-one 3-sodium sulfate (Organon)	
		$A^5 *S''Na_{3\beta}on_{17}$	
37 IM 501		3β-Hydroxy-5-androstene-17β-carboxylic acid (Roussel)	
		$A^5I''_{17\beta}ol_{3\beta}$	
38 IM 440		3β-Hydroxy-20-oxo-17α-pregn-5-ene-16β-carboxylic acid (Syntex)	
		$A^5I''_{16\beta}II_{17\alpha}/on_{//1}ol_{3\beta}$	
39 IM 500		3β,17β-Dihydroxy-5-pregnen-20-yne-21-carboxylic acid (Roussel)	
		$A^5III^{2,2''}_{17\alpha}ol_{3\beta,17}$	
40 IM 363	(10 mg)	1α,2α-Epoxy-4,6-androstadiene-3,17-dione (Linet)	
		$A^{4,6}on_{3,17}\,\theta_{1\alpha-2}$	
41 IM 498		3β-Acetoxy-5,15-androstadiene-17-carboxylic acid (Roussel)	
		$A^{5,15}I''_{17\beta} *II''_{3\beta}$	
42 IM 452		17β-Hydroxy-12α-13β-etiojerv-4-en-3-one (SC-19886)	
		$An18,nC,hoD^4I_{17\alpha}ol_{17\beta}on_3$	
43 IM 447		3β-Hydroxy-5α-pregnan-20-one (Steraloids)	
		$P\,5\alpha\ ol_{3\beta}on_{20}$	
44 IM 135		2β-(2'-Phenyl-ethylamino)-3α-hydroxy-5α-pregnan-20-one hydrochloride (Organon)	
		$P\,5\alpha\ ol_{3\alpha}on_{20}NH_{2\beta/II//Ph///2} \cdot HCl$	

Table 135 A (continued)

45 IM 82		2β-Piperidino-3α-hydroxy-5α-pregnan-20-one methobromide (Organon)
		$[P5\alpha \text{ ol}_{3\alpha}\text{on}_{20}\text{piperidino}_{2\beta/I//1}] \cdot Br^-$
46 IM 460		2β-Morpholino-3α-hydroxy-5α-pregnan-20-one hydrochloride (Organon)
		$P5\alpha \text{ ol}_{3\alpha}\text{on}_{20}\text{morpholino}_{2\beta} \cdot HCl$
47 IM 496		3β-Hydroxy-5α-pregnane-21,21-dicarboxylic acid (Roussel)
		$P5\alpha I''_{21,21}\text{ol}_{3\beta}$
48 IM 497		3β-Hydroxy-11-oxo-5β-pregnan-21-oic acid (Roussel)
		$P5\beta''_{21}\text{ol}_{3\alpha}\text{on}_{11}$
49 IM 545		3α-Acetoxy-23,24-bisnor-5β-cholan-22-oic acid (B.R.L.)
		$P5\beta I''_{20} *II''_{3\alpha}$
50 IM 544		3α-Acetoxy-23,24-bisnor-5β-cholan-22-al (B.R.L.)
		$P5\beta I \text{ al}_{20} *II''_{3\alpha}$
51 IM 436		3α-Hydroxy-11,20-dioxo-5β-pregnane-16α-carboxamide (U-35827)
		$P5\beta (CONH_2)_{16\alpha}\text{ol}_{3\alpha}\text{on}_{11,20}$
52 IM 557		21-Hydroxy-4-pregnene-3,11,20-trione (U-0569)
		$P^4\text{ol}_{21}\text{on}_{3,11,20}$

Table 135 A (continued)

#	ID	Name
53	IM 556	6β,11α-Dihydroxy-4-pregnene-3,20-dione diacetate (U-0471) P4 *II″$_{6\beta,11\alpha}$on$_{3,20}$
54	IM 561	4-Pregnene-3,11,20-trione (B.R.L.) P4on$_{3,11,20}$
55	IM 555	4-Pregnene-3,6,11,20-tetrone (U-0460) P4on$_{3,6,11,20}$
56	IM 546	22-Hydroxy-23,24-bisnorchol-4-en-3-one (B.R.L.) P4Iol$_{20}$on$_3$
57	IM 548	3-Oxo-23,24-bisnor-4-cholen-22-oic acid (B.R.L.) P4I″$_{20}$on$_3$
58	IM 416	3,20-Dioxo-4-pregnene-16α-carboxylic acid methyl ester (U-35258) P4I″$_{16\alpha}$/*Iol on$_{3,20}$
59	IM 547	3-Oxo-23,24-bisnor-4-cholen-22-al (B.R.L.) P4Ial$_{20}$on$_3$
60	IM 207	16α-Ethyl-20β-hydroxy-4-pregnen-3-one (Organon) P4II$_{16\alpha}$ol$_{20}$on$_3$

Table 135 A (continued)

#			
61 IM 524		5-Pregnen-3β-20β-diol 3-acetate (B.R.L.)	
		$P^5ol_{20\beta}$ *$II''_{3\beta}$	
62 IM 523		$3\beta,21$-Dihydroxy-5-pregnen-20-one diacetate (B.R.L.)	
		P^5 *$II''_{3\beta,21}on_{20}$	
63 IM 467		16β-Carboxy-5-pregnene-$3\beta,20\beta$-diol γ-lactone 3-acetate (SC-5634)	
		$P^5 I''\gamma lac_{16\beta-20}$*$II''_{3\beta}$	
64 IM 525		3,20-Dioxo-5-pregnene 3,3-20,20 bis-(ethylenedioxy) (B.R.L.)	
		$P^5\vartheta\vartheta II_{3,20}$	
65 IM 552		$9\xi,11\xi$-Epoxy-3β-hydroxy-5α-pregn-6-en-20-one-$5,8\alpha$-maleic anhydride adduct, acetate (U-0156)	
		$P5\alpha^6$ *$II''_{3\beta}on_{20}\theta_{9\xi-11}$ maleic anhydride adduct$_{5\alpha-8}$	
66 IM 465		16α-Carboxy-5-pregnene-$3\alpha,20$-diol diacetate (SC-5934)	
		$P^5I''_{16\alpha}$ *$II''_{3\alpha,20}$	
67 IM 415		20,20-(Ethylenedioxy)-3β-hydroxy-5-pregnene-16α-carboxylic acid (U-12872 E)	
		$P^5I''_{16\alpha}ol_{3\beta}\theta\theta II_{20}$	
68 IM 438		20,20-(Ethylenedioxy)-3β-hydroxy-5-pregnene-16α-carboxylic acid methyl ester (U-36548)	
		$P^5I''_{16\alpha/}*_Iol_{3\beta}\theta\theta II_{20}$	

Table 135 A (continued)

69	IM 437	20,20-(Ethylenedioxy)-3β-acetoxy-5-pregnene-16α-carboxylic acid (U-35939)	$P5I''_{16\alpha} *II''_{3\beta\theta\theta}II_{20}$
70	IM 71	3β-Hydroxy-16α-ethyl-5-pregnen-20-one (Organon)	$P5II_{16\alpha}ol_{3\beta}on_{20}$
71	IM 210	3β-Hydroxy-16α-isobutyl-5-pregnen-20-one (Organon)	$P5III_{16\alpha/I//20}ol_{3\beta}on_{20}$
72	IM 499	3α,17α-Dihydroxy-11-oxo-5β-pregn-20-ene-21-carboxylic acid (Roussel)	$P5\beta^{20}I''_{21}ol_{3\alpha,17}on_{11}$
73	IM 526	17,21-Dihydroxy-1,4-pregnadiene-3,11,20-trione *Prednisone* (B.R.L.)	$P^{1,4}ol_{17,21}on_{3,11,20}$
74	IM 503	17-Hydroxy-6-methyl-16-methylene-4,6-pregnadiene-3,20-dione acetate (U-21240)	$P^{4,6}I_6(CH_2)_{16} *II''_{17}on_{3,20}$
75	IM 553	3β-Hydroxy-5α-pregna-6,9(11)-dien-20-one-5,8α-maleic anhydride adduct, acetate (U-0157)	$P5\alpha^{6,9(11)}$ maleic anhydride adduct$_{5\alpha-8}$
76	IM 99	3β,21-Dihydroxy-5,16-pregnadien-20-one diacetate (Organon)	$P5,16 *II''_{3\beta,21}on_{20}$

Table 135 A (continued)

#			
77 IM 296		5β-Cholan-24-oic acid (Roussel)	
		$CH5\beta''_{24}$	
78 IM 493		3α-Hydroxy-5β-cholan-24-oic acid *Lithocholic acid* (Roussel)	
		$CH5\beta''_{24}ol_{3\alpha}$	
79 IM 485		3α,6α-Dihydroxy-5β-cholan-24-oic acid. *Hyodesoxylic acid* (Roussel)	
		$CH5\beta''_{24}ol_{3\alpha,6\alpha}$	
80 IM 492		3α,7α-Dihydroxy-5β-cholan-24-oic acid. *Chenodesoxylic acid* (Roussel)	
		$CH5\beta''_{24}ol_{3\alpha,7\alpha}$	
81 IM 490		3α,12α-Dihydroxy-5β-cholan-24-oic acid. *Desoxycholic acid* (Roussel)	
		$CH5\beta''_{24}ol_{3\alpha,12\alpha}$	
82 IM 488		3α,7α,12α-Trihydroxy-5β-cholan-24-oic acid. *Cholic acid* (Roussel)	
		$CH5\beta''_{24}ol_{3\alpha,7\alpha,12\alpha}$	
83 IM 487		3α-Hydroxy-11-oxo-5β-cholan-24-oic acid (Roussel)	
		$CH5\beta''_{24}ol_{3\alpha}on_{11}$	
84 IM 550		3α,7α,12α-Trihydroxy-5β-cholan-24-oic acid methyl ester (U-0021)	
		$CH5\beta''\ ol_{3\alpha,7\alpha,12\alpha}*I_{24}$	

Table 135 A (continued)

#			Name	Code
85 IM 541			3,7,12-Trioxo-5β-cholan-24-oic acid (B.R.L.)	$CH5\beta''_{24}on_{3,7,12}$
86 IM 491			3α-Hydroxy-5-cholen-24-oic acid (Roussel)	$CH5''_{24}ol_{3\alpha}$
87 IM 554			24,24-Diphenyl-5-cholene-3β,24-diol (U-0359)	$CH^5Ph_{24,24}ol_{3\beta,24}$
88 IM 198			3β-Hydroxy-5-cholestene 3-sodium sulphate (Organon)	$CHT^5 *S''Na_{3\beta}$
89 IM 532			5-Cholesten-3β-ol chloroformate (B.R.L.)	$CHT^5 *I''Cl_{3\beta}$
90 IM 530			5-Cholesten-3β-ol pelargonate (B.R.L.)	$CHT^5 *IX''_{3\beta}$
91 IM 531			5-Cholesten-3β-ol oleyl carbonate (B.R.L.)	$CHT^5 *XIX^{10''}{}_{3\beta}$
92 IM 529			3β-Chloro-5-cholestene (B.R.L.)	$CHT^5Cl_{3\beta}$

Table 135 A (continued)

93 IM 558		6-(Chloromercuri)-5-cholesten-3β-ol (U-0617)	
		$CHT^5ol_{3\beta}HgCl_6$	
94 IM 536	(0.1mg)	4,7,22-Ergostatrien-3-one (B.R.L.)	
		$ER^{4,7,22}on_3$	
95 IM 535		5,7,22-Ergostatrien-3β-ol **Ergosterol** (B.R.L.)	
		$ER^{5,7,22}ol_{3\beta}$	
96 IM 551		5,7,9(11),22-Ergostatetraen-3β-ol acetate (U-0025)	
		$ER^{5,7,9(11),22}\,{*II''}_{3\beta}$	
97 IM 537		3α-Hydroxy-5β-stigmast-22-ene (B.R.L.)	
		$ST5\beta^{22}ol_{3\alpha}$	
98 IM 538		3α-Hydroxy-5β-stigmast-22-ene acetate (B.R.L.)	
		$ST5\beta^{22}\,{*II''}_{3\alpha}$	
99 IM 533		5,22-Stigmastadien-3β-ol **Stigmasterol** (B.R.L.)	
		$ST^{5,22}ol_{3\beta}$	

Table 135 A (continued)

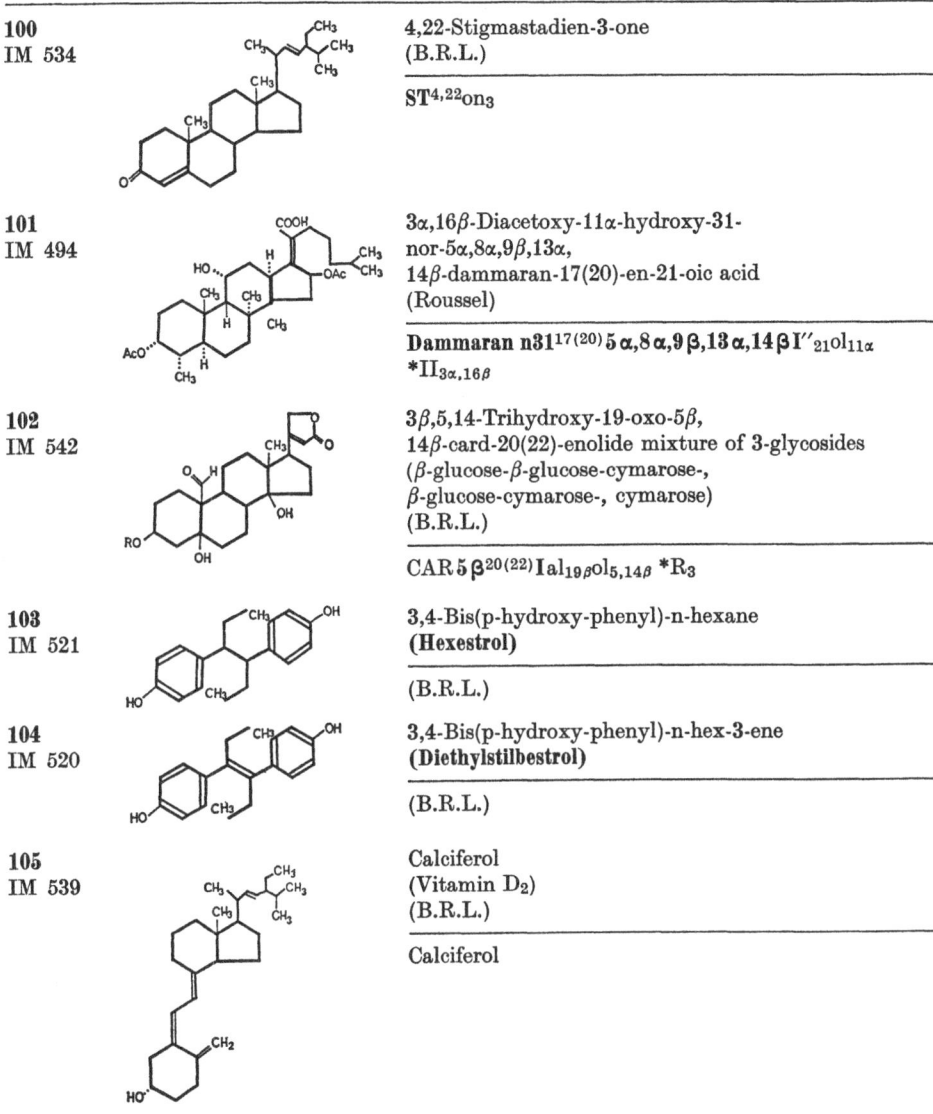

100 IM 534		4,22-Stigmastadien-3-one (B.R.L.) $ST^{4,22}on_3$
101 IM 494		$3\alpha,16\beta$-Diacetoxy-11α-hydroxy-31-nor-$5\alpha,8\alpha,9\beta,13\alpha$, 14β-dammaran-17(20)-en-21-oic acid (Roussel) **Dammaran n31$^{17(20)}$ 5α,8α,9β,13α,14β I″$_{21}$ol$_{11\alpha}$ *II$_{3\alpha,16\beta}$**
102 IM 542		$3\beta,5,14$-Trihydroxy-19-oxo-5β, 14β-card-20(22)-enolide mixture of 3-glycosides (β-glucose-β-glucose-cymarose-, β-glucose-cymarose-, cymarose) (B.R.L.) $CAR\,5\beta^{20(22)}Ial_{19\beta}ol_{5,14\beta}$ *R_3
103 IM 521		3,4-Bis(p-hydroxy-phenyl)-n-hexane **(Hexestrol)** (B.R.L.)
104 IM 520		3,4-Bis(p-hydroxy-phenyl)-n-hex-3-ene **(Diethylstilbestrol)** (B.R.L.)
105 IM 539		Calciferol (Vitamin D$_2$) (B.R.L.) Calciferol

eminently suitable for pharmaco-chemical correlation studies. It must be kept in mind, however, that these assessments of activity are subjective and hence only very high or essentially negative ratings deserve serious consideration as indexes of strong and negligible activity respectively. This is all the more true since, in many instances, the total number of rats had to be limited to five per group because the majority of the steroids tested were available only in small amounts. On the other hand, all compounds which are highly potent in increasing resistance to one or both of these toxicants were retested at lower dose levels.

Table 135B. *First step (ctd.): Synopsis of all 500 steroids tested for their ability to prevent digitoxin and indomethacin intoxication*

Group	SSS Name	Dose (mg)	Digi-toxin[a]	Indo-methacin[a]	Activity index[b]
1 IM 360	$G^4II_{13\alpha,17\alpha}ol_{17}on_3$ (d-Norbolethone)	10	3	3	**0.3**
2 IM 343	$G^4II_{13,17\alpha}ol_{17}on_3$ (d,l-Norbolethone)	10 0.5 0.1	3 0 0	3 0.5 —	0.3 **0.5** 0
3 IM 142	$E^4ol_{17\beta}$	10	0	3	**0.15**
4 IM 147	E^4on_{17}	10	0	2	**0.1**
5 IM 188	$E^4on_{3,17}$	10	1	2	**0.15**
6 IM 146	$E^4ol_{17\beta}on_3$ (Nortestosterone)	10	2	0	**0.1**
7 IM 522	$E^{4*}II''_{17\beta/Cl//2,2,2}on_3$	0.5	0	0	0
8 IM 340	$E^{4*}III''Ph_{17\beta}on_3$ (Nandrolonephenyl pr.)	10	0	0	0
9 IM 339	$E^{4*}X''_{17\beta}on_3$ (Nondrolone dec.)	10	0	0	0
10 IM 186	$E^{1(10),5}ol_{3\beta}on_{17}$	10	0	3	**0.15**
11 IM 33	$E^{1,3,5(10)}ol_{3,17\beta}$ (Estradiol)	10 1	0 0	— 0.5	0 **0.25**
12 IM 505	$E^{1,3,5(10)}ol_3{*}II''_{17\beta/Br//2,2,2}$	0.5	0	0	0
13 IM 504	$E^{1,3,5(10)}ol_3{*}II''_{17\beta/Cl//2,2,2}$	0.5	0	0	0

[a] As in the previously reported data the figures indicate the means of the statistical difference grades of protection ranging from "0" (no protection) to "3" (perfect protection). For further data concerning the techniques *cf.* p. VIII.

[b] Based on the formula $\frac{D+I}{2} \times \frac{1}{mg}$, where D = reading for digitoxin, I = indomethacin, mg = the dose tested.

It is noteworthy that, among the 500 steroids listed in Table 135B, only 20 exhibited an activity index of 10 or more. It is hardly coincidental that all compounds of this select group are 16α-carbonitriles, except for TMACN (Cpd. 149) which is a 2α-carbonitrile, the 16α-17-methyl-oxazolyl (Cpd. 329), CS-1 (Cpd. 191), and dexamethasone acetate (Cpd. 360). It may be significant that within this small group of exceptions we find: one steroid (Cpd. 149) which also carries a carbonitrile substituent on the ring, although in the 2α-position, two 9α-fluoro-compounds (CS-1 and dexamethasone), one steroid (Cpd. 329) substituted at 16α, although not by a carbonitrile. It will be interesting to see whether other 16α-substituted or halogenated steroids possess considerable catatoxic activity and whether the latter can be further increased by the introduction of several apparently advantageous substituents into the same molecule.

Table 135 B (continued)

Group	SSS Name	Dose (mg)	Digi-toxin[a]	Indo-methacin[a]	Activity index[b]
14 IM 506	$E^{1,3,5(10)}ol_3{*}II''_{17\beta/F//2,2,2}$	0.5	0	0	0
15 IM 513	$E^{1,3,5(10)}ol_3{*}III''_{17\beta/ol//2}$	0.5	0	0	0
16 IM 507	$E^{1,3,5(10)}ol_3{*}III''_{17\beta/I,ol//2}$	0.5	0	0	0
17 IM 509	$E^{1,3,5(10)}ol_3{*}V''_{17\beta}$	0.5	0	0	0
18 IM 510	$E^{1,3,5(10)}ol_3{*}VII''_{17\beta}$	0.5	0	0	0
19 IM 511	$E^{1,3,5(10)}ol_3{*}XVI''_{17\beta}$	0.5	0	0	0
20 IM 512	$E^{1,3,5(10)}ol_3{*}Bz''_{17\beta}$	0.5	0	0	0
21 IM 508	$E^{1,3,5(10)}ol_3{*}adamantoate_{17\beta}$	0.5	0	0	0
22 IM 518	$E^{1,3,5(10)}ol_{17\beta}{*}II''_{3/I//2,2,2}$	0.5	0	0	0
23 IM 519	$E^{1,3,5(10)}ol_{17\beta}{*}III''_{3/I,Br//2}$	0.1	0	0	0
24 IM 514	$E^{1,3,5(10)}{*}II''_{3/I//2,2,2}{*}II''_{17\beta/Cl//2,2,2}$	0.5	0	0	0
25 IM 516	$E^{1,3,5(10)}{*}II''_{3/I//2,2,2}{*}methyltartrate_{17\beta}$	0.1	0	0	0
26 IM 517	$E^{1,3,5(10)}{*}furoate_{3,17\beta}$	0.1	0	0	0
27 IM 21	$E^{1,3,5(10)}ol_3on_{17}$ (Estrone)	10	0	2.5	**0.125**
28 IM 515	$E^{1,3,5(10)}{*}II''_{17\beta/Cl//2,2,2}\theta III^2{}_3$	0.5	0	0	0
29 IM 194	$E^{1,3,5(10)}on_{17}\theta I_3$	10	0	1.5	**0.075**
30 IM 356	$E^{4,9,11}on_{3,17}$	10	0.5	0	**0.025**
31 IM 355	$E^{4,9,11}on_3\theta III^2{}_{17\beta/I//2}$	10 / 0.5	1.5 / —	3 / 0	**0.225** / 0
32 IM 435	$E\,5\beta\,CN_5II^{1-1}{}_{17\alpha}ol_{17}on_3$	0.5	0	0	0
33 IM 428	$E\,5\beta\,CN_5III^2{}_{17\alpha/I//2}ol_{17}on_3$	0.5	0	0	0

Table 135B (continued)

Group	SSS Name	Dose (mg)	Digi-toxin[a]	Indo-methacin[a]	Activity index[b]
34 IM 430	$E5\xi CN_5 III^2{}_{17\alpha/I//2} ol_{17} on_3$	0.5	0	0	0
35 IM 192	$E^4 I_{17\alpha} ol_{17} on_3$	10	3	3	**0.3**
		0.5	—	0	0
36 IM 79	$E^4 I_{17\alpha} ol_{4,17} on_3$	10	0	3	**0.15**
		0.5	—	0	0
37 IM 59	$E^4 II_{17\alpha} ol_{17}$ (Ethylestrenol)	10	3	3	**0.3**
		0.5	0	0	0
38 IM 76	$E^4 II_{17\alpha} ol_{17} * III''_{3\beta}$	10	0	3	**0.15**
39 IM 57	$E^4 II_{17\alpha} ol_{17} on_3$ (Norethandrolone)	10	3	0.5	**0.175**
40 IM 193	$E^4 II^1{}_{17\alpha} ol_{17} on_3$	10	1	2	**0.15**
41 IM 315	$E^4 III'' \gamma lac_{17\alpha} on_3$	10	3	2.5	**0.275**
42 IM 101	$E^4 III^2{}_{17\alpha} ol_{17}$ (Allylestrenol)	10	0	3	**0.15**
43 IM 338	$E^{5(10)} II^{1-1}{}_{17\alpha} ol_{17} on_3$ (Norethynodrel)	10	0	0	0
44 IM 392	$E^{1,3,5(10)} I_{16\alpha} CN_{16} * II''_{17\beta} \theta I_3$	0.5	0	0	0
45 IM 395	$E^{1,3,5(10)} I_{16\xi} CN_{16} on_{17} \theta I_3$	0.5	0	0	0
46 IM 35	$E^{1,3,5(10)} II^{1-1}{}_{17\alpha} ol_{3,17}$ (Ethynylestradiol)	10	0	0	0
47 IM 304	$E^{1,3,5(10)} II^{1-1}{}_{17\alpha} ol_{17} \theta I_{3\beta}$	10	0	3	**0.15**
		0.5	—	0	0
48 IM 168	$E^{1,3,5(10),7} furyl_{17\alpha/3} ol_{17} * II''_{3\beta}$	10	0	2.5	**0.125**
49 IM 169	$E^{1,3,5(10),7} furyl_{17\alpha/3} ol_{17} \theta cyc V/_{3\beta}$	10	0	3	**0.15**
50 IM 380	$E^{1,3,5(10),16} CN_{17} * II''_3$	0.5	0	0	0
51 IM 400	$E^{1,3,5(10),16} CN_{17} \theta I_3$	0.5	0	0	0
52 IM 326	$E(O_2)^{4,9(10)} ol_{17\beta} on_3$	10	3	0	**0.15**
		0.5	1	—	2
53 IM 328	$E(O_2)^{4,9,11} ol_{17\beta} on_3$	10	1.5	0.5	**0.1**

Table 135 B (continued)

Group	SSS Name	Dose (mg)	Digi-toxin[a]	Indo-methacin[a]	Activity index[b]
54 IM 336	$Eab^{10(5\to 4)}I_{7\alpha,17\alpha}ol_{17}on_{3,5}$	10	2	1.5	**0.175**
55 IM 196	$A5\alpha ol_{11\beta,17\beta}$	10	3	0	**0.15**
56 IM 183	$A5\alpha on_{3,17}$	10	3	0.5	**0.175**
57 IM 100	$A5\alpha ol_{17\beta}on_3$ (Androstanolone)	10	2	0	**0.1**
58 IM 191	$A5\alpha *S''Na_{3\alpha}on_{17}$	0.5	0	0	**0**
59 IM 327	$A5\alpha on_{17}\theta_{2\beta-19}Cl_{3\alpha}$	10	0	2	**0.1**
60 IM 252	$A5\alpha *II''_{3\beta}on_{17}Cl_{5,6\beta}$	10	0	0	**0**
61 IM 229	$A5\alpha NOH_{17}$	10	3	3	**0.3**
62 IM 213	$A5\alpha ol_{11\beta}NOH_{17}$	10	3	3	**0.3**
63 IM 224	$A5\alpha ol_{11\beta}(NH_2)_{17\beta}$	10	1.5	0	**0.075**
64 IM 246	$A5\alpha ol_{3\beta}sp\ imidazolidyl_{17/on//2,5}$	10	0	0	**0**
65 IM 319	$A5\alpha ol_{3\alpha}on_{17}(N_3)_{2\beta}$	10	0	0	**0**
66 IM 313	$A5\alpha ol_{2\beta}on_{17}NH_{3\alpha/I}\cdot HCl\ 15H_2O$	0.5	0	0	**0**
67 IM 140	$A5\alpha ol_{2\beta}on_{17}N_{3\alpha/I//1,1}\cdot HClH_2O$	0.5	0	0	**0**
68 IM 284	$[A5\alpha *II''_{3\alpha}on_{17}N_{2\beta/I,II,II}]Br^-$	0.5	0	0	**0**
69 IM 260	$[A5\alpha *II''_{3\alpha}on_{17}N_{2\beta/I,III,III}]Br^-$	0.5	0	0	**0**
70 IM 253	$A5\alpha *II''_{3\beta}on_{17}Cl_5(N_3)_{6\beta}$	10	0	0	**0**
71 IM 453	$A5\alpha *II''_{3\alpha,17\beta}piperidino_{2\beta,16\beta}\cdot\cdot 2\ HCl\ 15\ H_2O$	0.5	0	0	**0**
72 IM 361	$[A5\alpha *II''_{3\alpha,17\beta}piperidino_{2\beta,16\beta}]$ (Pancuronium Br) $\cdot 2\ Br^-H_2O$	10	0	1.5	**0.075**
73 IM 185	$[A5\alpha ol_{3\alpha}on_{17}piperidino_{2\beta,16\beta/I/1,1}]\cdot 2\ Br$	0.5	0	0	**0**

Table 135B (continued)

Group	SSS Name	Dose (mg)	Digi-toxin[a]	Indo-methacin[a]	Activity index[b]
74 IM 325	A5α*III''$_{17\beta/cycV//3}$S$_{2\alpha-3}$	10	0	0	0
75 IM 250	A5β*II''$_{3\beta}$on$_{17}\theta_{5\beta-6}$	10	0	0	0
76 IM 141	A^{4}on$_{3,17}$ (Androstenedione)	10	1	0.5	**0.075**
77 IM 8	A^{4}on$_{3,11,17}$ (Andrenosterone)	10	0	—	0
78 IM 53	A^{4}ol$_{17\beta}$on$_3$ (Testosterone)	10	3	0.5	**0.175**
		0.5	0	0	0
79 IM 131	A^4*II''$_{17\beta}$on$_3$ (Testosterone acetate)	10	0	0	0
80 IM 58	A^4*III''$_{17\beta}$on$_3$ (Testosterone pr.)	10	0	0	0
81 IM 199	A^4*S''Na$_{17\beta}$on$_3$	0.5	0	0	0
82 IM 226	A^4*II''$_{11\alpha,17\beta}$on$_3$	10	0	2	**0.1**
83 IM 563	A^{4}ol$_{11\alpha}$on$_{3,17}$	0.5	0	0	0
84 IM 187	A^{4}ol$_{19}$on$_{3,17}$	10	0	0	0
85 IM 358	A^4*cycVI''$_{17\beta}$on$_3$F$_{2\alpha}$	10	0	0	0
86 IM 216	A^4*III''$_{17\beta}$on$_3$F$_{6\alpha}$	10	0	0	0
87 IM 41	A^{4}ol$_{11\beta}$on$_{3,17}$F$_{9\alpha}$ (Fluorohydroxyandrostenedione)	10	0.5	1.5	**0.1**
88 IM 251	A^{4}ol$_{3\beta}$on$_{17}$(N$_3$)$_{6\beta}$	10	0	3	**0.15**
89 IM 17	A^{5}ol$_{3\beta,16\alpha}$ (Cetadiol)	10	0	0	0
90 IM 139	A^5*II''$_{3\beta}$*Bz''$_{17\beta}$	10	0	2.5	**0.125**
91 IM 31	A^{5}ol$_{3\beta}$on$_{17}$ (Dehydroepiandrosterone)	10	2	3	**0.25**
		0.5	0	0.5	0
92 IM 27	A^5*II''$_{3\beta}$on$_{17}$ (Dehydroepiandrosterone acetate)	10	0	3	**0.15**
		0.5	—	0	0
93 IM 362	A^5*S''Na$_{3\beta}$on$_{17}$	0.5	0	0	0

Table 135 B (continued)

Group	SSS Name	Dose (mg)	Digi-toxin[a]	Indo-methacin[a]	Activity index[b]
94 IM 184	$A^5ol_{3\beta,19}on_{17}$	10	0	0	0
95 IM 245	$A^5ol_{3\beta}sp\ imidazolidinyl_{17/on//2,5}$	10	0	0	0
96 IM 332	$A^5ol_{3\beta}$(2-Disopropylaminoethyl formamido)$_{17\beta}$	10	0	0	0
97 IM 321	$A^5ol_{3\beta}$(3-Dimethylaminopropyl methylamino)$_{17\beta} \cdot 2HCl$	10	0	0	0
98 IM 247	$A^{5*}II''_{3\beta}sp\ oxazolyl_{17/I//2}$	10	0	0	0
99 IM 363	$A^{4,6}on_{3,17}\theta_{1\alpha-2}$	10	0	0	0
100 IM 153	$A^{4,9(11)}ol_{17\beta}on_3$	10	0	1.5	**0.075**
101 IM 280	$A5\alpha I_{1\alpha}ol_{17\beta}on_3$	10	0.5	0	**0.025**
102 IM 189	$A5\alpha L_{4\alpha}ol_{17\beta}on_3$	10	3	0.5	**0.175**
103 IM 51/d	$A5\alpha I_{17\alpha}ol_{3\beta,11\beta,17}$ (Methyl-androstanetriol)	10	3	3	**0.3**
104 IM 190	$A5\alpha I_{17\alpha}ol_{17}on_3$	10	3	0	**0.15**
105 IM 163	$A5\alpha I_{17\alpha}ol_{11\beta,17}on_3$	10	3	3	**0.3**
106 IM 320	$A5\alpha I_{17\alpha}ol_{17}\theta I_{3\alpha}$	10 0.5	3 0	1.5 —	**0.225** 0
107 IM 419	$A5\alpha I_{17\alpha}ol_{3\alpha,17}SCN_{2\beta}$	0.5	0	0	0
108 IM 248	$A5\alpha I_{17\alpha}ol_{3\beta,5,17}(N_3)_{6\beta}$	10	0	0.5	**0.025**
109 IM 454	$A5\alpha I_{16\alpha,17\alpha}*II''_{3,17}$	10 0.5	3 0	— 0	**0.3** 0
110 IM 451	$A5\alpha CHOH_2ol_{17\beta}on_3$	0.5	0	0	0
111 IM 427	$A5\alpha CN_{1\alpha}ol_{17\beta}on_3$	0.5	0	0	0
112 IM 433	$A5\alpha CN_{1\alpha}*II''_{17\beta}on_3$	0.5	0	0	0
113 IM 424	$A5\alpha CN_{3\xi}ol_{17\beta}(NH_2)_3$	0.5	0	0	0

Table 135 B (continued)

Group	SSS Name	Dose (mg)	Digi-toxin[a]	Indo-methacin[a]	Activity index[b]
114 IM 434	$A\,5\alpha CN_5 ol_{17\beta} on_3$	0.5	0	0	0
115 IM 420	$A\,5\beta CN_5 ol_{17\beta} on_3$	10	0	0	0
		0.03	0	0	0
		0.015	0	0	0
		0.005	0	0	0
		0.001	0	0	0
116 IM 421	$A\,5\alpha CN_5{}^*III''_{17\beta} on_3$	0.5	0	0	0
117 IM 422	$A\,5\beta CN_5{}^*III''_{17\beta} on_3$	0.5	0	0	0
118 IM 442	$A\,5\alpha I_{17\alpha} Iol_{2\alpha} ol_{3\beta,17}$	0.5	0	0	0
119 IM 98/a	$A\,5\alpha I_{17\alpha} CHOH_2 ol_{17} on_3$ (Oxymetholone)	10	3	0	**0.15**
120 IM 443	$A\,5\alpha I_{17\alpha}(CHNH_2)_2 ol_{17} on_3$	0.5	0	0	0
121 IM 425	$A\,5\alpha I_{17\alpha} CN_5 ol_{17} on_3$	0.5	0	0	0
122 IM 382	$A\,5\alpha I_{16\beta} CN_{17} ol_{3\beta,17\xi}$	0.5	0	0	0
123 IM 275	$A\,5\alpha II_{17\alpha/on//1} ol_{3\beta} \theta_{16\beta-17}$	10	3	3	**0.3**
124 IM 276	$A\,5\alpha II_{17\alpha/on//1} on_3,11 \theta_{16\beta-17}$	10	2	3	**0.25**
125 IM 441	$A\,5\alpha I''_{16\beta} II_{17\alpha/on//1} ol_{3\beta}$	0.5	0	0	0
126 IM 432	$A\,5\alpha II^{1-1}{}_{17\alpha} CN_5 ol_{3\alpha,17}$	0.5	0	0	0
127 IM 335	$A\,5\alpha III_{17\alpha/I//2} ol_{3\beta,17}$	10	3	3	**0.3**
		0.5	—	0	0
128 IM 78	$A\,5\alpha^1 I_1{}^*II''_{17\beta} on_3$ (Methenolone acetate)	10	1.5	0	**0.075**
129 IM 77	$A\,5\alpha^1 I_1{}^*VII''_{17\beta} on_3$ (Methenolone oenonthate)	10	2.5	0	**0.125**
130 IM 318	$A\,5\alpha^2 I_{17\alpha} ol_{17}$	10	1.5	1	**0.125**
131 IM 365	$A\,5\alpha^2 CN_3 on_{17}$	10	2	2	**0.2**
		0.5	0	0	0
132 IM 150	$A\,5\alpha^2\|_{17\alpha} \text{isoxazolyl}_{2-3/3,4} ol_{17}$	10	1.5	0.5	**0.1**
		0.5	0	0	0

Table 135 B (continued)

Group	SSS Name	Dose (mg)	Digi-toxin[a]	Indo-methacin[a]	Activity index[b]
133 IM 249	$A5\beta I_{17\alpha}ol_{17}*II''_{3\beta}\theta_{5\beta-6}$	10	0	1.5	**0.075**
134 IM 165	$A5\beta I_{17\alpha}ol_{17}on_{3,11}F_{9\alpha}$	10	2	0.5	**0.125**
135 IM 357	$A5\beta Ial_{17\beta}ol_{3\alpha,17}on_{11}$	10	0	0	0
136 IM 386	$A5\beta CN_{17\beta}*II''_{3\alpha}$	0.5	0	0	0
137 IM 377	$A5\beta CN_{17}ol_{17\xi}*II''_{3\alpha}$	0.5	0	0	0
138 IM 426	$A5\beta I_{17\alpha}CN_5ol_{17}on_3$	0.5	0	0	0
139 IM 489	$A5\beta I_{17\beta/I''//1,1}ol_{3\alpha}on_{11}$	0.5	0	1.5	**1.5**
		0.03	—	0	0
140 IM 381	$A5\beta ICN_{17\beta}ol_{3\alpha}$	0.5	0	0	0
141 IM 385	$A5\beta ICN_{17\beta}*II''_{3\alpha}on_{11}$	0.5	0	0	0
142 IM 384	$A5\beta I_{17\beta/CN}\text{tetrahydropyranyl}_{3\beta/ol//2}$	0.5	0	0	0
143 IM 369	$A5\beta I_{17\beta/CN//1,1}CN_{17}ol_{3\alpha}on_{11}$	0.5	0	0	0
144 IM 495	$A5\beta$ benzyloxy methyl-dimethyl malonate $_{17\beta}ol_{3\alpha}on_{11}$	0.5	0	0	0
145 IM 368	$A5\beta^2CN_3ol_{17\beta}$	10	0.5	2	**0.125**
		0.5	0	0	0
146 IM 254	$A5\beta^2II_{3\beta/on//1}ol_{17\beta}$	10	0	0	0
147 IM 378	$A5\beta^{16}CN_{17}*II''_{3\alpha}$	0.5	0	0	0
148 IM 393	$A5\beta^{17(20)}ICN_{17\beta}*II''_{3\alpha}on_{11}$	0.5	0	1.5	**1.5**
149 IM 406	$A5\beta^{17(20)}I_{17\beta/CN//1,1}ol_{3\alpha}on_{11}$	0.5	0	0	0
150 IM 120	$A4I_{6\alpha}ol_{17\beta}on_3$ (Methyltestosterone)	10	2.5	3	**0.275**
151 IM 208	$A4I_{6\alpha}ol_{11\beta,17\beta}on_3$	10	3	3	**0.3**
		0.5	—	0	0
152 IM 55	$A4I_{17\alpha}ol_{17}on_3$ (Methyltestosterone)	10	3	1.5	**0.225**

Table 135B (continued)

Group	SSS Name	Dose (mg)	Digi-toxin[a]	Indo-methacin[a]	Activity index[b]
153 IM 90	$A^4I_{17\alpha}ol_{4,17}on_3$ (Oxymesterone)	10	0.5	3	**0.175**
154 IM 223	$A^4I_{17\alpha}ol_{6\beta,17}on_3$	10	0	1	**0.05**
155 IM 160	$A^4I_{17\alpha}ol_{11\alpha,17}on_3$	10	3	3	**0.3**
156 IM 241	$A^4I_{17\alpha}ol_{11\beta,17}on_3$	10	3	3	0.3
		0.5	2	—	**4.0**
157 IM 85	$A^4I_{17\alpha}ol_{17\beta}*SII''_{1\alpha,7\alpha}on_3$ (Emdabol)	10	2	1	0.15
		0.5	0.5	0	**0.5**
		0.1	0	—	0
158 IM 81	$A^4I_{17\alpha}ol_{11\beta,17}on_3F_{9\alpha}$ (Fluoxymesterone)	10	3	2	0.25
		0.5	3	0	**3.0**
		0.1	0	—	0
159 IM 162	$A^4I_{17\alpha}ol_{17}on_{3,11}F_{9\alpha}$	10	3	2	**0.25**
160 IM 502	$A^4I''_{17\beta}on_3$	0.5	0	0	0
161 IM 450	$A^4(CONH_2)_{7\beta}ol_{17\beta}on_3$	0.5	0	0	0
162 IM 391	$A^4CN_{17}*II''_{17\xi}on_3$	0.5	0	0	0
163 IM 374	$A^4CN_{17}ol_{17\xi}on_{3,11}$	0.5	0	0	0
164 IM 375	$A^4CN_{17}*II''_{17\xi}on_{3,11}$	0.5	0	0	0
165 IM 36	$A^4II^{1-1}_{17\alpha}ol_{17}on_3$ (Ethyltestosterone)	10	0	1	**0.05**
166 IM 10	$A^4III''K_{17\alpha}ol_{11\beta,17}on_3F_{9\alpha}$ (CS-1)	10	3	3	0.3
		0.5	3	3	6.0
		0.1	1	1.5	**12.5**
		0.03	0	0	0
167 IM 314	$A^4III''\gamma lac_{17\alpha}on_3$	10	3	3	**0.3**
		0.5	—	0	0
168 IM 9	$A^4III''\gamma lac_{17\alpha}*SII''_{7\alpha}on_3$ (Spironolactone)	10	3	3	0.3
		0.5	0	0	**1.5**
		0.1	—	0	0
169 IM 66	$A^4III''\gamma lac_{17\alpha}ol_{11\beta}on_3F_{9\alpha}$	10	3	2	0.25
		0.5	3	—	**6.0**

Table 135 B (continued)

Group	SSS Name	Dose (mg)	Digi-toxin[a]	Indo-methacin[a]	Activity index[b]
170 IM 342	A^4tetrahydrofuryl$_{17\alpha}$*SII''$_{7\alpha}$on$_3$ (Spiroxasone)	10	3	3	0.3
		0.5	0	1.5	1.5
		0.1	—	0.5	**5.0**
171 IM 312	A^4imidazolyl$_{17\beta/I/2}$on$_3$	10	0	1	**0.05**
172 IM 54	$A^5I_{17\alpha}ol_{3\beta,17}$ (Methylandrostenediol)	10	0	0	0
173 IM 159	$A^5I_{4,4}ol_{17\beta}on_3$	10	0	1.5	**0.075**
174 IM 501	$A^5I''_{17\beta}ol_{3\beta}$	0.5	0	0	0
175 IM 306	$A^5I''K_{17\beta}ol_{3\beta}(NH_2)_{17}$	10	0	0	0
176 IM 255	$A^5I''_{17\alpha/*I}$*II''$_{3\alpha}$NHII''$_{17}$	10	3	1	**0.2**
177 IM 390	$A^5CN_{17}ol_{17\alpha}\theta\theta II_3$	0.5	0	0	0
178 IM 182	$A^5I_{17\alpha}I''_{17/*I}ol_{3\beta}$	10	0	1.5	**0.075**
179 IM 568	$A^5I_{4,4}CN_{2\alpha}ol_{17}on_3$	0.5	2	0.5	**2.5**
		0.03	—	—	0
180 IM 364	$A^5I_{4,4,17\alpha}CN_{2\alpha}ol_{17}on_3$ (TMACN)	10	3	3	0.3
		0.5	2.5	3	5.5
		0.1	2	2	**20.0**
		0.03	0	0	0
181 IM 308	$A^5II_{17\alpha/on//1///ol////2}$*II''$_{3\beta}\theta_{16\beta-17}$	10	0	0	0
182 IM 448	$A^5I''_{16\beta}II_{17\alpha/ol//1}ol_{3\beta}$	0.5	1.5	3	**4.5**
		0.1	0.5	0	2.5
		0.03	0	0	0
183 IM 440	$A^5I''_{16\beta}II_{17\alpha/on//1}ol_{3\beta}$	0.1	0	0	0
184 IM 446	$A^5II_{17\alpha/on//1}(CONH_2)_{16\beta}ol_{3\beta}$	0.5	0	1.5	**1.5**
		0.1	0	0	0
185 IM 417	$A^5CN_{17}I_{17\beta/CN/1,1}ol_{3\beta}$	0.5	0	0	0
186 IM 118	$A^5II^{1-1}{}_{17\alpha}ol_{3\beta,17}$	10	0	0	0
187 IM 350	$A^5III''\gamma lac_{17\alpha}ol_{3\beta}$	10	0	3	**0.15**
		0.5	—	0	0

Table 135 B (continued)

Group	SSS Name	Dose (mg)	Digi-toxin[a]	Indo-methacin[a]	Activity index[b]
188 IM 351	$A^5III^{1''}\gamma lac_{17\alpha}ol_{3\beta}$	10 0.5	3 —	3 0.5	0.3 1
189 IM 354	$A^5III^{1-1''}{}_{17\alpha}ol_{3\beta,17}$	10	0	0	0
190 IM 500	$A^5III^{2-2''}{}_{17\alpha}ol_{3\beta,17}$	0.5	0	0	0
191 IM 217	$A^{1,4}I_{6\alpha}on_{3,11,17}$	10 0.5	3 —	3 1	0.3 2
192 IM 281	$A^{1,4}I_{17\alpha}ol_{17}on_3$	10	0.5	1	**0.075**
193 IM 164	$A^{1,4}I_{17\alpha}ol_{11\beta,17}on_3$	10	2	1.5	**0.175**
194 IM 323	$A^{4,6}III''K_{17\alpha}ol_{17}on_3$ (Aldadiene Kalium)	10 0.5	3 0	3 —	**0.3** 0
195 IM 316	$A^{4,6}III''\gamma lac_{17\alpha}ol_{17}on_3$ (Aldadiene)	10 0.5	3 0	3 —	**0.3** 0
196 IM 157	$A^{4,9(11)}I_{17\alpha}ol_{17}on_3$	10	3	3	**0.3**
197 IM 222	$A^{4,9(11)}I_{2\alpha,17\alpha}ol_{17}on_3$	10	3	1	**0.2**
198 IM 389	$A^{4,16}CN_{17}on_3$	0.5	0	0	0
199 IM 498	$A^{5,15}I''_{17\beta}*II''_{3\beta}$	0.5	0	0	0
200 IM 396	$A^{5,16}CN_{17}*II''_{3\beta}$	0.5	0	0	0
201 IM 322	$A(O_2)5\alpha I_{17\alpha}ol_{17}$	10	3	1.5	**0.225**
202 IM 80	$A(O_2)4I_{17\alpha}ol_{17}on_3$ (Oxandrolone)	10 0.5	3 0	3 0	**0.3** 0
203 IM 410	$A(N_4)II_{17\alpha}ol_{17}on_3$	10 0.5	1.5 0	3 0	**0.225** 0
204 IM 302	$AnA5\alpha on_{2,16}$	10	3	3	**0.3**
205 IM 126	$AnB^4ol_{17\beta}on_3$ (B-Nortestosterone)	10	0.5	1	**0.075**
206 IM 84	$AhoD(O_{17\alpha})^{1,4}on_{3,17}$	10	2	3	**0.25**
207 IM 452	$An18,nC,hoD^4I_{17\alpha}ol_{17}on_3$	0.5	0	0	0

Table 135 B (continued)

Group	SSS Name	Dose (mg)	Digi-toxin[a]	Indo-methacin[a]	Activity index[b]
208 IM 143	$A^{49}\beta,10\alpha ol_{17\beta}on_3$ (Retrotestosterone)	10	0	0.5	**0.025**
209 IM 145	$A^{49}\beta,10\alpha on_{3,17}$ (Retroandrostene-dione)	10	3	0.5	**0.175**
210 IM 243	$P5\alpha on_{3,20}$	10	0.5	0.5	0.05
211 IM 72	$P5\beta on_{3,20}$ (Pregnanedione)	10 0.5	0 —	2 0	0.1 0
212 IM 106	$P5\alpha on_{3,11,20}$	10	3	3	0.3
213 IM 115	$P5\beta on_{3,11,20}$	10 0.5	2.5 —	3 0	**0.275** 0
214 IM 447	$P5\alpha ol_{3\beta}on_{20}$	0.5	0	0	0
215 IM 261	$P5\alpha ol_{3\beta,16\alpha}on_{20}$	10	0	0.5	**0.025**
216 IM 136	$P5\alpha ol_{3\beta}on_{11,20}$	10	1.5	3	**0.225**
217 IM 301	$P5\beta ol_{3\beta}on_{11,20}$	10 0.5	3 —	3 0	0.3 0
218 IM 122	$P5\alpha ol_{3\beta,17}on_{11,20}$	10	3	3	0.3
219 IM 277	$P5\alpha ol_{3\beta}on_{11,20}\theta_{16\alpha-17}$	10	3	3	0.3
220 IM 272	$P5\alpha^{*}II''_{3\beta}on_{20}Cl_{5,6\beta}$	10	0	0.5	**0.025**
221 IM 273	$P5\alpha ol_{3\beta,17}on_{20}Cl_{5,6\beta}$	10	0	0.5	**0.025**
222 IM 215	$P5\alpha ol_5on_{3,20}F_{6\beta}$	10	0	0	0
223 IM 290	$P5\alpha^{*}II''_{3\beta,20}\theta_{5\alpha-6}$methyloxazolyl$_{16\alpha-17}$	10	2	3	**0.25**
224 IM 285	$P5\alpha^{*}II''_{3\beta}on_{11,20}$methyloxazolyl$_{16\alpha-17}$	10	0.5	1	**0.075**
225 IM 286	$P5\alpha^{*}III''_{3\beta}on_{11,20}$ethyloxazolyl$_{16\alpha-17}$	10	1	0.5	**0.075**
226 IM 331	$P5\alpha ol_{3\beta}$[N-(piperidinoethyl)-formamido]$_{20\beta}$	10	0.5	2.5	**0.15**
227 IM 82	$[P5\alpha ol_{3\alpha}on_{20}$piperidino$_{2\beta/I//1}]Br^-$	0.5	0	0	0

Table 135 B (continued)

Group	SSS Name	Dose (mg)	Digi-toxin[a]	Indo-methacin[a]	Activity index[b]
228 IM 135	$P5\alpha ol_{3\alpha}on_{20}NH_{2\beta/II//Ph///2} \cdot HCl$	0.5	0	0	0
229 IM 274	$P5\alpha ol_5*II''_{3\beta}on_{20}(N_3)_{6\beta}$	10	0	1.5	**0.075**
230 IM 283	$P5\alpha ol_{3\beta,17}on_{11,20}(N_2)_{16\beta}$	10	0	0	0
231 IM 282	$P5\alpha ol_{3\beta,16\alpha}on_{11,20}(N_3)_{17}$	10	2	1	**0.15**
232 IM 460	$P5\alpha ol_{3\alpha}on_{20}morpholino_{2\beta} \cdot HCl$	0.5	0	0	0
233 IM 269	$P5\alpha^{16}on_{3,11,20}$	10 0.5	0 —	3 0	**0.15** 0
234 IM 264	$P5\alpha^{16}*II''_{3\beta,11\alpha}on_{20}$	10	0	3	**0.075**
235 IM 263	$P5\alpha^{16}*III''_{3\beta}on_{11,20}$	10	0	0	0
236 IM 270	$P5\alpha^{16}on_{11,20}\theta I_{3,3}$	10 0.5	1.5 —	3 0	**0.225** 0
237 IM 265	$P5\alpha^{17(20)}*II''_{3\beta,20}$	10	0	3	**0.15**
238 IM 128	$P5\beta ol_{3\alpha,12\alpha,20}$	10 0.5	3 0	3 —	**0.3** 0
239 IM 129	$P5\beta ol_{3\alpha,20}on_{12}$	10	3	3	**0.3**
240 IM 113	$P5\beta*II''_{3\alpha,20}on_{12}$	10 0.5	3 0	3 0	**0.3** 0
241 IM 112	$P5\beta ol_{3\alpha}on_{20}$	10	0	3	**0.15**
242 IM 110	$P5\beta ol_{3\alpha}*II''_{12\alpha}on_{20}$	10	0	3	**0.15**
243 IM 127	$P5\beta*II''_{3\alpha,12\alpha}on_{20}$	10	0.5	3	**0.175**
244 IM 11	$P5\beta*suc''Na_{21}on_{3,20}$ (Hydroxydione Sodium)	10 0.5	2 0	0 —	**0.15** 0
245 IM 121	$P5\beta ol_{3\alpha}on_{11,20}$	10	3	1.5	**0.225**
246 IM 293	$P5\beta*II''_{3\alpha}on_{11,20}$	10 0.5	3 —	3 0	**0.3** 0
247 IM 294	$P5\beta ol_{3\alpha,17}on_{11,20}$	10 0.5	2 —	3 0	**0.25** 0

Table 135 B (continued)

Group	SSS Name	Dose (mg)	Digi-toxin[a]	Indo-methacin[a]	Activity index[b]
248 IM 303	$P5\beta ol_{3\alpha,17}*II''_{21}on_{11,20}$	10	0	1.5	**0.075**
249 IM 300	$P5\beta ol_{17}*II''_{3\alpha,21}on_{11,20}$	10	0	0	0
250 IM 305	$P5\beta ol_{17}*II''_{21}on_{3,11,20}$	10	0	0.5	**0.025**
251 IM 497	$P5\beta''_{21}ol_{3\alpha}on_{11}$	0.5	0	0	0
252 IM 116	$P5\beta ol_{3\alpha,20}\theta_{11\beta-12}$	10 0.5	3 —	3 0	**0.3** 0
253 IM 74	$P^4on_{3,20}$ (Progesterone)	10 0.5	1.5 0	3 0	**0.225** 0
254 IM 561	$P^4on_{3,11,20}$	0.5	0	0	0
255 IM 555	$P^4on_{3,6,11,20}$	0.5	0	0	0
256 IM 133	$P^4ol_{3\beta,16\alpha,17}on_{20}$	10	0	0	0
257 IM 119	$P^4ol_{11\alpha}on_{3,20}$ (Hydroxyprogesterone)	10 0.5	1.5 0	3 0	**0.225** 0
258 IM 47	$P^4ol_{17}on_{3,20}$ (Hydroxyprogesterone)	10	3	3	**0.3**
259 IM 73	$P^4*II''_{17}on_{3,20}$ (Acetoxyprogesterone)	10 0.5	3 0	3 0.5	0.3 **0.5**
260 IM 244	$P^4ol_{21}on_{3,20}$ (Desoxycorticosterone)	10	3	2	**0.25**
261 IM 25	$P^4*II''_{21}on_{3,20}$ (Desoxycorticosterone acetate)	10 0.5	1 —	0 0.5	**0.05 1.0**
262 IM 53	$P^4*II''_{6\beta,11\alpha}on_{3,20}$	0.5	0	0	0
263 IM 23	$P^4ol_{11\beta,21}on_{3,20}$ (Corticosterone, Kendall "Cpd. B")	10 0.5	3 0	3 0	**0.3** 0
264 IM 134	$P^4ol_{11\beta}*II''_{21}on_{3,20}$ (Corticosterone acetate)	10	2	1.5	**0.175**
265 IM 70	$P^4ol_{17,21}on_{3,20}$ (Hydroxydesoxy-corticosterone)	10	3	3	**0.3**
266 IM 235	$P^4ol_{11\alpha,17,21}on_{3,20}$	10	3	3	**0.3**

Table 135 B (continued)

Group	SSS Name	Dose (mg)	Digi-toxin[a]	Indo-methacin[a]	Activity index[b]
267 IM 45/a	$P^4ol_{11\beta,17,21}on_{3,20}$ (Hydrocortisone, Cortisol)	10	3	1	**0.2**
268 IM 45	$P^4ol_{11\beta,17}*II''_{21}on_{3,20}$ (Cortisol acetate)	10 0.5	3 0	0 0	**0.15** 0
269 IM 298	$P^4ol_{11\beta,17}*IV''_{21/I//3,3}on_{3,20}$ (Cortisol tetrabutylacetate)	10	0	0	0
270 IM 98	$P^4ol_{11\beta,17}*suc''_{21}on_{3,20}$ (Cortisol hemisuccinate)	10	0	0	0
271 IM 337	$P^4ol_{11\beta,17}*suc''Na_{21}on_{3,20}$ (Cortisol sodium succinate)	10	2	0.5	**0.125**
272 IM 256	$P^4ol_{14\alpha,17}*II''_{21}on_{3,20}$	10	1.5	2.5	**0.2**
273 IM 237	$P^4ol_{6\beta}on_{3,11,20}$	10	0.5	1.5	**0.1**
274 IM 557	$P^4ol_{21}on_{3,11,20}$	0.5	0	0	0
275 IM 102	$P^4ol_{17,21}on_{3,11,20}$ (Cortisone)	10 0.5	3 0	0 —	**0.15** 0
276 IM 22	$P^4ol_{17}*II''_{21}on_{3,11,20}$ (Cortisone acetate)	10 0.5	3 0	0 0	**0.15** 0
277 IM 43	$P^4ol_{11\beta,21}on_{3,20}al_{18}$ (Aldosterone)	10	0	0	0
278 IM 149	$P^4ol_{11\beta,21}on_{3,20}\theta\theta_{16\alpha-17I,I}$ (Cortisol acetonide)	10	3	0	**0.15**
279 IM 130	$P^4*II''_{21}on_{3,20}\theta_{16\alpha-17}$ (Epoxy-desoxycorticosterone)	10	0	1.5	**0.075**
280 IM 123	$P^4on_{3,20}\theta_{16\alpha-17}$ (Epoxyprogesterone)	10	0.5	3	**0.175**
281 IM 16	$P^4on_{3,11,20}Br_{9\alpha}$	10 0.5	1 —	1 3	**0.2** 0
282 IM 179	$P^4on_{3,20}Br_{17}$ (Bromoprogesterone)	10	0.5	3	**0.175**
283 IM 18	$P^4ol_{17}*II''_{21}on_{3,11,20}Cl_4$ (Chlorocortisone acetate)	10	0.5	—	**0.05**
284 IM 19	$P^4ol_{11\beta,17}*II''_{21}on_{3,20}Cl_{9\alpha}$ (Chlorocortisol acetate)	10	0	—	0

Table 135 B (continued)

Group	SSS Name	Dose (mg)	Digi-toxin[a]	Indo-methacin[a]	Activity index[b]
285 IM 230	$P^4ol_{11\alpha}on_{3,20}F_{6\alpha}$	10	2	3	**0.25**
286 IM 214	$P^4ol_{11\beta,17}*II''_{21}on_{3,20}F_{6\alpha}$ (Fluorohydrocortisone acetate)	10	0	1.5	**0.075**
287 IM 170	$P^4ol_{11\beta}*II''_{3\beta}on_{20}\theta\theta I_{16\alpha-17/I,I}F_{6\alpha}$	10	0	0	0
288 IM 173	$P^4ol_{11\beta}on_{3,20}\theta\theta I_{16\alpha-17/I,I}F_{6\alpha}$	10 0.5	3 0	1.5 —	**0.225** 0
289 IM 15	$P^4ol_{11\beta}on_{3,20}F_{9\alpha}$	10	3	3	**0.3**
290 IM 39	$P^4ol_{11\beta,17}*II''_{21}on_{3,20}F_{9\alpha}$ (Fluorocortisol acetate)	10	1.5	2.5	**0.2**
291 IM 174	$P^4ol_{11\beta}on_{3,20}\theta\theta I_{16\alpha-17/I,I}F_{6\alpha,9\alpha}$	10	0	0.5	**0.025**
292 IM 524	$P^5ol_{20\beta}*II''_{3\beta}$	0.5	0	0	0
293 IM 69	$P^5ol_{3\beta}on_{20}$ (Pregnenolone)	10	1	3	**0.2**
294 IM 125	$P^5*II''_{3\beta}on_{20}$	10	0	1	**0.05**
295 IM 195	$P^5ol_{3\beta,17}on_{20}$	10	0	0	0
296 IM 132	$P^5ol_{17}*II''_{3\beta}on_{20}$	10	0	0	0
297 IM 3	$P^5ol_{3\beta}*II''_{21}on_{20}$ (Acetoxypregnenolone)	10	0	1.5	**0.075**
298 IM 523	$P^5*II''_{3\beta,21}on_{20}$	0.5	0	0	0
299 IM 176	$[P^5*II''_{17}*S''_{3\beta}on_{20}]pyridinium^+$	10	1.5	3	**0.225**
300 IM 108	$P^5ol_{17}*II''_{3\beta,21}on_{20}$	10	0	1	**0.05**
301 IM 297	$P^5on_{20}\theta I_{3\beta}$	10 0.5	1 —	3 0	**0.2** 0
302 IM 525	$P^5O,OII_{3,20}$	0.5	0	0	0
303 IM 359	$P^5*I''_{11\alpha}O,OI_{17-20,20-21}O,OII_3$	10 0.5	0.5 —	3 0	**0.175** 0
304 IM 177	$P^5ol_{3\beta}on_{20}\theta_{16\alpha-17}$	10	0	0.5	**0.025**

Table 135 B (continued)

Group	SSS Name	Dose (mg)	Digi-toxin[a]	Indo-methacin[a]	Activity index[b]
305 IM 109	$P^5ol_{3\beta}*II''_{21}on_{20}\theta_{16\alpha-17}$	10	0	0.5	**0.025**
306 IM 178	$P^5ol_{3\beta}on_{20}Br_{17}$ (Bromopregnenolone)	10	0	0	**0.15**
307 IM 317	$P^{1,4}on_{3,15,20}$	10	3	3	**0.3**
308 IM 7	$P^{1,4}ol_{11\beta,17,21}on_{3,20}$ (Prednisolone)	10	3	0.5	**0.175**
309 IM 56	$P^{1,4}ol_{11\beta,17}*II''_{21}on_{3,20}$ (Prednisolone acetate)	10 0.5	2 0	3 0	**0.25** 0
310 IM 96	$P^{1,4}ol_{11\beta,17}*suc''_{21}on_{3,20}$ (Prednisolone hemisuccinate)	10 0.5	3 0	3 —	**0.3** 0
311 IM 97	$P^{1,4}ol_{11\beta,17}*Bz''_{21/S''Na//3}on_{3,20}$ (Prednisolone m-sulfobenzoate sodium)	10	3	1.5	**0.225**
312 IM 526	$P^{1,4}ol_{17,21}on_{3,11,20}$	0.5	0	0	0
313 IM 68/a	$P^{1,4}ol_{17}*II''_{21}on_{3,11,20}$ (Prednisone acetate)	10 0.5	3 0	3 —	**0.3** 0
314 IM 211	$P^{1,4}ol_{11\beta,17,21}on_{3,20}F_{6\alpha}$ (Fluoroprednisolone)	10	3	0.5	**0.175**
315 IM 32	$P^{1,4}ol_{11\beta,16\alpha,17,21}on_{3,20}F_{9\alpha}$ (Triamcinolone)	10 2	0 0	0 0	0 0
316 IM 148	$P^{1,4}ol_{11\beta,21}on_{3,20}\theta\theta I_{16\alpha-17/I,I}F_{9\alpha}$ (Triamcinolone acetonide)	10	0	0	0
317 IM 257	$P^{3,5}ol_{17}*II''_{3,21}on_{20}$	10 0.5	3 —	3 0	**0.3** 0
318 IM 288	$P^{3,5}*II''_{21}on_{20}\theta I_{3\beta}methyloxalolyl_{16\alpha-17}$	10 0.5	1.5 —	3 0	**0.225** 0
319 IM 171	$P^{4,6}*II''_{3\beta,17}on_{20}Cl_6$	10	2	1	**0.15**
320 IM 172	$P^{4,6}*II''_{17}on_{3,20}Cl_6$	10 0.5	3 0	3 0	**0.3** 0
321 IM 206	$P^{4,16}on_{3,20}$	10 0.5	2 —	3 0	**0.25** 0
322 IM 154	$P^{4,17(20)}ol_{11\beta,21}on_3$	10 0.5	3 0	3 0	**0.3** 0

Table 135B (continued)

Group	SSS Name	Dose (mg)	Digi-toxin[a]	Indo-methacin[a]	Activity index[b]
323 IM 240	$P^{4,17(20)}ol_{11\beta}*II''_{21}on_3$	10	1	0	0.05
324 IM 239	$P^{4,17(20)''}*I_{21}on_{3,11}$	10	3	3	0.3
		0.5	—	0	0
325 IM 156	$P^{4,17(20)}ol_{11\beta}on_3al_{21}$	10	0	0	0
326 IM 180	$P^{5,16}ol_{3\beta}on_{20}$ (Dehydropregnenolone)	10	0	3	0.15
327 IM 111	$P^{5,16}*II''_{3\beta}on_{20}$ (Dehydropregnenolone acetate)	10	0	1.5	0.075
328 IM 99	$P^{5,16}*II''_{3\beta,21}on_{20}$	0.5	0	0	0
329 IM 287	$P^{1,4,9(11)}*II''_{21}on_{3,20}$ methyloxazolyl$_{16\alpha-17}$	10	3	3	0.3
		0.5	3	3	6
		0.2	—	3	10.0
330 IM 161	$P^{1,4,17(20)}ol_{11\beta,21}on_3$	10	3	3	0.3
		0.5	0	—	0
331 IM 228	$P^{1,4,17(20)}ol_{11\beta}*II''_{21}on_3$	10	0	0.5	0.025
332 IM 231	$P^{1,4,17(20)}ol_{11\beta,16\alpha}*II''_{21}on_3$	10	3	2	0.25
333 IM 329	$P^{5,17(20),20}*II''_{3\beta,21}$	10	0	0	0
334 IM 330	$P^{5,17(20),20}*II''_{3\beta}(SO_2CH_3)_{21}$	10	1	0	0.05
335 IM 212	$P5\alpha I_{6\beta}ol_{5,11\alpha}on_{3,20}$	10	3	3	0.3
		0.5	0	0	0
336 IM 233	$P5\alpha I_{6\beta}ol_{5,11\beta,17}*II''_{21}on_{3,20}$	10	0	1.5	0.075
337 IM 262	$P5\alpha I_{16\alpha}ol_{17}*II''_{21}on_{3,20}$	10	0	0	0
338 IM 266	$P5\alpha I_{16\beta}ol_{3\beta}on_{20}$	10	0	0	0
339 IM 259	$P5\alpha I_{16\beta}ol_{11\alpha,17}*II''_{21}on_{3,20}$	10	3	3	0.3
		0.5	—	0.5	1
340 IM 258	$P5\alpha I_{16\beta}ol_{17}*II''_{21}on_{3,11,20}$	10	2	3	0.25
		0.5	—	0	0
341 IM 267	$P5\alpha I_{16\beta}ol_{3\beta,11\alpha}on_{20}\theta_{16\alpha-17}$	10	3	3	0.3
		0.5	0	0.5	0.5
342 IM 431	$P5\alpha CN_5*II''_{17}on_{3,20}$	0.5	0	0	0

Table 135B (continued)

Group	SSS Name	Dose (mg)	Digi-toxin[a]	Indo-methacin[a]	Activity index[b]
343 IM 449	$P5\alpha CN_6\beta ol_{3\beta,5}on_{20}$	0.5	0	0	0
344 IM 307	$P5\alpha(CH_2)_{16}ol_{17}*II''_{3\beta}on_{11,20}$	10	0.5	0	**0.025**
345 IM 496	$P5\alpha I''_{21,21}ol_{3\beta}$	0.5	0	0	0
346 IM 366	$P5\alpha^2 CN_3\theta\theta II_{20}$	10	0.5	2	0.125
		0.5	0	2	**2.0**
		0.03	—	0	0
347 IM 552	$P5\alpha^6$maleic anhydride adduct$_{5\alpha-8}$ $*II''_{3\beta}on_{20}\theta_{9\xi-11}$	0.5	0	0	0
348 IM 402	$P5\alpha^{20''}CN_{21}ol_{3\beta}*II_{21}$	0.5	0	0	0
349 IM 553	$P5\alpha^{6,9(11)}$maleic anhydride adduct$_{5\alpha-8}*II''_{3\beta}on_{20}$	0.5	0	0	0
350 IM 28	$P5\alpha^{6,9(11)}$maleic anhydrid adduct$_{5\alpha-8}*II''_{3\beta,21}on_{20}$	10	0	0	0
351 IM 166	$P5\beta I_{11\alpha}on_{3,20}$	10	0	1	**0.05**
352 IM 227	$P5\beta I_{11\alpha}ol_{11}NOH_{3,20} \cdot H_2O$	10	3	3	**0.3**
		0.5	0	—	0
353 IM 545	$P5\beta I''_{20}*II''_{3\alpha}$	0.5	0	0	0
354 IM 544	$P5\beta Ial_{20}*II_{3\alpha}$	0.5	0	0	0
355 IM 436	$P5\beta(CONH_2)_{16\alpha}ol_{3\alpha}on_{11,20}$	0.5	0	0	0
356 IM 418	$P5\beta CN_{16\alpha}*II''_{3\beta}on_{11,20}$	0.5	2.5	2	4.5
		0.1	2.5	2	22.5
		0.03	0	1.5	25.0
		0.015	0	1.5	50.0
357 IM 383	$P5\beta CN_{20}ol_{20\xi}*II''_{3\alpha}$	0.5	0	0	0
358 IM 388	$P5\beta CN_{20}ol_{20\xi}*II''_{3\beta,21}$	0.5	0	0	0
359 IM 403	$P5\beta CN_{20}ol_{20\xi}*II''_{3\alpha}on_{11}$	0.5	0	0	0
360 IM 398	$P5\beta''_{21}CN_{20}ol_{3\alpha}$	0.5	0	0	0
361 IM 399	$P5\beta CN_{21}ICN_{20}*II''_{3\alpha}$	0.5	0	0	0

Table 135 B (continued)

Group	SSS Name	Dose (mg)	Digi-toxin[a]	Indo-methacin[a]	Activity index[b]
362 IM 367	$P5\beta^2CN_3\theta\theta II_{20}$	10	0	0	0
363 IM 394	$P5\beta^{17(20)}CN_{20}*II''_{3\alpha}on_{11}$	0.5	0.5	1.5	**2.0**
364 IM 371	$P5\beta^{17(20)''}CN_{20}*II''_{3\alpha}*IIol_{21}$	0.5	0	0	0
365 IM 405	$P5\beta^{17(20)''}{}_{21}CN_{20}ol_{3\alpha}on_{11}$	0.5	0	0	0
366 IM 408	$P5\beta^{17(20)''}CN_{20}*II''_{3\alpha}*II_{21}on_{11}$	0.5	0	0	0
367 IM 499	$P5\beta^{20}I''_{21}ol_{3\alpha,17}ol_{3\alpha,17\alpha}on_{11}$	0.5	0	0	0
368 IM 370	$P5\beta^{20''}CN_{21}ol_{3\alpha}*II_{21}$	0.5	0	0	0
369 IM 158	$P^4I_{2\alpha}ol_{11\beta,17}*II''_{21}on_{3,20}$ (Methylcortisol acetate)	10	3	2.5	**0.275**
370 IM 51/h	$P^4I_{2\alpha}ol_{17}*II''_{21}on_{3,20}\theta_{9\beta-11}$	10 / 0.5	3 / 0	3 / 1.5	**0.3** / **1.5**
371 IM 51/j	$P^4I_{2\alpha}ol_{11\beta,17}*II''_{21}on_{3,20}Cl_{9\alpha}$	10	0	1.5	**0.075**
372 IM 51/f	$P^4I_{6\alpha}on_{3,11,20}$	10 / 0.5	3 / 0	3 / 0	**0.3** / 0
373 IM 51/c	$P^4I_{6\alpha}ol_{11\beta}on_{3,20}$	10 / 0.5	3 / 0	3 / —	**0.3** / 0
374 IM 220	$P^4I_{6\alpha}ol_{17}on_{3,20}$	10 / 0.5	3 / 0.5	3 / —	**0.3** / **1**
375 IM 219	$P^4I_{6\alpha}*II''_{17}on_{3,20}$	10 / 0.5	3 / 0	3 / —	**0.3** / 0
376 IM 51/i	$P^4I_{6\alpha}ol_{11\beta,17}on_{3,20}$	10 / 0.5	3 / 0	3 / —	**0.3** / 0
377 IM 242	$P^4I_{6\alpha}ol_{11\beta,17,21}on_{3,20}$ (Methylcortisol)	10	3	0	**0.15**
378 IM 209	$P^4I_{6\alpha}ol_{11\beta,17}*II''_{21}on_{3,20}$ (Methylcortisol acetate)	10	2	0.5	**0.125**
379 IM 546	$P^4Iol_{20}on_3$	0.5	0	0	0
380 IM 416	$P^4I''_{16\alpha/*I}on_{3,20}$	0.5	0	0	0
381 IM 155	$P^4Ial_{20\beta}on_3$	10	0.5	0	**0.025**

Table 135 B (continued)

Group	SSS Name	Dose (mg)	Digi-toxin[a]	Indo-methacin[a]	Activity index[b]
382 IM 547	$P^4Ial_{20}on_3$	0.5	0	0	0
383 IM 466	$P^4CN_{16\alpha}on_{3,20}$	0.1	3	0	**15.0**
		0.015	0	0	0
384 IM 475	$P^4CN_{16\alpha}on_3\theta\theta III_{20/I//2,2}$	0.5	1.5	3	4.5
		0.03	0.5	0	**8.33**
385 IM 225	$P^4I_{20\beta/NOH}NOH_3$	10	3	3	**0.3**
		0.5	0	—	0
386 IM 207	$P^4II_{16\alpha}ol_{20}on_3$	0.5	0	0	0
387 IM 472	$P^4ICN_{16\alpha/}on_{3,20}$	0.5	0	0	0
388 IM 105	$P^5I_{16\alpha}*II''_{3\beta}on_{20}$	10	0	0.5	**0.025**
389 IM 201	$P^5I_{16\alpha}ol_{3\beta,17}on_{20}$	10	0	0	0
390 IM 200	$P^5I_{16\beta}ol_{3\beta}on_{20}\theta_{16\alpha-17}$	10	3	2	**0.25**
391 IM 465	$P^5I''_{16\alpha}*II''_{3\alpha,20}$	0.5	0	0	0
392 IM 415	$P^5I''_{16\alpha}ol_{3\beta}\theta\theta II_{20}$	0.5	0	0	0
393 IM 437	$P^5I''_{16\alpha}*II''_{3\beta}\theta\theta II_{20}$	0.5	0	0	0
394 IM 438	$P^5I''_{16\alpha/*I}ol_{3\beta}\theta\theta II_{20}$	0.5	0	0	0
395 IM 352	$P^5(CH_2NH_2)_{16\alpha}ol_{3\beta}on_{20}$	2	0	0	0
396 IM 444	$P^5CN_{16\alpha}ol_{3\beta,20}$	0.5	1.5	3	4.5
		0.1	1	1.5	**12.5**
		0.03	0	0	0
397 IM 464	$P^5CN_{16\alpha}*II''_{3\beta,20\beta}$	0.1	0	2	**10.0**
		0.03	—	0	0
398 IM 346	$P^5CN_{16a}ol_{3\beta}on_{20}$ (Pregnenolone-16α-carbonitrile, PCN)	10	3	3	0.3
		1	3	3	3.0
		0.5	3	3	6.0
		0.2	3	3	15.0
		0.1	3	3	30.0
		0.03	2	3	**83.0**
		0.015	0	0	0

Table 135B (continued)

Group	SSS Name	Dose (mg)	Digi-toxin[a]	Indo-methacin[a]	Activity index[b]
399 IM 413	$P^5CN_{16\alpha}*II''_{3\beta}on_{20}$	0.5	2.5	2	4.5
		0.1	0.5	2	12.5
		0.03	1	1.5	**41.67**
		0.015	0	0	0
400 IM 479	$P^5CN_{16\alpha}*VII''_{3\beta}on_{20}$	0.5	3	3	6.0
		0.03	1	1.5	**41.67**
		0.015	0	0	0
401 IM 476	$P^5CN_{16\alpha}*suc''Na_{3\beta}on_{20}$ (PCN sodium hemisuccinate)	0.5	3	3	6.0
		0.03	2.5	3	91.67
		0.015	2	1.5	116.67
		0.005	0	2	**200.0**
402 IM 478	$P^5CN_{16\alpha}*adamantoate_{3\beta}on_{20}$	0.5	0.5	3	**3.5**
		0.03	—	0	0
403 IM 483	$P^5CN_{16\alpha}*S''(NH_4)_{3\beta}on_{20}$ (PCN ammonium sulfate)	0.5	3	3	6.0
		0.03	3	3	**100.0**
		0.015	1	0.5	50.0
404 IM 423	$P^5CN_{16\alpha}ol_{3\beta}on_{7,20}$	0.5	3	1.5	4.5
		0.03	0	0.5	**8.33**
405 IM 429	$P^5CN_{16\alpha}*II''_{3\beta}on_{7,20}$	0.5	3	2	5.0
		0.03	0	1.5	**25.0**
406 IM 411	$P^5CN_{16\alpha}on_{11,20}\theta\theta II_3$	0.5	2.5	2	4.5
		0.1	2.5	2	22.5
		0.03	0	1.5	25.0
		0.015	0	1 5	**50.0**
407 IM 414	$P^5CN_{16\alpha}ol_{3\beta}\theta\theta II_{20}$	0.5	2.5	2	4.5
		0.1	2	2	20.0
		0.03	0.5	1.5	**33.3**
		0.015	0	0	0
408 IM 412	$P^5CN_{16\alpha}on_{11}\theta\theta II_{3,20}$	0.5	2.5	2	4.5
		0.1	0	2	10.0
		0.03	0	1.5	**25.0**
		0.015	0	0	0
409 IM 461	$P^5CN_{16\alpha}ol_{3\beta}\theta\theta III_{20/I//2,2}$	0.5	2	3	5.0
		0.03	2	0	**33.3**
		0.015	0	—	0
410 IM 445	$P^5CN_{16\alpha}*II''_{3\beta}\theta\theta II_{20}$	0.5	1.5	3	4.5
		0.1	0	1.5	**7.5**
		0.03	0	0	0

Table 135 B (continued)

Group	SSS Name	Dose (mg)	Digi-toxin[a]	Indo-methacin[a]	Activity index[b]
411 IM 482	$P^5CN_{16\alpha}ol_{3\beta}(NOCH_3)_{20}$	0.5	1	1.5	2.5
		0.03	1.5	0	**25.0**
		0.015	0	—	0
412 IM 462	$P^5CN_{16\alpha}ol_{3\beta}NOH_{20}$	0.5	3	3	6.0
		0.03	2.5	3	**91.67**
		0.015	0.5	1	50.0
		0.010	—	0	0
413 IM 404	$P^{5''}CN_{20}{*}II''_{3\beta}{*}II_{21}$	0.5	0	0	0
414 IM 474	$P^5I_{4,4}CN_{16\alpha}on_{3,20}$	0.5	0.5	3	**3.5**
		0.03	—	0	0
415 IM 481	$P^5I_{4,4}CN_{16\alpha}on_3\theta\theta III_{20/I//2,2}$	0.5	0	0	0
416 IM 71	$P^5II_{16\alpha}ol_{3\beta}on_{20}$	0.5	0	0	0
417 IM 469	$P^5ICN_{16\alpha}ol_{3\beta}on_{20}$	0.5	0	0	0
418 IM 409	$P^5II''_{16\alpha/{*}II//CN///20}ol_{3\beta}on_{20}$	10	0	0	0
419 IM 210	$P^5III_{16\alpha/I//20}ol_{3\beta}on_{20}$	0.5	0	0	0
420 IM 467	$P^5I''\gamma lac_{16\beta-20}{*}II''_{3\beta}$	0.5	0	0	0
421 IM 52	$P^{1,4}I_{6\alpha}ol_{11\beta,17,21}on_{3,20}$ (Methylprednisolone)	10	3	3	**0.3**
		0.5	0	0	0
422 IM 52/a	$P^{1,4}I_{6\alpha}ol_{11\beta,17}{*}II''_{21}on_{3,20}$ (Methylprednisolone acetate)	10	3	2	0.25
		0.5	1	—	2.0
423 IM 221	$P^{1,4}I_{6\alpha}ol_{11\beta,17}{*}suc''Na_{21}on_{3,20}$	10	3	1.5	0.225
		0·5	0	—	0
424 IM 218	$P^{1,4}I_{6\alpha}ol_{11\beta,17}on_{3,20}F_{9\alpha}$	10	2	0	**0.1**
425 IM 51/e	$P^{1,4}I_{6\alpha}ol_{11\beta,17}on_{3,20}F_{9\alpha,21}$	10	1.5	—	**0.15**
426 IM 345	$P^{1,4}I_{16\alpha}ol_{11\beta,17}{*}II''_{21}on_{3,20}F_{6\alpha}$ (Methylprednisolone)	10	0.5	1.5	**0.1**
427 IM 152	$P^{1,4}I_{16\alpha}ol_{11\beta,17}{*}II''_{21}on_{3,20}F_{9\alpha}$ (Dexamethasone acetate)	10	3	0	0.15
		1	3	1.5	2.25
		0.5	2.5	0.5	3.0
		0.1	3	1	20.0
		0.03	3	0	**50.0**
		0.015	0	—	0

Table 135 B (continued)

Group	SSS Name	Dose (mg)	Digi-toxin[a]	Indo-methacin[a]	Activity index[b]
428 IM 527	$P^{1,4}I_{16\alpha}ol_{11\beta,17}*Bz''_{21/S''Na//3}on_{3,20}F_{9\alpha}$	0.5 0.03	0 —	1.5 0	1.5 0
429 IM 151	$P^{1,4}I_{16\beta}ol_{11\beta,17}*II''_{21}on_{3,20}F_{9\alpha}$ (Betamethasone acetate)	10 2 1 0.5 0.1	2 3 2 1.5 0	0 3 1.5 1.5 1	0.1 1.5 1.75 3.0 5.0
430 IM 95	$P^{1,4}I_{21}ol_{11\beta,17}*II''_{21}on_{3,20}F_{9\alpha}$ (Fluperolone acetate)	10 0.5	3 0	2 —	0.25 0
431 IM 289	$P^{3,5}Ial_6*II''_{21}on_{20}\theta I_{3\beta}$methyl-oxazolyl$_{16\alpha-17}$	10 0.5	2 —	3 0	0.25 0
432 IM 459	$P^{3,5}CN_6*II''_{16\alpha}on_{20}\theta I_3$	0.5	0	0	0
433 IM 458	$P^{3,5}CN_6ol_{11\beta,17\alpha}*II''_{21}on_{20}\theta I_3$	0.5	0	0	0
434 IM 455	$P^{3,5}CN_6*II''_{21}on_{11,20}\theta II_{3\beta/Cl//2}$ $\theta\theta I_{16\alpha-17/I,I}F_{9\alpha}$	0.5	0	1	1.0
435 IM 456	$P^{3,5}CN_6ol_{11\beta}*III''_{21/I//2,20}on_{20}\theta II_{3/Cl//2}$ $\theta\theta I_{16\alpha-17/I,I}F_{9\alpha}$	0.5	0	0	0
436 IM 457	$P^{3,5}CN_6ol_{11\beta}*II''_{21}on_{20}\theta II_{3/Cl//2}$ $\theta\theta I_{16\alpha-17/I,I}F_{9\alpha}$	0.5	0	0	0
437 IM 470	$P^{3,5}CN_{16\alpha}on_{7,20}$	0.1	0	0	0
438 IM 471	$P^{3,5}CN_{16\alpha}ol_3on_{7,20}$	0.1	0	—	0
439 IM 167	$P^{4,6}I_{17}*II''_{3\beta}on_{20}Cl_6$	10 0.5	3 —	3 0	0.3 0
440 IM 279	$P^{4,6}I_{1\alpha-2}*II''_{17}on_{3,20}Cl_6$ (Cyproterone acetate)	10 1 0.5 0.1	3 2.5 2 0	3 3 3 0.5	0.3 2.75 5.0 2.5
441 IM 175	$P^{4,6}I_{6,17}on_{3,20}$	10 0.5	3 0	3 1.5	0.3 1.5
442 IM 503	$P^{4,6}I_6(CH_2)_{16}*II''_{17}on_{3,20}$	0.5	0	0	0
443 IM 295	$P^{5,16}I_6*II''_{3\beta}on_{20}$	10	0	3	0.15
444 IM 268	$P^{5,16}I_6*I''_{3\beta}on_{20}$	10	3	1	2

Table 135B (continued)

Group	SSS Name	Dose (mg)	Digi-toxin[a]	Indo-methacin[a]	Activity index[b]
445 IM 373	P$^{5,17(20)}$"CN$_{20}$*II"$_{3\beta}$*II$_{21}$	0.5	0	0	0
446 IM 278	Pn19^4*VI"$_{17}$on$_{3,20}$ (Depostat)	10	3	3	0.3
		0.5	—	0	0
447 IM 407	Pn19^{4,9,11}CN$_{20\xi}$ol$_{20}$on$_3$	0.5	0	0	0
448 IM 477	P$^{3\alpha(5)}$5αCN$_{16\alpha}$ol$_{6\beta}$on$_{20}$	0.5	2	3	5.0
		0.03	0	0	0
449 IM 480	P$^{3\alpha(5)}$5αCN$_{16\alpha}$ol$_{6\beta}\theta\theta$III$_{20/I//2,2}$	0.5	1	3	4.0
		0.03	0	0	0
450 IM 144	P9β,10α^{4}on$_{3,20}$ (Retroprogesterone)	10	2	3	0.25
451 IM 349	CH5βol$_{3\alpha,12\alpha,24}$	10	0	1	0.05
452 IM 296	CH5β"$_{24}$ (Cholanic acid)	0.5	0	0	0
453 IM 493	CH5β"$_{24}$ol$_{3\alpha}$	0.5	0	0	0
454 IM 485	CH5β"$_{24}$ol$_{3\alpha,6\alpha}$	0.5	0	0	0
455 IM 492	CH5β"$_{24}$ol$_{3\alpha,7\alpha}$	0.5	0	0	0
456 IM 490	CH5β"$_{24}$ol$_{3\alpha,12\alpha}$	0.5	0	0	0
457 IM 488	CH5β"$_{24}$ol$_{3\alpha,7\alpha,12\alpha}$	0.5	0	0	0
458 IM 311	[CH5β"ol$_{3\alpha,12\alpha}$*II$_{24/N//I,II,II}$]Br$^-$	10	0	0	0
459 IM 550	CH5β"ol$_{3\alpha,7\alpha,12\alpha}$*I$_{24}$	0.5	0	0	0
460 IM 310	[CH5β"ol$_{3\alpha,7\alpha,12\alpha}$*II$_{24/N//I,II,II}$]Br$^-$	10	0	0	0
461 IM 541	CH5β"$_{24}$on$_{3,7,12}$	0.5	0	0	0
462 IM 487	CH5β"$_{24}$ol$_{3\alpha}$on$_{11}$	0.5	0	0	0
463 IM 117	CH5β"*I$_{24}$*II"$_{3\alpha,7\alpha}$on$_{12}$	10	0	0	0
464 IM 309	CH5β"*II$_{24/N//II,II}$on$_{3,12}$ · HCl	10	0	0	0
465 IM 491	CH$^{5"}$$_{24}ol_{3\alpha}$	0.5	0	0	0

Table 135 B (continued)

Group	SSS Name	Dose (mg)	Digi-toxin[a]	Indo-methacin[a]	Activity index[b]
466 IM 282	$CH^{5''}ol_{3\beta}*I_{24}$	10	0	0	0
467 IM 554	$CH^5Ph_{24,24}ol_{3\beta,24}$	0.5	0	0	0
468 IM 124	$CHn\,24\,5\,\beta''ol_{3\alpha,12\alpha}*I_{23}$ (Methyl nordeoxycholanate)	10 0.5	3 0	3 0	**0.3** 0
469 IM 376	$CHn(24)\,5\,\beta\,CN_{20}ol_{3\alpha}on_{11}(CONH_2)_{20}$	0.5	0	0	0
470 IM 401	$CHn(24)\,5\,\beta''CN_{20}*II''_{3\alpha}*II_{21}on_{11}$	0.5	0	0	0
471 IM 107	$CHT\,5\,\alpha\,ol_{3\beta}$ (Dihydrocholesterol)	10	0	0	0
472 IM 114	CHT^4on_3 (Cholestenone)	10	0	0	0
473 IM 104	$CHT^5*II''_{3\beta}$ (Cholesteryl acetate)	10	0	0	0
474 IM 530	$CHT^5*IX''_{3\beta}$	0.5	0	0	0
475 IM 531	$CHT^5*\,carbonate_{3\alpha/}\cdot XVIII^9$	0.5	0	0	0
476 IM 198	$CHT^5*S''Na_{3\beta}$	0.5	0	0	0
477 IM 348	$CHT^5ol_{3\beta}on_7$	10	3	0	**0.15**
478 IM 529	$CHT^5Cl_{3\beta}$	0.5	0	0	0
479 IM 532	$CHT^5*I''Cl_{3\beta}$	0.5	0	0	0
480 IM 558	$CHT^5ol_{3\beta}HgCl_6$	0.5	0	0	0
481 IM 138	$CHT^{5,7}*Bz''_{3\beta}$ (Dehydrocholesteryl benzoate)	10	0	0	0
482 IM 232	$CHT(NO_{25})^5ol_{3\beta}$	10	0	1.5	**0.075**
483 IM 341	$ER\,5\,\alpha^{22}ol_{3\beta}on_{11}$	10	0	0	0
484 IM 299	$ER\,5\,\alpha^{8,22}*II''_{3\beta}on_{11}$	10	0	0	0
485 IM 536	$ER^{4,7,22}on_3$	0.1	0	0	0

Table 135B (continued)

Group	SSS Name	Dose (mg)	Digi-toxin[a]	Indo-methacin[a]	Activity index[b]
486 IM 535	ER^{5,7,22}ol$_{3\beta}$	0.5	0	0	0
487 IM 551	ER$^{5,7,9(11),22}$*II''$_{3\beta}$	0.5	0	0	0
488 IM 537	ST5β^{22}ol$_{3\alpha}$	0.5	0	0	0
489 IM 538	ST5β^{22}*II''$_{3\alpha}$	0.5	0	0	0
490 IM 103	ST^{5}ol$_{3\beta}$ (β-Sitosterol)	10	0	0	0
491 IM 534	ST^{4,22}on$_3$	0.5	0	0	0
492 IM 533	ST^{5,22}ol$_{3\beta}$	0.5	0	0	0
493 IM 204	SP5α*II''$_{3\beta}$	10	0	0	0
494 IM 203	SP5α*II''$_{3\beta}$on$_{12}$	10	0	0	0
495 IM 205	SP5βol$_{3\beta}$	10	0	0	0
496 IM 137	SP^5*II''$_{3\beta}$	10	0	0	0
497 IM 202	SP^{5}ol$_{3\beta}$on$_{12}$	10	0	1.5	**0.075**
498 IM 291	SP5α$^{9(11)}$*II''$_{3\beta}$	10	0	0	0
499 IM 542	CAR5β$^{20(22)}$Ial$_{19\beta}$ol$_{5,14\beta}$*R$_3$	0.5	0	0	0
500 IM 494	Dammaran-n31$^{17(20)}$5α,8α,9β,13α,14β I''$_{21}$ol$_{11\alpha}$*II$_{3\alpha,16\beta}$	0.5	0	0	0

The "Activity Index" is based on the formula $\frac{D+I}{2} \times \frac{1}{mg}$ where D = reading for digitoxin, I = indomethacin, and mg = the dose tested. Thus, the index reflects overall activity against both substrates at any one dose level. The highest Activity Index reading for each steroid is emphasized by boldface numerals, but direct inter-comparisons are possible only at corresponding dose levels. Naturally, a compound tested only at the high level of 10 mg per dose could not reveal its full potency in this method of expression, but if it had little or no activity, lower doses were not tested.

On the other hand, steroids available only in very small amounts could be assayed only at dose levels too low for comparison with many other compounds.

For simplicity's sake the compounds are designated and sequentially enumerated according to the rules of the "SSS Nomenclature of Steroids" (*cf.* p. 774).

Second Step: Determination of "Protective Spectrum"

Having selected the most promising protective substances by first screening them for activity against digitoxin and indomethacin, we proceeded to appraise the "Protective Spectrums" of the most potent ones among them. These compounds were now tested against a heterogenous set of 10 pathogens, widely differing in their chemical structure and in the organ changes that they elicit.

The statistical significance of the results was computed (as outlined on p. 771) for the inhibition or aggravation of the changes produced by each of the 10 model toxicants. After this, the "Overall Protective Indexes" ("OPI") and the "Protective Spectrum Index" ("PSI") were calculated, as rough indications of the mean degree and the specificity of protection, that is of the quantitative and qualitative prophylactic potencies respectively. These data are summarized in Tables 136, p. 836 and 137.

For the 10 toxicants enumerated in the caption of Table 136 the techniques of administration and the manner in which protection is expressed have been described in an earlier paper (Selye G 70,420/71), as well as in the sections devoted to the effect of various steroids upon each toxicant in this monograph. Suffice it to recall that the highest possible degree of protection corresponds to grade "3", the "OPI" expresses the mean grade of protection, whereas the "PSI" gives the percentage of the toxicants tested against which significant protection is obtained (irrespective of the degree of significance). These two indexes — given in the last two vertical columns of Table 136 — do not run strictly parallel but the various compounds tested for protective potency are listed roughly in decreasing order of their OPIs. Whenever the material at our disposal permitted it, compounds active at a certain dose were retested at a lower dose level. Of course, the two indexes were not calculated for dose levels at which, because of toxicity or lack of material, not all protective compounds could be tested (marked with a dash); hence the OPI and PSI are listed only for the highest, but still well tolerated, dose of each protective compound. The last two horizontal lines in Table 136 list the indexes for the amenability of the toxicants to detoxication by the conditioning agents as explained on p. 772.

Perusal of Table 136 indicates that almost all **steroids** were active in offering protection, at least against some of the damaging agents; but this is so merely because most of the steroids tested here were included in this study precisely because they had shown some potency in preliminary tests.

It is noteworthy that among all steroids tested PCN (Cpd. 1), again exhibited the highest catatoxic activity as judged by both indexes. It was even more active than any of the other 16α-carbonitriles tested against all 10 substrates. CS-1, spironolactone, Cpds. 4, 5, cyproterone acetate, ethylestrenol, norbolethone, TMACN and Cpd. 10 were almost equally efficacious at the highest dose (10 mg), but at the 500 µg dose level, activity fell roughly in the order in which the compounds are mentioned here. Indomethacin and digitoxin are most readily detoxified by these steroids — in the case of PCN even at the dose level of 300 µg/kg. However, the general indexes of activity are not very meaningful at the low dose levels at which efficacy against other toxicants has not been examined; hence they are listed only for the optimal protective dose. It will be noted that usually this is 10 mg (the highest dose tested) but in the case of such compounds as the strong glucocorticoids or estradiol, inherent toxicity of heavy overdosage counteracts the protective effect against drugs by causing severe mortality. In these instances, lower dose levels were selected for the computation of the OPI and PSI (last two vertical columns at right).

On the other hand, Cpd. 34 and the steroids listed after it in Table 136 exhibit only negligible if any activity, with the exception of occasional strong inhibitory effects (grade 2 or 3) against individual toxicants (e.g., pregnanedione against parathion, hexobarbital and indomethacin; progesterone against indomethacin; 11α-hydroxyprogesterone against indomethacin, hydroxydione against digitoxin, DOC against nicotine). This singular specificity of protection among compounds having a very low, if any, protective effect against other substrates may well depend upon specific so-called "physiologic antagonisms" (e.g., the anesthetic effect of hydroxydione or the mineralocorticoid action of DOC), but further experiments will be necessary to prove this.

A glance at the OPI and PSI of the toxicants (last two horizontal lines at the bottom of Table 136) shows that digitoxin, dioxathion, hexobarbital, progesterone, indomethacin and DHT were most readily detoxified by the largest number of conditioning agents, whereas parathion, nicotine, zoxazolamine and especially the infarctoid cardiopathy produced by fluorocortisol + Na_2HPO_4 + corn oil were most resistant.

Among the **nonsteroidal agents** of Table 137 rather specific antagonisms were quite common. For example, ACTH increased resistance to the neuromuscular blocking action of zoxazolamine, although it had little if any effect against other agents.

Vitamin E offered some protection against DHT; whereas acetylsalicylic acid protected against progesterone anesthesia, zoxazolamine paralysis and indomethacin ulcers, but these compounds offered no noteworthy protection against other toxicants.

Bile duct ligature offered complete protection against DHT-induced calcinosis, the F-COL + Na_2HPO_4 + oil cardiopathy and indomethacin ulcers, but the mortality was not completely prevented and hence, the grade of protection — which reflects the mean inhibition of lesions plus mortality — is comparatively moderate. It is very likely that occlusion of the choledochus acts by preventing bile secretion, thereby interfering with lipid absorption and the enterohepatic circulation of drugs.

Digitoxin, indomethacin, vitamin A and vitamin D — all of which are readily detoxified under the influence of catatoxic steroids — do not act as inducers of protective enzymes against any of the substrates tested. Obviously, there is no relationship between amenability to detoxication by steroid-induced enzymes and the power to induce such enzymes.

As with the steroidal protective agents, indomethacin intoxication appears to be particularly easy to prevent, but digitoxin poisoning (which is likewise combated by virtually all catatoxic steroids) is singularly resistant to protection by nonsteroidal agents, with the exception of nicotine and phentolamine.

Among the nonsteroidal agents, the highest general protective indexes are exhibited by phetharbital, diphenylhydantion, phenobarbital and phenylbutazone, but at high dose levels, tolbutamide and compound W-1372 are also quite efficacious.

Table 136. Second step: "Protective Spectrums" of some steroidal agents

Group	Steroidal Conditioning Agent	Dose mg	Digitoxin	Dioxathion	Parathion	Nicotine	Hexobarbital	Progesterone	Zoxazolamine	Indomethacin	Fluorocortisol + Na_2HPO_4 + Corn oil	Dihydrotachysterol (DHT)	OPI	PSI %
1 IM 346a	3β-Hydroxy-20-oxo-5-pregnene-16α-carbonitrile PCN (SC-4674) $P^5CN_{16\alpha}O_{3\beta}ON_{20}$	10	3	3	2	2.5	3	3	3	3	1.5	2	2.6	100
		1	3	3	2.5	0	1	3	3	3	0.5	—		
		0.5	3	3	1.5	0	1	3	3	3	0	2		
		0.2	3	—	3	—	—	3	3	3	—	1.5		
		0.1	3	3	2	—	—	2	3	3	—	0		
		0.03	2	0.5	0	—	0	3	—	3	—	—		
		0.015	0	—	—	—	—	3	0	0	—	—		
		0.005	—	—	—	—	—	3	—	—	—	—		
		0.003	—	—	—	—	—	2	—	—	—	—		
		0.001	—	—	—	—	—	0	—	—	—	—		
2 IM 10	9α-Fluoro-11β,17-dihydroxy-3-oxo-4-androstene-17α-propionic acid potassium salt CS-1, (SC-11927) $A^4III''K_{17\alpha}Ol_{11\beta,17}ON_3F_{9\alpha}$	10	3	1.5	1.5	3	3	3	2	3	1.5	3	2.5	100
		0.5	3	3	0.5	0	0	3	1	3	0	1		
		0.1	1	1.5	—	—	—	2	0	1.5	—	0		
		0.03	0	0	—	—	—	0	—	0	—	—		
3 IM 9	17-Hydroxy-7α-thioacetyl-3-oxo-4-androstene-17α-propionic acid γ lactone Spironolactone (SC-9420) $A^4III''\gamma lac_{17\alpha}ON_3$ *$SII''_{7\alpha}$	10	3	1.5	2	3	3	3	1	3	2	2	2.4	100
		0.5	0	0	0	0	0	2	0	1.5	0	0		
		0.1	—	—	—	—	—	0	—	0	—	—		

#	Compound	Structure code																					
4 IM 423	16α-Cyano-3β-hydroxy-5-pregnene-7,20-dione (SC-6813) $P5CN_{16α}ol_{3β}on_{7,20}$		1	3	3	1.5	2.5	3	3	3	2	2	2	1.5	2.4	100
			0.5	3	2	2	0	2	2	2	0	1.5	1	1.5		
			0.03	0	–	0	–	0	0	0	–	2.5	0	–		
5 IM 414	3β-Hydroxy-20-oxo-5-pregnene-16α-carbonitrile, cyclic (ethylene acetal) (U-19653) $P5CN_{16α}ol_{3β}θII_{20}$		1	3	3	0.5	2	2	3	2	2	2	0	0.5	1.8	90
			0.5	3	2.5	–	0	3	3	3	3	3	–	–		
			0.1	1	0	–	–	–	–	–	1.5	1.5	–	–		
			0.03	1.5	–	–	–	3	3	–	0	1.5	–	–		
			0.015	0	–	–	–	–	–	–	–	0	–	–		
6 IM 279	6-Chloro-17-hydroxy-1α,2α-dihydro-2'H-cyclopropa(1,2)-4,6-pregnadiene-3,20-dione acetate Cyproterone acetate (Schering) $P4,6I_{1α-2}*II''_{17α}on_{3,20}Cl_6$		10	3	2	3	3	3	3	3	3	3	0	1.5	2.5	90
			1	2.5	3	1.5	0	1	3	3	3	3	–	–		
			0.5	2	2	0.5	–	0	3	2	2	3	–	0		
			0.1	0	0	–	–	–	2	2	0	0.5	–	–		
			0.03	0	–	–	–	–	0	0	–	–	–	–		
7 IM 59a	17α-Ethyl-4-estren-17-ol Ethylestrenol (Organon) $E^4II_{17α}ol_{17}$		10	3	1.5	2	3	3	3	2	3	3	0	3	2.4	90
			0.5	0	0	0	0.5	1	2	0	0	0	–	0.5		
			0.1	–	–	–	0	0	3	3	–	–	–	–		
			0.03	–	–	–	–	–	0	–	–	–	–	–		
8 IM 343	13,17α-Diethyl-17-hydroxy-4-gonen-3-one Norbolethone (Wy-3475) $G^4II_{13,17α}ol_{17}on_3$		10	3	1.5	1.5	3	3	3	0	3	3	1	3	2.2	90
			0.5	0	2	0	0	0	2	–	0.5	0.5	0	1		
			0.1	0	0	–	–	–	0	–	–	–	–	0		

[a] Underneath the serial number of the compounds, the "IM" numbers (for Institut de Médecine et de Chirurgie expérimentales) are mentioned. These identify steroids in our collection and remain the same in all Tables as well as in other publications from this Institute.

Table 136 (continued)

Group	Steroidal Conditioning Agent	Dose mg	Digitoxin	Dioxathion	Parathion	Nicotine	Hexobarbital	Progesterone	Zoxazolamine	Indomethacin	Fluorocortisol + Na_2HPO_4 + Corn oil	Dihydrotachy-sterol (DHT)	OPI	PSI %
9 IM 364	17β-Hydroxy-4,4,17-trimethyl-3-oxo-5-androstene-2α-carbonitrile TMACN (Winthrop) $A^5I_{4,4,17\alpha}CN_{2\alpha}ol_{17}on_3$	10 0.5 0.1 0.03 0.015	3 2.5 2 0 —	2.5 3 1.5 0 —	2 0.5 — — —	0 0 — — —	3 1 0 — —	3 3 3 3 0	3 1 0 — —	3 3 2 0 —	2 −0.5 — — —	2 1.5 0 — —	2.1	90
10 IM 267	16β-Methyl-16,17-epoxy-3β,11α-dihydroxy-5α-pregnan-20-one (Lepetit) $P5\alpha I_{16\beta}ol_{3\beta,11\alpha}on_{20}\theta_{16\alpha\to17}$	10 0.5 0.1	3 0 —	3 0 —	2 1 0	0 — —	1 0 —	3 1 0	3 0 —	3 0.5 —	0.5 0 —	1.5 0 —	2.0	90
11 IM 52a	6α-Methyl-11β,17,21-trihydroxy-1,4-pregnadiene-3,20-dione 6α-Methylprednisolone "Medrol" (Upjohn) $P^{1,4}I_{6\alpha}ol_{11\beta,17,21}on_{3,20}$	10 0.5 0.1 0.03 0.015	3 0 — — —	3 0 — — —	0.5 0 — — —	0 — — — —	3 2 2 3 0	3 1 0 — —	2 1 0 — —	3 0 — — —	0 — — — —	1.5 0.5 — — —	1.9	80
12 IM 81	9α-Fluoro-17α-methyl-11β,17-dihydroxy-4-androsten-3-one Fluoxymesterone (U-6040) $A^4I_{17\alpha}ol_{11\beta,17}on_3F_{9\alpha}$	10 0.5 0.1 0.03 0.015	3 3 0 — —	3 2 3 0.5 —	0 — — — —	1 0 — — —	2 3 3 3 0	3 3 3 0 —	3 0 — — —	2 0 — — —	0 — — — —	2 1 0 — —	1.9	80

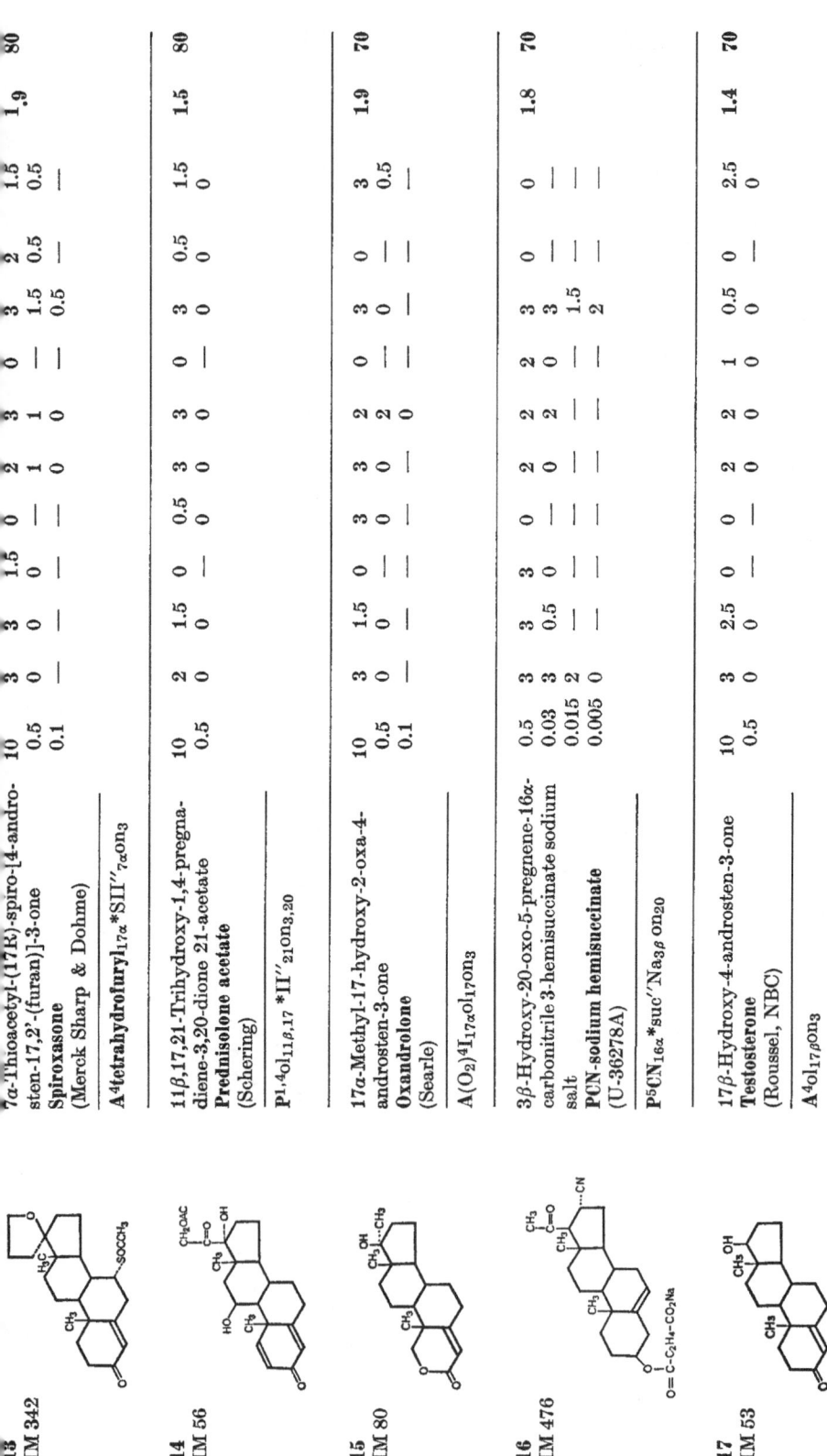

13 IM 342	7α-Thioacetyl-(17R)-spiro-[4-androsten-17,2'-(furan)]-3-one **Spiroxasone** (Merck Sharp & Dohme) A^4tetrahydrofuryl$_{17\alpha}$*SII''$_{7\alpha}$on$_3$	10 0.5 0.1	3 0 —	3 0 —	1.5 0 —	0 — —	2 1 0	3 1 0	0 — —	3 1.5 0.5	2 0.5 —	1.5 0.5 —	1.9	80
14 IM 56	11β,17,21-Trihydroxy-1,4-pregnadiene-3,20-dione 21-acetate **Prednisolone acetate** (Schering) $P^{1,4}ol_{11\beta,17}$*II''$_{21}$on$_{3,20}$	10 0.5	2 0	1.5 0	0 —	0.5 0	3 0	3 0	0 —	3 0	0.5 0	1.5 0	1.5	80
15 IM 80	17α-Methyl-17-hydroxy-2-oxa-4-androsten-3-one **Oxandrolone** (Searle) $A(O_2)^4I_{17\alpha}ol_{17}on_3$	10 0.5 0.1	3 0 —	1.5 0 —	0 — —	3 0 —	3 0 —	2 2 0	0 — —	3 0 —	0 — —	3 0.5 —	1.9	70
16 IM 476	3β-Hydroxy-20-oxo-5-pregnene-16α-carbonitrile 3-hemisuccinate sodium salt **PCN sodium hemisuccinate** (U-36278A) $P^5CN_{16\alpha}$*suc''Na$_{3\beta}$on$_{20}$	0.5 0.03 0.015 0.005	3 3 2 0	3 0.5 — —	3 0 — —	0 — — —	2 0 — —	2 2 — —	2 0 — —	3 3 1.5 2	0 — — —	0 — — —	1.8	70
17 IM 53	17β-Hydroxy-4-androsten-3-one **Testosterone** (Roussel, NBC) $A^4ol_{17\beta}on_3$	10 0.5	3 0	2.5 0	0 —	0 —	2 0	2 0	1 0	0.5 0	0 —	2.5 0	1.4	70

Table 136 (continued)

Group	Steroidal Conditioning Agent	Dose mg	Toxicant										OPI	PSI %
			Digitoxin	Dioxathion	Parathion	Nicotine	Hexobarbital	Progesterone	Zoxazolamine	Indomethacin	Fluorocortisol + Na_2HPO_4 + Corn oil	Dihydrotachysterol (DHT)		
18 IM 152	9α-Fluoro-16α-methyl-11β,17,21-trihydroxy-1,4-pregnadiene-3,20-dione 21-acetate **Dexamethasone acetate** (Schering) $P^{1,4}I_{16\alpha}ol_{11\beta,17}*II''_{21}on_{3,20}F_{9\alpha}$	10 1 0.5 0.1 0.03 0.015 0.005 0.003	3 3 2.5 3 3 0 — —	— 3 3 — — — — —	— −0.5 0 — — — — —	— — — — — — — —	2 3 1 2 2 2 0 —	— 3 3 — — — — —	— 0 — — — — — —	0 1.5 0.5 1 0 — — —	— 0 — — — — — —	1 0 0 0 — — — —	1.3	60
19 IM 85	17α-Methyl-17-hydroxy-1α,7α-dithio-4-androsten-3-one 1,7-diacetate **Emdabol** (Merck, Sharp & Dohme) $A^4I_{17\alpha}ol_{17}*SII''_{1\alpha,7\alpha}on_3$	10 0.5 0.1	2 0.5 0	2 0 —	0 — —	— — —	3 0 —	3 0 —	— — —	1 0 —	— — —	2 0 —	1.3	60
20 IM 23	11β,21-Dihydroxy-4-pregnene-3,20-dione **Corticosterone, Kendall "Cpd. B"** (Merck, Sharp & Dohme) $P^4ol_{11\beta,21}on_{3,20}$	10 0.5 0.1	3 0 —	0.5 — —	0.5 — —	0 — —	0 — —	3 1 0	— — —	3 0 —	— — —	2 0 —	1.2	60
21 IM 22	17,21-Dihydroxy-4-pregnene-3,11,20-trione 21-acetate **Cortisone acetate** (Upjohn) $P^4ol_{17}*II''_{21}on_{3,11,20}$	10 0.5	— —	— —	— —	0 −0.5	3 0	2 0	3 0	0 0	−1 0	1 0	1.2	60

#	Name	Structure code												
22 IM 429	16α-Cyano-3β-hydroxy-5-pregnene-7,20-dione acetate (SC-6703) $P^5CN_{16\alpha}*II''_{3\beta}on_{7,20}$	1 0.5 0.03	3 3 0	2	0	0.5	0	2	3 3	3 3	1.5 2 1.5	0	0	1.2 1.6 60
23 IM 412	3,11,20-Trioxo-5-pregnene-16α-carbonitrile, cyclic 3,20-bis(ethylene acetal) (U-35910) $P^5CN_{16\alpha}on_{11}\theta\theta II_{3,20}$	1 0.1 0.03 0.015	3 0 — —	3	0	0	1	3	2.5 1.5 1.5 0	0	0	1.6 60
24 IM 483	3β-Hydroxy-20-oxo-5-pregnene-16α-carbonitrile 3-sulfate ammonium salt PCN ammonium sulfate (U-37863C) $P^5CN_{16\alpha}*S''(NH_4)_{3\beta}on_{20}$	0.5 0.03 0.015	3 3 1	3 1.5 2	0	0	3	2 0	0	3 3 0.5	0	0.5	1.5 60
25 IM 461	3β-Hydroxy-20-oxo-5-pregnene-16α-carbonitrile, cyclic(2,2-dimethyltrimethylene acetal) (U-36961) $P^5CN_{16\alpha}ol_{3\beta}\theta\theta III_{20/1/2.2}$	0.5 0.03 0.015	2 2 0	3 0	0.5	0	1	3 0	0	3 0	0	0	1.3 60
26 IM 31	3β-Hydroxy-5-androsten-17-one Dehydroepiandrosterone (Ayerst) $A^5ol_{3\beta}on_{17}$	10 0.5 0.1	2 0 —	1 0	0	2 2 0		2 0		3 0.5	0	0	1.1 60

Table 136 (continued)

Group	Steroidal Conditioning Agent	Dose mg	Digitoxin	Dioxathion	Parathion	Nicotine	Hexobarbital	Progesterone	Zoxazolamine	Indomethacin	Fluorocortisol + Na$_2$HPO$_4$ + Corn oil	Dihydrotachysterol (DHT)	OPI	PSI %
27 IM 54	17α-Methyl-5-androstene-3β,17-diol Methylandrostenediol "MAD" (Organon) A^{5}I$_{17α}$Ol$_{3β,17}$	10 0.5	0 —	3 0	0 —	0 —	3 0	3 0	3 0	0 —	0 —	2 0	1.4	50
28 IM 477	6β-Hydroxy-20-oxo-3α,5α-cyclopregnane-16α-carbonitrile (U-36710) P$^{3(5)}$5αCN$_{16α}$Ol$_{6β}$ON$_{20}$	0.5 0.03 0.015	2 0 —	2 0 —	0 — —	0 — —	0 — —	3 1 0	3 0 —	3 0 —	0 — —	0 — —	1.3	50
29 IM 413	3β-Hydroxy-20-oxo-5-pregnene-16α-carbonitrile acetate PCN acetate (U-34889, Syntex) P^{5}CN$_{16α}$ *II''$_{3β}$ON$_{20}$	0.5 0.1 0.03 0.015	1.5 0.5 0 —	1 — — —	0 — — —	0 — — —	0 — — —	3 — 0 —	3 — — —	2 1.5 1.5 0	0 — — —	0 — — —	1.1	50
30 IM 73	17α-Hydroxy-4-pregnene-3,20-dione acetate 17-Acetoxyprogesterone (U-5533) P^4 *II''$_{17α}$On$_{3,20}$	10 0.5	3 0	1 0.5	0 —	0 —	0 —	2 0	0 —	3 0.5	0 —	2 0	1.1	50

No.	Compound	Dose													
31 IM 466	16α-Cyano-4-pregnene-3,20-dione Cyanoprogesterone (SC-4688)	0.5	—	1	0	0	1	3	2	—	0	—	0	0.9	50
		0.1	3	—	—	—	0	0	2	0	—	—	—		
		0.03	0	—	—	—	—	0	—	—	—	—	—		
	$P^4CN_{16\alpha}on_{3,20}$	0.015	0	—	—	—	—	—	—	—	—	—	—		
32 IM 151	9α-Fluoro-16β-methyl-11β,17,21-trihydroxy-1,4-pregnadiene-3,20-dione 21-acetate Betamethasone acetate (Schering)	10	2	—	—	—	—	—	—	—	—	—	—	0.8	50
		2	3	—	—	—	—	—	—	—	—	—	—		
		1	2	1	−1.5	0	3	3	0	1.5	0	1.5	—		
		0.5	1.5	0.5	0	—	0	3	0	1.5	0	0.5	—		
		0.1	0	0	0	—	0	1	—	—	−1	0	—		
	$P^{1,4}I_{16\beta}ol_{11\beta,17}*II''_{21}on_{3,20}F^{9\alpha}$	0.03	—	—	—	—	—	0	—	—	—	—	—		
33 IM 74	4-Pregnene-3,20-dione Progesterone (Roussel, Organon)	10	1.5	0.5	0	1	0	0	0	3	0	1.5	—	0.8	50
	$P^4on_{3,20}$	0.5	0	0.5	—	0	—	—	—	0	—	0	—		
34 IM 462	3β-Hydroxy-20-oxo-5-pregnene-16α-carbonitrile, 20-oxime (U-37722)	0.5	3	3	0	0	0	3	0	3	0	0	—	1.2	40
		0.03	2.5	0	—	—	—	0	—	3	—	—	—		
		0.015	0.5	—	—	—	—	—	—	1	—	—	—		
	$P^5CN_{16\alpha}ol_{3\beta}NOH_{20}$	0.01	0	—	—	—	—	—	—	—	—	—	—		
35 IM 479	3β-Hydroxy-20-oxo-5-pregnene-16α-carbonitrile 3-heptanoate PCN heptanoate (U-37001)	0.5	3	3	0	0	0	2	0	3	0	0	—	1.1	40
		0.03	1	0	—	—	—	0	—	1.5	—	—	—		
	$P^5CN_{16\alpha}*VII''_{3\beta}on_{20}$	0.015	0	—	—	—	—	—	—	0	—	—	—		

Table 136 (continued)

Group	Steroidal Conditioning Agent	Dose mg	Toxicant												IPO	PSI %
			Digitoxin	Dioxathion	Parathion	Nicotine	Hexobarbital	Progesterone	Zoxazolamine	Indomethacin	Fluorocortisol + Na_2HPO_4 + Corn oil	Dihydrotachy-sterol (DHT)				
36 IM 45	11β,17,21-Trihydroxy-4-pregnene-3,20-dione 21-acetate **Cortisol acetate** (Roussel) $P^4ol_{11\beta,17}$ *II″$_{21}on_{3,20}$	10 0.5 0.1 0.03	3 0 — —	0 0 — —	−0.5 0 — —	−0.5 0 — —	3 0 — —	0 3 2 0	3 2 1 0	0 0 — —	0 −0.5 0.5 — —	1.5 1 0 —	0.9	40
37 IM 72	5β-Pregnane-3,20-dione **Pregnanedione** (Searle) $P5\beta\ on_{3,20}$	10 0.5	0 —	1 0	2.5 0	0 —	2 0	0 —	0 —	2 0	0 —	0 —	0.8	40
38 IM 11	21-Hydroxy-5β-pregnane-3,20-dione hemisuccinate sodium salt **Hydroxydione sodium** (Schering, Pfizer) $P5\beta$ *suc″$Na_{21}\ on_{3,20}$	10 0.5	3 0	1.5 0	0.5 0	0.5 0	0 —	0 —	0 —	0 —	0 —	0 —	0.6	40
39 IM 25	21-Hydroxy-4-pregnene-3,20-dione acetate **Desoxycorticosterone acetate "DOC-Ac"** (Schering) P^4 *II″$_{21}on_{3,20}$	10 0.5	0 —	1.5 0	0 —	2 0	0 —	0 —	0 —	1 0.5	0 —	0.5 —	0.5	40

No.	Compound															
40 IM 33	1,3,5(10)-Estratriene-3,17β-diol Estradiol (Roussel) E1,3,5(10)ol3,17β	10 1 0.5 0.1 0.03	0 0 — — —	0 — 1.5 0.5 —	0 — —1.5 0 —	0 — 0 — —	— — 1 0 —	— — 1 0 —	0 — — — —	0 0.5 — — —	0.5 0 — — —	0.5 0 — — —	0 0 — — —	0.3	40
41 IM 119	11α-Hydroxy-4-pregnene-3,20-dione 11α-Hydroxyprogesterone (SKF, Ayerst) P4ol11αon3,20	10 0.5	1.5 0	0 —	0 —	0 —	2 0	2 0	0 —	3 0	0 —	0 —	0 —	0.7	30
42 IM 32	9α-Fluoro-11β,16α,17,21-tetra- hydroxy-1,4-pregnadiene-3,20-dione Triamcinolone (Lederle) P1,4ol11β,16α,17,21on3,20F9α	10 2 0.5 0.1	— 0 — —	— —1.5 0 —	— —0.5 0 —	0 0 — —	— 1 0 —	— 0 — —	0 — — —	— 0 — —	0.5 1 1.5 0	1.5 0 — —	0 — —	0.2	30
43 IM 124	3α,12α-Dihydroxy-24-nor-5β-cholan 23-oic acid methyl ester Methyl nordeoxycholanate (SKF) CHn24,5β″ol3α,12α *I23	10 0.5	3 0	0 —	0 —	—0.5 —	3 0	3 0	0 —	3 0	0 —	0 —	0 —	0.9	30
44 IM 480	6β-Hydroxy-20-oxo-3α,5α-cyclo- pregnane-16α-carbonitrile, cyclic(2′2′-dimethyltrimethylene acetal) (U-37483) P3(5)5αCN16αol6β∂∂III20/1/2,2	0.5 0.03	1 0	0 —	0 —	—0.5 —	2 0	2 0	0 —	3 0	0 —	0 —	0 —	0.6	30

Table 136 (continued)

Group	Steroidal Conditioning Agent	Dose mg	Digitoxin	Dioxathion	Parthion	Nicotine	Hexobarbital	Progesterone	Zoxazolamine	Indomethacin	Fluorocortisol + Na₃HPO₄ + Corn oil	Dihydrotachysterol (DHT)	OPI	PSI %
45 IM 474	4,4-Dimethyl-3,20-dioxo-5-prenene-16α-carbonitrile (U-35641)	0.5	0.5	0	0	0	1	0	0	3	0	0	0.5	30
	$P^5I_{4,4}CN_{16\alpha}on_{3,20}$	0.03	—	—	—	—	—	—	—	0	—	—		
46 IM 39	9α-Fluoro-11β,17,21-trihydroxy-4-pregnene-3,20-dione 21-acetate 9α-Fluorocortisol (F-COL) acetate (U-4845)	2 0.5 0.1	0 — —	0 — —	0 — —	−0.5 — —	2 0 0	0 — —	0 — —	0.5 0 —	0 — —	0 — —	0.2	20
	$P^4ol_{11\beta,17} *II'_{21}on_{3,20}F_{9\alpha}$													
47 IM 454	16α,17-Dihydro-3'H-cyclopropa(16,17)-5α-androstane-3β,17β-diol diacetate (SC-21940)	0.5	0	0	0	0	0	0	0	0	0	0	0	0
	$A5\alpha I_{16\alpha-17} *II''_{3\beta,17\beta}$													
OPI			2.2	1.6	0.6	0.6	1.5	2.1	1.2	2.1	0.3	1.0		
SPI%			80	80	40	30	70	80	50	90	20	60		

The infarctoid cardiopathy produced by fluorocortisol + Na_2HPO_4 + corn oil, which is inhibited by several steroids (particularly spironolactone and spiroxasone, among those listed in Table 136), was consistently resistant to prophylaxis by any of the nonsteroidal drugs in Table 137. Of course, potassium salts (e.g., KCl) or potassium-sparing agents (e.g., amiloride, triamterene) offer excellent protection against this cardiopathy, as shown by our previous investigations, and since spironolactone and spiroxasone likewise retain potassium, it is probable that here they also act primarily through this mechanism.

The relative amenability of the other toxicants to protection by nonsteroidal conditioning agents can be most readily appraised on the basis of the indexes listed in the last two horizontal lines of Table 137, p. 848. It will be seen that indomethacin and dioxathion have the highest PSI, but in general, the overall protective effect of these nonsteroidal agents falls far short of that of the steroids listed in Table 136. Indeed, whatever overall protective values can be ascribed to the set of nonsteroidal agents are mainly due to the comparatively high efficacy of phenobarbital, phetharbital, diphenylhydantoin, phenylbutazone, and to a lesser extent, of tolbutamide and W-1372; the other agents in this list are either inactive or offer protection only against very few toxicants.

Third Step: Identification of Damaging Agents Amenable to Prophylaxis

As previously stated, this third step of the screening procedure was designed primarily to identify the types of compounds that can be detoxified by steroids. However, for comparative purposes, we have also tested thyroxine and phenobarbital under identical conditions, as examples of nonsteroidal agents previously shown to influence resistance against many toxicants. The steroids included in this battery of tests were purposely selected to comprise proven syntoxic or catatoxic substances, as well as compounds which had never been shown to protect against any toxic agent.

The prophylactic steroids were administered, as outlined on p. VIII, in 1 ml water by a stomach tube, twice daily, from the first day until termination of the experiment, unless otherwise stated in the footnotes. Thyroxine was administered at the dose of 0.2 mg in 0.2 ml water s.c., once daily, and phenobarbital at the dose of 6 mg in 1 ml water p.o., twice daily, as described in Table 137. The treatment with the toxicants and the assessment of the lesions they produce was again expressed as outlined on p. 834. The results are summarized in Table 138, p. 850.

In this series of experiments, the "OPI" and "PSI" refer to the amenability of the individual damaging agents to the protective effect of the compounds listed in the caption of Table 138. In other words, in the two last vertical columns of Tables 135, 136, 137, these indexes were computed to express the protective action of many agents against a standard set of toxicants, whereas in Table 138 (as in the two last horizontal lines of Tables 136, 137) they are meant to reflect the amenability of diverse toxicants to inactivation by a standard set of potential prophylactic agents.

In Table 137, the damaging agents are listed merely in alphabetic order but a glance at the OPI column reveals that the **toxicants most amenable to prophylaxis** by diverse agents are: cocaine, cyclobarbital, cycloheximide, digitoxin, EPN, ethion, ethylmorphine, glutethimide, hexobarbital, indomethacin, methyprylon, nicotine,

848 Synopsis of Pharmaco-Chemical and Pharmaco-Pharmacologic Interrelations

Table 137. Second step (Ctd.): "Protective Spectrums" of some nonsteroidal agents

Nonsteroidal Conditioning Agent	Dose[a]	Digitoxin	Dioxathion	Parathion	Nicotine	Hexobarbital	Progesterone	Zoxazolamine	Indomethacin	Fluorocortisol + Na_2HPO_4 + Corn oil	Dihydro-tachysterol	OPI	PSI%
Phetharbital (Burroughs Wellcome) in 1 ml water, p.o., twice daily	10	2	3	2	2.5	3	3	3	3	0	2.5	2.4	90
	0.5	0	1.5	1	0	0	0	0	0	—	0		
	0.1	—	0	0	—	—	—	—	—	—	—		
Diphenylhydantoin (Eastman) in 1 ml water, p.o., twice daily	25	1.5	1.5	2	3	3	3	3	3	0	0.5	2.1	90
	6	0	2.5	3	0.5	3	2	2	3	—	0.5		
	1	0	0	1.5	0	0	—	0	0	—	0.5		
Phenobarbital sodium (BDH) in 1 ml water, p.o., twice daily	6	0	3	2.5	3	3	3	1	3	0	2	2.1	80
	0.5	0	2	1	0	3	3	0	3	—	0		
	0.1	0	0	0.5	—	1	1	0	0	—	—		
	0.03	—	—	—	—	0	—	—	—	—	—		
Phenylbutazone (Geigy) in 1 ml water, p.o., twice daily	10	0	3	1	3	3	3	0	3	0	0	1.6	60
	0.5	—	0	0	0	0	1	—	0	—	—		
	0.1	—	—	—	—	—	0	—	—	—	—		
Tolbutamide (Hoechst Pharmaceutical) in 1 ml water, p.o., twice daily	50	0	3	1	0	3	3	0	2	0	0.5	1.3	60
	10	—	0.5	0	—	0	2	—	0	—	—		
	5						0						
W-1872 (Wallace) in 1 ml corn oil, p.o., twice daily	10	0	3	0	0	3	3	3	3	0	0	1.5	50
	5	0	3	1	0	0	2	3	0	0	—		
	1	0	1.5	0.5	0	0	0	0	0	0	—		
	0.5	—	0.5	—	—	—	—	0	—	—	—		
Vitamin E (Distillation Products Ind.) in 1 ml corn oil, p.o., twice daily	50	0	1	0	0	1	1	0	0	0	1.5	0.5	40
	10	—	—	—	—	0	—	—	—	—	0		
Bile duct ligature	—	0	0.5	0.5	0	-3	-3	-3	1.5	1.5[b]	1.5	-0.4	40
Acetylsalicylic acid (Merck) in 2 ml water,	10	0	0	0	0	0	3	1	3	0	0	0.7	30

Compound	Dose									OPI	PSI %
Sodium salicylate (Fisher) in 1 ml water, p.o., twice daily	10	0	0	1	0	0	0	1	0	3	0
	0.5	—	—	0	—	—	—	0	—	0	0.5 / 30
Nicotine (Eastman Organic Chemical) in 1 ml water, p.o., twice daily	3	1	0.5	0	0	0	0	0	0	1.5	0.3
	0.15	0	—	—	—	—	—	—	—	0	0 / 30
ACTH (Nordic Biochemical Ltd.) in 0.2 ml water, s.c., twice daily	50 I.U.	0	0	0	0	0	0	2	0	0	1
	2.5 I.U.	—	—	—	—	—	—	1	—	0	0 / 0.3 / 20
Vitamin D_2 (Wander) in 0.5 ml corn oil, p.o., twice daily	0.025	0.5	0	0.5	0	0	0	0	0	0	0
											0.1 / 20
Vitamin A (Hoffmann-La Roche) in 0.5 ml corn oil, p.o., twice daily	2500 I.U.	0	0	0	0	0	0	0	0	0	0.5 / 0.1 / 10
Indomethacin (Merck Sharp & Dohme) in 0.2 ml water, s.c., twice daily	0.15	0	0	0	0	0	0	0	0	0	0 / 0 / 0
STH (C.H.Li) in 0.2 ml water, s.c., twice daily	1 / 0.05 / 0.01	0	0	0	0	0	0	2	0	0	0 / 0
Vitamin C (Fisher) in 1 ml water, p.o., twice daily	50	0	0	0	0	0	−1	0	0	0	−0.1 / 0
Digitoxin (Roussel) in 1 ml water, p.o., twice daily	0.15	0	0	0	0	0	0	0	0	−0.5	−0.1 / 0
L-Thyroxine (BDH) in 0.2 ml water, s.c., daily	0.2 / 0.01	−1.5 / 0	−2 / 0	0	0	0	0	0	0	0	−0.4 / 0
Phentolamine (Ciba) in 0.2 ml water, s.c., twice daily	3 / 0.5	2 / 0	1 / 0	—	—	0	—	—	0.5	—	—
OPI		0.4	0.9	0.4	0.6	0.8	1.1	0.5	1.3	0.1	0.5
PSI %		25	50	36	21	35	47	31	55	5	42

[a] Doses in international units (I.U.) are so indicated; all other dosages are expressed in milligrams.
[b] This inhibition may be spurious since all rats were moribund or dead by the end of the experiment, although they showed no cardiac necrosis.

850 Synopsis of Pharmaco-Chemical and Pharmaco-Pharmacologic Interrelations

Table 138. *Third step: Identification of damaging agents amenable to prophylaxis*

Toxicant	Pheno-barbital	PCN	Ethyl-estrenol	CS-1	Spirono-lactone	Nor-bolethone	Oxan-drolone	Predni-solone-Ac	Proges-terone	Triamci-nolone	DOC-Ac	Hydroxy-dione	Estradiol	Thyroxine	MPI[1]	OPI[2]	PSI[3]
Acetanilide	1.5	1.5	1.5	1.5	1.5	1.5	0	1.5	0	0	0	0	—1	1.5	0.8	12	60
Acrylamide	3	3	0	1.5	0.5	0	0	0	0	0	0	0	0	0	0.6	8	30
Aminoacetonitrile	0	0	0	0	0	0	0	3	1	3c	—1	—0.5	1b	3	0.9	12	40
o-Aminophenol HCl	0	—	0	0	0	0	0	0	0	0	0	0	0	—1.5	—0.2	0	0
Aminopyrine	1	2.5b	3	2.5	1	2.5	0	2.5	2.5	2.5	0	0	0	0	1.4	20	60
DL-Amphetamine	0	0	0.5	0	0	0	0	—0.5	0	—1.5	0	0	0	—1.5	—0.2	1	10
Arsenic pentoxide	—1	0	0	0	1	—1	0	—1.5	0	—0.5	0	0	—3	0	—0.2	2	10
Barbital	—2	0	0	—1	0	0	0	2	0	0a	—3	—1	—3b	0	—0.6	2	10
Bile duct ligature	—	—	1	1	2	0	2	—1	0	—1a	0	0	0b	0	—0.2	0	0
Bishydroxycoumarin	0	0	—0.5	0	0	1	0	0	—0.5	0a	0	0	3	0	0.7	10	40
Bromobenzene	—	—	0	0	0	0	0	—1	0	—1	0	0	0	0	—0.3	0	0
Bromopheniramine maleate	—	—	1	0	1	0	0	0	0	0a	0	0	0b	0	0	0	0
Cadmium chloride	0	1.5	0	0	0	0.5	0	2.5	0	1.5	0	0	2.5	1	0.8	12	60
Caramiphen HCl	0.5	1.5	1	0.5	2	0	0	1	—1	0	0.5	0	0	—1	0.3	5	40
Carisoprodol	0	1	1	3	1	0	0	2	0	0	—0.5	0	0	—1	0.5	9	40
Chlordiazepoxide	0	3	3	3	3	1	0	0	0	0	0	0	0b	0	0.8	11	40
Cinchophen	3	3	2	3	3	2	2	3	0	0a	0	0	3	0	1.1	16	40
Cocaine	3	3	3	3	3	2.5	2	3	1.5	0	0	1	3	0	2.0	28	80
Colchicine	2	3	1.5	3	3	0	2	0	0.5	0a	0.5	0	0b	0	1.1	16	60
DL-Coniine	0	2	0	0	0	0	0	1.5	0	2a	—0.5	0	2	0	0.5	8	30
Croton oil	0	2	0	0	3	0	0	2	0	2	0	0	0b	0	0.4	6	20
Cyclobarbital	3	3	3	3	3	3	3	3	3	3a	1	1	0b	0	1.9	27	60
Cycloheximide (100 µg)	3	3	3	3	3	3	3	0	3	0a	—1	1	0	0	1.9	26	70

Third Step: Identifikation of Damaging Agents Amenable to Prophylaxis

Conditioning agent	Algebraic sum[1]	Arithmetic sum[2]	Percentage[3]
DDT	0.04	2	10
DHT	1.7	24	80
Digitoxin	1.8	25	60
Digitoxin + Na_2HPO_4 + Oil	1.0	15	60
Diisopropylfluorophosphate "DFP"	0.1	2	60
Dimercaprol	−0.04	0	30
Dinitrophenol	−0.2	0	0
Dioxathion	0.9	16	80
Diphenylhydantoin	−0.3	3	20
Dipicrylamine	0.1	4	10
DOC-Ac + NaH_2PO_4	−0.3	2	10
Doxepin	0.1	1	10
E-coli endotoxin No. 08	0.2	5	10
Edrophonium chloride	0	0	10
Elementary yellow phosphorus	0	0	0
Emetine HCl	0.1	4	20
Ephedrine sulfate	−0.1	1	10
Epinephrine	−0.5	0	0
EPN	1.9	28	90
Estradiol + NaH_2PO_4	−0.3	1	10
Ethion	2	28	70
Ethyl alcohol	−0.1	0	0
Ethylene chlorohydrin	0.04	1	10
Ethylene glycol	0.3	6	20
Ethylmorphine	1.9	27	80
Fasting	0	0	0
Flufenamic acid	0.5	10	50
Fluorocortisol + $NaClO_4$ + Oil	0.4	7	40

a–c Administered at the dose level of: [a] 2 mg, [b] 1 mg, [c] 0.5 mg.

[1] Algebraic sum of all grades divided by numbers of toxicants tested.
[2] Arithmetic sum of all grades.
[3] Percentage of all positive grades taking grade "3" protection by all conditioning agents as 100%.

852 Synopsis of Pharmaco-Chemical and Pharmaco-Pharmacologic Interrelations

Table 138 (continued)

Toxicant	Conditioning Agent																MPI[1]	OPI[2]	PSI[3]
	Pheno-barbital	PCN	Ethyl-estrenol	CS-1	Spirono-lactone	Nor-bolethone	Oxan-drolone	Predni-solone-Ac	Proges-terone	Triamci-nolone	DOC-Ac	Hydroxy-dione	Estradiol	Thyroxine			
Fluorocortisol + Na₂HPO₄ + Oil	0	1.5	0	1.5	2	1	0	0.5	0	0.5	0	0	0.5	0	0.5	8	50
Fluorocortisol + Na₂HPO₄ + Restraint	1	2	0	1.5	2	0	0	—0.5	0	—0.5	0	1	0	0	0.5	8	40
Fluphenazine di HCl	0	3	1	3	0	0	1	1	0	0	1	0	2	0	0.6	9	40
Glutethimide	3	3	3	3	3	3	3	3	0	3	0	0	2	0	1.9	27	70
Glycerol	0.5	0	1.5	1	0	1	0.5	1.5	1	—2	0	0	0	1.5	0.5	9	60
Griseofulvin	0	0	0	0	0	0	0	0.5	0	0[a]	0	—0.5	0[b]	0	0	1	10
Guthion	3	3	3	3	3	3	3	1	0	0[a]	0	0	0[b]	0	1.6	22	60
Haloperidol	0	1.5	1.5	1.5	1.5	1.5	1.5	1.5	1	—1.5	0	0	—0.5	—1.5	0.6	12	60
Heptachlor	0	0	0	0	0	—0.5	0	0.5	—0.5	0	0	0	—0.5	—0.5	—0.1	1	10
Hexamethonium Cl	0	0	0	0	0	0	0	3	0	3	0	0	0	0	0.4	6	10
Hexobarbital	3	3	3	3	3	3	3	3	0	1[a]	0	0	1[b]	0	1.9	26	70
Homatropine HBr	—	2	0	1	0	0	0	0	0	0	0	0	0	0	0.2	2	20
Hydrazine	0.5	0	0	0	0	0	0	2	0	1.5	0	0	0	0.5	0.3	5	30
Hydroquinone	2	2	3	3	3	3	0	—1	0	—3	0	0	0	0	0.3	8	30
Imipramine	2.5	2	2	1.5	2	0	0	0	0	0	0	0	0.5	0	0.8	11	40
Indium trichloride	—	0	0	0	0	0	0	0	0	—0.5	0	0	0	—0.5	—0.1	0	0
Indomethacin	3	3	3	3	3	3	3	3	3	0[a]	1	0	0.5[b]	0	2.0	29	80
LSD	1	3	3	3	0	3	0	3	1	3	0	0	3	0	1.6	23	60
Mechlorethamine HCl	0	0	3	3	0	0	—1	—3	0	—3	0	—3	0	—3	—0.9	0	0
Mephenesin	0	3	3	3	3	3	0	1	0	0[a]	1	0	0	0	1.2	17	50
Meprobamate	3	3	3	3	3	3	3	3	0	0[a]	0	0	0[b]	0	1.7	24	60
Mercurio chloride (400 μg)	0	0	0.5	0	0	0	0	0.5	2	0	0	0	1	—0.5	0.5	7	40
Mersalyl (4 mg)	0	0	2	0	3	1.5	0.5	3	0.5	1	0	0	0	0	0.8	12	50

Third Step: Identifikation of Damaging Agents Amenable to Prophylaxis

n-Methylaniline	2	2b		0.5	0	0	0	0	0	0	0.5	0	0.3	7	40
Methylphenidate	0	0	1	0	0	0	−0.5	−2	0	0	−2	−1.5	−0.1	0	0
Methylsalicylate	0.5	1.5	1.5	1.5	1.5	0	0	0	0	0.5	0	−0.5	0.5	9	50
Methyprylon	3	3	3	3	3	3	3	3	3	0	2	0	2.4	33	90
Morphine sulfate	0	0	0	0	0	0	0	0	0	1	0	−0.5	−0.04	0	0
α-Naphthylisothiocyanate	3	3	3	2.5	0	0	0	0	0	0	0	0	0.9	12	40
Neostigmine Br	1.5	1.5	0.5	0.5	0	0	0.5	−0.5	−1.5	0	0	0	0	5	40
Nephrectomy	—	—	0	—			0	0	0	0	−1	−1.5	0	0	0
Nicotine	3	2.5	3	3	3	3	0.5	0	0	0.5	0	0	1.8	25	80
Nikethamide	1.5	1	1.5	1.5	1.5	0	0	1	1.5	1	1.5	−0.5	0.8	13	70
p-Nitroanisole	0	2	0.5	0	0.5	0	0	1.5	0	1.5	0.5	0	0.4	6	40
OMPA (1 mg)	0	0	0	0	0	0	0	0	2	0	−3	0	−0.2	0	0
Pancuronium Br	0	1.5	1	3	0	0	2.5	0	0	0	0	0.5	0.9	13	50
Parathion	2.5	2	2	1.5	2	3	0	0	1.5	0	−1.5b	−2	0.6	12	50
Pentylenetetrazol	1	3	0	0	0	0	0	2.5	−0.5a	0	0	0	0.6	9	30
Phenindione	3	1.5	3	3	3	3	2.5	1	0	0.5	0.5b	0	1.6	23	80
Phenyl isothiocyanate	3	3	2.5	0.5	0.5	0.5	3	0	0a	0	0	0	1.0	14	50
Phenyramidol	3	3	3	3	3	2	0	1.5	0	0	3	0	1.8	25	60
Physostigmine sulfate	0	0.5	1	1	0.5	0	2	0	0a	0	−1b	−2	0.04	4	40
Picrotoxin	3	3	3	3	3	3	0.5	0	0.5a	2	0b	0	2.2	31	90
Piperidine	3	0	3	3	0	3	3	3	3	1	3	1	1.9	26	70
Pipradol	—	1.5	0	0	0	0	0	0	0	3	0	−0.5	0.1	2	10
Pralidoxime Cl	0.5	0	1	0	0	0	2.5	2	2	0	1	0	0.5	8	40
Progesterone	3	3	3	3	3	2	3	0a	0a	0.5	1b	0	1.7	24	60
Propionitrile	0	−2.5	0	0	0	0	−2.5	0	−3	0	0.5	−3	−0.7	1	10
Propylthiouracil	2	2	1.5	2	1.5	2	0	0.5	−0.5	0	0	−0.5	0.9	13	60
Pyrilamine	—	—	0	0	0	0	0	0	0	0	0	0	0	0	0
SKF 525-A	1	2	1	3	3	3	3	3	3a	1	0b	0	1.7	24	80
Sodium perchlorate	0	0	0	0	1	0	−1	0	0a	0	0b	1.5	−0.1	2	10
Strychnine	3	0.5	0.5	−1.5	0	0	3	0	3	0	3	−0.5	0.9	14	50
Tetraethyl ammonium Cl	1.5	0	0	0	0.5	0	0.5	0.5	3	0	1	0.5	0.6	9	40
Thallium chloride	—	0	0	0	0	0	0	0.5	0.5	0	0.5	0	0.1	2	20

Table 138 (continued)

Toxicant	Conditioning Agent															MPI[1]	OPI[2]	PSI[3]
	Pheno-barbital	PCN	Ethyl-estrenol	CS-1	Spirono-lactone	Nor-bolethone	Oxan-drolone	Predni-solone-Ac	Proges-terone	Triamci-nolone	DOC-Ac	Hydroxy-dione	Estradiol	Thyroxine			
Theobromine	3	3	0	3	0	0	0	0	2.5	0	0	0	0	0	0.8	12	30
Theophylline	3	3	3	3	0.5	2	2	3	3	0	0.5	0.5	0	0	1.7	24	80
Thimerosal	0	1.5	1.5	1	1	2	0.5	1	0	0	0	0.5	2	0	0.8	11	60
Thioacetamide	−0.5	−2	0	−2	0	−0.5	−2	−2	−2	−1	−2	0	0	−2	−1.1	0	0
Thiopental	3	3	3	3	3	0	2	3	0	0[a]	0	0	0[b]	0	1.2	20	40
Tremorine	0	—	0	0.5	0	0	0	0.5	0	0	0	0	0	0	0.1	1	20
Triamcinolone	−1	3	3	3	2	2	0	−3	−1	−3[a]	−1	0	−3[b]	0	−0.1	10	30
Tribromoethanol	0	3	3	3	3	3	0	3	0	0[a]	−1	0	0[b]	0	1.1	18	60
Trichloroethanol	3	3	3	2	3	2	0	3	0	0	0	0	−2	1	1.3	20	60
3,3,5-Triiodo-L-thyronine	0	0	0.5	0	0	1	0	−1.5	0	−1	0	0	−0.5	0	−0.1	2	10
Tri-o-cresyl phosphate	−1	−1	0	0	0	−0.5	0	−0.5	0	−1	0	0	0	1	−0.2	1	10
d-Tubocurarine	0	3	3	3	3	2	0	3	2	3	0	0	0	0	1.6	22	60
Tyramine HCl	0	0	0.5	0	1	1	0	1	0	2	1	0	0	0	0.5	7	40
L-Tyrosine	3	3	3	3	2	1	0	1.5	1	1.5[a]	0	0	0.5	−1	0.6	18	60
W 1372 (40 mg)	2	3	1.5	1.5	3	1.5	1	0	1.5	0	1	0.5	2	0	1.4	20	80
Warfarin	0	0	0	1	0	0	0	0	0	0	0	0	0	0	0.1	1	10
Zoxazolamine	1	3	2	2	1	0	0	0	0	0	0	0	0	0	0.6	9	40

Third Step: Identification of Damaging Agents Amenable to Prophylaxis

phenyramidol, picrotoxin, and piperidine. The PSI of these toxicants runs roughly parallel to their OPI, that is to say the agents whose toxicity is most significantly impeded by various prophylactics are, in general, also detoxified by the largest number of potentially prophylactic substances.

Several substrates in Table 138 are very amenable to detoxication but only by few compounds; hence, despite their great activity in one or two respects, they have extremely low general protective indexes. For example, mercuric chloride is almost completely detoxified by spironolactone, yet its overall amenability to protection is very low, because its detoxication depends upon a steroid-borne thioacetyl group. In this series of conditioners, such a substituent occurs only in this particular steroid. Similarly, the intoxications amenable to protection by glucocorticoids only (lathyrogens, ganglioplegics, croton oil, E. coli, pralidoxime, strychnine, ethylene glycol), give comparatively low overall protective indexes, because only two of the prophylactic substances tested possess strong glucocorticoid potency.

Reading the columns in Table 138 vertically, we confirmed that the best **protection against the largest number of toxicants** is offered by the typical catatoxic steroids: PCN, ethylestrenol, CS-1, spironolactone, norbolethone, and oxandrolone.

Furthermore, some systemic toxicants (e.g., cyclobarbital, methyprylon, SKF 525-A, d-tubocurarine) are combated both by catatoxic steroids and by the two glucocorticoids included in this series. Several other drugs (e.g., barbital, cinchophen, cocaine, ethion, meprobamate, picrotoxin, thiopental, tribromoethanol, trichloroethanol) are well detoxified by prednisolone but not by triamcinolone, although the latter is the more potent glucocorticoid. Presumably, prednisolone possesses both catatoxic and syntoxic properties. Yet, here again we must remember that such in vivo tests can only determine whether a compound is or is not amenable to detoxication by steroids that have syntoxic or catatoxic actions with respect to other substrates. Further investigations will be required to identify the underlying mechanism.

DOC, hydroxydione, estradiol and thyroxine are comparatively **ineffective** both as regards the intensity and the spectrum of protection. In fact, in many cases, pretreatment with thyroxine results in toxication rather than detoxication. In the computation of the OPI and PSI, the results of toxication are not deducted from those of detoxication, but merely considered as "O"; hence the aggravating effect of thyroxine emerges only from the MPI.

In general, intoxications that can be inhibited by catatoxic steroids are also amenable to **prophylaxis by phenobarbital.** Yet, here again, there are exceptions: chlordiazepoxide, cyclophosphamide, digitoxin, digitoxin + Na_2HPO_4 + corn oil, haloperidol, mephenesin, triamcinolone, tribromoethanol, and tubocurarine, though readily detoxified by most catatoxic steroids, are virtually resistant to phenobarbital. In several other instances, phenobarbital is effective, but much less so than the most potent catatoxic steroids. The converse is rarely if ever the case; among the intoxications tested, only strychnine and piperidine poisoning responded much better to phenobarbital than to catatoxic steroids, but perhaps here, the hypnotic effect of the drug played a special role.

It must be emphasized that we cannot draw far-reaching conclusions as to the **specificity of catatoxic and syntoxic steroid actions** from this experimental series, since in some groups, the number of experimental animals may have been too small to compensate for individual variations in susceptibility. Furthermore, the conditioners were administered in fixed amounts; dose effect curves would be required in each case to make more meaningful comparisons. Still even these data suffice to show that there are qualitative differences in the prophylactic actions of the various conditioning agents.

In surveying Table 138, it is striking how few conditioning agents induced a considerable **decrease in resistance** ($-$ 2.5 or more) to the toxicants tested. This is all the more noteworthy since overdosage with two drugs (the toxicant and the conditioning agent) might be expected to be more difficult to resist than treatment with the toxicant alone. Most of the apparent decreases in resistance were seen after conditioning with prednisolone and triamcinolone, but of course here the toxic effect of heavy glucocorticoid overdosage (loss of body weight with a predisposition for spontaneous infections) was probably the decisive factor. In addition, when given in combination with DOC-Ac + NaH_2PO_4, the glucocorticoids notoriously sensitize to myocardial necrosis. Furthermore, when triamcinolone was used as a toxicant, it was obvious a priori that additional treatment with the same or another glucocorticoid would aggravate the overdosage syndrome. It is perhaps more remarkable that intoxication with hydroquinone was greatly accentuated by triamcinolone.

Among the other steroids, let us point out that PCN appears to sensitize to the toxic effects of propionitrile, whereas estradiol considerably aggravates poisoning with OMPA and triamcinolone. Thyroxine markedly diminishes resistance to epinephrine and propionitrile, but to a lesser extent, it also accentuates the toxicity of several other agents and rarely offers protection.

Synoptic "Diagram Table"

The "Diagram Table" (Table 139) graphically summarizes the highlights of Table 138 except that:

1. The results are registered only for inhibitions (not for aggravations) of intoxications.

2. Intermediates between the four basic grades (0, 1, 2 and 3) are disregarded in that:

$\square$ = 0.5 or less
◉ = 1
◢ = 1.5 to 2
■ = 2.5 to 3

The absence of any sign indicates that the corresponding experiment has not been done.

3. Here, the toxicants are listed according to decreasing "Total OPI" values.

When thus arranged, it becomes particularly obvious that among the hormonal conditioning agents, PCN is effective against the largest number of toxicants and its protective potency roughly parallels that of phenobarbital at the dose levels employed here. However — as mentioned in discussing Table 138 — the parallelism in the protective value of these two compounds is not absolute. Tables 138 and 139 clearly show furthermore that (in addition to PCN) ethylestrenol, CS-1, spironolactone and oxandrolone have high protective potencies, prednisolone and progesterone are much less active, whereas triamcinolone, DOC, hydroxydione, estradiol and thyroxine protect only against very few toxicants.

Synoptic "Diagram Table"

Table 139. *"Diagram Table"* a

[Table showing compounds (rows) versus substances (columns: Phenobarbital, PCN, Ethylestrenol, CS-1, Spironolactone, Norbolethone, Oxandrolone, Prednisolone-Ac, Progesterone, Triamcinolone, DOC-Ac, Hydroxydione, Estradiol, Thyroxine) with pictorial symbols indicating grading levels. Compounds listed: Methyprilon, Picrotoxin, Indomethacin, Ethion, Cocaine, EPN, Cyclobarbital, Glutethimide, Ethylmorphine, Hexobarbital, Cycloheximide, Piperidine, Nicotine, Digitoxin, Phenyramidol, Progesterone, Meprobamate, DHT, SKF 525-A, Theophylline, Phenindione, LSD, Guthion, d-Tubocurarine, Aminopyrine, Thiopental, W 1372, Trichloroethanol, Tribromoethanol, L-Tyrosine, Mephenesin, Dioxathion, Colchicine, Cinchophen, Dig+Na$_2$HPO$_4$+Oil, PIT, Strychnine.]

---

a In this Table the compounds are enumerated in the same order as in Table 138. However, in the latter, grades of 0.5 or less were also considered whereas here they were taken as 0 (□). Furthermore, no distinction is made here between 1.5 and 2 or 2.5 and 3. This explains the minor discrepancies between the grading judged by the pictorial symbols and the sequence in which the compounds are listed.

858 Synopsis of Pharmaco-Chemical and Pharmaco-Pharmacologic Interrelations

Table 139 (continued)

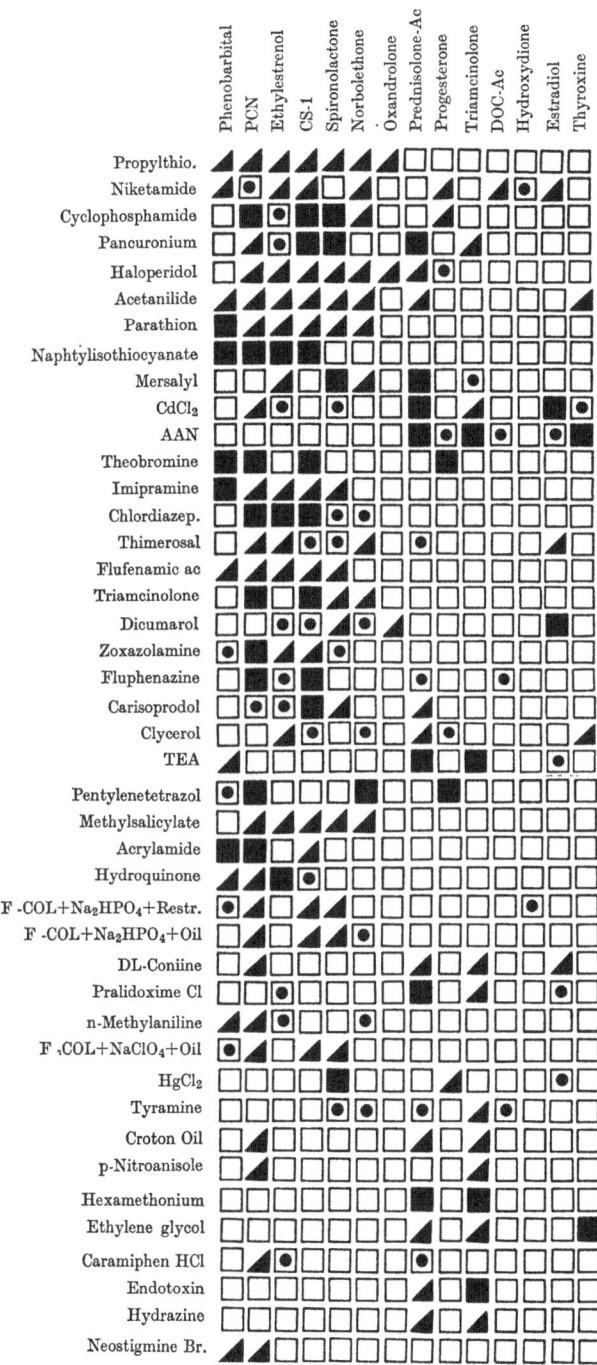

Table 139 (continued)

	Phenobarbital	PCN	Ethylestrenol	CS-1	Spironolactone	Norbolethone	Oxandrolone	Prednisolone-Ac	Progesterone	Triamcinolone	DOC-Ac	Hydroxydione	Estradiol	Thyroxine
Dipicrylamine	□	▲	□	▲	□	□	□	□	□	□	□	□	□	□
Emetin	□	▲	□	▲	□	□	□	□	□	□	□	□	□	□
Physostigmine	□	□	●	●	□	□	□	□	□	□	□	□	□	□
Diphenylhydantoin	●	□	□	●	●	□	□	□	□	□	□	□	□	□
DDT	▲	□	□	□	□	□	□	□	□	□	□	□	□	□
Pipradol	▲	□	□	□	□	□	□	□	□	□	□	□	□	□
Homatropine HBr	▲	□	□	□	□	□	□	□	□	□	□	□	□	□
Methadone	□	□	▲	□	□	□	□	□	□	□	□	□	□	□
Arsenic Pentoxide	●	□	□	□	□	●	□	□	□	□	□	□	□	□
DOC-Ac+NaH$_2$PO$_4$	□	□	□	□	□	□	□	□	□	□	□	□	□	▲
3,3,5-Triiodo-L-Thyronine	□	□	□	□	□	□	□	●	□	□	□	□	□	□
Barbital	□	□	□	□	□	□	□	□	▲	□	□	□	□	□
NaClO$_4$	□	□	□	□	□	□	□	□	□	□	□	□	□	▲
Doxepin	□	□	●	□	□	□	□	□	□	□	□	□	□	□
Warfarin	□	□	□	●	□	□	□	□	□	□	□	□	□	□
Tri-o-cresyl	□	□	□	□	□	□	□	□	□	□	□	□	□	●

No significant protection was obtained by any of the conditioners against:

DFP
TlCl
Propionitrile
Griseofulvin
DL-Amphetamine
Tremorine
Estradiol + NaH$_2$PO$_4$
Heptachlor
OMPA
Epinephrine
Mechlorethamine
o-Aminophenol
Fasting
Bile duct ligature
Bromobenzene
Brompheniramine
Dimercaprol
Dinitrophenol
Endrophonium
Yellow phosphorus
Ephedrine
Ethyl alcohol
Ethylene chlorohydrin
Nephrectomy
Methylphenidate
InCl$_3$
Morphine
Pyrilamine

Varia

Conney F88,649/67: A review of the literature on more than 200 drugs leads to the conclusion that "there is no apparent relationship between either their actions or structure and their ability to induce enzymes. It is of interest that most of the inducers are soluble in lipid at a physiological pH."

Moscona & Piddington F90,487/67: In retinal explants of 12-day chick embryos, glutamine synthetase activity can be induced by the addition of various corticoids to the culture medium. Cortisol, corticosterone and aldosterone are particularly active in this respect, whereas pregnenolone, progesterone, DOC, 11-desoxycortisol, 17α-hydroxyprogesterone, and 11α-hydroxyprogesterone had little activity. 11β-Hydroxyprogesterone and 11β,17α-dihydroxyprogesterone exhibited intermediate degrees of activity. Apparently, "the 11β-position is of primary significance in the activity of these molecules in inducing retinal glutamine synthetase in this system.

Table 140. *Effect of the standard conditioners upon body and organ weights*

Treatment[a]	Final body weight (g)	Liver weight (g)	Kidney weight (mg)	Preputial glands weight (mg)
None	131 ± 2	5.0 ± 0.1	533.1 ± 8.9	48.8 ± 1.9
PCN	130 ± 2 NS	7.4 ± 0.2 ***	518.4 ± 8.0 NS	51.4 ± 2.3 NS
CS-1	140 ± 3 *	6.4 ± 0.2 ***	528.7 ± 10.6 NS	68.9 ± 3.3 ***
Ethylestrenol	142 ± 3 **	5.8 ± 0.1 ***	512.8 ± 6.9 NS	106.5 ± 5.4 ***
Spironolactone	138 ± 2 **	5.9 ± 0.1 ***	484.9 ± 6.4 ***	47.1 ± 2.9 NS
Norbolethone	144 ± 3 ***	5.6 ± 0.2 **	529.0 ± 10.7 NS	99.7 ± 4.8 ***
Oxandrolone	135 ± 2 NS	5.1 ± 0.1 NS	520.1 ± 8.4 NS	88.0 ± 3.1 ***
Prednisolone-Ac	82 ± 1 ***	7.1 ± 0.2 ***	726.6 ± 12.2 ***	43.3 ± 2.9 NS
Triamcinolone (2 mg)	90 ± 2 ***	5.9 ± 0.2 ***	609.6 ± 10.4 ***	42.1 ± 2.8 NS
Progesterone	130 ± 3 NS	5.3 ± 0.1 NS	531.1 ± 6.3 NS	66.3 ± 2.6 ***
Estradiol	90 ± 3 ***	6.1 ± 0.3 ***	666.3 ± 17.0 ***	41.9 ± 4.6 NS
DOC-Ac	125 ± 2 NS	4.9 ± 0.1 NS	546.7 ± 8.3 NS	54.1 ± 2.5 NS
Hydroxydione	124 ± 2 *	4.9 ± 0.1 NS	546.5 ± 13.7 NS	56.9 ± 2.6 *
Thyroxine	127 ± 2 NS	5.7 ± 0.1 ***	618.7 ± 8.3 ***	54.8 ± 4.1 NS
Phenobarbital	129 ± 2 NS	6.8 ± 0.2 ***	554.7 ± 11.8 NS	62.0 ± 3.2 ***

[a] 25 ♀ 100 g rats per group. All treatments were given at the standard dose levels (*cf.* p. VIII) from the 1st to the 8th day. Final body weights were registered on the 9th day at which time the organs were fixed in formalin saturated with picric acid. All organ weights are listed as a percentage of the final body weight. (Student's t-test comparing all weights with the corresponding values of the untreated controls.)

For further details on technique of tabulation, *cf.* p. VIII.

This conclusion is further supported by the fact that cortisone, which has a ketone group in the 11-position, had no effect under these conditions."

Wattenberg et al. G71,805/68: In rats, the relationship between chemical structure and benzpyrene hydroxylase activity was studied on a large series of 2-phenylbenzothiazoles. "Introduction of an appropriate halogen into the 4'-phenyl position approximately doubles inducing activity compared to unsubstituted 2-phenylbenzothiazole. Other substitutions and modifications of the molecule result in either lesser increases in inducing activity or, in some instances, reduction or total loss of inducing activity. Most compounds show similar inducing effects on both lung and liver."

Selye G70,421/70: 304 Steroid were tested for their ability to protect rats against usually fatal intoxication with indomethacin or digitoxin. Using a "Simplified Activity Grading" system, 65 among these compounds were found to be active against indomethacin, 54 against digitoxin, and 23 against both substrates at a 10 mg dose level. But only 4 of these steroids were still capable of inhibiting one or both of these substrates at the 0.5 mg dose level. The only steroid still active against both substrates at the dose of 0.2 mg was pregnenolone carbonitrile "PCN" (3β-hydroxy-20-oxo-5-pregnene-16α-carbonitrile).

Selye G70,480/71: A review (28 pp., 111 refs.) on "Hormones and Resistance." The historic developments and present status of our concept of syntoxic and catatoxic steroids is summarized and the standard techniques for the in vivo bioassay of protective hormones are described at length.

Solymoss et al. G60,084/71: In rats, ethylestrenol, norbolethone, progesterone, triamcinolone, prednisolone and hydroxydione exhibited no antimineralocorticoid properties (Kagawa's test). Thus, the catatoxic effect of steroids appears to be unrelated to antimineralocorticoid potency.

Selye PROT. 43477: In otherwise untreated 100 g ♀ rats, the influence of the most commonly used conditioners upon the final body and organ weights (the latter expressed as a percentage of the body weight) has been determined for comparison with the experiments in which such conditioning agents were given conjointly with toxicants. After eight days of treatment, the final *body weight* was diminished

Table 140 (continued)

Uterus weight (mg)	Ovary weight (mg)	Thymus weight (mg)	Thyroid weight (mg)	Adrenal weight (mg)
149.6 ± 31.0	11.3 ± 0.8	244.5 ± 14.3	6.8 ± 0.2	14.2 ± 0.3
164.0 ± 27.1 NS	7.9 ± 0.8 **	267.2 ± 8.7 NS	9.0 ± 0.4 ***	15.9 ± 0.4 **
133.8 ± 13.0 NS	10.3 ± 0.7 NS	234.7 ± 19.4 NS	8.5 ± 0.4 **	12.4 ± 0.3 ***
183.4 ± 12.5 NS	8.5 ± 0.6 **	137.6 ± 9.2 ***	7.4 ± 0.6 NS	10.4 ± 0.3 ***
147.0 ± 26.3 NS	9.0 ± 0.7 *	253.2 ± 12.1 NS	7.3 ± 0.6 NS	12.2 ± 0.3 ***
168.6 ± 13.2 NS	7.0 ± 0.7 ***	157.5 ± 11.6 ***	8.2 ± 0.4 **	10.8 ± 0.4 ***
331.1 ± 29.9 ***	9.5 ± 0.5 NS	174.2 ± 8.9 ***	7.4 ± 0.4 NS	12.5 ± 0.3 ***
144.3 ± 8.4 NS	10.6 ± 0.6 NS	19.3 ± 1.5 ***	10.0 ± 0.6 ***	10.1 ± 0.5 ***
105.8 ± 12.7 NS	13.1 ± 0.9 NS	25.0 ± 2.0 ***	8.2 ± 0.4 *	10.6 ± 0.8 ***
144.5 ± 37.1 NS	7.8 ± 0.7 **	249.4 ± 16.8 NS	7.2 ± 0.5 NS	12.4 ± 0.3 ***
535.2 ± 98.4 **	14.7 ± 1.6 NS	63.7 ± 8.4 ***	8.3 ± 0.3 **	19.6 ± 0.8 ***
144.9 ± 37.1 NS	8.7 ± 0.7 *	217.9 ± 16.0 NS	8.0 ± 0.4 *	12.8 ± 0.4 *
155.3 ± 46.3 NS	8.4 ± 0.8 *	279.3 ± 23.3 NS	8.2 ± 0.5 *	15.0 ± 0.7 NS
74.5 ± 9.8 *	6.7 ± 0.7 ***	243.5 ± 17.5 NS	6.2 ± 0.4 NS	15.0 ± 0.6 NS
137.7 ± 31.3 NS	10.4 ± 0.8 NS	290.9 ± 14.9 *	10.0 ± 0.4 ***	15.5 ± 0.5 *

by prednisolone, triamcinolone and estradiol. To a lesser extent, hydroxydione also caused a decrease in body weight gain, but this may have been due to the prolonged daily anesthetic effect of this steroid. The rats treated with anabolics, particularly ethylestrenol and norbolethone, showed a body weight increase but this was not pronounced during this short time experiment. Although oxandrolone likewise proved to be anabolic in earlier experiments (in that it combated the catabolism produced by DHT or glucocorticoids) it did not cause an absolute increase in body weight. When organ weights were expressed as percentages of the final body weight, significant *hepatic* enlargement was obtained by PCN, CS-1, spironolactone, norbolethone, prednisolone, triamcinolone, estradiol and phenobarbital. This is of interest since triamcinolone and estradiol are virtually devoid of catatoxic potency. Among all steroids, PCN caused the greatest hepatic enlargement, exceeding even that elicited by phenobarbital. The percental increase in *renal* weight was especially conspicuous following treatment with prednisolone, triamcinolone, estradiol and thyroxine, although the glucocorticoids and estradiol markedly diminished the absolute final body weight of these same animals. Phenobarbital and PCN caused no renal enlargement. The *preputial glands* are only imperfect indicators of testoid activity. Our earlier experiments showed that ordinary pregnenolone (3β-hydroxy-5-pregnen-20-one) possesses a pronounced preputial gland stimulating effect, although it is virtually devoid of typical testoid actions upon the capon's comb or the castrate rat's seminal vesicles. The insignificant increase in preputial gland weight, observed under our experimental conditions following treatment with PCN, suggests that the attachment of the carbonitrile group to this molecule decreases rather than increases its preputial gland stimulating action. In any event, the compound is much less "virilizing" under these conditions than is progesterone. The preputial glands were most markedly enlarged following treatment with ethylestrenol, norbolethone and oxandrolone, but to a lesser extent also by CS-1, progesterone and phenobarbital, perhaps owing to the endogenous production of testoid metabolites. As expected, *uterine* enlargement was greatest after treatment with estradiol, but some increase in uterine weight was noted also under the influence of oxandrolone, whereas thyroxine had an inverse effect. None of the conditioners tested caused *ovarian* enlargement, but PCN, ethylestrenol, norbolethone, progesterone and thyroxine induced significant ovarian atrophy. The *thymus* weight was most markedly diminished by prednisolone, triamcinolone and estradiol, but to a lesser extent also by ethylestrenol, norbolethone and oxandrolone. Curiously, phenobarbital appears to have caused a barely significant and PCN a nonsignificant increase in thymus weight. Phenobarbital, prednisolone,

PCN, CS-1, norbolethone and estradiol also increased the weight of the *thyroid* approximately in decreasing order as enumerated. The most pronounced *adrenal* hypertrophy was elicited by estradiol, but minor degrees were also obtained by PCN and phenobarbital. Possibly, detoxication of endogenous corticoids might have led to a compensatory hypertrophy of this magnitude. On the other hand, CS-1, ethylestrenol, spironolactone, norbolethone, oxandrolone, prednisolone, triamcinolone, progesterone and DOC caused a diminution of the percental adrenal weight, *cf.* Table 140, p. 860.

Selye PROT. 22393: There appears to be no obligatory relationship between glucocorticoid and catatoxic activity. Thus, large doses of prednisolone offer excellent protection against the ulcerogenic effect of indomethacin, whereas triamcinolone, a much more potent glucocorticoid, is devoid of this protective effect over a broad dose range *cf.* Table 141.

Solymoss PROT. 42234: As judged by the Kagawa test, PCN is practically devoid of antimineralocorticoid activity. In male adrenalectomized adult rats, 6 μg of DOC s.c. produced a pronounced decrease in the urinary Na/K excretion, which could not be counteracted by 1 mg of PCN.

Table 141. *Glucocorticoid potency not responsible for inactivation of indomethacin by prednisolone*

Treatment (mg)[a]	Intestinal ulcers (%)[b]	Mortality (Dead/Total)[b]
None	100	5/5
Triamcinolone 0.1	100	5/5
Triamcinolone 0.5	100	5/5
Triamcinolone 10	100	5/5
Prednisolone 0.1	100	5/5
Prednisolone 0.5	100	4/5
Prednisolone 10	0	0/5

[a] In addition to the treatments listed in this column, the rats (100 g ♀) of all groups received indomethacin 1 mg in 0.2 ml water/day, s.c., on 4th day ff. Triamcinolone and prednisolone were given at the doses indicated in 1 ml water × 2/day, p.o., 1st day ff.

[b] Intestinal ulcers (% positive) and mortality on 10th day.

SUMMARY AND OUTLOOK

This treatise attempts to outline the history and present status of research on the regulation of resistance by hormones. It would obviously be impossible to give a meaningful résumé of this vast field here, but it may be helpful to summarize the highlights of the research with which our group has had personal experience, namely: the effect of natural and artificial steroids upon comparatively nonspecific resistance phenomena.

The protective agents are classified, according to their mechanism of action, into two main groups: 1. "syntoxic" compounds which improve tissue tolerance by permitting a symbiotic type of coexistence with the pathogen (e.g., by suppressing inflammatory reactions); 2. "catatoxic" substances which actually destroy the aggressor (e.g., through the induction of hepatic microsomal enzymes).

The syntoxic effects are virtually limited to glucocorticoids, and since these have received sufficient attention in the past, this monograph deals primarily with recent studies on catatoxic steroids.

We have tested more than 500 steroids, under comparable conditions, for their possible protective effect against numerous toxicants. The results of these studies are tabulated and their evaluation revealed the following principal facts:

1. **The catatoxic effect can manifest itself independently of all classic hormonal actions,** although it is frequently associated with anabolic, antimineralocorticoid or glucocorticoid properties.

2. Some of the most potent catatoxic steroids are **carbonitriles**; these also have an unusually broad "spectrum of activity", in that they protect against many toxicants.

3. The **16α-position of the —CN group** appears to be particularly advantageous for catatoxic activity. Its introduction into a virtually ineffective steroid, e.g., 5-pregnenolone, endows the latter with sufficient catatoxic potency to protect a rat, at dose levels as low as 300 μg/kg, against fatal digitoxin or indomethacin intoxication.

4. Steroids may serve as especially favorable **carriers** of pharmacologically active groups, for example of thioacetyl (for the detoxication of mercury), quaternary ammonium bases (for the induction of a neuromuscular block), oncolytic agents, etc.

5. Certain catatoxic steroids possess **abortifacient** properties and interfere with **lactation.**

6. It is not yet proven that effective amounts of catatoxic steroids are normally **secreted in response to a need** (as glucocorticoids are during stress). However, they certainly represent basic "**soil-factors**" determining normal resistance; for example testosterone in amounts secreted by the testis raises the resistance of male rats far above that of females or gonadectomized animals of either sex. Furthermore, corticosterone — the natural life-maintaining steroid of the rat — possesses catatoxic activity against several substrates and is undoubtedly secreted in response to a need during stress.

7. Certain substrates, which are not subject to inactivation by steroidal or nonsteroidal catatoxic compounds, can be "**opsonized**" (that is made amenable to this type of detoxication) by the addition of a radical. Thus, morphine is resistant, whereas ethylmorphine is highly sensitive, to inactivation by various compounds (catatoxic steroids, phenobarbital). This may well be due to a decrease in the polarity of the compound which may facilitate its penetration through membranes to the sites where enzymic detoxication can occur. It is interesting to speculate about the multitude of toxicants that might be made amenable to steroid-induced degradation if we learned how to stimulate their fat solubilization in vivo.

8. Many observations suggest that both syntoxic and catatoxic steroids may have important **clinical applications** in a variety of diseases caused by exogenous or endogenous toxicants. This is particularly true of maladies due to pathogens amenable to biotransformation by hepatic microsomal enzymes. In principle, here, enzyme induction would have to precede contact with the pathogen, and, hence, catatoxic steroids would be expected to have only prophylactic potency. Yet, if the pathogens act over a prolonged period (e.g., chronic indomethacin or digitoxin intoxication), curative effects have been obtained even when treatment was begun only after clinical manifestations of intoxication had become evident. Finally, if catatoxic steroids are important, "soil-factors" determining normal resistance, we should search for the possible existence of diseases caused by inadequate production of these compounds, or of disturbances in the responsiveness of the enzyme-inducing mechanisms which they regulate. Such maladies might be expected to result not only in deficient detoxication of exogenous pathogens but also in deficient or excessive degradation of endogenous chemical constituents of the body, such as hormones and metabolites.

As we have said in the Introduction to this monograph, animals are endowed with a complex hormonal defense system comparable in its scope to those based upon nervous, or immunologic reactions. Through conscious planning of defense, conditioned reflexes, or autonomic "emergency reactions," the body can adapt standard responses of its nervous system to defense against a multitude of specific injuries. Appropriate immunologic reactions can adjust the basic phenomenon of antibody formation to cope with a great variety of potential pathogens which possess antigenic properties.

The main purpose of this monograph was to show that there exists a third general adaptive system in which a group of hormones and hormone derivatives (particularly steroids) offer resistance to agents not easily combated through the first-mentioned two defensive mechanisms; here, syntoxic hormones help to tolerate a pathogen, whereas catatoxic substances destroy it.

The 35 years of research — from the first description of the defensive role of corticoids in combating stress, to the latest observations on the extraordinary catatoxic potency of steroid carbonitriles — represent only a rough outline of the introductory phase in the elucidation of the hormonal defense system. The many references cited in the preceding pages clearly show that even in this first sketch, our own observations provided only a small percentage of the established facts. We have raised more questions than we have answered; but perhaps, by providing an inventory of pertinent facts, this monograph will help others to clarify this new field, which appears to have implications in virtually all phases of homeostasis under physiologic and pathologic conditions.

REFERENCES

Abbott, D. D., Harrisson, W. E.: Further study of the effect of salicylates upon the osseous tissue of young rats. *Fed. Proc.* 24, 640 (1965). [F 36,510/65

Abderhalden, E.: Weitere Beiträge zur Kenntnis von Nahrungsstoffen mit spezifischer Wirkung. XXIII. Vergleichende Versuche über das Verhalten von schilddrüsenlosen Meerschweinchen und solchen, die Schilddrüsen besitzen, gegenüber einer Nahrung, die zum Skorbut führt. *Pflügers Arch. ges. Physiol.* 198, 164—168 (1923). [13,399/23

Abderhalden, E.: Der gegenwärtige Stand der Erforschung der Abwehrfermente (Abwehr-Proteinasen). In: *Schweizerischen medizinischen Jahrbuch 1933.* Basel: Benno Schwabe and Co. 1933. [67,622/33

Abderhalden, E., Wertheimer, E.: Versuche über den Einfluß des Geschlechts auf die Alkoholwirkung. *Biochem. Z.* 186, 252 (1927). [A 49,424/27

Abderhalden, E., Wertheimer, E.: Studien über die Wirkung des Thyroxins auf den tierischen Organismus und insbesondere auf die Wärmeregulation des Gleichwarmblüters. *Pflügers Arch. ges. Physiol.* 219, 588—608 (1928). [19,292/28

Abdul-Karim, R. W., Prior, J. T., Nesbitt, R. E. L. Jr.: Influence of maternal estrogen on fetal bone development in the rabbit. *Obstet. and Gynec.* 31, 346—353 (1968). [G 55,510/68

Abe, M., Langendorff, H.: Untersuchungen über einen biologischen Strahlenschutz. 60. Mitteilg.: Das Verhalten des Hodengewebes von Mäusen bei einmaliger oder wiederholter lokaler Bestrahlung unter Serotonin-Schutz. *Strahlentherapie* 125, 358—370 (1964). [G 23,763/64

Abelin, I.: Über die Beziehungen zwischen Carotin (Vitamin A) und Thyroxin. *Hoppe-Seylers Z. physiol. Chem.* 217, 109—114 (1933). [57,019/33

Abelin, I., Schönenberger, A.: Über den Antagonismus Dijodtyrosin: Thyroxin und über die Rolle der Diät bei der Hyperthyreose. *Z. ges. exp. Med.* 88, 528—542 (1933). [4,290/33

Abernathy, R.: The effect of cortisone on experimental brucellosis. *43rd Meet. Amer. Soc. clin. Invest.* p. 5 (1951). [B 57,911/51

Abernathy, R., Spink, W. W.: The influence of cortisone and adrenocorticotrophic hormone on brucellosis. I. Cortisone in experimentally infected animals. *J. clin. Invest.* 31, 947—957 (1952). [B 75,468/52

Abernathy, R. S., Spink, W. W.: Resistance to endotoxin after protection against initial lethal challenge with adrenocorticosteroids or chlorpromazine. *Proc. Soc. exp. Biol. (N.Y.)* 95, 580—581 (1957). [G 68,366/57

Abernathy, R. S., Spink, W. W.: Studies with brucella endotoxin in humans: the significance of susceptibility to endotoxin in the pathogenesis of brucellosis. *J. clin. Invest.* 37, 219—231 (1958). [C 48,635/58

Abraham, S., Kopelovich, L., Chaikoff, I. L.: Dietary and hormonal regulation of the hepatic citrate-cleavage enzyme. *Biochim. biophys. Acta (Amst.)* 93, 185—187 (1964). [G 20,214/64

Abrams, H. L.: Influence of age, body weight, and sex on susceptibility of mice to the lethal effects of X-radiation. *Proc. Soc. exp. Biol. (N.Y.)* 76, 729—732 (1951). [B 58,956/51

Adamkiewicz, V. W.: Insulin sensitization to the action of K-strophanthin. *Canad. J. Biochem.* 39, 9—13 (1961). [C 97,998/61

Adamkiewicz, V. W.: Glycemia and immune responses. *Canad. med. Ass. J.* 88, 806—811 (1963). [D 61,626/63

Adamkiewicz, V. W., Adamkiewicz, L. M.: Alloxan diabetes and dextran 'anaphylactoid' inflammation. *Amer. J. Physiol.* 197, 377—379 (1959). [C 73,760/59

Adamkiewicz, V. W., Kopacka, B., Fredette, V.: Rôle du diabète alloxanique dans la gangrène gazeuse expérimentale de la souris blanche. *Rev. canad. Biol.* 26, 153—157 (1967). [F 99,983/67

Adamkiewicz, V. W., Langlois, Y.: Sensitization by insulin to the dextran 'anaphylactoid' reaction. *Canad. J. Biochem.* 35, 251—256 (1957). [C 31,853/57

Adams, W. M., Wagner, W. C.: The role of corticoids in parturition. *Biol. Reprod.* **3**, 223—228 (1970). [G 80,309/70

Adelman, R. C.: Reappraisal of biological ageing. *Nature (Lond.)* **228**, 1095—1096 (1970). [H 32,850/70

Adlard, B. P. F., Lathe, G. H.: Breast milk jaundice: effect of 3α 20β-pregnanediol on bilirubin conjugation by human liver. *Arch. Dis. Childh.* **45**, 186—189 (1970). [G 74,759/70

Adler, T. K., Elliott, H. W., George, R.: Some factors affecting the biological disposition of small doses of morphine in rats. *J. Pharmacol. exp. Ther.* **119**, 475—487 (1957). [G 79,852/57

Adlercreutz, H.: Oestrogen metabolism in liver disease. *J. Endocr.* **46**, 129—163 (1970). [H 21,321/70

Adlersberg, D., Wang, C. I., Schaefer, L. E.: Extreme elevation of plasma lipids in the cholesterol-fed rabbit treated with cortisone and hydrocortisone. *J. clin. Invest.* **32**, 550 to 551 (1953). [B 82,951/53

Adolph, E. F.: Lethal limits of cold immersion in adult rats. *Amer. J. Physiol.* **155**, 378—387 (1948). [B 35,581/48

Agarkov, F. T., Maximovich, V. A., Namyatny, A. N.: The significance of adrenal glands for the thermal resistance of the body. (Russian text.) *Probl. Endokr. Gormonoter.* 8/15, 15—21 (1962). [D 40,496/62

Agarwal, M. K., Berry, L. J.: Effect of RES-active agents on tryptophan pyrrolase activity and endotoxin lethality. *J. reticuloendoth. Soc.* **3**, 223—235 (1966). [G 66,479/66

Agarwal, M. K., Berry, L. J.: Influence of reticuloendothelial-active agents on inducible liver enzymes in mice. *J. reticuloendoth. Soc.* **4**, 490—509 (1967). [G 66,480/67

Agarwal, M. K., Berry, L. J.: Reticuloendothelial response and liver enzyme induction in relation to endotoxicosis in mice. *Biochem. Med.* **2**, 274—285 (1969). [G 65,866/69

Agarwal, M. K., Hoffman, W. W., Rosen, F.: The effect of endotoxin and thorotrast on inducible enzymes in the isolated, perfused rat liver. *Biochim. biophys. Acta (Amst.)* **177**, 250—258 (1969). [G 65,716/69

Agduhr, E.: Ergosterin erhöht die Fruchtbarkeit bei den Versuchstieren, und die normalen sexuellen Funktionen steigern ihre Widerstandskraft gegenüber der Toxitität des Ergosterins. *Z. mikr.-anat. Forsch.* **36**, 576 bis 588 (1934). [52,908/34

Agduhr, E.: Ergosterol increases the prolific capacity of the experimental animals, and normal sexual functions intensify their resisting power against the toxicity of the ergosterol. *Z. Vitaminforsch.* **4**, 54—65 (1935). [70,849/35

Agduhr, E.: Sexual intercourse increases the resisting power of the organism against injurious factors. *Skand. Arch. Physiol.* **77**, 2—4 (1937). [A 51,257/37

Agduhr, E.: Internal secretion and resistance to injurious factors. *Acta med. scand.* **99**, 387—424 (1939). [75,856/39

Agduhr, E.: Till kännedomen om på hormonell väg åstadkommen resistensökning och mekanismen härvid (Swedish text with German summary: Studien über hormonale Resistenzsteigerung und ihren Mechanismus). *Hygiea (Stockh.)* **104**, 1587—1598 (1941). [G 37,252/41

Agduhr, E.: Einiges über Methoden und Ergebnisse bei Forschung über resistenzfördernde Wirkungen der Sexualfunktionen. *Z. mikr.-anat. Forsch.* **49**, 589—615 (1941). [A 39,060/41

Agduhr, E.: Contributions to the knowledge of the mechanism behind the heightened resistance brought about by the normal sexual functions. *Läk.-Fören. Förh.* **47**, 1—54 (1941). [E 70,688/41

Aggeler, P. M., O'Reilly, R. A.: Effect of heptabarbital on the response to bishydroxycoumarin in man. *J. Lab. clin. Med.* **74**, 229—238 (1969). [G 68,730/69

Agnoli, R. T.: Study of pituitary hormones. IV. Relation between hypophysis hormones and vitamin C. *J. Pharmacol. exp. Ther.* **44**, 47—53 (1932). [2,633/32

Agostini, L., Giagheddu, M.: The effect of hormones on experimental catalepsy induced by reserpine. IV. On testosterone, follicular hormone, corticosteroids and adrenaline. *Riv. Neurobiol.* 9/1, 32—40 (1963). [G 14,490/63

Aird, R. B.: The effect of desoxycorticosterone in epilepsy. *J. nerv. ment. Dis.* **99**, 501 to 510 (1944). [B 683/44

Aitio, A., Hänninen, O.: The activities of rat liver alanine, aspartate and tyrosine aminotransferases during the administration of cinchophen. *Ann. Med. exp. Fenn.* **45**, 239 to 242 (1967). [G 66,417/67

Akerrén, Y.: Prolonged jaundice in the newborn associated with congenital myxedema. A syndrome of practical importance. *Acta paediat. (Uppsala)* **43**, 411—425 (1954). [G 76,866/54

Akoev, I. G., Lagun, M. A., Klassovskii, Y. A.: Efficacy of hormone therapy of radiation effects. (Russian.) *Radiobiologiya* 5/6, 827—832 (1965). [F 73,202/65

Alam, S. Q., Boctor, A. M., Rogers, Q. R., Harper, A. E.: Some effects of amino acids and cortisol on tyrosine toxicity in the rat. *J. Nutr.* **93**, 317—323 (1967). [G 53,636/67

Albert, S.: Influence of testosterone on the morphogenetic actions of estradiol. *Endocrinology* **30**, 454—458 (1942). [A 37,132/42

Albert, S., Selye, H.: The effect of various pharmacological agents on the morphogenetic actions of estradiol. *J. Pharmacol. exp. Ther.* **75**, 308—315 (1942). [A 37,637/42

Aldrete, J. A., Homatas, J., Boyes, R. N., Starzl, T. E.: Effects of hepatectomy on the disappearance rate of lidocaine from blood in man and dog. *Anesth. Analg. Curr. Res.* **49**, 687—690 (1970). [G 78,399/70

Aldrete, J. A., Weber, M.: Le rôle du foie dans le métabolisme des agents anesthésiques; leur influence sur la physiopathologie hépatique. *Anest. Analg. Réanim.* **27**, 297—314 (1970). [G 75,396/70

Aldridge, W. N., Barnes, J. M.: Some problems in assessing the toxicity of the 'organophosphorus' insecticides towards mammals. *Nature (Lond.)* **169**, 345—347 (1952). [G 41,307/52

Alexander, C. S., Hunt, V. R.: Inhibition of aminonucleoside nephrosis in rats. II. Effect of nucleic acid precursors and L-triiodothyronine. *Proc. Soc. exp. Biol. (N.Y.)* **108**, 706—709 (1961). [D 20,284/61

Alexander, C. S., Hunt, V. R.: Evidence against immune mechanism in aminonucleoside nephrosis in rats. *J. Lab. clin. Med.* **62**, 103—108 (1963). [E 20,128/63

Allardyce, J., Fitch, F., Semple, R.: Amelioration of experimental hypertension. *Trans. roy. Soc. Can. Sect. 5*, **42**, 25—35 (1948). [B 29,416/48

Allegri, A., Campagnari, F., Paloschi, G.: Influenza del propionato di testosterone sulle lesioni epatiche indotte nei ratti da somministrazione prolongata di tetrachloruro di carbonio. *Arch. Sci. med.* **82**, 118—141 (1957). [C 31,532/57

Allegri, A., Ferrari, V.: Ormoni sessuali maschili e steatosi epatica. II. Azione del propionato di testosterone sulla steatosi epatica da fosforo. *Arch. Sci. med.* **88**, 440—453 (1949). [B 53,060/49

Allen, B. M., Ewell, L. M.: Resistance of X-irradiation by embryonic cells of the limbbuds of tadpoles. *J. exp. Zool.* **142**, 309—335 (1959). [C 92,110/59

Allison, A. C., Taylor, R. B.: Observations on thymectomy and carcinogenesis. *Cancer Res.* **27**, 703—707 (1967). [F 83,300/67

Alonso, A.: Efecto de la cicloheximida sobre la cancerizacion hepatica con dietilnitrosamina. *Rev. esp. Fisiol.* **26**, 347—364 (1970). [G 81,092/70

Alper, R., Rubulis, A., Prior, J. T., Ruegamer, W. R.: Effects of methylprednisolone on plasma lipids and aortic mucopolysaccharides of normal and cholesterol-fed rabbits. *Proc. Soc. exp. Biol. (N.Y.)* **129**, 623—627 (1968). [H 5,589/68

Alper, R., Ruegamer, W. R.: Hormonal effects on the acid mucopolysaccharide composition of the rat aorta. *J. Atheroscler. Res.* **10**, 19—32 (1969). [H 17,023/69

Altieri, N., Bazerque, P., Denti, A.: Influencia de la tiroides sobre la acción del aloxano en la rata. *Rev. Soc. argent. Biol.* **34**, 331—334 (1958). [C 71,565/58

Altucci, P., Coraggio, F., Pecori, V.: L'ormone somatotropo in alcune infezioni virali sperimentali in culture di cellule e in vivo. *G. Mal. infett.* **14**, 418—425 (1962). [D 65,819/62

Altucci, P., Coraggio, F., Pecori, V.: Il prednisolone ed i suoi derivati nelle infezioni virali sperimentali in culture di cellule in vitro ed in vivo nel topo. *G. Mal. infett.* **14**, 403—417 (1962). [D 65,818/62

Altura, B. M., Hsu, R., Mazzia, V. D. B., Hershey, S. C.: Effects of vasopressors on the microcirculation and on survival in bowel ischemia shock. *Fed. Proc.* **24**, 340. (1965). [F 36,124/65

Altura, B. M., Hsu, R., Mazzia, V. D. B., Hershey, S. G.: Influence of vasopressors on survival after traumatic, intestinal ischemia and endotoxin shock in rats. *Proc. Soc. exp. Biol. (N.Y.)* **119**, 389—393 (1965). [F 43,209/65

Amante, S.: Azione dell'ormone somatotropo ipofisario in condizioni sperimentali di shock e reazione di allarme. *Arch. Sci. med.* **106**, 702—719 (1958). [C 62,537/58

Amante, S., Mancini, M.: Antitiroidei e reazione d'allarme. (Ricerche sperimentali). *Gazz. int. Med. Chir.* **61**, 1146—1158 (1956). [C 21,222/56

Ambre, J. J.: The effect of prednisolone on the metabolism of 5-fluorouracil in vivo. (Abstr.). *Fed. Proc.* **29**, 610 (1970). [H 24,704/70

Ambrus, J. L., Ambrus, C. M., Leonard, C. A., Moser, C. E., Harrisson, J. W. E.: Synergism between histamine, antihistamines, and hypnotic drugs. *J. Amer. pharm. Ass. sci. Ed.* **41**, 606—608 (1952). [C 16,607/52

Amici, A.: Sul comportamento di Mus musculus trattati con iniezione contemporanea di dosi letali di stricnina e varie sostanze adrenalinosimili. *Riv. Biol.* **46**, 273—293 (1954).
[C 5,836/54

Anan, S.: Über den Einfluß des Schilddrüsenhormons auf die Giftwirkung von verschiedenen Opiumalkaloiden. *Folia pharmacol. jap.*, **8**, 17—41 (1929). [24,228/29

Anas, P., Neely, W. A., Hardy, J. D.: Effects of vasoactive drugs on oxygen consumption in endotoxin shock. *Arch. Surg.* **98**, 189—193 (1969). [G 64,139/69

Anderson, B. G.: Potency and duration of action of triiodothyronine and thyroxine in rats and mice. *Endocrinology* **54**, 659—665 (1954). [B 94,669/54

Anderson, R. E., Doughty, W. E., Leonard, L.: Parabiotic intoxication in neonatally thymectomized germ-free mice. *Arch. Path.* **87**, 469—473 (1969). [H 11,186/69

Anderson, T. A., Hubbert, F. Jr., Roubicek, C. B.: Effect of thyroxine, thiouracil and ambient temperature on the utilization of vitamin A by vitamin A-deficient rats. *J. Nutr.* **82**, 457—462 (1964). [G 11,709/64

Andersson, B., Ekman, L., Hökfelt, B., Jobin, M., Olsson, K., Robertshaw, D.: Studies of the importance of the thyroid and the sympathetic system in the defence to cold of the goat. *Acta physiol. scand.* **69**, 111—118 (1967).
[G 45,246/67

Andervont, H. B., Dunn, T. B.: Effect of castration and sex hormones on the induction of tumors in mice with o-aminoazotoluene. *J. nat. Cancer Inst.* **7**, 455—461 (1947).
[A 96,182/47

Andervont, H. B., Grady, H. G., Edwards, J. E.: Induction of hepatic lesions, hepatomas, pulmonary tumors, and hemangioendotheliomas in mice with o-aminoazotoluene. *J. nat. Cancer Inst.* **3**, 131—153 (1942). [A 94,080/42

Andreani, D.: Inibizione del fenomeno di Halpern e Martin mediante somministrazione di ACTH. *Boll. Soc. ital. Biol. sper.* **26**, 1603—1604 (1950). [B 63,732/50

Andreani, D., Marescotti, V., Giacomelli, F.: L'azione tossica della T.E.M. nei ratti trattati con corticotropina e cortisone. *Boll. Soc. med.-chir. Pisa* **23**, 593—606 (1955).
[C 14,628/55

Andrews, W. H. H.: The blood flow of the liver. *Brit. med. Bull.* **13**, 82—86 (1957). [D 94,471/57

Andriole, V. T., Cohn, G. L.: Estrogen and the pathogenesis of hematogenous pyelonephritis in the rat. *Clin. Res.* **11**, 408 (1963). [G 807/63

Angel, C., Burkett, M. L.: Adrenalectomy, stress and the bloodbrain barrier. *Dis. nerv. Syst.* **27**, 389—393 (1966). [G 39,712/66

Angela, G. C., Nola, F. di: Effetto del cortisone sullo sviluppo della Coxiella burnetii nell'uovo fecondato e nelle cavie. *G. Mal. infett.* **6**, 488—492 (1954). [C 12,561/54

Angelakos, E. T., Daniels, J. B.: Effect of catecholamine infusions on lethal hypothermic temperatures in dogs. *J. appl. Physiol.* **26**, 194—196 (1969). [G 64,739/69

Anonymous: Phenobarbitone and dicophane in jaundice. *Lancet* **1969 II**, 144—145. [H 19,246/69

Antona, G.: Rilievi preliminari sulle possibilità d'impiego della 5-ossitriptamina per la prevenzione del sanguinamento nel corso di interventi chirurgici. *Farmaco Ed. sci.* **10**, 86—90 (1955). [C 11,379/55

Antopol, W.: Anatomic changes produced in mice treated with excessive doses of cortisone. *Proc. Soc. exp. Biol. (N.Y.)* **73**, 262—265 (1950). [E 50,253/50

Appelmans, R.: Réponse à la note de Kepinow et Lanzenberg au sujet du phénomène de l'anaphylaxie chez les animaux thyroïdectomisés. *C. R. Soc. Biol. (Paris)* **88**, 1216 (1923).
[14,085/23

Aragona, F.: La capacità oncogena degli ormoni sessuali. II. Effetto delle sostanze androgene iniettate in animali con fegato leso. *Arch. De Vecchi Anat. pat.* **13**, 157—173 (1949). [B 53,747/49

Aragona, F.: Modificazioni ematiche e degli organi emopoietici in seguito a introduzione di ormoni estrogeni in animali con fegato leso. *Arch. E. Maragliano Pat. Clin.* **5**, 245—258 (1950). [B 53,056/50

Aragona, F., Barone, P.: Tiroide ed epatiti croniche sperimentali. *Arch. E. Maragliano Pat. Clin.* **8**, 511—534 (1953). [B 92,455/53

Araki, T.: The beneficial influence of corticotrophin, cortisol and nicotinamide on male mice exposed to cold stress, with special reference to the mode of action of nicotinamide. *J. Fac. Sci. (Tokyo)* **10**, 101—106 (1963).
[G 11,847/63

Arcasoy, M. M., Smuckler, E. A.: Acute effects of digoxin intoxication on rat hepatic and cardiac cells. Structural and functional changes in the endoplasmic reticulum. *Lab. Invest.* **20**, 190—201 (1969). [G 63,705/69

Arcuri, F., Fontana, G., de Lorenzi, F.: Considerazioni sull'associazione protidoanabolizzante alla terapia con steroidi di tipo cortisonico. *Minerva gastroent.* 8, 136—139 (1962). [D65,779/62]

Arias, I. M.: Effects of a plant acid (icterogenin) and certain anabolic steroids on the hepatic metabolism of bilirubin and sulfobromophthalein (BSP). *Ann. N.Y. Acad. Sci.* 104, 1014—1025 (1963). [D63,323/63]

Arias, I. M., Gartner, L. M.: Production of unconjugated hyperbilirubinaemia in full-term new-born infants following administration of pregnane-3(alpha), 20(beta)-diol. *Nature (Lond.)* 203, 1292—1293 (1964). [F21,711/64]

Arias, I. M., Gartner, L. M., Cohen, M., Ezzer, J. B., Levi, A. J.: Chronic nonhemolytic unconjugated hyperbilirubinemia with glucuronyl transferase deficiency. Clinical, biochemical, pharmacologic and genetic evidence for heterogeneity. *Amer. J. Med.* 47, 395—409 (1969). [G72,103/69]

Arias, I. M., Gartner, L. M., Seifter, S., Furman, M.: Neonatal unconjugated hyperbilirubinemia associated with breast-feeding and a factor in milk that inhibits glucuronide formation in vitro. (Abstr.). *J. clin. Invest.* 42, 913 (1963). [G76,756/63]

Arias, I. M., Gartner, L. M., Seifter, S., Furman, M.: Prolonged neonatal unconjugated hyperbilirubinemia associated with breast feeding and a steroid, pregnane-3(Alpha), 20(Beta)-Diol, in maternal milk that inhibits glucuronide formation in vitro. *J. clin. Invest.* 43, 2037 to 2047 (1964). [F24,502/64]

Ariëns, E. J.: Reduction of drug action by drug combination. *Fortschr. Arzneimittelforschg.* 14 11—58 (1970). [G79,943/70]

Arima, K.: Über den Einfluß des Thymusdrüsenhormons auf die Giftwirkung von einigen Opiumalkaloiden. *Folia Pharmacol. jap.* 21, 41—47 (1935). [60,156/35]

Ariyoshi, T., Takabatake, E.: Drug metabolism in ethionine induced fatty liver. *Life Sci.* 9, 371—377 (1970). [G75,246/70]

Arlander, T. R.: Actions of cortisone, vitamin B_{12}, and androgens on hearts, livers and kidneys of mice. *Anat. Rec.* 139, 203 (1961). [D5,055/61]

Arnold, H., Delbrück, A., Hartmann, F.: Beitrag zur Biochemie einer experimentellen Lebercirrhose und zur Möglichkeit, sie pharmakologisch zu beeinflussen. *Dtsch. Arch. klin. Med.* 209, 92—116 (1963). [E27,627/63]

Arnould, P., Lamarche, M., Jochum, F.: Influence de la cortisone sur la résistance à l'anoxémie chez le Cobaye non anesthésié. *C. R. Soc. Biol. (Paris)* 149, 557 (1955). [C12,257/55]

Aronsen, K. F., Grundsell, H., Ohlsson, E. G., Waldeskog, B.: Studies of the functional changes in the reticulo-endothelial and parenchymal cells of the liver following partial hepatectomy in dogs. *Acta chir. scand.* 135, 165—169 (1969). [H22,143/69]

Arora, R. B., Wig, K. L., Somani, P.: Effectiveness of hydrocortisone and hydrocortisone-antivenene combination against Echis carinatus snake venom. *Arch. int. Pharmacodyn.* 137, 299—306 (1962). [D27,786/62]

Arrigo, L., Pontremoli, S.: Azione dell'ormone corticotropo ipofisario sulla rigenerazione del fegato dopo parziale epatectomia. *Boll. Soc. ital. Biol. sper.* 26, 258—259 (1950). [B54,373/50]

Arrigo, L., Trasino, M.: Ormoni anteroipofisari e morfologia del pancreas esocrino. *Ormonologia* 15, 1—19 (1955). [C21,687/55]

Arrigoni-Martelli, E., Galimberti, P., Gerosa, V., Kramer, M., Melandri, M.: Synthesis and potentiating activity of some malonic and succinic derivatives. *Farmaco, Ed. sci.*, 15, 19—28 (1960). [G74,653/60]

Arrigoni-Martelli, E., Kramer, M.: Einfluß von Iproniazid und von Beta-phenylisopropylhydrazin (JB 516) auf die narkotische Wirkung und den Abbau von Hexobarbital und Thiopental. *Med. Exp.* (Basel) 1, 45—51 (1959). [G74,659/59]

Asagoe, T.: Biochemical studies on the development of experimental cirrhosis in albino rats induced by carbon tetrachloride. II. Study on the influence of cortisone upon the collagen contents in experimentally induced cirrhotic liver. (Japanese text.) *Jap. Arch. intern. Med.* 6, 1059—1064 (1959). [D13,524/59]

Asagoe, T.: Biochemical studies on the development of experimental cirrhosis in albino rats induced by carbon tetrachloride. III. Study on the influence of castration and testosterone propionate upon the collagen contents in experimentally induced cirrhotic liver. *Jap. Arch. intern. Med.* 7, 171—176 (1960). [D13,523/60]

Aschkenasy, A.: Protection exercée par la caséine contre l'ostéolathyrisme chez le rat mâle. Protection réduite chez le rat femelle et le rat mâle castré. *J. Physiol. (Paris)* 52, 10—11 (1960). [C90,362/60]

Aschkenasy, A.: Protection par la caséine alimentaire contre les lésions osseuses du lathyrisme chez le rat mâle. Protection réduite chez le rat femelle et le rat mâle castré. *C. R. Soc. Biol. (Paris)* 154, 556—560 (1960). [C91,685/60

Aschkenasy, A.: Action de la thyroxine et du propylthiouracile sur l'ostéolathyrisme du rat. *C. R. Soc. Biol. (Paris)* 156, 434—438 (1962). [D30,881/62

Aschkenasy, A.: Action de la surrénalectomie, de la cortisone et de l'hormone somatotrope sur l'ostéolathyrisme du rat. *C. R. Soc. Biol. (Paris)* 156, 470—475 (1962). [D30,892/62

Aschkenasy-Lelu, P.: L'hormone du sexe faible. Une étude critique des divers effets protecteurs des oestrogènes. *Rev. franç. Étud. clin. biol.* 9, 109—117 (1964). [G9,425/64

Asher, L., Wagner, H.: Untersuchungen über die Spezifität der Asherschen Methode der Prüfung der Schilddrüsenfunktion durch Sauerstoffmangel. *Z. ges. exp. Med.* 68, 32—81 (1929). [23,903/29

Ashford, A., Ross, J. W.: Toxicity of depressant and antidepressant drugs in hyperthyroid mice. *Brit. med. J.* 1968I, 217—218. [H2,686/68

Askew, B. M.: Hyperpyrexia as a contributory factor in the toxicity of amphetamine to aggregated mice. *Brit. J. Pharmacol.* 19, 245—257 (1962). [G72,695/62

Aspinall, R. L.: Differential effect of spironolactone on the ulcerogenic and antiinflammatory activities of indomethacin. *Proc. Soc. exp. Biol. (N.Y.)* 135, 561—564 (1970). [H32,269/70

Astarabadi, T.: The regression in the size of the hypertrophic remaining kidney after hypophysectomy in rats. *Quart. J. exp. Physiol.* 47, 93—97 (1962). [D8,815/62

Astarabadi, T. M., Essex, H. E.: Effect of epinephrine on male and female albino rats. *Amer. J. Physiol.* 171, 75—77 (1952). [B75,437/52

Astarabadi, T. M., Essex, H. E.: Effect of hypophysectomy on size of remaining kidney after ureteroduodenostomy and contralateral nephrectomy. *Proc. Soc. exp. Biol. (N.Y.)* 81, 25—28 (1952). [B75,446/52

Astarabadi, T. M., Essex, H. E.: Effect of hypophysectomy on compensatory renal hypertrophy after unilateral nephrectomy. *Amer. J. Physiol.* 173, 526—536 (1953). [B86,411/53

Aterman, K.: Effect of cortisone on early fibrosis of the liver in rats. *Lancet* 1950II, 517—519. [B52,265/50

Aterman, K.: Studies in fibrosis of the liver induced by carbon tetrachloride. II. A quantitative study of the effect of cortisone on fibrosis of the liver in rats. *Arch. Path.* 57, 12—25 (1954). [B92,038/54

Aterman, K.: The thyroid-adrenal relationship: the effect of cortisone and of thyroid hormone on hepatic necrosis of dietary origin in the rat. *Endocrinology* 60, 711—717 (1957). [C35,275/57

Aterman, K.: Aldosterone and experimental hepatic necrosis. *Nature (Lond.)* 182, 1324 (1958). [C61,786/58

Aterman, K.: Growth hormone and partial hepatectomy in diet-deficient rats. Effects on the hepatic necrosis produced in rats by a deficient diet. *Arch. Path.* 72, 666 (1961). [D15,536/61

Aterman, K., Ahmad, N. D.: Cortisone and liver function. *Lancet* 1953I, 71—73. [B76,967/53

Aterman, K., Howell, J. S.: The bromsulphthalein excretion test in hypothyroid rats. *Lab. Invest.* 8, 19—28 (1959). [C63,343/59

Atkinson, R. M., Pratt, M. A., Tomich, E. G.: A sex difference in sensitivity of GFF mice to an anaesthetic steroid. *J. Pharm. Pharmacol.* 14, 698 (1962). [D33,188/62

Aubert, C., Bohuon, C.: Dépigmentation produite chez le hamster doré par l'administration d'une dose per os de 9—10 diméthyl-1, 2-benzanthracène. Rôle de l'épiphysectomie. *C. R. Acad. Sci. (Paris)* 271, 281—284 (1970). [G77,483/70

Avant, W. E., Weatherby, J. H.: Effects of epinephrine on toxicities of several local anesthetic agents. *Proc. Soc. exp. Biol. (N.Y.)* 103, 353—356 (1960). [C81,325/60

Avezzu, G.: Alterazioni muscolari in corso di diabete allossanico ed interferenza del cloruro di cobalto. *Arch. Sci. med.* 103, 510—530 (1957). [C46,134/57

Avezzu, G., Fiaccadori, F., Scarpioni, L.: Su di alcune alterazioni morfologiche ed enzimatiche indotte nel rene mediante allossana e cortisone. *G. Clin. med.* 35, 1551—1577 (1954). [C12,653/54

Axelrod, J.: The enzymatic deamination of amphetamine (Benzedrine). *J. biol. Chem.* 214, 753—763 (1955). [E40,270/55

Axelrod, J.: The enzymatic N-demethylation of narcotic drugs. *J. Pharmacol. exp. Ther.* 116, 322—330 (1956). [D28,544/56

Axelrod, J.: The enzymic cleavage of aromatic ethers. *Biochem. J.*, 63, 634—639 (1956). [G 74,652/56

Axelrod, J.: Demethylation and methylation of drugs and physiologically active compounds. In: Brodie and Erdös; *Metabolic Factors Controlling Duration of Drug Action* 6, p. 97 to 110. New York: The MacMillan Co. 1962. [G 66,350/62

Axelrod, J.: Enzymatic formation of adrenaline and other catechols from monophenols. *Science* 140, 499—500 (1963). [D 64,159/63

Axelrod, J., Reichenthal, J., Brodie, B. B.: Mechanism of the potentiating action of β-diethylaminoethyl diphenylpropylacetate. *J. Pharmacol. exp. Ther.* 110, 49—54 (1954). [D 79,919/54

Aycock, W. L., Foley, G. E.: The enhancement of tuberculous infection in the guinea pig by steroid hormones. *J. clin. Endocr.* 5, 337—344 (1945). [B 773/45

Azarnoff, D. L., Grady, H. J., Svoboda, D. J.: The effect of DDD on barbiturate and steroid-induced hypnosis in the dog and rat. *Biochem. Pharmacol.* 15, 1985—1993 (1966). [G 42,999/66

Azarnoff, D. L., Svoboda, D. J.: Microbodies in experimentally altered cells. VI. Thyroxine displacement from plasma proteins and clofibrate effect. *Arch. int. Pharmacodyn.* 181, 386—393 (1969). [H 19,856/69

Baader, H., Girgis, S., Kiese, M., Menzel, H., Skrobot, L.: Der Einfluß des Lebensalters auf Umsetzungen von Phenacetin, p-Phenetidin, N-Acetyl-p-aminophenol, p-Aminophenol und Anilin im Hunde. *Naunyn-Schmiedebergs Arch. exp. pathol. Pharmak.* 241, 317—334 (1961). [D 43,960/61

Bächtold, H.: Die Beeinflussung des experimentellen Hochdrucks an der Ratte durch Methylthiouracil, Jod und Thyroxin. *Thesis.* Universität Basel (1950). [B 60,463/50

Bačić, M., Engström, L., Johannisson, E., Leideman, T., Diczfalusy, E.: Effect of F-6103 on implantation and early gestation in women. *Acta endocr. (Kbh.)* 64, 705—717 (1970). [H 28,711/70

Backman, A.: The influence of induced hyperthyroidism on experimental tuberculosis in mice. *Ann. Med. exp. Fenn.* 38, Suppl. 3, 1—56 (1960). [C 94,674/60

Backus, B., Cohn, V. H.: Genetic influences in metabolism of hexobarbital in mice. *Fed. Proc.* 25, 531 (1966). [D 92,313/66

Bacon, J. A., Patrick, H., Hansard, S. L.: Some effects of parathyroid extract and cortisone on metabolism of strontium and calcium. *Proc. Soc. exp. Biol. (N.Y.)* 93, 349—351 (1956). [C 26,675/56

Bacq, Z. M.: The amines and particularly cysteamine as protectors against roentgen rays. *Acta radiol. (Stockh.)* 41, 47—55 (1954). [D 77,006/54

Bacq, Z. M., Beaumariage, M. L.: Propriété radioprotectrice d'une préparation synthétique d'ocytocine (Syntocinon Sandoz) chez la souris. *Arch. int. Physiol.* 68, 516—518 (1960). [C 87,128/60

Bacq, Z. M., Herve, A., Lecomte, J., Fischer, P., Blavier, J., Dechamps, G., Le Bihan, H., Rayet, P.: Protection contre le rayonnement X par la β-mercaptoéthylamine. *Arch. int. Physiol.* 59, 442—447 (1951). [E 91,032/51

Badarau, L., Ristesco, G., Calinca, N.: L'effet nécrosant commun des stéroïdes ovariens et cortico-surrénaux sur le trophoblaste placentaire chez le rat, 'diminué ou annihilé' par l'injection des couples antagonistes des mêmes hormones. *Bull. Féd. Soc. Gynéc. Obstét. franç.* 20, 311—312 (1968). [G 69,247/68

Bader, G.: Elektronenmikroskopische Untersuchungen zur funktionellen Morphologie der regenerierenden Leberzelle nach partieller Hepatektomie. *Acta hepato-splenol. (Stuttg.)* 16, 281—297 (1969). [G 70,347/69

Baglioni, A., Console, V.: Insulina e beri-beri sperimentale del Colombo. *Arch. Fisiol.* 33, 564—577 (1934). [45,284/34

Bahr, C. von, Sjöqvist, F., Orrenius, S.: The inhibitory effect of hydrocortisone and testosterone on the plasma disappearance of nortriptyline in the dog and the perfused rat liver. *Europ. J. Pharmacol.* 9, 106—110 (1970). [H 21,089/70

Bailey, C. H.: The production of arteriosclerosis and glomerulonephritis in the rabbit by intravenous injections of diphtheria toxin. *J. exp. Med.* 25, 109—127 (1917). [A 1,154/17

Bailey, J. M., Butler, J., Macnamara, T., Roe, N.: Antiinflammatory steroids in experimental atherosclerosis. (Abstr.) *Fed. Proc.* 27, 440 (1968). [H 450/68

Baird, P. C. Jr., Cloney, E., Albright, F.: Effect of cortical hormone in preventing extreme drop in colonic temperature displayed by hypophysectomized rats upon exposure to cold with preliminary observations upon the effect of hypophyseal and other hormones. *Amer. J. Physiol.* 104, 489—501 (1933). [14,881/33

Baird, W. L. M.: Clinical experience with pancuronium. *Proc. roy. Soc. Med.* 63, 697 to 699 (1970). [H 27,487/70

Baird, W. L. M., Reid, A. M.: The neuromuscular blocking properties of a new steroid compound, pancuronium bromide. A pilot study in man. *Brit. J. Anaesth.* **39**, 775—780 (1967). [G 51,827/67

Baïsset, A., Boer, A., Montastruc, P.: Action des extraits post-hypophysaires dans la surcharge sodique prolongée. *C. R. Soc. Biol. (Paris)* **151**, 1253—1256 (1957). [C 55,475/57

Baïsset, A., Demonte, H., Montastruc, P.: Action des extraits post-hypophysaires et de la désoxycorticostérone dans la surcharge sodique. *Path. et Biol.* **7**, 815—827 (1958). [C 84,788/58

Baïsset, A., Montastruc, P.: Effet de l'hormone antidiurétique sur le besoin d'alcool créé par l'habitude. *C. R. Soc. Biol. (Paris)* **156**, 945—948 (1962). [D 34,473/62

Baïsset, A., Montastruc, P.: Effet de l'hormone antidiurétique sur la soif consécutive a l'ingestion d'alcool. *Ann. Endocr. (Paris)* **23**, 425—429 (1962). [D 37,918/62

Bajusz, E., Selye, H.: Effect of various hormones upon the muscular contractions induced by sodium perchlorate. *Acta pharmacol. (Kbh.)* **15**, 235—243 (1959). [C 57,180/59

Bajusz, E., Selye, H.: An experimental type of muscular dystrophy and role of chlorides in its prevention. *Proc. 2nd ann. Meet. Canad. Fed. Biol.* (Toronto) **2**, 5 (1959). [C 64,511/59

Baker, B. L., Ingle, D. J., Li, C. H., Evans, H. M.: The effect on liver structure of treatment with adrenocorticotropin under varied dietary conditions. *Amer. J. Anat.* **82**, 75—104 (1948). [B 26,490/48

Baker, B. L., Kent, J. F., Pliske, E. C.: Histological response of the duodenum to X-irradiation in hypophysectomized rats. *Radiat. Res.* **9**, 48—58 (1958). [C 56,998/58

Baker, R., Reaven, G., Sawyer, J.: Ground substance and calcification: the influence of dye binding on experimental nephrocalcinosis. *J. Urol. (Baltimore)* **71**, 511—522 (1954). [C 24,277/54

Balabanski, L., Dachev, G.: Le rôle du foie dans le métabolisme des hormones oestrogènes. *Rev. roum. Endocr.* **3**, 121—126 (1966). [F 68,584/66

Baldratti, G.: The biological evaluation of the anabolic activity. In: Martini and Pecile; *Hormonal Steroids, Biochemistry, Pharmacology and Therapeutics* 2, p. 173—180. New York, London: Academic Press Inc. 1965. [E 5,460/65

Baldratti, G., Sala, G., Mars, G.: Azione del 4-clorotestosterone acetate e del 4-cloro-19-nortestosterone acetate sull'ipotrofia surrenale indotta da cortisone. *Boll. Soc. ital. Biol. sper.* **33**, 342—345 (1957). [C 45,101/57

Bálint, R., Molnár, B.: Experimentelle Untersuchungen über gegenseitige Wechselwirkung innerer Secretionsprodukte. *Berl. klin. Wschr.* **48**, 289—292 (1911). [34,586/11

Ball, H. A., Samuels, L. T.: Hypophysis and detoxification. *Proc. Soc. exp. Biol. (N.Y.)* **30**, 26—27 (1932). [7,404/32

Ball, J. K., Dawson, D. A.: Biological effects of the neonatal injection of 7,12-dimethylbenz[a]anthracene. *J. nat. Cancer Inst.* **42**, 579—591 (1969). [G 67,723/69

Ballerini, G., Bosi, L.: Effects of serotonin, anti-serotonin and anti-histamine drugs on uracil-mustard intoxication. *Experientia (Basel)* **21**, 377—378 (1965). [G 31,956/65

Balner, H., Dersjant, H.: Neonatal thymectomy and tumor induction with methylcholanthrene in mice. *J. nat. Cancer Inst.* **36**, 513—521 (1966). [G 37,980/66

Baraldi, M.: Azione dell'elettrourto sul quadro isto-patologico prodotto dai 'tioureici' nei conigli. *Riv. sper. Freniat.* **74**, 3—14 (1950). [B 52,651/50

Barbazzo, M.: Tossina tifica e 17-idrossicorticosterone. *Ormonologia* **15**, 401 (1955). [C 13,021/55

Barbe, M.: Influence de la Δ'-déhydrocortisone sur le développement de l'oedème adrénalique expérimental. *C. R. Soc. Biol. (Paris)* **151**, 247—249 (1957). [C 46,902/57

Barbour, J. H., Seevers, M. H.: Narcosis induced by carbon dioxide at low environmental temperatures. *J. Pharmacol. exp. Ther.* **78**, 296 to 303 (1943). [84,296/43

Bardin, C. W., Bullock, L., Gram, T. E., Schroeder, D. H., Gillette, J. R.: End organ insensitivity to testosterone (T) in the pseudohermaphrodite rat (PS) (Abstr.). *Program 51st Meet. Endocr. Soc. New York, N.Y.*, p. 40 (1969). [H 12,120/69

Bardier, E., Stillmunkès, A.: Intoxication scorpionique et syncope adrénalino-chloroformique. *C. R. Soc. Biol. (Paris)* **88**, 559 a 561 (1923). [13,522/23

Bardier, E., Stillmunkès, A.: Syncope adrenaline-chloroformique et envenimations. (Venins de vipère et de scorpion.). *C. R. Soc. Biol. (Paris)* **94**, 1063—1064 (1926). [25,803/26

Barella, A.: Influenza della castrazione nell' ipertemia passiva. *Folia endocr. (Roma)* **18**,

121—129, 145—151, 169—175 (1940).
[B3,397/40

Bargeton, D., Krumm-Heller, C., de Fombelle, F.: Etude des conditions de dosage d'activité des corps à action antithyroidienne. *J. Physiol.* 41, 125—136 (1949). [B50,869/49

Bargon, G., Eger, W., Jr., Rittmeyer, K.: Die experimentelle Bestrahlungsnephritis unter Prednisolonbehandlung. *Strahlentherapie* 140, 192—203 (1970). [G78,255/70

Bar-Hay, J., Benderly, A., Rumney, G.: Treatment of a case of nontumorous Cushing's syndrome with o,p'DDD. *Pediatrics* 33, 239 to 244 (1964). [G1,283/64

Barker, E. A., Arcassoy, M., Smuckler, E. A.: A comparison of the effects of partial surgical and partial chemical (CCl_4) hepatectomy on microsomal cytochrome b_5 and P_{450} and oxidative N-demethylation. *Agents and Actions* 1, 27—34 (1969). [H13,059/69

Barksdale, B., Henson, E. C., Brunson, J. G.: Effects of epinephrine on the generalized Shwartzman reaction. *Arch. Path.* 89, 259—265 (1970). [H21,684/70

Barlow, J. C., Sellers, E. A.: The effect of growth hormone on recovery from exposure to X-radiation. *Radiat. Res.* 2, 461—466 (1955).
[C21,626/55

Bar-Maor, J. A., Ungar, J.: Effect of alpha-naphthyl -isothiocyanate (ANIT) on the mitotis rate of liver cells following partial hepatectomy. *Bull. Res. Coun. Israel E*, 9E, 79—96 (1961). [D41,800/61

Barnes, J. H., Lowman, D. M. R.: The effect of a monoamine oxidase inhibitor on radiation protection by 5-hydroxytryptophan. *Int. J. Radiat. Biol.* 14, 389—390 (1968). [G63,518/68

Barnes, J. H., Lowman, D. M. R.: Relative radioprotective abilities of 5-hydroxytryptophan and 5-hydroxytryptamine. *Int. J. Radiat. Biol.* 14, 87—88 (1969). [G64,917/69

Barnett, G. O., Teague, R. S.: The antagonism of salicylate to diethylstilbestrol upon liver glycogen in the rat. *Endocrinology* 63, 205—211 (1958). [C56,641/58

Baronofsky, I. D., Canter, J. W.: The effect of endocrinectomy on ascites with especial reference to adrenalectomy and thyroidectomy. *Amer. J. Surg.* 99, 512—518 (1960).
[C85,341/60

Barral, P., d'Arrac, C. H., Vairel, J.: Modifications de l'intensité du choc anaphylactique et du choc peptonique chez le cobaye préalablement insulinisé. *C. R. Soc. Biol. (Paris)* 109, 1363—1364 (1932). [8,858/32

Barral, P., Seguin, H., d'Arrac, C. H.: Importance de l'état glycémique préalable sur l'intensité du choc anaphylactique et du choc peptonique. Le glucose agent protecteur contre le choc. *C. R. Soc. Biol. (Paris)* 109, 1365—1366 (1932). [8,860/32

Barron, D. H.: Some factors influencing the susceptibility of albino rats to injections of sodium amytal. *Science* 77, 372—373 (1933).
[A42,858/33

Barta, L., Beregi, E.: Über Nebennierenblutung bei Alkoholintoxikation. *Z. ges. inn. Med.* 19, 785—787 (1964). [F24,783/64

Bartók, I., Varga, L., Varga, G.: Elektronenmikroskopische Veränderungen in der Rattenleber nach Verabreichung von dem oralen Antikonzeptionsmittel Lynestrenol. *Acta hepatosplenol. (Stuttg.)* 17, 1—10 (1970).
[G74,513/70

Basil, B., Somers, G. F., Woollett, E. A.: Measurement of thyroid activity by the mouse anoxia method. *Brit. J. Pharmacol.* 5, 315—322 (1950). [B53,039/50

Bates, R. R.: Sex hormones and skin tumorigenesis. I. Effect of the estrous cycle and castration on tumorigenesis by 7,12-dimethylbenz(a)anthracene. *J. nat. Cancer Inst.* 41, 559 to 563 (1968). [H13,409/68

Batliwalla, R. K., Deshpande, C. K.: Effects of cortisone in experimental diphtheritic myocarditis and diphtheritic intoxication in guinea-pigs. *Indian J. med. Sci.* 20, 780—789 (1966).
[G43,844/66

Batten, J. C., McCune, R. M. Jr.: The influence of corticotrophin and certain corticosteroids on populations of mycobacterium tuberculosis in tissues of mice. *Brit. J. exp. Path.* 38, 413—423 (1957). [C53,554/57

Baumann, C. A., Moore, T.: Thyroxine and hypervitaminosis-A. *Biochem. J.* 33, 1639 to 1644 (1939). [C38,599/39

Bauman, T. R., Turner, C. W.: The effect of varying temperatures on thyroid activity and the survival of rats exposed to cold and treated with L-thyroxine or corticosterone. *J. Endocr.* 37, 355—359 (1967). [F81,331/67

Bavetta, L. A., Bekhor, I., Nimni, M. E.: Effects of hormone administration on collagen biosynthesis in the rat. *Proc. Soc. exp. Biol. (N.Y.)* 110. 294—297 (1962). [D29,064/62

Bavetta, L. A., Bekhor, I., Shah, R., O'Day, P., Nimni, M. E.: Metabolic and anti-inflammatory properties of 6-methyl prednisolone alone and in combination with anabolic hormones. *Endocrinology* 71, 221—226 (1962).
[D29,035/62

Bavetta, L. A., Bernick, S., Ershoff, B. H.: Selective effects of growth hormone on rats fed a tryptophan-low diet. *Endocrinology* 59, 701 to 707 (1956). [C17,656/56

Bavetta, L. A., Bernick, S., Ershoff, B. H.: The influence of dietary thyroid on the bones and periodontium of rats on total and partial tryptophan deficiencies. *J. dent. Res.* 36, 13 to 20 (1957). [C47,327/57

Bavetta, L. A., Bernick, S., Ershoff, B. H.: Effects of growth hormone on the bone and periodontium of vitamin A-depleted rats. *Arch. Path.* 66, 610—617 (1958). [C60,277/58

Beach, E. F., Bradshaw, P. J., Blatherwick, N. R.: Alloxan diabetes in the albino rat as influenced by sex. *Amer. J. Physiol.* 166, 364—373 (1951). [B61,498/51

Bean, J. W., Bauer, R.: Thyroid in pulmonary injury induced by O_2 in high concentration at atmospheric pressure. *Proc. Soc. exp. Biol. (N.Y.)* 81, 693—694 (1952). [B76,951/52

Bean, J. W., Johnson, P.: Hypophyseal involvement in response to O_2 at high pressure. *Fed. Proc.* 11, 9 (1952). [B68,165/52

Bean, W. B., Ponseti, I. V.: Dissecting aneurysm produced by diet. *Circulation* 12, 185 to 192 (1955). [C29,403/55

Beaton, G. H., Beare, J., Ryu, M. H., McHenry, E. W.: Protein metabolism in the pregnant rat. *J. Nutr.* 54, 291—304 (1954). [A49,354/54

Beaton, G. H., Curry, D. M.: The resistance of pregnant rats to cortisone treatment. *Rev. canad. Biol.* 16, 465 (1957). [C42,333/57

Beaton, G. H., Curry, D. M., Veen, M. J.: Alanine-glutamic transaminase activity and protein metabolism. *Arch. Biochem.* 68, 288—290 (1957). [D83,636/57

Beaton, G. H., Ozawa, G., Beaton, J. R., McHenry, E. W.: Effect of anterior pituitary growth hormone on certain liver enzymes. *Proc. Soc. exp. Biol. (N.Y.)* 83, 781—784 (1953). [B86,367/53

Beaton, G. H., Ryu, M. H., McHenry, E. W.: Studies on the role of growth hormone in pregnancy. *Endocrinology* 57, 748—754 (1955). [C10,012/55

Beaton, J. R.: Previous dietary protein level and survival of starving rats in the cold. *Canad. J. Biochem.* 41, 171—178 (1963). [D55,998/63

Beatson, G. T.: On the treatment of inoperable cases of carcinoma of the mamma: suggestion for a new method of treatment with illustrative cases. *Lancet* 104, 162—165 (1896). [A50,749/1896

Beck, L. V.: Lethal and tumor-damaging effects of certain trivalent arsenicals, as modified by 2,3-dimercaptopropanol (BAL) and by adrenal extracts (Abstr.). *Cancer Res.* 10, 202 (1950). [B58,869/50

Beck, L. V.: Action of adrenal hormones on lethal toxicities of certain organic compounds. *Proc. Soc. exp. Biol. (N.Y.)* 78, 392—397 (1951). [B64,609/51

Beck, L. V., Voloshin, T.: Influence of adrenal hormones on toxic and tumor-damaging effects of certain substances. *Amer. J. Physiol.* 163, 696 (1950). [B58,271/50

Becker, F. F., Brenowitz, J. B.: The concentration of actinomycin D in hepatocyte nuclei as related to inhibition of ribonucleic acid synthesis. *Biochem. Pharmacol.* 19, 1457—1462 (1970). [G75,528/70

Becker, K.: Biochemische Untersuchungen zum Bindegewebsstoffwechsel bei menschlicher und experimenteller Leberzirrhose. *Dtsch. Z. Verdau.- u. Stoffwechselkr.* 28, 161 bis 162 (1968). [H22,471/68

Becker, K.: Der Einfluß von Cortison auf Proliferation und Stoffwechsel des Bindegewebes bei der experimentellen Leberzirrhose. *Ztschr. gesamt. exp. Med.* 151, 10—17 (1969). [H17,711/69

Beckett, A. H., Triggs, E. J.: Enzyme induction in man caused by smoking. *Nature (Lond.)* 216, 587 (1967). [G70,154/67

Behrman, R. E., Fisher, D. E.: Phenobarbital for neonatal jaundice. *J. Pediat.* 76, 945—948 (1970). [G75,312/70

Bein, H. J.: Aldosterone and alterations in circulatory reactivity following endotoxins. In: Shock; *An International Symposium*, p. 162—168. Berlin, Göttingen, Heidelberg: Springer-Verlag 1962. [D37,982/62

Bein, H. J., Desaulles, P. A., Loustalot, P.: Endokrine Faktoren bei der experimentellen renalen Hypertonie. *Bull. schweiz. Akad. med. Wiss.* 14, 223—230 (1958). [C57,714/58

Bein, H. J., Jaques, R.: The antitoxic effect of aldosterone. *Experientia (Basel)* 16, 24—26 (1960). [D41,862/60

Bekemeier, H.: Nephrocalcitopotrope Wirkung von Äthinylnortestosteron und Progesteron. *Naturwissenschaften* 52, 397 (1965). [G31,719/65

Bekemeier, H.: Beeinflussung von Kalkablagerungen in der Rattenniere durch Androgene. *Acta biol. med. germ.* **14**, 863—864 (1965). [F 53,774/65

Bekemeier, H.: Lokalisation des Kalkes in der Niere von Maus, Kaninchen, Hund und Mensch bei mit Östrogenen behandelter D-Hypervitaminose. *Z. Urol.* **60**, 145—148 (1967). [F 80,690/67

Bekemeier, H., Leiser, H.: Beeinflussen endogene Oestrogene und Androgene den Ort der durch Calcinosefaktor erzeugten Kalkablagerungen in der Niere? *Z. ges. exp. Med.* **135**, 281—284 (1961). [D 76,990/61

Bekemeier, H., Leiser, H.: Verschiebung des Ortes experimentell bedingter Kalkablagerungen in der Niere unter dem Einfluß von Oestrogenen. *Naunyn-Schmiedebergs Arch. Pharmak.* **241**, 146—148 (1961). [D 76,994/61

Bekemeier, H., Leiser, H.: Der Einfluß von Nebennieren- und Hypophysenentfernung auf das durch Calcinosefaktor erzeugte Verkalkungsbild der Rattenniere. *Naunyn-Schmiedebergs Arch. Pharmak.* **245**, 115—116 (1963). [D 65,289/63

Bekemeier, H., Leiser, H., Schottek, W.: The influence of testosterone on the location of renal calcification induced by a calcinosing factor. *Z. ges. exp. Med.* **135**/6, 541—544 (1962). [E 97,156/62

Bélanger, L. F., Migicovsky, B. B.: Comparative effects of vitamin D, calcium, cortisone, hydrocortisone, and norethandrolone on the epiphyseal cartilage and bone of rachitic chicks. *Develop. Biol.* **2**, 329—342 (1960). [C 95,269/60

Belaval, G. S., Widen, A. L.: Meprobamate toxicity. *U. S. armed Forces med. J.* **9**, 1691—1702 (1958). [C 76,528/58

Belding, D. L., Wyman, L. C.: The role of the suprarenal gland in the natural resistance of the rat to diphtheria toxin. *Amer. J. Physiol.* **78**, 50—55 (1926). [3,915/26

Bella, D. D., Rognoni, F., Teotino, U.: Effect of β-diethylaminoethyl 3,3-diphenylpropylacetate on the action of suxamethonium and other neuromuscular blocking drugs. *Brit. J. Pharmacol.* **18**, 563—571 (1962). [G 77,568/62

Benacerraf, B., Thorbecke, G. J., Jacoby, D.: Effect of zymosan on endotoxin toxicity in mice. *Proc. Soc. exp. Biol. (N.Y.)* **100**, 796 to 799 (1959). [C 67,852/59

Bendoc, C. C., Beskid, G., Wolferth, C. C. Jr., Howard, J. M., O'Malley, J. F.: Cardiovascular and antitoxic effects of aldosterone on cats in endotoxin shock. *Surg. Gynec. Obstet.* **114**, 43—46 (1962). [D 24,577/62

Benes, J., Zicha, B.: Effect of ionizing radiation on tryptophan oxygenase of rat liver. *Strahlentherapie* **137**, 612—619 (1969). [G 67,159/69

Benetato, G., Gaina, I., Oprisiu, C.: Influence de l'hypertrophie provoquée de la corticosurrénale et de l'extrait cortical sur la résistance à certaines intoxications. *C. R. Soc. Biol. (Paris)* **120**, 353—355 (1935). [33,773/35

Bengmark, S.: Liver regeneration. In: Pack, G. T., Islami, A. H.; *Tumor of the Liver. Recent Results in Cancer Research,* p. 187—212. Berlin, Heidelberg, New York: Springer-Verlag 1969. [G 74,917/69

Bengmark, S., Ekdahl, P.-H., Gottfries, A., Mobacken, H., Olsson, R., Rehnström, B., Schersten, T.: Influence of testosterone treatment in experimental nutritional hepatic cirrhosis in the rat. *Gastroenterologia* **105**, 301—315 (1966). [F 67,484/66

Bengmark, S., Hafström, L. O., Loughridge, B.: Studies of the influence of hepatic artery ligation on liver regeneration in partially hepatectomized rats. *Acta hepato.-splenol. (Stuttg.)* **16**, 349—355 (1969). [G 71,689/69

Bengmark, S., Olsson, R.: The effect of sex and of testosterone on toxic liver damage. *J. Endocr.* **25**, 293—297 (1962). [D 48,932/62

Bengmark, S., Olsson, R.: Effect of testosterone upon liver regeneration. *Bull. Soc. int. Chir.* No. 5—6, 451—457 (1963). [D 14,663/63

Bengmark, S., Olsson, R.: Experimental study of liver healing after partial hepatectomy. Special regard to the changes in content of liver glutamic pyruvic transaminase. *Acta hepato-splenol. (Stuttg.)* **10**, 282—293 (1963). [E 34,627/63

Bengmark, S., Olsson, R.: Effect of vitamin B_{12} on liver regeneration after partial hepatectomy. *Gastroenterologia (Basel)* **100**, 75—86 (1963). [E 34,736/63

Bengmark, S., Olsson, R.: The effect of testosterone on liver healing after partial hepatectomy. *Acta chir. scand.* **127**, 93—100 (1964). [D 6,135/64

Bengmark, S., Olsson, R.: The effect of castration and testosterone treatment on liver healing in male rats after carbon tetrachloride injury. *Path. et Microbiol. (Basel)* **27**, 167—174 (1964). [G 13,853/64

Benkö, A.: Die gemeinsame Wirkung des Nikotinsäureamids und Cortigens auf die Porphyrinurie bei Bleivergiftung. *Dtsch. med. Wschr.* **68**, 271—272 (1942). [95,966/42

Bennett, I. L., Jr., Beeson, P. B.: The effect of cortisone upon reactions of rabbits to bacterial endotoxins with particular reference to acquired resistance. *Bull. Johns Hopk. Hosp.* **93**, 290—308 (1953). [B95,351/53

Bennette, J. G.: Amethopterin: a toxic tumour growth inhibitor. *Brit. J. Cancer* **6**, 377—388 (1952). [D77,417/52

Bennison, B. E., Coatney, G. R.: The sex of the host as a factor in plasmodium gallinaceum infections in young chicks. *Science* **107**, 147—148 (1947). [B17,600/47

Benoit, J., Clavert, J.: Rôle de la glande thyroide dans l'ostéogénèse folliculinique chez les oiseaux. *Congr. Anat. (Strasbourg)*, No. 68, p. 68—75 (1948). [B27,669/48

Benton, D. A.: Regression of 3,4,9,10-dibenzpyrene induced tumors in mice following adrenalectomy. (Abstr.) *Proc. Amer. Ass. Cancer Res.* **3**, 303 (1962). [D22,526/62

Benveniste, J., Higounet, F., Salomon, J. C.: Effects of various doses of prednisolone on the phagocytic activity in axenic and holoxenic mice. *J. reticuloendothel. Soc.* **8**, 499—507 (1970). [G80,804/70

Berde, B., Takács, L.: Heat tolerance of castrated female rabbits. *Z. Vitamin-, Hormon- u. Fermentforsch.* **1**, 480—483 (1948). [B31,943/48

Berde, B. I., Takács, L.: Heat tolerance of castrated male rabbits. *Z. Vitamin-, Hormon- u. Fermentforsch.* **2**, 23—25 (1948). [B38,366/48

Berdjis, C. C.: Cortisone and radiation. III. Histopathology of the effect of cortisone on the irradiated rat kidney. *Arch. Path.* **69**, 431—439 (1960). [C83,954/60

Berdjis, C. C.: Influence of cortisone on hepatotoxic agents. *Fed. Proc.* **26**, 575 (1967). [F79,528/67

Berdjis, C. C., Brown, R. F.: Histopathology of the effect of cortisone on the irradiated rat lung. *Dis. Chest* **32**, 481 (1957). [C45,470/57

Berencsi, G., Krompecher, S.: Recent data concerning the connexion between thyroid and hepatic functions. *Acta anat. (Basel)* **64**, 235—244 (1966). [G43,712/66

Berencsi, G., Krompecher,S., Märcz, I.: Experimental data on the correlation between hepatic and thyroid functions. *Acta anat. (Basel)* **60**, 507—515 (1965). [G33,802/65

Bergen, J. R., Beisaw, N. E., Krus, D. M., Koella, W. P., Pincus, G.: Central nervous system and behavior: some properties of progesterone. In: Martini and Pecile; *Hormonal Steroids. Biochemistry, Pharmacology, and Therapeutics* **2**, p. 483—490. New York, London: Academic Press 1965. [E5,492/65

Bergen, J. R., Krus, D., Pincus, G.: Suppression of LSD-25 effects in rats by steroids. *Proc. Soc. exp. Biol. (N.Y.)* **105**, 254—256 (1960). [C97,551/60

Bergen, J. R., Pincus, G. G.: Steroid suppression of LSD induced behavior changes in rats. *Fed. Proc.* **19**, 20 (1960). [C82,720/60

Bergenstal, D. M., Hertz, R., Lipsett, M. B., Moy, R. H.: Chemotherapy of adrenocortical cancer with o,p′DDD. *Ann. intern. Med.* **53**, 672—682 (1960). [C94,436/60

Bergenstal, D. M., Lipsett, M. B., Moy, R. H., Hertz, R.: Regression of adrenal cancer and suppression of adrenal function in man by o,p′ DDD. *Trans. Ass. Amer. Phycns* **72**, 341—350 (1959). [G74,073/59

Berger, E.: Die experimentellen Voraussetzungen einer Behandlung der Diphtherie mit Vitamin C und Nebennierenrindenhormon. *Klin. Wschr.* **16**, 1177—1180 (1937). [95,075/37

Berglund, K.: Studies on factors which condition the effect of cortisone on antibody production. I. The significance of time of hormone administration in primary hemolysin response. *Acta pathol. microbiol. scand.* **38**, 311—328 (1956). [C16,832/56

Bergman, F., Linden, W. van der: Influence of D-thyroxine on gallstone formation in hamsters. *Acta chir. scand.* **129**, 547—552 (1965). [G30,642/65

Bergman, F., Linden, W. van der: Further studies on the influence of thyroxine on gallstone formation in hamsters. *Acta chir. scand.* **131**, 319—328 (1966). [G39,200/66

Bergman, F., Linden, W. van der: Influence of cholestyramine, a bile acid sequestrant, on gallstone formation in hamsters. *Acta chir. scand.* **132**, 724—730 (1966). [G43,913/66

Bergman, H. C., Rosenfeld, D. D., Hechter, O., Prinzmetal, M.: Ineffectiveness of adrenocortical hormones, thiamine, ascorbic acid, nupercaine, and post-traumatic serum in shock due to scalding burns. *Amer. Heart J.* **29**, 506—512 (1945). [B2,009/45

Berkovich, S., Ressel, M.: Effect of gonadectomy on susceptibility of the adult mouse to

coxsackie B1 virus infection. *Proc. Soc. exp. Biol. (N.Y.)* 119, 690—694 (1965).
[F46,105/65

Berlin, C. M., Schimke, R. T.: Influence of turnover rates on the responses of enzymes to cortisone. *Molec. Pharmacol.* 1, 149—156 (1965). [G37,616/65

Berliner, D. L., Keller, N., Dougherty, T. F.: Tissue retention of cortisol and metabolites induced by ACTH: an extra-adrenal effect. *Endocrinology* 68, 621—632 (1961).
[G75,988/61

Berliner, D. L., Keller, N., Dougherty, T. F.: Medicated and direct effects of ACTH and corticosteroids in stress. In: Bajusz; *Physiology and Pathology of Adaptation Mechanisms: Neural-Neuroendocrine-Humoral*, p. 204—213. Oxford, London, Edingburgh: Pergamon Press 1969. [E8,170/69

Berliner, D. L., Wiest, W. G.: The extrahepatic metabolism of progesterone in rats. *J. biol. Chem.* 221, 449—459 (1956). [C22,807/56

Berman, D.: Hormonal effects on fat deposition in the liver. *Thesis*. University of McGill (1946). [A46,758/46

Berman, D., Sylvester, M., Hay, E. C., Selye, H.: The adrenal and early hepatic regeneration. *Endocrinology* 41, 258—264 (1947).
[97,700/47

Berman, L. B.: Modification of protein catabolism in the anuric dog. *Proc. Soc. exp. Biol. (N.Y.)* 101, 809—811 (1959). [C74,922/59

Berman, M. L., Bochantin, J. F.: Nonspecific stimulation of drug metabolism in rats by methoxyflurane. *Anesthesiology* 32, 500—506 (1970). [G75,502/70

Bernard, C.: Leçons sur les phénomènes de la vie communs aux animaux et aux végétaux. Paris: Librairie J.-B. Baillière et Fils 1, 1878; 2, 1879. [E719/1878/79

Bernick, S., Ershoff, B. H., Sobel, H.: The effects of various hormones upon the bone changes induced by toxic doses of cortisone in rats. *Anat. Rec.* 139, 207 (1961). [D5,063/61

Bernick, S., Hyman, C., Paldino, R. L.: Histological studies of the sex difference in intrahepatic distribution of thorotrast and T-1824 in rabbits. *Anat. Rec.* 126, 213—223 (1956).
[C39,526/56

Berry, L. J.: Endotoxin lethality and tryptophan pyrrolase induction in cold-exposed mice. *Amer. J. Physiol.* 207, 1058—1062 (1964).
[F24,603/64

Berry, L. J.: Effects of endotoxins on the level of selected enzymes and metabolites. In: Landy and Braun; *Bacterial Endotoxins*, p. 151—159. New Brunswick, N.J.: Rutgers, State University 1964. [G68,858/64

Berry, L. J.: Effect of environmental temperature on lethality of endotoxin and its effect on body temperature in mice. *Fed. Proc.* 25, 1264—1270 (1966). [F69,416/66

Berry, L. J., Agarwal, M. K., Snyder, I. S.: Comparative effect of endotoxin and reticuloendothelial "blocking" colloids on selected inducible liver enzymes. In: Di Luzio and Paoletti; *The Reticuloendothelial System and Atherosclerosis*, p. 266—274. New York: Plenum Press 1967. [E7,069/67

Berry, L. J., Smythe, D. S.: Effects of bacterial endotoxin on metabolism. II. Protein-carbohydrate balance following cortisone. Inhibition of intestinal absorption and adrenal response to ACTH. *J. exp. Med.* 110, 407—418 (1959).
[C73,199/59

Berry, L. J., Smythe, D. S.: Effects of bacterial endotoxin on metabolism. VI. The role of tryptophan pyrrolase in response of mice to endotoxin. *J. exp. Med.* 118, 587—603 (1963).
[E28,203/63

Berry, L. J., Smythe, D. S.: Effects of bacterial endotoxins on metabolism. VII. Enzyme induction and cortisone protection. *J. exp. Med.* 120, 721—732 (1964). [D19,640/64

Berry, L. J., Smythe, D. S., Colwell, L. S.: Inhibition of inducible liver enzymes by endotoxin and actinomycin D. *J. Bact.* 92, 107—115 (1966). [G67,237/66

Berry, L. J., Smythe, D. S., Colwell, L. S., Chu, P. H. C.: Influence of hypoxia, glucocorticoid, and endotoxin on hepatic enzyme induction. *Amer. J. Physiol.* 215, 587—592 (1968). [H2,124/68

Berry, L. J., Smythe, D. S., Young, L. G.: Effects of bacterial endotoxin on metabolism. I. Carbohydrate depletion and the protective role of cortisone. *J. exp. Med.* 110, 389—405 (1959). [C73,198/59

Bertolotti, E., Giordano, S.: Il fenil-propionato di norandrostenolone nella intossicazione da vitamina "D." *Minerva pediat.* 14, 1175—1178 (1962). [D57,171/62

Besendorf, H., Pletscher, A.: Beeinflussung zentraler Wirkungen von Reserpin und 5-Hydroxytryptamin durch Isonicotinsäurehydrazide. *Helv. physiol. pharmacol. Acta* 14, 383 bis 390 (1956). [C31,623/56

Best, C. H., Solandt, D. Y.: Concentrated serum in treatment of traumatic and histamine shock in experimental animals. *Brit. med. J.* 1940 I, 799—802. [A33,635/40

Bettini, S., Cantore, G.: Sull'azione protettiva dell'ACTH, del cortisone, del gluconato di calcio, della pirilamina (Neoantergan), della prometazina (Fargan), della cloropromazina (Largactil) nel latrodectismo indotto nella cavia. *R. C. Ist. sup. Sanita* 18, 488—495 (1955). [C 21,801/55

Betz, E. H.: Contribution a l'étude du syndrome endocrinien provoqué par l'irradiation totale de l'organisme. *Thesis.* Université de Liège (1955). [C 13,907/55

Bevan, B. R., Holton, J. B., Lathe, G. H.: The effect of pregnanediol and pregnanediol glucuronide on bilirubin conjugation by rat liver slices. *Clin. Sci.* 29, 353—361 (1965).
[G 35,435/65

Bhagat, B.: The effects of a deficiency in thiamine and an excess of thyroid hormone on the analgesic action of morphine. *Arch. int. Pharmacodyn.* 148, 536—544 (1964).
[F 9,444/64

Bianchi, A., Maio, M. de: Ricerche sperimentali sul potenziamento della narcosi da 21-idrossipregnandione ad opera della serotonina, della reserpina e dell'esametonio. *G. ital. Chir.* 14, 280—289 (1958). [C 54,169/58

Biancifiori, C., Caschera, F., Giornell-Santilli, F. E., Bucciarelli, E.: The action of oestrone and four chemical carcinogens in intact and ovariectomised BALB/c/Cb/Se mice. *Brit. J. Cancer* 21, 452—459 (1967). [F 98,833/67

Bickel, M. H., Minder, R.: Metabolism and biliary excretion of the lipophilic drug molecules, imipramine and desmethylimipramine in the rat. I. Experiments in vivo and with isolated perfused livers. *Biochem. Pharmacol.* 19, 2425—2435 (1970). [G 77,613/70

Bickel, M. H., Minder, R.: Metabolism and biliary excretion of the lipophilic drug molecules, imipramine and desmethylimipramine in the rat. II. Uptake into bile micelles. *Biochem. Pharmacol.* 19, 2437—2443 (1970).
[G 77,614/70

Bidleman, K., Mannering, G. J.: Induction of drug metabolism V. Independent formation of cytochromes P-450 and P_1-450 in rats treated with phenobarbital and 3-methylcholanthrene simultaneously. *Molec. Pharmacol.* 6, 697—701 (1970). [G 80,042/70

Biebl, M., Essex, H. E., Mann, F. C.: Studies on the physiology of the liver. *Amer. J. Physiol.* 100, 167—172 (1932). [44,898/32

Biedl, A., Winterberg, H.: Beiträge zur Lehre von der Ammoniakentgiftenden Funktion der Leber. *Pflügers Arch. ges. Physiol.* 88, 140—200 (1901). [47,485/01

Bielschowsky, F.: The role of hormonal factors in the development of tumours induced by 2-aminofluorene and related compounds. *Acta Un. int. Cancr.* 17, 121—130 (1961).
[D 10,255/61

Bielschowsky, F., Hall, W. H.: Carcinogenesis in parabiotic rats. Tumours of the ovary induced by acetylaminofluorene in intact females joined to gonadectomized litter-mates and the reaction of their pituitaries to endogenous oestrogens. *Brit. J. Cancer* 5, 331—344 (1951). [G 71,797/51

Bielschowsky, F., Hall, W. H.: Carcinogenesis in the thyroidectomized rat. *Brit. J. Cancer* 7, 358—366 (1953). [C 194/53

Biezunski, N.: Action of warfarin injected into rats on protein synthesis in vitro by liver microsomes as related to its anticoagulating action. *Biochem. Pharmacol.* 19, 2645—2652 (1970).
[G 78,643/70

Biozzi, G., Benacerraf, B., Halpern, B. N.: The effect of Salm. typhi and its endotoxin on the phagocytic activity of the reticulo-endothelial system in mice. *Brit. J. exp. Path.* 36, 226—235 (1955). [E 22,483/55

Birchall, K., O'Day, W. G., Fajer, A. B., Burstein, S.: Urinary cortisol and 6β-hydroxycortisol in the monkey, Cebus albifrons: normal variation and the effects of ACTH and phenobarbital. *Gen. comp. Endocr.* 7, 352—362 (1966). [F 76,581/66

Birchmeier, P. J.: Quantitative changes in mouse liver ultrastructure following cortisone and insulin administration. *Austral. J. biol. Sci.* 22, 965—978 (1969). [G 69,512/69

Bird, C. C., Crawford, A. M., Currie, A. R.: Foetal adrenal necrosis induced by 7-hydroxymethyl-12-methylbenz(a)-anthracene and its prevention. *Nature (Lond.)* 228, 72—73 (1970).
[H 30,425/70

Bisetti, A., Barbolini, G.: Effetto degli ormoni corticotropo e somatotropo nella tubercolosi sperimentale del ratto ipofisectomizzato. *Rass. Fisiopat. clin. ter.* 33, 406—422 (1961).
[D 12,624/61

Bishop, R. F., Marshall, V.: The enhancement of Clostridium welchii infection by adrenaline-in-oil. *Med. J. Austral.* 2, 656—657 (1960).
[C 95,338/60

Biskind, G. R.: Inactivation of methyl testosterone in castrate male rats. *Proc. Soc. exp. Biol. (N.Y.)* 43, 259—261 (1940). [A 31,848/40

Biskind, G. R.: Inactivation of testosterone propionate by normal female rats. *Proc. Soc. exp. Biol. (N.Y.)* 46, 452—453 (1941). [A 35,907/41

Biskind, G. R.: The inactivation of estradiol and estradiol benzoate in castrate female rats. *Endocrinology* 28, 894—896 (1941). [A 36,315/41

Biskind, G. R.: Inactivation of estrone in normal adult male rats. *Proc. Soc. exp. Biol. (N.Y.)* 47, 266—268 (1941). [A 36,481/41

Biskind, G. R., Mark, J.: The inactivation of testosterone propionate and estrone in rats. *Bull. Johns Hopk. Hosp.* 65, 212—217 (1939). [A 31,656/39

Biskind, M. S., Biskind, G. R.: Effect of vitamin B complex deficiency on inactivation of estrone in the liver. *Endocrinology* 31, 109—114 (1942). [A 38,221/42

Bixler, D., Muhler, J. C., Shafer, W. G.: The effect of radioactive iodine on dental caries in the rat. *J. Amer. dent. Ass.* 53, 667—671 (1956). [E 99,118/56

Black, M., Sherlock, S.: Treatment of Gilbert's syndrome with phenobarbital. *Lancet* 1970 I, 1359—1362. [H 26,290/70

Blackham, A., Spencer, P. S. J.: The effects of oestrogens and progestins on the response of mice to barbiturates. *Brit. J. Pharmacol.* 37, 129—139 (1969). [G 69,913/69

Blackham, A., Spencer, P. S. J.: Interactions of oestrogenic and progestational steroids with dexamphetamine and fencamfamin in mice. *Brit. J. Pharmacol.* 37, 508—509 (1969). [G 76,301/69

Blackham, A., Spencer, P. S. J.: Response of female mice to anticonvulsants after pretreatment with sex steroids. *J. Pharm. Pharmacol.* 22, 304—305 (1970). [G 73,813/70

Black-Schaffer, B., Johnson, D. S., Gobbel, W. G., Jr.: Experimental total midzonal hepatic necrosis. *Amer. J. Path.* 26, 397—409 (1950). [B 55,142/50

Blackwell, B.: Tranylcypromine. *Lancet* 1963 II, 414. [E 65,708/63

Blatt, L. M., Slickers, K. A., Kim, K. H.: Effect of prolactin on thyroxine-induced metamorphosis. *Endocrinology* 85, 1213—1215 (1969). [H 19,832/69

Blaw, M. E., Good, R. A., Peterson, R. D. A.: Curare sensitivity in neonatally thymectomized mice. *Nature (Lond.)* 210, 129—130 (1966). [F 65,571/66

Bledsoe, T., Island, D. P., Ney, R. L., Liddle, G. W.: An effect of o,p'DDD on the extraadrenal metabolism of cortisol in man. *J. clin. Endocr.* 24, 1303—1311 (1964). [E 20,690/64

Bloch, E., Lew, M., Klein, M.: Studies on the inhibition of fetal androgen formation: testosterone synthesis by fetal and newborn mouse testes in vitro. *Endocrinology* 88, 41—46 (1971). [H 34,907/71

Bloch, R. G.: The effect of hyperthyroidism on tuberculosis in the guinea pig. *Amer. Rev. resp. Dis.* 87, 525—528 (1963). [D 61,174/63

Block, L. H., Lamy, P. P.: Therapeutic incompatibilities. *J. Amer. pharm. Ass.* 8, 66—68, 82—84 (1968). [G 81,054/68

Block, L. H., Lamy, P. P.: Drug interactions. *J. Amer. pharm. Ass.* 9, 202—206 (1969). [G 81,052/69

Blood, F. R., Glover, R. M., Henderson, J. B., D'Amour, F. E.: Relationship between hypoxia, oxygen consumption and body temperature. *Amer. J. Physiol.* 156, 62—66 (1949). [B 48,970/49

Bloodworth, J. M. B. Jr., Arscott, P., Hamwi, G. J., Morton, J. L.: Effect of somatotrophic hormone and chlortetracycline on weight and mortality of irradiated rats. *Fed. Proc.* 15, 508 (1956). [C 14,328/56

Blount, H. C., Jr., Smith, W.: The influence of thyroid and thiouracil on mice exposed to roentgen radiation. *Science* 109, 83—84 (1949). [B 30,000/49

Blum, F.: Neue, experimentell gefundene Wege zur Erkenntnis und Behandlung von Krankheiten, die durch Auto-Intoxicationen bedingt sind. *Virchows Arch. path. Anat.* 162, 375—406 (1900). [38,401/1900

Blum, F.: Neues und Altes zur Physiologie und Pathologie der Schilddrüse. *Verhandl. 23. Kongr. inn. Med. München,* p. 183—218 (1906). [38,405/06

Boatman, J. B.: Response of the normal and thyroidectomized cat to severe cold. *Amer. J. Physiol.* 196, 983—986 (1959). [C 68,449/59

Bóbr, J.: The effect of alloxan diabetes on experimental staphylococcal infection in mice. *J. Path. Bact.* 89, 749—752 (1965). [G 30,418/65

Bóbr, J., Ptak, W.: Hormones influencing resistance to crude staphylococcal α-toxin. *Postępy Mikrobiol.* 5, 309—312 (1966). [G 47,053/66

Bochner, F., Lloyd, H. M., Roeser, H. P., Thomas, M. J.: Effects of O,p'DDD and aminoglutethimide on metastatic adrenocortical carcinoma. *Med. J. Austral.* **56**, 809—812 (1969). [H31,656/69

Bock, F. G., Dao, T. L.: Factors affecting the polynuclear hydrocarbon level in rat mammary glands. *Cancer Res.* **21**, 1024—1029 (1961). [D11,892/61

Boctor, A. M., Rogers, Q. R., Harper, A. E.: The influence of thyroxine and thiouracil on rats fed excess tyrosine. *Proc. Soc. exp. Biol. (N.Y.)* **133**, 821—825 (1970). [H22,509/70

Bodaiji, S., Mori, Y.: Effect of cortisone on the experimental tuberculosis in rabbit. *Kobe J. med. Sci.* **3**, 89 (1957). [C35,586/57

Bodansky, M., Duff, V. B.: The influence of pregnancy on resistance to thyroxine, with data on the creatine content of the maternal and fetal myocardium. *Endocrinology* **20**, 537—540 (1936). [63,084/36

Bodo, R. D. de, Prescott, K. F.: The antidiuretic action of barbiturates (phenobarbital, amytal, pentobarbital) and the mechanism involved in this action. *J. Pharmacol. exp. Ther.* **85**, 222—233 (1945). [88,791/45

Boer, B. de: Factors affecting pentothal anesthesis in dogs. *Anesthesiology* **8**, 375—381 (1947). [A52,450/47

Boer, B. de: The effects of thiamine hydrochloride upon pentobarbital sodium ("Nembutal") hypnosis and mortality in normal, castrated, and fasting rats. *J. Amer. pharm. Ass., sci. Ed.* **37**, 302—307 (1948). [A48,817/48

Boer, B. de, Mukomela, A. E.: Thiopental and pentobarbital hypnosis in normal and castrate rats as modified by ACTH and cortisone. *Fed. Proc.* **14**, 332 (1955). [C5,245/55

Boeri, R.: Ormoni ipofiso-surrenalici e soglia convulsiva. *Minerva med.* **50**, 2813—2815 (1958). [C78,610/58

Bogdanovitch, S. B.: The effect of methylthiouracil on the toxicity of oxophenarsine. *Arch. int. Pharmacodyn.* **106**, 307—311 (1956). [C18,912/56

Bogdanovitch, S. B., Varagitch, V. M.: Influence of thyroidea hormone on the toxicity of dichlormapharsen. *Acta med. iugosl.* **8**, 196 to 199 (1954). [G71,534/54

Boggs, T. R., Jr., Hardy, J. B., Frazier, T. M.: Correlation of neonatal serum total bilirubin concentrations and developmental status at age eight months. A preliminary report from the collaborative project. *J. Pediat.* **71**, 553 to 560 (1967). [G71,887/67

Bois, P., Bélanger, L. F., Le Buis, J.: Effect of growth hormone and aminoacetonitrile on the mitotic rate of epiphysial cartilage in hypophysectomized rats. *Endocrinology* **73**, 507 to 509 (1963). [E29,177/63

Bojesen, E., Egense, J.: Elimination of endogenous corticosteroids in vivo. The effects of hepatectomy and total abdominal evisceration in the acutely adrenalectomized cat, and the effect of muscular exercise and insulin administration on the isolated hindquarter preparation. *Acta endocr. (Kbh.)* **33**, 347—369 (1960). [G75,996/60

Boler, R. K., Bibighaus, A. J., Brunson, J. G.: An electron microscopic study of the liver of endotoxin-shocked dogs treated with a combination of propiomazine and levarterenol. *Lab. Invest.* **20**, 319—325 (1969). [G65,722/69

Bolis, L.: Cardiovasculopatie sperimentali e gonadotropine. *Atti Soc. lombarda Sci. med.-biol.* **2**, 254—259 (1956). [E50,716/56

Bomskov, C., Hölscher, B., Hartmann, J.: Der Thymustod. *Pflügers Arch. ges. Physiol.* **245**, 483—492 (1942). [A56,954/42

Bond, E. J., Butler, W. H., Matteis, F. de, Barnes, J. M.: Effects of carbon disulphide on the liver of rats. *Brit. J. industr. Med.* **26**, 335—337 (1969). [H18,559/69

Bondoc, C. C., Beskid, G., Wolferth, C. C. Jr., Howard, J. M., O'Malley, J. F.: Cardiovascular and antitoxic effects of aldosterone on cats in endotoxin shock. *Surg. Gynec. Obstet.* **114**, 43—46 (1962). [D69,984/62

Bondurant, C. P., Campbell, C.: Adrenal cortex extract in the treatment of bromide eruption and bromide intoxication. *J. Amer. med. Ass.* **116**, 100—104 (1941). [A36,066/41

Bonetti, E., Guerzon, A. P., Stirpe, F.: Induction of tryptophan pyrrolase in rats after early injections of tryptophan or neonatal thymectomy. *Experientia (Basel)* **23**, 436—437 (1967). [G48,030/67

Bongiovanni, A. M., Eberlein, W. R., Goldman, A. S., New, M.: Disorders of adrenal steroid biogenesis. In: Pincus, G.; *Recent Progress in Hormone Research*, p. 375—449. New York, London: Academic Press 1967. [E7,039/67

Bonino, A.: Ovariectomia e tossicosi ganglioplegica. *Ormologia* **15**, 362—364 (1955). [C13,016/55

Bonino, A.: Sesso e tossicosi acetilcolinica. *Ormologia* **16**, 174—177 (1956). [C30,089/56

Bonino, A.: Sesso e ganglioplegici. *Ormologia* **16**, 256—260 (1956). [C30,099/56

Bonino, A.: Spasmo morfinico e gestazione. *Ormonologia* 17, 195—199 (1957). [C64,366/57

Bonmassar, E., Melan, F., Montagnani-Marelli, A.: Influsso di un ormone anabolizzante (dimetazina) sullo stato immunitario del topo verso il cancro ascite di Ehrlich. *Arch. ital. Pat.* 10, 37—40 (1967). [F85,891/67

Bonnycastle, D. D., Giarman, N. J., Paasonen, M. K.: Anticonvulsant compounds and 5-hydroxytryptamine in rat brain. *Brit. J. Pharmacol.* 12, 228—231 (1957). [C37,036/57

Bonta, I. L., Goorissen, E. M.: Different potency of pancuronium bromide on two types of skeletal muscle. *Europ. J. Pharmacol.* 4, 303—308 (1968). [G75,052/68

Bonta, I. L., Overbeek, G. A.: Experimental design for studying the pattern of central nervous activity of steroids. In: Martini and Pecile; *Hormonal Steroids, Biochemistry, Pharmacology and Therapeutics.* New York: Academic Press 1965. [E5,494/65

Bonta, I. L., Vargaftig, B. B., de Vos, C. J., Grijsen, H.: Haemorrhagic mechanisms of some snake venoms in relation to protection by estriol succinate of blood vessel damage. *Life Sci.* 8, 881—888 (1969). [G69,044/69

Bonta, I. L., de Vos, C. J., Delver, A.: Inhibitory effects of estriol-16,17-disodium succinate on local haemorrhages induced by snake venom in canine heart-lung preparations. *Acta endocr. (Kbh.)* 48, 137—146 (1965). [F28,544/65

Booth, J., Gillette, J. R.: The effect of anabolic steroids on drug metabolism by microsomal enzymes in rat liver. *J. Pharmacol. exp. Ther.* 137, 374—379 (1962). [D34,656/62

Boquet, P., Izard, Y., Grave, F., Delpuech, M.: Influence de l'acide ascorbique et de la cortisone sur les réactions homéostatiques des petits rongeurs expérimentalement intoxiqués par l'antigène typhique O. *Ann. Inst. Pasteur* 91, 292—311 (1956). [E52,759/56

Boquoi, E., Kreuzer, G.: Der Einfluß von Östrogen und gestagen wirkenden Hormonen auf die durch Diäthylnitrosamin erzeugten Leberveränderungen und Tumoren bei der Ratte. *Arch. Geschwulstforsch.* 26, 223—233 (1965). [F82,383/65

Borberg, H., Lücker, P.: Tierexperimentelle Untersuchungen über die antikatabole Wirkung des 1-Methyl-androst-1-en-17β-ol-3-on. (Primobolan Schering). *Acta endocr. (Kbh.)* 47, 231—236 (1964). [F24,271/64

Borchardt, W.: Fieber, Schilddrüse und Nebennieren. (Nach Versuchen an Katzen.) *Klin. Wschr.* 2, 1507—1509 (1928). [23,683/28

Borglin, N. E.: Oral contraceptives and liver damage. *Brit. med. J.* 1965 I, 1289—1290. [F40,990/65

Borglin, N. E., Mansson, B.: The effect of natural oestrogen on the toxic action of amidopyrine. *Acta endocr. (Kbh.)* 8, 81—89 (1951). [B62,206/51

Borgman, R. F.: Increased survival-time in dystrophic mice treated with methylandrostenediol dienanthoylacetate. *Nature (Lond.)* 197, 1304 (1963). [D62,710/63

Borgman, R. F., Haselden, F. H.: Cholelithiasis in rabbits: effects of bile constituents and hormones on dissolution of gallstones. *Amer. J. vet. Res.* 30, 107—112 (1969). [H29,947/69

Börner, H., Klinkmann, H., Tessmann, D., Wüstenberg, P. W.: Zur Testosteronbehandlung der Urämie. Kasuistik und tierexperimenteller Beitrag. *Wiss. Z. Univ. Rostock* 15, 157—161 (1966). [E85,972/66

Boroff, D. A.: Studies of the toxin of Clostridium botulinum. IV. Fluorescence of Clostridium botulinum toxin and its relation to toxicity. *Int. Arch. Allergy* 15, 74—90 (1959). [C75,371/59

Boroff, D. A., Fleck, U.: Effects of serotonin on the toxin of Clostridium botulinum. *J. Pharmacol. exp. Ther.* 157, 427—431 (1967). [F87,254/67

Borowsky, B. A., Kessner, D. M., Hartroft, W. S., Recant, L., Koch, M. B.: Aminonucleoside-induced chronic glomerulonephritis in rats. *J. Lab. clin. Med.* 57, 512—521 (1961). [D2,508/61

Borzelleca, J. F., Manthei, R. W.: Factors influencing pentobarbital sleeping time in mice. *Arch. int. Pharmacodyn.* 111, 296—307 (1957). [C40,953/57

Bosányi, A. de: Experimental studies on rickets. III. Protein substances as a factor in normal osteogenesis and in the healing of rickets. *Amer. J. Dis. Child.* 30, 780—798 (1925). [367/25

Bose, B. C., Saifi, A. Q., Bhagwat, A. W.: Effect of Cannabis indica on hexobarbital sleeping time and tissue respiration of rat brain. *Arch. int. Pharmacodyn.* 141, 520—524 (1963). [D58,773/63

Both, P. C. J.: Sur l'action préventive d'un dérivé de l'hormone mâle, dans la cancérisation des souris provoquée par des implants d'hormone femelle (action du pH). *Ann. Endocr. (Paris)* 25, Sup. 119—121 (1964). [F29,450/64

Bottiglioni, E., Orlandi, G., Sturani, P. L.: Aspetti istologici ed istochimici dell'apparato cardiovascolare e dei muscoli dell'attivà volontaria nel ratto in carenza di vitamina A; effetto della somministrazione di ormone somatotropo e di una frazione lipidica diencefalica. *Musc. Dystrophy Abstr.* **3**, 117 (1959). [C70,889/59

Bottiglioni, F., Pedrelli, P., Savorelli, M.: Studio dell'influenza di un antiandrogeno (il cyproterone) sull'attività steroidogenetica del testicolo di ratto in vitro. *Boll. Soc. ital. Biol. sper.* **45**, 993—996 (1969). [G76,203/69

Bourque, J. E., Haterius, H. O., Glassco, E.: Treatment of circulatory collapse of experimental venous occlusion: use of adrenal cortical extract and saline solution. *Proc. Soc. exp. Biol. (N.Y.)* **52**, 313—314 (1943). [A57,912/43

Bousquet, W. F.: Pharmacology and biochemistry of drug metabolism. *J. pharm. Sci.* **51**, 297—309 (1962). [H11,613/62

Bousquet, W. F., Rupe, B. D., Miya, T. S.: Morphine inhibition of drug metabolism in the rat. *Biochem. Pharmacol.* **13**, 123—125 (1964). [E39,107/64

Bousquet W. F., Rupe, B. D., Miya, T. S.: Endocrine modification of drug responses in the rat. *J. Pharmacol. Exp. Ther.* **147/3**, 376 to 379 (1965). [F35,073/65

Bouyard, P., Klein, M.: Action musculaire de l'ouabaïne chez le rat traité par la 9-α-fluoro, 16-β-méthyl, Δ-hydrocortisone. *C. R. Soc. Biol. (Paris)* **157**, 342—344 (1963). [D69,070/63

Bouyard, P., Klein, M.: Actions de divers corticoïdes anti-inflammatoires dans le 'choc hémorragique irréversible' expérimental. *Ann. Anesth. franç.* **7**, 569—573 (1966). [G41,843/66

Bowen, S. T., Gowen, J. W., Tauber, O. E.: Cortisone and mortality in mouse typhoid. I. Effect of hormone dosage and time of injection. *Proc. Soc. exp. Biol. (N.Y.)* **94**, 476—479 (1957). [C31,414/57

Bowen, S. T., Gowen, J. W., Tauber, O. E.: Cortisone and mortality in mouse typhoid. II. Effect of environmental temperature. *Proc. Soc. exp. Biol. (N.Y.)* **94**, 479—482 (1957). [C31,415/57

Bowen, S. T., Gowen, J. W., Tauber, O. E.: Cortisone and mortality in mouse typhoid. III. Effect of natural and acquired immunity. *Proc. Soc. exp. Biol. (N.Y.)* **94**, 482—485 (1957). [C31,416/57

Bowman, W. C., Osuide, G.: Interaction between the effects of tremorine and harmine and of other drugs in chicks. *Europ. J. Pharmocol.* **3**, 106—111 (1968). [F98,712/68

Bowman, W. C., Rand, M. J., West, G. B.: Textbook of Pharmacology, p. 1025. Oxford, Edinburgh: Blackwell Scientific Publ. 1968. [E714/68

Boyer, F., Chedid, L.: La cortisone dans les infections expérimentales de la souris. *Ann. Inst. Pasteur* **84**, 453—457 (1953). [C624/53

Boyland, E. and Jondorf, W. R.: The stimulation of ascorbic acid excretion in rats. *Brit. J. Cancer* **16**, 489—493 (1962). [D47,605/62

Bozzo, G. B.: Ricerche sperimentali sulla epatosteatosi dietetica in gravidanza. *Quad. Clin. ostet. ginec.* **4**, 206—213 (1949). [B50,296/49

Bracharz, H., Laas, H., Beitzien, G.: Die Wirkung von Aldactone auf die arterielle Hypertension. In: *Klinische Anwendung der Aldosteron-Antagonisten*, p. 89. Stuttgart: Georg Thieme Verlag 1962. [D37,973/62

Brachet, J., Jeener, R.: Phosphatase alcaline des noyaux et vitesse de remplacement du phosphore de l'acide thymonucléique. *C. R. Soc. Biol. (Paris)* **140**, 1121—1122 (1946). [B23,118/46

Bradford, R. H., Howard, R. P., Joel, W., Shetlar, M. R.: Antagonistic effects of parathyroid extract and cortisone. Effects on serum protein and glycoprotein fractions and on renal calcification. *Arch. Path.* **69**, 382—389 (1960). [D76,315/60

Bradley, G. M., Spink, W. W.: Acute hepatic necrosis induced by brucella infection in hyperthyroid mice. *J. exp. Med.* **110**, 791—800 (1959). [C76,042/59

Bradlow, H. L., Hellman, L., Zumoff, B., Gallagher, T. F.: Interaction of hormonal effects: influence of triiodothyronine on androgen metabolism. *Science* **124**, 1206—1207 (1956). [C27,897/56

Brainerd, H., Scaparone, M.: The effect of cortisone on the fixation and neutralization of diphtheria toxin. *Antibiot. et Chemother. (Basel)* **3**, 693—697 (1953). [B87,957/53

Braun-Menéndez, E.: Tiroides e hipertensión nefrógena experimental. *Rev. Soc. argent. Biol.* **30**, 138—147 (1954). [C4,927/54

Braun-Menéndez, E., Houssay, H. E. J.: Hipertrofia compensadora del riñon en la rata hipofisopriva. *Rev. Soc. argent. Biol.* **25**, 55—62 (1949). [B45,945/49

Brazda, F. G., Baucum, R.: The effect of nikethamide on the metabolism of pentobarbital by liver microsomes of the rat. *J. Pharmacol. exp. Ther.* **132**, 295—298 (1961). [D48,613/61

Brazda, F. G., Coulson, R. A.: The influence of coramine on the liver of the young rat. *Proc. Soc. exp. Biol. (N.Y.)* 67, 37—40 (1948). [B 32,015/48

Bremer, F., Titeca, J.: Action de l'adrénaline sur l'atonie musculaire du stade initial de la curarisation. *C. R. Soc. Biol. (Paris)* 99, 624—627 (1928). [23,673/28

Brena, S., D'Agostino, A.: Narcosi barbiturica e orchiectomia. *Ormonologia* 14, 1—8 (1954). [C 11,921/54

Brenk, H. A. S. van den: Radiation lethality in histamine depleted rats. *Brit. J. exp. Path.* 39, 300—306 (1958). [C 57,624/58

Brenk, H. A. S. van den, Elliott, K.: Radioprotective action of 5-hydroxytryptamine. *Nature (Lond.)* 182, 1506—1507 (1958). [C 76,268/58

Brenk, H. A. S. van den, Moore, R.: Effect of high oxygen pressure on the protective action of cystamine and 5-hydroxytryptamine in irradiated rats. *Nature (Lond.)* 183, 1530 to 1531 (1959). [C 71,353/59

Brenner, G., Korte, W., Puck, A.: Die Wirkung von Oestradiol-17 und Oestriol auf die experimentelle diätetische Lebernekrose der Ratte. *Endokrinologie* 42, 212—222 (1962). [D 24,411/62

Bresnick, E., Stevenson, J. G.: Microsomal N-demethylase activity in developing rat liver after administration of 3-methylcholanthrene (3MC). (Abstr.) *Biochem. Pharmacol.* 17, 1815 to 1822 (1968). [H 215/68

Brewster, W. R. Jr., Isaacs, J. P., Osgood, P. F., King, T. L.: The hemodynamic and metabolic interrelationships in the activity of epinephrine, norepinephrine and the thyroid hormones. *Circulation* 13, 1—20 (1956). [C 11,771/56

Brin, M., McKee, R. W.: Effects of X-irradiation, nitrogen mustard, fasting, cortisone and adrenalectomy on transaminase activity in the rat. *Arch. Biochem.* 61, 384—389 (1956). [C 31,261/56

Britton, S. W., Kline, R. F.: Age, sex, carbohydrate, adrenal cortex and other factors in anoxia. *Amer. J. Physiol.* 145, 190—202 (1945). [93,980/45

Britton, S. W., Myers, W. K.: The thyroid gland and the sensitivity of animals to insulin. *Amer. J. Physiol.* 84, 132—140 (1928). [18,695/28

Brock, N., Hohorst, H. J.: Über die Aktivierung von Cyclophosphamid im Warmblüterorganismus. *Naturwissenschaften* 49, 610—611 (1962). [G 71,533/62

Brodeur, J., Côté, J.-Y., Nantel, J., Auger, P.: Effects de l'âge, du sexe et de divers traitements hormonaux sur l'activité de la procaïnestérase du foie de rat in vitro. *Rev. canad. Biol.* 26, 135—140 (1967). [F 99,981/67

Brodeur, J., Du Bois, K. P.: Comparison of acute toxicity of anticholinesterase insecticides to weanling and adult male rats. *Proc. Soc. exp. Biol. (N.Y)* 114, 509—511 (1963). [E 33,487/63

Brodeur, J., DuBois, K. P.: Mechanisms of age difference in malathion toxicity. *Proc. canad. Fed. biol. Soc.* 8, 18 (1965). [F 40,590/65

Brodeur, J., DuBois, K. P.: Studies on factors influencing the acute toxicity of malathion and malaoxon in rats. *Canad. J. Physiol. Pharmacol.* 45, 621—631 (1967). [F 85,072/67

Brodie, B. B.: Pathways of drug metabolism. *J. Pharm. Pharmacol.* 8, 1—17 (1956). [C 12,157/56

Brodie, B. B.: Drug metabolism—subcellular mechanisms. In: Mongar and de Reuck; *Ciba Foundation Symposium on Enzymes and Drug Action*, p. 317—343. London: J. & A. Churchill Ltd. 1962. [G 55,013/62

Brodie, B. B.: Some prospects in toxicology. *Environm. Res.* 2, 368—372 (1969). [G 72,492/69

Brodie, B. B., Axelrod J., Cooper, J. R., Gaudette, L., La Du, B. N., Mitoma C., Udenfriend, S.: Detoxication of drugs and other foreign compounds by liver microsomes. *Science* 121, 603—604 (1955). [G 66,772/55

Brodie, B. B., Cosmides, G. J., Rall, D. P.: Toxicology and the biomedical sciences. *Science* 148, 1547—1554 (1965). [F 42,949/65

Brodie, B. B., Gillette, J. R., La Du, B. N.: Enzymatic metabolism of drugs and other foreign compounds. *Ann. Rev. Biochem.* 27, 427—454 (1958). [E 92,717/58

Brodie, B. B., Maickel, R. P.: Comparative biochemistry of drug metabolism. In: Brodie and Erdös; *Metabolic Factors Controlling Duration of Drug Action* 6, p. 299—324. New York: The Macmillan Co. 1962. [G 67,800/62

Brodie, B. B., Maickel, R. P., Jondorf, W. R.: Termination of drug action by enzymatic inactivation. *Fed. Proc.* 17, 1163—1174 (1958). [E 92,716/58

Brodie, B. B., Reid, W. D., Cho, A. K., Sipes, G., Krishna, G., Gillette, J. R.: Possible mechanism of liver necrosis caused by aromatic organic compounds. *Proc. nat. Acad. Sci. (Wash.)* 68, 160—164 (1971). [G 80,473/71

Brodie, D. A., Cook, P. G., Bauer, B. J., Dagle, G. E.: Indomethacin-induced intestinal lesions in the rat. *Toxicol. appl. Pharmacol.* 17, 615 to 624 (1970). [G 67,797/70

Brody, S.: Mechanism of growth. II. The influence of p-dimethylaminoazobenzene on rat liver regeneration after partial hepatectomy. *Cancer Res.* 20, 1469—1473 (1960). [G 71,680/60

Brooke, M. S., Hechter, O., Kass, E. H.: Antiendotoxic activity of corticosteroids. *Endocrinology* 69, 867—869 (1961). [D 11,627/61

Brooks, G. T., Harrison, A.: The oxidative metabolism of aldrin and dihydroaldrin by houseflies, housefly microsomes and pig liver microsomes and the effect of inhibitors. *Biochem. Pharmacol.* 18, 557—568 (1969). [G 65,297/69

Brouet, G., Marche, J., Chrétien, J., Mallet, J., Quichaud, J.: Hormone somatotrope et infection tuberculeuse. Données expérimentales et cliniques. *Therapie* 11, 584—631 (1956). [G 72,418/56

Brown, A. K.: Studies on the neonatal development of the glucuronide conjugating system. *J. Dis. Child.* 94, 510—512 (1957). [H 28,215/57

Brown, B. B.: Lysergic acid diethylamide antagonism of certain drugs. *Ann. N.Y. Acad. Sci.* 66, 677—685 (1957). [C 31,328/57

Brown, I. N., Allison, A. C., Taylor, R. B.: Plasmodium berghei infections in thymectomized rats. *Nature (Lond.)* 219, 292—293 (1968). [H 1,304/68

Brown, J. H., Schwartz, N. L.: Interaction of lysosomes and anti-inflammatory drugs. *Proc. Soc. exp. Biol. (N.Y.)* 131, 614—620 (1969). [H 14,096/69

Brown, J. H. U., Smith, R. B., Griffin, J. B., Jacobs, J.: The influence of cortisone on the action of an adrenocorticolytic drug. *Endocrinology* 61, 106—109 (1957). [C 37,523/57

Brown, J. R.: The effect of environmental and dietary stress on the concentration of 1,1-bis(4-chlorophenyl)-2,2,2-trichloroethane in rats. *Toxicol. appl. Pharmacol.* 17, 504—510 (1970). [G 78,684/70

Brown, P. S., Wells, M.: Factors which influence assays of gonadotrophin based on the induction of ovulation in mice. *J. Endocr.* 33, 507—514 (1965). [F 57,759/65

Brown, R. R., Miller, J. A., Miller, E. C.: The metabolism of methylated aminoazo dyes. IV. Dietary factors enhancing demethylation in vitro. *J. biol. Chem.* 209, 211—222 (1954). [G 57,030/54

Brown, T. G. Jr., Evangelista, B. S., Green, T. J., Gwilt, D. J.: Experimental study of current therapeutic approaches to endotoxin shock. (Abstr.). *Fed. Proc.* 27, 447 (1968). [H 456/68

Brown, W. D., Johnson, A. R., O'Halloran, M. W.: The effect of the level of dietary fat on the toxicity of phenolic antioxidants. *Austral. J. exp. Biol. med. Sci.* 37, 533—547 (1959). [G 69,691/59

Brown, W. R., Boon, W. H.: Ethnic group differences in plasma bilirubin levels of full-term, healthy Singapore newborns. *Pediatrics* 36, 745 to 751 (1965). [G 78,957/65

Bruce, J. A., Brunson, J. G.: Use of propiomazine and levarterenol in endotoxin shock. *Fed. Proc.* 26, 690 (1967). [F 79,682/67

Brück, K., Wünnenberg, W., Zeisberger, E.: Comparison of cold adaptive metabolic modifications in different species, with special reference to the miniature pig. *Fed. Proc.* 28, 1035—1041 (1969). [H 13,180/69

Bruckner, W. L., Barenfus, M., Snow, H. D., Longmire, W. P., Jr.: Abrasive ablation: a new experimental surgical technique to study nonparenchymal aspects of hepatic regeneration. *J. surg. Res.* 9, 461—469 (1969). [H 34,704/69

Brues, A. M., Drury, D. R., Brues, M. C.: A quantitative study of cell growth in regenerating liver. *Arch. Path.* 22, 658—673 (1936). [A 45,962/36

Brues, A. M., Marble, B. B.: An analysis of mitosis in liver restoration. *J. exp. Med.* 65, 15—28 (1937). [A 47,729/37

Bruger, M., Fitz, F.: Experimental atherosclerosis. I. Effect of prolonged administration of the thyrotropic factor of the anterior lobe of the pituitary on experimental atherosclerosis in rabbits. *Arch. Path.* 65, 637—642 (1938). [A 15,324/38

Brühl, P., Schmidt, H. J.: Die Wirkung von Nalidixinsäure auf den Ablauf der experimentellen Pyelonephritis unter dem Einfluß resistenzbeeinflussender Pharmaka. *Zbl. Bakt., I. Abt. Ref.* 212, 517—526 (1970). [G 76,086/70

Brunson, J. G., Kalina, R. E., Eckman, P. L.: Studies on experimental shock. Effects of vasopressor amines and phenothiazine derivatives. *Amer. J. Path.* 35, 1149—1167 (1959). [C 78,005/59

Brust, A. A., Assali, N. S., Ferris, E. B.: Evaluation of neurogenic and humoral factors in blood pressure maintenance in normal and toxemic pregnancy using tetraethylammonium chloride. *J. clin. Invest.* **27**, 717—726 (1948). [B 18,590/48

Brust, A. A., Ransohoff, W., Reiser, M. F.: Blood pressure responses to ACTH and cortisone in normotensive and hypertensive subjects in the resting state and during autonomic blockade with tetraethylammonium chloride. *Program 43rd Meet. Amer. Soc. clin. Invest.*, p. 9 (1951). [B 57,917/51

Brust, A. A., Ransohoff, W., Reiser, M. F., Ferris, E. B.: Vascular response to ACTH and alterations in sodium intake. In: Mote, J. R.; *Proceedings of the second clinical ACTH conference. I. Research*, p. 177—195. New York, Philadelphia, Toronto: The Blakiston Co. 1951. [B 58,739/51

Buchel, L.: Influence de l'âge des rats sur leur sensibilité à quelques hypnotiques. *Anesth. et Analg.* **10**, 526—545 (1953). [D 59,654/53

Buchel, L.: Influence des glandes sexuelles sur la sensibilité des rats blancs à quelques hypnotiques. *Anesth. et Analg.* **11**, 229—251 (1954). [D 73,669/54

Buchel, L.: Influence des hormones sexuelles sur l'activité de l'hexobarbital chez le rat. Durée du séjour de cet hypnotique dans l'organisme du rat. *Anesth. et Analg.* **11**, 268—279 (1954). [G 67,326/54

Buchel, L., Levy, J.: Induction des hydroxylases des microsomes du foie. I. Présence, reversibilité, reproducibilité de l'induction chez la souris prétraitée par le phénobarbital. *Thérapie* **25**, 91—106 (1970). [G 74,850/70

Buchel, L., Levy, J.: Induction des hydroxylases des microsomes du foie. II. Reversibilité, reproducibilité de l'induction chez le rat, prétraité par le phénobarbital. *Thérapie* **25**, 107—123 (1970). [G 74,851/70

Buchel, L., Liblau, L.: Contribution à l'étude du métabolisme de l'hexobarbital chez le rat blanc, suivant le sexe. *Arch. Sci. physiol.* **16**, 227—235 (1962). [E 87,108/62

Buchel, L., Liblau, L.: Contribution à l'étude du métabolisme de l'hexobarbital chez la souris. *Arch. Sci. physiol.* **17**, 255—259 (1963). [E 89,233/63

Bucher, N. L. R.: Regeneration of mammalian liver. *Int. Rev. Cytol.* **15**, 245—300 (1963). [G 68,621/63

Bucher, N. L. R., McGarrahan, K.: The biosynthesis of cholesterol from acetate-1-C^{14} by cellular fractions of rat liver. *J. biol. Chem.* **222**, 1—15 (1956). [G 67,470/56

Bucher, N. L. R., Swaffield, M. N.: Ribonucleic acid synthesis in relation to precursor pools in regenerating rat liver. *Biochim. biophys. Acta (Amst.)* **174**, 491—502 (1969). [H 21,579/69

Bucher, N. L. R., Schrock, T. R., Moolten, F. L.: An experimental view of hepatic regeneration. *Johns Hopk. med. J.* **125**, 250—257 (1969). [G 72,546/69

Bucher, N. L. R., Scott, J. F., Aub, J. C.: Regeneration of the liver in parabiotic rats. *Cancer Res.* **11**, 457—465 (1951). [D 42,066/51

Buckett, W. R.: The pharmacology of pancuronium bromide: a new non-depolarising neuromuscular blocking agent. *Irish J. med. Sci.* **1**, 565—568 (1968). [G 75,531/68

Buckett, W. R., Marjoribanks, C. E. B., Marwick, F. A., Morton, M. B.: The pharmacology of pancuronium bromide (Org. NA 97), a new potent steroidal neuromuscular blocking agent. *Brit. J. Pharmacol.* **32**, 671—682 (1968). [G 56,175/68

Bugbee, L. M., Like, A, A., Stewart, R. B.: The effects of cortisone on intradermally induced vaccinia infection in rabbits. *J. infect. Dis.* **106**, 166—173 (1960). [C 84,115/60

Bull, L. B., Dick, A. T., McKenzie, J. S.: The acute toxic effects of heliotrine and lasiocarpine, and their N-oxides, on the rat. *J. Path. Bact.* **75**, 17—25 (1958). [C 49,278/58

Bullock, G. R., Delaney, V. B., Sawyer, B. C., Slater, T. F.: Biochemical and structural changes in rat liver resulting from the parenteral administration of a large dose of sodium salicylate. *Biochem. Pharmacol.* **19**, 245—253 (1970). [G 73,358/70

Burberi, S., Cioli, V., Piccinelli, D.: Effects of benzydamine on experimental gastric ulcers produced by indomethacin and reserpine. *Pharmacol. Res. Commun.* **2**, 91—95 (1970). [G 80,224/70

Burckhardt, D., LaDue, J. S.: Östrogenähnliche Wirkung von Digitalis. Seine Wirkung auf die Gonadotropinausscheidung bei postklimakterischen Frauen. *Schweiz. med. Wschr.* **98**, 1250—1252 (1968). [H 15,071/68

Burger, A., Laudat, P., Bricaire, H.: Determination de la transcortine plasmatique au cours de diverses endocrinopathies. *Acta endocr. (Kbh.)* **64**, 602—609 (1970). [H 28,702/70

Burger, P. C., Herdson, P. B.: Phenobarbital-induced fine structural changes in rat liver. *Amer. J. Path.* **48**, 793—809 (1966). [G 66,499/66

Burns, J. J.: Implications of enzyme inductions for drug therapy. *Amer. J. Med.* 37, 327—331 (1964). [G41,546/64

Burns, J. J., Conney, A. H.: Therapeutic implications of drug metabolism. *Semin. Hemat.* 1, 375—400 (1964). [G71,448/64

Burns, J. J., Conney, A. H.: Enzyme stimulation and inhibition in the metabolism of drugs. *Proc. Roy. Soc. Med.* 58, 955—960 (1965). [F56,503/65

Burns, J. J., Welch, R. M., Conney, A. H.: Drug effects on enzymes. In: Siegler and Moyer; *Animal and Clinical Pharmacologic Techniques in Drug Evaluation* 2, p. 67—75. Chicago, Ill.: Year Book Medical Publication Inc. 1967. [G66,103/67

Burrill, M. W., Greene, R. R.: The liver and endogenous androgens. *Proc. Soc. exp. Biol. (N.Y.)* 44, 273—276 (1940). [A32,956/40

Burrill, M. W., Greene, R. R.: Effect of rat's liver on activity of testosterone and methyl testosterone. *Endocrinology* 31, 73—77 (1942). [A38,214/42

Burstein, S.: Determination of initial rates of cortisol 2α- and 6β-hydroxylation by hepatic microsomal preparations in guinea pigs: effect of phenobarbital in two genetic types. *Endocrinology* 82, 547—554 (1968). [F95,565/68

Burstein, S., Bhavnani, B. R.: Effect of phenobarbital administration of the in vitro hydroxylation of cortisol and on over-all substrate and product metabolism in the guinea pig and rat. *Endocrinology* 80, 351—356 (1967). [F77,040/67

Burstein, S., Klaiber, E. L.: Phenobarbital-induced increase in 6β-hydroxycortisol excretion: clue to its significance in human urine. *J. clin. Endocr.* 25, 293—296 (1965). [F31,533/65

Burton, R. R., Smith, A. H., Carlisle, J. C., Sluka, S. J.: Role of hematocrit, heart mass, and high-altitude exposure in acute hypoxia tolerance. *J. appl. Physiol.* 27, 49—52 (1969). [G67,617/69

Buschke, A.: Thallium und thymus. *Klin. Wschr.* 12, 311 (1933). [4,823/33

Buschke, A., Spanier, F., Pleger: Versuche zu einer Modifikation der Thalliumepilation. *Dermat. Wschr.* 96, 226—229 (1933). [43,284/33

Busfield, D., Child, K. J., Basil, B., Tomich, E. G.: The influence of sex on the catabolism of griseofulvin. *J. Pharm.* 12, 539—543 (1960). [D10,983/60

Busfield, D., Child, K. J., Tomich, E. G.: An effect of phenobarbitone on griseofulvin metabolism in the rat. *Brit. J. Pharmacol.* 22, 137—142 (1964). [G74,680/64

Bush, G. H., Stead, A. L.: The use of d-tubocurarine in neonatal anaesthesia. *Brit. J. Anaesth.* 34, 721—728 (1962). [G78,967/62

Busso, R.-R.: Sensibilité des animaux éthyroïdés a l'égard de certains toxiques. *C. R. Soc. Biol. (Paris)* 92, 820—821 (1925). [26,684/25

Butler, T. C., Mahaffee, D., Mahaffee, C.: The role of the liver in the metabolic disposition of mephobarbital. *J. Pharmacol. exp. Ther.* 106, 364—369 (1952). [G76,364/52

Buttle, G. A. H., Squires, S.: A method of assessing ACTH by means of the antagonism of histamine intoxication. *J. Endocr.* 7, xxvii to xxviii (1951). [B59,985/51

Buu-Hoi, N. P., Hien, D. P.: Zoxazolamine-hydroxylase inducing effect of polycyclic aromatic hydrocarbons; relationships between structure and activity, and degree of correlation with carcinogenicity. *Biochem. Pharmacol.* 18, 741—748 (1969). [G66,135/69

Byerrum, R. U.: Influence of dietary iodine on Susceptibility of rats to alpha naphthylthiourea poisoning. *Proc. Soc. exp. Biol. (N.Y.)* 62, 328—330 (1946). [B1,322/46

Byerrum, R. U., DuBois, K. P.: The influence of Diet on the Susceptibility of rats to Alpha-Naphathylthiourea. *J. Pharmacol. Exp. Ther.* 90, 321—329 (1947). [B3,076/47

Byrne, J. J.: The sympathetic nervous system and pulmonary embolism. *Arch. Surg.* 73, 936—938 (1956). [C46,341/56

Byrom, F. B.: The effect of oestrogenic and other sex hormones: on the response of the rat to vasopressin. *Lancet* 1839 I, 129—131. [A9,905/38

Cabibbe, F., Paracchi, G., Lanzara, D.: Azione di alcuni psicofarmaci sulla triptofano-pirrolasi epatica di ratti in stato di stress post-operatorio. *Boll. Soc. ital. Biol. sper.* 43, 1183—1186 (1967). [G52,346/67

Cahn, J., Georges, G., Herold, M., Pierre, R.: Influence de la sérotonine sur le métabolisme cérébral et la narcose barbiturique au cours des 24 heures suivant l'injection intraveineuse de 12,5 mg/kg chez le lapin in vivo. *Therapie* 13, 62—65 (1958). [C64,625/58

Cahn, J., Georges, G., Pierre, R.: Essais d'anesthésie prolongée par la 5-hydroxytryptamine (séronine) et contrôlée des drogues à action neurovégétative. II. Etude chez le rat. *C. R. Soc. Biol. (Paris)* **150**, 162—164 (1956). [C19,722/56

Cahn, J., Herold, M.: Importance des groupes sulfhydryles en biologie. Physiopathologie des dérivés sulfhydryles. *Agressologie* **1**, 157—171 (1960). [G72,124/60

Cahn, J., Pierre, R., Georges, G.: Essais d'anesthésie prolongée par la 5-hydroxytryptamine (sérotonine) et contrôlée par des drogues à action neurovégétative. II. Etude chez le lapin. *C. R. Soc. Biol. (Paris)* **150**, 290—292 (1956). [G71,537/56

Calabro, G.: Richerche sperimentali e considerazioni sull'azione epatoprotettiva della colina in gravidanza. *Quad. Clin. ostet. ginec.* **4**, 228—232 (1949). [B48,121/49

Calandi, C., Calzolari, C., Di Maria, M., Pierro, U.: Poisoning due to vitamin D in early infancy. (12 case reports). *Riv. Clin. pediat.* **77/1**, 3—18 (1966). [F75,662/66

Calcagno, A., Quercio, M.: Modificazioni della reattività alla ibernazione in rapporto al tipo di trauma sperimentale chirurgico. *Pathologica* **57**, 367 (1965). [G46,022/65

Caldwell, W. L., Thomassen, R. W., Bosch, A.: Unfavourable response of radiation nephritis to administration of L-triiodothyronine. *Nature (Lond.)* **197**, 200—201 (1963). [D54,096/63

Calhoun, F. J., Tolson, W. W., Schrogie, J. J.: Effects of various drugs on the uterotropic response to mestranol and norethynodrel in the rat. *Proc. Soc. exp. Biol. (N.Y.)* **136**, 47—50 (1971). [H34,806/71

Calof, N. S., Smith, C. M.: Effect of α and β adrenergic agonists on traumatic shock in the rat. (Abstr.). *Fed. Proc.* **28**, 611 (1969). [H10,412/69

Calvert, D. N., Brody, T. M.: Role of the sympathetic nervous system in CCl_4 hepatotoxicity. *Amer. J. Physiol.* **198**, 669—676 (1960). [C82,653/60

Calvert, D. N., Brody, T. M.: The effects of hyperthyroidism and hypothyroidism on the hepatotoxicity produced by CCl_4. *Fed. Proc.* **19**, 133 (1960). [C82,829/60

Calvert, D. N., Brody, T. M.: The effects of thyroid function upon carbon tetrachloride hepatotoxicity. *J. Pharmacol. exp. Ther.* **134**, 304—310 (1961). [D61,412/61

Camargo, A. C. M., Cornicelli, J., Cardoso, S. S.: Alteration in lipid content of the liver in the rat after partial hepatectomy. *Proc. Soc. exp. Biol. (N.Y.)* **122**, 1151—1154 (1966). [F72,052/66

Cameron, A. T., Carmichael, J.: A note on tetany in thyroid-fed rats and the supposed antagonism between thymus and parathyroid. *Trans. Roy. Soc. Can. Sect. V* **19**, 53—56 (1925). [27,015/25

Cameron, A. T., Carmichael, J.: Sudden atmospheric changes as contributory factors in the production of tetany. *Trans. Roy. Soc. Can., Sect. V* **20**, 277—296 (1926). [42,188/26

Cameron, A. T., Moore, A.: The effect of thyroid feeding on rats on a vitamin-deficient diet. *Trans. Roy. Can., Sect. V* **15**, 29—36 (1921). [57,815/21

Cameron, G. R.: Liver regeneration and biliary obstruction. *J. Path. Bact.* **41**, 283—288 (1935). [A48,168/35

Cameron, G. R.: Some recent work on barbiturates. *Proc. Roy. Soc. Med. (Sect. Anaesth.)* **32**, 309—314 (1939). [A34,503/39

Cameron, G. R., Cooray, G. H., De, S. N.: The effect of castration on the action of some barbiturates. *J. Path. Bact.* **60**, 239—246 (1948). [B45,221/48

Cameron, G. R., Saram, G. S. W. de: The effect of liver damage on the action of some barbiturates. *J. Path. Bact.* **48**, 49—54 (1939). [G72,101/39

Cameron, J. M., Pirie, T. G., Robb, R. A.: The protective action of certain hormones and vitamins against lathyrogenic drugs. *Brit. J. exp. Path.* **43**, 496—505 (1962). [D38,527/62

Campanacci, L. Jr., Pieragnoli, E., Tura, S.: Neurosecreto, epatopatia sperimentale ed ormone somatotropo. Azione dell'STH sulla neurosecrezione ipotalamo-ipofisaria e sul fegato, nel ratto, in condizioni normali e nell intossicazione cronica sperimentale da CCl_4. (Ricerche istochimiche). *Folia endocr. (Roma)* **9**, 381—401 (1956). [C20,086/56

Campbell, J. A.: Oxygen poisoning and the thyroid gland. *J. Physiol. (Lond.)* **90**, 91P—92P (1937). [A14,903/37

Campbell, J. G.: Studies on the influence of sex hormones on the avian liver. III. Oestrogen-induced regeneration of the chronically damaged liver. *J. Endocr.* **15**, 351—354 (1957). [C38,327/57

Campbell, R. A., Bern, H. A., DeOme, K. B.: The adverse effect of oestrogen on the resistance of mice to stress. *Acta endocr. (Kbh.)* **23**, 49—59 (1956). [C23,145/56

Campbell, R. M., Cuthbertson, D. P., Pullar, J. D.: The effects of betamethasone and fracture on nitrogen metabolism. *Quart. J. exp. Physiol.* **49**, 141—150 (1964). [G9,081/64

Campbell, W. C., Collette, J. V.: Effect of cortisone upon infection with Trichuris muris in albino mice. *J. Parasit.* **48**, 933—934 (1962). [D 61,500/62

Câmpeanu, L., Vrăbiescu, A., Comsa, E.: Induced arteriosclerosis in female white rats related to age. *Excerpta med. (Amst.), Int. Congr. Ser.* No. 57, p. 10 (1963). [G 21,413/63

Canadell, J. M., Valdecasas, F. G.: Action inhibitrice du thiouracil sur la carotine. *Experientia (Basel)* **3**, 35 (1947). [B 25,697/47

Canal, N., Maffei-Faccioli, A.: Induction of tryptophan-peroxydase-oxydase in rat liver by reserpine. *Naturwissenschaften* **46**, 494 (1959). [G 66,306/59

Candole, C. A. de: Successful use of pressor drugs in paraoxon poisoning. *Proc. Canad. Physiol. Soc. 20th Ann. Meet. Montreal*, p. 13 (1956). [C 25,237/56

Cannon, W. B.: The Wisdom of the Body. New York: W. W. Norton and Co. 1939. [B 14,905/39

Cantarow, A., Paschkis, K. E., Stasney, J., Rothenberg, M. S.: The influence of sex hormones upon the hepatic lesions produced by 2-acetaminofluorene. *Cancer Res.* **6**, 610—616 (1946). [B 18,774/46

Canter, J. W., Kreel, I., Segal, R. L., Frankel, A., Baronofsky, I. D.: Influence of thyroidectomy on experimental ascites. *Proc. Soc. exp. Biol. (N.Y.)* **100**, 771—774 (1959). [C 67,855/59

Cantin, M.: Inhibition de la néphrocalcinose expérimentale par la parathyroïdectomie. *Proc. 30th Congress ACFAS Montreal*, p. 37 (1962). [D 36,815/62

Cantin, M.: Role of the parathyroid and of the thyroid in the production of experimental nephrocalcinosis. *Fed. Proc.* **23**, 545 (1964). [F 5,681/64

Cantrell, W.: Cortisone and the course of trypanosoma equiperdum infection in the rat. *J. infect. Dis.* **104**, 71—77 (1959). [C 64,728/59

Canzanelli, A., Guild, R., Rapport, D.: Pituitary and adreno-cortical relationships to liver regeneration and nucleic acids. *Endocrinology* **45**, 91—95 (1949). [B 37,729/49

Čapek, R.: Some effects of bradykinin on the central nervous system. *Biochem. Pharmacol.* **10**, 61—64 (1962). [D 54,290/62

Capitolo, G.: Sugli effetti della tiroparatiroidectomia nel colpo di calore. Resistenza dell'organismo e andamento termico. *Arch. Sci. med.* **62**, 587—595 (1936). [A 1,730/36

Caprino, G., Gallina, F.: Azione del 19-norandrostenolone fenilpropionato sul recupero negli animali panirradiati. *Boll. Soc. ital. Biol. sper.* **39**, 1687—1691 (1963). [G 10,521/63

Caprino, G., Gallina, F.: Effetto del propiltiouracile nell'animale panirradiato. *Boll. Soc. ital. Biol. sper.* **39**, 1691—1692 (1963). [G 13,680/63

Carbone, J. V., Grodsky, G. M., Hjelte, V.: Effect of hepatic dysfunction on circulating levels of sulfobromophthalein and its metabolites. *J. Clin. Invest.* **38**, 1989—1995 (1959). [C 77,294/59

Careddu, P., Sereni, L. P., Giunta, A., Sereni, F.: Sulla possibilità di attivare i processi di coniugazione e di escrezione epatica della bilirubina mediante alcuni farmaci. Ricerche sperimentali con la dietilamide dell'acido nicotinico (Coramina) e con l'acido fenil-etil-barbiturico (Gardenale). *Minerva med.* **55**, 2559—2562 (1964). [G 21,332/64

Caren, L. D., Rosenberg, L. T.: The role of complement in resistance to endogenous and exogenous infection with a common mouse pathogen, Corynebacterium kutscheri. *J. exp. Med.* **124**, 689—699 (1966). [G 41,288/66

Caridroit, F., Arvy, L.: Action favorisante de la thyroxine sur le développement des vésicules séminales des souris castrées traitées par le propionate de testostérone. *C. R. Soc. Biol. (Paris)* **136**, 3—5 (1942). [A 57,397/42

Carlo, F. J. Di, Haynes, L. J., Coutinho, C. B., Phillips, G.: Pentobarbital sleeping time and RES stimulation in mice. *J. reticuloendoth. Soc.* **2**, 360—361 (1965). [F 74,536/65

Carlson, G. P., DuBois, K. P.: Studies on the toxicity and biochemical mechanism of action of 6-methyl-2,3-quinoxalinedithiol cyclic carbonate (Morestan). *J. Pharmacol. exp. Ther.* **173**, 60—70 (1970). [H 24,653/70

Carmichael, E. B.: Nembutal anesthesia. III. The median lethal dose of nembutal (pentobarbital sodium) for young and old rats. *J. Pharmacol. exp. Ther.* **62**, 284—291 (1938). [D 68,076/38

Carmichael, R. H., Wilson, C., Martz, B. L.: Effect of anabolic steroids on liver function tests in rabbits. *Proc. Soc. exp. Biol. (N.Y.)* **113**, 1006—1008 (1963). [E 28,041/63

Carrasco, R., Vargas, L.: Hormonas esteroideas y estilbestrol en el tratamiento de la diabetes aloxánica. *Bol. Soc. Biol. Santiago* **6**, 61—62 (1949). [B 50,792/49

Carrasco-Formiguera, R., Escobar, I.: Influence of previous injection of epinephrine upon diabetogenic effect of alloxan in rabbits. *Amer. J. Physiol.* **152**, 609—614 (1948). [B19,877/48

Carrier, R. N., Buday, P. V.: Augmentation of toxicity of monoamine oxidase inhibitor by thyroid feeding. *Nature (Lond.)* **191**, 1107 (1961). [D11,237/61

Carrier, R. N., Buday, P. V.: The influence of thyroid feeding on the pharmacologic actions of some monoamine oxidase inhibitors. *Arch. int. Pharmacodyn.* **145**, 18—35 (1963).
[E28,887/63

Carroll, K. K., Noble, R. L.: Resistance induced by anti-thyroid compounds and by goitrogenic diets against experimental pulmonary edema in rats. *Fed. Proc.* **8**, 22 (1949). [B32,718/49

Carroll, R.: Temporary hepatic ischaemia in the rabbit. *J. Path. Bact.* **85**, 67—75 (1963).
[G71,190/63

Carroll, R.: The extent and distribution of experimental hepatic infarcts. *J. Path. Bact.* **85**, 349—355 (1963). [G71,191/63

Carstensen, B., Paulsen, F., Rudberg-Roos, I.: Some experiments with somatotropin (STH) and insulin in tuberculosis. Preliminary report. *Acta tuberc. scand.* **31**, 225—235 (1955).
[C12,300/55

Cartner, L. M., Arias, I. M.: Developmental pattern of glucuronide formation in rat and guinea pig liver. *Amer. J. Physiol.* **205**, 663 to 666 (1963). [E28,857/63

Caskey, M. W.: Effect of adrenalin on the temperature of skeletal muscle before and after ligation of the hepatic artery and the portal vein. *Amer. J. Physiol.* **80**, 381—390 (1927).
[20,936/27

Cassidy, G. J., Dworkin, S., Finney, W. H.: Insulin and the mechanism of hibernation. *Amer. J. Physiol.* **73**, 417—428 (1925).
[24,604/25

Cassidy, G. J., Dworkin, S., Finney, W. H.: The action of insulin on the domestic fowl. *Amer. J. Physiol.* **75**, 609—615 (1926).
[26,459/26

Castells, S., Bransome, E. D., Jr.: Effects of ACTH and an inhibitor of 3β-hydroxysteroid dehydrogenase on the synthesis of adrenocortical mitochondrial proteins. *Endocrinology* **86**, 444—447 (1970). [H21,283/70

Caster, W. O., Wade, A. E., Greene, F. E., Meadows, J. S.: Effect of different levels of corn oil in the diet upon the rate of hexobarbital, heptachlor and aniline metabolism in the liver of the male white rat. *Life Sci.* **9**, 181—190 (1970). [G73,426/70

Castro, J. A., Gillette, J. R.: Species and sex differences in the kinetic constants for the N-demethylation of ethyl-morphine by liver microsomes. *Biochem. biophys. Res. Commun.* **28**, 426—430 (1967). [G77,558/67

Castro, J. A., Greene, F. E., Gigon, P., Sasame, H., Gillette, J. R.: Effect of adrenalectomy and cortisone administration on components of the liver microsomal mixed function oxygenase system of male rats which catalyzes ethylmorphine metabolism. *Biochem. Pharmacol.* **19**, 2461 to 2467 (1970). [G77,615/70

Catton, D. V.: The injection of epinephrine during methoxyflurane anesthesia. *Anesth. Analg. Curr. Res.* **48**, 900—905 (1969).
[G71,124/69

Catz, C., Yaffe, S. J.: Individual variation in drug response. *J. Dis. Child.* **102**, 579—580 (1961). [G37,059/61

Catz, C., Yaffe, S. J.: Pharmacological modification of bilirubin conjugation in the newborn. *J. Dis. Child.* **104**, 516—517 (1962).
[G71,888/62

Catz, C., Yaffe, S. J.: Barbiturate enhancement of bilirubin conjugation and excretion in young and adult animals. *Pediat. Res. (Basel)* **2**, 361 to 370 (1968). [H14,471/68

Cauwenberge, H. van, Jaques, L. B.: Haemorrhagic effect of ACTH with anticoagulants. *Canad. med. Ass. J.* **79**, 536—540 (1958).
[C58,521/58

Cauwenberge, H. van, Jaques, L. B.: Prothrombin time and hemorrhagic death in dicumarolized rats receiving pituituary and adrenal hormones. *Thrombos. Diathes. haemorrh. (Stuttg.)* **3**, 45—58 (1959). [C72,748/59

Cauwenberge, H. van, Lecomte, J., Palem Vliers, M.: Effects de l'amino-acétonitrile administré chez le rat adulte seul ou en association avec des médications anti-inflammatoires. *Path. et Biol.* **7**, 547—551 (1959). [C78,726/59

Cauwenberge, H. van, Lefebvre, P.: De l'étude des médications anti-inflammatoires à celle des propriétés biologiques du glucagon. *Bull. Acad. Roy. Méd. Belg., Ser. 7* **4**, 267—311 (1964). [G58,189/64

Cavalca, G.-G.: Experimentelle Myopathien nach Behandlung mit Prednisolon und Schilddrüsenpräparaten. *Wien. klin. Wschr.* **79**, 308 bis 313 (1967). [F83,698/67

Cavallero, C.: Influence of hormones on infection. In: Asboe-Hansen, G.; *Connective Tissue in Health and Disease*, p. 214—224. Copenhagen: Ejnar Munksgaard Publ. 1954.
[C829/54

Cavallero, C., Sala, G., Amira, A. Borasi, M.: Effects of cortisone on early fibrosis of the liver in rats. *Lancet* **1951** I, 55. [B54,229/51

Cavallero, C., Sala, G., Ballabio, C. B.: Experimental studies with cortisone. *Bull. schweiz. Akad. med. Wiss.* **8**, 116—118 (1952).
[B69,181/52

Cavallot, A., Einaudi, G.: Estratto pancreatico desulinizzato e roentgen irradiazione a dose letale. *Ormonologia* **16**, 118—127 (1956).
[C30,084/56

Caviles, A., Jr.: Abnormalities in liver function in the course of massive dosage of stanozolol. (Abstr.) *Excerpta med. (Amst.)* **24**, Sect. 6, 163 (1970). [H30,761/70

Cawthorne, M. A., Bunyan, J., Sennitt, M. V., Green, J., Grasso, P.: Vitamin E and hepatotoxic agents. 3. Vitamin E, synthetic antioxidants and carbon tetrachloride toxicity in the rat. *Brit. J. Nutr.* **24**, 357—384 (1970).
[H26,441/70

Cedrangolo, F.: L'adattamento come problema di enzimologia. *Pubb. Staz. Zool. Napoli* **21**, Sup., 28—59 (1949). [B46,622/49

Cervini, C., Longo, C.: L'influenza del cortisone sugli effetti della pan-irradiazione sperimentale. *Nunt. radiol. (Roma)* **21**, 348—359 (1955). [C9,357/55

Chaffee, R. R. J., Tichy, R., Foucrier, J.: A comparison of cold resistance between thyroidectomized hamsters (Mesocricetus auratus) and rats. (Abstr.). *Amer. Zool.* **3**, 538—539 (1963). [G71,307/63

Chahovitch, X.: Béribéri experimental et insuline. *C. R. Soc. biol. (Paris)* **93**, 652—655 (1925). [26,462/25

Chahovitch, X.: Action de l'insuline sur le béribéri expérimental du pigeon. *C. R. Soc. Biol. (Paris)* **93**, 1333—1335 (1925). [26,685/25

Chamberlin, P. E., Hall, V. E.: Sex-difference in susceptibility to dinitrophenol intoxication in anesthetized cats. *Proc. Soc. exp. Biol. (N.Y.)* **34**, 385—388 (1936). [66,611/36

Chambon, M., Bouvet, G.: Sur l'action de l'hyposulfite de soude dans l'intoxication oxycarbonée. *C. R. Soc. Biol. (Paris)* **114**, 45—46 (1933). [A48,279/33

Chambon, Y., Picard, F., Gourvès, M.: Influence du sexe et des glandes sexuelles sur l'hyperplasie régénératrice du foie chez le rat. *C. R. Soc. Biol. (Paris)* **160**, 2415 (1966).
[F80,788/66

Chamorro, A.: Action narcotique de la progestérone et de l'acétate de désoxycorticostérone. *C. R. Soc. Biol. (Paris)* **136**, 391—392 (1942). [A57,215/42

Chan, S.-K., Cohen, P. P.: A comparative study of the effect of hydrocortisone injection on tyrosine transaminase activity of different vertebrates. *Arch. Biochem.* **104**, 335—337 (1964). [D18,552/64

Chandler, A. B., Nordöy, A.: Adenosine diphosphate induced thrombosis in hypothyroid rats. *Scand. J. Haemat.* **1**, 89—93 (1964).
[G22,017/64

Chandler, H. L., Collins, W. V., Minsky, G. R., Athans, J. C., Mallory, K. C., Byrne, J. J.: Cortisone in experimental obstructive jaundice. *Ann. Surg.* **146**, 195—206 (1957). [C39,998/57

Chandler, R. L.: Infection of laboratory animals with Mycobacterium johnei. I. Infection in Swiss white mice and its modification by suramin and cortisone. *J. comp. Path.* **71**, 118 to 130 (1961). [D5,239/61

Chandler, R. L.: Infection of laboratory animals with Mycobacterium johnei. II. Infection in white rats; effect of cortisone treatment. *J. comp. Path.* **71**, 131—134 (1961). [D5,240/61

Chang, C. T., Lei, H. P.: Pharmacology of 17 α-methyl-5α-androstan-17β-ol. (Chinese.) *Acta pharm. sin.* **12**/11, 734—739 (1965).
[F78,943/65

Chang, S. I., McGinnis, J.: Vitamin D deficiency in adult quail and chickens and effects of estrogen and testosterone treatments. *Proc. Soc. exp. Biol. (N.Y.)* **124**, 1131—1135 (1967).
[F83,363/67

Chany, E., Boy, J.: Influence de la cortisone sur le délai de cancérisation du foie chez le rat normal ou surrénaloprivé. *C. R. Acad. Sci. (Paris)* **250**, 3752—3754 (1960). [D2,278/60

Chaouki, K., Viljoen, J. F., Kellner, G. A.: Pancuronium bromide. A new non-depolarizing muscle relaxant. Preliminary report on its use in fifty patients. *Cleveland Clin. Quart.* **37**, 133—137 (1970). [G77,223/70

Chaplin, H., Jr., Cassell, M.: Studies on the possible relationships of tolbutamide to dicumarol in anticoagulant therapy. *Amer. J. med. Sci.* **235**, 706—716 (1958). [D99,463/58

Chaplin, M. D., Mannering, G. J.: Role of phospholipids in the hepatic microsomal drug metabolizing system. *Molec. Pharmacol.* **6**, 631—640 (1970). [G75,976/70

Chappel, C. I., Rona, G., Gaudry, R.: Relationship between thyroid function and cardiotoxic properties of isoproterenol. *Endocrinology* **65**, 208—215 (1959). [C71,409/59

Chappel, C. I., Rona, G., Gaudry, R.: The influence of adrenal cortical steroids on cardiac necrosis produced by isoproterenol. *Acta endocr. (Kbh.)* **32**, 419—424 (1959). [C76,910/59

Charbon, G. A.: The development of resistance to tolbutamidum in dogs. *Arch. int. Pharmacodyn.* **130**, 207—210 (1961). [G76,685/61

Chase, R. E., Saidman, L. J.: The effect of spironolactone on altering the anesthetic action of cyclopropane in the rat. (Abstr.) *Fed. Proc.* **30**, 541 (1971). [H35,774/71

Chatterjee, A.: The role of cortisone in the prevention of gonadal inhibition in chlorpromazinized female rats. *Acta anat. (Basel)* **65**, 606 to 609 (1966). [G48,145/66

Chatterton, R. T., Jr., Chatterton, A. J., Hellman, L.: Metabolism of progesterone by the rabbit liver. *Endocrinology* **87**, 941—950 (1970). [H31,456/70

Chaturvedi, U. C.: Influence of sex on hepatic injury in albino rats. *Indian J. med. Sci.* **23**, 374—379 (1969). [G69,350/69

Chedid, L.: Actions comparées de la prométhazine, de la chlorpromazine et de la cortisone chez la souris recevant des doses mortelles d'une endotoxine bactérienne. *C. R. Soc. Biol. (Paris)* **148**, 1039—1043 (1954). [C622/54

Chedid, L.: Disparition de l'action antiendotoxique de la cortisone chez la souris immunisée par le bacille de Bordet-Gengou (Hemophilus Pertussis). *Ann. Endocr. (Paris)* **15**, 746—750 (1954). [C1,930/54

Chedid, L., Boyer, F.: Hypercorticisme gravidique et résistance aux salmonelloses expérimentales. *Ann. Endocr. (Paris)* **16**, 467—471 (1955). [C10,098/55

Chedid, L., Boyer, F.: Etude comparative du pouvoir antitoxique de la cortisone et de la chlorpromazine. *Ann. Inst. Pasteur* **88**, 336 a 346 (1955). [C17,612/55

Chedid, L., Boyer, F., Pophillat, F., Parant, M.: Etude de la toxicité d'une endotoxine radioactive (^{51}Cr) injectée à des parabiontes normaux et hypophysectomisés. *Ann. Inst. Pasteur* **104**, 197—207 (1963). [D57,924/63

Chedid, L., Boyer, F., Saviard, M.: Action de la cortisone vis-à-vis de l'infection expérimentale avec Salmonella typhi chez la souris. *C. R. Acad. Sci. (Paris)* **233**, 713—716 (1951). [B91,160/51

Chedid, L., Boyer, F., Saviard, M.: Surrénales et infection. *Ann. Inst. Pasteur* **83**, 213—231 (1952). [B91,161/52

Chedid, L., Boyer, F., Saviard, M.: Nouveaux aspects de l'action antitoxique de la cortisone. *Ann. Inst. Pasteur* **86**, 347—355 (1954). [B99,547/54

Chedid, L., Boyer, F., Saviard, M.: Disparition de différents effets de la cortisone chez la femelle gestante du rat. *C. R. Acad. Sci.* **238**, 156—158 (1954). [C621/54

Chedid, M. L., Parant, M.: Effets de la reserpine sur la résistance aux endotoxines bactériennes du rat et de la souris traités à la cortisone. Influence de la surrénalectomie et de l'hypophysectomie. *Ann. Endocr.* **22**, 117—125 (1961). [D6,761/61

Chedid, L., Parant, M., Boyer, F., Skarnes, R. C.: Nonspecific host responses in tolerance to the lethal effect of endotoxins. In: Landy and Braun; *Bacterial Endotoxins*, p. 500—516. New Brunswick, N. J.: Institute of Microbiology, Rutgers, The State University 1964. [E8,476/64

Chen, G., Wickel, A.: Protective effect of steroids against acute egg-white toxicity in adrenalectomized rats. *Endocrinology* **51**, 21 to 25 (1952). [B74,534/52

Chenderovitch, J.: Stop-flow analysis of bile secretion. *Amer. J. Physiol.* **214**, 86—93 (1968). [G80,059/68

Cheng, K. K.: A technique for total hepatectomy in the rat and its effect on toxicity of octamethyl pyrophosphoramide. *Brit. J. exp. Path.* **32**, 444—447 (1951). [G71,450/51

Chernozemski, I. N., Warwick, G. P.: Liver regeneration and induction of hepatomas in B6AF$_1$ mice by urethan. *Cancer Res.* **30**, 2685 to 2690 (1970). [H33,929/70

Cherrick, G. R., Stein, S. W., Leevy, C. M., Davidson, C. S.: Indocyanine green: observations on its physical properties, plasma decay, and hepatic extraction. *J. clin. Invest.* **39**, 592—600 (1960). [E98,251/60

Cherry, J. W.: Endotoxin shock. *Surg. Clin. N. Amer.* **50**, 403—408 (1970). [G74,846/70

Chesler, A., LaBelle, G. C., Himwich, H. E.: A study of the comparative toxic effects of morphine on the fetal, newborn and adult rats. *J. Pharmacol. exp. Ther.* **75**, 363—366 (1942). [A52,010/42

Cheverie, J. C., Lynn, W. G.: High temperature tolerance and thyroid activity in the teleost fish, tanichthys albonubes. *Biol. Bull.* **124**, 153—162 (1963). [D68,411/63

Cheymol, J., Pfeiffer, A.: Atteinte de la surrénale au cours de l'intoxication phalloïdienne. Essai de traitement par les hormones cortico-surrénales. *Arch. int. Pharmacodyn.* **79**, 273—281 (1949). [B 54,350/49

Cheymol, J., Quinquaud, A.: Sur la baisse de la calcemie du chien privé d'appareil thyroidïen. Influence de l'anesthésie au chloralosane. *C. R. Soc. Biol. (Paris)* **110**, 528—530 (1932).
[3,531/32

Chiancone, F. M.: I dati piu recenti sulla triptofano pirrolasi epatica. *Acta vitamin. (Milano)* **21**, 37—62 (1967). [F 85,259/67

Chiesara, E., Conti, F., Meldolesi, J.: Influence of partial hepatectomy on the induction of liver microsomal drug-metabolizing enzymes produced by phenobarbital. A biochemical and ultrastructural study. *Lab. Invest.* **22**, 329 to 338 (1970). [G 75,314/70

Chiodi, H., Sammartino, R.: Renotrophic action of lead in the rat. *Acta physiol. lat.-amer.* **1**, 33—45 (1950). [B 52,225/50

Chirico, G.: Données expérimentales sur quelques activités biologiques de l'hormone somatrope. *Rev. Path. gen.* **56**, 1041—1072 (1956). [C 24,381/56

Chirico, G., Zangaglia, O., Petronio, L.: Influenza della tiroxina sulla malattia tbc. del 'Mus musculus' albino. *Arch. Sci. med.* **107**, 225—240 (1959). [C 67,012/59

Chirico, G., Zangaglia, O., Viola, S.: Somatotropina (STH) e tubercolosi. Ricerche sperimentali. *Arch. Sci. med.* **98**, 1—20 (1954).
[C 5,040/54

Chivers, B. R., Raick, A. N., Ritchie, A. C.: Some effects of 9,12-dimethyl(a)benzanthracene and corn oil on mitoses in mouse liver after partial hepatectomy. (Abstr.) *Proc. Canad. Fed. biol. Soc. Montreal, Que.* **13**, 110 (1970). [H 25,819/70

Choi, Y., Thrasher, K., Werk, E., Sholiton, L., Olinger, C.: Enhancement of tissue uptake and turnover of cortisol by diphenylhydantoin (DPH). *Program 51st Meet. Endocr. Soc., New York, N.Y.,* p. 130 (1969).
[H 12,299/69

Choisy, H., Potron, G.: Etude comparée de l'action de la thyroxine et du métronidazole sur la vitesse de disparition de l'éthanol dans le sang du lapin. *Thérapie* **23**, 903—918 (1968).
[H 28,010/68

Christensen, B. G., Jacobsen, E.: Studies on liver regeneration. *Acta med. scand. Sup.* **243**, 103—108 (1949). [A 49,204/49

Christian, H. A.: Study XV. Hepatic lesions associated with experimental cardiac lesions. *Arch. intern. Med.* **8**, 547—551 (1911).
[D 1,675/11

Christian, H. A., Smith, R. M., Walker, I. C.: Experimental cardiorenal disease. *Arch. intern. Med.* **8**, 468—551 (1911). [C 81,653/11

Christoforov, B., Deraedt, R., Foliot, A., Petite, J. P.: Effets du phénobarbital sur l'hyperbilirubinémie provoquée chez les rats Gunn hétérozygotes et Wistar. *Path. et Biol.* **18**, 663—667 (1970). [G 77,086/70

Chury, Z., Kasparek, M.: Syndrom podobny progerii po DHT u kastrovanych krysich samecku. (Progeria-like syndrome occurring after DHT administration in castrated male rats.) *Cs. Pat.* **5**, 23—28 (1969). [H 29,730/69

Chury, Z., Nevrtal, M.: Die Herz- und Ekg-Veränderungen bei dem progerieähnlichen Syndrom der Ratte. *Ztschr. gesamt. inn. Med.* **25**, 923—928 (1970). [H 33,801/70

Ciampolini, M.: Terapia con barbiturici degli itteri da difettosa coniugazione della bilirubina. *Minerva pediat.* **21**, 2440—2446 (1969).
[G 81,416/69

Cicardo, V. H.: Sensibilidad convulsivante de los animales adrenoprivos, hipofisoprivos e inyectados con desoxicorticoesterona. *Rev. Soc. argent. Biol.* **12**, 207—213 (1945).
[B 964/45

Cicchini, T., Cao-Pinna, M., De Carlo, M.: Azione del 4-clorotestosterone acetato sulle lesioni epatiche degenerative provocate nei ratti dalla dieta di Handler. (Abstr.) *Minerva med.* **49**, 1848 (1958). [C 57,934/58

Cier, A., Maigrot, J. C., Nofre, C.: Effets synergiques de quelques substances douées d'une activité radioprotectrice. *C. R. Soc. Biol. (Paris)* **161**, 360—363 (1967).
[F 85,815/67

Cilli, V., Scuro, L. A., Castrucci, G., Barboni, E., Guercio, P. del, Ippolito, A.: Ormoni ipofisari (STH e ACTH) e desametazone nell fisiopatologia delle infezioni virale. Contributo sperimentale sulla infezione da virus del vaiolo ovino. *G. Mal. infett.* **13**, 225—250 (1961).
[D 12,192/61

Cîrstea, M., Suhaciu, G.: Incercări de terapie experimentală în şocul anafilactic la cîine. (Essais de thérapie expérimentale du choc anaphylactique du chien.) *Stud. Cercet. Fiziol.* **8**, 631—641 (1963). [G 2,471/63

Cittadini, G., Lanfredini, L., Mancini, G.: Fattori che influenzano la formazione di colonie ematopoietiche endogene nella milza del topo dopo panirradiazone. II. Effetti dello stress da freddo e dell'ormone adrenocorticotropo. *Boll. Soc. ital. Biol. sper.* **46**, 91—94 (1970).
[G 76,028/70

Ciulla, U., Razzini, M.: Ormoni gonadotropi urinari ed intossicazione da tossina difterica. Atti 36 Congr. Soc. ital. Ostet. Ginec. Torino, p. 3—10 (1939). [B50,987/39

Civen, M., Knox, W. E.: Induced synthesis of tryptophan peroxidase in rat liver slices. Fed. Proc. 16, 165 (1957). [E53,175/57

Civen, M., Knox, W. E.: The independence of hydrocortisone and tryptophan inductions of tryptophan pyrrolase. J. Biol. Chem. 234, 1787—1790 (1959). [E64,178/59

Civen, M., Wilson, C., Brown, C. B., Granner, D.: Diurnal variations in liver tyrosine α-ketoglutarate transaminase: the relationship between changes in catalytic and antigenic activity. Program 51st Meet. Endocr. Soc. New York, N.Y., p. 65 (1969). [H12,169/69

Clark, J. H., Jr., Pesch, L. A.: Effects of cortisone upon liver enzymes and protein synthesis. J. Pharmacol. exp. Ther. 117, 202—207 (1956). [C18,864/56

Clark, J. M., Higginbotham, R. D.: Influence of adrenalectomy and/or cortisol treatment on resistance to moccasin (Agkistrodon P. piscivorous) venom. Toxicon (Oxford) 8, 25—32 (1970). [G77,169/70

Clark, M. B., Pennock, J., Kalu, D. N., Bordier, P., Doyle, F. H., Foster, G. V.: Effects of calcitonin on metabolically-induced bone changes in rats. (Abstr.) Calc. Tiss. Res. 2, Sup. 18 (1968). [H5,009/68

Clark, W. C., Blackman, H. J., Preston, J. E.: Certain factors in aggregated mice damphetamine toxicity. Arch. int. Pharmacodyn. 170, 350—363 (1967). [F92,621/67

Clark, W. G., Barnes, R. H.: Effects of salts and adrenal cortical extracts upon toxicity of drugs. Proc. Soc. exp. Biol. (N.Y.) 44, 340 to 344 (1940). [A33,441/40

Clark, W. G., MacKay, E. M.: Effect of l-epinephrine and l-arterenol on egg white edema in the rat. Proc. Soc. exp. Biol. (N.Y.) 71, 86—87 (1949). [B36,925/49

Clarke, E. L.: The antagonism between steroid anesthesia and picrotoxin. Proc. canad. physiol. Soc. (7th Ann. Meet., Montebello), p. 5 (1941). [A36,747/41

Claude, A.: Microsomes, endoplasmic reticulum and interactions of cytoplasmic membranes. In: Gillette, J. R., Conney, A. H., et al.; Microsomes and Drug Oxidations, p. 3 to 39. New York, London: Academic Press Inc. 1969. [E8,217/69

Claus, J. L., Trunnell, J. B., Llaurado, J. G.: Thyroid and adrenal changes in rats bearing an experimentally induced fibrosarcoma and their influences upon the growth of the tumour. Acta endocr. (Kbh.) 40, 584—603 (1962). [D29,754/62

Cleghorn, R. A.: Studies of shock produced by muscle trauma. III. The effect of serum isinglass, glucose, certain salts, and adrenal cortical hormones on survival. Canad. J. Res. 25, 86—99 (1947). [B2,571/47

Clodi, P. H., Schnack, H.: Tierexperimentelle Untersuchungen über den sekretionshemmenden Einfluß anabol wirkender Steroide auf die Bromsulphophthaleinausscheidung durch die Leber. Wien. Z. inn. Med., 43, 50—59 (1962). [D41,569/62

Clouet, D. H., Ratner, M.: The effect of altering liver microsomal N-demethylase activity on the development of tolerance to morphine in rats. J. Pharmacol. exp. Ther. 144, 362—372 (1964). [F14,837/64

Cochin, J., Axelrod, J.: Biochemical and pharmacological changes in the rat following chronic administration of morphine, nalorphine and normorphine. J. Pharmacol. exp. Ther. 125, 105—110 (1959). [G67,795/59

Cochin, J., Sokoloff, L.: Effects of administration of L-thyroxin on liver N-demethylating activity in normal and morphine-treated rats. Proc. Soc. exp. Biol. (N.Y.) 104, 504—506 (1960). [D29,487/60

Cody, D. T. R., Code, C. F.: Protection of the rat against anaphylaxis by removal of the spleen and thymus. Fed. Proc. 22, 379 (1963). [G4,417/63

Cohen, J. L., Jao, J. Y.: Enzymatic basis of cyclophosphamide activation by hepatic microsomes of the rat. J. Pharmacol. exp. Ther. 174, 206—210 (1970). [H27,933/70

Cohen, M. B., Wasserman, P., Rudolph, J. A.: Observations on the influence of certain drugs on edema of paraphenylenediamine. J. Pharmacol. exp. Ther. 48, 235—239 (1933). [92,880/33

Cohen, P. P., Hekhuis, G. L.: Transamination in tumors, fetal tissues, and regenerating liver. Cancer Res. 1, 620—626 (1941). [93,220/41

Cohn, K. E., Agmon, J., Gamble, O. W.: The effect of glucagon on arrhythmias due to digitalis toxicity. Amer. J. Cardiol. 25, 683–689 (1970). [H26,723/70

Coker, C. M.: Cellular factors in acquired immunity to Trichinella spiralis as indicated by cortisone treatment of mice. J. infect. Dis. 98, 187—197 (1956). [C48,693/56

Coker, C. M.: Effect of cortisone on natural immunity to Schistosoma mansoni in mice. *Proc. Soc. exp. Biol. (N.Y.)* **96**, 1—3 (1957). [C 42,296/57

Colafranceschi, M., Tosi, P.: Sull'azione adrenocorticolitica nel ratto del 7,12-dimetilbenz (alfa)antracene. I. Può la funzione gonadica influenzare la suscettibilità surrenalica al tossico? *Arch. De Vecchi Anat. pat.* **49**, 541 a 564 (1967). [G 59,115/67

Colafranceschi, M., Tosi, P.: Sull'azione adrenocorticolitica nel ratto del 7,12-dimetilbenz (a) antracene. II. Influenza dell'intossicazione acuta da CCl_4, dell'epatectomia parziale e di una dieta steatogena sulla suscettibilità corticosurrenalica al tossico. *Arch. De Vecchi Anat. pat.* **50**, 681 (1967). [G 61,860/67

Colás, A.: The 16α-hydroxylation of dehydroepiandrosterone (3β-hydroxyandrost-5-en-17-one) by rat-liver slices. *Biochem. J.* **82/3**, 390—394 (1962). [D 20,925/62

Colby, H. D., Brownie, A. C.: In vivo interaction of metyrapone with adrenal cortical mitochondrial cytochrome P-450. *Arch. Biochem.* **138**, 632—639 (1970). [G 75,695/70

Cole, L. J., Foley, W. A.: Modification of urethan-lung tumor incidence by low X-radiation doses, cortisone, and transfusion of isogenic lymphocytes. *Radiat. Res.* **39**, 391—399 (1969). [H 35,251/69

Cole, L. J., Habermeyer, J. G., Bond, V. P.: Recovery from acute radiation injury in mice following administration of rat bone marrow. *J. nat. Cancer Inst.* **16**, 1—9 (1955). [C 14,411/55

Cole, V. V.: A possible method for the determination of prolonged action of barbiturates. *J. Pharmacol. exp. Ther.* **78**, 170—173 (1943). [A 30,204/43

Cole, V. V., Hulpieu, H. R.: Effect of epinephrine on toxicity of procaine. *Fed. Proc.* **8**, 283 (1949). [B 32,910/49

Cole, V. V., Hulpieu, H. R.: Influence of epinephrine and related drugs on toxicity of procaine used intravenously in dogs. *Curr. Res. Anesth.* **29**, 235—238 (1950). [B 57,578/50

Colfer, H. F.: Studies of the relationship between electrolyte of the cerebral cortex and the mechanism of convulsions. *Res. Publ. Ass. nerv. ment. Dis.* **26**, 98—117 (1947). [A 47,355/47

Collins, E. J.: Steroid-induced adrenal-pituitary hypofunction. *Proc. Soc. exp. Biol. (N.Y.)* **89**, 443—445 (1955). [C 7,486/55

Collins, E. J.: Steroid-induced adrenal-pituitary hypofunction II. *Proc. Soc. exp. Biol. (N.Y.)* **91**, 336—338 (1956). [C 12,721/56

Collins, E. J.: Steroid-induced adrenal-pituitary hypofunction. *Endocrinology* **58**, 777—780 (1956). [C 17,662/56

Collip, J. B., Kutz, R. L., Long, C. N. H., Thomson, D. L., Toby, G., Selye, H.: Acute fatty liver following partial hepatectomy. *Canad. med. Ass. J.* **33**, 689 (1935). [36,231/35

Collip, J. B., Selye, H., Thomson, D. L.: The antihormones. *Biol. Rev.* **15**, 1 (1940). [A 32,156/40

Combes, B., Shibata, H., Adams, R., Mitchell, B. D., Trammell, V.: Alterations in sulfobromophthalein sodium-removal mechanisms from blood during normal pregnancy. *J. clin. Invest.* **42**, 1431—1442 (1963). [E 26,415/63

Common, R. H., Bolton, W., Rutledge, W. A.: The influence of gonadal hormone on the composition of the blood and liver of the domestic fowl. *J. Endocr.* **5**, 263—273 (1948). [B 23,003/48

Common, R. H., Keefe, T. J., Burgess, R., Maw, W. A.: Modification of the biochemical responses of the immature pullet to oestrogen by means of dietary aureomycin. *Nature (Lond.)* **166**, 992 (1950). [B 59,914/50

Common, R. H., Moo-Young, A. J., McCully, K. A.: Some effects of dietary thiouracil and dietary iodine supplementation on the responses of the immature pullet to estrogen. *Canad. J. biochem.* **39**, 1441—1450 (1961). [D 12,509/61

Conney, A. H.: Enzyme induction and drug toxicity. In: Brodie and Gillette; *Drugs and Enzymes* (Proc. 2nd int. pharmacol. Meet.) **4**, p. 277. New York: MacMillan Co. 1965. [G 41,879/65

Conney, A. H.: Pharmacological implications of microsomal enzyme induction. *Pharmacol. Rev.* **19**, 317—366 (1967). [F 88,649/67

Conney, A. H.: Stimulatory effect of drugs on drug metabolism. (Abstr.) *Pharmacologist* **9**, 77 (1967). [G 69,760/67

Conney, A. H.: Drug metabolism and therapeutics. *New Engl. J. Med.* **280**, 653—660 (1969). [H 8,988/69

Conney, A. H.: Environmental factors influencing drug metabolism. In: *Fundamentals of Drug Metabolism and Drug Disposition* (in press). [G 70,316

Conney, A. H., Burns, J. J.: Factors influencing drug metabolism. *Advanc. Pharmacol.* **1**, 31—38 (1962). [G 67,166/62

Conney, A. H., Burns, J. J.: Induced synthesis of oxidative enzymes in liver microsomes by polycyclic hydrocarbons and drugs. In: Weber; *Advances in Enzyme Regulation*, 1, p. 189—214. New York: The MacMillan Co. 1963. [G 66,473/63

Conney, A. H., Garren, L.: Effects of thyroxin on the metabolism of zoxazolamine and hexobarbital (Abstr.). *Pharmacologist* 2, 82 (1960). [D 78,956/60

Conney, A. H., Garren, L.: Contrasting effects of thyroxin on zoxazolamine and hexobarbital metabolism. *Biochem. Pharmacol.* 6, 257—262 (1961). [D 93,666/61

Conney, A. H., Ikeda, M., Levin, W., Cooper, D., Rosenthal, O., Estabrook, R.: Carbon monoxide inhibition of steroid hydroxylation in rat liver microsomes. *Fed. Proc.* 26, 462 (1967). [F 79,331/67

Conney, A. H., Jacobson, M., Levin, K., Scheidman, K., Kuntzman, R.: Decreased central depressant effect of progesterone and other steroids in rats pretreated with drugs and insecticides. *J. Pharmacol. exp. Ther.* 154, 310—318 (1966). [F 73,731/66

Conney, A. H., Jacobson, M., Schneidman, K., Kuntzman, R.: Induction of liver microsomal cortisol 6β-hydroxylase by diphenylhydantoin or phenobarbital: an explanation for the increased excretion of 6-hydroxycortisol in humans treated with these drugs. *Life Sci.* 4, 1091—1098 (1965). [G 29,083/65

Conney, A. H., Klutch, A.: Increased activity of androgen hydroxylases in liver microsomes of rats pretreated with phenobarbital and other drugs. *J. biol. Chem.* 238, 1611—1617 (1963). [D 65,813/63

Conney, A. H., Kuntzman, R.: Metabolism of normal body constituents by drug-metabolizing enzymes in liver microsomes. In: *Concepts in Biochem. Pharmacol.* (in press). [G 70,540

Conney, A. H., Levin, W., Ikeda, M., Kuntzman, R., Cooper, D. Y., Rosenthal, O.: Inhibitory effect of carbon monoxide on the hydroxylation of testosterone by rat liver microsomes. *J. biol. Chem.* 243, 3912—3915 (1968). [G 67,773/68

Conney, A. H., Levin, W., Jacobson, M., Kuntzman, R., Cooper, D. Y., Rosenthal, O.: Specificity in the regulation of the 6β, 7α- and 16α-hydroxylation of testosterone by rat liver microsomes. In: Gillette, J. R., Conney, A. H. et al.; *Microsomes and Drug Oxidations*, p. 279—302. New York, London: Academic Press Inc. 1969. [E 8,232/69

Conney, A. H., Michaelson, I. A., Burns, J. J.: Stimulatory effect of chlorcyclizine on barbiturate metabolism. *J. Pharmacol. exp. Ther.* 132, 202—206 (1961). [D 52,543/61

Conney, A. H., Miller, E. C., Miller, J. A.: The metabolism of methylated aminoazo dyes. V. Evidence for induction of enzyme synthesis in the rat by 3-methyl-cholanthrene. *Cancer Res.* 16, 450—459 (1956). [D 87,867/56

Conney, A. H., Schneidman, K.: Enhanced androgen hydroxylase activity in liver microsomes of rats and dogs treated with phenylbutazone. *J. Pharmacol. exp. Ther.* 146, 225—235 (1964). [F 24,913/64

Conney, A. H., Schneidman, K.: Decreased hypnotic action of progesterone and other steroids in rats pretreated with drugs that stimulate steroid metabolism. *Fed. Proc.* 24, 152 (1965). [F 35,870/65

Conney, A. H., Schneidman, K., Jacobson, M., Kuntzman, R.: Drug-induced changes in steriod metabolism. *Ann. N.Y. Acad. Sci.* 123, 98—109 (1965). [G 65,135/65

Conney, A. H., Welch, R. M., Kuntzman, R., Burns, J. J.: Effects of pesticides on drug and steroid metabolism. *Clin. Pharmacol. Ther.* 8, 2—10 (1967). [G 43,018/67

Connolly, J. E.: The use of adrenal cortical compounds in hemorrhagic shock. *Lancet* 1959 I, 460—463. [C 78,861/59

Connolly, J. E., Bruns, D. L., Stofer, R. C.: The use of intravenous hydrocortisone in hemorrhagic shock. *Surg. Forum* 9, 17—22 (1958). [D 57,333/58

Connor, R. C. R.: Causes of disseminated sclerosis. *Lancet* 1970 I, 724—725. [H 23,400/70

Connors, T. A., Elson, L. A.: Reduction of the toxicity of 'radiomimetic' alkylating agents in rats by thiol pretreatment. *Biochem. Pharmacol.* 11, 1221—1232 (1962). [G 2,440/62

Connors, T. A., Elson, L. A., Leese, C. L.: The effect of glucose pretreatment on the antitumour action of Mannitol Myleran. *Biochem. Pharmacol.* 13, 963—968 (1964). [G 17,080/64

Constantin, B., Bouyard, P.: Relations du bichlorhydrate de diallylnortoxiférine avec l'effet anticurare de l'adrénaline chez le lapin anesthésié. *C. R. Soc. Biol. (Paris)* 163, 478—481 (1969). [H 15,750/69

Constantinides, P., Gordon, M. L.: The effect of some synthetic steroids on the morphogenetic action of stilbestrol, in the rat. *Rev. Canad. Biol.* 9, 107—112 (1950). [B 41,764/50

Constantinides, P., Gutmann-Auersperg, N., Hospes, D., Williams, K.: Estriol and prednisolone in rabbit atherosclerosis. *Arch. Path.* 73, 277—280 (1962). [D 21,813/62

Conti, M., Neglia, V.: Funzionalità epatica e ovulostatici orali. *Ann. ostet. Ginec.* 90, 554 to 560 (1968). [H 30,753/68

Contreras, E., Tamayo, L., Quijada, L.: Analgesic effect of ergonovine in male and female rats. *Med. Pharmacol. exp. (Basel)* 16, 159 to 164 (1967). [F 81,599/67

Cook, J. W., Blake, J. R., Williams, M. W.: The enzymic hydrolysis of malathion and its inhibition (ethyl p-nitrophenyl phenyl- and other organic phosphorus phosphonothionate) compounds. *J. Ass. Offic. Agricult. Chem.* 40, 664—665 (1957). [G 74,655/57

Cook, L., Macko, E., Fellows, E. J.: The effect of β-diethylaminoethyldiphenylpropylacetate hydrochloride on the action of a series of barbiturates and C.N.S. depressants. *J. Pharmacol. exp. Ther.* 112, 382—386 (1954). [E 34,395/54

Cook, L., Navis, G., Fellows, E. J.: Enhancement of the action of certain analgetic drugs by β-diethylaminoethyldiphenylpropylacetate hydrochloride. *J. Pharmacol. exp. Ther.* 112, 473—479 (1954). [D 94,204/54

Cook, L., Toner, J. J., Fellows, E. J.: The effect of β-diethylaminoethyldiphenylpropylacetate hydrochloride (SKF No. 525-A) on hexobarbital. *J. Pharmacol. exp. Ther.* 111, 131—141 (1954). [D 23,923/54

Cooper, D. Y., Rosenthal, O.: Acceleration by noradrenaline of hydroxylation of steroids by adrenocortical homogenates. *Arch. Biochem.* 96, 327—330 (1962). [D 20,337/62

Cooper, D. Y., Rosenthal, O.: Action of noradrenaline and ascorbic acid on C-21 hydroxylation of steroids by adrenocortical microsomes. *Arch. Biochem.* 96, 331—335 (1962). [D 20,338/62

Cooper, J., Gutstein, W. H.: Calcific aortic atherosclerosis of the rabbit after cholesterol and pitressin treatment. *J. Atheroscler. Res.* 6, 75—86 (1966). [F 61,290/66

Cooper, J. R., Axelrod, J., Brodie, B. B.: Inhibitory effects of β-diethylaminoethyl diphenylpropylacetate on a variety of drug metabolic pathways in vitro. *J. Pharmacol. exp. Ther.* 112, 55—63 (1954). [H 25,117/54

Cope, O., Graham, J. B., Mixter, G., Jr., Ball, M. R.: Threshold of thermal trauma and influence of adrenal cortical and posterior pituitary extracts on the capillary and chemical changes. An experimental study. *Arch. Surg.* 59, 1015—1069 (1949). [B 52,084/49

Coppo, M.: Ricerche sperimentali sui rapporti tra ormoni e vitamine, con speciale riguardo al timo e all'ergosterina irradiata. *Arch. int. Pharmacodyn.* 43, 123—185 (1932). [3,642/32

Coraggio, F., Coto, V., Oriente, P., Longis, G. de, Galeota, C. A.: Influenza del 19-nor-androstenolone sulla produzione di anticorpi antimorbillosi nel coniglio. *Boll. Soc. ital. Biol. sper.* 38, 1316—1317 (1962). [D 58,058/62

Coraggio, F., Pecori, V., Altucci, P., de Marco, G.: L'aldosterone nelle infezioni virali sperimentali. — III) Attività nell'infezione da virus vaccinico in culture di cellule di rene umano. *Boll. Soc. ital. Biol. sper.* 37, 714—717 (1961). [D 12,550/61

Cori, G.: Über den Einfluß der Schilddrüse auf die Wärmeregulation. Zugleich eine Bemerkung zu P. Schenk: Über den Einfluß der Schilddrüse auf den Stoffwechsel mit besonderer Berücksichtigung des Wärmehaushaltes. *Naunyn-Schmiedebergs Arch. Pharmak.* 95, 378 bis 380 (1922). [17,210/22

Corn, M.: Effect of phenobarbital and glutethimide on biological half-life of warfarin. *Thrombos. Diathes. haemorrh. (Stuttg.)* 16, 606 to 612 (1966). [H 33,065/66

Cornelius, C. E.: Studies on ovine urinary biocolloids and phosphatic calculosis. *Ann. N.Y. Acad. Sci.* 104, 638—657 (1963). [D 58,739/63

Cornforth, J. W., Long, D. A.: Influence of carbohydrate metabolism on bacterial allergy. Its relation to cortisone desensitisation. *Lancet* 1953 I, 160—164. [B 77,176/53

Correll, J. T., Lyth, L. F., Long, S., Vanderpoel, J. C.: Some physiologic responses to 5-hydroxytryptamine creatinine sulfate. *Amer. J. Physiol.* 169, 537—544 (1952). [E 57,669/52

Cort, J. H., Hammer, J., Ulrych, M., Piša, Z., Douša, T., Rudinger, J.: Synthetic extended-chain analogues of vasopressin and oxytocin in the treatment of experimental haemorrhagic shock. *Lancet* 1964 II, 840—841. [F 23,086/64

Cort, J. H., Jeanjean, M. F., Thomson, A. E., Nickerson, M.: Effects of 'hormonogen' forms of neurohypophysial peptides in hemorrhagic shock in dogs. *Amer. J. Physiol.* 214, 455—462 (1968). [F 96,105/68

Cosmides, G. J., Miya, T. S., Carr, C. J.: A study of the effects of certain lactones on digitoxin toxicity. *J. Pharmacol. Exp. Ther.* 118, 286—295 (1956). [G45,832/56

Costa, A., Smorlesi, L.: Il ripristino del fegato e la reversione rapida della cirrosi da CCl₄ dopo asportazione di larga parte del fegato cirrotico. *Arch. De Vecchi Anat. pat.* 16, 49—70 (1951). [E34,570/51

Côté, G., Gabbiani, G., Tuchweber, B.: Inhibition de l'hyperparathyroïdisme expérimental. *Un. méd. Can.* 96, 1489—1501 (1967). [G46,713/67

Côté, G., Gabbiani, G., Tuchweber, B., Déziel, C.: Effect of thyrocalcitonin and thyroxine on experimental metastatic calcification. *Acta endocr. (Kbh.)* 59, 362—370 (1968). [G46,741/68

Cournot, L., Halpern, B. N.: La testostérone a-t-elle une action protectrice contre la néphrite mercurielle chez la souris? *C. R. Soc. Biol. (Paris)* 144, 936—938 (1950). [B54,669/50

Courrier, R.: Endocrinologie de la gestation. Paris: Masson et Co. pp. 396 (1945). [86,924/45

Cox, E., Wright, S. E.: The hepatic excretion of digitalis glycosides and their genins in the rat. *J. Pharmacol. exp. Ther.* 126, 117—122 (1959). [G66,614/59

Cox, F. E. G.: The effect of betamethasone on acquired immunity to Plasmodium vinckei in mice. *Ann. trop. Med. Parasit.* 62, 295—300 (1968). [G64,797/68

Crabtree, D. G., Ward, J. C., Welch, J. F.: Sex differences in albino rats to toxic doses of powdered red squill. *Endocrinology* 25, 629—632 (1939). [A19,999/39

Craig, C. R.: Anticonvulsant activity of steroids: separability of anticonvulsant from hormonal effects. *J. Pharmacol. exp. Ther.* 153, 337—343 (1966). [F69,385/66

Craig, C. R., Deason, J. R.: Anticonvulsant activity of steroids, specificity of structure. *Arch. int. Pharmacodyn.* 172, 366—372 (1968). [F99,058/68

Crainiceanu, A., Copelman, L.: Recherches expérimentales sur l'action antitoxique de la sécrétion interne de l'ovaire. *Bull. Mem. Sect. Endocr.* 1, 92 (1935). [67,918/35

Crane, M., Loring, J., Villee, C. A.: Progesterone metabolism in regenerating rat liver. *Endocrinology* 87, 80—83 (1970). [H25,068/70

Crawford, J. S., Rudofsky, S.: Placental transmission and neonatal metabolism of promazine. *Brit. J. Anaesth.* 37, 303—309 (1965). [G78,958/65

Crawford, J. S., Rudofsky, S.: The mode of administration of promazine as a factor in determining the extent of placental transmission. *Brit. J. Anaesth.* 37, 310—313 (1965). [G78,959/65

Crawford, J. S., Rudofsky, S.: Some alterations in the pattern of drug metabolism associated with pregnancy, oral contraceptives, and the newly-born. *Brit. J. Anaesth.* 38, 446—454 (1966). [G42,454/66

Creaven, P. J., Parke, D. V., Williams, R. T.: Differential stimulation of the o- and p-hydroxylation of biphenyl by liver microsomes. *Biochem. J.* 91, 12P—13P (1964). [G77,565/64

Cremer, N., Watson, D. W.: Influence of stress on distribution of endotoxin in RES determined by fluorescein antibody technic. *Proc. Soc. exp. Biol. (N.Y.)* 95, 510—513 (1957). [C37,986/57

Crevier, M., d'Iorio, A., Robillard, E.: Influence des glandes sexuelles sur la désintoxication du pentobarbital par le foie. *Rev. canad. Biol.* 9, 336—343 (1950). [B54,151/50

Crigler, J. F., Jr.: Phenobarbital, hormones, and bilirubin. *Johns Hopk. med. J.* 125, 245—249 (1969). [G72,545/69

Crigler, J. F., Jr., Gold, N. I.: Sodium phenobarbital-induced decrease in serum bilirubin in an infant with congenital nonhemolytic jaundice and kernicterus. (Abstr.) *J. clin. Invest.* 45, 998—999 (1966). [G68,552/66

Crigler, J. F., Jr., Gold, N. I.: Effect of sodium phenobarbital on the metabolism of bilirubin-³H and ¹⁴C in an infant with congenital nonhemolytic jaundice and kernicterus. (Abstr.). *J. clin. Invest.* 46, 1047 (1967). [G68,705/67

Crigler, J. F., Jr., Gold, N. I.: Effect of sodium phenobarbital on bilirubin metabolism in an infant with congenital, nonhemolytic, unconjugated hyperbilirubinemia, and kernicterus. *J. clin. Invest.* 48, 42—55 (1969). [H7,119/69

Crispens, C. G., Rey, I. F.: Additional studies on the effects of neonatal thymectomy and lactate dehydrogenase virus infection on mice. *Experientia (Basel)* 23, 681—683 (1967). [F87,332/67

Cronin, R. F. P., Tan, E. H.: The inotropic effect of 1-noradrenaline in experimental cardiogenic shock. *Canad. J. Physiol. Pharmacol.* 43, 55—68 (1965). [F29,408/65

Cronkite, E. P., Shellabarger, C. J., Bond, V. P., Lippincott, S. W.: Studies on radiation-induced mammary gland neoplasia in the rat.

I. The role of the ovary in the neoplastic response of the breast tissue to total- or partial-body-X-irradiation. *Radiat. Res.* 12, 81—93 (1960). [C 81,609/60

Cruickshank, E. M., Kodicek, E.: The antagonism between cortisone and vitamin D: experiments on hypervitaminosis D in rats. *J. Endocr.* 17, 35—40 (1958). [C 53,881/58

Cruveilhier, J.: Anatomie pathologique du corps humain. Bailliere, Paris (1933). [A 73,454/33

Cucinell, S. A., Conney, A. H., Sansur, M., Burns, J. J.: Drug interactions in man. I. Lowering effect of phenobarbital on plasma levels of bishydroxycoumarin (Dicumarol) and diphenylhydantoin (Dilantin). *Clin. Pharmacol. Ther.* 6, 420—429 (1965). [G 66,286/65

Cueto, C., Jr.: Cardiovascular effects of o,p'-DDD. *Industr. Med. Surg.* 39, 31—32 (1970). [G 72,544/70

Cullberg, G., Lundström, R., Stenram, U.: Jaundice during treatment with an oral contraceptive, Lyndiol. *Brit. med. J.* 1965 I, 695—697. [F 34,942/65

Cullen, S. I., Catalano, P. M.: Griseofulvin-warfarin antagonism. *J. Amer. med. Ass.* 199, 582—583 (1967). [G 68,707/67

Culliford, D., Hewitt, H. B.: The influence of sex hormone status on the susceptibility of mice to chloroform-induced necrosis of the renal tubules. *J. Endocr.* 14, 381—393 (1957). [C 28,738/57

Cummings, M. M., Hudgins, P. C.: Symposium on cortisone and ACTH. The influence of cortisone on experimental tuberculosis. *Trans. 47. Ann. Meet. nat. Tuberc. Ass.*, p. 1—11 (1951). [B 66,423/51

Cunningham, M. D., Mace, J. W., Peters, E. R.: Clinical experience with phenobarbitone in icterus neonatorum. *Lancet* 1969 I, 550—551. [G 77,715/69

Curreri, P. W., Kothari, H. V., Bonner, M. J., Miller, B. F.: Increased activity of lysosomal enzymes in experimental atherosclerosis, and the effect of cortisone. *Proc. Soc. exp. Biol. (N.Y.)* 130, 1253—1256 (1969). [H 11,525/69

Currie, A. R., Helfenstein, J. E., Young, S.: Massive adrenal necrosis in rats caused by 9,10-dimethyl-, 2-benzanthracene and its inhibition by metyrapone. *Lancet* 1962 II, 1199 to 1200. [D 48,292/62

Curry, D. M., Beaton, G. H.: Glucagon administration in pregnant rats (Abstr.). *Endocrinology* 63, 252—254 (1958). [C 56,647/58

Cutts, J. H.: Protective action of diethylstilbestrol on the toxicity of vinblastine in rats. *J. nat. Cancer Inst.* 41, 919—922 (1968). [H 22,100/68

Czarnecki, E., Kiersz, J.: Der Verlauf des experimentellen Schocks nach Schilddrüsen- und Nebenschilddrüsenentfernung. *Arch. int. Pharmacodyn.* 134, 189—197 (1961). [D 15,579/61

Czeizel, E., Palkovits, M., Palkovich, I.: Die Wirkung der natürlichen Oestrogene auf die Funktion der gesunden und geschädigten Leber der Ratten. *Endocrinologie* 46, 288—298 (1964). [F 23,802/64

Dagradi, A., Candia, G. de: In tema di biologia comparata della rigenerazione epatica dopo resezione del fegato. *Chir. Pat. sper.* 10, 351—366 (1962). [D 56,609/62

Dagradi, A., Galanti, G.: Esperimenti di resezioni epatiche ripetute. *Chir. Pat. sper.* 10, 447—467 (1962). [D 62,332/62

Dairman, W., Balazs, T.: Comparison of liver microsome enzyme systems and barbiturate sleep times in rats caged individually or communally. *Biochem. Pharmacol.* 19, 951 to 955 (1970). [G 78,636/70

Dallemagne, M. J.: L'accoutumance expérimentale a l'évipan et au numal. *Arch. int. Pharmacodyn.* 65, 52—62 (1941). [A 47,748/41

Dallner, G., Siekevitz, P., Palade, G. E.: Phospholipids in hepatic microsomal membranes during development. *Biochem. biophys. Res. Commun.* 20, 142—148 (1965). [G 74,691/65

Dallner, G., Siekevits, P., Palade, G. E.: Synthesis of microsomal membranes and their enzymic constituents in developing rat liver. *Biochem. biophys. Res. Commun.* 20, 135—141 (1965). [G 74,693/65

Dallner, G., Siekevits, P., Palade, G. E.: Biogenesis of endoplasmic reticulum membranes. II. Synthesis of constitutive microsomal enzymes in developing rat hepatocyte. *J. Cell. Biol.* 30, 97—117 (1966). [G 78,599/66

Danielsson, H., Tchen, T. T.: Steroid metabolism. In: Greenberg, D. M.; *Metabolic Pathways. II. Lipids, Steroids, and Carotenoids*, p. 117—168. New York, London: Academic Press Inc. 1968. [G 72,327/68

Danysz, A., Kocmierska-Grodzka, D.: The investigations on the new ways of chemical radioprotection. *Agressologie* 8, 277—290 (1967). [F 84,845/67

Danysz, A., Panek, R.: Ocena działania radio-ochronnego metyloandrostenolonu w przebiegu choroby popromiennej wywołanej różnymi dawkami promieni RTG. *Acta physiol. pol.* **16**, 893—902 (1965). [F 61,858/65

Danysz, A., Panek, R.: Untersuchungen über die Strahlenschutzwirkung des Methandrostenolon bei Rattenweibchen. *Strahlentherapie* **135**/4, 459—463 (1968). [G 57,847/68

Danysz, A., Panek, R., Proniewski, H., Kruszewska, J.: Untersuchungen über den Wirkungsmechanismus der Strahlenschutzsubstanz Methandrostenolon. Teil I und II. *Strahlentherapie* **128**, 419—424, 610—616 (1965). [G 38,389/65

Dao, T. L.: The role of ovarian hormones in initiating the induction of mammary cancer in rats by polynuclear hydrocarbons. *Cancer Res.* **22**, 973—981 (1962). [D 36,011/62

Dao, T. L.: Some considerations on molecular structures of polynuclear hydrocarbons and inhibition of adrenal necrosis in rats. *Cancer Res.* **24**, 1238—1242 (1964). [F 19,168/64

Dao, T. L.: Carcinogenesis of mammary gland in rat. *Progr. exp. Tumor Res. (Basel)* **5**, 157—216 (1964). [G 37,357/64

Dao, T. L., Bock, F. G., Greiner, M. J.: Mammary carcinogenesis by 3-methylcholanthrene. II. Inhibitory effect of pregnancy and lactation on tumor induction. *J. nat. Cancer Inst.* **25**, 991—1003 (1960). [E 57,368/60

Dao, T. L., Greiner, M. J.: Mammary carcinogenesis by 3-methylcholanthrene. III. Induction of mammary carcinoma and milk secretion in male rats bearing ovarian grafts. *J. nat. Cancer Inst.* **27**, 333—349 (1961). [D 91,850/61

Dao, T. L., Sunderland, H.: Mammary carcinogenesis by 3-methylcholanthrene. I. Hormonal aspects in tumor induction and growth. *J. nat. Cancer Inst.* **23**, 567—585 (1959). [D 79,860/59

Dao, T. L., Tanaka, Y.: Inhibitory effect of 3-methylcholanthrene on induction of massive necrosis of adrenal cortex by 7,12-dimethylbenz(a)anthracene. *Proc. Soc. exp. Biol. (N.Y.)* **113**, 78—81 (1963). [D 67,132/63

Dao, T. L., Tanaka, Y.: Inhibitory effect of polynuclear hydrocarbons and amphenone analogs on induction of acute adrenal necrosis by 7,12-dimethylbenz(a)anthracene. *Cancer Res.* **23**, 1148—1152 (1963). [E 29,709/63

Dao, T. L., Yogo, H.: Effects of polynuclear aromatic hydrocarbons on benzpyrene hydroxylase activity in rats. *Proc. Soc. exp. Biol. (N.Y.)* **116**, 1048—1050 (1964). [F 21,633/64

Darcis, L., Brisbois, A.-M.: Influence de la thyroxine et du propionate de testostérone sur la réponse de l'intestin grêle du rat à une irradiation roentgénienne localisée. *Ann. Endocr. (Paris)* **18**, 1042—1045 (1957). [C 50,953/57

D'Arcy-Hart, P., Rees, R. J. W.: Enhancing effect of cortisone on tuberculosis in the mouse. *Lancet* **1950 II**, 391—395. [B 50,249/50

D'Arcy, P. F., Spurling, N. W.: The effect of cortisol and corticotrophin on amphetamine toxicity in mice under crowded and non-crowded conditions. *J. Endocr.* **22**, xxxv—xxxvi (1961). [D 8,818/61

Dardachti, D., Garg, B. D., Khandekar, J. D., Kovacs, K.: L'effet du metyrapone sur l'ultrastructure hépatique chez le rat surrénalectomisé. *Ann. Anat. path. (in press).* [G 79,006/

Da Rocha Lagoa, F., *cf.* Rocha Lagoa, F. da [B 49,008/47

Das, R. P., Kar, A. B.: Effect of corticoids on the testis of cadmium chloride treated rats. *Proc. nat. Inst. Sci. India B*, **27**, 46—51 (1961). [D 14,801/61

Dashputra, P. G., Sharma, M. L., Rajapurkar, M. V.: Modification of metrazol induced convulsions in rats by adrenal cortical steroids. *Arch. int. Pharmacodyn.* **150**, 483—488 (1964). [F 19,871/64

Dasler, W.: Protective action of glutamine, cysteine and other substances against experimental lathyrism in the rat. *Proc. Soc. exp. Biol. (N.Y.)* **91**, 554—557 (1956). [C 15,943/56

Dasler, W.: Experimental lathyrism. *Chic. Med. Sch. Quart.* **18**, 1—10 (1957). [C 36,068/57

D'Aste, G., Ardau, B.: Sulfotiazolo, penicillina, streptomicina, metiltiouracile, neoantergan e loro influenza sullo shock sperimentale. *Riv. Chir. Med.* **1**, 91—123 (1949). [B 56,421/49

Datta, D. V., Isselbacher, K. J.: Effect of corticosteroids on mouse hepatitis virus infection. *Gut* **10**, 522—529 (1969). [G 68,822/69

Datta, P. R.: In vivo detoxication of p,p'-DDT via p,p'-DDE to p,p'-DDA in rats. *Industr. Med. Surg.* **39**, 190—194 (1970). [G 75,362/70

Dau, W., Weber, H. G.: Chemisch-hormonelle Stoffwechselbeeinflussung und Verlängerung der Wiederbelebungszeit. *Langenbecks Arch. klin. Chir.* **302**, 779—784 (1963). [G 20,433/63

Daugharty, D. A., Sullivan, J. F., Gantner, G. E.: Effect of cortisone on ethionine-induced pancreatitis in the rat. *Proc. Soc. exp. Biol. (N.Y.)* 101, 826—829 (1959). [C74,925/59

Dautrebande, L.: L'action du benzol sur le système vaso-moteur. La syncope adrénalinobenzolique. *C. R. Soc. Biol. (Paris)* 111, 218—220 (1932). [8,083/32

da Vanzo, J. P., *cf.* **Vanzo, J. P. da**
[F19,865/64

Davenport, V. D.: Relation between brain and plasma electrolytes and electroshock seizure thresholds in adrenalectomized rats. *Amer. J. Physiol.* 156, 322—327 (1949). [B36,663/49

Davidow, B., Frawley, J. P.: Tissue distribution, accumulation and elimination of the isomers of benzene hexachloride. *Proc. Soc. exp. Biol. (N.Y.)* 76, 780—783 (1951).
[H27,655/51

Davidson, A., Owen, J., Thomas, C. G., Jr.: Further studies on the role of altered thyroid function on experimentally induced breast cancer in Sprague-Dawley rats. (Abstr.) *Proc. Amer. Ass. Cancer Res.* 10, 17 (1969). [H10,206/69

Davies, D. S., Gigon, P. L., Gillette, J. R.: Sex differences in the kinetic constants for the N-demethylation of ethylmorphine by rat liver microsomes. *Biochem. Pharmacol.* 17, 1865 to 1872 (1968). [H22,054/68

Davies, D. S., Gigon, P. L., Gillette, J. R.: Species and sex differences in electron transport systems in liver microsomes and their relationship to ethylmorphine demethylation. *Life Sci.* 8, 85—91 (1969). [G76,865/69

Davies, J. E., Edmundson, W. F., Carter, C. H., Barquet, A.: Effect of anticonvulsant drugs on dicophane (D.D.T.) residues in man. *Lancet* 1969 II, 7—9. [G77,532/69

Davis, D. A., Medline, N. M.: Spironolactone (aldactone) bodies: concentric lamellar formations in the adrenal cortices of patients treated with spironolactone. *Amer. J. clin. Path.* 54, 22—32 (1970). [G76,611/70

Davis, N. C., Whipple, G. H.: The influence of drugs and chemical agents on the liver necrosis of chloroform anesthesia. Paper II. *Arch. intern. Med.* 23, 636—654 (1919).
[58,731/19

Davis, V. E.: Effect of cortisone and thyroxine on aromatic amino acid decarboxylation. *Endocrinology* 72, 33—38 (1963). [D92,322/63

Davis, W. M., Su, M. Q.: Effects of adrenalectomy and repeated convulsions on responses of rats to flurothyl. *Int. J. Neuropharmacol.* 8, 55—59 (1969). [H31,927/69

Davison, A. N.: The conversion of schradan (OMPA) and parathion into inhibitors of cholinesterase by mammalian liver. *Biochem. J.* 61, 203—209 (1955). [A49,341/55

Davydova, S. A.: Effect of sex hormones on course of acute radiation sickness. *Fed. Proc.* 23/2, T1166—T1168 (1964). [F23,736/64

Dayton, P. G., Tarcan, Y., Chenkin, T., Weiner, M.: The influence of barbiturates on coumarin plasma levels and prothrombin response. *J. clin. Invest.* 40, 1797—1802 (1961).
[D42,366/61

Dearing, W. H., Barnes, A. R., Essex, H. E.: Experiments with calculated therapeutic and toxic doses of digitalis. I. Effects on the myocardial cellular structure. *Amer. Heart J.* 25, 648—664 (1943). [C41,482/43

Dearing, W. H., Barnes, A. R., Essex, H. E.: Myocardial lesions produced by digitalis in the presence of hyperthyroidism; an experimental study. *Circulation* 1, 394—403 (1950).
[B53,571/50

DeBaun, J. R., Miller, E. C., Miller, J. A.: N-hydroxy-2-acetylaminofluorene sulfotransferase: its probable role in carcinogenesis and in protein-(methion-S-yl) binding in rat liver. *Cancer Res.* 30, 577—595 (1970). [H26,701/70

Debias, D. A.: Hormonal factors in the rat's tolerance to altitude. *Amer. J. Physiol.* 203, 818—820 (1962). [D41,419/62

Debias, D. A.: Thyroid-adrenal relationship in altitude tolerance. *Fed. Proc.* 25, 1227—1229 (1966). [F69,410/66

Debias, D. A., Wang-Yen: The effect of hormones on the rat's tolerance to simulated altitude. *Fed. Proc.* 21, 186 (1962).
[D22,848/62

de Boer, B., *cf.* **Boer, B. de** [A48,817/48

de Boer, B., Mukomela, A. E., *cf.* **Boer, B. de, Mukomela, A. F.** [C5,245/55

Debry, G.: Influence du terrain endocrinien sur les infections. (Etudes clinique et expérimentale). Ses conséquences en médecine sociale. Tome II. *Thèse,* Université de Nancy 1956.
[C30,870/56

Debry, G., Berger, H., Jolibois, C.: Le rôle de la thyroïde dans l'infection tuberculeuse expérimentale. *Rev. Tuberc. (Paris)* 26, 311—325 (1962). [D34,828/62

Decken, A. von der, Hultin, T.: The enzymatic composition of rat liver microsomes during liver regeneration. *Exp. Cell. Res.* 19, 591—604 (1960). [G37,124/60

Decken, A. von der, Hultin, T.: Inductive effects of 3-methylcholanthrene on enzyme activities and amino acid incorporation capacity of rat liver microsomes. *Arch. Biochem.* **90**, 201—207 (1960). [G 68,039/60

De Dominicis, G., *cf.* Dominicis, G. De [B 3,412/42

DeFeo, J. J., Baumel, I., Lal, H.: Drug environment interactions: acute hypoxia and chronic isolation. *Fed. Proc.* **29**, 1985—1990 (1970). [H 32,863/70

Dehnen, W., Tomingas, R., Schagholi, H.: Abbau von Benzo(a)pyren durch Enzyme der Rattenlebermikrosomen in vitro in Abhängigkeit vom Alter und Geschlecht der Versuchstiere. *Z. Krebsforsch.* **73**, 363—370 (1970). [G 74,165/70

Deichmann, W. B., Dees, J. E., Keplinger, M. L., Farrell, J. J., MacDonald, W. E., Jr.: Toxicity of crotalus adamanteus (Rattlesnake) venom and the antidotal effects of hydrocortisone. *Fed. Proc.* **16**, 291 (1957). [C 33,188/57

Deichmann, W. B., Radomski, J. L., Farrell, J. J., MacDonald, W. E., Keplinger, M. L.: Acute toxicity and treatment of intoxications due to crotalus adamanteus (Rattlesnake venom). *Amer. J. med. Sci.* **236**, 204—207 (1958). [C 73,854/58

Deichmann, W. B., Witherup, S., Kitzmiller, K. V.: The toxicity of DDT. Experimental observations. *Prev. Med. and Industr. Health, Coll. Med.*, p. 71 (1950). [D 98,307/50

DeLeon, A., Gartner, L. M., Arias, I. M.: The effect of phenobarbital on hyperbilirubinemia in glucuronyl transferase deficient rats. *J. Lab. clin. Med.* **70**, 273—278 (1967). [G 71,826/67

Delfini, C.: Influenza dell'elettro-schok sull'arteriosclerosi sperimentale da adrenalina. *G. Psichiat. Neuropat.* **78**, 305—325 (1950). [B 52,659/50

DeLorimier, A. A., Gordan, G. S., Lowe, R. C., Carbone, J. V.: Methyltestosterone, related steroids, and liver function. *Arch. intern. Med.* **116**, 289—294 (1965). [G 31,525/65

DeLuca, H. F.: Vitamin D. *New Engl. J. Med.* **281**, 1103—1104 (1969). [H 17,327/69

De Marchi, G., *cf.* Marchi, G. De [A 30,837/38

De Mitri, T., *cf.* Mitri, T. De [D 64,042/63

Denef, C., de Moor, P.: The "puberty" of the rat liver. II. Permanent changes in steroid metabolizing enzymes after treatment with a single injection of testosterone propionate at birth. *Endocrinology* **83**, 791—798 (1968). [H 3,569/68

Denef, C., de Moor, P.: "Puberty" of the rat liver. IV. Influence of estrogens upon the differentiation of cortisol metabolism induced by neonatal testosterone. *Endocrinology* **85**, 259—269 (1969). [H 15,811/69

Denison, M. E., Zarrow, M. X.: The effect of cold on survival and reproductive activities in the rat. *Anat. Rec.* **113**, 531 (1952). [B 77,713/52

Dent, C. E., Richens, A., Rowe, D. J. F., Stamp, T. C. B.: Osteomalacia with long-term anticonvulsant therapy in epilepsy. *Brit. med. J.* **1970 II**, 69—72. [H 30,946/70

Deplano, P.: Il comportamento degli acidi nucleinici nel fegato dopo epatectomia parziale nel ratto normale e nel ratto sottoposto a trattamento cortisonico. *Atti Acad. med. lombarda* **23**, 741—748 (1968). [H 23,483/68

Deplano, P., Fornara, C. F.: Il comportamento della fosfatasi alcalina nel fegato dopo epatectomia parziale nel ratto normale e nel ratto sottoposto a trattamento cortisonico. *Atti Acad. med. lombarda* **23**, 749—754 (1968). [H 23,484/68

Deppe, H. D., Lutzmann, L.: Einfluß eines anabolen Steroids auf die cytostatisch gehemmte Antikörperbildung bei der Ratte. *Z. Hyg. Infekt.-Kr.* **149**, 401—406 (1964). [G 14,653/64

Deringer, M. K., Dunn, T. B., Heston, W. E.: Results of exposure of strain C3H mice to chloroform. *Proc. Soc. exp. Biol. (N.Y.)* **83**, 474—479 (1953). [G 64,723/53

Derom, P., van Hoydonck, J.: Influence de l'A.C.T.H. et de la cortisone sur la leptospirose expérimentale du cobaye. *Rev. belge Path.* **24**, 207—208 (1955). [C 17,095/55

Dérot, M., Tutin, M.: Néphropathie aiguë après ingestion de nitrate mercurique. (Considérations sur le traitement des néphropathies mercurielles). *Bull. Soc. méd. Hôp. Paris* **73**, 1039—1044 (1957). [C 67,130/57

Dési, I., Szold, E., Olasz, J.: Die Verlängerung der Lebensdauer urämischer Tiere mit einem neuen Hormonpräparat. *Z. Urol.* **54**, 161—164 (1961). [D 11,138/61

Dési, I., Szold, A., Weisz, P., Kádas, T., Zalán, J.: Wirkung des somatotropen Hormons auf experimentelle Urämie. *Z. ges. inn. Med.* **14**, 299—300 (1959). [C 69,045/59

DesMarais, A., Dugal, L. P.: Circulation périphérique et teneur des surrénales en adrénaline et en artgrénol (nor-adrénaline) chez le rat blanc exposé au froid. *Proc. Canad.*

Physiol. Soc., 14th Ann. Meet., Ottawa, p. 11 (1950). [B 51,093/50]

DesMarais, A., Dugal, L. P.: Influence de l'administration d'adrénaline et d'arténol, sur l'hypertrophie de la surrénale au froid. *Canad. J. med. Sci.* **29**, 104—107 (1951). [B 64,359/51]

Despopoulos, A.: Excretion of sulfobromophthalein by perfused rat liver as influenced by steroidal hormones. *J. Pharmacol. exp. Ther.* **173**, 37—42 (1970). [H 24,651/70]

Despopoulos, A.: Hepatic and renal excretory metabolism of bile salts a background for understanding steroid-induced cholestasis. *J. Pharmacol. exp. Ther.* **176**, 273—283 (1971). [H 35,471/71]

Dessau, F.: Nebennierenwirkungen bei der akuten Acetonitrilvergiftung der Ratte. *Acta brev. neerl. Physiol.* **5**, 1—2 (1935). [34,845/35]

de Valderrama, J. A. F., Munuera, L. M., *cf.* Valderrama, J. A. F. de, Munuera, L. M. [E 6,008/66]

Dewaide, J. H.: Species differences in hepatic drug oxidation in mammals and fishes in relation to thermal acclimation. *Comp. gen. Pharmacol.* **1**, 375—384 (1970). [G 80,406/70]

Dewar, A. D.: The nature of the weight gain induced by progesterone in mice. *Quart. J. exp. Physiol.* **49**, 151—161 (1964). [G 9,079/64]

Dewhurst, F.: The effect of 1:2:5:6 dibenzanthracene (D.B.A.) upon the metabolism of β-naphthylamine in the rat. *Naturwissenschaften* **50**, 404—405 (1963). [G 76,687/63]

Dewhurst, F., Kitchen, D. A.: The effect of prolonged pretreatment with 6-substituted benzo pyrene derivatives upon zoxazolamine paralysis times in mice. *Biochem. Pharmacol.* **19**, 615—617 (1970). [G 73,848/70]

Dhunèr, K. G., Nordqvist, P.: Sleep reinduced by cortisone and glucose in patients intoxicated with barbiturates and related drugs. *Acta anaesth. scand.* **1**, 55—62 (1957). [D 98,693/57]

Diaz, C. J., Vivanco, F., Ramos, F., Martin, J. A. S.: Ulteriores estudios sobre el latirismo experimental de la rate (odoratismo). *Rev. clin. exp.* **67**, 295—304 (1957). [C 50,497/57]

Diaz, C. J., Vivanco, F., Ramos, F., Martin, J. A. S.: Further studies of experimental lathyrism in rats (odoratism). *Bull. Inst. med. Res. (Madr.)* **11**, 23—40 (1958). [D 99,329/58]

Di Carlo, F. J., et al., *cf.* Carlo, F. J. Di, et al. [F 74,536/65]

Dick, E. C., Greenberg, S. M., Herndon, J. F., Jones, M., van Loon, E. J.: Hypocholesteremic effect of β-diethylaminoethyl diphenylpropylacetate hydrochloride (SKF No. 525-A) in the dog. *Proc. Soc. exp. Biol. (N.Y.)* **104**, 523—526 (1960). [G 74,672/60]

Dick, W., Droh, R., Frey, R., Hadjidimos, M., Halmagyi, M., Heymer, G., Oettel, P.: Experimentelle und klinische Untersuchungen mit dem Muskelrelaxans Pancuroniumbromid. *Anaesthesist* **19**, 248—250 (1970). [G 77,777/70]

Dieckhoff, J., Bartel, J., Hoppe, E.: Zur Pathogenese und Therapie des Waterhouse-Friderichsen-Syndroms. *Dtsch. med. Wschr.* **93**, 1397—1401 (1968). [H 1,991/68]

Diengott, D., Ungar, H.: Effect of cortisone on carbon tetrachloride cirrhosis in rats. *Arch. Path.* **58**, 449—454 (1954). [E 84,645/54]

Dietrich, L. S.: Effect of hyperphysiological levels of steroid hormones on nicotinamide deamidase and NAD synthesis in mouse liver tissue. *Biochem. Pharmacol.* **14**, 467—472 (1965). [G 28,103/65]

Dietrich, L. S., Franklin, L., Farinas, B.: Effect of hyperphysiological levels of hexestrol on the hepatic metabolism of nicotinate in the mouse. *Proc. Soc. exp. Biol. (N.Y.)* **133**, 160—163 (1970). [H 19,763/70]

Dietrich, L. S., Yero, I. L.: Endocrine involvement in the suppression of NAD synthesis produced by hyperphysiological levels of steroid hormones. *Biochim. biophys. Acta (Amst.)* **97**, 385—388 (1965). [G 26,959/65]

Dietrich, W. C., Beutner, R.: The mechanism of action of thiouracil. *Proc. Soc. exp. Biol. (N.Y.)* **57**, 35—36 (1944). [B 20,412/44]

Dille, J. M.: Studies on barbiturates. IX. The effect of barbiturates on the embryo and on pregnancy. *J. Pharmacol. exp. Ther.* **52**, 129 to 136 (1934). [45,154/34]

Dille, J. M., Seeberg, V. P.: Preliminary report on the elimination of metrazol. *Pharm. Arch.* **12**, 9 (1941). [84,277/41]

Dingell, J. V., Heimberg, M.: The effect of aliphatic halogenated hydrocarbons on hepatic drug metabolism. *Biochem. Pharmacol.* **17**, 1269—1278 (1968). [G 72,112/68]

Discher, R., Laaff, H., Creutzfeldt, W., Kühn, H. A.: Untersuchungen über die therapeutische Beeinflußbarkeit experimenteller Lebercirrhosen bei der Ratte. III. Die Tetrachlorkohlenstoff-Cirrhose der Ratte und ihre therapeutische Beeinflussung durch Glucocorticoide mit und ohne gleichzeitige Verabreichung von

Antibiotica und Androgenen. *Z. ges. exp. Med.* 136, 500—516 (1963). [D 64,428/63

Dixon, R. L., Fouts, J. R.: Inhibition of microsomal drug metabolic pathways by chloramphenicol. *Biochem. Pharmacol.* 11, 715—720 (1962). [E 53,752/62

Dixon, R. L., Hart, L. G., Fouts, J. R.: The metabolism of drugs by liver microsomes from alloxan diabetic rats. *J. Pharmacol. Exp. Ther.* 133/1, 7—11 (1961). [D 9,331/61

Dixon, R. L., Hart, L. G., Rogers, L. A., Fouts, J. R.: The metabolism of drugs by liver microsomes from alloxan-diabetic rats: long term diabetes. *J. Pharmacol. exp. Ther.* 142, 312—317 (1963). [E 35,705/63

Dixon, R. L., Rogers, L. A., Fouts, J. R.: The effects of norepinephrine treatment on drug metabolism by liver microsomes from rats. *Biochem. Pharmacol.* 13, 623—631 (1964). [G 11,757/64

Dixon, R. L., Shultice, R. W., Fouts, J. R.: Factors affecting drug metabolism by liver microsomes. IV. Starvation. *Proc. Soc. exp. Biol. (N.Y.)* 103, 333—335 (1960). [G 65,886/60

Dixon, R. L., Willson, V. J.: Metabolism of hexobarbital and zoxazolamine by placentae and fetal liver supernatant fraction and response to phenobarbital and chlordane treatment. *Arch. int. Pharmacodyn.* 172, 453—466 (1968). [H 30,692/68

Dmitriev, V. N.: The hormone prophylaxis of dyshormonal hyperplasias of the mammary glands in mice. (Russian text.) *Vop. Onkol.* 15/1, 59—61 (1969). [H 28,154/69

Dmowski, W. P., Scholer, H. F. L., Mahesh, V. B., Greenblatt, R. B.: Danazol: a synthetic steroid derivative with interesting physiologic properties. *Fertil. and Steril.* 22, 9—18 (1971). [G 80,777/71

Dobrescu, D., Coeugniet, E., Coeugniet, A.: Influența prednisolonului și testosteronului asupra toleranței la morfină. (Influence de la prednisolone et de la testostérone sur la tolérance envers la morphine.) *Stud. Cercet. Fiziol.* 15, 163—169 (1970). [H 26,899/70

Dobrev, P.: Experimentelle Studien zur Pathogenese der Tuberkulose bei Diabetikern. *Beitr. Klin. Tuberk.* 129, 153—157 (1964). [G 23,362/64

Dobrokhotova, L. P.: Effect of methylthiouracil on haemorrhagic shock under the influence of trauma to the nervous system. (Russian text with Engl. summary.) *Doklady Akad. nauk. SSSR.* 114, 1320—1321 (1957). [C 55,431/57

Dobrolvolskaïa-Zavadskaïa, N., Vérotennikoff, M. S., Rodzévitch, M.: La survie des souris, de lignée et d'âge differents, aprés une seule irradiation totale par les rayons X. *C. R. Acad. Sci.* 213, 704—706 (1941). [86,799/41

Dodd, J. M., Dent, J. N.: Thyroid gland and temperature tolerance relationships in cold-blooded vertebrates. *Nature (Lond.)* 199, 299 (1963). [E 21,585/63

Dolfini, E., Kobayashi, M.: Studies with amphetamine in hyper- and hypothyroid rats. *Europ. J. Pharmacol.* 2, 65—66 (1967). [F 91,611/67

Dolgova, Z. Y., Dolgov, E. G.: Effect of thyroid hormone on the internal organs in rats as revealed by vital staining of the tissues. (Russian text.) *Bull. exp. Biol. Med.* 58, 1246—1248 (1964). [G 33,058/64

Dominicis, G. De: Tricloroetilene, estratti corticali e vitamina C. *Folia endocr. (Roma)* 20, 97—106 (1942). [B 3,412/42

Domschke, W., Domagk, G. F., Domschke, S., Erdmann, W. D.: Hemmung der Soman-induzierten Enzymbiosynthese in der Rattenleber durch Äthionin. *Arch. Toxikol.* 26, 142—148 (1970). [G 74,897/70

Donatelli, L.: Età, sesso e barbiturismo acuto. Contributo clinico e sperimentale. *Arch. int. Pharmacodyn.* 74, 90—111 (1947). [B 38,172/47

Donatelli, L.: Età, sesso ed idrargirismo acuto. Contributo clinico e sperimentale. *Arch. int. Pharmacodyn.* 74, 193—211 (1947). [B 38,554/47

Done, A. K.: Developmental pharmacology. *Clin. Pharmacol. Ther.* 5, 432—479 (1964). [G 81,518/64

Done, A. K.: Perinatal pharmacology. *Ann Rev. Pharmacol.* 6, 189—208 (1966). [G 81,512/66

Donomae, I., Hori, M., Hattori, S., Mishima, J.: Histochemical studies on the experimental tuberculous cavity formation of the rabbit lung: effect of ACTH administration on the cavity formation. *Med. J. Osaka Univ.* 6, 463—478 (1955). [C 22,935/55

Dontenwill, W., Mancini, A. M.: IV. Experimentelle Untersuchungen über hormonale Beeinflussung des Knochenwachstums beim Kaninchen. *Beitr. pathol. Anat.* 117, 50—64 (1957). [C 35,119/57

Dooley, E. S., Holtman, D. F.: Effect of the administration of cortisone on the response of chicks to the endotoxin of salmonella pullorum. *J. Bact.* **78**, 562—566 (1959). [C84,689/59

Dorfman, R. I.: Steroids and tissue oxidation. In: Harris, R.S., *Vitamins and Hormones*, p. 331. New York: Academic Press Inc. Publ. 1952. [B76,571/52

Dorrance, S. S., Thorn, G. W., Tyler, F. H., Katzin, B.: Work performance of normal rats under conditions of anoxia. *Endocrinology* **31**, 209—216 (1942). [A38,460/42

Dosne, C.: The effect of dosage and duration of administration on the anti-uremic effect of desoxycorticosterone. *Amer. J. Physiol.* **134**, 71—73 (1941). [A35,924/41

Dossena, P.: Recherches sur l'influence des hormones sexuelles dans l'intoxication expérimentale par le venin de naja flava (Cape cobra). *Acta trop. (Basel)* **6**, 263—267 (1949). [B47,510/49

Dotti, L. B.: The response of the rabbit to insulin. *Amer. J. Physiol.* **114**, 538—550 (1936). [34,994/36

Dougherty, J. H., Dougherty, T. F.: Acute effect of 4-aminopteroylglutamic acid on blood lymphocytes and the lymphatic tissue of intact and adrenalectomized mice. *J. Lab. clin. Med.* **35**, 271—279 (1950). [G77,517/50

Douglas, A. C.: Treatment of radiation pneumonitis with prednisolone. *Brit. J. Dis. Chest* **53**, 346—355 (1959). [C78,775/59

Douglas, B.: Action protectrice de l'adrénaline. Syncope adrénalino-chloro-formique. *C. R. Soc. Biol. (Paris)* **91**, 1419—1420 (1924). [20,147/24

Douglas, B.: Action empêchante de l'adrénaline sur l'absorption du venin de cobra par la peau. *C. R. Soc. Biol. (Paris)* **91**, 1223—1224 (1924). [21,321/24

Douglas, B. H., Clower, B. R.: Hepatotoxic effect of carbon tetrachloride during pregnancy. *Amer. J. Obstet. Gynec.* **102**, 236—239 (1968). [H20,791/68

Doull, J., Tricou, B. J.: Studies on the radioprotective effect of serotonin in mice. *Fed. Proc.* **20**, 400 (1961). [D4,271/61

Dowben, R. M.: Prolonged survival of dystrophic mice treated with 17α-ethyl-19-nortestosterone. *Nature (Lond.)* **184**, 1966—1967 (1959). [C79,563/59

Dowben, R. M.: Anabole Steroide bei Myopathien. In: Beckmann; *Myopathien*, p. 242—251. Stuttgart: Georg Thieme Verlag 1965. [E80/65

Dowben, R. M., Gordon, P.: Effects of steroids on the survival of dystrophic mice. *Fed. Proc.* **20**, 302 (1961). [D4,188/61

Dowben, R. M., Zuckerman, L., Gordon, P., Sniderman, S. P.: Effect of steroids on the course of hereditary muscular dystrophy in mice. *Amer. J. Physiol.* **206**, 1049—1056 (1964). [F10,902/64

Dowling, J. N., Feldman, H. A.: Quantitative biological assay of bacterial endotoxins. *Proc. Soc. exp. Biol. (N.Y.)* **134**, 861—864 (1970). [H31,139/70

Downs, A. W., Eddy, N. B.: The effect of repeated doses of cocaine on the rat. *J. Pharmacol. exp. Ther.* **46**, 199—200 (1932). [58,426/32

Drabkin, D. L.: The effect of thyroidectomy and of thiouracil on cytochrome c metabolism and liver regeneration. *Fed. Proc.* **7**, 151 (1948). [B17,795/48

Drabkin, D. L.: Cytochrome c metabolism and liver regeneration. Influence of adrenalectomy. *J. biol. Chem.* **182**, 351—357 (1950). [B53,844/50

Drabkin, D. L.: Cytochrome c metabolism and liver regeneration. Influence of thyroid gland and thyroxine. *J. biol. Chem.* **182**, 335—349 (1950). [D18,388/50

Drachman, R. H., Root, R. K., Wood, W. B. Jr.: Studies on the effect of experimental nonketotic diabetes mellitus on antibacterial defense. I. Demonstration of a defect in phagocytosis. *J. exp. Med.* **124**, 227—240 (1966). [F81,617/66

Dragstedt, L. R., Peacock, S. C.: Studies on the pathogenesis of tetany. I. The control and cure of parathyroid tetany by diet. *Amer. J. Physiol.* **64**, 424—434 (1923). [17,556/23

Dragstedt, L. R., Phillips, K., Sudan, A. C.: Studies on the pathogenesis of tetany. II. The mechanism involved in recovery from parathyroid tetany. *Amer. J. Physiol.* **65**, 368—378 (1923). [17,561/23

Draize, J. H., Tatum, A. L.: A method for the study of the biological potency of thyroid preparations. *J. Pharmacol. exp. Ther.* **42**, 262 (1931). [3,901/31

Draize, J. H., Tatum, A. L.: Experimental thyrotoxicosis. *Arch. int. Pharmacodyn.* **43**, 237—245 (1932). [3,657/32

Drawkins, M. J. R.: Carbon tetrachloride poisoning in the liver of the new-born rat. *J. Path. Bact.* **85**, 189—196 (1963). [G78,605/63

Drews, J.: Klinische und biochemische Wirkungen der Glukokortikoide, dargestellt am

Beispiel des Cushing-Syndroms. *Med. Klin.* 64, 773—789 (1969). [H 12,100/69

Drews, J., Brawerman, G.: Alterations in the nature of ribonucleic acid synthesized in rat liver during regeneration and after cortisol administration. *J. biol. Chem.* 242, 801—808 (1967). [G 52,150/67

Driever, C. W., Bousquet, W. F.: Stress drug interactions: evidence for rapid enzyme inductions. *Life Sci.* 4, 1449—1454 (1965). [G 31,872/65

Driever, C. W., Bousquet, W. F., Miya, T. S.: Stress stimulation of drug metabolism in the rat. *Int. J. Neuropharmacol.* 5, 199—205 (1966). [F 73,812/66

Druskemper, H. L.: Anabolic Steroids, pp. 236. New York, London: Academic Press Inc. 1968. (Originally published in German) Stuttgart: George Thieme Verlag 1963. [E 933/63

Dryden, L. P., Hartman, A. M.: Unidentified nutrients required by the hyperthyroid rat. *Fed. Proc.* 18, 523 (1959). [C 66,416/59

DuBois, K. P.: Inhibition by radiation of the development of drug-detoxification enzymes. *Radiat. Res.* 30, 342—350 (1967). [G 77,578/67

DuBois, K. P., Doull, J., Coon, J. M.: Studies on the toxicity and pharmacological action of octamethyl pyrophosphoramide (OMPA: Pestox III). *J. Pharmacol. exp. Ther.* 99, 376 to 393 (1950). [D 92,992/50

DuBois, K. P., Doull, J., Salerno, P. R., Coon, J. M.: Studies on the toxicity and mechanism of action of p-nitrophenyl diethyl thionophosphate (parathion). *J. Pharmacol. exp. Ther.* 95, 79—91 (1949). [G 66,495/49

DuBois, K. P., Herrmann, R. G., Erway, W. F.: Studies on the mechanism of action of thiourea and related compounds. III. The effect of acute poisoning on carbohydrate metabolism. *J. Pharmacol. exp. Ther.* 89, 186—195 (1947). [B 3,089/47

DuBois, K. P., Holm, L. W., Doyle, W. L.: Studies on the mechanism of action of thiourea and related compounds. I. Metabolic changes after acute poisoning by alpha-naphthylthiourea. *J. Pharmacol. exp. Ther.* 87, 53—62 (1946). [B 3,103/46

DuBois, K. P., Kinoshita, F.: Modification of the anticholinesterase action of 0,0-diethyl 0-(4-methylthio-m-tolyl) phosphorothioate (DMP) by drugs affecting hepatic microsomal enzymes 1. *Arch. int. Pharmacodyn.* 156, 418—431 (1965). [G 66,247/65

DuBois, K. P., Kinoshita, F.: Stimulation of detoxification of 0-ethyl 0-(4-nitrophenyl) phenylphosphonothioate (EPN) by nikethamide and phenobarbital. *Proc. Soc. exp. Biol. (N.Y.)* 121, 59—62 (1966). [H 24,226/66

DuBois, K. P., Kinoshita, F. K.: Influence of induction of hepatic microsomal enzymes by phenobarbital on toxicity of organic phosphate insecticides. *Proc. Soc. exp. Biol. (N.Y.)* 129, 699—702 (1968). [G 66,349/68

DuBois, K. P., Puchala, E.: Studies on the sex difference in toxicity of a cholinergic phosphorothioate. *Proc. Soc. exp. Biol. (N.Y.)* 107, 908—911 (1961). [D 43,878/61

Dubos, R. J.: Effect of metabolic factors on the susceptibility of albino mice to experimental tuberculosis. *J. exp. Med.* 101, 59—84 (1955). [D 93,317/55

Dubos, R. J.: Biochemical determinants of infection. *Bull. N. Y. Acad. Med.* 31, 5—19 (1955). [G 71,484/55

Dubos, R. J., Smith, J. M., Schaedler, R. W.: Metabolic disturbances and infection. *Proc. Roy. Soc. Med.* 48, 911—918 (1955). [C 21,520/55

Ducheneau, L.: Action de l'insuline sur les lapins ethyroidés. *C. R. Soc. Biol. (Paris)* 90, 248—249 (1924). [20,846/24

Ducommun, P., Ducommun, S.: Sur l'action de la somatotrophine hypophysaire dans la prévention des infections favorisées par le surdosage en cortisone. *Ann. Endocr. (Paris)* 14, 765—771 (1953). [B 70,251/53

Ducommun, P., Ducommun, S., Baquiche, M.: Comparaison entre l'action du 17-ethyl-19-nortestosterone et du propionate de testosterone chez le rat adulte et immature. *Acta endocr. (Kbh.)* 30, 78—92 (1959). [C 62,099/59

Ducommun, P., Ducommun, S., Baquiche, M.: Etude expérimentale des actions antagonistes d'un spirolactone (Aldactone) et de la désoxycorticostérone. *Schweiz. med. Wschr.* 90, 607—611 (1960). [C 91,529/60

Duffy, B. J., Jr., Morgan, H. R.: ACTH and cortisone aggravation or suppression of the febrile response of rabbits to bacterial endotoxin. *Proc. Soc. exp. Biol. (N.Y.)* 78, 687 to 689 (1951). [B 65,399/51

Dufour, D., Dugal, L. P.: Effet de l'hormone somatotrope sur la résistance du rat exposé au froid. *C. R. Soc. Biol. (Paris)* 149, 2056 à 2060 (1955). [C 15,508/55

Dufour, D., Dugal, L. P.: Effet de l'association STH-vitamine C sur la résistance du rat blanc au froid. *Ann. ACFAS* 23, 83 (1957). [C 26,092/57

Dufour, D., Dugal, L. P., Desmarais, A.: Effet de l'hormone somatotrope chez le rat surrénalectomisé exposé au froid. *C. R. Soc. Biol. (Paris)* 149, 1722—1725 (1955). [C12,151/55

Dugal, L. P., Dufour, D.: Maintien, par l'hormone somatotrope, de la croissance normale du rat exposé au froid. *C. R. Soc. Biol. (Paris)* 148, 1521—1523 (1954). [C8,603/54

Dugal, L. P., Ross, S.: Effet de l'ablation partielle du foie sur l'activité spontanée du rat blanc. *Rev. Canad. Biol.* 2, 435—441 (1943). [84,992/43

Dugal, L. P., Saucier, G.: Cryptorchidisme et effet nocif du testostérone chez le rat mâle, après une longue exposition au froid. *Proc. Canad. Fed. Biol. Soc., First Ann. Meet.*, Kingston, p. 15 (1958). [C53,333/58

Dugal, L. P., Saucier, G.: Cryptorchidisme et toxicité du testostérone chez le rat mâle, longuement exposé au froid. *Ann. ACFAS* 24, 70—71 (1958). [C77,621/58

Duncan, G. W., Lyster, S. C., Clark, J. J., Lednicer, D.: Antifertility activities of two diphenyldihydronaphthalene derivatives. *Proc. Soc. exp. Biol. (N.Y.)* 112, 439—442 (1963). [D58,473/63

Dunn, T. B.: Morphologic changes preceding virus-induced leukemia in rodents. *Acta Un. int. Cancr.* 19, 665—667 (1963). [E29,253/63

Dunn, T. B., Green, A. W.: Morphology of BALB/c mice inoculated with Rauscher virus. *J. nat. Cancer Inst.* 36, 987—1001 (1966). [G40,311/66

Dunning, W. F., Curtis, M. R., Friedgood, C. E.: The incidence of benzpyrene-induced sarcomas in alloxan-diabetic rats. *Cancer Res.* 8, 83—89 (1948). [A48,770/48

Dunphy, T. W.: The pharmacist's role in the prevention of adverse drug interactions. *Amer. J. Hosp. Pharm.* 26, 367—377 (1969). [G77,712/69

Duran, M.: Beiträge zur Physiologie der Drüsen. Nr. 44. Das Verhalten von normalen, mit Schilddrüsensubstanz gefütterten und schilddrüsenlosen Ratten gegen reinen Sauerstoffmangel. *Biochem. Z.* 106, 254—274 (1920). [A10,045/20

Duran-Reynals, M. L.: Combined effects of methylcholanthrene and vaccinia virus in cortisone-treated and untreated mice. *Acta Un. int. Cancr.* 19, 792—796 (1963). [E29,252/63

Durham, W. F., Cueto, C., Jr., Hayes, W. J., Jr.: Hormonal effects on DDT storage in the white rat. *Fed. Proc.* 15, 419 (1956). [C14,264/56

Durham, W. F., Cueto, C., Jr., Hayes, W. J., Jr.: Hormonal influences on DDT metabolism in the white rat. *Amer. J. Physiol.* 187, 373 to 377 (1956). [C27,425/56

Durham, F. M., Gaddum, J. H., Marchal, J. E.: Toxicity tests for novarsenobenzene (neosalvarsan). *Spec. Rep. Ser. med. Res. Counc. (Lond.)* 128, 6—40 (1929). [A49,445/29

Duru, S., Türker, R. K.: Effect of prostaglandin E_1 on the strychnine-induced convulsion in the mouse. *Experientia (Basel)* 25, 275 (1969). [H10,307/69

Dury, A.: Effect of cortisone on lipid metabolism of plasma, liver and aorta and on retrogression of atherosclerosis in the rabbit. *Amer. J. Physiol.* 187, 66—74 (1956). [C25,675/56

Dutta, S., Marks, B. H.: Distribution of ouabain and digoxin in the rat and guinea pig. *Life Sci.* 5, 915—920 (1966). [G73,208/66

Dutton, G. J.: Glucuronide synthesis in foetal liver and other tissues. *Biochem. J.* 71, 141 to 148 (1959). [G70,064/59

Dutton, G. J.: Variations in glucuronide formation by perinatal liver. *Biochem. Pharmacol.* 15, 947—951 (1966). [G78,598/66

Dutz, H., Voigt, K., Wendler, J.: Über die Beeinflußbarkeit der experimentellen Rattennephritis durch Testosteron, Oestradiol, Kastration und somatotropes Hormon. *Z. ges. inn. Med.* 11, 1115—1120 (1956). [C31,646/56

Dworetzky, M., Code, C. F., Higgins, G. M.: Effect of cortisone and ACTH on eosinophils and anaphylactic shock in guinea pigs. *Proc. Soc. exp. Biol. (N.Y.)* 75, 201—206 (1950). [B52,246/50

Dzyubinskaya, T. K.: Nonspecific changes in the course of tuberculosis due to administration of 6-methylthiouracil. (Russian text). *Probl. Endokr. Gormonoter.* 6/5, 14—20 (1960). [C97,348/60

Eades, C. H., Jr., Hsu, I. C., Ekholm, C. A., Harrsch, F.: Antithyroid agents as antihypertensive agents in unilaterally nephrectomized meat-fed rats. (Abstr.) *Fed. Proc.* 28, 394 (1969). [H9,590/69

Eades, C. H., Jr., Hsu, I. C., Ekholm, C. A., Harrsch, F., Phillips, G. E.: Prevention of coronary atherosclerosis by propylthiouracil in unilaterally nephrectomized meat-fed rats. (Abstr.) *Circulation* 36, Sup. 2, II-9—II-10 (1967). [F89,204/67

East, J., Parrott, D. M. V., Seamer, J.: The ability of mice thymectomized at birth to survive infection with lymphocytic choriomeningitis virus. *Virology* **22**, 160—162 (1964). [E 38,279/64

Ebert, R. V., Borden, C. W., Hall, W. H., Gold, D.: A study of hypotension (shock) produced by meningococcus toxin. *Circulat. Res.* **3**, 378—384 (1955). [E 56,239/55

Eckhardt, E. T.: The influence of methylphenidate (MP) on the capacity of the liver to limit DL-7-H³-norepinephrine (NE) pressor responses in the rat. (Abstr.) *Fed. Proc.* **24**, 265 (1965). [F 36,030/65

Eckhardt, E. T., Armstrong, C. B.: Some effects observed following an acute liver bypass in the rat. (Abstr.) *Fed. Proc.* **26**, 682 (1967).
[F 79,670/67

Eddy, N. B.: Studies of morphine, codeine and their derivatives. XIV. The variation with age in the toxic effects of morphine, codeine and some of their derivatives. *J. Pharmacol. exp. Ther.* **66**, 182—201 (1939). [A 50,050/39

Edgren, R. A.: On the endocrine basis of sexual-differences in hexobarbital sleeping-time in rats. *Experientia* **13**, 86—87 (1957).
[C 45,010/57

Efron, D. H.: Reserpine toxicity and 'nonspecific stress'. *Life Sci.* **1**, 561—564 (1962).
[D 59,758/62

Eger, W.: Osteodystrophia fibrosa generalisata, Epithelkörperchen und Nieren. *Frankfurt. Z. Path.* **56**, 369—450 (1942). [B 35,694/42

Eger, W., Schulz, E., Stratakis, K.: Die durch Allylalkohol oder Thiocetamid experimentell erzeugte Leberzirrhose unter dem Einfluß von Prednisolon. *Medizinische* **28**, 871—872 (1959).
[E 58,108/59

Eger, W., Stratakis, K.: Über den Einfluß des Prednisolon auf die Bindegewebsentwicklung der experimentell erzeugten Leberzirrhose. *Z. ges. exp. Med.* **129**, 559—572 (1958).
[D 89,546/58

Ehrlich, H. P., Hunt, T. K.: Effects of cortisone and vitamin A on wound healing. *Ann. Surg.* **167**, 324—328 (1968). [G 55,237/68

Ehrlich, H. P., Hunt, T. K.: The effects of cortisone and anabolic steroids on the tensile strength of healing wounds. *Ann. Surg.* **170**, 203—206 (1969). [G 68,785/69

Eichholtz, F.: Über rektale Narkose mit Avertin (E 107). Pharmakologischer Teil. *Dtsch. med. Wschr.* **53**, 710—712 (1927).
[A 27,018/27

Eichholtz, F., Hotovy, R., Collischonn, P., Knauer, H.: Beeinflussung der Entgiftungszeiten von Avertin und Pentothal-Natrium an der nebennierenlosen Ratte durch Nebennieren-Rindenhormon (Pentothal-Natrium-test). *Arch. exp. Pathol. Pharmacol.* **207**, 576—585 (1949). [B 45,516/49

Einer-Jensen, N.: Antifertility properties of two diphenylethenes. *Acta pharmacol. (Kbh.)* **26**, Sup. 1, 97 (1968). [G 75,787/68

Einhauser, M.: Giftwirkung der Schlafmittel und Nebennierenrinde. *Klin. Wschr.* **18**, 423—427 (1939). [A 19,483/39

Einheber, A., Munan, L. P., Leese, C. E.: Survival rates in experimental burn shock. *Fed. Proc.* **11**, 42 (1952). [B 68,195/52

Einheber, A., Wren, R. E., Klobukowski, C. J.: Interference of hepatic drug metabolism in plasmodium berghei-infected mice and its therapeutic modification: a study of hexobarbital sleeping time and phenobarbital-induced liver stimulation. *Exp. Parasit.* **27**, 424—443 (1970). [G 75,665/70

Einhorn, S. L., Hirschberg, E., Gellhorn, A.: Effects of cortisone on regenerating rat liver. *J. gen. Physiol.* **37**, 559—573 (1954).
[E 55,369/54

Eisalo, A.: Liver function tests during treatment with contraceptive pills. (Abstr.) *Excerpta med. (Amst.)*, Int. Congr. Ser. No. 210, p. 67. (1970) 3rd Int. Congr. on Hormonal steroids, Hamburg. [H 29,326/70

Eisalo, A., Järvinen, P. A., Luukkainen, T.: Hepatic impairment during the intake of contraceptive pills: clinical trial with postmenopausal women. *Brit. med. J.* **1964 II**, 426—427.
[F 18,828/64

el-Denshary, E. S. M., Scott, P. M., el-Masri, A. M.: Studies on the protective effectiveness of drugs against the hepatic toxicity of primaquine diphosphate in rabbits. *J. Egypt. med. Ass.* **52**, 552—560 (1969). [G 77,356/69

Elder, T. D., Baker, R. D.: Pulmonary mucormycosis in rabbits with alloxan diabetes. Increased invasiveness of fungus during acute toxic phase of diabetes. *Arch. Path.* **61**, 159 to 168 (1956). [C 12,831/56

Elgee, N. J., Williams, R. H.: Degradation of insulin-I^{131} by liver and kidney in vivo. *Proc. Soc. exp. Biol. (N.Y.)* **87**, 352—355 (1954).
[C 430/54

Eling, T. E., Harbison, R. D., Becker, B. A., Fouts, J. R.: Kinetic changes in microsomal drug metabolism with age and diphenylhydantoin treatment. *Europ. J. Pharmacol.* **11**, 101 to 108 (1970). [H 27,047/70

Ellinger, F.: Acetonitril test for thyroid according to Reid Hunt and irradiation with ultraviolet light. *Radiologica* 3, 195—200 (1938). [78,163/38

Ellinger, F.: Protective action of desoxycorticosterone acetate against X-ray-induced liver changes. *Science* 104, 502—503 (1946). [93,367/46

Ellinger, F.: Some effects of desoxycorticosterone acetate on mice irradiated with X-rays. *Proc. Soc. exp. Biol. (N.Y.)* 64, 31—35 (1947). [93,953/47

Ellinger, F.: Influence of pharmacological agents on effects of irradiation. *Radiology* 50, 234—243 (1948). [B 24,015/48

Ellinger, F.: The use of adrenal cortical hormone in radiation sickness. *Radiology* 51, 394—399 (1948). [B 57,402/48

Ellinger, F.: Some effects of testosterone propionate on mice irradiated with X-rays. *Proc. Soc. exp. Biol. (N.Y.)* 74, 616—619 (1950). [B 49,654/50

Ellinger, F.: Endocrine influences on radiosensitivity. *Radiol. clin. (Basel)* 23, 182—190 (1954). [B 95,888/54

Ellinger, F., Roswit, B., Glasser, S. M.: The treatment of radiation sickness with adrenal cortical hormone (desoxycorticosterone acetate): A preliminary report on fifty cases. *Amer. J. Roentgenol.* 61, 387—396 (1949). [B 44,439/49

Ellinwood, E. H.: Paradoxical effect of dichloroisoproterenol on pentobarbital sleep time in hyperthyroid mice. *Nature (Lond.)* 209, 1250—1251 (1966). [F 64,417/66

Ellinwood, E. H., Jr., Prange, A. J., Jr.: Effect of epinephrine pretreatment on pentobarbital sleeping time of mice with altered thyroid status. *Nature (Lond.)* 201, 305—306 (1964). [E 39,187/64

Emans, J. B., Jones, A. L.: Hypertrophy of liver cell smooth surfaced reticulum following progesterone administration. *J. Histochem. Cytochem.* 16, 561—571 (1968). [H 20,754/68

Emerson, W. J., Zamecnik, P. C., Nathanson, I. T.: The effect of sex hormones on hepatic and renal lesions induced in rats by a cholinedeficient diet. *Endocrinology* 48, 548—559 (1951). [B 59,636/51

Emmens, C. W.: Steroid anaesthesia. *J. Endocr.* 5, xii (1946). [A 46,574/46

Emmens, C. W., Cox, R. I., Martin, L.: Antiestrogens. In: Pincus; *Recent Progr. Hormone Res.* 18, 415—466 (1962). (The Proceedings of the Laurentian Hormone Conference, 1961.) New York, London: Academic Press. [D 25,360/62

Emmens, C. W., Parkes, A. S.: Assay of thyroidal activity by a closed vessel technique. *J. Endocr.* 5, 186—206 (1947). [B 4,928/47

Englhardt-Gölkel, A.: Untersuchungen über die antagonistischen Wirkungen von Methylandrostendiol und Cortisonacetat auf den Eiweißhaushalt beim Menschen. *Z. klin. Med.* 153, 222—229 (1955). [C 42,792/55

English, J. M.: A case of probable phosgene poisoning. *Brit. med. J.* 1964 I, 38. [F 399/64

Epple, A., Jørgensen, C. B., Rosenkilde, P.: Effect of hypophysectomy on blood sugar, fat, glycogen, and pancreatic islets in starving toads (Bufo bufo L.). *Gen. comp. Endocr.* 7, 197—202 (1966). [F 76,569/66

Epstein, S. S., Andrea, J., Clapp, P., Mackintosh, D.: Enhancement by piperonyl butoxide of acute toxicity due to Freons, benzo (α) pyrene, and griseofulvin in infant mice. *Toxicol. appl. Pharmacol.* 11, 442—448 (1967). [G 77,545/67

Epstein, S. S., Andrea, J., Joshi, S., Mantel, N.: Hepatocarcinogenicity in griseofulvin following parenteral administration to infant mice. *Cancer Res.* 27, 1900—1906 (1967). [H 30,997/67

Epstein, S. S., Joshi, S., Andrea, J., Clapp, P., Falk, H., Mantel, N.: Synergistic toxicity and carcinogenicity of 'Freons' and piperonyl butoxide. *Nature (Lond.)* 214, 526—528 (1967). [H 29,385/67

Eriksson, M.: Salicylate-induced foetal damage during late pregnancy in mice. The modifying effect of repeated administration and dosage. *Acta paediat. scand.* 59, 517—522 (1970). [H 30,468/70

Ershoff, B. H.: Deleterious effects of pancreas in the hyperthyroid rat. *Proc. Soc. exp. Biol. (N.Y.)* 69, 122—124 (1948). [B 24,883/48

Ershoff, B. H.: Potentiating effects of reserpine on thyrotoxicity in the rat. *Proc. Soc. exp. Biol. (N.Y.)* 99, 189—192 (1958). [C 60,006/58

Ershoff, B. H.: Unidentified nutritional factors and resistance to stress. *J. dent. Med.* 16, 71—75 (1961). [D 5,818/61

Ershoff, B. H., Deuel, H. J., Jr.: The effect of growth hormone on the vitamin A-deficient rat. *Endocrinology* 36, 280—282 (1945). [B 14,516/45

Erspamer, V.: Influence of 5-hydroxytryptamine (enteramine) on the course of the acute lethal sublimate intoxication in the rat. *Experientia (Basel)* IX/5, 186 (1953). [B 84,587/53

Erspamer, V.: Peripheral physiological and pharmacological actions of indolealkylamines. In: Eichler, O., Farah, A,: *Handbuch der experimentellen Pharmakologie*, p. 245—359. Berlin, Heidelberg, New York: Springer-Verlag 1966. [E 5,915/66

Ertel, I. J., Newton, W. A., Jr.: Therapy in congenital hyperbilirubinemia: phenobarbital and diethylnicotinamide. *Pediatrics* 44, 43—48 (1969). [G 68,390/69

Ertuganova, Z. A.: The influence of cortisone, desoxicorticosterone, largactyl and phenergan on the course and issue of pneumococcal infection. (Russian text.) *Farmakol. i. Toksikol.* 23, 348—349 (1960). [C 97,404/60

Eschenbrenner, A. B.: Induction of hepatomas in mice by repeated oral administration of chloroform, with observations on sex differences. *J. nat. Cancer Inst.* 5, 251—255 (1945). [93,202/45

Eschenbrenner, A. B., Miller, E.: Sex differences in kidney morphology and chloroform necrosis. *Science* 102, 302—303 (1945). [94,309/45

Estabrook, R. W., Franklin, M. R., Cohen, B., Shigamatzu, A., Hildebrandt, A. G.: Influence of hepatic microsomal mixed function oxidation reactions on cellular metabolic control. *Metabolism* 20, 187—199 (1971). [H 34,125/71

Estabrook, R. W., Hildebrandt, A. G., Baron, J., Netter, K. J., Leibman, K.: A new spectral intermediate associated with cytochrome P-450 function in liver microsomes. *Biochem. biophys. Res. Commun.* 42, 132—139 (1971). [G 81,261/71

Etoh, H., Egami, N.: Effect of hypophysectomy and adrenalectomy on the length of survival time after X-irradiation in the goldfish, Carassius auratus. *Proc. Jap. Acad.* 39, 503—506 (1963). [G 11,664/63

Eufinger, H., Wiesbader, H.: Reid Huntsche Reaktion und Schwangerschaft. II. Mitt. *Arch. Gynäk.* 142, 662—667 (1930). [4,663/30

Eufinger, H., Wiesbader, H., Focsaneanu, L.: Reid Huntsche Reaktion und Schwangerschaft. *Arch. Gynäk.* 136, 12—18 (1929). [22,082/29

Euler, H. von, Klussmann, E.: Carotin (Vitamin A) und Thyroxin. *Hoppe-Seylers Z. physiol. Chem.* 213, 21—34 (1932). [4,928/32

Evangelista, B. S., Green, T. J., Gwilt, D. J., Brown, T. G., Jr.: An experimental study of current therapeutic approaches to endotoxin shock. *Arch. int. Pharmacodyn.* 180, 57—67 (1969). [H 16,824/69

Evans, D. G., Miles, A. A., Niven, J. S. F.: The enhancement of bacterial infections by adrenaline. *Brit. J. exp. Path.* 29, 20—39 (1948). [B 65,652/48

Evans, E. A., Eisenlord, G., Hine, C. H.: Studies in detoxication by means of the isolated perfused liver. *Toxicol. appl. Pharmacol.* 5, 129—141 (1963). [G 65,279/63

Eversole, W. J.: Inhibition of Azo dye carcinogenesis by adrenalectomy and treatment with desoxycorticosterone trimethylacetate. *Proc. Soc. exp. Biol. (N.Y.)* 96, 643—646 (1957). [C 45,823/57

Eversole, W. J., Edelmann, A., Gaunt, R.: Effect of adrenal cortical transplants on life-maintenance and "water intoxication." *Anat. Rec.* 76, 271—281 (1940). [78,679/40

Eversole, W. J., Gaunt, R.: Methods of administering desoxycorticosterone and the problem of its inactivation by the liver. *Endocrinology* 32, 51—56 (1943). [A 56,551/43

Evonuk, E., Hannon, J. P.: Cardiovascular and pulmonary effects of noradrenaline in the cold-acclimatized rat. *Fed. Proc.* 22, 911—916 (1963). [E 21,027/63

Evropeitzeva, N. V.: The effect of thiourea on development of the thyroid in coregonous lafaretus ludoga. *Dokl. Akad. Nauk. SSSR, Otd. Biokh.* 68, 977—980 (1949). [A 49,151/49

Ewing, P. L., Tree, H. G., Emerson, G. A.: Nonspecific factors in chemotherapy of trypanosomiases. *Fed. Proc.* 9, 270 (1950). [B 50,244/50

Faber, H. von: Über die Beeinflussung der Nebenschilddrüse durch Verabreichung von Stilboestrol allein und kombiniert mit Thyroxin, bzw. Testosteronpropionat an Hähne. *Endokrinologie* 32, 295—302 (1955). [C 6,925/55

Fabrikant, J. I.: Cell proliferation in the regenerating liver of continuously irradiated mice; effect of a radiation-free interval. *Brit. J. Radiol.* 41, 369—374 (1968). [H 8,091/68

Fahim, M. S., Dement, G., Hall, D. G., Fahim, Z.: Induced alterations in the hepatic metabolism of androgens in the rat. *Amer. J. Obstet. Gynec.* 107, 1085—1091 (1970). [G 77,345/70

Fahim, M. S., Hall, D. G., Jones, T. M., Fahim, Z., Whitt, F. D.: Drug-steroid interaction in the pregnant rat, fetus, and neonate. *Amer. J. Obstet. Gynec.* **107**, 1250—1258 (1970). [G 77,383/70

Fahim, M. S., Ishaq, J., Hall, D. G., Jones, T.: Induced alteration in the biologic activity of estrogen by DDT. *Amer. J. Obstet. Gynec.* **108**, 1063—1067 (1970). [G 81,358/70

Fahim, M. S., King, T. M., Hall, D. G.: Induced alterations in the biologic activity of estrogen. *Amer. J. Obstet. Gynec.* **100**, 171—175 (1968). [G 67,772/68

Fahim, M. S., King, T. M., Venson, V., Norwich, C., Bolt, D. J.: Uterotropic action of estrogens in phenobarbital-treated mice. *Fertil. and Steril.* **20**, 344—350 (1969). [G 65,075/69

Fairchild, E. J.: Neurohumoral factors in injury from inhaled irritants. *Arch. environm. Hlth.* **6**, 79—86 (1963). [G 71,531/63

Fairchild, E. J., Graham, S. L.: Thyroid influence on the toxicity of respiratory irritant gases, ozone and nitrogen dioxide. *J. Pharmacol. exp. Ther.* **139**, 177—184 (1963). [D 56,574/63

Fairchild, E. J., Graham, S. L., Stokinger, H. E.: Pharmacologic aspects of humoral mechanisms in the toxic response to pulmonary irritant gases. *Biochem. Pharmacol.* **12**, Suppl. 158 (1963). [E 32,187/63

Fairchild, E. J., Stokinger, H. E.: The thyroid in pulmonary injury of acute ozone poisoning. *Fed. Proc.* **20**, 203 (1961). [D 4,088/61

Falk, R.: Antagonisme entre les extraits testiculaires et certaines substances hypno-anesthésiques. *C. R. Soc. Biol. (Paris)* **123**, 779—781 (1936). [A 337/36

Falta, W., Jvcovic, L.: Adrenalin als Antidot. *Berl. klin. Wschr.* **46**, 1929—1930 (1909). [A 1,273/09

Falutz, S. E.: Action of catecholamines and some precursors on tremorine-induced tremor in cats. *Proc. Canad. Fed. biol. Soc. (Montreal)* **10**, 139 (1967). [F 85,463/67

Fanfani, M., Dini, S.: Le modificazioni istopatologiche del miocardio nella paramiloidosi sperimentale da caseinato sodico. *Arch. De Vecchi Anat. pat.* **26**, 327—363 (1957). [C 48,253/57

Farah, A., Smuskowicz, E.: The effect of liver damage on the activity of g-strophanthin in the rat. *J. Pharmacol. exp. Ther.* **96**, 139—144 (1949). [A 49,134/49

Farber, E., Koch-Weser, D., Popper, H.: Influence of steroid hormone on fatty livers. *Fed. Proc.* **9**, 329 (1950). [B 47,283/50

Farber, E., Koch-Weser, D., Popper, H.: The influence of sex and of testosterone upon fatty liver due to ethionine. *Endocrinology* **48**, 205—212 (1951). [D 24,923/51

Farber, E., Segaloff, A.: Effect of androgens and growth and other hormones on ethionine fatty liver in rats. *J. biol. Chem.* **216**, 471—477 (1955). [D 95,996/55

Farese, R. V.: Inhibition of cholesterol side chain cleavage by cyanoketone (2α-cyano-4,4,17α-trimethyl-17β-hydroxyandrost-5-en-3-one). *Steroids* **15**, 245—250 (1970). [H 27,025/70

Farnell, D. R.: Functional and structural effects of magnesium deficiency and cortisone treatment in mice. *Amer. J. vet. Res.* **29**, 1695—1706 (1968). [H 15,528/68

Farrar, W. E., Jr., Magnani, T. J.: Endotoxin susceptibility following hepatic injury by carbon tetrachloride. *Proc. Soc. exp. Biol. (N.Y.)* **115**, 596—601 (1964). [F 6,647/64

Farson, D. B., Carr, C. J., Krantz, J. C., Jr.: Anesthesia. XXIV. The effect of cholesterol on pentothal and ether anesthesia. *J. Pharmacol. exp. Ther.* **89**, 222—226 (1947). [A 49,680/47

Fasold, H., Heidemann, E. R.: Über die Gelbfärbung der Milch thyreopriver Ziegen. *Z. ges. exp. Med.* **92**, 53—56 (1933). [16,518/33

Fasold, H., Peters, H.: Über den Antagonismus zwischen Thyroxin und Vitamin. *Z. ges. exp. Med.* **92**, 57—62 (1933). [A 54,337/33

Fastier, F. N.: Prolongation of hypnosis by 5-hydroxytryptamine (serotonin). *Experientia (Basel)* **12**, 351 (1956). [D 95,950/56

Fastier, F. N., Speden, R. N., Waal, H.: Prolongation of chloral hydrate sleeping time by 5-hydroxytryptamine and by certain other drugs. *Brit. J. Pharmacol.* **12**, 251—256 (1957). [C 37,038/57

Fautrez, J., Pisi, E., Cavalli, G.: Activité mitotique provoquée par la thiourée et teneur en acide désoxyribonucléique de la cellule hépatique. *Exp. Cell. Res.* **9**, 189—192 (1955). [C 23,124/55

Fazekas, I. G.: Die Wirkung von Corticosteoridfraktionen auf die Alkoholdehydrogenaseaktivität der Leber. *Arch. Toxikol.* **19**, 388—395 (1962). [D 55,397/62

Fazekas, I. G.: Corticosterone content of peripheric blood and alcoholdehydrogenase activity of the liver after adrenalectomy. *Folia endocr. (Roma)* **16**, 600—607 (1963). [G 9,347/63

Fazekas, I. G.: Alkoholabbau und Nebennierenrinde. *Acta Med. leg. soc. (Liège)* 17, 77—80 (1964). [F 71,641/64

Fazekas, I. G., Rengei, B.: Die Wirkung von Adrenalektomie und Alkohol auf die Alkoholdehydrogenase-Aktivität von Rattenorganen. *Enzymologia* 34, 226—230 (1968). [G 58,271/68

Fazekas, I. G., Rengei, B.: Über den NAD- und NADH$_2$-Gehalt in Leber, Herz und Nieren adrenalektomierter und alkoholbehandelter Ratten. *Enzymologia* 36, 59—64 (1969).
[G 64,534/69

Fazekas, I. G., Rengei, B., Fazekas, A. G.: Die Wirkung der Nebennierenrindenfunktion auf die Aktivität der Alkoholdehydrogenase der Leber. *Arch. Toxicol.* 19, 229—236 (1961).
[D 22,442/61

Fazio, M., Oddone, I., Boglione, F.: Ricerche sperimentali sull'influenza dell'ACTH e del cortisone sui processi infettivi. II. Infezione streptococcica del ratto. *G. Mal. infett.* 8, 168—173 (1956). [C 34,111/56

Feigelson, M., Gross, P. R., Feigelson, P.: Early effects of cortisone on nucleic acid and protein metabolism of rat liver. *Biochim. biophys. Acta (Amst.)* 55, 495—504 (1962).
[G 68,042/62

Feigelson, P.: Comparison of the mechanisms of substrate and hormonal induction of rat liver tryptophan pyrrolase. *Fed. Proc.* 20, 223 (1961). [D 4,122/61

Feigelson, P., Dashman, T., Margolis, F.: The half-lifetime of induced tryptophan peroxidase in vivo. *Arch. Biochem.* 85, 478—482 (1959).
[G 67,768/59

Feigelson, P., Feigelson, M.: Studies on the mechanism of regulation by cortisone of the metabolism of liver purine and ribonucleic acid. *J. Biol. Chem.* 238, 1073—1077 (1963).
[D 59,123/63

Feigelson, P., Feigelson, M., Greengard, O.: Comparison of the mechanisms of hormonal and substrate induction of rat liver tryptophan pyrrolase. In: Pincus; *Recent Progr. Hormone Res.* 18, 491—512 (1962). (The Proceedings of the Laurentian Hormone Conference, 1961.) New York, London: Academic Press.
[D 25,364/62

Feigelson, P., Greengard, O.: Immuno chemical evidence for increased titers of liver tryptophan pyrrolase during substrate and hormonal enzyme induction. *J. biol. Chem.* 237, 3714 to 3717 (1962). [D 46,319/62

Feinstein, R. N., Seaholm, J. E.: Effect of a serotonin antagonist on radiation lethality. *Proc. Soc. exp. Biol. (N.Y.)* 114, 247—248 (1963). [E 29,638/63

Feldman, S. A., Tyrrell, M. F.: A new steroid muscle relaxant Dacuronium-NB. 68 (Organon). *Anaesthesia* 25, 349—355 (1970). [G 76,666/70

Fell, H. B.: The direct action of cortisol on skeletal tissue in organ culture. In: *Proc. 2nd int. Congr. Endocr. Part II*, p. 922—927. London: Excerpta Medica Foundation 1964.
[F 48,679/64

Fell, H. B., Thomas, L.: The influence of hydrocortisone on the action of excess vitamin A on limb bone rudiments in culture. *J. exp. Med.* 114, 343—361 (1961). [D 10,358/61

Feller, D. R., Gerald, M. C.: Possible liver microsomal induction in mice by spironolactone. (Abstr.) *Fed. Proc.* 29, 346 (1970).
[H 22,744/70

Fellinger, K., Hochstädt, O.: Über die Beeinflussung des Reid-Huntschen Versuches durch Antithyreoidale Schutzstoffe. *Klin. Wschr.* 14, 1250—1251 (1935). [63,744/35

Felsher, B. F., Barretto, F. T., Redeker, A. G.: Effect of caloric intake and phenobarbital on serum bilirubin (SB). (Abstr.) *Clin. Res.* 19, 175 (1971). [H 34,479/71

Felsher, B. F., Craig, J. R., Carpio, N. M.: Hepatic glucuronyl transferase (GT) and betaglucuronidase (BG) in Gilbert's syndrome (GS). (Abstr.) *Clin. Res.* 19, 175 (1971). [H 34,480/71

Fenu, G.: Intorno alla capacità dell'adrenalina di potenziare l'azione narcotica del pentotal. *Minerva otorinolaring.* 4, 91—93 (1954).
[C 17,650/54

Ferguson, C. C., Rogers, C. S., Vars, H. M.: Liver regeneration in the presence of common bile duct obstruction. *Amer. J. Physiol.* 159, 343—350 (1949). [G 71,528/49

Ferraris, F.: Ovariectomia e tossicosi isoniazidica. *Chemoterapia* 8 (1954). [C 27,552/54

Ferraris, F.: Ovariectomia e tossicosi isoniazidica. *Ormonologia* 16, 235—238 (1956).
[C 30,097/56

Ferret, P.: The effect of diet on oestrogen inactivation by the liver. *Brit. J. exp. Path.* 31, 590—596 (1950). [E 50,456/50

Ferris, B. G., Jr., Affeldt, J. E., Kriete, H. A., Whittenberger, J. L.: Pulmonary function in patients with pulmonary disease treated with ACTH. *Arch. industr. Hyg.* 3, 603—616 (1951).
[B 65,475/51

Ferruccio, S.: Eliminazione urinaria dei 17-chetosteroidi nella steatosi sperimentale da colesterina e nella steatosi da colesterina trattata con sostanze metilanti, testosterone e vit. E (Ricerche sperimentali). *Chir. Pat. sper.* **12**, 695—711 (1964). [F 62,336/64

Feuer, G.: Induction of drug-metabolising enzymes of rat liver by derivatives of coumarin. *Canad. J. Physiol. Pharmacol.* **48**, 232—240 (1970). [H 24,218/70

Feuer, G., Golberg, L.: Stimulation of liver processing enzymes by derivatives of coumarin. *Biochem. J.* **103**, 13P (1967). [G 76,853/67

Feuer, G., Liscio, A.: Origin of delayed development of drug metabolism in the newborn rat. *Nature (Lond.)* **223**, 68—70 (1969). [H 14,579/69

Feyel, P.: L'action trophique des hormones sexuelles sur le rein chez la souris. *Ann. Endocr.* **4**, 93—110 (1943). [99,416/43

Fiala, S., Fiala, A. E.: Hormonal dependence of cytotoxic action of actidione (cycloheximide). *Proc. Amer. Ass. Cancer Res.* **6**, 18 (1965). [F 33,398/65

Fiala, S., Fiala, E.: Hormonal dependence of actidione (cycloheximide) action. *Biochim. biophys. Acta (Amst.)* **103**, 699—701 (1965). [F 70,819/65

Fiala, S., Fiala, E.: Induction of tyrosine transaminase in rat liver by actidione. *Nature (Lond.)* **210**, 530—531 (1966). [F 65,983/66

Fiegelson, E. B., Drake, J. W., Recant, L.: Experimental aminonucleoside nephrosis in rats. *J. Lab. clin. Med.* **50**, 437—446 (1957). [D 96,580/57

Field, J. B., Ershoff, B. H., Dolendo, E., Mireles, A.: The effect of endocrine agents on the toxicity of anti-cancer drugs. (Abstr.) *Proc. Amer. Ass. Cancer Res.* **8**, 17 (1967). [F 78,812/67

Field, J. B., Mireles, A., Dolendo, E. C.: Effect of androgens on survival of mice treated with anti-cancer drugs. *Proc. Amer. Ass. Cancer Res.* **6**, 19 (1965). [F 33,399/65

Figueroa, M. A., Yañez, J. A.: Hepatectomía parcial experimental. Técnica en dos tiempos operatorios. *Pren. méd. argent.* **56**, 925—927 (1969). [H 18,495/69

Filipp, G., Mess, B.: Role of the adrenocortical system in suppressing anaphylaxis after hypothalamic lesion. *Ann. Allergy* **27**, 607—610 (1969). [G 71,129/69

Filner, P., Wray, J. L., Varner, J. E.: Enzyme induction in higher plants. Environmental or developmental changes cause many enzyme activities of higher plants to rise or fall. *Science* **165**, 358—367 (1969). [H 15,309/69

Finch, C. E., Foster, J. R., Mirsky, A. E.: Ageing and the regulation of cell activities during exposure to cold. *J. gen. Physiol.* **54**, 690—712 (1969). [G 71,208/69

Finch, C. E., Huberman, H. S., Mirsky, A. E.: Regulation of liver tyrosine aminotransferase by endogenous factors in the mouse. *J. gen. Physiol.* **54**, 675—689 (1969). [G 71,207/69

Findlay, G. M., Howard, E. M.: The effects of cortisone and adrenocorticotrophic hormone on poliomyelitis and on other virus infections. *J. Pharm. Pharmacol.* **4**, 37—42 (1952). [B 81,142/52

Fine, J., Fishmann, J., Frank, H. A.: The effect of adrenal cortical hormones in hemorrhage and shock. *Surgery* **12**, 1—13 (1942). [A 56,268/42

Fine, J., Palmerio, C., Rutenburg, S.: New developments in therapy of refractory traumatic shock. *Arch. Surg.* **96**, 163—175 (1968). [G 53,608/68

Finger, H.: Möglichkeiten der Unterdrückung paralytischer Komplikationen nach antirabischer Schutzimpfung. *Arb. Paul-Ehrlich-Inst.* **57**, 63—79 (1962). [E 26,273/62

Fingl, E., Olsen, L. J., Harding, B. W., Cockett, A. T., Goodman, L. S.: Effects of chronic anticonvulsant administration upon cortisone-induced brain hyperexcitability. *J. Pharmacol. exp. Ther.* **105**, 37—45 (1952). [D 38,091/52

Finney, D. J.: The Fischer-Yates test of significance in 2×2 contingency tables. *Biometrika* **35**, 145—156 (1948). [D 31,291/48

Fiore-Donati, L., Chieco-Bianchi, L., Bertaccini, G.: Effetto protettivo della 5-idrossitriptamina sul danno epatocellulare da tetracloruro di carbonio nel ratto. *Arch. int. Pharmacodyn.* **123**, 115—131 (1959). [C 78,953/59

Fiore-Donati, L., Maiorano, G., Chieco-Bianchi, L.: Interferenza della 5-idrossitriptamina sullo sviluppo della cirrosi sperimentale da CCl_4. *Boll. Soc. ital. Biol. sper.* **34**, 1493—1494 (1958). [C 62,200/58

Fiorentino, M.: Diagnosi biologica di tubercolosi, accelerata con ormone corticotropo. *Riv. Anat. pat.* **16**, 78—84 (1959). [D 8,379/59

Firkin, F. C., Linnane, A. W.: Biogenesis of mitochondria. 8. The effect of chloramphenicol on regenerating rat liver. *Exp. Cell. Res.* **55**, 68—76 (1969). [H 31,607/69

Firschein, H. E., DeVenuto, F., Fitch, W. M., Pearce, E. M., Westphal, U.: Distribution of injected cortisol-4-C^{14} in normal and shocked rats. *Endocrinology* 60, 347—358 (1957). [C30,553/57

Fishel, C. W., Szentivanyi, A., Talmage, D. W.: Adrenergic factors in Bordetella pertussis-induced histamine and serotonin hypersensitivity of mice. In: Landy, M., Braun, W.; *Bacterial Endotoxins*, p. 474—481. New Brunswick, N.J.: Institute of Microbiology, Rutgers, The State University 1964. [E8,474/64

Fischer, E., Ludmer, R. I., Sabelli, H. C.: The antagonism of phenylethylamine to catecholamines on mouse motor activity. *Acta physiol. lat.-amer.* 17, 15—21 (1967). [G48,517/67

Fischer, E. R., Fisher, B.: Experimental studies of factors influencing development of hepatic metastases. XVII. Role of thyroid. *Cancer Res.* 26, 2248—2253 (1966). [F74,176/66

Fischer, H.: Zum Ausbau der tierexperimentellen Forschung in der Psychiatrie. *Mschr. Psychiat. Neurol.* 48, 181—192 (1920). [50,723/20

Fisher, B., Fisher, E. R.: Experimental studies of factors influencing hepatic metastases. II. Effect of partial hepatectomy. *Cancer* 12, 929—932 (1959). [G72,106/59

Fisher, E. R., Fisher, B.: Nephrotoxic serum nephritis in thymectomized rats. *Proc. Soc. exp. Biol. (N.Y.)* 115, 156—160 (1964). [E690/64

Fisher, E. R., Gruhn, J.: Aminonucleoside nephrosis. Effect of adrenalectomy, cortisone, hypophysectomy and saline ingestion. *Arch. Path.* 71, 23—30 (1961). [D12,898/61

Fister, V.: Effect of carbutamide BZ-55 treatment on the resistance to hypoxia in albino rats. *Rev. argent. Endocr.* 5, 191 (1959). [C97,077/59

Fitzhugh, O. G., Nelson, A. A.: The chronic oral toxicity of DDT (2,2-bis (p-Chlorophenyl-1,1,1-Trichloroethane). *J. Pharmacol. exp. Ther.* 89, 18—30 (1947). [A47,885/47

Fitzhugh, O. G., Nelson, A. A., Bliss, C. I.: The chronic oral toxicity of selenium. *J. Pharmacol. exp. Ther.* 80, 289—299 (1944). [A45,940/44

Fitzhugh, O. G., Nelson, A. A., Calvery, H. O.: The chronic toxicity of ergot. *J. Pharmacol. exp. Ther.* 82, 364—376 (1944). [A46,537/44

Fiumara, A., Nuciforo, G., Gafa, L., Condorelli, B.: Differente intensita' delle lesioni arteriose da intossicazione acuta con di-idrotachisterolo nei ratti giovani maschi e femmine. *Riv. Anat. pat.* 33, XXXVIII—XLVI (1968). [H34,170/68

Flaks, A.: Observation of the action of the thymus on the induction of lung tumours by 9,10-dimethyl-1,2-benzanthracene (DMBA) in new-born A mice. *Brit. J. Cancer* 21, 390—392 (1967). [F95,414/67

Flaks, J.: Influence of testosterone propionate on the induction of subcutaneous tumours in mice by 20-methylcholanthrene. *Brit. J. Cancer* 2, 386—394 (1948). [B35,572/48

Fleischer, J., Riedel, H.: Histologische Organveränderungen beim Kaninchen nach Gaben von Prednisolon und Endoxan. *Folia haemat. (Frankfurt)* 82, 23—39 (1964). [G20,778/64

Fleischmann, W., Kann, S.: Untersuchungen über die Beziehungen zwischen dem Schilddrüsenhormon und dem Vitamin A. *Wien. klin. Wschr.* 49, 1488—1489 (1936). [67,360/36

Fleisher, M. S., Wilhelmj, C. M.: The influence of thyroidectomy on anaphylaxic shock. *Z. Immun.-Forsch.* 51, 115—125 (1927). [23,337/27

Flemming, K., Langendorff, M.: Untersuchungen über einen biologischen Strahlenschutz. 66. Mitteilung: Das Pro-Östrogen Chlortrianisen (Tace) als Strahlenschutzsubstanz. *Strahlentherapie* 128, 109—118 (1965). [G38,381/65

Fletcher, H. P., Miya, T. S., Bousquet, W. F.: Influence of estradiol on the disposition of chlorpromazine in the rat. *J. pharm. Sci.* 54, 1007—1009 (1965). [F44,604/65

Flint, M., Lathe, G. H., Ricketts, T. R., Silman, G.: Development of glucuronyl transferase and other enzyme systems in the newborn rabbit. *Quart. J. exp. Physiol.* 49, 66—73 (1964). [G78,603/64

Flückiger, E., Verzar, F.: Senkung und Restitution der Körpertemperatur bei niedrigem atmosphärischen Druck und der Einfluß von Thyreoidea, Hypophyse und Nebennierenrinde auf dieselbe. *Helvet. physiol. pharmacol. Acta* 10, 349—359 (1952). [B86,489/52

Fogelman, M. J., Ivy, A. C.: Effect of thiouracil on liver regeneration. *Amer. J. Physiol.* 153, 397—401 (1948). [B23,357/48

Foglia, V. G., Penhos, J. C.: Diferencia sexual en la diabetes pancreática de ratas castradas al nacer. *Rev. Soc. argent. Biol.* 28, 143—148 (1952). [B79,957/52

Földes, P., Szeri, I., Bános, Z., Anderlik, P., Balázs, M.: LCM infection of mice thymectomized in newborn age. *Acta microbiol. Acad. Sci. hung.* 11, 277—282 (1965). [G 29,263/65

Foley, E. J.: Therapeutic effect of chlortetracycline and oxytetracycline in immunized mice treated with cortisone. *Antibiot. and Chemother.* 5, 1—5 (1955). [C 13,263/55

Foley, E. J., Morgan, W. A., Greco, G.: Effect of prednisone and prednisolone on Streptococcus infections in mice treated with chlortetracycline. *Antibiot. and Chemother.* 7, 65—69 (1957). [C 31,073/57

Foley, G. E., Aycock, W. L.: Alterations in the autarceologic susceptibility of the mouse to experimental poliomyelitis by estrogenic substances. *Endocrinology* 37, 245—251 (1945). [B 764/45

Fontan, M., Cotlenko, V., Barberis, D.: Effet protecteur du noyau cyclo-pentano-phénantrène vis-à-vis de l'intoxication par le Di-isopropyl-fluoro-phosphate (D.F.P.). *Lille méd.* 13, 299—302 (1968). [F 98,752/68

Fontan, M., Cotlenko, V., Cheval, P., Barberis, D.: Interactions spironolactone/di-iso-propylfluoro-phosphate (D.F.P.). *Lille méd.* 10, 780—784 (1965). [F 55,419/65

Fonts, J. M., Martinez, J. M., D'Angeli, S. R.: Contribución al estudio de la acción anestésica de la progesterona y del acetato de desoxicorticoesterona. *An. Med. Cir. (Barcelona)* 27, 353—356 (1950). [B 54,459/50

Fonzo, D., Bosso, P., Dogliotti, L., Lauro, R., Martinis, C. de: Osservazioni preliminari sulle differenze della distribuzione e deiodazione della tiroxina-1-125 tra ratti maschi e femmine di razza wistar. *Boll. Soc. ital. Biol. sper.* 46, 328 to 331 (1970). [G 77,635/70

Forabosco, A., Bratina, F., Narducci, P.: Sulla rigenerazione epatica nel ratto timectomizzato in età adulta. V. Attività istochimica di alcune deidrogenasi alla 30ª ora di rigenerazione. *Boll. Soc. ital. Biol. sper.* 45, 363—365 (1969). [G 70,749/69

Forabosco, A., Guli, F.: Sulla rigenerazione epatica nel ratto timectomizzato in età adulta. IV. La ricostituzione della massa epatica alla 30ª ora del processo rigenerativo. *Boll. Soc. ital. Biol. sper.* 45, 361—363 (1969). [G 70,748/69

Forabosco, A., Narducci, P.: Sulla rigenerazione epatica nel ratto timectomizzato in età adulta. II. L'attività mitotica alla 30ª ora di rigenerazione. *Boll. Soc. ital. Biol. sper.* 45, 356—359 (1969). [G 70,746/69

Forabosco, A., Toni, G.: Sulla rigenerazione epatica nel ratto timectomizzato in età adulta. III. L'attività di sintesi di DNA alla 30ª ora di rigenerazione. *Boll. Soc. ital. Biol. sper.* 45, 359—361 (1969). [G 70,747/69

Forbes, R. M.: Mineral utilization in the rat. V. Effects of dietary thyroxine on mineral balance and tissue mineral composition with special reference to magnesium nutriture. *J. Nutr.* 86, 193—200 (1965). [G 30,402/65

Forchielli, E., Brown-Grant, K., Dorfman, R. I.: Steroid 4-hydrogenases of rat liver. *Proc. Soc. exp. Biol. (N.Y.)* 99, 594—596 (1958). [D 75,874/58

Forchielli, E., Dorfman, R. I.: Separation of Δ^4-5α- and Δ^4-5β-hydrogenases from rat liver homogenates. *J. biol. Chem.* 223, 443—448 (1956). [G 66,498/56

Ford, E. J. H.: The fate of mycobacterium johnei in young mice and guinea-pigs. *J. Path. Bact.* 73, 363—374 (1957). [G 67,455/57

Ford, E., Huggins, C.: Selective destruction in testis induced by 7,12-dimethylbenz(a)anthracene. *J. exp. Med.* 118, 27—40 (1963). [D 69,790/63

Fornaroli, P.: Sull'effetto potenziante l'attività dei narcotici della 5-ossitriptamina. In: Various Authors; Scritti Medici in Onore di Luigi Villa, p. 363—374. Milano: C.E.A. 1957. [C 47,728/57

Forsander, O. A., Hillbom, M. E., Lindros, K. O.: Influence of thyroid function on the acetaldehyde level of blood and liver of intact rats during ethanol metabolism. *Acta pharmacol. (Kbh.)* 27, 410—416 (1969). [G 71,697/69

Fortune, P. Y.: Comparative studies of the thyroid function in teleosts of tropical and temperate habitats. *J. exp. Biol.* 32, 504—513 (1955). [C 17,485/55

Fortune, P. Y.: An inactive thyroid gland in Carassius auratus. *Nature (Lond.)* 178, 98 (1956). [C 21,670/56

Fournier, G.: Détoxification du métrazol. *J. Hôtel-Dieu Montréal* 2, 112—115 (1943). [84,151/43

Fournier, G., Selye, H.: Concerning the site of pentamethylenetetrazol (metrazol) detoxification. (Abstr.) *Fed. Proc.* 1, 25 (1942). [81,980/42

Fouts, J. R.: The metabolism of drugs by subfractions of hepatic microsomes. *Biochem. biophys. Res. Commun.* 6, 373—378 (1961). [G 79,654/61

Fouts, J. R.: Interaction of drugs and hepatic microsomes. *Fed. Proc.* **21**, 1107—1111 (1962). [D43,347/62

Fouts, J. R.: Physiological impairment of drug metabolism. In: Brodie, B. B., Erdös, E. G.; *Metabolic Factors Controlling Duration of Drug Action*, p. 257—275. New York: MacMillan Co. 1962. [G77,514/62

Fouts, J. R.: Factors affecting hepatic microsomal enzyme systems involved in drug metabolism. In: Weber, G.; *Advances in Enzyme Regulation*, p. 225—233. New York: MacMillan Co. 1963. [G76,304/63

Fouts, J. R.: Drug interactions: effects of drugs and chemicals on drug metabolism. *Gastroenterology* **46**, 486—490 (1964). [G77,566/64

Fouts, J. R.: Some effects of insecticides on hepatic microsomal enzymes in various animal species. *Rev. Canad. Biol.* **29**, 377—389 (1970). [G76,868/70

Fouts, J. R.: The stimulation and inhibition of hepatic microsomal drug-metabolizing enzymes with special reference to effects of environmental contaminants. *Toxicol. appl. Pharmacol.* **17**, 804—809 (1970). [G79,537/70

Fouts, J. R., Adamson, R. H.: Drug metabolism in the newborn rabbit. *Science* **129**, 897—898 (1959). [H24,325/59

Fouts, J. R., Brodie, B. B.: Inhibition of drug metabolic pathways by the potentiating agent, 2,4-dichloro-6-phenylphenoxyethyl diethylamine. *J. Pharmacol. exp. Ther.* **113**, 68—73 (1955). [D83,597/55

Fouts, J. R., Brodie, B. B.: On the mechanism of drug potentiation by iproniazid (2-isopropyl-1-isonicotinyl hydrazine). *J. Pharmacol. exp. Ther.* **116**, 480—485 (1956). [D95,674/56

Fouts, J. R., Dixon, R. L., Shultice, R. W.: The metabolism of drugs by regenerating liver. *Biochem. Pharmacol.* **7**, 265—270 (1961). [G68,041/61

Fouts, J. R., Rogers, L. A.: Morphological changes in the liver accompanying stimulation of microsomal drug metabolizing enzyme activity by phenobarbital, chlordane, benzpyrene or methylcholanthrene in rats. *J. Pharmacol. exp. Ther.* **147**, 112—119 (1965). [F29,497/65

Fowler, J. S. L.: Carbon tetrachloride metabolism in the rabbit. *Brit. J. Pharmacol.* **37**, 733—737 (1969). [G70,865/69

Fox, S. L.: Potentiation of anticoagulants caused by pyrazole compounds. *J. Amer. med. Ass.* **188**, 320—321 (1964). [F8,079/64

Franchimont, P., Lefebvre, P., Cauwenberge, H. van: Effets de la sérotonine, d'un de ses inhibiteurs, l'UML 491, et du glucagon sur l'ostéolathyrisme expérimental du rat. *C. R. Soc. Biol.* **155**, 427—431 (1961). [D13,136/61

Franco, M.: Edema polmonare sperimentale adrenalinico e testosterone. *Ormonologia* **14**, 389—403 (1954). [C27,538/54

Franke, H., Klinger, W.: Untersuchungen zum Mechanismus der Enzyminduktion. IX. Die Wirkung von Barbital auf die Substruktur der Leberzellen gravider Ratten und ihrer Foeten. *Acta biol. med. Germanica* **17**, 507—526 (1966). [H31,874/66

Franken, F. H., Hagelskamp, W.: Barbiturate und Leber. *Dtsch. med. Wschr.* **95**, 1613—1616 (1970). [H28,823/70

Franklin, M.: Studies on the N-demethylation of morphine and other compounds. *Canad. J. Biochem.* **43**, 1053—1062 (1965). [G32,826/65

Fraser, H. F., Isbell, H., Wikler, A., Eisenman, A. I., Kornetsky, C. H.: Cortisone therapy in barbiturate abstinence syndrome. *Fed. Proc.* **10**, 296—297 (1951). [B57,226/51

Frawley, J. P., Hagan, E. C., Fitzhugh, O. G.: A comparative pharmacological and toxicological study of organic phosphate-anticholinesterase compounds. *J. Pharmacol. exp. Ther.* **105**, 156—165 (1952). [G69,644/52

Frawley, T. F., Roche, M., Jenkins, D., Thorn, G. W.: The role of the pituitary adrenocortical system in the response to anoxia. *43rd Meet. Amer. Soc. clin. Invest.*, p. 17 (1951). [B57,930/51

Fredericq, L.: Influence du milieu ambiant sur la composition du sang des animaux aquatiques. *Arch. Zool. exp. gén.* **3**, XXXIV à XXXVIII (1885). [A5,288/1885

Freedland, R. A.: Urea cycle adaptations in intact and adrenalectomized rats. *Proc. Soc. exp. Biol. (N.Y.)* **116**, 692—696 (1964). [F17,044/64

Freedland, R. A.: Effects of thyroid hormones on metabolism. Effect of thyroxine and iodinated casein on liver enzyme activity. *Endocrinology* **77**, 19—27 (1965). [F46,702/65

Freedland, R. A.: Effect of hypophysectomy on urea cycle enzyme adaptations. *Life Sci.* **4**, 899 (1965). [G28,270/65

Freedland, R. A., Avery, E. H.: Studies on threonine and serine dehydrase. *J. biol. Chem.* **239**, 3357—3360 (1964). [G67,766/64

Freedland, R. A., Avery, E. H., Taylor, A. R.: Effect of thyroid hormones on metabolism. II. The effect of adrenalectomy or hypophysectomy on responses of rat liver enzyme activity to L-thyroxine injection. Canad. J. Biochem. 46, 141—150 (1968). [G 55,808/68

Freedland, R. A., Krakowski, M. C., Waisman, H. A.: Effect of age, sex, and nutrition on liver phenylalanine hydroxylase activity in rats. Amer. J. Physiol. 202, 145—148 (1962). [G 66,662/62

Freedland, R. A., Murad, S., Hurvitz, A. I.: Relationship of nutritional and hormonal influences on liver enzyme activity. Fed. Proc. 27, 1217—1222 (1968). [H 2,949/68

Freeman, S., Svec, M.: Effect of complete hepatectomy upon plasma concentration and urinary excretion of eighteen amino acids. Amer. J. Physiol. 167, 201—205 (1951). [B 64,175/51

Fregly, M. J.: Prevention of salt hypertension by propylthiouracil treatment in rats. Proc. Soc. exp. Biol. (N.Y.) 102, 299—302 (1959). [C 77,939/59

Fregly, M. J.: Effect of changes of ambient temperature on spontaneous activity of hypothyroid rats. Canad. J. Biochem. 39, 1085—1096 (1961). [D 5,800/61

Fregly, M. J.: Effect of chlorothiazide and hydrochlorothiazide on blood pressure and thyroid activity of hypertensive rats. Amer. J. Cardiol. 8, 890—898 (1961). [D 15,796/61

Fregly, M. J.: Comments on cross-adaptation. Environm. Res. 2, 435—441 (1969). [G 72,594/69

Fregly, M. J., Baker, M. I., Gennaro, J. F., Jr.: Effect of certain anti-thyroid treatments on development or renal hypertension in rats. Fed. Proc. 18, 48 (1959). [C 66,042/59

Fregly, M. J., Baker, M. I., Gennaro, J. F., Jr.: Comparison of effects of thyroidectomy with propylthiouracil treatment on renal hypertension in rats. Amer. J. Physiol. 198, 4—12 (1960). [C 80,398/60

Fregly, M. J., Black, B. A.: Effect of methylphenidate on spontaneous activity, food intake, and cold tolerance of propylthiouracil-treated rats. Canad. J. Physiol. Pharmacol. 42, 415—429 (1964). [F 15,674/64

Fregly, M. J., Cook, K. M.: Role of the thyroid gland in development and maintenance of renal hypertension in rats. Acta endocr. (Kbh.) 34, 411—429 (1960). [C 88,371/60

Frenkel, J. K.: Effects of hormones on the adrenal necrosis produced by besnoitia jellisoni in golden hamsters. J. exp. Med. 103, 375—398 (1956). [C 13,371/56

Frenkel, J. K.: Effects of cortisone, total body irradiation and nitrogen mustard on chronic, latent toxoplasmosis. Amer. J. Path. 33, 618—619 (1957). [C 34,875/57

Frenkel, J. K.: Evaluation of immunity-depressing effects of anti-inflammatory corticoids. Fed. Proc. 17, 437 (1958). [C 52,043/58

Frenkel, J. K.: Evaluation of infection-enhancing activity of modified corticoids. Proc. Soc. exp. Biol. (N.Y.) 103, 552—555 (1960). [C 84,036/60

Freund, H.: Digitaliswirkung und Stoffwechsel. Naunyn-Schmiedebergs Arch. Pharmak. 167, 73—76 (1932). [A 26,153/32

Friedgood, C. E., Vars, H. M., Zerbe, J. W.: Role of adrenal cortex in liver regeneration. Amer. J. Physiol. 163, 354—363 (1950). [B 52,238/50

Friedlaender, S., Friedlaender, A. S.: The effect of pituitary adrenocorticotrophic hormone (ACTH) on histamine intoxication and anaphylaxis in the guinea pig. J. Allergy 21, 303—309 (1950). [B 55,467/50

Friedman, M., Bine, R., Jr., Byers, S. O.: Urinary excretion of digitoxin in the rat. Proc. Soc. exp. Biol. (N.Y.) 71, 406—407 (1949). [A 49,249/49

Friedman, S. M., Friedman, C. L.: A screening test to indicate opposition to the cardiovascular-renal effects of desoxycorticosterone acetate in the rat: the effect of adrenal cortical extract. Endocrinology 46, 367—374 (1950). [B 48,306/50

Friedrich, F., Kovac, W., Swoboda, W.: Die Beeinflussung der Vitamin-D-Wirkung auf die experimentelle Rattenrachitis durch Durabolin. Z. Kinderheilk. 92, 249—263 (1965). [F 39,223/65

Frölén, H.: Effects of some radioprotective substances upon prenatal survival of offspring to roentgen irradiated male mice. Acta radiol. (Stockh.) -Therapy- 4, 373—384 (1966). [G 43,045/66

Frommel, E. von, Ledebur, I., Béguin, M.: De l'action pseudomorphinique de la cortisone en administration unique et de son effet amphétaminolike en administration répétée. Expérimentation animale. Schweiz. med. Wschr. 92, 1265—1269 (1962). [E 37,967/62

Fudema, J. J., Oester, Y. T., Proctor, C. D.: Effect of I^{131} thyroid suppression on nutritional muscular dystrophy in rabbits. *Fed. Proc.* 21, 313 (1962). [D 23,102/62

Fujii, K., Jaffe, H., Bishop, Y., Arnold, E., MacKintosh, D., Epstein, S. S.: Structure-activity relations for methylenedioxyphenyl and related compounds on hepatic microsomal enzyme function as measured by prolongation of hexobarbital narcosis and zoxazolamine paralysis in mice. *Toxicol. appl. Pharmacol.* 16, 482—494 (1970). [G 77,242/70

Fujii, K., Jaffe, H., Epstein, S. S.: Factors influencing the hexobarbital sleeping time and zoxazolamine paralysis time in mice. *Toxicol. Appl. Pharmacol.* 13, 431—438 (1968).
[H 28,618/68

Fujimoto, J. M., Blickenstaff, D. E., Schueler, F. W.: Urethan induced acceleration of hexobarbital metabolism. *Proc. Soc. exp. Biol. (N.Y.)* 103, 463—465 (1960). [D 78,955/60

Fujimoto, J. M., Eich, W. F., Nichols, H. R.: Enhanced sulfobromophthalein disappearance in mice pretreated with various drugs. *Biochem. Pharmacol.* 14, 515—524 (1965).
[G 30,289/65

Fujita, T., Orimo, H., Ohata, M., Yoshikawa, M., Kataumi, S., Lehr, D.: Effect of age and thyrocalcitonin on myocardial changes induced by sodium sulfaacetylthiazole. *Endocr. jap.* 15, 247—249 (1968). [H 2,733/68

Fujiwara, K., Takagaki, Y., Maejima, K., Kato, K., Naiki, M., Tajima, Y.: Tyzzer's disease in mice: pathologic studies on experimentally infected animals. *Jap. J. exp. Med.* 33, 183—202 (1963). [E 34,642/63

Fujiwara, K., Takagaki, Y., Naiki, M., Maejima, K., Tajima, Y.: Tyzzer's disease in mice. Effects of corticosteroids on the formation of liver lesions and the level of blood transaminases in experimentally infected animals. *Jap. J. exp. Med.* 34, 59—75 (1964).
[F 17,247/64

Fukui, G. M.: Some factors affecting endotoxin-induced "nonspecific" resistance. In: Landy, Braun; *Bacterial Endotoxin*, p. 373 to 381. New Brunswick, N. J.: Institute of Microbiology, Rutgers, The State University 1964. [E 8,467/64

Fuller, G. C., Olshan, A., Puri, S. K., Lal, H.: Induction of hepatic drug metabolism in rats by methylchloroform inhalation. *J. Pharmacol. exp. Ther.* 175, 311—317 (1970). [H 31,807/70

Fuller, R. W.: Differences in the regulation of tyrosine aminotransferase in brain and liver. *J. Neurochem.* 17, 539—543 (1970).
[G 75,131/70

Fumarola, D., Giordano, D.: Influenza della timectomia e della ipertimizzazione sulla insorgenza e sullo sviluppo del sarcoma da 3,4-benzopirene nel ratto. *Tumori* 48, 5—12 (1962).
[D 33,779/62

Funahashi, H.: Ultrastructural changes in liver cells. I. Electronmicroscopic observations on human and rat liver in hyperthyroidism (Jap. text). *Jap. Arch. intern. Med.* 14, 1—16 (1967). [F 98,400/67

Furner, R. L., McCarthy, J. S., Stitzel, R. E., Anders, M. W.: Stereoselective metabolism of the enantiomers of hexobarbital. *J. Pharmacol. exp. Ther.* 169, 153—158 (1969). [H 17,931/69

Furner, R. L., Stitzel, R. E.: Stress-induced alterations in microsomal drug metabolism in the adrenalectomized rat. *Biochem. Pharmacol.* 17, 121—127 (1968). [G 54,558/68

Furstman, L., Bernick, S., Zipkin, I.: The effect of hydrocortisone and fluoride upon the rat's mandibular joint. *J. oral Therap. Pharmacol.* 1, 515—525 (1965). [G 31,603/65

Furukawa, T.: Role of endocrine glands and sympathetic nerves in fatty liver due to carbon tetrachloride. *Wakayama med. Rep.* 9, 203 to 210 (1965). [F 71,711/65

Fuwa, M., Waugh, D.: Experimental renal papillary necrosis. Effects of diuresis and antidiuresis. *Arch. Path.* 85, 404—409 (1968).
[F 96,546/68

Gabay, S., Vivanco, F., Ramos, F., Diaz, C. J.: Influence of DL-thyroxine and cortisone on femurs of rats with odoratism. *Arch. Biochem.* 92, 87—93 (1961). [D 98,867/61

Gabbiani, G.: Inibizione della calcifilassi per mezzo del metiltestosterone. *Sperimentale* 112, 457—466 (1962). [D 32,379/62

Gabbiani, G., Selye, H., Tuchweber, B.: Adrenal localization of a thrombohemorrhagic phenomenon. *Endocrinology* 77, 177—182 (1965).
[G 19,450/65

Gabbiani, G., Tuchweber, B.: Prevention by calcitonin of metallic salt intoxications. *Calc. Tiss. Res.* 4, Sup., 144—145 (1970).
[G 70,453/70

Gabbiani, G., Tuchweber, B., Côté, G.: Action of thyroxine on experimental parathyroid extract overdosage. *Endocrinology* 81, 798 to 802 (1967). [G 39,934/67

Gabbiani, G., Tuchweber, B., Côté, G., Lefort, P.: Action of thyroxine and calcitonin on experimental soft-tissue calcification. *Calc. Tiss. Res.* 2, 30—37 (1968). [G 46,731/68

Gabbiani, G., Tuchweber, B., Côté, G., Pahk, U. S., Selye, H.: Influence of thyroparathyroid apparatus on experimental soft-tissue calcification. *Int. Congr. Ser. No. 159* p. 485—498 (1968). [G 46,730/68

Gabler, E.: Die therapeutische Wirkung von Adrenalin und Alupent nach letaler Röntgenganzkörperbestrahlung. *Experientia (Basel)* **22**, 542—543 (1966). [G 40,828/66

Gaddum, J. H.: Recent work on 5-hydroxytryptamine and lysergic acid derivatives. *20th Congr. int. Physiol., Brussels*, p. 442—455 (1956). [C 25,117/56

Gaetani, G. F. de: Modificazioni della pressione arteriosa e del ritmo cardiaco e respiratorio nell'assideramento sotto l'influenza della adrenalina. *Riv. Pat. sper.* **15**, 201—211 (1935). [33,111/35

Gaines, T. B.: Acute toxicity of pesticides. *Toxicol. appl. Pharmacol.* **14**, 515—534 (1969). [G 67,102/69

Gallagher, T. F., Kappas, A.: Estrogen effects on BSP metabolism in rats. (Abstr.) *Fed. Proc.* **24**, 144 (1965). [F 35,850/65

Gallagher, T. F., Mueller, M. N., Kappas, A.: Estrogen pharmacology. IV. Studies on the structural basis for estrogen-induced impairment of liver function. *Medicine (Baltimore)* **45**, 471—479 (1966). [F 86,156/66

Galletti, F., Bruni, G.: Eteri steroidali; effetto anticatabolico di uno steroide anabolizzante non 17α-alchilato in ratti trattati con prednisone. *Boll. Soc. ital. Biol. sper.* **39**, 1898—1902 (1963). [G 16,710/63

Galliard, H., Buttner, A., Bourcart, N.: Effet de l'hormone somatotrope sur une trypanosomose mortelle pour Rana esculenta L., due au Trypanosoma inopinatum sergent, 1904 (souche algérienne). *C. R. Soc. Biol. (Paris)* **147**, 1695—1698 (1953). [G 70,892/53

Galliard, H., Lapierre, J.: Effets neutralisants de la somatotrophine hypophysaire, dans les infections à Plasmodium berghei chez la souris. *C. R. Acad. Sci. (Paris)* **237**, 477—479 (1953). [E 82,642/53

Galliard, H., Lapierre, J., Murard, J.: Inhibition de l'infection à Plasmodium berghei chez la souris et le rat par l'hormone hypophysaire de croissance (S.T.H.). *Ann. Parasit. hum. comp.* **29**, 167—178 (1954). [D 89,408/54

Gallut, J.: Du rôle de la glande surrénale dans l'intoxication cholérique expérimentale de la souris. *C. R. Soc. Biol. (Paris)* **149**, 1414 (1955). [C 14,519/55

Gandini, S., Gandini-Collodel, E.: Azione del 4-Clorotestosterone sul metabolismo proteico della cellula nervosa. Studio istochimico delle fosfatasi alcaline in animali affaticati. *Boll. Soc. ital. Biol. sper.* **38**, 1329—1331 (1962). [D 58,657/62

Ganesan, D.: Influence of female sex hormones on pentobarbitone sodium anaesthesia in rats. *Arch. int. Pharmacodyn.* **177**, 88—91 (1969). [H 12,504/69

Ganguli, N. C., Roy, S. C., Guha, B. C.: Studies on the biosynthesis of L-ascorbic acid by the rat. I. Effect of adenosine triphosphate and other compounds on the synthesis stimulated by chloretone. *Arch. Biochem.* **61**, 211—219 (1956). [G 71,669/56

Ganley, O. H.: Studies of the prevention of sensitization by Bordetella pertussis in alloxan diabetic mice. *Canad. J. Biochem.* **40**, 1179 to 1183 (1962). [D 31,168/62

Ganley, O. H., Balch, H. H., Pulaski, E. J.: Effect of ACTH and adrenocortical hormones on experimental gas gangrene toxemia. *Proc. Soc. exp. Biol. (N.Y.)* **89**, 485—487 (1955). [C 7,489/55

Ganley, O. H., Robinson, H. J.: Influence of alloxan on sensitizing properties of B. pertussis in the mouse. *Fed. Proc.* **18**, 392 (1959). [C 66,305/59

Ganong, W. F.: Review of Medical Physiology, p. 298. Los Altos, Calif.: Lange Medical Publ., 3rd ed. (1967). [G 74,587/67

Ganong, W. F.: Review of Medical Physiology, Los Altos, Calif.: Lange Medical Publ., 4th ed., Sect. IV (1969). [G 74,400/69

Gans, H., Stern, R., Tan, B. H.: Effect of hepatectomy on thrombin clearance. *Ann. Surg.* **170**, 937—946 (1969). [G 71,042/69

Garattini, S., Gaiardoni, P., Mortari, A., Palma, V.: Increased toxicity of serotonin in adrenalectomized animals. *Nature (Lond.)* **190**, 540—541 (1961). [D 4,913/61

Garattini, S., Valzelli, L.: Sostanze interferenti sulla attività potenziante gli ipnotici svolta dalla serotonina. *Boll. Soc. ital. Biol. sper.* **32**, 292—295 (1956). [G 71,229/56

Gardell, C., Blascheck, J. A., Kovács, K.: Action de la norboléthone sur le réticulum endoplasmique hépatique du rat. *J. Micr.* **9**, 133—138 (1970). [G 60,062/70

Gardell, C., Blascheck, J. A., Kovács, K.: Protection par la spironolactone contre la cardiopathie expérimentale causée par la digitoxine, le phosphate disodique et l'huile. *Path. et Biol.* **18**, 141—146 (1970). [G 60,065/70

Gardell, C., Somogyi, A., Kovács, K.: Influence de la dl-méthionine sur l'action protectrice de la spironolactone lors d'intoxication à la digitoxine chez le rat. *Europ. J. Toxicol.* 3, No. 2, 107 a 109 (1970). [G 60,076/70

Gardell, C., Tuchweber, B., Hatakeyama, S., Kovács, K.: Steroïdes et cardiopathie de néphrectomie. *Rev. Canad. Biol.* 29, No. 2, 181—185 (1970). [G 70,430/70

Gardner, W. U., Pfeiffer, C. A.: Inhibition of estrogenic effects on the skeleton by testosterone injections. *Proc. Soc. exp. Biol. (N.Y.)* 38, 599—602 (1938). [72,281/38

Garg, B. D., Blascheck, J. A., Kovács, K.: A comparative ultrastructural study on drug-induced proliferation of smooth-surfaced endoplasmic reticulum in hepatocytes. *Tohoku J. exp. Med.* (in press). [G 70,495/

Garg, B. D., Khandekar, J. D., Dardachti, D. F., Kovacs, K.: Effect of betamethasone and dexamethasone on the liver ultrastructure in rats. *Indian J. med. Res. (in press)*. [G 79,011/

Garg, B. D., Khandekar, J. D., Tuchweber, B., Kovacs, K.: Influence of dactinomycin on the ultrastructural changes induced in rat hepatocytes by spironolactone and pregnenolone-16α-carbonitrile. *Agressologie (in press)*. [G 79,030/

Garg, B. D., Kovács, K., Blascheck, J. A., Selye, H.: Ultrastructural changes in hepatocytes induced by a steroid carbonitrile. *Folia endocr. (Roma)* 23, 357—363 (1970). [G 60,031/70

Garg, B. D., Kovács, K., Blascheck, J. A., Selye, H.: Ultrastructural changes induced by pregnenolone nitrile in the rat liver. *J. Pharm. Pharmacol.* 22, 872—873 (1970). [G 70,474/70

Garg, B. D., Solymoss, B., Tuchweber, B.: Effect of spironolactone on the distribution and excretion of $^{203}HgCl_2$ in the rat. *Arzneimittel-Forsch.* 22, 872—873 (1970). [G 60,078/70

Garg, B. D., Szabo, S., Khandekar, J. D., Kovacs, K.: Effect of hypophysectomy on pregnenolone-16α-carbonitrile-induced ultrastructural changes in rat liver. *Naunyn-Schmiedebergs Arch. Pharmak.* 269, 7—14 (1971). [G 79,002/71

Garg, B. D., Szabo, S., Khandekar, J. D., Kovacs, K.: Ultrastructural changes caused by pregnenolone-16α-carbonitrile in the liver of hypophysectomized rats. (Abstr.) *8th Acta endocr. Congr. Copenhagen*, July 4—8, 1971. [G 79,008/71

Garren, L. D., Conney, A. H., Tomkins, G. M.: Stimulatory effect of phenobarbital on steroid metabolism. *J. clin. Invest.* 40, 1041 (1961). [G 66,660/61

Garren, L. D., Howell, R. R., Tomkins, G. M.: Mammalian enzyme induction by hydrocortisone. The possible role of RNA. *J. molec. Biol.* 9, 100—108 (1964). [G 19,151/64

Garren, L. D., Howell, R. R., Tomkins, G. M., Crocco, R. M.: A paradoxical effect of actinomycin D: the mechanism of regulation of enzyme synthesis by hydrocortisone. *Proc. nat. Acad. Sci. (Wash.)* 52, 1121—1129 (1964). [G 28,021/64

Garrido, C. M.: Acción de distintas substancias en la resistencia al frío de ratas blancas suprarrenoprivas y normales. *Rev. Soc. argent. Biol.* 35, 96—102 (1959). [C 77,562/59

Garrido, C. M.: Thyroïde et résistance au froid. *C. R. Soc. Biol. (Paris)* 154, 2378 (1960). [D 8,112/60

Garvin, P. J., Jr., Jennings, R. B., Gesler, R. M.: Some comparative effects of sodium D- and sodium L-thyroxine administered chronically to rats and dogs. *Toxicol. appl. Pharmacol.* 4, 276—285 (1962). [D 21,160/62

Gasic, G.: Local resistance to a lethal dose of formalin. *Proc. Soc. exp. Biol. (N.Y.)* 66, 579—582 (1947). [B 17,561/47

Gass, G. H., Umberger, E. J.: Lack of effect of two 17-substituted testosterones on hepatic sulfobromophthalein clearance in dogs. *Toxic. appl. Pharmac.* 1, 545—547 (1959). [C 94,624/59

Gastinel, P., Collart, P., Vaisman, A., Hamelin, A., Dunoyer, F.: A propos des résultats obtenus par l'emploi de la cortisone en syphilis expérimentale. *Ann. Derm. Syph. (Paris)* 87, 612—617 (1960). [D 8,309/60

Gaudette, L. E., Brodie, B. B.: Relationship between the lipid solubility of drugs and their oxidation by liver microsomes. *Biochem. Pharmacol.* 2, 89—96 (1959). [E 90,437/59

Gaunt, R.: Protection of normal rats against death from water intoxication with adrenal cortical substances. *Proc. Soc. exp. Biol. (N.Y.)* 54, 19—21 (1943). [A 63,323/43

Gaunt, R.: The effect of thyroxin on water diuresis and water intoxication in the rat. *Fed. Proc.* 3, 12 (1944). [84,566/44

Gaunt, R., Howell, C., Antonchek, N.: The effect of other steroids on the response to cortisone. *J. clin. Endocr.* 12, 957 (1952). [B 71,987/52

Gaunt, R., Steinets, B. G., Chart, J. J.: Pharmacologic alteration of steroid hormone functions. *Clin. Pharmacol. Ther.* 9, 657—681 (1968). [G63,202/68]

Gaunt, R., Tuthill, C. H., Antonchak, N., Leathem, J. H.: Antagonists to cortisone: an ACTH-like action of steroids. *Endocrinology* 52, 407—423 (1953). [B82,200/53]

Gautieri, R. F., Mann, D. E., Jr.: Effect of gonadectomy and estradiol benzoate administration on the minimal carcinogenic dose$_{50}$ of methylcholanthrene on mouse epidermis. *J. Pharm. Sci.* 50, 556—560 (1961). [H30,506/61]

Gavosto, F., Pileri, A., Brusca, A.: Increased transaminase activity in the liver after administration of cortisone. *Biochim. biophys. Acta (Amst.)* 24, 250—254 (1957). [C34,243/57]

Gayet-Hallion, T., Bouvet, P.: Action du sang de cheval éthyroïdé sur la toxicité de groupe de l'amphétamine. Comparaison avec le sang de cheval normal et avec la réserpine. *C. R. Soc. Biol. (Paris)* 158, 269—271 (1964). [F16,484/64]

Gaylord, C., Hodge, H. C.: Duration of sleep produced by pentobarbital sodium in normal and castrate female rats. *Proc. Soc. exp. Biol. (N.Y.)* 55, 46—48 (1944). [B11,425/44]

Gedalia, I., Frumkin, A., Zukerman, H.: Effects of estrogen on bone composition in rats at low and high fluoride intake. *Endocrinology* 75, 201—205 (1964). [F17,787/64]

Gelboin, H. V.: Drugs and protein synthesis. *Exp. Med. Surg.* 23, 85—103 (1965). [F62,759/65]

Gelboin, H. V.: Carcinogens, enzyme induction, and gene action. *Advanc. Cancer Res.* 10, 1—81 (1967). [G53,802/67]

Gelboin, H. V., Miller, J. A., Miller, E. C.: Studies on hepatic protein-bound dye formation in rats given single large doses of 3′-methyl-4-dimethylaminoazobenzene. *Cancer Res.* 18, 608—617 (1958). [D81,074/58]

Gelehrter, T. D., Tomkins, G. M.: The role of RNA in the hormonal induction of tyrosine aminotransferase in mammalian cells in tissue culture. *J. molec. Biol.* 29, 59—76 (1967). [G51,315/67]

Geller, E., Yuwiler, A., Schapiro, S.: Comparative effects of a stress and cortisol upon some enzymatic activities. *Biochim. biophys. Acta (Amst.)* 93, 311—315 (1964). [G22,722/64]

Geller, E., Yuwiler, A., Schapiro, S.: Tyrosine aminotransferase: activation or repression by a stress. *Proc. Soc. exp. Biol. (N.Y.)* 130, 458—461 (1969). [H8,414/69]

Geller, P., Merrill, E. R., Jawetz, E.: Effects of cortisone and antibiotics on lethal action of endotoxins in mice. *Proc. Soc. exp. Biol. (N.Y.)* 86, 716—719 (1954). [B98,147/54]

Gellhorn, E.: Schilddrüse und Nitrilvergiftung. *Pflügers Arch. ges. Physiol.* 200, 571—582 (1923). [16,839/23]

Gemmill, C. L.: Comparison of activity of thyroxine and 3,5, 3′-triiodothyronine. *Amer. J. Physiol.* 172, 286—290 (1953). [B85,291/53]

Genitis, V. E., Borkon, E. L., Templeton, R. D.: The influence of temperature on parathyroid tetany in the albino rat. *Amer. J. Physiol.* 113, 48 (1935). [68,723/35]

Georgii, A., Mehnert, H., Prosiegel, R., Kastein, H., Stock, G.: Tierexperimentelle Leberbefunde nach langfristigen Sulfonylharnstoffgaben (D 860) und gleichzeitiger Leberschädigung mit Thioacetamid. *Z. ges. exp. Med.* 131, 181—190 (1959). [C69,388/59]

Gerald, M. C., Feller, D. R.: Evidence for spironolactone as a possible inducer of liver microsomal enzymes in mice. *Biochem. Pharmacol.* 19, 2529—2532 (1970). [G74,092/70]

Gerald, M. C., Feller, D. R.: A comparison of spironolactone (SL) and a major metabolite (SC-9376) as inducers of hepatic microsomal enzyme systems in male and female mice. *Pharmacologist* 12, 279 (1970). [G74,396/70]

Gerald, M. C., Feller, D. R.: Stimulation of barbiturate metabolism by spironolactone in mice. *Arch. int. Pharmacodyn.* 187, 120—124 (1970). [G78,804/70]

Gerber, W., Cottier, P.: Zur Wirkung anaboler Hormone auf die Azotämie bei Nierenversagen. *Helv. med. Acta* 28/3, 197—215 (1961). [D12,775/61]

Gerlich, N.: Experimentelle Studien über die Beziehungen zwischen Schilddrüse und Krampfbereitschaft. *Naunyn-Schmiedebergs Arch. Pharmak.* 207, 159—172 (1949). [B49,124/49]

Germer, W. D., Regoeczi, E.: Ein experimenteller Beitrag zur Testosteron-Wirkung bei toxischen Leberschäden. *Dtsch. Arch. klin. Med.* 205, 343—361 (1958). [C64,975/58]

Germuth, F. G., Jr., Ottinger, B., Oyama, J.: The influence of cortisone on the evolution of acute infection and the development of immunity. *Bull. Johns Hopk. Hosp.* 91, 22—48 (1952). [D77,106/52]

Gersh, I., Wagner, C. E.: Metabolic factors in oxygen poisoning. *Amer. J. Physiol.* 144, 270—277 (1945). [B1,140/45

Gershbein, L. L.: Pregnancy and liver regeneration in partially hepatectomized rats. *Proc. Soc. exp. Biol. (N.Y.)* 99, 716—717 (1958). [G71,666/58

Gershbein, L. L.: Effect of carcinogenic and noncarcinogenic hydrocarbons and hepatocarcinogens on rat liver regeneration. *J. nat. Cancer Inst.* 21, 295—310 (1958). [G71,667/58

Gershbein, L. L.: Transplanted tumor growth and liver regeneration in the rat. *J. nat. Cancer Inst.* 31, 521—528 (1963). [E71,030/63

Gershbein, L. L.: Effects of various agents on liver regeneration and Walker tumor growth in partially hepatectomized rats. *Cancer Res.* 26, 1905—1908 (1966). [F71,304/66

Gershbein, L. L.: Effect of insecticides on rat liver regeneration. *Res. Commun. chem. Path. Pharmacol.* 1, 740—748 (1970). [H31,893/70

Gershoff, S. N., Vitale, J. J., Antonowicz, I., Nakamura, M., Hellerstein, E. E.: Studies of interrelationships of thyroxine, magnesium and vitamin B_{12}. *J. biol. Chem.* 231, 849—854 (1958). [C54,255/58

Geschwind, I. I., Li, C. H.: Influence of hypophysectomy and of adrenocorticotropic hormone on a mammalian adaptive enzyme system. *Nature* 172, 732—733 (1953). [B95,517/53

Geschwind, I. I., Li, C. H.: Endocrine control of an induced hepatic enzyme system. *J. clin. Endocr.* 14, 789—790 (1954). [B93,277/54

Gessner, T., Acara, M., Baker, J. A., Edelman, L. L.: Effects of sex hormones on the duration of drug action in mice. *J. pharm. Sci.* 56, 405—407 (1967). [F77,776/67

Geyer, G.: Erfolgreiche Behandlung eines Falles von Cushing-Syndrom mit o,p-DDD [2,2-bis (2-chlorphenyl-4-chlorophenyl)-1,1-Dichloroäthan.] *Acta endocr. (Kbh.)* 40, 332—348 (1962). [D27,915/62

Geyer, G., Schüller, E.: Über den Einfluß von o,p-DDD [2,2-bis (2-chlorphenyl-4-chlorphenyl)-1,1-Dichloräthan] auf die Steroidausscheidung im Harn bei Nebennieren-gesunden und bei einigen Fällen typischer adrenocorticaler Funktionsstörung. *Klin. Wschr.* 40, 734—740 (1962). [D38,170/62

Geyer, R. P., Bryant, J. E., Bleisch, V. R., Peirce, E. M., Stare, F. J.: Effect of dose and hormones on tumor production in rats given emulsified 9,10-dimethyl-1,2-benzanthracene intravenously. *Cancer Res.* 13, 503—506 (1953). [H31,923/53

Ghedini, Ollino: Influence de la situation endocrinique sur l'action des médicaments cardio-vasculaires. *C. R. Soc. Biol. (Paris)* 76, 659—660 (1914). [A21,128/14

Ghione, M.: Azione antiinfettiva di steroidi anabolizzanti. *Sperimentale* 107, 182—195 (1957). [D87,868/57

Ghione, M.: Anti-infective action of an anabolic steroid. *Proc. Soc. exp. Biol. (N.Y.)* 97, 773—775 (1958). [C51,954/58

Ghione, M., Turolla, E.: Steroidi anabolizzanti e processi infettivi. *G. ital. Chemioter.* 10, 290—302 (1964). [G18,525/64

Ghiringhelli, L.: Influenza dell'ormone somatropo sulla produzione di anticorpi antiovalbumina in animali da esperimento. *Folia endocr. (Roma)* 13, 416—421 (1960). [C90,609/60

Ghys, R.: Action radiomodificatrice de la testostérone chez des rats soumis à l'action de neutrons rapides ou à l'irradiation interne par rayons béta du 32 P. *Rev. canad. Biol.* 21, 95—103 (1962). [D30,012/62

Ghys, R.: Action radiomodificatrice des hormones sexuelles chez le rat. II. Influence du traitement hormonal combiné à l'irradiation chez le rat hypophysectomisé. *J. belge Radiol.* 45, 67—82 (1962). [D70,483/62

Ghys, R.: L'influence des facteurs métaboliques sur la radiosensibilité. *Laval méd.* 34, 69—79 (1963). [D54,640/63

Ghys, R., Loiselle, J. M.: Les facteurs influençant les réactions des animaux soumis à une irradiation totale non fractionnée. *Rev. canad. Biol.* 19, 53—79 (1960). [C83,564/60

Giberti, A., Ponzoni, R., Spampinato, V.: Sulla morte precoce delle cavie in corso di trattamento aureomicinico. Tentativi di protezione con vitamine dei gruppi B e C e con cortisone. Nota II. Ricerche istologiche. *Boll. Ist. sieroter. Milan* 32, 246—255 (1953). [B90,116/53

Giberti, A., Vecchiati, R., Belluzzi, V.: Il propiltiuracile sulla rigenerazione epatica. *Folia endocr. (Roma)* 6, 267—272 (1953). [B82,948/53

Gibson, J. E., Becker, B. A.: Demonstration of enhanced lethality of drugs in hypoexcretory animals. *J. pharm. Sci.* 56, 1503—1505 (1967). [E65,709/67

Gigante, D., Scopinaro, D.: Sulla fisiopatologia dei vasi sanguigni nei congelamenti. III. Azione del propionato di testosterone sulla pressione arteriosa e venosa, sull'osciliometria e sulla temperatura cutanea nei congelati. *Ormonologia* 4, 65—76 (1946). [B 67,617/46

Gigon, P. L., Gram, T. E., Gillette, J. R.: Effect of drug substrates on the reduction of hepatic microsomal cytochrome P-450 by NADPH. *Biochem. biophys. Res. Commun.* 31, 558—562 (1968). [G 76,365/68

Gigon, P. L., Gram, T. E., Gillette, J. R.: Studies on the rate of reduction of hepatic microsomal cytochrome P-450 by reduced nicotinamide adenine dinucleotide phosphate: effect of drug substrates. *Molec. Pharmacol.* 5. 109—122 (1969). [G 66,216/69

Gilger, A. P., Potts, A. M., Johnson, L. V.: Studies on the visual toxicity of methanol. II. The effect of parenterally administered substances on the systemic toxicity of methyl alcohol. *Amer. J. Ophthal.* 35, 113—126 (1952). [B 73,737/52

Gillett, J. W.: Microsomal epoxidation: effect of age and duration of exposure to dietary DDT on induction. *Bull. environm. Contam. Toxicol.* 4, 160—168 (1969). [G 74,480/69

Gillette, J. R.: Oxidation and reduction by microsomal enzymes. In: Brodie and Erdös; *Metabolic Factors Controlling Duration of Drug Action* (Proc. of the 1. int. pharmacol. Meet. Vol. 6), p. 13—29. New York: MacMillan Co. 1962. [E 52,874/62

Gillette, J. R.: Metabolism of drugs and other foreign compounds by enzymatic mechanisms. *Fortschr. Arzneimittel-Forsch.* 6, 11—73 (1963). [G 51,908/63

Gillette, J. R.: Factors that affect the stimulation of the microsomal drug enzymes induced by foreign compounds. In: Weber; *Advances in Enzyme Regulation*, Vol. 1, p. 215—223. New York: MacMillan Co. 1963. [G 66,248/63

Gillette, J. R.: Drug toxicity as a result of interference with physiological control mechanisms. *Ann. N.Y. Acad. Sci.* 123, 42—54 (1965). [G 66,246/65

Gillette, J. R.: Biochemistry of drug oxidation and reduction by enzymes in hepatic endoplasmic reticulum. In: Garattini, S., Shore, P. A.; *Advances in Pharmacology*, p. 219—261. New York, London: Academic Press 1966. [E 7,538/66

Gillette, J. R.: Individually different responses to drugs according to age, sex and functional or pathological state. In: Wolstenholme, Porter; *Ciba Foundation Symposium on Drug Responses in Man*, p. 24—49. London: J. and A. Churchill Ltd. 1967. [G 67,333/67

Gillette, J. R.: Theoretical aspects of drug interaction. In: Siegler, P. E., Moyer, J. H.; *Animal and Clinical Pharmacologic Techniques in Drug Evaluation*, 2, p. 48—66. Chicago: Year Book Medical Publ. Inc. 1967. [G 78,390/67

Gillette, J. R.: Effect of various inducers on electron transport system associated with drug metabolism by liver microsomes. *Metabolism* 20, 215—227 (1971). [H 34,126/71

Gillette, J. R., Conney, A. H., Cosmides, G. J., Estabrook, R. W., Fouts, J. R., Mannering, G. J.: Microsomes and drug oxidations (*Symp. on Microsomes and Drug Oxidations*, Bethesda, Md. 1968). New York, London: Academic Press Inc. 1969, p. 547. [E 8,216/69

Gillissen, G., Busanny-Caspari, W.: Über den Einfluß der Hypophysektomie auf die experimentelle Tuberkulose. *Z. Hyg. Infekt.-Kr.* 137, 516—517 (1953). [C 6,858/53

Gillman, J., Gilbert, C.: Periarteritis and other forms of necrotising angeitis produced by vitamin D in thyroximised rats with an assessment of the aetiology of those vascular lesions. *Brit. J. exp. Path.* 37, 584—596 (1956). [C 31,076/56

Ginoulhiac, E.: Attività comparativa del prednisolone, del dexametasone e di altri derivati fluorurati del prednisolone sulla triptofano-perossidasi-ossidasi. *Acta vitamin (Milano)* 13, 149—154 (1959). [G 67,780/59

Giordano, P. L., Invernizzi, G.: Tierexperimentelle Untersuchungen über die Wirkung niedriger Röntgendosen auf das Zentralnervensystem und Strahlenschutzversuche mit Arzneimitteln. *Arzneimittel-Forsch.* 18, 1417 bis 1420 (1968). [H 5,873/68

Giotti, A., Donatelli, L.: Influenza dello stato gravidico sulla narcosi barbiturica. *Boll. Soc. ital. Biol. sper.* 24, 711—712 (1948). [B 39,580/48

Girard, G.: Cortisone et pasteurella pestis (souches de virulence affaiblie) chez la souris blanche. *Gaz. Hôp. (Paris)* 128, 863 (1956). [C 22,665/56

Girkin, G., Kampschmidt, R. F.: Effect of thiouracil on liver enlargement in tumor-bearing rats. *Amer. J. Physiol.* 200, 61—63 (1961). [C 99,934/61

Girolami, M.: Treatment of ascitic atrophic cirrhosis of the liver with high dosages of testosterone propionate. *J. Amer. Geriat. Soc.* 6, 306—323 (1958). [C 55,043/58

Giroud, P., Capponi, M., Dumas, N.: De la maladie inapparente à la maladie mortelle chez le rat blanc infecté par Toxoplasma gondi et traité aux stéroïdes synthétiques. *Bull. Soc. Path. exot.* **55**, 335—339 (1962). [D 68,563/62

Gish, C. D., Chura, N. J.: Toxicity of DDT to Japanese quail as influenced by body weight, breeding condition, and sex. *Toxicol. appl. Pharmacol.* **17**, 740—751 (1970). [G 80,046/70

Gispen, W. H., Greidanus, T. B. van W., Wied, D. de: Effects of hypophysectomy and ACTH$_{1-10}$ on responsiveness to electric shock in rats. *Physiol. and Behav.* **5**, 143—146 (1970). [G 77,128/70

Giuliani, L.: La rispota prostatica a variazioni dell'equilibrio ormonico sessuale nel quadro di un danno epatico irreversibile. *Folia endocr. (Roma)* **8**, 933—952 (1955). [C 15,153/55

Giunta, F., Rath, J.: Effect of environmental illumination in prevention of hyperbilirubinemia of prematurity. *Pediatrics* **44**, 162—167 (1969). [H 35,532/69

Giuseppe, O.: Edema polmonare sperimentale adrenalinico ed estrogeni. *Ormonologia* **14**, 219—236 (1954). [C 27,530/54

Glaser, R. J., Berry, J. W., Loeb, L. H., Wood, W. B., Jr.: The effect of cortisone on acute bacterial infections. *3rd Meet. Amer. Soc. clin. Invest.* p. 19 (1951). [B 57,933/51

Glaser, R. J., Berry, J. W., Loeb, L. H., Wood, W. B., Jr.: The effect of cortisone in streptococcal lymphadenitis and pneumonia. *J. Lab. clin. Med.* **38**, 363—373 (1951). [B 65,298/51

Glaser, R. J., Berry, J. W., Loeb, L. H., Wood, W. B., Jr., Daughaday, W. H.: Effect of ACTH and cortisone in experimental streptococcal and pneumococcal infections. *J. Lab. clin. Med.* **36**, 826 (1950). [B 58,299/50

Glaubach, S., Pick, E. P.: Über die Beeinflussung der Temperaturregulierung durch Thyroxin. I. Mitteilg. *Naunyn-Schmiedebergs Arch. Pharmak.* **151**, 341—370 (1930). [11,431/30

Glaubach, S., Pick, E. P.: Über die Beeinflussung der Temperaturregulierung durch Thyroxin. II. Mitteilg. Kokain, Perkain und Novokainwirkung bei thyroxinvorbehandelten Tieren. *Naunyn-Schmiedebergs Arch. Pharmak.* **162**, 537—550 (1931). [6,241/31

Glaubach, S., Pick, E. P.: Über den Einfluß der Schilddrüse auf die Arzneiempfindlichkeit. *Schweiz. med. Wschr.* **64**, 1115 (1934). [30,481/34

Glees, P.: Experimentelle Markscheidendegeneration durch Tri-ortho-kresylphosphat und ihre Verhütung durch Cortisonacetat. *Dtsch. med. Wschr.* **86**, 1175—1178 (1961). [D 7,966/61

Glees, P.: Central nerve fibre degeneration caused by tri-ortho-cresyl phosphate and its arrest by the action of cortisone acetate. *Germ. med. Mth.* **6**, 245—247 (1961). [D 14,872/61

Glenn, E. M., Lyster, S. C., Bowman, B. J., Richardson, S. L.: Potentiation of biological activities of steroids by carcinogenic hydrocarbons. *Endocrinology* **64**, 419—430 (1959). [C 64,744/59

Glenn, E. M., Richardson, S. L., Bowman, B. J., Lyster, S. C.: Steroids and experimental mammary cancer. In: Pincus, G.; *Biological Activities of Steroids in Relation to Cancer*, p. 257—305. New York, N. Y.: Academic Press Inc. 1960. [G 70,204/60

Glenn, T. M., Lefer, A. M.: Anti-toxic action of methylprednisolone in hemorrhagic shock. *Europ. J. Pharmacol.* **13**, 230—238 (1971). [H 34,576/71

Glickman, I., Selye, H., Smulow, J. B.: Systemic factors that influence the manifestations of osteolathyrism in the periodontium. *J. dent. Res.* **42**, 835—841 (1963). [E 24,104/63

Glock, G. E.: Thiourea and the suprarenal cortex. *Nature (Lond.)* **156**, 508 (1945). B 23,056/45

Glogner, P., Ermert A.: Untersuchung zum Metabolismus von Phenacetin. *Arzneimittel-Forsch.* **20**, 636—637 (1970). [H 27,073/70

Glover, E. L., Reuber, M. D.: Chronic thyroiditis in Buffalo rats with carbon tetrachloride-induced cirrhosis. *Endocrinology* **80**, 361—364 (1967). [F 77,043/67

Glover, E. L., Reuber, M. D., Grollman, S.: Influence of age and sex on thyroiditis in rats injected subcutaneously with 3-methylcholanthrene. *Path. et Microbiol. (Basel)* **32**, 314—320 (1968). [H 12,898/68

Gluck, T.: Über die Bedeutung physiologisch-chirurgischer Experimente an der Leber. *Langenbecks Arch. klin. Chir.* **29**, 139—145 (1883). [A 5,289/1883

Glucksmann, A., Cherry, C. P.: The effect of oestrogens, testosterone and progesterone on the induction of cervico-vaginal tumours in intact and castrate rats. *Brit. J. Cancer* **22**, 545—562 (1968). [H 19,200/68

Glucksmann, A., Cherry, C. P.: The effect of increased numbers of carcinogenic treatments on the induction of cervico-vaginal and vulval tumours in intact and castrate rats. *Brit. J. Cancer* **24**, 333—351 (1970). [G 77,810/70

Godfraind, T., Godfraind-De Becker, A.: Action des glucosides cardiotoniques sur l'iléon de cobaye et sa modification par la désoxycorticostérone. Arch. int. pharmacodyn. 130/3—4, 435—436 (1961). [D45,080/61

Goedbloed, J. F., Vos, O.: Influences on the incidence of secondary disease in radiation chimeras: thymectomy and tolerance. Transplantation (Baltimore) 3, 603—609 (1965). [G33,427/65

Gogolák, G., Liebeswar, G., Stumpf, C.: Durch Nicotin und Pentetrazol ausgelöste EEG-Veränderungen an normalen und hypothyreotischen Kaninchen. Naunyn-Schmiedebergs Arch. Pharmak. 258, 383—390 (1967). [G51,384/67

Goldberg, L., Störtebecker, T. P.: Antinarcotic effect of estrone on alcohol intoxication. Acta physiol. scand. 5, 289—296 (1943). [B31,834/43

Golden, J. B., Sevringhaus, E. L.: Inactivation of estrogenic hormone of the ovary by the liver. Proc. Soc. exp. Biol. (N.Y.) 39, 361—362 (1938). [A37,808/38

Goldenthal, E. I.: A compilation of LD50 values in newborn and adult animals. Toxicol. appl. Pharmacol. 18, 185—207 (1971). [G81,411/71

Goldenthal, E. I., D'Aguanno, W., Lynch, J. F.: Hormonal modification of the sex differences following monocrotaline administration. Toxicol. appl. Pharmacol. 6, 434—441 (1964). [G18,384/64

Goldfischer, S., Arias, I. M., Essner, E., Novikoff, A. B.: Cytochemical and electron microscopic studies of rat liver with reduced capacity to transport conjugated bilirubin. J. exp. Med. 115, 467—474 (1962). [D20,605/62

Goldhaber, P.: Bone-resorption factors, cofactors, and giant vacuole osteoclasts in tissue culture. In: Gaillard, Talmage, Budy; The Parathyroid Glands: Ultrastructure, Secretion, and Function, p. 153—169. Chicago: The University of Chicago Press 1965. [E5,596/65

Goldin, A., Greenspan, E. M., Goldberg, B., Schoenbach, E. B.: Studies on the mechanism of action of chemotherapeutic agents in cancer. I. A sex difference in toxicity to the folic acid analogue, 4-amino-pteroylglutamic acid. Cancer (Philad.) 3, 849—855 (1950). [D76,907/50

Goldman, A. S.: Experimental congenital adrenocortical hyperplasia; persistent postnatal deficiency in activity of 3β-hydroxysteroid dehydrogenase produced in utero. J. clin. Endocr. 27, 1041—1049 (1967). [F85,342/67

Goldman, A. S.: Stoichiometric inhibition of various 3β-hydroxysteroid dehydrogenases by a substrate analogue. J. clin. Endocr. 27, 325—332 (1967). [F78,224/67

Goldman, A. S.: Maternal and fetal effects of two inhibitors of 3β-hydroxysteroid dehydrogenase and $\varDelta^{5-4}$, 3-ketosteroid isomerase in the rat. Endocrinology 85, 325—329 (1969). [H15,818/69

Goldman, A. S.: Experimental congenital lipoid adrenal hyperplasia: prevention of anatomic defects produced by aminoglutethimide. Endocrinology 87, 889—893 (1970). [H31,449/70

Goldman, A. S., Bongiovanni, A. M., Yakovac, W. C.: Production of congenital adrenal cortical hyperplasia, hypospadias, and clitoral hypertrophy (adrenogenital syndrome) in rats by inactivation of 3β-hydroxysteroid dehydrogenase. Proc. Soc. exp. Biol. (N.Y.) 121, 757—766 (1966). [F64,070/66

Goldman, A. S., Bongiovanni, A. M., Yakovac, W. C.: Experimental adrenal cortical hyperplasia produced by persistent inhibition of fetal 3β-hydroxysteroid dehydrogenase (3β-enzyme). (Abstr.). Excerpta med. (Amst.), Int. Congr. Ser. No. 111, p. 177. (1966). 2nd Int. Congr. on hormonal steroids, Milan, Italy. [G73,456/66

Goldman, A. S., Neumann, F.: Differentiation of the mammary gland in experimental congenital adrenal hyperplasia due to inhibition of $\varDelta^5,3\beta$-hydroxysteroid dehydrogenase in rats. Proc. Soc. exp. Biol. (N.Y.) 132, 237—241 (1969). [H18,122/69

Goldman, A. S., Yakovac, W. C.: The enhancement of salicylate teratogenicity by maternal immobilization in the rat. J. Pharmacol. exp. Ther. 142, 351—357 (1963). [E35,710/63

Goldsmith, E. D., Gordon, A. S., Charipper, H. A.: Estrogens, thiourea, thiouracil, and the tolerance of rats to simulated high altitudes (low atmospheric pressures). Endocrinology 36, 364—369 (1945). [B333/45

Goldstein, A., Aronow, L., Kalman, S. M.: Principles of Drug Action. The Basis of Pharmacology, p. 206—279. New York, Evanston, London: Harper and Row Publ. 1968. [E165/68

Goldstein, L., Stella, E. J., Knox, W. E.: The effect of hydrocortisone on tyrosine-α-ketoglutarate transaminase and tryptophan pyrrolase activities in the isolated, perfused rat liver. J. biol. Chem. 237, 1723—1726 (1962). [D70,931/62

Gonzalez, C. A., de Anda, L. B., Roel, R. G., Pisanty, O. J., Rodriguez, M.: Shock bacterémico en gineco-obstetricia. *Ginec. Obstet. Méx.* 22, 1153—1163 (1967). [F88,028/67

González-Angulo, A., Aznar-Ramos, R., Márquez-Monter, H., Bierzwinsky, G., Martínez-Manautou, J.: The ultrastructure of liver cells in women under steroid therapy. I. Normal pregnancy and trophoblastic growths. *Acta endocr. (Kbh.)* 65, 193—206 (1970).
[H30,301/70

Gonzalez, R.: Influencia de la hipófisis sobre la hipertrofía renal compensadora. *Rev. Soc. argent. Biol.* 14, 173—183 (1938). [79,025/38

Gonzalez, R.: Action de l'hypophyse sur l'hypertrophie rénale compensatrice chez les batraciens. *C. R. Soc. Biol. (Paris)* 129, 1270—1271 (1938). [A34,057/38

Good, E. E., Ware, G. W.: Effects of insecticides on reproduction in the laboratory mouse. IV. Endrin and dieldrin. *Toxicol. appl. Pharmacol.* 14, 201—203 (1969). [G76,670/69

Goodall, C. M.: Effect of cortisone on hepatoma formation in rats. *A. R. Brit. Emp. Cancer Campgn.* 40, 548—549 (1962). [G77,088/62

Goodall, C. M.: Hepatic carcinogenesis in thyroidectomized rats: apparent blockade at the stage of initiation. *Cancer Res.* 26, 1880—1883 (1966). [F71,302/66

Goodsell, E. B.: Ethanol intoxication in adrenocorticosteroid-treated mice. *Fed. Proc.* 20, 170 (1961). [D3,916/61

Gorby, C. K., Leonard, C. A., Ambrus, J. L., Harrison, J. W. E.: The effects of cortisone and desoxycorticosterone on the toxicity of barbiturates. *J. Amer. Pharm. Ass.* 42, 213—214 (1953). [B84,489/53

Gordeyeva, K. V.: The effect of insulin and glucose on the glucogen content of the liver in X-ray sickness. (Russian text.) *Vop. med. Khim.* 6/4, 408—411 (1960). [C97,407/60

Gordon, A. S., Goldsmith, E. D., Charipper, H. A.: Effects of para aminobenzoic acid and thiouracil on thyroid function and resistance to low pressures. *Endrocrinology* 37, 223—229 (1945). [B761/45

Gordon, D., Kobernick, S. D., McMillan, G. C., Duff, G. L.: The effect of cortisone on the serum lipids and on the development of experimental cholesterol atherosclerosis in the rabbit. *J. exp. Med.* 99, 371—386 (1954). [B95,119/54

Gordon, G. G., Southren, A. L., Tochimoto, S., Olivo, J., Altman, K., Rand, J., Lemberger, L.: Effect of medroxyprogesterone acetate (Provera) on the metabolism and biological activity of testosterone. *J. clin. Endocr.* 30, 449—456 (1970). [H24,106/70

Gordon, P., Linton, M. A.: Beneficial effect of serotonin and compound F on E. coli endotoxin mortality in mice. (Abstr.) *Fed. Proc.* 16, 301 (1957). [C33,200/57

Gordon, P., Lipton, M. A.: Hormonal modification of endotoxin mortality in mice. *Proc. Soc. exp. Biol. (N.Y.)* 105, 162—164 (1960).
[C94,649/60

Goss, J. E., Dickhaus, D. W.: Increased bishydroxycoumarin requirements in patients receiving phenobarbital. *New Engl. J. Med.* 273, 1094—1095 (1965). [F53,987/65

Goswami, M. N. D., Sripati, C. E., Khouvine, Y.: Effet de la 8-azaguanine sur l'adaptation de la tyrosine aminotransférase (EC 2.6.1.5) hépatique de rats adultes surrénalectomisés et traités par la L-tyrosine. *C. R. Acad. Sci. (Paris)* 266, 724—727 (1968). [G55,570/68

Goth, A., Nash, W. L., Nagler, M., Holman, J.: Inhibition of histamine release in experimental diabetes. *Amer. J. Physiol.* 191, 25—28 (1957). [C43,836/57

Göthe, C. J.: Effect of cortisol on lymphatic lung clearance and on experimental silicosis. A study in rats. *Acta endocr. (Kbh.)* 63, 313—324 (1970). [H20,084/70

Göthe, C. J.: Effect of different doses of prednisolone and adrenocorticotrophic hormone (ACTH) on lymphatic lung clearance and on experimental silicosis. A study in rats. *Acta endocr. (Kbh.)* 63, 325—337 (1970).
[H20,085/70

Govier, W. C.: Reticuloendothelial cells as the site of sulfanilamide acetylation in the rabbit. *J. Pharmacol. exp. Ther.* 150, 305—308 (1965). [F57,820/65

Govier, W. C., Lovenberg, W.: Induction of tyrosine aminotransferase by phentolamine. *Biochem. Pharmacol.* 18, 2667—2672 (1969).
[G70,841/69

Grab, W.: Die funktionelle Bedeutung der Bauelemente der Schilddrüse. *Naunyn-Schmiedebergs Arch. Pharmak.* 172, 586—629 (1933). [44,536/33

Grad, B., Leblond, C. P.: Role of the liver in the thyroxine metabolism of the albino rats. *Proc. Canad. Physiol. Soc. 12th Ann. Meet. Laval Univ. Québec*, 1948, p. 320—321.
[B23,328/48

Grad, B., Leblond, C. P.: Effect of thyroxine on oxygen consumption and heart rate follow-

ing bile duct ligation and partial hepatectomy. *Amer. J. Physiol.* **162**, 17—23 (1950).
[B 49,686/50

Grafov, A. A.: The effect of ACTH on the clinical course of acute radiation sickness in hypophysectomized rats. (Russian text.) *Probl. Endokr. Gormonoter.* 8/2, 57—64 (1962).
[D 20,890/62

Graham, A. B., Werder, A. A., Syverton, J. T., Friedman, J.: Synergistic effect of roentgen radiation and cortisone upon pathogenicity of Coxsackie virus. *Fed. Proc.* **11**, 470 (1952).
[B 68,455/52

Graham, J. B., Graham, R. M.: Pharmacological modification of resistance to radiation — A preliminary report. *Proc. nat. Acad. Sci. (Wash.)* **35**, 102—106 (1949). [A 49,307/49

Graham, J. B., Graham, R. M.: The modification of resistance to ionizing radiation by humoral agents. *Cancer (Philad.)* **3**, 709—717 (1950). [B 58,164/50

Graham, J. B., Graham, R. M., Graffeo, A. J.: The influence of adrenal cortical hormones on sensitivity of mice to ionizing radiations. *Endocrinology* **46**, 434—440 (1950).
[B 48,335/50

Graham, J. S.: Adrenal cortex and blood pressure response to carbon arc irradiation. *Amer. J. Physiol.* **139**, 604—611 (1943).
[A 61,343/43

Graham, W. D., Carmichael, E. J., Allmark, M. G.: The in vivo potentiation of barbiturates by tetraethylthiuram disulphide. *J. Pharm. Pharmacol.* **3**, 497—500 (1951). [G 77,527/51

Gram, T. E., Guarino, A. M., Greene, F. E., Gigon, P. L., Gillette, J. R.: Effect of partial hepatectomy on the responsiveness of microsomal enzymes and cytochrome P-450 to phenobarbital or 3-methylcholanthrene. *Biochem. Pharmacol.* **17**, 1769—1778 (1968). [G 62,231/68

Gram, T. E., Guarino, A. M., Schroeder, D. H., Gillette, J. R.: Changes in certain kinetic properties of hepatic microsomal aniline hydroxylase and ethylmorphine demethylase associated with postnatal development and maturation in male rats. *Biochem. J.* **113**, 681—685 (1969). [G 68,711/69

Gran, F. C.: Structure and function of the endoplasmic reticulum in animal cells. *FEBS Symp. Oslo (1967)*, **14**, pp. 100 (1968). [G 80,994/68

Grandpierre, R., Robert, A. M.: Inhibition de l'action oestrogénique par des extraits de foie. *C. R. Soc. Biol. (Paris)* **163**, 1731—1733 (1969). [H 22,252/69

Grangaud, R., Conquy, T.: Vitamine A et progestérone. *C. R. Soc. Biol. (Paris)* **152**, 1230—1234 (1958). [G 71,675/58

Grangaud, R., Conquy, T.: Effets de la progestérone administrée en injection à la femelle du rat blanc carencée en vitamine A. *C. R. Acad. Sci. (Paris)* **246**, 3274—3277 (1958).
C 71,751/58

Grangaud, R., Conquy, T., Nicol, M.: Progestérone et accroissement pondéral chez la jeune ratte albinos carencée en vitamine A. *C. R. Soc. Biol. (Paris)* **153**, 1327—1330 (1959).
[C 97,508/59

Grangaud, R., Conquy, T., Nicol, M.: Action de la progestérone chez le rat mâle carencé en vitamine A. *C. R. Soc. Biol. (Paris)* **154**, 115—118 (1960). [C 88,406/60

Grangaud, R., Conquy, T., Nicol, M.: Vitamine A et hormones stéroïdes. *Arch. Sci. physiol.* **14**, 131—142 (1960). [C 89,715/60

Granitsas, A. N., Leathem, J. H.: Response of the rat kidney to steroids. *Bull. Nat. Inst. Sci. India* **19**, 148—151 (1962). [D 25,514/62

Granner, D. K., Hayashi, S. I., Thompson, E. B., Tomkins, G. M.: Stimulation of tyrosine aminotransferase synthesis by dexamethasone phosphate in cell culture. *J. molec. Biol.* **35**, 291—301 (1968). [H 11,721/68

Grant, G., Roe, F. J. C., Pike, M. C.: Effect of neonatal thymectomy on the induction of papillomata and carcinomata by 3,4-benzopyrene in mice. *Nature (Lond.)* **210**, 603—604 (1966).
[F 66,117/66

Grassi, B., Cagianelli, M. A., Spremolla, G.: Rene e intossicazione sperimentale da tetracloruro di carbonio. Rilievi istologici in corso di trattamento prednisolonico e steroideo in ratti albini. *Minerva nefrol.* **6**, 81—94 (1959).
[E 58,693/59

Grassi, B., Spremolla, G.: Il fegato nella deplezione potassica. (Ricerche sperimentali in ratti albini.) *Rass. Fisiopat. clin. ter.* **36**, 379—391 (1964). [F 28,126/64

Graubard, M., Pincus, G.: The oxidation of estrogens by phenolases. *Proc. nat. Acad. Sci. (Wash.)* 149—152 (1941). [80,931/41

Graul, E. H., Rüther, W.: The question of the efficiency of radiation-protection substances after exposure to fast neutrons. *Proc. Int. Conf. Radiation Biology, Kyoto*, p. 97—105 (1967).
[G 66,718/67

Gray, J. L., Moulden, E. J., Tew, J. T., Jensen, H.: Attempts to prevent or reduce radiation injury by pharmacological means. *Fed. Proc.* **11**, 221 (1952). [B 68,316/52

Gray, J. L., Moulden, E. J., Tew, J. T., Jensen, H.: Protective effect of pitressin and of epinephrine against total body x-irradiation. Proc. Soc. exp. Biol. (N.Y.), 79, 384—387 (1952). [B 69,100/52

Gray, J. L., Tew, J. T., Jensen, H.: Protective effect of serotonin and of p-aminopropiophenone against lethal doses of X-radiation. Proc. Soc. exp. Biol. (N.Y.) 80, 604—607 (1952). [B 92,332/52

Grayhack, J. T., Scott, W. W.: Observation on the in vivo inactivation of testosterone propionate by the liver of the white rat. Endocrinology 48, 453—461 (1951). [B 58,923/51

Grazia, A. di, Sardo, M.: Insulina e colpo di calore. Biochim. Terap. sper. 21, 176—184 (1934). [27,853/34

Greaves, J. D., Schmidt, C. L. A.: Studies on the vitamin A requirements of the rat. Amer. J. Physiol. 116, 456—467 (1936). [A 48,725/36

Green, A. R., Curzon, G.: Decrease of 5-hydroxytryptamine in the brain provoked by hydrocortisone and its prevention by allopurinol. Nature (Lond.) 220, 1095—1097 (1968). [H 5,891/68

Green, D. M.: Mechanisms of desoxycorticosterone action: effects of liver passage. Endocrinology 43, 325—328 (1948). [B 28,239/48

Greenberg, J., Nadel, E. M., Coatney, G. R.: The influence of strain, sex and age of mice on infection with Plasmodium berghei. J. infect. Dis. 93, 96—100 (1953). [G 70,739/53

Greenberg, L. A.: Acetoin not a product of the metabolism of alcohol. Quart. J. Stud. Alcohol 3, 347—350 (1942). [A 48,342/42

Greenberg, S. R.: Glomerular changes in chronic alloxan diabetes. Arch. Path. 73, 263—273 (1962). [D 21,811/62

Greenberger, N. J., MacDermett, R. P., Martin, J. F., Dutta, S.: Intestinal absorption of six tritium-labeled digitalis glycosides in rats and guinea pigs. J. Pharmacol. exp. Ther. 167, 265 to 273 (1969). [H 13,503/69

Greene, A. E., Ambrus, J. L., Gershenfeld, L.: Effect of cortisone and desoxycorticosterone on infection with tetanus spores and upon the toxicity of tetanus toxin. Antibiot. and Chemother. 3, 1121—1124 (1953). [B 94,257/53

Greengard, O., Feigelson, P.: Immunochemical evidence of increased liver tryptophan pyrrolase amounts following induction in vivo. Biochem. J. 84, 111P (1962). [G 67,329/62

Greengard, O., Gordon, M.: The cofactor-mediated regulation of apoenzyme levels in animal tissues. I. The pyridoxine-induced rise of rat liver tyrosine transaminase level in vivo. J. Biol. Chem. 238, 3708—3710 (1963). [G 15,572/63

Greengard, O., Smith, M. A., Acs, G.: Relation of cortisone and synthesis of ribonucleic acid to induced and developmental enzyme formation. J. biol. Chem. 238, 1548—1551 (1963). [D 63,145/63

Greengard, O., Weber, G., Singhal, R. L.: Glycogen deposition in the liver induced by cortisone; dependence on enzyme synthesis. Science 141, 160—161 (1963). [E 20,258/63

Greengard, P., Kalinsky, H., Manning, T. J., Zak, S. B.: Prevention and remission by adrenocortical steroids of nicotinamide deficiency disease. II. A study of the mechanism. J. biol. Chem. 243, 4216—4221 (1968). [G 63,690/68

Greengard, P., Quinn, G. P., Landrau, M. A., Hormonal effects on DPN concentration in rat liver. Biochim. biophys. Acta (Amst.) 47, 614—616 (1961). [D 12,966/61

Greengard, P., Sigg, E. B., Fratta, I., Zak, S. B.: Prevention and remission by adrenocortical steroids of nicotinamide deficiency disorders and of 6-aminonicotinamide toxicity in rats and dogs. J. Pharmacol. exp. Ther. 154, 624—631 (1966). [F 74,421/66

Greenman, D. L., Wicks, W. D., Kenney, F. T.: Stimulation of ribonucleic acid synthesis by steroid hormones. II. High molecular weight components. J. biol. Chem. 240, 4420—4426 (1965). [G 35,063/65

Gregerman, R. I.: Estimation of thyroxine secretion rate in the rat by the radioactive thyroxine turnover technique: Influence of age, sex and exposure to cold. Endocrinology 72, 382—392 (1963). [D 57,876/63

Gregoriadis, G., Sourkes, T. L.: Regulation of hepatic copper in the rat by the adrenal gland. Canad. J. Biochem. 48, 160—163 (1970). [G 72,808/70

Gregorio, G. de, Armellini, C.: Proprietà cardiotrofiche di alcuni ormoni e principi enzimatici. Azione protettiva sulla cardiopatia sperimentale emetinica. Acta. med. ital. Med. trop. 19, 122—132 (1964). [G 64,277/64

Greig, A.: Massive doses of vitamin D. Vet. Rec. 75, 981 (1963). [G 68,415/63

Greig, M. E., Gibbons, A. J.: An antidote to cycloheximide (actidione) poisoning. Toxicol. appl. Pharmacol. 1, 598—601 (1959). [C 94,626/59

Greig, M. E., Gibbons, A. J., Elliott, G. A.: A comparison of the effects of melengestrol acetate and hydrocortisone acetate on experimental allergic encephalomyelitis in rats. *J. Pharmacol. exp. Ther.* **173**, 85—93 (1970). [H 24,654/70

Greig, W. R., Crooks, J., Macgregor, A. G., McIntosh, J. A. R.: The radioprotective effect of methylthiouracil on the thyroid gland of the rat. *Brit. J. Radiol.* **38**, 72—74 (1965). [E 60,304/65

Greim, H.: Toxizität und therapeutische Anwendbarkeit des DDT und seiner Metaboliten. *Ärztl. Forsch.* **24**, 197—201 (1970). [G 76,366/70

Greim, H.: Therapeutische Möglichkeiten durch die Induzierbarkeit arzneimittelabbauender Enzyme. *Dtsch. med. Wchschr.* **95**, 2196—2199 (1970). [H 32,018/70

Greisman, S. E., Woodward, C. L.: Mechanisms of endotoxin tolerance. VII. The role of the liver. *J. Immunol.* **105**, 1468—1476 (1970). [G 80,339/70

Grella, P.: Ipofunzione corticosurrenalica da fluossimesterone. *Attual. Ostet. Ginec.* **9**, 231—239 (1963). [E 21,538/63

Gresham, P. A., Pover, W. F. R.: Neuroendocrine reactions and the radiation-induced variations in rat intestinal alkaline ribonuclease levels. *Radiat. Res.* **34**, 256—264 (1968). [G 58,354/68

Grether, I., Naugler, W. E., Kuzell, W. C.: The effect of phenylbutazone (Butazolidin) and cortisone acetate on gold toxicity. (Abstr.) *Stanf. med. Bull.* **10**, 322 (1952). [C 12,471/52

Greuel, H., Schäfer, E. L.: Die Bedeutung einer Vor-Behandlung mit ACTH, Cortison bzw. Doca für den Ablauf der experimentellen Meerschweinchentuberkulose. *Z. Tuberk.* **108**, 321—326 (1956). [E 54,859/56

Grewe, H. E.: Experimentelle Untersuchungen der geschlechtsverschiedenen Wirksamkeit von Barbitursäurederivaten zur Narkose. *Z. ges. exp. Med.* **121**, 497—502 (1953). [D 35,140/53

Griffin, A. C., Richardson, H. L., Robertson, C. H., O'Neal, M. A., Spain, J. D.: The role of hormones in liver carcinogenesis. *J. nat. Cancer Inst.* **15**, Sup., 1623—1628 (1955). [C 14,406/55

Griffin, A. C., Rinfret, A. P., Corsigilia, V. F.: The inhibition of liver carcinogenesis with 3-methyl-4-dimethylaminoazobenzene in hypophysectomized rats. *Cancer Res.* **13**, 77—79 (1953). [B 77,163/53

Griffin, M. J., Cox, R. P.: Studies on the mechanism of hormone induction of alkaline phosphatase in human cell cultures. II. Rate of enzyme synthesis and properties of base level and induced enzymes. *Proc. nat. Acad. Sci. (Wash.)* **56**, 946—953 (1966). [F 86,851/66

Griffith, J. Q., Jr., Comroe, B. I.: Reduced tolerance to ergotamine tartrate in hyperthyroidism. An experimental study. *J. Pharmacol. exp. Ther.* **69**, 34—36 (1940). [A 33,738/40

Griffith, W. H.: Choline metabolism. IV. The ralation of the age, weight and sex of young rats to the occurrence of hemorrhagic degeneration on a low choline diet. *J. Nutr.* **19**, 437—448 (1940). [A 33,347/40

Grinnell, E. H., Johnson, J. R., Rhone, J. R., Tillotson, A., Noffsinger, J., Huffman, M. N.: Oestrogen protection against acute digitalis toxicity in dogs. *Nature (Lond.)* **190**, 1117 to 1118 (1961). [D 10,545/61

Grinnell, E. H., Smith, P. W.: Effect of estrogens on myocardial sensitivity to toxic effects of digoxin. *Proc. Soc. exp. Biol. (N.Y.)* **94**, 524—526 (1957). [C 31,428/57

Griswold, D. P., Jr., Green, C. H.: Observations on the hormone sensitivity of 7,12-dimethylbenz(a)anthracene-induced mammary tumors in the Sprague-Dawley rat. *Cancer Res.* **30**, 819—826 (1970). [H 26,709/70

Grob, H. S., Gordon, A. S., Kupperman, H. S.: Estrogen-parathyroid extract interaction in the albino rat. In: *The Endocrine Society, Program of 45th Meeting*, p. 55 (1963). [E 20,745/63

Grognot, P., Senelar, R.: Etudes expérimentales sur les réactions histologiques précoses du poumon après inhalation d'oxygène. *Rev. méd. Nancy* **82**, 925—931 (1957). [C 41,294/57

Groppetti, A., Costa, E.: Factors affecting the rate of disappearance of amphetamine in rats. *Int. J. Neuropharmacol.* **8**, 209—215 (1969). [H 31,959/69

Gross, A.: L'épine irritative broncho-pulmonaire dans l'asthme (étude expérimentale). *Gaz. Hôp. (Paris)* **127**, 953—956 (1955). [C 30,649/55

Grossman, A., Boctor, A. M., Lane, B.: Dependence of pancreatic integrity on adrenal and ovarian secretions. *Endocrinology* **85**, 956—959 (1969). [H 18,545/69

Grossman, A., Mavrides, C.: Studies on the regulation of tyrosine aminotransferase in rats. *J. biol. Chem.* **242**, 1398—1405 (1967). [G 46,206/67

Grossman, M. S., Penrod, K. E.: The thyroid and high oxygen poisoning in rats. *Amer. J. Physiol.* 156, 182—184 (1949). [B36,303/49

Groza, P., Buzoianu, V., Constantinescu, F., Ionescu, S.: Actiunea aldosteronului asupra ulcerului experimental atofanic. *Stud. Cercet. Fiziol.* 13, 391—395 (1968). [H6,695/68

Gruber, C. M., Crawford, W. M., Greene, W. W., Drayer, C. S.: The effect of sodium phenobarbital and the antagonism of morphine to phenobarbital and to pituitary extract in intact intestine in non-anesthetized dogs. *J. Pharmacol. exp. Ther.* 42, 27—34 (1931). [2,199/31

Gruber, C. M., Jr., Lashichenko, Z., Lee, K. S.: The effect of orally administered antabuse on the sleeping time of mice, rats, and rabbits given barbiturates, ether, chloroform, urethane, chloral hydrate, alcohol, or acetaldehyde by injection. *Arch. int. Pharmacodyn.* 97, 79—97 (1954). [D41,363/54

Grunberg, E., Titsworth, E.: The effect of cortisone on infection of white mice with Histoplasma capsulatum. *Amer. Rev. resp. Dis.* 87, 911—913 (1963). [D67,985/63

Grunert, R. R., Phillips, P. H.: Sodium and its relation to alloxan diabetes and glutathione. *J. biol. Chem.* 181, 821—827 (1949). [B48,993/49

Grunt, J. A., Higgins, J. T., Jr., Hammond, C. B.: Effects of ethionine on neonatally castrated male rats. *J. Nutr.* 70, 459—462 (1960). [C84,696/60

Grushina, A. A., Sorkina, J. A., Presnova, Z. F.: Effect of desoxycorticosterone on antitumor activity of thiophosphamide in intact and adrenalectomized rats with sarcoma 45. (Russian text.) *Vop. Onkol.* 15/2, 61—65 (1969). [H31,216/69

Gualandi, G., Lusiani, G. B., Pederzini, A.: Castrazione e ateromasia sperimentale nel ratto albino. *52e Congr. Soc. ital. Med. intern. Roma, Ott.*, p. 6 (1951). [C7,736/51

Guarino, A. M., Gram, T. E., Schroeder, D. H., Call, J. B., Gillette, J. R.: Alterations in kinetic constants for hepatic microsomal aniline hydroxylase and ethylmorphine N-demethylase associated with pregnancy in rats. *J. Pharmacol. exp. Ther.* 168, 224—228 (1969). [H15,843/69

Guérois, M. F. M., De Oliveira, H. L., Da Silva, A. C.: Ação agravante da cortisone na lesão hepática produzida pelo tetracloreto de carbone. *Rev. Hosp. Clin.* 11, 101—106 (1957). [C58,363/57

Guerra, L., Siccardi, A.: Il ricambio delle catecolamine nel fegato sottoposto a mutilazioni chirurgiche. *Arch. De Vecchi Anat. pat.* 37, 789—798 (1962). [D69,656/62

Guerrero, S., Gallardo, A., Munoz, C.: Influencia de las gonadas sobre la diferencia sexual en la resistencia a los efectos tóxicos de la cocaina en ratas. *Arch. Biol. Med. exp. (Santiago)* 2, 51—54 (1965). [F70,995/65

Guillermand, J., Duché, G., Falcoz, J.: L'apport de l'hormone somatotrope hypophysaire dans le traitement de la tuberculose pulmonaire. *Rev. Tuberc. (Paris)* 19, 1386—1391 (1955). [C15,540/55

Gunn, S. A., Gould, T. C., Anderson, W. A. D.: Protective effect of estrogen against vascular damage to the testis caused by cadmium. *Proc. Soc. exp. Biol. (N.Y.)* 119, 901—905 (1965). [F46,162/65

Günther, G., Hübner, K., Schneider, E.: Die quantitative Bedeutung der Mitosen beim kompensatorischen Wachstum der Leber und der Nebennierenrinde. *Beitr. pathol. Anat.* 139, 261—274 (1969). [H18,480/69

Gupta, D. das, Giroud, C. J. P.: Effect of an aldosterone antagonist on the fluid retention of aminonucleoside nephrosis. *Endocrinology*, 65, 500—503 (1959). [C73,800/59

Guttman, P. H.: Effect of thymectomy and splenectomy on the course of X-ray induced progressive intercapillary glomerulosclerosis in the mouse kidney. *Int. Arch. Allergy* 31, 163—173 (1967). [G45,255/67

Guze, L. B., Beeson, P. B.: The effect of cortisone on experimental hydronephrosis following ureteral ligation. *J. Urol. (Baltimore)* 78, 337—342 (1957). [C43,020/57

Gwee, M. C. E., Lim, H. S.: An interaction between hydrocortisone and hemicholiniums in mice. *J. Pharm. Pharmacol.* 23, 63—64 (1971). [G81,043/71

Gyermek, L., Pataky, G.: Die Wirkung des Histamins auf den Stoffwechsel. *Acta. physiol. Hung.* 2, 179—188 (1950). [B65,706/50

György, P.: Inactivation of estrone by liver. Assay method in vivo for dietary hepatic injury in rats. *Proc. Soc. exp. Biol. (N.Y.)* 60, 344—349 (1945). [E86,573/45

György, P., Goldblatt, H.: Thiouracil in the prevention of experimental dietary cirrhosis of liver. *Science* 102, 451—452 (1945). [G71,898/45

György, P., Rose, C. S.: The lipotropic effect of estrogenic hormones in inbred rats. *Proc. Soc. exp. Biol. (N.Y.)* 71, 552—555 (1949). [A48,519/49

György, P., Rose, C. S., Goldblatt, H.: Prevention of experimental dietary hepatic cirrhosis by goitrogenic substances. Proc. Soc. exp. Biol. (N.Y.) 67, 67—70 (1948). [G 71,701/48

György, P., Rose, C. S., Shipley, R. A.: Activity of estrone as a lipotropic factor. Arch. Biochem. 12, 125—133 (1947). [A 47,909/47

György, P., Rose, C. S., Shipley, R. A.: The effect of steroid hormones on the fatty liver induced in rats by dietary means. Arch. Biochem. 21, 108—118 (1949). [D 77,819/49

György, P., Seifter, J., Tomarelli, R. M., Goldblatt, H.: Influence of dietary factors and sex on the toxicity of carbon tatrachloride in rats. J. exp. Med. 83, 449—462 (1946). [E 86,574/46

Haam, E. von, Rosenfeld, I.: The effect of the various sex hormones upon experimental pneumococcus infections in mice. J. infect. Dis. 70, 243—247 (1942). [A 44,924/42

Haas, J.: Die Corticosteroidtherapie nach Intoxikation mit Schlangengiften, sowie eigene Beobachtungen bei der Behandlung eines Bisses von Bothrops nasutus. Z. Tropenmed. Parasit. 17, 26—35 (1966). [G 38,758/66

Haber, M. H., Jennings, R. B.: Sex differences in renal toxicity of mercury in the rat. Nature (Lond.) 201, 1235—1236 (1964). [G 10,684/64

Hagan, E. C., Woodard, G.: Toxicological properties of hexaethyl tetraphosphate (Abstr.). Fed. Proc. 6, 335 (1947). [A 48,819/47

Hagen, A. A., Troop, R. C.: Influence of age, sex and adrenocortical status on hepatic reduction of cortisone in vitro. Endocrinology 67, 194—203 (1960). [G 77,512/60

Hager, C. B., Kenney, F. T.: Regulation of tyrosine-α-ketoglutarate transaminase in rat liver. VII. Hormonal effects on synthesis in the isolated, perfused liver. J. biol. Chem. 243, 3296—3300 (1968). [G 58,950/68

Hagino, N., Ramaley, J. A., Gorski, R. A.: Inhibition of estrogen-induced precocious ovulation by pentobarbital in the rat. Endocrinology 79, 451—454 (1966). [F 69,360/66

Hahn, P., Koldovský, O.: Development of metabolic processes and their adaptations during postnatal life. In: Bajusz; Physiology and Pathology of Adaptation Mechanisms: Neural-Neuroendocrine-Humoral, p. 48—73. Oxford, London, Edingburgh: Pergamon Press 1969. [E 8,164/69

Hahn, T. J., Birge, S. J., Scharp, S. C., Avioli, L. V.: Vitamin D metabolism and phenobarbital therapy. (Abstr.) Clin. Res. 19, 50 (1971). [H 34,347/71

Hajdu, A., Chappel, C. I., Rona, G.: The influence of estrogens on scorbutic bone lesions in guinea-pigs. Experientia (Basel) 21, 466 (1965). [G 32,889/65

Hakstian, R. W., Hampson, L. G., Gurd, F. N.: Pharmacological agents in experimental hemorrhagic shock. A controlled comparison of treatment with hydralazine, hydrocortisone, and levarterenol (l-Norepinephrine). Arch. Surg. 83, 335—347 (1961). [D 10,396/61

Halac, E., Jr., Sicignano, C.: Re-evaluation of the influence of sex, age, pregnancy, and phenobarbital on the activity of UDP-glucuronyl transferase in rat liver. J. Lab. clin. Med. 73, 677—685 (1969). [G 77,576/69

Halberg, F., Spink, W. W., Bittner, J. J.: Protection by aldosterone and 11,17-oxycorticoids against effects of Brucella somatic antigen in adrenalectomized mice. Endocrinology 59, 380—383 (1956). [G 68,353/56

Haldane, J. S.: Respiration. New Haven: Yale University Press 1922. [E 715/22

Hale, H. B.: Cross-adaptation. Environm. Res. 2, 423—434 (1969). [G 72,522/69

Hale, H. B., Mefferd, R. B., Jr.: Effects of adrenocorticotropin on temperature- and pressure-dependent metabolic functions. Amer. J. Physiol. 197, 1291—1296 (1959). [C 79,669/59

Haley, T. J., Flesher, A. M., Komesu, N.: Muscle fatigue in X-irradiated rats (Abstr.). Fed. Proc. 17, 374 (1958). [C 51,851/58

Haley, T. J., Mann, S., Dowdy, A. H.: A comparison of the response of normal and hypothyroid mice to acute whole body roentgen radiation. Science 112, 333—334 (1950). [B 49,990/50

Haley, T. J., Mann, S., Dowdy, A. H.: The effect of reontgen ray irradiation on normal, hypothyroid and hyperthyroid rats. Endocrinology 48, 365—369 (1951). [B 58,913/51

Haley, T. J., Mann, S., Dowdy, A. H.: The inability of thiourea to modify roentgen ray irradiation mortality in rats. Science 114, 153—154 (1951). [B 60,616/51

Haley, T. J., Mann, S., Dowdy, A. H.: The effect of roentgen ray irradiation on rats premedicated with thyroxin and thiouracil derivatives. J. Amer. pharm. Ass. sci. Ed. 41, 39—41 (1952). [G 71,834/52

Halmagyi, D. F. J., Starzecki, B., Horner, G. J.: Mechanism and pharmacology of endotoxin shock in sheep. J. appl. Physiol. 18, 544—552 (1963). [D 68,121/63

Halmagyi, D. F. J., Starzecki, B., Horner, G. J.: Mechanism and pharmacology of shock due to rattlesnake venom in sheep. *J. appl. Physiol.* 20, 709—718 (1965). [G 31,584/65

Halpern, B. N., Drudi-Baracco, C., Bessirard, D.: Exaltation de la toxicité de l'amphétamine par la DL-thyroxine. *C. R. Soc. Biol. (Paris)* 157, 1879—1882 (1963). [G 11,305/63

Halpern, B. N., Drudi-Baracco, C., Bessirard, D.: Aggravation par la thyroxine des réactions émotionelles induites par des amines sympathomimétiques et objectivées par la 'toxicité de groupe'. *C. R. Acad. Sci. (Paris)* 257, 1641—1643 (1963). [G 63,588/63

Halpern, B. N., Drudi-Baracco, C., Bessirard, D.: Exaltation de la toxicité absolue de certaines amines sympathomimétiques par la thyroxine. *C. R. Acad. Sci (Paris)* 257, 1559—1562 (1963). [G 67,689/63

Halpern, B. N., Drudi-Baracco, C., Bessirard, D.: Exaltation of toxicity of sympathomimetic amines by thyroxine. *Nature (Lond.)* 204, 387—388 (1964). [F 24,137/64

Halpern, B. N., Drudi-Baracco, C., Bessirard, D.: Potentialisation de la toxicité absolue et de la toxicité de groupe de la L-éphédrine par la thyroxine. *C. R. Soc. Biol. (Paris)* 158, 1284—1289 (1964). [F 27,643/64

Hamburgh, M., Lynn, E.: The influence of temperature on skeletal maturation of hypothyroid rats. *Anat. Rec.* 150, 163—171 (1964). [G 21,782/64

Hamburgh, M., Vicari, E.: Physiological mechanisms underlying susceptibility to audiogenic seizures in mice. *Anat. Rec.* 132, 450 (1958). [C 71,704/58

Hamburgh, M., Vicari, E.: A study of some physiological mechanisms underlying susceptibility to audiogenic seizures in mice. *J. Neuropath. exp. Neurol.* 19, 461—472 (1960). [D 11,010/60

Hamilton, K. F., Sacher, G. A., Grahn, D.: A sex difference in mouse survival under daily gamma irradiation and its modification by gonadectomy. *Radiat. Res.* 18, 12—16 (1963). [D 64,060/63

Hammer, W., Sjöqvist, F.: Plasma levels of monomethylated tricyclic antidepressants during treatment with imipramine-like compounds. *Life Sci.* 6, 1895—1903 (1967). [G 79,581/67

Hámori, A., Nemes, T., Hal, T.: Effect of prednisolone on the development of cinchophen ulcer in the dog. *Acta med. Acad. Sci. hung.* 25, 315—321 (1968). [G 65,054/68

Hámori, A., Nemes, T., Illyés, T.: Effect of desoxycorticosterone acetate and cortisone on the development of cinchophen ulcer in the dog. *Acta med. Acad. Sci. hung.* 26, 391—395 (1969). [G 72,363/69

Hamprecht, B.: Regulation der Cholesterol-Synthese. *Naturwissenschaften* 56, 398—405 (1969). [G 69,560/69

Hamre, C. J., Yaeger, V. L.: Influence of cortisone acetate on formation of exostoses by rats fed Lathyrus odoratus. *Anat. Rec.* 124, 405 to 406 (1956). [D 76,147/56

Hänninen, O., Hartiala, K.: The induction of liver tyrosine 2-oxoglutarate transaminase in rats by immobilization. *Acta endocr. (Kbh.)* 54, 85—90 (1967). [F 76,119/67

Hannon, J. P., Larson, A. M.: The site and mechanism of norepinephrine-calorigenesis in the cold acclimatised rat. *Fed. Proc.* 20, 209 (1961). [D 4,112/61

Hanssler, H.: Über den Einfluß der Nebennierenrinde auf das Knochenwachstum Vitamin D-frei ernährter Ratten. *Klin. Wschr.* 34, 646—647 (1956). [C 18,293/56

Hanssler, H.: Experimentelle Untersuchungen über die Rachitisbeeinflussung durch Nebennierenrinden-Hormone. *Z. ges. exp. Med.* 128, 76—86 (1956). [C 45,007/56

Hanzlik, P. J.: A study of the toxicity of the salicylates based on clinical statistics. *J. Amer. med. Ass.* 60, 957 (1913). [A 49,483/13

Hanzlik, P. J., Karsner, H. T.: A comparison of the prophylactic effects of atropine and epinephrine in anaphylactic shock and anaphylactoid phenomena from various colloids and arsphenamine. *J. Pharmacol. exp. Ther.* XIV, 425—447 (1920). [10,286/20

Haque, M. E., Lillie, R. J., Shaffner, C. S., Briggs, G. M.: Effects of vitamin deficiencies in New Hampshire chicks injected with high doses of thyroxine. *Endocrinology* 42, 273—278 (1948). [B 19,204/48

Harada, T., Okuda, H., Fujii, S.: Effect of citrate on acyl-CoA synthetase of rat liver. *J. Biochem. (Tokyo)* 65, 497—501 (1969). [H 15,156/69

Harbison, R. D., Becker, B. A.: Barbiturate mortality in hypothyroid and hyperthyroid rats. *J. pharm. Sci.* 58, 183—185 (1969). [H 10,917/69

Harding, H. R., Potts, G. O.: The anticatabolic activity of anabolic steroids based on the suppression of cortisone acetate (EAc) induction of liver tryptophan pyrrolase (TPO). *Excerpta med. (Amst.)* No. 99, E155 (1965). [F55,311/65

Harding, H. R., Rosen, F., Nichol, C. A.: Inhibition of hepatic alanine transaminase activity in response to treatment with 11-desoxycorticosterone. *Proc. Soc. exp. Biol. (N.Y.)* 108, 96—99 (1961). [D14,355/61

Hardinge, M., Peterson, D. I.: The effects of exercise and limitation of movement on amphetamine toxicity. *J. Pharmacol. exp. Ther.* 141, 260—265 (1963). [E26,072/63

Hargreaves, T., Holton, J. B.: Jaundice of the newborn due to novobiocin. *Lancet* 1962 I, 839. [H30,986/62

Hargreaves, T., Lathe, G. H.: Inhibitory aspects of bile secretion. *Nature (Lond.)* 200, 1172—1176 (1963). [G81,289/63

Hári, P.: Beiträge zur Physiologie der Schilddrüse. Eine kritische Studie. *Pflügers Arch. ges. Physiol.* 176, 123—167 (1919). [51,049/19

Hári, P.: Entgegnung auf G. Mansfelds Abwehr, p. 32. Esztergom, Ungarn: Gustav Buzarovits 1921. [40,209/21

Harke, H. P., Frahm, B., Schultz, C., Dontenwill, W.: Abbau von Nikotin bei Hamster und Ratte. *Biochem. Pharmacol.* 19, 495—498 (1970). [G73,847/70

Harkness, R. D.: Changes in the liver of the rat after partial hepatectomy. *J. Physiol. (Lond.)* 117, 267—277 (1952). [E80,279/52

Harkness, R. D.: Regeneration of liver. *Brit. med. Bull.* 13, 87—93 (1957). [E57,419/57

Harman, D.: Atherosclerosis: effect of anti-inflammatory steroids prednisone and dexamethasone. *Circulation* 32, Sup. 2, II—16 (1965). [F59,112/65

Harris, C.: The role of the adrenal in toxicity in rats caused by dimethylbenzanthracene. *Cancer Res.* 28, 764—768 (1968). [F98,166/68

Harrison, H. C., Harrison, H. E., Park, E. A.: Vit. D and citrate metabolism. Inhibition of Vit. D effect by cortisol. *Proc. Soc. exp. Biol. (N.Y.)* 96, 768—773 (1957). [C45,829/57

Hart, L. G., Adamson, R. H.: Effect of microsomal enzyme modifiers on toxicity and therapeutic activity of cyclophosphamide in mice. *Arch. int. Pharmacodyn.* 180, 391—401 (1969). [G69,481/69

Hart, L. G., Adamson, R. H., Dixon, R. L., Fouts, J. R.: Stimulation of hepatic microsomal drug metabolism in the newborn and fetal rabbit. *J. Pharmacol. exp. Ther.* 137, 103—106 (1962). [D27,689/62

Hart, L. G., Fouts, J. R.: Studies of the possible mechanisms by which chlordane stimulates hepatic microsomal drug metabolism in the rat. *Biochem. Pharmacol.* 14, 263—272 (1965). [G27,102/65

Hart, L. G., Shultice, R. W., Fouts, J. R.: Stimulatory effects of chlordane on hepatic microsomal drug metabolism in the rat. *Toxicol. appl. Pharmacol.* 5, 371—386 (1963). [G69,761/63

Hartshorn, E. A.: Drug interaction. 2. How drugs interact. *Drug Intelligence* 2, 58—65 (1968). [G78,178/68

Hartshorn, E. A.: Drug interaction. I. General considerations. *Drug Intelligence* 2, 4—7 (1968). [G81,056/68

Hartshorn, E. A.: Drug interaction. *Drug Intelligence* 2, 174—180 (1968). [G81,057/68

Hartshorn, E. A.: Drug interactions. III. Classes of drugs and their interactions. Anti-infective agents. Part two. *Drug Intelligence* 3, 131 to 137 (1969). [G81,055/69

Hartveit, F., Andersen, K.: Reticuloendothelial activity related to age and sex in mice. *Acta path. microbiol. scand.* 76, 161—163 (1969). [G67,345/69

Hasegawa, A. T., Landahl, H. D.: Studies on spleen oxygen tension and radioprotection in mice with hypoxia, serotonin, and p-aminopropiophenone. *Radiat. Res.* 31, 389—399 (1967). [G48,428/67

Hass, G. M., Henson, D. E., Scott, R. A., McClain, E. C., Hemmens, A.: Influence of cirrhosis on production of atheroarteriosclerosis and thromboarteritis with vitamin D and dietary cholesterol. *Amer. J. Path.* 57, 405 to 429 (1969). [H19,697/69

Hasselblatt, A., Bastian, G.: Vergleichende Untersuchungen über die krampferregende Wirkung von Insulin und N_1-(4-Methyl-benzolsulfonyl)-N_2-butylharnstoff an der Maus unter normalen und nach einer Behandlung mit Thyroxin veränderten Stoffwechselverhältnissen. *Arzneimittel-Forsch.* 8, 590—594 (1958). [C59,171/58

Hasselblatt, A., Hukuhara, T.: Beeinflussung der Elimination von Bromsulphalein (Leberfunktionstest) durch Tolbutamid. *Naunyn-Schmiedebergs Arch. Pharmak.* 243, 307—308 (1962). [G77,523/62

Hässler, A., Bräunlich, H., Ankermann, H.: Die Bedeutung der Aufzuchtbedingungen für die Wirkungsdauer von Hexobarbital und deren individuelle Variation bei Ratten. *Acta biol. med. Germanica* **23**, 831—842 (1969). [H23,853/69]

Hay, E. C.: Hepato- and nephrotoxic effect of glycine. *Fed. Proc.* **6**, 26 (1947). [93,491/47]

Hayaishi, O.: Enzymic hydroxylation. *Ann. Rev. Biochem.* **38**, 21—44 (1969). [H13,776/69]

Hayakawa, T., Kanai, N., Yamada, R., Kuroda, R., Higashi, H., Mogami, H., Jinnai, D.: Effect of steroid hormone on activation of endoxan (cyclophosphamide). *Biochem. Pharmacol.* **18**, 129—135 (1969). [G64,146/69]

Hayasaka, H., Howard, J. M.: Mechanism of action of D-aldosterone in endotoxin shock. *Surgery* **54**, 761—763 (1963). [E31,136/63]

Hayasaka, H., Howard, J. M.: Studies on the mechanism of action of aldosterone in endotoxic shock. *Surg. Forum* **14**, 23—24 (1963). [G10,112/63]

Hayasaka, H., O'Malley, J. F., Howard, J. M.: Antitoxic effect of aldosterone on cats in endotoxic shock. Further studies. *Arch. Surg.* **87**, 861—865 (1963). [E31,522/63]

Hayasaki, N., Tsukada, K.: Increased activity of deoxyribonuclease inhibitor in rat serum after partial hepatectomy. *Biochim. biophys. Acta (Amst.)* **204**, 255—256 (1970). [G73,554/70]

Hayashida, T.: Effect of pituitary adrenocorticotropic and growth hormones on the resistance of rats infected with Pasteurella pestis. *J. exp. Med.* **106**, 127—143 (1957). [C37,366/57]

Hayashida, T., Li, C. H.: The influence of adrenocorticotropic and growth hormones on antibody formation. *J. exp. Med.* **105**, 93—98 (1957). [C29,987/57]

Haydu, G. G., Wolfson, A. H.: Effect of temperature extremes and cortisone on toxicity of diphosphopyridine nucleotide in mice. *Proc. Soc. exp. Biol. (N.Y.)* **102**, 325—327 (1959). [C77,942/59]

Hayes, W. J., Jr.: The pharmacology and toxicology of DDT. In: Müller; *The Insecticide DDT and its Significance*. Basel: Birkhäuser vol. 2, 59. [E53,090/59]

Hayes, W. J., Jr., Dale, W. E., Pirkle, C. I.: Evidence of safety of long-term, high, oral doses of DDT for men. *A. M. A. Arch. environm. Hlth.* **22**, 119—135 (1971). [G80,268/71]

Heaney, R. P., Whedon, G. D.: Impairment of hepatic bromsulphalein clearance by two 17-substituted testosterones. *J. Lab. Clin. Med.* **52**, 169—175 (1958). [C56,394/58]

Heather, A. J.: Treatment of osteoporosis with an anabolic compound and L-lysine. *Delaware med. J.* **35**, 245—249 (1963). [G67,332/63]

Heboyan, M., Messeri, E.: Variazioni immunitarie in ratti tenuti a dieta normale e a dieta di Handler, vaccinati con salmonella typhi e trattati con 4-idrossi-19 nortestosterone-17 ciclopentil propionato. *Rass. ital. Gastroent.* **8**, 590—598 (1962). [G69,057/62]

Hedwall, P., Heeg, E.: Die Beeinflussung einer Staphylokokken-Infektion der Rattenniere durch Analgetica. *Arzneimittel-Forsch.* **11**, 909—912 (1961). [D14,804/61]

Heikel, T. A. J.: Effect of steroid drugs on biliary secretion: intrahepatic cholestasis. *Biochem. J.* **103**, 63P—64P (1967). [G81,287/67]

Heikel, T. A. J., Lathe, G. H.: The effect of oral contraceptive steroids on bile secretion and bilirubin Tm in rats. *Brit. J. Pharmacol.* **38**, 593—601 (1970). [G73,162/70]

Heim, W. G., Ellenson, S. R.: Adrenal cortical control of the appearance of rat slow alpha$_2$-globulin. *Nature (Lond.)* **213**, 1260—1261 (1967). [F77,887/67]

Heim, W. G., Kerrigan, J. M.: Appearance of slow a_2-globulin after interference with the liver. *Nature (Lond.)* **199**, 1100—1101 (1963). [G68,369/63]

Heiman, R., Heuson, J. C., Coune, A.: Tumors developing in oophorectomized Sprague-Dawley rats after a single gastric instillation of 7,12-dimethylbenz(a)anthracene. *Cancer Res.* **28**, 309—313 (1968). [F95,958/68]

Heimburg, A. von, Schmidt, L.: Experimenteller Beitrag zur Klärung der verschiedenen Widerstandskraft männlicher und weiblicher Ratten gegen die chronische Quecksilber-Vergiftung. *Arzneimittel-Forsch.* **9**, 321—324 (1959). [C69,587/59]

Heinonem, J., Takki, S., Jarho, L.: Plasma lidocaine levels in patients treated with potential inducers of microsomal enzymes. *Acta anaesth. scand.* **14**, 89—95 (1970). [G80,898/70]

Heinrichs, W. L., Colas, A.: The selective stimulation, inhibition and physicochemical alteration of the 7- and 16a-hydroxylases of 3β-hydroxyandrost-5-en-17-one and drug-metabolizing enzymes in hepatic microsomal fractions. *Biochemistry* **7**, 2273—2280 (1968). [H11,717/68]

Heinrichs, W. L., Feder, H. H., Colas, A.: The steroid 16a-hydroxylase system in mammalian liver. *Steroids* **7**, 91—98 (1966). [F72,860/66

Helfenstein, J. E., Young, S.: Effect of 2-methyl-1,2-bis-(3-pyridyl)-1-propanone (metyrapone) on the production of mammary tumours induced in rats by oral feeding with dimethylbenzanthracene. *Nature (Lond.)* **200**, 1113—1114 (1963). [G 76,331/63

Heller, B., Saavedra, J. M., Fischer, E.: Influence of adrenergic blocking agents upon morphine and catecholamine analgesic effect. *Experientia (Basel)* **24**, 804—805 (1968). [H 2,707/68

Heller, B., Saavedra, J. M., Lumbreras, N. de L. A.: Les relations entre mécanismes adrénergiques et effets analgésiques. *C. R. Soc. Biol. (Paris)* **162**, 2025—2026 (1968). [H 13,896/68

Heller, C. G.: Metabolism of the estrogens. The effect of liver and uterus upon estrone, estradiol and estriol. *Endocrinology* **26**, 619—630 (1940). [A 32,137/40

Heller, J. H., Meier, R. M., Zucker, R., Mast, G. W.: The effect of natural and synthetic estrogens on reticuloendothelial system function. *Endocrinology* **61**, 235—241 (1957). [C 40,073/57

Hellman, L., Weitzman, E. D., Roffwarg, H., Fukushima, D. K., Yoshida, K., Zumoff, B., Gallagher, T. F.: Effect of o,p'-DDD on cortisol secretory pattern in Cushing's syndrome. *J. clin. Endocr.* **31**, 227—230 (1970). [H 28,347/70

Hellman, L., Zumoff, B., Fishman, J., Gallagher, T. F.: Estradiol metabolism in total extrahepatic biliary obstruction. *J. clin. Endocr.* **30**, 161—165 (1970). [H 21,323/70

Hemingway, J. T., Cater, D. B.: Effects of pituitary hormones and cortisone upon liver regeneration in the hypophysectomized rat. *Nature (Lond.)* **181**, 1065—1066 (1958). [C 56,780/58

Hempel, R.: Der Einfluß eines Antiandrogens auf die Schlafdauer männlicher und weiblicher Mäuse und Ratten nach Hexobarbitalgabe. *Naunyn-Schmiedebergs Arch. Pharmak.* **257**, 27 (1967). [F 84,763/67

Hempel, R.: Zur hormonellen Beeinflussung des Hexobarbitalschlafes der Ratte. *Naunyn-Schmiedebergs Arch. Pharmak.* **259**, 413—418 (1968). [G 57,828/68

Henane, R.: Effet d'inhibiteur de l'aldostérone sur l'épuisement musculaire en ambiance chaude. *C. R. Soc. Biol. (Paris)* **159**, 878—881 (1965). [F 52,022/65

Henane, R., Laurent, F.: Nouvelles observations sur l'inhibition de l'aldostérone, lors de l'acclimatement à la chaleur, chez le rat blanc. *C. R. Soc. Biol. (Paris)* **160**, 733—736 (1966). [F 71,731/66

Henderson, P. T., Kersten, K. J.: Metabolism of drugs during rat liver regeneration. *Biochem. Pharmacol.* **19**, 2343—2351 (1970). [G 77,181/70

Henneman, D.: Estradiol inhibition of lathyritic effect of nitriles on skin and bone collagen (Abstr.). *Program 51st Meet. Endocr. Soc.*, New York, N.Y., p. 106 (1969). [H 12,251/69

Henriques, O. B., Henriques, S. B., DeGrandpré, R., Selye, H.: Influence of amino-acids on adrenal enlargement, nephrosclerosis and hypertension by anterior pituitary preparations. *Proc. Soc. exp. Biol. (N.Y.)* **69**, 591—593 (1948). [B 24,140/48

Henry, B., Fahlberg, W. J.: The potentiating effect of hydrocortisone acetate and tetracycline on monilial infection in mice. *Antibiot. and Chemother.* **10**, 114—120 (1960). [C 81,623/60

Henschler, D., Jacob, K. O.: Prednisolon zur Therapie von Reizgaslungenödemen. *Klin. Wschr.* **36**, 684 (1958). [C 56,126/58

Henschler, D., Reich, E.: Zum Mechanismus der ödemhemmenden Wirkung von Prednisolon bei toxischen Lungenödemen. *Klin. Wschr.* **37**, 716—717 (1959). [C 71,216/59

Hepler, O. E., Simonds, J. P.: Mechanism of shock. Effects of intravenous injection of salt solution in collapse induced by mechanical impounding of blood in the splanchnic region in normal and in hyperthyroid dogs. *Arch. Path.* **25**, 149—159 (1938). [A 15,174/38

Herbert, I. V., Becker, E. R.: Effect of cortisone and X-irradiation on the course of Trypanosoma lewisi infection in the rat. *J. Parasit.* **47**, 304—308 (1961). [G 63,454/61

Herbeuval, R., Debry, G., Cuny, G.: Action de l'acétate de testostérone sur la septicémie à staphylocoque doré du lapin. *Ann. Endocr. (Paris)* **19**, 408—411 (1958). [C 55,674/58

Herbeuval, R., Debry, G., Cuny, G.: Influence de l'extrait somatotrope sur la septicémie à staphylocoque doré du lapin. *Ann. Endocr. (Paris)* **19**, 412—417 (1958). [C 55,675/58

Herbeuval, R., Debry, G., Cuny, G.: Influence de la cortisone et de la désoxycorticostérone sur la septicémie à staphylocoque doré du lapin. *Ann. Endocr. (Paris)* **19**, 418—427 (1958). [C 55,676/58

Herken, H., Maibauer, D., Neubert, D.: Der Einfluß von Äthionin und anderen Lebergiften auf Fermentsysteme der Lebermikrosomen. *Naunyn-Schmiedebergs Arch. Pharmak.* **233**, 139—150 (1958). [G 74,662/58

Herken, H., Senft, G., Schwarz, W., Merker, H.: Glomerular structure and function after glucocorticoid action in nephrosis induced by aminonucleoside. *Arch. Exp. Path. Pharmak.* 245/2, 289—304 (1963). [G 15,041/63

Herlant, M.: Influence du thiouracyl sur l'hypertrophie compensatrice du rein. *Bull. Acad. Roy. Belg. Cl. Sci.* 33, 567—576 (1947). [B 30,957/47

Herlant, M.: Actions comparées de la thyroxine sur le rein normal et sur le rein en hypertrophie compensatrice. *Bull. Acad. Roy. Belg. Cl. Sci.*, Séance 10 Jan., 85—96 (1948). [B 30,956/48

Hermann, H., Portes, F., Jourdan, F.: Syncopes adrenalino-mono-, di-, et tetrachlorométhaniques. *C. R. Soc. Biol. (Paris)* 107, 1541—1542 (1931). [10,215/31

Hermann, H., Vial, J.: Nouvelles syncopes cardiaques par association toxique de l'adrénaline et de divers produits organiques volatils. *C. R. Soc. Biol. (Paris)* 119, 1316—1317 (1935). [32,885/35

Herrick, E. H., Mead, E. R., Egerton, B. W., Hughes, J. S.: Some effects of cortisone on vitamin C-deficient guinea pigs. *Endocrinology* 50, 259—263 (1952). [B 69,259/52

Herrmann, M.: Einfluß von Testosteron auf die Wiederaufnahme der Nebennierenrindenfunktion nach langfristiger Cortisonvorbehandlung beim Meerschweinchen. *Ztschr. Mikrosp.-anat. Forschg.* 68, 393—401 (1962). [D 34,026/62

Herrmann, M., Winkler, G.: Abkürzungen der Restitutionsphase der Nebennierenrinde beim Meerschweinchen nach langfristiger Vorbehandlung mit Cortison durch gleichzeitige Zufuhr von Methandrostenolon. *Arzneimittel-Forsch.* 12, 82—85 (1962). [D 20,550/62

Herrmann, M., Winkler, G.: Über den Einfluß von Oestradiol auf die Restitutionsphase der Nebennierenrinde nach langfristiger Cortisonvorbehandlung. *Acta endocr. (Kbh.)* 40, 410 to 420 (1962). [D 27,922/62

Hershey, S. G., Mazzia, V. D. B., Gyure, L., Singer, K.: Influence of a synthetic analogue of vasopressin on survival after hemorrhagic shock in rats. *Proc. Soc. exp. Biol. (N.Y.)* 115, 325—328 (1964). [F 2,455/64

Hertogh, R. de, Ekka, E., Vanderheyden, I., Hoet, J. J.: Metabolic clearance rates and the interconversion factors of estrone and estradiol-17β in the immature and adult female rat. *Endocrinology* 87, 874—880 (1970). [H 31,447/70

Hertz, R.: Interference with estrogen-induced tissue growth in the chick genital tract by a folic acid antagonist. *Science* 107, 300 (1948). [B 18,379/48

Hervé, A.: Semi-carbazone de l'adrénochrome et rayons X. *Arch. int. Pharmacodyn.* 85, 242—244 (1951). [B 61,654/51

Hervé, A.: Action radioprotectrice de l'ocytocine chez la souris. *Arch. int. Physiol.* 62, 136—137 (1954). [D 78,167/54

Hervé, A., Lecomte, J.: Action de la semicarbazone de l'adrénochrome sur les pétéchies provoquées par le rayonnement X. *Arch. int. Pharmacodyn.* 79, 109—112 (1949). [B 46,855/49

Hess, K.: Beitrag zur Lehre von den traumatischen Leberrupturen. *Virchows Arch. pathol. Anat.* 121, 154—175 (1890). [E 74,646/1890

Heuser, G.: Hormones and the nervous system. Experimental anesthesia and convulsions with steroids. *Thesis*, University of Montreal (1957). [C 33,938/57

Heuser, G.: Experimental anesthesia and convulsions with steroids. *Rev. canad. Biol.* 17, 229 (1958). [C 54,451/58

Heuson, J. C.: Nouvelle influence hormonale dans le cancer mammaire. Rôle de l'insuline in vitro et in vivo. *C. R. Soc. franç. Gynéc.* 40, 85—93 (1970). [G 78,138/70

Hewett, C. L., Savage, D. S., Lewis, J. J., Sugrue, M. F.: Anticonvulsant and interneuronal blocking activity in some synthetic amino-steroids. (Letter to the editor.) *J. Pharm. Pharmacol.* 16, 765—767 (1964). [D 19,834/64

Hewitt, H. B.: Renal necrosis in mice after accidental exposure to chloroform. *Brit. J. exp. Path.* 37, 32—39 (1956). [C 41,385/56

Hewitt, H. B.: A sensitive method for the assay of androgens based on their power to alter the reactions of the mouse kidney to chloroform. *J. Endocr.* 14, 394—399 (1957). [C 28,739/57

Heymann, G., Jandl, G.: Experimentelle Untersuchungen zur Wertbemessung von Typhus-Impfstoffen. I. Mitteilg. Die Schutzwirkung von humoralen Antikörpern verschiedener Spezifität bei der weißen Maus. *Z. Immun.-Forsch.* 119, 279—294 (1960). [C 94,285/60

Hiestand, W. A., Stemler, F. W., Wiebers, J. E., Rockhold, W. T.: Alcohol toxicity as related to (alloxan) diabetes, insulin, epinephrine and glucose in mice. *Fed. Proc.* 12, 67 (1953). [B 78,576/53

Hietbrink, B. E., DuBois, K. P.: Influence of X-radiation on development of enzymes responsible for desulfuration of an organic phosphorothioate and reduction of p-nitrobenzoic acid in the livers of male rats. *Radiat. Res.* 22, 598—605 (1964). [G 26,464/64

Hietbrink, B. E., DuBois, K. P.: Influence of partial-body X-irradiation on development of phosphorothioate oxidase in the livers of male rats. *Radiat. Res.* 27, 669—675 (1966).
[F 65,296/66

Higginbotham, R. D.: Influence of adrenalectomy and cortisol on resistance of mice to histamine, serotonin, anaphylactic and endotoxin shocks. *J. Allergy* 33, 35—44 (1962).
[D 21,395/62

Higginbotham, R. D., Dougherty, T. F.: Potentiation of polymyxin B toxicity by ACTH. *Proc. Soc. exp. Biol. (N.Y.)* 96, 466—470 (1957). [C 44,529/57

Higgins, G. M.: Experimental pathology of the liver. XII. Effects of feeding desiccated thyroid gland on restoration of the liver. *Arch. Path.* 16, 226—231 (1933). [9,809/33

Higgins, G. M., Anderson, R. M.: Experimental pathology of the liver. I. Restoration of the liver of the white rat following partial surgical removal. *Arch. Path.* 12, 186—202 (1931).
[597/31

Higgins, G. M., Woods, K. A.: The influence of the adrenal gland on some of the changes induced in the animal organisms by the folic acid analogue, aminoteropterin. *Proc. Mayo Clin.* 24, 533—537 (1949). [B 40,212/49

Highman, B., Altland, P. D., Hanks, A. R., Rantanen, N. W.: Bacterial endocarditis. Effect of dimethyl sulfoxide in X-irradiated and non-irradiated rats. *Arch. Path.* 88, 645—652 (1969). [H 19,382/69

Hildebrandt, A. G., Leibman, K. C., Estabrook, R. W.: Metyrapone interaction with hepatic microsomal cytochrome P-450 from rats treated with phenobarbital. *Biochem. biophys. Res. Commun.* 37, 477—485 (1969). [G 69,992/69

Hilf, R., Goldenberg, H., Bell, C.: Effect of actidione (cycloheximide) on estrogen-induced biochemical changes in R 3230 AC mammary tumors, uteri, and mammary glands. *Cancer Res.* 27, 1485—1493 (1967). [F 88,514/67

Hines, J. R., Roncoroni, M.: Acute hepatic ischemia in dogs. *Surg. Gynec. Obstet.* 102, 689—694 (1956). [G 72,976/56

Hines, J. R., Roncoroni, M.: Acute hepatic ischemia in ACTH treated dogs. *Surg. Gynec. Obstet.* 105, 39—48 (1957). [C 40,870/57

Hines, W. J. W.: The effect of two synthetic steroids on the ultrastructure of the liver of Rattus norvegicus L. *J. Pharm. Pharmacol.* 21, 509—513 (1969). [G 68,829/69

Hinshaw, L. B., Solomon, L. A., Reins, D. A., Freeny, P. C.: Peripheral and pulmonary vascular actions of the steroid methylprednisolone in endotoxin shock (Abstr.). *Fed. Proc.* 25, 634 (1966). [F 65,403/66

Hinton, W. E., Evers, C. G., Brunson, J. G.: The influence of adrenal medullary hormones on nephrotoxic nephritis in rabbits. *Lab. Invest.* 13, 1374—1380 (1964). [G 21,390/64

Hirano, T., Ruebner, B. H.: Studies on the mechanism of destruction of lymphoid tissue in murine hepatitis virus (MHV$_3$) infection. I. Selective prevention of lymphoid necrosis by cortisone and puromycin. *Lab. Invest.* 15, 270—282 (1966). [G 38,763/66

Hirokawa, T.: Studies on the poisoning by benzol and its homologues. IV. Experimental studies on the sexual differences of blood picture. *Jap. J. med. Sci. Biol.* 8, 275—281 (1955).
[G 71,106/55

Hirschfelder, A. D., Maxwell, H. C.: Effect of insulin in experimental intoxication with alcohol and acetone. *Amer. J. Physiol.* 70, 520—523 (1924). [26,930/24

Hirschlerowa, Z.: Rola gruczołu tarczykowego przy toskoplasmozie. *Wiad. Parazyt.* 2, Sup., 63—64 (1956). [C 35,235/56

Hirvonen, J. I., Karlsson, L. K. J., Ojala, K.: Zum Einfluß von Äthanol auf die Zona glomerulosa und Zona fasciculata der Rattennebennierenrinde bei gleichzeitiger Belastung mit Insulin und hypertonischer Kochsalzlösung. *Dtsch. Ztschr. gesamt. gerichtl. Med.* 62, 232—238 (1968). [G 59,966/68

Hitachi, M.: Some observations on the effect of nicotinamide on the adrenal cortex in methylcholanthrene-treated mice. *J. Fac. Sci. Univ. Tokyo, Sect. IV*, 10, 459—465 (1965).
[F 67,866/65

Hjort, A. M., deBeer, E. J., Fassett, D. W.: The hypnotic effect of repeated injections of unsymmetrical ethyl-0-ethylphenylurea in albino rats and the influence of sex thereon. *J. Pharmacol. exp. Ther.* 68, 62—68 (1940).
[A 32,832/40

Hoak, J. C., Connor, W. E., Stone, D. B.: Hypophysectomy and blood lipids in aminonucleoside nephrosis (Abstr.). *Clin. Res.* 13, 308 (1965). [F 61,136/65

Hoch, F. L.: Biochemical actions of thyroid hormones. *Physiol. Rev.* 42, 605—673 (1962).
[D 25,881/62

Hoch-Ligeti, C.: Effect of cortisone administration on induced and transplanted hepatomas. *J. nat. Cancer Inst.* **15**, 1633—1636 (1955). [C14,407/55

Hochwald, A.: Anaphylaktischer Shock und Vitamin C. II. Mitteilg. *Z. ges. exp. Med.* **98**, 578—582 (1936). [36,114/36

Hoene, R., Coutu, L., Horava, A., Procopio, J., Robert, A., Salgado, E.: Influence of ACTH on anaphylactic shock in guinea pigs. *J. Allergy* **23**, 343—351 (1952). [B68,152/52

Hoene, R., Rindani, T. H., Michon, J.: Study on the influence of somatotropic hormone upon the effect of X-irradiation on antibody formation. *Rev. canad. Biol.* **13**, 11—17 (1954). [B92,374/54

Holck, H. G. O.: Influence of preliminary administration of insulin or of epinephrine hydrochloride upon fatal dose of Sodium Evipal in albino mice. *J. Amer. pharm. Ass., sci. Ed.* **37**, 86—87 (1948). [B42,745/48

Holck, H. G. O.: Studies on sex variation to picrotoxin in the albino rat. *J. Amer. pharm. Ass., sci. Ed.* **38**, 604—610 (1949). [D28,543/49

Holck, H. G. O., Cannon, P. R.: On the cause of the delayed death in the rat by isopropyl betabromallyl barbituric acid (nostal) and some related barbiturates. *J. Pharmacol. exp. Ther.* **57**, 289—309 (1936). [A55,846/36

Holck, H. G. O., Fink, L. D.: Influence of sex life upon resistance to nostal and pentobarbital. *J. Amer. Pharmac. Ass.* **29**, 475—480 (1940). [A35,663/40

Holck, H. G. O., Hillyard, I. W., Malone, M. H.: The influence of experimental hypo-and hyperthyroidism on the effects of Nostal, thiopental sodium, and hexobarbital sodium in the adult albino rat. *J. Amer. pharm. Ass., sci. Ed.* **43**, 276—282 (1954). [B95,270/54

Holck, H. G. O., Kanân, M. A.: Intravenous lethal doses of amytal in the dog and rabbit and a table of animal dosages compiled from the literature. *J. Lab. clin. Med.* **19**, 1191—1205 (1934). [A43,097/34

Holck, H. G. O., Kanân, M. A.: Sex difference in white rat in tolerance to certain barbiturates. *Proc. Soc. exp. Biol. Med.* **32**, 700—701 (1935). [31,302/35

Holck, H. G. O., Kanân, M. A., Mills, L. M., Smith, E. L.: Effects of castration and of male hormone administration upon the responses of the rat to certain barbiturates. *49th Ann. Meet. Proc. Amer. Physiol. Soc., Memphis. Tenn.*, p. 82 (1937). [68,297/37

Holck, H. G. O., Kanân, M. A., Mills, L. M., Smith, E. L.: Studies upon the sex-differences in rats in tolerance to certain barbiturates and to nicotine. *J. Pharmacol. exp. Ther.* **60**, 1—24 (1937). [A8,011/37

Holck, H. G. O., Kimura, K. K.: Influence of sex upon resistance to ouabain in the rat. *Fed. Proc.* **3**, 75 (1944). [84,604/44

Holck, H. G. O., Kimura, K. K.: Studies on sex difference in resistance to ouabain in the albino rat. *J. Amer. pharm. Ass., sci. Ed.* **40**, 327—332 (1951). [D99,625/51

Holck, H. G. O., Mathieson, D. R.: Resistance to slowly increasing doses of sodium pentobarbital in the white rat: Duration of higher tolerance after parturition and effects of age, sex, castration and administration of testosterone propionate. *Proc. Amer. physiol. Soc.* p. 144 (1941). [80,435/41

Holck, H. G. O., Mathieson, D. R.: Effects of age, sex, castration and interval of time after parturition upon the ability of the albino rat to build up tolerance to and to detoxify pentobarbital sodium. *J. Amer. pharm. Ass., sci. Ed.* **33**, 174—176 (1944). [B644/44

Holck, H. G. O., Mathieson, D. R., Smith, E. L., Fink, L. D.: Effects of testosterone acetate and propionate and of estradiol dipropionate upon the resistance of the rat to evipal sodium, nostal, pernostan and pentobarbital sodium. *J. Amer. pharm. Ass. Sect. Ed.* **31**, 116—123 (1942). [A55,755/42

Holck, H. G. O., Weeks, J. R., Mathieson, D. R., Duis, B.: Effects of age and sex upon the margin of safety of "delvinal" sodium vinbarbital and of calcium 5-ethyl 5-(2-butyl) N-methyl barbituric acid in the albino rat. *J. Amer. Pharm. Ass.* **32**, 180—182 (1943). [84,766/43

Hollander, W., Wilkins, R. W.: The pharmacology and clinical use of rauwolfia, hydralazine; thiazides, and aldosterone antagonists in arterial hypertension. *Progr. cardiovasc. Dis.* **8**, 291—318 (1966). [G37,370/66

Holman, R. L., Jones, C. K.: Protective influence of pregnancy on experimental collagen disease lesions. *Arch. Path.* **56**, 231—237 (1953). [B93,771/53

Holmes, W. L., Bentz, J. D.: Inhibition of cholesterol biosynthesis in vitro by β-diethylaminoethyl diphenylpropylacetate hydrochloride (SKF 525-A). *J. biol. Chem.* **235**, 3118 to 3122 (1960). [G74,656/60

Holten, C. H., Larsen, V.: The potentiating effect of benactyzine derivatives and some other compounds on evipal anaesthesia in mice. *Acta pharmacol. (Kbh.)* **12**, 346—363 (1956). [G74,395/56

Holtman, D. F.: The effect of thiouracil and thyroactive substances on mouse susceptibility to poliomyelitis virus. *Science* 104, 50—51 (1946). [B 1,287/46]

Holton, J. B., Lathe, G. H.: Inhibitors of bilirubin conjugation in new-born infant serum and male urine. *Clin. Sci.* 25, 499—509 (1963). [E 35,112/63]

Holtz, P., Balzer, H., Westermann, E.: Beeinflussung der Narkosedauer durch Hemmung der Cholinesterase des Gehirns. *Naunyn-Schmiedebergs Arch. Pharmak.* 233, 438—467 (1958). [C 76,300/58]

Holtz, P., Balzer, H., Westermann, E., Wezler, E.: Beeinflussung der Evipannarkose durch Reserpin, Iproniazid und biogene Amine. *Naunyn-Schmiedebergs Arch. Pharmak.*, 231, 333—348 (1957). [D 98,342/57]

Holzmann, H., Korting, G. W., Morsches, B.: Bestimmung der Myokinase und der Kreatin-Phosphokinase im Serum bei experimentellem Lathyrismus, bei Dermatomyositis und bei progressiver Sklerodermie. *Arch. klin. exp. Dermat.* 223, 319—327 (1965). [F 56,165/65]

Holzmann, H., Korting, G. W., Morsches, B.: Bestimmung von Sorbit-Dehydrogenase und Creatin-Phosphokinase im Serum von lathyritischen und mit Prednison behandelten lathyritischen Ratten. *Naturwissenschaften*, 52, p. 499 (1965). [G 33,879/65]

Homburger, E., Etsten, B., Himwich, H. E.: Some factors affecting the susceptibility of rats to various barbiturates. The effect of age and sex. *J. Lab. clin. Med.* 32, 540—547 (1947). [E 61,371/47]

Homburger, F., Kasdon, S. C., Fishman, W. H.: Methylandrostenediol, a non-virilizing steroid hormone with testosterone-like effects. *42nd Meet. Amer. Soc. clin. Invest.*, p. 33, May (1950). [B 47,878/50]

Homburger, F., Kelley, T., Jr., Baker, T. R., Russfield, A. B.: Sex effect on hepatic pathology from deficient diet and safrole in rats. *Arch. Path.* 73, 118—125 (1962). [E 94,913/62]

Homburger, F., Pettengill, O.: The protein anabolic and other effects of testosterone propionate in mice: effects of nutrition and interrelationship of biologic activities of the hormone. *Endocrinology* 57, 296—301 (1955). [C 8,310/55

Honjo, I., Kozaka, S.: Extensive resection of the liver in two stages. *Rev. int. Hépat.* 15, 309—319 (1965). [E 51,472/65

Hook, J. B., Williamson, H. E.: Addition of the natruretic action of SKF 525-A to the action of certain other natruretic agents. *J. Pharmacol. exp. Ther.* 146, 265—269 (1964). [F 24,917/64]

Hoosier, G. L. van, Jr., Gist, C., Trentin, J. J.: Facilitation, by thymectomy, of tumor formation by weakly oncogenic adenoviruses. *Proc. Amer. Ass. Cancer Res.* 8, 70 (1967). [F 78,860/67]

Hoosier, G. L. van, Jr., Kirschstein, R. L., Abinanti, F. R., Hottle, G. A., Baron, S.: The safety test for poliomyelitis vaccine. I. An evaluation of variable factors in the monkey and cell culture systems. *Amer. J. Hyg.* 74, 209—219 (1961). [D 12,216/61]

Horák, J., Hůlek, P., Šimek, J.: Changes of the blood volume, plasma volume and blood cell mass after partial hepatectomy. *Sborn. véd. Praci lék. Fak. Hradci Králové* 11, 773—774 (1968). [G 71,097/68]

Horava, A., Selye, H.: Sur les effets de l'administration de l'hydrocortisone et de l'hormone somatotrope. *Ann. Endocr. (Paris)* 14, 772—778 (1953). [B 70,249/53]

Hori, S., Masumura, S., Ono, K.: Effect of aldosterone on angiotensin-induced glycosuria. *Mie med. J.* 19, 61—66 (1969). [G 72,331/69]

Horinaga, T.: Über den sexuellen Empfindlichkeitsunterschied gegen Narkotika. *Hukuoka Acta Med.* 34, 2—3 (1941). [A 36,414/41]

Horton, H. R., Franz, J. M.: Effect of ethionine on the cortisone-evoked stimulation of tryptophan peroxidase-oxidase activity. *Endocrinology* 64, 258—261 (1959). [C 63,790/59]

Horváth, E., Kovács, K., Blascheck, J. A., Somogyi, A.: Ultrastructural changes induced in the liver of rats by various steroid compounds. *Virchows Arch. Abt. B Zellpath.* 29, 756 (1970). [G 70,490/70]

Horváth, E., Kovács, K., Tuchweber, B., Blascheck, J. A., Gardell, C., Somogyi, A.: Effects of various steroids on the ultrastructure of the liver (Abstr.). *Fed. Proc.* 29, 756 (1970). [G 70,408/70]

Horváth, E., Somogyi, A., Kovács, K.: Einfluß von Spironolacton auf das Regenerationsvermögen der Leber bei Ratten. *Klin. Wschr.* 48, 385—387 (1970). [G 70,405/70]

Horváth, E., Somogyi, A., Kovács, K.: Effect of estradiol on 7,12-dimethylbenz(a)anthracene-induced adrenocortical necrosis. A histochemical study. *Arch. Geschwulstforsch.* (in press). [G 70,443/

Horváth, F., Horváth, J.: Untersuchungen zur Verminderung von Strahlenschädigungen der

Ossifikationszonen bei in Entwicklung begriffenen Kaninchen durch Verabreichung von Durabolin, Vitamin D_2 und Eierschalenpulver. *Strahlentherapie* **135**/1, 38—47 (1968). [G 55,076/68]

Hoshino, J., Kröger, H.: Properties of L-serine dehydratase purified from rat liver after induction by fasting or feeding casein hydrolysate. *Hoppe-Seylers Z. physiol. Chem.* **350**, 595—602 (1969). [H 13,867/69]

Hotchin, J., Sikora, E.: Protection against the lethal effect of lymphocytic choriomeningitis virus in mice by neonatal thymectomy. *Nature (Lond.)* **202**, 214—215 (1964). [F 8,620/64]

Hotterbeex, P., Darcis, L.: Action du phénylpropionate de testostérone sur la sensibilité de la muqueuse rectale de la rate à une irradiation locale. *Ann. Endocr. (Paris)* **20**, 366—370 (1959). [C 75,318/59]

Houchin, O. B., Smith, P. W.: Cardiac insufficiency in the vitamin E deficient rabbit. *Amer. J. Physiol.* **141**, 242—248 (1944). [B 6,967/44]

Houck, J. C., Jacob, R. A.: Connective tissue. VIII. Factors inhibiting the dermal chemical response to cortisol. *Proc. Soc. exp. Biol. (N. Y.)* **113**, 692—698 (1963). [E 21,446/63]

Houssay, B. A.: Action of sulphur compounds on carbohydrate metabolism and on diabetes. *Amer. J. med. Sci.* **219**, 353—367 (1950). [B 60,812/50]

Houssay, B. A., Busso, R. R.: Sensibilité des animaux éthyroïdés vis-à-vis de l'insuline. *C. R. Soc. Biol. (Paris)* **91**, 1037—1038 (1924). [20,601/24]

Houssay, B. A., Cisneros, A. D.: Le choc anaphylactique et peptonique chez les chiens éthyroïdés. *C. R. Soc. Biol. (Paris)* **93**, 886 a 887 (1925). [26,936/25]

Houssay, B. A., Houssay, A. B., Cardeza, A. F.: Acción de la radioyodotiroidectomia sobre la diabetes aloxánica del perro. *Rev. Soc. argent. Biol.* **31**, 213—222 (1955). [C 15,702/55]

Houssay, B. A., Rietti, C. T.: Hipófisis y tiroides. VIII. Extracto de lóbulo anterior de hipófisis y sensibilidad a la anoxemia. *Rev. Soc. argent. Biol.* **8**, 53—57 (1932). [3,187/32]

Houssay, B. A., Rietti, C. T.: Hypophyse et thyroïde. Extrait de lobe antérieur d'hypophyse et sensibilité à l'anoxémie. *C. R. Soc. Biol. (Paris)* **110**, 144—145 (1932). [3,283/32]

Houssay, B. A., Rietti, C. T.: Hipófisis y tiroides. X. Nuevos experimentos sobre extracto de lóbulo anterior de hipófisis y resistencia a la anoxemia. *Rev. Soc. argent. Biol.* **8**, 249—253 (1932). [5,793/32]

Houssay, B. A., Sara, J.: Tiroides y sensibilidad al aloxano. *Rev. Soc. argent. Biol.* **21**, 81—85 (1945). [B 727/45]

Houssay, B. A., Sordelli, A.: Sensibilité des animaux éthyroïdés envers les toxines et le bacille diphtérique. Formation d'anticorps chez les animaux éthyroïdés. *C. R. Soc. Biol. (Paris)* **85**, 677, 679, 1220 (1921). [A 48,113/21]

Houssay, B. A., Sordelli, A.: Thyroïde et anaphylaxie. *C. R. Soc. Biol. (Paris)* **87**, 354—356 (1923). [13,430/23]

Howard, R. G., Maeir, D. M., Zaiman, H.: Experimental trichinous myocarditis: effect of cortisone. *Fed. Proc.* **21**, 134 (1962). [D 22,789/62]

Hoyrup, E., Vinten-Johansen, E.: Acut phenemal—og difhydanforgiftning. (Acute phenobarbital and diphenylhydantoin poisoning.) *Nord. Med.* **47**, 283—285 (1952). [B 84,197/52]

Hrůza, Z.: Sex differences in the circulatory reaction of rats traumatized in the Noble-Collip drum. *Physiol. bohemoslov.* **8**, 300—306 (1958). [C 74,576/58]

Hrůza, Z.: Sexual differences in resistance to trauma in the Noble-Collip drum and during adaptation to trauma and the effect of castration. *Physiol. bohemoslov.* **10**, 173—180 (1961). [D 5,993/61]

Hrůza, Z., Poupa, O.: Studies on the adaptation of metabolism. V. A method of experimental traumatization in the Noble-Collip drum. *Physiol. bohemoslov.* **6**, 179—187 (1957). [C 44,659/57]

Hrůza, Z., Stetson, C. A., Jr.: Protective effect of depot catecholamines in traumatic and endotoxin shock (Abstr.). *Fed. Proc.* **27**, 447 (1968). [H 455/68]

Hrůza, Z., Zweifach, B. W.: Catecholamines and dibenzyline in trauma and adaptation to trauma. *J. Trauma* **10**, 412—419 (1970). [G 77,195/70]

Hsia, D. Y. Y., Dowben, R. M., Shaw, R., Grossman, A.: Inhibition of glucuronosyl transferase by progestational agents from serum of pregnant women. *Nature* **187**, 693—694 (1960). [C 90,465/60]

Hsieh, A. C. L.: The role of the thyroid in rats exposed to cold. *J. Physiol. (Lond.)* **161**, 175—188 (1962). [D 20,969/62]

Hsieh, A. C. L.: Thyroid hormone requirement in rats exposed to cold. *Gunma Symp. Endocr.* **3**, 239—248 (1966). [F 71,817/66]

Hsu, H. S.: Cellular basis of cortisone-induced host susceptibility to tuberculosis. *Amer. Rev. resp. Dis.* **100**, 677—684 (1969). [G 70,576/69]

Hucker, H. B., Zacchei, A. G., Cox, S. V., Brodie, D. A., Cantwell, N. H. R.: Studies on the absorption, distribution and excretion of indomethacin in various species. *J. Pharmacol. exp. Ther.* **153**, 237—249 (1966). [G 67,791/66

Huebener, H. J., Amelung, D.: Enzymatische Umwandlungen von Steroiden. II. Mittlg. Geschlechtsunterschiede der enzymatischen Leberleistungen. *Hoppe-Seylers Z. physiol. Chem.* **293**, 137—141 (1953). [B 91,352/53

Hueper, W. C.: Experimental studies in cardiovascular pathology. VII. Chronic nicotine poisoning in rats and in dogs. *Arch. Path.* **35**, 846—856 (1943). [91,722/43

Huggins, C., Briziarelli, G., Sutton, H., Jr.: Rapid induction of mammary carcinoma in the rat and the influence of hormones on the tumors. *J. exp. Med.* **109**, 25—42 (1959). [C 62,178/59

Huggins, C., Fukunishi, R.: Cancer in the rat after single exposures to irradiation or hydrocarbons. Age and strain factors. Hormone dependence of the mammary cancers. *Radiat. Res.* **20**, 493—503 (1963). [E 35,442/63

Huggins, C., Fukunishi, R.: Induced protection of adrenal cortex against 7,12-dimethylbenz-(a)anthracene. Influence of ethionine. Induction of menadione reductase. Incorporation of thymidine-H^3. *J. exp. Med.* **119**, 923—942 (1964). [G 14,366/64

Huggins, C., Fukunishi, R.: Molecular structure of aromatics related to their ability to induce adrenal protection. *Arzneimittel-Forsch.* **14**, 834—836 (1964). [F 18,350/64

Huggins, C., Grand, L. C., Brillantes, F. P.: Mammary cancer induced by a single feeding of polynuclear hydrocarbons and its suppression. *Nature (Lond.)* **189**, 204—207 (1961). [C 99,772/61

Huggins, C., Morii, S.: Selective adrenal necrosis and apoplexy induced by 7,12-dimethylbenz(a)-anthracene. *J. exp. Med.* **114**, 741—760 (1961). [D 13,007/61

Huggins, C., Yang, N. C.: Induction and extinction of mammary cancer. *Science* **137**, 257—262 (1962). [D 27,549/62

Huggins, C. B., Grand, L.: Neoplasms evoked in male Sprague-Dawley rat by pulse doses of 7,12-dimethylbenz(a)anthracene. *Cancer Res.* **26**, 2255—2258 (1966). [F 74,177/66

Huggins, C. B., Sugiyama, T.: Production and prevention of two distinctive kinds of destruction of adrenal cortex. *Nature (Lond.)* **206**, 1310—1314 (1965). [F 44,582/65

Hughes, P. E.: Mitotic responses to partial hepatectomy in preneoplastic rat liver. *Chem.-Biol. Interaction* **1**, 315—320 (1970). [G 74,311/70

Huizenga, K. A., Brofman, B. L., Wiggers, C. J.: Ineffectiveness of adreno-cortical preparations in standardized hemorrhagic shock. *Proc. Soc. exp. Biol. (N.Y.)* **52**, 77 (1943). [A 54,816/43

Huizenga, K. A., Brofman, B. L., Wiggers, C. J.: The ineffectiveness of adrenal cortex extracts in standardized hemorrhagic shock. *J. Pharmacol. exp. Ther.* **78**, 139—153 (1943). [A 59,447/43

Hulka, J. F., Mohr, K.: Interference of cortisone-induced homograft survival by progestins. *Amer. J. Obstet. Gynec.* **97**, 407—410 (1967). [G 44,272/67

Hulth, A., Westerborn, O.: Effect of cortisone on the epiphysial cartilage. A histologic and autoradiographic study. *Virchows Arch. pathol. Anat.* **336**, 209—219 (1963). [D 56,601/63

Hunt, C. E., Carlton, W. W.: Neural-lathyrism in white Pekin duck. *Fed. Proc.* **23**, 128 (1964). [F 3,186/64

Hunt, R.: The influence of thyroid feeding upon poisoning by acetonitrile. *J. biol. Chem.* **1**, 1—12 (1905). [60,064/05

Hunt, R.: The relation of iodin to the thyroid gland. *J. Amer. med. Ass.* **49**, 1323—1329 (1907). [49,716/07

Hunt, R.: The probable demonstration of thyroid secretion in the blood in exophthalmic goiter. *J. Amer. med. Ass.* **49**, 240—241 (1907). [49,717/07

Hunt, R.: The effects of a restricted diet and of various diets upon the resistance of animals to certain poisons. *Hyg. Lab., Bull.* No. 69, pp. 93 (1910). [50,349/10

Hunt, R.: Experiments on the relation of the thyroid to diet. *J. Amer. med. Ass.* **57**, 1032 to 1033 (1911). [49,718/11

Hunt, R.: The acetonitril test for thyroid and of some alterations of metabolism. *Amer. J. Physiol.* **63**, 257—299 (1923). [13,889/23

Hunt, R., Seidell, A.: Studies on thyroid. I. The relation of iodine to the physiological activity of thyroid preparations. *Hyg. Lab. Bull.* **47**, 1—115 (1909). [50,346/09

Hunt, R., Seidell, A.: Thyreotropic iodine compounds. *J. Pharmacol. exp. Ther.* **2**, 15—47 (1910). [46,617/10

Hunter, J., Maxwell, J. D., Carrella, M., Stewart, D. A., Williams, R.: Urinary D-glucaric-acid excretion as a test for hepatic enzyme induction in man. *Lancet* **1971 I**, 572—575. [H 36,993/71

Hurd, E. L., Bass, F. K., DeGraff, A. C., Kupperman, H. S.: The effect of cortisone upon the fatty liver and kidney changes of choline-deficient rats. *J. clin. Endocr.* 13, 839—840 (1953). [B83,869/53]

Hurst, E. W.: Sexual differences in the toxicity and therapeutic action of chemical substances. In: Walpole and Spinks; *A Symposium on the Evaluation of Drug Toxicity*, p. 12—25. London: J. & A. Churchill Ltd. 1958. [D33,743/58]

Hurst, E. W., Melvin, P. A., Thorp, J. M.: The influence of sex on equine encephalomyelitis in the mouse and on its treatment with mepacrine. *J. comp. Path.* 70, 346—360 (1960). [C94,088/60]

Hurst, E. W., Melvin, P. A., Thorp, J. M.: The influence of cortisone, ACTH, thyroxine and thiouracil on equine encephalomyelitis in the mouse and on its treatment with mepacrine. *J. comp. Path.* 70, 361—373 (1960). [C94,089/60]

Hussar, D. A.: Therapeutic incompatibilities: drug interactions. *Hosp. Pharm. (Philad.)* 3, 14—24, 32 (1968). [G81,059/68]

Hussar, D. A.: Mechanisms of drug interactions. *J. Amer. pharm. Ass.* 9, 208—209, 213 (1969). [G81,053/69]

Hutchinson, A. H.: Amelioration of experimental hypertension. *Trans. roy. Soc. Can., Sect. V* 42, 25—35 (1948). [B29,416/48]

Hutchinson, L. A., Andrews, G. A., Kniseley, R. M.: Influence of cortisone on toxicity of nitrogen mustard in rats. *Proc. Soc. exp. Biol. (N.Y.)* 83, 376—377 (1953). [B84,257/53]

Hutter, A. M., Jr., Kayhoe, D. E.: Adrenal cortical carcinoma. Results of treatment with o,p'DDD in 138 patients. *Amer. J. Med.* 41, 581—592 (1966). [F74,271/66]

Hutterer, F., Bacchin, P. G., Raisfeld, I. H., Schenkman, J. B., Schaffner, F., Popper, H.: Alteration of microsomal biotransformation in the liver in cholestasis. *Proc. Soc. exp. Biol. (N.Y.)* 133, 702—706 (1970). [G75,925/70]

Hutterer, F., Klion, F. M., Wengraf, A., Schaffner, F., Popper, H.: Hepatocellular adaptation and injury. Structural and biochemical changes following dieldrin and methyl butter yellow. *Lab. Invest.* 20, 455—464 (1969). [G66,323/69]

Hutterer, F., Rubin, E., Gall, E., Popper, H.: Cortisone effect in stages of hepatic injury. A cytochemical, autoradiographic, and histologic study. *Exp. molec. Path.* 1, 85—95 (1962). [E54,152/62]

Hutterer, F., Rubin, E., Singer, E. J., Popper, H.: Quantitative relation of cell proliferation and fibrogenesis in the liver. *Cancer Res.* 21, 205—215 (1961). [D902/61]

Huttunen, J. K., Miettinen, T. A.: Glucuronidation in rats of different ages and strains. *Acta physiol. scand.* 63, 133—140 (1965). [G27,972/65]

Hyde, P. M., Elliott, W. H., Doisy, E. A., Jr., Doisy, E. A.: Synthesis and metabolic studies of 17α-methyl-C^{14}-Δ^5-androstene-3β, 17β-diol. *J. biol. Chem.* 207, 287—294 (1954). [D99,140/54]

Hyde, P. M., Williams, R. H.: Absorption and metabolism of hydrocortisone-4-C^{14}. *J. biol. Chem.* 227, 1063—1081 (1957). [C40,540/57]

Hyde, T. A.: The effect of nephrectomy and renal ischaemia on liver regeneration. *J. Path. Bact.* 96, 131—136 (1968). [H15,523/68]

Hyde, T. A., Davis, J. C.: The effects of cortisol and chlorazanil on the mitotic rate in mouse liver and skin. *Europ. J. Cancer* 2, 227—230 (1966). [F82,461/66]

Hyman, G. A., Ragan, C., Turner, J. C.: Effect of cortisone and adrenocorticotropic hormone (ACTH) on experimental scurvy in the guinea pig. *Proc. Soc. exp. Biol. (N.Y.)* 75, 470—475 (1950). [B53,374/50]

Hyman, G. A., Ragan, C., Turner, J. C.: The effect of cortisone and ACTH on experimental scurvy in the guinea pig. *Trans. N.Y. Acad. Sci.* 13, 167—168 (1951). [B57,989/51]

Ichii, S., Yago, N.: Hormonal regulation of aminopyrine N-demethylase system in rat liver. *J. Biochem. (Tokyo)* 65, 597—601 (1969). [H15,158/69]

Igić, R., Jeličić, J., Nikulin, E., Stern, P.: Myotropischer Effekt des Metenolazetat auf die experimentelle Muskeldystrophie der Ratte. *Endokrinologie* 54, 103—106 (1969). [H13,355/69]

Ilavsky, J., Foley, E. J.: Studies on the effect of cortisone with chemotherapeutic agents on tuberculous peritonitis in mice. *Antibiot. and Chemother.* 4, 1068—1074 (1954). [C7,577/54]

Imamura, T.: Studies upon the relation between hormones and bacterial toxins, especially on the influence of follicle liquid of the ovarium on tetanus toxin in relation to the uterine hormone. *Acta med. Keijo* 12, 249—285 (1929). [14,567/29]

Infante, R., Turchetto, E., Rabbi, A.: Influenza della tiroxina sulla attività lipotropa della vitamina B_{12}. *Boll. Soc. ital. Biol. sper.* 31, 157—159 (1955). [C17,520/55]

Ingbar, S. H., Freinkel, N.: Intrinsic factors affecting radiation mortality in the mouse (Abstr.). *Fed. Proc.* **11**, 77 (1952). [B 68,221/52

Ingle, D. J.: The survival of non-adrenalectomized rats in shock with and without adrenal cortical hormone treatment. *Amer. J. Physiol.* **139**, 460—463 (1943). [A 59,854/43

Ingle, D. J.: The effect of adrenal cortical extract on the resistance of non-adrenalectomized rats to peptone shock. *Amer. J. Physiol.* **142**, 191—194 (1944). [85,588/44

Ingle, D. J.: The resistance of non-adrenalectomized rats to diphtheria toxin with and without adrenal cortical hormone treatment. *Exp. Med. Surg.* **5**, 375—378 (1947).
[B 42,751/47

Ingle, D. J.: The technique of evisceration in the rat. *Exp. Med. Surg.* **7**, 34—36 (1949).
[B 39,012/49

Ingle, D. J., Baker, B. L.: Histology and regenerative capacity of liver following multiple partial hepatectomies. *Proc. Soc. exp. Biol. (N.Y.)* **95**, 813—815 (1957). [C 40,980/57

Ingle, D. J., Kuizenga, M. H.: The survival of non-adrenalectomized rats in burn shock with and without adrenal cortical hormone treatment. *Amer. J. Physiol.* **145**, 203—205 (1945).
[96,155/45

Ingle, D. J., Nezamis, J. E.: Effect of insulin and glucose upon survival time of eviscerated rats. *Proc. Soc. exp. Biol. (N.Y.)* **69**, 441—442 (1948). [B 28,601/48

Ingle, D. J., Nezamis, J. E.: Infection as a factor causing death in the eviscerate rat. *Proc. Soc. exp. Biol. (N.Y.)* **71**, 438—439 (1949).
[B 37,742/49

Ingle, D. J., Nezamis, J. E.: Effect of antibiotics upon survival of the eviscerate rat. *Amer. J. Physiol.* **166**, 349—353 (1951).
[B 65,286/51

Ingle, D. J., Nezamis, J. E., Kuizenga, M. H.: The effects of epinephrine and of adrenal cortex extract upon the survival of eviscerated rats. *Exp. Med. Surg.* **5**, 379—382 (1947).
[B 42,752/47

Ingle, D. J., Nezamis, J. E., Prestrud, M. C.: The effect of diethylstilbestrol upon alloxan diabetes in the male rat. *Endocrinology* **41**, 207—212 (1947). [B 3,163/47

Ingle, D. J., Prestrud, M. C., Nezamis, J. E., Kuizenga, M. H.: Effect of adrenal cortex extract upon the tolerance of the eviscerated rat for intravenously administered glucose. *Amer. J. Physiol.* **150**, 423—427 (1947).
[B 2,737/47

Inscoe, J. K., Axelrod, J.: Some factors affecting glucuronide formation "in vitro". *J. Pharmacol. exp. Ther.* **129**, 128—131 (1960).
[D 1,700/60

Inscoe, J. K., Daly, J., Axelrod, J.: Factors affecting the enzymatic formation of O-methylated dihydroxy derivatives. *Biochem. Pharmacol.* **14**, 1257—1263 (1965). [F 70,325/65

Ippolito, A., Pagliari, M., Manno, G., De Santis, R.: La prevenzione dell'ulcera gastro-duodenale da cortisonici mediante trattamento associato con idrossido di alluminio ed anabolizzanti. *Rass. Fisiopat. clin. ter.* **34**, 486—494 (1962). [D 57,498/62

Isacson, S., Nilsson, I. M.: Effect of treatment with combined phenformin and ethyloestrenol on the coagulation and fibrinolytic systems. *Scand. J. Haemat.* **7**, 404—408 (1970).
[G 80,478/70

Ishikawa, E., Ninagawa, T., Suda, M.: Hormonal and dietary control of serine dehydratase in rat liver. *J. Biochem. (Tokyo)* **57**, 506—513 (1965). [F 41,763/65

Ishimura, Y., Ullrich, V., Peterson, J. A.: Oxygenated cytochrome P-450 and its possible role in enzymic hydroxylation. *Biochem. biophys. Res. Commun.* **42**, 140—146 (1971).
[G 81,262/71

Ishizaki, A., Tanabe, S., Matsuda, S., Sakamoto, M.: Experimental study on the chronic cadmium poisoning in relation to calcium deficiency. (Japanese text.) *Jap. J. Hyg.* **20**, 398—404 (1966). [F 94,533/66

Israel, S. L., Meranze, D. R., Johnston, C. G.: The inactivation of estrogen by the liver. Observations on the fate of estrogen in heart-lung and heart-lung-liver perfusion systems. *Amer. J. med. Sci.* **194**, 835—843 (1937).
[A 16,424/37

Issekutz, B. von, Issekutz, B. von, Jr.: Wirkungsort des Thyroxins. *Naunyn-Schmiedebergs Arch. Pharmak.* **177**, 442—449 (1935).
[45,261/35

Ito, T.: Study on the sex difference in benzene inhalation. (Japanese text.) *Showa med. J.* **22**/7, 25—29 (1962). [E 44,788/62

Ito, T., Hoshino, T., Sawauchi, K.: Effect of gonadectomy and adrenalectomy on development of urethan-induced thymic lymphoma in mice. *Gann* **57**, 201—204 (1966). [G 42,670/66

IUPAC Commission on the Nomenclature of Organic Chemistry (CNOC) and IUPAC-IUB Commission of Biochemical Nomenclature (CBN): The nomenclature of steroids. Revised tentative rules. *European J. Biochem.* **10**, 1—19 (1969). [G 82,068/69

Izzo, R. A., Cicardo, V. H.: Influencia de la tiroides sobre la tuberculosis experimental. *Publ. Cent. Invest. tisiol. (B. Aires)* 11, 237—247 (1947). [B 23,261/47

Izzo, R. A., Cicardo, V. H.: Effect of thyroid on experimental tuberculosis. *Amer. Rev. Tuberc.* 56, 52—58 (1947). [B 67,482/47

Jabbari, M., Leevy, C. M.: Protein anabolism and fatty liver of the alcoholic. *Medicine (Baltimore)* 46, 131—139 (1967). [G 45,526/67

Jackson, E. B., Smadel, J. E.: The effects of cortisone and ACTH on toxins of Rickettsiae and Salmonella typhosa. *J. Immunol.* 66, 621—625 (1951). [B 77,408/51

Jackson, E. B., Smadel, J. E.: Cortisone and ACTH on toxins of Rickettsiae and Salmonella typhosa (Abstr.). *Bact. Proc.* 92—93 (1951). [E 52,720/51

Jackson, G. J.: The effect of cortisone on Plasmodium berghei infections in the white rat. *J. infect. Dis.* 97, 152—159 (1955). [C 11,604/55

Jacob, D., Morris, J. M.: The estrogenic activity of postcoital antifertility compounds. *Fertil. and Steril.* 20, 211—222 (1969). [G 73,856/69

Jacob, M., Forbes, R. M.: A study of the relative potency of L- and D-thyroxine in preventing kidney calcification associated with magnesium deficiency. *J. Nutr.* 99, 152—156 (1969). [G 69,934/69

Jacob, S. T., Sajdel, E. M., Munro, H. N.: Regulation of nucleolar RNA metabolism by hydrocortisone. *Europ. J. Biochem.* 7, 449—453 (1969). [G 64,812/69

Jacobsen, J., Broderseen, R., Trolle, D.: Patterns of bilirubin conjugation in the newborn. *Scand. J. clin. Lab. Invest.* 20, 249—251 (1967). [H 30,765/67

Jaffe, J. J.: Diurnal mitotic periodicity in regenerating rat liver. *Anat. Rec.* 120, 935—954 (1954). [G 77,570/54

Jahkola, M., Atanasiu, P., Duplan, J. F.: Evolution de la maladie due à un virus cytomégalique chez des radiochimères thymiprivés isogéniques. *Ann. Inst. Pasteur* 112, 781—797 (1967). [G 47,813/67

Jandásek, L.: Einfluß des Thyroxins auf die experimentelle Zeckenenzephalitis der infantilen Ratte. *Z. Immun.-Forsch.* 119, 365—369 (1960). [C 88,870/60

Jandásek, L.: Einfluß des Thyroxins auf die experimentelle Zeckenenzephalitis der Maus. *Scr. med. Fac. Med. Brün.* 33, 35—40 (1960). [C 92,117/60

Janes, R. G., Brady, J.: Thiamine deficiency in normal rats and in rats made diabetic with alloxan. *Amer. J. Physiol.* 153, 417—424 (1948). [B 23,359/48

Janes, R. G., Brady, J. M.: Thiamine deficiency in adult normal and diabetic rats as studied under paired-feeding conditions (Abstr.). *Fed. Proc.* 6, 136 (1947). [98,541/47

Jannuzzi, C., Bassetti, D., Frigerio, G.: Ricerche cliniche controllate sull'effetto di steroidi anabolizzanti nell'epatite virale. *Minerva med.* 61, 1902—1911 (1970). [H 27,335/70

Jannuzzi, C., Bassi, A.: Ormoni steroidei ed anticorpopoiesi. Nota III. Potenziamento della vaccinazione antidifterica nel bambino da parte di ormoni 'anabolizzanti'. *Boll. Ist. sieroter. milan.* 41, 221—226 (1962). [G 68,895/62

Janoff, A.: Alterations in lysosomes (intracellular enzymes) during shock; effects of preconditioning (tolerance) and protective drugs. In: Hershey; *Shock* 2, p. 251—269. Boston, Mass.: Little, Brown & Co. 1964. [G 68,991/64

Janoff, A., Kaley, G.: Studies on lysosomes in tolerance, shock, and local injury induced by endotoxin. In: Landy and Braun; *Bacterial Endotoxin*, p. 631—647. New Brunswick, N.J.: Institute of Microbiology, Rutgers, The State University, 1964. [E 8,484/64

Janoff, A., Weissmann, G., Zweifach, B. W., Thomas, L.: Pathogenesis of experimental shock. IV. Studies on lysosomes in normal and tolerant animals subjected to lethal trauma and endotoxemia. *J. exp. Med.* 116, 451—466 (1962). [D 35,553/62

Janoski, A. H., Shaver, J. C., Christy, N. P., Rosner, W.: On the pharmacologic actions of 21-carbon hormonal steroids ('glucocorticoids') of the adrenal cortex in mammals. In: Eichler, Farah et al.; *Handbuch der Experimentellen Pharmakologie*, 14/3, p. 256. Berlin, Heidelberg, New York: Springer-Verlag 1968. [E 7,896/68

Januschke, H.: Adrenalin ein Antidot gegen Strychnin? *Wien. klin. Wschr.* 23, 284—286 (1910). [50,228/10

Japundžić, M. M.: The goitrogenic effect of phenobarbital-Na on the rat thyroid. *Acta anat. (Basel)* 74, 88—96 (1969). [G 74,862/69

Jaques, L. B.: Effects of hormones and drugs on hemostasis (Proc. 3. Int. Pharmacol. Meet. July 24—30, 1966.) In: *Drugs in Relation to Blood Coagulation, Haemostasis and Throm-*

bosis, p. 25—55. Oxford & New York: Pergamon Press 1968. [G70,979/68

Jaques, R.: The protection afforded by a benzyl glucofuranoside and hydrocortisone against lethal wasp venom shock in the guinea-pig. *Pharmacology (Basel)* **2**, 21—26 (1969).
[H13,146/69

Jarcho, L. W., Eyzaguirre, C., Lilienthal, J. L., Jr.: Sex difference in the response of rats to sodium pentobarbital. *Proc. Soc. exp. Biol. (N.Y.)* **74**, 332—333 (1950). [B59,706/50

Jasmin, G.: Production expérimentale chez le rat de lésions ressemblant à l'éclampsie. *Rev. Canad. Biol.* **12**, 89 (1953). [B80,596/53

Jasmin, G.: Action of hormones on the progression of magnesium deficiency syndrome in rats. In: Jasmin, G., *Endocrine Aspects of Disease Processes*, p. 356—381. St. Louis, Missouri: Warren H. Green Inc. 1968.
[E7,631/68

Jasmin, G., Bajusz, E., Mongeau, A.: Influence du sexe et de la castration sur la production de tumeurs musculaires chez le rat par le sulfure de nickel. *Rev. canad. Biol.* **22**, 113—114 (1963). [D68,263/63

Jasmin, G., Bois, P.: Myotoxic action of dimethyl-phenylenediamine. *Proc. Canad. Fed. biol. Soc. 2nd. Ann. Meet. Toronto*, p. 32 (1959). [G73,640/59

Jasmin, G., Bois, P.: Effect of various agents on the development of kidney infarcts in rats treated with serotonin. *Lab. Invest.* **9**, 503—515 (1960). [C92,099/60

Jasmin, G., Bois, P.: Experimental muscular dystrophy induced in rats by dimethyl-p-phenylenediamine. *Fed. Proc.* **19**, 254 (1960).
[G83,058/60

Jasmin, G., Bois, P., Mongeau, A.: Effect of cortisol and norethandrolone on inflammation and tumor growth. *Experientia (Basel)* **16**, 212 to 213 (1960). [C89,132/60

Jasmin, G., Riopelle, J. L.: Nephroblastomas induced in ovariectomized rats by dimethylbenzanthracene. *Cancer Res.* **30**, 321—326 (1970). [H23,587/70

Jay, G. E., Jr.: Variation in response of various mouse strains to hexobarbital (Evipal). *Proc. Soc. exp. Biol. (N.Y.)* **90**, 378—380 (1955). [G71,140/55

Jayle, M. F., Pasqualini, J. R.: Implication of conjugation of endogenous compounds—Steroids and thyroxine. In: Dutton, G. J.; *Glucuronic Acid. Free and Combined Chemistry, Biochemistry, Pharmacology and Medicine*, p. 507—543. New York, London: Academic Press Inc. 1966. [G67,284/66

Jean, C.: Développement somatique embryonnaire et post-natal après traitement oestrogénique prénatal. *C. R. Soc. Biol. (Paris)* **164**, 784 à 791 (1970). [H33,486/70

Jean, C., Jean, C.: Influence des oestrogènes injectés à la mère gravide sur la mortalité du foetus et du nouveau-né. *C. R. Soc. Biol. (Paris)* **164**, 779—783 (1970). [H33,485/70

Jeffries, C. D.: Liver carbohydrate levels in mice treated with endotoxin, cortisone, and eliptene. *Proc. Soc. exp. Biol. (N.Y.)* **132**, 540—542 (1969). [H19,361/69

Jelínek, J., Křeček, J.: The effect of age and pinealectomy on the hypertension produced by adrenal regeneration. *Experientia (Basel)* **24**, 912—913 (1968). [H2,778/68

Jelínek, J., Mikulášková, J., Pelc, B.: The action of some steroid compounds on $HgCl_2$-nephrosis in mouse and rat kidney. *Acta biol. med. Germanica* **13**, 204—208 (1964).
[F20,543/64

Jelínek, J., Mikulášková, J., Veselá, H., Jelínek, V., Pelc, B.: The effect of some steroid compounds on compensatory hypertrophy and regenerative processes. *Biochem. Pharmacol.* **12**, 219 (1963). [E32,261/63

Jelínek, J. M.: The effect of some androgenic steroids on anesthesia. *Acta biol. med. Germanica* **20**, 495—501 (1968). [H1,518/68

Jelínek, V., Zikmund, E.: Variations sexuelles de l'action vasculaire de l'acide nicotinique. *C. R. Soc. Biol. (Paris)* **142**, 1044—1047 (1949). [B52,661/49

Jelliffe, R. W., Blankenhorn, D. H.: Effect of phenobarbital on digitoxin metabolism. *Clin. Res.* **14**, 160 (1966). [E65,188/66

Jellinck, P. H., Cox, J.: Effect of spermine on the kinetics of estradiol hydroxylation by rat liver microsomes. *Experientia (Basel)* **26**, 1066 (1970). [H32,603/70

Jellinck, P. H., Garland, M., McRitchie, D.: Effect of metopirone and 3-(1,2,3,4-tetrahydro-1-oxo-2-naphthyl)-pyridine on the metabolism of corticosteroids and DMBA in relation to adrenal necrosis. *Experientia (Basel)* **24**, 124 to 125 (1968). [F96,053/68

Jellinck, P. H., Lucieer, I.: Sex differences in the metabolism of oestrogens by rat liver microsomes. *J. Endocr.* **32**, 91—98 (1965).
[F37,592/65

Jenkins, V. K., Upton, A. C., Odell, T. T., Jr.: Effect of estradiol on splenic repopulation by endogenous and exogenous hemopoietic cells in irradiated mice. *J. cell. Physiol.* **73**, 149—157 (1969). [H 27,688/69

Jensen, D., Chaikoff, I. L., Tarver, H.: The ethionine-induced fatty liver: dosage, prevention, and structural specificity. *J. biol. Chem.* **192**, 395—403 (1951). [D 83,567/51

Jensen, H., Grattan, J. F.: The identity of the glycotropic (antiinsulin) substance of the anterior pituitary gland. *Amer. J. Physiol.* **128**, 270—275 (1940). [77,887/40

Jeremy, R., Towson, J.: Interaction between aspirin and indomethacin in the treatment of rheumatoid arthritis. *Med. J. Austral.* **2**, 127—129 (1970). [G 77,324/70

Jöchle, W., Langecker, H.: Biologische Wirkungen des 1-Methyl-Δ'-androsten-17β-ol-3-on-17-acetats und -17-önanthats (Methenolon-acetat und Methenolon-önanthat): Wachstumsstimulierung, Zusammensetzung des Tierkörpers und Fermenthaushalt. *Arzneimittel-Forsch.* **12**, 218 bis 223 (1962). [D 22,258/62

Johnson, A. D., Gomes, W. R., Demark, N. L. van: Early actions of cadmium in the rat and domestic fowl testis. I. Testis and body temperature changes caused by cadmium and zinc. *J. Reprod. Fertil.* **21**, 383—393 (1970). [H 23,801/70

Johnson, A. E., Eckman, M., Lowenstein, B. E.: Effect of adrenal cortical extract on the altitude tolerance of normal and of adrenalectomized rats. *War Med. (Chic.)* **4**, 318—323 (1943). [96,626/43

Johnson, A. R., Hewgill, F. R.: The effect of the antioxidants, butylated hydroxy anisole, butylated hydroxy toluene and propyl gallate on growth, liver and serum lipids and serum sodium levels of the rat. *Austral. J. exp. Biol. med. Sci.* **39**, 353—360 (1961). [E 51,900/61

Johnson, H. A.: Liver regeneration and the "critical mass" hypothesis. *Amer. J. Path.* **57**, 1—15 (1969). [H 18,571/69

Johnson, S., Siebert, W. J.: Experimental myocarditis. *Amer. Heart J.* **3**, 279—286 (1928). [C 91,021/28

Johnson, S., Siebert, W. J.: Experimental myocarditic lesions in the rabbit. Their effect on myocardial abscess from intravenous injection of staphylococci. *Arch. Path.* **6**, 54—66 (1928). [C 91,037/28

Johnston, A. D., Follis, R. H., Jr.: Bone destruction associated with aminonucleoside administration. *J. Bone Jt Surg.* **43**-A, 865 to 875 (1961). [D 12,799/61

Johnston, L. C., Grieble, H. G.: Treatment of arterial hypertensive disease with diuretics. V. Spironolactone, and aldosterone antagonist. *Arch. intern. Med.* **119**, 225—231 (1967). [F 94,590/67

Jondorf, W. R., Maickel, R. P., Brodie, B. B.: Inability of newborn mice and guinea pigs to metabolize drugs. *Biochem. Pharmacol.* **1**, 352—354 (1958). [E 90,586/58

Jones, A. L., Armstrong, D. T.: Increased cholesterol biosynthesis following phenobarbital induced hypertrophy of agranular endoplasmic reticulum in liver. *Proc. Soc. exp. Biol. (N.Y.)* **119**, 1136—1139 (1965). [F 51,262/65

Jones, B.: Glucuronyl transferase inhibition by steroids. *J. Pediat.* **64**, 815—821 (1964). [G 19,777/64

Jones, B. J., Roberts, D. J.: The effects of intracerebroventricularly administered noradnamine and other sympathomimetic amines upon leptazol convulsions in mice. *Brit. J. Pharmacol.* **34**, 27—31 (1968). [G 60,654/68

Jones, J. H.: Further observations on the possible interrelationship between the physiological actions of the parathyroid glands and vitamin D. *J. biol. Chem.* **111**, 155—161 (1935). [33,139/35

Jones, R. K., Shapiro, A. P.: Increased susceptibility to pyelonephritis during acute hypertension by angiotensin II and norepinephrine. *J. clin. Invest.* **42**, 179—186 (1963). [D 55,793/63

Jones, W. A., Cohen, R. B.: The effect of estrogen on the liver in murine viral hepatitis. *Amer. J. Path.* **42**, 237—249 (1963). [D 55,380/63

Jori, A., Bianchetti, A., Prestini, P. E.: Effect of contraceptive agents on drug metabolism. *Europ. J. Pharmacol.* **7**, 196—200 (1969). [H 17,070/69

Jori, A., Bianchetti, A., Prestini, P. E.: Relations between barbiturate brain levels and sleeping time in various experimental conditions. *Biochem. Pharmacol.* **19**, 2687—2694 (1970). [G 81,674/70

Jori, A., Pugliatti, C.: An interaction between the antidepressant drugs desipramine and modaline sulphate. *J. Pharm. Pharmacol.* **19**, 853—855 (1967). [G 70,112/67

Joshi, U. M., Rao, S. S.: Potentiation by a progestational agent of liver damage induced by a hepatotoxic agent. *Indian J. exp. Biol.* **7**, 79—81 (1969). [G 72,489/69

Jost, J. P., Khairallah, E. A., Pitot, H. C.: Studies on the induction and the repression of enzymes in rat liver. *J. Biol. Chem.* **243**, 3057—3066 (1968). [H 11,724/68

Jouppila, P., Suonio, S.: The effect of phenobarbital given to toxaemic and normal parturients on the serum bilirubin concentration of newborn infants. *Ann. clin. Res.* **2**, 209—213 (1970). [G 78,916/70

Juchau, M. R., Cran, R. L., Plaa, G. L., Fouts, J. R.: The induction of benzpyrene hydroxylase in the isolated perfused rat liver. *Biochem. Pharmacol.* **14**, 473—482 (1965). [E 50,728/65

Juchau, M. R., Fouts, J. R.: Effects of norethynodrel and progesterone on hepatic microsomal drug-metabolizing enzyme systems. *Biochem. Pharmacol.* **15**, 891—898 (1966). [G 40,275/66

Jude, A., Laborit, H., Leroux, R.: Action de l'hormone somatotrope sur la toxi-infection typhoïdique expérimentale de la souris blanche. *Rev. Immunol.* **19**, 58—63 (1955). [C 16,220/55

Julius, H. W.: The action of the gonadotropic extract of urine, Pregnyl on tar carcinoma. *Acta brev. neerl. Physiol.* **4**, 74 (1934). [29,127/34

Jull, J. W.: The effect of infection, hormonal environment, and genetic constitution on mammary tumor induction in rats by 7,12-dimethylbenz(a)anthracene. *Cancer Res.* **26**, 2368—2373 (1966). [F 74,180/66

Jull, J. W., Streeter, D. J., Sutherland, L.: The mechanism of induction of ovarian tumors in the mouse by 7,12-dimethylbenz-(a)anthracene. I. Effect of steroid hormones and carcinogen concentration in vivo. *J. nat. Cancer Inst.* **37**, 409—420 (1966). [G 41,663/66

Kabelik, J.: L'action antianaphylactique du sérum au thiosulfate. *C. R. Soc. Biol. (Paris)* **110**, 397—400 (1932). [9,032/32

Kádas, L., Zsámbéky, P.: The hormonal therapy of mercury bichloride poisoning. *Acta med. Acad. Sci. hung.* **9**, 363—379 (1956). [C 26,265/56

Kádas, L., Zsámbéky, P.: Neue experimentelle Angaben zur Hormontherapie der Sublimatvergiftung. *Endokrinologie* **35**, 127—137 (1957). [C 49,522/57

Kadzielawa, K., Widy-Tyszkiewicz, E.: Shortening of hexobarbital sleeping time after p-chlorophenylalanine. *Arch. int. Pharmacodyn.* **180**, 368—372 (1969). [H 18,469/69

Kaeser, H. E., Wüthrich, R.: Versuch zur Beeinflussung einer experimentellen Myopathie mit einer anabolen Substanz. *Med. Pharmacol. exp. (Basel)* **16**, 365—370 (1967). [F 80,357/67

Kagawa, C. M.: Anti-Aldosterones. In: Dorfman; *Methods in Hormone Research* **3**, 351 to 414. New York, London: Academic Press 1964. [E 4,593/64

Kagawa, C. M.: Action of antialdosterone compounds in the laboratory. In: Martini et al.; *Hormonal Steroids* **1**, 445—456. New York, London: Academic Press 1964. [E 4,772/64

Kagawa, C. M., Sturtevant, F. M., van Arman, C. G.: Pharmacology of a new steroid that blocks salt activity of aldosterone and desoxycorticosterone. *J. Pharmacol. exp. Ther.* **126**, 123—130 (1959). [D 88,974/59

Kahl, G. F.: Zur Wirkung von Metyrapon auf Elektronentransportvorgänge in der Leberzelle. *Naunyn-Schmiedebergs Arch. Pharmak.* **264**, 251—252 (1969). [G 69,105/69

Kahlson, G.: A place for histamine in normal physiology. *Lancet* **1960 I**, 67—71. [G 52,949/60

Kaczak, M., Gutowska-Grzegorczyk, G., Madyk, E.: The effect of chronic administration of acetylsalicylic acid on the rabbit's liver. *Pol. med. J.* **9**, 128—134 (1970). [G 75,716/70

Kalnins, V., Ledina, H.: Die Wirkung des Epithelkörperchenhormons auf Zähne und Knochen normaler und skorbutischer Meerschweinchen. *Upsala Läk.-Fören. Förh.* **52**, 235—276 (1947). [B 19,372/47

Kalow, W.: Pharmacogenetics. Heredity and the response to drugs. Philadelphia, London: W. B. Saunders Co., pp. 231 (1962). [E 695/62

Kalser, S. C., Kunig, R.: Effect of varying periods of cold exposure on the action and metabolism of hexobarbital. *Biochem. Pharmacol.* **18**, 405—412 (1969). [G 65,211/69

Kalter, H.: The effect of cortisone on the food consumption of pregnant mice. *Canad. J. Biochem.* **33**, 767—772 (1955). [C 8,008/55

Kalter, S. S., Stuart, D. C., Jr., Tepperman, J.: Alterations in rate of influenza virus proliferation produced by growth hormone and testosterone. *Proc. Soc. exp. Biol. (N.Y.)* **74**, 605—607 (1950). [B 49,656/50

Kaltiala, E. H.: Drug metabolism by liver microsomes after partial hepatectomy. *Ann. Med. exp. Fenn.* **48**, 184—187 (1970). [G 79,608/70

Kalyanpur, S. G., Naik, S. R., Pahujani, S., Sheth, U. K.: Anti-convulsant action of anabolic steroids. *Biochem. Pharmacol.* **18**, 957—959 (1969). [G 66,147/69

Kalyanpur, S. G., Naik, S. R., Sheth, U. K.: Study of some factors affecting pentobarbital sleeping time. *Arch. int. Pharmacodyn.* **173**, 1—10 (1968). [F 99,270/68

Kamikubo, A.: The influence of alloxan on the distribution of zinc in animals bearing malignant tumours. (Japanese text.) *Advanc. Obst. & Gynaec.* **11**, 182 (1959). [D 7,362/59

Kampioni, B.: The effect of ACTH on the pleura of a tuberculous guinea pig. *Pol. med. J.* **3**, 1074—1077 (1964). [G 33,098/64

Kandror, V. I.: The role of the hypophysial-adrenal system in the development of symptoms originating from radiation pathology (Literature survey). (Russian text.) *Probl. Endokr. Gormonoter.* **9**, 109—117 (1963).
[E 27,416/63

Kaneko, A., Sakamoto, S., Morita, M., Onoé, T.: Morphological and biochemical changes in rat liver during the early stages of ethyl chlorophenoxyisobutyrate administration. *Tohoku J. exp. Med.* **99**, 81—101 (1969).
[H 19,398/69

Kaplan, H. S., Nagareda, C. S., Brown, M. B.: V. The role of hormones in blood and blood-forming organs. Endocrine factors and radiation-induced lymphoid tumors in mice. In: *Recent Progress in Hormone Research* **10**, p. 293—338. New York: Academic Press Inc. 1954. [B 98,601/54

Kappas, A.: Estrogens and the liver. *Gastroenterology* **52**, 113—116 (1967). [G 43,772/67

Kappas, A.: Studies in endocrine pharmacology. Biologic actions of some natural steroids on the liver. *New Engl. J. Med.* **278**, 378—384 (1968). [F 94,299/68

Kar, A. B., De, N. N.: Experimental heat stress and the adrenal hormones. *Bull. nat. Inst. Sci. India*, No. 10B, 41—43 (1955).
[C 72,791/55

Kar, A. B., Karkun, J. N., De, N. N.: The effect of 19-nortestosterone on the adrenal cortex of the rat. *Acta endocr. (Kbh.)* **25**, 238—248 (1957). [G 79,565/57

Kar, A. B., Roy, A. C., Chakravarty, R. N.: The effect of testosterone propionate on glycogen content and histopathology of the liver of experimental hypothyroid rats. *Indian J. med. Res.* **43**, 217—222 (1955). [C 17,531/55

Karásek, F.: Teoretické předpoklady chininové léčby srdce při thyreotoxikose. (Bases théoriques de la médication quinique de coeur au cours de l'hyperthyroidisme.) *Čas. lék. čes.* **76**, 105—146 (1937). [B 52,652/37

Karim, M. F., Taylor, W.: Steroid metabolism in the cat. Biliary and urinary excretion of metabolites of [4-^{14}C] oestradiol. *Biochem. J.* **117**, 267—270 (1970). [G 74,179/70

Karlson, P., Sekeris, C. E.: Biochemical mechanisms of hormone action. *Acta endocr. (Kbh.)* **53**, 505—518 (1966). [F 73,338/66

Karnofsky, D. A., Hamre, P. J., Hysom, G.: Toxicity of progesterone in the newborn mouse. *Proc. Soc. exp. Biol. (N.Y.)* **79**, 641—643 (1952). [B 69,772/52

Kass, E. H.: Effect of corticosteroids and of hormones of pregnancy on the lethal action of bacterial endotoxin. *Ann. N.Y. Acad. Sci.* **88**, 107—115 (1960). [D 35,079/60

Kass, E. H., Finland, M.: Effect of ACTH on induced fever. *New Engl. J. Med.* **243**, 693—695 (1950). [B 54,130/50

Kass, E. H., Finland, M.: The role of adrenal steroids in infection and immunity. *New Engl. J. Med.* **244**, 464—470 (1951). [B 59,076/51

Kass, E. H., Finland, M.: Adrenocortical hormones in infection and immunity. *Ann. Rev. Microbiol.* **7**, 361—388 (1953).
[C 80,582/53

Kass, E. H., Finland, M.: Adrenocortical hormones and the management of infection. *Ann. Rev. Med.* **8**, 1—18 (1957). [E 56,566/57

Kass, E. H., Finland, M.: Corticosteroids and infections. *Advanc. intern. Med.* **9**, 45—80 (1958). [D 87,314/58

Kass, E. H., Ingbar, S. H., Lundgren, M. M., Finland, M.: The effect of ACTH and cortisone on pneumococcal and influenza viral infections in the white mouse. *J. Lab. clin. Med.* **37**, 780—788 (1951). [B 69,981/51

Kass, E. H., Lundgren, M. M., Finland, M.: The effect of adrenal steroids, corticotropin and growth hormone on resistance to experimental infections. *J. exp. Med.* **99**, 89—104 (1954). [B 95,353/54

Katabuchi, H.: On the production of typhoid antitoxic substance and its relation with hormones. *Acta med. Keijo* **12**, 105—146 (1929).
[44,803/29

Katine, F., Hurd, E. L., Kupperman, H. S., DeGraff, A. C.: Prevention of fatty liver changes by cortisone in choline deficient rats (Abstr.). *J. Pharmacol. exp. Ther.* **106**, 399 to 400 (1952). [B 80,347/52

Kato, R.: An antagonism between 3—4 dioxyphenylalanine (DOPA) and 5-hydroxytryptophan (5-HTP). *Experientia (Basel)* **15**, 424—425 (1959). [C 78,047/59

Kato, R.: Un pretrattamento, eseguito 48 ore prima, con svariate sostanze può diminuire gli effetti farmacologici del nembutal. *Atti Soc. lombarda Sci. med.-biol.* 14, 777—780 (1959). [E60,785/59

Kato, R.: Reduced sensitivity to some drugs 48 h after chlorpromazine treatment. *Experientia (Basel)* 16, 427—428 (1960). [E87,340/60

Kato, R.: Modifications of the toxicity of strychnine and octomethylpyrophosphoramide (OMPA) induced by pretreatment with phenaglycodol and thiopental. *Arzneimittel-Forsch.* 11/8, 797—798 (1961). [D46,405/61

Kato, R.: Possible role of P-450 in the oxidation of drugs in liver microsomes. *J. Biochem. (Tokyo)* 59, 574—583 (1966). [G74,104/66

Kato, R.: Effects of starvation and refeeding on the oxidation of drugs by liver microsomes. *Biochem. Pharmacol.* 16, 871—881 (1967). [G66,471/67

Kato, R., Chiesara, E.: Diversa capacità di metabolizzazione della stricnica in rapporto al sesso. *Atti Accad. med. lombarda* 15, 397—401 (1960). [G68,581/60

Kato, R., Chiesara, E., Frontino, G.: Induction of hepatic carisoprodol-metabolizing enzyme by pretreatment with some neuropsychotropic drugs in rats. *Jap. J. Pharmacol.* 11, 31—36 (1961). [G74,632/61

Kato, R., Chiesara, E., Frontino, G.: Induced increase of meprobamate metabolism in rats pretreated with phenobarbital or phenaglycodol in relation to age. *Experientia (Basel)* 17, 520—521 (1961). [H27,665/61

Kato, R., Chiesara, E., Frontino, G.: Influence of sex difference on the pharmacological action and metabolism of some drugs. *Biochem. Pharmacol.* 11, 221—227 (1962). [G64,325/62

Kato, R., Chiesara, E., Vassanelli, P.: Metabolic differences of carisoprodol in the rat in relation to sex. *Med. exp. (Basel)* 4, 387—392 (1961). [G66,023/61

Kato, R., Chiesara, E., Vassanelli, P.: Increased activity of microsomal strychnine-metabolizing enzyme induction by phenobarbital and other drugs. *Biochem. Pharmacol.* 11, 913—922 (1962). [G74,030/62

Kato, R., Chiesara, E., Vassanelli, P.: Stimulating effect of some inhibitors of the drug metabolisms (SKF 525 A, Lilly 18947, Lilly 32391 and MG 3062) on excretion of ascorbic acid and drug metabolisms. *Med. exp. (Basel)* 6, 254—260 (1962). [D27,768/62

Kato, R., Chiesara, E., Vassanelli, P.: Metabolic differences of strychnine in the rat in relation to sex. *Jap. J. Pharmacol.* 12, 26—33 (1962). [D38,983/62

Kato, R., Chiesara, E., Vassanelli, P.: Further studies on the inhibition and stimulation of microsomal drug-metabolizing enzymes of rat liver by various compounds. *Biochem. Pharmacol.* 13, 69—83 (1964). [E47,494/64

Kato, R., Gillette, J.: Differences in the effects of starvation and sucrose feeding on TPNH-dependent enzymes in liver microsomes of rats. *Fed. Proc.* 23, 538 (1964). [F5,638/64

Kato, R., Gillette, J. R.: Effect of starvation on NADPH-dependent enzymes in liver microsomes of male and female rats. *J. Pharmacol. exp. Ther.* 150, 279—284 (1965). [F57,816/65

Kato, R., Gillette, J. R.: Sex differences in the effects of abnormal physiological states on the metabolism of drugs by rat liver microsomes. *J. Pharmacol. exp. Ther.* 150, 285—291 (1965). [F57,817/65

Kato, R., Onoda, K.: Effect of morphine administration on the activities of microsomal drug-metabolizing enzyme systems in liver of different species. *Jap. J. Pharmacol.* 16, 217 to 219 (1966). [G68,411/66

Kato, R., Onoda, K.: Studies on the regulation of the activity of drug oxidation in rat liver microsomes by androgen and estrogen. *Biochem. Pharmacol.* 19, 1649—1660 (1970). [G75,544/70

Kato, R., Onoda, K. I., Omori, Y.: Mechanism of thyroxine-induced increase in steroid Δ^4-reductase activity in male rats. *Endocr. jap.* 17, 215—219 (1970). [H31,735/70

Kato, R., Takahashi, A.: Thyroid hormone and activities of drug-metabolizing enzymes and electron transport systems of rat liver microsomes. *Molec. Pharmacol.* 4, 109—120 (1968). [G55,715/68

Kato, R., Takahashi, A.: Effect of phenobarbital on the activities of drug-metabolizing enzymes and electron transport system of liver microsomes in alloxan diabetes and thyroxine treated rats. *Jap. J. Pharmac.* 19, 45—52 (1969). [H11,853/69

Kato, R., Takahashi, A.: Decreased hydroxylation of steroid hormones by liver microsomes from rats bearing walker carcinosarcoma 256. *Cancer Res.* 30, 2346—2352 (1970). [H30,605/70

Kato, R., Takahashi, A., Ohshima, T., Hosoya, E.: Effect of morphine administration on the hydroxylation of steroid hormones by rat liver microsomes. *J. Pharmacol. exp. Ther.* **174**, 211 to 220 (1970). [H 27,934/70

Kato, R., Takahashi, A., Omori, Y.: Effect of androgen and estrogen on the hydroxylation of steroid hormones by rat liver microsomes. *Endocr. jap.* **16**, 653—663 (1969). [H 25,499/69

Kato, R., Takahashi, A., Omori, Y.: The mechanism of sex differences in the anesthetic action of progesterone in rats. *Europ. J. Pharmacol.* **13**, 141—149 (1971). [H 34,571/71

Kato, R., Takahashi, A., Onoda, K. I., Omori, Y.: Effect of adrenalectomy on the substrate interaction with cytochrome P-450 in the hydroxylation of steroid hormones by liver microsomes. *Endocr. jap.* **17**, 207—213 (1970). [H 31,734/70

Kato, R., Takanaka, A.: Effect of starvation on the in vivo metabolism and effect of drugs in female and male rats. *Jap. J. Pharmacol.* **17**, 208—217 (1967). [F 88,660/67

Kato, R., Takanaka, A., Omori, Y.: Factors affecting toxicity and metabolisms of OMPA (octamethylpyrophosphoramide) in rats. *Jap. J. Pharmacol.* **17**, 509—518 (1967). [H 34,342/67

Kato, R., Takanaka, A., Onoda, K.: Species and sex differences in aminopyrine N-demethylating activity of liver microsomes under unphysiological conditions. *Jap. J. Pharmacol.* **18**, 516—517 (1968). [G 80,897/68

Kato, R., Takanaka, A., Onoda, K.: Individual difference in the effect of drugs in relation to the tissue concentration of drugs. *Jap. J. Pharmacol.* **19**, 260—267 (1969). [H 15,635/69

Kato, R., Takanaka, A., Shoji, H.: Inhibition of drug-metabolizing enzymes of liver microsomes by hydrazine derivatives in relation to their lipid solubility. *Jap. J. Pharmacol.* **19**, 315—322 (1969). [H 15,638/69

Kato, R., Takanaka, A., Takahashi, A., Onoda, K.: Species differences in the alteration of drug-metabolizing activities of liver microsomes by thyroxine treatment. *Jap. J. Pharmacol.* **19**, 5—18 (1969). [H 11,851/69

Kato, R., Takayanaghi, M.: Differences among the action of phenobarbital, methylcholanthrene and male sex hormone on microsomal drug-metabolizing enzyme systems of rat liver. *Jap. J. Pharmacol.* **16**, 380—390 (1966). [F 76,403/66

Kato, R., Takayanagi, M., Oshima, T.: Differences in the oxidative metabolism of drugs by liver microsomes. *Jap. J. Pharmacol.* **19**, 53—62 (1969). [H 11,854/69

Kato, R., Vassanelli, P.: Induction of increased meprobamate metabolism in rats pretreated with some neurotropic drugs. *Biochem. Pharmacol.* **11**, 779—794 (1962). [D 40,237/62

Kato, R., Vassanelli, P., Frontino, G., Chiesara, E.: Variation in the activity of liver microsomal drug-metabolizing enzymes in rats in relation to the age. *Biochem. Pharmacol.* **13**, 1037—1051 (1964). [G 17,077/64

Kato, Y.: Factors elevating liver tyrosine: 2-oxoglutarate aminotransferase activity in tumor-bearing mice. *Nagoya J. med. Sci.* **30**, 211—223 (1967). [G 54,276/67

Kaufmann, G.: Tetrachlorkohlenstoff-Zirrhose und Restauration der Leber. *Beitr. pathol. Anat.* **113**, 253—270 (1953). [E 60,536/53

Kawashima, S., Ueda, T.: Protective effect of ethylcarbamate on the sensitized rats to hypoxia by insulin. (Japanese text.) *J. Nara med. Ass.* **17**, 219—223 (1966). [F 68,970/66

Kay, J. H., Balla, G. A., Lamb, W.: Effect of certain antihistaminic and steroid compounds on appendical peritonitis. *Proc. Soc. exp. Biol. (N.Y.)* **76**, 496—497 (1951). [B 60,579/51

Kedrova, E. M., Krekhova, M. A.: Absence of summation of protective effect of cysteine and ACTH in irradiation of rats by X-ray. (Russian text.) *Med. Radiol. (Mosk.)* **4/1**, 60—63 (1959). [G 71,665/59

Keil, A. M.: Effects of oxytocin on the response to suxamethonium in rabbits, sheep and pigs. *Brit. J. Anaesth.* **34**, 306—308 (1692). [D 27,254/62

Kellaway, P. E., Hoff, H. E., Leblond, C. P.: The response to thyroxine after subtotal hepatectomy. *Endocrinology* **36**, 272—279 (1945). [B 14,515/45

Kelly, A. R., Shideman, F. E.: Liver as the major organ involved in the detoxication of thiopental by the dog (Abstr.). *Fed. Proc.* **8**, 306 (1949). [A 49,706/49

Kelly, L. S., Brown, B. A., Dobson, E. L.: Cell division and phagocytic activity in liver reticulo-endothelial cells. *Proc. Soc. exp. Biol. (N.Y.)* **110**, 555—559 (1962). [D 32,495/62

Kemény, T., Filipp, G., Csalay, L., Kelenhegyi, M.: Gonadok, thymus és anaphylaxia. *Kiserl. Orvostad.* **3**, 145—147 (1951). [B 66,729/51

Keminger, K.: Thyreotoxische Krisen in der Chirurgie. *Klin. Med. (Wien)* **21**, 1—34 (1966). [G 42,501/66

Kemmer, C., Müller, M.: Morphologische und histochemische Leberveränderungen weib-

licher Mäuse nach Oestrastilben D-Applikation. *Frankfurt. Z. Path.* **77**, 235—244 (1967).
[F 89,190/67

Kennedy, B. J., Pare, J. A. P., Pump, K. K., Beck, J. C., Johnson, L. G., Epstein, N. B., Venning, E. H., Browne, J. S. L.: Effect of adrenocorticotropic hormone (ACTH) on beryllium granulomatosis and silicosis. *Amer. J. Med.* **10**, 134—155 (1951). [B 59,278/51

Kennedy, W. P.: Sodium salt of C-C-cyclohexenylmethyl-N-methyl barbituric acid (Evipan) anaesthesia in laboratory animals. *J. Pharmacol. exp. Ther.* **50**, 347—353 (1934).
[A 43,060/34

Kenney, F. T.: On the nature of adrenocorticoid-induced increase in tyrosine-α-ketoglutarate transaminase activity of rat liver. *Biochem. biophys. Res. Commun.* **2**, 333—335 (1960). [D 98,193/60

Kenney, F. T.: Induction of tyrosine-α-ketoglutarate transaminase in rat liver. III. Immunochemical analysis. *J. biol. Chem.* **237**, 1610—1614 (1962). [E 89,716/62

Kenney, F. T.: Induction of tyrosine-α-ketoglutarate transaminase in rat liver. IV. Evidence for an increase in the rate of enzyme synthesis. *J. biol. Chem.* **237**, 3495—3498 (1962). [E 98,787/62

Kenney, F. T.: Regulation of tyrosine-α-ketoglutarate transaminase in rat liver. V. Repression in growth hormone-treated rats. *J. biol. Chem.* **242**, 4367—4371 (1967).
[G 50,810/67

Kenney, F. T., Albritton, W. L.: Repression of enzyme synthesis at the translational level and its hormonal control. *Proc. nat. Acad. Sci. (Wash.)* **54**, 1693—1698 (1965). [G 64,557/65

Kenney, F. T., Flora, R. M.: Induction of tyrosine-α-ketoglutarate transaminase in rat liver. I. Hormonal nature. *J. Biol. Chem.* **236**, 2699—2702 (1961). [D 12,237/61

Kenney, F. T., Holten, D., Hager, C. B.: Hormonal regulation of enzyme synthesis. *Gunna Symp. Endocr.* **5**, 31—41 (1968).
[H 4,503/68

Kenney, F. T., Kull, F. J.: Hydrocortisone-stimulated synthesis of nuclear RNA in enzyme induction. *Proc. nat. Acad. Sci. (Wash.)* **50**, 493—499 (1963). [G 22,373/63

Képinow, L.: Anaphylaxie chez les animaux éthyroïdés nourris avec de la thyroïde. *C. R. Soc. Biol. (Paris)* **87**, 409—411 (1922).
[13,298/22

Képinow, L.: Glande thyroïde et anaphylaxie. Influence de la glande thyroïde sur le choc anaphylactique lors de son administration per os peu de temps avant l'injection déchaînante. *C. R. Soc. Biol. (Paris)* **88**, 846—847 (1923).
[13,941/23

Képinow, L., Lanzenberg, A.: Glande thyroïde et anaphylaxie. *C. R. Soc. Biol. (Paris)* **86**, 906—908 (1922). [13,258/22

Képinow, L., Metalnikow, S.: Glande thyroïde et sensibilité des animaux tuberculeux envers la tuberculine. *C. R. Soc. Biol. (Paris)* **87**, 210 à 212 (1922). [40,285/22

Kepl, M., Caldwell, G., Ochsner, A.: Use of adrenal cortical hormone in Cl. welchii infections in guinea pigs. *Proc. Soc. exp. Biol. (N.Y.)* **52**, 25—26 (1943). [A 56,633/43

Keplinger, M. L., Lanier, G. E., Deichmann, W. B.: Effects of environmental temperature on the acute toxicity of a number of compounds in rats. *Toxicol. app. Pharmacol.* **1**, 156—161 (1959). [G 70,208/59

Kepp, R., Hofmann, D.: Über den Einfluß der weiblichen Keimdrüsen auf die allgemeine und lokale Strahlenempfindlichkeit. *Strahlentherapie* **108**, 34—42 (1959). [C 65,530/59

Kerman, E. F.: Experimental catalepsy in the rat produced by a steroid hormone: Desoxycorticosterone acetate, and the antagonistic effect of pentamethylenetetrazol (Metrazol). *Dis. nerv. Syst.* **8**, 313—317 (1947).
[A 43,330/47

Kersten, H., Staudinger, H.: Der Einfluß von Butazolidin auf die Cortisoninaktivierung in Leberhomogenaten. *Klin. Wschr.* **34**, 523—525 (1956). [G 67,796/56

Kessler, F. J., Krüskemper, H. L., Noell, G.: Tierexperimentelle Vergleichsuntersuchungen zur Wirkung von D-Thyroxin und D-Trijodthyronin bei alimentär gestörtem Lipidstoffwechsel. *Arzneimittel-Forsch.* **17**, 1190 bis 1195 (1967). [F 89,469/67

Ketkar, M. B., Sirsat, S. M.: Mast cells in experimental skin carcinogenesis in relation to hormonal stress. *Indian J. med. Sci.* **19**, 477 to 484 (1965). [G 32,601/65

Khandekar, J. D.: Catatoxic steroids. *J. Indian med. Ass.* **56**, 59 (1971). [G 70,492/71

Khandekar, J. D., Garg, B. D., Dardachti, D., Tuchweber, B., Kovacs, K.: Effect of cycloheximide on the ultrastructural changes produced by spironolactone and pregnenolone-16α-carbonitrile in the rat liver. *Beitr. Pathol.* (in press). [G 79,026

Khandekar, J. D., Garg, B. D., Kovacs, K.: Effect of N-y-phenylpropyl-N-benzyloxy acetamide (W-1372) on the liver ultrastructure in rats. *A. M. A. Arch. Path.* (in press) [G 79,016

Khandekar, J. D., Garg, B. D., Tuchweber, B., Kovacs, K.: Influence of cycloheximide on the ultrastructural changes in rat hepatocytes caused by spironolactone (SNL) and pregnenolone-16α-carbonitrile (PCN). (Abstr.) *5th Ann. Meet. Europ. Soc. clin. Invest., Scheveningen, Netherlands*, April 22—24, p. 48 (1971). [G 79,014/71

Khogali, A.: Quantitative studies on the suppression of the skeletal lesions of β-aminopropionitrile by L- and D-triiodothyronine. *J. Physiol.* 158, 29P—30P (1961). [D 10,840/61

Khogali, A.: Bone strength and calcium retention of rats in hypervitaminosis-A. *Quart. J. exp. Physiol.* 51, 120—129 (1966). [F 73,238/66

Khoobyarian, N., Walker, D. L.: Effect of cortisone on mouse resistance to intravenous toxicity of influenza virus. *Proc. Soc. exp. Biol. (N.Y.)* 94, 295—298 (1957). [C 30,210/57

Khrabrova, O. P.: Specific features in the reaction to shockogenic stimulus following aminazine administration. (Russian text.) *Byull. eksp. Biol. Med.* 51/2, 23—27 (1961). [D 49,985/61

Khrabrova, O. P.: On the application of ACTH and cortisone in experimental shock. (Russian text.) *Probl. Endokr. Gormonoter.* 8, 16—18 (1962). [D 33,557/62

Kilbourne, E. D.: Paradoxical effects of cortisone on influenza B virus infection of the chick embryo (Abstr.). *Amer. Soc. clin. Invest.* 34 (1952). [B 69,376/52

Kilbourne, E. D., Horsfall, F. L., Jr.: Increased virus in eggs injected with cortisone. *Proc. Soc. exp. Biol. (N.Y.)* 76, 116—118 (1951). [B 55,005/51

Kilbourne, E. D., Horsfall, F. L., Jr.: Lethal infection with Coxsackie virus of adult mice given cortisone. *Proc. Soc. exp. Biol. (N.Y.)* 77, 135—138 (1951). [B 65,487/51

Kim, U., Furth, J.: Relation of mammary tumors to mammotropes. II. Hormone responsiveness of 3-methylcholanthrene induced mammary carcinomas. *Proc. Soc. exp. Biol. (N.Y.)* 103, 643—645 (1960). [H 31,205/60

Kimbrough, R. D., Gaines, T. B., Linder, R. E.: The ultrastructure of livers of rats fed DDT and dieldrin. *A. M. A. Arch. environm. Hlth.* 22, 460—467 (1971). [G 81,969/71

Kimeldorf, D. J., Jones, D. C., Fishler, M. C.: The effect of exercise upon the lethality of roentgen rays for rats. *Science* 112, 175—176 (1950). [B 49,240/50

Kimura, A.: An electron microscopic study on regenerating rat liver after partial hepatectomy. I. Ultrastructural alterations of hepatocytes in early post-operative stage. (Japanese text.) *Sapporo med. J.* 35, 265—288 (1969). [G 75,331/69

Kind, L. S.: Inhibition of histamine death in pertussis-inoculated mice by cortisone and neoantergan. *J. Allergy* 24, 52—59 (1953). [B 81,943/53

Kind, L. S.: The altered reactivity of mice after inoculation with Bordetella pertussis vaccine. *Bact. Rev.* 22, 173—182 (1958). [E 67,787/58

King, J. E.: Sex differences in the response of rats to pentobarbital sodium. IV. Pentobarbital levels in pregnant and nonpregnant rats. *Amer. J. Obstet. Gynec.* 89, 1019—1025 (1964). [G 78,963/64

King, J. E., Becker, R. F.: The influence of sex on response of rat to pentobarbital. *Anat. Rec.* 136, 223 (1960). [E 38,612/60

King, J. E., Becker, R. F.: Differential response of pregnant rats to pentobarbital. *Anat. Rec.* 139, 245 (1961). [D 5,106/61

King, J. E., Becker, R. F.: Sex differences in the response of rats to pentobarbital sodium. I. Males, nonpregnant females, and pregnant females. *Amer. J. Obstet. Gynec.* 86, 856—864 (1963). [G 78,964/63

King, T. M., Burgard, J. K.: Drug interaction. *Amer. J. Obstet. Gynec.* 98, 128—134 (1967). [G 46,498/67

King, T. M., Fahim, M. S., Bolt, D. J.: Androgen response in phenobarbital-treated orchiectomized rats. *Amer. J. Obstet. Gynec.* 101, 850 to 852 (1968). [H 16,446/68

Kinoshita, F. K., Du Bois, K. P.: Induction of hepatic microsomal enzymes by Herban, Diuron, and other substituted urea herbicides. *Toxicol. appl. Pharmacol.* 17, 406—417 (1970). [G 78,681/70

Kinoshita, F. K., Frawley, J. P., Du Bois, K. P.: Quantitative measurement of induction of hepatic microsomal enzymes by various dietary levels of DDT and toxaphene in rats. *Toxicol. appl. Pharmacol.* 9, 505—513 (1966). [G 71,863/66

Kinsell, L. W., Zillesson, F. O., Smith, A. M., Palmer, J.: Protective action of cardiac glycosides and adrenal cortical hormone against thyroxin. *Endocrinology* 20, 221—226 (1942). [A 37,369/42

Kinsey, V. E.: Use of sodium pentobarbital for repeated anesthesia in the white rat. *J. Amer. Pharm. Ass.* 29, 387—390 (1940). [A 39,742/40

Kirby, A. H. M.: The combined action of 2-acetylaminofluorene and sex hormones in the Wistar rat. *Brit. J. Cancer* 1, 68—79 (1947). [B 30,101/47

Kirschbaum, A., Shapiro, J. R., Mixer, H. W.: Synergistic action of leukemogenic agents. *Cancer Res.* 13, 262—268 (1953). [H 27,666/53

Kirsteins, A.: Survival of cortisone- and corticotropin-treated rats during exposure to cold. *Surgery* 40, 337—348 (1956). [C 41,958/56

Klaassen, C. D.: Plasma disappearance and biliary excretion of sulfobromophthalein and phenol-3,6-dibromphthalein disulfonate after microsomal enzyme induction. *Biochem. Pharmacol.* 19, 1241—1249 (1970). [G 75,506/70

Klaassen, C. D., Plaa, G. L.: Studies on the mechanism of phenobarbital-enhanced sulfobromophthalein disappearance. *J. Pharmacol. exp. Ther.* 161, 361—366 (1968). [F 99,395/68

Klain, G. J., Hannon, J. P.: Gluconeogenesis in cold-exposed rats. *Fed. Proc.* 28, 965—968 (1969). [H 13,174/69

Klärner, P., Klärner, R.: Die Beeinflussung induzierter Lungentumoren durch Hitze, Alloxan-Diabetes, Thyroxin und andere Agentien. *Z. Krebsforsch.* 62, 297—301 (1958). [C 45,812/58

Klatskin, G.: Toxic and drug-induced hepatitis. In: Schiff, L.; *Diseases of the Liver*, 3rd ed., p. 498—601. Philadelphia, Toronto: J. B. Lippincott Company 1969. [G 65,221/69

Klein, M.: Development of hepatomas in inbred albino mice following treatment with 20-methylcholanthrene. *Cancer Res.* 19, 1109—1113 (1959). [G 76,354/59

Kleinbaum, H.: Vitamin D_2-Intoxikation im Kindesalter. *Dtsch. Gesundh.-Wesen* 17, 35—37 (1962). [E 23,570/62

Kleiner, G. J., Kresch, L., Arias, I. M.: Studies of hepatic excretory function. II. The effect of norethynodrel and mestranol on bromsulfalein sodium metabolism in women of childbearing age. *New Engl. J. Med.* 273, 420—423 (1965). [F 47,209/65

Kleinsorg, H., Loeser, A.: Schilddrüse und kompensatorische Hypertrophie der Niere bei Nephrektomie. *Arch. int. Pharmacodyn.* 79, 83—96 (1949). [B 41,137/49

Klevay, L. M.: Dieldrin excretion by the isolated perfused rat liver: a sexual difference. *Toxicol. appl. Pharmacol.* 17, 813—815 (1970). [G 80,049/70

Kligman, A. M., Baldridge, G. D., Rebell, G., Pillsbury, D. M.: The effect of cortisone on the pathologic responses of guinea pigs infected cutaneously with fungi, viruses, and bacteria. *J. Lab. clin. Med.* 37, 615—620 (1951). [G 64,164/51

Kline, E. M., Inkley, S. R., Pritchard, W. H.: Five cases from the fluorescent lamp industry. Treatment of chronic beryllium poisoning with ACTH and cortisone. *Arch. industr. Hyg.* 3, 549—564 (1951). [B 65,488/51

Kline, R. F., Britton, S. W.: Age and sex differences in resistance to anoxia (Abstr.). *Fed. Proc.* 4, 41 (1945). [85,856/45

Klinenberg, J. R., Miller, F.: Effect of corticosteroids on blood salicylate concentration. *J. Amer. med. Ass.* 194, 601—604 (1965). [F 54,504/65

Klinger, R.: Über den angeblichen Antagonismus von Schilddrüse und Milz. *Biochem. Z.* 92, 376—384 (1918). [51,094/18

Klinger, W.: Untersuchungen zum Mechanismus der Enzyminduktion bei Ratten und Mäusen. VII. Der Einfluß der Schilddrüse auf die Askorbinsäure-Normausscheidung und ihre Steigerung sowie auf die Hexobarbitalschlafzeit und ihre Verkürzung durch Barbital. *Acta biol. med. germ.* 16, 404—414 (1966). [F 66,416/66

Klinger, W.: Toxizität, narkotische Wirkung, Aufwachkonzentration im Blut, Elimination aus dem Blut und Biotransformation von Hexobarbital bei Ratten unterschiedlichen Alters nach Induktion mit Barbital und nach CCl_4-Schädigung. *Arch. int. Pharmacodyn.* 184, 5—18 (1970). [H 25,517/70

Klinger, W., Elger, J., Franke, H., Reinicke, C., Traeger, A., Volkmann, H., Wahrenberg, I., Ankermann, H.: Untersuchungen zum Mechanismus der Enzyminduktion. XV. Induktionsmuster und submikroskopische Veränderungen in der Leber nach Applikation von Phenylbutazon bei unterschiedlich alten Ratten. *Acta biol. med. germ.* 24, 463—482 (1970). [H 28,896/70

Klinger, W., Koch, M., Kramer, B.: Untersuchungen zum Mechanismus der Enzyminduktion bei Ratten und Mäusen. V. Der Einfluß der Keimdrüsen auf die L-Askorbinsäure-Normausscheidung und ihre Steigerung sowie auf die Hexobarbitalschlafzeit und ihre

Verkürzung durch Barbital. *Acta biol. med. germ.* **15**, 700—706 (1965). [F 62,929/65

Klinger, W., Zwacka, G., Ankermann, H.: Untersuchungen zum Mechanismus der Enzyminduktion. XIII. Die Übertragung eines zytoplasmatischen Hemmfaktors der Entwicklung mikrosomaler Leberenzyme aus der Leber von Rattenfoeten auf infantile Ratten. *Acta biol. med. germ.* **20**, 137—145 (1968). [H 30,598/68

Klinkmann, H., Hübel, A.: Testosteron-Behandlung bei schwerer intravenöser Sublimat-Intoxikation. *Münch. med. Wschr.* **106**, 1466 bis 1468 (1964). [F 19,820/64

Klotz, H. P.: Le rôle du terrain préalable dans l'accoutumance à l'alcool. *C. R. Soc. Biol. (Paris)* **124**, 23—25 (1937). [A 96,052/37

Klug, W.: Klinische Erfahrungen mit dem anabol wirkenden Testosteronderivat Nerobol. *Dtsch. Gesundh.-Wesen* **19**, 1360—1363 (1964). [G 19,783/64

Knaab, I.: Reid Hunt-Reaktion und Leberglykogen. *Naunyn-Schmiedebergs Arch. Pharmak.* **171**, 65—72 (1933). [14,828/33

Knigge, K. M.: Neuroendocrine mechanisms influencing ACTH and TSH secretion and their role in cold acclimation. *Fed. Proc.* **19**, Sup. 5, 45—50 (1960). [C 97,819/60

Knox, A. W.: Influence of pregnancy in mice on the course of infection with murine poliomyelitis virus. *Proc. Soc. exp. Biol. (N.Y.)* **73**, 520—523 (1950). [B 47,631/50

Knox, W. E.: Two mechanisms which increase in vivo the liver tryptophan peroxidase activity: specific enzyme adaptation and stimulation of the pituitary-adrenal system. *Brit. J. exp. Path.* **32**, 462—469 (1951). [B 71,418/51

Knox, W. E.: Adaptive enzymes in the regulation of animal metabolism. In: Prosser; *Physiological Adaptation*, p. 107—125. Washington, D.C.: Amer. Physiol. Soc. 1958. [G 67,799/58

Knox, W. E.: Adaptive enzymes in animals. In: Mongar and de Reuck; *Ciba Found. Symp. for Symp. on Drug Action on Enzymes and Drug Action*, p. 275, London: J. & A. Churchill Ltd. 1962. [G 51,969/62

Knox, W. E.: The adaptive control of tryptophan and tyrosine metabolism in animals. *Trans. N.Y. Acad. Sci.* **25**, 503—512 (1963). [D 66,995/63

Knox, W. E.: Substrate-type induction of tyrosine transaminase, illustrating a general adaptive mechanism in animals. In: Weber; *Advances in Enzyme Regulation* 2, p. 311—318. New York: MacMillan Co. 1964. [G 65,171/64

Knox, W. E., Auerbach, V. H.: The hormonal control of tryptophan peroxidase in the rat. *J. biol. Chem.* **214**, 307—313 (1955). [E 76,825/55

Knox, W. E., Auerbach, V. H., Lin, E. C. C.: Enzymatic and metabolic adaptations in animals. *Physiol. Rev.* **36**, 164—254 (1956). [E 83,471/56

Kobayashi, K.: Experimental analysis of skin cancer production in mice thymectomized at adult age. *J. Fac. Sci. Tokyo., Sect. 4*, **11**, 537—540 (1969). [H 27,113/69

Kobayashi, K.: Effect of thymus extract injection and thymus cell transfusion on papilloma production due to DMBA, in mice thymectomized as adults. *J. Fac. Sci. Tokyo., Sect. 4*, **11**, 541—544 (1969). [H 27,114/69

Kobayashi, S., Nakamura, W., Eto, H.: Protective effect of 5-hydroxytryptophan against lethal doses of X-radiation in mice. *Int. J. Radiat. Res.* **11**, 505—508 (1966). [G 73,566/66

Kobayashi, T., Danjo, H., Hata, K.: Fine structural changes in the liver cells of Gilbert's and Dubin-Johnson's syndrome induced by phenobarbital. (Japanese text.) *Jap. J. clin. Elect. Micr.* **2**, 418—419 (1970). [H 28,794/70

Kobrin, S., Seifter, J.: ω-Amino acids and various biogenic amines as antagonists to pentylenetetrazol. *J. Pharmacol. exp. Ther.* **154**, 646—651 (1966). [F 74,422/66

Koch, P., Guy, R., Venne, L.: Influence du Somatron, de l'Acton et du Duracton sur l'évolution du trauma thermique chez le rat. *Un. méd. Can.* **86**, 515—518 (1957). [C 33,922/57

Koch, R.: Untersuchungen über einen biologischen Strahlenschutz. 80. Mitteilg. Über quantitative Beziehungen des chemischen Strahlenschutzes zu seinem Wirkungsmechanismus. *Strahlentherapie* **134**, 102—109 (1967). [G 51,862/67

Kochmann, M.: Standardisierung des Parathyreoideahormons und seine antagonistische Wirkung gegenüber dem Oxalation. *Dtsch. med. Wschr.* **60**, 406 (1934). [55,946/34

Kochmann, M.: Zur Wertbestimmung des Parathyreoideahormons mittels Natriumfluorid. *Dtsch. med. Wschr.* **60**, 1062—1063 (1934). [55,947/34

Koch-Weser, J.: Potentiation by glucagon of the hypoprothrombinemic action of warfarin. *Ann. intern. Med.* **72**, 331—335 (1970). [G 73,494/70

Kocsár, L. T., Bertók, L., Várterész, V.: Effect of bile acids on the intestinal absorption of endotoxin in rats. *J. Bact.* **100**, 220—223 (1969). [G 69,983/69]

Kodama, M., Moore, G. E.: The role of the thymus in polyoma virus infection. *J. nat. Cancer Inst.* **30**, 225—238 (1963). [D 56,877/63]

Kodicek, E.: Discussion. In: Wolstenholme & O'Connor; *Bone Structure and Metabolism*, p. 201—205. London: J. and A. Churchill Ltd. 1956. [C 32,412/56]

Kodoma, Y., Bock, F. G.: Benzo(α)pyrene-metabolizing enzyme activity of livers of various strains of mice. *Cancer Res.* **30**, 1846—1849 (1970). [H 28,307/70]

Kodousková, V., Kodousek, R., Dušek, J.: Calcification of the Islets of Langerhans and renal corticol tubular epithelium in alloxan treated calciphylactic rats. *Experientia (Basel)* **19**, 314 (1963). [D 69,797/63]

Koerner, D. R.: Assay and substrate specificity of liver 11β-hydroxysteroid dehydrogenase. *Biochim. biophys. Acta (Amst.)* **176**, 377—382 (1969). [G 65,718/69]

Koff, R. S., Carter, E. A., Lui, S., Isselbacher, K. J.: Prevention of the ethanol-induced fatty liver in the rat by phenobarbital. *Gastroenterology* **59**, 50—61 (1970). [G 76,179/70]

Kohn, H. I., Corbascio, A. N., Gultman, P. H.: Estradiol treatment and the X-ray-induced acceleration of the age-specific mortality rate. *J. nat. Cancer Inst.* **29**, 853—862 (1962). [D 42,858/62]

Kohn, H. I., Corbascio, A. N., Gultman, P. H., Ludwig, F. C.: Effect of X-ray dose and estradiol treatment on the chronic mortality rate of adult female mice. *Radiation Res.* **14**, 479 (1961). [D 9,831/61]

Kohn, H. I., Kallman, R. F.: The influence of strain on acute X-ray lethality in the mouse. 1. LD_{50} and death rate studies. *Radiat. Res.* **5**, 309—317 (1956). [C 25,371/56]

Kohn, R. R., Rivera-Velez, J. M.: Function of collagen: blood pressure in lathyritic rats. *Nature (Lond.)* **207**, 537 (1965). [F 73,678/65]

Köhnlein, H. E., Rehn, J.: Der Einfluß von Androgenen auf die ischaemisierte Rattenniere. *Arzneimittel-Forsch.* **12**, 1112—1116 (1962). [D 44,607/62]

Köhnlein, H. E., Rehn, J., Berneker, G. C.: Der Einfluß des Wachstumshormons auf die ischaemisierte Rattenniere. *Arzneimittel-Forsch.* **12**, 957—963 (1962). [D 38,961/62]

Koike, K., Otaka, T., Okui, S.: Repressive effect of cortisone administration on protein synthesis of mouse liver in vitro. *J. Biochem. (Tokyo)* **63**, 709—715 (1968). [H 15,766/68]

Koivisto, M., Ojala, A., Järvinen, P. A.: The effect of neonatal bilirubin levels of oestrogen given to the mother before delivery. *Ann. clin. Res.* **2**, 204—208 (1970). [G 78,915/70]

Kolb, K. H., Kimbel, K. H., Schulze, P. E.: Der Einfluß verschiedener anabol wirksamer Steroide auf die Farbstoffausscheidung in die Rattengalle. *Arzneimittel-Forsch.* **12**, 228—230 (1962). [D 22,260/62]

Koller, M.: Sulla dipendenza dal sesso dell'attività di steroidi ad azione anestetica. *Boll. Soc. ital. Biol. sper.* **32**, 78—80 (1956). [C 19,288/56]

Komiya, A.: Effect of adrenocortical hormones on the concentration of barbital in mouse brain. *Gunma J. med. Sci.* **4**, 87 (1955). [C 7,045/55]

Komiya, A.: Effects of the administration of adrenocortical hormones and ACTH on the barbital anesthesia. *Gunma J. med. Sci.* **4**, 175 (1955). [C 8,533/55]

Komiya, A., Machida, J., Kosuge, M., Fukushima, K.: The effect of the administration of cortisone acetate on barbital anesthesia in male rabbits. *Gunma J. med. Sci.* **5**, 71 (1956). [D 26,331/56]

Komiya, A., Shibata, K.: Effect of adrenalectomy and replacement with adrenocortical steroids on barbital anesthesia in mice. *J. Pharmacol. exp. Ther.* **116**, 98—106 (1956). [C 13,129/56]

Komiya, A., Shibata, K.: Effect of adrenocortical steroids and ACTH administration on barbital anesthesia in normal mice. *J. Pharmacol. exp. Ther.* **117**, 68—74 (1956). [C 16,708/56]

Komiya, A., Shibata, K., Kosuge, M.: Effects of epinephrine and norepinephrine on barbiturates anesthesia in mice. *Endocr. jap.* **2**, 221—228 (1956). [C 21,326/56]

König, M. P.: Androgentherapie und Antiandrogene. *Schweiz. med. Wschr.* **99**, 744—747 (1969). [G 66,684/69]

Konishi, G.: Change in Δ^4-steroid hydrogenase activity in rat liver after tumor implantation. *Bull. Tokyo med. dent. Univ.* **16**, 37—46 (1969). [H 14,720/69]

Korenchevsky, V.: I. The influence of removal of sexual glands on the skeleton of animals kept on normal or rickets-producing diets. II. Spontaneous rickets in rats. *J. Path. Bact.* **26**, 207—223 (1923). [14,032/23]

Korenchevsky, V.: Treatment of senescent male rats with cortisone acetate alone or together with sex and thyroid hormones. *J. Geront.* **11**, 261—267 (1956). [C 18,714/56

Korenchevsky, V., Dennison, M., Kohn-Speyer, A.: Simultaneous administration of testicular hormone with antuitrin and prolan or with desiccated thyroid. *Biochem. J.* **27**, 1513—1516 (1933). [16,451/33

Korényi, Z., Hajdu, I.: Die Rolle der Nebenniere im physiologischen Mechanismus des Trainings. *Arbeitsphysiol.* **12**, 31—43 (1942). [A 56,945/42

Korpássy, B., Kovács, K., Sztanojevits, A.: Influence of sex and dietary casein content upon lethal and liver injurious effect of tannic acid. Ineffectiveness of certain so-called liver protecting substances. *Acta physiol. Acad. Sci. hung.* **3**, 233—241 (1952). [B 74,333/52

Korteweg, R., Thomas, F.: Tumor induction and tumor growth in hypophysectomized mice. *Amer. J. Cancer* **37**, 36—44 (1939). [A 33,075/39

Korting, G. W., Holzmann, H., Morsches, B.: Enzymatic determination in serum of lathyritic and prednisone-treated lathyritic rats. *Nature (Lond.)* **209**, 1130 (1966). [F 63,363/66

Kory, R. C., Bradley, M. H., Watson, R. N., Callahan, R., Peters, B. J.: A six-month evaluation of an anabolic drug, norethandrolone in underweight persons. II. Bromsulphalein (BSP) retention and liver function. *Amer. J. Med.* **26**, 243—248 (1959). [C 75,742/59

Kosdoba, A. S.: Zur Frage nach den pathologisch-anatomischen Begründungen Zusammenhanges einiger chirurgischer Erkrankungen des Blutgefäßsystems mit Nikotinismus. *Mitt. Grenzgeb. Med. Chir.* **41**, 687—699 (1929—30). [A 39,432/29—30

Koss, L. G., Lavin, P.: Effects of a single dose of cyclophosphamide on various organs in the rat. II. Response of urinary bladder epithelium according to strain and sex. *J. nat. Cancer Inst.* **44**, 1195—1200 (1970). [G 75,309/70

Kostowski, W., Nowacka, M.: Influence of some adrenal steroids on hexobarbital and hydroxydione anaesthesia. *Arch. int. Pharmacodyn.* **184**, 362—365 (1970). [H 26,526/70

Kostrubiak, W., Howard, J. M.: Studies of the effect of aldosterone in the experimental toxemia with the alpha-toxin of Clostridium welchii. *J. Trauma* **4**, 814—818 (1964). [G 57,804/64

Kostrubiak, W., Howard, J. M.: The protective effect of aldosterone against the toxin of clostridium tetani. *Surg. Gynec. Obstet.* **121**, 59—62 (1965). [F 43,646/65

Kotin, P., Edmondson, H. A., Falk, H. L.: The inhibiting effect of estrogens on the development of cirrhosis and hepatocellular carcinoma in rats on a choline deficient diet. *Amer. J. Path.* **32**, 633—634 (1956). [C 16,597/56

Kottke, F. J., Taylor, C. B., Kubicek, W. G., Erickson, D. M., Evans, G. T.: Adrenal cortex and altitude tolerance. *Amer. J. Physiol.* **153**, 16—20 (1948). [B 25,989/48

Kottra, J., Kappas, A.: Steroid effects on hepatic function: recent observations. *Ann. Rev. Med.* **18**, 325—332 (1967). [F 79,911/67

Kottra, L. L., Kappas, A.: Estrogen pharmacology. III. Effect of estradiol on plasma disappearance rate of sulfobromophthalein in man. *Arch. intern. Med.* **117**, 373—376 (1966). [G 37,574/66

Koudstaal, J., Hardonk, M. J.: Histochemical demonstration of enzymes related to NADPH-dependent hydroxylating systems in rat liver after phenobarbital treatment. *Histochemie* **20**, 68—77 (1969). [G 69,482/69

Koudstaal, J., Hardonk, M. J.: Histochemical demonstration of enzymes in rat liver during post-natal development. Enzymes related to NADPH-dependent hydroxylating systems and to sex-difference. *Histochemie* **23**, 71—81 (1970). [G 78,115/70

Kovách, A. G. B., Takács, L., Moháscsi, A., Kaldor, V., Kalmar, Z.: Effect of metabolism-increasing or -decreasing substances on the susceptibility of rats to shock. *Acta physiol. Acad. Sci. hung.* **11**, 181—188 (1957). [C 50,699/57

Kovács, I. B., Görög, P.: Bronchoconstrictor effect of endotoxin in guinea-pig; the protective effect of antihistamine and antiinflammatory compounds. *Europ. J. Pharmacol.* **4**, 91—95 (1968). [H 2,570/68

Kovács, K.: Effect of androgenisation on the development of mammary tumours in rats induced by the oral administration of 9,10-dimethyl-1,2-benzanthracene. *Brit. J. Cancer* **19**, 531—537 (1965). [G 34,582/65

Kovács, K.: Effect of spironolactone on the liver and of 7,12-dimethylbenz(a)anthracene on the adrenal cortex. An electronmicroscopic study. Workshop on DMBA Activity, Laval Univ. Quebec City, p. 57—62 (1969). [G 70,404/69

Kovács, K., Blascheck, J. A., Gardell, C.: Spironolactone-induced proliferation of smooth-surfaced endoplasmic reticulum in the liver of rats. *Z. ges. exp. Med.* **152**, 104—110 (1970). [G 60,045/70

Kovács, K., Blascheck, J. A., Garg, B. D., Somogyi, A.: Effect of cyproterone acetate on the liver ultrastructure in rats. *Horm. metab. Res.* **3**, 44—47 (1971). [G 70,476/71

Kovács, K., Garg, B. D., Khandekar, J. D.: Hepatic injury caused by N-y-phenylpropyl-N-benzyloxy acetamide (W-1372). A light and electron microscopic study. *J. Pharm. Sci.* (in press). [G 79,003

Kovács, K., Khandekar, J., Dardachti, D., Garg, B. D., Tuchweber, B.: Ultrastructural changes in rat liver cells after intramuscular implantation of a Walker tumor. *Experientia (Basel)* (in press). [G 46,737

Kovács, K., Khandekar, J. D., Dardachti, D., Garg, B. D., Tuchweber, B.: Alteraciones ultraestructurales producidas por la pregnenolona-16α-carbonitrilada en hepatocitos de ratas portadoras de un tumor Walker. *Rev. argent Med. intern.* (in press). [G 79,033

Kovács, K., Somogyi, A.: Prevention by spironolactone of 7,12-dimethylbenz(a)anthracene-induced adrenal necrosis. *Proc. Soc. exp. Biol. (N.Y.)* **131**, 1350—1352 (1969). [G 60,025/69

Kovács, K., Somogyi, A.: Abolition by Dl-ethionine of the protective effect of spironolactone on 7,12-dimethylbenz(a)anthracene-induced adrenal necrosis in rats. *Biochim. Biol. sper.* **8**, 227—230 (1969). [G 60,060/69

Kovács, K., Somogyi, A.: Suppression by spironolactone of 7,12-dimethylbenz(a)anthracene-induced mammary tumors. *Europ. J. Cancer* **6**, 195—201 (1970). [G 60,089/70

Kovács, K., Szijj, I.: Effect of alloxan diabetes and insulin administration on the incidence of pituitary necrosis caused by hexadimethrine bromide in rats. *Experientia (Basel)* **24**, 257—258 (1968). [F 96,892/68

Kowalewski, K.: Uptake of radiosulphur in growing bones of cockerels treated with cortisone and 17-ethyl-19-nortestosterone. *Proc. Soc. exp. Biol. (N.Y.)* **97**, 432—434 (1958). [C 48,527/58

Kowalewski, K.: Comparison of the effects of cortisone and certain anabolic-androgenic steroids on the uptake of radiosulfur in a healing fractured bone. *Endocrinology* **62**, 493—497 (1958). [C 50,864/58

Kowalewski, K.: Uptake of radiosulfate in growing bones of cockerels treated with cortisone and certain anabolic-androgenic steroids. *Endocrinology* **63**, 759—764 (1958). [C 61,936/58

Kowalewski, K.: Effect of certain androgenic steroids and cortisone on gastric ulcerogenesis in fasting rats. *Proc. Soc. exp. Biol. (N.Y.)* **101**, 147—150 (1959). [C 68,938/59

Kowalewski, K.: Effect of steroids on bone formation. In: Gross; *Protein Metabolism (An Inter. Symp.)*, p. 238—262. Berlin, Göttingen, Heidelberg: Springer Verlag 1962. [G 41,978/62

Kowalewski, K., Bain, G. O.: Prevention of post-histaminic gastric ulcers in guinea pigs by posterior pituitary extract. *Acta gastro-ent. belg.* **17**, 539—551 (1954). [C 3,897/54

Kowalewski, K., Couves, C. M., Lang, A.: Protective action of 17-ethyl-19-nortestosterone against the inhibition of bone repair in the lathyrus-fed rat. *Acta endocr. (Kbh.)* **30**, 268—272 (1959). [C 63,273/59

Kowalewski, K., Emery, M. A.: Effect of a lathyrus factor and of an anabolic steroid on healing of fractures in rats studied by ^{35}S uptake method. *Acta endocr. (Kbh.)* **34**, 317—322 (1960). [C 86,516/60

Kowalewski, K., Gort, J.: An anabolic androgen as a stimulant of bone healing in rats treated with cortisone. *Acta endocr. (Kbh.)* **30**, 273 to 276 (1959). [C 63,274/59

Kozlowski, H., Hrabowska, M.: Über den Einfluß anaboler Steroide auf die Entwicklung der experimentellen Amyloidose bei Mäusen. *Zbl. allg. Path. path. Anat.* **112**, 184—193 (1969). [H 14,243/69

Kozuka, S.: Inhibiting effect of reserpine and female sensitivity in hepatic tumor induction with 2,7-diacetamidofluorene in SMA/Ms strain mice. *Cancer Res.* **30**, 1384—1386 (1970). [H 27,469/70

Kracht, J., Meissner, G.: Wachstumshormon und Cortison bei experimenteller Tuberkulose mit unterschiedlicher Keimvirulenz. *Frankfurt. Z. Path.* **67**, 391—405 (1956). [C 21,867/56

Krahe, M., Heinen, G.: Über den proteinanabolen Effekt von Methandrostenolon auf das Yoshida-Sarkom und das Walker-256-Carcinosarkom. *Klin. Wschr.* **40**, 913—916 (1962). [D 35,677/62

Krahe, M., Künkel, H.-A.: Die Strahlenempfindlichkeit der Ratten bei erhöhtem Grundumsatz. *Strahlentherapie* **106**, 260—262 (1958). [C 77,236/58

Kramer, M., Arrigoni-Martelli, E.: Die Verstärkung des narkotischen Effekts und die Abbauhemmung von Hexobarbital durch Malonsäurederivate. *Naunyn-Schmiedebergs Arch. Pharmak.* **237**, 264—275 (1959). [G 74,673/59]

Kratter, V., Martelli, O. F.: Ricerche sperimentali sul comportamento di conigli stimizzati in rapporto alle infezioni provocate. *Sperimentale* **99**, 453—470 (1949). [B 60,263/49]

Krawczak, J. J., Brodie, B. B.: Effect of adrenalectomy and complete blockade of adrenergic function on mortality from histamine, endotoxin, formation and tourniquet stress in rats. *Pharmacology (Basel)* **3**, 65—75 (1970). [H 25,296/70]

Kreek, M. J., Peterson, R. E., Sleisenger, M. H., Jeffries, G. H.: Influence of ethinyl estradiol-induced cholestasis on bile flow and biliary excretion of estradiol and bromsulfophthalein by the rat. (Abstr.) *J. clin. Invest.* **46**, 1080 (1967). [F 83,145/67]

Kreek, M. J., Sleisenger, M. H.: Reduction of serum-unconjugated-bilirubin with phenobarbitone in adult congenital non-haemolytic unconjugated hyperbilirubinaemia. *Lancet* **1968 II**, 73—78. [G 71,811/68]

Kreek, M. J., Sleisenger, M. H.: Estrogen induced cholestasis due to endogenous and exogenous hormones. *Scand. J. Gastroent.*, Sup. 7, 123—131 (1970). [G 77,590/70]

Kreek, M. J., Sleisenger, M. H., Jeffries, G. H.: Recurrent cholestatic jaundice of pregnancy with demonstrated estrogen sensitivity. *Amer. J. Med.* **43**, 795—803 (1967). [G 51,605/67]

Kreek, M. J., Weser, E., Sleisenger, M. H., Jeffries, G. H.: Idiopathic cholestasis of pregnancy. The response to challenge with the synthetic estrogen, ethinyl estradiol. *New Engl. J. Med.* **277**, 1391—1395 (1967). [F 92,343/67]

Krems, A. D., Martin, A. W., Dille, J. M.: Experimental study of tolerance to sulfanilamide in the albino rat. *J. Pharmacol. exp. Ther.* **71**, 215—221 (1941). [A 46,116/41]

Kritchevsky, D., Tepper, S. A., Staple, E., Whitehouse, M. W.: Influence of sex and sex hormones on the oxidation of cholesterol-26-C^{14} by rat liver mitochondria. *J. Lipid Res.* **4**, 188—192 (1963). [G 16,024/63]

Krizek, T. J., Davis, J. H.: The effect of diabetes on experimental infection. *Surg. Forum* **15**, 60—61 (1964). [F 14,734/64]

Kříženecký, J.: Über den Einfluß der Hyperthyreoidisation und der Hyperthymisation auf das Gewicht der ausgewachsenen Vögel. Ein fünfter Beitrag zum Studium der entwicklungsmechanisch-antagonistischen Wirkung der Thymus und der Thyreoidea. *Z. vergl. Physiol.* **8**, 16—36 (1928). [4,176/28]

Kříženecký, J.: Recherches sur l'antagonisme du thymus et du corps thyroide au point de vue de leur influence sur le poids du corps. *C. R. Soc. Biol. (Paris)* **98**, 1031—1033 (1928). [23,688/28]

Kříženecký, J.: Nouvelles recherches sur l'antagonisme du thymus et du corps thyroïde. *C. R. Soc. Biol. (Paris)* **106**, 325—327 (1930). [277/30]

Kříženecký, J., Podhradský, J.: Zur Frage der entwicklungsmechanisch-antagonistischen Wirkung der Thymus und der Thyreoidea. (Versuche an Kaulquappen.) *Wilhelm Roux' Arch. Entwickl. Mechanik. Organis.* **108**, 68—86 (1926). [4,186/26]

Kröger, H., Kotulla, W., Hoshino, J.: Zur Rolle des Substrats bei der Cortison-Induktion von Enzymen in der Leber. *Z. Naturforsch.* **24 b**, 229—233 (1969). [G 66,240/69]

Kroneberg, G.: Über den Einfluß des Thyroxins auf die Wirkungen von Adrenalin und Arterenol. *Naunyn-Schmiedebergs Arch. Pharmak.* **216**, 240—249 (1952). [B 87,448/52]

Kroneberg, G., Hüter, F.: Der Einfluß von Thyroxin auf die Toxicität des Adrenalins und Arterenols. *Klin. Wschr.* **29**, 649 (1951). [B 69,838/51]

Kroneberg, G., Pötzsch, E.: Über die Toxizität des Flexner-Endotoxins und den Endotoxinkollaps an thyroxinbehandelten Mäusen. *Naunyn-Schmiedebergs Arch. Pharmak.* **216**, 233 bis 239 (1952). [E 54,858/52]

Krupa, P. L., Hamburgh, M., Zaiman, H.: Effect of hypothyroidism on resistance of mice to infection with Trichinella spiralis. *J. Parasit.* **53**, 126—129 (1967). [G 45,694/67]

Krus, D. M., Wapner, S., Bergen, J., Freeman, H.: The influence of progesterone on behavioral changes induced by lysergic acid diethylamide (LSD-25) in normal males. *Psychopharmacologia (Berlin)* **2**, 177—184 (1961). [G 78,688/61]

Krüskemper, H. L.: Anabolic Steroids, pp. 236. New York, London: Academic Press, Inc. 1968. (Originally published in the German Language. Stuttgart: George Thieme Verlag 1963.) [E 933/68]

Krüskemper, H. L., Noell, G.: Liver toxicity of a new anabolic agent: methyltrienolone (17α-methyl-4,9,11-estratriene-17β-ol-3-one). *Steroids* **8**, 13—24 (1966). [G 48,300/66]

Kubota, D. C., Bernstein, A.: Adrenocorticotropic hormone (ACTH) in the treatment of barbiturate poisoning. *Illinois med. J.* 111, 80—83 (1957). [C 52,401/57

Kucharik, J., Telbisz, A.: Die Rolle der Nebenniere in der Pathologie und Behandlung der Senfgasvergiftungen. *Schweiz. med. Wschr.* 75, 996—997 (1945). [96,165/45

Küchmeister, H., Schuhmacher, H. H., Herrning, G., Pentz, U. von: Die Wirkung des ACTHs auf die Reaktionsweise der Leber nach Allylformiatvergiftung. *Z. ges. exp. Med.* 120, 215—220 (1953). [B 84,244/53

Kuck, N. A.: The effect of triamcinolone, prednisolone, and hydrocortisone on dosage requirements of tetracycline for control of a streptococcus infection in mice. In: Welch and Marti-Ibanez; *Antibiotics Annual 1958—1959*, p. 234—238. New York: Medical Encyclopedia Inc. 1959. [C 69,754/59

Kudo, M., Mutai, S., Uraguchi, K.: The effects of cortisone, cortate, parotin and adrenalectomy on Japanese encephalitis virus infection in mice. *Yokohama med. Bull.* 5, 337—344 (1954). [C 11,417/54

Kuhlmann, K., Oduah, M., Coper, H.: Über die Wirkung von Barbituraten bei Ratten verschiedenen Alters. *Naunyn-Schmiedebergs Arch. Pharmak.* 265, 310—320 (1970). [G 74,362/70

Kühn, H. A., Creutzfeldt, W., Discher, R., Röttger, P.: Untersuchungen über die therapeutische Beeinflußbarkeit experimenteller Lebercirrhosen bei der Ratte. I. Beobachtungen an gesunden Ratten nach alleiniger und kombinierter Gabe von Glucocorticoiden, Androgenen, Leberextrakten, Lipocaic, Antibiotica und Sulfonamidderivaten. *Z. ges. exp. Med.* 136, 162—168 (1962). [D 64,992/62

Kuhn, L. A., Page, L. B., Turner, J. K., Frieden, J.: Effect of cold exposure on resistance to hemorrhage in dogs. *Amer. J. Physiol.* 196, 715—718 (1959). [C 67,681/59

Kuipers, F., Ely, R. S., Kelley, V. C.: Metabolism of steroids: the removal of exogenous 17-hydroxycorticosterone from the peripheral circulation in dogs. *Endocrinology* 62, 64—74 (1958). [C 48,349/58

Kulagin, V. K.: The use of certain hormones of hypophysis and adrenals for shock prophylaxis and therapy in prolonged crush syndrome. (Russian text.) *Byul. eksper. biol. i med.* 49, 35—39 (1960). [D 236/60

Kulcsár, A., Földes, I., Kulcsár-Gergely, J.: Importance of mucopolysaccharides in the development of the protective hepatotropic effect of hypothyrosis. *Tohoku J. exp. Med.* 97, 373—384 (1969). [H 14,649/69

Kulcsár, A., Kulcsár-Gergely, J.: Über Leberschutz durch Kastration bei experimenteller Leberläsion. *Naturwissenschaften* 47, 183 (1960). [C 94,710/60

Kulcsár, A., Kulcsár-Gergely, J.: The influence of hormonal disturbances on the survival of liver-damaged animals. *Tohoku J. exp. Med.* 89, 315—320 (1966). [F 74,930/66

Kulcsár, A., Kulcsár-Gergely, J., Dan, S., Sari, B.: Functional adaptation of the liver in thyroidal disturbances. *Rev. int. Hepat.* 19, 359 to 364 (1969). [G 72,002/69

Kulcsár, A., Kulcsár-Gergely, J., Daroczy, A.: Influence of thyroid function on experimental liver injuries. *Tohoku J. exp. Med.* 101, 251 to 256 (1970). [H 24,478/70

Kulcsár-Gergely, J., Kulcsár, A.: Toxic actions of oestrogens on the liver. *J. Pharm. Pharmacol.* 12, 312—316 (1960). [C 99,083/60

Kulcsár-Gergely, J., Kulcsár, A.: Leberfunktion während der Hypothyreose. *Naturwissenschaften* 49, 610 (1962). [G 71,532/62

Kulcsár-Gergely, J., Kulcsár, A.: Über die Leberschutzwirkung der Hypothyreose. *Naturwissenschaften* 50, 693 (1963). [E 33,917/63

Kulcsár-Gergely, J., Kulcsár, A.: Über die hepatoendokrinen Zusammenhänge des Eierstockes und der Schilddrüse. *Naturwissenschaften* 51, 43 (1964). [G 1,372/64

Kulcsár-Gergely, J., Kulcsár, A., Dévényi, I.: The protective effect of thyroidectomy and ovariectomy on experimental liver lesion. *Tohoku J. exp. Med.* 84, 256—258 (1964). [F 32,037/64

Kumagai, A., Otomo, M., Yano, S., Takeuchi, N., Nishino, K., Ueda, H., Ko, S., Kitamura, M.: Inhibitors of the corticoid metabolism in vitro. *Endocr. jap.* 5, 122—126 (1958). [C 57,345/58

Kumagai, A., Otomo, M., Yano, S., Takeuchi, N., Nishino, K., Ueda, H., Ko, S., Kitamura, M.: Inhibition of cortisol metabolism in the liver by other steroids. *Endocr. jap.* 6, 86—92 (1959). [C 73,732/59

Kunde, M. M., Williams, L. A.: Experimental cretinism. II. The influence of the thyroid gland on the production and control of experimental rickets. *Amer. J. Physiol.* 83, 245—249 (1927). [18,960/27

Kuntzman, R.: Drugs and enzyme induction. *Ann. Rev. Pharmacol.* 9, 21—36 (1969). [G 64,989/69

Kuntzman, R., Jacobson, M.: Effect of drugs on the metabolism of progesterone by liver microsomal enzymes from various animal species. *Fed. Proc.* **24**, 152 (1965). [F35,869/65

Kuntzman, R., Jacobson, M., Conney, A. H.: Effect of phenylbutazone on cortisol metabolism in man (Abstr.). *Pharmacologist* **8**, 195 (1966). [G67,761/66

Kuntzman, R., Jacobson, M., Levin, W., Conney, A. H.: Stimulatory effect of n-phenylbarbital (phetharbital) on cortisol hydroxylation in man. *Biochem. Pharmacol.* **17**, 565—571 (1968). [G57,741/68

Kuntzman, R., Jacobson, M., Schneidman, K., Conney, A. H.: Similarities between oxidative drug-metabolizing enzymes and steroid hydroxylases in liver microsomes. *J. Pharmacol. exp. Ther.* **146**, 280—285 (1964). [F27,893/64

Kuntzman, R., Klutch, A., Tsai, I., Burns, J. J.: Physiological distribution and metabolic inactivation of chlorcyclizine and cyclizine. *J. Pharmacol. exp. Ther.* **149**, 29—35 (1965). [F45,464/65

Kuntzman, R., Lawrence, D., Conney, A. H.: Michaelis constants for the hydroxylation of steroid hormones and drugs by rat liver microsomes. *Molec. Pharmacol.* **1**, 163—167 (1965). [E55,528/65

Kuntzman, R., Levin, W., Jacobson, M., Conney, A. H.: Studies on microsomal hydroxylation and the demonstration of a new carbon monoxide binding pigment in liver microsomes. *Live Sci.* **7**, 215—224 (1968). [G71,857/68

Kuntzman, R., Mark, L. C., Brand, L., Jacobson, M., Levin, W., Conney, A. H.: Metabolism of drugs and carcinogens by human liver enzymes. *J. Pharmacol. exp. Ther.* **152**, 151 to 156 (1966). [H30,992/66

Kuntzman, R., Sansur, M., Conney, A. H.: Effect of drugs and insecticides on the anesthetic action of steroids. *Endocrinology* **77**, 952 to 954 (1965). [F55,537/65

Kuntzman, R., Welch, R., Conney, A. H.: Factors influencing steroid hydroxylases in liver microsomes. In: Weber; *Advances in Enzyme Regulation* **4**, p. 149—160. Oxford, London, Edinburgh: Pergamon Press 1966. [G66,245/66

Künzel, B., Müller-Oerlinghausen, B.: Wirkung von Testosteron und einem Anti-Androgen (Cyproteronacetat) auf die Glucuronidbildung in der Rattenleber. *Naunyn-Schmiedebergs Arch. Pharmak.* **262**, 112—123 (1969). [G64,178/69

Kupfer, D., Peets, L.: The effect of o,p′DDD on cortisol and hexobarbital metabolism. *Biochem. Pharmacol.* **15**, 573—581 (1966). [G40,053/66

Kupfer, D., Peets, L.: Potentiation of cortisol induction of hepatic tyrosine transaminase by β-diethylaminoethyl diphenylpropylacetate. *Nature (Lond.)* **215**, 637—638 (1967). [F85,854/67

Kupferberg, H. J., Way, E. L.: Pharmacologic basis for the increased sensitivity of the newborn rat to morphine. *J. Pharmacol. exp. Ther.* **141**, 105—112 (1963). [E21,867/63

Kupperman, H. S., de Graff, A. C.: Effect of hypoadrenalcorticoidism and excessive doses of desoxycorticosterone acetate and thyroid upon response of rat to cardiac glycosides. *Fed. Proc.* **9**, 293 (1950). [B47,267/50

Kusama, J.: Studies on carbohydrate metabolism of Graves' disease. Part 3. On glycogen of thyroid-fed rats. (Japanese text.) *Shinshu med. J.* **6**, 395—398 (1957). [C58,473/57

Kutner, F. R., Schwartz, S. I., Adams, J. T.: The effect of adrenergic blockade on lymph flow in endotoxin shock. *Ann. Surg.* **165**, 518—527 (1967). [G46,379/67

Laatikainen, T.: Excretion of neutral steroid hormones in human bile. *Ann. clin. Res.* **2**, Sup. 5, 7—28 (1970). [G78,706/70

Labbé, H., Théodoresco, B.: Recherches sur l'antagonisme physiologique de la caféine et de l'insuline. *Ann. Méd.* **16**, 211—217 (1924). [17,831/24

Laborit, H., Broussolle, B., Perrimond-Trouchet, R.: Essais pharmacologiques concernant le mécanisme des convulsions dues a l'oxygène pur en pression chez la souris. *J. Physiol. (Paris)* **49**, 953—962 (1957). [C48,371/57

Laborit, H., Broussolle, B., Perrimond-Trouchet, R.: Action protectrice de la 5-hydroxytryptamine contre les accidents convulsifs de l'oxygène sous pression chez la souris. *C. R. Soc. Biol. (Paris)* **151**, 930—933 (1958). [C52,731/58

Laborit, H., Niaussat, P., Broussolle, B., Jouanu, J. M.: Exposé de résultats expérimentaux concernant certaines propriétés originales de la sérotonine. *Med. exp. (Basel)* **1**, 27—33 (1959). [C77,964/59

Labrie, F., Korner, A.: Growth hormone inhibition of hydrocortisone induction of tyrosine transaminase and tryptophan pyrrolase and its reversal by amino acids. *J. biol. Chem.* **243**, 1120—1122 (1968). [G56,018/68

Lacassagne, A., Chamorro, A., Hurst, L., Giao, N. B.: Effet de l'éphysectomie sur l'hépatocancérogenèse chimique, chez le rat. *C. R. Acad. Sci. (Paris)* **269**, 1043—1046 (1969). [G74,931/69

Lacassagne, A., Hurst, L.: The effect of desoxycorticosterone and of hydrocortisone on the development of cancer in the rat liver under the influence of p-dimethylaminoazobenzene (DAB). *C. R. Acad. Sci. (Paris)* **257**, 1576—1580 (1963). [G12,688/63

Lacassagne, A., Hurst, L.: Influence de sulfamides hypo- ou hyperglycémiants sur la cancérisation du foie du rat par le 2-acétylaminofluorène. *Bull. Cancer* **56**, 397—410 (1969). [G78,530/69

Lacassagne, A., Jayle, M. F., Hurst, L.: Action des stéroïdes en C 21 sur la cancérisation du foie du rat par le paradiméthyl-aminoazobenzène (DAB). *C. R. Acad. Sci. (Paris)* **268**, 740—743 (1969). [G74,932/69

Lacassagne, A., Jayle, M. F., Hurst, L., Pasqualini, J. R.: Influence de differents corticostéroïdes sur la cancérisation du foie du rat par le p-diméthylaminoazobenzène (DAB). *C. R. Acad. Sci. (Paris)* **262**, 2117—2119 (1966). [G39,677/66

Lacassagne, A., Nyka, W.: Influence de la privation d'hypophyse sur le développement des tumeurs chez le lapin. *C. R. Soc. Biol. (Paris)* **121**, 822—824 (1936). [59,016/36

Lacassagne, A., Tuchmann-Duplessis, H.: Atténuation de la radiosensibilité du rat et du cobaye par l'hormone de croissance antéhypophysaire. *C. R. Acad. Sci. (Paris)* **236**, 440 a 443 (1953). [E53,832/53

Lack, C. H.: Increased vascular permeability, chondrolysis and cortisone. *Proc. Roy. Soc. Med.* **55**, 5—8 (1962). [D54,382/62

Laddu, A. R., Sanyal, R. K.: Effects of newer glucocorticoids on anaphylactic shock in the rat and the mouse. *Int. Arch. Allergy* **33**, 593—597 (1968). [G60,298/68

Ladner, H. A., Wollschläger, G., Schneider, J. Zur Strahlenschutzwirksamkeit von Serotonin bei Ratten. *Naturwissenschaften* **52**, 393 (1965). [G31,673/65

LaDu, B. N., Trousof, N., Brodie, B. B.: Enzymatic dealkylation of aminopyrine and other alkylamines in vitro. *Fed. Proc.* **12**, 339 (1953). [G74,654/53

Lage, G. L., Spratt, J. L.: Antagonism of intravenous digitoxigenin lethality by reserpine pretreatment in the mouse. *Proc. Soc. exp. Biol. (N.Y.)* **125**, 580—583 (1967). [F86,237/67

Lagôa, F. R.: Infecções experimentais pelo virus da influenza e corticoesteróides. *Brasil-méd.* **76**, 187—192 (1962). [D58,191/62

Lagrange, E.: L'action des ultrasons sur la bilharziose expérimentale de la souris. *C. R. Soc. Biol. (Paris)* **156**, 1725—1727 (1962). [D57,434/62

Lagrange, E.: A la recherche de stéroïdes de synthèse à action antibilharzienne. *C. R. Soc. Biol. (Paris)* **157**, 425—427 (1963). [D69,093/63

Lal, H., Puri, S. K., Fuller, G. C.: Impairment of hepatic drug metabolism by carbon tetrachloride inhalation. *Toxicol. appl. Pharmacol.* **16**, 35—39 (1970). [G77,285/70

Lalich, J. L., Turner, H.: Dilatation of colon induced in rats by β-aminopropionitrile feeding. *Exp. Molecul. Path.* **6**, 1—10 (1967). [G44,676/67

Lamanna, C., Jensen, W. I., Bross, I. D. J.: Body weight as a factor in the response of mice to botulinal toxins. *Amer. J. Hyg.* **62**, 21—28 (1955). [G60,750/55

Lamarche, M., Pluche, B.: Etude de l'action de l'acide triiodothyroacétique sur la résistance à l'anoxie aiguë. *C. R. Soc. Biol. (Paris)* **160**, 367—368 (1966). [F68,410/66

Lamson, P. D., Greig, M. E., Hobdy, C. J.: Modification of barbiturate anesthesia by glucose, intermediary metabolites and certain other substances. *J. Pharmacol. exp. Ther.* **103**, 460—470 (1951). [C14,547/51

Lamson, P. D., Greig, M. E., Williams, L.: Potentiation by epinephrine of the anesthetic effect in chloral and barbiturate anesthesia. *J. Pharmacol. exp. Ther.* **106**, 219—225 (1952). [B89,712/52

Lancker, J. L. van: Control of DNA synthesis in regenerating liver. *Fed. Proc.* **29**, 1439—1442 (1970). [H28,381/70

Lane, E. A., Mavrides, C.: Hormonal-dietary interactions in the regulation of tyrosine aminotransferase. *Proc. Canad. Fed. biol. Soc. Edmonton, Alta* **12**, 78 (1969). [H12,953/69

Lane, M., Liebelt, A., Calvert, J., Liebelt, R. A.: Effect of partial hepatectomy on tumor incidence in BALB/c mice treated with urethan. *Cancer Res.* **30**, 1812—1816 (1970). [H28,306/70

Lang, D. J.: Polyoma virus infection in neonatally thymectomized hamster. *Arch. ges. Virusforsch.* **22**, 159—170 (1968). [G55,002/68

Lange, G.: Verschiedene Induktion der mikrosomalen N- und p-Hydroxylierung von Anilin und N-Äthylanilin bei Kaninchen. *Naunyn-Schmiedebergs Arch. Pharmak.* 257, 230—256 (1967). [G 78,593/67

Lange, K., Gold, M. M. A., Weiner, D., Kramer, M.: Factors influencing resistance to cold environments. *Bull. U. S. Army med. Dep.* 8, 849—859 (1948). [B 23,962/48

Langendorff, H.: Grundlagen und Möglichkeiten eines biologisch-chemischen Strahlenschutzes bei äußerer Strahleneinwirkung. *Arzneimittel-Forsch.* 15, 463—472 (1965). [F 42,481/65

Langendorff, H., Catsch, A., Koch, R.: Untersuchungen über einen biologischen Strahlenschutz. XIX Mitteilg. Weitere Untersuchungen über die Strahlenempfindlichkeit und den Cysteaminschutz bei gonadektomierten männlichen Mäusen. *Strahlentherapie* 102, 291—297 (1957). [C 36,885/57

Langendorff, H., Koch, R.: Untersuchungen über einen biologischen Strahlenschutz. VI. Mitteilg. Über die Absterbeordnung röntgenbestrahlter Mäuse, die Unterschiede des Geschlechtes und den Einfluß der Keimdrüsen auf die Strahlenempfindlichkeit. *Strahlentherapie* 94, 250—257 (1954). [B 98,043/54

Langendorff, H., Koch, R.: Untersuchungen über einen biologischen Strahlenschutz. XVIII. Mitteilg. Die Wirkung zentralerregender Pharmaka auf das bestrahlte Tier. *Strahlentherapie* 102, 58—64 (1957). [C 36,881/57

Langendorff, H., Koch, R., Beisinghoff, G.: The influence of chemical protective agents on the radioiron utilization of irradiated animals. *Int. J. appl. Radiat.* 16, 521—522 (1965). [G 34,793/65

Langendorff, H., Langendorff, M.: Untersuchungen über einen biologischen Strahlenschutz. 68. Mitteilg. Strahlenempfindlichkeit und Schutzwirkung des Serotonins bei Mäusen verschiedener Altersstufen. *Strahlentherapie* 129, 425—431 (1966). [G 38,396/66

Langendorff, H., Langendorff, M.: Untersuchungen über einen biologischen Strahlenschutz. 72. Mitteilg. Die Wirksamkeit verschiedener Strahlenschutzsubstanzen bei fraktionierter Röntgenbestrahlung von Mäusen. *Strahlentherapie* 131, 37—50 (1966). [G 42,801/66

Langendorff, H., Melching, H. J., Ladner, H. A.: Untersuchungen über einen biologischen Strahlenschutz. XXX. Mitteilg. über die Strahlenschutzwirkung des 5-Hydroxytryptamin im Tierversuch. *Strahlentherapie* 108, 251—256 (1959). [C 69,396/59

Langendorff, H., Melching, H. J., Messerschmidt, O., Streffer, C.: Untersuchungen über Kombinationsschäden. 3. Mitteilg. Zur Wirksamkeit von Strahlenschutzsubstanzen bei einer Kombination von Strahlenbelastung und Hautwunde. *Strahlentherapie* 128, 264—272 (1965). [G 38,385/65

Langendorff, H., Messerschmidt, O.: Strahlenbelastung und Wunde (tierexperimenteller Beitrag zur Frage der Kombinationsschäden). *Nippon Acta Ragior.* 3, 289—297 (1966). [G 45,424/66

Lannigan, R.: The production of chronic renal disease in rats by a single intravenous injection of aminonucleoside of pyromycin and the effect of low dosage continuous hydrocortisone. *Brit. J. exp. Path.* 44, 326—333 (1963). [D 69,709/63

Lansing, A. M., Stevenson, J. A. F., Gowdey, C. W.: The effect of noradrenaline on the survival of rats subjected to hemorrhagic shock. *Canad. J. Biochem.* 35, 93—101 (1957). [C 30,227/57

Lanzenberg, A., Képinow, L.: Glande thyroide et anaphylaxie. *C. R. Soc. Biol. (Paris)* 86, 204—205 (1922). [13,117/22

Lanzetta, A.: Tiroxina, 2—4 DPN e narcosi da barbiturici. *Boll. Soc. ital. Biol. sper.* 34, 1955—1956 (1958). [C 68,990/58

Larizza, P., Ventura, S.: Hanno anche gli estrogeni un'azione antisteatogena? *Rif. med.* 63, 457—463 (1949). [B 38,397/49

Laroche, M. J., Brodie, B. B.: Lack of relationship between inhibition of monoamine oxidase and potentiation of hexobarbital hypnosis. *J. Pharmacol. exp. Ther.* 130, 134—137 (1960). [H 21,467/60

Laron, Z., Boss, J. H.: Failure of 19-nor-androstenolone phenylpropionate (durabolin) to prevent the alterations produced by cortisone on the growing bone in rats. *Endocrinology* 69, 608—612 (1961). [D 10,620/61

Laron, Z., Canlas, B. D., Jr., Crawford, J. D.: The action of cortisone on the teeth of rachitic rats. *Arch. Path.* 61, 177—180 (1956). [C 12,833/56

Laron, Z., Canlas, B. D., Jr., Crawford, J. D.: The interaction of cortisone and vitamin D on bones of rachitic rats. *Arch. Path.* 65, 403—406 (1958). [C 50,634/58

Laron, Z., Laufer, A.: Effect of cortisone on the development of nephrocalcinosis and ectopic bone in the ischemic rat kidney. *Endocrinology* 70, 437—441 (1962). [D 20,687/62

Laron, Z., Muhlethaler, J. P., Klein, R.: The interrelationship between cortisone and parathyroid extract in rats. *Arch. Path.* **65**, 125 to 130 (1958). [C 47,872/58

Larsh, J. E., Jr.: The effect of thyroid and thiouracil on the natural resistance of mice to infection with Hymenolepsis. (Abstr.) *J. Parasit.* **33**, Sup. 24—25 (1947). [A 47,571/47

Larson, R. E., Plaa, G. L.: A correlation of the effects of cervical cordotomy, hypothermia, and catecholamines on carbon tetrachloride-induced hepatic necrosis. *J. Pharmacol. exp. Ther.* **147**, 103—111 (1965). [F 29,496/65

Larsson-Cohn, U.: The 2 hour sulfobromophthalein retention test and the transaminase activity during oral contraceptive therapy. *Amer. J. Obstet. Gynec.* **98**, 188—193 (1967). [G 46,952/67

Larsson-Cohn, U.: The serum alanine aminotransferase activity and the two-hour sulphobromophthalein retention test during daily low-dose gestagen oral-contraceptive treatment. *Acta Soc. Med. upsalien.* **74**, 283—288 (1969). [G 74,875/69

Laszt, L., Verzár, F.: Hemmung des Wachstums durch Jodessigsäure und antagonistische Beeinflussung durch Vitamin B_2 sowie Nebennierenrinden-Hormon. *Pflügers Arch. ges. Physiol.* **236**, 693—704 (1935). [34,843/35

Lathe, G. H., Walker, M.: Inhibition of bilirubin conjugation in rat liver slices by human pregnancy and neonatal serum and steroids. *Quart. J. exp. Physiol.* **43**, 257—265 (1958). [C 55,335/58

Lathe, G. H., Walker, M.: The synthesis of bilirubin glucuronide in animal and human liver. *Biochem. J.* **70**, 705—712 (1958). [G 78,969/58

Latvalahti, J.: Experimental studies on the influences of certain hormones on the development of amyloidosis. *Thesis*, University of Helsinki (1953). [B 88,191/53

Lauber, H. J.: Hormonwirkung bei akuten Infektionen. *Bruns Beitr. Klin. Chir.* **154**, 613—634 (1932). [9,102/32

Laufer, A., Tal, C., Kolander, N.: Experimental amyloidosis and the effect of cortisone treatment. *Path. Microbiol.* **31**, 85—92 (1968). [H 13,434/68

Laufman, H., Freed, S. C.: Observations on the transudate in intestinal strangulation. I. The effect of adrenal cortical extract on its toxicity. *Surg. Gynec. Obstet.* **77**, 605—609 (1943). [88,861/43

Laug, E. P., Nelson, A. A., Fitzhugh, O. G., Kunze, F. M.: Liver cell alteration and DDT storage in the fat of the rat induced by dietary levels of 1 to 50 p.p.m. DDT. *J. Pharmacol. exp. Ther.* **98**, 268—273 (1950). [A 94,356/50

Lauria, P., Sharma, V. N.: Effects of three recently synthesized indole derivatives on central nervous system. *Indian J. med. Res.* **54**, 374—382 (1966). [F 67,259/66

Lavelle, G. C., Starr, T. J.: Relationship of phagocytic activity to pathogenicity of mouse hepatitis virus as affected by triolein and cortisone. *Brit. J. exp. Path.* **50**, 475—480 (1969). [H 18,566/69

Leathem, J. H.: The influence of antithyroid drugs and testosterone propionate on the organ weights of rats. *Exp. Med. Surg.* **6**, 428—433 (1948). [B 38,768/48

Leathem, J. H.: Influence of sex on 2-acetylaminofluorene-induced liver tumors in rats and mice (Abstr.). *Cancer Res.* **11**, 266 (1951). [G 74,736/51

Leathem, J. H., Oddis, L.: Hyperthyroidism and hepatic tumor induction. (Abstr.) *Proc. Amer. Ass. Cancer Res.* **3**, 243 (1961). [D 2,742/61

Leber, H. W., Rawer, P., Schütterle, G.: Beeinflussung mikrosomaler Enzyme der Rattenleber durch Spironolacton, Etacrynsäure und Furosemid. *Klin. Wschr.* **49**, 116—118 (1971). [H 35,676/71

Leblanc, J., Pouliot, M.: Direct evidence for a role of noradrenaline in cold adaptation. *Fed. Proc.* **23**, 368 (1964). [F 4,622/64

Leblond, C. P.: Detoxification of pregnanediol in the liver (Abstr.). *Fed. Proc.* **1**, 49 (1942). [82,066/42

Leblond, C. P.: Detoxification of progesterone derivatives in the liver. *Amer. J. med. Sci.* **204**, 566—570 (1942). [A 55,928/42

Lecannelier, S., Quevedo, M.: Analgesic effect of salicylic and pyrazolon derivatives associated with morphine. *Arch. Biol. Med. exp. (Santiago)* **4**, 150—153 (1967). [H 8,759/67

Lecomte, J.: Sur les facteurs surrénaliens qui conditionnent la résistance du rat intoxiqué par l'histamine. 1e partie: l'histamine exogène. *Arch. int. Physiol.* **69**, 563—581 (1961). [D 12,212/61

Lecomte, J., Sodovez, J. C.: Sur les facteurs surrénaliens qui conditionnent la résistance du rat intoxiqué par l'histamine. IIe partie: L'histamine endogène. *Arch. int. Physiol. Biochim.* **70**, 16—26 (1962). [D 20,641/62

Lecoq, R.: Action comparée des effets de l'hormone adrénocorticotrope (A.C.T.H.) et de la cortisone avec quelques facteurs enzymatiques sur l'intoxication alcoolique expérimentale. *C. R. Soc. Biol. (Paris)* **145**, 1600—1603 (1951). [B 79,754/51

Lecoq, R., Chauchard, P., Mazoué, H.: Vitamines, sécrétions endocrines et métabolisme de l'alcool. Déductions sur le rôle de ces substances dans l'intoxication et la désintoxication des alcooliques. *Int. Z. Vitamin-Forsch.* **23**, 141 a 163 (1951). [B 66,406/51

Leduc, E. H.: Regeneration of the liver. In: Rouiller, C.; *The Liver. Morphology, Biochemistry, Physiology* **2**, p. 63—89. New York, London: Academic Press Inc. 1964. [G 79,104/64

Lee, N. D., Baltz, B. E.: Tryptophan pyrrolase induction and the influence of adrenocorticoids. *Endocrinology* **70**, 84—87 (1962). [D 16,649/62

Lee, Y. C.: Experimental studies on the relation between nicotine and sexual hormone. I. *J. Severance Un. Med. Coll.* **2**, 80 (1935). [32,854/35

Lees, M. H., Ruthven, C. R. J.: The effect of triiodothyronine in neonatal hyperbilirubinaemia. *Lancet* **1959 II**, 371—373. [C 74,543/59

Leevy, C. M., Paumgartner, G.: Jaundice in Alcoholism. Int. Symp. on Jaundice, Friesburg, p. 205—210 (1968). [G 72,234/68

Lefer, A. M., Martin, J.: Mechanism of the protective effect of corticosteroids in hemorrhagic shock. *Amer. J. Physiol.* **216**, 314—320 (1969). [H 7,806/69

Lefort, P., Déziel, C., Côté, G., Tuchweber, B., Gabbiani, G.: Action de la thyroxine et de la thyrocalcitonine (TCT) chez l'animal néphrectomisé. *Ann. ACFAS 35e Congr.* 3 et 4 Nov. (1967). [G 46,725/67

Leger, J., Leith, W., Rose, B.: Effect of adrenocorticotrophic hormone on anaphylaxis in the guinea pig. *Proc. Soc. exp. Biol. (N.Y.)* **69**, 465—467 (1948). [A 48,766/48

Lehmann, P., Thierree, R. A., Metzger, Mlle: Sur des nouvelles techniques de radio-protection de l'organisme. Action favorable de la cortisone. *J. Radiol. Electrol.* **37**, 480—483 (1956). [C 46,970/56

Lehmann, W. D., Breuer, H.: Einfluß der Schilddrüse auf den Stoffwechsel von Östron in der Leber. In: Kracht, J.; *Nebenschilddrüse und endokrine Regulationen des Calciumstoffwechsels Spontan-Hypoglykämie Glucagon*, p. 286—288. Berlin, Heidelberg, New York: Springer-Verlag 1968. [E 8,112/68

Lehmann, W. D., Breuer, H.: Wirkung des Funktionszustandes der Schilddrüse auf den Stoffwechsel der Östrogene in der Mikrosomen-Fraktion der Rattenleber. *Acta endocr. (Kbh.)* **61**, 461—476 (1969). [H 15,110/69

Lehmann, W. D., Schütz, M.: Oestronstoffwechsel in der Mikrosomenfraktion der Leber von menschlichen Feten und von einem erwachsenen Mann. *Arch. Gynäk.* **207**, 539—549 (1969). [H 14,215/69

Lehr, D.: Causative relationships of parathyroid hormone to renogenic and reniprival cardiovascular disease. *Ann. N.Y. Acad. Sci.* **72**, 901—969 (1959). [C 84,326/59

Lehr, D., Krukowski, M.: Protection by pregnancy against the sequalae of acute hyperparathyroidism. *Naunyn-Schmiedebergs Arch. Pharmak.* **242**, 143—167 (1961). [D 22,446/61

Lehr, D., Krukowski, M.: Prevention of myocardial necrosis by advanced pregnancy. *J. Amer. med. Ass.* **178**, 823—826 (1961). [D 81,044/61

Lehr, D., Krukowski, M.: About the mechanism of protection by advanced pregnancy against experimental myocardial necrosis. *Rev. Canad. Biol.* **22**, 281—295 (1963). [E 21,312/63

Lehr, D., Martin, C.: Prevention of cardiovascular and smooth muscle necrosis in the albino rat by parathyroidectomy. *J. Pharmacol. exp. Ther.* **116**, 38 (1956). [C 13,119/56

Lehr, D., Martin, C. R.: Prevention of severe cardiovascular and smooth muscle necrosis in the rat by thyro-parathyroidectomy. *Endocrinology* **59**, 273—288 (1956). [C 23,011/56

Leibman, K. C.: Effects of metyrapone on liver microsomal drug oxidations. *Molec. Pharmacol.* **5**, 1—9 (1969). [G 66,210/69

Lemonde, P.: Etude sur les facteurs hormonaux dans les infections. *These*, Université de Montréal (1954). [C 310/54

Lemonde, P.: S.T.H. and tuberculosis. *Brit. med. J.* **1955 I**, 537. [C 6,400/55

Lemonde, P., Jasmin, G., Mongeau, A.: Action de la noréthandrolone sur la tuberculose expérimentale chez le rat. *ACFAS*, 28. Congr., p. 28 (1960). [C 95,984/60

Lemonde, P., Panisset, M., Dobija, M., Selye, H.: Protection by somatotropic hormone (STH) against experimental tuberculosis. *J. clin. Endocr.* **12**, 973—974 (1952). [B 69,349/52

Lemonde, P., Panisset, M., Dobija, M., Selye, H.: Influence de la somatotrophine sur la tuberculose expérimentale chez le rat et la souris. *Ann. Endocr. (Paris)* **13**, 897—904 (1952). [B 70,248/52

Lemonde, P., Panisset, M., Selye, H.: Somatotrophic hormone in tuberculosis. *Amer. Rev. Tuberc.* **71**, 319—321 (1955). [C 526/55

Lennon, H. D.: Effect of several anabolic steroids on sulfobromophthalein (BSP) retention in rabbits. *Steroids* **5**, 361—373 (1965). [F 69,077/65

Lennon, H. D.: Relative effects of 17-alkylated anabolic steroids on sulfobromophthalein (BSP) retention in rabbits. *J. Pharmacol. exp. Ther.* **151**, 143—150 (1966). [F 63,769/66

Léonard, A., Maisin, J. R.: Effets de la β-aminoéthylisothiourée (AET) sur les mutations induites chez la souris par les rayons X. II. Diminution du taux de létalité dominante induite chez les spermatozoïdes irradiés avec des fortes doses de rayons X. *C. R. Soc. Biol. (Paris)* **157**, 913—915 (1963). [E 26,654/63

Léonard, A., Maisin, J. R., Mattelin, G.: Effect of a mixture of chemical protectors against X-irradiation induced testis injury in mice. *Strahlentherapie* **138**, 614—618 (1969). [G 71,644/69

Leonard, C. A., Gorby, C. K., Ambrus, J. L., Harrisson, J. W. E.: A note on the effect of cortisone and desoxycorticosterone on metrazol convulsions in mice. *J. Amer. pharm. Ass. sci. Ed.* **42**, 444—445 (1953). [B 86,814/53

Leone, G., Rinaldi, L.: Effetti della talidomide sull'ossificazione endomidollare del piccione (Columba livia Gm.) adulto. *R. C. Cl. Sci. fis. nat e nat. Ser. VIII* **38**, 578—581 (1965). [G 44,123/65

LePage, G. A., Kaneko, T.: Effective means of reducing toxicity without concomitant sacrifice of efficacy of carcinostatic therapy. *Cancer Res.* **29**, 2314—2318 (1969). [H 22,380/69

Lepri, G., Fornaro, L.: Considerazioni sull' azione dell'A.C.T.H. et del cortisone nella tubercolosi oculare sperimentale. *Boll. Oculist.* **33**, 725—736 (1954). [D 91,865/54

Lerner, L. J., Holthaus, F. J., Jr., Thompson, C. R.: A non-steroidal estrogen antagonist 1-(p-2-diethylaminoethoxyphenyl)-1-phenyl-2-p-methoxyphenyl ethanol. *Endocrinology* **63**, 295—318 (1958). [C 57,905/58

Lesca, S., Mosca, L.: Possibili rapporti tra rigenerazione epatica funzionalitá tiroidea. *Atti Soc. Ital. Pat.* **1**, 223—226 (1949). [B 48,329/49

Letov, V. N.: The effect of noradrenaline on radiation injury of proliferative pilary follicles. (Russian text.) *Vop. Onkol.* **14**, 63—66 (1968). [H 19,253/68

Lettré, H., Landschütz, C., Nobel, J.: Über Synergisten von Mitosegiften. 10. Nebennierenrindenhormone und Colchicin. *Klin. Wschr.* **29**, 555 (1951). [B 63,159/51

Leung, P. M.-B., Rogers, O. R., Harper, A. E.: Effect of cortisol on growth, food intake, dietary preference and plasma amino acid pattern of rats fed amino acid imbalanced diets. *J. Nutr.* **96**, 139—151 (1968). [G 60,800/68

Levaditi, C., Haber, P.: Influence de certaines glandes endocrines sur la réceptivité des Simiens à l'égard du virus poliomyélitique et sur leur immunité acquise. *C. R. Soc. Biol. (Paris)* **119**, 16—17 (1935). [33,069/35

Levens, P., Swann, H. G.: Obesity in the rat. *Proc. Amer. physiol. Soc.* p. 173 (1941). [80,483/41

Levey, R. H., Trainin, N., Law, L. W., Black, P. H., Rowe, W. P.: Lymphocytic choriomeningitis infection in neonatally thymectomized mice bearing diffusion chambers containing thymus. *Science* **142**, 483—485 (1963). [E 30,471/63

Levi, A. J., Sherlock, S., Walker, D.: Phenylbutazone and isoniazid metabolism in patients with liver disease in relation to previous drug therapy. *Lancet* **1968 I**, 1275. [F 99,523/68

Levin, G. E., McMullin, G. P., Mobarak, A. N.: Controlled trial of phenobarbitone in neonatal jaundice. *Arch. Dis. Childh.* **45**, 93—96 (1970). [G 73,664/70

Levin, L.: Physical stress and liver fat content of the fasted mouse (Abstr.). *Fed. Proc.* **8**, 218—219 (1949). [B 32,877/49

Levin, L.: The possible involvement of the adrenal cortex and thyroid in mobilization of fat to the liver. *Ass. Study Int. Secr. 31st Meet. Atlantic City, N.J.*, June 3 and 4, p. 16 (1949). [B 35,913/49

Levin, S. S., Cooper, D. Y., Vars, H. M., Parkins, W. M.: Adrenal corticoids in ischemic shock induced by temporary occlusion of the thoracic aorta in dogs. *Fed. Proc.* **19**, 102 (1960). [C 82,785/60

Levin, W., Conney, A. H.: Effect of phenobarbital on the uterine response to estradiol-17B (Abstr.). *Fred. Proc.* **25**, 251 (1966). [F 64,557/66

Levin, W., Welch, R. M., Conney, A. H.: Effect of chronic phenobarbital treatment on the liver microsomal metabolism and uterotropic action of 17β-estradiol. *Endocrinology* **80**, 135—140 (1967). [F 75,365/67

Levin, W., Welch, R. M., Conney, A. H.: Effect of phenobarbital and other drugs on the metabolism and uterotropic action of estradiol-17β and estrone. *J. Pharmacol. exp. Ther.* **159**, 362—371 (1968). [F94,711/68

Levin, W., Welch, R. M., Conney, A. H.: Decreased uterotropic potency of oral contraceptives in rats pretreated with phenobarbital. *Endocrinology* **83**, 149—156 (1968). [H894/68

Levin, W., Welch, R. M., Conney, A. H.: Inhibitory effects of phenobarbital or chlordane pretreatment on the androgen-induced increase in seminal vesicle weight in the rat. *Steroids* **13**, 155—161 (1969). [G64,184/69

Levin, W., Welch, R. M., Conney, A. H.: Effect of carbon tetrachloride and other inhibitors of drug metabolism on the metabolism and action of estradiol-17β and estrone in the rat. *J. Pharmacol. exp. Ther.* **173**, 247—255 (1970). [H26,593/70

Levine, W. G.: Effect of SKF 525-A on biliary function. Influence of body temperature. *Life Sci.* **9**, 437—442 (1970). [G75,350/70

Levine, W. G.: The role of microsomal drug-metabolizing enzymes in the biliary excretion of 3,4-benzpyrene in the rat. *J. Pharmacol. exp. Ther.* **175**, 301—310 (1970). [H31,806/70

Levine, W. G., Millburn, P., Smith, R. L., Williams, R. T.: The role of the hepatic endoplasmic reticulum in the biliary excretion of foreign compounds by the rat. The effect of phenobarbitone and SKF 525-A (diethylaminoethyl diphenylpropylacetate). *Biochem. Pharmacol.* **19**, 235—244 (1970). [G73,357/70

Levitan, I. B., Webb, T. E.: Modification by 8-azaguanine of the effects of hydrocortisone on the induction and inactivation of tyrosine transaminase of rat liver. *J. biol. Chem.* **244**, 341—347 (1969). [G64,051/69

Levitan, I. B., Webb, T. E.: Posttranscriptional control in the steroid-mediated induction of hepatic tyrosine transaminase. *Science* **167**, 283—285 (1970). [H20,594/70

Levitin, H., Kendrick, M. I., Kass, E. H.: Effect of route of administration on protective action of corticosterone and cortisol against endotoxin. *Proc. Soc. exp. Biol. (N.Y.)* **93**, 306 to 309 (1956). [C26,683/56

Levy, E. Z., North, W. C., Wells, J. A.: Modification of traumatic shock by adrenergic blocking agents. *J. Pharmacol. exp. Ther.* **112**, 151—157 (1954). [C10,848/54

Levy, R. P., Moir, T. W., Miller, M.: BAL and testosterone propionate in the treatment of mercuric chloride poisoning. *Proc. Soc. exp. Biol. (N.Y.)* **73**, 498—500 (1950). [B47,634/50

Lewis, D. A., Symons, A. M., Ancill, R. J.: The stabilization-lysis action of anti-inflammatory steroids on lysosomes. *J. Pharm. Pharmacol.* **22**, 902—908 (1970). [G80,342/70

Lewis, J. J., Martin-Smith, M., Muir, T. C., Ross, H. H.: Steroidal monoquaternary ammonium salts with non-depolarizing neuromuscular blocking activity. *J. Pharm. Pharmacol.* **19**, 502—508 (1967). [F95,691/67

Lewis, J. T.: Sensibilité des rats privés de surrénales envers les toxiques. *C. R. Soc. Biol. (Paris)* **84**, 163—164 (1921). [12,272/21

Lewis, J. T.: Sensibility to intoxication in albino rats after double adrenalectomy. *Amer. J. Physiol.* **64**, 506—511 (1923). [61,803/23

Leybold, K., Staudinger, H.: Geschlechtsunterschiede im Steroidstoffwechsel von Rattenlebermikrosomen. *Biochem. Z.* **331**, 389—398 (1959). [C77,908/59

Leybold, K., Staudinger, H.: Geschlechtsunterschied im Steroidstoffwechsel von Rattenlebercytoplasma. *Med. exp.* **2**, 46—53 (1960). [C88,830/60

Leybold, K., Staudinger, H.: Wirkung von Pharmaka auf den Steroidstoffwechsel von Rattenlebermikrosomen. *Klin. Wschr.* **39**, 952—953 (1961). [D11,904/61

Li, B. N., Sos, J.: The effect of thyroidectomy on the increase in blood pressure caused by p N oxyphenyl glycine. (Abstr.) *Kisérl. Orvostud.* **20**, 588—590 (1968). [H30,786/68

Li, C. H., Evans, H. M.: I. Hormones in growth and metabolism. The biochemistry of pituitary growth hormone. In: Pincus, G.; *Recent Progress in Hormone Research.* Proc. Laur. Horm. Conf., p. 3. New York: Acad. Press. Inc. Publ. 1948. [B29,320/48

Li, C. H., Ingle, D. J., Evans, H. M., Prestruda, M. C., Nezamis, J. E.: Effect of adrenocorticotrophic hormone upon liver fat and urinary phosphorus in normal force-fed rat. *Proc. Soc. exp. Biol. (N.Y.)* **70**, 753—756 (1949). [B34,773/49

Li, C. P., Prescott, B., Chi, L. L., Martino, E. C.: Antiviral and antibacterial activity of thymus extracts. *Proc. Soc. exp. Biol. (N.Y.)* **114**, 504—509 (1963). [E33,523/63

Liashenko, V. A.: The influence exerted by cortisone on the therapeutic effect of levomycetin employed in treatment of acute experimental infections. (Russian text.) *Antibiotiki* **5**, 41—44 (1960). [D51,368/60

Liashenko, V. A.: Effect of cortisone on the therapeutic action of levomycetin at different stages of experimental infection in connection with the hormone's action on phagocytosis. (Russian text.) *Antibiotiki* 6, 504—507 (1961). [D 50,402/61]

Liddle, G. W.: Specific and non-specific inhibition of mineralocorticoid activity. *Metabolism* 10, 1021—1030 (1961). [D 14,432/61]

Lieberman, J.: Papain-induced emphysema in hamsters and the role of progesterone and stilbesterol in prevention. (Abstr.) *Clin. Res.* 19, 192 (1971). [H 34,495/71]

Lieberman, M., Pollikoff, R., Pascale, A. M.: Effect of concomitant treatment by cortisone and N-ethylisatin β-thiosemicarbazone on neurovaccinia virus infected mice. *Proc. Soc. exp. Biol. (N.Y.)* 122, 484—489 (1966). [F 67,288/66]

Lieberman, M. W.: Early developmental stress and later behavior. *Science* 141, 824—825 (1963). [E 24,883/63]

Lien, W. M., McCormick, J. R., Davies, M. W., Egdahl, R. H.: Corticosteroid clearance by the gastrointestinal tract in dogs and monkeys. *Endocrinology* 87, 206—208 (1970). [H 25,091/70]

Liling, M., Gaunt, R.: Acquired resistance to water intoxication. *Amer. J. Physiol.* 144, 571—577 (1945). [89,147/45]

Lillehei, R. C., Dietzman, R. H., Movsas, S., Bloch, J. H.: Treatment of septic shock. In: Kuhn and Abramson; *Modern Treatment*, p. 321—346. New York: Hoeber Medical Division, Harper & Row 1967. [G 45,335/67]

Lillehei, R. C., Longerbeam, J. K., Bloch, J. H.: Physiology and therapy of bacteremic shock. Experimental and clinical observations. *Amer. J. Cardiol.* 12, 599—613 (1963). [E 31,273/63]

Lillehei, R. C., Longerbeam, J. K., Bloch, J. H., Manax, W. G.: The modern treatment of shock based on physiologic principles. *Clin. Pharmacol. Ther.* 5, 63—101 (1964). [E 37,842/64]

Lillehei, R. C., MacLean, L. D.: The intestinal factor in irreversible endotoxin shock. *Ann. Surg.* 148, 513—525 (1958). [D 59,725/58]

Lillehei, R. C., MacLean, L. D.: Physiological approach to successful treatment of endotoxin shock in the experimental animal. *Arch. Surg.* 78, 464—471 (1959). [D 84,873/59]

Lim, H. S., Davenport, H. T., Robson, J. G.: The response of infants and children to muscle relaxants. *Anesthesiology* 25, 161—168 (1964). [G 78,962/64]

Limperos, G.: Effects of varying oxygen tension on mortality of x-rayed mice. *J. Franklin Inst.* 249, 513—514 (1950). [E 50,944/50]

Limperos, G., Mosher, W. A.: Protection of mice against X-radiation by thiourea. *Science* 112, 86—87 (1950). [B 49,737/50]

Lin, C. D., Hoshino, K.: Testosterone dependency of the lethal factor in mouse submandibular gland isografts. *Canad. J. Physiol. Pharmacol.* 47, 335—338 (1969). [H 9,995/69]

Lin, E. C. C., Knox, W. E.: Adaptation of the rat liver tyrosine-α-ketoglutarate transaminase. *Biochim. biophys. Acta (Amst.)* 26, 85—88 (1957). [E 63,521/57]

Lin, E. C. C., Knox, W. E.: Specificity of the adaptive response of tyrosine-α-ketoglutarate transaminase in the rat. *J. biol. Chem.* 233, 1186—1189 (1958). [C 73,824/58]

Lin, E. C. C., Rivlin, R. S., Knox, W. E.: Effect of body weight and sex on activity of enzymes involved in amino acid metabolism. *J. Physiol.* 196, 303—306 (1959). [C 96,929/59]

Lindegren, C. C.: The receptor-hypothesis of induction of gene-controlled adaptive enzymes. *J. theor. Biol.* 5, 192—210 (1963). [G 66,494/63]

Lindegren, C. C.: The receptor hypothesis of gene action. In: Bajusz, E.; *Physiology and Pathology of Adaption Mechanisms: Neural-Neuroendocrine-Humoral*, p. 452—461. Oxford, London, Edinburgh: Pergamon Press 1969. [E 8,182/69]

Lindner, A., Stoklaska, E.: Über den Einfluß des Cortisons auf die Digitoxinwirkung. *Wien. klin. Wschr.* 68, 516—519 (1956). [C 35,550/56]

Linet, O.: Interactions between androgenic-anabolic steroids and glucocorticoids. *Fortschr. Arzneimittel-Forsch.*, 14, 139—195 (1970). [G 79,963/70]

Linet, O., Hava, M., Jakubovic, A., Mikulaskova, J.: On the pharmacology of 1,2α-oxydoandrostan-3,17-dione (OAD). *Arch. int. Pharmacodyn.* 158, 222—233 (1965). [F 58,620/65]

Linet, O., Mikulašková, J.: On the problem of gastric ulcer formation by glucocorticoids in rats and the effect of androgenic-anabolic steroid on them. *Endokrinologie* 51, 224—233 (1967). [F 86,027/67]

Lippman, R. W., Marti, H. U., Jacobs, E. E.: Sex differences in pathogenesis of nephrotoxic globulin (NTG) nephritis. *Fed. Proc.* 11, 96 (1952). [B 68,238/52]

Lissák, K.: Beiträge zur Frage der Beziehung zwischen Tetanie und Tetanus. *Naunyn-Schmiedebergs Arch. Pharmak.* 176, 425—428 (1934). [29,256/34

Little, K.: Interaction between catabolic and anabolic steroids. *Curr. ther. Res.* 12, 658—676 (1970). [G 78,533/70]

Litwack, G., Nemeth, A. M.: Development of liver tyrosine aminotransferase activity in the rabbit, guinea pig, and chicken. *Arch. Biochem.* 109, 316—320 (1965). [G 26,050/65]

Llanos, J. M. E., Saffe, I. E.: Acción promotora de la regeneración posthepatectomía sobre los hepatomas espontáneos de C3H/mza machos. *Rev. Soc. argent. Biol.* 37, 240—249 (1961). [G 71,663/61]

Llaurado, J. G., Trunnell, J. B., Claus, J. L.: Some effects of simultaneous administration of norethandrolone and cortisone in the rat. *Acta endocr. (Kbh.)* 32, 536—544 (1959). [G 79,936/59]

Locatelli, P.: Alterazioni delle cellule epatiche in seguito ad avvelenamento da tossina difterica. Influenza della tiroidectomia. *Boll. Soc. med.-chir. Pavia* 48, 405—410 (1934). [28,678/34]

Lockwood, J. E., Hartman, F. A.: Relation of the adrenal cortex to vitamins A, B_1 and C. *Endocrinology* 17, 501 (1933). [15,573/33]

Loewe, L., Lenke, S. E.: The use of estrogenic hormone in experimental peripheral gangrene. *J. Pharmacol. exp. Ther.* 63, 93—98 (1938). [A 43,451/38]

Loewit, K.: Über den Einfluß anaboler Hormone auf die Folgen einer Strahlenschädigung bei der weißen Maus. *Strahlentherapie* 125, 281—298 (1964). [G 23,765/64]

Logaras, G., Drummond, J. C.: Vitamin A and the thyroid. *Biochem. J.* 32, 964—968 (1938). [A 16,392/38]

Loggie, J. M. H., Privitera, P. J., Sugarman, S., Gaffney, T. E.: Effects of hydrocortisone on survival in neonatal beagles given endotoxin. *Proc. Soc. exp. Biol. (N.Y.)* 128, 326—329 (1968). [F 99,839/68]

Long, D. A.: The influence of the thyroid gland upon immune responses of different species to bacterial infection. In: Wolstenholme and Millar; *Ciba Foundation Colloquia on Endocrinology*, Vol. 10, 287—297. London: J. & A. Churchill Ltd. 1957. [C 32,348/57]

Long, D. A., Miles, A. A.: Opposite actions of thyroid and adrenal hormones in allergic hypersensitivity. *Lancet* 1950 I, 492—495. [D 41,973/50]

Long, D. A., Miles, A. A., Perry, W. L. M.: Influence of thyroxine on the desensitizing action of A.C.T.H. and of cortisone in B.C.G.-infected guinea-pigs. *Lancet* 1951 I, 1392—1394. [B 60,189/51]

Long, D. A., Miles, A. A., Perry, W. L. M.: Action of ascorbic acid on tuberculin-sensitivity in guinea-pigs and its modification by dietary and hormonal factors. *Lancet* 1951 I, 1085—1088. [D 85,907/51]

Long, D. A., Miles, A. A., Perry, W. L. M.: The action of dehydroascorbic acid and alloxan on tuberculin-sensitivity in guinea pigs. *Lancet* 1951 II, 902—904. [B 63,843/51]

Long, D. A., Shewell, J.: The influence of the thyroid gland on sensitivity to tuberculin in guinea-pigs. *Brit. J. exp. Path.* 35, 503—506 (1954). [G 71,833/54]

Long, D. A., Shewell, J.: The influence of the thyroid gland on the production of antitoxin in the guinea-pig. *Brit. J. exp. Path.* 36, 351—356 (1955). [G 71,832/55]

Long, P. L., Rose, M. E.: Extended schizogony of Eimeria mivati in betamethasone-treated chickens. *Parasitology* 60, 147—155 (1970). [G 72,642/70]

Longenecker, H. E., Fricke, H. H., King, C. G.: The effect of organic compounds upon vitamin C synthesis in the rat. *J. biol. Chem.* 135, 497—510 (1940). [A 47,520/40]

Longerbeam, J. K., Lillehei, R. C.: The effects of various pharmacological agents on the canine intestinal hemodynamics during endotoxin shock (Abstr.). *Fed. Proc.* 20, 116 (1961). [D 3,868/61]

Longley, L. P.: Effect of treatment with testosterone propionate on mercuric chloride poisoning in rats. *J. Pharmacol. exp. Ther.* 74, 61—64 (1942). [A 37,552/42]

Loosli, C. G., Hull, R. B., Berlin, B. S., Alexander, E. R.: The influence of ACTH on the course of experimental influenza virus type A infections. *J. Lab. Clin. Med.* 37, 464—476 (1950). [B 58,316/50]

Lopez-Lomba, J.: Prolongation de la survie dans le scorbut chez les cobayes thymectomisés. *C. R. Soc. Biol. (Paris)* 89, 370—371 (1923). [17,165/23]

Loschiavo, F.: Potere battericida del sangue in convalescenti d'ileo-tifo sottoposti alla vaccinazione antitifica e trattati con 4-idrossi-19-nortestosterone-17-ciclopentilpropionato. *G. Mal. infett.* 17, 59—65 (1965). [G 28,338/65]

Lostroh, A. J.: Relationship of steroid and pituitary hormones to myocardial calcification in the mouse. *Proc. Soc. exp. Biol. (N.Y.)* 98, 84—88 (1958). [C 54,348/58]

Louria, D. B., Fallon, N., Browne, H. G.: The influence of cortisone on experimental fungus infections in mice. *J. clin. Invest.* **39**, 1435 to 1449 (1960). [C 91,764/60

Lowenstein, B. E., Zwemer, R. L.: Resistance of rats to potassium poisoning after administration of thyroid or of desoxycorticosterone acetate. *Endocrinology* **33**, 361—365 (1943). [A 74,481/43

Lowenthal, J., Fisher, L. M.: The effect of thyroid function on the prothrombin time response to Warfarin in rats. *Experientia (Basel)* **8**, 253—254 (1957). [C 40,044/57

Lu, A. Y., Junk, K. W., Coon, M. J.: Resolution of the cytochrome P-450 containing ω-hydroxylation system of liver microsomes into three components. *J. biol. Chem.* **244**, 3714—3721 (1969). [G 67,623/69

Lu, A. Y. H., Coon, M. J.: Role of hemoprotein P-450 in fatty acid ω-hydroxylation in a soluble enzyme system from liver microsomes. *J. biol. Chem.* **243**, 1331—1332 (1968). [G 71,879/68

Lu, A. Y. H., Strobel, H. W., Coon, M. J.: Hydroxylation of benzphetamine and other drugs by a solubilized form of cytochrome P-450 from liver microsomes: lipid requirement for drug demethylation. *Biochem. biophys. Res. Commun.* **36**, 545—551 (1969). [G 68,802/69

Lübke, A.: Leberveränderungen thyreotoxischer Mäuse nach Überwärmung und akutem Hitzekollaps. *Zbl. allg. Path. path. Anat.* **94**, 365—372 (1956). [C 12,952/56

Lucey, J. F.: Nursery illumination as a factor in neonatal hyperbilirubinemia. *Pediatrics* **44**, 155—157 (1969). [H 35,539/69

Lucherini, T., Schiavetti, L., Marino, T., Lucchesi, M.: Influenza del cortisone E della somatotropina (STS) sulla infezione tubercolare sperimentale della cavia. *Policlinico Sez. med.* **60**, 358—369 (1953). [B 89,088/53

Ludewig, S.: The effect of partial hepatectomy on the liver lipids. *Proc. Amer. Soc. biol. Chem. Toronto, Can.*, 33. Meet. LX11. (1939). [74,865/39

Lüders, D.: Bilirubin distribution studies in Gunn rats following the injection of sodium dehydrocholate. *Biol. Neonat. (Basel)* **15**, 329—341 (1970). [G 81,789/70

Lüders, D.: Das Für und Wider der Luminalbehandlung von Hyperbilirubinämien. *Monatschr. Kinderheilk.* **118**, 94—102 (1970). [H 24,062/70

Lüders, D.: Einfluss von Phenobarbital auf den Bilirubinstoffwechsel bei Gunnratten. Versuche mit inaktivem und ^{14}C-markiertem Bilirubin. *Ztschr. Kinderheilk.* **109**, 149—168 (1970). [H 34,593/70

Luhby, A. L., Davis, P., Murphy, M., Gordon, M., Brin, M., Spiegel, H.: Pyridoxine and oral contraceptives. *Lancet* **1970 II**, 1083. [H 32,376/70

Lum, B. K. B.: Protection against potassium intoxication by nicotine and by epinephrine (Abstr.). *Fed. Proc.* **29**, 476 (1970). [H 22,940/70

Lumper, L., Zahn, H.: Chemie und Biochemie des Disulfidaustausches. *Advanc. Enzymol.* **27**, 199—237 (1965). [G 72,128/65

Lund, C. C., Benedict, E. B.: The influence of the thyroid gland on the action of morphine. *New Engl. J. Med.* **201**, 345—353 (1929). [A 14,206/29

Lund, H.: Corticosteroid osteoporosis and treatment with anabolic hormone. *Acta med. scand.* **174**, 735—738 (1963). [E 38,261/63

Lungu, M., Petrescu, A., Tonescu, T.: Anti-influenza vaccination in mice with experimental hyper- and hypothyroidism. *Rev. roum. Endocr.* **3**, 127—132 (1967). [F 84,406/67

Luongo, M. A., Reid, D. H., Weiss, W. W.: The effect of ACTH in trichinosis; a clinical and experimental study. *New Engl. J. Med.* **245**, 757—760 (1951). [B 69,505/51

Lupulescou, A.: Les effets des hormones oestrogènes, de la noradrénaline et de l'hormone corticotrope (ACTH) sur le myocarde de cobaye. *Folia endocr. (Roma)* **16**, 91—104 (1963). [E 21,838/63

Lupuleseu, A., Potorac, E., Vasilescu, T., Pop, A., Merculiev, E., Oprisan, R., Oprisan, A.: Effects of the anabolic steroid (4-chlorotestosterone) on antibody production in hyper- and hypothyroid rabbits. *Path. et Microbiol. (Basel)* **29**, 800—810 (1966). [F 77,999/66

Lurie, M. B.: On the role of hormones in experimental tuberculosis. *Advanc. Tuberc. Res.* **6**, 18—48 (1955). [C 14,768/55

Lurie, M. B., Abramson, S., Allison, M. J.: Constitutional factors in resistance to infection. I. The effect of estrogen and chorionic gonadotropin on the course of tuberculosis in highly inbred rabbits. *Amer. Rev. Tuberc.* **59**, 168—185 (1949). [B 31,931/49

Lurie, M. B., Abramson, S., Heppleston, A. G., Allison, M. J.: Constitutional factors in resistance to infection. III. On the mode of action of estrogen and gonadotropin on the progress of tuberculosis. *Amer. Rev. Tuberc.* 59, 198—218 (1949). [B31,933/49

Lurie, M. B., Abramson, S., Heppleston, A. G., Dannenberg, A. M., Jr.: Immunological and hormonal studies on the nature of genetic resistance to tuberculosis (Abstr.). *Fed. Proc.* 11, 475 (1952). [B68,457/52

Lurie, M. B., Harris, T. N., Abramson, S., Allison, J. M.: Constitutional factors in resistance to infection. II. The effect of estrogen on tuberculin skin sensitivity and on the allergy of the internal tissues. *Amer. Rev. Tuberc.* 59, 186—197 (1949). [B31,932/49

Lurie, M. B., Ninos, G. S.: Effect of triiodothyronine and propyl thiouracil on native resistance to tuberculosis. *Fed. Proc.* 15, 601 (1956). [C14,387/56

Lurie, M. B., Zappasodi, P., Blaker, R. G., Levy, R. S.: On the role of the thyroid in native resistance to tuberculosis. II. The effect of hypothyroidism. The mode of action of thyroid hormones. *Amer. Rev. Tuberc.* 79, 180—203 (1959). [C64,295/59

Lurie, M. B., Zappasodi, P., Dannenberg, A. M., Jr., Swartz, I. B.: Constitutional factors in resistance to infection: The effect of cortisone on the pathogenesis of tuberculosis. *Science* 113, 234—237 (1951). [B55,625/51

Lurie, M. B., Zappasodi, P., Levy, R. S., Blaker, R. G.: Role of thyroid in native resistance to tuberculosis (Abstr.). *Fed. Proc.* 17, 447 (1958). [C52,055/58

Lurie, M. B., Zappasodi, P., Levy, R. S., Blaker, R. G.: On the role of the thyroid in native resistance to tuberculosis. I. The effect of hyperthyroidism. *Amer. Rev. Tuberc.* 79, 152—179 (1959). [C65,610/59

Lurie, M. B., Zappasodi, P., Levy, R. S., Twisdom, J. M., Ninos, G. S.: On the effect of levo-triiodothyronine and propylthiouracil on native resistance to tuberculosis (Abstr.). *J. clin. Endocr.* 16, 979 (1956). [C14,963/56

Luther, I. G., Heistad, G. T., Sparber, S. B.: Effect of ovariectomy and of estrogen administration upon gastric ulceration induced by cold-restraint. *Psychosom. Med.* 31, 389—392 (1969). [G70,681/69

Lutzmann, L., Schmidt, C. G.: Anabole Steroide und zytostatische Therapie. *Med. Welt (Stuttg.)* Nr. 47, 2644—2646 (1965). [F57,784/65

Macco, G. di: Azione della tirossina nell'ipertermia passiva. *Boll. Soc. ital. Biol. sper.* 10, 904—905 (1935). [34,121/35

MacDonald, R. A., Guiney, T., Tank, R.: Regeneration of the liver in Tirturus viridescens. *Proc. Soc. exp. Biol. (N.Y.)* 111, 277—280 (1962). [D41,743/62

MacGillivray, M. H., Crawford, J. D., Robey, J. S.: Congenital hypothyroidism and prolonged neonatal hyperbilirubinemia. *Pediatrics* 40, 283—286 (1967). [G48,968/67

Machinist, J. M., Dehner, E. W., Ziegler, D. M.: Microsomal oxidases. III. Comparison of species and organ distribution of dialkylarylamine N-oxide dealkylase and dialkylarylamine N-oxidase. *Arch. Biochem.* 125, 858—864 (1968). [H15,503/68

Mack, L., Smith, E. A.: Methylene blue in illuminating gas poisoning. *Proc. Soc. exp. Biol. (N.Y.)* 31, 1031—1032 (1934). [45,162/34

MacKay, E. M., Carne, H. O.: Influence of adrenalectomy and choline on the fat content of regenerating liver during fasting. *Proc. Soc. exp. Biol. (N.Y.)* 38, 131—133 (1938). [A14,767/38

MacKay, E. M., MacKay, L. L.: The relation of natural morphine tolerance to age and sex and the weight of the adrenal glands. *Arch. int. Pharmac. therap.* 52, 363—367 (1936). [56,167/36

MacKenzie, J. B., MacKenzie, C. G.: Production of pulmonary edema by thiourea in the rat, and its relation to age. *Proc. Soc. exp. Biol. (N.Y.)* 54, 34—37 (1943). [A49,024/43

Maddaloni, F.: Ormone cortico-surrenale ed ipertermia passiva. Ricerche sperimentali. *Arch. ital. Med. sper.* 2, 1 (1938). [A18,244/38

Maddock, W. O., Rankin, V. M., Youmans, W. B.: Prevention of the anti-curare action of epinephrine by dibenamine. *Proc. Soc. exp. Biol. (N.Y.)* 67, 151—153 (1948). [B18,670/48

Maekawa, K., Hosoyama, Y.: Protective effects of steroidal hormones on rat testis against injurious actions of cadmium. (Japanese text). *Zool. Mag.* 74, 17—23 (1965). [G79,815/65

Maekawa, K., Tsunenari, Y.: Mechanism involved in selective injurious effect of cadmium on the testis. *Gunma Symp. Endocr.* 4, 161—169 (1967). [H1,627/67

Maekawa, K., Tsunenari, Y., Yoshitoshi, K.: Estrogen and destructive effect of cadmium on testicular tissue. (Japanese text). *Zool. Mag.* 76, 84—90 (1967). [G79,814/67

Magalhães, M. M., Magalhães, M. C.: Ultrastructural alterations produced in rat liver by metopiron. *J. Ultrastruct. Res.* 32, 32—42 (1970). [G 76,648/70

Magara, M.: Sur l'action défensive de l'hormone sexuelle contre l'infection. *C. R. Soc. Biol. (Paris)* 121, 1193—1194 (1936). [35,283/36

Maibauer, D., Neubert, D., Rottka, H.: Pharmakologische Untersuchungen bei der experimentellen Leberverfettung. *Naunyn-Schmiedebergs Arch. Pharmak.* 234, 474—489 (1958). [G 74,663/58

Maickel, R. P., Brodie, B. B.: Increase in rat liver tryptophan peroxidase as a response to pituitary-adrenal stimulation by various centrally acting drugs. *Fed. Proc.* 19, 267 (1960). [C 83,071/60

Maickel, R. P., Bush, M. T., Jondorf, W. R., Miller, F. P., Gillette, J. R.: Factors influencing the metabolism and distribution of corticosterone-1,2-^{3}H in the rat. *Molec. Pharmacol.* 2, 491—495 (1966). [G 41,515/66

Mairesse, M., Darcis, L.: Influence de la castration et de la testostérone sur la radiosensibilité de la muqueuse jugale de la Lapine. *C. R. Soc. Biol. (Paris)* 156, 407—409 (1962). [D 27,579/62

Maisin, J., Desmedt, P., Jacqmin, L.: Influence de la castration sur l'éclosion et l'évolution du cancer du goudron chez la souris blanche. *C. R. Soc. Biol. (Paris)* 94, 769—770 (1926). [25,708/26

Maisin, J., Pourbaix, Y., Rijckaert, G.: Influence du propionate de testostérone sur l'évolution du cancer au benzopyrène chez la souris. *C. R. Soc. Biol. (Paris)* 130, 109—112 (1939). [A 30,500/39

Maisin, J. R., Doherty, D. G.: Chemical protection of mammalian tissues. *Fed. Proc.* 19, 564—572 (1960). [C 91,781/60

Maisin, J. R., Léonard, A., Lambiet, M., Mattelin, G.: Action de la 2-β-aminoéthylisothiourée (AET) et de la 5-hydroxytryptamine (sérotonine) sur l'intestin grêle et le système hématopoïétique des souris irradiées. *C. R. Soc. Biol. (Paris)* 157, 1525—1529 (1963). [E 36,751/63

Maisin, J. R., Mattelin, G.: Reduction in radiation lethality by mixtures of chemical protectors. *Nature (Lond.)* 214, 207—208 (1967). [F 78,796/67

Maisin, J. R., Mattelin, G.: Radioprotecteurs et radiothérapie des cancers. *Bull. Cancer* 54, 149—158 (1967). [H 719/67

Maisin, J. R., Mattelin, G., Fridman-Manduzio, A., Parren, J. van der: Reduction of short- and long-term radiation lethality by mixtures of chemical protectors. *Radiat. Res.* 35, 26—44 (1968). [G 59,894/68

Mäkinen, E., Näätänen, E., Similä, S.: The role of androgens in inducing experimental electrolyte-steroid-cardiopathy. *Ann. Med. exp. Fenn.* 40, 401—408 (1963). [E 20,847/63

Makino, Y.: Effects of hepatic periarterial neurectomy upon hepatic blood flow and regeneration of the liver after partial hepatectomy in the dog. *Arch. jap. Chir.* 37, 485—502 (1968). [H 19,101/68

Malhotra, O. P., Reber, E. F.: Effects of hormones and strain of rat on the incidence of the hemorrhagic syndrome in male rats fed irradiated beef. *Fed. Proc.* 19, 421 (1960). [C 83,177/60

Malhotra, O. P., Reber, E. F.: Methionine and testosterone effect on occurrence of hemorrhagic diathesis in rats. *Amer. J. Physiol.* 205, 1089—1092 (1963). [E 36,906/63

Malik, Z.: Pokusy s experimentálnou vnímavostou kurčiat voči mikróbu erysipelothrix rhusiopathiae. *Vet. Cas.* 11, 89—94 (1962). [D 34,701/62

Malkiel, S.: The influence of ACTH and cortisone on histamine and anaphylactic shock in the guinea pig. *J. Immunol.* 66, 379—384 (1951). [G 71,451/51

Malkiel, S., Hargis, B. J.: Histamine sensitivity and anaphylaxis in the pertussis-vaccinated rat. *Proc. Soc. exp. Biol. (N.Y.)* 81, 689—691 (1952). [D 27,396/52

Mallov, S.: Effect of sex hormones on ethanol induced fatty infiltration of liver in rats. *Proc. Soc. exp. Biol. (N.Y.)* 97, 226—229 (1958). [C 47,222/58

Maloney, A. H., Fitch, R. H., Tatum, A. L.: Picrotoxin as an antidote in acute poisoning by the shorter acting barbiturates. *J. Pharm. exp. Ther.* 41, 465—482 (1931). [61,235/31

Maloney, A. H., Froix, C., Booker, W. M.: Further studies on effect of pentobarbital sodium on adrenalectomized rats. *Fed. Proc.* 11, 398 (1952). [E 48,771/52

Mancini, R. T., Gautieri, R. F., Mann, D. E., Jr.: Effect of cortisone on the minimal carcinogenic dose$_{50}$ of methylcholanthrene in albino mice. *J. pharm. Sci.* 53, 385—388 (1964). [D 18,183/64

Mandel, L., Wintzerith, M., Mandel, P.: Action du propylthiouracile sur l'évolution biochimique de l'hypertrophie rénale compensatrice. *C. R. Soc. Biol. (Paris)* 154, 2125—2128 (1960). [D6,027/60

Mangum, J. H., Klingler, M. D., North, J. A.: The purification of a soluble cytochrome from pig kidney with spectral properties similar to those of microsomal cytochrome b_5. *Biochem. biophys. Res. Commun.* 40, 1520—1525 (1970). [G81,296/70

Man'ko, Y. K.: Toxicity of dopan, chlorambucil and endoxan by reduced serotonin. *Fed. Proc.* 25, T1073—T1075 (1966). [F74,715/66

Man'ko, Y. K.: Decrease of dopan, chlorambucil and endoxan toxic effect on animals by means of treatment with serotonin. (Russian text.) *Vop. Onkol.* 12/1, 52—56 (1966). [F82,459/66

Mann, F. D., Fishback, F. C., Gay, J. G., Green, G. F.: Experimental pathology of the liver. *Arch. Pathol.* 12, 787 (1931). [712/31

Mannering, G. J.: Significance of stimulation and inhibition of drug metabolism in pharmacological testing. In: Burger, A.; *Selected Pharmacological Testing Methods* 3, p. 51—119. New York: Marcel Dekker Inc. 1968. [G71,818/68

Mannering, G. J.: Significance of stimulation and inhibition of drug metabolism in pharmacologic testing. In: Tedeschi and Tedeschi; *Importance of Fundamental Principles in Drug Evaluation*, p. 105—127. New York: Raven Press 1968. [G75,980/68

Mannering, G. J.: Stimulation and inhibition of drug metabolism. In: Cerletti, A. and Bové F. J.; *The Present Status of Psychotropic Drugs*, p. 107—110. Excerpta med. Found. 1969. [G75,979/69

Mannering, G. J.: Properties of cytochrome P-450 as affected by environmental factors: qualitative changes due to administration of polycyclic hydrocarbons. *Metabolism* 20, 228—245 (1971). [H34,127/71

Mannering, G. J.: Microsomal enzyme systems which catalyze drug metabolism. In: LaDu et al.; *Fundamentals of Drug Metabolism and Disposition*. Baltimore, Md.: Williams and Wilkins (in press). [G74,558

Mannering, G. J.: Inhibition of drug metabolism. In: Brodie and Gillette; *Handbook of Experimental Pharmacology*. Berlin, Heidelberg, New York: Springer-Verlag (in press). [G74,572

Mannering, G. J.: Drug interactions. In: Epstein and Lederberg; *Chronic Non-Psychiatric Hazards of Abuse*. U. S. Government Printing Office (in press). [G74,881

Mannering, G. J.: Role of substrate binding to P-450 hemoproteins in drug metabolism. In: Michich; *Drugs and Cell Regulation*. New York: Academic Press (in press). [G78,898

Mansfeld, G.: Beiträge zur Physiologie der Schilddrüse. IX. Mitteilg. (Zur Abwehr). *Pflügers Arch. gesamt. Physiol.* 181, 249—270 (1920). [11,881/20

Mansfeld, G., Müller, F.: Beiträge zur Physiologie der Schilddrüse. I. Mitteilg. Die Ursache der gesteigerten Stickstoffausscheidung infolge Sauerstoffmangels. *Pflügers Arch. gesamt. Physiol.* 143, 157—174 (1911). [35,416/11

Manso, C., Friend, C., Wroblewsky, F.: The influence of 17-hydrocorticosterone on viral hepatitis of mice. *J. Lab. clin. Med.* 53, 729—736 (1959). [C68,152/59

Manston, R.: Calcium and phosphorus metabolism in cows after simultaneous injection of vitamin D_3 with vitamin A or thyroxine. *Brit. vet. J.* 125, 177—182 (1969). [G69,733/69

Mantegazza, P., Naimzada, K. M., Riva, M.: Activity of amphetamine in hypothyroid rats. *Europ. J. Pharmacol.* 5, 10—16 (1968). [H7,676/68

Mantegazza, P., Riva, M.: Attività della amfetamina in animali ipotiroidei. *Atti Acad. med. lombarda* 20, 10—15 (1965). [F47,703/65

Mantegazzini, P.: Alcune osservazioni circa l'azione di forti dosi di 5HT sul sistema nervoso centrale. *Boll. Soc. ital. Biol. sper.* 32, 839—841 (1956). [C33,637/56

Manunta, G.: Azione del benzoato di estradiolo sulla sopravvivenza dei ratti maschi tiroparatiroidectomizzati. *R. C. Accad. naz. Lincei, Cl. Sci. fis. mat. nat.* Ser. VIII, 12, 104—107 (1952). [B73,160/52

Maral, R.: Etude comparée de l'action du 4.560 R.P. (chlorpromazine) et de la cortisone sur certaines toxines. *Atti 6e Congr. int. Microbiol. Roma* 1, 615—618 (1953). [C17,604/53

Maral, R., Cosar, C.: Etude de l'action de la chlorpromazine, de la prométhazine et de la cortisone vis-à-vis de diverses infections expérimentales. *Arch. int. Pharmacodyn.* 102, 1—16 (1955). [C14,760/55

Marañón, G., Aznar, C.: Sobre la acción protectora de diferentes extractos de órganos contra la estricnina. *Bol. Soc. esp. Biol.* 302—305 (1915). [46,926/15

Marbé, S.: Les opsonines dans les états thyroïdiens. I. Les opsonines des animaux hyperthyroïdés. *C. R. Soc. Biol. (Paris)* 64, 1058 a 1060 (1908). [A4,623/08

Marbé, S.: Les opsonines dans les états thyroïdiens. II. Les opsonines des animaux éthyroïdés. *C. R. Soc. Biol. (Paris)* **64**, 1113—1115 (1908). [A 4,624/08

Marbé, S.: Les opsonines dans les états thyroïdiens. III. Les opsonines et la phagocytes chez les myxoedémateux. *C. R. Soc. Biol. (Paris)* **65**, 612—614 (1908). [A 4,625/08

Marbé, S.: Les opsonines et la phagocytose dans les états thyroïdiens. IV. Action directe, in vitro, du corps thyroïde. *C. R. Soc. Biol. (Paris)* **66**, 432—433 (1909). [A 4,626/09

Marbé, S.: Les opsonines et la phagocytose dans les états thyroïdiens. V. La phagocytose chez les animaux hyperthyroïdés et éthyroïdés. L'indice phagocytaire. *C. R. Soc. Biol. (Paris)* **66**, 1073—1075 (1909). [A 4,627/09

Marbé, S.: Les opsonines et la phagocytose dans les états thyroïdiens. VI. Le nombre des leucocytes et la formule leucocytaire chez les animaux hyperthyroïdés et chez les éthyroïdés. Rapport entre la formule leucocytaire et la phagocytose. *C. R. Soc. Biol. (Paris)* **67**, 44—46 (1909). [A 23,010/09

Marbé, S.: Les opsonines et la phagocytose dans les états thyroïdiens. VII. La phagocytose non microbienne dans les états thyroïdiens. Sur la chimiotaxie. *C. R. Soc. Biol. (Paris)* **67**, 111—113 (1909). [A 23,011/09

Marbé, S.: Les opsonines et la phagocytose dans les états thyroïdiens. VIII. Aspect et réaction du sérum et des leucocytes des animaux hyperthyroïdés et éthyroïdés. Rapport entre la réaction du sérum et l'indice opsonique. *C. R. Soc. Biol. (Paris)* **67**, 293—295 (1909). [A 23,012/09

Marbé, S.: Les opsonines et la phagocytose dans les états thyroïdiens. IX. L'indice phago-opsonique, la formule leucocytaire et la réaction du sérum dans la maladie de Basedow. Sur la pathogénie de la maladie de Basedow. *C. R. Soc. Biol. (Paris)* **67**, 362—364 (1909). [A 23,013/09

Marbé, S.: Les opsonines et la phagocytose dans les états thyroïdiens. XII. L'influence de la thyratoxine sur le pouvoir opsonique normal des animaux. *C. R. Soc. Biol. (Paris)* **69**, 355—357 (1910). [A 23,016/10

Marbé, S.: Hypersensibilisation générale thyroïdienne. III. La recherche des leucocytes dans le liquide péritonéal, et la formule leucocytaire des cobayes hyperthyroïdés et infectés avec le bacille d'Eberth. *C. R. Soc. Biol. (Paris)* **68**, 468—470 (1910). [A 23,018/10

Marbé, S.: Hypersensibilisation générale thyroïdienne. I. Sur la diminution de la résistance des cobayes hyperthyroïdés vis-à-vis de l'infection éberthienne expérimentale. *C. R. Soc. Biol. (Paris)* **68**, 351—353 (1910). [34,320/10

Marbé, S.: Hypersensibilisation générale thyroïdienne. II. Sur la diminution de la résistance des cobayes pesteux et hyperthyroïdés, ainsi que de ceux soumis même au traitement spécifique. *C. R. Soc. Biol. (Paris)* **68**, 412—414 (1910). [34,321/10

Marbé, S.: Les opsonines et la phagocytose dans les états thyroïdiens. XIII. Les inhibines phagocytaires d'origine thyroïdienne. *C. R. Soc. Biol. (Paris)* **69**, 387—389 (1910). [34,561/10

Marbé, S.: Hypersensibilisation générale thyroïdienne. VI. Sur la diminution de la résistance des cobayes hyperthyroïdés vis-à-vis de l'intoxication diphtérique, but de ces expériences. *C. R. Soc. Biol. (Paris)* **71**, 357—358 (1911). [35,374/11

Marbé, S.: L'hypersensibilisation générale thyroïdienne. VII. Exaltation et atténuation du bacille typhus muyium dans les milieux de culture thyroïdés. *C. R. Soc. Biol. (Paris)* **72**, 710—712 (1912). [A 23,015/12

Marc, V., Morselli, P. L.: Metabolism of exogenous cortisol in the rat in various experimental conditions. *J. Pharm. Pharmacol.* **21**, 864—866 (1969). [G 71,617/69

March, C. H., Elliott, H. W.: Distribution and excretion of radioactivity after administration of morphine-N-methyl C^{14} to rats. *Proc. Soc. exp. Biol. (N.Y.)* **86**, 494—497 (1954). [G 77,519/54

March, C. H., Gordan, G. S., Way, E. L.: The effect of castration and of testosterone on the action and distribution of dl-methadone in the rat. *Arch. int. Pharmacodyn.* **83**, 270—276 (1950). [B 58,376/50

Marchal, C., Benichoux, R.: Histoire de la régénération hépatique expérimentale. *Lyon chir.* **58**, 47—55 (1962). [D 37,572/62

Marchant, J.: The influence of sex and castration on the induction of skin tumours in mice by methyl cholanthrene. *Brit. J. Cancer* **13**, 106—114 (1959). [C 69,830/59

Marchi, G. de: Ricerche sull'azione della vitamina C e dell'estratto corticosurrenale nell'intossicazione difterica sperimentale, con particolare riguardo alle lesioni cardiache. *Accad. med.* **53**, 254—262 (1938). [A 30,837/38

Marie, A.: Glandes surrénales et toxi-infections. (Troisième note.) *C. R. Soc. Biol. (Paris)* 74, 221—223 (1913). [37,085/13

Marie, A.: Glandes surrénales et toxi-infections. *Ann. Inst. Pasteur* 32, 97—110 (1918). [32,348/18

Marie, A.: Du mode d'action de l'adrénaline vis-à-vis des toxines solubles. *C. R. Soc. Biol. (Paris)* 82, 581—583 (1919). [37,087/19

Marino, A., Bianchi, A., Giaquinto, S., Casola, L.: Induzione e trattamento della cardiopatia sperimentale da stress psicologico e pitressina. *Arch. int. Pharmacodyn.* 141, 377—395 (1963). [D 58,761/63

Markova, I. V.: Age sensitivity to barbiturates and its dependence on the development of the hypophyseal adrenal system. (Russian text.) *Byull. eksp. Biol. Med.* 50, 87—91 (1960). [D 49,769/60

Markova, I. V.: Underdevelopment of the hypophyseo-adrenal system in the newborn animals as a cause of reduced morphine resistance. (Russian text.) *Probl. Endokr. Gormonoter.* 8, 3—8 (1962). [D 47,081/62

Marmo, E., Miele, E.: Effetti di associazioni fra steroidi anabolizzanti e thiotepa su diverse neoplasie sperimentali. *Boll. Soc. ital. Biol. sper.* 37, 1474—1477 (1961). [D 27,478/61

Marmorston-Gottesman, J., Perla, D.: Immunological studies in relation to the suprarenal gland. III. The effect of injections of epinephrine on the hemolysin formation in normal rats. *J. exp. Med.* 48, 225—233 (1928). [23,446/28

Maros, T., Hadnagy, C., Seress-Sturm, L., Csiky, M., Kovács, I.: Die Wirkung von Vitamin B_{12} und von Cortison auf die Regeneration der Rattenleber. *Int. Z. Vitamin-Forsch.* 31, 303—307 (1961). [D 12,784/61

Marquardt, G. H., Fisher, C. I., Levy, P., Dowben, R. M.: Effect of anabolic steroids on liver function tests and creatine excretion. *J. Amer. med. Ass.* 175, 851—853 (1961). [D 82,860/61

Marshall, R. T., Freeman, S.: Effect of 'thyroidectomy' on nephrectomized dogs and rats. *Fed. Proc.* 11, 101 (1952). [B 68,239/52

Marshall, R. T., Freeman, S.: The effect of hypothyroidism on the development of experimental uremia. *Endocrinology* 55, 205—211 (1954). [B 96,575/54

Marsilii, G., Simone, M. de: Su alcuni aspetti submicroscopici del fegato rigenerante. *Boll. Soc. ital. Biol. sper.* 38, 1034—1036 (1962). [G 1,552/62

Martin, J. M.: Necrosis hepática por aloxano y cloroformo. Factores agravantes y protectores. *Rev. Soc. argent. Biol.* 29, 103—107 (1953). [B 88,524/53

Martin, L. G., Bullard, R. W.: Thyroxine-enhanced susceptibility of mice to Klebsiella pneumoniae. *Proc. Soc. exp. Biol. (N.Y.)* 131, 824—827 (1969). [H 15,263/69

Martin, S. J., Herrlich, H. C., Clark, B. B.: The effect of various tissues on the detoxification of evipal in the dog. *Anesthesiology* 1, 153—157 (1940). [A 48,575/40

Martinengo, L., Beghelli, G.: Dijodotirosina e ipertermia passiva. *Folia Ther.* 17, 35—50 (1939). [B 3,426/39

Martinez, C.: Tiroids y sensibilidad al aloxano endovanoso. *Rev. Soc. argent. Biol.* 21, 254—258 (1945). [B 15,837/45

Martinez, C.: Acción del tiouracilo sobre la diabetes aloxánica y pancreática en la rata. *Rev. Soc. argent. Biol.* 22, 135—146 (1946). [B 2,342/46

Martinez, C.: The SH groups in experimental diabetes. *Acta physiol. lat.-amer.* 2, 135—162 (1951). [B 61,239/51

Martinez-Manautou, J., Aznar-Ramos, R., Bautista-O'Farrill, J., Gonzáles-Angulo, A.: The ultrastructure of liver cells in women under steroid therapy. II. Contraceptive therapy. *Acta endocr. (Kbh.)* 65, 207—221 (1970). [H 30,302/70

Maruyama, M., Fujita, T., Ohata, M.: Purification and properties of a microsomal endopeptidase from rat kidney preferentially hydrolyzing parathyroid hormone. *Arch. Biochem.* 138, 245—253 (1970). [G 74,893/70

Marver, H. S., Schmid, R., Schützel, H.: Heme and methemoglobin: naturally occurring repressors of microsomal cytochrome. *Biochem. biophys. Res. Commun.* 33, 969—974 (1968). [G 76,839/68

Maśliński, C.: The effect of thyroid gland on the course of experimental tuberculosis. *Bull. Acad. pol. Sci.* 4, 273—278 (1956). [C 50,519/56

Maśliński, C.: The course of tuberculous infection on the ground of the existing hyperfunction or hypofunction of the thyroid gland. *Bull. Acad. pol. Sci.* 4, 279—282 (1956). [C 50,520/56

Maśliński, C.: Tarczyca a gruźlica doświadczalna. (Thyroid gland and experimental tuberculosis) *Rozpr. Wydz. Nauk Med.* 2/1, 137—192 (1957). [C 48,845/57

Mason, H. S., North, J. C., Vanneste, M.: Microsomal mixed-function oxidations: the metabolism of xenobiotics. *Fed. Proc.* 24, 1172—1180 (1965). [F51,528/65

Mason, R. C., Johnson, D. H., Robinson, H. J.: Comparative effects of corticosterone and cortisone on experimental corynebacterium infection of mice. *Fed. Proc.* 15, 456 (1956). [C14,288/56

Massalski, W., Kulejewska, M.: Działanie ACTH w doświadczalnym tezcu. (Influence of ACTH in experimental tetanus.) *Pol. Tyg. lék.* 12, 252—254 (1957). [C52,338/57

Massei, G., Villani, C., Caturegli, G.: Effetti del propionato di testosterone a forti dosi nella epatopatia sperimentale da CCl$_4$. *Arch. Sci. med.* 108, 811—852 (1959). [D2,594/59

Masson, G.: Influence des traits hypophysaires sur la résistance à l'anesthésie. *Rev. canad. Biol.* 4, 121—124 (1945). [B275/45

Masson, G.: Effects of proteins on the resistance to anesthesia produced by barbiturates. *Fed. Proc.* 5, 72 (1946). [A95,888/46

Masson, G.: Influence de préparations hypophysaires sur la résistance à l'anesthésie produite par les barbiturates. *Rev. canad. Biol.* 5, 400—406 (1946). [B1,217/46

Masson, G.: Non-spécificité de l'action de préparations hypophysaires sur la résistance au nembutal. *Rev. canad. Biol.* 6, 26—35 (1947). [94,205/47

Masson, G.: Action de la thyroxine sur l'effet testoïde de la testostérone. *Rev. canad. Biol.* 6, 355—358 (1947). [96,171/47

Masson, G.: Inhibition de l'action hépatotoxique du tétrachlorure de carbone. *Rev. canad. Biol.* 6, 362—366 (1947). [96,335/47

Masson, G., Beland, E.: Studies on the detoxification of barbiturates. *Fed. Proc.* 3, 32 (1944). [A72,286/44

Masson, G., Corcoran, A. C., Page, I. H.: Dietary and hormonal influences in experimental uremia. *J. Lab. clin. Med.* 34, 925—931 (1949). [B40,204/49

Masson, G., Hoffman, M. M.: Studies on the role of the liver in the metabolism of progesterone. *Endocrinology* 37, 111—116 (1945). [B513/45

Masson, G. M. C., Beland, E.: Influence of the liver and the kidney on the duration of anesthesia produced by barbiturates. *Anesthesiology* 6, 483—491 (1945). [B344/45

Masson, G. M. C., Page, I. H., Corcoran, A. C.: Vascular reactivity of rats and dogs treated with desoxycorticosterone acetate. *Proc. Soc. Exp. Biol. (N.Y)* 73, 434—436 (1950). [B47,635/50

Masson, M. C., Corcoran, A. C., Page, H.: Experimental vascular diseases due to desoxycorticosterone acetate and anterior pituitary extract. 1. Comparison of functional changes. *J. Lab. clin. Med.* 34, 1416—1426 (1949). [B48,694/49

Matsumura, F., Wang, C. M.: Reduction of dieldrin storage in rat liver: factors affecting in situ. *Bull. environm. Contam. Toxicol.* 3, 203—210 (1968). [G74,472/68

Matthews, S. A., Austin, W. C.: The effect of the blood calcium level on the tolerance to magnesium. Some observations on hypercalcemia induced by the parathyroid hormone. *Amer. J. Physiol.* 79, 708—718 (1927). [21,067/27

Matthies, H., Schmidt, J.: Die Beeinflussung der Hexobarbitalnarkose durch intracerebrale Injektion biogener Amine nach Reserpinvorbehandlung. *Naunyn-Schmiedebergs Arch. Pharmak.* 241, 508—509 (1961). [D84,334/61

Matzen, R. N.: Effect of vitamin C and hydrocortisone on the pulmonary edema produced by ozone in mice. *J. appl. Physiol.* 11, 105—109 (1957). [C39,985/57

Maurer, H. M.: New concepts in the management of neonatal jaundice: use of enzyme induction and phototherapy. *Med. Coll. Va Quart.* 6, 79—86 (1970). [H29,765/70

Maurer, H. M., Wolff, J. A., Finster, M., Poppers, P. J., Pantuck, E., Kuntzman, R., Conney, A. H.: Reduction in concentration of total serum-bilirubin in offspring of women treated with phenobarbitone during pregnancy. *Lancet* 1968 II, 122—124. [G71,810/68

Mayer, J., Goddard, J. W.: Effects of administration of gonadotropic hormone on vitamin A deficient rats. *Proc. Soc. exp. Biol. (N.Y.)* 76, 149—151 (1951). [B55,008/51

Mayer, J., Truant, A. P.: Effects of administration of testosterone on vitamin A-deficient rats. *Proc. Soc. exp. Biol. (N.Y.)* 72, 436—438 (1949). [B43,456/49

Mayer, R. L., Hays, H. W., Brousseau, D., Mathieson, D., Rennick, B., Yonkman, F. F.: Pyribenzamine (N'-pyridyl-N'-benzyl-N-dimethylethylene-diamine HCL), an antagonist of histamine. *J. Lab. clin. Med.* 31, 749—751 (1946). [B3,674/46

Mayewski, R. J., Litwack, G.: ^{3}H-cortisol radioactivity in hepatic smooth endoplasmic reticulum. *Biochem. biophys. Res. Commun.* 37, 729—735 (1969). [G 70,720/69

Mazel, P., Bush, M. T.: Pharmacological studies of the bloodbrain barrier. *Fed. Proc.* 20, 306 (1961). [D 4,194/61

Mazel, P., Bush, M. T.: Brain barbital levels and anesthesia as influenced by physostigmine and epinephrine. *Biochem. Pharmacol.* 18, 579—586 (1969). [G 65,299/69

McArthur, J. N., Dawkins, P. D., Smith, M. J. H.: The binding of indomethacin, salicylate and phenobarbitone to human whole blood in vitro. *J. Pharm. Pharmacol.* 23, 32—36 (1971). [G 81,040/71

McCallum, H. M.: Lathyrism in mice. *Nature (Lond.)* 182, 1169—1170 (1958). [C 61,614/58

McCann, S. M., Matsumura, Y., Dimick, M. K., Pencharz, R., Lepkovsky, S.: Effect of hypothalamic lesions on tryptophan peroxidase of the liver. *Proc. Soc. exp. Biol. (N.Y.)* 100, 586—588 (1959). [E 93,864/59

McCarthy, J. L., Rietz, C. W., Wesson, L. K.: Inhibition of adrenal corticosteroidogenesis in the rat by cyanotrimethylandrostenolone, a synthetic androstane. *Endocrinology* 79, 1123 to 1129 (1966). [F 74,065/66

McCarthy, J. S., Furner, R. L., Dyke, K. van, Stitzel, R. E.: Effect of malarial infection on host microsomal drug-metabolizing enzymes. *Biochem. Pharmacol.* 19, 1341—1349 (1970). [G 75,511/70

McClure, D. J., Cleghorn, R. A.: Suppression studies in affective disorders. *Canad. psychiat. Ass. J.* 13, 477—488 (1968). [G 76,696/68

McCluskey, R. T., Thomas, L.: The removal of cartilage matrix in vivo by papain. Prevention of recovery with cortisone, hydrocortisone and prednisolone by a direct action on cartilage. *Amer. J. Path.* 35, 819—833 (1959). [C 71,485/59

McColl, J. D., Robinson, S., Sagritalo, G. M.: Enhancement of postcoital antifertility activity of estrogens by dimenhydrinate in the rat. (Abstr.) *Fed. Proc.* 29, 781 (1970). [H 24,915/70

McColl, J. D., Sacra, P.: Alteration in toxicity and action of hypoglycemic agents in the rat by sex hormones. *Toxicol. appl. Pharmacol.* 4, 631—637 (1962). [D 34,973/62

McCormack, C. E., Meyer, R. K.: Ovulating hormone release in gonadotropin treated immature rats. *Proc. Soc. exp. Biol. (N.Y.)* 110, 343—346 (1962). [D 29,101/62

McCormack, C. E., Meyer, R. K.: Minimal age for induction of ovulation with progesterone in rats: evidence for neutral control. *Endocrinology* 74, 793—799 (1964). [F 9,493/64

McDonagh, J. E. R.: The active principle of the parathyroid glands, tetany and calcium metabolism. *Amer. Med. (Philad.)* 34, 36—49 (1928). [19,285/28

McEuen, C. S., Selye, H., Collip, J. B.: Effect of testosterone on somatic growth. *Proc. Soc. exp. Biol. (N.Y.)* 36, 390—394 (1937). [39,157/37

McFarlane, E. S., Embil, J. A., Jr.: Effect of gonadectomy on adenovirus-12 oncogenesis in Syrian hamsters. *Canad. J. Microbiol.* 14, 1013—1014 (1968). [H 18,880/68

McFarland, L. Z., Lacy, P. B.: Physiologic and endocrinologic effects of the insecticide kepone in the Japanese quail. *Toxicol. appl. Pharmacol.* 15, 441—450 (1969). [G 68,855/69

McGill, H. C., Parrish, L. E., Holman, R. L.: Influence of alloxan diabetes of cholesterol atherosclerosis in the rabbit. *Fed. Proc.* 8, 361 (1949). [B 32,954/49

McGrath, E. J.: Experimental peripheral gangrene. *J. Amer. med. Ass.* 105, 854—856 (1935). [A 29,208/35

McGrath, E. J., Herrmann, L. G.: Influence of estrogens on the peripheral vasomotor mechanism. *Ann. Surg.* 120, 607—616 (1944). [B 500/44

McGraw, J. Y.: La régulation de la résistance capillaire. IV. Influence de traitements vitaminiques et hormonaux sur la croissance et la résistance capillaire du cobaye. *Laval méd.* 27, 660—710 (1959). [C 68,484/59

McGraw, J. Y.: La régulation de la résistance capillaire. VII. Influence de la thyroïde et des surrénales sur la croissance et la résistance capillaire. *Laval méd.* 28, 643—698 (1959). [C 80,136/59

McGuire, J. S., Jr., Hollis, V. W., Jr., Tomkins, G. M.: Some characteristics of the microsomal steroid reductases (5α) of rat liver. *J. biol. Chem.* 235, 3112—3117 (1960). [D 82,559/60

McGuire, J. S., Jr., Tomkins, G. M.: The effects of thyroxin administration on the enzymic reduction of Δ^4-3-ketosteroids. *J. biol. Chem.* 234, 791—794 (1959). [E 90,938/59

McGuire, J. S., Jr., Tomkins, G. M.: The heterogeneity of Δ^4-3-ketosteroid reductases (5α). *J. biol. Chem.* 235, 1634—1638 (1960). [D 5,722/60

McGuire, J. S., Tomkins, G. M.: The multiplicity and specificity of Δ^4-3-ketosteroid hydrogenases (5α). *Arch. Biochem.* 82, 475—477 (1959). [E 91,579/59

McIver, A. K.: Drug incompatibilities. *Pharm. J.* 195, 609—612 (1965). [G 78,391/65

McIver, A. K.: Drug interactions. *Pharm. J.* 199, 205—210 (1967). [G 77,708/67

McIver, M. A.: Increased susceptibility to chloroform poisoning produced in the albino rat by injection of crystalline thyroxin. *Proc. Soc. exp. biol. (N.Y.)* 45, 201—206 (1940). [A 35,431/40

McIver, M. A., Winter, E. A.: Deleterious effects of anoxia on the liver of the hyperthyroid animal. *Arch. Surg.* 46, 171—185 (1943). [B 33,399/43

McKenna, J. M., Zweifach, B. W.: Reticuloendothelial system in relation to drum shock. *Amer. J. Physiol.* 187, 263—268 (1956). [C 27,414/56

McLean, E. K., McLean, A. E. M., Sutton, P. M.: Instant cirrhosis. An improved method for producing cirrhosis of the liver in rats by simultaneous administration of carbon tetrachloride and phenobarbitone. *Brit. J. exp. Path.* 50, 502—506 (1969). [H 18,569/69

McLean, S., Marchand, C.: The effect of SKF 525-A on drug concentration in the blood. *Life Sci.* 9/I, 1075—1080 (1970). [G 78,253/70

McLoughlin, D. K.: The influence of dexamethasone on attempts to transmit Eimeria meleagrimitis to chickens and E. tenella to turkeys. *J. Protozool.* 16, 145—148 (1969). [G 73,149/69

McLuen, E. F., Fouts, J. R.: The effect of obstructive jaundice on drug metabolism in rabbits. *J. Pharmacol. exp. Ther.* 131, 7—11 (1961). [E 99,285/61

McMullin, G. P.: Phenobarbitone and neonatal jaundice. *Lancet* 1968 II, 978—979. [G 77,713/68

McMullin, G. P., Hayes, M. F., Arora, S. C.: Phenobarbitone in rhesus haemolytic disease. A controlled trial. *Lancet* 1970 II, 949—952. [H 31,772/70

McQueen-Williams, M., Thompson, K. W.: The effect of ablation of the hypophysis upon the weight of the kidney of the rat. *Yale J. Biol. Med.* 12, 531—541 (1940). [A 33,938/40

Medina, M. A., Merritt, J. H.: Drug metabolism and pharmacologic action in mice exposed to reduced barometric pressure. *Biochem. Pharmacol.* 19, 2812—2816 (1970). [G 81,699/70

Medlinsky, J. T., Napier, C. D., Gurney, C. W.: The use of an antiandrogen to further investigate the erythropoietic effects of androgens. *J. Lab. clin. Med.* 74, 85—92 (1969). [G 67,839/69

Medvedeva, G. I.: Correlations of direct and indirect calorimetry data during recovery from hypothermia in healthy rabbits and in experimental hypothyroidism. *Probl. Endokr.* 14/1, 105—110 (1968). [F 96,027/68

Meer, C. van der, Bekkum, D. W. van: The mechanism of radiation protection by histamine and other biological amines. *Int. J. Radiat. Biol.* 1, 5—23 (1959). [G 71,673/59

Mehrotra, R. M. L., Mangalik, V. S., Nayak, N. C.: An experimental study of the effect of doca on the development of ascites in CCl_4 cirrhosis. *Indian J. med. Res.* 45, 183—190 (1957). [C 54,806/57

Mehrotra, R. M. L., Sarna, S.: Thyroid hormone and paraaminosalicylate-induced liver changes. *J. Path. Bact.* 82, 522—526 (1961). [D 14,287/61

Meier, H.: Experimental pharmacogenetics. Physiopathology of heredity and pharmacologic responses. New York, London: Academic Press, Inc., pp. 213 (1963). [E 690/63

Meier, R., Neipp, L.: Verstärkung der chemotherapeutischen Wirkung von Sulfonamiden durch zusätzliche Behandlung mit chemotaktisch wirkenden Polysacchariden aus Harn und Bakterien. *Schweiz. med. Wschr.* 86, 249 bis 251 (1956). [C 37,215/56

Meissner, R.: Über Paraphenylendiamin. *Naunyn-Schmiedebergs Arch. Pharmak.* 84, 181 bis 222 (1919). [E 52,567/19

Meister, V. von: Recreation des Lebergewebes nach Abtragung ganzer Leberlappen. Experimentelle Untersuchung. *Beitr. path. Anat.* 15, 1—116 (1894). [A 25,263/1894

Meites, J., Feng, Y. S. L., Wilwerth, A. M.: The effects of endocrine imbalances on vitamin requirements. *Amer. J. clin. Nutr.* 5, 381—392 (1957). [C 39,753/57

Mejia, R. H., Rennis, M. A., Bolo, H. J.: Influence of adrenal glands on the survival time of hypovolemic shock. *Acta physiol. lat.-amer.* 18, 151—156 (1968). [G 60,637/68

Melby, J. C., Bradley, G. M., Spink, W. W.: The influence of triiodothyronine on the lethal effect of bacterial endotoxin and infection due to Br. melitensis. *Clin. Res.* 6, 280 (1958). [C 86,232/58

Melby, J. C., Egdahl, R. H., Bossenmaier, I. C., Spink, W. W.: Suppression by cortisol of increased serum-transaminase induced by endotoxin. *Lancet* 1959 I, 441—444. [C 65,221/59

Melby, J. C., Spink, W. W.: Enhancement of lethal action of endotoxin in mice by triiodothyronine. *Proc. Soc. exp. Biol. (N.Y.)* **101**, 546—547 (1959). [C 72,440/59

Melcher, G. W., Jr., Blunt, J. W., Ragan, C.: Occurrence of hepatitis in cortisone-treated rats following inoculation with human infectious hepatitis serum. *Amer. Soc. clin. Invest. 44th Ann. Meet. Atlantic City*, p. 40 (1952).
[B 69,381/52

Melching, H. J., Langendorff, M., Ladner, H. A.: Über die Abhängigkeit der Strahlenschutzwirksamkeit des 5-Hydroxytryptamins von Konzentration und Zeitfaktor. *Naturwissenschaften* **45**, 545 (1958). [C 76,527/58

Meldolesi, J.: On the significance of the hypertrophy of the smooth endoplasmic reticulum in liver cells after administration of drugs. *Biochem. Pharmacol.* **16**, 125—129 (1967). [G 66,053/67

Meldolesi, J., Vincenzi, L., Bassan, P., Morini, M. T.: Effect of carbon tetrachloride on the synthesis of liver endoplasmic reticulum membranes. *Lab. Invest.* **19**, 315—323 (1968).
[G 69,793/68

Mellette, S. J.: Interrelationships between vitamin K and estrogenic hormones. *Amer. J. clin. Nutr.* **9**, 109—116 (1961). [D 7,939/61

Melnik, M.: Contribution à l'étude des relations entre les glandes à sécrétion interne et l'immunité. Le corps thyroïde et le bacilli de Shiga. *C. R. Soc. Biol. (Paris)* **92**, 474—475, 944—945 (1925). [26,134/25

Menguy, R., Masters, Y. F.: The effects of parathyroid extract on the stomach. *Physiologist* **7**, 205 (1964). [F 17,447/64

Menguy, R., Masters, Y. F.: Role of the liver in the glycoprotein mobilizing property of parathyroid extract (Abstr.). *Clin. Res.* **13**, 257 (1965). [F 61,098/65

Mercier-Parot, L., Tuchmann-Duplessis, H.: Propriétés embryotoxique et tératogène d'une méthylhydrazine antitumorale: influence de la progestérone. *C. R. Acad. Sci. (Paris)* **270**, 1153—1156 (1970). [G 73,572/70

Merli, G. M., Gandini, A.: Richerche sperimentali sulla resistenza alla intossicazione latirogenica da n-butilamina in ratti epatectomizzati. *Biochem. Biol. sper.* **111**, 289 (1964).
[F 32,684/64

Messina, C.: Effetti del trattamento con H.C.G. e con ergotamina in ratti integri ed ipofisectomizzati. *Boll. Soc. ital. Biol. sper.* **40**, 439—442 (1964). [G 18,016/64

Messini, M., Coppo, M.: Ricerche sui rapporti fra ormoni e vitamine. Studio sul meccanismo d'azione della vitamina antirachitica nell'organismo come contributo alla conoscenza della fisiopatologia del timo. *Arch. Ist. biochim. ital.* **7**, 195—232 (1935). [31,827/35

Metzenberg, R. L., Marchall, M., Paik, W. K., Cohen, P. P.: The synthesis of carbamyl phosphate synthetase in thyroxin-treated tadpoles. *J. Biol. Chem.* **36**, 162—165 (1961).
[D 86,024/61

Metzler, A. von: Die Wirkung von Desoxycorticosteron auf den Blutdruck bei der Ratte nach vorheriger Behandlung mit 3-Methylcholanthren. *Klin. Wschr.* **48**, 695—696 (1970).
[H 27,243/70

Metzler, A. von, Hergott, J.: Über den Einfluß des Percortens auf toxische Strophanthindosen am Froschherzen in situ. *Klin. Wschr.* **29**, 91—92 (1951). [B 63,494/51

Méwissen, D. J., Lagneau, L. E.: Le rôle du thymus sur la survie des souris après irradiation totale, avec ou sans protection chimique. *Acta clin. belg.* **19**, 71—72 (1964). [G 14,713/64

Méwissen, D. J., Rust, J. H., Lagneau, L. E.: Le rôle du thymus dans la survie de la souris C57 BL irradiée, avec ou sans protection chimique. *C. R. Soc. Biol. (Paris)* **159**, 240—242 (1965). [F 45,017/65

Meyer, B. J., Karel, L.: The effects of iodides, l-thiosorbitol, and twenty-five other compounds on alphanaphthylthiourea (ANTU) toxicity in rats. *J. Pharmacol. exp. Ther.* **92**, 15—31 (1948). [B 18,102/48

Meyer, B. J., Vos, A. C.: The effect of lathyrus odoratus meal, cholesterol and various hormones on the structure of the aorta and coronary arteries. *S. Afr. J. med. Sci.* **22**, 29—36 (1957). [C 41,429/57

Meyer, D. L., Forbes, R. M.: Effects of thyroid hormone and phosphorus loading on renal calcification and mineral metabolism of the rat. *J. Nutr.* **93**, 361—367 (1967). [G 53,688/67

Meyers, F. H., Peoples, D.: The positive role of the liver in the rapid metabolism of thiopental. *Anesthesiology* **15**, 146—149 (1954).
[G 70,570/54

Meyers, K. P.: Implantation and deciduoma formation after administration of antiestrogenic compounds. *Biol. Reprod.* **3**, 61—66 (1970). [G 77,432/70

Mezzano, M., Peluffo, G.: Elettività cardiotropa nel sinergismo endotossina noradrenalina. *Pathologica* **52**, 369—377 (1960).
[D 9,328/60

Michael, M., Jr., Cummings, M. M., Bloom, W. L.: Course of experimental tuberculosis in the albino rat as influenced by cortisone. *Proc. Soc. exp. Biol. (N.Y.)* **75**, 613—616 (1950). [B 53,378/50

Michalek, L., Slaughter, D., Harshfield, R.: Morphine addiction and cortone (Abstr.). *J. Pharmacol. exp. ther.* **103**, 354—355 (1951). [B 91,619/51

Michalovà, G.: The effect of ACTH on experimental silicosis, with special respect to neurohumoral regulation. *Acta physiol. Acad. Sci.* **14**, 79—87 (1958). [C 56,094/58

Michel, R., Truchot, R.: Sur la concentration hépatique du cholestérol chez le rat traité par la thyroxine. *C. R. Soc. Biol. (Paris)* **153**, 572—574 (1959). [C 79,107/59

Middleton, W. R. J., Isselbacher, K. J.: The stimulation of intestinal cholesterogenesis in the rat by phenobarbital. *Proc. Soc. exp. Biol. (N.Y.)* **131**, 1435—1437 (1969). [H 17,133/69

Mikes, A., Todorović, D.: Effet de la 6-aminonicotamide sur le foie du cobaye. Effet protecteur de la nicotamide et de la prednisolone. I. Intoxication aiguë. *Rev. int. Hépat.* **9**, 759—767 (1959). [C 86,716/59

Mikuni, C., Ujiie, T., Ibayashi, J.: Electron micrographs of biligraphin in rat's hepatic tissue. (Japanese text.) *Jap. J. clin. Elect. Micr.* **2**, 474 (1970). [H 28,797/70

Millen, J. W., Woollam, D. H. M.: Influence of cortisone on teratogenic effects of hypervitaminosis-A. *Brit. med. J.* **1957 II**, 196—197. [C 38,328/57

Miller, J. F. A. P.: Rôle du thymus dans les processus immunitaires. *Ann. Inst. Pasteur* **105**, 1007—1016 (1963). [E 37,260/63

Miller, J. W., George, R., Elliott, H. W., Sung, C. Y., Way, E. L.: The influence of the adrenal medulla in morphine analgesia. *J. Pharmacol. exp. Ther.* **113**, 43—50 (1955). [G 73,877/55

Miller, V. L., Bearse, G. E., Russell, T. S., Csonka, E.: The effect of several hormones and sodium thiomalate on retention of mercury by two strains of chicks. *Poultry Sci.* **48**, 613 to 620 (1969). [G 77,153/69

Miller, W. L., Jr., Baumann, C. A.: Basal metabolic rate and liver tumors due to azo dyes. *Cancer Res.* **11**, 634—639 (1951). [G 74,552/51

Milošević, M. P.: The action of sympathomimetic amines on intravenous anesthesia in rats. *Arch. int. Pharmacodyn.* **106**, 437—446 (1956). [C 39,053/56

Milošević, M. P.: Uticaj reserpina i 5-hidroksitriptamina (serotonina) na toksičnost adrenalina. [The toxicity of adrenaline as influenced by reserpine and 5-hydroxytryptamine (serotonin).] *Acta med. jugosl.* **11**, 180—185 (1957). [C 41,594/57

Mims, C. A.: The haemorrhagic enteritis syndrome in mice. *Brit. J. exp. Path.* **53**, 24—30 (1962). [G 68,101/62

Mincis, M.: A ação do álcool sôbre o fígado. *Rev. Ass. méd. bras.* **16**, 157—166 (1970). [H 30,210/70

Minkowitz, S., Berkovich, S.: Hepatitis produced by Coxsackie-virus B1 in adult mice. *Arch. Path.* **89**, 427—433 (1970). [H 23,844/70

Minz, B., Domino, E. F.: Effects of epinephrine and norepinephrine on electrically induced seizures. *J. Pharmacol. exp. Ther.* **107**, 204 to 218 (1953). [B 81,852/53

Mirand, E. A., Reinhard, M. C., Goltz, H. L.: Protective effect of adrenal steroid administration on irradiated mice. *Proc. Soc. exp. Biol. (N.Y.)* **81**, 397—400 (1952). [B 76,197/52

Mistry, P. B., Monnot, P., Duplan, J. F.: Stimulation de la leucémogenèse AKR par des irradiations X fractionnées: action inhibitrice de l'hydrocortisone. *C. R. Soc. Biol. (Paris)* **164**, 697—700 (1970). [H 33,481/70

Mitchell, M. L., Girerd, R. J.: Effect of growth hormone and antibiotics upon nitrogen mustard treated rats. *Proc. Soc. exp. Biol. (N.Y.)* **83**, 615—618 (1953). [B 82,866/53

Miti, L., Memeo, S. A.: Influenza dell'aldosterone sulla rigenerazione epatica. *G. Geront.* **10**, 281—286 (1962). [D 27,223/62

Mitoma, C.: Response to drugs by rats showing long or short hexobarbital-induced sleep. *Arch. int. Pharmacodyn.* **184**, 124—128 (1970). [H 25,522/70

Mitoma, C., LeValley, S. E.: Effect of newborn rats of perinatal exposure to phenobarbital. *Arch. int. Pharmacodyn.* **187**, 155—162 (1970). [H 31,720/70

Mitoma, C., Neubauer, S. E., Badger, N. L., Sorich, T. J.: Hepatic microsomal activities in rats with long and short sleeping times after hexobarbital: a comparison. *Proc. Soc. exp. Biol. (N.Y.)* **125**, 284—288 (1967). [G 69,268/67

Mitoma, C., Yasuda, D., Tagg, J. S., Neubauer, S. E., Calderoni, F. J., Tanabe, M.: Effects of various chemical agents on drug metabolism and cholesterol biosynthesis. *Biochem. Pharmacol.* **17**, 1377—1383 (1968). [G 72,113/68

Mitri, T. de, Felisati, D., Bastianini, L.: Influence of cortisone on the evolution of experimental bronchopneumonia due to Candida albicans. Pract. oto-rhino-laryng. (Basel) 25, 15—22 (1963). [D 64,042/63

Mitropoulos, K. A., Myant, N. B.: The metabolism of cholesterol in the presence of liver mitochondria from normal and thyroxine treated rats. Biochem. J. 94, 594—603 (1965). [G 26,978/65

Mitznegg, P., Säbel, M., Heim, F.: Inhibition of estrogen-induced radioprotection of placental nucleic acids and proteins by the antiestrogen clomiphene. Life Sci. 9/II, 815—820 (1970). [G 77,075/70

Miura, M.: The effects of thyroid, thyroxin and other iodine compounds upon the acetonitrile tests. J. Lab. clin. Med. 7, 349—356 (1922). [13,081/22

Miyaji, T., Moszkowski, L. I., Senoo, T., Ogata, M., Oda, T., Kawai, K., Sayama, Y., Ishida, H., Matsuo, H.: Inhibition of 2-acetylaminofluorene tumors in rats with simultaneously fed 20-methylcholanthrene, 9: 10-dimethyl-1: 2-benzanthracene and chrysene, and consideration of sex difference in tumor genesis with 2-acetylaminofluorene. Gann 44, 281—283 (1953). [D 24,881/53

Mizumoto, R., Wexler, M., Slapak, M., Kojima, Y., McDermott, W. V., Jr.: The effect of hepatic artery inflow on regeneration, hypertrophy, and portal pressure of the liver following 50 per cent hepatectomy in the dog. Brit. J. Surg. 57, 513—517 (1970). [H 28,787/70

Mody, J. K.: Influence of testosterone in intact and mammectomised female mice. Gann 58, 291—295 (1967). [G 49,656/67

Mody, M. R., Anjaria, P. D., Golwalla, A. F.: Intravenous hydrocortisone in the toxaemia of typhoid fever. Antiseptic 53, 866—868 (1956). [C 45,962/56

Mogabgab, W. J., Thomas, L.: The effects of cortisone on bacterial infection. J. Lab. Clin. Med. 39, 271—289 (1952). [B 72,457/52

Mohammed, A. H., Rohayem, H., Zaky, O.: The action of scorpion toxin on blood sodium and potassium. J. trop. Med. Hyg. 57, 85—87 (1954). [C 7,579/54

Moir, W. M.: The influence of age and sex on the repeated administration of sodium pentobarbital to albino rats. J. Pharmacol. exp. Ther. 59, 68—85 (1937). [E 54,544/37

Mole, R. H., Philpot, J. S. L., Hodges, G. R. V.: Reduction in lethal effect of X-radiation by pretreatment with thiourea or sodium ethane dithiophosphonate. Nature (Lond.) 166, 515 (1950). [D 96,011/50

Molimard, R., Benozio, M.: Étude de la rate au cours de la régénération hépatique après hépatectomie partielle. Path. et Biol. 18, 429—432 (1970). [G 75,048/70

Moll, T.: The susceptibility of weaned mice to Escherichia coli and Salmonella typhimurium endotoxins during, and subsequent to, cortisone treatment. Amer. J. vet. Res. 17, 786—788 (1956). [D 38,913/56

Moll, T.: The susceptibility of weaned mice to Escherichia coli during, and subsequent to, cortisone treatment. Amer. J. vet. Res. 17, 795—798 (1956). [D 38,927/56

Møller-Christensen, E.: Investigations on the inactivation of vasopressin in the liver. Acta Endocr. (Kbh.) 6, 153—160 (1951). [B 56,243/51

Molomut, N.: The effect of hypophysectomy on immunity and hypersensitivity in rats with a brief description of the operative technic. J. Immunol. 37, 113—131 (1939). [76,648/39

Molteni, A., Brownie, A. C., Skelton, F. R.: Potentiation of methylandrostenediol hypertension by ACTH administration (Abstr.). Circulation, 38, Sup. 6, VI-140 (1968). [H 4,919/68

Money, W. L.: The interrelation of the thyroid and the adrenals. In: Edelmann; The Thyroid, p. 137—168. Brookhaven Symp. in Biol., Brookhaven National Laboratory 1954. [C 5,393/54

Montgomery, E. H.: The role of thyroid and of diet in the acetonitrile test. Yale J. Biol. Med. 6, 101—110 (1933). [18,184/33

Montuori, E.: Action de la cortisone sur la toxicité du salicylate de soude. C. R. Soc. Biol. (Paris) 148, 1640—1642 (1954). [G 60,881/54

Moolten, F. L., Oakman, N. J., Bucher, N. L. R.: Accelerated response of hepatic DNA synthesis to partial hepatectomy in rats pretreated with growth hormone or surgical stress. Cancer Res. 30, 2353—2357 (1970). [H 30,606/70

Moon, H. D., Simpson, M. E., Evans, H. M.: Inhibition of methylcholanthrene carcinogenesis by hypophysectomy. Science 116, 331 (1952). [B 74,251/52

Moon, R. J., Berry, L. J.: Role of tryptophan pyrrolase in endotoxin poisoning. J. Bact. 95, 1247—1253 (1968). [G 57,245/68

Moor, P. de, Hendrikx, A., Hinnekens, M.: Extra-adrenal influence of corticotropin (ACTH) on cortisol metabolism. *J. clin. Endocr.* 21, 106—109 (1961). [G 75,989/61]

Moore, H. C.: The effect of oxytocin on the kidneys of weanling, adult non-pregnant and pregnant rats receiving progesterone and oestrogens. *J. Obstet. Gynaec. Brit. Cwlth.* 71, 272—276 (1964). [G 11,771/64]

Moore, K. E.: Amphetamine toxicity and thyroid hormones. *Fed. Proc.* 24, 518 (1965). [F 36,358/65]

Moore, K. E.: Amphetamine toxicity in hyperthyroid mice: effects on endogenous catecholamines. *Biochem. Pharmacol.* 14, 1831 to 1837 (1965). [G 36,616/65]

Morcos, S. R.: The effect of the protein value of the diet on the neurological manifestations produced in rats by β,β-iminodipropionitrile. *Brit. J. Nutr.* 21, 269—274 (1967). [F 80,855/67]

Moreno, O. M., Brodie, D. A.: Effects of drugs on gastric hemorrhages produced by the administration of polymyxin B. *J. Pharmacol. exp. Ther.* 135, 259—264 (1962). [D 20,261/62]

Morgan, L. M., Binnion, P. F.: The distribution of 3H-digoxin in normal and acutely hyperkalaemic dogs. *Cardiovasc. Res.* 4, 235—241 (1970). [G 76,782/70]

Morii, S.: Adrenocortical damage induced by 7,12-dimethylbenz(α) anthracene and its implication in carcinogenesis. *Acta path. jap.* 15, 93—110 (1965). [G 34,628/65]

Morii, S., Huggins, C.: Adrenal apoplexy induced by 7,12-dimethylbenz(a)anthracene related to corticosterone content of adrenal gland. *Endocrinology* 71, 972—976 (1962). [D 45,369/62]

Morii, S., Kuwahara, I.: The effect of 7,12-dimethylbenz(α) anthracene upon the adrenal cortex of mammals (Japanese text). *J. Kansai Med. Sch.* 230—234 (1963). [G 33,213/63]

Moritsch, H.: Virologische Untersuchungen über den Einfluß von Penicillin und Cortison auf die experimentelle Infektion der Maus mit Psittakosisvirus. *Wien. klin. Wschr.* 68, 80—83 (1956). [C 15,606/56]

Morris, D. M., Mokal, A.: Effect of nutrition on survival time of thyroidectomized rats bearing a transplantable leukemia. *J. nat. Cancer Inst.* 30, 847—854 (1963). [D 65,803/63]

Morrison, J., Kilpatrick, N.: Low urinary oestriol excretion in pregnancy associated with oral prednisone therapy. *J. Obstet. Gynaec. Brit. Cwlth.* 76, 719—720 (1969). [G 69,282/69]

Morrow, D. H.: Anesthesia and digitalis toxicity. II. Effect of norepinephrine infusion on ouabain tolerance. *Anesth. Analg. Curr. Res.* 46, 319—323 (1967). [G 47,272/67]

Morselli, P. L., Marc, V., Garattini, S., Zaccala, M.: Metabolism of exogenous cortisol in humans. Influence of phenobarbital treatment on plasma cortisol disappearance rate. *Rev. europ. Etud. clin. biol.* 15, 195—198 (1970). [G 76,129/70]

Morton, D. M., Chatfield, D. H.: The effects of adjuvant-induced arthritis on the liver metabolism of drugs in rats. *Biochem. Pharmacol.* 19, 473—481 (1970). [G 73,681/70]

Mosbach, E. H., Bevans, M.: Biological studies of dihydrocholesterol. V. Effect of androgens upon the biologic disposition of dihydrocholesterol in the rabbit. *Arch. Path.* 75, 558—563 (1963). [D 65,362/63]

Moscona, A. A., Piddington, R.: Enzyme induction by corticosteroids in embryonic cells: steroid structure and inductive effect. *Science* 158, 496—497 (1967). [F 90,487/67]

Moses, S. W., Levin, S., Chayoth, R., Steinitz, K.: Enzyme induction in a case of glycogen storage disease. *Pediatrics* 38, 111—121 (1966). [G 40,253/66]

Moss, L. D., Dury, A.: Influences of adrenal hormones on aortic histopathology in relation to blood lipoproteins in rabbits. *J. Mt Sinai Hosp.* 24, 1047—1054 (1957). [C 44,068/57]

Motsay, G. J., Alho, A., Jaeger, T., Dietzman, R. H., Lillehei, R. C.: Effects of corticosteroids on the circulation in shock: experimental and clinical results. *Fed. Proc.* 29, 1861—1873 (1970). [H 32,852/70]

Moudgil, L. R.: Possible protective action of antialdosterone compounds in myocardial necrosis in rats. *Brit. J. Pharmacol.* 35, 558—562 (1969). [G 65,314/69]

Mouriquand, G., Michel, P.: Accidents du type scorbutique chez des animaux à une alimentation normale, non carencée, soumis à l'action de l'extrait thyroïdien. *C. R. Soc. Biol. (Paris)* 84, 43—45 (1921). [12,231/21]

Mowat, A. P., Arias, I. M.: Liver function and oral contraceptives. *J. reprod. Med.* 3, 19—29 (1969). [G 74,246/69]

Mrozikiewicz, A., Strzyzewski, W.: Wpływ ACTH i niektórych hormonów kory nadnerczy na drgawki wywołane hydrazydem kwasu izonikotynowego. *Przegl. lek.* 22, 543—544 (1966). [G 68,152/66]

Mrozikiewicz, A., Strzyzewski, W.: Effect of long-term administration of ACTH and adrenocortical hormones on the course of hydrazide convulsions. *Arch. Immunol. Ther. exp.* **15**, 909—911 (1967). [H 7,524/67

Mückter, H., Frankus, E., Moré, E.: Experimental investigations with 1-(morpholinomethyl)-4-phthalimido-piperidindione-2, 6 and drostanolone propionate in dimethylbenzanthracene induced tumors of Sprague-Dawley rats. *Cancer Res.* **30**, 430—438 (1970). [H 23,589/70

Mudge, G. H.: Drugs affecting renal function and electrolyte metabolism. In: Goodman, L. S.; A. Gilman; *The Pharmacological Basis of Therapeutics*, 3rd ed., p. 820. Toronto, Canada: Collier-Macmillan Canada Ltd. 1965. [E 4,490/65

Mueller, G. C., Rumney, G.: Formation of 6-β-hydroxy and 6-keto derivatives of estradiol-16-C^{14} by mouse liver microsomes. *J. Amer. Chem. Soc.* **79**, 1004 (1957). [C 30,708/57

Mueller, M. N., Kappas, A.: Estrogen pharmacology. I. The influence of estradiol and estriol on hepatic disposal of sulfobromophthalein (BSP) in man. *J. clin. Invest.* **43**, 1905—1914 (1964). [F 22,282/64

Mueller, M. N., Kappas, A.: Impairment of hepatic excretion of sulfobromophthalein (BSP) by natural estrogens. *Trans. Ass. Amer. Phycns.* **77**, 248—258 (1964). [G 81,288/64

Muftic, M., Redmann, U.: Wachstumsförderung und Wachstumshemmung von Mycoplasma gallisepticum durch Steroide. *Zbl. Bakt., I. Abt. Orig.* **206**, 228—237 (1968). [G 58,918/68

Mullen, J. O., Juchau, M. R., Fouts, J. R.: Studies of interactions of 3,4-benzpyrene, 3-methylcholanthrene, chlordane, and methyltestosterone as stimulators of hepatic microsomal enzyme systems in the rat. *Biochem. Pharmacol.* **15**, 137—144 (1966). [G 37,764/66

Müller, L.: Recherches sur le lieu et le mode d'origine des cytolysines naturelles (alexines et ambocepteurs normaux) et les moyens d'en provoquer l'hypersécrétion. *Zbl. Bakt., I. Abt. Orig.* **57**, 577—656 (1911). [A 47,855/11

Müller-Oerlinghausen, B., Jahns, R., Künzel, B., Hasselblatt, A.: Die Wirkung von Tolbutamid auf Blutglucose und Glucuronsäurekonjugation im Lebergewebe normaler und adrenalektomierter Mäuse. *Naunyn-Schmiedebergs Arch. Pharmak.* **262**, 17—28 (1969). [G 64,175/69

Müller-Oerlinghausen, B., Schinke, G.: Wirkung eines Insulinmangels auf die Bilirubinausscheidung in der Galle, *Naunyn-Schmiedebergs Arch. Pharmak.* **266**, 3—17 (1970). [G 79,199/70

Mullins, L. J., Adler, T. K., Fenn, W. O.: The effect of adrenocortical extracts on the distribution of injected potassium (Abstr.). *Fed. Proc.* **2**, 36 (1943). [83,885/43

Munan, L. P., Einheber, A.: Greater resistance of the female to experimental burns following starvation. *Science* **116**, 425—427 (1952). [B 74,511/52

Munan, L. P., Einheber, A.: The effect of sex on survival following standardized burn shock. *Endocrinology* **52**, 484—485 (1953). [B 82,207/53

Muñoz, C., Guerrero, S., Paeile, C., Campos, I.: Sexual differences in the toxicity of procaine in rats. *Toxicol. appl. Pharmacol.* **3**, 445—454 (1961). [G 68,223/61

Muñoz, J.: Hypersensitivity reactions induced in mice treated with Bordetella pertussis. In: Landy and Braun; *Bacterial Endotoxins*, p. 460—473. New Brunswick, N.J.: Institute of Microbiology, Rutgers, The State University 1964. [E 8,473/64

Muñoz, J., Schuchardt, L. F.: Effect of H. pertussis on sensitivity of mice to cold stress. *Proc. Soc. exp. Biol. (N.Y.)* **94**, 186—190 (1957). [C 28,986/57

Muñoz, J. M.: El fluor de los huesos y dientes en la fluorosis. *Rev. Soc. argent. Biol.* **12**, 50—56 (1936). [67,126/36

Munson, A. E., Barnes, D., Regelson, W., Wooles, W. R.: The relationship between drug metabolism and the reticuloendothelial (RE) activity (Abstr.). *Fed. Proc.* **29**, 411. (1970). [H 22,843/70

Murakami, H., Kowalewski, K.: Effects of cortisone and an anabolic androgen on the fractured humerus in guinea pigs: clinical and histological study over a six-week period of fracture healing. *Canad. J. Surg.* **9**, 425—434 (1966). [G 41,228/66

Murnaghan, M. F., Mazurkiewicz, I. M.: Some pharmacological properties of 4-methyltropolone. *Rev. canad. Biol.* **22**, 99—102 (1963). [D 68,260/63

Muro, P. de, Rowinski, P.: The role of sex in the hypertensive action of desoxycorticosterone acetate (DCA). *Acta med. scand.* **141**, 70—76 (1951). [B 66,413/51

Murphy, S. D., Anderson, R. L., DuBois, K. P.: Potentiation of toxicity of malathion by triorthotolyl phosphate. *Proc. Soc. exp. Biol. (N.Y.)* **100**, 483—487 (1959). [G 74,671/59

Murphy, S. D., DuBois, K. P.: Quantitative measurement of inhibition of the enzymatic detoxification of malathion by EPN (ethyl p-nitrophenyl thionobenzenephosphonate). *Proc. Soc. exp. Biol. (N.Y.)* 96, 813—818 (1957). [G 74,670/57

Murphy, S. D., DuBois, K. P.: The influence of various factors on the enzymatic conversion of organic thiophosphates to anticholinesterase agents. *J. Pharmacol. Exp. Ther.* 124, 194—202 (1958). [D 28,546/58

Murphy, S. D., Malley, S.: Effect of carbon tetrachloride on induction of liver enzymes by acute stress or corticosterone. *Toxicol. appl. Pharmacol.* 15, 117—130 (1969). [G 68,408/69

Murphy, W. H., Jr., Wiens, A. L., Watson, D. W.: Impairment of innate resistance by triiodothyronine. *Proc. Soc. exp. Biol. (N.Y.)* 99, 213—215 (1958). [C 60,008/58

Murray, F. J.: Outbreak of unexpected reactions among epileptics taking isoniazid. *Amer. Rev. resp. Dis.* 86, 729—732 (1962). [G 77,553/62

Murray, R., Branham, S. E.: Effect of cortisone and ACTH on adrenals in experimental diphtheria, Shiga, and Meningococcus intoxication. *Proc. Soc. exp. Biol. (N.Y.)* 78, 750—753 (1951). [B 65,414/51

Myers, D. K., Hemphill, C. A., Townsend, C. M.: Deoxycytidylate deaminase levels in regenerating rat liver. *Canad. J. Biochem.* 39/6, 1043—1054 (1961). [D 48,663/61

Myers, H. B., Ferguson, C.: Iodine poisoning counteracted by thiosulphate. *Proc. Soc. exp. Biol. (N.Y.)* 25, 784—785 (1928). [A 48,023/28

Nadasdi, M.: Effect of a steroid spirolactone on the cardiovascular changes produced by renal ischemia. *Endocrinology* 69, 246—249 (1961). [D 9,288/61

Nadel, E. M., Young, B., Hilgar, A., Mandell, A.: Effects of adrenocorticotropin and endotoxin on adrenal stimulation and resistance to infection. *Amer. J. Physiol.* 201, 551—553 (1961). [D 12,681/61

Nagata, K., Baba, T., Nagasawa, Y., Takagi, K., Hara, K.: Effect of cortisone on the course of Schistosoma japonicum infection in mice, particularly of the hepatic tissue. *Gunma J. med. Sci.* 5, 24—36 (1956). [D 26,285/56

Naguib, M., Robson, J. M.: The effect of cortisone alone and in combination with isoniazid on experimental murine leprosy in mice. *Brit. J. Pharmacol.* 11, 326—329 (1956). [C 23,199/56

Naidu, N. V., Reddi, O. S.: Effect of post-treatment with erythropoietin(s) on survival and erythropoietic recovery in irradiated mice. *Nature (Lond.)* 214, 1223—1224 (1967). [F 80,336/67

Nair, V.: Modification of pharmacological activity following X-irradiation. *Radiat. Res.* 30, 359—373 (1967). [G 67,247/67

Nair, V., Bau, D.: Inhibition of a hepatic microsomal enzyme system after head X-irradiation of rats. *Proc. Soc. exp. Biol. (N.Y.)* 126, 853—856 (1967). [G 67,246/67

Nair, V., Bau, D., Siegel, S.: Effects of prenatal X-irradiation: studies on the mechanism of X-irradiation-induced inhibition of microsomal enzyme development in rat liver. *Radiat. Res.* 36, 493—507 (1968). [G 67,245/68

Nair, V., Bau, D., Siegel, S.: X-irradiation effects on the ontogenic vs. drug induced increase in the activity of a hepatic microsomal enzyme system. *Radiat. Res.* 35, 559 (1968). [G 67,304/68

Nair, V., Brown, T., Bau, D., Siegel, S.: Evidence for hypothalamic regulation of hepatic hexobarbital oxidase in rats. *Pharmacologist* 11, 252 (1969). [G 67,250/69

Nair, V., Brown, T., Bau, D., Siegel, S.: Hypothalamic regulation of hepatic hexobarbital metabolizing enzyme system. *Europ. J. Pharmacol.* 9, 31—40 (1970). [H 21,083/70

Nair, V., DuBois, K. P.: Prenatal and early postnatal exposure to environmental toxicants. *Chic. med. Sch. Quart.* 27, 75—89 (1968). [G 67,244/68

Nair, V., Finer, S., Shah, D.: Interactive effects of X-irradiation and barbiturates. *Proc. Soc. exp. Biol. (N.Y.)* 120, 246—252 (1965). [F 53,576/65

Nair, V., Zeitlin, E.: Impairment of the development of a liver microsomal enzyme system (hexobarbital metabolizing system) after in-utero and early postnatal exposure to X-irradiation. *Radiat. Res.* 31, 609—610 (1967). [G 65,099/67

Nakagawa, Y., Kanda, Y.: Studies on the influence upon the susceptibility of mice to virus. III. Report. Effect of cortisone on the susceptibility of mice to virus. *Kurume med. J.* 2, 1—18 (1955). [C 8,165/55

Nakagawa, Y., Kanda, Y.: Studies on the influence upon the susceptibility of mice to virus. III. Report. Effect of cortisone on the susceptibility of mice to virus. *Kurume med. J.* 2, 92—109 (1955). [C 9,941/55

Nakamura, T., Nakamura, S., Sugawara, K., Katakura, Y., Takizawa, T., Isono, T.: On renal injuries in young rats on choline deficiencies. *Tohoku J. exp. Med.* **66**, 1—6 (1957). [C41,067/57

Nakanishi, S., Masamura, E., Tsukada, M., Akabane, J.: Effects of different types of stress on hepatic drug-metabolizing enzyme activity in the rat. *Med. J. Shinshu Univ.* **15**, 71—76 (1970). [G79,299/70

Nakano, K., Kishi, T., Kurita, N., Ashida, K.: Effect of dietary amino acids on amino acid-catabolizing enzymes in rat liver. *J. Nutr.* **100**, 827—836 (1970). [G76,247/70

Nash, C. B., Alley, J. H., Manley, E. S.: The suppression of ouabain toxicity by oxytocin and reserpine. *Toxicol. appl. Pharmacol.* **6**, 163—167 (1964). [G9,641/64

Nasio, J.: Influence of some vitamins and hormones in the prevention of experimental cinchophen peptic ulcer. *Rev. Gastroent.* **13**, 195—204 (1946). [97,932/46

Nasio, J.: Acción del estilbestrol en la prevención de la úlcera péptica cincofénica en perros castrados. *Pren. méd. argent.* **33**, 1603—1605 (1946). [B34,100/46

Nasio, J.: Tratamiento médico de la úlcera gastroduodenal experimental, pp. 151. Buenos Aires: La Prensa Médica Argentina 1946. [B77,063/46

Nassi, L.: Ricerche radiologiche ed emochimiche sull'effetto svolto dall'estratto liposolubile di timo nel rachitismo sperimentale. *Boll. Soc. ital. Biol. sper.* **38**, 678—681 (1962). [G1,107/62

Nassi, L.: Ricerche istologiche sull'effetto svolto dall'estratto liposulubile del timo nel rachitismo sperimentale. *Boll. Soc. ital. Biol. sper.* **38**, 681—683 (1962). [G1,108/62

Nayak, N. C., Chopra, P., Ramalingaswami, V.: The role of liver cell endoplasmic reticulum and microsomal enzymes in carbon tetrachloride toxicity: an in vivo study. *Life Sci.* 9/I, 1431—1439 (1970). [G80,728/70

Neal, P. A., Oettingen, W. F. von, Dunn, R. G., Sharpless, N. E.: Toxicity and potential dangers of aerosols and residues from such aerosols containing three percent DDT. (Second report.) *Publ. Hlth Res. Sup.* 183, 1—32 (1945). [17,438/45

Neal, R. A., DuBois, K. P.: Studies on the mechanism of detoxification of cholinergic phosphorothioates. *J. Pharmacol. exp. Ther.* **148**, 185—192 (1965). [F40,198/65

Neal, W. B., Jr., Woodward, E. R., Kark, A. E., Zubiran, J. M., Montalbetti, J. A.: Effect of ACTH, cortisone, and DOCA on survival of burned rat. *Arch. Surg.* **65**, 774—782 (1952). [B80,371/52

Neale, M. G., Parke, D. V.: The effect of pregnancy on the hydroxylation and reduction of drugs and cytochrome P-450 content of rat liver microsomes. *Biochem. J.* **113**, 12P-13P (1969). [G67,965/69

Nebert, D. W., Gelboin, H. V.: Substrate-inducible microsomal aryl-hydroxylase in mammalian cell culture. I. Assay and properties of induced enzyme. *J. biol. Chem.* **243**, 6242—6249 (1968). [H23,691/68

Nebert, D. W., Gelboin, H. V.: Substrate-inducible microsomal aryl hydroxylase in mammalian cell culture. II. Cellular responses during enzyme induction. *J. biol. Chem.* **243**, 6250—6261 (1968). [H23,692/68

Nebert, D. W., Gelboin, H. V.: Drugs and microsomal enzyme formation in vivo and in mammalian cell culture. In: Gillette, Conney et al.; *Microsomes and Drug Oxidations*, p. 389—429. New York, London: Academic Press 1969. [E8,237/69

Negrete, J. M.: Influencia de la progesterona sobre la "anestesia" producida por desoxicorticosterona. *Bol. Inst. Estud. Med. Biol. (Mex.)* **13**, 135—137 (1955). [C23,001/55

Nelson, R. S., Lanza, F. L.: Steroid therapy in massive hepatic necrosis due to viral hepatitis. *Sth. med. J. (Bgham, Ala.)* **63**, 1436—1439 (1970). [G80,151/70

Németh, Š., Vigaš, M.: Endocrine glands and metabolic background of trauma resistance. I. Resistance of rats with different hormonal states traumatized in the Noble-Collip drum. *Endocr. exp.* **2**, 39—44 (1968). [F98,055/68

Netter, K. J.: Die Hemmung der Procainhydrolyse durch die Diäthylaminoäthanolester der Diphenylpropylessigsäure (SKF 525-A) und der Diphenylessigsäure ('Trasentin'). *Naunyn-Schmiedebergs Arch. Pharmak.* **235**, 498—512 (1959). [G74,665/59

Netter, K. J.: Eine Methode zur direkten Messung der 0-Demethylierung in Lebermikrosomen und ihre Anwendung auf die Mikrosomenhemmwirkung von SKF 525-A. *Naunyn-Schmiedebergs Arch. Pharmak.* **238**, 292—300 (1960). [G74,666/60

Netter, K. J.: Drugs as inhibitors of drug metabolism. In: Brodie and Erdös; *Metabolic Factors Controlling Duration of Drug Action* (Proc.

1. int. pharmacol. Meet. Vol. 6), p. 213—233. New York: The Macmillan Company 1962. [E 52,768/62

Netter, K. J., Jenner, S., Kajuschke, K.: Über die Wirkung von Metyrapon auf den mikrosomalen Arzneimittelabbau. *Naunyn-Schmiedebergs Arch. Pharmak. exp. Pathol.* 259, 1—16 (1967). [G 53,255/67

Netter, K. J., Kahl, G. F., Magnussen, M. P.: Kinetic experiments on the binding of metyrapone to liver microsomes. *Naunyn-Schmiedebergs Arch. Pharmak.* 265, 205—215 (1969). [G 71,785/69

Neubaur, J., Hollmann, S.: Die Aktivität der Glucuronyltransferase in der Leber des menschlichen Feten und Frühgeborenen. *Klin. Wschr.* 44, 723—724 (1966). [H 30,996/66

Neubert, D.: Enzymatische Leistungen der Lebermikrosomen bei der Äthioninvergiftung. *Naunyn-Schmiedebergs Arch. Pharmak.* 232, 235—237 (1957). [G 74,661/57

Neubert, D., Herken, H.: Wirkungssteigerung von Schlafmitteln durch den Phenyldiallylessigsäureester des Diäthylaminoäthanols. *Naunyn-Schmiedebergs Arch. Pharmak.* 225, 453—462 (1955). [G 74,660/55

Neubert, D., Hoffmeister, I.: Mitochondrienatmung und Atmungskettenphosphorylierung bei erhöhtem intramitochondralen Gehalt an Gesamtfetten. *Naunyn-Schmiedebergs Arch. Pharmak.* 238, 348—357 (1960). [G 74,667/60

Neubert, D., Maibauer, D.: Vergleichende Untersuchungen der oxydativen Leistungen von Mitochondrien und Mikrosomen bei experimenteller Leberschädigung. *Naunyn-Schmiedebergs Arch. Pharmak.* 235, 291—300 (1959). [G 74,664/59

Neubert, D., Schaefer, J., Stein, F.: Eigenwirkungen radioaktiven Phosphates (P^{32}) auf oxydative Leistungen von Mitochondrien und Mikrosomen der Rattenleber. *Naunyn-Schmiedebergs Arch. Pharmak.* 239, 245—255 (1960). [G 74,787/60

Neubert, D., Timmler, R.: Einfluß einiger Phenylessigsäurederivate (CFT 1201, SKF 525 A) auf den Einbau von 1-C^{14}-dl-Alanin in Mikrosomenproteine. *Naunyn-Schmiedebergs Arch. Pharmak.* 238, 358—363 (1960). [G 74,668/60

Neuman, M.: Intéractions médicamenteuses. (I). *Presse méd.* 78, 1938—1940 (1970). [G 80,018/70

Neuman, M.: Intéractions médicamenteuses. (II). *Presse méd.* 78, 2023—2025 (1970). [G 80,550/70

Neumann, F., Elger, W., von Berswordt-Wallrabe, R.: Intersexualität männlicher Feten und Hemmung androgenabhängiger Funktionen bei erwachsenen Tieren durch Testosteronblocker. *Dtsch. med. Wschr.* 92, 360—366 (1967). [F 78,500/67

Neumann, F., Goldman, A. S.: Prevention of mammary gland defects in experimental congenital adrenal hyperplasia due to inhibition of 3 β-hydroxysteroid dehydrogenase in rats. *Endocrinology* 86, 1169—1171 (1970). [H 25,234/70

Neuweiler, W.: Reid Hunt'sche Reaktion und Schwangerschaft. *Zbl. Gynäk.* 56, 2936—2938 (1932). [43,582/32

Neville, A. M., Engel, L. L.: Inhibition of 3 β- and 3 α-hydroxysteroid dehydrogenases and of steroid Δ-isomerase by anabolic steroids (Abstr.). *Program 49th Ann. Meet. Endocr. Soc.* Bal Harbour, Fla., p. 67 (1967). [F 83,477/67

Newberne, P. M., Williams, G.: Inhibition of aflatoxin carcinogenesis by diethylstilbestrol in male rats. *Arch. environm. Hlth* 19, 489—498 (1969). [G 69,601/69

Newman, A. J., Gross, S.: Hyperbilirubinemia in breast-fed infants. *Pediatrics* 32, 995—1001 (1963). [G 75,237/63

Nicák, A.: The influence of serotonine and amphetamine on analgesic effect of morphine after reserpine premedication in rats and mice. *Med. Pharmacol. exp. (Basel)* 13, 43—48 (1965). [F 47,918/65

Nichol, C. A., Rosen, F.: Induction of drug-metabolizing and cortisol-responsive enzymes. *Fed. Proc.* 23, 386 (1964). [F 4,729/64

Nicholas, J. S., Barron, D. H.: The use of sodium amytal in the production of anesthesia in the rat. *J. Pharm. exp. Ther.* 46, 125—129 (1932). [62,223/32

Nicol, M., Grangaud, R.: Vitamine A et progestérone chez le rat traité au thiouracile. *C. R. Soc. Biol. (Paris)* 155, 1634—1638 (1961). [D 20,176/61

Nicol, T., Bilbey, D. L. J., Charles, L. M., Cordingley, J. L., Vernon-Roberts, B.: Oestrogen: the natural stimulant of body defence. *J. Endocr.* 30, 277—291 (1964). [F 25,320/64

Nicol, T., Brownlee, G., Druce, C., Ware, C. C.: Effect of three compounds related to diethylstilboestrol on the phagocytic activity of the reticulo-endothelial system. *Nature (Lond.)* 187, 1032—1033 (1960). [C 92,079/60

Nicol, T., Vernon-Roberts, B., Quantock, D. C.: Protective effect of oestrogens against the toxic decomposition products of tribromoethanol. *Nature (Lond.)* **208**, 1098—1099 (1965). [F 58,460/65

Nicol, T., Vernon-Roberts, B., Quantock, D. C.: Effect of orchidectomy and ovariectomy on survival against lethal infections in mice. *Nature (Lond.)* **211**, 1091—1092 (1966). [F 70,028/66

Nicola, C. de: El choque peptónico en los perros sin hígado. *Rev. Sco. argent. Biol.* **6**, 437 (1930). [43,101/30

Nichols, J., Hennigar, G.: Studies on DDD, 2,2,-Bis (parachlorophenyl)-1,1-dichloroethane. *Exp. Med. Surg.* **15**, 310—316 (1957). [C 48,736/57

Nicolette, J. A., Gorski, J.: Cortisol effects on the uterine response to estrogen. *Endocrinology* **74**, 955—959 (1964). [F 12,788/64

Nicolis, F. B., Ginoulhiac, E.: La determinazione della triptofanpirrolasi come test biologico di attività dei derivati prednisonici. *Boll. Soc. ital. Biol. sper.* **37**, 1534 (1961). [D 27,485/61

Nicolis, F. B., Ginoulhiac, E.: Studio delle variazioni della triptofano-pirrolasi epatica indotte da differenti corticosteroidi nel ratto. *Acta vitamin (Milano)* **23**, 19—26 (1969). [H 14,045/69

Nienstedt, W., Hartiala, K.: Steroid metabolism by the canine intestine. I. Qualitative experiments with progesterone. *Scand. J. Gastroent.* **4**, 483—488 (1969). [G 69,886/69

Nikki, P.: Arecoline and halothane shivering in thyroxine-treated mice. *Ann. Med. exp. Fenn.* **47**, 191—196 (1969). [G 71,573/69

Nikki, P., Rosenberg, P.: Halothane shivering in mice after injection of catecholamines and 5 HT into the cerebral ventricles. *Ann. Med. exp. Fenn.* **47**, 197—202 (1969). [G 71,574/69

Nimni, M. E., Geiger, E.: Non-suitability of levator ani method as an index of anabolic effect of steroids. *Proc. Soc. exp. Biol. (N.Y.)* **94**, 606—610 (1957). [C 31,438/57

Nishikawa, T.: The effect of cortisone acetate on the oral inoculation with Candida albicans in the germ-free mice. *Keio J. Med.* **18**, 47—57 (1969). [G 73,894/69

Nishimura, S., Nitta, K.: Über das Knochenwachstum bei B-Avitaminose und besonders den Einfluß der Schilddrüse auf dasselbe. I. Mitteilg. Über den Einfluß der Fütterung mit kleinen Mengen von Schilddrüsensubstanz auf das Knochenwachstum der B-avitaminösen Ratten. *Folia endocr. jap.* **4**, 83—84 (1929). [1,171/29

Noble, G. A.: Leishmania braziliensis: physical and chemical stress in hamsters. *Exp. Parasit.* **29**, 30—32 (1971). [G 81,736/71

Noble, R. L.: Effects of synthetic oestrogens and carcinogens when administered to rats by subcutaneous implantation of crystals or tablets. *J. Endocr.* **1**, 216—229 (1939). [A 30,160/39

Noble, R. L.: The effect of adrenergic blocking agents on drum shock. *Proc. Canad. Physiol. Soc.* 19th Ann. Meet., 13th—15th Oct., p. 47. London 1955. [C 10,541/55

Noble, R. L., Collip, J. B.: Adrenal and other factors affecting experimental traumatic shock in the rat. *Quart. J. exp. Physiol.* **31**, 201—210 (1942). [A 56,107/42

Nocke, L., Breuer, H., Lichton, J. I.: Effect of aldactone on the urinary excretion of total oestrogens, 17-hydroxycorticosteroids and 17-oxosteroids in pregnant women. (Abstr.) *Excerpta med. (Amst.),* Int. Congr. Ser. No. 210, p. 183. (1970) 3rd Int. Congr. on Hormonal Steroids, Hamburg. [H 29,580/70

Nola, F. di, Angela, G. C., Salassa, M. R., Rapellini, M.: Intossicazione difterica sperimentale in cavie pretrattate con cortisone. *Arch. Sci. med.* **103**, 242—248 (1957). [C 33,308/57

Nola, F. di, Salassa, M. R., Rapellini, M., Sardi, P.: Intossicazione difterica sperimentale nella cavia pretrattata con ACTH. *Arch. Sci. med.* **104**, 554—560 (1957). [C 43,232/57

Nolan, J. P.: Protective action of oestrogen against the lethal effect of endotoxin in the rat. *Nature (Lond.)* **213**, 201—202 (1967). [F 75,232/67

Nolan, J. P., Ali, M. V.: Time related effect of estrogen administration on the sensitivity of rats to endotoxin. *Fed. Proc.* **26**, 628 (1967). [F 79,610/67

Nolan, J. P., Ali, M. V.: Late effect of estrogen on endotoxin response in the rat. *J. Lab. clin. Med.* **71**, 501—510 (1968). [G 55,490/68

Nolan, J. P., Ali, M. V., Bistany, T. S.: Comparison of endotoxin blockade by estrogenic substances and hydrocortisone. *J. reticuloendothel. Soc.* **5**, 9—21 (1968). [H 5,204/68

Nomura, J., Maeda, M., Nakazawa, K., Hatotani, N.: Experimental studies on cerebrohepatic relationship-effects of several conditions on enzyme activities in rat liver and brain, and on estrogen inactivation in rat liver. *Folia psychiat. neurol. jap.* **19**, 156—166 (1965). [G 33,405/65

Noordhoek, J., Rümke, C. L.: Sex differences in the rate of drug metabolism in mice. *Arch. int. Pharmacodyn.* 182, 401 (1969). [H 21,660/69

Norman, G. F., Mittler, A.: Interrelationship of vitamin D and the sex hormones in calcium and phosphorus metabolism of rats. *Proc. Soc. exp. Biol. (N.Y.)* 67, 104—111 (1948). [B 18,001/48

Norton, P. R. E.: Some endocrinological aspects of barbiturate dependence. *Brit. J. Pharmacol.* 41, 317—330 (1971). [G 80,572/71

Novelli, A., Marinari, U. M., Cottalasso, D.: Riduzione della componente fibrotica in granulomi silicotici polmonari di ratti sottoposti a parziale epatectomia. *Pathologica* 61, 111 a 117 (1969). [H 24,185/69

Novelli, A., Mor, M. A. D.: Behaviour of normal and regenerated liver mitochondria after small doses of carbon tetrachloride. *Ital. J. Biochem.* 11, 47—53 (1962). [D 36,206/62

Novelli, A., Zinnari, A.: Inibizione della produzione di fibre collagene nel granuloma da carragenina nel ratto durante la rigenerazione del fegato dopo parziale epatectomia. *Pathologica* 60, 115—120 (1968). [H 8,990/68

Novick, W. J., Jr., Stohler, C. M., Swagzdis, J.: The influence of steroids on drug metabolism in the mouse. *J. Pharmacol. exp. Ther.* 151, 139—142 (1966). [F 63,768/66

Nutter, J. E., Gemmill, C. L., Myrvik, Q. N.: The influence of 3,3',5-triodo-L-thyronine on the survival time of mice with tuberculosis and pneumococcosis. *Amer. Rev. Tuberc.* 79, 339 to 343 (1959). [C 65,285/59

Nuzhdin, N. I., Shapiro, N. I., Chudinovskaia, G. A., Pankova, N. V.: Action of protective substances on mammalian gonads. (Russian text). *Zh. Obshchei Biol.* 21/6, 430—438 (1960). [D 5,866/60

Nyfors, A.: The influence of cortico-steroids on the allergic skin wheal reaction and the delayed-type reaction (Mantoux). *Acta allerg. (Kbh.)* 25, 53—62 (1970). [G 76,097/70

Nymark, M., Rasmussen, J.: Effect of certain drugs upon amitriptyline induced electrocardiographic changes. *Acta pharmacol. (Kbh.)* 24, 148—156 (1966). [G 42,054/66

Oehlert, W., Hämmerling, W., Büchner, F.: Der zeitliche Ablauf und das Ausmaß der Desoxyribonukleinsäure-Synthese in der regenerierenden Leber der Ratte nach Teilhepatektomie. (Autoradiographische Untersuchungen unter Verwendung von H³-Thymidin). *Beitr. pathol. Anat.* 126, 91—112 (1962). [D 36,669/62

Oehme, C., Paal, H.: Die Reid-Hunt-Reaktion. Klinisches und Experimentelles. *Ergebn. inn. Med. Kinderheilk.* 44, 214—256 (1932). [62,442/32

Oester, Y. T.: Adrenal medullary hormones and arteriosclerosis. *Ann. N.Y. Acad. Sci.*, 72, 885—895 (1959). [C 84,324/59

Oester, Y. T., Davis, O. F., Friedman, B.: Progesterone and alpha tocopherol in experimental epinephrine-thyroxine arteriosclerosis and in cholesterol-induced atherosclerosis. *Circulation* 12, 505 (1955). [C 8,951/55

Oettel, H., Franck, E.: Über die Beeinflussung von Leberschäden durch Desoxycorticosteronacetat. *Z. ges. exp. Med.* 110, 535—547 (1942). [A 72,420/42

Ogandzhanyan, E. E., Pareishvili, E. A., Batikyan, I. G.: The effect of some hormones on the hemopoiesis and survival of irradiated black mice of the $C_{57/6}$ strain. (Russian text.) *Probl. Endokr. Gormonoter.* 10, 107—110 (1964). [F 7,045/64

O'Gara, R. W., Ards, J.: Incidence of leukemia and other tumors in thymectomized irradiated mice bearing thymic transplants. *J. nat. Cancer Inst.* 27, 299—309 (1961). [D 12,341/61

Ogawa, H.: Studies on protective effects of corticosteroids against Habuvenom shock of rats. *Gunma J. med. Sci.* 14, 60—85 (1965). [F 54,550/65

Okada, H., Fuwa, H., Kato, T.: Effects of cortisone upon guinea pigs inoculated with BCG or bole bacilli. *Nagoya J. med. Sci.* 18, 168—176 (1955). [C 18,328/55

Okano, K., Fujita, T., Orimo, H., Yoshikawa, M.: Age and calcium metabolism in relation to cardiovascular changes induced by renal injury with sodium sulfaacetylthiazole. *J. Amer. Geriat. Soc.* 18, 458—470 (1970). [H 25,894/70

Okonogi, T., Fukai, K., Yamaguchi, K., Kato, K., Suda, A.: Studies on the haemophilus pertussis. XIV. The effects of ACTH, cortisone and adrenaline on the morbid changes on the experimental pertussis. *Gunma J. med. Sci.* 5, 304—309 (1956). [C 34,465/56

Olds, W. H., Jr.: The effects of thyroidectomy on the resistance of rats to morphine poisoning. *Amer. J. Physiol.* 26, 354—360 (1910). [34,544/10

O'Leary, J. A., Davies, J. E., Feldman, M.: Spontaneous abortion and human pesticide residues of DDT and DDE. *Amer. J. Obstet. Gynec.* 108, 1291—1292 (1970). [G 80,260/70

Oliva, L., Valli, P.: Influenza degli ormoni sessuali sugli effetti delle radiazioni ionizzanti. Studio sperimentale. *Attual. Ostet. Ginec.* 4, 155—166 (1958). [C50,803/58

Olivecrona, T., Fex, G.: Metabolism of plasma lipids in partially hepatectomized rats. *Biochim. biophys. Acta (Amst.)* 202, 259—268 (1970). [G74,083/70

Oliveira, H. L. de, Patricio, L. D., Cintra, A. de U., Mattar, E.: O propionato de testosterona no tratamento da intoxicação mercurial aguda. *Rev. Hosp. Clin. Fac. Med. S. Paulo* 2, 15—22 (1947). [B43,032/47

Oliver, M. F., Roberts, S. D., Hayes, D., Pantridge, J. F., Suzman, M. M., Bersohn, I.: Effect of atromid and ethyl chlorophenoxyisobutyrate on anticoagulant requirements. *Lancet* 1963 I, 143—144. [D54,029/63

Oliver, W. J., Kelsch, R. C.: Effect of hypophysectomy upon edema formation in aminonucleoside nephrosis. *Endocrinology* 75, 973 to 974 (1964). [F25,772/64

Olivier, L., Cheever, A. W.: Comparison of the effect of cortisone and of trichinella spiralis infection on injury to rats by encephalomyocarditis virus infection. *Amer. J. trop. Med. Hyg.* 12/4, 675—677 (1963). [G15,789/63

Olson, J. A. Jr., Lindberg, M., Bloch, K.: On the demethylation of lanosterol to cholesterol. *J. biol. Chem.* 226, 941—956 (1957). [G61,438/57

Omura, T., Sato, R., Cooper, D. Y., Rosenthal, O., Estabrook, R. W.: Function of cytochrome P-450 of microsomes. *Fed. Proc.* 24, 1181 to 1189 (1965). [F51,529/65

O'Neal, M. A., Griffin, A. C.: Pituitary association with diacetylaminofluorene. (Abstr.) *Proc. Amer. Ass. Cancer Res.* 2, 236 (1957). [C31,971/57

Oppenheim, E., Bruger, M.: The effect of cortisone and ACTH on experimental cholesterol atherosclerosis in rabbits. *Program Proc. 6th Ann. Meet., Amer. Soc. Arterioscl.* Chicago, Nov. 9—10, p. 470—471 (1952). [B74,288/52

Oppenheimer, J. H., Bernstein, G., Surks, M. I.: Increased thyroxine turnover and thyroidal function after stimulation of hepatocellular binding of thyroxine by phenobarbital. *J. clin. Invest.* 47, 1399—1406 (1968). [F99,583/68

Oppenheimer, J. H., Wise, H. M., Lasley, D. A.: The role of the thyroid gland in experimental traumatic shock. *J. clin. Invest.* 37, 380—388 (1958). [C50,563/58

Oppenheimer, M. J., Flock, E. V.: Alkaline phosphatase levels in plasma and liver following partial hepatectomy. *Amer. J. Physiol.* 149, 418—421 (1947). [B4,738/47

Orimo, H., Fujita, T., Yoshikawa, M., Hayano, K.: A progeria-like syndrome produced by dihydrotachysterol: its prevention by conjugated estrogens (Premarin). *J. Amer. Geriat. Soc.* 18, 11—23 (1970). [H20,265/70

Orione, G.: Adrenalin e tossicosi da ganglioplegici. *Ormonologia* 16, 202—212 (1956). [C37,851/56

Orlova, L. V., Klimova, S. P., Rodionov, V. M.: Radioprotective effect of ACTH. (Russian text.) *Med. Radiol.* 9, 19—22 (1963). [G22,562/63

Orlova, L. V., Rodionov, V. M.: The time of histone synthesis in regenerating rat liver. *Exp. Cell Res.* 59, 329—333 (1970). [G73,079/70

Orrenius, S.: Further studies on the induction of the drug-hydroxylating enzyme system of liver microsomes. *J. Cell Biol.* 26, 725—733 (1965). [G74,389/65

Orrenius, S., Das, M., Gnosspelius, Y.: Overall biochemical effects of drug induction on liver microsomes. In: Gillette, Conney et al.; *Microsomes and Drug Oxidations,* p. 251—277. New York, London: Academic Press 1969. [E8,231/69

Orrenius, S., Ericsson, J. L. E., Ernster, L.: Phenobarbital-induced synthesis of the microsomal drug-metabolizing enzyme system and its relationship to the proliferation of endoplasmic membranes. *J. Cell Biol.* 25, 627—639 (1965). [G66,249/65

Ortega, P.: Light and electron microscopy of dichlorodiphenyltrichloroethane (DDT) poisoning in the rat liver. *Lab. Invest.* 15, 657 to 679 (1966). [G76,671/66

Ortega, P.: Partial hepatectomy in rats fed dichlorodiphenyltrichloroethane (DDT). *Amer. J. Path.* 56, 229—249 (1969). [H15,674/69

Ortega, P., Hayes, W. J., Jr., Durham, W. F., Mattson, A. M.: *Publ. Hlth. Monogr. No. 43* (1956). [E40,218/56

Osipovich, V. V.: The effect of hormones on compensatory hypertrophy of the kidneys. (Russian text.) *Byull. eksp. Biol. Med.* 43/3, 37—39 (1957). [C58,570/57

Osment, L. S.: The many effects of griseofulvin. *Ala. J. med. Sci.* 6, 392—398 (1969). [G72,369/69

Osorio, J. A.: Influencia de la hormona tiroidea sobre la reactividad vascular a la acción de sustáncias vasoactivas en la rata. *Rev. Soc. argent. Biol.* **32**, 29—35 (1956). [C31,059/56

Osumi, Y.: Effects of 3,5,3'-triiodothyroinine on the experimental atheromatosis caused by cholesterol feeding in rabbits. *Jap. J. Pharmacol.* **15**, 280—294 (1965). [G34,534/65

Ouzelatz, V. S.: Etude sur l'influence des crises hypoglycémiques dans le processus évolutif de l'ulcère gastrique. *Presse méd.* **65**, 1118 a 1119 (1957). [C36,618/57

Ove, P., Jenkins, M. D., Laszlo, J.: DNA replication and degradation in mammalian tissue. I. Changes in DNA polymerase and nuclease during rat liver regeneration. *Biochim. biophys. Acta (Amst.)* **174**, 629—635 (1969).
[H23,725/69

Overbeek, G. A.: Anabole Steroide. Chemie und Pharmakologie, pp. 80. Berlin, Heidelberg, New York: Springer-Verlag 1966. [E8,318/66

Overbeek, G. A., Bonta, I. L.: Steroids that act on the nervous system. In: Martini et al.; *Hormonal Steroids* **1**, p. 493—500. New York, London: Academic Press 1964. [E4,775/64

Overman, R. R., Bass, A. C., Davis, A. K., Golden, A.: II. The effect of lipo-adrenal extract on ionic balance in fatal simian malaria. *Amer. J. clin. Path.* **19**, 907—917 (1949).
[B49,805/49

Owens, J. C., Neely, W. B., Owen, W. R.: Effect of sodium dextrothyroxine in patients receiving anticoagulants. *New Engl. J. Med.* **266**, 76—99 (1962). [D21,725/62

Oya, J. C. de, Rio, A. del, Noya, M., Villanueva, A.: Phenobarbitone in posthepatitic unconjugated hyperbilirubinaemia. *Lancet* **1970 II**, 521. [H28,966/70

Paal, H.: Schilddrüsenfunktion und die Reaktion nach Reid Hunt. *Naunyn-Schmiedebergs Arch. Pharmak.* **148**, 232—245 (1930).
[22,603/30

Paal, H.: Zur Technik der Acetonitrilreaktion nach Reid Hunt. *Klin. Wschr.* **12**, 1988—1989 (1933). [18,183/33

Paeile, C., Guerrero, S., Campos, I., Muñoz, E., Novoa, L., Muñoz, C.: Estudios sobre el mecanismo de las diferencias sexuales en la sensibilidad a la procaina en ratas. *Arch. Biol. Med. exp. (Santiago)* **1**, 152—156 (1964).
[F52,633/64

Paeile, C., Guerrero, S., Gallardo, A., Muñoz, C.: Comparación de la toxicidad de diversos anestésicos locales en ratas machos y hembras. *Arch. Biol. Med. exp.* **2**, 48—50 (1965).
[G75,994/65

Page, I. H., Taylor, R. D.: Sensitization to the pressor action of epinephrine ("adrenalin"). A warning concerning the use of epinephrine as an antidote after the administration of tetraethyl ammonium chloride. *J. Amer. med. Ass.* **135**, 348—349 (1947). [B24,841/47

Painter, E. E., Brues, A. M.: The radiation syndrome. *New Engl. J. Med.* **240**, 871—876 (1949). [B39,627/49

Pallotta, A. J., Kelly, M. G., Rall, D. P., Ward, J. W.: Toxicology of acetoxycycloheximide as a function of sex and body weight. *J. Pharmacol. exp. Ther.* **136**, 400—405 (1962).
[D26,380/62

Palmerio, C., Fine, J.: The nature of resistance to shock. *Arch. Surg.* **98**, 679—684 (1969).
[G66,810/69

Paluszka, D. J., Hamilton, L. H.: Effect of heparin on the metabolic and leukocyte responses to hydrocortisone injections in rats. *Physiologist* **2**, 92—93 (1959). [C72,116/59

Palva, I. P., Mustala, O. O.: Oral contraceptives and liver damage. *Brit. med. J.* **1964 II**, 688—689. [F21,067/64

Pan, F., Lee, S. C., Chang, G. G., Sing-Fie, C.: Gonadal hormones in the regulation of methionine adenosyltransferase levels in rat liver. *Proc. Soc. exp. Biol. (N.Y.)* **129**, 161—165 (1968). [H3,934/68

Panisset, J. C., Beaulnes, A., Bois, P.: Effect of thyroxine on the sensitivity of the rat smooth muscle to 5-hydroxytryptamine. *Rev. canad. Biol.* **25**, 155—159 (1966). [F71,775/66

Pannella, A., Gasparrini, G.: Azione del testosterone e degli estrogeni sull'insorgenza dei tumori sperimentali da 20-metilcolantrene. *Arch. Pat. Clin. med.* **39**, 198—218 (1963).
[D64,636/63

Parant, M.: Action de la chlorpromazine, de la cortisone et de l'ACTH vis-à-vis d'une endotoxine bactérienne injectée à la souris hypophysectomisée. *Ann. Inst. Pasteur* **102**, 85—91 (1962). [D82,116/62

Parfentjev, I. A.: The use of hypersensitive mice for standardization of new drugs. *Ann. N.Y. Acad. Sci.* **111**, 712—714 (1964).
[F10,707/64

Parhon, C., Urechia, C.: L'influence de la castration sur les phénomènes de l'intoxication strychnique. *C. R. Soc. Biol. (Paris)* **70**, 610—612 (1911). [A23,732/11

Parhon, C., Urechia, C. I.: Recherches sur l'influence des glandes endocrines sur l'excitabilité des centres nerveux. *Bull. Soc. Med. ment. Belg.* No. 166, 5—35 (1913). [62,361/13

Parhon, C. I., Ballif, L.: Sur l'anaphylaxie chez les animaux éthymisés et thyréoprives. *C. R. Soc. Biol. (Paris)* 88, 544—545 (1923). [13,548/23

Parhon, C. I., Ballif, L.: Nouvelles recherches sur l'anaphylaxie chez les animaux éthyroïdés éthymisés. *C. R. Soc. Biol. (Paris)* 89, 1063 a 1065 (1923). [17,302/23

Parhon, C. I., Werner, G.: Recherches expérimentales sur la tétanie guanidinique et sur les effets des injections de guanidine, chez les animaux thyroparathyroidectomisés. La biochimie du sang à la suite des injections de guanidine. *Bull. Mem. Sect. endocr.* 1, 188—193 (1935). [34,844/35

Parhon, C.-J., Parhon, C.: Note sur l'hyperthyroïdisation chez les oiseaux et sur la résistance des animaux ainsi traités aux infections spontanées. *C. R. Soc. Biol. (Paris)* 76, 662—663 (1914). [36,340/14

Parized, J.: Sterilization of the male by cadmium salts. *J. Reprod. Fertil.* 1, 294—309 (1960). [D23,927/60

Parized, J.: The peculiar toxicity of cadmium during pregnancy; an experimental 'toxaemia of pregnancy' induced by cadmium salts. *J. Reprod. Fertil.* 9, 111—112 (1965). [F31,959/65

Pařízek, J., Ošťádalová, I., Beneš, I., Pitha, J.: The effect of a subcutaneous injection of cadmium salts on the ovaries of adult rats in persistent oestrus. *J. Reprod. Fertil.* 17, 559—562 (1968). [H7,672/68

Parker, R. T., Snyder, M. J., Merideth, A. M.: Effect of various antibiotics and cortisone upon botulinum, tetanal and diphtherial toxins in vivo (Abstr.). *Amer. J. Med.* 14, 753 (1953). [D77,476/53

Parkes, A. S.: Some factors affecting resistance to anoxia in mice. *J. Endocr.* 7, lxii—lxiii (1951). [B63,024/51

Parks, H. F.: Electron microscopic investigation of the source and direction of movement of lipid granules appearing in the hepatic perisinusoidal space following partial hepatectomy. *Amer. J. Anat.* 124, 513—529 (1969). [H28,647/69

Parmer, L. G.: Effect of desoxycorticosterone on the development of rats treated with thiouracil. *Proc. Soc. exp. Biol. (N.Y.)* 66, 574—575 (1947). [B17,568/47

Paroli, E.: Influenza degli estrogeni sulla tolleranza alla morfina nel ratto. *Arch. ital. Sci. Farmacol.* (Ser. 3/4), 309—310 (1954). [G14,277/54

Paroli, E.: Morfina ed estrogeni. I. Riduzione della resistenza alla morfina nel ratto per opera di estrogeni. *Arch. Ist. biochim. ital.* 18, 35—44 (1957). [C62,998/57

Paroli, E.: Morfina ed estrogeni. II. Influenza degli estrogeni sull'analgesia morfinica, il quadro dell'intossicazione acuta e l'escrezione urinaria della morfina nel ratto. *Arch. Ist. biochim. ital.* 18/2, 1—5 (1957). [C63,939/57

Paroli, E.: Morfina ed estrogeni. III. Effetto dell'estradiolo, dello stilbestrolo, dell'esestrolo sulla assuefazione del ratto alla azione analgesica della morfina. *Arch. Ist. biochim. ital.* 18/2, 6—8 (1957). [C63,938/57

Paroli, E.: Effetto del D.O.C.A. sul quadro dell'avitaminosi B_1 nel colombo. *Boll. Soc. ital. Biol. sper.* 33, 1393—1396 (1957). [C63,940/57

Paroli, E.: Indagini sull'effetto antimorfinico dell'ACTH. — II. Influenza dell'idrocortisone, del prednisolone e del desametazone sugli effetti analgesico e respiratorio della morfina. *Boll. Soc. ital. Biol. sper.* 40, 23—25 (1963). [G12,543/63

Paroli, E., De Arcangelis, A.: Influenza del progesterone, del pregnandiolo, del pregnandione e del pregnenolone sull'effetto analgesico della morfina nel ratto. *Arch. Ist. biochim. ital.* 18/2, 8—10 (1957). [C63,937/57

Parratt, J. R., West, G. B.: Hypersentitivity and the thyroid gland. *Int. Arch. Allergy* 16, 288—302 (1960). [D235/60

Paschkis, K. E., Cantarow, A., Stasney, S.: Pregnancy in partially hepatectomized rats. *Fed. Proc.* 15, 141—142 (1956). [C14,122/56

Paschkis, K. E., Cantarow, A., Stasney, J., Hobbs, J. H.: Tumor growth in partially hepatectomized rats. *Cancer Res.* 15, 579—582 (1955). [C8,982/55

Pasley, J. N., Chadwick, G. G., Krueger, H.: Thyroxine antagonism of pentachlorophenol poisoning in cichlid fish. *Proc. West. pharmacol. Soc.* 11, 129—132 (1968). [G67,522/68

Pasquariello, C., Mainardi, L.: Effetto di replicazione ravvicinata di un trattamento cortisonico sulla linea triptofano-acido nicotinico nell'uomo. *Acta vitamin. (Milano)* 24, 11—14 (1970). [H28,663/70

Passow, H., Rothstein, A., Clarkson, T. W.: The general pharmacology of the heavy metals. *Pharmacol. Rev.* 13, 185—224 (1961). [G38,172/61

Pataki, A.: Experimentelle Nebennierenrindennekrosen durch massive intravasale Gerinnung und ihre Beeinflussung durch ACTH. Z. ges. exp. Med. 142, 75—86 (1967). [F 75,591/67

Patel, A. A., Rao, S. S.: Action of adrenaline on tetanus toxin. Indian J. med. Sci. 19, 818—820 (1965). [G 36,076/65

Patrick, R. S.: The influence of cortisone and ACTH on experimental zonal necrosis of the liver. J. Path. Bact. 70, 377—385 (1955). [C 12,967/55

Patrignani, A.: Incorporazione dell'acidoΔ-amino levulinico 4-^{14}C nella bilirubina biliare del ratto: modificazioni indotte dal trattamento con testosterone. Riv. Farmacol. Ter. 1, 337—345 (1970). [H 32,792/70

Patt, H. M., Smith, D. E., Tyree, E. B., Straube, R. L.: Further studies on modification of sensitivity to X-rays by cysteine. Proc. Soc. exp. Biol. (N.Y.) 73, 18—21 (1950). [B 54,522/50

Patt, H. M., Straube, R. L., Tyree, E. B., Swift, M. N., Smith, D. E.: Influence of estrogens on the acute x-irradiation syndrome. Amer. J. Physiol. 159, 269—280 (1949). [B 43,570/49

Patt, H. M., Swift, M. N., Straube, R. L., Tyree, E. B., Smith, D. E.: Influence of a conditioning injection of estrogen on the hematologic and organ weight response to X-irradiation. Fed. Proc. 8, 124 (1949). [B 32,806/49

Patt, H. M., Swift, M. N., Tyree, E. B., Straube, R. L.: X-irradiation of the hypophysectomized rat. Science 108, 475—476 (1948). [B 33,711/48

Patt, H. M., Tyree, E. B., Straube, R. L., Smith, D. E.: Cysteine protection against X irradiation. Science 110, 213—214 (1949). [B 54,521/49

Patton, C. L., Clark, D. T.: Trypanosoma lewisi infections in normal rats and in rats treated with dexamethasone. J. Protozool. 15, 31—35 (1968). [G 73,195/68

Pavlovic-Hournac, M., Andjus, R. K.: Survie en milieu froid des rats thyroïdectomisés porteurs de greffes intraoculaires de thyroïdes. C. R. Soc. Biol. (Paris) 157, 1201—1203 (1963). [E 33,972/63

Pawlowski, Z.: The hormonal homeostasis of the host and the development of the parasite. Helminthologia (Bratisl.) 9, 463—466 (1968). [G 65,301/68

Payne, J. M.: The pathogenesis of experimental brucellosis in virgin heifers with and without continuous progesterone treatment. J. Endocr. 20, 345—354 (1960). [C 89,814/60

Payne, J. M., Belyavin, G.: The experimental infection of pregnant rats with the virus of enzootic abortion of sheep. J. Path. Bact. 80, 215—223 (1960). [C 95,892/60

Payne, R. W.: Studies on the fat-mobilizing hormone of the anterior pituitary gland (Abstr.). Fed. Proc. 125—126 (1949). [B 32,809/49

Peakall, D. B.: Pesticide-induced enzyme breakdown of steroids in birds. Nature (Lond.) 216, 505—506 (1967). [F 90,310/67

Pecori, V., Altucci, P., Cimino, R., Buonanno, G. A.: Steroidi a tipo prednisonico nelle infezioni sperimentali da virus. I. Studio comparativo delle modificazioni indotte dal prednisolone e dal triamcinolone nel quadro della epatite da virus MHV-3 del topo. G. Mal. infett. 11, 1144—1146 (1959). [C 89,118/59

Pecori, V., Altucci, P., Coraggio, F., De Martino, E., Guarino, G.: L'aldosterone nelle infezioni virali sperimentali. II. Attività nell'infezione da virus vaccinico nel coniglio. B. D. S. Italiana 37, 711—714 (1961). [D 12,549/61

Pecori, V., Cimino, R., Buonanno, G. A., Altucci, P.: Il prednisolone e l'ormone somatotropo nell'epatite del topo da virus MHV-3. G. Mal. infett. 11, 1148—1150 (1959). [C 89,121/59

Pekárek, J., Vrána, M.: The effect of hormones on histamine shock in rats sensitized with pertussis vaccine. Acta allerg. (Kbh.) 17, 387—399 (1962). [D 52,098/62

Pelissier, N. A., Burgee, S. L., Jr.: Guide to incompatibilities. Hosp. Pharm. (Philad.) 3, 15—28, 32 (1968). [G 79,655/68

Pellanda, E. B.: Eclampsia experimental. Rev. Med. Rio Grande do Sul 11, 247—266 (1955). [C 7,961/55

Pellerin, J., D'Iorio, A., Robillard, E.: Influence des hormones sexuelles et l'hépatectomie partielle sur l'anesthésie au pentobarbital. Rev. Canad. Biol. 13, 257—263 (1954). [B 98,672/54

Pelouze, P. S., Rosenberger, R. C.: The interesting behavior of tuberculous guinea-pigs under parathyroid and calcium administration. A preliminary report. Amer. J. med. Sci. 168, 546—553 (1924). [62,508/24

Peltola, P.: The effect of thyroid powder on the lethal dose of adrenaline. Ann. Med. exp. Fenn. 28, Sup., pp. 59 (1950). [B 57,468/50

Penhos, J. C.: Effect of triamcinolone, dexamethasone and aminopterin on the growth of rats. Acta physiol. lat.-amer. 12, 329—341 (1962). [G 8,997/62

Penhos, J. C., Blaquier, J. A.: Toxicidad de la fenetildiguanida (DBI). Rev. Soc. argent. Biol. 34, 21—28 (1958). [C 59,755/58

Peraino, C., Lamar, C., Pitot, H. C.: Studies on the induction and repression of enzymes in rat liver. IV. Effects of cortisone and phenobarbital. *J. biol. Chem.* 241, 2944—2948 (1966). [G 40,083/66]

Peräsalo, O., Latvalahti, J.: Amyloid degeneration in the light of clinical and experimental studies. *Acta path. microbiol. scand.* 34, 208 to 217 (1954). [C 9,661/54]

Perelmuter, C., Miletzkaja, S.: Interaction between thyroid gland and vitamin B. (Russian text.) *Probl. zootech. exp. Endocr.* 1, 283—305 (1934). [78,650/34]

Pérez, V.: Higado y drogas. Buenos Aires: Editorial Paidos, pp. 270 (1969). [E 8,836/69]

Pérez, V., Gorosdisch, S., de Martire, J., Nicholson, R., di Paola, G.: Oral contraceptives: long-term use produces fine structural changes in liver mitochondria. *Science* 165, 805—807 (1969). [H 14,794/69]

Pérez-Tamayo, R., Romero, R.: Role of the spleen in regeneration of the liver. *Lab. Invest.* 7, 248—257 (1958). [D 38,897/58]

Perla, D., Freiman, D. G., Sandberg, M., Greenberg, S. S.: Prevention of histamine and surgical shock by cortical hormone (desoxy-corticosterone acetate and cortin) and saline. *Proc. Soc. exp. Biol. (N.Y.)* 43, 397—404 (1940). [A 31,863/40]

Perla, D., Marmorston-Gottesman, J.: Immunological studies in relation to the suprarenal gland. IV. The effect of repeated injections of epinephrine on the hemolysin formation in suprarenalectomized rats. *J. exp. Med.* 50, 87—92 (1929). [16,042/29]

Perla, D., Marmorston-Gottesman, J.: Further studies on T. lewisi infection in albino rats. I. The effect of splenectomy on T. lewisi infection in albino rats and the protective action of splenic autotransplants. II. The effect of thymectomy and bilateral gonadectomy on T. lewisi infection in albino rats. *J. exp. Med.* 52, 601—616 (1930). [810/30]

Perla, D., Marmorston-Gottesman, J.: Injections of cortin on resistance of suprarenalectomized rats. Biological assay of extracts of suprarenal cortex. *Proc. Soc. exp. Biol. (N.Y.)* 28, 475—477 (1931). [10,865/31]

Perry, A. S.: Studies on microsomal cytochrome P-450 in resistant and susceptible houseflies. *Life Sci.* 9, 335—350 (1970). [G 74,358/70]

Perry, D. J.: The effect of adrenalectomy on the development of tumours induced by 2-acetylaminofluorene. *Brit. J. Cancer* 15, 284—290 (1961). [D 10,864/61]

Pesch, L. A., Segal, S., Topper, Y. J.: Progesterone effects on galactose metabolism in prepubertal patients with congenital galactosemia and in rats maintained on high galactose diets. *J. clin. Invest.* 39, 178—184 (1960). [C 79,957/60]

Peterkofsky, B., Tomkins, G. M.: Effect of inhibitors of nucleic acid synthesis on steroid-mediated induction of tyrosine aminotransferase in hepatoma cell cultures. *J. molec. Biol.* 30, 49—61 (1967). [G 52,839/67]

Peters, J. M., Boyd, E. M.: The influence of sex and age in albino rats given a daily oral dose of caffeine at a high dose level. *Canad. J. Physiol. Pharmacol.* 45, 305—311 (1967). [F 77,819/67]

Petty, W. C., Karler, R.: The influence of aging on the activity of anticonvulsant drugs. *J. Pharmacol. exp. Ther.* 150, 443—448 (1965). [F 58,540/65]

Petzold, H.: Der Einfluß von Turinabol auf die Tetrachlorkohlenstoff-Fibrose des Kaninchens. *Z. ges. inn. Med.* 20, 191—193 (1965). [F 61,425/65]

Petzold, H., Matzkowski, H., Burckhardt, M.: Der Einfluß von Oral-Turinabol auf die 'Thioacetamidzirrhose' der Rattenleber. *Dtsch. Z. Verdau.- u. Stoffwechselkr.* 29, 127—132 (1969). [H 20,651/69]

Petzold, H., Meincke, K.: Die Wirkung von 6-Methylprednisolon auf Gewebsenzyme der Tierleber bei chronischer Tetrachlorkohlenstoffschädigung. *Dtsch. Z. Verdau.- u. Stoffwechselkr.* 22, 150—157 (1962). [D 39,959/62]

Petzold, H., Ziegler, A.: Der Einfluß von Prednison und Turinabol auf Gewebsphosphatasen der experimentellen Fettleber der Ratte. *Z. ges. inn. Med.* 22, 654—657 (1967). [F 92,832/67]

Peyster, F. A. de, Jobgen, E. A., Petravicius, M. A.: Humoral accelerating effect of regeneraing liver on distant tumor take and growth in rats. *Surg. Forum* 12, 149—150 (1961). [G 71,671/61]

Pfeifer, A. K., György, L., Fodor, M.: Role of catecholamines in the central effects of amphetamine. *Acta med. Acad. Sci. hung.* 25, 441—450 (1968). [G 65,057/68]

Pfeifer, A. K., Pataky, I., Sátory, E., Vértes, P.: Observations on the early pharmacological effects of thyroxine. *Arch. int. Pharmacodyn.* 127, 44—57 (1960). [D 12,952/60]

Pfeiffer, H.: Über den Einfluß des Schilddrüsenverlustes auf die Wärmeregulation des Meerschweinchens. *Naunyn-Schmiedebergs Arch. Pharmak.* **98**, 253—256 (1923). [16,694/23

Pflüger, E.: Die teleologische Mechanik der lebendigen Natur. *Pflügers Arch. ges. Physiol.* **15**, 57—103 (1877). [A 4,877/1877

Phansalkar, A. G., Joglekar, G. V., Balwani, J. H.: A study of digoxin, thyroxine and reserpine interrelationship. *Arch. int. Pharmacodyn.* **182**, 44—48 (1969). [H 20,555/69

Phillips, P. H., English, H., Hart, E. B.: The augmentation of the toxicity of fluorosis in the chick by feeding desiccated thyroid. *J. Nutr.* **10**, 399—407 (1935). [34,798/35

Piantoni, L.: Azione del cortisone sulle infezioni sperimentali da lieviti asporigeni avirulenti e virulenti. *G. Mal. infett.* **7**, 1—47 (1955). [C 38,892/55

Piantoni, L.: Azione del cortisone sulle infezioni sperimentali da actinomiceti avirulenti e virulenti. *Biol. lat. (Milano)* **8**, 1095—1117 (1955). [C 38,895/55

Picha, E.: Neue Gesichtspunkte zur Anwendung anaboler Steroide in der gynäkologischen Strahlentherapie. *Strahlentherapie* **138**, 300 bis 322 (1969). [G 70,118/69

Pichler, E.: Behandlung eines Cushing-Syndroms auf Grund einer Nebennierenrindenhyperplasie bei einem 7jährigen Mädchen mit dem Nebennierenrindenblocker opDDD. *Helv. paediat. Acta* **21**, 447—474 (1966). [G 43,794/66

Pierce, A. E., Long, P. L.: Studies on acquired immunity to coccidiosis in bursaless and thymectomized fowls. *Immunology* **9**, 427—439 (1965). [G 36,006/65

Pieroni, R. E., Broderick, E. J., Bundeally, A., Levine, L.: A simple method for the quantitation of submicrogram amounts of bacterial endotoxin. *Proc. Soc. exp. Biol. (N.Y.)* **133**, 790—794 (1970). [H 31,137/70

Pieroni, R. E., Levine, L.: Enhancing effect of insulin on endotoxin lethality. *Experientia (Basel)* **25**, 507—508 (1969). [G 68,105/69

Pierre, R.: Influence de la sérotonine, de dérivés de la phénothiazine, de stéroïds, de tranquillisants sur l'EEG du lapin intoxiqué par la diéthylamide de l'acide lysergique. I. Action sur l'intoxication chronique par la LSD. *C. R. Soc. Biol. (Paris)* **151**, 890—892 (1957). [C 52,727/57

Pierre, R.: Influence de la sérotonine, de dérivés de la phénothiazine, de stéroïdes, de tranquillisants sur l'EEG du lapin intoxiqué par le diéthylamide de l'acide lysergique. II. Action sur la réaction d'éveil produite par la LSD. *C. R. Soc. Biol. (Paris)* **151**, 1135—1137 (1957). [C 55,459/57

Pierre, R., Cahn, J.: Essais d'anesthésie prolongée par la 5-hydroxytryptamine. *C. R. Soc. Biol. (Paris)* **149**, 1406—1407 (1955). [C 24,570/55

Pierre, R., Cahn, J., Herold, M., Georges, G.: Actions de la 21-hydroxyprégnanedione et du méthyl-androstanolone sur le système nerveux central. *Presse méd.* **65**, 1621 (1957). [C 46,326/57

Pinchot, G. B., Close, V. P., Long, C. N. H.: Adrenal changes produced in rats by infection with B. Tularense and B. Coli. *Endocrinology* **45**, 135—142 (1949). [B 39,038/49

Pincus, G.: The Control of Fertility. New York, London: Academic Press Inc., pp. 360 (1965). [E 689/65

Pincus, G., Martin, D. W.: Liver damage and estrogen inactivation. *Endocrinology* **27**, 838 to 839 (1940). [A 34,939/40

Pines, I., Salazar, E., Lopez, T.: On the influence of the intravenous injections of glucocorticoids upon the electrocardiogram. An experimental study. *Arch. int. Pharmacodyn.* **122**, 1—14 (1959). [C 87,661/59

Pinto, M. I. M.: Estudos sobre epidemiologia experimental. I.—Acção da cortisona na infestação do rato albino pelo cestodo Hymenolepis nana, Tipo "M". *An. Inst. Med. trop.* **17**, 83—97 (1960). [D 23,719/60

Pirani, C. L., Stepto, R. C., Sutherland, K.: Effects of cortisone on normal and ascorbic acid-deficient guinea pigs. *Fed. Proc.* **10**, 368 (1951). [B 57,272/51

Pisanty, J., Toscano, S.: Adrenal cortex performance in shock. *Amer. J. Physiol.* **187**, 622 (1956). [C 30,049/56

Pitot, H. C.: Substrate and hormonal interactions in the regulations of enzyme levels in rat hepatomas. *Advanc. Enzyme Regul.* **1**, 309 to 319 (1963). [G 65,475/63

Pitot, H. C., Peraino, C., Morse, P. A., Jr., Potter, V. R.: Hepatomas in tissue culture compared with adapting liver in vivo. *Nat. Cancer Inst. Monogr.* **13**, 229—245 (1964). [G 37,125/64

Pizzi, P. T., Chemke, S. J.: Acción de la cortisona sobre la infección experimental de la rata por Trypanosoma cruzi. *Biologica* **21**, 31—48 (1955). [C 34,555/55

Plaa, G. L.: Biliary and other routes of excretion of drugs. In: Ladu, B., Way, E. L., and Mandell, H. G.: *Fundamentals of Drug Metabolism* *and Drug Disposition* Baltimore: Williams and Wilkins Co. (in press). [G 73,820

Plaa, G. L., Becker, B. A.: Demonstration of bile stasis in the mouse by a direct and an indirect method. *J. appl. Physiol.* 20, 534—537 (1965). [G 76,082/65

Plagge, J. C., Marasso, F. J., Zimmerman, H. J.: Estrogen inhibition of nutritional fatty liver. *Metabolism* 7, 154—161 (1958). [C 50,216/58

Plotka, C., Jequier, R., Velluz, L.: Sur un effet protecteur de l'adrénostérone dans l'athérome expérimental a l'adrénaline. *C. R. Acad. Sci. (Paris)* 244, 264—265 (1957). [C 51,239/57

Podwyssozki, W.: Über die Regeneration der Epithelien der Leber, der Niere, der Speichel- und Meibom'schen Drüsen unter pathologischen Bedingungen. Vorläufige Mitteilung. *Fortschr. Med.* 3 (1885). [E 77,767/1885

Poe, C. F., Suchy, J. F.: Effect of vitamin B_1 on the toxicity of strychnine. *Arch. int. Pharmacodyn.* 86, 449—453 (1951).
[D 75,977/51

Poe, C. F., Suchy, J. F., Witt, N. F.: Toxicity of strychnine for male and female rats of different ages. *J. Pharmacol. exp. Ther.* 58, 239—242 (1936). [A 45,388/36

Poe, R. H., Davis, T. R. A.: Cold exposure and acclimation in alloxan-diabetic rats. *Amer. J. Physiol.* 202, 1045—1048 (1962). [D 27,155/62

Poe, R. H., White, J. W., Davis, T. R. A.: Alloxan-diabetic rats during acclimation to cold. *Amer. J. Physiol.* 205, 184—188 (1963). [E 21,412/63

Poel, W. E.: Progesterone enhancement of mammary tumor development as a model of co-carcinogenesis. *Brit. J. Cancer* 22, 867 to 873 (1968). [H 23,662/68

Pohl, H., Hart, J. S.: Thermoregulation and cold acclimation in a hibernator, Citellus tridecemlineatus. *J. appl. Physiol.* 20, 398 to 404 (1965). [F 62,568/65

Pohle, K., Bekemeier, H.: Antagonistische Beeinflussung der Rattenniere durch Oestrogene und Nebennierenrindenhormone. *Endokrinologie* 51, 314—318 (1967). [F 91,972/67

Pokrajac, N., Osterman, J., Bilic, N.: The tolerance to massive doses of insulin in adrenalectomized and cortisol-treated rats. *Diabetologia (Berlin)* 3, 361—367 (1967). [G 49,275/67

Poland, A., Smith, D., Kuntzman, R., Jacobson, M., Conney, A. H.: Effect of intensive occupational exposure to DDT on phenylbutazone and cortisol metabolism in human subjects. *Clin. Pharmacol. Ther.* 11, 724—732 (1970).
[G 78,061/70

Polemann, G., Froitzheim, G.: Tierexperimentelle Untersuchungen zur Therapie der D_2-Hypervitaminose. *Z. Vitamin-, Hormon- u. Fermentforsch.* 5, 329—357 (1953). [B 87,589/53

Polishuk, Z. W., Wassermann, M., Wassermann, D., Groner, Y., Lazarovici, S., Tomatis, L.: Effects of pregnancy on storage of organochlorine insecticides. *A. M. A. Arch. environm. Hlth.* 20, 215—217 (1970). [G 72,380/70

Poll, M., Seitchik, M. W., Canter, J. W., Segal, R. L., Baronofsky, I. D.: The effect of thyroidectomy on experimental ascites. *Surgery* 49, 636 to 640 (1961). [D 4,775/61

Polliack, A., Charuzy, I., Levij, I. S.: The effect of oestrogen on 9, 10-dimethyl-1,2-benzanthracene (DMBA)-induced cheek pouch carcinoma in castrated and non-castrated male Syrian golden hamsters. *Brit. J. Cancer* 23, 781—786 (1969). [G 72,389/69

Polliack, A., Charuzy, I., Levij, I. S.: The effect of testosterone on chemical carcinogenesis in the buccal pouches of castrated and intact male hamsters. *Path. et Microbiol. (Basel)* 35, 348 to 354 (1970). [H 31,578/70

Poloni, A.: Serotonia e schizofrenia. Rilievi sperimentali in favore dell'ipotesi di una tossicosi da 5-idrossitriptamina della schizofrenia. *Cervello* 31, 231—242 (1955).
[D 95,333/55

Poloni, A.: Serotonina e schizofrenia. Azione della serotonia (S.) sola e associata ai barbiturici (Ba.), alla dietilamide dell'acido lisergico (LSD. 25), alla mescalina (M.) e alla bulbocapnina (B.) sul tracciato EEG. di schizofrenici, epilettici e altri ammalati di mente. *Cervello* 31, 355—382 (1955). [D 99,472/55

Pomp, H., Schnoor, M., Netter, K. J.: Untersuchungen über die Arzneimitteldemethylierung in der fetalen Leber. *Dtsch. med. Wschr.* 94, 1232, 1237—1240 (1969). [H 14,237/69

Ponchon, G., Kennan, A. L., DeLuca, H. F.: "Activation" of vitamin D by the liver. *J. clin. Invest.* 48, 2032—2037 (1969).
[H 18,243/69

Ponfick, E.: Experimentelle Beiträge zur Pathologie der Leber. *Virchows Arch. pathol. Anat.* 118, 209—249 (1889). [A 24,568/1889

Ponseti, I. V.: Lesions of the skeleton and of other mesodermal tissues in rats fed sweet-pea (lathyrus odoratus) seeds. *J. Bone Jt Surg.* 36-A, 1031—1058 (1954). [D 49,845/54

Ponseti, I. V.: Prevention of aminonitrile lesions in rats with L-triiodothyronine. *Proc. Soc. exp. Biol. (N.Y.)* 96, 14—17 (1957).
[E 54,643/57

Ponseti, I. V.: Studies of the suppression of aminonitrile lesions in rats by thyroxine analogues. *Endocrinology* **64**, 795—806 (1959). [C 68,050/59

Ponseti, I. V.: Studies on the nature of skeletal lesions produced by aminonitriles. *Bull. Hosp. Dis. (N.Y.)* **20**, 1—8 (1959). [C 78,321/59

Ponseti I. V., Aleu, F.: Fracture healing in rats treated with aminoacetonitrile. *J. Bone Surg.* **40-A**, 1093—1102 (1958). [C 61,715/58

Pontremoli, S., Arrigo, L.: Effetti dell'asportazione della milza sulla 'rigenerazione' del fegato dopo parziale epatectomia. *Boll. Soc. ital. Biol. sper.* **26**, 355—357 (1950). [D 63,528/50

Popper, H., Stein, R., Kent, G., Bruce, C.: Hepatic interstitial cell reaction in experimental liver damage. *Fed. Proc.* **16**, 369 (1957). [C 33,264/57

Porrazzi, L. C., Vecchione, R., Cali, A.: Effetti del DOCA sull'aterogenesi da colesterolo nel coniglio. *Riv. Anat. pat.* **33**, 351—367 (1968). [H 34,157/68

Porto, A., Donato, A.: Estudos sobre a regeneracao hepatica experimental. *Medico (Porto)* **51**, 11—25 (1969). [H 34,703/69

Poser, W., Jahns, R.: Eine vereinfachte Methode zur funktionellen Hepatektomie. *Pflügers Arch. gesamt. Physiol.* **297**, 196 (1967). [F 90,235/67

Posner, H. S., Graves, A., King, C. T. G., Wilk, A.: Experimental alteration of the metabolism of chlorcyclizine and the incidence of cleft palate in rats. *J. Pharmacol. exp. Ther.* **155**, 494—505 (1967). [H 31,661/67

Pospíšil, M., Novák, L.: Effect of thyroid pretreatment on the mortality of X-irradiated mice. *Nature (Lond.)* **182**, 1603—1604 (1958). [C 67,534/58

Post, J., Himes, M. B., Klein, A., Hoffman, J.: Responses of the liver to injury. Effects of growth hormone upon acute carbon tetrachloride poisoning. *Arch. Path.* **64**, 278—283 (1957). [C 40,180/57

Potop, I., Boeru, V., Biener, J.: L'influence d'un extrait lipoprotéique isolé du thymus sur le développement des tumeurs expérimentales. *Rev. roum. Endocr.* **2**, 41—48 (1965). [F 38,309/65

Potop, I., Lupulesco, A., Biener, J.: Modifications morphologiques et biochimiques dans le foie des rats après administration de diète cancérigène et d'extrait thymique. *Acta biol. med. Germ.* **8**, 230—237 (1962). [E 39,894/62

Potter, J. L.: On papain and flop-eared rabbits. *Arthr. and Rheum.* **4**, 389—399 (1961). [D 23,805/61

Potvliege, P. R.: Hypervitaminosis D_2 in gravid rats. Study of its influence on fetal parathyroid glands and a report of hitherto undescribed placental alterations. *Arch. Path.* **73**, 371—382 (1962). [E 98,323/62

Powell, J., Waterhouse, J., Culley, P., Wood, B.: Effect of phenobarbitone and pre-eclamptic toxaemia on neonatal jaundice. *Lancet* **1969 II**, 802. [H 17,195/69

Pozo, E. C. del, Negrete, J.: Effects of cortisone on muscular contraction. *Fed. Proc.* **11**, 32 (1952). [B 68,183/52

Pradhan, S. N., Achinstein, B., Shear, M. J.: Potentiation of urethan anesthesia by epinephrine. *Proc. Soc. exp. Biol. (N.Y.)* **92**, 146—149 (1956). [C 13,632/56

Prange, A. J., Jr., Lipton, M. A.: Enhancement of imipramine mortality in hyperthyroid mice. *Nature (Lond.)* **196**, 588—589 (1962). [D 42,869/62

Prange, A. J., Jr., Lipton, M. A.: Effects of propylthiouracil and thyroid feeding on the response of mice to injected convulsant barbiturate. *Nature (Lond.)* **208**, 791—792 (1965). [F 56,756/65

Prange, A. J., Jr., Lipton, M. A., Love, G. N.: Diminution of imipramine mortality in hypothyroid mice. *Nature (Lond.)* **197**, 1212—1213 (1963). [D 62,707/63

Prange, A. J., Jr., Lipton, M. A., Love, G. N.: Effect of altered thyroid status on desmethylimipramine mortality in mice. *Nature (Lond.)* **204**, 1204—1205 (1964). [F 29,162/64

Prange, A. J., Jr., Lipton, M. A., Shearin, R. B., Love, G. N.: The influence of thyroid status on the effects and metabolism of pentobarbital and thiopental. *Biochem. Pharmacol.* **15**, 237 to 248 (1966). [G 40,154/66

Prange, A. J., Jr., Wilson, I. C., Knox, A., McClane, T. K., Lipton, M. A.: Enhancement of imipramine by thyroid stimulating hormone: clinical and theoretical implications. *Amer. J. Psychiat.* **127**, 191—199 (1970). [G 76,612/70

Prange, A. J., Jr., Wilson, I. C., Lipton, M. A., Rabon, A. M., McLae, T. K., Knox, A. E.: Use of a thyroid hormone to accelerate the action of imipramine. *Psychosomatics* **11**, 442—444 (1970). [H 31,796/70

Prange, A. J., Jr., Wilson, I. C., Rabon, A. M., Lipton, M. A.: Enhancement of imipramine antidepressant activity by thyroid hormone. *Amer. J. Psychiat.* **126**, 457—469 (1969). [G69,595/69]

Prasad, A. S., Oberleas, D., Wolf. P., Horwitz, J. P.: Effect of growth hormone on nonhypophysectomized zinc-deficient rats and zinc on hypophysectomized rats. *J. Lab. clin. Med.* **73**, 486—494 (1969). [G64,823/69]

Prasad, M. R. N., Singh, S. P., Rajalakshmi, M.: Fertility control in male rats by continuous release of microquantities of cyproterone acetate from subcutaneous silastic capsules. *Contraception* **2**, 165—178 (1970). [G78,450/70]

Pratt, T. W.: A comparison of the action of pentobarbital (Nembutal) and sodium barbital in rabbits as related to the detoxicating power of the liver. *J. Pharmacol. exp. Ther.* **48**, 285 (1933). [G71,897/33]

Pratt, T. W., Vanlandingham, H. W., Talley, E. E., Nelson, J. M., Johnson, E. O.: Studies of the liver function of dogs. *Amer. J. Physiol.* **102**, 148—152 (1932). [G72,105/32]

Preisig, R., Morris, T. Q., Shaver, J. C., Christy, N. P.: Volumetric, hemodynamic, and excretory characteristics of the liver in acromegaly. *J. clin. Invest.* **45**, 1379—1387 (1966). [F70,515/66]

Prellwitz, W., Bässler, K. H.: Veränderungen an Proteinen der Leber und des Blutes bei experimenteller Lebercirrhose und nach Behandlung mit Decortin und einem anabolen Steroid. *Klin. Wschr.* **41**, 1125—1139 (1963). [E36,762/63]

Prescott, L. F.: Pharmacokinetic drug interactions. *Lancet* **1969** II, 1239—1243. [H19,333/69]

Preusse, H.: Zur Frage der Alkoholentgiftung durch Thyroxin. *Thesis*, University of Halle-Wittenberg (1933). [26,352/33]

Previte, J. J., Berry, L. J.: Studies on the potentiation of endotoxin in mice by exposure to cold. *J. infect. Dis.* **113**, 43—51 (1963). [E89,101/63]

Prewitt, R., Musacchia, X. J.: Mechanisms of radio-protection by sympathomimetics. *Physiologist* **12**, 330 (1969). [H16,155/69]

Preziosi, P., Scapagnini, U., Nistico, G.: Toxicite d'esters de la bétaméthasone seuls ou associés à des anabolisants chez le rat nouveau-né. *Arch. int. Pharmacodyn.* **166**, 208—213 (1967). [F78,520/67]

Pribram, B. O.: Die Steuerungsmöglichkeit der Avertinnarkose durch Thyroxin. *Zbl. Chir.* **56**, 3138—3142 (1929). [A47,677/29]

Priestly, B. G., Plaa, G. L.: Temporal aspects of carbon tetrachloride-induced alteration of sulfobromophthalein excretion and metabolism. *Toxicol. appl. Pharmacol.* **17**, 786—794 (1970). [G80,048/70]

Priestley, J. T., Markowitz, J., Mann, F. C.: Studies on the physiology of the liver. XX. The detoxicating function of the liver with special reference to strychnine. *Amer. J. Physiol.* **96**, 696—708 (1931). [9,158/31]

Prioreschi, P.: Stress e anestesia da bromuro di sodio. *Atti Soc. lombarda Sci. med.-biol.* **14**, 215—217 (1959). [C68,485/59]

Proulx, L., D'Iorio, A., Beznak, M.: The metabolism of catecholamines in hyperthyroid and vitamin B_{12} deficient rats. *Canad. J. Biochem.* **44**, 1577—1585 (1966). [G43,289/66]

Pulkkinen, M. O.: Sulphate conjugation during development, in human, rat and guinea pig. *Acta physiol. scand.* **66**, 115—119 (1966). [G39,295/66]

Pyatnitskaya, T. M.: Hepatic changes in methylthiouracil treatment (Russian text). *Probl. Endokr. Gormonoter.* 2/4, 96—100 (1956). [C43,809/56]

Pyörälä, K., Kekki, M.: Decreased anticoagulant tolerance during methandrostenolone therapy. *Scand. J. clin. Lab. Invest.* **15**, 367—374 (1963). [E31,756/63]

Pyörälä, K., Seppälä, T., Punsar, S.: Effect of corticoids, adrenocorticotrophic hormone, thyroxine and thyrotrophic hormone on aortic lesions in experimental lathyrism. *Acta path. microbiol. scand.* **45**, 37—48 (1959). [G67,833/59]

Quadri, G.: Sulla funzione antitossica delle paratiroidi. Ricerche sperimentali. *Gazz. med. ital.* **51**, 61—72 (1906). [45,920/06]

Quattrocchi, G., Foresti, A.: Influenza del trattamento con PTE sullo shock anafilattico e sul fenomeno di Sanarelli-Schwartzman. *Boll. Soc. ital. Biol. sper.* **42**, 1093—1095 (1966). [G43,535/66]

Querci, V., Massari, L., Barni, I.: Sul metabolismo e l'azione tossica del parathion in ratti pretrattati con CCl_4. *Boll. Soc. ital. Biol. sper.* **45**, 404—406 (1969). [G70,597/69]

Quevauviller, A., Podevin, R.: Activité hypnotique et métabolisme du thiopental chez la souris rendue diabétique par l'alloxanne. *Anesth. Analg. Réanim.* **25**, 45—52 (1968). [G57,209/68]

Quimby, F. H.: Effects of hormone, vitamin and liver supplements on the appetite and growth of the young rat during recovery from chronic starvation. *Amer. J. Physiol.* **166**, 566—571 (1951). [B 62,481/51

Quinn, G. P., Axelrod, J., Brodie, B. B.: Species and sex differences in metabolism and duration of action of hexobarbital (Evipal). *Fed. Proc.* **13**, 396 (1954). [G 67,327/54

Quinn, G. P., Axelrod, J., Brodie, B. B.: Species, strain and sex differences in metabolism of hexobarbitone, amidopyrine, antipyrine and aniline. *Biochem. Pharmacol.* **1**, 152—159 (1958). [E 89,993/58

Qureshi, S. A., Zaman, H.: The effect of small doses of prednisolone on the incidence of subcutaneous sarcomas induced by 3-methylcholanthrene in virgin female Swiss mice. *Cancer Res.* **26**, 1516—1519 (1966). [F 68,389/66

Raab, K. H., Webb, T. E.: Inhibition of DNA synthesis in regenerating rat liver by hydrocortisone. *Experientia (Basel)* **25**, 1240—1242 (1969). [H 20,502/69

Rabboni, F., Milazzo, S.: Modificazioni anatomo-istologiche dei reni in seguito a tiroidectomia. *Boll. Soc. ital. Biol. sper.* **23**, 6—8 (1947). [B 18,975/47

Rabes, H., Tuczek, H. V.: Topik der Leberregeneration nach Teilhepatektomie bei Allylformiat-vergifteten Ratten (Demonstration). *Verh. dtsch. path. Ges.* **52**, 449—453 (1968). [H 30,729/68

Rabes, H., Tuczek, H. V.: Quantitative autoradiographische Untersuchung zur Heterogenität der Leberzellproliferation nach partieller Hepatektomie. *Virchows Arch. Abt. B Zellpathol.* **6**, 302—312 (1970). [H 33,839/70

Radomski, J. L., Fuyat, H. N., Nelson, A. A., Smith, P. K.: The toxic effects, excretion and distribution of lithium chloride. *J. Pharmacol. exp. Ther.* **100**, 429—444 (1950). [B 63,492/50

Radouco-Thomas, S., Radouco-Thomas, C., LeBreton, E.: Action de la Noradrénaline et de la Réserpine sur l'analgésie expérimentale. *Naunyn-Schmiedeberg's Arch. exp. Pathol. Pharmak.* **232**, 279—281 (1957). [E 60,201/57

Radzialowski, F. M., Bousquet, W. F.: Circadian rhythm in hepatic drug-metabolizing activity in the rat. *Life Sci.* **6**, 2545—2548 (1967). [G 53,591/67

Radzialowski, F. M., Bousquet, W. F.: Daily rhythmic variation in hepatic drug metabolism in the rat and mouse. *J. Pharmacol. exp. Ther.* **163**, 229—238 (1968). [H 2,264/68

Raffucci, F. L.: The effects of temporary occlusion of the afferent hepatic circulation in dogs. *Surgery* **33**, 342—351 (1953). [B 83,148/53

Raffucci, F. L., Wangensteen, O. H.: Tolerance of dogs to occlusion of entire afferent vascular inflow to the liver. *Surg. Forum* **1**, 191—195 (1951). [G 33,029/51

Räihä, N. C. R., Kekomäki, M. P.: Studies on the development of ornithine-keto acid aminotransferase activity in rat liver. *Biochem. J.* **108**, 521—525 (1968). [G 68,114/68

Raisfeld, I. H., Bacchin, P., Hutterer, F., Schaffner, F.: The effect of 3-amino-1,2,4-triazole on the phenobarbital-induced formation of hepatic microsomal membranes. *Molec. Pharmacol.* **6**, 231—239 (1970). [G 75,045/70

Raitschew, R.: Significance of hormonal factors in inducing melanoma in hamsters with DMBA. *Z. Krebsforsch.* **74**, 115—121 (1970). [G 76,731/70

Rall, D. P.: Screening procedures and preclinical pharmacology relating to antineoplastic agents. In: Nodine and Siegler; *Animal and Clinical: Pharmacologic Techniques in Drug Evaluation*, p. 624—631. Chicago: Year Book Med. Publ. Inc. 1964. [G 72,239/64

Ramboer, C., Thompson, R.P.H., Williams, R.: Controlled trials of phenobarbitone therapy in neonatal jaundice. *Lancet* **1969 I**, 966—968. [H 12,643/69

Ramos, A., Silverberg, M., Stern, L.: Pregnanediols and neonatal hyperbilirubinemia. *A.M.A.J. Dis. Child.* **111**, 353—356 (1966). [G 38,868/66

Ramseyer, W. F., Smith, C. A. H., McCay, C. M.: Effect of sodium fluoride administration on body changes in old rats. *J. Geront.* **12**, 14—19 (1957). [C 29,608/57

Ranney, R. E., Drill, V. A.: The ability of 17-ethyl-19-nortestosterone to block ethionine-induced fatty liver in rats. *Endocrinology* **61**, 476—477 (1957). [C 41,986/57

Rapoport, M. I., Lust, G., Beisel, W. R.: Host enzyme induction of bacterial infection. *Arch. intern. Med.* **121**, 11—16 (1968). [G 53,334/68

Räsänen, T., Taskinen, E.: Protection of the gastric mucosa against the lesions caused by reserpine through degranulation of mucosal mast cells. *Acta physiol. scand.* **71**, 96—104 (1967). [G 51,026/67

Ratnoff, O. D., Mirick, G. S.: Influence of sex upon the lethal effects of an hepatotoxic alkaloid, monocrotaline. *Bull. Johns Hopk. Hosp.* **84**, 507—525 (1949). [B 48,154/49

Ratschow, M., Klostermann, H. C.: Experimentelle Befunde zur Gefäßwirkung der Sexualhormone und ihre Beziehungen zur Klinik der peripheren Durchblutungsstörungen. *Z. klin. Med.* **135**, 198—211 (1938). [A 19,494/38

Ratsimamanga, A. R.: Fonction du cortex surrénal au cours du travail musculaire. *J. Physiol. (Paris)* **42**, 81—112 (1950). [B 48,447/50

Ratsimamanga, A. R., Buu-Hoi, N. P.: Toxicité et non-saturation des molécules. IV. Action des substances polycycliques cancérigènes sur la fonction cortico-surrénales. *Bull. Soc. Chim. Biol. (Paris)* **29**, 325—329 (1947). [B 33,923/47

Ravdin, I. S., Vars, H. M., Goldschmidt, S.: The non-specificity of suspensions of sodium zanthine in protecting the liver against injury by chloroform, and the probable cause of its action. *J. clin. Invest.* **18**, 633—640 (1939). [B 25,566/39

Recknagel, R. O.: Carbon tetrachloride hepatotoxicity. *Pharmacol. Rev.* **19**, 145—208 (1967). [F 85,043/67

Redmond, W. B.: Influence of cortisone on natural course of malaria in the pigeon. *Proc. Soc. exp. Biol. (N.Y.)* **79**, 258—261 (1952). [B 67,882/52

Regniers, P., Demeulenaere, L., Wieme, R. J.: Les modalités évolutives des lésions hépatiques provoquées par le tetrachlorure de carbone administré à dose cirrhogène sous l'influence de la cortisone. *Acta clin. belg.* **10**, 88—100 (1955). [C 7,634/55

Reichard, S. M., Edelmann, A., Gordon, A. S.: Endocrine influences upon the uptake of colloidal thorium by reticulo-endothelial organs. *Res. Bull.* **2**, 34—39 (1956). [C 32,593/56

Reid, E.: Growth hormone and adrenocortical hormones in relation to experimental tumors: a review. *Cancer Res.* **14**, 249—266 (1954). [B 93,930/54

Reid, E.: Membrane systems. In: Roodyn, D. B.; *Enzyme Cytology*, p. 321—406. London, New York: Academic Press Inc. 1967. [G 71,333/67

Reif, A. E., Brown, R. R., Potter, V. R., Miller, E. C., Miller, J. A.: Effect of diet on the antimycin titer of mouse liver. *J. biol. Chem.* **209**, 223—226 (1954). [D 97,006/54

Reifenstein, E. C., Jr.: Control of corticoid-induced protein depletion and osteoporosis by anabolic steroid therapy. *Metabolism* **7**, 78—89 (1958). [C 47,377/58

Reinhard, J. F.: Prolongation of hypnosis by epinephrine and insulin. *Proc. Soc. exp. Biol. (N.Y.)* **58**, 210—211 (1945). [B 283/45

Reinmuth, O. M., Smith, D. T.: The effect of ACTH on pneumonia induced with tuberculin in sensitized rabbits. *Trans. nat. Ass. Tuberc. (Lond.)* 47th Ann. Meet. 1951, p. 1—7. [B 60,585/51

Reis, G. von: Stora doser noradrenalin vid akuta barbituratin-toxikationer. (Large doses of norepinephrine in the treatment of acute barbiturate intoxications.) *Opuscula med. (Stockh.)* **4**, 50—52 (1959). [C 76,244/59

Reisfield, D. R., Leathem, J. H.: The closed vessel technic for testing thyroid activity in mice. *Endocrinology* **46**, 122—124 (1950). [B 46,491/50

Reiss, M., Sideman, M. B., Plichta, E. S.: Influence of anabolic hormones on phenylalanine metabolism: II. Studies in animals. *J. ment. Defic. Res.* **10**, 130—140 (1966). [F 81,632/66

Remmer, H.: Der Einfluss von Steroidhormonen auf den Abbau von Evipan bei der Ratte. *Naunyn-Schmiedebergs Arch. Pharmak.* **232**, 268—269 (1957). [G 79,941/57

Remmer, H.: Die Wirkung der Nebennierenrinde auf den Abbau von Pharmaka in den Lebermikrosomen. *Naturwissenschaften* **45**, 522 (1958). [C 73,857/58

Remmer, H.: Die Verstärkung der Abbaugeschwindigkeit von Evipan durch Glykocorticoide. *Naunyn-Schmiedebergs Arch. Pharmak.* **233**, 184—191 (1958). [D 86,728/58

Remmer, H.: Geschlechtsspezifische Unterschiede in der Entgiftung von Evipan und Thiopental bei Ratten. *Naunyn-Schmiedebergs Arch. Pharmak.* **233**, 173—183 (1958). [D 86,916/58

Remmer, H.: Der beschleunigte Abbau von Pharmaka in den Lebermikrosomen unter dem Einfluß von Luminal. *Naunyn-Schmiedebergs Arch. Pharmak.* **235**, 279—290 (1959). [E 52,112/59

Remmer, H.: Die Beschleunigung des Abbaues als Ursache der Gewöhnung an Barbiturate. *Naturwissenschaften* **46**, 580—581 (1959). [E 61,211/59

Remmer, H.: Drug tolerance. In: Mongar and de Reuck; *Ciba Foundation Symposium on Enzymes and Drug Action*, p. 276—300. London: J. & A. Churchill Ltd. 1962. [G 66,542/62

Remmer, H.: Drugs as activators of drug enzymes. In: Brodie and Erdös; *Metabolic Factors Controlling Duration of Drug Action* 6, p. 235—256. New York: MacMillan Co. 1962. [G67,788/62

Remmer, H.: Drug-induced formation of smooth endoplasmic reticulum and of drug-metabolizing enzymes. In: *Some Factors Affecting Drug Toxicity*, 4, p. 57—77. Amsterdam, New York, London: Excerpta Medica Foundation. Int. Congr. Ser. 81. 1964. [G67,786/64

Remmer, H.: Gewöhnung an Hexobarbital durch beschleunigten Abbau. *Arch. int. Pharmacodyn.* 152, 346—359 (1964). [F31,499/64

Remmer, H.: The fate of drugs in the organism. *Ann. Rev. Pharmacol.* 5, 405—428 (1965). [G78,385/65

Remmer, H.: Die Induktion arzneimittelabbauender Enzyme im endoplasmatischen Retikulum der Leberzelle durch Pharmaka. *Dtsch. med. Wschr.* 92, 2001—2008 (1967). [F90,864/67

Remmer, H., Alsleben, B.: Die Aktivierung der Entgiftung in den Lebermikrosomen während der Gewöhnung. *Klin. Wschr.* 36, 332—333 (1958). [G67,790/58

Remmer, H., Merker, H.-J.: Enzyminduktion und Vermehrung von endoplasmatischem Retikulum in der Leberzelle während der Behandlung mit Phenobarbital (Luminal). *Klin. Wschr.* 41, 276—283 (1963). [D61,064/63

Remmer, H., Merker, H.-J.: Drug-induced changes in the liver endoplasmic reticulum. Association with drug-metabolizing enzymes. *Science* 142, 1657—1658 (1963). [E36,389/63

Remmer, H., Merker, H.-J.: Evaluation and mechanisms of drug toxicity. Part II. Metabolic aspects of the toxicity of drugs. Effect of drugs on the formation of smooth endoplasmic reticulum and drug-metabolizing enzymes. *Ann. N. Y. Acad. Sci.* 123, 79—97 (1965). [G66,868/65

Remmer, H., Siegert, M.: Kumulation und Elimination von Phenobarbital. *Naunyn-Schmiedebergs Arch. Pharmak.* 243, 479—494 (1962). [G74,636/62

Remmer, H., Siegert, M., Merker, H.-J.: Vermehrung arzneimitteloxydierender Enzyme durch Tolbutamid. *Naunyn-Schmiedebergs Arch. Pharmak.* 249, 71—84 (1964). [D19,894/64

Renaud, S.: The influence of weather, climate and season on the effect of pharmacological treatment. In: Tromp; *Medical Biometeorology. Weather, Climate and the Living Organism*, p. 585—930. Amsterdam, London, New York: Elsevier Publ. Co. 1963. [C77,620/63

Renaud, S., Allard, C., Latour, J. G.: The prevention by glucocorticoids of endotoxin-initiated thrombosis in rat, in relation to fibrinolysis, coagulation, and lipemia. *Amer. Heart J.* 72, 797—805 (1966). [F74,449/66

Renaud, S., Latour, J. G.: Effect of prolonged glucocorticoid administration on lipemia, coagulation and thrombosis in rat. *Proc. Soc. exp. Biol. (N.Y.)* 128, 32—35 (1968). [F99,806/68

Renovanz, H. D.: Der Einfluß des Paraoxypropiophenons auf den Tuberkulose-Ablauf im Tierversuch. *Ärztl. Wschr.* 14, 524—529 (1959). [C78,772/59

Repke, K.: Über Spaltung und Hydroxylierung von Digitoxin bei der Ratte. *Naunyn-Schmiedebergs Arch. Pharmak.* 237, 34—48 (1959). [D27,189/59

Replogle, R. L., Gazzaniga, A. B., Gross, R. E.: Use of corticosteroids during cardiopulmonary bypass: possible lysosome stabilization. *Circulation* 33, 86—92 (1966). [G40,447/66

Reuber, M. D.: Accentuation of Ca edetate nephrosis by cortisone. *Arch. Path.* 76, 382 to 386 (1963). [E27,340/63

Reuber, M. D.: The role of the thyroid gland in hepatic carcinogenesis. (Abstr.) *Fed. Proc.* 23, 336 (1964). [F4,431/64

Reuber, M. D.: The influence of thyroid hormone and testosterone on the induction of carcinoma and cirrhosis of the liver in female Wistar rats ingesting N-2-fluorenyldiacetamide. *Fed. Proc.* 24, 431 (1965). [F36,234/65

Reuber, M. D.: Thyroiditis in rats given subcutaneous injections of trypan blue. *Toxicol. appl. Pharmacol.* 14, 108—113 (1969). [G64,737/69

Reuber, M. D.: Influence of age and sex on dietary-induced cirrhosis. An experimental study in the rat. *Arch. environm. Hlth.* 18, 792—797 (1969). [H29,035/69

Reuber, M. D.: Influence of age and sex on chronic thyroiditis in rats given subcutaneous injections of trypan blue. *Toxicol. appl. Pharmacol.* 17, 60—66 (1970). [G77,295/70

Reuber, M. D.: Hepatic vein thrombosis. Increased incidence in rats given methylchol-

anthrene and carbon tetrachloride. *A. M. A Arch. environm. Hlth.* **20**, 458—461 (1970).
[G 73,605/70]

Reuber, M. D., Glover, E. L.: Thyroiditis in rats injected subcutaneously with 3-methylcholanthrene. *Proc. Soc. exp. Biol. (N.Y.)* **129**, 509—511 (1968). [H 5,582/68]

Reuber, M. D., Grollmann, S., Glover, E. L.: Effect of 3-methyl-cholanthrene on experimentally induced cirrhosis. A study using rats of varying ages. *A. M. A. Arch. Path.* **89**, 531 to 536 (1970). [H 26,492/70]

Reyes, H., Levi, A. J., Gatmaitan, Z., Arias, I. M.: Organic anion-binding protein in rat liver: drug induction and its physiologic consequence. *Proc. nat. Acad. Sci. (Wash.)* **64**, 168—170 (1969). [G 71,233/69]

Ribble, J. C., Zalesky, M., Braude, A. I.: Distribution of Cr^{51}-labelled endotoxin in cortisone-treated mice. *Bull. Johns Hopk. Hosp.* **105**, 272—283 (1959). [C 92,576/59]

Rice, A. J., Roberts, R. J., Plaa, G.L.: The effect of carbon tetrachloride, administered in vivo, on the hemodynamics of the isolated perfused rat liver. *Toxicol. appl. Pharmacol.* **11**, 422—431 (1967). [G 55,767/67]

Richards, R. K.: Toxicity of hypnotics as affected by temperature, thyroxin and adrenalectomy. *Anesthesiology* **2**, 37—43 (1941).
[79,646/41]

Richards, R. K., Appel, M.: The barbiturates and the liver. *Anesth. Analg. Curr. Res.* **20**, 64—77 (1941). [A 48,718/41]

Richards, R. K., Taylor, J. D.: Some factors influencing distribution, metabolism and action of barbiturates: a review. *Anesthesiology* **17**, 414—458(1956). [H 19,235/56]

Richardson, H. L., Griffin, A. C., Rinfret, A. P.: Adrenal histological change and liver tumor inhibition in hypophysectomized rats fed the azo dye, 3-methyl-4-methylaminoazobenzene. *Cancer (Philad.)* **6**, 1025—1029 (1953).
[C 2,406/53]

Richardson, H. L., O'Neal, M. A., Robertson, C. H., Griffin, A. C.: The role of hormones in azo-dye induction of liver cancer and the adrenal-lipoid response in hypophysectomized rats. *Cancer (Philad.)* **7**, 1044—1047 (1954).
[B 99,907/54]

Richardson, H. L., Stier, A. R., Borsos-Nachtnebel, E.: Liver tumor inhibition and adrenal histologic responses in rats to which 3-methyl-4-dimethylaminoazobenzene and 20-methylcholanthrene were simultaneously administered. *Cancer Res.* **12**, 356—361 (1952).
[B 70,382/52]

Richardson, K. E.: Endogenous oxalate synthesis in male and female rats. *Toxicol. appl. Pharmacol.* **7**, 507—515 (1965).
[D 88,284/65

Richardson, K. E.: Effects of vitamin-B_6, glycolic acid, testosterone, and castration on the synthesis, deposition and excretion of oxalic acid in rats. *Toxicol. appl. Pharmacol.* **10**, 40—53 (1967). [G 45,620/67]

Richens, A., Rowe, D. J. F.: Disturbance of calcium metabolism by anticonvulsant drugs. *Brit. med. J.* 1970 II, 73—76. [H 30,947/70]

Richet, C.: Dictionnaire de Physiologie. Paris: Félix Alcan, Edit. 1900. [E 1,101/1900]

Ridder, C.: Pentamethylentetrazol (Cardiazol). IV. Mitteilung: Wird Cardiazol in der Leber entgiftet? *Naunyn-Schmiedebergs Arch. Pharmak.* **120**, 126—128 (1927).
[A 47,894/27]

Riedel, H.: Tierexperimentelle Untersuchungen über Hirnveränderungen bei akuter und chronischer Hyperthyreose und ihre Wandelbarkeit durch Sauerstoffmangel. *Z. ges. inn. Med.* **19**, 718—726 (1964). [F 22,473/64]

Riegelman, S., Rowland, M., Epstein, W. L.: Griseofulvin-phenobarbital interaction in man. *J. Amer. med.Ass.* **213**, 426—431 (1970).
[H 27,268/70]

Rigat, L.: Il trattamento ormonico dell' organismo esposto all'azione delle radiozioni ionizzanti. *Radioter. Radiobiol. Fis. med.* **10**, 87—136 (1955). [C 10,747/55]

Rigatuso, J.L., Legg, P.G., Wood, R.L.: Microbody formation in regenerating rat liver. *J. Histochem. Cytochem.* **18**, 893—900 (1970).
[G 80,722/70]

Rîmniceanu, C., Schneider, F., Dema, E.: Actiunea cortizonului asupra metabolismului celulei hepatice- intactă, intoxicată şi protejată de vitamin B_{12}. (Action of cortisone on the metabolism of the intact, intoxicated or protected by vitamin B_{12} liver cell.) *Morfol. norm. si pat.* **12**, 301—308 (1967). [F 98,503/67]

Rîmniceanu, C., Schneider, F., Dema, E.: The action of cortisone on the metabolism of the normal, intoxicated, or vitamin-B_{12} protected liver cell. *Rom. med. Rev.* **12**, 11—16 (1968).
[G 66,073/68

Rinaudo, M. T., Lattes, M. G., Guardabassi, A.: Effetti degli ormoni somatotropo e lattotropo su alcune reazioni della glicolisi anaerobia nel fegato di girini di Bufo bufo. *Arch. Sci. biol. (Bologna)* 51, 79—84 (1967). [F95,471/67

Rinne, U. K., Näätänen, E. K.: The effect of norandrostenolone-phenylpropionate on the atrophy of the adrenal cortex and inhibition of growth induced by cortisone acetate. *Acta endocr. (Kbh.)* 27, 423—431 (1958). [C50,335/58

Ritterson, A. L.: Innate resistance of species of hamsters to Trichinella spiralis and its reversal by cortisone. *J. infect. Dis.* 105, 253—266 (1959). [C78,122/59

Rivlin, R. S., Knox, W. E.: Effects of age, body size and growth hormone on level of tryptophan peroxidase-oxidase in rat liver. *Amer. J. Physiol.* 197, 65—67 (1959). [C71,249/59

Rivlin, R. S., Wolf, G.: Diminished responsiveness to thyroid hormone in riboflavin-deficient rats. *Nature (Lond.)* 223, 516—517 (1969). [H13,055/69

Rixon, R. H., Baird, K. M.: The therapeutic effect of serotonin on the survival of X-irradiated rats. *Radiat. Res.* 33, 395—402 (1968). [G55,192/68

Rixon, R. H., Whitfield, J. F., Youdale, T.: Increased survival of rats irradiated with X-rays and treated with parathyroid extract. *Nature (Lond.)* 182, 1374 (1958). [C61,789/58

Rizzo, A. J., Webb, T. E.: Concurrent changes in the concentration of monomeric ribosomes and the rate of ribosome synthesis in rat liver. *Biochim. biophys. Acta (Amst.)* 169, 163—174 (1968). [H21,587/68

Roach, M. K., Reese, W. N., Jr., Creaven, P. J.: Ethanol oxidation in the microsomal fraction of rat liver. *Biochem. biophys. Res. Commun.* 36, 596—602 (1969). [G68,807/69

Robert, A., Nezamis, J. E.: Polymyxin ulcers: effect of fluid intake and of corticoids (Abstr.). *Fed. Proc.* 21, 264 (1962). [D23,064/62

Robert, A., Nezamis, J. E.: Effect of a histamine releaser on steroid induced ulcers. *Proc. Soc. exp. Biol. (N.Y.)* 109, 698—700 (1962). [D23,289/62

Robert, A., Northam, J. I., Nezamis, J. E., Phillips, J. P.: Exertion ulcers in rats. *Amer. J. dig. Dis.* 15, 497—507 (1970). [G74,748/70

Roberts, P., Turnbull, M. J., Winterburn, A.: Diurnal variation in sensitivity to and metabolism of barbiturate in the rat: lack of correlation between in vivo and in vitro findings. *Europ. J. Pharmacol.* 12, 375—377 (1970). [H31,840/70

Roberts, R. J., Plaa, G. L.: Effect of norethandrolone, acetohexamide, and Enovid on α-naphthylisothiocyanate-induced hyperbilirubinemia and cholestasis. *Biochem. Pharmacol.* 15, 333—341 (1966). [G39,694/66

Roberts, R. J., Plaa, G. L.: Studies on bilirubin production and excretion in mice and rats treated with phenobarbital, chlorpromazine, norethandrolone, acetohexamide or Enovid. *Toxicol. app. Pharmacol.* 15, 483—492 (1969). [G69,070/69

Roberts, R. J., Shriver, S. L., Plaa, G. L.: Effect of norethandrolone on the biliary excretion of bilirubin in the mouse and rat. *Biochem. Pharmacol.* 17, 1261—1268 (1968). [H8,328/68

Roberts, S.: The influence of the adrenal cortex on the mobilization of tissue protein. *J. biol. Chem.* 200, 77—88 (1953). [B97,023/53

Roberts, S., Szego, C. M.: The early reduction in uterine response to alpha-estradiol in the partially-hepatectomized rat, and the subsequent enhancement during active liver regeneration. *Endocrinology* 40, 73—85 (1947). [A49,254/47

Robertson, C. H., O'Neal, M. A., Griffin, A. C., Richardson, H. L.: Pituitary and adrenal factors involved in azo dye liver carcinogenesis. *Cancer Res.* 13, 776—779 (1953). [B88,672/53

Robertson, C. H., O'Neal, M. A., Richardson, H. L., Griffin, A. C.: Further observations on the role of the pituitary and the adrenal gland in azo dye carcinogenesis. *Cancer Res.* 14, 549—553 (1954). [E61,212/54

Robertson, T.: Multiple injections of potassium as a test for adrenocortical function, with modifications induced by desoxycorticosterone. *Fed. Proc.* 8, 366 (1949). [B32,963/49

Robertson, T.: A sex difference in the tolerance of wistar rats for potassium. *Endocrinology* 50, 569—573 (1952). [B70,810/52

Robillard, E., Crevier, M., D'Iorio, A.: Influence of sex glands on the detoxication of pentobarbital by the liver in the rat. *Proc. Canad. Physiol. Soc. 14th Ann. Meet. Ottawa*, p. 38 (1950). [B51,110/50

Robillard, E., Guénel, J., Pellerin, J., D'Iorio, A., Crevier, M.: Influence de la thyroïde sur la désintoxication du pentobarbital par le foie. *Rev. canad. Biol.* 10, 472—478 (1951). [B66,661/51

Robillard, E., D'Iorio, A., Pellerin, J.: Influences endocriniennes sur la désintoxication hépatique du pentobarbital. *Un. méd. Can.* 83, 853—860 (1954). [G67,325/54

Robillard, E., Pellerin, J.: Influence of the adrenals on pentobarbital anaesthesia. *Proc. Canad. Physiol. Soc., 16th Ann. Meet.*, Oct. 10—11, Quebec, p. 54 (1952). [B75,692/52

Robinson, D. S., MacDonald, M. G.: The effect of phenobarbital administration on the control of coagulation achieved during warfarin therapy in man. *J. Pharmacol. exp. Ther.* 153, 250—253 (1966). [F69,377/66

Robinson, H. J.: Effects of cortisone on intradermal pneumococcal infections in rabbits. *Fed. Proc.* 10, 332 (1951). [B57,249/51

Robinson, H. J., Phares, H. F., Siegel, H., Graessle, O. E.: Comparative effect of indomethacin and hydrocortisone on experimental tuberculosis in mice. *Amer. Rev. resp. Dis.* 97, 32—37 (1968). [G53,271/68

Robinson, S., Kincaid, R. K., Rhamy, R. K.: Effects of desoxycorticosterone acetate on acclimatization of men to heat. *J. appl. Physiol.* 2, 399—406 (1950). [B56,828/50

Rocha Lagoa, F. da: O potássio plasmático em infecções bacterianas experimentais. *Mem. Inst. Osw. Cruz* 45, 41—57 (1947). [B49,008/47

Roche, G. La, Leblond, C. P.: Destruction of thyroid gland of atlantic salmon (Salmo salar L.) by means of radio-iodine. *Proc. Soc. exp. Biol. (N.Y.)* 87, 273—276 (1954). [C434/54

Rodin, A. E., Kowalewski, K.: Histological and histochemical effects of cortisone and an anabolic androgen on long bones of young cockerels and rats. *Canad. J. Surg.* 6, 229—236 (1963). [D60,272/63

Rodriguez-Olleros, A., Galindo, L.: Acción de la cortisona y ACTH sobre la gastritis y úlceras experimentales. *Bol. Asoc. méd. P. Rico* 48, 65—79 (1956). [C17,868/56

Rodriguez-Olleros, A., Galindo, L.: The action of cortisone and anterior corticotropic hormone on experimental gastritis and gastric ulcers. *Gastroenterology* 32, 675—688 (1957). [C38,499/57

Roe, J. H., Coover, M. O.: Role of the thyroid gland in urinary pentose excretion in the rat. *Proc. Soc. exp. Biol. (N.Y.)* 75, 818—819 (1951). [B54,246/51

Roger, A. E., Shaka, J. A., Pechet, G., MacDonald, R. A.: Regeneration of the liver. Absence of a 'humoral factor' affecting hepatic regeneration in parabiotic rats. *Amer. J. Path.* 39, 561—578 (1961). [E93,548/61

Rogers, L. A., Alcantara, G. A., Fouts, J. R.: p-Aminosalicylic acid-induced prolongation of hexobarbital sleeping time. *J. Pharmacol. exp. Ther.* 142, 242—247 (1963). [E31,897/63

Rogers, L. A., Dixon, R. L., Fouts, J. R.: The effects of SKF 525-A on hepatic glycogen and rate of hepatic drug metabolism. *Biochem. Pharmacol.* 12, 341—348 (1963). [D64,023/63

Rogers, L. A., Fouts, J. R.: Some of the interactions of SKF 525-A with hepatic microsomes. *J. Pharmacol. exp. Ther.* 146, 286—293 (1964). [F27,894/64

Rogoff, J. M., DeNecker, J.: The influence of the adrenals on the toxicity of morphine. *J. Pharmacol. exp. Ther.* 26, 243—258 (1925). [63,527/25

Rohr, H. P., Strebel, J., Bianchi, L.: Ultrastrukturell-morphometrische Untersuchungen an der Rattenleberparenchymzelle in der Frühphase der Regeneration nach partieller Hepatektomie. *Beitr. path. Anat.* 141, 52—74 (1970). [H30,433/70

Rolf, L. L. Jr., Campbell, L. A.: Thiobarbiturate anesthesia: a comparative study and statistical analysis in the dog. *Arch. int. Pharmacodyn.* 180, 350—359 (1969). [H18,467/69

Romeo, F., Squadrito, G., Ceruso, D.: Effetti proepatici di alcuni anabolizzanti: risultati clinici e sperimentali. *Fegato* 13, 313—314 (1967). [F91,552/67

Romeo, F., Squadrito, G., Ceruso, D.: Effetti proepatici degli steroidi anabolizzanti. Risultati clinici e sperimentali. *Fegato* 14, 153—172 (1968). [H7,930/68

Rona, G.: Experimental studies on the mechanism of equine estrogens on pathological epiphyseal ossification. *Proc. canad. Fed. biol. Soc.* 5, 67 (1962). [D26,276/62

Rona, G., Chappel, C. I.: Protection of scorbutic bone lesions of the guinea pig by equine estrogen. *Endocrinology* 72, 1—10 (1963). [D48,101/63

Róna, G., Kerényi, N., Oblatt, E., Bretán, M.: Einfluß des Methylandrostendiol (Neosteron) auf die bei experimentellem Steroid-Diabetes auftretenden vaskulären Veränderungen. *Z. ges. exp. Med.* 128, 87—102 (1956). [C39,946/56

Rondell, P.: Follicular processes in ovulation. *Fed. Proc.* 29, 1875—1879 (1970). [H32,853/70

Ronzoni, G., Alquati, P., Pola, P., Alcini, E.: Studio sulla carcinogenesi prostatica con 20-metil-colantrene, nel ratto albino. *Chir. Pat. sper.* 16, 435—444 (1968). [H18,409/68

Ronzoni, G., Pirozzi, V., Zucchetti, E., Alcini, E., Wiel Marin, A.: Sulle epatosclerosi: L'OHprolina nelle epatectomie subtotali di ratti con cirrosi sperimentale (Nota I). *Chir. Pat. sper.* 16, Sup., 62—70 (1968). [H 18,986/68

Rooks, W. H.: Irradiation protection. In: Dorfman; *Methods in Hormone Research,* p. 127—137. New York, London: Academic Press 1964. [E 4,589/64

Rooks, W. H., Dorfman, R. I.: Steroid-induced increase in survival of tumor-bearing rats. *Cancer Res.* 26, 338—339 (1966). [F 62,099/66

Root, G. T., Mann, F. C.: An experimental study of shock with special reference to its effect on the capillary bed. *Surgery* 12, 861 to 877 (1942). [A 57,542/42

Rosadini, G., Bernardini, G.: Ricerche sperimentali sui rapporti tra steroidi sessuali femminili ed epilessie — I. Azione del progesterone e dell-estrone solfato nel test metrazolico. *Boll. Soc. ital. Biol. sper.* 38, 1294—1297 (1962). [D 58,047/62

Rose, D. F., Cramp, D. G.: Reduction of plasma tyrosine by oral contraceptives and oestrogens: a possible consequence of tyrosine aminotransferase induction. *Clin. chim. Acta* 29, 49—53 (1970). [G 75,215/70

Rose, D. P., Braidman, I. P.: Oral contraceptives, depression, and aminoacid metabolism. *Lancet* 1970I, 1117—1118.
[H 25,726/70

Rose, M. E.: Immunity to coccidiosis: effect of betamethasone treatment of fowls on Eimeria mivati infection. *Parasitology* 60, 137—146 (1970). [G 73,104/70

Rose, M. E., Long, P. L.: Resistance to Eimeria infections in the chicken: the effects of thymectomy, bursectomy, whole body irradiation and cortisone treatment. *Parasitology* 60, 291—299 (1970). [G 74,020/70

Rose, W. C., Bradley, S. G.: Retardation by methylprednisolone of the synergistic toxicity of endotoxin with sparsomycin or pactamycin. *Proc. Soc. exp. Biol. (N.Y.)* 132, 729—731 (1969). [H 19,375/69

Rose, W.C., Bradley, S.G.: Enhanced toxicity for mice of bacterial endotoxin with daunomycin or sparsomycin (in press). [G 79,576

Rosen, A., Moran, N. C.: Comparison of the action of ouabain on the heart in hypothyroid, euthyroid and hyperthyroid dogs. *Circulat. Res.* 12, 479—486 (1963). [D 65,414/63

Rosen, F., Harding, H. R., Milholland, R. J., Nichol, C. A.: Glucocorticoids and transaminase activity. VI. Comparison of the adaptive increases of alanine- and tyrosine-α-ketoglutarate transaminases. *J. biol. Chem.* 238, 3725 to 3729 (1963). [E 32,653/63

Rosen, F., Milholland, R. J.: Induction of tryptophan pyrrolase (TPO) and tyrosine-α-ketoglutarate transaminase (TKT) by tryptophan and its analogues in intact and adrenalectomized rats. *Fed. Proc.* 21, 237 (1962).
[D 23,053/62

Rosen, F., Milholland, R. J.: Glucocorticoids and transaminase activity. VII. Studies on the nature and specificity of substrate induction of tyrosine-α-ketoglutarate transaminase and tryptophan pyrrolase. *J. biol. Chem.* 238, 3730 to 3735 (1963). [E 32,652/63

Rosen, F., Roberts, N. R., Budnick, L. E., Nichol, C. A.: An enzymatic basis for the gluconeogenic action of hydrocortisone. *Science* 127, 287—288 (1958). [C 47,568/58

Rosen, F., Roberts, N. R., Budnick, L. E., Nichol, C. A.: Specificity of the stimulatory effect of hydrocortisone on glutamic-pyruvic transaminase. *Proc. Amer. Ass. Cancer Res.* 2, 339—340 (1958). [C 50,741/58

Rosen, F., Roberts, N. R., Budnick, L. E., Nichol, C. A.: Corticosteroids and transaminase activity: the specificity of the glutamic-pyruvic transaminase response. *Endocrinology* 65, 256—264 (1959). [C 71,414/59

Rosen, F., Roberts, N. R., Nichol, C. A.: Glucocorticosteroids and transaminase activity. I. Increased activity of glutamic-pyruvic transaminase in four conditions associated with gluconeogenesis. *J. biol. Chem.* 234, 476—480 (1959). [G 66,496/59

Rosen, R., Nichol, C. A.: Corticosteroids and enzyme activity. In: Harris and Wool; *Vitamins and Hormones. Advances in Research and Applications* 21, p. 135—214. New York, London: Academic Press 1963. [E 3,837/63

Rosenbaum, P., Obrinsky, W.: Effect of cortisone on diphtheria intoxication and the Schick test in guinea pigs. *Proc. Soc. exp. Biol. (N.Y.)* 83, 502—506 (1953).
[B 85,352/53

Rosenblum, I.: Interaction of vasopressin with adrenocorticotrophic hormone, cortisone and somatotrophic hormone; possible relation to eclamptic convulsions. *Proc. Soc. exp. Biol. (N.Y.)* 89, 84—85 (1955). [C 5,974/55

Rosene, G. L., Jr.,: Alteration of tumor cell and hepatic parenchymal cell mitotic rates in tumor-injected partially hepatectomized mice. *Cancer Res.* 28, 1469—1477 (1968).
[G 71,661/68

Rosenfeld, G.: Potentiation of the narcotic action and acute toxicity of alcohol by primary aromatic monoamines. *Quart. J. Stud. Alcohol.* 21, 584—596 (1960). [G 72,151/60

Rosenfeld, R., Kvapilová, I., Steiglová, J., Rosenfeldová, A.: Sensitization of challenger effect of iron following partial hepatectomy. *Physiol. bohemoslov.* 16, 577—580 (1967). [G 55,854/67

Rosenfeld, R., Kvapilová, I., Steiglová, J., Rosenfeldová, A.: Neobvyklý pohled na výnzam jater pro challengerový účinek železa při kalcifylaxi. (Abstr.) *Čs. Fysiol.* 16, 273 (1967). [G 67,785/67

Rosenfeldová, A., Steiglová, J., Kvapilová, I., Rosenfeld, R.: Enhanced toxic effect of pharmacological doses of calciferol in rats after partial hepatectomy. *Physiol. bohemoslov.* 16, 581 (1967). [G 55,855/67

Rosenthal, S. M.: Experimental chemotherapy of burns and shock. III. Effects of systemic therapy on early mortality. *Publ. Hlth. Rep. (Wash.)* 58, 513—522 (1943). [B 26,228/43

Ross, L. E., van Wagtendonk, W. J., Wulzen, R.: Evidence for a steroid compound in cane juice possessing antistiffness activity. *Proc. Soc. exp. Biol. (N.Y.)* 71, 281—283 (1949). [B 37,268/49

Rossi, G. B., Oriente, P., Porrazzi, L. C., Vecchione, A., Cerqua, R.: Deoxycorticosterone acetate and experimental atherosclerosis in cholesterol-fed rabbits. *Nature (Lond.)* 203, 252—254 (1964). [F 18,184/64

Rosta, J., Makói, Z., Fehér, T., Korányi, G.: Steroid inhibition of glucuronization. *Acta paediat. Acad. Sci. hung.* 11, 67—69 (1970). [G 77,094/70

Roth, F. J., Jr., Friedman, J., Syverton, J. T.: Effects of roentgen radiation and cortisone on susceptibility of mice to Candida albicans. *J. Immunol.* 78, 122—127 (1956). [C 32,916/56

Rothlin, E.: Sur la thérapeutique de l'intoxication par le phosgène. *C. R. gén. XIme Congr. int. Méd. Pharm. milit.*, p. 1—10 (1947). [B 30,696/47

Rothlin, E., Schalch, W. R.: Zur Pharmakologie und Toxikologie des Scillirosids und des Scillirosidins. *Helv. physiol. pharmacol. Acta* 10, 427—437 (1952). [G 75,565/52

Rotter, W.: Untersuchungen über den Einfluß gesteigerter Schilddrüsentätigkeit auf die Höhenfestigkeit im Tierexperiment. *Arch. Kreisl.-Forsch.* 9, 226—257 (1942). [A 63,564/42

Röttger, P., Nolte, F., Kühn, H. A., Creutzfeldt' W.: Untersuchungen über die therapeutische Beeinflußbarkeit experimenteller Lebercirrhosen bei der Ratte. II. Die Thioacetamid-Cirrhose der Ratte und ihre Beeinflussung durch Glucocorticoide, Androgene und Tolbutamid. *Z. ges. exp. Med.* 136, 486—499 (1963). [D 64,427/63

Rous, P., Larimore, L. D.: Relation of the portal blood to liver maintenance. A demonstration of liver atrophy conditional on compensation. *J. exp. Med.* 31, 609—632 (1920). [D 88,911/20

Rowe, W. P., Black, P. H., Levey, R. H.: Protective effect of neonatal thymectomy on mouse LCM infection. *Proc. Soc. exp. Biol. (N.Y.)* 114, 248—251 (1963). [E 29,673/63

Rowinski, P., De Muro, P., Manunta, G.: Ipertensione sperimentale da desossicorticosterone (D.C.A.) e sesso. *Boll. Soc. ital. Biol. sper.* 27, 1 — 2 (1951). [B 64,142/51

Rowinski, P., Manunta, G.: Influenza dell'ovaio sulla sopravivenza di ratti paratiroidectomizzati. *R. C. Accad. naz. Lincei, Cl. Sci. fis. mat. nat.*, Ser. *VIII*, 10, 495—499 (1951). [B 64, 144/51

Roy, A. B.: The enzymic synthesis of aryl sulphamates. 2. The effect of 3β-methoxyandrost-5-en-17-one on arylamine sulphokinase. *Biochem. J.* 79, 253—261 (1961). [D 5,284/61

Rubin, A., Stohler, C. M., Novick, W. J.: Inhibition of testosterone stimulation of microsomal hexobarbital metabolism by 17α-methyl-B-nortestosterone (SK&F 7690). *Biochem. Pharmacol.* 14, 1898—1899 (1965). [F 73,811/65

Rubin, A., Tephly, T. R., Mannering, G. J.: Kinetics of drug metabolism by hepatic microsomes. *Biochem. Pharmacol.* 13, 1007 to 1016 (1964). [G 58,057/64

Rubin, A., Tephly, T. R., Mannering, G. J.: Inhibition of hexobarbital metabolism by ethylmorphine and codeine in the intact rat. *Biochem. Pharmacol.* 13, 1053—1057 (1964). [G 58,747/64

Rubin, B. L.: Sex differences in orientation of reduction products of 30keto-C_{19} steroids by rat liver homogenates. *J. biol. Chem.* 227, 917—927 (1957). [G 76,315/57

Rubin, B. L., Strecker, H. J.: Further studies on the sex difference in 3β-hydroxysteroid dehydrogenase activity of rat livers. *Endocrinology* 69, 257—267 (1961). [D 9,290/61

Rubin, E., Hutterer, F.: Quantitation of cortisone effect on hepatic fibrosis. *Fed. Proc.* **20**, 289 (1961). [D4,173/61

Rubino, F., Giacalone, O.: Sul decorso della ipoalimentazione calorica dei ratti trattati con 17α-metil-17β-idrossiandrosta-1-4-dien-3-one. *Boll. Soc. ital. Biol. sper.* **39**, 154—155 (1963). [E36,677/63

Rubio, M.: Influencia del acetato de cortisona sobre la virulencia y localizacion tisular de una nueva cepa de Trypanosoma cruzi. Estudio de la persistencia de los cambios observados. *Biologica* **21**, 75—89 (1955). [C34,556/55

Rubio, M.: Mitosis en celulas parasitadas por Trypanosoma cruzi. Estudio en animales de laboratorio. *Biologica (Chile)* **22**, 51—62 (1956). [C41,052/56

Rudas, B., Weissel, W.: Frühketonämie bei Alloxandiabetes, zugleich ein Beitrag zur Durabolinwirkung. *Wien. klin. Wschr.* **75**, 846—848 (1963). [E34,762/63

Rudofsky, S., Crawford, J. S.: Some alterations in the pattern of drug metabolism associated with pregnancy, oral contraceptives and the newly-born. *Pharmacologist* **8**, 181 (1966). [E58,989/66

Ruebner, B. H., Hirano, T., Slusser, R. J.: Electron microscopy of the hepatocellular and Kupffercell lesions of mouse hepatitis, with particular reference to the effect of cortisone. *Amer. J. Path.* **51**, 163—189 (1967). [G48,873/67

Rugh, R., Clugston, H.: Radiosensitivity with respect to the estrous cycle in the mouse. *Radiat. Res.* **2**, 227—236 (1955). [C11,209/55

Rugh, R., Skaredoff, L., Makay, C.: Postirradiation castration of the male and enhanced survival. *Proc. Soc. exp. Biol. (N.Y.)* **116**, 1110—1114 (1964). [F21,653,64

Rugh, R., Wolff, J.: Relation of gonad hormones to X-irradiation sensitivity in mice. *Proc. Soc. exp. Biol. (N.Y.)* **92**, 408—410 (1956). [C19,209/56

Rümke, C. L.: Enhancing and decreasing effects of drugs on the convulsant action of bemegride. *Acta physiol. pharmacol. neerl.* **10**, 288—289 (1962). [G76,692/62

Rümke, C. L.: Die Verlängerung der Hexobarbitalnarkose durch kurz vorher intraperitoneal oder subcutan verabreichtes Serotonin. *Naunyn-Schmiedebergs Arch. Pharmak.* **243**, 298 (1962). [G76,693/62

Rümke, C. L.: The influence of drugs on the duration of hexobarbital and hydroxydione narcosis in mice. *Naunyn-Schmiedebergs Arch. Pharmak.* **244**, 519—530 (1963). [G69,768/63

Rümke, C. L.: Unterschiedliche Dauer der Hexobarbitalnarkose bei männlichen und weiblichen Mäusen. *Naunyn-Schmiedebergs Arch. Pharmak.* **255**, 64—65 (1966). [G68,532/66

Rümke, C. L.: A difference between the duration of hexobarbital narcosis in male and female mice? *Arzneimittel-Forsch.* **18**, 60—62 (1968). [G71,098/68

Rümke, C. L., Bout, J.: Die Beeinflussung der Hexobarbitalnarkose durch vorher verabfolgte Pharmaka. *Naunyn-Schmiedebergs Arch. Pharmak.* **240**, 218—223 (1960). [G74,669/60

Rümke, C. L., Noordhoek, J.: The influence of pretreatment with lynestrenol on the anticonvulsant effect of phenobarbitone and phenytoin in mice. *Acta physiol. pharmacol. neerl.* **15**, 66 (1969). [G76,850/69

Rümke, C. L., Noordhoek, J.: The influence of lynestrenol on the rate of metabolism of phenobarbital, phenytoin and hexobarbital in mice. *Europ. J. Pharmacol.* **6**, 163—168 (1969). [H14,039/69

Rümke, C. L., Noordhoek, J.: Sex differences in the duration of hexobarbital narcosis and in serum MUP content in mice. *Arch. int. Pharmacodyn.* **182**, 399—400 (1969). [H21,659/69

Rummel, W.: Zur Abhängigkeit der Narkoseschwelle von metabolischen, hormonellen und pharmakologischen Einflüssen. *Anaesthesist* **8**, 328—332 (1959). [C79,429/59

Rummel, W., Jacobi, H., Kreutzer, F. J., von der Brelie, E.: Abhängigkeit der N₂O-Narkoseschwelle von Erregungszustand und Stoffwechsel. *Naunyn-Schmiedebergs Arch. Pharmak.* **231**, 141—148 (1957). [D89,013/57

Rummel, W., Wellensiek, H. J.: Der Einfluß von Thyroxin und 2,4-Dinitrophenol auf die N₂O-Narkoseschwelle schilddrüsenloser Ratten. *Naturwissenschaften* **45**, 266—267 (1958). [D96,909/58

Rummel, W., Wellensiek, H. J., Puder, D.: Über die Wirkung von Steroidhormonen auf die N₂O-Narkoseschwelle der Ratte. *Arch. int. Pharmacodyn.* **122**, 329—338 (1959). [C80,035/59

Rumsfeld, H. W., Jr., Miller, W. L., Jr., Baumann, C. A.: A sex difference in the development of liver tumors in rats fed 3'-methyl-4-dimethylaminoazobenzene or 4'-fluoro-4-dimethylaminoazobenzene. *Cancer Res.* **11**, 814—819 (1951). [G73,677/51

Rupe, B. D., Bousquet, W. F., Miya, T. S.: Stress modification of drug response. *Science* **141**, 1186—1187 (1963). [E 26,910/63

Rupp, E., Knackstedt, R.: Zur Frage der experimentellen Gonokokkeninfektion der weißen Maus unter dem Einfluß von Cortison. *Dermat. Wschr.* **136**, 932—936 (1957). [C 42,998/57

Rusakov, V. I., Chernov, V. N.: Another way of preventing the adhesion disease. (Russian text.) *Eksp. Khir.* **14/1**, 28—32 (1969). [H 9,072/69

Russell, F. E., Emery, J. A.: Effects of corticosteroids on lethality of Ancistrodon contortrix venom. *Amer. J. med. Sci.* **241**, 507—511 (1961). [D 2,497/61

Rutsch, W.: Der Einfluß der Schilddrüse auf die Erregbarkeit des Zentralnervensystems, geprüft mit einer Methode quantitativer Narkose. *Z. Biol.* **93**, 283—292 (1933). [7,744/33

Rybová, R., Janáček, K.: A sex-dependent effect of aldosterone on frog bladder. *Naturwissenschaften* **57**, 459—460 (1970). [G 78,569/70

Rydin, H.: Action de la chlorophylle et de la thyroxine sur la sensibilité de l'organisme à l'égard d'une raréfaction de l'oxygène. *C. R. Soc. Biol. (Paris)* **99**, 1685—1686 (1928). [22,940/28

Saarnivaara, L.: A possible role of 5-hydroxytryptamine in morphine analgesia in rabbits. *Scand. J. clin. Lab. Invest.* **21**, Sup. 101, 85—86 (1968). [H 2,855/68

Saarnivaara, L.: Effect of 5-hydroxytryptamine on morphine analgesia in rabbits. *Ann. Med. exp. Fenn.* **47**, 113—123 (1969). [G 71,565/69

Sackler, M. D., Sackler, A. M., Martin, C. R., Sackler, R. R.: Gonadectomy and histamine tolerance. *Fed. Proc.* **12**, 363 (1953). [B 78,749/53

Sacra, P., McColl, J. D.: Modification of acute toxicity of hypoglycemics by hormones. *Proc. Canad. Fed. Biol. 2nd Ann. Meet. 9—11 June, Toronto*, p. 58 (1959). [C 73,654/59

Sacra, P. J., Adamkiewicz, V. W.: Glycemia and the activity of compound 48—80 in the rat. *Arch. int. Pharmacodyn.* **156**, 255—260 (1965). [F 49,352/65

Saggers, V. H., Hariratnajothi, N., McLean, A. E. M.: The effect of diet and phenobarbitone on quinine metabolism in the rat and in man. *Biochem. Pharmacol.* **19**, 499—503 (1970). [G 73,683/70

Saidi, P., Hoag, M. S., Aggeler, P. M.: Transplacental transfer of bishydroxycoumarin in the human. *J. Amer. med. Ass.* **191**, 761—763 (1965). [F 32,236/65

Saini, V. C., Patrick, S. J.: Effect of estrone on conversion of cholesterol to bile acids. *Biochim. biophys. Acta (Amst.)* **202**, 556—559 (1970). [G 74,405/70

Saint Omer, F. B., Mincione, G.: La rigenerazione epatica dopo ampia epatectomia nel corso della steatosi da dieta ipocolinica. *Arch. De Vecchi Anat. pat.* **33**, 597—618 (1960). [D 53,460/60

Saint-Omer, F. B., Tosi, P., Colafranceschi, M., Bruscagli, G.: Le modificazioni della rigenerazione epatica dopo epatectomia parziale in topi inoculati con carcinoma-ascite di Ehrlich e con mastocitoma-ascite. *Arch. De Vecchi Anat. pat.* **53**, 165—190 (1968). [G 71,148/68

Saito, S. et al.: Antipicrotoxin-convulsion effects of catecholamines caused by the intracerebral in mice and the role of brain catecholamines, 5 HT and GABA. (Japanese text.) *Keio J. Med.* **8**, 879—899 (1963). [E 27,616/63

Sakamoto, A., Prasad, K. N.: Radioprotective action of β-melanocyte-stimulating hormone (MSH) in rodents exposed to whole-body X-irradiation. *Int. J. Radiat. Biol.* **12**, 97—99 (1967). [F 95,441/67

Saksena, S. K., Chaudhury, R. R.: Androgenic, anti-androgenic and anabolic activity of azasteroids on immature castrated rats. *Indian J. med. Res.* **58**, 513—518 (1970). [G 78,486/70

Sakurai, K.: Über die Rückbildung des Met-Hämoglobins. III. Mitteilg.: Versuche am lebenden Tier. *Naunyn-Schmiedebergs Arch. Pharmak.* **109**, 214—232 (1925). [E 67,662/25

Sala, E., Perris, C.: Ricerche sull'attivita della 5-idrossitriptamina a livello della giunzione neuromuscolare (Abstr.). *Musc. Dystrophy. Abstr.* **3**, Nr. 1179, p. 331 (1959). [C 78,420/59

Salgado, E. D., Mulroy, M. I.: The role of the pituitary and thyroid in DCA-induced cardiovascular disease in the rat. *Ann. N. Y. Acad. Sci.* **72**, 854—862 (1959). [C 84,321/59

Salmoiraghi, G. C., Page, I. H.: Effects of LSD 25, BOL 148, bufotenine, mescaline and ibogaine on the potentiation of hexobarbital hypnosis produced by serotonin and reserpine. *J. Pharmacol. exp. Ther.* **120**, 20—25 (1957). [C 38,518/57

Salmoiraghi, G. C., Sollero, L., Page, I. H.: Blockade by brom-lysergic-acid-diethylamide (BOL) of the potentiating action of serotonin and reserpine on hexobarbital hypnosis. *J. Pharmacol. exp. Ther.* **117**, 166—168 (1956). [C 21,596/56

Salva, S. de: Effects of centrally acting drugs in intact and hypophysectomized rats on EST. *Arch. int. Pharmacodyn.* **137**, 267—271 (1962). [D 27,783/62

Salva, S. de: Effect of drugs on EST in various endocrine deficient states. *Arch. int. Pharmacodyn.* **142**, 361—365 (1963). [D 66,176/63

Salva, S. de: EST effects of diphenylhydantoin in hypophysectomized rats. *Arch. int. Pharmacodyn.* **142**, 366—370 (1963). [D 66,177/63

Salva, S. de, Evans, R., Johson, C., Schauer, W.: EST and drug effects in endocrine deficiencies. *Fed. Proc.* **17**, 363 (1958). [C 51,842/58

Salvador, R. A., Atkins, C., Haber, S., Conney, A. H.: Changes in the serum concentration of cholesterol, triglycerides and phospholipids in the mouse and rat after administration of either chlorcyclizine or phenobarbital. *Biochem. Pharmacol.* **19**, 1463—1469 (1970). [G 75,529/70

Salvador, R. A., Atkins, C., Haber, S., Kozma, C., Conney, A. H.: Effect of phenobarbital and chlorcyclizine on the development of atheromatosis in the cholesterol-fed rabbit. *Biochem. Pharmacol.* **19**, 1975—1981 (1970). [G 74,397/70

Salvador, R. A., Conney, A. H., Kozman, C.: Inhibitory effect of phenobarbital on cholesterol-induced atherosclerosis in the rabbit (Abstr.). *Pharmacologist* **9**, 254 (1967). [G 68,113/67

Salvin, S. B., Peterson, R. D. A., Good, R. A.: The thymus gland and resistance to infectious agents. *Fed. Proc.* **24**, 160 (1965). [F 35,876/65

Salvin, S. B., Peterson, R. D. A., Good, R. A.: The role of the thymus in resistance to infection and endotoxin toxicity. *J. Lab. clin. Med.* **65**, 1004—1022 (1965). [G 30,533/65

Salzberg, D. A., Griffin, A. C.: Inhibition of azo dye carciogenesis in the alloxan-diabetic rat (Abstr.). *Cancer Res.* **12**, 294 (1952). [B 68,802/52

Samaras, S. C., Dietz, N., Jr.: Precipitation of prolonged convulsions in stressed rats and mice. *Physiologist* **1**, 68 (1958). [C 56,733/58

Sambhi, M. P., Weil, M. H., Udhoji, V. N., Shubin, H.: Adrenocorticoids in the management of shock. In: Hershey; *Shock 2*, p. 421 to 433. Boston, Mass.: Little, Brown & Co. 1964. [G 68,985/64

Samiy, A. E.: Effect of thyroxin pretreatment on decarboxylation of dihydroxyphenylalanine (dopa) and production of sustained hypertension. *Fed. Proc.* **11**, 136 (1952). [B 68,269/52

Sammalisto, L.: Blood sugar and alcohol intoxication in the rat. *Acta physiol. scand.* **55**, 313—318 (1962). [G 76,362/62

Samuels, L. T., Eik-Nes, K. B.: Metabolism of steroid hormones. In: Greenberg, D. M.; *Metabolic Pathways. II. Lipids, Steroids, and Carotenoids*, p. 169—220. New York, London: Academic Press Inc. 1968. [G 73,454/68

Sananès, N., Psychoyos, A.: Effet de l'actinomycine-D sur le développement du déciduome chez la ratte. *C. R. Acad. Sci. (Paris)* **271**, 430—433 (1970). [G 78,230/70

Sandberg, F.: The effect of hepatectomy and nephrectomy on the anaesthetic activity of some N-substituted barbiturates. *Acta physiol. scand.* **28**, 1—5 (1953). [G 71,886/53

Sandhu, D. K., Sandhu, R. S., Damodaran, V. N., Randhawa, H. S.: Effect of cortisone on bronchopulmonary aspergillosis in mice exposed to spores of various Aspergillus species. *Sabouraudia* **8**, 32—38 (1970). [G 75,603/70

Sandri, O., Gallarate, L., Ballarin, G.: Azione dell'ipofisi sulla ipertrofia renale compensatoria nei ratti. *Atti Soc. lombarda Sci. med. biol.* **10**, 480—484 (1955). [C 13,150/55

Sanfilippo, E.: Ipotermia passiva e ormone paratiroideo. *Rass. terap. Patol. clin.* **7**, 465—480 (1935). [56,085/35

Sanfilippo, E., Ricca, S.: Influenza dell'ormone tiroideo nell'assideramento. Resistenza dell'organismo, temperatura e peso degli organi. *Riv. Pat. sper.* **4**, 303—317 (1935). [31,704/35

Santo, E.: Die histologischen Grundlagen der Reid Hunt-Reaktion an der Schilddrüse der weißen Maus. *Z. ges. exp. Med.* **93**, 793—802 (1934). [27,439/34

Sanyal, R. K.: Chemical mediators of adrenaline-induced pulmonary oedema. *Int. Arch. Allergy* **33**, 59—64 (1968). [G 55,044/68

Sanyal, R. K., Spencer, P. S. J., West, G. B.: Insulin and hypersensitivity. *Nature (Lond.)* **184**, 2020 (1959). [C 79,555/59

Sarre, H.: Zur Pathogenese und Therapie des nephrotischen Syndroms. *Dtsch. med. Wschr.* **79**, 1652—1654, 1713—1717 (1954). [B 99,950/54

Sas, M., Herczeg, J.: Das Verhalten der Steroidausscheidung und des Serum-Bilirubinspiegels bei Neugeborenen nach C_{19}-Steroid-Belastung. *Arch. Gynäk.* **209**, 50—57 (1970). [H 27,522/70

Sas, M., Herczeg, J.: Serum-Bilirubinwerte und Steroidausscheidung bei mit 3α, 20α- und 3α, 20β-Pregnandiol belasteten Neugeborenen. *Arch. Gynäk.* 209, 58—70 (1970). [H 27,523/70

Sas, M., Herczeg, J.: Serum bilirubin level and steroid excretion following progesterone loads in new-born infants. *Acta paediat. Acad. Sci. hung.* 11, 35—40 (1970). [G 77,093/70

Sasame, H. A., Castro, J. A., Gillette, J. R.: Studies on the destruction of liver microsomal cytochrome P-450 by carbon tetrachloride administration. *Biochem. Pharmacol.* 17, 1759 to 1768 (1968). [G 72,114/68

Sátori, O., Szabó, G.: Über die Wirkung von Dexamethason beim Tourniquet-Schock. *Z. ges. exp. Med.* 137, 47—51 (1963). [E 21,902/63

Satoskar, R. S., Trivedi, J. C.: Effect of hydrocortisone on acute pentobarbital toxicity in mice. *Proc. Soc. exp. Biol. (N.Y.)* 89, 695 to 696 (1955). [C 8,678/55

Saviano, M.: Azione della follicolina nel rachitismo sperimentale. *Arch. Sci. biol. (Bologna)* 21, 579—607 (1935). [60,155/35

Savini, E., Savini, T.: Thyroïde et anaphylaxis. *C. R. Soc. Biol. (Paris)* 78, 198—199 (1915). [A 24,559/15

Savoie, L., Krajny, M., Kleiman, B.: Digitoxin induced cardiac necrosis and its inhibition. *Cardiologia (Basel)* 54, 287—294 (1969). [G 60,080/69

Savoie, L., Krajny, M., Selye, H.: Prophylactic action of spironolactone in digitoxin poisoning (Abstr.). *Proc. Canad. Fed. biol. Soc., Edmonton, Alta* 12, 58 (1969). [G 60,028/69

Savoldi, F., Maggi, G. C., Noli, S.: Azione dell'adrenalina e della noradrenalina sull'attività elettrica corticale del coniglio in narcosi barbiturica. *Boll. Soc. ital. biol. sper.* 36, 545 a 547 (1960). [C 92,984/60

Scaffidi, L., Arrigo, F.: Studio comparativo sugli effetti di HCG e di HMG sulla cardiopatia sperimentale da emetina. *Boll. Soc. ital. Biol. sper.* 44, 991—993 (1968). [G 62,941/68

Scaffidi, L., Fidecaro, A.: Azione protettiva della cocarbossilasi e della gonadotropina corionica sulla miocardiopatia difterica sperimentale. *Arch. Atti Soc. med.-chir. Messina* 9, 3—23 (1965). [G 51,129/65

Scaffidi, L., Fidecaro, A.: Azione protettiva della cocarbossilasi e della gonadotropina corionica sulla miocardiopatia difterica sperimentale. *Boll. Soc. ital. Biol. sper.* 42, 1284—1286 (1966). [G 43,543/66

Scarborough, E. M.: The influence of thyroid feeding on nembutal poisoning. *J. Physiol. (Lond.)* 86, 183—189 (1936). [34,971/36

Scarinci, V.: Ricerche farmacologiche sulla idrossitriptamina. I. Azione sull'epilessia riflessa. *Arch. ital. Sci. farmacol.* 5, 265—270 (1955). [G 66,316/55

Schachter, H., Sidlofsky, S., Baker, D. G., Hamilton, J. R., Haist, R. E.: The effect of previous exposure to cold on shock secondary to limb ischaemia. *Canad. J. Biochem.* 37, 211—223 (1959). [C 63,544/59

Schachter, R. J., Huntington, J.: Use of orally administered desiccated thyroid in production of traumatic shock. *Proc. Soc. exp. Biol. (N.Y.)* 44, 66—68 (1940). [A 32,970/40

Schäfer, E. L.: Tuberkulose und innere Sekretion. *Ergebn. ges. Tuberk.-Forsch.* 12, 209—327 (1954). [B 99,955/54

Schäfer, E. L.: Tierexperimentelle Untersuchungen zur Frage der Bedeutung des Mineralstoffwechsels für die Tuberkulose. *Beitr. Klin. Tuberk.* 110, 409—425 (1954). [G 58,597/54

Schäfer, E. L., Greuel, H.: Orale Antidiabetika und experimentelle Meerschweinchen-Tuberkulose. *Tuberk.-Arzt* 16, 589—595 (1962). [D 54,900/62

Schapiro, S.: Adrenal cortical hormones and resistance to histamine stress in the infant rat. *Acta endocr. (Kbh.)* 48, 249—252 (1965). [F 31,856/65

Schapiro, S.: Interaction between growth hormone and cortisol on the regulation of liver tyrosine transaminase activity. *Endocrinology* 83, 475—478 (1968). [H 2,360/68

Schapiro, S., Geller, E., Yuwiler, A.: Differential effects of a stress on liver enzymes in adult and infant rats. *Neuroendocrinology (Basel)* 1, 138—143 (1965/66). [F 65,746/65/66

Schapiro, S., Geller, E., Yuwiler, A.: Interaction of STH and corticoids in enzyme regulation during stress and development. *Program 51st Meet. Endocr. Soc., New York, N. Y.*, p. 186 (1969). [H 12,411/69

Schapiro, S., Yuwiler, A., Geller, E.: Stress-activated inhibition of the cortisol effect on hepatic transaminase. *Life Sci.* 3, 1221—1226 (1964). [G 21,848/64

Schapiro, S., Yuwiler, A., Geller, E.: Maturation of a stress-activated mechanism inhibiting induction of tyrosine transaminase. *Science* 152, 1642 (1966). [F 67,227/66

Scharf, J.-H., Ehrenbrand, F., Goliah, S.: Veränderungen des Zellbildes des Hypophysenvorderlappens der Ratte unter getrennter und kombinierter Verabreichung von Methylthiouracil, p-Oxypropiophenon und 2,3-Dithiopropanol. *Z. mikr.-anat. Forsch.* **66**, 251—265 (1960). [C 91,620/60

Scharf, J.-H., Wichmann, T., Marzotko, D., Schmidt, R.: Vergleiche zwischen den Lebern antithyreoidal, antadenohypophysär und contrainsular behandelter weißer Ratten. *Z. mikr.-anat. Forsch.* **74**, 482—522 (1966).
[F 69,957/66

Schatzmann, H. J.: Kompetitiver Antagonismus zwischen g-Strophanthin und Corticosteron an isolierten Streifen von Rattenaorten. *Experientia* **15/2**, 73—74 (1959).
[C 73,682/59

Schauer, A., Kunze, E., Burkhard, B., Rosnitschek, J.: Beeinflussung der Cancerisierung der Rattenleber durch Steroidhormone. *Naturwissenschaften* **57**, 676—677 (1970). [G 81,318/70

Schechet, I. A.: The effect of desiccated thyroid, iodinated casein on a rachitogenic diet. *Science* **113**, 60—61 (1951). [B 61,419/51

Scheer, B. T., Mumbach, M. W., Cox, B. L.: Hormonal regulation of salt balance in frogs. *Fed. Proc.* **20**, 177 (1961). [D 3,935/61

Scheffler, J., Westphal, W.: Die Beeinflussung der Leberregeneration bei Ratten durch ein Gemisch von Purinen und Orotsäure. *Arzneimittel-Forsch.* **13**, 75—76 (1963). [D 56,080/63

Scheifley, C. H.: Pentothal sodium: its use in the presence of hepatic disease. *Anesthesiology* **7**, 263—267 (1946). [A 48,124/46

Scheifley, C. H., Higgins, G. M.: The effect of partial hepatectomy on the action of certain barbiturates and a phenylurea derivative. *Amer. J. med. Sci.* **200**, 264—268 (1940).
[48,633/40

Schenkman, J. B., Frey, I., Remmer, H., Estabrook, R. W.: Sex differences in drug metabolism in rat liver microsomes. *Molec. Pharmacol.* **3**, 516—525 (1967). [G 67,777/67

Scherb, J., Kirschner, M., Arias, I.: Studies of hepatic excretory function. The effect of 17α-ethyl-19-nortestosterone on sulfobromophthalein sodium (BSP) metabolism in man. *J. clin. Invest.* **42**, 404—408 (1963). [D 58,943/63

Scherr, G. H.: The influence of hormones on experimental moniliasis. *Monogr. Therap.* **2**, 80—82 (1957). [C 39,263/57

Schimke, R. T.: Studies on factors affecting the levels of urea cycle enzymes in rat liver. *J. biol. Chem.* **238**, 1012—1018 (1963). [D 39,880/63

Schimke, R. T., Doyle, D.: Control of enzyme levels in animal tissues. *Ann. Rev. Biochem.* **39**, 929—958 (1970). [G 75,997/70

Schimke, R. T., Sweeney, E. W., Berlin, C. M.: An analysis of the kinetics of rat liver tryptophan pyrrolase induction: the significance of both enzyme synthesis and degradation. *Biochem. biophys. Res. Commun.* **15**, 214—219 (1964). [G 11,062/64

Schimke, R. T., Sweeney, E. W., Berlin, C. M.: The roles of synthesis and degradation in the control of rat liver tryptophan pyrrolase. *J. biol. Chem.* **240**, 322—331 (1965). [G 24,293/65

Schimmelpfennig, W., Hagemann, I., Korte, G.: Über den Einfluß von 4-Chlortestosteronazetat (Turinabol) auf das akute Nierenversagen der Ratte. *Acta biol. med. germ.* **17**, 298—306 (1966).
[F 74,978/66

Schlesinger, K., Boggan, W. O., Griek, B. J.: Pharmacogenetic correlates of pentylenetetrazol and electroconvulsive seizure thresholds in mice. *Psychopharmacologia (Berlin)* **13**, 181 to 188 (1968). [G 61,802/68

Schlesinger, K., Stavnes, K. L., Boggan, W. O.: Modification of audiogenic and pentylenetetrazol seizures with gamma-aminobutyric acid, norepinephrine and serotonin. *Psychopharmacologia (Berlin)* **15**, 226—231 (1969).
[G 69,565/69

Schmid, K., Cornu, F., Imhof, P., Keberle, H.: Die biochemische Deutung der Gewöhnung an Schlafmittel. *Schweiz. med. Wschr.* **94**, 235—240 (1964). [G 34,008/64

Schmid, R., Buckingham, S., Mendilla, G. A., Hammaker, L.: Bilirubin metabolism in the foetus. *Nature (Lond.)* **183**, 1823—1824 (1959).
[G 76,338/59

Schmid, R., Marver, H. S., Hammaker, L.: Enhanced formation of rapidly labeled bilirubin by phenobarbital: hepatic cytochromes as a possible source. *Biochem. biophys. Res. Commun.* **24**, 319—328 (1966). [G 68,199/66

Schmidinger, H., Kröger, H.: Zur Hunger-Induktion der Serin-Dehydratase in der Rattenleber. *Hoppe-Seylers Z. physiol. Chem.* **348**, 1367—1371 (1967). [F 92,031/67

Schmidt, E., Schmidt, F. W.: Enzyme activities in human liver. *Enzymol. biol. clin. (Basel)* **11**, 67—129 (1970). [G 73,170/70

Schmidt, H.: Versuche zur therapeutischen Beeinflussung der Diphtheriegiftwirkung beim Meerschweinchen durch C-Vitamin und Nebennierenrindenhormon-Präparate. *Dtsch. med. Wschr.* **63**, 1003—1006 (1937). [94,670/37

Schmidt, J.: Über die gegenseitige pharmakologische Beeinflussung von Serotonin und Noradrenalin. *Biochem. Pharmacol.* **12**, Sup. 163 (1963). [E 32,188/63]

Schmidt, J., Matthies, H.: Die Beeinflussung der Pentetrazol-Krampfschwelle durch intracerebrale Injektion von Reserpin und biogenen Aminen. *Acta biol. med. germ.* **8**, 426—436 (1962). [D 34,219/62]

Schmidt, L., Bernauer, W.: Die chronische Lithiumvergiftung an Ratten unter besonderer Berücksichtigung der Veränderungen im Steroidgehalt der Nebennierenrinde. *Naunyn-Schmiedebergs Arch. Pharmak.* **245**, 112 (1963). [D 65,293/63]

Schmidt, L. H.: The effect of thyroxine ingestion on the toxicity of certain bile salts. *Amer. J. Physiol.* **108**, 613—620 (1934). [27,511/34]

Schmuñis, G., Weissenbacher, M., Parodi, A. S.: Tolerance to Junin virus in thymectomized mice. *Arch. ges. Virusforsch.* **21**, 200—204 (1967). [G 55,003/67]

Schneiberg, K., Gorski, T.: X-ray irradiation and thymectomy as the factors enhancing the chemical cancerogenesis in mouse skin. *Pol. med. J.* **8**, 647—653 (1969). [G 68,745/69]

Schneiberg, K., Jonecko, A., Bartnikowa, W.: Thymus-organe hématopoïétique? I. L'âge et la saison comme facteurs déterminants. L'influence du thymus sur la radiorésistance naturelle chez la souris. *Folia haemat. (Lpz.)* **88**, 253—259 (1967). [G 56,009/67]

Schneiberg, K., Jonecko, A, Bartnikowa, W.: Der Thymus — ein hämatopoetisches Organ? III. Der Einfluß von Thymusgewebe in Diffusionskammern auf das Überleben und das blutbildende System von Mäusen nach subletaler Ganzkörperbestrahlung. *Folia haemat. (Lpz.)* **89**, 265—282 (1968). [G 69,791/68]

Schneiberg, K., Koziol-Bartnikowa, W., Jonecko, A.: Serum protein changes in acute radiation disease in thymectomized mice. *Arch. Immunol. Ther. exp.* **16**, 85—91 (1968). [G 58,579/68]

Schneiberg, K., Stiller-Winkler, R., Jonecko, A.: Regeneration of peripheral blood in thymectomized mice after sublethal whole-body irradiation. *Pol. med. J.* **6**, 1163—1179 (1967). [G 58,580/67]

Schneider, E., Widman, E.: Die hepatohormonale Steuerung des Vitamin-A-Umsatzes und die Ätiologie der Ostitis deformans Paget. *Klin. Wschr.* **14**, 1786—1790 (1935). [33,725/35]

Schnitzer, A.: Klinische und experimentelle Untersuchungen zur Pathogenese der Karzinome. *Oncologia (Basel)* **9**, 301—309 (1956). [C 32,871/56]

Schoen, H. R., Voss, R.: Der Einfluß einer Vorbehandlung mit Thyroxin, anorganischem Jod und essentiellen Phospholipiden auf die Tetanustoxin-Empfindlichkeit des Meerschweinchens. *Klin. Wschr.* **39**, 972—973 (1961). [D 11,906/61]

Schoenfield, L. J., Foulk, W. T.: Studies of sulfobromophthalein sodium (BSP) metabolism in man. II. The effect of artificially induced fever, norethandrolone (Nilevar), and iopanoid acid (Telapaque). *J. clin. Invest.* **43**, 1419—1423 (1964). [F 16,168/64]

Schoental, R.: Hepatotoxic activity of retrorsine, senkirkine and hydroxysenkirkine in newborn rats, and the role of epoxides in carcinogenesis by pyrrolizidine alkaloids and aflatoxins. *Nature (Lond.)* **227**, 401—402 (1970). [H 27,417/70]

Scholler, K. L.: Augmentation ou suppression de l'hépatotoxicité du chloroforme. *Cah. Anesth.* **18**, 223—230 (1970). [G 75,794/70]

Scholtz, H. G.: Beeinflussung von experimentellem Hyperparathyroidismus durch Thymuspräparate. *Z. ges. exp. Med.* **85**, 547—558 (1932). [4,272/32]

Schönbaum, E., Sellers, E. A., Johnson, G. E.: Heat production and noradrenaline. *Fed. Proc.* **22**, 917—919 (1963). [E 21,028/63]

Schoor, W. P.: Effect of anticonvulsant drugs on insecticide residues. *Lancet* **1970 II**, 520 to 521. [H 28,965/70]

Schopp, R. T., Kreutter, W. F., Guzak, S. V.: Neuromyal blocking action of mescaline. *Amer. J. Physiol.* **200**, 1226—1228 (1961). [E 92,442/61]

Schopp, R. T., Rife, E. M.: Neuromuscular actions of serotonin following partial curarization. *Physiologist* **6**, 269 (1963). [E 24,636/63]

Schor, J. M., Frieden, E.: Induction of tryptophan peroxidase of rat liver by insulin and alloxan. *J. Biol. Chem.* **233**, 612—618 (1958). [C 57,994/58]

Schottek, W., Bekemeier, H.: Beeinflussung experimentell erzeugter Kalkablagerungen in der Niere durch Hormone. *Acta biol. med. germ.* **10**, Sup. 2, 237—239 (1963). [E 39,551/63]

Schöttler, W. H. A.: Antihistamine, ACTH, cortisone, hydrocortisone and anesthetics in snake bite. *Amer. J. trop. Med. Hyg.* **3**, 1083 to 1091 (1954). [C 10,890/54

Schöttler, W. H. A.: On the therapeutic value of ACTH and cortisone in experimental burns. *Endocrinology* **57**, 445–449 (1955). [C8,455/55

Schou, J.: Absorption of drugs from subcutaneous connective tissue. *Pharmacol. Rev.* **13**, 441–464 (1961). [E92,436/61

Schreiber, E. C.: The metabolic alteration of drugs. *Ann. Rev. Pharmacol.* **10**, 77–98 (1970). [G73,539/70

Schreiber, H.: Über die Bedeutung von Schwefel in Form von SH- bzw. SS-Gruppen enthaltenden Stoffen für den Organismus. *Ergebn. Hyg. Bakt.* **14**, 271–296 (1933). [A48,020/33

Schreiber, V.: Experimentalni příspěvek k poznání vlivu strumigenů na vegetativní nervový systém. *Fysiologie* **3**, 400–401 (1954). [C3,482/54

Schriefers, H., Ghraf, R., Brodesser, M.: Geschlechtsspezifika der Biosynthese von Steroidglucuroniden in der mit Testosteron perfundierten Rattenleber. *Acta endocr. (Kbh.)* **63**, 59–68 (1970). [H21,007/70

Schriefers, H., Wassmuth, E.: Das Ausmaß der Cortison-Hydrierung durch Rattenleberschnitte in seiner geschlechtsspezifischen Abhängigkeit von der mikrosomalen Δ^4-5α-Hydrogenase-Aktivität. *Hoppe-Seylers Z. physiol. Chem.* **338**, 100–104 (1964). [G23,742/64

Schrogie, J. J., Solomon, H. M.: The anticoagulant response to bishydroxycoumarin. II. The effect of D-thyroxine, clofibrate, and norethandrolone. *Clin. Pharmacol. Ther.* **8**, 70–77 (1966). [G43,019/66

Schulte, F. J., Bruggencate, H. G. ten.: Die Wirkung von Nebennierenrindenhormon auf einzelne Nervenzellen im Rückenmark der Katze. Ein experimenteller Beitrag zum Wirkungsmechanismus des Prednisolon in der Therapie zentralnervöser Erkrankungen. *Klin. Wschr.* **40**, 865–872 (1962). [D32,457/62

Schultz, J.: Influence of the presence of a sterile abscess on the detoxication of brombenzene as mercapturic acid. *Fed. Proc.* **7**, 185 (1946). [B18,183/46

Schultz, M. P.: The induction of carditis by the combined effects of infection and hyperthyroidism. *Trans. 3rd Int. Goiter Conf. Amer. Ass. Study Goiter*, Washington, p. 355–358 (1938). [99,001/38

Schultz, M. P., Rose, E. J.: Induction of carditis by the treatment of infected guinea pigs with insulin. *U.S. publ. Health Repts.* **54**, 527–532 (1939). [B31,347/39

Schulz, K.-D., Stutzer, H., Bettendorf, G.: Die Wirkung von Clomid auf die Aktivität der mikrosomalen NAD-spezifischen 17-β-Hydroxysteroiddehydrogenase in der Leber weiblicher infantiler Meerschweinchen. *Endokrinologie* **55**, 22–27 (1969). [H19,404/69

Schumer, W.: Dexamethasome in oligenic shock. Physiochemical effects in monkeys. *Arch. Surg.* **98**, 259–261 (1969). [G64,570/69

Schuurmans, R.: De invloed van de zwangerschap op ontstaan en verloop van het aneurysma dissecans. *Geneesk. Gids* **40**, 138–141 (1962). [D23,829/62

Schwartz, H. L., Kozyreff, V., Surks, M. I., Oppenheimer, J. H.: Increased deiodination of L-thyroxine and L-triiodothyronine by liver microsomes from rats treated with phenobarbital. *Nature (Lond.)* **221**, 1262–1263 (1969). [H9,326/69

Schwartz, H. L., Shapiro, H. C., Surks, M. I., Oppenheimer, J. H.: Dissociation between metabolism and action of L-thyroxine T4. (Abstr.) Program 52nd Meet. Endocr. Soc., St. Louis Miss., p. 92 (1970). [H26,012/70

Schwartz, K.: Inhibitory effect of cortisone on dietary necrotic liver degeneration in the rat. *Science* **113**, 485–486 (1951). [B57,985/51

Schweizer, W.: Studies on the effect of l-tyrosine on the white rat. *J. Physiol.* **106**, 167–176 (1947). [B3,047/47

Schweppe, J. S., Jungmann, R. A.: The effect of hormones on hepatic cholesterol ester synthesis in vitro. *Proc. Soc. exp. Biol. (N.Y.)* **131**, 868–870 (1969). [H15,266/69

Schweppe, J. S., Jungmann, R. A.: Hormones and cholesterol ester metabolism. *J. Amer. Geriat. Soc.* **17**, 740–754 (1969). [H15,978/69

Schwetz, B. A., Plaa, G. L.: Catecholamine potentiation of carbon tetrachloride-induced hepatotoxicity in mice. *Toxicol. appl. Pharmacol.* **14**, 495–509 (1969). [G67,000/69

Scilabra, G. A., Pugliese, F.: L'influsso della noradrenalina sulla reversione controllata della xantomatosi viscerale. *Arch. De Vecchi Anat. pat.* **51**, 883–902 (1968). [G68,796/68

Scott, E. B., Dynes, T. F.: The effects of growth hormone on phenylalanine-tyrosine deficient and pairfed rats. *Growth* **21**, 115–128 (1957). [C53,564/57

Scott, W. J. M.: The influence of the adrenal glands on resistance. I. The susceptibility of adrenalectomized rats to morphine. *J. exp. Med.* **38**, 543–560 (1923). [16,870/23

Scott, W. J. M.: The influence of the adrenal glands on resistance. II. The toxic effect of killed bacteria in adrenalectomized rats. *J. exp. Med.* **39**, 457–471 (1924). [17,400/24

Scott, W. J. M., Bradford, W. L., Hartman, F. A., McCoy, O. R.: The influence of adrenal cortex extract on the resistance to certain infections and intoxications. *Endocrinology* **17**, 529—536 (1933). [15,446/33

Sealy, W. C.: Role of infection in the pathogenesis of liver necrosis in hyperthyroidism. *Ann. Surg.* **116**, 851—859 (1942). [A56,716/42

Sealy, W. C., Lyons, C. K.: Necrosis of the liver produced by the combination of experimental hyperthyroidism and inflammation. *Arch. Surg.* **59**, 1319—1326 (1949). [B46,719/49

Segal, H. L., Beattie, D. S., Hopper, S.: Purification and properties of liver glutamic-alanine transaminase from normal and corticoid-treated rats. *J. biol. Chem.* **237**, 1914—1920 (1962). [G67,774/62

Segal, H. L., Kim, Y. S.: Glucocorticoid stimulation of the biosynthesis of glutamic-alanine transaminase. *Proc. nat. Acad. Sci. (Wash.)* **50**, 912—918 (1963). [G67,769/63

Segal, H. L., Rosso, R. G., Hopper, S., Weber, M. M.: Direct evidence for an increase in enzyme level as the basis for the glucocorticoid-induced increase in glutamic-alanine transaminase activity in rat liver. *J. biol. Chem.* **237**, 3303—3305 (1962). [D45,899/62

Segaloff, A., Maxfield, W. S.: The synergism between radiation and estrogen in the production of mammary cancer in the rat. *Cancer Res.* **31**, 166—168 (1971). [H36,188/71

Seguy, Dayot, Napie: Cancer provoqué au benzopyrène chez la rate. Etude de l'action des stimulines hypophysaires et des oestrogènes. Etude particulière de l'oestrus pendant la cancérisation. *Bull. Acad. nat. Méd. (Paris)* **145**, 181—186 (1961). [D5,238/61

Seidman, I., Teebor, G. W., Becker, F. F.: Hormonal and substrate induction of tryptophan pyrrolase in regenerating rat liver. *Cancer Res.* **27**, 1620—1625 (1967). [F88,452/67

Seifter, J., Rauzzino, F., Kramer, S. Z.: The effect of some indoles in chicks (Abstr.). *Pharmacologist* **5**, 246 (1963). [G71,087/63

Seller, M. J., Spector, R. G.: Effect of aldosterone and cortisol on leptazol-induced seizures in rats. *Brit. J. Pharmacol.* **19**, 271—273 (1962). [D36,979/62

Sellers, E. A., Reichman, S., Thomas, N.: Acclimatization to cold: natural and artificial. *Amer. J. Physiol.* **167**, 644—650 (1951). [B65,310/51

Sellers, E. A., You, R. W.: Propylthiouracil, thyroid, and dietary liver injury. *J. Nutr.* **44**, 513—535 (1951). [B68,641/51

Sellers, E. A., You, R. W., Ridout, J. H., Best, C. H.: Partial protection by cortisone against renal lesions produced by hypolipotropic diets. *Nature (Lond.)* **166**, 514 (1950). [B52,716/50

Sellers, M. I.: Studies in the entry of viruses into the central nervous system of mice via the circulation. Differential effects of vasoactive amines and CO_2 on virus infectivity. *J. exp. Med.* **129**, 719—746 (1969). [H10,893/69

Selye, H.: A syndrome produced by diverse nocuous agents. *Nature (Lond.)* **138**, 32 (1936). [36,031/36

Selye, H.: Studies on adaptation. *Endocrinology* **21**, 169—188 (1937). [38,798/37

Selye, H.: The effect of the alarm reaction on the absorption of toxic substances from the gastro-intestinal tract. *J. Pharmacol. exp. Ther.* **64**, 138—145 (1938). [A8,052/38

Selye, H.: On the toxicity of oestrogens with special reference to diethylstilboestrol. *Canad. med. Ass. J.* **41**, 48—49 (1939). [A18,206/39

Selye, H.: Morphological changes in female mice receiving large doses of testosterone. *J. Endocr.* **1**, 208—215 (1939). [A18,308/39

Selye, H.: The effect of testosterone on the kidney and on the general condition of uremic animals. *Canad. med. Ass. J.* **42**, 189 (1940). [A30,863/40

Selye, H.: On the protective action of testosterone against the kidney damaging effect of sublimate. *J. Pharmacol. exp. Ther.* **68**, 454 to 457 (1940). [A31,126/40

Selye, H.: On the protective action of testosterone against the kidney-damaging effect of sublimate. *Canad. med. Ass.* **42**, 173—174 (1940). [A31,128/40

Selye, H.: The beneficial action of desoxycorticosterone acetate in uraemia. *Canad. med. Ass. J.* **43**, 333—335 (1940). [A34,190/40

Selye, H.: Anesthetic effect of steroid hormones. *Proc. Soc. exp. Biol. (N.Y.)* **46**, 116—121 (1941). [A35,003/41

Selye, H.: On the role of the liver in the detoxification of steroid hormones and artificial estrogens. *J. Pharmacol. exp. Ther.* **71**, 236 to 238 (1941). [A35,150/41

Selye, H.: Acquired adaptation to the anesthetic effect of steroid hormones. *J. Immunol.* **41**, 259—268 (1941). [A35,410/41

Selye, H.: The anesthetic effect of steroid hormones. *Amer. J. Physiol.* **133**, 442 (1941). [A35,659/41

Selye, H.: Studies concerning the anesthetic action of steroid hormones. *J. Pharmacol. exp. Ther.* **73**, 127—141 (1941). [A 36,210/41

Selye, H.: The antagonism between anesthetic steroid hormones and pentamethylenetetrazol (Metrazol). *J. Lab. clin. Med.* **27**, 1051—1053 (1942). [A 36,443/42

Selye, H.: Studies concerning the correlation between anesthetic potency, hormonal activity and chemical structure among steroid compounds. *Anesth. Analg. Curr. Res.* **21**, 42 (1942). [A 36,447/42

Selye, H.: Mechanism of parathyroid hormone action. *Arch. Path.* **34**, 625—632 (1942). [A 36,715/42

Selye, H.: Correlations between the chemical structure and the pharmacological actions of the steroids. *Endocrinology* **30**, 437 (1942). [A 36,744/42

Selye, H.: The pharmacology of steroid hormones and their derivatives. *Rev. canad. Biol.* **1**, 577—632 (1942). [A 37,822/42

Selye, H.: Morphological changes in the fowl following chronic overdosage with various steroids. *J. Morph.* **73**, 401—421 (1943). [A 56,607/43

Selye, H.: Encyclopedia of Endocrinology. Section I. The steroids. Montréal: A.W.T. Franks Publ. Co. 1943. [A 57,606/43

Selye, H.: Experimental investigations concerning the role of the pituitary in tumorigenesis. *Surgery* **16**, 33—46 (1944). [A 60,638/44

Selye, H.: Role of the hypophysis in the pathogenesis of the diseases of adaptation. *Canad. med. Ass. J.* **50**, 426—433 (1944). [A 75,044/44

Selye, H.: Textbook of Endocrinology, 2nd ed., p. 914. Montreal, Canada: *Acta Endocrinologica Inc.* 1947, 1949. [94,572/49

Selye, H.: Further studies concerning the participation of the adrenal cortex in the pathogenesis of arthritis. *Brit. med. J.* **1949 II**, 1129 to 1135. [B 39,702/49

Selye, H.: Stress, p. 822. Montreal: Acta Inc., Med. Publ. 1950. [B 40,000/50

Selye, H.: Interactions between the adrenocorticotrophic hormone (ACTH) and the somatotrophic hormone (STH) in respect to their effects upon the kidney and the cardiovascular apparatus. In: Mote, J. R.; *Proceedings of the second clinical ACTH conference*, p. 95—107. New York, Philadelphia, Toronto: The Blakiston Co. 1951. [B 53,934/51

Selye, H.: Production par la somatotrophine hypophysaire (STH) d'hyalinose expérimentale. Inhibition par la cortisone, aggravation par la désoxycorticostérone. *Rev. canad. Biol.* **9**, 473—474 (1951). [B 53,940/51

Selye, H.: Inhibition par une substance folliculoide de la néphrosclérose normalement produite par la désoxycorticostérone. *Rev. canad. Biol.* **9**, 474 (1951). [B 53,941/51

Selye, H.: The influence of STH, ACTH and cortisone upon resistance to infection. *Canad. med. Ass. J.* **64**, 489—494 (1951). [B 57,451/51

Selye, H.: First Annual Report on Stress, p. 644. Montreal, Canada: Acta Inc. Med. Publ. 1951. [B 58,650/51

Selye, H.: Role of somatotrophic hormone (STH) in body defense against infection. *Fed. Proc.* **11**, 144 (1952). [B 65,065/52

Selye, H.: The Story of the Adaptation Syndrome, p. 225. Montreal, Canada: Acta Inc. Med. Publ. 1952. [B 71,000/52

Selye, H.: Prevention of cortisone overdosage effects with the somatotrophic hormone (STH). *Amer. J. Physiol.* **171**, 381—384 (1952). [B 75,329/52

Selye, H.: Effets d'un traitement simultané à la STH et à une substance folliculoïde. *Ann. Endocr. (Paris)* **14**, 378—384 (1953). [B 70,245/53

Selye, H.: Use of "granuloma pouch" technic in the study of antiphlogistic corticoids. *Proc. Soc. exp. Biol. (N.Y.)* **82**, 328—333 (1953). [B 76,060/53

Selye, H.: On the mechanism through which obstructive jaundice influences inflammatory processes. *Ann. rheum. Dis.* **13**, 102—108 (1954). [B 90,556/54

Selye, H.: Anticortisol action of aldosterone. *Science* **121**, 368—369 (1955). [B 98,268/55

Selye, H.: The Stress of Life, p. 324. New York, Toronto, London: McGraw-Hill Book Co. 1956. [C 19,000/56

Selye, H.: Protection by pregnancy against the development of experimental arteriosclerosis and metastatic calcification. *Amer. J. Obstet. Gynec.* **74**, 289—294 (1957). [C 25,011/57

Selye, H.: Über die humorale Beeinflussung des experimentellen Lathyrismus. *Arch. exp. Path. Pharmacol.* **230**, 155—160 (1957). [C 25,013/57

Selye, H.: Skeletal lesions produced by chronic treatment with somatotrophic hormone (STH) and aminoacetonitrile (AAN). *J. Geront.* **12**, 270—278 (1957). [C 25,910/57

Selye, H.: Effect of castration upon arteriosclerosis produced by dihydrotachysterol (AT-10) in male rats. *Lab. Invest.* **6**, 301–304 (1957). [C27,682/57

Selye, H.: Effect of various hormones upon the syndrome of dihydrotachysterol (AT-10) intoxication. *Acta endocr. (Kbh.)* **25**, 83–90 (1957). [C27,735/57

Selye, H.: Über den Einfluß lokaler Faktoren bei der Entstehung von Nierensteinen und Gewebsverkalkungen. *Z. Urol.* **50**, 440–444 (1957). [C27,736/57

Selye, H.: Lathyrism. *Rev. canad. Biol.* **16**, 1–82 (1957). [C31,369/57

Selye, H.: Participation of the adrenals in the effect of various hormones upon experimental osteolathyrism. *Arch. int. Physiol.* **65**, 391–395 (1957). [C31,790/57

Selye, H.: Prevention by thyroxine of the ocular changes normally produced by $\beta\beta'$-iminodipropionitrile (IDPN). *Amer. J. Ophthal.* **44**, 763–765 (1957). [C36,049/57

Selye, H.: Prevention of vitamin A overdosage by somatotrophic hormone. *J. Endocr.* **16**, 231–235 (1957). [C36,050/57

Selye, H.: Effect of sex hormones upon hypervitaminosis-A. *Rev. suisse Zool.* **64**, 757–761 (1957). [C37,276/57

Selye, H.: Sensitization by oestradiol to the production of experimental nephrocalcinosis. *Nature (Lond.)* **180**, 1420–1421 (1957). [C38,401/57

Selye, H.: Effect of corticoids upon skeletal and renal changes produced by stylomycin aminonucleoside. *Proc. Soc. exp. Biol. (N.Y.)* **96**, 544–547 (1957). [C38,594/57

Selye, H.: Influence of various hormones and vitamin-D preparations upon established bone lathyrism. *Acta anat. (Basel)* **33**, 146–156 (1958). [C28,810/58

Selye, H.: Prevention of the ECC syndrome by thyroxin. *J. clin. exp. Psychopath.* **19**, 97–101 (1958). [C36,069/58

Selye, H.: Sensitization of the skeleton to vitamin-A overdosage by cortisol. *Arthr. and Rheum.* **1**, 87–90 (1958). [C36,386/58

Selye, H.: Prevention of experimental nephrocalcinosis with thyroxine (Abstr.). *Endocrinology* **62**, 227–229 (1958). [C38,627/58

Selye, H.: Participation of ovarian hormones in the development of nephrocalcinosis. *Gynaecologia (Basel)* **145**, 161–167 (1958). [C38,768/58

Selye, H.: Schutzwirkung der Hypophysektomie gegenüber einer experimentellen Nephrocalcinose. *Endokrinologie* **35**, 193–196 (1958). [C39,319/58

Selye, H.: Protection by pregnancy against the development of "infarctoid cardiopathy" and nephrocalcinosis. *J. Obstet. Gynaec. Brit. Emp.* **65**, 588–589 (1958). [C44,470/58

Selye, H.: The Chemical Prevention of Cardiac Necroses, p. 235. New York: The Ronald Press Co. 1958. [C50,810/58

Selye, H.: Wechselwirkungen zwischen Stress, Elektrolyten und Steroiden beim Entstehen verschiedener Kardiopathien und Myopathien. *Endokrinologie* **38**, 195–217 (1959). [C61,814/59

Selye, H.: Protection by a steroid-spirolactone against certain types of cardiac necroses. *Proc. Soc. exp. Biol. (N.Y.)* **104**, 212–213 (1960). [C82,516/60

Selye, H.: The Pluricausal Cardiopathies, p. 438. Springfield, Ill.: Charles C Thomas Publ. 1961. [C92,918/61

Selye, H.: Nonspecific Resistance. *Ergebn. allg. Pathol. pathol. Anat.* **41**, 208 (1961). [C95,972/61

Selye, H.: Calciphylaxis, p. 552. Chicago, Ill.: The University of Chicago Press 1962. [D15,540/62

Selye, H.: The Mast Cells, p. 498. London: Butterworths 1965. [G19,425/65

Selye, H.: Thrombohemorrhagic Phenomena, p. 337. Springfield, Ill.: Charles C Thomas Publ. 1966. [E5,986/66

Selye, H.: Anaphylactoid Edema, p. 318. St. Louis, Miss.: Warren H. Green Inc. 1968. [G46,715/68

Selye, H.: Spironolactone actions, independent of mineralocorticoid blockade. *Steroids* **13**, 803 to 808 (1969). [G60,003/69

Selye, H.: Catatoxic Steroids. *Canad. med. Ass. J.* **101**, 51 (1969). [G60,039/69

Selye, H.: Prevention of indomethacin-induced intestinal ulcers by spironolactone and norbolethone. *Canad. J. Physiol. Pharmacol.* **47**, 981–983 (1969). [G60,046/69

Selye, H.: Role of the liver in the prevention of indomethacin-induced intestinal ulcers by spironolactone. *Acta hepato-splenol. (Stuttg.)* 59–74 (1969). [G60,058/69

Selye, H.: Inhibition of anesthesia by steroids. *J. Pharmacol. exp. Ther.* **174**, 478–486 (1970). [G60,044/70

Selye, H.: Prevention of various forms of metabolic myocardial necrosis by catatoxic steroids. *J. molec. Cell. Cardiol.* **1**, 91—99 (1970). [G 60,064/70

Selye, H.: Adaptive steroids: retrospect and prospect. (Russian text). *Pat. Fiziol. éksp. Ter.*, (in press). [G 70,410/71

Selye, H.: Adaptive steroids: retrospect and prospect. *Perspect. Biol. Med.* **13**, 343—363 (1970). [G 60,070/70

Selye, H.: Experimental Cardiovascular Diseases, p. 1120. Berlin, Heidelberg, New York: Springer 1970. [G 60,083/70

Selye, H.: Prevention of mephenesin intoxication by catatoxic steroids. *Acta pharmacol. (Kbh.)* **28**, 145—148 (1970). [G 60,086/70

Selye, H.: Resistance to picrotoxin poisoning induced by catatoxic steroids. *Agents and Actions* **1**, 133—135 (1970). [G 60,087/70

Selye, H.: Protection by catatoxic steroids against phenindione overdosage. *Thrombos. Diathes. haemorrh. (Stuttg.)* xxiv, No. 1, p. 77 (1970). [G 60,094/70

Selye, H.: Protection against methyprylon overdosage by catatoxic steroids. *Canad. Anaesth. Soc. J.* **17**, 107 (1970). [G 60,097/70

Selye, H.: Prevention of colchicine intoxication by catatoxic steroids. *Endocr. exp.* **4**, 71—76 (1970). [G 60,098/70

Selye, H.: Les stéroïdes catatoxiques: rétrospective et perspective. *Rev. Méd. fonct.* p. 163—199 (1970). [G 60,100/70

Selye, H.: Protection by catatoxic steroids against cycloheximide intoxication. *Toxicol. appl. Pharmacol.* **17**, 721—725 (1970). [G 70,403/70

Selye, H.: Pharmaco-chemical interrelations among catatoxic steroids. *Rev. canad. Biol.* **29**, 49—102 (1970). [G 70,421/70

Selye, H.: Mercury poisoning: prevention by spironolactone. *Science* **169**, 775—776 (1970). [G 70,426/70

Selye, H.: Steroids and nonspecific resistance. *Image* 12, No. 5, p. 3 (1970). [G 70,427/70

Selye, H.: Conditioning of catatoxic steroid actions by the thyroid. *J. Med. exp. clin.* **1**, 43—55 (1970). [G 70,428/70

Selye, H.: Resistance to various pesticides induced by catatoxic steroids. *Arch. environm. Hlth.* **21**, 706—710 (1970). [G 70,435/70

Selye, H.: Hormone und Widerstandsfähigkeit. *Münch. med. Wschr.* **31**, 1401—1407 (1970). [G 70,447/70

Selye, H.: Protection by glucocorticoids against ganglioplegics. *Res. Commun. chem. Path. Pharmacol.* **1**, No. 4, 572—579 (1970). [G 70,448/70

Selye, H.: Stress, hormones and cardiovascular disease. *Proc. 3rd Ann. Meet. Int. Study Group in Cardiac Metab.* Stowe, Vt. (1970). [G 70,465/70

Selye, H.: Protection by catatoxic steroids against cyclophosphamide-induced organ lesions, *Virchows Arch. Pathol. Anat.* **351**, 248 to 259 (1970). [G 70,466/70

Selye, H.: Catatoxic steroids. *G. Clin. med.* **51**, 619—625 (1970). [G 70,491/70

Selye, H.: Neue Ergebnisse der Streßforschung: Katatoxische Steroide. In: Jubilee Volume of German Society for the Advancement of Medical Science, p. 69—77 (1971). [G 79,017/71

Selye, H.: Steroids influencing the toxicity of l-tyrosine. *J. Nutr.* **101**, 515—524 (1971). [G 70,468/71

Selye, H.: Hormones and resistance. *J. pharm. Sci.* **60**, 1—28 (1971). [G 70,480/71

Selye, H.: Prevention of indomethacin-induced intestinal ulcers by various catatoxic steroids. *Exp. Med. Surg.* (in press). [G 60,066

Selye, H.: Protection by catatoxic steroids against cocaine poisoning. *Int. J. Psychobiol.* (in press). [G 70,471

Selye, H.: Influence of various catatoxic steroids upon chronic dihydrotachysterol intoxication. *Hormones* (in press). [G 70,467

Selye, H.: Steroids and resistance. *Jubilee volume of Prof. A. I. Strukov, Medicina (Kaunas)*, (in press). [G 79,021

Selye, H., Bajusz, E.: Effect of various stressors on muscular contraction induced by NaH$_2$PO$_4$ and NaClO$_4$. *Amer. J. Physiol.* **196**, 681—684 (1959). [C 55,656/59

Selye, H., Beland, E., Stone, H.: Effet des hormones hypophysaires, thyroïdienne et corticosurrénale sur la structure rénale. *Rev. canad. Biol.* **4**, 120 (1945). [B 229/45

Selye, H., Bois, P.: Experimental studies on the influence of corticoids and STH upon the course of obstructive jaundice. *Gastroenterologia (Basel)* **82**, 193—209 (1954). [B 97,074/54

Selye, H., Bois, P.: Morphologische Studien über den Synergismus zwischen dem somatotrophen Hormon und den Mineralocorticoiden. *Virchows Arch. pathol. Anat.* **327**, 235—252 (1955). [C 1,718/55

Selye, H., Bois, P.: On the role of the adrenal cortex in the production of renal calcification. *Proc. Roy. Soc. Can.* **50**, app. C., 54 (1956). [C 12,616/56

Selye, H., Bois, P.: Effect of corticoids on the resistance of the kidney to an excess of phosphates. *Amer. J. Physiol.* **187**, 41—44 (1956). [C 13,141/56

Selye, H., Bois, P.: On the participation of the adrenal cortex in the production of experimental nephrocalcinosis. *Acta endocr. (Kbh.)* **22**, 330—334 (1956). [C 13,168/56

Selye, H., Bois P.: Anticortisol action of 2-methyl-9(α)-fluorocortisol. *Proc. Soc. exp. Biol. (N.Y.)* **92**, 362—364 (1956). [C 14,534/56

Selye, H., Bois, P.: On the influence of various hormones upon the development of experimental lathyrism. *Rev. canad. Biol.* **15**, 281 (1956). [C 18,280/56

Selye, H., Bois, P.: Effect of corticoids upon the resistance of the kidney to sublimate intoxication. *J. Lab. clin. Med.* **49**, 263—266 (1957). [C 14,441/57

Selye, H., Bois, P.: On the role of corticoids in conditioning the gastric mucosa to certain toxic actions of ergocalciferol. *Brit. J. Nutr.* **11**, 18 to 22 (1957). [C 16,506/57

Selye, H., Bois, P.: Effet des hormones adaptives sur le lathyrisme expérimental du rat. *Ann. ACFAS* **23**, 80 (1957). [C 22,712/57

Selye, H., Bois, P.: Effect of STH on experimental lathyrism. *Proc. Soc. exp. Biol. (N.Y.)* **94**, 133—137 (1957). [C 23,297/57

Selye, H., Bois, P.: Effect of corticoids upon experimental lathyrism. *Endocrinology* **60**, 507 to 513 (1957). [C 23,298/57

Selye, H., Bois, P.: Anaphylaktoide Entzündung und Magengeschwüre bei mit Serotonin behandelten Ratten. *Allergie u. Asthma* **3**, 11—15 (1957). [C 23,958/57

Selye, H., Bois, P., Ventura, J.: Inhibition of experimental nephrocalcinosis by hypophysectomy. *Proc. Soc. exp. Biol. (N.Y.)* **92**, 488 to 493 (1956). [C 16,047/56

Selye, H., Cantin, M.: Hormonal bedingte Dissoziation der Wirkung eines Lathyrogens auf Knochen und Herz. *Beitr. pathol Anat.* **124**, 175—182 (1961). [C 88,878/61

Selye, H., Clarke, E.: Potentiation of a pituitary extract with Δ^5-pregnenolone and additional observations concerning the influence of various organs on steroid metabolism. *Rev. canad. Biol.* **2**, 319 to 328 (1943). [55,978/43

Selye, H., Collip, J. B., Thomson, D. L.: Some interrelations between water and fat metabolism in relation to disturbed liver function. *Lancet* **1935 II**, 297. [32,783/35

Selye, H., Dosne, C.: Inhibition by cortin of the blood sugar changes caused by adrenalin and insulin. *Proc. Soc. exp. Biol. (N.Y.)* **42**, 580 to 583 (1939). [A 30,701/39

Selye, H., Dosne, C.: Effect of cortin after partial and after complete hepatectomy. *Amer. J. Physiol.* **128**, 729—735 (1940). [A 30,702/40

Selye, H., Dosne, C.: Treatment of wound shock with corticosterone. *Lancet* **1940 I**, 70—71. [A 33,299/40

Selye, H., Dosne, C.: Physiological significance of compensatory adrenal atrophy. *Endocrinology* **30**, 581—584 (1942). [A 37,249/42

Selye, H., Dosne, G., Bassett, L., Whittaker, J.: On the therapeutic value of adrenal cortical hormones in traumatic shock and allied conditions. *Canad. med. Ass. J.* **43**, 1—8 (1940). [A 32,768/40

Selye, H., Friedman, S. M.: The beneficial action of testosterone in experimental renal atrophy caused by ligature of the ureter. *Endocrinology* **29**, 80—81 (1941). [A 35,722/41

Selye, H., Gabbiani, G., Jean, P.: Inhibition by hypophysectomy of organ lesions normally produced by parathyroid hormone or dihydrotachysterol. *Lab. Invest.* **11**, 1332—1339 (1962). [D 25,666/62

Selye, H., Gabbiani, G., Tuchweber, B.: Beteiligung der Hypophyse bei dem durch Dihydrotachysterin und Chromchlorid erzeugten calciphylaktischen Syndrom. *Endokrinologie* **43**, 241—252 (1962). [D 20,710/62

Selye, H., Gabbiani, G., Tuchweber, B.: Factors influencing topical calcinosis induced by trauma following intravenous injection of lead acetate. *Arch. int. Pharmacodyn.* **145**, 254—264 (1963). [D 25,657/63

Selye, H., Gabbiani, G., Tuchweber, B.: Organ lesions produced by hexadimethrine and their modification by various agents. *Med. exp. (Basel)* **8**, 74—82 (1963). [D 25,745/63

Selye, H., Gabbiani, G., Tuchweber, B.: Effect of parathyroidectomy and ferric dextrin upon calciphylactic sensitization by uremia. *J. Urol. (Baltimore)* **90**, 120—124 (1963). [D 32,610/63

Selye, H., Gentile, G.: Erzeugung calciphylaktischer Speicheldrüsenveränderungen durch Serotonin. *Naturwissenschaften* **48**, 671 (1961). [D 6,950/61

Selye, H., Goldie, I., Strebel, R.: Effect of anabolic hormones and ferric dextran upon the progeria-like syndrome produced by dihydrotachysterol. *Gerontologia (Basel)* 7, 94−104 (1963). [D30,544/63

Selye, H., Grasso, S., Padmanabhan, N.: Protection by anti-mineralocorticoid against an otherwise fatal dihydrotachysterol intoxication. *Lancet* 1960 II, 1350−1351. [C93,892/60

Selye, H., Heuser, G.: Fourth annual report on stress, p. 749. Montreal, Canada: *Acta Inc. Med. Publ.* 1954. [C1,001/54

Selye, H., Heuser, G.: Fifth annual report on stress, p. 815. Montreal, Canada: *Acta Inc., Med. Publ.* 1956. [C9,000/56

Selye, H., Horava, A.: Second annual report on stress, p. 526. Montreal, Canada: *Acta Inc., Med. Publ.* 1952. [B87,000/52

Selye, H., Horava, A.: Third annual report on stress, p. 637. Montreal, Canada: *Acta Inc., Med. Publ.* 1953. [B90,100/53

Selye, H., Jean, P., Bajusz, E.: Résistance croisée et prévention des cardiopathies expérimentales produites par un dérivé de la vitamine D. *Path. et Biol.* 9, 331−335 (1961). [C91,680/61

Selye, H., Jean, P., Cantin, M.: Prevention by stress and cortisol of gastric ulcers normally produced by 48/80. *Proc. Soc. exp. Biol. (N.Y.)* 103, 444−446 (1960). [C78,128/60

Selye, H., Jelinek, J., Krajny, M.: Prevention of digitoxin poisoning by various steroids. *J. pharm. Sci.* 58, 1055 (1969). [G60,023/69

Selye, H., Kovacs, K., Horvath, E., Yeghiayan, E., Blascheck, J. A., Gardell, C.: Lipoid hyperplasia of the adrenal cortex induced in rats by aniline. (Abstr.) *Program 52nd Meet. Endocr. Soc., St. Louis, Miss.*, p. 203 (1970). [G70,424/70

Selye, H., Krajny, M., Savoie, L.: Digitoxin poisoning: prevention by spironolactone. *Science* 164, 842−843 (1969). [G46,800/69

Selye, H., Lefebvre, F.: Détoxification du W-1372 (N-y-phénylpropyl-N-benzyloxy acétamide) par les stéroïdes cataxoxiques. *Arch. Anat. Path.* (in press). [G79,005

Selye, H., Lemire, Y., Cantin, M.: Topical blockade of carbon angiotaxis by cortisol. *Med. exp. (Basel)* 1, 11−16 (1959). [C70,942/59

Selye, H., Mandeville, R., Yeghiayan, E.: On the cataxoxic effect of antimineralocorticoids. *Naunyn-Schmiedebergs Arch. Pharmak.* 266, 34−42 (1970). [G60,050/70

Selye, H., Masson, G.: Effect of pituitary anterior lobe preparations on the action of anesthetics. *Canad. med. Ass. J.* 51, 579 (1944). [A97,571/44

Selye, H., Mécs, I.: Blockade of cataxoxic steroid actions by metyrapone. *Acta physiol. Acad. Sci. hung.* 37, 141−144 (1970). [G60,095/70

Selye, H., Mécs, I., Savoie, L.: Inhibition of anesthetics and sedative actions by spironolactone. *Anesthesiology* 31, 261 (1969). [G60,016/69

Selye, H., Mécs, I., Szabó, S.: Prevention of mercurial poisoning by steroids (Abstr.). *Proc. Canad. Fed. Biol. Soc.* 13, 10 (1970). [G70,432/70

Selye, H., Mécs, I., Szabó, S.: Protection by steroids against acute $HgCl_2$ poisoning. *Urol. and Nephrol.* 2, 287−301 (1970). [G70,440/70

Selye, H., Mécs, I., Szabó, S.: Sensitization by estrogens to the toxic effect of octamethyl pyrophosphamide (OMPA). *Arzneimittel-Forsch.* 10, 1488−1490 (1970). [G70,457/70

Selye, H., Mécs, I., Tamura, T.: Effect of spironolactone and norbolethone on the toxicity of digitalis compounds in the rat. *Brit. J. Pharmacol.* 37, 485−488 (1969). [G60,042/69

Selye, H., Mishra, R. K.: On the ability of methyltestosterone to counteract catabolism in diverse conditions of stress. *Arch. int. Pharmacodyn.* 117, 444−451 (1958). [C38,201/58

Selye, H., Mishra, R. K.: Protection by thyroxine against intoxication with elementary yellow phosphorus. *Acta pharmacol. (Kbh.)* 14, 359−362 (1958). [C40,183/58

Selye, H., Mortimer, H., Thomson, D. L., Collip, J. B.: Effect of parathyroid extract on the bones of the hypophysectomized rat. A histologic study. *Arch. Path.* 18, 878−880 (1934). [30,634/34

Selye, H., Nielsen, K.: Action of desoxycorticosterone on non-protein nitrogen content of blood during experimental uremia. *Proc. Soc. exp. Biol. (N.Y.)* 46, 541−542 (1941). [A35,723/41

Selye, H., Nielsen, K.: On the renotropic action of an anterior pituitary extract. *Endocrinology* 35, 207 (1944). [84,644/44

Selye, H., Padmanabhan, N., Walsh, J. T.: Schutzwirkung der Hypophysektomie gegenüber der sogenannten 'dystrophischen Gewebsverkalkung'. *Virchows Arch. pathol. Anat.* 335, 12−20 (1962). [D8,010/62

Selye, H., Pentz, E. I.: Pathogenetical correlations between periarteritis nodosa, renal hypertension and rheumatic lesions. *Canad. med. Ass. J.* 49, 264−272 (1943). [A59,789/43

Selye, H., Prioreschi, P., Cantin, M.: Factors that determine the production of cardiovascular and renal lesions by polymyxin. *Antibiot. and Chemother.* 11, 12—25 (1961). [C83,616/61

Selye, H., Renaud, S.: On the anticatabolic and anticalcinotic effects of 17-ethyl-19-nortestosterone. *Amer. J. med. Sci.* 235, 1—6 (1958). [C40,518/58

Selye, H., Rowley, E. M.: Prevention of experimental nephrosclerosis with methyl-testosterone. *Fed. Proc.* 3, 41 (1944). [A72,287/44

Selye, H., Rowley, E. M.: Prevention of experimental nephrosclerosis with methyl-testosterone. *J. Urol.* 51, 439—442 (1944). [A72,302/44

Selye, H., Savoie, L., Sayegh, R.: Inhibition of anesthetic and sedative actions by norbolethone. *Pharmacology (Basel)* 2, 265 (1969). [G60,020/69

Selye, H., Solymoss, B.: Protection by catatoxic steroids against meprobamate. *Int. J. Neuropharmacol.* 9, No. 4, 327—332 (1970). [G70,402/70

Selye, H., Stehle, R. L., Collip, J. B.: Recent advances in the experimental production of gastric ulcers. *Canad. med. Ass. J.* 34, 339 (1936). [58,020/36

Selye, H., Stevenson, J.: The toxic effect of oestrogens as influenced by progesterone. *Canad. med. Ass. J.* 42, 190 (1940). [77,177/40

Selye, H., Strebel, R., Mikulaj, L.: A progeria-like syndrome produced by dihydrotachysterol and its prevention by methyltestosterone and ferric dextran. *J. Amer. Geriat. Soc.* 11, 1—16 (1963). [D28,648/63

Selye, H., Sylvester, O., Hall, C. E., Leblond, C. P.: Hormonal production of arthritis. *J. Amer. med. Ass.* 124, 201—207 (1944). [A72,284/44

Selye, H., Szabo, S., Tache, Y., Kouroumakis, P., Szablowska, M.: Tentative rules for the SSS nomenclature of steroids. (in press). (1971). [G79,034

Selye, H., Tuchweber, B.: El concepto de los esteroides catatoxicos: sus implicaciones clinicas. *Rev. argent. Med. Interna* (in press). [G70,494

Selye, H., Tuchweber, B., Caruso, P. L.: Protection against neurotropic mastocalcergy. *Exp. Neurol.* 10, 451—461 (1964). [G11,123/64

Selye, H., Tuchweber, B., Gabbiani, G.: Beeinflussung der Indiumvergiftung durch Nebenschilddrüsenhormon und Dihydrotachysterin. *Naunyn-Schmiedebergs Arch. Pharmak.* 244, 109—116 (1962). [D25,667/62

Selye, H., Tuchweber, B., Gabbiani, G.: Further studies on anacalciphylaxis. *J. Amer. Geriat. Soc.* 12, 207—214 (1964). [E24,117/64

Selye, H., Tuchweber, B., Jacqmin, M.: Protection by various anabolic steroids against dihydrotachysterol-induced calcinosis and catabolism. *Acta endocr. (Kbh.)* 49, 589—602 (1965). [G19,426/65

Selye, H., Tuchweber, B., Jahnke, V.: Schutzwirkung der Fesselung gegen Serotoninintoxikation in Abwesenheit der Nebennieren. *Acta biol. med. germ.* 13, 198—203 (1964). [E24,146/64

Selye, H., Tuchweber, B., Ortega, M. R.: Prevention by methyltestosterone of parathyroid cyst formation. *Endocrinology* 75, 619—621 (1964). [G11,109/64

Selye, H., Ventura, J.: Effect of hypophysectomy and substitution therapy with STH upon experimental bone lathyrism. *Amer. J. Path.* 33, 919—929 (1957). [C27,684/57

Selye, H., Yeghiayan, E., Mandeville, R.: Protection by catatoxic steroids against dihydrotachysterol intoxication. *J. Atheroscler. Res.* 11, 321—331 (1970). [G60,055/70

Selye, H., Yeghiayan, E., Mécs, I.: Prevention of nicotine intoxication by catatoxic steroids. *Arch. int. Pharmacodyn.* 183, No. 2, p. 235 (1970). [G60,069/70

Semenov, L. F.: The testing of indoleamine compounds in the prevention of radiation sickness. (Russian text.) *Med. Radiol. (Mosk.)* 5/5, 47—52 (1960). [D7,087/60

Sen, H. G., Joshi, U. N., Seth, D.: Effect of cortisone upon Ancylostoma caninum infection in albino mice. *Trans. Roy. Soc. trop. Med. Hyg.* 59, 684—689 (1965). [F76,261/65

Sereni, F., Kenney, F. T., Kretchmer, N.: Factors influencing the development of tyrosine-α-ketoglutarate transaminase activity in rat liver. *J. biol. Chem.* 234, 609—612 (1959). [C80,562/59

Serkes, K. D., Berman, W., Lang, S.: Hydrocortisone and lysosomal enzymes in tourniquet shock. *Proc. Soc. exp. Biol. (N.Y.)* 126, 362 to 365 (1967). [F92,105/67

Serrone, D. M., Fujimoto, J. M.: Inhibition of the metabolism of hexobarbital in vitro. *Biochem. Pharmacol.* 5, 263—264 (1960). [D83,863/60

Serrone, D. M., Fujimoto, J. M.: The diphasic effect of N-methyl-3-piperidyl-(N',N')-diphenyl carbamate HCl (MPDC) on the metabolism of hexobarbital. *J. Pharmacol. exp. Ther.* 133/1, 12—17 (1961). [D48,610/61

Serrone, D. M., Fujimoto, J. M.: The effect of certain inhibitors in producing shortening of hexobarbital action. *Biochem. Pharmacol.* **11**, 609—615 (1962). [D80,098/62

Sethy, V. H., Naik, S. R., Sheth, U. K.: Effect of stress on pentobarbital sleeping time in rats. *Indian J. med. Res.* **58**, 352—357 (1970).
[G77,511/70

Severi, F., Rondini, G., Zaverio, S., Vegni, M.: Prolonged neonatal hyperbilirubinemia and pregnane-3(α),20(β)-diol in maternal milk. *Helv. paediat. Acta* **25**, 517—521 (1970).
[G82,341/70

Severin, V. N., Bashkurov, E. P.: The clinical picture and treatment of acute poisoning with methyl alcohol. (Russian text.) *Klin. Med. (Mosk.)* **45**, 125—129 (1967). [G49,801/67

Shafer, R. B., Adicoff, A.: Digitalis antagonism by a specific lactone. *Curr. ther. Res.* **12**, 755 to 758 (1970). [G80,179/70

Sharpless, S. K.: Hypnotics and sedatives. I. The barbiturates. In: Goodman, L. S. and Gilman, A.; *The Pharmacological Basis of Therapeutics*, p. 98—120. New York: McMillan Co. 1970. [E8,852/70

Shaw, F. H., Shankley, K. H.: Factors affecting the duration of Nembutal anaesthesia in rats. *Austral. J. exp. Biol. med. Sci.* **26**, 481—491 (1948). [A52,203/48

Shay, H., Aegerter, E. A., Gruenstein, M., Komarov, S. A.: Development of adenocarcinoma of the breast in the Wistar rat following the gastric instillation of methyl-cholanthrene. *J. nat. Cancer Inst.* **10**, 255—266 (1949).
[H26,763/49

Shay, H., Gruenstein, M., Kessler, W. B.: Estrogenic inhibition of methylcholanthrene-induced breast cancer in the rat. (Abstr.) *Proc. Amer. Ass. Cancer Res.* **3**, 268 (1961). [D2,760/61

Shay, H., Harris, C., Gruenstein, M.: Influence of sex hormones on the incidence and form of tumors produced in male or female rats by gastric instillation of methylcholanthrene. *J. nat. Cancer Inst.* **13**, 307—331 (1952).
[H31,719/52

Sheehan, H. L., Summers, V. K., Nichols, J.: D.D.D. therapy in Cushing's syndrome. *Lancet* **1953I**, 312—314. [B77,668/53

Sheldon, W. H., Bauer, H.: The role of predisposing factors in experimental fungus infections. *Lab. Invest.* **11**, 1184—1191 (1962).
[D46,962/62

Shellabarger, C. J., Aponte, G. E., Cronkite, E. P., Bond, V. P.: Studies on radiation-induced mammary gland neoplasia in the rat. VI. The effect of changes in thyroid function, ovarian function, and pregnancy. *Radiat. Res.* **17**, 492—507 (1962). [D39,218/62

Shelton, E.: Production of liver tumors in mice with 2-amino-5-azotoluene (Abstr.). *Proc. Amer. Ass. Cancer Res.* **1**, 44 (1954).
[G76,339/54

Sherlock, S.: Primary biliary cirrhosis (chronic intrahepatic obstructive jaundice). *Gastroenterology* **37**, 574—586 (1959). [G79,591/59

Sherman, I. W., Ruble, J. A.: Virulent Trypanosoma lewisi infections in cortisone-treated rats. *J. Parasit.* **53**, 258—262 (1967). [G49,628/67

Sherwin-Weidenreich, R., Herrmann, F.: Hair cycle and chemically induced epidermal carcinogenesis in mice receiving tri-iodothyronine. I. Findings after single application of 9,10-dimethyl-1,2-benzanthracene. *J. invest. Derm.* **40**, 225—232 (1963). [D67,842/63

Shiba, S., Matsuyoshi, H., Miyatake, M.: Tryptophan pyrrolase in the isolated perfused liver of a tumor-bearing animal. *Gann* **56**, 121—126 (1965). [G31,114/65

Shibata, H., Mizuta, M., Combes, B.: Hepatic glucuronyl transferase activity and bilirubin T_m in pregnancy in the rat. *Amer. J. Physiol.* **211**, 967—970 (1966). [G80,058/66

Shibata, K., Komiya, A.: Effect of adrenocortical steroids on duration of pentothal anesthesia in adrenalectomized mice. *Proc. Soc. exp. Biol. (N.Y.)* **84**, 308—310 (1953).
[B88,660/53

Shibata, K., Komiya, A., Machida, J., Fukushima, K.: Effect of cortisone acetate on barbital anesthesia in normal rabbits. *Endocr. jap.* **4**, 28—34 (1957). [C49,533/57

Shideman, F. E., Kelly, A. R., Adams, B. J.: The role of the liver in the detoxication of thiopental (Pentothal) and two other thiobarbiturates. *J. Pharmacol. exp. Ther.* **91**, 331—339 (1947). [E60,046/47

Shigei, M.: Effects of adrenalectomy and hydrocortisone administration on the fine structure of parenchymal cells of normal and regenerating rat liver. *J. Fac. Sci. Tokyo, Sect. 4*, **11**, 511—536 (1969). [H27,112/69

Shih-Chi, L., Hsiu-Yuan, C., Chen-Yu, S.: Effects of thyroxine and propylthiouracil on the toxicity of trivalent ammonium antimonyl gluconate and the distribution and excretion of antimony after administration of the compound. (Chinese text with English summary.) *Acta physiol. sinica* **22**, 289—293 (1958).
[C72,194/58

Shimamoto, T.: Experimental study on atherosclerosis. An attempt at its prevention and treatment. *Acta path. jap.* 19, 15–43 (1969). [G70,917/69

Shimazu, T.: Biological mechanism of the effect of 20-methylcholanthrene on the induction of dimethylaminoazobenzene-demethylase activity of rat liver. *Gann* 56, 143–149 (1965). [G31,110/65

Shimazu, T.: Response to 20-methylcholanthrene of hepatic aniline- and acetanilide 4-hydroxylase of rats with hypothalamic lesions *Biochim. biophys. Acta (Amst.)* 105, 377–380 (1965). [G34,311/65

Shimazu, T., Suda, M.: Mechanism of 20-methylcholanthrene on the induction of DAB-demethylase in rat liver. *Gann* 50, Sup. 65–66 (1959). [G76,684/59

Shipley, R. A., Chudzik, E. B., György, P., Rose, C. S.: Mechanism of the lipotropic action of estrogen. *Arch. Biochem.* 25, 309–315 (1950). [B50,163/50

Shipley, R. A., György, P.: Effect of dietary hepatic injury on inactivation of estrone. *Proc. Soc. exp. Biol. (N.Y.)* 57, 52–55 (1944). [20,418/44

Shirasu, Y., Grantham, P. H., Weisburger, E. K., Weisburger, J. H.: Effects of adrenocorticotropic hormone and growth hormone on the metabolism of N-hydroxy-N-2-fluorenylacetamide and on physiologic parameters. *Cancer Res.* 27, 81–87 (1967). [F76,819/67

Shirasu, Y., Grantham, P. H., Yamamoto, R. S., Weisburger, J. H.: Effects of pituitary hormones and prefeeding N-hydroxy-N-2-fluorenylacetamide on the metabolism of this carcinogen and on physiologic parameters. *Cancer Res.* 26, 600–606 (1966). [F65,704/66

Shisa, H.: Studies on the mechanism of 7, 12-dimethylbenz [α] anthracene leukemogenesis in mice. III. Acceleration of DMBA leukemogenesis in mice by pretreatment of cortisone acetate. *Mie med. J.* 19, 111–121 (1969). [G72,582/69

Shklar, G.: Cortisone and hamster buccal pouch carcinogenesis. *Cancer Res.* 26, 2461 to 2463 (1966). [F74,973/66

Shleser, I. H., Asher, R.: Efficacy of adrenal cortical extract and of paredrine in the prevention of experimental shock following venous occlusion of a limb. *Amer. J. Physiol.* 138, 1–6 (1942). [A56,711/42

Shmelev, N. A., Uvarova, O. A.: The effect of ACTH on the course of experimental TB. (Russian text.) *Probl. Endokr. Gormonoter.* 2/6, 38–43 (1956). [C53,553/56

Sholiton, L. J., Werk, E. E., Jr., MacGee, J.: The in vitro effect of 5,5'-diphenylhydantoin on the catabolism of cortisol by rat liver. *Metabolism* 13, 1382–1392 (1964). [F23,871/64

Shore, P. A., Silver, S. L., Brodie, B. B.: Interaction of serotonin and lysergic acid diethylamide (LSD) in the central nervous system. *Experientia (Basel)* 11, 272 (1955). [C18,383/55

Shou, L., Pan, F., Chin, S. F.: Pancreatic hormones and hepatic methionine adenosyltransferase in the rat. *Proc. Soc. exp. Biol. (N.Y.)* 131, 1012–1018 (1969). [H15,277/69

Shrotri, D. S., Bhadkamkar, U. A., Balwani, J. H.: Modification of hexobarbitone action by insulin. *Indian J. med. Res.* 50, 446–448 (1962). [D27,239/62

Shubik, P., Ritchie, A. C.: Sensitivity of male dba mice to the toxicity of chloroform as a laboratory hazard. *Science* 117, 285 (1953). [D67,964/53

Shuster, L.: Metabolism of drugs and toxic substances. *Ann. Rev. Biochem.* 33, 571–596 (1964). [F38,575/64

Shwartzman, G.: Enhancing effect of cortisone upon poliomyelitis infection (Strain MEFI) in hamsters and mice. *Proc. Soc. exp. Biol. (N.Y.)* 75, 835–838 (1950). [B54,248/50

Shwartzman, G.: Enhancement of susceptibility to experimental poliomyelitis by means of cortisone (Abstr.). *Amer. J. Path.* 27, 714 (1951). [B66,955/51

Shwartzman, G.: Poliomyelitis infection in cortisone-treated hamsters induced by the intraperitoneal route. *Proc. Soc. exp. Biol. (N.Y.)* 79, 573–576 (1952). [B69,778/52

Shwartzman, G., Aronson, S. M.: Poliomyelitis infection by parenteral routes made possible by cortisone. *Ann. N.Y. Acad. Sci.* 56, 793–797 (1953). [B84,833/53

Shwartzman, G., Fisher, A.: Alteration of experimental poliomyelitis infection in the Syrian hamster with the aid of cortisone. *J. exp. Med.* 95, 347–362 (1952). [B69,580/52

Sidransky, H.: Sex difference in induction of fatty liver in the rat by dietary orotic acid. *Endocrinology* 72, 709–714 (1963). [D64,556/63

Sidransky, H., Farber, E.: Sex difference in induction of periportal fatty liver by methionine deficiency in the rat. *Proc. Soc. exp. Biol. (N.Y.)* 98, 293–297 (1958). [C55,020/58

Sidransky, H., Verney, E., Egan, R. F.: The influence of testosterone on the induction of fatty liver by methionine deficiency. *Lab. Invest.* 16, 858—863 (1967). [G 48,110/67]

Sidransky, H., Verney, E., Lombardi, B.: Factors influencing orotic acid-induced fatty liver. *Fed. Proc.* 22, 371 (1963). [G 4,364/63]

Sidransky, H., Wagle, D. S., Verney, E.: Hepatic protein synthesis in rats force-fed a threonine-devoid diet and treated with cortisone acetate or threonine. *Lab. Invest.* 20, 364—370 (1969). [G 65,724/69]

Sidransky, H., Wagner, B. P., Morris, H. P.: Sex difference in liver tumorigenesis in rats ingesting N-2 fluorenylacetamide. *J. nat. Cancer Inst.* 26, 151—187 (1961). [C 99,347/61]

Siegel, B. V., Aird, R. B., Anderson, W. W.: Effect of trypan red on Columbia-SK virus pathogenicity. *Neurology (Minneap.)* 11, 982 to 988 (1961). [D 13,002/61]

Siegel, S.: Nonparametric Statistics for the Behavioral Sciences, p. 270. New York, Toronto, London: McGraw-Hill Book Co. Inc. 1956. [G 67,296/56]

Siegel, W. V., Shklar, G.: The effect of dimethyl sulfoxide and topical triamcinolone on chemical carcinogenesis of hamster buccal pouch. *Oral Surg.* 27, 772—779 (1969). [H 35,238/69]

Siegert, M., Alsleben, B., Liebenschütz, W., Remmer, H.: Unterschiede in der mikrosomalen Oxydation und Acetylierung von Arzneimitteln bei verschiedenen Arten und Rassen. *Naunyn-Schmiedebergs Arch. Pharmak.* 247, 509—521 (1964). [G 71,866/64]

Siegler, R., Duran-Reynals, M. L.: Observations on the pathogenesis of experimental skin tumors. A study of the mechanism by which papillomas develop. *J. nat. Cancer Inst.* 29, 653—673 (1962). [D 54,814/62]

Silberberg, R., Silbergber, M.: Strain differences in skeletal growth and ageing of mice fed a high fat diet. *Fed. Proc.* 9, 344 (1950). [B 48,364/50]

Silk, M. R.: The effect of progesterone on cats administered endotoxin. *J. surg. Res.* 7, 35—40 (1967). [F 95,477/67]

Silvestri, F.: Eliminazione urinaria dei 17-chetosteroidi nella steatosi sperimentale da colesterine e nella steatosi da colesterina trattata con sostanze metilanti, testosterone e vit. E. (Ricerche sperimentali). *Chir. Pat. sper.* 12, 695—711 (1964). [F 62,336/64]

Šimek, J., Erbenová, Z., Deml, F., Dvořáčková, I.: Liver regeneration after partial hepatectomy in rats exposed before the operation to the stress stimulus. *Experientia (Basel)* 24, 1166—1167 (1968). [H 13,837/68]

Šimek, J., Husáková, A., Erbenová, Z., Dvořáčková, I.: The relationship of glucocorticoids to the early changes of liver triglycerides content after partial hepatectomy in rats. *Sborn. ved. Praci lék. Fak. Hradci Králové* 11, 5—7 (1968). [G 71,089/68]

Šimek, J., Husáková, A., Erbenová, Z., Kanta, J.: The role of the adrenals in changes of liver triglycerides content after partial hepatectomy in rats of different ages. *Physiol. bohemoslov.* 563—567 (1968). [H 22,183/68]

Simionovici, M., Winter, D., Sterescu, N.: Sur le rôle des amines biogènes dans l'antagonisme de certains phénomènes réserpiniques centraux chez la souris. *Rev. roum. Physiol.* 2, 43—48 (1965). [F 43,099/65]

Simmons, D. J., Pankovich, A. M., Budy, A. M.: Osteolathyrism in mice and inhibition of the endosteal bone reaction in estrogen-treated mice by aminoacetonitrile. *Amer. J. Anat.* 116, 387—399 (1965). [G 28,592/65]

Simmons, F., Boyle, J. D.: Effect of heterologous serum albumin on liver regeneration after partial hepatectomy. *Arch. Surg.* 98, 369—371 (1969). [H 22,141/69]

Simon, A.: Über die Wertbestimmung des Parathyreoideahormons mit Magnesiumsulfat. *Naunyn-Schmiedebergs Arch. Pharmak.* 178, 57—63 (1935). [31,369/35]

Simon, E. R., Pesch, L. A., Topper, Y. J.: Localization of the steroid hormone effect on galactose metabolism. *Biochem. biophys. Res. Commun.* 1, 6—8 (1959). [C 84,793/59]

Simpson, L. L.: The interaction between 5-hydroxytryptamine and botulinum toxin type A. *Toxicol. appl. Pharmacol.* 12, 249—259 (1968). [G 60,451/68]

Simpson, L. L.: Evidence for the non-specificity of the interaction between 5-hydroxytryptamine and botulinum toxin. *Toxicon* 5, 239—246 (1968). [H 5,300/68]

Simpson, W. L., Bond, B., Leithauser, G., Yamaguchi, I., Horeglad, S.: Effects of thymectomy on the response of Sprague-Dawley rats to a single feeding of 7-12 dimethylbenzanthracene (Abstr.) *Proc. Amer. Ass. Cancer Res.* 5, 58 (1964). [F 2,965/64]

Simpson-Herren, L., Griswold, D. P., Jr.: Studies of the kinetics of growth and regression of 7,12-dimethylbenz(α)anthracene-induced mammary adenocarcinoma in Sprague-Dawley rats. *Cancer Res.* 30, 813—818 (1970). [H 26,708/70

Sinclair, K. B.: The effect of corticosteroid on the pathogenicity and development of Fasciola Hepatica in lambs. *Brit. vet. J.* **124**, 133—139 (1968). [G65,622/68

Sindram, I.: Der Einfluß von Cortin auf die Empfindlichkeit für Narkotika. *Acta brev. neerl. Physiol.* **5**, 29—30 (1935). [52,504/35

Singer, E.: Experimental studies on the combined sulphanilamide and serum treatment of gas gangrene infections. *Med. J. Austral.* **2**, 275—279 (1940). [B316/40

Singer, S., Mason, M.: Tyrosine-α-ketoglutarate transaminase effect of the administration of sodium benzoate and related compounds on the hepatic enzyme level. *Biochim. biophys. Acta (Amst.)* **110**, 370—379 (1965). [G66,500/65

Singh, I., Sehra, K. B., Bhargaya, S. P.: Tolbutamide in cirrhosis of the liver. *Lancet* **1961 I**, 1144. [D6,799/61

Singhal, R. L., Valadares, J. R. E., Ling, G. M.: Influence of chronic phenobarbitone treatment on uterine phosphorfructokinase induction. *J. Pharm. Pharmacol.* **19**, 545—547 (1967). [G67,770/67

Singhal, R.L., Valadares, J.R.E., Schwark, W.S.: Inhibition by phenobarbitone of oestrogen-stimulated increases in uterine enzymes. *J. Pharm. Pharmacol.* **21**, 194—195 (1969). [G78,387/69

Sirsat, S.M., Ketkar, M.B.: Influence of DOC on induced epidermal cancers in mice. *J. invest. Derm.* **46**, 331—340 (1966). [F65,926/66

Skalka, M.: Nebennierenfunktion und Veränderungen der Leber nach Röntgenbestrahlung. *Experientia (Basel)* **15/4**, 153—155 (1959). [C71,368/59

Skanse, B.: The effect of altered sexual functions on the storage of arsenic in mice. *Upsala Läk.-Fören. Förh.* **47**, 55—79 (1941). [A72,698/41

Skanse, B., Nyman, G. E., Törnegren, L.: Electroencephalographic abnormalities in vitamin D intoxication and the effect of cortisone. *Acta endocr. (Kbh.)* **31**, 282—290 (1959). [C69,514/59

Skinhøj, P., Quaade, F.: Intracutaneous serotonin test in dysthyroid and normal persons. *Acta allerg. (Kbh.)* **24**, 280—283 (1969). [G72,600/69

Sklower, A.: Über Beziehungen zwischen Schilddrüse und Thymus. *Z. vergl. Physiol.* **6**, 150—166 (1927). [25,299/27

Skobba, T., Miya, T. S.: Hyperthermic responses and toxicity of chlorpromazine in L-thyroxine sodium-treated rats. *Toxicol. appl. Pharmacol.* **14**, 176—181 (1969). [G64,738/69

Skuratova, N. A.: A comparative study of the ACTH and the growth hormone effect on the resistance of albino mice to diphtheria toxin. (Russian text.) *Probl. Endokr. Gormonoter.* **8/2**, 38—43 (1962). [D20,887/62

Sladek, N.E., Mannering, G.J.: Induction of drug metabolism. I. Differences in the mechanisms by which polycyclic hydrocarbons and phenobarbital produce their inductive effects on microsomal N-demethylating systems. *Molec. Pharmacol.* **5**, 174—185 (1969). [G66,219/69

Sladek, N. E., Mannering, G. J.: Induction of drug metabolism. II. Qualitative differences in the microsomal N-demethylating systems stimulated by polycyclic hydrocarbons and by phenobarbital. *Molec. Pharmacol.* **5**, 186—199 (1969). [G66,220/69

Slebodzinski, A., Srebro, Z.: The course of radiation disease in hyper and hypothyreotic rats. *Folia Biol. (Krakow)* **17**, 145—158 (1969). [H29,972/69

Slocombe, A. G.: Effects of lysergic acid diethylamide and related amines on the electrical activity of the rat brain. *Fed. Proc.* **15**, 172 (1956). [C14,144/56

Sloper, J. C., Pegrum, G. D.: Regeneration of crushed mammalian skeletal muscle and effects of steroids. *J. Path. Bact.* **93**, 47—63 (1967). [G49,073/67

Smart, K. M., Kilbourne, E. D.: The influence of cortisone on experimental viral infection. VII. Kinetics of interferon formation and its inhibition with hydrocortisone in relation to viral strain and virulence. *J. exp. Med.* **123**, 309 to 325 (1966). [G33,810/66

Smiecinski, W., Gorski, T.: The induction of uterine cervical carcinoma in thymectomised mice. *Folia biol. (Krakow)* **16**, 211—212 (1968). [H20,765/68

Smith, A. U.: Further observations on the closed vessel technique for testing thyroid activity. *J. Endocr.* **5**, lxiv (1947). [B4,939/47

Smith, A. U., Emmens, C. W., Parkes, A. S.: Assay of thyroidal activity by a closed vessel technique. *J. Endocr.* **5**, 186—206 (1947). [B4,928/47

Smith, C. W., Bean, J. W., Bauer, R.: Thyroid influence in reactions to O_2 at atmospheric pressure. *Amer. J. Physiol.* **199**, 883—888 (1960). [C95,244/60

Smith, D. C. W.: The role of the endocrine organs in the salinity tolerance of trout. In:

Jones, I. C., and Eckstein, P.: *The Comparative Endocrinology of Vertebrates, Part II*, p. 83 to 101. Toronto: MacMillan Co. Canada Ltd. 1956. [C46,496/56

Smith, D. E., Tyree, E. B.: Influence of X-irradiation upon water consumption by the rat. *Amer. J. Physiol.* 184, 127—133 (1956). [C12,045/56

Smith, E., McMillan, E., Mack, L.: Factors influencing the lethal action of illuminating gas. *J. industr. Hyg.* 17, 18—20 (1935). [45,163/35

Smith, I. M., Lindell, S. S., Hazard, E. C.: Inhibitory action of the testosterone and liver extract on staphylococcal infections in mice. *Nature (Lond.)* 211, 722—723 (1966). [F68,892/66

Smith, J. M., Dubos, R. J.: The effect of dinitrophenol and thyroxin on the susceptibility of mice to staphylococcal infections. *J. exp. Med.* 103, 119—126 (1956). [C12,130/56

Smith, J. M., Murphy, J. S., Mirick, G. S.: Effect of adrenal hormones on infection of mice with pneumonia virus of mice (PVM). *Proc. Soc. exp. Biol. (N.Y.)* 78, 505—510 (1951). [B64,635/51

Smith, L. C., Dugal, L. P.: Effect of food and water consumption, liver function, and thyroid function on the spontaneous running activity of white rats. *Canad. J. Physiol. Pharmacol.* 44, 455—464 (1966). [F65,692/66

Smith, L. L., Muller, W., Hinshaw, D. B.: The management of experimental endotoxin shock. The circulatory effects of levarterenol, hydrocortisone, phenoxybenzamine hydrochloride, and blood volume expansion. *Arch. Surg.* 89, 630—636 (1964). [D18,862/64

Smith, M. W.: The effect of hyaluronidase and cortisol on the inactivation of vasopressins by rat kidney slices. *J. Endocr.* 24, 415—424 (1962). [D27,805/62

Smith, O. W., Smith, G. van S.: Menstrual discharge of women. I. It's toxicity in rats. *Proc. Soc. exp. Biol. (N.Y.)* 44, 100—104 (1940). [A32,972/40

Smith, R. T., Thomas, L.: Lethal action of gram-negative bacterial endotoxins on the chick embryo. *Fed. Proc.* 14, 478 (1955). [C5,334/55

Smith, R. T., Thomas, L.: The letal effect of endotoxins on the chick embryo. *J. exp. Med.* 104, 217—231 (1956). [C97,047/56

Smith, W. W.: The effect of thyroid hormone and radiation on the mitotic index of mouse epidermis. *J. cell. comp. Physiol.* 38, 41—49 (1951). [B66,170/51

Smith, W. W., Alderman, I. M., Schneider, C., Cornfield, J.: Sensitivity of irradiated mice to bacterial endotoxin. *Proc. Soc. exp. Biol. (N.Y.)* 113, 778—781 (1963). [E21,486/63

Smith, W. W., Dooley, R., Thompson, E. C.: Simulated high altitude following whole-body radiation of mice. *J. Aviat. Med.* 19, 227—237 (1948). [B48,252/48

Smith, W. W., Smith, F.: Effect of thyroid hormone on radiation lethality. *Amer. J. Physiol.* 165, 639—650 (1951). [B60,347/51

Smith, W. W., Smith, F.: Effects of thyroid and radiation on sensitivity to hypoxia, basal rate of O_2 consumption and tolerance to exercise. *Amer. J. Physiol.* 165, 651—661 (1951). [B60,348/51

Smith, W. W., Smith, F., Thompson, E. C.: Failure of cortisone or ACTH to reduce mortality in irradiated mice. *Proc. Soc. exp. Biol. (N.Y.)* 73, 529—531 (1950). [B47,642/50

Smoake, J. A., Mulvey, P. F., Jr.: Factors influencing tolerance time in rats exposed to severe hypoxia (33,000 ft.) (Abstr.). *Fed. Proc.* 29, 581 (1970). [H23,262/70

Smookler, H. H., Buckley, J. P.: Effect of drugs on animals exposed to chronic environmental stress. *Fed. Proc.* 29, 1980—1984 (1970). [H32,862/70

Smuckler, E. A.: Structural and functional alteration of the endoplasmic reticulum during CCl_4 intoxication. *FEBS Symp. Oslo (1967)* 14, 13—55 (1968). [G80,996/68

Snyder, F., Cress, E. A., Kyker, G. C.: Liver lipid response to intravenous rare earths in rats. *J. Lipid. Res.* 1, 125—131 (1959). [C99,417/59

Soave, O. A.: Reactivation of rabbits virus in a guinea pig with adrenocorticotropic hormone. *J. infect. Dis.* 110, 129—131 (1962). [D22,275/62

Sobel, H., Sideman, M., Arce, R.: Effect of cortisone on survival of morphine treated guinea pigs under decompression hypoxia. *Proc. Soc. exp. Biol. (N.Y.)* 104, 31—32 (1960). [C90,836/60

Sobis, H.: Pathomorphological changes in the lungs of mice in experimental influenza. *Pol. med. J.* 3/2, 287—307 (1964). [G29,127/64

Soffer, L. J.: Bilirubin excretion as a test for liver function during normal pregnancy. *Bull. Johns Hopk. Hosp.* 52, 365—375 (1933). [7,166/33

Soiva, K., Grönroos, M., Aho, A. J., Rinne, U.: Über die Einwirkung von "Stress" auf die Geschlechtsorgane und -funktionen der schwangeren und nichtschwangeren Ratten. *Geburtsh. Frauenheilk.* **20**, 505—508 (1960). [C97,218/60

Solanki, B. R., Junnarkar, R. V.: Influence of thyroid gland on tuberculosis; studies on mode of action. *Indian J. med. Res.* **49**, 1063—1074 (1961). [D21,370/61

Solomon, H. M., Schrogie, J. J.: Change in receptor site affinity: a proposed explanation for the potentiating effect of D-thyroxine on the anticoagulant response to warfarin. *Clin. Pharmacol. Ther.* **8**, 797—799 (1968).
[H1,868/68

Solotorovsky, M., Gregory, F. J., Stoerk, H. C.: Loss of protection by vaccination following cortisone treatment in mice with experimentally induced tuberculosis. *Proc. Soc. exp. Biol. (N.Y.)* **76**, 286—288 (1951). [B56,305/51

Solymoss, B.: The effect of various steroids, partial hepatectomy, SKF 525-A and cycloheximide on the plasma digitoxin level. *Proc. on Drug metabolism in man.* New York 1970.
[G70,484/70

Solymoss, B.: A máj-microsomális enzymek szerepe a szervezet védedezőreactióiban. Budapest: Medicina (in press). [G79,009

Solymoss, B., Classen, H. G., Varga, S.: Increased hepatic microsomal activity induced by spironolactone and other steroids. *Proc. Soc. exp. Biol. (N.Y.)* **132**, 940—942 (1969).
[G60,054/69

Solymoss, B., Classen, H. G., Varga, S.: The role of electrolyte disturbances and extracellular alkalosis in metabolic cardiac necrosis and the preventive effect of amiloride. *Amer. J. Cardiol.* **26**, 46—51 (1970). [G60,053/70

Solymoss, B., Krajny, M., Varga, S.: Independence of antimineralocorticoid and catatoxic effects of various steroids. *J. pharm. Sci.* **59**, 712—714 (1970). [G60,084/70

Solymoss, B., Krajny, M., Varga, S., Werringloer, J.: Suppression by nucleic acid- and protein-synthesis inhibitors of drug detoxication induced by spironolactone or ethylestrenol. *J. Pharmacol. exp. Ther.* **174**, 473 to 477 (1970). [G70,412/70

Solymoss, B., Selye, H.: Protection by catatoxic steroids against chronic digitoxin and indomethacin intoxication (Abstr.). *Fed. Proc.* **29**, 833 (1970). [G70,409/70

Solymoss, B., Somogyi, A., Kovács, K.: Effect of spironolactone and SKF 525-A on 7,12-dimethylbenz(α)anthracene-induced hematologic changes. *Haematologia* (in press). [G70,445

Solymoss, B., Tóth, S., Varga, S., Krajny, M.: Enhancement of digitoxin biotransformation by spironolactone and other steroids (Abstr.). *Proc. 3rd Ann. Meet. int. Study group for Res. in cardiac metabolism*, Stowe, Vt., p. 66 (1970).
[G70,461/70

Solymoss, B., Tóth, S., Varga, S., Krajny, M.: The influence of spironolactone and other steroids on the plasma level of digitoxin. *Proc. 3rd Ann. Meet. int. Study group for Res. in cardiac metabolism*, Stowe, Vt., p. 71 (1970).
[G70,463/70

Solymoss, B., Tóth, S., Varga, S., Krajny, M.: The influence of spironolactone on its own biotransformation. *Steroids* **16**:3, 263—275 (1970). [G70,464/70

Solymoss, B., Tóth, S., Varga, S., Selye, H.: Protection by spironolactone and oxandrolone against chronic digitoxin or indomethacin intoxication. *Toxicol. appl. Pharmacol.* **18**, 586 to 592 (1971). [G70,441/71

Solymoss, B., Tóth, S., Varga, S., Werringloer, J.: Effect of spironolactone and ethylestrenol on benzo(α)pyrene-hydroxylase and other chemical constituents of hepatic microsomes. *Canad. J. Physiol. Pharmacol.* (in press). [G70,488

Solymoss, B., Varga, S.: Spironolacton és egyéb steroidok hatása bishydroxycumarin enxymaticus lebontására és alvadásgátlo hatására. *Orvosképzée* (in press). [G70,500

Solymoss, B., Varga, S., Classen, H. G.: Effect of various steroids on microsomal aliphatic hydroxylation and N-pealkylation. *Europ. J. Pharmacol.* **10**, 127—130 (1970). [G60,075/70

Solymoss, B., Varga, S., Krajny, M.: Increased drug metabolism induced by various steroids and its suppression by SKF 525-A. *Acta physiol. Acad. Sci. hung.* **37**, 145—149 (1970).
[G60,099/70

Solymoss, B., Varga, S., Krajny, M.: Effect of spironolactone, norbolethone, progesterone, hydroxydione and SKF 525-A on the disappearance rate of indomethacin from blood. *Arzneimittel-Forsch.* **21**, 384 (1971).
[G60,093/71

Solymoss, B., Varga, S., Krajny, M., Werringloer, J.: Influence of spironolactone and other steroids on the enzymatic decay and anticoagulant activity of bishydroxycoumarin. *Thrombos. Diathes. haemorrh. (Stuttg.)* XXIII, No. 3, p. 562—568 (1970). [G70,423/70

Solymoss, B., Werringloer, J., Toth, S.: The influence of pregnenolone-16α-carbonitrile on hepatic mixed-function oxygenases. *Steroids* **17**/4, 427—433 (1971). [G79,015/71

Solymoss, B., Zsigmond, G., Werringloer, J.: Stimulation of sulfobromophthalein sodium (BSP) metabolism and bile flow by spironolactone, pregnenolone-16α-carbonitrile and other steroids. (Abstr.) *Proc. canad. Fed. biol. Soc.* 14, 110 (1971). [G79,007/71

Solymoss, B., Zsigmond, G., Werringloer, J.: Increased sulfobromophthalein sodium (BSP) metabolism and bile flow induced by spironolactone and other steroids. *J. Lab. clin. Med.* (in press). [G79,023

Somlyo, A. P.: The Toxicology of Digitalis. *Amer. J. Cardiol.* 5, 523—533 (1960). [G62,791/60

Sommer, S.: Experimenteller Beitrag zur Reid Hunt-Reaktion mit besonderer Berücksichtigung der Sera von Schwangeren, Eklamptischen und Karzinomkranken und Extrakte aus Schwangerenharn. *Zbl. Gynäk.* 58, 385—388 (1934). [44,648/34

Sommer, S.: Zum Einfluß von somatotropem Hormon und Cortison auf den Verlauf einer experimentellen Trypanosomeninfektion (Trypanosoma cruzi). *Arch. exp. Pathol. Pharm.* 626, 527—531 (1955). [C9937/55

Somogyi, A.: Inhibition of DMBA-induced adrenal necrosis by spironolactone. Workshop on DMBA Activity, Laval Univ. Quebec City, p. 55—56 (1969). [G70,406/69

Somogyi, A.: The effect of various steroids on certain biologic actions 7,12-dimethylbenz(α)anthracene. *Thesis*, University of Montreal (1970). [G70,416/70

Somogyi, A., Kovács, K.: Inhibition by spironolactone of 7-hydroxymethyl-12-methylbenz(α)anthracene-induced adrenal necrosis in rats. *Endokrinologie* 56, 245—247 (1970). [G60,061/70

Somogyi, A., Kovács, K.: Effect of various steroids on the adrenal necrosis induced by 7,12-dimethylbenz(α)anthracene in rats. *Rev. canad. Biol.* 29, 169—180 (1970). [G60,074/70

Somogyi, A., Kovács, K.: Effect of stress on the adrenocorticolytic and carcinogenic action of 7,12-dimethylbenz(α)anthracene. *Z. Krebsforsch.* 75, 288—295 (1971). [G70,482/71

Song, C. S., Kappas, A.: The influence of estrogens, progestins and pregnancy on the liver. *Vitam. and Horm.* 26, 147—195 (1968). [G68,413/68

Song, C. S., Kappas, A.: The influence of hormones on hepatic function. In: Popper, H. and Schaffner, F., Progress in liver diseases., pp. 89—109. New York, London: Grune and Stratton, 3, 1970. [G80,521/70

Song, C. S., Rifkind, A. B., Gillette, P. N., Kappas, A.: Hormones and the liver. The effect of estrogens, pogrestins, and pregnancy on hepatic function. *Amer. J. Obstet. Gynec.* 105, 813—847 (1969). [G70,575/69

Soriano, L.: Etude sur la différenciation in vitro de l'épithélium oesophagien embryonnaire de souris. Action de la vitamine A et de l'hydrocortisone. *J. Embryol. exp. Morph.* 17, 247—261 (1967). [G44,574/67

Soroff, H. S., Rozin, R. R., Mooty, J., Lister, J., Raben, M. S.: Role of human growth hormone in the response to trauma. I. Metabolic effects following burns. *Ann. Surg.* 166, 739—752 (1967). [G52,127/67

Sotaniemi, E., Arvela, P., Hakkarainen, H., Huhti, E.: The clinical significance of microsomal enzyme induction in the therapy of epileptic patients. *Ann. clin. Res.* 2, 223—227 (1970). [G78,917/70

Souda, S.: Correlation between mitotic activity and DPN content of regenerating liver in normal and cortisone-treated rats. *J. Fac. Sci. Univ. (Tokyo)* 9, 379 (1962). [D62,846/62

Southam, C. M., Babcock, V. I.: Effect of cortisone, related hormones, and adrenalectomy, on susceptibility of mice to virus infections. *Proc. Soc. exp. Biol. (N.Y.)* 78, 105—109 (1951). [B63,662/51

Southren, A. L., Gordon, G. G.: Studies in androgen metabolism. *Mt. Sinai J. Med.* 37, 516—527 (1970). [G77,117/70

Southren, A. L., Gordon, G. G., Altman, K.: Inhibition of cortisol induction of rat liver tryptophan pyrrolase by 6β-hydroxycortisol. *Program 48th Meet. Endocr. Soc.*, June, Chicago, Ill., p. 101, 1966. [F66,647/66

Southren, A. L., Gordon, G. G., Tochimoto, S., Krikun, E., Krieger, D., Jacobson, M., Kuntzman, R.: Effect of N-phenylbarbital (phetharbital) on the metabolism of testosterone and cortisol in man. *J. clin. Endocr.* 29, 251—256 (1969). [H8,265/69

Southren, A. L., Tochimoto, S., Isurugi, D., Gordon, G. G., Drikun, E., Stypulkowski, W.: The effect of 2,2-bis (2 chlorophenyl-4 chlorophenyl)-1, 1-dichloroethane (o,p′-DDD) on the metabolism of infused cortisol 7-3H. *Steroids* 7, 11—29 (1966). [F73,262/66

Southren, A. L., Tochimoto, S., Strom, L., Ratuschni, A., Ross, H., Gordon, G.: Remission in Cushing's syndrome with o,p′-DDD. *J. clin. Endocr.* 26, 268—278 (1966). [F63,163/66

Soyka, L. F.: Determinants of in vitro binding of barbiturates by rat hepatic subcellular fractions. *Proc. Soc. exp. Biol. (N.Y.)* **128**, 322—325 (1968). [H 30,981/68

Soyka, L. F.: Determinants of hepatic aminopyrine demethylase activity. *Biochem. Pharmacol.* **18**, 1029—1038 (1969). [G 66,626/69

Soyka, L. F., Campbell, P., Gyermek, L.: Metabolism and distribution of pregnanolone, a pharmacologically active metabolite of progesterone. (Abstr.) *Clin. Res.* **18**, 125 (1970). [H 33,315/70

Soyka, L. F., Gyermek, L., Campbell, P.: A study of the mechanism responsible for the sensitivity of newborn rats to pregnanolone. *J. Pharmacol. exp. Ther.* **175**, 276—282 (1970). [H 31,803/70

Spain, D. M.: Symposium on cortisone and ACTH studies on the effect of cortisone on the guinea pig's resistance to tuberculosis. *Trans. nat. Ass. Tuberc. (Lond.)* 47th Ann. Meet. May 14—18, p. 41—46 (1951). [B 69,019/51

Spain, D. M., Molomut, N.: Effects of cortisone on the development of tuberculous lesions in guinea pigs and on their modification by streptomycin therapy. *Amer. Rev. Tuberc.* **62**, 337—344 (1950). [B 60,878/50

Spain, D. M., Molomut, N.: The effect of cortisone-streptomycin on experimental tuberculosis in guinea pigs. *Proc. N. Y. St. Ass. Publ. Hlth Lab.* **30**, 7—8 (1950). [B 80,256/50

Sparano, B. M.: Sex difference in chlortetracycline-induced fatty livers in rats. *Lab. Invest.* **14**, 1931—1938 (1965). [F 71,594/65

Specchia, G.: Azione del Luminal sull'ittero anemolitico a bilirubinemia indiretta dell' adulto: descrizione di un caso. *Minerva Med.* **61**, 2068—2071 (1970). [H 27,907/70

Specht, O.: Weitere Untersuchungen an Meerschweinchen über den Einfluß endokriner Drüsen auf die Krampffähigkeit und die elektrische Erregbarkeit. *Bruns' Beitr. klin. Chir.* **128**, 25—53 (1923). [13,475/23

Speck, L. B.: Toxicity and effects of increasing doses of mescaline. *J. Pharmacol. exp. Ther.* **119**, 78—84 (1957). [C 31,193/57

Speirs, R. S.: Effect of oxytetracycline upon cortisone-induced pseudotuberculosis in mice. *Antibiot. and Chemother.* **6**, 395—399 (1956). [C 34,744/56

Spencer, P. S. J., Waite, R.: Barbiturate-induced sleep in hyperthyroid mice. *Europ. J. Pharmacol.* **11**, 392—394 (1970). [H 30,100/70

Spencer, P. S. J., West, G. B.: Further observations on the relationship between the thyroid gland and the anaphylactoid reaction in rats. *Int. Arch. Allergy* **20**, 321—343 (1962). [D 32,617/62

Spiegel, E.: Anticonvulsant effects of desoxycorticosterone, testosterone and progesterone. *Fed. Proc.* **2**, 47 (1943). [83,892/43

Spiegel, E., Wycis, H.: Anticonvulsant effects of steroids. *J. Lab. clin. Med.* **30**, 947—953 (1945). [93,925/45

Spiess-Bertschinger, A.: Die Bedeutung der Schilddrüse für die Reaktionsweise der Leber bei experimenteller Schädigung. *Virchows Arch. pathol Anat.* **312**, 601—615 (1944). [B 40,585/44

Spigolon, G.: Ascite sperimentale da legatura lenta della vena porta associata a,'tiroidectomia chimica da tioureici'. *Ormonologia* **11**, 201—208 (1949). [B 52,689/49

Spinelli, A.: Influenza della tiroide sull' avvelenamento acuto da istamina. *Boll. Soc. ital. Biol. sper.* **4**, 937—941 (1929). [14,294/29

Spinelli, A.: Ricerche sulle variazioni di sensibilità verso alcune sostanze tossiche, conseguenti alla ablazione della tiroide nella cavia (Abstr.). *Riv. Pat. sper.* **7**, 294—323 (1931). [10,086/31

Spinelli, A.: Osservazioni intorno ai rapporti tra funzione tiroidea e anafilassi. I. Influenza della tiroidectomia sullo shock anafilattico nella cavia. *Riv. Pat. sper.* **9**, 212—221 (1932). [7,369/32

Spinelli, A.: Azione protettiva della tiroide contro l'intossicazione guanidinica nella cavia. *Arch. Fisiol.* **31**, 598—608 (1932). [7,409/32

Spink, W. W.: The pathogenesis and management of shock due to infection. *Arch. intern. Med.* **106**, 433—442 (1960). [C 91,027/60

Spink, W. W.: Endotoxin shock. *Ann. intern. Med.* **57**, 538—552 (1962). [D 39,028/62

Spink, W. W., Anderson, D.: Experimental studies on the significance of endotoxin in the pathogenesis of brucellosis. *J. clin. Invest.* **33**, 540—548 (1954). [B 95,168/54

Spink, W. W., Vick, J.: Evaluation of plasma, metaraminol and hydrocortisone in experimental endotoxin shock. *Circulat. Res.* **9**, 184—188 (1961). [C 98,717/61

Spink, W. W., Vick, J. A.: Reversal of experimental endotoxin shock with a combination of aldosterone and metaraminol. *Proc. Soc. exp. Biol. (N.Y.)* **107**, 777—779 (1961). [D 12,885/61

Spink, W. W., Vick, J. A., Melby, J. C., Finstad, J.: Influence of aldosterone and angiotensin II on endotoxin shock in the primate. *Proc. Soc. exp. Biol. (N.Y.)* 112, 795—799 (1963). [D 61,007/63

Spinks, A., Burn, J. H.: Thyroid activity and amine oxidase in the liver. *Brit. J. Pharmacol.* 7, 93—98 (1952). [B 72,891/52

Spode, E.: Über den Stoffwechsel von Radio-Quecksilber (^{203}Hg) im Organismus der weißen Maus unter Berücksichtigung von Dekorporationsmaßnahmen. *Z. ges. inn. Med.* 15, 603 bis 609 (1960). [G 72,979/60

Spremolla, G., Grassi, B.: Nefropatia da deplezione potassica. Rilievi istologici ed umorali in corso di trattamento con steroidi anabolizzanti. *Minerva nefrol.* 10, 5—11 (1963). [G 68,941/63

Sprunt, D. H., McDearman, S.: Studies on the relationship of sex hormones to infection. III. A quantitative study of the increased resistance to vaccinial infection produced by the estrogenic hormone and pseudopregnancy. *J. Immunol.* 38, 81—95 (1940). [A 33,321/40

Srebro, Z., Slebodzinski, A., Szirmai, E.: Radiation disease in hypo- and hyperthyreotic rats. *Agressologie* 11, 343—356 (1970). [H 32,848/70

Srinivasan, S., Balwani, J. H.: Effect of thyroxine on thioacetamide hepatotoxicity. *Acta pharmacol. (Kbh.)* 26, 475—481 (1968). [G 64,503/68

Srinivasan, S., Srinivasan, U., Balwani, J. H.: Effect of thyroxine, reserpine and serotonin on allyl alcohol induced hepatotoxicity in rats. *Acta pharmacol. (Kbh.)* 28, 338—345 (1970). [G 78,977/70

Srivastava, P. N., Etoh, H., Hyodo, Y., Egami, N.: Thyroid activity and radiosensitivity relationship in goldfish, Carassius auratus L. *Strahlentherapie* 125, 305—308 (1964). [G 23,764/64

Stahnke, H. L.: Stress and the toxicity of venoms. *Science* 150, 1456—1457 (1965). [F 57,253/65

Stalhandske, T.: Effects of increased liver metabolism of nicotine on its uptake, elimination and toxicity in mice. *Acta physiol. scand.* 80, 222—234 (1970). [G 80,388/70

Stalhandske, T., Slanina, P.: Effect of nicotine treatment on the metabolism of nicotine in the mouse liver in vitro. *Acta pharmacol. (Kbh.)* 28, 75—80 (1970). [G 73,544/70

Stamler, J., Pick, R., Katz, L. N.: Prevention of coronary atherosclerosis by estrogen-androgen administration in the cholesterol-fed chick. *Circulat. Res.* 1, 94—98 (1953). [B 91,353/53

Stamler, J., Pick, R., Katz, L. N.: Further observations on the effects of thyroid hormone preparations on cholesterolemia and atherogenesis in cholesterol-fed cockerels. *Circulat. Res.* 6, 825—829 (1958). [C 81,655/58

Stämpfli, H.: Der Einfluß der Thymusdrüse auf die Empfindlichkeit gegen Sauerstoffmangel mit besonderer Berücksichtigung des Atmungszentrums. *Biochem. Z.* 185, 192—204 (1927). [931/27

Stanbury, J. B., Morris, M. L., Corrigan, H. L., Lassiter, W. E.: Thyroxine deiodination by a microsomal preparation requiring FE, oxygen, and cysteine or glutathione. *Endocrinology* 67, 353—362 (1960). [C 90,693/60

Starnes, W. R.: Metabolism of dexamethasone by rat liver. *Ala. J. med. Sci.* 6, 149—151 (1969) [G 68,434/69

Starr, T. J., Pollard, M.: Susceptibility of cortisone-treated mice to infection with mouse hepatitis virus. *Proc. Soc. exp. Biol. (N.Y.)* 99, 108—110 (1958). [C 60,012/58

Stasney, J., Paschkis, K. E., Cantarow, A., Rothenberg, M. S.: Neoplasms in rats with 2-acetaminofluorene and sex hormones. *Cancer Res.* 7, 356—362 (1947). [B 26,653/47

Staudinger, H., Degkwitz, E., Ullrich, V.: Oxidativer Arzneimittelabbau. *Med. Welt (Stuttg.)* 20, 2747—2754 (1969). [H 20,267/69

Stavinoha, W. B., Emerson, G. A., Nash, J. B.: The effects of some sulfur compounds on thallotoxicosis in mice. *Toxicol. appl. Pharmacol.* 1, 638—646 (1959). [C 94,628/59

Stearner, S. P., Christian, E. J. B., Brues, A. M.: Protective action of low oxygen tension and epinephrine against X-ray mortality in the chick. *Amer. J. Physiol.* 176, 455—460 (1954). [B 92,163/54

Stechschulte, D. J.: Plasmodium berghei infection in thymectomized rats. *Proc. Soc. exp. Biol. (N.Y.)* 131, 748—752 (1969). [H 15,256/69

Steelman, S. L., Brooks, J. R., Morgan, E. R., Patanelli, D. J.: Antiandrogenic activity of spironolactone. *Steroids* 14, 449—450 (1969). [G 69,340/69

Stein, R. J., Kent, G., Popper, H.: Effect of cortisone and growth hormone upon ductular cell proliferation in liver ethionine intoxication. *Proc. Soc. exp. Biol. (N.Y.)* 99, 24—28 (1958). [C 59,992/58

Steinbach, M. M.: Experimental tuberculosis in the albino rat. The comparative effects of avitaminosis, suprarenalectomy and thyroid-parathyroidectomy on experimental tuberculosis. *Amer. Rev. Tuberc.* **26**, 52—76 (1932). [92,528/32

Steinbach, M. M., Duca, C. J., Molomut, N.: Experimental tuberculosis in hypophysectomized rats. *Amer. Rev. Tuberc.* **49**, 105—108 (1944). [B 7,316/44

Steiner, A., Davidson, J. D., Kendall, F. E.: Further studies on the production of arteriosclerosis in dogs by cholesterol and thiouracil feeding. *Amer. Heart J.* **36**, 13 (1948). [B 28,166/48

Steiner, P. E., Martinez, B.: Effects on the rat liver of bile duct, portal vein and hepatic artery ligations. *Amer. J. Path.* **39**, 257—289 (1961). [D 40,903/61

Steinetz, B.G., Leathem, J.H.: Effects of methylandrostenediol on weight and cholesterol content of adrenals of cortisone or thiouraciltreated rats. *Proc. Soc. exp. Biol. (N.Y.)* **108** 113—115 (1961). [D 14,466/61

Stender, H. S., Hornykiewytsch, T.: Der Einfluß der O_2-Spannung auf die Strahlenempfindlichkeit bei Ganzkörperbestrahlung. *Strahlentherapie* **96**, 445—452 (1955). [C 37,079/55

Stender, H. S., Hornykiewytsch, T.: Die Abhängigkeit des Dosiseffektes von der Sauerstoffspannung und Reaktionslage bei Ganzkörperbestrahlung. *Z. Naturforsch.* **10**, 32—34 (1955). [C 37,086/55

Stenger, R.J.: Organelle pathology of the liver. The endoplasmic reticulum. *Gastroenterology* **58**, 554—574 (1970). [G 74,578/70

Stenger, R.J., Miller, R.A., Williamson, J.N.: Effects of phenobarbital pretreatment on the hepatotoxicity of carbon tetrachloride. *Exp. molec. Path.* **13**, 242—252 (1970). [G 78,940/70

Stenram, U.: The effect of vitamin B_{12} and the animal protein factor on thyroid-fed rats, with special reference to liver cytology. *Exp. Cell. Res.* **3**, 147—153 (1952). [B 69,173/52

Stenram, U.: The ultrastructure of the liver in thyroid-fed rats. *Z. Zellforsch.* **100**, 402—410 (1969). [G 70,339/69

Stenram, U., Nordgren, H., Willén, R.: Liver ultrastructure and RNA labelling after partial hepatectomy in protein-fed and protein-deprived rats. *Virchows Arch. Abt. B Zellpathol.* **6**, 12—23 (1970). [H 30,015/70

Sterental, A., Dominguez, J.M., Weissman, C., Pearson, O.H.: Pituitary role in the estrogen dependency of experimental mammary cancer. *Cancer Res.* **23**, 481—484 (1963). [D 61,608/63

Stern, E., Mickey, M.R.: Neural mechanism in induction of dioestrus and tumor in the androgen sterile rat. *Nature (Lond.)* **216**, 185—187 (1967). [F 89,080/67

Stern, L., Khanna, N. N., Levy, G., Yaffe, S. J.: Effect of phenobarbital on hyperbilirubinemia and glucuronide formation in newborns. *Amer. J. Dis. Child.* **120**, 26—31 (1970). [G 76,135/70

Stewart, R. B.: The effect of cortisone on the lethality of psittacosis virus for the chick embryo. *J. infect. Dis.* **103**, 129—134 (1958). [C 59,979/58

St. George, S., Bine, R., Jr., Friedman, M.: Role of the liver in excretion and destruction of digitoxin. *Circulation* **6**, 661—665 (1952). [G 71,843/52

Stitzel, R. E., Furner, R. L.: Stress-induced alterations in microsomal drug metabolism in the rat. *Biochem. Pharmacol.* **16**, 1489—1494 (1967). [G 48,920/67

Stöcker, E.: Autoradiographische Untersuchungen zum zellulären Proliferationsstoffwechsel im Parenchym von Leber und Niere der Ratte. *Acta histochem. (Jena)*, Sup. 8, 205—229 (1968). [G 76,916/68

Stoerk, H. C., Boeninghaus, J., Celozzi, E.: Interactions of parathormone and hydrocortisone on endochondral ossification. *Fed. Proc.* **22**, 546 (1963). [G 5,410/63

Stoffel, W.: Biosynthesis of polyenoic fatty acids. *Biochem. biophys. Res. Commun.* **6**, 270 to 273 (1961). [G 66,819/61

Stolk, A.: Effect of castration on experimental liver lesion in Iguana iguana. *Nature (Lond.)* **190**, 93 (1961). [D 2,285/61

Stoppani, A. O. M., Brignone, C. M. C. de, Brigone, J. A.: Structural requirements for the action of steroids as inhibitors of electron transfer. *Arch. Biochem.* **127**, 463—475 (1968). [H 19,278/68

Störtebecker, T. P.: Further results concerning the acute antinarcotic effect of estrone. *Skand. Arch. Physiol.* **77**, 78 (1937). [69,765/37

Störtebecker, T. P.: Die Antinarkotische Wirkung von Follikulin und Testishormon. *Klin. Wschr.* **16**, 302—303 (1937). [A 1,993/37

Störtebecker, T. P.: Hormones and resistance. An acute antinarcotic and antitoxic effect of the estrogenic hormones. *Acta path. microbiol. scand.* Sup. 41, 294 (1939). [76,398/39

Stowe, C. M., Plaa, G. L.: Extrarenal excretion of drugs and chemicals. *Ann. Rev. Pharmacol.* **8**, 337—356 (1968). [G 73,241/68

Straube, R. L., Patt, H. M., Swift, M. N.: Influence of estrogens on x-ray toxicity. *Amer. J. Physiol.* 155, 471 (1948). [B33,113/48]

Straube, R. L., Patt, H. M., Tyree, E. B., Smith, D. E.: Influence of level of adrenal cortical steroids on sensitivity of mice to X-irradiation. *Proc. Soc. exp. Biol. (N.Y.)* 71, 539—541 (1949). [B39,082/49]

Strebel, R. F., Dickinson, E. O., Payan, H., Bouverot, M.: Effect of pregnancy and lactation on an aging-like syndrome of rats (Abstr.). *Fed. Proc.* 24, 165 (1965). [F35,901/65]

Strebel, R. F., Payan, H., House, E. L., Pansky, B., Barath, M.: Sex differences in a progeria-like syndrome. *Proc. Soc. exp. Biol. (N.Y.)* 117, 583—586 (1964). [F25,229/64]

Strebel, R. F., Payan, H., Levine, S.: Thymic calcification in the neonatal rat. *Proc. Soc. exp. Biol. (N.Y.)* 118, 617—620 (1965). [F34,734/65]

Street, J. C., Chadwick, R. W., Wang, M., Phillips, R. L.: Insecticide interactions affecting residue storage in animal tissues. *J. agric. Food. Chem.* 14, 545—549 (1966). [G75,678/66]

Streffer, C., Langendorff, H., Allert, U.: Untersuchungen über einen biologischen Strahlenschutz. 83. Mitteilg. Über die Schutzwirksamkeit des 5-Hydroxytryptamins bei Teilkörperbestrahlung. *Strahlentherapie* 135, 76—82 (1968). [G55,078/68]

Strehler, E., Sollberger, H.: Der Einfluß von Cholesterin, Mais und Tetramethylthioharnstoff auf die Entstehung und Form der Masuginephritis des Kaninchens. *Helv. med. Acta* 17, 79—90 (1950). [B54,646/50]

Streicher, E., Garbus, J.: The effect of age and sex on the duration of hexobarbital anesthesia in rats. *J. Geront.* 10, 441—444 (1955). [G76,681/55]

Streuli, H.: Das Verhalten von schilddrüsenlosen, milzlosen, schilddrüsen- und milzlosen Tieren bei O_2-Mangel, zugleich ein Beitrag zur Theorie der Bergkrankheit. *Biochem. Z.* 87, 359—417 (1918). [32,220/18]

Stripp, B., Hamrick, M., Zampaglione, N.: Effect of spironolactone treatment of rats on the oxidation of drugs by liver microsomes (Abstr.). *Fed. Proc.* 29, 346 (1970). [H22,743/70]

Stripp, B., Hamrick, M. E., Zampaglione, N. C., Gillette, J. R.: The effect of spironolactone on drug metabolism by hepatic microsomes. *J. Pharmacol. exp. Ther.* 176, 766—771 (1971). [G79,538/71]

Strittmatter, C. F., Umberger, F. T.: Oxidative enzyme components of avian liver microsomes. Changes during embryonic development and the effects of phenobarbital administration. *Biochim. biophys. Acta (Amst.)* 180, 18—27 (1969). [G66,629/69]

Ströder, J., Garbe, A., Hiller, H.: Rachitisheilung unter Cortison. *Klin. Wschr.* 40, 1014 bis 1015 (1962). [D36,990/62]

Stromberg, K., Reuber, M. D.: Influence of age and sex on hepatic lesions induced by chemical carcinogenesis: ingestion of N-4-(4'-fluorobiphenyl)acetamide by Buffalo strain rats. *J. nat. Cancer Inst.* 44, 1047—1054 (1970). [G75,306/70]

Strong, F. M.: Deleterious compounds in foods. *Amer. J. clin. Nutr.* 11, 500—501 (1962). [G73,964/62]

Strong, F. M., Lalich, J. J., Lipton, S. H., Sievert, H. W., Garbutt, J. T.: Aminonitriles related to rat lathyrism (odoratism). (Abstr.). *4th Int. Congr. Biochem. Wien*, p. 100 (1958). [G61,885/58]

Strubelt, O., Sieger, C. P., Breining, H.: Der Einfluß von Noradrenaline auf die Hepatotoxicität von Tetrachlorkohlenstoff und Allylalkohol. *Arch. Toxikol.* 27, 53—66 (1970). [G80,282/70]

Strubelt, O., Steffen, J., Stutz, U.: Der Einfluß der Schilddrüsenfunktion auf die chronotropen und einige metabolische Wirkungen von Theophyllin und Coffein. *Naunyn-Schmiedebergs Arch. Pharmak.* 267, 135—154 (1970). [G78,572/70]

Studer, A.: Zur Frage der Angriffsorte von Compound E (Cortison). Eine experimentelle Studie. *Z. ges. exp. Med.* 121, 287—418 (1953). [B89,161/53]

Stuhlfauth, K., Englhardt-Gölkel, A.: Über die Beeinflussung der Schlafzeit nach Pentothal-Natrium bei normalen und nebennierenlosen Ratten durch Glucose und Fructose. *Naunyn-Schmiedebergs Arch. Pharmak.* 221, 328—335 (1954). [G78,396/54]

Stumpf, H. H., Wilens, S. L.: Inhibitory effect of cortisone hyperlipemia on arterial lipid deposition in cholesterol-fed rabbits. *Proc. Soc. exp. Biol. (N.Y.)* 86, 219—223 (1954). [G95,325/54]

Stupfel, M., Bouley, G., Romary, F., Magnier, M., Champsavin, M. de, Polianski, J.: Facteurs sexuels et résistance à l'hypoxie expérimentale. *C. R. Acad. Sci. (Paris)* 272, 1120—1122 (1971). [G82,171/71]

Sturtevant, F. M.: The vascular reactivity of normotensive and metacorticoid hypertensive rats. *Anat. Rec.* **122**, 479 (1955). [C9,089/55

Sturtevant, F. M.: Studies on vascular reactivity in normotensive and metacorticoid hypertensive rats. *Amer. Heart J.* **52**, 410—418 (1956). [C21,591/56

Sturtevant, F. M.: Prolongation of hexobarbital-hypnosis in mice by iproniazid, serotonin, and reserpine. *Naturwissenschaften* **43**, 67—68 (1956). [D87,568/56

Sturtevant, F. M.: Antihypertensive effects of an aldosterone antagonist. *Science* **127**, 1393 to 1394 (1958). [C54,613/58

Suchowsky, G. K., Junkmann, K.: Über zwei neue anabol wirksame Steroide. *Klin. Wschr.* **39**, 369—371 (1961). [D2,674/61

Sugihara, R.: The ultrastructure of regenerating parenchymal cells of the albino rat liver. (Japanese text.) *Jap. J. clin. Elect. Micr.* **1**, 143—157 (1969). [H18,030/69

Sugiura, K.: Chemotherapy of induced skin tumors in mice. *Gann* **59**, 367—376 (1968). [G64,932/68

Suhrmann, R.: Weitere Versuche über die Temperaturadaptation der Karauschen (Carassius vulgaris NILS.) *Biol. Ztrbl.* **74**, 432 bis 448 (1955). [D76,901/55

Šulcová, J., Stárka, L.: Extrahepatic 7α-hydroxylation of dehydroepiandrosterone. *Experientia (Basel)* **19**, 632—633 (1963). [E37,298/63

Sulman, F. G., Khazan, N., Steiner, J. E.: Biotransformation of prednisone by "trained" blocked and "untrained" liver enzymes. *Arch. int. Pharmacodyn.* **122**, 180—189 (1959). [C79,823/59

Sulser, F., Kunz, H. A., Gantenbein, R., Wilbrandt, W.: Zur Frage einer antagonistischen Wirkung zwischen Herzglykosiden und Corticosteroiden auf die Elektrolytausscheidung der Niere. *Naunyn-Schmiedebergs Arch. Pharmak.* **235**, 400—411 (1959). [D96,543/59

Sundaresan, P. R., Winters, V. G., Therriault, D. G.: Effect of low environment temperature on the metabolism of vitamin A (retinol) in the rat. *J. Nutr.* **92**, 474—478 (1967). [G50,127/67

Sunderman, F. W., Jr.: Effect of nickel carbonyl upon incorporation of ^{14}C-leucine into hepatic microsomal proteins. *Res. Commun. chem. Path. Pharmacol.* **1**, 161—168 (1970). [G73,628/70

Sunderman, F. W., Jr., Leibman, K. C.: Nickel carbonyl inhibition of induction of aminopyrine demethylase activity in liver and lung. *Cancer Res.* **30**, 1645—1650 (1970). [H28,301/70

Sung, C. Y., Way, E. L.: The effect of altered thyroid function on the actions and fate of DL-methadone. *J. Pharmacol. exp. Ther.* **108**, 1—10 (1953). [B91,323/53

Sure, B., Buchanan, K. S.: Antithyrogenic action of crystalline vitamin B. *J. Nutr.* **13**, 513—519 (1937). [A6,259/37

Sure, B., Buchanan, K. S.: Influence of hyperthyroidism on vitamin A reserves of the albino rat. *J. Nutr.* **13**, 521—524 (1937). [A48,611/37

Süssmann, H.: Experimentelle Studien mit Parathormone-Collip an weißen Mäusen. *Z. ges. exp. Med.* **56**, 817—830 (1927). [24,462/27

Sutherland, J. M., Keller, W. H.: Novobiocin and neonatal hyperbilirubinemia. An investigation of the relationship in an epidemic of neonatal hyperbilirubinemia. *A. M. A. Amer. J. Dis. Child.* **101**, 447—453 (1961). [G78,607/61

Suzman, M. M., Freed, C. C., Prag, J. J.: Studies on experimental peripheral vascular disease, with special reference to thromboangeitis obliterans. The effect of ovarian follicular hormone and of castration on the development of the trophic changes produced by ergotamine tartrate in albino rats. *S. Afr. J. med. Sci.* **3**, 29—39 (1938). [A44,452/38

Suzue, K., Sano, A., Yosida, H.: Über die Beziehungen der Schilddrüsenfunktionsstörungen zur Bildung der sogenannten Xanthominseln durch Fettüberfütterung. *Trans. Soc. Path. jap.* **26**, 480—483 (1936). [38,509/36

Svedmyr, N.: The influence of thyroxine treatment and thyroidectomy on the calorigenic and some other metabolic effects of adrenaline and noradrenaline in experiments on fasted rabbits. *Acta physiol. scand.* **66**, 257—268 (1966). [G39,171/66

Svirbely, J. L.: The effect of desiccated thyroid, α-dinitrophenol, and cortical hormone extract on the vitamin C content of some organs of the guinea pig fed graded doses of ascorbic acid. *J. biol. Chem.* **111**, 147—154 (1935). [33,140/35

Svoboda, D., Azarnoff, D., Reddy, J.: Microbodies in experimentally altered cells. II. The relationship of microbody proliferation to endocrine glands. *J. Cell Biol.* **40**, 734—746 (1969). [G64,564/69

Swann, H. E., Jr., Woodson, G. S., Ballard, T. A.: The acute toxicity of intramuscular parathion in rats and the relation of weight, sex and sex hormones to this toxicity. *Amer. industr. Hyg. J.* **19**, 190—195 (1958). [C73,379/58

Swann, H. G.: The relation of morphine withdrawal symptoms in the rat to the thyroid gland. *Proc. Amer. physiol. Soc.*, 53rd Ann. Meet., Chicago, Ill., p. 279 (1941). [80,669/41

Swanson, H. E.: Interrelations between thyroxin and adrenalin in the regulation of oxygen consumption in the albino rat. *Endocrinology* 59, 217—225 (1956). [C 22,149/56

Swartz, F. J.: Polyploidization of liver after partial hepatectomy in the dwarf mouse and hypophysectomized rat; effect of extended regenerative periods. *Exp. Cell. Res.* 48, 557 to 568 (1967). [G 53,670/67

Swedberg, B.: Studies in experimental tuberculosis. An investigation of some problems of immunity and resistance. *Acta med. scand.* 139, Sup. 254, 1—120 (1951). [B 59,988/51

Swedberg, B., Dahlström, G., Luft, R.: The effect of adrenocorticotrophic hormone (ACTH) on experimental tuberculosis in mice; preliminary report. *Acta endocr. (Kbh.)* 6, 215—220 (1951). [B 58,412/51

Swensson, A., Ulfarson, U.: Experiments with different antidotes in acute poisoning by different mercury compounds. Effects on survival and on distribution and excretion of mercury. *Int. Arch. Gewerbepathol. Gewerbehygiene* 24, 12—50 (1967). [F 89,451/67

Swingle, W. W., Overman, R. R., Remington, J. W., Kleinberg, W., Eversole, W. J.: Ineffectiveness of adrenal cortex preparations in the treatment of experimental shock in non-adrenalectomized dogs. *Amer. J. Physiol.* 139, 481—489 (1943). [A 61,337/43

Swinyard, E. A., Schiffman, D. O., Goodman, L. S.: Effect of variations in extracellular sodium concentration on the susceptibility of mice to pentylenetetrazole (metrazol)-induced seizures. *J. Pharmacol. exp. Ther.* 114, 160 to 166 (1955). [C 17,213/55

Swinyard, E. A., Weaver, L. C., Goodman, L. S.: Effect of liver injury and nephrectomy on the anti-convulsant activity of clinically useful hydantoins. *J. Pharmacol. exp. Ther.* 104, 309—316 (1952). [G 74,657/52

Swyer, G. I. M., Little, V.: Absence of hepatic impairment in long-term oral-contraceptive users. *Brit. med. J.* 1965 I, 1412—1414. [F 42,188/65

Symeonidis, A.: Inibizione della formazione dei tumori epatici nei topi C 3 Hf surrenalectomizzati. *Minerva med.* 61, 1863—1868 (1970). [H 27,336/70

Symeonidis, A., Mulay, A. S., Burgoyne, F. H.: Effect of adrenalectomy and of desoxycorticosterone acetate on the formation of liver lesions in rats fed p-dimethylaminoazobenzene. *J. nat. Cancer Inst.* 14, 805—817 (1954). [B 93,003/54

Symons, A. M., Lewis, D. A., Ancill, R. J.: The uptake of anti-inflammatory steroids by lysosomes. *J. Pharm. Pharmacol.* 22, 944—945 (1970). [G 80,345/70

Szablowska, M., Selye, H.: L'Influence des hormones sur l'intoxication par l'ethylène glycol (Abstr.). *Ann. ACFAS* (38e Congr.) Sup. 37, 12 (1970). [G 70,499/70

Szablowska, M., Selye, H.: Hormonal influences upon ethylene glycol poisoning. *Arch. environm. Hlth* 23, 13—17 (1971). [G 70,475/71

Szabó, G., Sátori, O. Grandtner, G.: Prevention and treatment of shock with corticosteroids. Effect of prednisolone in norepinephrine- and epinephrine-induced shock. *Acta med. Acad. Sci. hung.* 23, 49—52 (1966). [G 44,867/66

Szabó, S.: Catatoxic steroids. 10th *Med. Days*, Subotica, Yugoslavia, June 24—28 (1970). [G 70,456/70

Szabó, S.: Katatoksični steroidi. In: Perčič, V.: *Zbornik Radova Internistickih Dana* (in press). [G 70,498

Szabó, S., Kovacs, K., Garg, B. D., Khandekar, J. D., Selye, H.: Effect of pregnenolone-16α-carbonitrile upon drug intoxication and hepatic ultrastructure in hypophysectomized rats. (Abstr.) *Proc. canad. Fed. biol. Soc.* 14, 135 (1971). [G 79,024/71

Szabó, S., Selye, H.: L'effet de l'hypophysectomie et des stéroïdes catatoxiques sur la toxicité du parathion et du navadel (Abstr.). *Ann. ACFAS* (38e Congr.) Sup., 37, 12 (1970). [G 70,497/70

Szabó, S., Selye, H.: Inhibition by hypophysectomy of nephrocalcinosis produced by mercuric chloride. *Urol. int. (Basel)* 26, 39—44 (1971). [G 70,478/71

Szabó, S., Selye, H.: Adrenal apoplexy and necrosis produced by acrylonitrile. *Endokrinologie* (in press). [G 70,493

Szabó, S., Selye, H.: Adrenal apoplexy produced by acrylonitrile and its prevention by ACTH and hypophysectomy. (Abstr.) *Fed. Proc.* 30, 307 (1971). [G 79,010/71

Szabó, S., Selye, H., Mecs, I.: Katatoxikus steroidok hatasa az indomethacin és digitoxin mérgezésre hörcsögökben. *Kisérl. Orvostud.* (in press). [G 79,013

Szarvas, F., Kovács, K.: Die Untersuchung der Serotoninwirkung bei der mit Hormonen hervorgerufenen Nierenrindennekrose bei Ratten. *Med. exp. (Basel)* 9, 241—248 (1963). [E 34,633/63

Szeberényi, S., Fekete, G.: Influence of spironolactone on the action and metabolism of various drugs. (Abstr.) *Excerpta med.* (Amst.), Int. Congr. Ser. No. 210, p. 182—183 (1970) 3rd. Int. Congr. on Hormonal steroids, Hamburg. [H 29,579/70]

Szeberényi, S., Garattini, S.: Effect of metopirone on the rate of cortisol disappearance from plasma. *Biochem. Pharmacol.* 18, 927 to 928 (1969). [G 66,140/69]

Szeberényi, S., Szalay, K. S., Garattini, S.: Removal of plasma metyrapone in rats submitted to previous pharmacological treatment. *J. Pharm. Pharmacol.* 21, 201—202 (1969). [G 64,752/69]

Szego, C. M., Roberts, S.: Steroid action and interaction in uterine metabolism. *Recent Progr. Hormone Res.* 8, 419—469 (1953). [B 73,573/53]

Szeri, I., Bános, Z., Anderlik, P., Balázs, M., Földes, P.: Pathogenesis of the wasting syndrome following neonatal thymectomy. *Acta microbiol. Acad. Sci. hung.* 13, 255—262 (1966). [G 56,565/66]

Szilágyi, T., Csernyánszky, H., Csernyánszky, I., Szabó, E., Csaba, B.: Effect of hypothermia on the adrenaline-chloroform syncope. *Acta physiol. Acad. Sci. hung.* 20, 149—153 (1961). [D 21,498/61]

Szilágyi, T., Tóth, S., Miltényi, L., Jóna, G.: Oxygen poisoning and thyroid function. *Acta physiol. Acad. Sci. hung.* 35, 59—61 (1969). [G 68,248/69]

Szold, A., Weisz, P., Dési, I., Kádas, T.: Wirkung des Methylandrostendiols und Norandrostenolons auf experimentelle Urämie. *Z. Urol.* 52, 652—658 (1959). [C 79,889/59]

Szold, E., Gimes, B., Erdös, B.: Anabolic steroids and radiation damage. *Lancet* 1960 I, 289—290. [C 80,607/60]

Szold, E., Szendröi, Z., Weisz, P., Pintér, I., Dési, I., Kádas, T.: Anabolic steroids in uraemia. *Lancet* 1959 I, 368. [C 64,498/59]

Szontagh, F. E., Kovacs, L.: Post-coital contraception with dienoestrol. *Med. Gynaec. Sociol.* 4, 36—37 (1969). [G 73,899/69]

Tabachnick, I. I. A., Parker, R. E., Wagner, J., Anthony, P. Z.: A re-evaluation of the calorigenic action of the L- and D-isomers of thyroxine. *Endocrinology* 59, 153—158 (1956). [C 22,161/56]

Tabachnick, I. I. A., Thorstad, J. A., Wagner, J., Parker, R. F.: A partial pharmacologic profile of the response to neuromuscular blocking agents as modified by sodium l-thyroxine. *Arch. int. Pharmacodyn.* 114, 210—216 (1958). [C 50,317/58]

Taber, K. W.: Counteracting the acute radiation syndrome with corticotropin (ACTH). *Amer. J. Roentgenol.* 73, 259—264 (1955). [C 10,417/55]

Tabusse, L., Curveille, J., Olsen, O.: Modifications de la tolérance à l'anoxémie par la cortisone. *C. R. Soc. Biol. (Paris)* 148, 567 (1954). [C 10,563/54]

Tada, H.: Studies on the relation between steroid hormones and the liver. (Japanese.) *Jap. J. Gastroent.* 57/3, 373—397 (1960). [E 96,131/60]

Tainter, M. L.: Prevention of the edema of paraphenylenediamine by drugs acting on the adrenals. *J. Pharmacol. exp. Ther.* 27, 201—229 (1926). [25,429/26]

Tainter, M. L.: Comparative antiedemic efficiency of epinephrine and related amines and pituitary in experimental edemas. *J. Pharmacol. exp. Ther.* 33, 129—146 (1928). [23,737/28]

Takabatake, E.: Metabolism of drugs. XI. The relationship between hypnotic activity and metabolism of ethylhexabital. (2) The effect of sex hormones. *Pharm. Bull. (Tokyo)* 5, 266 to 271 (1957). [G 76,713/57]

Takabatake, E., Ariyoshi, T.: Biochemical studies on the drug metabolism. II. The effects of some steroids on the metabolism of cyclobarbital. *Endocr. jap.* 9, 193—200 (1962). [D 48,245/62]

Takács, L., Kovách, A. G. B., Mohácsi, A., Káldor, V., Kalmár, Z.: Die Wirkung von Stoffwechselveränderungen auf die Schockempfindlichkeit. *Acta physiol. hung. Sup.* 5, 30—31 (1954). [C 29,459/54]

Takagaki, Y., Naiki, M., Fujiwara, K., Tajima, Y.: Maladie de Tyzzer expérimentale de la souris traitée avec la cortisone. *C. R. Soc. Biol. (Paris)* 157, 438—441 (1963). [D 69,101/63]

Takahashi, A., Kato, R.: Effect of toxohormone on microsomal cytochromes and hydroxylating systems of rat liver. *J. Biochem. (Tokyo)* 65, 325—327 (1969). [H 15,250/69]

Takemori, A. E., Mannering, G. J.: Metabolic N- and O-demethylation of morphine- and morphinan-type analgesics. *J. Pharmacol. exp. Ther.* 123, 171—179 (1958). [H 24,294/58]

Takens, H.: Vitamin D_2 (calciferol) intoxication. An experimental investigation. *Acta med. scand.* 163, 417—428 (1959). [C 69,439/59]

Tanabe, K.: Hypersensitive toxicity of 5-n-butyl-1-cyclohexyl-2,4,6-trioxoperhydropyrimidine in the pregnant rat. *Jap. J. Pharmacol.* 17, 381–392 (1967). [F92,176/67

Tanabe, S.: Experimental study of chronic cadmium poisoning especially about the accumulation in the bodies of rats. No. 3. An experiment of giving some drinking water including 300 ppm Cd. (Japanese text). *J. Juzen med. Soc.* 76, 34–14–34–17 (1968). [G72,457/68

Tanabe, T., Cafruny, E. J.: Adrenal hypertrophy in rats treated chronically with morphine. *J. Pharmacol. exp. Ther.* 122, 148–153 (1958). [C48,625/58

Tanaka, Y., Dao, T. L.: Effect of hepatic injury on induction of adrenal necrosis and mammary cancer by 7,12-dimethylbenz[α]anthracene in rats. *J. nat. Cancer Inst.* 35, 631–640 (1965). [G34,593/65

Tanret, P., Thomas, J., Cottenot, F.: Evolution des dépôts oxaliques et lipidiques au cours de la lithiase rénale expérimentale par l'éthylène-glycol et l'acide oxalique. *C. R. Soc. Biol. (Paris)* 155, 1025–1027 (1961). [G68,367/61

Tanret, P., Thomas, J., Thomas, E., Cottenot, F.: Influence du sexe sur les formations de dépôts d'oxalate de calcium dans les reins chez le rat intoxiqué par l'éthylène-glycol. *C. R. Soc. Biol. (Paris)* 156, 1285–1287 (1962). [D44,140/62

Tao, L., Nakamura, A., Sakurai, H.: Study on susceptibility of hamster to various strains of mycobacteria. Report IV. Influence of cortisone administration upon tuberculous lesion of hamster. *Jap. J. Tuberc.* 7, 62–75 (1959). [C82,168/59

Tarantino, C., Natali, P.: Modificazioni indotte dall'ACTH sul quadro ateromatoso sperimentale da colesterina. *Folia endocr. (Roma)* 5, 279–288 (1952). [B71,460/52

Tardiff, R. G., DuBois, K. P.: Inhibition of hepatic microsomal enzymes by alkylating agents. *Arch. int. Pharmacodyn.* 177, 445–456 (1969). [H11,752/69

Tarján, G., Czeizel, E., Görgényi, F., Székesi, J.: Medikamentöse Prävention der Endotoxin-bedingten Mortalität trächtiger Tiere. *Zbl. Gynäk.* 89, 1420–1427 (1967). [G54,411/67

Tarnowski, W., Seitz, H. J., Lierse, W.: A critical experimental contribution concerning the value of CCl_4-intoxicated liver in metabolic studies. *Biochem. Pharmacol.* 19, 1409–1417 (1970). [G75,524/70

Tatum, H. J., Kozelka, F. L.: Distribution, excretion and rate and site of detoxification of metrazol. *J. Pharmacol. exp. Ther.* 72, 284 to 290 (1941). [81,376/41

Tauber, H., Garson, W.: Effect of cortisone, properdin and reserpine on Neisseria gonorrhoea endotoxin activity. *Proc. Soc. exp. Biol. (N.Y.)* 97, 886–888 (1958). [C51,966/58

Tavassoli, M., Crosby, W. H.: The fate of fragments of liver implanted in ectopic sites. *Anat. Rec.* 166, 143–151 (1970). [G73,038/70

Tawara, S.: Du mode d'action de l'adrénaline et des acides vis-à-vis des toxines bactériennes. *C. R. Soc. Biol (Paris)* 85, 401–402 (1921). [12,478/21

Taylor, A., Carmichael, N.: Male mice tolerate dosages of pteroylglutamic acid lethal to females. *Proc. Soc. exp. Biol. (N.Y.)* 71, 544 to 545 (1949). [A49,002/49

Taylor, D. W.: Effects of adrenalectomy on oxygen poisoning in the rat. *J. Physiol. (Lond.)* 140, 23–36 (1958). [C47,861/58

Taylor, W.: Steroid metabolism in the rabbit. Biliary and urinary excretion of metabolites of [4-^{14}C] cortisone. *Biochem. J.* 117, 263–265 (1970). [G74,178/70

Tchen, T. T., Bloch, K.: On the conversion of squalene to lanosterol in vitro. *J. biol. Chem.* 226, 921–930 (1957). [G66,130/57

Tedeschi, G., Gualandi, G.: Azione del metil-androstendiolo sulla steatosi epatica di ratti digiunanti trattati con etionina. *Boll. Soc. ital. Biol. sper.* 32, 628–629 (1956). [C33,614/56

Teilum, G., Engbaek, H. C., Harboe, N., Simonsen, M.: Effects of cortisone on experimental glomerulonephritis. *J. clin. Path.* 4, 301–315 (1951). [B62,687/51

Telivuo, L., Louhimo, I.: Experimental haemorrhagic shock in rabbits. The effect of nor-adrenaline and hydrocortisone on survival and acid base balance. *Acta anaesth. scand.* 10, 1–8 (1966). [G39,506/66

Temple, T. E., Jr., Jones, D. J., Jr., Liddle, G. W., Dexter, R. N.: Treatment of Cushing's disease. Correction of hypercortisolism by o,p'DDD without induction of aldosterone deficiency. *New Engl. J. Med.* 281, 801–805 (1969). [H17,091/69

Templeton, R. D., Patras, M. C.: Effects of thyroparathyroidectomy and of thyroid feeding in rats on limited intake of vitamin B. *Amer. J. Physiol.* 105, 95 (1933). [9,640/33

Tenhunen, R., Marver, H. S., Schmid, R.: The enzymatic catabolism of hemoglobin: stimulation of microsomal heme oxygenase by hemin. *J. Lab. clin. Med.* 75, 410–421 (1970). [G73,193/70

Tentori, L., Toschi, G., Vivalci, G.: L'effetto dell'ipertiroidismo sperimentale sulla comparsa di lesioni muscolari nel ratto mantenuto ad una dieta carente di vitamina E. *R. C. Ist. sup. Sanita* **17**, 106—114 (1954). [C 7,904/54

Teodorovic, S., Ingalls, J. W., Greenberg, L.: Effects of corticosteroids on experimental amoebiasis. *Nature* **197**, 86—87 (1963).
[D 52,087/63

Tephly, T. R., Mannering, G. J.: Inhibition of microsomal drug metabolism by steroid hormones (Abstr.). *Pharmacologist* **6**, 186 (1964).
[G 67,764/64

Tephly, T. R., Mannering, G. J.: Inhibition of drug metabolism. V. Inhibition of drug metabolism by steroids. *Molec. Pharmacol* **4**, 10—14 (1968). [G 53,874/68

Terawaki, A., Yasui, O., Yamanouchi, M., Fukuyama, T., Nakajima, S.: Phenylalanine hydroxylase in tumor-bearing animals. *Gann*. **58**, 177—183 (1967). [G 50,735/67

Terayama, H., Takata, A.: Effect of adrenal hormones, methylcholanthrene and ionizing irradiation upon aminoazo dye N-demethylating activity in regenerating rat liver. *J. Biochem. (Tokyo)* **60**, 1—11 (1966).
[F 69,475/66

Terragna, A.: Azione di ormoni proteino-anabolici sul decorso dell'infezione sperimentale da virus influenzale APR 8. *G. Mal. infett.* No. 12, 1—16 (1963). [G 36,765/63

Terragna, A., Jannuzzi, C.: Ormoni steroidei e anticorpopoiesi. Nota II: Valutazione comparativa di vari ormoni anabolizzanti. *G. Mal. infett.* **15**, 360—362 (1963). [G 2,778/63

Terragna, A., Jannuzzi, C.: Valutazione degli effetti dell'ormone somatotropo ipofisario sull'anticorpopoiesi. *Minerva med.* **57**, 367—369 (1966). [F 62,290/66

Terragna, A., Jannuzzi, C., Giovanelli, A.: Decorso dell'epatite virale trattata con steroidi anabolizzanti. Studio bioptico e funzionale. *G. Mal. infett.* **16**, 484—489 (1964). [G 25,811/64

Terragna, A., Jannuzzi, C., Quazza, G. F.: Studio istologico (con particolare riguardo all'apparato mitocondriale) in casi di epatite virale trattati con steroidi proteinoanabolici. *Minerva pediat.* **17**, 772—776 (1965). [36,590/65

Terragna, A., Roscioli, B., Chiossi, F. M.: Azione degli steroidi proteino-anabolici sul decorso dell'intossicazione difterica sperimentale della cavia. *Boll. Ist. sieroter. ital.* **45**, 407 to 416 (1966). [E 66,111/66

Terragna, A., Roscioli, B., Chiossi, F. M.: Azione degli steroidi proteino-anabolici nella intossicazione da lipopolisaccaride di E. coli O 127: B 8. Studio sperimentale. *Pathologica* **58**, 567 a 571 (1966). [F 86,979/66

Tessmann, D.: Zur Frage des Prednisoneffekts bei akuter Leberschädigung (Tetrachlorkohlenstofftest an der Rattenleber). *Z. ges. inn. Med.* **19**, 204—209 (1964). [F 8,084/64

Tessmann, D.: Elektronenmikroskopische und enzymhistochemische Untersuchungen über den Einfluß des Testosterons auf die ischämisierte Mäuse- und Rattenniere. *Exp. Pathol.* **1**, 363—378 (1967). [H 5,695/67

Tessmann, D.: Über den Einfluß des Testosterons auf die tubuläre Regeneration der Mäuse- und Rattenniere nach Sublimatintoxikation. Histologische und enzymhistochemische Untersuchungen. *Z. ges. inn. Med.* **23**, 174—178 (1968). [G 65,320/68

Tessmann, D., Nicsovics, K., Holtz, M.: Histologische und enzymhistochemische Untersuchungen über den Prednisoneffekt auf die Bindegewebsentwicklung der Kaninchenleber bei chronischer Allylalkoholvergiftung unter Einbeziehung quantitativer Bindegewebsbestimmungen. *Zbl. allg. Pathol. pathol. Anat.* **107**, 370—377 (1965). [G 38,224/65

Tessmann, D., Ziegler, P. F.: Experimentelle Vergleichsuntersuchungen zur Frage des Prednisoneffektes auf die akute Leberschädigung bei unterschiedlicher Kortikoidapplikation. *Z. ges. inn. Med.* **21**, 45—48 (1966). [F 64,393/66

Thaler, M. M., Dallman, P. R., Goodman, J. R.: Effect of phenobarbital on microsomal enzyme induction and biliary excretion in man (Abstr.). *Program Amer. Soc. clin. Invest. Inc.*, 62nd Ann. Meet., Atlantic City, p. 95a—96a (1970).
[H 23,990/70

Thatcher, J. S., Radike, A. W.: Tolerance to potassium intoxication in the albino rat. *Amer. J. Physiol.* **151**, 138—146 (1947). [B 4,515/47

Theile, H., Reich, J.: Die Wirkung von Phenobarbital auf den Bilirubinspiegel bei Frühgeborenen. *Helv. paediat. Acta* **25**, 77—82 (1970). [G 73,421/70

Theologides, A., Zaki, G. F.: Mitotic index in the regenerating liver of tumor-bearing mice. *Cancer Res.* **29**, 1913—1915 (1969).
[H 19,577/69

Thibault, O., Lachaze, A.: Recherches sur la nature de la 'thyroxine active'. Renforcement immédiat par la thyroxamine des effets de l'adrénaline sur divers muscles lisses. *C. R. Soc. Biol. (Paris)* **145**, 797—800 (1951).
[B 69,990/51

Thiéblot, L., Berthelay, J., Lavarenne-Vannier, J.: Action de la thyroxine sur l'excitabilité réflexe sympathique. *J. Physiol. (Paris)* 48, 718—720 (1956). [C18,452/56

Thier, D., Gravenstein, J. S.: Thyroxin and reserpin on rate of atrial contraction. *Fed. Proc.* 19, 294 (1960). [C83,115/60

Thiersch, J. B.: Effect of 2,4,6,triamino-"S"-triazine (TR), 2,4,6 "Tris" (ethyleneimino)-"S"-triazine (TEM) and N,N′,N″-triethylenephosphoramide (TEPA) on rat litter in utero. *Proc. Soc. exp. Biol. (N.Y.)* 94, 36—40 (1957). [C28,993/57

Thiersch, J. B., Conroy, L., Stevens, A. R., Jr., Finch, C. A.: Adverse effect of cortisone on marrow regeneration following irradiation. *J. Lab. clin. Med.* 40, 174—181 (1952) [B76,313/52

Thoenes, F., Schröter, P.: Nebennierenrindenhormone und Rachitis. *Z. Kinderheilk.* 81, 239 bis 260 (1958). [C56,987/58

Thomas, C. S., Brockman, S. K.: Steroids in endotoxin shock. *Clin. Res.* 14, 96 (1966). [F82,789/66

Thomas, L.: The physiological disturbances produced by endotoxins. *Ann. Rev. physiol.* 16, 467—490 (1954). [B92,009/54

Thomas, L.: Reversible collapse of rabbit ears after intravenous papain, and prevention of recovery by cortisone. *J. exp. Med.* 104, 245 to 252 (1956). [C20,800/56

Thomas, L.: The effects of papain, vitamin A and cortisone on cartilage matrix in vivo. *Biophys. J.* 4, 207—213 (1964). [E37,875/64

Thomas, L., McCluskey, R. T., Li, J.: Prevention of vitamin A-induced depletion of cartilage matrix in rabbits by cortisone (Abstr.). *Fed. Proc.* 21, 467 (1962). [D23,234/62

Thomas, L., McCluskey, R. T., Li, J., Weissmann, G.: Prevention by cortisone of the changes in cartilage induced by an excess of vitamin A in rabbits. *Amer. J. Path.* 42, 271—283 (1963). [D57,729/63

Thomas, L, Mogabgab, W. J., Good, R. A.: The effects of cortisone on experimental bacterial infection and on the tissue damage produced by bacterial toxins. *Amer. Soc. clin. Invest.* (43rd Meet.), p. 57. (1951). [B57,977/51

Thomas, L, Smith, R. T.: Effect of cortisone on response to endotoxin in mature rabbits. *Proc. Soc. exp. Biol. (N.Y.)* 86, 810—813 (1954). [E23,202/54

Thomas, R. M.: Sex hormone therapy in experimental peripheral gangrene. *Yale J. Biol. Med.* 12, 415—418 (1940). [A33,372/40

Thomas, W. C., Jr., Morgan, H. G.: The effect of cortisone in experimental hypervitaminosis D. *Endocrinology* 63, 57—64 (1958). [C55,688/58

Thompson, E. B., Tomkins, G. M., Curran, J. F.: Induction of tyrosine α-ketoglutarate transaminase by steroid hormones in a newly established tissue culture cell line. *Proc. nat. Acad. Sci. (Wash.)* 56, 296—303 (1966). [F81,633/66

Thompson, G. E., Scheel, L. D.: Alteration of lung pathology from diisocyanate by glycemic or sensitizing agents. *Arch. environm. Hlth* 16, 363—370 (1968). [G55,229/68

Thompson, J. S., Crawford, M. K., Reilly, R. W., Severson, C. D.: The effect of estrogenic hormones on immune responses in normal and irradiated mice. *J. Immunol.* 98, 331—335 (1967). [G44,654/67

Thompson, J. S., Gurney, C. W., Kirsten, W. H.: The tumor-inhibitory effects of 3-methylcholanthrene on transplantable and 3-methylcholanthrene-induced tumors in C3H mice. *Cancer Res.* 20, 1214—1219 (1960). [C92,646/60

Thompson, J. S., Simmons, E. L., Crawford, M. K., Severson, C. D.: Studies on the mechanisms of estradiol-induced radioprotection. *Radiat. Res.* 40, 70—84 (1969). [G70,145/69

Thompson, R. P. H., Eddleston, A. L. W. F., Williams, R.: Low plasma-bilirubin in epileptics on phenobarbitone. *Lancet* 1969 I, 21 to 22. [G71,802/69

Thompson, R. P. H., Pilcher, C. W. T., Robinson, J., Stathers, G. M., McLean, A. E. M., Williams, R.: Treatment of unconjugated jaundice with dicophane. *Lancet* 1969 II, 4—6. [G71,801/69

Thompson, R. P. H., Williams, R.: Treatment of chronic intrahepatic cholestasis with phenobarbitone. *Lancet* 1967 II, 646—648. [G71,813/67

Thomson, D. L., Collip, J. B., Selye, H.: The effect of parathyroid hormone on the bones of hypophysectomized rats. *Proc. Roy. Soc. Can.* 28, 124 (1934). [A239/34

Thomson, D. L., Collip, J. B., Selye, H.: The antihormones. *J. Amer. med. Ass.* 116, 132 (1941). [A35,782/41

Thomson, J. F., Mikuta, E. T.: Effect of total body X-irradiation on the tryptophan peroxidase activity of rat liver. *Proc. Soc. exp. Biol. (N.Y.)* 85, 29—32 (1954). [B90,975/54

Thomson, J. F., Mikuta, E. T.: The effect of cortisone and hydrocortisone on the tryptophan peroxidase-oxidase activity of rat liver. *Endocrinology* **55**, 232—233 (1954). [B 96,579/54]

Thorn, G. W., Clinton, M., Jr., Davis, B. M., Lewis, R. A.: Effect of adrenal cortical hormone therapy on altitude tolerance. *Endocrinology* **36**, 381—390 (1945). [B 335/45]

Tillotson, C., Kochakian, C. D.: Effect of castration and testosterone on weight of organs and individual muscles of the fasting guinea pig. *Fed. Proc.* **15**, 187 (1956). [C 14,153/56]

Timar, M., Hädrich, I., Botez, A., Vrejoiu, G.: Rôle de la fonction granulopexique du système réticulo-histiocytaire (SRH) dans le mécanisme d'installation de l'accoutumance au phénobarbital. *Med. Pharmacol. exp. (Basel)* **16**, 193—198 (1967). [F 82,696/67]

Timiras, P. S., Koch, P.: Modifications chimiques et morphologiques induites par la cortisone et l'acétate de desoxycorticostérone au niveau du foie du lapin. *Rev. canad. Biol.* **9**, 481—482 (1951). [B 53,947/51]

Timiras, P. S., Koch, P.: Morphological and chemical changes elicited in the liver of the rabbit by cortisone and desoxycorticosterone acetate. *Anat. Rec.* **113**, 349—363 (1952). [B 54,551/52]

Timmler, R.: Die Bedeutung der N-Demethylierung für die Gewöhnung an Morphin und morphinähnlich wirkende Verbindungen. *Thesis.* University of Berlin (1960). [E 48,422/60]

Tinacci, F.: L'azione di alcune sostanze antitiroidee (Tiuracile, Metiltiuracile e Aminotiazolo) sul Mustelus Laevis. *Publ. Staz. Zool. Napoli* **21**, 124—131 (1947). [B 28,546/47]

Tindall, V. R., Beazley, J. M.: An assessment of changes in liver function during normal pregnancy using a modified bromsulphthalein test. *J. Obstet. Gynaec. Brit. Cwlth.* **72**, 717—737 (1965). [G 34,865/65]

Tinel, J., Ungar, G.: Epilepsie expérimentale par l'adrénaline chez le cobaye préparé par la yohimbine, l'ergotamine ou la peptone. *C. R. Soc. Biol. (Paris)* **112**, 542—543 (1933). [14,897/33]

Tinozzi, F. P., Pannella, A.: Influenza del diabete da allossana sui tumori sperimentali da 20-metilcolantrene. *Arch. De Vecchi Anat. pat.* **36**, 311—327 (1961). [D 54,092/61]

Toberentz, H.: Über einige Wirkungsbedingungen der Basisnarkotika. Narkosebreite, Streuung der Empfindlichkeit und Weckbarkeit. *Naunyn-Schmiedebergs Arch. exp. Path. Pharmak.* **171**, 346—362 (1933). [A 51,399/33]

Tobian, L., Jr., Strauss, E.: Effect of adrenal cortical extract on recovery from severe pneumococcic infection in mice. *Proc. Soc. exp. Biol. (N.Y.)* **69**, 529—531 (1948). [B 28,613/48]

Todd, A. C.: Thyroactive iodocasein and thiouracil in the diet, and growth of parasitized chicks. *Poultry Sci.* **27**, 818—821 (1948). [G 71,890/48]

Todd, A. C.: Thyroid condition of chickens and development of parasitic nematodes. *J. Parasit.* **35**, 255—260 (1949). [B 40,185/49]

Todd, R. S., Laine, J. B., Howard, J. M., Singh, L. M., Vega, R. E.: Effects of aldosterone on prolongation of renal homografts in dogs. *Surg. Forum* **14**, 501—502 (1963). [G 10,342/63]

Toivanen, P.: Effect of estrogens and progestins on the susceptibility of mice to experimental staphylococcal infection. *Ann. Univer. Turk.* (Ser. A/II), No. 35, p. 7—27 (1966). [G 59,609/66]

Toivanen, P.: Enhancement of staphylococcal infection in mice by estrogens. I. Effect of the timing, quantity and quality of the hormone. *Ann. Med. exp. Fenn.* **45**, 138—146 (1967). [G 49,847/67]

Toivanen, P.: Enhancement of staphylococcal infection in mice by estrogens. II. Effect of the inoculum size and the strain variation of bacteria and mice. *Ann. Med. exp. Fenn.* **45**, 147 to 151 (1967). [G 49,848/67]

Tolckmitt, W.: Über den Einfluß von Steroidpräparaten mit Hormonwirksamkeit auf den Umsatz von L-Tryptophan beim Säugling. *Arch. Kinderheilk.* **181**, 158—168 (1970). [G 77,793/70]

Tolentino, P.: Protein anabolic steroid hormones and antibody formation. *Ann. paediat. (Basel)* **199**, 467—471 (1962). [D 34,052/62]

Tolentino, P., Terragna, A., Jannuzzi, C.: Ormoni steroidei e anticorpopoiesi. Nota I. Blocco enzimatico della 11-idrossilasi surrenalica. Effetto della somministrazione di androgeni. *G. Mal. infett.* **13**, 561—563 (1961). [D 16,593/61]

Tolentino, P., Terragna, A., Jannuzzi, C.: Ormoni steroidei ed anticorpopoiesi. Mancata azione di stimolo da parte di steroidi proteinoanabolici nella somministrazione distanziata dall'antigene 'O' nella risposta anamnestica. *Ann. Sclavo* **6**, 439—444 (1964). [G 70,136/64]

Tomich, E. G., Woollett, E. A., Pratt, M. A.: Some biological actions of iodo-1-thyronines. *J. Endocr.* **20**, 65—68 (1960). [C 83,307/60]

Tomkins, G. M.: The enzymatic reduction of Δ^4-3-ketosteroids. *J. Biol. Chem.* **225**, 13—24 (1957). [C32,526/57]

Tomkins, G. M., Garren, L. D., Howell, R. R., Peterkofsky, B.: The regulation of enzyme synthesis by steroid hormones: the role of translation. *J. cell. comp. Physiol.* **66**, Sup. 1, 137—152 (1965). [G35,353/65]

Tomkins, G. M., Gelehrter, T. D., Granner, D., Martin, D., Jr., Samuels, H. H., Thompson, E. B.: Control of specific gene expression in higher organisms. Expression of mammalian genes may be controlled by repressors acting on the translation of messenger RNA. *Science* **166**, 1474—1480 (1969). [H19,499/69]

Tomkins, G. M., Thompson, E. B., Hayashi, S., Gelehrter, T., Granner, D., Peterkofsky, B.: Tyrosine transaminase induction in mammalian cells in tissue culture. *Symp. Quant. Biol. (Cold Spring Harbor)* **31**, 349—360 (1966). [G49,588/66]

Tomlinson, G. A., Yaffe, S. J.: The formation of bilirubin and p-nitrophenyl glucuronides by rabbit liver. *Biochem. J.* **99**, 507—512 (1966). [G76,303/66]

Tonutti, E.: Toxische Gewebsschäden, Entstehungsmechanismus und Folgerungen. *Langenbecks Arch. klin. Chir.* **264**, 61—68 (1950). [B48,892/50]

Tonutti, E.: Desoxycorticosteron und Cortison bei Diphtherietoxinvergiftung, insbesondere ihre Wirkungsunterschiede hinsichtlich des allgemeinen Resistenzvermögens. *Arzneimittel-Forsch.* **2**, 97—102 (1952). [B69,136/52]

Tonutti, E., Fetzer, S.: Einfluß von Desoxycorticosteron und Cortison auf das Resistenzvermögen gegen Giftstoffe des Tuberkelbazillus. *Münch. med. Wschr.* **94**, 2161—2168 (1952). [B75,190/52]

Torda, C., Wolff, H. G.: Effect of cortisone and ACTH on the threshold of convulsions induced by pentamethylene tetrazol. *Fed. Proc.* **10**, 137 (1951). [B57,149/51]

Torda, C., Wolff, H. G.: Effects of various concentrations of adrenocorticotrophic hormone on electrical activity of brain and on sensitivity to convulsion-inducing agents. *Amer. J. Physiol.* **168**, 406—413 (1952). [B69,986/52]

Tormey, J., Lasagna, L.: Relation of thyroid function to acute and chronic effects of amphetamine in the rat. *J. Pharmacol. exp. Ther.* **128**, 201—209 (1960). [C80,689/60]

Torrence, J.L., Bauer, G.E.: Protection from 7,12-dimethylbenz(a)anthracene-induced adrenal apoplexy and necrosis by Celite. *Endocrinology* **88**, 1069—1071 (1971). [H37,366/71]

Tournade, A., Raymond-Hamet: Syncope noradrénalino-chloroformique. *C. R. Soc. Biol. (Paris)* **111**, 897—900 (1932). [7,436/32]

Tourniaire, A., Blum, J., Guyot, R., Madignier, M.: L'hyperexcitabilité myocardique des cardiopathies décompensées. Effet de la spironolactone. *Sem. Hôp. Paris* **45**, 1388—1392 (1969). [G66,481/69]

Traeger, A., Klinger, W.: Der Einfluß von Triorthokresylphosphat auf die Hexobarbitalseitenlagenzeit verschieden alter Ratten. *Acta biol. med. germ.* **23**, 925—928 (1969). [H23,856/69]

Traina, V.: Adrenotropic hormone (ACTH), aminopterin and eosinophil count. *Nature (Lond.)* **168**, 250 (1951). [B72,887/51]

Trainin, N.: Adrenal imbalance in mouse skin carcinogenesis. *Cancer Res.* **23**, 415—419 (1963). [D61,599/63]

Trasino, M.: Effetti della splenectomia in varie condizioni sperimentali. *Boll. Soc. ital. Biol. sper.* **26**, 1152—1154 (1950). [B56,794/50]

Travis, J. W., Keyl, A. C., Dragstedt, C. A.: The effect of pancreatectomy on the toxicity of k-strophanthin in the dog. *J. Pharmacol. exp. Ther.* **117**, 148—150 (1956). [C18,863/56]

Treadwell, A. de G., Gardner, W. U., Lawrence, J. H.: Effect of combining estrogen with lethal doses of roentgen-ray in Swiss mice. *Endocrinology* **32**, 161—164 (1943). [A56,593/43]

Trentini, G. P., Scilabra, G. A., Botticelli, A., Pugliese, F.: Il quadro arterioso e splancnico del coniglio trattato con 5-HT e colesterolo, e con 5-HT, colesterolo e tween 80. *Arch. De Vecchi Anat. pat.* **53**, 455—471 (1968). [G71,152/68]

Trinci, M.: Effetti della stimolazione surrenalica con ormone corticotropo, in ratti irradiati su tutto il corpo con raggi γ del Co^{60}. *Nunt. radiol. (Roma)* **32**, 437—453 (1966). [G45,713/66]

Triner, L., Mráz, M., Chmelařová, M.: The effect of glucose and glucose together with insulin on the resistance of fasted rats to trauma in the Noble-Collip drum. *Physiol. bohemoslov.* **12**, 136 to 144 (1963). [D65,801/63]

Tripi, H. B., Kuzell, W. C., Gardner, G. M.: Thiouracil administration and thyroidectomy in experimental polyarthritis of rats. *Ann. rheum. Dis.* **8**, 125—131 (1949). [B12,732/49]

Trnavský, K., Trnavská, Z., Cebecauer, L.: Attempt to influence the increased solubility of

collagen in lathyrism by hydrocortisone. *Nature (Lond.)* **207**, 993—994 (1965).
[F 49,077/65

Trnavská, Z., Trnavský, K.: Effect of antirheumatic drugs on experimental lathyrism. *Biochem. Pharmacol.* **17**, 71—74 (1968).
[G 54,556/68

Trojanová, M.: The effect of thyroidectomy and parathyroidectomy during the early postnatal period upon survival of the respiratory centre in the rat in anoxia. *Physiol. bohemoslov.* **15**, 454—458 (1966). [G 42,905/66

Trolle, D.: Phenobarbitone and neonatal icterus. *Lancet* **1968 I**, 251—252. [G 71,807/68

Trolle, D.: Decrease of total serum-bilirubin concentration in newborn infants after phenobarbitone treatment. *Lancet* **1968 II**, 705—708.
[G 71,809/68

Trolle, D.: A possible drop in first-week-mortality rate for low-birth-weight infants after phenobarbitone treatment. *Lancet* **1968 II**, 1123 to 1124. [G 77,159/68

Trotter, N. L.: The effect of partial hepatectomy in subcutaneously transplanted hepatomas in mice. *Cancer. Res.* **21**, 778—782 (1961).
[E 90,324/61

Trotter, N. L.: A fine structure study of lipid in mouse liver regenerating after partial hepatectomy. *J. Cell Biol.* **21**, 233—244 (1964).
[G 71,660/64

Tsuru, C.: Influence of endocrinous medicine upon the formation of Rhodan compound. (Japanese text p. 619—639.) *J. orient. Med.* **19**, 47 (1933). [44,467/33

Tuchmann-Duplessis, H., Mercier-Parot, L.: Essais de prévention des effets embryotoxique et tératogène de l'actinomycine D. I. Action de la progestérone ou d'une association progestérone folliculine. *C. R. Soc. Biol. (Paris)* **164**, 6—10 (1970). [H 28,871/70

Tuchmann-Duplessis, H., Mercier-Parot, L.: Essais de prévention des effets embryotoxique et tératogène de l'actinomycine D. II. Influence de l'hormone lactogène. *C. R. Soc. Biol. (Paris)* **164**, 60—63 (1970). [H 28,876/70

Tuchweber, B., Gabbiani, G., Côté, G.: Effect of thyroxine and calcitonin on experimental hyperparathyroidism. Present. Nat. Found. Conf. *Hormones in Development*, Nottingham University, Sept. 9—12, 1968. [G 46,759/68

Tuchweber, B., Gabbiani, G., Selye, H.: Einfluß des Hypophysen-Nebennierenrindensystems auf die durch Hexadimethrin hervorgerufenen Organveränderungen. *Med. Welt (Stuttg.)* No. 45, 2272—2275 (1963). [G 27,884/63

Tuchweber, B., Gabbiani, G., Selye, H.: Effect of vitamin E and methyltestosterone upon the progeria-like syndrome produced by dihydrotachysterol. *Amer. J. clin. Nutr.* **13**, 238—242 (1963). [D 65,261/63

Tuchweber, B., Garg, B. D.: Protection by spironolactone and various anabolic steroids against vitamin-A overdosage (Abstr.). *Proc. Canad. Fed. Biol. Soc.* Montreal, Quebec, **13**, 10 (1970). [G 70,434/70

Tuchweber, B., Garg, B. D., Hatakeyama, S.: Prevention of hypervitaminosis-A by spironolactone and anabolic steroids. *Int. Z. Vitaminforsch.* **40**, 575—584 (1970). [G 70,477/70

Tuchweber, B., Kovacs, K.: Influence of phenobarbital and various steroids on CCl$_4$ hepatotoxicity. *Arch. Toxikol.* **27**, 159—167 (1971).
[G 70,489/71

Tuchweber, B., Kovacs, K., Khandekar, J. D., Garg, B. D.: Intramitochondrial lamellar formations induced by pregnenolone-16α-carbonitrile in the hepatocytes of pregnant rats. *J. Ultrastruct. Res.* (in press). [G 79,031

Tuchweber, B., Solymoss, B., Khandekar, J. D., Garg, B. D., Kovacs, K.: Effect of pregnenolone-16α-carbonitrile on the liver ultrastructure and microsomal enzyme activity in pregnant rats. (Abstr.) Program 52nd Meet. Endocr. Soc. St. Louis, Miss., (in press). [G 79,020

Tullio, P.: Il tasso glicemico come indice della resistenza dell'organismo al raffreddamento. *Arch. Sci. biol. (Bologna)* **14**, 379—390 (1930).
[22,671/30

Tuohy, G. F.: Drugs: reactions and interactions. *S. Dak. J. Med.* **22**, 19—22 (1969).
[G 66,351/69

Turcotte, J. G., Haines, R. F., Brody, G. L., Meyer, T. J., Schwartz, S. A.: Immunosuppression with medroxyprogesterone acetate. *Transplant. Bull.* **6**, 248—260 (1968). [G 56,529/68

Tureman, J., Maloney, A. H., Booker, W. M., Froix, C., Jones, W.: Further studies on the depressant action of pentobarbital sodium on adrenalectomized rats (Abstr.). *J. Pharmacol. exp. Ther.* **106**, 420 (1952). [B 80,379/52

Turner, K. B., De Lamater, A.: Effect of thyrotropic hormone on blood cholesterol of thyroidectomized rabbits. *Proc. Soc. exp. Biol. (N.Y.)* **49**, 150—152 (1942). [A 37,602/42

Turner, M. M., Berry, L. J.: Inhibition of gastric emptying in mice by bacterial endotoxin. *Amer. J. Physiol.* **205**, 1113—1116 (1963).
[E 36,911/63

Turner, T. B., Hollander, D. H.: Cortisone in experimental syphilis (a preliminary note). *Bull. Johns Hop. Hosp.* 87, 505—509 (1950). [B 55,488/50

Tyce, G. M., Flock, E. V., Owen, C. A., Jr., Stobie, G. H. C., David, C.: 5-Hydroxyindole metabolism in the brain after hepatectomy. *Biochem. Pharmacol.* 16, 979—992 (1967). [G 47,432/67

Tyce, G. M., Stobie, G. H. C., Flock, E. V., Bollman, J. L.: 5-Hydroxytryptamine content of the brain after hepatectomy. *Fed. Proc.* 21, 301 (1962). [D 23,092/62

Tyler, F.H., West, C.D., Jubiz, W., Meikle, A.W.: Dilantin and metyrapone: a clinically significant example of enzyme induction. *Trans. Amer. clin. climat. Ass.* 81, 213—219 (1969). [G 79,955/69

Tyree, E. B., Swift, M. N., Patt, H. M.: X irradiation of the hypophysectomized rat. *Amer. J. Physiol.* 155, 473 (1948). [B 33,116/48

Tyslowitz, R., Astwood, E. B.: The effect of corticotrophin on the resistance of hypophysectomized rats to low environmental temperatures. *Proc. Amer. physiol. Soc. 53rd Ann. Meet. Chicago, Ill.* P 284—P 285 (1941). [80,678/41

Uehleke, H.: Extrahepatic microsomal drug metabolism. In: Baker and Tripod; *Sensitization to Drugs.* Int. Congr. Ser. No. 181, 10, p. 94—100. Amsterdam: Excerpta Medica Foundation 1969. [G 70,915/69

Uehleke, H., Greim, H.: Stimulierung der Oxydation von Fremdstoffen in Nierenmikrosomen durch Phenobarbital. *Naunyn-Schmiedebergs Arch. Pharmak.* 261, 152—161 (1968). [G 70,906/68

Uete, T.: Mode of action of adrenal cortical hormones. *J. Biochem (Tokyo)* 65, 513—521 (1969). [H 15,157/69

Ulmansky, M., Sela, J.: Changes in the epiphyseal cartilages of mice treated with parathormone, fluoride and copper. *J. comp. Path.* 79, 367—370 (1969). [G 70,273/69

Ungváry, G., Demeter, J., Hudák, A., Tari, J.: Changes in the vascular structure of the liver following subtotal hepatectomy in the rat. *Acta morph. Acad. Sci. hung.* 17, 143—155 (1969). [G 72,366/69

Urist, M. R., Deutsch, N. M., Pomerantz, G., McLean, F. C.: Interrelations between actions of parathyroid hormone and estrogens on bone and blood in avian species. *Amer. J. Physiol.* 199, 851—855 (1960). [C 95,236/60

Uroić, B., Rabadjija, M., Supek, Z.: Toxicity of a nucleotoxic agent, mustine hydrochloride, and its enhancement by 5-hydroxytryptamine pretreatment. *J. Pharm. Pharmacol.* 16, 61—62 (1964). [E 37,637/64

Uspenskaya, G. S.: Role of the thyroid gland in thallium intoxication. (Russian text.) *Vestn. Vener. Derm.*, No. 2—3, 78—80 (1939). [D 34,628/39

Usuelli, F., Piana, G., Mainardi, B.: Testosterone e digiuno. *Folia endocr. (Roma)* 2, 31—39 (1949). [B 34,756/49

Uyldert, I. E.: The effect of DOCA and of adrenal cortical extract on hepatic regeneration in adrenalectomized rats. *Acta physiol. pharmacol. neerl.* 1, 359—362 (1950). [G 76,358/50

Vacek, L.: Studie o steroidní anestesii: 3. Desoxykortikosteron a krecove latky. *Scr. med. Fac. Med. Brun.* 31, 323—328 (1958). [C 63,230/58

Vacek, L.: Studie o steroidní anestesii: 6. Vliv serotoninu a jeho antagonistû na centrál ne tlumivý účinek hydroxypregnandionu.(A study of steroid anesthesia: 6. The influence of serotonin and its antagonists on the central inhibitive effect of hydroxypregnandion). *Scr. med. Fac. Med. Brun.* 34, 65—72 (1961). [D 10,919/61

Vácha, J., Pošpísil, M.: Individual differences in the stress respone of mice and their relationship to the differences in radiation tolerance. *Med. exp. (Basel)* 19, 58—63 (1969). [H 17,170/69

Vakilzadeh, J., Vandiviere, M. R.: Hormones in experimental tuberculoimmunity. *Acta tuberc. pneumol. scand.* 43, 170—180 (1963). [E 32,626/63

Valderrama, J. A. F. de, Munuera, L. M.: The effect of cortisone and anabolic agents on bone. In: Fleisch, Blackwood and Owen; *Calcified Tissues* (Proc. 3. europ. Symp.), p. 245—249. Berlin, Heidelberg, New York: Springer 1966. [E 6,008/66

Valeriote, F. A., Auricchio, F., Tomkins, G. M., Riley, D.: Purification and properties of rat liver tyrosine aminotransferase. *J. biol. Chem.* 244, 3618—3624 (1969). [G 67,621/69

Vallecalle, E., Soto-Rivera, A., de Armas, T. G., Luque, A. G.: Influencia de las hormonas sexuales sobre la excitabilidad del sistema nervioso central. *Acta endocr. (Kbh.)* 51, 99 to 100 (1960). [C 93,280/60

Valori, P.: Influenza della tiroidectomia sopra l'ipertrofia di compenso e l'attività metabolica del rene superstite a nefrectomia monolaterale. *Arch. Fisiol.* **48**, 196—203 (1948). [B 46,667/48

Valtin, H., Tenney, S. M.: Respiratory and circulatory adaptation to hyperthyroidism in rats at rest and during exercise. *Fed. Proc.* **18**, 162 (1959). [C 66,148/59

Vanamee, P., Winawer, S.J., Sherlock, P., Sonenberg, M., Lipkin, M.: Decreased incidence of restraint-stress induced gastirc erosions in rats treated with bovine growth hormone. *Proc. Soc. exp. Biol. (N.Y.)* **135**, 259—262 (1970). [H 32,254/70

Van Cauwenberge, H., Jaques, L. B., *cf.* **Cauwenberge, H. van, Jaques, L. B.** [C 58,521/58

Van Cauwenberge, H., Jaques, L. B., *cf.* **Cauwenberge, H. van, Jaques, L. B.** [C 72,748/59

Van den Brenk, H. A. S., *cf.* **Brenk, H. A. S. van den** [C 57,624/58

Vanderlinde, R. E., Westerfeld, W. W.: The inactivation of estrone by rats in relation to dietary effects on the liver. *Endocrinology* **47**, 265—273 (1950). [B 51,537/50

Vandestrate, M.: Action du chlorure de manganèse et de l'hyposulfite de soude sur l'intoxication tuberculinique et sur la sensibilité du derme à la tuberculine chez le cobaye tuberculeux. *C. R. Soc. Biol. (Paris)* **112**, 357—359 (1933). [A 48,036/33

Vanha-Perttula, T. P. J., Näätänen, E. K.: The effect of cortisone on cardiovascular sclerosis induced in rats with cholesterol and vitamin D. *Acta endocr. (Kbh.)* **35**, 20—33 (1960). [90,637/60

Vanzo, J. P. da: Effect of 2-methyl-9α-fluorohydrocortisone on survival of tourniquet-shocked rats. *Arch. int. Pharmacodyn.* **150**, 442 to 446 (1964). [F 19,865/64

Varga, F., Fischer, E.: Hexobarbital sleeping time in male rats with hepatic injury. *Acta physiol. Acad. Sci. hung.* **36**, 431—439 (1969). [G 76,189/69

Vargas, M. V.: Antagonismo farmacologico del propionato de testosterona y bicloruro de hidrargirio. *Crón. méd. (Lima)* **65**, 57—72 (1948). [B 44,689/48

Various authors: Application of metabolic data to the evaluation of drugs. A report prepared by the Committee on Problems of Drug Safety of the Drug Research Board, National Academy of Sciences—National Research Council. *Clin. Pharmacol. Ther.* **10**, 607—634 (1969). [G 68,203/69

Vauthey, P., Vauthey, M.: Effet protecteur de la vitamine C contre les intoxications. *J. Méd. Lyon* **28**, 305—308 (1947). [A 48,670/47

Velluda, C. C., Russu, I. G.: Le système réticuloendothélial et la syncope adrénalino-chloroformique. *J. Physiol. Path. gén.* **34**, 815—823 (1936). [38,782/36

Venkatesan, N., Argus, M.F., Arcos, J.C.: Mechanism of 3-methyl-cholanthrene-induced inhibition of dimethylnitrosamine demethylase in rat liver. *Cancer. Res* **30**, 2556—2562 (1970). [H 31,273/70

Vennet, K. V., Schneewind, J. H.: The effect of steroids on mortality in experimental traumatic shock. *Proc. Soc. exp. Biol. (N.Y.)* **109**, 674 to 675 (1962). [D 23,294/62

Ventura, J., Richer, C. L., Selye, H.: Effect of hypophysectomy upon the leukemoid organ infiltrations in Walker tumor-bearing rats. *Cancer Res.* **17**, 215—217 (1957). [C 23,299/57

Ventura, J., Selye, H.: Inverse 'conditioning' by hypophysectomy of mineralocorticoid and glucocorticoid activities of 9(α)-chlorocortisol. *Amer. J. Physiol.* **189**, 412—414 (1957). [C 24,231/57

Verbin, R. S., Sullivan, R. J., Farber, E.: The effects of cycloheximide on the cell cycle of the regenerating rat liver. *Lab. Invest.* **21**, 179—182 (1969). [G 70,538/69

Verne, J., Hébert, S., Barbarin, Y.: Action de la cortisone sur l'intoxication par le cyanure de potassium. *Presse méd.* **62**, 1101 (1954). [B 99,912/54

Verne, J., Roth, P.C.J.: The preventive effect of norandrostenolone phenylpropionate on carcinogenesis. *Bull. Cancer* **50**, 49—52 (1963). [E 48,050/63

Vernikos-Danellis, J., Marks, B. H.: Pituitary inhibitory effects of digitoxin and hydrocortisone. *Proc. Soc. exp. Biol. (N.Y.)* **109**, 10—14 (1962). [D 21,210/62

Vesell, E. S.: Induction of drug-metabolizing enzymes in liver microsomes of mice and rats by softwood bedding. *Science* **157**, 1057—1058 (1967). [F 88,031/67

Vesselinovitch, S. D., Mihailovich, N.: The effect of gonadectomy on the development of hepatomas induced by urethan. *Cancer Res.* **27**, 1788—1791 (1967). [F 91,584/67

Vest, M., Signer, E., Weisser, K., Olafsson, A.: A double blind study of the effect of phenobarbitone on neonatal hyperbilirubinaemia and frequency of exchange transfusion. *Acta paediat. scand.* **59**, 681—684 (1970). [H 32,456/70

Vest, M., Wyler, F., Girard, J.: Zur Entwicklungsphysiologie der Leber. *Praxis* **57**, 1693 bis 1695 (1968). [H 14,687/68

Viale, L. C. San M. de, Viale, A. A., Nacht, S., Grinstein, M.: Experimental porphyria induced in rats by hexachlorobenzene. A study of the porphyrins excreted by urine. *Clin. chim. Acta* 28, 13—23 (1970). [G 74,147/70

Vick, J.: Interaction of ionizing radiation and E. coli endotoxin. *Fed. Proc.* 26, 628 (1967). [F 79,609/67

Vick, J., Spink, W. W.: Supplementary role of hydralazine in reversal of endotoxin shock with metaraminol and hydrocortisone. *Proc. Soc. exp. Biol. (N.Y.)* 106/2, 280—283 (1961). [D 43,929/61

Vick, J. A.: Physiological and pharmacological studies on the reversibility of endotoxin shock in dogs (Abstr.). *J. clin. Invest.* 39, 1037 (1960). [C 84,708/60

Vick, J. A.: Use of isoproterenol and phenoxybenzamine in treatment of endotoxin shock. *Physiologist* 8, 296 (1965). [F 48,509/65

Vick, J. A., Ciuchta, H. P., Manthei, J. H.: Use of isoproterenol and phenoxybenzamine in treatment of endotoxin shock. *J. Pharmacol. exp. Ther.* 150, 382—388 (1965). [F 58,531/65

Vick, J. A., Lafave, J. W., MacLean, L. D.: Effect of treatment of endotoxin shock on renal hemodynamics and survival. *Surgery* 54, 78—85 (1963). [E 20,146/63

Vilchez, C. A., Sadnik, I. L., Bade, E. G.: Influence of starvation on liver regeneration in the mouse. *Naturwissenschaften* 55, 392—393 (1968). [H 15,524/68

Vincent, V., Motin, J.: Intoxication volontaire associant insuline et barbituriques. *Lyon méd.* 218, 407—408 (1967). [G 51,414/67

Visconti, J. A.: Use of drug interaction information in patient medication records. *Amer. J. Hosp. Pharm.* 26, 378—387 (1969). [G 77,709/69

Vittorio, P. V., Mars, H., Johnston, M. J.: Effect of X-irradiation on normal, hypothyroid, and hyperthyroid rabbits. *Canad. J. Biochem.* 37, 1271—1275 (1959). [C 76,156/59

Vittorio, P. V., Watkins, E. A., Dziubalo-Blehm, S.: The effect of erythropoietin on survival in irradiated polycythemic mice. *Canad. J. Physiol. Pharmacol.* 47, 221—223 (1969). [H 7,759/69

Vittorio, P. V., Wight, E. W., Sinnott, B. E.: A study of the protective action of serotonin (5-hydroxytryptamine) against whole-body X-irradiation in mice with the aid of chromium 51. *Canad. J. Biochem.* 41, 347—360 (1963). [D 56,243/63

Vivan, A., Braito, E.: Ricerche sperimentali sul ruolo del fegato nella patogenesi degli itteri emolitici. *Attual. Ostet. Ginec.* 8, 113—120 (1962). [D 22,638/62

Vivanco, F., Gabay, S., Martin, J. A. S., Ramos, F.: Effect of DL-thyroxine on the PBI and BMR of rats poisoned with aminonitriles. *Endocrinology* 69, 654—658 (1961). [D 10,627/61

Vivanco, F., Ramos, F., Jimenez-Diaz, C.: Determination of γ-aminobutyric acid and other free amino acids in whole brains of rats poisoned with α, γ'-iminodipropionitrile and β, β-diaminobutyric acid with, or without, administration of thyroxine. *J. Neurochem.* 13, 1461—1467 (1966). [G 43,566/66

Vivanco, F., Sanchez-Martin, J. A., Diaz, C. J.: Neuronal degeneration, electroencephalographic disturbances and polyserositis in rats produced by iminodipropionitrile and prevented by l-thyroxine. *Endocrinology* 69, 1111—1116 (1961). [D 15,606/61

Vizet, J.: De quelques relations de perméabilité de la barrière hémo-encéphalique et de pénétration des dérivés barbituriques dans les tissus nerveux centraux. *Biol. méd. (Paris)* 56, 1 to 107 (1967). [F 77,760/67

Vodicka, I., Dostál, M.: Ein Beitrag zur Wirkungsanalyse der anabolen Steroide bei der akuten Strahlenkrankheit von Ratten. *Strahlentherapie* 135/6, 739—744 (1968). [G 69,171/68

Vogel, R. A., Michael, M., Jr., Timpe, A.: Cortisone in experimental histoplasmosis. *Amer. J. Path.* 31, 535—543 (1955). [C 10,597/55

Vogt, O., Tissières, A., Verzár, F.: Einfluß der Thymektomie auf die Empfindlichkeit von Ratten gegenüber A und D Vitamin Mangel sowie eiweißarme Diät. *Int. Z. Vitamin-forsch.* 20, 44—60 (1948). [B 36,750/48

Voigt, W., Fernandez, E. P., Hsia, S. L.: P-450 level and taurochenodeoxycholate 6β-hydroxylase system of rat liver microsomes. *Proc. Soc. exp. Biol. (N.Y.)* 133, 1158—1161 (1970). [H 25,247/70

Vollmer, E. P., Hurlbut, H. S.: Ineffectiveness of cortisone therapy in mice infected with Japanese B encephalitis and the adverse effect of high doses. *J. infect. Dis.* 89, 103—106 (1951). [B 66,973/51

Vollmer, H., Buchholz, C.: Untersuchungen über die Giftempfindlichkeit weißer Mäuse nach Vorbehandlung mit oxydationssteigernden Substanzen. *Naunyn-Schmiedebergs Arch. Pharmak.* 155, 185—218 (1930). [A 48,810/30

Volterrani, U.: ACTH, cortisone e ipossia. *Ormonologia* 17, 415—424 (1957). [C 64,384/57

Volterrani, U.: Ipossia e cortisone. *Ormonologia* 17, 425—435 (1957). [C 64,385/57

von der Decken, A., *cf.* Decken, A. von der [G 68,039/60

Von Rummel, W., *cf.* Rummel, W. von [C 79,429/59

Von Zwehl, T., *cf.* Zwehl, T. von [25,477/26

Vorhaus, E. F., Vorhaus, L. J.: Protective effects of pretreatment with cortisone, aureomycin, and folic acid in carbon tetrachloride-induced hepatic injury in rats. *Gastroenterology* 26, 887—894 (1954). [B 97,869/54

Voss, J.: Pentamethylentetrazol (Cardiazol). III. Mitteilung über die Wirkung von Cardiazol bei peroraler Applikation. *Naunyn-Schmiedebergs Arch. Pharmak.* 118, 259—266 (1926). [A 47,860/26

Voss, R., Walther, D.: Einfluß der Drosselung endokriner Leistungen auf die Wiederbelebungszeit des Rückenmarks. *Langenbecks Arch. klin. Chir.* 293, 616—622 (1960). [E 53,093/60

Vunder, P. A., Lapshina, V. F.: Strumous action of paraaminosalicylic acid. (Russian text). *Probl. Endokr. Gormonoter.* 2/4, 76—81 (1956). [D 34,912/56

Wada, F., Hirata, K., Nakao, K., Sakamoto, Y.: Participation of the microsomal electron transport system involving cytochrome P-450 in 7 α-hydroxylation of cholesterol. *J. Biochem. (Tokyo)* 66, 699—703 (1969). [H 19,993/69

Wada, F., Hirata, K., Sakamoto, Y.: Relation of cholesterol synthesis and NADPH oxidation by microsomal electron transport system involving P-450. *Biochim. biophys. Acta (Amst.)* 143, 273—275 (1967). [G 67,771/67

Wada, F., Hirata, K. Sakamoto, Y.: Possible participation of cytochrome P-450 in cholesterol synthesis. *J. Biochem. (Tokyo)* 65, 171 to 175 (1969). [H 15,247/69

Wada, F., Shimakawa, H., Takasugi, M., Kotake, T., Sakamoto, Y.: Effects of steroid hormones on drug-metabolizing enzyme systems in liver microsomes. *J. Biochem. (Tokyo)* 64, 109—113 (1968). [H 15,468/68

Wada, J. A., Ikeda, H., McGeer, E. G.: The susceptibility to audiogenic stimuli of rats treated with methionine sulfoximine and various psychoactive agents. *Exp. Neurol.* 18, 327 to 337 (1967). [G 48,380/67

Waelsch, H., Selye, H.: Beiträge zur Entgiftung im tierischen Organismus. III. Mitteilung: Bedeutung der Leber bei Avertin- und Magnesium-narkosen. *Naunyn-Schmiedebergs Arch. Pharmak.* 161, 115—118 (1931). [3,972/31

Wagner, W. H., Lammers, L.: Cortison und Prednison bei der experimentellen Mäusetuberkulose. In: Various Authors; *Medizin und Chemie* 6, p. 225—248. Weinheim, Bergstr.: Verlag Chemie GmbH 1958. [C 83,426/58

Wajda, I., Lehr, D., Krukowski, M.: Sex difference in aortic rupture induced by lathyrus odoratus in immature rats. *Fed. Proc.* 16, 343 (1957). [C 33,241/57

Wajda, I., Lehr, D., Krukowski, M.: Influence of sex hormones upon incidence of dissecting aortic aneurysm in immature rats on a sweet pea seed diet. *J. Pharmacol. exp. Ther.* 122, 79 A—80 A (1958). [C 48,618/58

Wakabayashi, I., Arimura, A., Schally, A. V.: Effect of adrenocortical hormones on plasma radioimmunoassayable growth hormone (RIA-GH) in rats (Abstr.). *Physiologist* 13, 332 (1970). [H 27,784/70

Wakim, K. G., McKenzie, B. F., McGuckin, W. F., Brown, A. L., Jr.: The effects of heparin, nicotinic acid and ACTH on experimental nephrosis. *Amer. J. med. Sci.* 245, 259—276 (1963). [D 39,883/63

Walden, B., Brunson, J. G.: A study on tolerance to experimental shock in rabbits. *Fed. Proc.* 22, 639 (1963). [G 5,968/63

Walker, D. G., Wirtschafter, Z. T.: Resorption of embryos in rats on Lathyrus odoratus diet. *J. Nutr.* 58, 147—160 (1956). [C 29,985/56

Walker, J. M., Parry, C. B. W.: The effect of hepatectomy on the action of certain anaesthetics in rats. *Brit. J. Pharmacol.* 4, 93—97 (1949). [B 46,639/49

Walker, W., Hughes, M. I., Barton, M.: Barbiturate and hyperbilirubinaemia of prematurity. *Lancet* 1969 I, 548—550. [G 77,714/69

Wall, M. E., Abernethy, G. S., Jr., Carroll, F. I., Taylor, D. J.: The effects of some steroidal alkylating agents on experimental animal mammary tumor and leukemia systems. *J. med. Chem.* 12, 810—818 (1969). [G 69,969/69

Wallace, E. Z., Silverstein, J. N., Villadolid, L. S., Weisenfeld, L. S.: Cushing's syndrome due to adrenocortical hyperplasia. Treatment with an inhibitor of adrenocortical secretions. *New Engl. J. Med.* 265, 1088—1093 (1961). [E 89,875/61

Wallon, D., Browaeys, J.: Aplasie éosinophile de la moelle après corticothérapie massive chez le rat. *Sang*, No. 6, 587—595 (1959). [C 78,322/59

Walser, A.: Untersuchungen über die antikatabole Wirkung anaboler Steroide. *Schweiz. med. Wschr.* **92**, 396—398 (1962). [D33,753/62]

Walther, D., Voss, R.: Über die Verlängerung der Wiederbelebungszeit des Rückenmarks nach vorheriger Schilddrüsenbehandlung mit Endojodin. *Langenbecks Arch. klin. Chir.* **295**, 800—804 (1960). [G71,664/60]

Waltman, R., Bonura, F., Nigrin, G., Pipat, C.: Ethanol in prevention of hyperbilirubinaemia in the newborn. A controlled trial. *Lancet* 1969 II, 1265—1267. [H19,551/69]

Waltregny, A., Mesdjian, E.: Hypoglycémie et seuil pentétrazolique. *C. R. Soc. Biol. (Paris)* **160**, 1912—1914 (1966). [F78,025/66]

Waltregny, A., Mesdjian, E.: Etude polygraphique des crises d'épilepsie induites par surcharge hydrique chez le chat. *C. R. Soc. Biol. (Paris)* **161**, 389—394 (1967). [F85,818/67]

Waltz, H., Bartels, M., Matthies, H.: Zur Wirkung von ACTH, DOCA, Testosteronpropionat und Thyroxin auf die Pentothal-Schlafzeit hypophysektomierter Ratten. *Arch. exp. Pathol. Pharmakol.* **224**, 523—527 (1955). [C11,847/55]

Wang, C.-I., Schaefer, L. E., Adlersberg, D.: Tissue permeability — a factor in atherogenesis. Studies with cortisone and hyaluronidase. *Circulat. Res.* **3**, 293—296 (1955). [E83,672/55]

Ward, J.C., Crabtree, D.G.: Strychnine. X. Comparative accuracies of stomach tube and intraperitoneal injection methods of bioassay. *J. Amer. pharm. Ass., sci. Ed.* **31**, 113—115 (1942). [A29,199/42]

Ward, K. A., Pollak, J. K.: The composition of rat liver microsomes. The structural proteins of rat liver microsomes. *Biochem. J.* **114**, 41—48 (1969). [G69,320/69]

Wardle, E.N., Wright, N.A.: Endotoxin and acute renal failure associated with obstructive jaundice. *Brit. med. J. Nov.* 21, 472—474 (1970). [H32,903/70]

Wasielewski, E. von, Knick, B.: Experimenteller Beitrag zur Cortisonwirkung am Tier nach Inoculation pathogener und apathogener Mikroorganismen. *Z. ges. exp. Med.* **129**, 548 bis 558 (1958). [G68,292/58]

Wassermann, M., Wassermann, D., Lazarovici, S.: Effects of thyroidectomy on the storage of organochlorine insecticides. *Bull. environm. Contam. Toxicol.* **4**, 327—336 (1969). [G74,485/69]

Wasz-Höckert, O., Backman, A.: An attempt at shortening the diagnostic guinea-pig test. *Ann. Med. exp. Fenn.* **34**, 433—437 (1956). [C30,700/56]

Wasz-Höckert, O., Backman, A.: Effect of somatotropic hormone on the course of experimental guinea pig tuberculosis. *Ann. Paediat. Fenn.* **2**, 150—155 (1956). [C34,801/56]

Wasz-Höckert, O., Backman, A., Poppius, H.: Influence of hyperthyroidism and hypothyroidism on guinea-pig tuberculosis. *Ann. Med. exp. Fenn.* **34**, 411—419 (1956). [C30,699/56]

Wasz-Höckert, O., McCune, R.M.: The influence of somatotropin on growth and chronic tuberculosis in mice. *Amer. Rev. resp. Dis.* **88**, 680 to 688 (1963). [E31,145/63]

Wattenberg, L. W., Leong, J. L.: Effects of phenothiazines on protective systems against polycyclic hydrocarbons. *Cancer Res.* **25**, 365 to 370 (1965). [F38,140/65]

Wattenberg, L. W., Leong, J. L., Strand, P. J.: Benzpyrene hydroxylase activity in the gastrointestinal tract. *Cancer Res.* **22**, 1120—1125 (1962). [D40,287/62]

Wattenberg, L. W., Page, M. A., Leong, J. L.: Induction of increased benzpyrene hydroxylase activity by 2-phenylbenzothiazoles and related compounds. *Cancer Res.* **28**, 2539—2544 (1968). [G71,805/68]

Waugh, D., Pearl, M.J.: Serotonin-induced acute nephrosis and renal cortical necrosis in rats. A morphologic study with pregnancy correlations. *Amer. J. Path.* **36**, 431—455 (1960). [C83,389/60]

Weatherall, J. A. C.: Anaesthesia in new-born animals. *Brit. J. Pharmacol.* **15**, 454—457 (1960). [G76,306/60]

Weber, G., Allard, C., Lamirande, G. de, Cantero, A.: Liver glucose-6-phosphatase activity and intracellular distribution after cortisone administration. *Endocrinology* **58**, 40—50 (1956). [C11,010/56]

Weber, G., Marconi, G., Serrâo, D.: Ricerche sperimentali sopra la rigenerazione epatica. I. La rigenerazione epatica dopo ampia epatectomia nel corso della colostasi da legatura del coledoco. *Arch. De Vecchi Anat. pat.* **30**, 923 to 944 (1960). [G71,819/60]

Webster, D. E., Gentile, G.: Effect of chemical thymectomy on skin homografts. A preliminary report. *Canad. med. Ass. J.* **89**, 914—916 (1963). [E30,434/63]

Wei, E., Wilson, J.T.: Stress-mediated decrease in liver hexobarbital metabolism: the role of corticosterone and somatotropin. *J. Pharmacol. exp. Ther.* **177**, 227—233 (1971). [H37,417/71]

Weidenreich-Sherwin, R., Herrmann, F.: Hair cycle and chemically induced epidermal carcinogenesis in mice receiving Liothyronine. II. Findings after multiple applications of methylcholanthrene. *Dermatologica (Basel)* 128, 483 to 490 (1964). [F 16,179/64

Weihe, W. H.: Influence of age, physical activity and ambient temperature on acclimatization of rats to high altitude. *Fed. Proc.* 25, 1342—1347 (1966). [F 69,421/66

Weil, M. H.: Experimental studies on the treatment of shock produced by endotoxin. *Clin. Res.* 8, 124 (1960). [C 91,305/60

Weil, M. H.: Adrenocortical steroid for therapy of acute hypotension. *Amer. Practit.* 12, 162 to 168 (1961). [G 68,214/61

Weil, M. H., Allen, K. S.: The effect of steroids on shock due to endotoxin. In: Mills and Moyer; *Inflammation and Diseases of Connective Tissue*, p. 768—778. Philadelphia, London: W. B. Saunders Co. 1961. [D 7,883/61

Weil, M. H., Allen, K. S.: A comparison of the effectiveness of hydrocortisone and its analogues against lethal effects of endotoxin. *Clin. Res.* 12, 94 (1964). [F 14,091/64

Weil, M. H., Miller, B. S.: Studies on the effects of a vasopressor agent, sympatholytic drugs, and corticosteroid in shock caused by bacterial toxin. *Circulation* 22, 830 (1960). [D 97,273/60

Weil, M. H., Shubin, H., Allen, K. S.: Superiority of prednisolone over cortisol against lethal effects of endotoxin. *Fed. Proc.* 23/1, 416 (1964). [F 4,907/64

Weil, M. H., Shubin, H., Whigham, H.: Reversal of hemorrhagic shock with pharmacological doses of cortico-steroid (Abstr.). *Clin. Res.* 13, 233 (1965). [F 61,024/65

Weil, M. H., Spink, W. W.: A comparison of shock due to endotoxin with anaphylactic shock. *J. Lab. clin. Med.* 50, 501—515 (1957). [D 96,274/57

Weil, M. H., Udhoji, V. N., Sambhi, M. P., Rosoff, L.: Hemodynamic studies on the mechanism and treatment of bacteremic shock (Abstr.). *Circulation* 26, 801 (1962). [G 68,706/62

Weil, M. H., Whigham, H.: Experimental observations on the effects of corticosteroid hormones for the treatment of 'irreversible' hemorrhagic shock. *Circulation* 30, Sup. 3, 176 (1964). [F 13,600/64

Weil, M. H., Whigham, H.: Corticosteroids for reversal of hemorrhagic shock in rats. *Amer. J. Physiol.* 209, 815—818 (1965). [F 52,838/65

Weil, M. H., Whigham, H., Marbach, E. P.: Mechanism of corticosteroid reversal of fatal shock after blood loss. *Physiologist* 8, 302 (1965). [F 48,510/65

Weil, P. G., Rose, B., Browne, J. S. L.: The reduction of mortality from experimental traumatic shock with adrenal cortical substances. *Canad. med. Ass. J.* 43, 8—11 (1940). [78,692/40

Weinbren, K.: The effect of bile duct obstruction on regeneration of the rat's liver. *Brit. J. exp. Path.* 34, 280—289 (1953). [B 90,949/53

Weinbren, K.: Regeneration of the liver. *Gastroenterology* 37, 657—668 (1959). [D 95,941/59

Weinbren, K., Billing, B. H.: Hepatic clearance of bilirubin as an index of cellular function in the regenerating rat liver. *Brit. J. exp. Path.* 37, 199—204 (1956). [G 76,309/56

Weiner, I. M.: Mechanisms of drug absoption and excretion. The renal excretion of drugs and related compounds. *Ann. Rev. Pharmacol.* 7, 39—56 (1967). [G 74,032/67

Weiner, M., Blake, D. A., Buterbaugh, G. G.: The possible involvement of cyclic AMP in altered hepatic drug metabolism produced by diabetes or starvation. (Abstr.) *Fed. Proc.* 29, 804 (1970). [H 24,942/70

Weiner, M., Siddiqui, A. A., Bostanci, N., Dayton, P. G.: Drug interactions: the effect of combined administration of the half-life of coumarin and pyrazolone drugs in man. *Fed. Proc.* 24, 153 (1965). [F 35,871/65

Weinstein, L.: Further studies on the prophylaxis of experimental infections and intoxications with various hormone preparations. *Yale J. Biol. Med.* 12, 549—557 (1940). [A 33,940/40

Weinstein, L.: Prophylaxis of experimental anthrax infection with various hormone preparations. LT *Yale J. Biol. Med.* 11, 369—392 (1939). [B 15,029/39

Weintraub, S., Kraus, S. D., Wright, L. T.: Influence of sex hormones on tolerance to aminopterin. *Proc. Soc. exp. Biol. (N.Y.)* 74, 609—612 (1950). [B 49,800/50

Weisburger, E. K., Yamamoto, R., Glass, R., Grantham, P. H., Weisburger, J. H.: Hormonal status of rats and liver cancer induction by N-hydroxy-N-2-fluorenyl acetamide. *Proc. Amer. Ass. Cancer Res.* 8, 71 (1967). [F 78,862/67

Weisburger, E. K., Yamamoto, R. S., Glass, R. M., Grantham, P. H., Weisburger, J. H.: Effect of neonatal androgen and estrogen injection on liver tumor induction by N-hydroxy-

N-2-fluorenylacetamide and on the metabolism of the carcinogen in rats. *Endocrinology* **82**, 685—692 (1968). [F 97,904/68

Weisburger, J. H., Grantham, P. H., Weisburger, E. K.: Metabolism of N-2-fluorenylacetamide in the hamster. *Toxicol. appl. Pharmacol.* **6**, 427—433 (1964). [G 79,387/64

Weisburger, J. H., Pai, S. R., Yamamoto, R. S.: Pituitary hormones and liver carcinogenesis with N-hydroxy-N-2-fluorenylacetamide. *J. nat. Cancer Inst.* **32**, 881—904 (1964).
[D 18,583/64

Weisburger, J. H., Schmehl, E. A., Pai, S. R.: Liver damage by the carcinogen N-hydroxy-N-2-fluorenylacetamide. Pentobarbital sleeping time and liver morphology. *Toxicol. appl. Pharmacol.* **7**, 579—587 (1965). [G 78,956/65

Weisburger, J. H., Yamamoto, R. S., Korzis, J., Weisburger, E. K.: Liver cancer: neonatal estrogen enhances induction by a carcinogen. *Science* **154**, 673—674 (1966). [F 72,720/66

Weiss, A. K.: Tissue responses in the cold-exposed rat. *Amer. J. Physiol.* **188**, 430—434 (1957). [C 34,561/57

Weiss, A. K.: Effects of aging on adaptation to cold. *Fed. Proc.* **18**, 168 (1959) [C 66,153/59

Weiss, A. K.: Artificial acclimatization of aging rats. *Excerpta med. (Amst.) Int. Congr. Ser.* No. 57, p. 37 (1963). [G 21,456/63

Weiss, C. F., Glazko, A. J., Weston, J. K.: Chloramphenicol in the newborn infant. A physiologic explanation or its toxicity when given in excessive doses. *New Engl. J. Med.* **262**, 787 to 794 (1960). [H 33,308/60

Weisskopf, A., Burn, H. F., Schoenholz, W. K.: Protective action of estrogen against streptococcal infection in mice, and its relation to connective tissues. *Laryngoscope* (St. Louis) **71**, 788—799 (1961). [D 35,320/61

Weissmann, G.: Changes in connective tissue and intestine caused by vitamin A in amphibia, and their acceleration by hydrocortisone. *J. exp. Med.* **114**, 581—592 (1961). [D 10,768/61

Weissmann, G.: The effects of steroids and drugs on lysosomes. In: Dingle, J. T. and Fell, H. B., Lysosomes in biology and pathology, p. 276—295. Amsterdam, London: North-Holland Publ. Co. 1969. [G 79,855/69

Weissmann, G., Bell, E., Thomas, L.: Prevention by hydrocortisone of changes in connective tissue induced by an excess of vitamin A acid in amphibia. *Amer. J. Path.* **42**, 571—585 (1963). [D 64,001/63

Weissmann, G., Dingle, J.: Release of lysosomal protease by ultraviolet irradiation and inhibition by hydrocortisone. *Exp. Cell Res.* **25**, 207 to 210 (1961). [D 14,268/61

Weissmann, G., Fell, H. B.: The effect of hydrocortisone on the response of fetal rat skin in culture to ultraviolet irradiation. *J. exp. Med.* **116**, 365—380 (1962). [D 46,242/62

Weissmann, G., Thomas, L.: Studies on lysosomes. The effect of cortisone and endotoxin. *Annual Meet. Amer. Soc. clin. Invest.*, Inc., Atlantic City, April 30, p. 75 (1962)
[D 23,630/62

Weissman, G., Thomas, L.: Studies on lysosomes. I. The effects of endotoxin, endotoxin tolerance, and cortisone on the release of acid hydrolases from a granular fraction of rabbit-liver. *J. exp. med.* **116**, 443—450 (1962).
[D 35,555/62

Weissmann, G., Thomas, L.: Studies on lysosomes. II. The effect of cortisone on the release of acid hydrolases from a large granule fraction of rabbit liver induced by an excess of vitamin A. *J. clin. Invest.* **42**, 661—669 (1963).
[D 65,709/63

Weissmann, G., Thomas, L.: The effects of corticosteroids upon connective tissue and lysosomes. In: Pincus; *Recent Progress in Hormone Research* **20**, p. 215—245. New York, London: Academic Press 1964. [E 4,216/64

Weissmann, G., Thomas, L.: On a mechanism of tissue damage by bacterial endotoxins. In: Landy and Braun; *Bacterial Endotoxins*, p. 602 to 609. New Brunswick, N. J.: Institute of Microbiology, Rutgers, The State University 1964. [E 8,482/64

Welch, R. M., Conney, A. H.: Organophosphate insecticide inhibition and phenobarbital stimulation of testosterone hydroxylase in rat liver microsomes. *Fed. Proc.* **24**, 639 (1965).
[F 36,508/65

Welch, R. M., Harrison, Y. E., Burns, J. J.: Implications of enzyme induction in drug toxicity studies. *Toxicol. appl. Pharmacol.* **10**, 340—351 (1967). [G 47,232/67

Welch, R. M., Harrison, Y. E., Gommi, B. W., Poppers, P. J., Finster, M., Conney, A. H.: Stimulatory effect of cigarette smoking on the hydroxylation of 3,4-benzpyrene and the N-demethylation of 3-methyl-4-monomethylaminoazobenzene by enzymes in human placenta. *Clin. Pharmacol. Ther.* **10**, 100—109 (1969). [G 65,788/69

Welch, R. M., Levin, W., Conney, A. H.: Insecticide inhibition and stimulation of steroid hydroxylases in rat liver. *J. Pharmacol. exp. Ther.* **155**, 167—173 (1967). [F 76,642/67

Welch, R. M., Levin, W., Conney, A. H.: Stimulatory effect of phenobarbital on the metabolism in vivo of estradiol-17 B and estrone in the rat. *J. Pharmacol. exp. Ther.* **160**, 171—178 (1968). [F 96,172/68

Welch, R. M., Levin, W., Conney, A. H.: Estrogenic action of DDT and its analogs. *Toxicol. appl. Pharmacol.* **14**, 358—367 (1969).
[G 65,737/69

Weller, O.: Die antikatabole Wirkung des I Methyl-Δ1 androstenolons (Methenolon). *Med. Welt. (Stuttg.)* Nr. **40**, 2073—2078 (1961).
[D 13,995/61

Weller, O.: Klinische Untersuchungen mit dem oral anwendbaren Methenolon-acetat. *Arzneimittel-Forsch.* **12**, 234—240 (1962).
[D 22,262/62

Wellmann, K. F., Volk, B. W., Lazarus, S. S.: Renal changes in experimental hypercholesterolosis in normal and subdiabetic rabbits (Abstr.). *Fed. Proc.* **28**, 368 (1969). [H 9,536/69

Wells, J. A., Anderson, L. H.: Mechanism of increased susceptibility to ergot gangrene in thyrotoxicosis. *Proc. Soc. exp. Biol. (N.Y.)* **74**, 374—377 (1950). [G 74,995/50

Weltman, A. S., Sackler, A. M.: Effects of thymectomy on the resistance of rats to drowning and histamine stress. *Nature (Lond.)* **192**, 460 to 461 (1961). [D 14,302/61

Wendt, H.: Natriumthiosulfat in der Therapie. Äußerliche Wirkung als Schwefel in statu nascendi, innerliche Wirkung als chemisches Antidot und als Antiallergikum. *Fortschr. Therap.* **14**, 88—96, 147—154, 202—207 (1938).
[A 48,250/38

Wenzel, D. G., Keplinger, M. L.: Central depressant properties of uracil and related oxypyrimidines. *J. Amer. pharm. Ass., sci. Ed.* **44**, 56—59 (1955). [G 76,357/55

Wenzel, M., Pollow-Hanisch, B., Pollow, K.: Änderung der Sexualspezifität bei der Androstendionreduktion durch Östradiol-17 β-Wasserstoff in Rattenleber nach Feminisierung durch Cyproteronacetat. *Hoppe-Seylers Z. physiol. Chem.* **350**, 791—792 (1969). [H 14,785/69

Werboff, J., Hedlund, L., Havlena, J.: Audiogenic seizures in adult female ovariectomized rats (Sprague-Dawley) treated with sex hormones. *J. Endocr.* **29**, 39—46 (1964).
[F 10,255/64

Werder, E. A., Yaffe, S. J.: Glucuronyl transferase activity in experimental neonatal hypothyroidism. *Biol. Neonat. (Basel)* **6**, 8—15 (1964). [G 12,065/64

Werk, E. E., MacGee, J., Sholiton, L. J.: Effect of diphenylhydantoin on cortisol metabolism in man. *J. clin. Invest.* **43**, 1824—1835 (1964).
[F 20,780/64

Werk, E. E., Jr., Sholiton, L. J., Olinger, C. P.: Amelioration of non-tumorous Cushing's syndrome by diphenylhydantoin (Abstr.). *2nd Int. Congr. on Hormonal steroids* Milan, Italy, p 301 (1966). [G 67,762/66

Werle, E. Lentzen, J.: Über die Beeinflussung der Injektionsnarkose durch kreislaufaktive Stoffe. *Naunyn-Schmiedebergs Arch. Pharmak.* **190**, 328—340 (1938). [A 28,007/38

Westermann, E. O., Maickel, R. P., Brodie, B. B.: Some biochemical effects of reserpine mediated by the pituitary. *Fed. Proc.* **19**, 268 (1960). [C 83,072/60

Westfall, B. A.: Pyruvic acid antagonism to barbiturate depression. *J. Pharmacol. exp. Ther.* **87**, 33—37 (1946). [B 31,306/46

Westfall, B. A., Boulos, B. M., Shields, J. L., Garb, S.: Sex differences in pentobarbital sensitivity in mice. *Proc. Soc. exp. Biol. (N.Y.)* **115**, 509—510 (1964). [F 2,504/64

Westmoreland, B., Bass, N. H.: Diphenylhydantoin intoxication during pregnancy. A chemical study of drug distribution in the albino rat. *A. M. A. Arch. Neurol. (Chic.)* **24**, 158—164 (1971). [G 80,590/71

Westphal, F., Hagen, U.: Strahlenschutz und Strahlensensibilisierung an den Chromosomen lymphatischer Zellen. *Strahlentherapie* **132**, 284—295 (1967). [G 45,683/67

Wheatley, D. N.: Action of drugs affecting the functioning of the adrenal cortex on adrenal necrosis induced by 7, 12-dimethylbenz(α) anthracene and its 7-hydroxymethyl derivative in rats. *Endocrinology* **82**, 1217—1222 (1968).
[F 98,919/68

Wheatley, D. N., Kernohan, I. R., Currie, A. R.: Liver injury and the prevention of massive adrenal necrosis from 9,10-dimethyl-1,2-benzanthracene in rats. *Nature (Lond.)* **211**, 387 to 389 (1966). [F 68,548/66

Wheeler, R. S., Hoffmann, E., Barber, C. W.: The effect of thiouracil-induced hypothyroidism on the resistance of chicks artificially infected with Eimeria tenella. *J. Amer. vet. med. Ass.* **112**, 473—474 (1948). [A 48,602/48

Wheeler, R. S., Perkinson, J. D., Jr.: Influence of induced hypo- and hyperthyroidism on vitamin E requirement of chicks. *Amer. J. Physiol.* **159**, 287—290 (1949). [B 43,572/49

Whigham, H.: Effect of corticosteroids on the progression of hemorrhagic shock in rats. *Calif. Med.* **106**, 10—11 (1967). [F 75,787/67

White, M. R., Finkel, A. J., Schubert, J.: Effect of adrenocorticotrophic hormone on tissue distribution and acute toxicity of beryllium. *Proc. Soc. exp. Biol. (N.Y.)* 80, 603–604 (1952). [B 74,079/52

Whitfield, C. F., Tidball, M. E.: Estrogen effect on skeletal muscle and degenerative signs of experimental Mg deficiency (Abstr.). *Fed. Proc.* 27, 498 (1968). [H 549/68

Wiancko, K. B., Kowalewski, K.: Strength of callus in fractured humerus of rat treated with anti-anabolic and anabolic compounds. *Acta endocr. (Kbh.)* 36, 310–318 (1961). [D 270/61

Wiberg, G. S., Carter, J. R., Stephenson, N. R.: The bioassay of thyroactive materials by the mouse anoxia test and goitre-prevention response in the same experimental animals. *Acta endocr. (Kbh.)* 43, 609–617 (1963). [E 23,265/63

Wicher, K., Jakubowski, A.: Effect of cortisone on the course of experimental syphilis in the guinea-pig. I. Effect of previously-administered cortisone on guinea-pigs infected with Treponema pallidum intradermally, intratesticularly, and intravenously. *Brit. J. vener. Dis.* 40, 213–216 (1964). [G 26,810/64

Wicks, W. D., Greenman, D. L., Kenney, F. T.: Stimulation of ribonucleic acid synthesis by steroid hormones. I. Transfer ribonucleic acid. *J. biol. Chem.* 240, 4414–4419 (1965). [G 35,046/65

Wiesbader, H.: Reid Hunt reaction and the thyrotropic hormone. *Endocrinology* 20, 100 to 102 (1936). [68,823/36

Wiese, C. E., Mehl, J. W., Deuel, H. J., Jr.: Studies on carotenoid metabolism. IX. Conversion of carotene to vitamin A in the hypothyroid rat. *J. biol. Chem.* 175, 21–28 (1948). [B 39,257/48

Wietek, H. F., Taupitz, E.: Der Einfluß lyophilisierter Placenta auf die experimentelle Arteriosklerose von Ratten. *Arzneimittel-Forsch.* 7, 479–485 (1957). [C 40,028/57

Wilbrandt, W., Weiss, E. M.: Antagonismus zwischen Herzglykosid und Corticosteroiden am Froschhautpotential. *Arzneimittel-Forsch.* 10, 409–412 (1960). [C 88,230/60

Wilgram, G. F.: Cardiovascular changes induced in choline-deficient rats by growth hormone. *Ann. N.Y. Acad. Sci.* 72, 863–869 (1959). [C 84,322/59

Wilgram, G. F., Best, C. H., Blumenstein, J.: Effect of growth hormone and testosterone on induction of cardiovascular changes in choline-deficient rats. *Proc. Soc. exp. Biol (N.Y.)* 91, 620–622 (1956). [C 15,960/56

Wilgram, G. F., Hartroft, W. S.: Pathogenesis of fatty and sclerotic lesions in the cardiovascular system of choline-deficient rats. *Brit. J. exp. Path.* 36, 298–305 (1955). [C 14,392/55

Williams, D. J., Rabin, B. R.: The effects of aflatoxin B_1 and steroid hormones on polysome binding to microsomal membranes as measured by the activity of an enzyme catalysing disulphide interchange. *FEBS Lett.* 4, 103–107 (1969). [G 77,164/69

Williams, R. H.: Textbook of Endocrinology, 4th ed., pp. 1258. Philadelphia, London, Toronto: W. B. Saunders Co. 1968. [E 8,139/68

Williams, R. T.: Detoxication Mechanisms. The Metabolism and Detoxication of Drugs, Toxic Substances and Other Organic Compounds, 2nd ed., pp. 796. New York: John Wiley and Sons Inc. 1959. [E 906/59

Williams, R. T.: Detoxication mechanisms in vivo. In: Brodie, B. B., Erdös, E. G., Metabolic factors controlling duration of drug action. (Proc. 1st int. Pharmacol. Meet. 'Mode of action of drugs', Stockholm, 1961). p. 1–12. New York: MacMillan Co., 1962. [G 73,007/62

Williams, R. T.: Detoxication mechanisms in man. *Clin. Pharmacol. Ther.* 4, 234–254 (1963). [G 77,567/63

Willmer, H. A.: The disappearance of phosphatase from the hydronephrotic kidney. *J. exp. Med.* 78, 225–230 (1943). [A 48,603/43

Willmer, J. S., Foster, T. S.: Enzymatic and metabolic adaptions. II. Changes in adrenalectomized rats subjected to dietary modifications. *Canad. J. Biochem.* 40, 961–972 (1962). [D 28,163/62

Wilson, G., Care, A. D., Anderson, C. K.: The effect of cortisone on vitamin D_2-induced nephrocalcinosis in the rat. *Clin. Sci.* 16, 181–185 (1957). [C 33,679/57

Wilson, J. L., Ashburn, A. D., Williams, W. L.: Effects of sex hormones on diet-induced atrial thrombosis. *Anat. Res.* 168, 331–337 (1970). [G 79,508/70

Wilson, J. T.: Prevention of the normal postnatal increase in drug-metabolizing enzyme activity in rat liver by a pituitary tumor. *Pediat. Res. (Basel)* 2, 514–518 (1968). [G 63,125/68

Wilson, J. T.: Identification of somatotropin as the hormone in a mixture of somatotropin, adrenocorticotropic hormone and prolactin which decreased liver drug metabolism in the rat. *Biochem. Pharmacol.* 18, 2029—2031 (1969). [G 69,098/69

Wilson, J. T.: Alteration of normal development of drug metabolism by injection of growth hormone. *Nature (Lond.)* 225, 861 to 863 (1970). [H 21,345/70

Wilson, J. T.: Altered rat hepatic drug metabolism after implantation of a pituitary mammotropic tumor (MtT), Walker carcinosarcoma or adenocarcinoma and after removal of the MtT. *Endocrinology* 88, 185—194 (1971). [H 34,926/71

Wilson, J. W., Leduc, E. H.: The effect of coramine on mitotic activity and growth in the liver of the mouse. *Growth* 14, 31—48 (1950). [E 43,062/50

Wilson, S. G. F., Pfefer, J., Nash, G., Heymann, W.: Aminonucleoside nephrosis in rats. *J. Dis. Child.* 94, 572 (1957). [C 45,755/57

Wilson, W. S.: Metabolism of digitalis. *Progr. cardiovasc. Dis.* 11, 479—487 (1969). [G 71,238/69

Wimberly, J. E., Martin, C. E., Foster, J. H.: Temporary hepatic inflow occlusion in dogs treated with methylprednisolone and antibiotics. *Amer. Surg.* 35, 271—273 (1969). [G 65,769/69

Winberg, J., Zetterström, R.: Cortisone treatment in vitamin D intoxication. *Acta paediat. (Scand.)* 45, 96—101 (1956). [C 12,829/56

Windorfer, A.: Über die Phenobarbitalbehandlung des Neugeborenenikterus. *Dtsch. med. Wschr.* 95, 1617—1619 (1970). [H 28,824/70

Winter, C. A., Flataker, L.: The effect of cortisone, desoxycorticosterone, and adrenocorticotrophic hormone upon the responses of animals to analgesic drugs. *J. Pharmacol. exp. Ther.* 103, 93—105 (1951). [B 62,935/51

Winter, C. A., Flataker, L.: The effect of cortisone, desoxycorticosterone, adrenocorticotrophic hormone and diphenhydramine upon the responses of albino mice to general anesthetics. *J. Pharmacol. exp. Ther.* 105, 358 (1952). [B 73,509/52

Winter, C. A., Hollings, H. L., Stebbins, R. B.: The effect of androgenic hormones upon the adrenal atrophy produced by cortisone injections and upon the anti-inflammatory action of cortisone. *Endocrinology* 52, 123—134 (1953). [B 79,381/53

Winter, D.: Le rôle du terrain thyroïdien dans la modification de la réactivité de l'organisme aux médicaments. Recherches expérimentales de pathopharmacologie. *Prod. Prob. pharm.* 20, 591—595 (1965). [G 71,836/65

Winter, D.: Toxizitätsveränderung neurotroper Pharmaka bei Versuchstieren mit experimentell hervorgerufener Hyperthyreoidie. *Med. Pharmacol. exp. (Basel)* 14, 391—394 (1966). [F 64,465/66

Winter, D.: The thyroid and the reactivity of the organism to drugs. *Rev. roum. Physiol.* 5, 89—96 (1968). [F 98,019/68

Winter, H.: Conditions influencing the course of steroid hormone anesthesia. *Endocrinology* 29, 790—792 (1941). [A 36,333/41

Winter, H., Bélanger, L. F.: On the protective action of testosterone against the kidney-damaging effect of phlorhizin. *Proc. Canad. physiol. Soc.* (7th Ann. Meet., Montebello), p. 17 (1941). [A 36,751/41

Winter, H., Selye, H.: Conditions influencing the course of steroid hormone anesthesia. *Amer. J. Physiol.* 133, 495 (1941). [A 35,658/41

Winternitz, M. C., Waters, L. L.: The effect of hypophysectomy on compensatory renal hypertrophy in dogs. *Yale J. Biol. Med.* 12, 705—709 (1940). [A 34,910/40

Winton, F. R.: The rat-poisoning substance in red squills. *J. Pharmacol. exp. Ther.* 31, 123 to 136 (1927). [A 42,964/27

Wirtheimer, C.: A propos de l'accélération par les hormones gonadotrophiques de l'apparition des manifestations ulcéreuses postréserpiniques. *C. R. Soc. Biol. (Paris)* 153, 1284—1285 (1959). [D 10,158/59

Wishart, M. B., Pritchett, I. W.: Experimental studies in diabetes. Ser. II. The internal pancreatic function in relation to body mass and metabolism. 6. Gas bacillus infections in diabetic dogs. *Amer. J. Physiol.* 54, 382—387 (1920). [12,285/20

Wiśniewski, K.: Influence of insulin on the action of analgesics. *Biochem. Pharmacol.* 12, Sup. 5 (1963). [E 32,005/63

Wiśniewski, K., Buczko, W.: The central pharmacological effect of chlorpromazine in rats with alloxan-diabetes. *Biochem. Pharmacol.* 16, 2227—2230 (1967). [G 51,489/67

Wiśniewski, K., Danysz, A.: The study on the insulin controlling and directing of chlorpromazine action and level in brain tissue. *Biochem. Pharmacol.* 15, 669—673 (1966). [G 40,054/66

Wiśniewski, K., Zarebski, M.: Insulin-dependent transport of drugs in vivo and in vitro.

(Abstr. 27th. Ann. Meet. Amer. Diabetes Ass.) *Diabetes* **16**, 515 (1967). [F85,977/67

Wiśniewski, K., Zarebski, M.: Effect of insulin on the transport and the analgesic action of sodium salicylates. *Metabolism* **17**, 212—217 (1968). [F96,973/68

Witzel, H.: Über anaesthetisch wirksame Steroide. *Z. Vitamin-, Hormon- u. Fermentforsch.* **10**, 46—75 (1959). [C68,395/59

Wohl, M. G., Feldman, J. B.: Vitamin A deficiency in disease of the thyroid gland: its detection by dark adaptation. *Endocrinology* **24**, 389—396 (1939). [A30,107/39

Wohl, M. G., Robertson, H. F.: Bromide intoxication: some observations on its treatment with sodium chloride and desoxycorticosterone. *Penn. med. J.* **47**, 802—808 (1944). [93,481/44

Wolbach, S. B., Maddock, C. L.: Vitamin-A acceleration of bone growth sequences in hypophysectomized rats. *Arch. Path.* **53**, 273—278 (1952). [B83,297/52

Wolbach, S. B., Maddock, C. L., Cohen, J.: The hypervitaminosis — A syndrome in adrenalectomized rats. *Arch. Path.* **60**, 130—135 (1955). [C14,796/55

Wolfram, J., Zwemer, R. L.: Cortin protection against anaphylactic shock in guinea pigs. *J. exp. Med.* **61**, 9—15 (1935). [30,809/35

Wollenberger, A., Karsh, M. L.: A note on the influence of sex upon the response of the rat heart to ouabain. *J. Amer. pharm. Ass., sci. Ed.* **40**, 637—638 (1951). [D95,331/51

Wong, D. T., Terriere, L. C.: Epoxidation of aldrin, isodrin, and heptachlor by rat liver microsomes. *Biochem. Pharmacol.* **14**, 375—377 (1965). [G77,538/65

Wood, J. S., Jr., Knox, W. E.: Studies on liver tryptophan peroxidase in mice bearing a transplantable sarcoma. *Proc. Amer. Ass. Cancer Res.* **1**, 52—53 (1954). [D81,779/54

Wood, S., Jr., Rivlin, R. S., Knox, W. E.: Biphasic changes of tryptophan peroxidase level in tumor-bearing mice and in mice subjected to growth hormone and stress. *Cancer Res.* **16**, 1053—1058 (1956). [C27,721/56

Woodbury, D. M.: Effect of hormones on brain excitability and electrolytes. In: *Recent Progress in Hormone Research* **10**, p. 65—107. New York: Academic Press Inc. 1954.
  [B98,594/54

Woodbury, D. M., Cheng, C.-P., Sayers, G., Goodman, L. S.: Antagonism of adrenocorticotrophic hormone and adrenal cortical extract to desoxycorticosterone: electrolytes and electroshock threshold. *Amer. J. Physiol.* **160**, 217—227 (1950). [B46,344/50

Woodbury, D. M., Davenport, V. D.: Brain and plasma cations and experimental seizures in normal and desoxycorticosterone-treated rats. *Amer. J. Physiol.* **157**, 234—240 (1949).
  [B37,243/49

Woodbury, D. M., Hurley, R. E., Lewis, N. G., McArthur, M. W., Copeland, W. W., Kirschvink, J. F., Goodman, L. S.: Influence of thyroidectomy, propylthiouracil and thyroxin on brain excitability. *Fed. Proc.* **11**, 404 (1952).
  [B68,423/52

Woodbury, D. M., Rosenberg, C. A., Sayers, G.: Antagonism of adrenocorticotrophic hormone (ACTH) and adrenal cortical extract (ACE) to desoxycorticosterone (DCA): pathological changes. *Fed. Proc.* **9**, 139 (1950).
  [B47,201/50

Woodbury, D. M., Timiras, P. S., Vernadakis, A.: Influence of adrenocortical steroids on brain function and metabolism. In: Hoagland, H.; *Hormones, Brain Function, and Behavior*, p. 27—54. New York: Acad. Press Inc. Publ. 1957. [C34,538/57

Wooles, W. R., Borzelleca, J. F.: Prolongation of barbiturate sleeping time in mice by stimulation of the reticuloendothelial system (RES). *J. reticuloendoth. Soc.* **3**, 41—47 (1966).
  [F93,374/66

Wooles, W.R., Munson, A.E.: The effect of stimulants and depressants of reticuloendothelial activity on drug metabolism. *J. reticuloendothel. Soc.* (in press). [G78,975

Woollam, D. H. M., Millen, J. W.: Influence of 4-methyl-2-thiouracil on the teratogenic activity of hypervitaminosis-A. *Nature (Lond.)* **181**, 992—993 (1958). [C64,432/58

Woolley, D. E., Timiras, P. S., Srebnik, H. H., Silva, A.: Threshold and pattern of electroshock convulsions during estrous cycle in the rat. *Fed. Proc.* **20**, 198 (1961). [D4,062/61

Wragg, L. E., Speirs, R. S.: Strain and sex differences in response of inbred mice to adrenal cortical hormones. *Proc. Soc. exp. Biol. (N,Y.)* **80**, 680—684 (1952). [B74,080/52

Wright, D. H.: The effect of neonatal thymectomy on the survival of golden hamsters infected with Plasmodium berghei. *Brit. J. exp. Path.* **49**, 379—384 (1968). [H1,836/68

Wulf, H. de, Hers, H. G.: The stimulation of glycogen synthesis and of glycogen synthetase in the liver by glucocorticoids. *Europ. J. Biochem.* **2**, 57—60 (1967). [G53,099/67

Wulfsohn, N. L., Politzer, W. M.: 5-Hydroxytryptamine in anaesthesia. *Anaesthesia* 17, 64 to 68 (1961). [D 22,421/61

Wurtman, R. J., Axelrod, J.: Sex steroids, cardiac ³H-norepinephrine, and tissue monoamine oxidase levels in the rat. *Biochem. Pharmacol.* 12, 1417—1419 (1963). [E 36,478/63

Wurtman, R. J., Axelrod, J., Anton-Tay, F.: Inhibition of the metabolism of H³-melatonin by phenothiazines. *J. Pharmacol. exp. Ther.* 161, 367—372 (1968). [F 99,396/68

Wüstenberg, P. W., Börner, H., Tessmann, D., Holtz, M.: Tierexperimentelle Untersuchungen zur Frage des Testosteroneinflusses bei akuter toxischer Nierenschädigung. *Zbl. allg. Pathol. pathol. Anat.* 107, 378—388 (1965).
[G 38,225/65

Wuth, O.: Über biologische Wirkungen proteinogener Amine. Zugleich ein Beitrag zur Frage der Acetonitrilreaktion. *Biochem. Z.* 116, 237—245 (1921). [A 48,026/21

Wyler, R., Kradolfer, F., Gross, F.: Entgiftende Wirkung von Dexamethason und Aldosteron gegenüber bakteriellen Lipopolysacchariden. *Helv. physiol. pharmacol. Acta* 18, 357—365 (1960). [D 5,696/60

Wynn, J., Gibbs, R., Royster, B.: Thyroxine degradation. I. Study of optimal reaction conditions of a rat liver thyroxine-degrading system. *J. biol. Chem.* 237, 1892—1897 (1962).
[G 67,767/62

Yaffe, S. J., Levy, G., Matsuzawa, T., Baliah, T.: Enhancement of glucuronide-conjugating capacity in a hyperbilirubinemic infant due to apparent enzyme induction by phenobarbital. *New. Engl. J. Med.* 275, 1461—1466 (1966).
[G 67,125/66

Yam, K. M., DuBois, K. P.: Effects of X-irradiation on the hexobarbital-metabolizing enzyme system of rat liver. *Radiat. Res.* 31, 315 to 326 (1967). [G 58,163/67

Yamada, A., Osada, Y., Takayama, S., Akimoto, T., Ogawa, H., Oshima, Y., Fujiwara, K.: Tyzzer's disease syndrom in laboratory rats treated with adrenocorticotropic hormone. *Jap. J. exp. Med.* 39, 505—518 (1969).
[H 24,079/69

Yamamoto, S., Lin, K., Bloch, K.: Some properties of the microsomal 2,3-oxidosqualene sterol cyclase. *Proc. nat. Acad. Sci. (Wash.)* 63, 110—117 (1967). [G 67,939/67

Yanagimoto, Y.: Liver circulation and function. Cyto- and biochemical studies of liver glycogen on a liver lobe ligation. *Ann. Histochim.* 14, 265 to 273 (1969). [G 71,560/69

Yanagimoto, Y., Nakahama, S., Noda, Y.: Liver circulation and function. Changes in lipids of rat liver following ligation of liver lobe. *Ann. Histochim.* 14, 215—223 (1969). [G 71,328/69

Yang, T. L., Lissak, K.: The effect of various temperatures and ACTH on physical performance. *Acta physiol. Acad. Sci. hung.* 16, 47 to 49 (1959). [C 77,913/59

Yano, R., Nobunaga, M.: Experimental study on the significance of serum β-glucuronidase activity in liver diseases. *Jap. J. Med.* 2, 308 to 309 (1963). [E 21,714/63

Yaoi, H., Goto, N., Yamasawa, R., Nagata, A.: Studies on the rabies vaccine XIVth report: On the effects of PVL and cortisone upon immunizing power of anti-rabies vaccine. *Yokohama med. Bull.* 7, 371—382 (1956).
[C 34,360/56

Yates, F. E., Herbst, A. L., Urquhart, J.: Sex difference in rate of ring A reduction of Δ^4-3-keto-steroids in vitro by rat liver. *Endocrinology* 63, 887—902 (1958). [C 61,952/58

Yates, F. E., Urquhart, J., Herbst, A. L.: Effect of thyroid hormones on ring A reduction of cortisone by liver. *Fed. Proc.* 17, 174 (1958).
[C 51,744/58

Yates, F. E., Urquhart, J., Herbst, A. L.: Impairment of the enzymatic inactivation of adrenal cortical hormones following passive venous congestion of the liver. *Amer. J. Physiol.* 194, 65—71 (1958). [C 56,413/58

Yeh, S. Y., Woods, L. A.: The effect of tolerance and withdrawal on the in vivo metabolism of N-C¹⁴-methyl-dihydromorphine in the rat. *J. Pharmacol. exp. Ther.* 169, 168—174 (1969).
[H 17,933/69

Yesair, D. W., Remington, L., Callahan, M., Kensler, C. J.: Comparative effects of salicylic acid, phenylbutazone, probenecid and other anions on the metabolism, distribution and excretion of indomethacin by rats. *Biochem. Pharmacol.* 19, 1591—1600 (1970).
[G 75,388/70

Yeung, C. Y., Field, C. E.: Phenobarbitone therapy in neonatal hyperbilirubinaemia. *Lancet* 1969 II, 135—139. [G 73,821/69

Ying, S. Y., Meyer, R. K.: Effect of steroids on neuropharmacologic blockade of ovulation in pregnant mare's serum (PMS)-primed immature rats. *Endocrinology* 84, 1466—1474 (1969).
[H 13,672/69

Yohn, D. S., Funk, C. A.: Sex-related resistance in hamsters to adenovirus-12 oncogenesis. IV. Gonadal hormone influences. *J. nat. Cancer Inst.* 43, 133—139 (1969). [G 68,339/69

Yohn, D. S., Funk, C. A., Grace, J. T., Jr.: Sex-related resistance in hamsters to adenovirus-12 oncogenesis. III. Influence of immunologic impairment by thymectomy or cortisone. *J. Immunol.* 100, 771—780 (1968). [G 57,790/68

Yokoi, Y., Kuwamura, T., Muto, Y.: A new explanation for the biphasic pattern of fever induced by bacterial pyrogen. *Jap. J. Physiol.* 11, 270—280 (1961). [D 8,839/61

You, S. S., Sellers, E. A.: Effect of desoxycorticosterone acetate and adrenal cortical extracts on survival of adrenalectomized and intact rats after burning. *Amer. J. Physiol.* 160, 83—88 (1950). [B 46,218/50

Youmans, G. P., Youmans, A. S.: The effect of hormonal preparations on the survival of mice injected intravenously with virulent, attenuated, and avirulent mycobacteria. *Amer. Rev. Tuberc.* 69, 790—796 (1954). [B 95,169/54

Young, A. G., Taylor, F. H. L.: Studies of the effect of sodium thiosulphate on mercury intoxication (Abstr.). *J. Pharmacol. exp. Ther.* 39, 248 (1930). [A 48,227/30

Young, A. G., Taylor, F. H. L.: The effect of sodium thiosulphate on mercury poisoning. *J. Pharmacol. exp. Ther.* 42, 185—195 (1931). [A 48,535/31

Young, S., Cowan, D. M., Davidson, C.: The production of mammary carcinomas in rats by 9,10-dimethyl-1,2-benzanthracene and its relationship to the oestrous cycle. *Brit. J. Cancer* 24, 328—332 (1970). [G 77,809/70

Young, S., Helfenstein, J. E., Baker, R. A.: Relationship of adrenocortical insufficiency to spontaneous regression in mammary tumours induced in rats by oral administration of dimethylbenzanthracene. *Nature (Lond.)* 203, 1079—1080 (1964). [F 20,579/64

Yousef, M. K., Chaffee, R. R. J., Robertson, W. D., Johnson, H. D.: Cold survival of surgically- and radio-thyroidectomized hamsters (Abstr.). *Physiologist* 10, 354 (1967). [F 86,757/67

Yousef, M. K., Chaffee, R. R. J., Robertson, W. D., Johnson, H. D.: Significance of thyroid in cold survival of hamsters. *Proc. Soc. exp. Biol. (N.Y.)* 127, 829—831 (1968). [F 98,470/68

Yu, C. A., Gunsalus, I. C.: Crystalline cytochrome P-450 cam. *Biochem. biophys. Res. Commun.* 40, 1431—1436 (1970). [G 81,295/70

Yun, I. S., Lee, Y. C.: Experimental studies on the relation between nicotine and sexual hormone. *Folia endocr. Jap.* 11, 9—12 (1935). [34,178/35

Yuwiler, A., Geller, E., Schapiro, S.: Response differences in some steroid-sensitive hepatic enzymes in the fasting rats. *Canad. J. Physiol. Pharmacol.* 47, 317—328 (1969). [H 9,994/69

Zacco, M., Pratesi, G.: Lo choc papainico. *Boll. Soc. ital. Biol. sper.* 23, 553—555 (1947). [B 37,559/47

Zackheim, H. S.: Effect of castration on the induction of epidermal neoplasms in male mice by topical methylcholanthrene. *J. invest. Derm.* 54, 479—482 (1970). [H 26,549/70

Zaltzman, S.: Efecto de la esplenectomía sobre la regeneración hepática. *Thesis.* University of Mexico (1956). [D 92,764/56

Zanowiak, P., Rodman, M. J.: A study of LSD-serotonin central interaction. *J. Amer. pharm. Ass., sci. Ed.* 48, 165—168 (1959). [C 85,018/59

Zapata-Ortiz, V., de la Mata, R. C.: The influence of aldosterone on hemorrhagic shock. *Arzneimittel-Forsch.* 12, 953—954 (1962). [D 37,373/62

Zárday, I., Weiner, P.: A thyroxin és az altatószerek között fennálló antagonismusról, különös tekintettel a constitutióra. *Orv. Hetil.* 78, 682—684 (1934). [A 52,879/34

Zárday, I., Weiner, P.: Barbitursäure und Schilddrüse. Zugleich ein Beitrag zur Kenntnis der funktionellen Konstitution. *Wien. Arch. inn. Med.* 26, 353—362 (1935). [53,715/35

Zarrow, M. X., Hiestand, W. A., Stemler, F. W., Wiebers, J. E.: Comparison of effects of experimental hyperthyroidism and hypothyroidism on resistance to anoxia in rats and mice. *Amer. J. Physiol.* 167, 171—175 (1951). [B 63,316/51

Zarrow, M. X., Money, W. L.: Involution of the adrenal cortex of rats treated with thiouracil. *Endocrinology* 44, 345—358 (1949). [B 27,880/49

Zarrow, M. X., Quinn, D. L.: Super ovulation in the immature rat following treatment with PMS alone and inhibition of PMS-induced ovulation. *J. Endocr.* 26, 181—188 (1963). [E 20,351/63

Zauder, H. L.: The effect of certain analgesic drugs and adrenal cortical hormones on the brain of normal and hypophysectomized rats as measured, by the thiobarbituric acid reagent. *J. Pharmacol. exp. Ther.* 101, 40—46 (1951). /B 57,611/51

Zauder, H. L.: The effect of prolonged morphine administration on the in vivo and in vitro conjugation of morphine by rats. *J. Pharmacol. exp. Ther.* 104, 11—19 (1952). [G 75,347/52

Zbinden, G.: Modification of the irritant effects of intraperitoneally administered phenylbutazone in rats after prolonged treatment with the same drug or phenobarbital. *Toxicol. appl. Pharmacol.* 9, 319—323 (1966). [G 66,033/66

Zeckwer, I.T.: Compensatory renal hypertrophy after unilateral nephrectomy in thyroidectomized rats, considered in relation to histological changes in the pituitary. *Fed. Proc.* 3, 53—54 (1944). [84,592/44

Zeisberger, E., Brück, K.: Quantitative Beziehung zwischen Noradrenalin-Effekt und Ausmaß der zitterfreien Thermogenese beim Meerschweinchen. *Pflügers Arch. ges. Physiol.* 296, 263—275 (1967). [F 89,184/67

Zeisberger, E., Brück, K., Wünnenberg, W., Wietasch, C.: Das Ausmaß der zitterfreien Thermogenese des Meerschweinchens in Abhängigkeit vom Lebensalter. *Pflügers Arch. ges. Physiol.* 296, 276—288 (1967). [F 89,185/67

Zelioli-Lanzini, F.: Differenza dell'azione degli estratti epatici e di quella delle piccole dosi di raggi Röntgen sull'attività mitotica del fegato parzialmente epatectomizzato. *Osped. Ital-Chir.* 20, 523—527 (1969). [H 19,493/69

Zeller, J., Margaretten, W., McKay, D. G.: Effect of saline infusion and norepinephrine on response of the kidney to bacterial endotoxin. *Proc. Soc. exp. Biol. (N.Y.)* 126, 446—449 (1967). [F 92,117/67

Zicha, L., Heck, K.-J.: Untersuchungen über die Beeinflussung der glukokortikoidbedingten Hemmung von Histamin-, Serotonin- und Azetylcholinwirkungen durch anabole Steroide. *Allergie u. Asthma* 12, 303—308 (1967). [F 78,128/67

Ziegler, D.M., Pettit, F.H.: Microsomal oxidases. I. The isolation and dialkylarylamine oxygenase activity of pork liver microsomes. *Biochemistry* 5, 2932—2938 (1966). [G 79,382/66

Zilberstein, R. M.: Effects of reserpine, serotonin and vasopressin on the survival of cold-stressed rats. *Nature (Lond.)* 185, 249 (1960). [C 80,282/60

Zimel, H., Macrineanu, A.: Recherches sur l'action hépatotrope de certaines substances hormonocytostatiques. *Rev. roum. Endocr.* 1, 335—341 (1964). [F 35,084/64

Zondek, B.: Über das Schicksal des Follikelhormons (Follikulin) im Organismus. *Skand. Arch. Physiol.* 70, 133—167 (1934). [30,531/34

Zondek, B., Sulman, F., Sklow, J.: Inactivation of stilbestrol by liver in vitro. *Endocrinology* 33, 333—336 (1943). [A 74,477/43

Zondek, H.: Die Beeinflussung des Blutdrucks der akuten experimentellen Nephritis des Kaninchens durch Pankreasextrakt. *Dtsch. Arch. klin. Med.* 115, 1—46 (1914). [36,326/14

Zsigmond, G., Solymoss, B.: Influence of 3β-hydroxy-20-oxo-5-pregnene-16α-carbonitrile (PCN) on the anesthetic effect and hepatic microsomal metabolism of progesterone. (Abstr.) *Proc. canad. Fed. biol. Soc.* 14, 80 (1971). [G 79,025/71

Zuchlewski, A. C., Gaebler, O. H.: Changes in the activity of transaminases and L-glutamic acid dehydrogenase induced by growth hormone. *Arch. Biochem.* 66, 463—473 (1957). [D 91,862/57

Zumoff, B., Fishman, J., Cassouto, J., Gallagher, T. F., Hellman, L.: Influence of age and sex on normal estradiol metabolism. *J. clin. Endocr.* 28, 937—941 (1968). [H 1,151/68

Zumoff, B., Fishman, J., Levin, J., Gallagher, T. F., Hellman, L.: Reversible reproduction of the abnormal estradiol metabolism of biliary obstruction by administration of norethandrolone. *J. clin. Endocr.* 30, 598—601 (1970). [H 25,277/70

Zwadyk, P., Jr., Harrison, E. F.: Comparison of the protective properties of soterenol and isoproterenol against endotoxin lethality. *Proc. Soc. exp. Biol. (N.Y.)* 133, 66—68 (1970). [H 19,753/70

Zwehl, T. von: Beiträge zur Wirkung des Dijodtyrosins im Säugetierversuch. *Arch. Entwickl.-Mech. Org.* 107, 456—480 (1926). [25,477/26

Zweifach, B. W., Thomas, L.: The relationship between the vascular manifestations of shock produced by endotoxin, trauma, and hemorrhage. I. Certain similarities between the reactions in normal and endotox intolerant rats. *J. exp. Med.* 106, 385—401 (1957). [D 91,826/57

Zwemer, R. L., Jungeblut, C. W.: Effect of various corticoadrenal extracts on diphtheria toxin in vivo and in vitro. *Proc. Soc. exp. Biol. (N.Y.)* 32, 1583—1588 (1935). [53,287/35

Zwemer, R. L., Truszkowski, R.: The importance of corticoadrenal regulation of potassium metabolism. *Endocrinology* 21, 40—49 (1937). [A 2,330/37

Zykov, A. A.: The influence of adrenocorticotropic hormone, hormone preparations of the adrenals and adrenalectomy on the course and issue of the dicain intoxication in mice. (Russian text.) *Eksp. Khir. Anest.* 14/6, 70—72 (1969). [H 21,879/69

INDEX

To facilitate the use of this index, boldface numerals refer to my own comments (single column, large type in text), the others to abstracts (double column, small print in text).

Greek letters, numbers and prefixes (p–, o–, m–) in chemical compounds are neglected in determining the alphabetic position of entries.

When a "target" A (drug or hormone) is influenced by an "agent" B (drug, hormone, surgical interventions or external environment), this is indicated by an arrow pointing from B to A, thus: A ← B, and the reverse entry B → A.

If two agents (B and C) act conjointly upon the same target, this is indexed thus: A ← B + C; B → A ← C; C → A ← B; that is each agent and the target appear once in the first position. The same rule applies when there are three or more agents.

The following group names are used: Anaphylactoidogenic agents, Antibiotics, Anticoagulants, Barbiturates, Carcinogens, Carcinolytics, Digitalis, Lathyrogens, Steroids in general, Corticoids, Folliculoids, Luteoids, Testoids. Pesticides and Vitamins are listed individually. However, entries for drugs or hormones belonging to any of these groups, should also be consulted individually.

Since most experiments have been performed on rats, this is not specifically mentioned; other species are identified at the end of the entry thus: A ← B/Mouse.

Salts of electrolytes are listed under the presumably most important ion; for example, instead of indium chloride (InCl₃), we write "indium", instead of sodium phosphates (NaH$_2$PO$_4$, Na$_2$HPO$_4$), "phosphates".

AAN; *cf. also* Lathyrogens
  ← CS-1 *Table 73* 257
  ← DOC *Table 73* 257
  ← estradiol *Table 73* 257
  ← ethylstrenol *Table 73* 257
  ← hydroxydione *Table 73* 257
  ← norbolethone *Table 73* 257
  ← oxandrolone *Table 73* 257
  ← PCN *Table 73* 257
  ← phenobarbital *Diagram Table 139* 857 to 859; *Tables 73, 139* 257, 850—854
  ← prednisolone *Table 73* 257
  ← progesterone *Table 73* 257
  ← spironolactone *Table 73* 257
  ← steroids *Diagram Table 139* 857—859; *Table 138* 850—854
  ← thyroxine *Diagram Table 139* 857—859; *Tables 73, 138* 257, 850—854
  ← triamcinolone *Table 73* 257
Abortifacient action of hepatic microsomal enzyme inducers **722**
  properties of catatoxic steroids **863**
"Abrasive ablation", methods **20**
Absorption of drugs **768**
Abstracting ***VII***

"Abwehrfermente" **27**
Acetaldehyde ← ACTH 408
  ← steroids 175
  ← thyroid hormones 470
2-Acetaminofluorene; *cf.* Carcinogens
Acetanilide ← CS-1 *Table 24* 176
  ← DOC *Table 24* 176
  ← ethylstrenol *Table 24* 176
  ← estradiol *Table 24* 176
  ← hydroxydione *Table 24* 176
  ← norbolethone *Table 24* 176
  ← oxandrolone *Table 24* 176
  ← PCN *Table 24* 176
  ← phenobarbital *Diagram Table 139* 857 to 859; *Tables 24, 138* 176, 850—854
  ← prednisolone *Table 24* 176
  ← progesterone *Table 24* 176
  ← spironolactone *Table 24* 176
  ← starvation/mouse *Table 3* 81
  ← steroids 176; *Diagram Table 139* 857 to 859; *Table 138* 850—854
  ← thyroxine *Diagram Table 139* 857—859; *Tables 24, 138* 176, 850—854
  ← triamcinolone *Table 24* 176
Acetone ← pancreatic hormones 522

Acetonitrile ← anterior pituitary preparations
    436, **437**
  ← epinephrine 533
  ← histamine 555
  ← pancreatic hormones 522
  ← posterior pituitary preparations 441
  ← species-dependent factors **674**, **675**
  ← steroids 175
  ← thyroid hormones **466**, **471**
  ← thyroid hormones/guinea pig 470
  ← thyroid hormones/mouse 470
Acetoxypregnenolone → steroids 133
Acetylcholine ← sex 635
Acetylsalicylic acid → F-COL *Table 137*
    848—849
  → DHT *Table 137* 848—849
  → digitoxin *Table 137* 848—849
  → dioxathion *Table 137* 848—849
  → hepatic microsomal drug metabolism in man **709**
  → hexobarbital *Table 137* 848—849
  → indomethacin *Table 137* 848—849
  → nicotine *Table 137* 848—849
  → parathion *Table 137* 848—849
  → progesterone *Table 137* 848—849
  → zoxazolamine *Table 137* 848—849
Aconitine (a highly poisonous plant alkaloid)
  ← thyroid hormones 471
Acrylamide ← CS-1 *Table 25* 176
  ← DOC *Table 25* 176
  ← estradiol *Table 25* 176
  ← ethylestrenol *Table 25* 176
  ← hydroxydione *Table 25* 176
  ← norbolethone *Table 25* 176
  ← oxandrolone *Table 25* 176
  ← PCN *Table 25* 176
  ← phenobarbital *Diagram Table 139* 857—859; *Tables 25, 138* 176, 850—854
  ← prednisolone *Table 25* 176
  ← progesterone *Table 25* 176
  ← spironolactone *Table 25* 176
  ← steroids 176; *Diagram Table 139* 857—859; *Table 138* 850—854
  ← thyroxine *Diagram Table 139* 857—859; *Tables 25, 138* 176, 850—854
  ← triamcinolone *Table 25* 176
Acrylonitrile ← ACTH 408
  ← CS-1 *Table 26* 177
  ← DOC *Table 26* 177
  ← estradiol *Table 26* 177
  ← ethylestrenol *Table 26* 177
  ← hydroxydione *Table 26* 177
  ← hypophysectomy 447
  ← norbolethone *Table 26* 177
  ← oxandrolone *Table 26* 177
  ← PCN *Table 26* 177
  ← phenobarbital *Table 26* 177

Acrylonitrile ← prednisolone *Table 26* 177
  ← progesterone *Table 26* 177
  ← spironolactone *Table 26* 177
  ← steroids 176
  ← STH **426**
  ← thyroxine *Table 26* 177
  ← triamcinolone *Table 26* 177
ACTH → acetaldehyde 408
  → acrylonitrile 408
  → allylformiate 408
  → aminocaproic acid 408
  → aminopterin 408
  → anaphylactoidogenic agents **406**, **408**
  → anticoagulants **406**, **408**
  → arboviruses **415**
  → arsenic 408
  → Bacillus piliformis (Tyzzer's disease) 416
  → bacteria **415**, **416**
  → bacterial toxins **415**, **416**, **419**
  → bacterial toxins/dog **416**, **419**
  → bacterial toxins/guinea pig **415**, **419**
  → bacterial toxins/man **416**, **419**
  → bacterial toxins/mouse **415**, **418**
  → bacterial toxins/rabbit **415**, **418**
  → barbiturates **406**, **409**
  → beryllium 409
  → breeding, repeated **422**, **423**
  → carcinogens **407**, **410**
  → carcinolytics 410
  → casein **407**, **410**
  → CCl₄ 410
  → cholesterol **407**, **410**
  → cholesterolase **424**
  → cinchophen 411
  → Clostridium tetani **415**, **416**
  → F-COL *Table 137* 848—849
  → complex diets **414**
  → Corynebacterium diphtheriae **415**, **416**
  → DHT **408**, **414**; *Fig. 16* 305; *Table 137* 848—849
  → diets, complex **414**
  → digitoxin *Table 137* 848—849
  → dioxathion *Table 137* 848—849
  → Diplococcus pneumoniae 416
  → diphenylhydantoin 411
  → DOC **405**
  → drugs **406**
  → electric stimuli 423
  → encephalomyelitis **415**
  → enzymes, hepatic **423**
  → EST **422**
  ← estradiol 137
  → ethanol 411
  → ethionine 411
  → formaldehyde 411
  → ganglioplegics **407**, **411**; *Table 60C* 246
  → GPT **424**

ACTH → hepatic enzymes **423**
  → hepatic lesions **420, 421**
  → hexadimethrine **411**
  → hexobarbital *Table 137* **848–849**
  → histamine **405, 406**
  → hormone-like substances **405**
  → hormones, nonsteroidal **405**
  → 5-HT **405, 406**
  → hyperoxygenation **421, 422**
  → hypoxia **421, 422**
  → immune reactions **419, 420**
  → immune reactions/guinea pig **419, 420**
  → immune reactions/rabbit **419, 420**
  → indomethacin *Table 137* **848–849**
  → influenza **415**
  → insulin **405, 406**
  → ionizing rays **421, 422**
  → isoniazid **412**
  → isoproterenol **412**
  → lathyrogens **407, 412**
  → leptospira **415, 416**
  → MAD **405**
  → meprobamate **412**
  → mercury **412**
  → microorganisms **415**
  → morphine **407, 412**
  → muscular performance **422, 423**
  → mustard powder **413**
  → Mycobacterium tuberculosis **415, 416**
  → nicotine *Table 137* **848–849**
  → nonsteroidal hormones **405**
  → osmosis **423**
  → parasites **415, 417**
  → parathion *Table 137* **848–849**
  → Pasteurella pestis **415, 417**
  → pentylenetetrazol **413**
  → plasmocid **413**
  → pneumococci **415**
  → poliomyelitis **415**
  → potassium **413**
  → progesterone *Table 137* **848–849**
  → puromycin aminonucleoside **413**
  → pyruvate **413**
  → rabies **415**
  → renal lesions **420, 421**
  → repeated breeding **422, 423**
  → RES-blocking agents **413**
  → resistance **405**
  → rickettsia **415, 417**
  → salinity tolerance **422**
  → "saprophytosis" **415, 417**
  ← sex **631**
  → steroids **405**
  ← steroids **137**
  → staphylococci **415, 417**
  → streptococci **415, 417**
  → tannic acid **413**

ACTH → TEA *Table 60C* **246**
  → temperature variations **422**
  → temperature variations/mouse **422**
  → tetracaine **413**
  → thyroxine **406**
  → TKT **423, 424**
  → TPO **423, 424**
  → trauma **422, 423**
  → Trichinella spiralis **415**
  → tumors **423**
  → Tyzzer's disease **416**
  → vaccines **415, 416**
  → variola **415**
  → venoms **416, 419**
  → viruses **415, 417**
  → vitamin C **407, 414**
  → vitamin D **408, 414**
  → zoxazolamine **414**; *Table 137* **848–849**
Actidione; *cf.* Cycloheximide
Actinomycetes ← steroids **316, 319**
Actinomycin **73**; *cf. also* Antibiotics, Blockers *under* Pharmacology
  ← anterior pituitary preparations **437**
  ← barbiturates **75**
  ← cortisol **74, 75**
  ← cortisone **73**
  ← diet, protein-deficient **74**
  ← endotoxin **74, 75**
  ← ethylestrenol **75**
  → glucagon **75**
  → insulin **75**
  → ionizing rays **75**
  reversal of antagonist action **84, 92**
  → spironolactone **75**
  → starvation **74**
  → stress **74**
  → tyrosine **74**
Activity index of steroids **863**
"Activity spectrums of hormones" **15**
Acylation reactions **47**
Adaptation to hormones, history **34**
  to steroid anesthesia **133**
Adaptive enzyme formation ← thymectomy **552**
  hormones **12**
Adenosine diphosphate ← thyroid hormones **471**
Adenovirus-12 ← steroids **325**
  ← thymectomy **551**
Adenoviruses ← steroids **327**
Adrenalectomy → amino acid enzymes **399**
  → bacterial toxins **336, 346**
  → barbiturates **150, 191**
  → barbiturates/guinea pig **193**
  → barbiturates/mouse **193**
  → carcinogens **212**
  → electric stimuli **375**

Adrenalectomy → enzymes 393, 399
 → hepatic lesions 354, 357
 → hepatic tissue 725, 729
 → hyperoxygenation 371
 → hypoxia 371
 → immune reactions 351, 353
 → indomethacin ← spironolactone *Tables 68
  —71* 252—254
 → indomethacin ← spironolactone + corticoids *Tables 68—71* 252—254
 → ionizing rays 362, 365
 → steroids 127
 → systemic trauma 377, 380
 → temperature variations 373, 374
 → TKT 393
 → TPO 393
 → vitamin D 303
Adrenaline; *cf.* Epinephrine
Adrenal necrosis ← DMBA + spironolactone *Fig. 2, 3* 213, 214
 ← DMBA + stress *Fig. 29* 693
 morphology 740
Adrenals, history 26, 33
Adrenal tumors ← aminoglutethimide 720
 ← barbiturates 715, 720
 ← DDD 715, 720
Adrenal weight ← CS-1 *Table 140* 860—861
 ← DOC *Table 140* 860—861
 ← estradiol *Table 140* 860—861
 ← ethylestrenol *Table 140* 860—861
 ← hydroxydione *Table 140* 860—861
 ← norbolethone *Table 140* 860—861
 ← oxandrolone *Table 140* 860—861
 ← PCN *Table 140* 860—861
 ← phenobarbital *Table 140* 860—861
 ← prednisolone *Table 140* 860—861
 ← progesterone *Table 140* 860—861
 ← spironolactone *Table 140* 860—861
 ← thyroxine *Table 140* 860—861
 ← triamcinolone *Table 140* 860—861
Adrenochrome → resistance 571
Adrenocortical hyperplasia with sexual anomalies ← steroids 382, 383
Aflatoxin; *cf.* Carcinogens
Agar ← stressors 689, 690
Age → aminopyrine 667, 669
 → barbiturates 667, 669
 → carcinogens 670
 → digitoxin ← PCN *Table 50* 232
 → drugs 667, 669
 → enzymes 673
 → hepatic enzymes 667, 672
 → hepatic lesions 672
 → indomethacin 667, 671
 → indomethacin ← PCN *Table 72* 254
 → meperidine 671
 → pesticides 667, 671

Age → pethidine 671
 → phenylbutazone 671
 → promazine 671
 → resistance 666
 → steroids 666, 668
 → strychnine 667, 671
 → TKT 667, 672
 → TPO 667, 672
Alanine; *cf. also* GPT *under* Influence of Steroids upon Enzymes
 ← SKF 525-A, 61
"Alarm reaction" 33
Alcohol dehydrogenase, chemistry 45
 oxidation 45
Aldadiene (SC-9376) → steroids 122, 123
Aldehyde oxidation 45
Aldosterone → barbiturates 196
 → endotoxin *Table 123* 348
Alloxan ← epinephrine 531, 532
Allyl alcohol ← norepinephrine 534
 → resistance 571
 ← steroids 176
 ← thyroid hormones 471
Allylformiate ← ACTH 408
 ← hepatic lesions 604
 ← steroids 177
 ← thyroid hormones 471
Ameba ← steroids 330, 331
Amiloride (potassium-sparing diuretic) → resistance 567, 571
Amino acid enzymes ← adrenalectomy 399
 ← corticoids 390
 ← hypophysectomy 460
Amino acids ← hepatic lesions 602, 604
Aminocaproic acid ← ACTH 408
Aminoglutethimide → adrenal tumors 720
 → Cushing's syndrome 720
 ← steroids 177
6-Aminonicotinamide ← steroids 177
o-Aminophenol ← phenobarbital *Diagram Table 139* 857—859; *Table 138* 850—854
 ← steroids 177; *Diagram Table 139* 857—859; *Table 138* 850—854
 ← thyroxine *Diagram Table 139* 857—859; *Table 138* 850—854
Aminopterin (antimetabolite, follic acid antagonist) ← ACTH 408
 ← sex 635
 ← steroids 177
4-Aminopyrazolopyrimidine ← enzymes, normal *Table 134* 759
Aminopyrine (antipyretic, analgesic) ← age 667, 669
 ← CCl_4 79
 ← CS-1 *Table 27* 179
 ← DOC *Table 27* 179

Aminopyrine ← estradiol *Table 27* 179
  ← ethylestrenol *Table 27* 179
  ← hydroxydione *Table 27*, 179
  ← oxandrolone *Table 27* 179
  ← norbolethone *Table 27* 179
  ← PCN *Table 27* 179
  ← phenobarbital *Diagram Table 139* 857–859; *Tables 27, 138* 176, 850–854
  ← prednisolone *Table 27* 179
  ← progesterone *Table 27* 179
  ← sex 635, 655
  ← SKF 525-A 60, 61
  ← spironolactone *Table 27* 179
  ← starvation/mouse *Table 3* 81
  ← steroids 178; *Diagram Table 139* 857–859, *Table 138* 850–854
  ← STH **426**
  ← stressors 690
  ← thyroxine *Diagram Table 139* 857–859; *Tables 27, 138* 179, 850–854
  ← triamcinolone *Table 27* 179
Aminopyrine-metabolizing enzymes ← tumors 704
p-Aminosalicylate ← thyroid hormones 471
p-Aminosalicylic acid **70**
  ← SKF 525-A 63
3-Amino-1,2,4-triazole 81, 82
Amitriptyline (antidepressant) ← norepinephrine 534
Ammonium chloride ← steroids 179
AMP (cyclic) ← steroids 179
Amphenone → resistance 571
Amphetamine (sympathomimetic, CNS stimulant) ← phenobarbital *Diagram Table 139* 857–859; *Table 138* 850–854
  → resistance 591
  ← sex 635
  ← SKF 525-A 61
  ← steroids 179; *Diagram Table 139* 857–859; *Table 138* 850–854
  ← stressors 689, 690
  ← thyroid hormones 466, 472
  ← thyroid hormones/mouse 472
  ← thyroxine *Diagram Table 139* 857–859; *Table 138* 850–854
Amyl nitrate (vasodilator) ← steroids 180
  ← thyroid hormones 472
Amyloid; *cf.* Casein
Anabolic steroids **9**
  → folliculoids 115, 119
  → glucocorticoids 114, 115
  → gluco-mineralocorticoids 114, 118
  → luteoids 114, 118
  → mineralocorticoids 114, 118
  → steroids 114, 119
Analytico-synthetic style **V, VIII**

Anaphylactoid edema; *cf.* Anaphylactoidogenic Agents
"Anaphylactoidogenic agents" **406**
  ← ACTH **406**, 408
  ← anterior pituitary preparations 437
  ← corticoids 180
  ← epinephrine **532**, 534
  ← folliculoids 180
  ← 5-HT 558
  ← norepinephrine **532**, 534
  ← pancreatic hormones **521, 522**, 523
  ← parathyroids 516
  ← pregnancy 661
  ← steroids 148, 180
  ← STH **426**
  ← stressors **689**, 690
  ← thyroid hormones 467, 472
Ancylostoma caninum ← steroids **330**, 332
Androgenic steroids; *cf.* Testoids
Andromimetic steroids; *cf.* Testoids
Androstano-5β-carbonitrile (ACN) → hemorrhages, multiple *Fig. 37* 741
Androsterone → barbiturates 197
Anesthetic steroids **9**
Anesthetics (various); *cf. also* Individual Anesthetics
  ← catatoxic steroids 180
Angiotensin → resistance 564
  ← thyroid hormones 466
Aniline ← sex 655, 690
  ←steroids 180
ANIT; *cf.* α-Naphthylisothiocyanate
Anoxia ← posterior pituitary preparations **441**
  ← sex **657**
Antabuse; *cf.* Disulfiram
"Antagonisms, physiologic" **15, 707**
Antagonisms, specific, classification 17
Antagonists, reversal of actions 84, 92
Anterior lobe extracts ← steroids **138**
  pituitary preparations → acetonitrile **436**, 437
    → actinomycin 437
    → anaphylactoidogenic agents 437
    → bacteria **436**, 439
    → bacterial toxins 440
    → barbiturates 437
    → BSP 440
    → cadmium 438
    → *Candida albicans* **437**
    → carcinogens **436**, 438
    → carcinoma transplants 440
    → CCl₄ **436**, 438
    → cholesterol **436**, 438
    → cold 440
    → diet 440
    → diphtheria toxin **437**
    → drugs **436**, 437

Anterior lobe extracts, pituitary preparations →
  → emetine **436**, 438
  → enzymes, hepatic 440
  → ergotamine **436**, 439
  → ethionine 439
  → glycine 439
  → hepatic enzymes 440
  → hepatic regeneration 440
  → hepatic tissue 726, 735
  → hormones 437
  → hypoxia **437**, 440
  → ionizing rays 440
  → lathyrogens **436**, 439
  → microorganisms **436**, 439
  → morphine 439
  → nephrectomy, partial 440
  → p-nitrobenzoic acid 439
  → pentobarbital **436**
  → progesterone 436
  → reserpine 439
  → resistance **436**
  → salinity tolerance 440
  → tumor transplants 440
  → vitamin A **436**, 439
  → vitamin C 439
"Anti-anaphylaxis" 589
Antiandrogens; cf. Antitestoids
Antibiotics; cf. also Clinical Implications; Individual Antibiotics
  ← epinephrine 534
  ← norepinephrine 534
  ← parathyroids 516
  → resistance 571
  ← sex 635
  ← steroids 181
  ← stressors **689**
Anticatatoxic compounds, antagonists **57**
  blockers 57
  competitors **57**
  inhibitors 57
Anticoagulants 82; cf. also Clinical Implications
  ← ACTH **406**, 408
  ← barbiturates 575
  ← epinephrine 534
  ← pregnancy 661
  → resistance 571
  ← SKF 525-A 63, 64
  ← species-dependent factors 675
  ← steroids 148, 181
  ← STH **426**
  ← stressors **689**, 690
  ← thyroid hormones 473
Antifolliculoids 54
Antiglucocorticoids 54
Antihistamines → resistance 571
Antihormones, history **27**

Antiluteoids 54
Antimineralocorticoid **9**, 54
  → barbiturates 150, 186
  → steroids **121**, 122
Antimony ← thyroid hormones 473
Antipyrine (antipyretic, analgesic) ← steroids 183
Antitestoids 54
  → hepatic tissue 726, 734
  → steroids **126**
"Antitoxic factor" **564**
ANTU; cf. 1-(Naphthyl)-2-thiourea under Thioureas
Appendical peritonitis ← steroids 325
Arboviruses ← ACTH 408, **415**
  ← steroids **325**, 327
Arsenic ← epinephrine 534
  pentoxide ← phenobarbital *Diagram Table 139* 857—859; *Table 138* 850—854
    ← steroids *Diagram Table 139* 857—859; *Table 138* 850—854
    ← thyroxine *Diagram Table 139* 857 to 859; *Table 138* 850—854
  ← pregnancy 661
  ← sex 635
  ← steroids 183
  ← thyroid hormones 473
As; cf. Arsenic
"Asher's method" **506**
Aspartate; cf. GOT under Influence of Steroids upon Enzymes
Atherosclerosis **716**
Atophane; cf. Cinchophen
Atropine ← hypophysectomy 447
  → resistance 572, 591
  ← thyroid hormones 473
Audiogenic convulsions ← steroids 383
Azaestranes → barbiturates 196
8-Azaguanine ← enzymes, normal *Table 134* 759
Azo reduction **45**
Azuridine ← enzymes, normal *Table 134* 759

Bacillus anthracis ← steroids **316**, 319
  anthracis ← thyroid hormones 497
  pertussis ← steroids **316**
    vaccine ← histamine 556
  piliformis (Tyzzer's disease) ← ACTH 416
    ← steroids **316**, 319
Bacteria ← ACTH **415**, 416
  ← anterior pituitary preparations 436, 439
  ← epinephrine **541**
  ← hypoxia 685
  ← pancreatic hormones **527**
  ← parathyroids **518**, 519
  Plasmodium berghei 81, 82
  ← pregnancy 666

Bacteria ← posterior pituitary preparations 442
→ resistance 595
← sex **656**
← steroids **316**
← STH 430
← stressors 699
← thymectomy **549**, 550
← thyroid hormones **496**, 497
Bacterial endotoxins ← stressors **698**, 699
toxins; *cf. also* Microorganisms, Vaccines and Parasites
 ← ACTH **415**, 416, 419
 ← ACTH/dog **416**, 419
 ← ACTH/guinea pig **415**, 419
 ← ACTH/man **416**, 419
 ← ACTH/mouse **415**, 418
 ← ACTH/rabbit **415**, 418
 ← adrenalectomy **336**, 346
 ← anterior pituitary preparations 440
 ← corticoids **335**, 343
 ← corticoids/cat **333**, 337
 ← corticoids/chicken **333**, 337
 ← corticoids/dog **333**, 338
 ← corticoids/guinea pig **333**, 339
 ← corticoids/man **335**, 344
 ← corticoids/monkey **333**, 339
 ← corticoids/mouse **333**, 340
 ← corticoids/rabbit **335**, 342
 ← corticoids/sheep 344
 ← epinephrine **541**
 ← folliculoids **337**, 347
 ← hepatic lesions **618**, 619
 ← histamine **555**, 556
 ← hormone-like substances 563
 ← 5-HT 561
 ← hypophysectomy **453**
 ← luteoids **336**, 346
 ← norepinephrine **541**
 ← pancreatic hormones 528
 ← parathyroids **518**, 519
 ← posterior pituitary preparations **441**, 442
 ← pregnancy 666
 → resistance 596
 ← sex **618**
 ← species-dependent factors 681
 ← steroids **333**, 337, 347
 ← STH **432**
 ← temperature variations 687
 ← testoids **337**, 347
 ← thymectomy 551
 ← thyroid hormones 497, 500
Barbital; *cf. also* Barbiturates
 ← CS-1 *Table 34* 198
 ← estradiol *Table 34* 198
 ← ethylestrenol *Table 34* 198

Barbital ← DOC *Table 34* 198
 ← hydroxydione *Table 34* 198
 ← norbolethone *Table 34* 198
 ← oxandrolone *Table 34* 198
 ← PCN *Table 34* 198
 ← phenobarbital *Diagram Table 139* 857 to 859; *Tables 34, 138,* 198, 850—854
 ← prednisolone *Table 34* 198
 ← progesterone *Table 34* 198
 ← spironolactone *Table 34* 198
 ← steroids 198; *Diagram Table 139* 857 to 859; *Table 138* 850—854
 ← thyroxine *Diagram Table 139* 857—859; *Tables 34, 138, 198* 850—854
 ← triamcinolone *Table 34* 198
Barbiturates; *cf. also* Individual Barbiturates
 ← ACTH **406**, 409
 ← actinomycin 75
 ← adrenalectomy **150**, 191
 ← adrenalectomy/guinea pig 193
 ← adrenalectomy/mouse 193
 → adrenal tumors **715**, 720
 ← age **667**, 669
 ← aldosterone 196
 ← androsterone 197
 ← anterior pituitary preparations 437
 ← anticoagulants 575
 ← antimineralocorticoids **150**, 186
 ← azaestranes 196
 → carbon disulfide 575
 ← barbiturates 575
 → bile pigments 575
 → bromobenzene 575
 ← CCl_4 79
 → CCl_4 575
 ← 4-chlorotestosterone 196
 → cholesterol 576
 → corticoids 572
 ← cortisol 197
 → Cushing's syndrome **715**, 720
 → cyclophosphamide 576
 ← cyproterone 196
 → DHT 578
 ← diet **592**
 → diphenylhydantoin 576
 ← diurnal variations 705
 ← DOC 196
 → drugs 578
 → dyes 576
 ← epinephrine **532**, 536
 ← epinephrine/dog 534
 ← epinephrine/guinea pig 534
 ← epinephrine/mouse 534
 ← epinephrine/rabbit 535
 ← estradiol 197
 → ethanol 576
 ← ethionine 79

Barbiturates ← ethylestrenol 197
  → folliculoids 573
  ← folliculoids 150, 190
  ← genetic factors 675
  ← glucocorticoids 149, 184
  ← glucocorticoids/man 185
  ← glucocorticoids/mouse 184
  ← glucocorticoids/rabbit 185
  ← gluco-mineralocorticoids 150, 185
  ← gonadectomy 151, 193
  ← gonadectomy/guinea pig 196
  ← gonadectomy/mouse 195
  → hepatic enzymes 578
  ← hepatic lesions 602, 605
  ← hepatic lesions/dog 604
  ← hepatic lesions/mouse 605
  ← hepatic lesions/rabbit 606
  → hepatic microsomal drug metabolism in man 708, 712
  → hepatic tissue 727, 736
  ← histamine 555
  → hormone-like substances 575
  ← 5-HT 556, 559
  ← 5-HT/man 558
  ← 5-HT/mouse 558
  ← 5-HT/rabbit 558
  ← hydroxydione 196, 198
  → hyperbilirubinemia 714, 717
  ← hypophysectomy 445, 447
  ← hypoxia 685
  ← ionizing rays 683
  → lidocaine 577
  ← luteoids 150, 189
  ← 17α-methyl-17β-hydroxy-4-aza-estran-3-one 196
  ← mineralocorticoids 150, 185
  → nicotine 577
  → nonsteroidal hormones 575
  ← norbolethone 197
  ← norepinephrine 532, 536
  ← norepinephrine/man 536
  ← norepinephrine/mouse 534
  ← norepinephrine/rabbit 535
  ← pancreatic hormones 522, 523
  ← parathyroids 516
  ← PCN 198
  → pesticides 577
  → phenylbutazone 577
  → picrotoxin 577
  ← posterior pituitary preparations 441
  ← pregnancy 661
  → pregnancy 578
  ← progesterone 197
  → quinine 577
  ← renal lesions 622, 623, 624
  → resistance 567, 572
reversal of substrate action 93

Barbiturates ← SC-5233 197
  ← sex 632, 636, 655
  ← sex/dog 633
  ← sex/guinea pig 633
  ← sex/mouse 635
  ← sex/rabbit 633
  ← SKF 525-A 60, 61, 62, 63
  ← species-dependent factors 675
  ← spironolactone 197
  → steroids 574
  ← steroids 149, 184
  ← STH 426
  ← stilbestrol 196
  ← stressors 689, 690
  → strychnine 577
  tabulation of Table 11 107
  ← temperature variations 686
  → testoids 572
  ← testoids 150, 187
  ← testoids/guinea pig 189
  ← testoids/mouse 189
  ← testosterone 197
  ← thyroid hormones 467, 474, 475
  ← thyroid hormones/cat 473
  ← thyroid hormones/frog 473
  ← thyroid hormones/mouse 473
  ← thyroid hormones/rabbit 474
  toxicants 105, 109
  → vitamin C 578
  → vitamin D 578
Basic principles of SSS steroid terminology 774
"Basophilic bone globules" Fig. 16 305
BCP ← pregnancy 662
  ← sex 640
Benactyzine (anticholinergic, ataraxic) 81; cf. also Phenothiazines
  ← hypophysectomy 448
Benzene ← sex 640
  ← steroids 198
Benzol ← epinephrine 536
Benzpyrene; cf. also Carcinogens
  → hepatic tissue 739
Benzydamine → resistance 578
Benzylamine ← enzymes, normal Table 134 759
Beryllium ← ACTH 409
  ← parathyroids 515, 516
  ← steroids 199
Besnoitia ← steroids 330, 331
Betamethasone; cf. also Corticoids
  → digitoxin Table 128 630, 631
  → dioxathion Table 128 630, 631
  → endotoxin Table 120 344
  → hexamethonium Table 60B 246
  → hexobarbital Table 128 630, 631
  → indomethacin Table 128 630, 631

Betamethasone → mercury *Table 81*   269
  → nicotine *Table 128*   630, 631
  → parathion *Table 128*   630, 631
  → pentolinium *Table 60B*   246
  → progesterone *Table 128*   630, 631
  → TEA *Table 60B*   246
  → zoxazolamine *Table 128*   630, 631
Bile-duct, common; *cf. also* Choledochus
  ligature → F-COL *Table 137*   848—849
    → DHT *Table 137*   848—849
    → digitoxin *Table 137*   848—849
    → dioxathion *Table 137*   848—849
    → hepatic tissue   739
    → hexobarbital *Table 137*   848—849
    → indomethacin *Table 137*   848—849
    → nicotine *Table 137*   848—849
    → parathion *Table 137*   848—849
    ← phenobarbital *Diagram Table 139*   857—859
    → progesterone *Table 137*   848—849
    ← steroids *Diagram Table 139*   857—859; *Table 138*   850—854
    ← thyroxine *Diagram Table 139*   857—859; *Table 138*   850—854
    → zoxazolamine *Table 137*   848—849
  ligatures, methods   **19, 21**
Bile, extrahepatic conditioning   103
  fistulas, methods   **19, 21**
  flow ← cholecystokinin-pancreozymin/dog *Table 10*   99
    ← epinephrine/dog *Table 10*   99
    ← ethinylestradiol *Table 10*, 99
    ← gastrin/dog *Table 10*, 99
    ← hormones *Table 10*, 99
    ← insulin/dog *Table 10*, 99
    ← norepinephrine/dog *Table 10*, 99
    ← norethandrolone/rabbit *Table 10*, 99
    ← secretin/dog *Table 10*, 99
  pigments; *cf. also* Clinical Implications
    ← barbiturates   575
    ← pregnancy   662
  secretion ← corticoids *Fig. 20*   356
Bilharzia; *cf.* Schistosomiasis
Biliary excretion   **97**
Bilirubin; *cf. also* α-Naphthylisothiocyanate (ANIT)
  ← genetic factors   677
  ← hepatic lesions   607
  ← pancreatic hormones   524
  ← steroids   **152**, 199
"Biologic stress"   **25**
Biosynthesis, corticoids   105; *Graph*   106
Bishydroxycoumarin; *cf. also* Anticoagulants
  ← cholesterol *Table 28*   182
  ← CS-1 *Table 28*   182
  ← DOC *Table 28*   182
  ← estradiol *Table 28*   182

Bishydroxycoumarin ← ethylestrenol *Table 28*   182
  ← hydroxydione *Table 28*   182
  ← norbolethone *Table 28*   182
  ← oxandrolone *Table 28*   182
  ← PCN *Table 28*   182
  ← phenobarbital *Diagram Table 139*   857—859; *Tables 28, 138*   182, 850—854
  ← prednisolone *Table 28*   182
  ← progesterone *Table 28*   182
  ← spironolactone *Table 28*   182
  ← steroids *Table 138*   850—854
  ← thyroxine *Tables 28, 138*   182, 850—854
  ← triamcinolone *Table 28*   182
Blockade of the sympathetic nervous system ← epinephrine   **545**
Blockers of enzyme induction   **72**
  actinomycin   **73**
  3-amino- 1,2,4-triazole   81
  benactyzine   81
  CCl_4 78
  classification   **72**
  cycloheximide   77
  ethionine   78
  hepatotoxic substances   78
  lynestrenol   80
  6-mercaptopurine   81
  mestranol   80
  methandrostenolone   80
  methylenedioxyphenyl compounds   81
  metyrapone   81
  nickel carbonyl   81
  Plasmodium berghei   81
  puromycin   **75**
  starvation   81
  steroids   80
  steroids C_{21}, C_{19}, C_{18} 80
  thorotrast   81
Blood, extrahepatic conditioning   103
Blood-vessel ligatures ← thyroid hormones   504
Body weight ← CS-1 *Table 140*   860—861
  ← DOC *Table 140*   860—861
  ← estradiol *Table 140*   860—861
  ← ethylestrenol *Table 140*   860—861
  ← hydroxydione *Table 140*   860—861
  ← norbolethone *Table 140*   860—861
  ← oxandrolone *Table 140*   860—861
  ← PCN *Table 410*   860—861
  ← phenobarbital *Table 140*   860—861
  ← prednisolone *Table 140*   860—861
  ← progesterone *Table 140*   860—861
  ← spironolactone *Table 140*   860—861
  ← thyroxine *Table 140*   860—861
  ← triamcinolone *Table 140*   860—861
Bone explants/chicken   **172**
  explants/mouse   **172**

Bone fracture → TEA *Table 60C* 246
Bordetella pertussis; *cf. also* Histamine and Vaccine
　← pancreatic hormones 527
　← steroids 319
Botulinum toxin ← 5-HT **557**
　← histamine 556
Bradykinin; *cf. also* Hormone-Like Substances
　→ resistance 564
Brain, extrahepatic conditioning 102
Breeding, repeated ← ACTH **422, 423**
Bromide ← steroids 199
　← stressors 692
Bromobenzene ← barbiturates 575
　← phenobarbital *Diagram Table 139* 857−859
　→ resistance 579
　← steroids 200; *Diagram Table 139* 857−859; *Table 138* 850−854
　← stressors 692
　← thyroxine *Diagram Table 139* 857−859; *Table 138* 850−854
Bromoethylamine hydrobromide ← posterior pituitary preparations 441
Brompheniramine; *cf. also* Parabromdylamine
　← phenobarbital *Diagram Table 139* 857−859
　← steroids *Diagram Table 139* 857−859; *Table 138* 850−854
　← thyroxine *Diagram Table 139* 857−859; *Table 138* 850−854
Bronchopulmonary aspergillosis ← steroids 330
Brucella ← pregnancy **665**
　← steroids **316**, 319
Brucella melitensis ← thyroid hormones 497
BSP ← anterior pituitary preparations 440
　← CCl₄ 80
Burns ← sex **657**
n-Butylamine ← hepatic lesions 607

"Cabbage factor" **350, 419**
Cadmium ← anterior pituitary preparations 438
　← CS-1 *Table 35* 200
　← DOC *Table 35* 200
　← estradiol *Table 35* 200
　← ethylestrenol *Table 35* 200
　← hydroxydione *Table 35* 200
　← hypophysectomy 448
　← norbolethone *Table 35* 200
　← oxandrolone *Table 35* 200
　← PCN *Table 35* 200
　← phenobarbital *Diagram Table 139* 857−859; *Tables 35, 138* 200, 850−854
　← prednisolone *Table 35* 200
　← pregnancy 662

Cadmium ← progesterone *Table 35* 200
　← sex 641
　← spironolactone *Table 35* 200
　← steroids 200; *Diagram Table 139* 857 to 859; *Table 138* 850−854
　← thyroxine *Diagram Table 139* 857−859; *Tables 35, 138* 200, 850−854
　← triamcinolone *Table 35* 200
Caffeine ← epinephrine 536
　← pancreatic hormones 524
　← sex 526, 641
　← steroids 200
　← thyroid hormones 475
Calcification, vascular ← DHT + pregnancy *Fig. 27* 664
　← DHT + stress *Figs. 31, 32* 696, 697
Calcitonin → digitoxin 520
　→ drugs **520**
　→ holmium **520**
　→ indium **520**
　→ lead **520**
　→ mercury **520**
　→ parathyroid hormone **520**
　→ renal lesions **520**, 521
　→ resistance **520**
　→ sulfa compounds **520**
　→ vitamin A **520**, 521
Calcium ← stressors 692
Cancers, hormone-dependent **716**
Candida albicans ← anterior pituitary preparations **437**
　← steroids **329**, 330
　← STH **430**
　← thymectomy **550**
Caramiphen ← CS-1 *Table 36* 201
　← DOC *Table 36* 201
　← estradiol *Table 36* 201
　← ethylestrenol *Table 36* 201
　← hydroxydione *Table 36* 201
　← norbolethone *Table 36* 201
　← oxandrolone *Table 36* 201
　← PCN *Table 36* 201
　← phenobarbital *Diagram Table 139* 857 to 859; *Tables 36, 138* 201, 850−854
　← prednisolone *Table 36* 201
　← progesterone *Table 36* 201
　← spironolactone *Table 36* 201
　← steroids 200; *Table 138* 850−854
　← thyroxine *Diagram Table 139* 857−859; *Tables 36, 138* 201, 850−854
　← triamcinolone *Table 36* 201
Carbon dioxide ← thyroid hormones 475
　disulfide (industrial solvent) ← barbiturates 576
　monoxide ← sex 641
　　← steroids 201
　　← thyroid hormones **467**, 475

Carbon tetrachloride; *cf.* CCl₄
Carbonitriles 862
Carcinogens ← ACTH 407, 410
  ← adrenalectomy 212
  ← age 670
  ← anterior pituitary preparations 436, 438
  ← corticoids 203
  ← diet 592, 593
  ← ethionine 78, 79
  ← folliculoids 205
  ← gonadectomy 210
  ← hepatic lesions 602, 607
  ← 5-HT 567
  ← hypophysectomy 446, 448
  ← ionizing rays 683
  ← luteoids 207
  ← pancreatic hormones 524
  ← pinealectomy 554
  ← pregnancy 662
  → resistance 568, 579
  ← sex 633, 641
  ← steroids 153, 213
  ← STH 425, 427
  ← stressors 692
  ← testoids 207
  ← thymectomy 548
  ← thyroid hormones 467, 476
Carcinolytics; *cf. also* Individual Carcinolytic Agents
  ← ACTH 410
  ← 5-HT 559
  ← posterior pituitary preparations 441
  ← sex 633, 643
  ← steroids 215
Carcinoma transplants ← anterior pituitary preparations 440
Cardiac diseases 721
  necrosis ← F-COL + spironolactone *Fig. 1* 123
Cardiopathy ← CS-1 + digitoxin *Fig. 5* 229
  ← digitoxin + spironolactone *Fig. 36* 733
Carisoprodol (skeletal muscle relaxant, sedative) ← CS-1 *Table 37* 216
  ← DOC *Table 37* 216
  ← estradiol *Table 37* 216
  ← ethylestrenol *Table 37* 216
  ← genetic factors 678
  ← hydroxydione *Table 37* 216
  ← norbolethone *Table 37* 216
  ← oxandrolone *Table 37* 216
  ← PCN *Table 37* 216
  ← phenobarbital *Diagram Table 139* 857—859; *Tables 37, 138* 216, 850—854
  ← prednisolone *Table 37* 216
  ← progesterone *Table 37* 216
  → resistance 591
  ← sex 644, 655

Carisoprodol ← SKF 525-A 61
  ← species-dependent factors 675, 678
  ← spironolactone *Table 37* 216
  ← steroids 215; *Diagram Table 139* 857 to 859; *Table 138* 850—854
  ← thyroxine *Diagram Table 139* 857—859; *Table 138* 850—854
  ← triamcinolone *Table 37* 216
Carotene; *cf.* Vitamin A
Carrageenin ← stressors 692
Casein; *cf. also* Amyloid
  ← ACTH 407, 410
  ← steroids 216
Cat 155, 233, 333, 337, 369, 374, 375, 377, 380, 473, 508, 511
Catatoxic compounds (agonists) 53, 54
  compounds, "structure-function" 53
  drugs 567
  effect 862
  hormones 6, 707
  steroids 9, 13; *cf. also* Steroids
    abortifacient properties 863
    → anesthetics (various) 180
    classification 16
    clinical applications 863
    → ganglioplegics *Table 60* 246
    → hepatic tissue 726, 734
    history 31, 40
    interference with lactation 863
    opsonization 863
    protection against toxicants 855
    reviews 3
    secretion in response to a need 863
    ← SKF 525-A 63, 64
    specificity of actions 855
"Catatoxic" substances 862
Catecholamines ← hepatic lesions 599, 601
  ← pregnancy 661
  ← sex 631
  ← stressors 688
  ← thyroid hormones 463
CCl₄ 78; *cf. also* Blockers *under* General Pharmacology
  ← ACTH 410
  → aminopyrine 79
  ← anterior pituitary preparations 436, 438
  → barbiturates 79
  ← barbiturates 575
  → BSP 80
  ← diet 593
  → diphenylhydantoin 79
  ← epinephrine 532, 536
  → estradiol 80
  → estrone 80
  ← hepatic lesions 602, 607
  → hepatic tissue 727, 737
  ← 5-HT 559, 567

CCl₄ → hydroxyproline 79
  ← hypophysectomy **446**, 448
  ← norepinephrine **532**, 536
  ← pancreatic hormones 524
  → paraoxon 79
  → parathion 79
  ← pregnancy 662
  → procaine 79
  → resistance **568**
  ← sex **633**, 641
  ← SKF 525-A 63
  ← steroids **152**, 201, 203
  ← steroids/guinea pig 203
  ← steroids/mouse 203
  ← steroids/rabbit 203
  ← STH **425**, 427
  ← stressors 692
  ← temperature variations **686**
  ← thyroid hormones **467**, 476
  toxicants 108, 110
Cd; cf. Cadmiun
Cedar chips → resistance **569**, 579
Cerium ← hypophysectomy 450
  ← sex 644
  ← steroids 216
CFT 1201 **64**
  reversal of antagonist actions 84
Chemical interactions between drugs **768**
  methods 18, 19
Chemistry **42**
  alcohol dehydrogenase **45**
  cholesterolase 50
  corticoidases 49
  cytochrome b₅ 50
  cytochrome P-450 50
  diamine oxidase **45**
  enzymes 52
  enzymes and resistance in general 48
  folliculoidases 49
  hepatic microsomal enzymes **43**
  monoamine oxidase **45**
  NADPH cytochrome c reductase 50
  steroidases in general 49
  testoidases 49
  thyroxynase 50
Chicken 172, **173**, 174, 238, 258, **333**, 337
Chloral hydrate (sedative, hypnotic) ← epinephrine 536
  ← hepatic lesions 607
  ← histamine **555**
  ← 5-HT **557**, 559
  ← norepinephrine 536
  ← posterior pituitary preparations 441
  ← sex 644
  ← SKF 525-A 60
  ← steroids 216
  ← stressors 692

Chloral hydrate ← temperature variations 687
  ← thyroid hormones **467**, 477
Chloralose ← thyroid hormones 477
Chloramphenicol (antimicrobial) **67**; cf. also
    Inhibitors *under* General Pharmacology
  ← hepatic lesions 608
Chlorazanil → hepatic tissue **727**, 737
Chlorcyclizine; cf. also Antihistamines
  → hepatic tissue 739
  → resistance 591
Chlordane; cf. also Pesticides
  → hepatic tissue 739
  → resistance 591
Chlordecone ← steroids 216
Chlordiazepoxide (tranquilizer) ← CS-1 *Table*
    38 217
  ← DOC *Table 38* 217
  ← estradiol *Table 38* 217
  ← ethylestrenol *Table 38* 217
  ← hydroxydione *Table 38* 217
  ← norbolethone *Table 38* 217
  ← oxandrolone *Table 38* 217
  ← PCN *Table 38* 217
  ← phenobarbital *Diagram Table 139* 857 to
    859; *Tables 38, 138* 217, 850—854
  ← prednisolone *Table 38* 217
  ← progesterone *Table 38* 217
  ← SKF 525-A 63
  ← spironolactone *Table 38* 217
  ← steroids **153**, 216 *Diagram Table 139*
    857—859; *Table 138* 850—854
  ← thyroid hormones **467**, 477
  ← thyroxine *Diagram Table 139* 857—859;
    Tables 38, 138 217, 850—854
  ← triamcinolone *Table 38* 217
Chloretone → resistance 591
  ← SKF 525-A 62
Chlorides ← stressors 693
Chloroform ← diet **592**, 593
  ← epinephrine **533**, 537
  ← genetic factors 678
  ← 5-HT **557**, 559
  ← norepinephrine 537
  ← sex **633**, 644
  ← species-dependent factors **675**
  ← steroids **153**, 217
  ← stressors 693
  ← thymus 549
  ← thyroid hormones **468**, 478
Chloropicrin (insecticide, war gas) ← steroids
    217
4-Chlorotestosterone → barbiturates 196
Chlorpromazine (sedative, antiemetic) ← pancreatic hormones 524
  ← posterior pituitary preparations 441
  → resistance 580, 591
  ← SKF 525-A 62

Chlorpromazine ← starvation/mouse *Table 3* 81
  ← steroids 217
  ← STH 427
  ← stressors 697
  ← thyroid hormones 478
Chlortetracycline (antimicrobial) ← steroids 218
Chlorzoxazone (skeletal muscle relaxant) ← steroids 218
Cholecystokinin-pancreozymin → bile flow/dog *Table 10* 99
Choledochus ← corticoids *Fig. 20* 356
  ligature; *cf. also* Hepatic Lesions
    → DHT *Figs. 24, 25* 614, 615
    → digitoxin *Table 126* 600
    → digitoxin ← spironolactone *Table 126* 600
    → dioxathion *Table 126* 600
    → dioxathion ← spironolactone *Table 126* 600
    → hexobarbital *Table 126* 600
    → hexobarbital ← spironolactone *Table 126* 600
    → indomethacin *Table 126* 600
    → indomethacin ← spironolactone *Table 126* 600
    → mercury *Fig. 23* 611
    → nephrocalcinosis ← mercury *Fig. 23* 611
Cholesterol ← ACTH 407, 410
  ← anterior pituitary preparations 436, 438
  ← barbiturates 576
  → bishydroxycoumarin *Table 28* 182
  → croton oil *Table 43* 223
  → cyclobarbital *Table 33* 198
  → cycloheximide *Table 44* 224
  → diphenylhydantoin *Table 53* 235
  ← diurnal variations 704, 705
  ← DOC 154
  → endotoxin *Table 123* 348
  ← epinephrine 537
  → EPN *Table 99* 284
  → ethylene glycol *Table 56* 243
  ← folliculoids 154
  ← glucocorticoids 154
  → guthion *Table 93* 281
  ← hepatic lesions 608
  → hexobarbital *Table 32* 197
  ← 5-HT 559
  ← norepinephrine 537
  ← pancreatic hormones 525, 530
  → pralidoxime *Table 104* 288
  ← pregnancy 663
  ← posterior pituitary preparations 441
  ← progesterone 154
  → resistance 580

Cholesterol ← sex 644
  → SKF 525-A *Table 106* 291
  ← SKF 525-A 61
  ← steroids 154, 218
  ← stressors 693
  → strychnine *Table 107* 292
  ← temperature variations 687
  → thiopental *Table 31* 197
  ← thyroid hormones 468, 478
  toxicants 105
  → tyrosine *Table 116* 299
Cholesterolase ← ACTH 424
  chemistry 50
Choline deficiency; *cf. also* Ethionine
  ← corticoids 219
  ← folliculoids 220
  ← gonadectomy 220
  ← testoids 219
Choline ← hepatic lesions 602, 608
  ← pregnancy 663
  ← sex 633, 645
  ← steroids 154
  ← STH 425, 427
  ← thyroid hormones 477
Chromium ← pancreatic hormones 525
Cinchophen (uricosuric, analgesic) ← ACTH 411
  ← CS-1 *Table 39* 221
  ← DOC *Table 39* 221
  ← estradiol *Table 39* 221
  ← ethylestrenol *Table 39* 221
  ← hydroxydione *Table 39* 221
  ← norbolethone *Table 39* 221
  ← oxandrolone *Table 39* 221
  ← PCN *Table 39* 221
  ← phenobarbital *Diagram Table 139* 857 to 859; *Tables 39, 138* 221, 850—854
  ← prednisolone *Table 39* 221
  ← progesterone *Table 39* 221
  → resistance 580
  ← spironolactone *Table 39* 221
  ← steroids 154, 220; *Diagram Table 139* 857—859; *Table 138* 850—854
  ← thyroxine *Diagram Table 139* 857—859; *Tables 39, 138* 221, 850—854
  ← triamcinolone *Table 39* 221
"Circulatory stress" 377
Classification 5, 8
  catatoxic steroids 16
  competitive inhibition 17
  enzyme inducers 16
  specific antagonism 17
  steroid hormones 16
  syntoxic steroids 16
Clinical applications of catatoxic steroids 863
  applications of syntoxic steroids 863
  implications 707, 710

Clinical implications, history **32**, 41
summary **724**
Clofibrate (antihypercholesterolemic) → hepatic tissue **727**, **737**
← thyroid hormones 478
"Closed vessel technique" **506**
Clostridium tetani ← ACTH **415**, **416**
← steroids 319
Clostridium welchii ← pancreatic hormones 527
← steroids **316**, 319
CoA-synthetase ← pancreatic hormones 530
Cobalt ← pancreatic hormones 525
→ resistance 580
Cobra venom ← hypophysectomy **453**
Cocaine (local anesthetic) ← CS-1 *Table 40* 221
← DOC *Table 40* 221
← epinephrine 537
← estradiol *Table 40* 221
← ethylestrenol *Table 40* 221
← hydroxydione *Table 40* 221
← norbolethone *Table 40* 221
← oxandrolone *Table 40* 221
← PCN *Table 40* 221
← phenobarbital *Diagram Table 139* 857–859; *Tables 40, 138* 221, 850–854
← prednisolone *Table 40* 221
← progesterone *Table 40* 221
← sex 645
← spironolactone *Table 40* 221
← steroids *Diagram Table 139* 857–859; *Table 138* 850–854
← thyroid hormones **468**, 478
← thyroxine *Diagram Table 139* 857–859; *Tables 40, 138* 221, 850–854
← triamcinolone *Table 40* 221
Codeine (analgesic, antitussive, narcotic)
← SKF 525-A 60, 61
← steroids 221, 222
← stressors 697
← thyroid hormones 479
← thymectomy **548**
F-COL; *cf. also* Corticoids
← acetylsalicylic acid *Table 137* 848–849
← ACTH *Table 137* 848–849
← bile duct ligation *Table 137* 848–849
→ cardiac necrosis, infarctoid ← spironolactone *Fig. 1* 123
← CS-1 *Tables 12, 13, 14* 133, 134
← digitoxin *Table 137* 848–849
← diphenylhydantoin *Table 137* 848–849
← DOC *Tables 12, 13, 14* 133, 134
← estradiol *Tables 12, 13, 14* 133, 134
← ethylestrenol *Tables 12, 13, 14* 133, 134
← hydroxydione *Tables 12, 13, 14* 133, 134
← indomethacin *Table 137* 848–849

F-COL → nephrocalcinosis ← spironolactone *Fig. 1* 123
← nicotine *Table 137* 848–849
← norbolethone *Tables 12, 13, 14* 133, 134
← oxandrolone *Tables 12, 13, 14* 133, 134
← PCN *Tables 12, 13, 14* 133, 134
← phenobarbital *Diagram Table 139* 857–859; *Tables 12, 13, 14, 137, 138* 133, 134, 848–849, 850–854
← phentolamine *Table 137* 848–849
← phenylbutazone *Table 137* 848–849
← phetharbital *Table 137* 848–849
← prednisolone *Tables 12, 13, 14* 133, 134
← progesterone *Tables 12, 13, 14* 133, 134
← salicylate *Table 137* 848–849
← spironolactone *Fig. 1* 123; *Tables 12, 13, 14* 133, 134
← steroids *Diagram Table 139* 857–859; *Tables 136, 138* 836–846, 850–854
← STH *Table 137* 848–849
← thyroxine *Diagram Table 139* 857–859; *Tables 12, 13, 14, 137, 138* 133, 134, 848 849, 850–854
← tolbutamide *Table 137* 848–849
← triamcinolone *Tables 12, 13, 14* 133, 134
← vitamin A *Table 137* 848–849
← vitamin C *Table 137* 848–849
← vitamin D *Table 137* 848–849
← vitamin E *Table 137* 848–849
← W-1372 *Table 137* 848–849
Colchicine (uricosuric in gout) ← CS-1 *Table 41* 222
← DOC *Table 41* 222
← estradiol *Table 41* 222
← ethylestrenol *Table 41* 222
← hydroxydione *Table 41* 222
← norbolethone *Table 41* 222
← oxandrolone *Table 41* 222
← PCN *Table 41* 222
← phenobarbital *Diagram Table 139* 857–859; *Tables 41, 138* 222, 850–854
← prednisolone *Table 41* 222
← progesterone *Table 41* 222
← spironolactone *Table 41* 222
← steroids **155**, 222; *Diagram Table 139*, 857–859; *Table 138* 850–854
← thyroid hormones 479
← thyroxine *Diagram Table 139* 857–859; *Tables 41, 138* 222, 850–854
← triamcinolone *Table 41* 222
Cold; *cf. also* Temperature Variations
← anterior pituitary preparations 440
← corticoids **372**, **373**
← corticoids/mouse **372**
← epinephrine **544**
← epinephrine/dog **544**
← epinephrine/minipig **544**

Cold ← hepatic lesions 618, 619
  ← histamine 555, 556
  ← 5-HT 557, 563
  ← hypophysectomy 456
  ← norepinephrine 544
  ← norepinephrine/dog 544
  ← norepinephrine/ground squirrel 544
  ← norepinephrine/minipig 544
  ← pancreatic hormones 528, 529
  ← parathyroids 520
  ← posterior pituitary preparations 441, 443
  ← sex 657
  ← STH 432
  ← TEA *Table 60C* 246
  ← thymectomy 553
"Cold stress" 372, 373
Collection of literature VII
Columbia-SK virus ← steroids 327
Competition between substrates 70
Competitive inhibition, classification 17
Complete hepatectomy 28; *cf. also* Hepatic Lesions
  history 35
  methods 18, 20
Complex diets ← ACTH 331, 414
  ← hepatic lesions 615
  ← thyroid hormones 495
Compound MO-911 ← thyroid hormones 479
Compounds, foreign, metabolized by "normal" enzymes *Table 134* 759
Conditioners, standard; *cf.* "Standard Conditioners"
Conditioning, extrahepatic; *cf.* Extrahepatic Conditioning
"Conditioning" mechanisms 688
Conditioning, specificity 95
DL-Coniine ← CS-1 *Table 42* 222
  ← DOC *Table 42* 222
  ← estradiol *Table 42* 222
  ← ethylstrenol *Table 42* 222
  ← hydroxydione *Table 42* 222
  ← norbolethone *Table 42* 222
  ← oxandrolone *Table 42* 222
  ← parathyroids 516
  ← PCN *Table 42* 222
  ← phenobarbital *Diagram Table 139* 857–859; *Tables 42, 138* 222, 850–854
  ← prednisolone *Table 42* 222
  ← progesterone *Table 42* 222
  ← spironolactone *Table 42* 222
  ← steroids 222; *Diagram Table 139* 857–859; *Table 138* 850–854
  ← thyroxine *Diagram Table 139* 857–859; *Tables 42, 138* 222, 850–854
  ← triamcinolone *Table 42* 222
Conjugation reactions 47
Contents XVII

Contraceptives → hepatic microsomal drug metabolism in man 708, 710
Convulsions, audiogenic ← steroids 383
Copper ← parathyroids 515, 516
  ← steroids 222
Corpus luteum-hormone-like; *cf.* Luteoid
Corticoidases, chemistry 49
Corticoids; *cf. also* Adrenocortical Hormones, Glucocorticoids, Mineralocorticoids and *under* Names of Individual Corticoids
  → amino acid enzymes 390
  → anaphylactoidogenic agents 180
  anti-inflammatory activity *Table 2* 54
  → bacterial toxins 335, 343
  → bacterial toxins/cat 333, 337
  → bacterial toxins/chicken 333, 337
  → bacterial toxins/dog 333, 338
  → bacterial toxins/guinea pig 333, 339
  → bacterial toxins/man 335, 344
  → bacterial toxins/monkey 333, 339
  → bacterial toxins/mouse 333, 340
  → bacterial toxins/rabbit 335, 342
  → bacterial toxins/sheep 344
  ← barbiturates 572
  → bile secretion *Fig. 20* 356
  biosynthesis 105; *Graph* 106
  → carcinogens 203
  → choledochus *Fig. 20* 356
  → choline deficiency 219
  → cold 372, 373
  → cold/mouse 372
  → diet, choline deficiency 219
  → DNA-polymerase 392
  → electric stimuli 374, 375
  → electric stimuli/cat 374, 375
  → electric stimuli/mouse 374, 375
  → enzymes 385, 392
  → epinephrine 144
  → GOT (aspartate) 390
  → G-6-P-ase 392
  → GPT (alanine) 390
  → heat 372, 373
  → heat/dog 372
  → heat/man 372
  → heat/mouse 372
  → heat/rabbit 372
  → hepatic lesions 354, 355
  → hepatic tissue 725, 728
  → hyperoxygenation 370, 371
  → hyperoxygenation/guinea pig 370, 371
  → hyperoxygenation/man 370, 371
  → hyperoxygenation/mouse 370, 371
  → hypoxia 370, 371
  → hypoxia/guinea pig 370, 371
  → hypoxia/man 370, 371
  → hypoxia/mouse 370, 371
  → immune reactions 349, 350, 351

Corticoids → immune reactions/dog **350**
  → immune reactions/guinea pig **350**
  → immune reactions/mouse **350**
  → immune reactions/rabbit **350**
  → indomethacin ← spironolactone + adrenalectomy *Tables 68—71* 252—254
  → ionizing rays **362, 363**
  → ionizing rays/guinea pig **362, 364**
  → ionizing rays/man **362, 364**
  → ionizing rays/mouse **361, 363**
  → ionizing rays/rabbit **362, 364**
  → lathyrogens 255
  → local trauma **381**
  → methionine 390
  → norepinephrine 144
  → OKT (ornithine) 390
  → parathyroid hormones 142
  → phosphatases 392
  → renal lesions **359**, 360
  → RNA-polymerase 392
  → SDH (serine) 390
  sodium retaining *Table 2* 54
  ← STH 425
  ← stressors 688
  → systemic trauma **376, 378**
  → systemic trauma/cat **377**, 380
  → systemic trauma/dog 380
  → systemic trauma/goat **377**, 380
  → systemic trauma/man **377**, 380
  → systemic trauma/mouse 380
  → systemic trauma/rabbit **377**, 380
  → TDH (threonine) 390
  ← thyroid hormones **461**
  → thyroid hormones 139
  → TKT (tyrosine) 385
  → TKT (tyrosine)/mouse 389
  → TPO (tryptophan) 385
  → TPO (tryptophan)/mouse 389
  → UDP-ase 392
  → urea-cycle enzymes 392
"Corticoids life-maintaining" **13**
Corticosterone, anti-inflammatory activity *Table 122* 345
  → endotoxin *Table 122* 345
"Cortin" **354**
Cortisol; *cf. also* Corticoids
  ← actinomycin 74, 75
  anti-inflammatory activity *Table 122* 345
  → barbiturates 197
  ← cycloheximide 77
  ← endotoxin *Tables 120—122* 344, 345
  → endotoxin ← cycloheximide *Table 121* 345
  → endotoxin ← dactinomycin *Table 121* 345
  → endotoxin ← ethionin *Table 121* 345
  → endotoxin ← metyrapone *Table 121* 345

Cortisol → endotoxin ← puromycin aminonucleoside *Table 121* 345
  → digitoxin ← spironolactone *Table 49* 231
  → hexamethonium *Table 60 B* 246
  → mercury *Table 81* 269
  → pentolinium *Table 60 B* 246
  → puromycin 76
  ← SKF 525-A 62
  → TEA *Table 60 B, C* 246
Cortisone; *cf. also* Corticoids
  ← actinomycin 73
  → endotoxin *Tables 120, 123* 344, 348
  → hexamethonium *Table 60 B* 246
  → mercury *Table 81* 269
  → parathyroid hormones **141**
  → pentolinium *Table 60 B* 246
  → resistance 591
  → steroids 133
  → TEA *Table 60 B* 246
Corynebacteria ← steroids **317**, 319
  ← STH 430
Corynebacterium diphtheriae ← ACTH **415**, 416
  diphtheriae ← steroids **317**
  kutscheri ← steroids **317**
Coxsackie ← steroids **325**, 327
Critique **VIII**
"Cross-resistance" **25, 688**
  nonspecific **698**
Croton oil ← cholesterol *Table 43* 223
  ← CS-1 *Table 43* 223
  ← DOC *Table 43* 223
  ← estradiol *Table 43* 223
  ← ethylestrenol *Table 43* 223
  ← hydroxydione *Table 43* 223
  ← norbolethone *Table 43* 223
  ← oxandrolone *Table 43* 223
  ← PCN *Table 43* 223
  ← phenobarbital *Diagram Table 139* 857—859; *Tables 43, 138* 223, 850—854
  ← prednisolone *Table 43* 223
  ← progesterone *Table 43* 223
  ← spironolactone *Table 43* 223
  ← steroids 222; *Diagram Table 139* 857—859; *Table 138* 850—854
  ← thyroxine *Diagram Table 139* 857—859; *Tables 43, 138* 223, 850—854
  ← triamcinolone *Table 43* 223
CS-1 → AAN *Table 73* 257
  → acetanilide *Table 24* 176
  → acrylamide *Table 25* 176
  → acrylonitrile *Table 26* 177
  → adrenal, weight *Table 140* 860—861
  → aminopyrine *Table 27* 179
  → barbital *Table 34* 198
  → bishydroxycoumarin *Table 28* 182
  → body weight *Table 140* 860—861

CS-1 → cadmium *Table 35* 200
→ caramiphen *Table 36* 201
→ cardiopathy ← digitoxin *Fig. 5* 229
→ carisoprodol *Table 37* 216
→ chlordiazepoxide *Table 38* 217
→ cinchophen *Table 39* 221
→ cocaine *Table 40* 221
→ F-COL *Tables 12, 13, 14* 133, 134
→ colchicine *Table 41* 222
→ DL-coniine *Table 42* 222
→ croton oil *Table 43* 223
→ cyclobarbital *Table 33* 198
→ cycloheximide *Tables 44, 45* 224
→ cyclophosphamide *Fig. 4(H)* 227; *Table 46* 225
→ DHT *Fig. 17* 308; *Table 117* 309
→ digitoxin *Fig. 5* 229; *Tables 47, 48* 230
→ digitoxin/mouse *Table 130* 677
→ dioxathion *Table 91* 280
→ dioxathion/mouse *Table 132* 680
→ diisopropyl fluorophosphate *Table 52* 234
→ diphenylhydantoin *Table 53* 235
→ dipicrylamine *Table 54* 235
→ DOC *Table 15* 135
→ emetine *Table 55* 238
→ endotoxin *Table 123*, 348
→ epinephrine *Table 23* 144
→ EPN *Table 99* 284
→ estradiol *Table 16* 135
→ ethion *Table 92* 281
→ ethylene glycol *Table 56* 243
→ ethylmorphine *Table 57* 244
→ flufenamic acid *Table 58* 245
→ fluphenazine *Table 59* 245
→ glutethimide *Table 63* 248
→ glycerol *Table 64* 249
→ guthion *Table 93* 281
→ heptachlor *Table 98* 283
→ hexamethonium *Tables 60 A, 61* 246, 247
→ hexobarbital *Tables 9, 32* 96, 197
→ hydroquinone *Table 65* 249
→ imipramine *Table 66* 250
→ indomethacin *Table 67* 250
→ kidney, weight *Table 140* 860—861
→ liver weight *Table 140* 860—861
→ LSD *Table 74* 258
→ mechlorethamine *Table 75* 260
→ meprobamate *Table 77* 261
→ mercury *Table 78* 267
→ mersalyl *Tables 79, 80* 268
→ methadone *Table 82* 269
→ methylaniline *Table 83* 270
→ methyprylon *Table 84* 270
→ NaClO₄ *Table 90* 278
→ α-naphthylisothiocyanate *Table 85* 273
→ nicotine *Table 86* 274
→ nikethamide *Table 87* 274

CS-1 → p-nitroanisole *Table 88* 275
→ OMPA *Table 94* 282
→ ovary, weight *Table 140* 860—861
→ pancuronium *Table 19* 136
→ parathion *Table 95* 282
→ pentobarbital/mouse *Table 129* 677
→ pentylenetetrazol *Table 89* 277
→ phenindione *Table 29* 183
→ phenyramidol *Table 100* 284
→ physostigmine *Table 101* 285
→ picrotoxin *Table 102* 286
→ piperidine *Table 103* 287
→ pralidoxime *Table 104* 288
→ preputial glands, weight *Table 140* 860—861
→ progesterone *Tables 9, 17* 96, 136
→ propionitrile *Table 105* 289
→ propylthiouracil *Tables 21, 22* 140, 141
repeated doses → dioxathion *Table 7* 90, 91
→ hexobarbital *Table 7* 90, 91
→ parathion *Table 7* 90, 91
→ progesterone *Table 7* 90, 91
→ zoxazolamine *Table 7* 90, 91
single dose → digitoxin *Table 6* 88, 89
→ dioxathion *Table 6* 88, 89
→ hexobarbital *Table 6* 88, 89
→ indomethacin *Table 6* 88, 89
→ nicotine *Table 6* 88, 89
→ parathion *Table 6* 88, 89
→ progesterone *Table 6* 88, 89
→ zoxazolamine *Table 6* 88, 89
→ SKF 525-A *Table 106* 291
→ steroids **122**, 124
→ strychnine *Table 107* 292
→ T3 *Table 20* 140
→ TEA *Tables 60 A, 62* 246, 248
→ theobromine *Table 108* 293
→ theophylline *Table 109* 293
→ thimerosal *Table 110* 294
→ thiopental *Table 31* 197
→ thymus, weight *Table 140* 860—861
→ thyroid, weight *Table 140* 860—861
→ triamcinolone *Table 18* 136
→ β-tribromoethanol *Table 111* 295
→ β-trichloroethanol *Table 112* 295
→ tri-o-cresyl phosphate *Table 113* 296
→ D-tubocurarine *Table 114* 296
→ tyramine *Table 115* 297
→ tyrosine *Table 116* 299
→ uterus, weight *Table 140* 860—861
→ W-1372 *Table 118* 309
→ zoxazolamine *Tables 9, 119*, 96, 313
Cu; *cf.* Copper
Curare (skeletal muscle relaxant) ← epinephrine **533**, 537
← 5-HT **557**, 559
← steroids 223

Curare ← thymectomy 549
  ← thyroid hormones 479
Cushing's syndrome ← aminoglutethimide 720
  ← barbiturates 715, 720
  ← DDD 715, 720
Cyanide metabolism 48
Cyanide ← steroids 223
Cyano-compounds ← thyroid hormones 468, 479
Cyclobarbital; cf. also Barbiturates
  ← cholesterol Table 33 198
  ← CS-1 Table 33 198
  ← DOC Table 33 198
  ← estradiol Table 33 198
  ← ethylestrenol Table 33 198
  ← hydroxydione Table 33 198
  ← norbolethone Table 33 198
  ← oxandrolone Table 33 198
  ← PCN Table 33 198
  ← phenobarbital Diagram Table 139 857 to 859; Tables 33, 138 198, 850—854
  ← prednisolone Table 33 198
  ← progesterone Table 33 198
  ← spironolactone Table 33 198
  ← steroids 198; Diagram Table 139 857 to 859; Table 138 850—854
  ← thyroxine Diagram Table 139 857—859; Tables 33, 138 198, 850—854
  ← triamcinolone Table 33 198
Cycloheximide (fungicide, inhibitor of protein synthesis) 77; cf. also Antibiotics, Blockers under Pharmacology
  ← cholesterol Table 44 224
  → cortisol 77
  ← CS-1 Tables 44, 45 224
  → 4-6-dienone, dethioacetylated 77
  ← DOC Tables 44, 45 224
  → endotoxin ← cortisol Table 121 345
  → estradiol 77
  ← estradiol Tables 44, 45 224
  → ethylestrenol 77
  ← ethylestrenol Tables 44, 45 224
  ← hydroxydione Tables 44, 45 224
  ← hypophysectomy 450
  ← norbolethone Tables 44, 45 224
  → norbolethone 77
  ← oxandrolone Tables 44, 45 224
  → PCN 78
  ← PCN Tables 44, 45 224
  ← phenobarbital Diagram Table 139 857—859; Tables 44, 45, 138 224, 850—854
  ← prednisolone Tables 44, 45, 224
  ← progesterone Tables 44, 45 224
  → progesterone 78
  → resistance 580
  ← spironolactone Tables 44, 45 224
  → spironolactone 77

Cycloheximide ← steroids 155, 223; Diagram Table 139 857—859; Table 138 850 to 854
  → steroids 77
  ← thyroid hormones 479
  ← thyroxine Diagram Table 139 857—859; Tables 44, 45, 138 224, 850—854
  ← triamcinolone Tables 44, 45 224
Cyclohexylamine ← epinephrine 537
Cyclophosphamide (alkylating antineoplastic)
  ← barbiturates 576
  ← CS-1 Fig. 4(H) 227; Table 46 225
  ← DOC Table 46 225
  ← estradiol Table 46 225
  ← ethylestrenol Fig. 4(A, C) 225, 226; Table 46 225
  ← hepatic lesions 608
  ← hydroxydione Table 46 225
  ← norbolethone Table 46 225
  ← oxandrolone Table 46 225
  ← PCN Fig. 4(B, D, F, J) 225—227; Table 46 225
  ← phenobarbital Diagram Table 139 857 to 859; Tables 46, 138 225, 850—854
  ← prednisolone Table 46 225
  ← progesterone Table 46 225
  ← SKF 525-A 62, 63
  ← spironolactone Table 46 225
  ← steroids 155, 223; Diagram Table 139 857—859; Table 138 850—854
  ← thyroid hormones 479
  ← thyroxine Fig. 22 480; Diagram Table 139 857—859; Tables 46, 138 225, 850—854
  ← triamcinolone Table 46 225
Cyclopropane ← steroids 224
Cyproterone → barbiturates 196
  → steroids 126
  ← thyroid hormones 480
Cytochrome b_5, chemistry 50
Cytochrome P-450, chemistry 50
Cytomegalic inclusion virus ← thymectomy 551
"Cytoplasmic repressor" 84

Dactinomycin; cf. also Antibiotics
  → endotoxins ← cortisol Table 121 345
Damaging agents amenable to prophylaxis, identification of 847
DAO; cf. Diamine Oxidase
Data, previously unpublished VIII
DDD (causes adrenocortical necrosis in dogs)
  → adrenal tumors 715, 720
  → Cushing's syndrome 715, 720
  → hyperbilirubinemia 719
  ← steroids 225
DDT (pediculicide, insecticide) → hyperbilirubinemia 714, 719

DDT ← phenobarbital *Diagram Table 139* 857; *Table 138* 850
 → resistance 591
 ← steroids 164; *Diagram Table 139* 857; *Table 138* 850
 ← thyroxine *Diagram Table 139* 857; *Table 138* 850
Decamethonium ← thyroid hormones 480
Decrease in resistance 856
Defense against "natural" vs. "foreign" compounds, Theories 758
Defense, first line 145
Defensive enzymes, history 27
 enzymes ← stressors 698
Dehalogenation 45
Desipramine (antidepressant) → resistance 569, 580
Detoxication, nonspecific 764
 specific 764
Dexamethasone; *cf. also* Corticoids
 → endotoxin *Table 120* 344
 → hexamethonium *Table 60 B* 246
 → mercury *Table 81* 269
 → pentolinium *Table 60 B* 246
 ← puromycin 76
 → TEA *Table 60 B* 246
Dexamphetamine ← steroids 225
DHT; *cf. also* Vitamin D
 ← acetylsalicylic acid *Table 137* 848
 ← ACTH 408, 414; *Fig. 16* 305; *Table 137* 848
 ← barbiturates 578
 ← bile duct ligature *Table 137* 848
 → calcification, vascular ← pregnancy *Fig. 27* 664
 → calcification, vascular ← stress *Figs. 31, 32* 696, 697
 ← choledochus ligature *Figs. 24, 25* 614, 615
 ← CS-1 *Fig. 17* 308
 ← digitoxin *Table 137* 848
 ← diphenylhydantoin *Table 137* 848
 ← epinephrine 540
 ← estradiol *Fig. 16* 306
 ← folliculoids 173
 ← hepatic lesions 604, 613
 ← 5-HT 557, 561
 ← hypophysectomy 446, 452
 ← indomethacin *Table 137* 848
 ← methyltestosterone *Fig. 16* 305, 306
 ← mineralocorticoids 173
 ← nicotine *Table 137* 848
 ← norepinephrine 540
 ← orchidectomy *Fig. 15* 304
 ← parathyroids 516, 518
 ← phenobarbital *Diagram Table 139* 857; *Tables 117, 137, 138* 309, 848, 850

DHT ← phentolamine, phenylbutazone, phetharbital *Table 137* 848
 ← pregnancy 661, 665; *Fig. 27* 664
 ← sex 635, 654
 ← salicylate *Table 137* 848
 ← steroids 172; *Fig. 16* 305, 306; *Diagram Table 139* 857; *Tables 117, 136, 138* 309, 836, 850
 ← steroids/rabbit 174
 ← STH 426, 428; *Fig. 16* 305; *Table 137* 848
 ← stress *Figs. 31, 32* 696, 697
 ← testoids 174
 ← thyroid hormones 494
 ← thyroxine *Diagram Table 137* 857; *Tables 117, 137, 138* 309, 848, 850
 ← tolbutamide *Table 137* 848
 ← triamcinolone *Table 117* 309
 ← vitamin A, C, D, E *Table 137* 848
 ← W-1372 *Table 137* 848
"Diagram table" 772, 856
Diamine oxidase, chemistry 45
α-Diaminobutyric acid ← thyroid hormones 480
2:6-Diaminopurine ← enzymes, normal *Table 134* 759
Diazepam; *cf. also* Chlordiazepoxide
 → resistance 591
 ← SKF 525-A 63
Dibucaine (local anesthetic) ← sex 645
 ← thyroid hormones 480
2,4-Dichloro-6-phenylphenoxyethyl diethylamine; *cf.* Lilly 18947
Dicumarol ← phenobarbital *Diagram Table 139* 857
 ← steroids *Diagram Table 139* 857
 ← thyroxine *Diagram Table 139* 857
Dieldrin; *cf.* Pesticides
4-6-Dienone, dethioacetylated ← cycloheximide 77
 ← SKF 525-A 64
Diet ← anterior pituitary preparations 440
 → barbiturates 592
 → carcinogens 592, 593
 → CCl₄ 593
 → chloroform 592, 593
 choline deficient ← corticoids 219
  ← gonadectomy 220
  ← folliculoids 220
  ← testoids 219
 complex ← stressors 698
 → digitoxin 593
 → drugs 592, 594
 fat ← steroids 315
 → folliculoid-inactivating system of the liver 592
 gallstone producing ration ← steroids 315
 → hepatic enzymes 594

Diet → hepatic enzyme systems 592
  → indomethacin 592, 593
  ← parathyroids 518
  → partial hepatectomy 592, 594
  → pesticides 592, 593
  ← pregnancy 665
  protein-deficient ← actinomycin 74
    ← steroids 313, 314
  → resistance 592
  ← sex 659
  skim milk powder ← steroids 315
  ← steroids 313
  → steroids 592
  ← STH 430
Dietary constituents, individual ← hepatic lesions 602
β-Diethylaminoethyl diphenylpropylacetate; cf. SKF 525-A
Diethylnitrosamine (n-nitrosodiethylamine) ← steroids 228
Diets, complex ← ACTH 414
  ← hepatic lesions 615
  ← thyroid hormones 495
Digitalis; cf. also Clinical Implications
  compounds, toxicants 105, 108
  ← epinephrine 537
  ← hepatic lesions 602, 608
  → hepatic tissue 737
  ← hypophysectomy 450
  ← norepinephrine 533, 537
  ← pancreatic hormones 522, 525
  ← posterior pituitary preparations 442
  → resistance 581
  ← sex 634, 645
  ← species 678
  ← steroids 155, 156, 228
  ← steroids/cat, dog, frog, guinea pig, hamster, mouse 155, 233, 234
  ← thyroid hormones 468, 481
Digitoxin ← acetylsalicylic acid Table 137 848
  ← ACTH Table 137 848
  ← betamethasone Table 128 630
  ← bile duct ligature Table 137 848
  ← calcitonin 520; Table 124 482
  → cardiopathy ← CS-1 Fig. 5 229
  → cardiopathy ← spironolactone Fig. 36 733
  ← choledochus ligature Table 126 600
  → F-COL Table 137 848
  ← CS-1 Fig. 5 229; Tables 47, 48 230
  ← CS-1/mouse Table 130 677
  ← CS-1, single dose Table 6 88, 89
  → DHT Table 137 848
  ← diet 593
  ← digitoxin Table 137 848
  → dioxathion Table 137 848
  ← diphenylhydantoin Table 137 848
  ← DOC/mouse Table 130 677

Digitoxin ← estradiol/mouse Table 130 677
  ← ethylestrenol Table 128 630
  ← ethylestrenol/mouse Table 130 677
  → hepatic tissue 728
  → hexobarbital Table 137 848
  ← hydroxydione/mouse Table 130 677
  → indomethacin Table 137 848
  ← indomethacin Table 137 848
  ← metyrapone + spironolactone Table 51 232
  → nicotine Table 137 848
  ← nicotine Table 137 848
  ← norbolethone Table 8 94
  ← norbolethone/mouse Table 130 677
  ← oxandrolone/mouse Table 130 677
  → parathion Table 137 848
  ← parathyroids 516; Table 124 482
  ← partial hepatectomy Table 126 600
  ← partial nephrectomy Table 126 600
  ← PCN Tables 124, 128 482, 630
  ← PCN + age Table 50 232
  ← PCN + parathyroidectomy Table 124 482
  ← PCN + propylthiouracil Table 124 482
  ← PCN, single dose Table 6 88, 89
  ← PCN + thyroidectomy Table 124 482
  ← phenobarbital Diagram Table 139 857; Tables 47, 48, 128, 137, 138 230, 630, 848, 850
  ← phenobarbital, single dose Table 6 88, 89
  ← phentolamine Table 137 848
  ← phenylbutazone Tables 128, 137 630, 848
  ← phetharbital Table 137 848
  ← prednisolone/mouse Table 130 677
  → progesterone Table 137 848
  ← progesterone/mouse Table 130 677
  ← propylthiouracil Table 124 482
  protection against 772
  ← renal lesions 626
  ← salicylate Table 137 848
  ← species 675
  ← spironolactone, Figs. 6, 36 233, 733; Tables 8, 126, 128 94, 600, 630
  ← spironolactone + choledochus ligature Table 126 600
  ← spironolactone + cortisol, DOC Table 49 231
  ← spironolactone, duration of pretreatment Table 4 85
  ← spironolactone/mouse Table 130 677
  ← spironolactone + partial hepatectomy Table 126 600
  ← spironolactone + partial nephrectomy Table 126 600
  ← spironolactone + steroids Table 49 231
  ← spironolactone, withdrawal Table 5 86

Digitoxin ← steroids **793**; *Diagram Table 139* 857; *Tables 47, 48, 135, 135 B, 136, 138* 230, 779, 807, 836, 850
  ← steroids (inactive) *Table 135 A* 794
  ← STH *Table 137* 848
  ← thyroidectomy *Table 124* 482
  ← thyroxine *Diagram Table 137* 857; *Tables 47, 48, 124, 137, 138* 230, 482, 848, 850
  ← thyroxine/mouse *Table 130* 677
  ← tolbutamide *Table 137* 848
  ← triamcinolone/mouse *Table 130* 677
  ← vitamin A, C, D, E *Table 137* 848
  ← W-1372 *Table 137* 848
  → zoxazolamine *Table 137* 848
Digoxin ← renal lesions 626
Dihydroxyphenylalanine ← thyroid hormones 481
Diisopropyl fluorophosphate (parasympathomimetic, miotic) ← phenobarbital *Diagram Table 139* 857; *Tables 52, 138* 234, 850
  ← steroids 234; *Diagram Table 139* 857; *Tables 52, 138* 234, 850
  ← thyroid hormones 481
  ← thyroxine *Diagram Table 139* 857; *Tables 52, 138* 234, 850
Dimenhydrinate; *cf.* Antihistamines
Dimercaprol (chelating agent) ← phenobarbital *Diagram Table 139* 857
  ← steroids 234; *Diagram Table 139* 857; *Table 138* 850
  ← thyroxine *Diagram Table 139* 857; *Table 138* 850
Dimethyl sulfoxide (DMSO) → resistance 581
Dinitrophenol (metabolic stimulant, causes fever) ← phenobarbital *Diagram Table 139* 857
  ← sex 646
  ← steroids 234; *Diagram Table 139* 857; *Table 138* 850
  ← temperature variations 687
  ← thyroid hormones 687
  ← thyroxine *Diagram Table 139* 857; *Table 138* 850
Dioxathion; *cf. also* Pesticides
  ← acetylsalicylic acid *Table 137* 848
  ← ACTH *Table 137* 848
  ← betamethasone *Table 128* 630
  ← bile duct ligature *Table 137* 848
  ← choledochus ligature *Table 126* 600
  ← CS-1, repeated doses *Table 7* 90, 91
  ← CS-1, single dose *Table 6* 88, 89
  ← digitoxin *Table 137* 848
  ← diphenylhydantoin *Table 137* 848
  ← ethylestrenol *Table 128* 630
  ← indomethacin *Table 137* 848
  ← nicotine *Table 137* 848

Dioxathion ← partial hepatectomy *Table 126* 600
  ← partial nephrectomy *Table 126* 600
  ← PCN *Table 128* 630
  ← PCN, repeated doses *Table 7* 90, 91
  ← PCN, single dose *Table 6* 88, 89
  ← phenobarbital *Diagram Table 139* 857; *Tables 91, 128, 137, 138* 280, 630, 848, 850
  ← phenobarbital, repeated doses *Table 7* 90, 91
  ← phenobarbital, single dose *Table 6* 88, 89
  ← phentolamine *Table 137* 848
  ← phenylbutazone *Tables 128, 137* 630, 848
  ← phetharbital *Table 137* 848
  ← prednisolone, repeated doses *Table 7* 90, 91
  ← renal lesions 626
  ← salicylate *Table 137* 848
  ← spironolactone *Tables 126, 128* 600, 630
  ← spironolactone + choledochus ligature *Table 126* 600
  ← spironolactone + partial hepatectomy *Table 126* 600
  ← spironolactone + partial nephrectomy *Table 126* 600
  ← spironolactone, repeated doses *Table 7* 90, 91
  ← steroids **165**; *Diagram Table 139* 857; *Tables 91, 136, 138* 280, 836, 850
  ← steroids/mouse *Table 132* 680
  ← STH *Table 137* 848
  ← thyroxine *Diagram Table 139* 857; *Tables 91, 137, 138* 280, 848, 850
  ← thyroxine/mouse *Table 132* 680
  ← tolbutamide *Table 137* 848
  ← vitamin A, C, D, E *Table 137* 848
  ← W-1372 *Table 137* 848
Diphenylhydantoin (anticonvulsant, anti-epileptic); *cf. also* Clinical Implications
  ← ACTH 411
  ← barbiturates 576
  ← CCl$_4$ 79
  ← cholesterol *Table 53* 235
  → F-COL *Table 137* 848
  → DHT *Table 137* 848
  → digitoxin *Table 137* 848
  → hepatic microsomal drug metabolism in man **708**, 713
  → hexobarbital *Table 137* 848
  ← hypophysectomy 450
  → indomethacin *Table 137* 848
  → nicotine *Table 137* 848
  → parathion *Table 137* 848
  ← phenobarbital *Diagram Table 139* 857; *Tables 53, 138* 235, 850
  → resistance **569**, 581, 591
  ← SKF 525-A 62, 63

Diphenylhydantoin ← steroids 234; *Diagram Table 139* 857; *Tables 53, 137, 138* 235, 848, 850
  ← thyroxine *Diagram Table 139* 857; *Tables 53, 138* 235, 850
  → zoxazolamine *Table 137* 848
Diphenhydramine ← hypophysectomy 450
Diphosphopyridine nucleotide (DPN)
  ← steroids 235
Diphtheria toxin ← anterior pituitary preparations 437
Dipicrylamine (reagent for K determination)
  ← phenobarbital *Diagram Table 139* 857 *Tables 54, 138* 235, 850
  ← steroids 235; *Diagram Table 139* 857; *Tables 54, 138* 235, 850
  ← thyroxine *Diagram Table 139* 857; *Tables 54, 138* 235, 850
Diplococcus pneumoniae ← ACTH 416
  ← steroids 320
Diseases 714
Distribution of drugs 768
Disulfiram (anti-alcoholic) 68; *cf. also* Ethanol, Pharmacology (Inhibitors)
  → resistance 581
  ← steroids 235
  ← thyroid hormones 481
Diurnal variations → barbiturates 705
  → cholesterol 704, 705
  → hepatic enzymes 705
  → hexobarbital 704
  → resistance 704, 705
  → TKT 704
DMBA → adrenal necrosis ← spironolactone *Figs. 2, 3* 213, 214
  → adrenocortical necrosis ← stress *Fig. 29* 693
  ← SKF 525-A 63
  ← spironolactone *Figs. 2, 3* 213, 214
  ← splenectomy 553
  ← stress *Fig. 29* 693
DMP; *cf. also* Phosphothioates
  ← steroids 165
DNA-polymerase ← corticoids 392
  ← hepatic lesions 621
  ← stressors 699, 703
DNA, theories 749
DOC; *cf. also* Corticoids
  → AAN *Table 73* 257
  → acetanilide *Table 24* 176
  → acrylamide *Table 25* 176
  → acrylonitrile *Table 26* 177
  ← ACTH 405
  → adrenal, weight *Table 140* 860
  → aminopyrine *Table 27* 179
  anti-inflammatory activity *Table 122* 345
  → barbital *Table 34* 198

DOC → barbiturates 196
  → bishydroxycoumarin *Table 28* 182
  → body weight *Table 140* 860
  → cadmium *Table 35* 200
  → caramiphen *Table 36* 201
  → carisoprodol *Table 37* 216
  → chlordiazepoxide *Table 38* 217
  → cholesterol 154
  → cinchophen *Table 39* 221
  → cocaine *Table 40* 221
  → F-COL *Tables 12, 13, 14* 133, 134
  → colchicine *Table 41* 222
  → DL-coniine *Table 42* 222
  → croton oil *Table 43* 223
  → cyclobarbital *Table 33* 198
  → cycloheximide *Tables 44, 45* 224
  → cyclophosphamide *Table 46* 225
  → DHT *Table 117* 309
  → digitoxin *Tables 47, 48* 230
  → digitoxin/mouse *Table 130* 677
  → digitoxin ← spironolactone *Table 49* 231
  → diisopropyl fluorophosphate *Table 52* 234
  → dioxathion *Table 91* 280
  → dioxathion/mouse *Table 132* 680
  → diphenylhydantoin *Table 53* 235
  → dipicrylamine *Table 54* 235
  → emetine *Table 55* 238
  → endotoxin *Tables 122, 123* 345, 348
  → epinephrine *Table 23* 144
  → EPN *Table 99* 284
  → estradiol *Table 16* 135
  → ethion *Table 92* 281
  → ethylene glycol *Table 56* 243
  → ethylmorphine *Table 57* 244
  → flufenamic acid *Table 58* 245
  → fluphenazine *Table 59* 245
  → glutethimide *Table 63* 248
  → glycerol *Table 64* 249
  → guthion *Table 93* 281
  → heptachlor *Table 98* 283
  → hexamethonium *Tables 60A, 61* 246, 247
  → hexobarbital *Table 32* 197
  → hydroquinone *Table 65* 249
  → imipramine *Table 66* 250
  → indomethacin *Table 67* 250
  → indomethacin/mouse *Table 131* 678
  → kidney, weight *Table 140* 860
  → liver, weight *Table 140* 860
  → LSD *Table 74* 258
  → mechlorethamine *Table 75* 260
  → mephenesin *Table 76* 260
  → meprobamate *Table 77* 261
  → mercury *Table 78* 267
  → mersalyl *Tables 79, 80* 268
  → methadone *Table 82* 269
  → methylaniline *Table 83* 270
  → methyprylon *Table 84* 270

DOC ← metyrapone *Table 125* 584
 → NaClO₄ *Table 90* 278
 → α-naphthylisothiocyanate *Table 85* 273
 → nicotine *Table 86* 274
 → nikethamide *Table 87* 274
 → p-nitroanisole *Table 88* 275
 → norepinephrine 143
 → OMPA *Table 94* 282
 → ovary, weight *Table 140* 860
 → pancreatic hormones 142
 → pancuronium *Table 19* 136
 → parathion *Table 95* 282
 → parathyroid hormones 141
 → pentobarbital/mouse *Table 129* 677
 → pentylenetetrazol *Table 89* 277
 → phenindione *Table 29* 183
 ← phenobarbital *Diagram Table 139* 857; *Tables 15, 138* 135, 850
 → phenyramidol *Table 100* 284
 → physostigmine *Table 101* 285
 → picrotoxin *Table 102* 286
 → piperidine *Table 103* 287
 → pralidoxime *Table 104* 288
 → preputial glands, weight *Table 140* 860
 → progesterone *Table 17* 136
 → propionitrile *Table 105* 289
 → propylthiouracil *Tables 21, 22* 140, 141
 → resistance 591
 → SKF 525-A *Table 106* 291
 ← steroids *Diagram Table 139* 857; *Tables 15, 138* 135, 850
 → strychnine *Table 107* 292
 → T3 *Table 20* 140
 → TEA *Tables 60A, 62* 246, 248
 → theobromine *Table 108* 293
 → theophylline *Table 109* 293
 → thimerosal *Table 110* 294
 → thiopental *Table 31* 197
 → thymus, weight *Table 140* 860
 → thyroid, weight *Table 140* 860
 ← thyroxine *Diagram Table 139* 857; *Tables 15, 138* 135, 850
 → triamcinolone *Table 18* 136
 → β-tribromoethanol *Table 111* 295
 → β-trichloroethanol *Table 112* 295
 → tri-o-cresyl phosphate *Table 113* 296
 → D-tubocurarine *Table 114* 296
 → tyramine *Table 115* 297
 → tyrosine *Table 116* 299
 → uterus, weight *Table 140* 860
 → W-1372 *Table 118* 309
 → zoxazolamine *Table 119* 313
Dog 139, 155, 157, 232, 238, **333**, 338, **350**, **369**, 372, 380, 416, 419, **506**, 534, 544, 604, 630, **633**; *Table 10* 99
Dose and route of administration 93

Dose, repeated, CS-1 → toxicants *Table 7* 90, 91
 repeated, phenobarbital → toxicants *Table 7* 90, 91
  prednisolone → toxicants *Table 7* 90, 91
  PCN → toxicants *Table 7* 90, 91
  spironolactone → toxicants *Table 7* 90, 91
 single, CS-1 → toxicants *Table 6* 88, 89
  PCN → toxicants *Table 6* 88, 89
  phenobarbital → toxicants *Table 6* 88, 89
Doxepin ← phenobarbital *Diagram Table 139* 857; *Table 138* 850
 ← steroids 236; *Diagram Table 139* 857; *Table 138* 850
 ← thyroxine *Diagram Table 139* 857; *Table 138* 850
Drug absorption 768
 antagonisms, specific 15
"Drug effects on enzymes", review 591
Drug excretion 768
 interactions in general 769
  various forms 768
 metabolism by hydrolysis 47
  in man, hepatic microsomal; *cf.* Hepatic Microsomal Drug Metabolism in Man
 metabolizing enzymes 768
Drugs; *cf. also* Individual Drugs, Toxicants
 absorption rate 14
 ← ACTH 406
 ← age 667, 669, 672
 ← anterior pituitary preparations 436, 437
 ← barbiturates 578
 ← calcitonin 520
 catatoxic 567
 chemical interactions 768
 ← diet 592, 594
 distribution 14, 768
 ← epinephrine 532
 ← genetic factors 674
 ← hepatic lesions 602
 → hepatic tissue 727, 728, 736
 ← histamine 555
 ← hormone-like substances 563
 ← 5-HT 556, 558
 ← hypophysectomy 445
 increased elimination 14
 ← ionizing rays 682
 ← norepinephrine 532
 ← pancreatic hormones 522
 ← parathyroids 515
 pharmacologic interactions 768
 ← posterior pituitary preparations 441
 ← pregnancy 661
 → resistance 567
 ← sex 632
 ← species 674
 ← splenectomy 553
 ← steroids 148

Drugs ← STH **425**
  ← stressors **689**
  syntoxic **567**
  ← temperature variations **686**
  ← thymectomy **547**
  ← thyroid hormones **462, 466**
Duck **484**
Duration of effect after withdrawal of conditioner **83, 85**
  of pretreatment, spironolactone → digitoxin *Table 4* **85**
Dyes; *cf. also* Bilirubin, Clinical Implications (for BSP), RES-blocking Agents
  ← barbiturates **576**
  ← hepatic lesions **603, 609**
  ← pancreatic hormones **525**
  ← pregnancy **663**
  ← sex **646**
  ← steroids **157, 237, 238**
  ← steroids/chicken, dog, man, rabbit **157, 236, 237, 238**
  ← thyroid hormones **481**

Eck fistula, methods **19**
E. coli No 08; *cf.* Endotoxin
Edrophonium (parasympathomimetic, muscle stimulant) ← phenobarbital *Diagram Table 139* **857**
  ← steroids **238**; *Diagram Table 139* **857**; *Table 138* **850**
  ← thyroxine *Diagram Table 139* **857**; *Table 138* **850**
EDTA (calcium disodium ethylenediaminetetraacetide) ← steroids **238**
Effect of steroids upon resistance **111**
Eimeria mivati ← steroids **330, 331**
  tenella ← thymectomy **550, 551**
Electric stimuli ← ACTH **423**
  ← adrenalectomy **375**
  ← corticoids **374, 375**
  ← corticoids/cat, mouse **374, 375**
  ← epinephrine **545, 546**
  ← folliculoids **375, 376**
  ← gonadectomy **375, 376**
  ← histamine **555, 556**
  ← 5-HT **557, 563**
  ← hypophysectomy **456**
  ← luteoids **375, 376**
  ← norepinephrine **545, 546**
  ← posterior pituitary preparations **441, 443**
  ← sex **658**
  ← steroids **374, 376**
  ← testoids **375, 376**
  ← thyroid hormones/guinea pig, mouse **511, 512**
Emdabol → mercury **162**
"Emergency reactions" **26, 531, 863**

Emetine (amebicide) ← anterior pituitary preparations **436, 438**
  ← phenobarbital *Diagram Table 139* **857**; *Tables 55, 138* **238, 850**
  ← steroids **239**; *Diagram Table 139* **857**; *Tables 55, 138* **238, 850**
  ← thyroxine *Diagram Table 139* **857**; *Tables 55, 138* **238, 850**
Encephalomyelitis ← ACTH **415**
  equine ← steroids **326**
  Japanese ← steroids **325**
  ← steroids **327**
Encephalomyocarditis ← steroids **326**
Endocrine glands, morphology **740**
"Endocrine kidney" **359**
"Endotheliomyelosis" ← STH **430**
Endotoxin ← actinomycin **74, 75**
  ← cholesterol *Table 123* **348**
  ← cortisol + cycloheximide, dactinomycin, ethionine, metyrapone, puromycin aminonucleoside *Table 121* **345**
  ← ethionine **78**
  ← glucocorticoids *Tables 120, 122* **344, 345**
  ← hypophysectomy **453**
  ← ionizing rays **684**
  ← pancreatic hormones **527**
  ← phenobarbital *Diagram Table 139* **857**; *Tables 123, 138* **348, 850**
  ← pregnancy **665**
  → resistance **595**
  shock **716, 722**
  ← species **681**
  ← steroids *Diagram Table 139* **857**; *Tables 120, 122, 123, 138* **344, 345, 348, 850**
  ← sympathectomy **554**
  ← thymectomy **550**
  ← thyroxine *Diagram Table 139* **857**; *Tables 123, 138* **348, 850**
Endoxan; *cf.* Cyclophosphamide
Enzyme formation, adaptive ← thymectomy **552**
  inducers, "aromatic hydrocarbon type" **15**
    classification **16**
    "phenobarbital type" **15, 16**
    "polycyclic hydrocarbon type" **16**
  induction by hormones, reviews **3**
    in general, reviews **1**
  inhibitors, p-aminosalicylic acid **70**
    CFT 1201 **64**
    chloramphenicol **67**
    disulfiram **68**
    EPB **66**
    EPDA **66**
    JB 516 **66**
    Lilly 18947 **65**
    MPDC **66**
    of **57**

Enzyme inhibitors, Sch 5705 **66**
    Sch 5712 **66**
    SKF 525-A 58
  systems, hepatic ← diet **592**
Enzymes ← adrenalectomy 393, 401
  ← age 673
  amino acid ← hypophysectomy 460
  and adaptation, reviews 3
  and resistance in general, chemistry 48
  chemistry 52
  ← corticoids 385, 392
  ← corticoids, reviews 385
  defensive, history 27
  defensive ← stressors **698**
  drug-metabolizing **768**
  ← folliculoids 402
  ← gonadectomy 403
  hepatic ← ACTH **423**
    ← age 667, 672
    ← anterior pituitary preparations 440
    ← barbiturates 578
    ← diet 594
    ← diurnal variations 705
    ← epinephrine 547
    ← genetic factors 682
    ← hepatic lesions **620**, 621
    ← hypophysectomy 457
    ← hypoxia 685
    ← ionizing rays **684**
    ← norepinephrine 547
    ← pancreatic hormones **529**
    ← pregnancy 666
    ← sex 659
    ← species 682
    ← STH **433**, 434
    ← STH/mouse **433**
    ← stressors 700
    ← temperature variations 687
    theories **743**
    ← thymectomy 553
    ← thyroid hormones 514
  ← luteoids 402
  microsomal, hepatic *Table 1* 46
    theories 746
  normal → 4-aminopyrazolopyrimidine *Table 134* 759
    → 8-azaguanine *Table 134* 759
    → azuridine *Table 134* 759
    → benzylamine *Table 134* 759
    → 2:6-diaminopurine *Table 134* 759
    → 6-mercaptopurine *Table 134* 759
    metabolizing foreign compounds *Table 134* 759
    → p-nitrobenzaldehyde *Table 134* 759
    → p-nitrobenzyl alcohol *Table 134* 759
    → procaine *Table 134* 759
    → succinylcholine *Table 134* 759

Enzymes normal → 6-thioxanthine *Table 134* 759
  ← sex **657**
  ← steroids **383**, 403
  ← stressors 703
  ← testoids 403
Enzymologic references **IX**
EPB **66**
EPDA **66**
Ephedrine (sympathomimetic, vasoconstrictor) ← hypophysectomy 450
  ← phenobarbital *Diagram Table 139* 857; *Table 138* 850
  ← SKF 525-A 60
  ← steroids 239; *Diagram Table 139* 857; *Table 138* 850
  ← thyroid hormones **468**
  ← thyroxine *Diagram Table 139* 857; *Table 138* 850
Epinephrine; *cf. also* Catecholamines
  → acetonitrile 533
  → alloxan **531**, 532
  → anaphylactoidogenic agents **532**, 534
  → antibiotics 534
  → anticoagulants 534
  → arsenic 534
  → bacteria **541**
  → bacterial toxins **541**
  → barbiturates **532**, 536
  → barbiturates/dog, guinea pig, mouse, rabbit 534, 535
  → benzol 536
  → bile flow/dog *Table 10* 99
  → blockade of the sympathetic nervous system 545
  → caffeine 536
  → CCl_4 **532**, 536
  → chloral hydrate 536
  → chloroform **533**, 537
  → cholesterol 537
  → cocaine 537
  → cold **544**
  → cold/dog, minipig **544**
  ← corticoids 144
  → curare **533**, 537
  → cyclohexylamine 537
  → DHT 540
  → digitalis 537
  → drugs **532**
  → electric stimuli **545**, 546
  ← epinephrine **531**, 532
  → ergotamine 537
  → ethanol 537
  ← folliculoids 144
  → formaldehyde 538
  → ganglioplegics **533**, 538
  ← glucocorticoids **143**

Epinephrine → hepatic enzymes 547
 → histamine 531, 532
 → hormone-like substances 531
 ← hydroxydione *Table 23* 144
 → hypoxia 545, 546
 → immune reactions 543
 → ionizing rays 543
 → ionizing rays/mouse 543
 → lead 538
 ← luteoids 144
 → mescaline 533, 538
 → methoxyflurane 538
 → methyltropolone 538
 → microorganisms 541
 → morphine 538
 → nicotine 539
 → nonsteroidal hormones 531
 → occlusion of the portal vein 545
 → papain 539
 → paraphenylenediamine 533, 539
 ← parathyroids 515
 → pentylenetetrazol 533, 539
 → peptone 539
 → pesticides 539
 ← phenobarbital *Diagram Table 139* 857; *Tables 23, 138* 144, 850
 → phenylethylamine 539
 → picrotoxin 533, 539
 → portal vein, occlusion of 545
 → potassium 540
 → reserpine 533
 → resistance 531, 540, 591
 ← sex 630
 ← steroids 143; *Diagram Table 139* 857; *Tables 23, 138* 144, 850
 → steroids 531
 → sparteine 533, 540
 ← stilbestrol 143
 → stressors 545
 ← stressors 689
 → strychnine 533, 540
 → sympathetic nervous system, blockade of 545
 ← testoids 143, 144
 → thyroid hormones 531, 532
 ← thyroid hormones 465, 482
 ← thyroxine *Diagram Table 139* 857; *Tables 23, 138* 144, 850
 → trauma 545
 → tremorine 540
 → urethan 540
 → vaccines 541
 → venoms 541, 542
 → viruses 541
 → vitamin D 533, 540
 → yohimbine 540
EPN; *cf. also* Pesticides

EPN ← cholesterol *Table 99* 284
 ← phenobarbital *Diagram Table 139* 857; *Tables 99, 138* 284, 850
 ← steroids 165; *Diagram Table 139* 857; *Tables 99, 138* 284, 850
 ← thyroxine *Diagram Table 139* 857; *Tables 99, 138* 284, 850
1,2α-Epoxy-androstan-3,17-dione → steroids 133
Equine encephalomyelitis ← steroids 326
Ergot (oxytocic) ← hypophysectomy 450
 ← sex 646
 ← steroids 157, 239
 ← thyroid hormones 482
Ergotamine ← anterior pituitary preparations 436, 439
 ← epinephrine 537
 → resistance 591
 ← sex 634
Erysipelothrix rhusiopathiae ← steroids 317, 320
Erythropoietin → resistance 563, 564
Escherichia coli ← pancreatic hormones 527
 endotoxin ← cholesterol *Table 123* 348
 ← phenobarbital *Table 138* 850
 ← steroids 317, 320; *Tables 123, 138* 348, 850
 ← thyroxine *Tables 123, 138* 348, 850
ESCN; *cf.* F-COL
EST ← ACTH 422
 ← hypophysectomy 456
 ← sex 657
 ← STH 433, 434
Estradiol; *cf. also* Folliculoids
 → AAN *Table 73* 257
 → acetanilide *Table 24* 176
 → acrylamide *Table 25* 176
 → acrylonitrile *Table 26* 176
 → ACTH 137
 → adrenal, weight *Table 140* 860
 → aminopyrine *Table 27* 179
 "antirachitic" 173
 → barbital *Table 34* 198
 → barbiturates 197
 → bishydroxycoumarin *Table 28* 182
 → body weight *Table 140* 860
 → cadmium *Table 35* 200
 → caramiphen *Table 36* 201
 → carisoprodol *Table 37* 216
 ← CCl₄ 80
 → chlordiazepoxide *Table 38* 217
 → cinchophen *Table 39* 221
 → cocaine *Table 40* 221
 → F-COL *Tables 12, 13, 14* 133, 134
 → colchicine *Table 41* 222
 → DL-coniine *Table 42* 222
 → croton oil *Table 43* 223

Estradiol → cyclobarbital *Table 33* 198
 ← cycloheximide 77
 → cycloheximide *Tables 44, 45* 224
 → cyclophosphamide *Table 46* 225
 → DHT *Fig. 16* 306; *Table 117* 309
 → digitoxin 230
 → digitoxin/mouse *Table 130* 677
 → digitoxin ← spironolactone *Table 49* 231
 → diisopropyl fluorophosphate *Table 52* 234
 → dioxathion *Table 91* 280
 → dioxathion/mouse *Table 132* 680
 → diphenylhydantoin *Table 53* 235
 → dipicrylamine *Table 54* 235
 → DOC *Table 15* 135
 → emetine *Table 55* 238
 → endotoxin *Table 123* 348
 → epinephrine *Table 23* 144
 → EPN *Table 99* 284
 → ethion *Table 92* 281
 → ethylene glycol *Fig. 7* 242; *Table 56* 243
 → ethylmorphine *Table 57* 244
 → flufenamic acid *Table 58* 245
 → fluphenazine *Table 59* 245
 → glutethimide *Table 63* 248
 → glycerol *Table 64* 249
 → guthion *Table 93* 281
 → heptachlor *Table 98* 283
 → hexamethonium *Tables 60A, 61* 246, 247
 → hexobarbital *Tables 9, 30, 32* 96, 195, 197
 → hexobarbital ← orchidectomy *Table 30* 195
 → hydroquinone *Table 65* 249
 → imipramine *Table 66* 250
 → indomethacin *Table 67* 250
 → indomethacin/mouse *Table 131* 678
 → kidney, weight *Table 140* 860
 → LSD *Table 74* 258
 → mechlorethamine *Table 75* 260
 → mephenesin *Table 76* 260
 → meprobamate *Table 77* 261
 → mercury *Table 78* 267
 → mersalyl *Tables 79, 80* 268
 → methadone *Table 82* 269
 → methylaniline *Table 83* 270
 → methyprylon *Table 84* 270
 → $NaClO_4$ *Table 90* 278
 → α-naphthylisothiocyanate *Table 85* 273
 → nicotine *Table 86* 274
 → nikethamide *Table 87* 274
 → p-nitroanisole *Table 88* 275
 → OMPA *Table 94* 282
 → ovary, weight *Table 140* 860
 → pancuronium *Table 19* 136
 → parathion *Table 95* 282
 → parathyroid hormones 142
 → pentobarbital/mouse *Table 129* 677

Estradiol → pentylenetetrazol *Table 89* 277
 → phenindione *Table 29* 183
 ← phenobarbital *Diagram Table 139* 857; *Tables 16, 138* 135, 850
 → phenyramidol *Table 100* 284
 → physostigmine *Table 101* 285
 → picrotoxin *Table 102* 286
 → piperidine *Table 103* 287
 → pralidoxime *Table 104* 288
 → preputial glands, weight *Table 140* 860
 → progesterone *Tables 9, 17* 96, 136
 → propionitrile *Table 105* 289
 → propylthiouracil *Tables 21, 22* 140, 141
 ← SKF 525-A 62
 → SKF 525-A *Table 106* 291
 ← steroids *Diagram Table 139* 857; *Tables 16, 138* 135, 850
 → steroids 133
 → strychnine *Table 107* 292
 → T3 *Table 20* 140
 → TEA *Tables 60A, 62* 246, 248
 → theobromine *Table 108* 293
 → theophylline *Table 109* 293
 → thimerosal *Table 110* 294
 → thiopental *Table 31* 197
 → thymus, weight *Table 140* 860
 → thyroid, weight *Table 140* 860
 ← thyroxine *Diagram Table 139* 857; *Tables 16, 138* 135, 850
 → triamcinolone *Table 18* 136
 → β-tribromoethanol *Table 111* 295
 → β-trichloroethanol *Table 112* 295
 → tri-o-cresyl phosphate *Table 113* 296
 → D-tubocurarine *Table 114* 296
 → tyramine *Table 115* 297
 → tyrosine *Table 116* 299
 → uterus, weight *Table 140* 860
 → W-1372 *Table 118* 309
 → zoxazolamine *Tables 9, 119* 96, 313
Estrogenic steroids; *cf.* Folliculoids
Estromimetic steroids; *cf.* Folliculoids
Estrone ← CCl_4 80
 ← SKF 525-A 63
Ethanol ← ACTH 411
 ← barbiturates 576
 ← epinephrine 537
 ← ethionine 79
 ← genetic factors 678
 ← hepatic tissue 737
 ← 5-HT 557, 559
 ← pancreatic hormones 525
 ← posterior pituitary preparations 442
 → resistance 581
 ← steroids/man, mouse, rabbit 158, 239, 240
 ← STH 427
 ← stressors 693
 ← thyroid hormones 482

Ether ← 5-HT **557**, 560
  ← sex 646, 647
  ← steroids 240
  ← thyroid hormones 483
"Ethereal sulphates" 47
Ethion; *cf. also* Pesticides
  ← phenobarbital *Diagram Table 139* 857; *Tables 92, 138* 281, 850
  ← steroids **165**; *Diagram Table 139* 857; *Tables 92, 138* 281, 850
  ← thyroxine *Diagram Table 139* 857; *Tables 92, 138* 281, 850
Ethionine (inhibitor of protein biosynthesis) 78; *cf. also* Blockers *under* General Pharmacology
  ← ACTH 411
  ← anterior pituitary preparations 439
  → barbiturates 79
  → carcinogens 78, 79
  → endotoxin 78
  → endotoxin ← cortisol *Table 127* 345
  → ethanol 79
  ← glucocorticoids 241
  ← gonadal steroids 241
  → metyrapone 79
  → "19-nortestosterone derivatives" 78
  ← sex **634**, 646
  → soman 79
  → spironolactone 79
  ← steroids **158**
  ← steroids, gonadal 241
  ← STH 427
  → Su 9055 79
  → Su 10603 79
p-Ethoxyacetanilide ← SKF 525-A 61
Ethyl alcohol ← phenobarbital *Diagram Table 139* 857; *Table 138* 850
  ← steroids *Diagram Table 139* 857; *Table 138* 850
  ← thyroxine *Diagram Table 139* 857; *Table 138* 850
Ethylene chlorohydrin (toxic solvent, causes renal damage) ← phenobarbital *Diagram Table 139* 857
  ← steroids 241; *Diagram Table 139* 857; *Table 138* 850
  ← thyroxine *Diagram Table 139* 857; *Table 138* 850
Ethylene glycol (toxic antifreeze) ← cholesterol *Table 56* 243
  ← phenobarbital *Diagram Table 139* 857; *Tables 56, 138* 243, 850
  ← sex **634**, 647
  ← steroids 241; *Fig. 7* 242; *Diagram Table 139* 857; *Tables 56, 138* 243, 850
  ← thyroxine *Diagram Table 139* 857; *Tables 56, 138* 243, 850

Ethylestrenol; *cf. also* Testoids
  → AAN *Table 73* 257
  → acetanilide *Table 24* 176
  → acrylamide *Table 25* 176
  → acrylonitrile *Table 26* 177
  ← actinomycin 75
  → adrenal, weight *Table 140* 860
  → aminopyrine *Table 27* 179
  → barbital *Table 34* 198
  → barbiturates 197
  → bile flow *Table 10* 99
  → bishydroxycoumarin *Table 28* 182
  → body weight *Table 140* 860
  → cadmium *Table 35* 200
  → caramiphen *Table 36* 201
  → carisoprodol *Table 37* 216
  → chlordiazepoxide *Table 38* 217
  → cinchophen *Table 39* 221
  → cocaine *Table 40* 221
  → F-COL *Tables 12, 13, 14* 133, 134
  → colchicine *Table 41* 222
  → DL-coniine *Table 42* 222
  → croton oil *Table 43* 223
  → cyclobarbital *Table 33* 198
  ← cycloheximide 77
  → cycloheximide *Tables 44, 45* 224
  → cyclophosphamide *Fig. 4(A, C)* 225, 226; *Table 46* 225
  → DHT *Table 117* 309
  → digitoxin *Tables 47, 48, 128, 130* 228, 230, 630, 677
  → diisopropyl fluorophosphate *Table 52* 234
  → dioxathion *Tables 91, 128* 280, 630
  → dioxathion/mouse *Table 132* 680
  → diphenylhydantoin *Table 53* 235
  → dipicrylamine *Table 54* 235
  → DOC *Table 15* 135
  → emetine *Table 55* 238
  → endotoxin *Table 123* 348
  → epinephrine *Table 23* 144
  → EPN *Table 99* 284
  → estradiol *Table 16* 135
  → ethion *Table 92* 281
  → ethylene glycol *Table 56* 243
  → ethylmorphine *Table 57* 244
  → flufenamic acid *Table 58* 245
  → fluphenazine *Table 59* 245
  → glutethimide *Table 63* 248
  → glycerol *Table 64* 249
  → guthion *Table 93* 281
  → heptachlor *Table 98* 283
  → hexamethonium *Tables 60A, 61* 246, 247
  → hexobarbital *Tables 9, 32, 128* 96, 197, 630
  → hydroquinone *Table 65* 249
  → imipramine *Table 66* 250

Ethylestrenol → indomethacin *Tables 67, 128* 250, 630
 → indomethacin/mouse *Table 131* 678
 → kidney, weight *Table 140* 860
 → lathyrogens *Fig. 9* 256
 → liver, weight *Table 140* 860
 → LSD *Table 74* 258
 → mechlorethamine *Table 75* 260
 → mephenesin *Table 76* 260
 → meprobamate *Table 77* 261
 → mercury *Table 78* 267
 → mersalyl *Fig. 10* 262; *Tables 79, 80* 268
 → methadone *Table 82* 269
 → methylaniline *Table 83* 270
 → methyprylon *Table 84* 270
 → NaClO$_4$ *Table 90* 278
 → α-naphthylisothiocyanate *Table 85* 273
 → nephrocalcinosis ← mersalyl *Fig. 10* 262
 → nicotine *Tables 86, 128* 274, 630
 → nikethamide *Table 87* 274
 → p-nitroanisole *Table 88* 275
 → OMPA *Table 94* 282
 → ovary, weight *Table 140* 860
 → pancuronium *Table 19* 136
 → parathion *Tables 95, 128* 282, 630
 → pentobarbital/mouse *Table 129* 677
 → pentylenetetrazol *Table 89* 277
 → phenindione *Table 29* 183
 → phenyramidol *Table 100* 284
 → physostigmine *Table 101* 285
 → picrotoxin *Table 102* 286
 → picrotoxin/mouse *Table 133* 680
 → piperidine *Table 103* 287
 → pralidoxime *Table 104* 288
 → preputial glands, weight *Table 140* 860
 → progesterone *Tables 9, 17, 128* 96, 136, 630
 → propionitrile *Table 105* 289
 → propylthiouracil *Tables 21, 22* 140, 141
 ← puromycin 76
 → SKF 525-A *Table 106* 291
 ← SKF 525-A 63, 64
 → strychnine *Table 107* 292
 → T3 *Table 20* 140
 → TEA *Tables 60A, 62* 246, 248
 → theobromine *Table 108* 293
 → theophylline *Table 109* 293
 → thimerosal *Table 110* 294
 → thiopental *Table 31* 197
 → thymus, weight *Table 140* 860
 → thyroid, weight *Table 140* 860
 → triamcinolone *Table 18* 136
 → β-tribromoethanol *Table 111* 295
 → β-trichloroethanol *Table 112* 295
 → tri-o-cresyl phosphate *Table 113* 296
 → D-tubocurarine *Table 114* 296
 → tyramine *Table 115* 297

Ethylestrenol → tyrosine *Table 116* 299
 → uterus, weight *Table 140* 860
 → W-1372 *Table 118* 309
 → zoxazolamine *Tables 9, 119, 128* 96, 313, 630
Ethyl-O-ethylphenylurea ← hepatic lesions 609
 ← sex 647
Ethylmorphine (narcotic, analgesic, antitussive); *cf. also* Morphine
 ← phenobarbital *Diagram Table 139* 857; *Tables 57, 138* 244, 850
 ← sex 647
 ← steroids **163**, 243; *Diagram Table 139* 857; *Tables 57, 138* 244, 850
 ← thyroxine *Diagram Table 139* 857; *Tables 57, 138* 244, 850
Ethyl urethan ← sex 648
"Eucorton" 254
Evisceration, extrahepatic conditioning 103
Excretion of drugs **768**
"Experimental pharmacogenetics" monograph 655
Extrahepatic conditioning **100**, 103
 conditioning, blood 103
  brain 102
  evisceration 103
  gastrointestinal tract 101, 103
  heart 102
  kidney 100, 102, 103
  lung 102
  milk 103
  muscle 103
  pancreas 103
  placenta 102
  reproductive tract 103
  RES 102, 103
  serum proteins 103
  spleen 102
  splenectomy 103
  sweat 103
  tears 103
  thymectomy 103
  thymus 103
 tissues, morphology **740**

Fasciola hepatica ← steroids **330**, 332
Fasting ← phenobarbital *Diagram Table 139* 857
 ← steroids **313**, 314; *Diagram Table 139* 857; *Table 138* 850
 → TEA *Table 60C* 246
 ← thyroxine *Diagram Table 139* 857
Fatty acids ← stressors 694
Fencamfamine (CNS stimulant) ← steroids 244
Ferric dextran → resistance 581
"First line of defense" **145**
First screening 771

Fish 505, 506, **509**, 511
Flufenamic acid (antihypotensive) ← phenobarbital *Diagram Table 139* 857; *Tables 58, 138* 245, 850
 ← steroids 244; *Diagram Table 139* 857; *Tables 58, 138* 245, 850
 ← thyroxine *Diagram Table 139* 857; *Tables 58, 138* 245, 850
N-2-Fluorenyldiacetamide; *cf.* Carcinogens
Fluoride ← parathyroids **516**
 ← sex 648
 ← steroids 244
 ← thyroid hormones 483
9α-Fluorohydrocortisone; *cf.* F-COL *under* COL
5-Fluorouracil ← steroids 245
Fluphenazine ← phenobarbital *Diagram Table 139* 857; *Tables 59, 138* 245, 850
 ← steroids 245; *Diagram Table 139* 857; *Tables 59, 138* 245, 850
 ← thyroxine *Diagram Table 139* 857; *Tables 59, 138* 245, 850
Flurothyl ← steroids 245
Follicle-hormone-like; *cf.* Folliculoids
Folliculoidases, chemistry 50
Folliculoid-inactivating system of the liver ← diet 592
Folliculoids **9**
 ← anabolic steroids **115**, 119
 → anaphylactoidogenic agents 180
 → bacterial toxins **337**, 347
 → barbiturates **150**, 190
 ← barbiturates 573
 → carcinogens 205
 → cholesterol **154**
 → choline deficiency 220
 → DHT **173**
 → diets, choline deficiency 220
 → electric stimuli **375**, 376
 → enzymes 402
 → epinephrine 144
 → hepatic lesions **354**, 358
 → hepatic tissue **725**, 729
 → hyperoxygenation **371**, 372
 → hypoxia **371**, 372
 → immune reactions **351**, 353
 → ionizing rays **362**, 367
 → ionizing rays/mouse **362**, 366
 → lathyrogens 255
 metabolism ← folliculoids *Graph* 125
  ← thyroid hormones *Graph* 125
 → norepinephrine 144
 → OMPA *Table 96* 283
 ← posterior pituitary preparations **441**
 → renal lesions **359**, 361
 ← steroids **124**
 ← STH **425**
 → systemic trauma **378**, 381

Folliculoids → temperature variations **373**, 374
 ← testoids **115**, 119
 → testoids, metabolism 125
 ← thyroid hormones **461**, 462
 → vitamin D **173**, 304
Food consumption ← steroids **314**, 315
Foreign compounds metabolized by "normal" enzymes *Table 134* 759
 compounds ← SKF 525-A 61
"Foreign" compounds, theories **758**
Formaldehyde ← ACTH 411
 ← epinephrine 538
 ← steroids 245
 ← stressors 693
 ← sympathectomy 554
 → TEA *Table 60C* 246
Frog **155**, 233, 473, 629
Fungi ← steroids **329**
 ← STH 432
 ← thymectomy 551

Galactosemia **716**, 722
Gallstone producing ration ← steroids 315
Ganglioplegics ← ACTH **407**, 411; *Table 60C* 246
 ← epinephrine **533**, 538
 ← glucocorticoids *Table 60* 246
 ← steroids **159**, 245
 ← steroids, catatoxic *Table 60* 246
 ← steroids/guinea pig **159**
 ← stressors 693; *Table 60* 246
G.A.S. 5, 6
Gastrin → bile flow/dog *Table 10* 99
Gastrointestinal tract, extrahepatic conditioning 101, 103
α-GDPH ← thyroid hormones 514
"General Adaptation Syndrome"; *cf.* G.A.S.
General pharmacology **53**
Genetic factors → barbiturates 675
 → bilirubin 677
 → carisoprodol 678
 → chloroform 678
 → drugs **674**
 → ethanol 678
 → hepatic enzymes 682
 → hepatic lesions 682
 → hexobarbital 675
 → morphine 680
 → pesticides **675**, 680
 → picrotoxin 680
 → resistance **673**
 → steroids **673**
 → strychnine **675**, 681
 → TKT 682
 → TPO 682
 → zoxazolamine **675**, 681

Gestogenic steroids; cf. Luteoids
v. Gierke's glycogen storage disease **716, 722**
Glossary **XIII**
Glucagon ← actinomycin 75
   ← pregnancy **660**
Glucocorticoids **9**
   ← anabolic steroids **114, 115**
   anti-inflammatory activity *Table 122* 345
   → barbiturates **149, 184**
   → barbiturates/man, mouse, rabbit **184**
   → cholesterol **154**
   → endotoxin *Tables 120, 121* 344, 345
   → epinephrine **143**
   → ethionine **241**
   → ganglioplegics *Table 60* 246
   → mercury **162**; *Table 81* 269
   → pancreatic hormones **142**
   ← pregnancy **660**
   → steroids **111, 112**
   → STH **137**
   ← testoids **114, 115**
   → vitamin D **302**
   → vitamin D/chicken, man, mouse **173**
Gluco-mineralocorticoids ← anabolic steroids **114, 118**
   → barbiturates **150, 185**
   ← pregnancy **660**
   → steroids **113**
   ← testoids **114, 118**
D-Glucose-6-phosphate; cf. G-6-P-ase and *under* Influence of Steroids upon Enzymes
Glucose → resistance **569, 581**
Glucuronidase ← hepatic lesions **621**
   ← sex **659**
Glucuronide ← pancreatic hormones **531**
   synthesis **47**
Glutamic acid ← steroids **247**
"Glutathiokinase" **47**
Glutethimide → hepatic microsomal drug metabolism in man **709, 713**
   ← phenobarbital *Diagram Table 139* 857; *Tables 63, 138* 248, 850
   → resistance **591**
   reversal of substrate actions **93**
   ← SKF 525-A **62**
   ← steroids **247**; *Diagram Table 139* 857; *Tables 63, 138* 248, 850
   ← thyroxine *Diagram Table 139* 857; *Tables 63, 138* 248, 850
Glycerol ← phenobarbital *Diagram Table 139* 857; *Tables 64, 138* 249, 850
   ← steroids **248**; *Diagram Table 139* 857; *Tables 64, 138* 249, 850
   ← thyroxine *Diagram Table 139* 857; *Tables 64, 138* 249, 850
Glycine ← anterior pituitary preparations **439**
Glycogen, hepatic, theories **757**

Glycolic acid (irritant to skin) ← sex **648**
   ← steroids **248**
Gold ← steroids **248**
Gonadal steroids → ethionine **241**
Gonadectomy → barbiturates **151, 193**
   → barbiturates/guinea pig, mouse **195, 196**
   → carcinogens **210**
   → choline deficiency **220**
   → diets, choline deficiency **220**
   → electric stimuli **375, 376**
   → enzymes **403**
   → hyperoxygenation **371, 372**
   → hypoxia **371, 372**
   → immune reactions **351, 353**
   → ionizing rays **362, 367**
   → renal lesions **359, 361**
   → steroids **129**
   → systemic trauma **378, 381**
   → temperature variations **373, 374**
   → temperature variations/rabbit **373**
   → vitamin D **303**
Gonococci; cf. Neisseria Gonorrhoeae
GOT ← hepatic lesions **621**
   ← hypophysectomy **459**
   ← pancreatic hormones **530**
   ← stressors **699, 703**
GOT (aspartate) ← corticoids **390**
G-6-P-ase ← corticoids **392**
GPT ← ACTH **424**
   ← hepatic lesions **621**
   ← hypophysectomy **459**
   ← pancreatic hormones **530**
   ← stressors **699, 703**
   ← thyroid hormones **514**
GPT (alanine) ← corticoids **390**
Griseofulvin; cf. also Antibiotics
   → hepatic microsomal drug metabolism in man **709, 713**
   ← phenobarbital *Diagram Table 139* 857; *Table 138* 850
   ← steroids *Diagram Table 139* 857; *Table 138* 850
   ← thyroxine *Diagram Table 139* 857; *Table 138* 850
   toxicants **110**
Guanidine (formerly in myasthenia gravis)
   ← parathyroids **516, 517**
   ← thyroid hormones **483**
Guinea pig **139, 155, 159, 164, 172, 189, 193, 196, 203, 233, 322, 333, 339, 350, 362, 364, 370, 371, 415, 419, 420, 470, 497, 506, 508, 511, 534, 633**
Guthion; cf. also Pesticides
   ← cholesterol *Table 93* 281
   ← phenobarbital *Diagram Table 139* 857; *Tables 93, 138* 281, 850

Guthion ← steroids **165**; *Diagram Table 139* **857**; *Tables 93, 138* **281, 850**
— ← thyroxine *Diagram Table 139* **857**; *Tables 93, 138* **281, 850**
Gynecogenic steroids; *cf.* Folliculoids

Haldranolone; *cf.* Corticoids
Haloperidol ← phenobarbital *Diagram Table 139* **857**; *Table 138* **850**
— ← steroids *Diagram Table 139* **857**; *Table 138* **850**
— ← thyroxine *Diagram Table 139* **857**; *Table 138* **850**
Halothane (inhalation anesthetic) ← 5-HT **557, 560**
— ← norepinephrine **538**
— ← thyroid hormones **483**
Hamster **234, 509, 511**
Harmine ← 5-HT **557, 560**
Heart, extrahepatic conditioning **102**
Heat; *cf. also* Temperature Variations
— ← corticoids **372, 373**
— ← corticoids/dog, man, mouse, rabbit **372**
— ← pancreatic hormones **529**
"Heat stress" **372, 373**
Heliotrine; *cf.* Plant Extracts
Hemorrhage ← norepinephrine **546**
— ← posterior pituitary preparations **441, 443**
— ← steroids **369, 370**
— ← steroids/cat, dog, monkey, rabbit **369, 370**
— → TEA *Table 60C* **246**
— ← thyroid hormones **512, 513**
Hemorrhages, multiple ← androstanolone-5β-carbonitrile (ACN) *Fig. 37* **741**
— multiple, morphology **740**
"Hemorrhagic death syndrome" **408, 426**
Hemorrhagic shock, "irreversible" **369**
— ← norepinephrine **545**
"Hemorrhagic stress syndrome" **148, 181, 534**
"Hemorrhagic syndrome of Jaques" **689**
Hepatectomy, complete; *cf.* Complete Hepatectomy
— partial; *cf.* Partial Hepatectomy
— subtotal; *cf.* Subtotal Hepatectomy
Hepatic; *cf. also* Liver, Microsomes
— changes ← hepatic lesions **615**
— ← pancreatic hormones **529**
— denervation, methods **19, 22**
— enzymes ← ACTH **423**
— ← age **667, 672**
— ← anterior pituitary preparations **440**
— ← barbiturates **578**
— ← diet **594**
— ← diurnal variations **705**
— ← epinephrine **547**

Hepatic enzymes ← genetic factors **682**
— ← hepatic lesions **620, 621**
— ← hypophysectomy **457**
— ← hypoxia **685**
— ← ionizing rays **684**
— ← norepinephrine **547**
— ← pancreatic hormones **529**
— ← pregnancy **666**
— ← sex **659**
— ← species **682**
— ← STH **433, 434**
— ← STH/mouse **433**
— ← stressors **700**
— ← temperature variations **687**
— theories **743**
— ← thymectomy **553**
— ← thyroid hormones **514**
— enzyme systems ← diet **592**
— extracts → resistance **564, 565**
— glycogen, theories **757**
— lesions **716, 722**; *cf. also* "Hepatic Lesions" as Agents
— ← ACTH **420, 421**
— ← adrenalectomy **354, 357**
— ← age **672**
— → allylformiate **604**
— → amino acids **602, 604**
— → ANIT (α-naphthylisothiocyanate) **604**
— → bacterial toxins **618, 619**
— → barbiturates **602, 605**
— → barbiturates/dog, mouse, rabbit **604, 605, 606**
— → bilirubin **607**
— → n-butylamine **607**
— → carcinogens **602, 607**
— → catecholamines **599, 601**
— → CCl₄ **602, 607**
— → chloral hydrate **607**
— → chloramphenicol **608**
— → cholesterol **608**
— → choline **602, 608**
— → cold **618, 619**
— → complex diets **615**
— ← corticoids **354, 355**
— → cyclophosphamide **608**
— → DHT **604, 613**
— → dietary constituents, individual **602**
— → diets, complex **615**
— → digitalis **602, 608**
— → DNA-polymerase **621**
— → drugs **602**
— → dyes **603, 609**
— → enzymes, hepatic **620**
— → ethyl-o-ethylphenylurea **609**
— ← folliculoids **354, 358**
— ← genetic factors **682**
— → glucuronidase **621**

Hepatic lesions ← gonadectomy 371
   → GOT 621
   → GPT 621
   → hepatic changes 615
   → hepatic enzymes 620, 621
   → hepatic regeneration 623
   → hepatic tissue 738
   → hexadimethrine 609
   → hormone-like substances 599
   → 5-HT 600, 601
   ← hypophysectomy 454
   → immune reactions 618, 620
   → indomethacin 609
   → insulin 599, 601
   ← ionizing rays 684
   → lathyrogens 603, 610
   → lead 610
   → lidocaine 610
   → mercury 603, 610
   → muscular performance 618, 619
   → nephrectomy 618
   → nicotine 610
   → nonsteroidal hormones 599
   → OKT 621
   → parathyroids 601
   → pentylenetetrazol 603, 610
   → peptone 610
   → pesticides 603, 612
   → phalloidin 612
   → phlogogens 612
   → phosphatase 621
   → pregnancy 619, 620
   ← pregnancy 666
   → renal lesions 619
   → RES-blockers 612
   → resistance 596
   ← sex 657
   → silica 612
   ← species 682
   ← steroids 354, 358
   → steroids 596
   ← STH 432, 433
   → strychnine 603, 612
   ← testoids 354, 358
   → tetrahydronaphthylamine 613
   → thrombin 621
   ← thymectomy 552
   ← thyroid hormones 502, 503
   → thyroid hormones 601
   → thyroxine 599
   → TKT 620
   → TPO 620
   → tribromoethanol 603, 613
   → tumors 618, 619
   → urethan 613
   → vasopressin 601
   → vitamin D 604, 613

Hepatic lesions → W-1372 613
  microsomal drug metabolism in man 707
    ← acetylsalicylic acid 709
    ← barbiturates 708, 712
    ← contraceptives 708, 710
    ← DDD; cf. "Cushing's Disease"
    ← diphenylhydantoin 708, 713
    ← glutethimide 709, 713
    ← griseofulvin 709, 713
    ← phenylbutazone 709, 713
    ← salicylates 713
    ← steroids 711
    ← thyroxine 714
  microsomal enzyme inducer, abortifacient action 722
  enzyme induction, history 30, 36
  microsomal enzymes Table 1 46
  chemistry 43
  microsomes ← starvation Table 3 81
  participation, theories 743
  regeneration ← anterior pituitary preparations 440
    ← ionizing rays 684
    ← renal lesions 623, 624
    ← tumors 704
  tissue ← adrenalectomy 725, 729
    ← anterior pituitary hormones 726, 735
    ← antitestoids 726, 734
    ← barbiturates 727, 736
    ← benzpyrene 739
    ← bile duct ligation 739
    ← catatoxic steroids 726, 734
    ← CCl_4 727, 737
    ← chlorazanil 727, 737
    ← chlorcyclizine 739
    ← chlordane 739
    ← clofibrate 727, 737
    ← corticoids 725, 728
    ← digitalis 737
    ← digitoxin 728
    ← drugs 727, 728, 736
    ← ethanol 737
    ← folliculoids 725, 729
    ← hepatic lesions 738
    ← hexachlorocyclohexane 739
    ← hormone-like substances 726, 735
    ← luteoids 726, 729
    ← methylcholanthrene 739
    ← metyrapone 728, 737
  monograph 739
  morphology 725
    ← nonsteroidal hormones 726, 735
    ← nikethamide 739
    ← phenobarbital 739
    ← phenylbutazone 738
    ← pancreatic hormones 727, 736
    ← pesticides 728, 737

Hepatic tissue, review 739
  ← salicylates 728, 738
  ← sex 739
  ← steroids 725, 726, 728, 735
  ← testoids 726, 734
  ← thyroid hormones 727, 736
  ← tumors 739
  vessel ligatures, methods 19, 21
Hepatitis, virus ← steroids 326, 327
Hepatocytes, SER in ← norbolethone *Fig. 33* 730
  SER in ← spironolactone *Fig. 34* 731
  ultrastructural changes ← PCN *Fig. 35* 732
Hepatotoxic substances 78
Hepatotoxins, history 35
Heptachlor; *cf. also* Pesticides
  ← phenobarbital *Diagram Table 139* 857; *Tables 98, 138* 283, 850
  ← steroids *Diagram Table 139* 857; *Tables 98, 138* 283, 850
  ← thyroxine *Diagram Table 139* 857; *Tables 98, 138* 283, 850
Heroin ← thymectomy 548
  ← thyroid hormones 483
Hexachlorobenzene (fungicide, skin irritant) ← sex 648
Hexachlorocyclohexane → hepatic tissue 739
Hexadimethrine (heparin neutralizer) ← ACTH 411
  ← hepatic lesions 609
  ← hypophysectomy 451
  ← pancreatic hormones 525
  ← steroids 248
Hexaethyl tetraphosphate ← sex 648
Hexamethonium; *cf. also* Ganglioplegics
  ← phenobarbital *Diagram Table 139* 857; *Tables 61, 138* 247, 850
  ← sex 648
  ← steroids *Diagram Table 139* 857; *Tables 60A, B, 61, 138* 246, 247, 850
  ← thyroxine *Diagram Table 139* 857; *Tables 61, 138* 247, 850
Hexobarbital; *cf. also* Barbiturates
  ← acetylsalicylic acid *Table 137* 848
  ← ACTH *Table 137* 848
  ← betamethasone *Table 128* 630
  ← bile duct ligature *Table 137* 848
  ← choledochus ligature *Table 126* 600
  ← cholesterol *Table 32* 197
  ← CS-1 *Table 9* 96
  ← CS-1, repeated doses *Table 7* 90, 91
  ← CS-1, single dose *Table 6* 88, 89
  ← digitoxin *Table 137* 848
  ← diphenylhydantoin *Table 137* 848
  ← diurnal variations 704
  ← estradiol *Tables 9, 30* 96, 195
  ← estradiol + orchidectomy *Table 30* 195

Hexobarbital ← ethylestrenol *Tables 9, 32, 128* 96, 197, 630
  ← genetic factors **675**
  ← indomethacin *Table 137* 848
  → metabolizing enzymes ← tumors **704**
  ← methyltestosterone *Table 30* 195
  ← methyltestosterone + orchidectomy *Table 30* 195
  ← nicotine *Table 137* 848
  ← norbolethone *Table 9* 96
  ← partial hepatectomy *Table 126* 600
  ← partial nephrectomy *Table 126* 600
  ← PCN *Tables 9, 30, 128* 96, 195, 630
  ← PCN + orchidectomy *Table 30* 195
  ← PCN, repeated doses *Table 7* 90, 91
  ← PCN, single dose *Table 6* 88, 89
  ← phenobarbital *Diagram Table 139* 857; *Tables 9, 32, 128, 137, 138* 96, 197, 630, 848, 850
  ← phenobarbital, repeated doses *Table 7* 90, 91
  ← phenobarbital, single dose *Table 6* 88, 89
  ← phentolamine *Table 137* 848
  ← phenylbutazone *Tables 128, 137* 630, 848
  ← phetharbital *Table 137* 848
  ← prednisolone, repeated doses *Table 7* 90, 91
  ← progesterone *Table 30* 195
  ← progesterone + orchidectomy *Table 30* 195
  ← renal lesions 623, 626
  ← sex 655
  ← salicylate *Table 137* 848
  ← spironolactone *Tables 9, 126, 128* 96, 600, 630
  ← spironolactone + choledochus ligature, partial hepatectomy, partial nephrectomy *Table 126* 600
  ← spironolactone, repeated doses *Table 7* 90, 91
  ← splenectomy 553
  ← starvation/mouse *Table 3* 81
  ← steroids *Diagram Table 139* 857; *Tables 32, 136, 138* 197, 836, 850
  ← STH *Table 137* 848
  ← stressors 697
  ← thyroxine *Diagram Table 139* 857; *Tables 32, 137, 138* 197, 848, 850
  ← tolbutamide *Table 137* 848
  ← vitamin A, C, D, E *Table 137* 848
  ← W-1372 *Table 137* 848
Hg; *cf.* Mercury
"Hilar pedicle" ligature, methods 22
Histamine → acetonitrile 555
  ← ACTH **405, 496**

Histamine → Bacillus pertussis vaccine 556
  → bacterial toxins 555, 556
  → barbiturates 555
  → botulinum toxin 556
  → chloral hydrate 555
  → cold 555, 556
  → drugs 555
  → electric stimuli 555, 556
  ← epinephrine 531, 532
  → hyperoxygenation 555, 556
  → ionizing rays 555, 556
  → lead 555
  → microorganisms 556
  → nereis toxin 556
  ← pancreatic hormones 521
  ← parathyroids 515
  → pentylenetetrazol 556
  ← posterior pituitary preparations 441
  → reserpine 556
  → resistance 555, 591
  ← sex 631
  ← steroids 145
  ← stressors 689
  ← sympathectomy 554
  ← thymectomy 547
  ← thyroid hormones 464, 466
  → vaccines 555, 556
Histoplasma capsulatum ← steroids 329, 330
History 24
  adaptation to hormones 34
  adrenals 26, 33
  antihormones 27
  catatoxic steroids 31, 40
  clinical implications 32, 41
  complete hepatectomy 35
  defensive enzymes 27
  hepatic microsomal enzyme induction 30, 36
  hepatotoxins 35
  hormones and resistance 33
  liver 28, 36
  partial hepatectomy 35
  sex differences 34
  smooth endoplasmic reticulum 40
    in hepatocytes 31
  syntoxic steroids 31, 40
  thyroid 26, 33
Holmium ← calcitonin 520
Homatropine hydrobromide (anticholinergic, mydriatic) ← steroids 249; *Diagram Table 139* 857; *Table 138* 850
  ← thyroxine *Diagram Table 139* 857; *Table 138* 850
"Homeostasis" 24
Homeostasis, theories 763
Hormonal defense system 26

Hormone-dependent cancers 716
  -like substances ← ACTH 405
    → bacterial toxins 563
    ← barbiturates 575
    → drugs 563
    ← epinephrine 531
    ← hepatic lesions 599
    → hepatic tissue 726, 735
    ← 5-HT 556, 558
    ← hypophysectomy 444, 445
    ← pancreatic hormones 521
    ← parathyroids 515
    ← posterior pituitary preparations 441
    ← pregnancy 660
    ← sex 631
    ← steroids 137
    → stress 563
    ← stress 688
    ← thymectomy 547
    ← thyroid hormones 462
  -producing neoplasms 716
Hormones, "activity spectrums" 15
  adaptive; *cf.* Adaptive Hormones
  and resistance, history 33
  ← anterior pituitary preparations 437
  → bile flow *Table 10* 99
  "catatoxic" 6
  nonsteroidal ← ACTH 405
    ← hypophysectomy 444, 445
    → resistance 405
    ← sex 631
    ← steroids 137
    ← thyroid hormones 463
  ← parathyroids 515
  ← posterior pituitary preparations 441
  prerequisites for the protective actions 770
  protective actions 770
  "syntoxic" 6
  ← thymectomy 547
5-HT ← ACTH 405, 406
  → anaphylactoidogenic agents 558
  → bacterial toxins 561
  → barbiturates 556, 559
  → barbiturates/man, mouse, rabbit 558
  → botulinum toxin 557
  → carcinogens 567
  → carcinolytics 559
  → CCl_4 557, 559
  → cholesterol 559
  → chloral hydrate 557, 559
  → chloroform 557, 559
  → cold 557, 563
  → curare 557, 559
  → DHT 557, 561
  → drugs 556, 558
  → electric stimuli 557, 563
  → ethanol 557, 559

5-HT→ ether 557, 560
- → halothane 557, 560
- → harmine 557, 560
- ← hepatic lesions 600, 601
- → hormone-like substances 556, 558
- → hyperoxygenation 557, 563
- ← hypophysectomy 444, 445
- → ionizing rays 557, 563
- → ionizing rays/mouse 562
- → lathyrogens 557, 560
- → lead 560
- → LSD 557, 560
- → mephenesin 557, 560
- → meprobamate 557, 560
- → mercury 560
- → methionine sulfoximine 558, 560
- → microorganisms 557, 561
- → morphine 557, 560
- → nitrogen mustard 557, 560
- → nonsteroidal hormones 556, 558
- ← pancreatic hormones 521
- → paraphenylenediamine 557, 560
- → pentylenetetrazol 557, 560
- → picrotoxin 557, 561
- → plasmocid 561
- ← posterior pituitary preparations 441
- ← pregnancy 660, 661
- → reserpine 557, 561
- → resistance 556, 591
- → sound 558, 563
- → steroids 558
- ← steroids 146
- ← stressors 689
- → stressors 557, 563
- → strychnine 557, 561
- ← thyroid hormones 464, 466
- → tremorine 561
- → tween 80 561
- → urethan 561
- → vitamin D 561

Hydrazine ← phenobarbital *Diagram Table 139* 857; *Table 138* 850
- → resistance 581
- ← steroids *Diagram Table 139* 857; *Table 138* 850
- ← thyroxine *Diagram Table 139* 857; *Table 138* 850

Hydroquinone (photographic reducer) ← phenobarbital *Diagram Table 139* 857; *Table 138* 850
- ← steroids 249; *Diagram Table 139* 857; *Tables 65, 138* 249, 850
- ← thyroid hormones 483
- ← thyroxine *Diagram Table 139* 857; *Tables 65, 138* 249, 850

Hydroxydione → AAN *Table 73* 257
- → acetanilide *Table 24* 176

Hydroxydione → acrylamide *Table 25* 176
- → acrylonitrile *Table 26* 177
- → adrenal weight *Table 140* 860
- → aminopyrine *Table 27* 179
- → barbital *Table 34* 198
- → barbiturates 196, 198
- → bishydroxycoumarin *Table 28* 182
- → body weight *Table 140* 860
- → cadmium *Table 35* 200
- → caramiphen *Table 36* 201
- → carisoprodol *Table 37* 216
- → chlordiazepoxide *Table 38* 217
- → cinchophen *Table 39* 221
- → cocaine *Table 40* 221
- → F-COL *Tables 12, 13, 14* 133, 134
- → colchicine *Table 41* 222
- → DL-coniine *Table 42* 222
- → croton oil *Table 43* 223
- → cyclobarbital *Table 33* 198
- → cycloheximide *Tables 44, 45* 224
- → cyclophosphamide *Table 46* 225
- → DHT *Table 117* 309
- → diisopropyl fluorophosphate *Table 52* 234
- → digitoxin *Tables 47, 48* 230
- → digitoxin/mouse *Table 130* 677
- → dioxathion *Tables 91, 132* 280, 680
- → diphenylhydantoin *Table 53* 235
- → dipicrylamine *Table 54* 235
- → DOC *Table 15* 135
- → emetine *Table 55* 238
- → endotoxin *Table 123* 348
- → epinephrine *Table 23* 144
- → EPN *Table 99* 284
- → estradiol *Table 16* 135
- → ethion *Table 92* 281
- → ethylene glycol *Table 56* 243
- → ethylmorphine *Table 57* 244
- → flufenamic acid *Table 58* 245
- → fluphenazine *Table 59* 245
- → glutethimide *Table 63* 248
- → glycerol *Table 64* 249
- → guthion *Table 93* 281
- → heptachlor *Table 98* 283
- → hexamethonium *Tables 60A, 61* 246, 247
- → hexobarbital *Table 32* 197
- → hydroquinone *Table 65* 249
- → imipramine *Table 66* 250
- → indomethacin *Table 67* 250
- → indomethacin/mouse *Table 131* 678
- → kidney, weight *Table 140* 860
- → liver, weight *Table 140* 860
- → LSD *Table 74* 258
- → mechlorethamine *Table 75* 260
- → mephenesin *Table 76* 260
- → meprobamate *Table 77* 261
- → mercury *Table 78* 267
- → mersalyl *Tables 79, 80* 268

Hydroxydione → methadone *Table 82* 269
  → methylaniline *Table 83* 270
  → methyprylon *Table 84* 270
  ← metyrapone *Table 125* 584
  → $NaClO_4$ *Table 90* 278
  → α-naphthylisothiocyanate *Table 85* 273
  → nicotine *Table 86* 274
  → nikethamide *Table 87* 274
  → p-nitroanisole *Table 88* 275
  → OMPA *Table 94* 282
  → ovary, weight *Table 140* 860
  → pancuronium *Table 19* 136
  → parathion *Table 95* 282
  → pentobarbital/mouse *Table 129* 677
  → pentylenetetrazol *Table 89* 277
  → phenindione *Table 29* 183
  → phenyramidol *Table 100* 284
  → physostigmine *Table 101* 285
  → picrotoxin *Table 102* 286
  → piperidine *Table 103* 287
  → pralidoxime *Table 104* 288
  → preputial glands, weight *Table 140* 860
  → propionitrile *Table 105* 289
  → propylthiouracil *Tables 21, 22* 140, 141
  ← SKF 525-A 62
  → strychnine *Table 107* 292
  → T3 *Table 20* 140
  → TEA *Tables 60A, 62* 246, 248
  → theobromine *Table 108* 293
  → theophylline *Table 109* 293
  → thimerosal *Table 110* 294
  → thiopental *Table 31* 197
  → thymus, weight *Table 140* 860
  → thyroid, weight *Table 140* 860
  → triamcinolone *Table 18* 136
  → β-tribromoethanol *Table 111* 295
  → β-trichloroethanol *Table 112* 295
  → tri-o-cresyl phosphate *Table 113* 296
  → D-tubocuranine *Table 114* 296
  → tyramine *Table 115* 297
  → tyrosine *Table 116* 299
  → uterus, weight *Table 140* 860
  → W-1372 *Table 118* 309
  → zoxazolamine *Table 119* 313
Hydroxylation reactions 44
N-(p-Hydroxyphenyl)glycine ← thyroid hormones 483
11-α-Hydroxyprogesterone, anti-inflammatory activity *Table 122* 345
  → endotoxin *Table 122* 345
Hydroxyproline ← CCl_4 79
Hymenolepis nana ← steroids 330, 332
Hyperbilirubinemia; *cf. also* Bilirubin *under* Drugs
  ← barbiturates 714, 717
  ← DDD 719
  ← DDT 714, 719

Hyperbilirubinemia ← light 720
  ← milk 715
  ← pregnancy 720
  ← steroids 715, 719
  ← thyroid 715, 720
Hyperoxygenation ← ACTH 421, 422
  ← adrenalectomy 371
  ← corticoids/guinea pig, man, mouse 370, 371
  ← epinephrine 545, 546
  ← folliculoids 371, 372
  ← gonadectomy 371, 372
  ← histamine 555, 556
  ← 5-HT 557, 563
  ← hypophysectomy 456
  ← pancreatic hormones 529
  ← posterior pituitary preparations 441, 443
  ← steroids 370
  ← stressors 700
  ← testoids 371, 372
  ← thyroid hormones 508
  ← thyroid hormones/cat 508
"Hypoexcretory states" 624
Hypophyseal hormones ← stressors 689
  ← thyroid hormones 464
Hypophysectomy → acrylonitrile 447
  → amino acid enzymes 460
  → atropine 447
  → bacterial toxins 453
  → barbiturates 445, 447
  → benactyzine 448
  → cadmium 448
  → carcinogens 446, 448
  → CCl_4 446, 448
  → cerium 450
  → cobra venom 453
  → cold 456
  → cycloheximide 450
  → DHT 446, 452
  → digitalis 450
  → diphenhydramine 450
  → diphenylhydantoin 450
  → drugs 445
  → electric stimuli 456
  → endotoxin 453
  → enzymes, amino acid 460
  → ephedrine 450
  → ergot 450
  → EST 456
  → GOT 459
  → GPT 459
  → hepatic enzymes 457
  → hepatic lesions 454
  → hexadimethrine 451
  → hormone-like substances 444, 445
  → hormones, nonsteroidal 444, 445

Hypophysectomy → 5-HT **444, 445**
 → hyperoxygenation **456**
 → immune reactions **454**
 → indomethacin **451**
 → ionizing rays **455, 456**
 → lathyrogens **446, 451**
 → magnesium **451**
 → meprobamate **451**
 → mercury **446, 451**
 → microorganisms **453**
 → morphine **451**
 → nonsteroidal hormones **444, 445**
 → oxygen tension **456**
 → ozone **451**
 → parathyroid extract **444**
 → parathyroid hormone **445**
 → partial hepatectomy **454**
 → partial nephrectomy **454**
 → pesticides **446, 452**
 → phenaglycodol **452**
 → phenyltoloxamine **452**
 → phosphates **446, 452**
 → puromycin aminonucleoside **446, 452**
 → renal lesions **454, 455**
 → reserpine **452**
 → resistance **443**
 → steroids **444**
 → stressors **455**
 → temperature variations **456**
 → TKT **457**
 → TPO **457**
 → tuberculosis **453**
 → tumors **457**
 → tumor transplants **456**
 → venoms **453, 454**
 → vitamin A **446, 452**
 → vitamin D **452**
 → zoxazolamine **447, 453**
Hypothalamic lesions → resistance **443**
Hypoxia ← ACTH **421, 422**
 ← adrenalectomy **371**
 ← anterior pituitary preparations **437, 440**
 → bacteria **685**
 → barbiturates **685**
 ← corticoids/guinea pig, man, mouse **370, 371**
 ← epinephrine **545, 546**
 ← folliculoids **371, 372**
 ← gonadectomy **372**
 → hepatic enzymes **685**
 → ionizing rays **685**
 ← pancreatic hormones **528, 529**
 ← posterior pituitary preparations **443**
 → resistance **685**
 ← sex **658**
 ← steroids **370**
 ← stressors **700**

Hypoxia ← testoids **371, 372**
 ← thyroid hormones/cat, dog, fish, guinea pig, mouse, rabbit **506**

Identification of damaging agents amenable to prophylaxis **847**
Imipramine (antidepressant) ← phenobarbital *Diagram Table 139* **857**; *Tables 66, 138* **250, 850**
 ← steroids **249**; *Diagram Table 139* **857**; *Tables 66, 138* **250, 850**
 ← thyroid hormones **468, 483**
 ← thyroxine *Diagram Table 139* **857**; *Tables 66, 138* **250, 850**
Immune reactions **13**
 ← ACTH/guinea pig, rabbit **419, 420**
 ← adrenalectomy **351, 353**
 ← corticoids/dog, guinea pig, mouse, rabbit **349, 350, 351**
 ← epinephrine **543**
 ← folliculoids **351, 353**
 ← gonadectomy **351, 353**
 ← hepatic lesions **618, 620**
 ← hypophysectomy **454**
 ← luteoids **351, 353**
 ← norepinephrine **543**
 ← pancreatic hormones **528**
 ← parathyroids **519**
 → resistance **596**
 ← sex **618**
 ← steroids **325, 349**
 ← STH **432, 433**
 ← stressors **700**
 ← temperature variations **687**
 ← testoids **351, 353**
 ← thymectomy **551**
 ← thyroid hormones **500**
Index, protective **771**
Indium **520**
 ← parathyroids **516, 517**
 ← phenobarbital *Diagram Table 139* **857**
 ← steroids **249**; *Diagram Table 139* **857**; *Table 138* **850**
 ← thyroxine *Diagram Table 139* **857**; *Table 138* **850**
Indocyanine green ← SKF 525-A **63**
Indomethacin (antiphlogistic) ← acetylsalicylic acid *Table 137* **848**
 ← ACTH *Table 137* **848**
 ← age **667, 671**
 ← betamethasone *Table 128* **630**
 ← bile duct ligature *Table 137* **848**
 ← choledochus ligature *Table 126* **600**
 → F-COL *Table 137* **848**
 ← CS-1, single dose *Table 6* **88, 89**
 → DHT *Table 137* **848**
 ← diet **592, 593**

Indomethacin → digitoxin *Table 137* 848
  ← digitoxin *Table 137* 848
  → dioxathion *Table 137* 848
  ← diphenylhydantoin *Table 137* 848
  ← ethylstrenol *Table 128* 630
  ← hepatic lesions 609
  → hexobarbital *Table 137* 848
  ← hypophysectomy 451
  ← indomethacin *Table 137* 848
  ← metyrapone + spironolactone *Table 51* 232
  ← nicotine *Table 137* 848
  → nicotine *Table 137* 848
  → parathion *Table 137* 848
  ← partial hepatectomy *Table 126* 600
  ← partial nephrectomy *Table 126* 600
  ← PCN *Table 128* 630
  ← PCN + age *Table 72* 254
  ← PCN, single dose *Table 6* 88, 89
  ← phenobarbital *Diagram Table 139* 857; *Tables 67, 128, 137, 138* 250, 630, 848, 850
  ← phenobarbital, single dose *Table 6* 88, 89
  ← phentolamine *Table 137* 848
  ← phenylbutazone *Tables 128, 137* 630 848
  ← phetharbital *Table 137* 848—849
  ← prednisolone *Table 141* 862
  ← progesterone *Table 137* 848
  protection against 772
  → pyloric ulcer/rabbit *Fig. 28* 679
  ← renal lesions 626
  → resistance 582
  ← sex 648
  ← salicylate *Table 137* 848
  ← species 675, 679
  ← spironolactone *Fig. 8* 251; *Tables 70, 71, 126, 128* 253, 254, 600, 630
  ← spironolactone + adrenalectomy *Tables 68, 69, 70, 71* 252, 253, 254
  ← spironolactone + adrenalectomy + corticoids *Tables 68, 69, 70, 71* 252, 253, 254
  ← spironolactone + choledochus ligature, partial hepatectomy, partial nephrectomy *Table 126* 600
  ← steroids 159, 250, 793; *Diagram Table 139* 857; *Tables 67, 135, 135B, 136, 138* 250, 779, 807, 836, 850
  ← steroids (inactive) *Table 135A* 794
  ← steroids/mouse 160; *Table 131* 678
  ← STH *Table 137* 848
  ← stressors 694
  ← thyroid hormones 468, 484
  ← thyroxine *Diagram Table 139* 857; *Tables 67, 137, 138* 250, 848, 850
  ← thyroxine/mouse *Table 131* 678

Indomethacin ← tolbutamide *Table 137* 848
  toxicants 108, 110
  ← triamcinolone *Table 141* 862
  → ulcers, intestinal ← spironolactone *Fig. 8* 251
  ← vitamin A, C, D, E, *Table 137* 848
  ← W-1372 *Table 137* 848
  → zoxazolamine *Table 137* 848
Inducers, interactions 56
  primary 73, 75, 388
  reversal of actions 83, 87
  secondary 73, 75, 388
Infections ← posterior pituitary preparations 441
  ← steroids 325
Influenza ← ACTH 415
  ← steroids 326, 328
  ← STH 430
Inhibition, competitive, classification 14
Inhibitors of enzymes 57
  of enzymes, classification 57
Insulin ← ACTH 405, 406
  ← actinomycin 75
  → bile flow/dog *Table 10* 99
  ← hepatic lesions 599, 601
  ← pancreatic hormones 522
  ← parathyroids 515
  ← sex 630
Interactions between inducers 56
Intersecting dose effect curves, law of 111, 112
Interventions, surgical ← thyroid hormones 502
Iodides ← thyroid hormones 484
Iodine → resistance 569, 582
Iodoacetate ← steroids 254
Ionizing rays ← ACTH 421, 422
  ← actinomycin 75
  ← adrenalectomy 362, 365
  ← anterior pituitary preparations 440
  → barbiturates 683
  → carcinogens 683
  ← corticoids/guinea pig, man, mouse, rabbit 362, 363, 364
  → drugs 682
  → endotoxin 684
  → enzymes 684
  ← epinephrine 543
  ← epinephrine/mouse 543
  ← folliculoids 362, 367
  ← folliculoids/mouse 362, 366
  ← gonadectomy 362, 367
  → hepatic lesions 684
  → hepatic regeneration 684
  ← histamine 556
  ← 5-HT 557, 563
  ← 5-HT/mouse 562
  ← hypophysectomy 455, 456

Ionizing rays ← hypoxia 685
  ← luteoids 362, 365
  → microorganisms 684
  ← norepinephrine 543
  ← norepinephrine/mouse 543
  ← pancreatic hormones 528, 529
  ← parathyroids 520
  → pesticides 683
  ← posterior pituitary preparations 441, 443
  ← pregnancy 666
  → resistance 682
  ← sex 657
  ← splenectomy 553, 554
  ← steroids 361, 368
  ← steroids, reviews 368
  ← STH 432, 434
  ← stressors 698, 700
  ← testoids/mouse, rabbit 362, 364, 365
  ← thymectomy 552
  ← thyroid hormones/fish, goldfish, mouse, rabbit, toad 504, 505, 506
  → TKT 684
  → TPO 684
Iproniazid (MAO inhibitor, antidepressant, tuberculostatic) 68; cf. also Inhibitors under General Pharmocology, MAO-Inhibitors
  → resistance 569
  ← thyroid hormones 484
Isocarboxazid 68; cf. MAO-Inhibitors
Isoniazid (antituberculous agent, CNS stimulator) ← ACTH 412
  ← steroids 254
  ← thyroid hormones 484
Isoproterenol (sympathomimetic bronchodilator) ← ACTH 412
  → resistance 582
  ← sex 648
  ← steroids 160, 255
  ← stressors 694
  ← thyroid hormones 484

Japanese encephalomyelitis ← steroids 325
JB 516 66

K; cf. Potassium
Kallikrein → resistance 563
Kidney, extrahepatic conditioning 100, 102
  weight ← phenobarbital Table 140 860
    ← steroids Table 140 860
    ← thyroxine Table 140 860
Klebsiella pneumoniae ← steroids 320
  ← thyroid hormones 497
KMnO$_4$; cf. Permanganate

Lactate dehydrogenase virus ← thymectomy 551

Lactation 863
Lactone → resistance 582
Lasiocarpine; cf. Plant Extracts
Lathyrism; cf. Lathyrogens
Lathyrogens ← ACTH 407, 412
  ← anterior pituitary preparations 436, 439
  ← corticoids 255
  ← ethylestrenol Fig. 9 256
  ← folliculoids 255
  ← hepatic lesions 603, 610
  ← 5-HT 557, 560
  ← hypophysectomy 446, 451
  ← norepinephrine 538
  ← pancreatic hormones 525
  ← prednisolone Fig. 9 256
  ← pregnancy 661, 663
  ← sex 634, 648
  ← steroids 160, 255
  ← steroids/chicken, mouse 258
  ← STH 426, 427
  ← testoids 255
  ← thyroid hormones 468, 484
  ← thyroid hormones/duck 484
  ← thyroxine Fig. 9 256
"Law of intersecting dose-effect curves" 111, 112
Lead ← calcitonin 520
  ← epinephrine 538
  ← hepatic lesions 610
  ← histamine 555
  ← 5-HT 560
  ← steroids 258
  ← thyroid hormones 485
Length of pretreatment necessary for conditioning 82, 85
Leptospira ← ACTH 415, 416
  ← steroids 317, 320
Li; cf. Lithium
Lidocaine ← barbiturates 577
  ← hepatic lesions 610
  ← sex 648
Ligature of hepatic vessels, methods 19, 21
Light → hyperbilirubinemia 720
Lilly 18947 65
Lipid solubility 769
Lipids ← stressors 694
Literature, collection of VII
Lithium ← sex 648
  ← steroids 258
Liver, fractions 36
  history 28
  perfusion 31, 40
    methods 18, 19
    regeneration 20, 21
  slices 36
    methods 22

Liver ← W-1372 *Figs. 18, 19* 310, 311
  ← W-1372 + PCN *Figs. 18, 19* 310, 311
  ← W-1372 + phenobarbital *Fig. 19* 311
  ← W-1372 + progesterone *Fig. 18* 310
  weight ← phenobarbital *Table 140* 860
    ← steroids *Table 140* 860
    ← thyroxine *Table 140* 860
Local trauma ← corticoids 381
  ← steroids 381
"Long-sleepers" 675
LSD (psychomimetic agent) ← 5-HT 557, 560
  ← phenobarbital *Diagram Table 139* 857; *Tables 74, 138* 258, 850
  ← steroids 161, 258; *Diagram Table 139* 857; *Tables 74, 138* 258, 850
  ← thyroxine *Diagram Table 139* 857; *Tables 74, 138*, 258, 850
Lung, extrahepatic conditioning 102
Luteoids 9
  ← anabolic steroids 114, 118
  → bacterial toxins 336, 346
  → barbiturates 150, 189
  → carcinogens 207
  → electric stimuli 375, 376
  → enzymes 402
  → epinephrine 144
  → hepatic tissue 726, 729
  → immune reactions 351, 353
  → ionizing rays 362, 365
  → norepinephrine 144
  → renal lesions 359, 361
  → steroids 120, 121
  → systemic trauma 378, 381
  ← testoids 114, 118
Lymphocytic choriomeningitis ← thymectomy 549, 550
Lynestrenol 80
  ← SKF 525-A 62
Lysosomal hydrolases ← stressors 699, 702
Lysosomes, theories 753

MAD ← ACTH 405
Magnesium ← hypophysectomy 451
  ← parathyroids 516, 517
  ← sex 648
  ← steroids 161, 259
  ← stressors 694
  ← temperature variations 687
  ← thyroid hormones 468, 485
Malaria (P. berghei) → resistance 595
Malathion ← steroids 165
Male-hormone-like; *cf.* Testoids
Malonic acid derivatives; *cf.* Sch 5712, Sch 5705
Man 139, 157, 173, 185, 235, 240, 335, 344, 362, 364, 370, 371, 372, 377, 380, 416, 419, 536, 558, 630; *cf. also* Clinical Implications, Genetic and Species-Dependent Factors

MAO, chemistry 45
  -inhibitors 68
    ← sex 648
    ← steroids 259
"Mean overall protective index" 771
Measles ← steroids 328
Mecamylamine; *cf.* Ganglioplegics
Mechanism of drug oxidation, *Graph* 49
Mechlorethamine (war gas) ← phenobarbital *Diagram Table 139* 857; *Tables 75, 138* 260, 850
  ← steroids 259; *Diagram Table 139* 857; *Tables 75, 138* 260, 850
  ← thyroxine *Diagram Table 139* 857; *Tables 75, 138* 260, 850
"Membrane systems" 48
Methionine sulfoximine ← 5-HT 560
Mepacrine ← sex 649
Meperidine (narcotic, analgesic) ← age 671
  ← norepinephrine 538
  ← pregnancy 661, 663
  ← SKF 525-A 60
  ← steroids 259
  ← thyroid hormones 486
Mephenesin (muscle relaxant) ← 5-HT 557, 560
  ← phenobarbital *Diagram Table 139* 857; *Tables 76, 138* 260, 850
  ← SKF 525-A 61
  ← steroids 161, 260; *Diagram Table 139* 857; *Tables 76, 138* 260, 850
  ← thyroxine *Diagram Table 139* 857; *Tables 76, 138* 260, 850
Meprobamate (tranquilizer) ← ACTH 412
  ← 5-HT 557, 560
  ← hypophysectomy 451
  ← norepinephrine 538
  ← phenobarbital *Diagram Table 139* 857; *Tables 77, 138* 261, 850
  → resistance 591
  ← SKF 525-A 62
  ← steroids 161, 260; *Diagram Table 139* 857; *Tables 77, 138* 261, 850
  ← stressors 697
  ← thyroid hormones 468, 486
  ← thyroxine *Diagram Table 139* 857; *Tables 77, 138* 261, 850
MER-25 (antifolliculoid) ← steroids 261
6-Mercaptopurine 81, 82
  ← enzymes, normal *Table 134* 759
Mercapturic acid formation 47
Mercury ← ACTH 412
  ← calcitonin 520
  ← choledochus ligature *Fig. 23* 611
  ← emdabol 162
  ← glucocorticoids 162; *Table 81* 269
  ← hepatic lesion 603, 610

Mercury ← 5-HT 560
  ← hypophysectomy **446**, 451
  ← nephrectomy, partial *Table 127* 624
  → nephrocalcinosis ← choledochus ligature *Fig. 23* 611
  → nephrocalcinosis ← spironolactone *Figs. 11, 12* 263—266
  → nephrocalcinosis ← ureter ligature, temporary *Fig. 26* 625
  ← pancreatic hormones 526
  ← phenobarbital *Diagram Table 139* 857; *Tables 78, 138* 267, 850
  ← renal lesions **623**, 624
  ← sex 649
  ← spironolactone **162**; *Figs. 11, 12* 263, 266
  ← spiroxasone **162**
  ← steroids **162**; *Diagram Table 139* 857; *Tables 78, 81, 138* 267, 269, 850
  ← testoids **162**, 261
  ← thyroxine *Diagram Table 139* 857; *Tables 78, 138* 267, 850
  toxicants **108**, 110
  ← ureter ligature, temporary *Fig. 26* 625; *Table 127* 624
  ← ureter ligature, temporary + partial nephrectomy *Table 127* 624
Mersalyl ← ethylestrenol *Fig. 10* 262
  → nephrocalcinosis ← ethylestrenol *Fig. 10* 262
  ← phenobarbital *Diagram Table 139* 857; *Tables 79, 80, 138* 268, 850
  ← steroids *Diagram Table 139* 857; *Tables 79, 80, 138* 268, 850
  ← thyroxine *Diagram Table 139* 857; *Tables 79, 80, 138* 268, 850
Mescaline ← epinephrine **533**, 538
Mestranol 80
  → OMPA *Table 97* 283
  → resistance 591
  ← SKF 525-A 62
Methadone (narcotic, analgesic) ← phenobarbital *Diagram Table 139* 857; *Tables 82, 138* 269, 850
  ← SKF 525-A 60
  ← steroids 268; *Diagram Table 139* 857; *Tables 82, 138* 269, 850
  ← thyroid hormones 486
  ← thyroxine *Diagram Table 139* 857; *Tables 82, 138* 269, 850
Methandrostenolone 80
Methanol ← norepinephrine 538
  ← steroids 269
Methionine; *cf. also* Choline, Diet (choline)
  adenosyl transferase ← pancreatic hormones 531
  ← corticoids 390

Methionine sulfoximine ← 5-HT **558**
Methods **5**, 17
  "abrasive ablation" 20
  Asher's (for thyroid hormone determination) 506
  bile-duct ligatures **19**, 21
  bile fistulas **19**, 21
  chemical **18**, 19
  complete hepatectomy **18**, 20
  Eck fistula **19**
  hepatic denervation **19**, 22
  "hilar pedicle" ligature 22
  ligature of hepatic vessels **19**, 21
  liver slices 22
  partial hepatectomy **15**, 18, 19, 20
  perfusion of the liver **19**, 22
  renal interventions **19**, 23
  surgical **18**, 19
Methorphinan ← SKF 525-A 60
Methotrexate; *cf.* Carcinolytic Agents
Methoxamine → resistance 591
Methoxyflurane (anesthetic) ← epinephrine 538
  → resistance 582
Methyl alcohol; *cf.* Methanol
Methylandrostenediol; *cf. also* Testoids
  → digitoxin ← spironolactone *Table 49* 231
Methylaniline ← phenobarbital *Diagram Table 139* 857; *Tables 38, 138* 270, 850
  ← sex 655
  ← SKF 525-A 61
  ← steroids 269; *Diagram Table 139* 857; *Tables 83, 138* 270, 850
  ← thyroxine *Diagram Table 139* 857; *Tables 83, 138* 270, 850
Methylation, N-, O-, S- **47**
Methylcholanthrene → hepatic tissue 739
  → resistance 591
Methyleneaminoacetonitrile; *cf.* MAAN
Methylenedioxyphenyl compounds **81**, 82
  → resistance 582
17α-Methyl-17β-hydroxy-4-aza-estran-3-one
  → barbiturates 196
3-Methyl-4-monomethyl-aminoazobenzene
  ← SKF 525-A 61
Methylparafynol ← SKF 525-A 60
Methylphenidate (CNS stimulant, antidepressant) ← phenobarbital *Diagram Table 139* 857; *Table 138* 850
  ← steroids 269; *Diagram Table 139* 857; *Table 138* 850
  ← thyroid hormones 486
  ← thyroxine *Diagram Table 139* 857; *Table 138* 850
6-Methylprednisolone; *cf.* Corticoids
6-α-Methylprednisone, anti-inflammatory activity *Table 122* 345
  → endotoxin *Table 122* 345

α-Methyl-p-tyrosine ← thyroid hormones 486
Methylsalicylate ← phenobarbital *Diagram Table 139* 857; *Table 138* 850
 ← steroids *Diagram Table 139* 857; *Table 138* 850
 ← thyroxine *Diagram Table 139* 857; *Table 138* 850
Methyltestosterone; *cf. also* Testoids
 → DHT *Fig. 16* 305, 306
 → digitoxin ← spironolactone *Table 49* 231
 → hexobarbital *Table 30* 195
 → hexobarbital ← orchidectomy *Table 30* 195
Methyltropolone ← epinephrine 538
α-Methyltyrosine ← stressors 694
Methyprylon (sedative, hypnotic) ← phenobarbital *Diagram Table 139* 857; *Tables 84, 138* 270, 850
 ← species 679
 ← steroids 162, 270; *Diagram Table 139* 857; *Tables 84, 138* 270, 850
 ← thyroxine *Diagram Table 139* 857; *Table 84, 138* 270, 850
Metrazol; *cf.* Pentylenetetrazol
Metyrapone (inhibitor of corticoid biosynthesis) 81
 → digitoxin ← spironolactone *Table 51* 232
 → DOC *Table 125* 584
 → endotoxin ← cortisol *Table 121* 345
 ← ethionine 79
 → indomethacin ← spironolactone *Table 51* 232
 → progesterone *Table 125* 584
 → resistance 569, 582
 reversal of antagonist actions 84
 ← steroids 270
 → hepatic tissue 728, 737
 → hydroxydione *Table 125* 584
Mg; *cf.* Magnesium
Microorganisms ← ACTH 415
 ← anterior pituitary preparations 436, 439
 ← epinephrine 541
 ← histamine 556
 ← 5-HT 557, 561
 ← hypophysectomy 435
 ← ionizing rays 684
 ← norepinephrine 541
 ← pancreatic hormones 527
 ← pregnancy 665, 666
 → resistance 595
 ← sex 656
 ← splenectomy 553
 ← STH 430
 ← stressors 698, 699
 ← steroids 315
 ← thymectomy 549
 ← thyroid hormones 496

Microsomal drug metabolism in man; *cf.* Hepatic Microsomal Drug Metabolism in Man
 enzyme induction, history 30
 enzymes, chemistry 43
 hepatic *Table 1* 46
 theories 746
Microsomes, hepatic ← starvation *Table 3* 81
 theories 747
"Milieu intérieur" 24, 25, 33
Milk, extrahepatic conditioning 103
 → hyperbilirubinemia 715
Mineralocorticoid hypertension 716
Mineralocorticoids 9
 ← anabolic steroids 114, 118
 → barbiturates 150, 185
 → DHT 173
 ← pregnancy 660
 → steroids 113
 → STH 137
 ← testoids 114, 118
 → vitamin D 303
Minipig 544
Mitomycin (antineoplastic, antibiotic) ← steroids 270
Moloney virus ← splenectomy 553
 ← thymectomy 551
Monkey 333, 339, 369, 370
Monoamine oxidase, *cf.* MAO
Monobutyl-4-aminoantipyrine ← SKF 525-A 61
Monocrotaline (toxic principle of C. spectabilis)
 ← sex 649
 ← steroids 162, 271
Monograph, hepatic tissue 793
Monomethyl-4-aminoantipyrine ← SKF 525-A 60, 61
Morestan ← steroids 165
Morphine (narcotic, analgesic); *cf. also* Ethylmorphine
 ← ACTH 407, 412
 ← anterior pituitary preparations 439
 ← epinephrine 538
 ← genetic factors 680
 ← 5-HT 557, 560
 ← hypophysectomy 451
 ← norepinephrine 538
 ← pancreatic hormones 526
 ← phenobarbital *Diagram Table 139* 857; *Table 138* 850
 ← posterior pituitary preparations 442
 ← pregnancy 663
 ← sex 649
 ← SKF 525-A 60
 ← steroids 163, 271; *Diagram Table 139* 857; *Table 138* 850
 ← stressors 694
 ← thymectomy 548, 549

Morphine ← thyroid hormones 468, 486
  ← thyroxine *Diagram Table 139* 857;
    Table 138 850
Morphology 725
  endocrine glands 740
  extrahepatic tissues 740
  hepatic tissue 725
  multiple hemorrhages 740
  myocardial necroses 740
  tissues 740
  uterus 740
Mouse 155, 158, 160, 164, 167, 172, 173, 184, 189, 193, 195, 203, 233, 240, 258, 321, **333**, 340, **350**, **361**, **362**, 363, 364, 366, **370**, 371, **372**, **374**, 375, 380, 389, 415, 418, **422**, **433**, 470, 472, 498, **504**, 505, 507, **509**, 511, **512**, 534, **543**, 558, 562, 605, **627**, 629, 635; *Tables 3, 129, 133* 81, 677, 678, 680
MPDC 66
  reversal of antagonist actions 84
Mucormycosis ← pancreatic hormones 527
Mumps ← steroids 328
Murine bone explants 171
Muscle, extrahepatic conditioning 103
Muscular dystrophy ← steroids **382**, 383
  performance ← ACTH **422**, 423
    ← hepatic lesions 618, 619
    ← sex **657**
    ← thyroid hormones **512**, 513
Mushrooms ← steroids 349
Mustard gas (war gas, vesicant) ← steroids 272
  powder ← ACTH 413
    ← steroids 272
Mycobacterium lepraemurium ← steroids **317**, 320
  paratuberculosis (johnei) ← steroids **317**, 321
  tuberculosis ← ACTH 415, 416
    ← pancreatic hormones 527
    ← steroids/guinea pig, mouse, rabbit **317**, 321, 322
    ← STH 431
    ← thyroid hormones/guinea pig, mouse, rabbit 497, 498
Mycoplasma ← steroids 322
  ← thyroid hormones 498
Myocardial necroses, morphology 740
Myoneural blockers 55
"Myotrophic" activity of testoid anabolics **313**

Na; *cf.* Sodium
NaClO$_4$ ← phenobarbital *Diagram Table 139* 857; *Tables 90, 138* 278, 850
  ← steroids *Diagram Table 139* 857; *Tables 90, 138* 278, 850
  ← thyroxine *Diagram Table 139* 857

NADPH cytochrome c reductase, chemistry 50
NADPH-linked electron transport ← pancreatic hormones 530
Naphthalene (intestinal antiseptic) ← steroids 272
α-Naphthylisothiocyanate (causes fever and kidney damage); *cf. also* Bilirubin
  ← hepatic lesions 604
  ← phenobarbital *Diagram Table 139* 857; *Table 85, 138* 273, 850
  ← steroids 273; *Diagram Table 139* 857; *Tables 85, 138* 273, 850
  ← thyroxine *Diagram Table 139* 857; *Tables 85, 138* 273, 850
1-1-Naphthyl-2-thiourea (ANTU); *cf.* Thioureas
Narcotics ← SKF 525-A 61
"Natural" vs. "foreign" compounds, theories 758
Navadel; *cf.* Dioxathion *under* Pesticides
Neisseria gonorrhoeae ← steroids 322
Nembutal; *cf.* Pentobarbital *under* Barbiturates
Neoplasms, hormone-producing 716
Neoprontosil ← sex 655
  ← starvation/mouse *Table 3* 81
Neostigmine ← phenobarbital *Diagram Table 139* 857; *Table 138* 850
  ← steroids *Diagram Table 139* 857; *Table 138* 850
  ← thyroid hormones 487
  ← thyroxine *Diagram Table 139* 857; *Table 138* 850
Neotetrazolium ← sex 655
Nephrectomy; *cf. also* Renal Lesions
  ← hepatic lesions 618
  partial; *cf.* Partial Nephrectomy
  ← phenobarbital *Diagram Table 139* 857
  ← pregnancy **665**
  ← steroids *Diagram Table 139* 857; *Table 138* 850
  ← thyroxine *Diagram Table 139* 857; *Table 138* 850
Nephrocalcinosis ← F-COL + spironolactone *Fig. 1* 123
  ← mercury + choledochus ligature *Fig. 23* 611
  ← mercury + ureter ligature, temporary *Fig. 26* 625
  ← mersalyl + ethylestrenol *Fig. 10* 262
  ← spironolactone + mercury *Figs. 11, 12* 263—266
Nereis toxin ← histamine 556
Nervous lesions → resistance 704, 705
"Neurocalcergy" **555**
Nialamide **68**; *cf.* MAO-Inhibitors

Nickel carbonyl 81, 82
  sulfide ← sex 650
    ← steroids 273
Nicotinamide; cf. Vitamin B
Nicotine (agricultural insecticide) ← acetylsalicylic acid Table 137 848
  ← ACTH Table 137 848
  ← barbiturates 577
  ← betamethasone Table 128 630
  → bile duct ligature Table 137 848
  → F-COL Table 137 848
  ← CS-1, single dose Table 6 88, 89
  → DHT Table 137 848
  ← digitoxin Table 137 848
  → digitoxin Table 137 848
  → dioxathion Table 137 848
  ← diphenylhydantoin Table 137 848
  ← epinephrine 539
  ← ethylestrenol Table 128 630
  ← hepatic lesions 610
  ← hexobarbital Table 137 848
  → indomethacin Table 137 848
  ← indomethacin Table 137 848
  ← nicotine Table 137 848
  → parathion Table 137 848
  ← PCN Table 128 630
  ← PCN, single dose Table 6 88, 89
  ← phenobarbital Diagram Table 139 857; Tables 86, 128, 137, 138 274, 630, 848, 850
  ← phenobarbital, single dose Table 6 88, 89
  ← phentolamine Table 137 848
  ← phenylbutazone Table 128, 137 630, 848
  ← phetharbital Table 137 848
  → progesterone Table 137 848
  → resistance 584
  ← sex 634, 650, 655
  ← salicylate Table 137 848
  ← spironolactone Table 128 630
  ← steroids 163, 273; Diagram Table 139 857; Tables 86, 136, 138 274, 836, 850
  ← STH Table 137 848
  ← stressors 694
  ← thyroid hormones 487
  ← thyroxine Diagram Table 139 857; Tables 86, 136, 138 274, 848, 850
  → tolbutamide Table 137 848
  toxicants 108, 110
  ← vitamin A, C, D, E Table 137 848
  ← W-1372 Table 137 848
  → zoxazolamine Table 137 848
Nicotinic acid (vasodilator, antipellagra factor)
  ← steroids 274
Nikethamide (diethylamide of nicotinic acid)
  ← phenobarbital Diagram Table 139 857; Tables 87, 138 274, 850
  → hepatic tissue 739

Nikethamide → resistance 584, 591
  ← SKF 525-A 62
  ← steroids 275; Diagram Table 139 857; Tables 87, 138 274, 850
  ← thyroxine Diagram Table 139 857; Tables 87, 138 274, 850
o-Nitroanisole ← SKF 525-A 61
p-Nitroanisole ← phenobarbital Diagram Table 139 857; Tables 88, 138 275, 850
  ← splenectomy 553
  ← steroids 275; Diagram Table 139 857; Tables 88, 138 275, 850
  ← thyroxine Diagram Table 139 857; Tables 88, 138 275, 850
p-Nitrobenzaldehyde ← enzymes, normal Table 134 759
p-Nitrobenzoate ← sex 655
p-Nitrobenzoic acid ← anterior pituitary preparations 439
  ← starvation/mouse Table 3 81
  ← stressors 697
p-Nitrobenzyl alcohol ← enzymes, normal Table 134 759
Nitrogen dioxide (highly toxic gas) ← thyroid hormones 487
  mustard ← 5-HT 557, 560
    → resistance 585
    ← steroids 275
    ← STH 426, 428
    ← thyroid hormones 488
Nitro reduction 45
Nitrose gas; cf. Ozone
Nitrous oxide (inhalation anesthetic, analgesic)
  ← steroids 275
  ← thyroid hormones 488
Noble — Collip drum 545
Nocardia asteroides ← steroids 317, 322
Nonhormonal factors → resistance 567
"Nonspecific cross-resistance" 698
Nonspecific detoxication 764
  resistance 25
  stress 452
  toxication 764
Nonspecificity of steroid-induced resistance, theories 763
Nonsteroidal agents, "protective spectrum" 835
  hormones ← ACTH 405
  ← barbiturates 575
  ← hepatic lesions 599
  → hepatic tissue 726, 735
  ← 5-HT 556, 558
  ← hypophysectomy 444, 445
  ← pancreatic hormones 521
  ← pregnancy 660
  ← sex 631
  ← steroids 137

Nonsteroidal agents, hormones ← stressors 688
  ← thyroid hormones 463
Noradrenaline; cf. Norepinephrine
Norbolethone; cf. also Testoids
  → AAN *Table 73* 257
  → acetanilide *Table 24* 176
  → acrylamide *Table 25* 176
  → acrylonitrile *Table 26* 177
  → adrenal weight *Table 140* 860
  → aminopyrine *Table 27* 179
  → barbital *Table 34* 198
  → barbiturates 197
  → body weight *Table 140* 860
  → bishydroxycoumarin *Table 28* 182
  → cadmium *Table 35* 200
  → caramiphen *Table 36* 201
  → carisoprodol *Table 37* 216
  → chlordiazepoxide *Table 38* 217
  → cinchophen *Table 39* 221
  → cocaine *Table 40* 221
  → F-COL *Tables 12, 13, 14* 133, 134
  → colchicine *Table 41* 222
  → DL-coniine *Table 42* 222
  → croton oil *Table 43* 223
  → cyclobarbital *Table 33* 198
  → cycloheximide *Tables 44, 45* 224
  ← cycloheximide 77
  → cyclophosphamide *Table 46* 225
  → digitoxin *Tables 8, 47, 48* 94, 230
  → digitoxin/mouse *Table 130* 677
  → diisopropyl fluorophosphate *Table 52* 234
  → dioxathion *Table 91* 280
  → dioxathion/mouse *Table 132* 680
  → diphenylhydantoin *Table 53* 235
  → dipicrylamine *Table 54* 235
  → DHT *Table 117* 309
  → DOC *Table 15* 135
  → emetine *Table 55* 238
  → endotoxin *Table 123* 348
  → epinephrine *Table 23* 144
  → EPN *Table 99* 284
  → estradiol *Table 16* 135
  → ethion *Table 92* 281
  → ethylene glycol *Table 56* 243
  → ethylmorphine *Table 57* 244
  → flufenamic acid *Table 58* 245
  → fluphenazine *Table 59* 245
  → glutethimide *Table 63* 248
  → glycerol *Table 64* 249
  → guthion *Table 93* 281
  → heptachlor *Table 98* 283
  → hexamethonium *Tables 60A, 61* 246, 247
  → hexobarbital *Tables 9, 32* 96, 197
  → hydroquinone *Table 65* 249
  → imipramine *Table 66* 250
  → indomethacin *Table 67* 250
  → indomethacin/mouse *Table 131* 678

Norbolethone → kidney, weight *Table 140* 860
  → liver, weight *Table 140* 860
  → LSD *Table 74* 258
  → mechlorethamine *Table 75* 260
  → mephenesin *Table 76* 260
  → meprobamate *Table 77* 261
  → mercury *Table 78* 267
  → mersalyl *Tables 79, 80* 268
  → methadone *Table 82* 269
  → methylaniline *Table 83* 270
  → methyprylon *Table 84* 270
  → $NaClO_4$ *Table 90* 278
  → α-naphthylisothiocyanate *Table 85* 273
  → nicotine *Table 86* 274
  → nikethamide *Table 87* 274
  → p-nitroanisole *Table 88* 275
  → OMPA *Table 94* 282
  → ovary, weight *Table 140* 860
  → pancuronium *Table 19* 136
  → parathion *Table 95* 282
  → pentobarbital/mouse *Table 129* 677
  → pentylenetetrazol *Table 89* 277
  → phenindione *Table 29* 183
  → phenyramidol *Table 100* 284
  → physostigmine *Table 101* 285
  → picrotoxin *Table 102* 286
  → piperidine *Table 103* 287
  → pralidoxime *Table 104* 288
  → preputial glands, weight *Table 140* 860
  → progesterone *Tables 9, 17* 96, 136
  → propionitrile *Table 105* 289
  → propylthiouracil *Tables 21, 22* 140, 141
  → SER in hepatocytes *Fig. 33* 730
  → SKF 525-A *Table 106* 291
  → strychnine *Table 107* 292
  → T3 *Table 20* 140
  → TEA *Tables 60A, 62* 246, 248
  → theobromine *Table 108* 293
  → theophylline *Table 109* 293
  → thimerosal *Table 110* 294
  → thiopental *Table 31* 197
  → thymus, weight *Table 140* 860
  → thyroid, weight *Table 140* 860
  → triamcinolone *Table 18* 136
  → tribromoethanol *Table 111* 295
  → trichloroethanol *Table 112* 295
  → tri-o-cresyl phosphate *Table 113* 296
  → D-tubocurarine *Table 114* 296
  → tyramine *Table 115* 297
  → tyrosine *Table 116* 299
  → uterus, weight *Table 140* 860
  → W-1372 *Table 118* 309
  → zoxazolamine *Tables 9, 119* 96, 313
Norepinephrine; cf. also Catecholamines
  → allyl alcohol 534
  → amitriptyline 534
  → anaphylactoidogenic agents **532**, 534

Norepinephrine → antibiotics 534
  → bacterial toxins 541
  → barbiturates/man, mouse, rabbit 532, 536
  → bile flow/dog *Table 10* 99
  → CCl$_4$ 532, 536
  → chloral hydrate 536
  → chloroform 537
  → cholesterol 537
  → cold/dog, ground squirrel, minipig 544
  ← corticoids 144
  → DHT 540
  → digitalis 533, 537
  ← DOC 143
  → drugs 532
  → electric stimuli 545, 546
  ← folliculoids 144
  → halothane 538
  → hemorrhagic shock 545, 546
  → hepatic enzymes 547
  → immune reactions 543
  → ionizing rays 543
  → ionizing rays/mouse 543
  → lathyrogens 538
  → luteoids 144
  → meperidine 538
  → meprobamate 538
  → methanol 538
  → microorganisms 541
  → morphine 538
  → occlusion of the portal vein 545
  → papain 539
  → paraoxon 539
  → pentylenetetrazol 533, 539
  → pesticides 539
  → plasmocid 539
  → portal vein, occlusion of 545
  → resistance 531, 591
  → shock, hemorrhagic 545, 546
  → steroids 531
  ← steroids 143
  → stressors 545
  → strychnine 540
  ← testoids 144
  → thyroid hormones 531, 532
  ← thyroid hormones 465
  → tremorine 540
  → tween 80 533, 540
  → urethan 540
  → vaccines 541
  → venoms 541
  → viruses 541
  → vitamin D 533
Norethandrolone → bile flow/rabbit *Table 10* 99
  → steroids 133
Norethynodrel → resistance 591

"Normal" enzymes metabolizing foreign compounds *Table 134* 759
"19-Nortestosterone derivatives" ← ethionine 78
Nortriptyline (antidepressant) ← steroids 275
Novocaine ← thyroid hormones 488

Octamethyl pyrophosphamide (OMPA); *cf.* Pesticides
pyrophosphoramide; *cf.* Pesticides
Occlusion of the portal vein ← epinephrine 545
  ← norepinephrine 545
OKT ← hepatic lesions 621
OKT (ornithine) ← corticoids 390
OMPA; *cf. also* Pesticides
  ← folliculoids *Table 96* 283
  ← mestranol *Table 97* 283
  ← phenobarbital *Diagram Table 139* 857; *Tables 94, 138* 282, 850
  ← sex 655
  ← steroids 165; *Diagram Table 139* 857; *Tables 94, 138* 282, 850
  ← thyroxine *Diagram Table 139* 857; *Tables 94, 138* 282, 850
"Operative stress" 740
OPI (Overall Protective Indexes) 834
Orchidectomy → DHT *Fig. 15* 304
  → hexobarbital ← steroids *Table 30* 195
Ornithine; *cf.* OKT *under* Influence of Steroids upon Enzymes
Ornithosis ← steroids 323
Orotic acid (food supplement, promotes growth of calves) ← sex 634, 670
  ← steroids 276
Osmosis ← ACTH 423
Osteomalacia 722
Osteoporosis 716, 722
Outlook 862
Ovary, weight ← phenobarbital *Table 140* 860
  ← steroids *Table 140* 860
  ← thyroxine *Table 140* 860
Overall Protective Indexes ("OPI") 834
Oxalate ← thyroid hormones 488
Oxandrolone; *cf. also* Testoids
  → AAN *Table 73* 257
  → acetanilide *Table 24* 176
  → acrylamide *Table 25* 176
  → acrylonitrile *Table 26* 177
  → adrenal, weight *Table 140* 860
  → aminopyrine *Table 27* 179
  → barbital *Table 34* 198
  → bishydroxycoumarin *Table 28* 182
  → body weight *Table 140* 860
  → cadmium *Table 35* 200
  → caramiphen *Table 36* 201
  → carisoprodol *Table 37* 216
  → cinchophen *Table 39* 221

Oxandrolone → chlordiazepoxide *Table 38* 217
  → cocaine *Table 40* 221
  → F-COL *Tables 12, 13, 14* 133, 134
  → colchicine *Table 41* 222
  → DL-coniine *Table 42* 222
  → croton oil *Table 43* 223
  → cyclobarbital *Table 33* 198
  → cycloheximide *Tables 44, 45* 224
  → cyclophosphamide *Table 46* 225
  → DHT *Table 117* 309
  → digitoxin *Tables 47, 48* 230
  → digitoxin/mouse *Table 130* 677
  → diisopropyl fluorophosphate *Table 52* 234
  → dioxathion *Table 91* 280
  → dioxathion/mouse *Table 132* 680
  → diphenylhydantoin *Table 53* 235
  → dipicrylamine *Table 54* 235
  → DOC *Table 15* 135
  → emetine *Table 55* 238
  → endotoxin *Table 123* 348
  → epinephrine *Table 23* 144
  → EPN *Table 99* 284
  → estradiol *Table 16* 135
  → ethion *Table 92* 281
  → ethylene glycol *Table 56* 243
  → ethylmorphine *Table 57* 244
  → flufenamic acid *Table 58* 245
  → fluphenazine *Table 59* 245
  → glutethimide *Table 63* 248
  → glycerol *Table 64* 249
  → guthion *Table 93* 281
  → heptachlor *Table 98* 283
  → hexamethonium *Tables 60 A, 61* 246, 247
  → hexobarbital *Table 32* 197
  → hydroquinone *Table 65* 249
  → imipramine *Table 66* 250
  → indomethacin *Table 67* 250
  → indomethacin/mouse *Table 131* 678
  → kidney, weight *Table 140* 860
  → liver, weight *Table 140* 860
  → LSD *Table 74* 285
  → mechlorethamine *Table 75* 260
  → mephenesin *Table 76* 260
  → meprobamate *Table 77* 261
  → mercury *Table 78* 267
  → mersalyl *Tables 79, 80* 268
  → methadone *Table 82* 269
  → methylaniline *Table 83* 270
  → methyprylon *Table 84* 270
  → NaClO$_4$ *Table 90* 278
  → α-naphthylisothiocyanate *Table 85* 273
  → nicotine *Table 86* 274
  → nikethamide *Table 87* 274
  → p-nitroanisole *Table 88* 275
  → OMPA *Table 94* 282
  → ovary, weight *Table 140* 860
  → pancuronium *Table 19* 136

Oxandrolone → parathion *Table 95* 282
  → parathyroids 517
  → pentobarbital/mouse *Table 129* 677
  → pentylenetetrazol *Table 89* 277
  → phenindione *Table 29* 183
  → phenyramidol *Table 100* 284
  → physostigmine *Table 101* 285
  → picrotoxin *Table 102* 286
  → piperidine *Table 103* 287
  → pralidoxime *Table 104* 288
  → preputial glands, weight *Table 140* 860
  → progesterone *Table 17* 136
  → propionitrile *Table 105* 289
  → propylthiouracil *Tables 21, 22* 140, 141
  → SKF 525-A *Table 106* 291
  → strychnine *Table 107* 292
  → T3 *Table 20* 140
  → TEA *Tables 60 A, 62* 246, 248
  → theobromine *Table 108* 293
  → theophylline *Table 109* 293
  → thimerosal *Table 110* 294
  → thiopental *Table 31* 197
  → thymus, weight *Table 140* 860
  → thyroid, weight *Table 140* 860
  → triamcinolone *Table 18* 136
  → β-tribromoethanol *Table 111* 295
  → trichloroethanol *Table 112* 295
  → tri-o-cresyl phosphate *Table 113* 296
  → D-tubocurarine *Table 114* 296
  → tyramine *Table 115* 297
  → tyrosine *Table 116* 299
  → uterus, weight *Table 140* 860
  → W-1372 *Table 118* 309
  → zoxazolamine *Table 119* 313
Oxidation of drugs, mechanism of, *Graph* 313
Oxidations not mediated by hepatic microsomes 45
Oxygen tension ← hypophysectomy 456
Ozone ← hypophysectomy 451
  ← steroids 276
  ← thyroid hormones **469**, 488

P; cf. Phosphorus
Pancreas, extrahepatic conditioning 103
Pancreatectomy, partial ← steroids **361**
Pancreatic hormones → acetone 522
  → acetonitrile 522
  → anaphylactoidogenic agents **521, 522,** 523
  → bacteria **527**
  → bacterial toxins 528
  → barbiturates **522,** 523
  → bilirubin 524
  → Bordetella pertussis 527
  → caffeine 524
  → carcinogens 524
  → CCl$_4$ 524
  → chlorpromazine 524

Pancreatic hormones → cholesterol 525
   → cholesterol palmitate 530
   → chromium 525
   → Clostridium welchii 527
   → CoA synthetase 530
   → cobalt 525
   → cold 528, 529
   → digitalis 522, 525
   ← DOC 142
   → drugs 522
   → dyes 525
   → endotoxins 527
   ← epinephrine 531
   → Escherichia coli 527
   → ethanol 525
   ← glucocorticoids 142
   → glucuronide 531
   → GOT 530
   → GPT 530
   → 5-HT 521
   → heat 529
   → hepatic changes 529
   → hepatic enzymes 529
   → hepatic tissue 727, 736
   → hexadimethrine 525
   → histamine 521
   → hormone-like substances 521
   → hyperoxygenation 529
   → hypoxia 528, 529
   → immune reactions 528
   → insulin 522
   → ionizing rays 528, 529
   → lathyrogens 525
   → mercury 526
   → methionine adenosyl transferase 531
   → microorganisms 527
   → morphine 526
   → mucormycosis 527
   → mycobacterium tuberculosis 527
   → NADPH-linked electron transport 530
   → nonsteroidal hormones 521
   → parasites 527
   → pentylenetetrazol 526
   → peptone 526
   → pesticides 526
   → pneumococci 527
   ← pregnancy 660
   ← progesterone 142
   → progesterone 521
   → resistance 521
   → salicylates 526
   → SDH 530
   ← sex 631
   → staphylococci 527
   ← steroids 142
   → steroids 521
   ← stilbestrol 142

Pancreatic hormones → streptococci 527
   → stressors 528
   ← testoids 142
   → TDH 530
   → thioacetamide 526
   → thiouracil 526
   → thyroid hormones 521
   ← thyroid hormones 463, 464
   → TKT 530
   → toluene diisocyanate 526
   → TPO 530
   → trauma 529
   → Trypanosoma equiperdum 528
   → uranium 526
   → vaccines 527
   → vitamin B_1 522
   → vitamin-B-complex 526
   → vitamin D 522, 526
   → Welchia perfringens 527
   → zinc 526

Pancuronium ← phenobarbital *Diagram Table 139* 857; *Tables 19, 138* 136, 850
   ← steroids *Diagram Table 139* 857; *Tables 19, 138* 136, 850
   ← thyroxine *Diagram Table 139* 857; *Tables 19, 138* 136, 850

Papain (protein digestant, anthelmintic)
   ← epinephrine 539
   ← norepinephrine 539
   ← pregnancy 663
   ← steroids 163, 276
   ← stress 694; *Fig. 30* 695
   → "tigroid" necrosis ← stress *Fig. 30* 695

Parabiosis → partial hepatectomy 703
   → resistance 703, 704
   ← thymectomy 552, 553

Parabromdylamine (antihistaminic) ← steroids 276

Paraldehyde ← thyroid hormones 488

Paraoxon ← CCl_4 79
   ← norepinephrine 539

Paraphenylenediamine ← epinephrine 533, 539
   ← 5-HT 557, 560
   ← posterior pituitary preparations 442
   ← thyroid hormones 488

Parasites ← ACTH 413, 415, 417
   ← pancreatic hormones 527
   → resistance 595
   ← steroids 315, 330
   ← STH 430, 432
   ← stressors 698
   ← thymectomy 549, 551
   ← thyroid hormones 496, 499

Parathion; *cf. also* Pesticides
   ← acetylsalicylic acid *Table 137* 848
   ← ACTH *Table 137* 848

Parathion ← betamethasone *Table 128* 630
  ← bile duct ligature *Table 137* 848
  ← CCl$_4$ 79
  ← CS-1, repeated doses *Table 7* 90, 91
  ← CS-1, single dose *Table 6* 88, 89
  ← digitoxin *Table 137* 848
  ← diphenylhydantoin *Table 137* 848
  ← ethylestrenol *Table 128* 630
  ← indomethacin *Table 137* 848
  ← nicotine *Table 137* 848
  ← PCN *Table 128* 630
  ← PCN, repeated doses *Table 7* 90, 91
  ← PCN, single dose *Table 6* 88, 89
  ← phenobarbital *Diagram Table 139* 857; *Tables 95, 128, 137, 138* 282, 630, 848, 850
  ← phenobarbital, repeated doses *Table 7* 90, 91
  ← phenobarbital, single dose *Table 6* 88, 89
  ← phentolamine *Table 137* 848
  ← phenylbutazone *Table 128, 137* 630, 848
  ← phetharbital *Table 137* 848
  ← prednisolone, repeated doses *Table 7* 90, 91
  ← salicylate *Table 137* 848
  ← spironolactone *Table 128* 630
  ← spironolactone, repeated doses *Table 7* 90, 91
  ← splenectomy 553
  ← steroids 165; *Diagram Table 139* 857; *Tables 95, 136, 138* 282, 836, 850
  ← STH *Table 137* 848
  ← thyroxine *Diagram Table 139* 857; *Tables 95, 137, 138* 282, 848, 850
  ← tolbutamide *Table 137* 848
  ← vitamin A, C, D, E *Table 137* 848
  ← W-1372 *Table 137* 848
Parathyroidectomy → digitoxin ← PCN *Table 124* 482
  ← steroids 361
Parathyroid extract; *cf. also* Parathyroids
  extract ← hepatic lesions 601
    ← hypophysectomy 444
    ← renal lesions 623
    ← thymectomy 547
    ← thyroid hormones 463
  hormones; *cf. also* Parathyroids
    ← calcitonin 520
    ← corticoids 142
    ← cortisone 141
    ← DOC 141
    ← estradiol 142
    ← hepatic lesions 601
    ← hypophysectomy 445
    ← pregnancy 660
    ← sex 631
    ← steroids 141

Parathyroid hormones ← stressors 688, 689
  ← thyroid hormones 464
Parathyroids → anaphylactoidogenic agents 516
  → antibiotics 516
  → bacteria 518, 519
  → bacterial toxins 518, 519
  → barbiturates 516
  → beryllium 515, 516
  → cold 520
  → coniine 516
  → copper 515, 516
  → DHT 516, 518
  → diet 518
  → digitoxin 516
  → drugs 515
  → epinephrine 515
  → fluoride 516
  → guanidine 516, 517
  → histamine 515
  → hormone-like substances 515
  → hormones 515
  → immune reactions 519
  → indium 516, 517
  → insulin 515
  → ionizing rays 520
  → magnesium 516, 517
  → oxalate 517
  → peptone 517, 520
  → perchlorates 517
  → permanganate 517
  → phosphate 516, 517
  → picrotoxin 517
  → potassium 517
  → puromycin aminonucleoside 517
  → renal lesions 518, 519
  → resistance 515
  → salicylates 517
  → steroids 515
  → stressors 519
  → strychnine 517
  → sulfa drugs 516, 517
  → trypan blue 520
  → uranium 516, 518
  → vitamin C 518
  → vitamin D 516, 518
Pargyline (MAO inhibitor, antihypertensive); *cf.* MAO-Inhibitors
Paroxypropionine (GTH inhibitor) ← thyroid hormones 488
Partial hepatectomy 28; *cf. also* Effect of Partial Hepatectomy upon Nutritional Disorders, Hepatic Lesions
  hepatectomy ← diet 592, 594
    → digitoxin *Table 126* 600
    → digitoxin ← spironolactone *Table 126* 600

Partial hepatectomy → dioxathion *Table 126* 600
  → dioxathion ← spironolactone *Table 126* 600
  → hexobarbital *Table 126* 600
  → hexobarbital ← spironolactone *Table 126* 600
  history 35
  ← hypophysectomy 454
  → indomethacin *Table 126* 600
  → indomethacin ← spironolactone *Table 126* 600
  methods 18, 19
  ← parabiosis **703**
  ← pregnancy **665**
  ← puromycin 76
  ← splenectomy **553, 554**
  → tumors **704**
nephrectomy; *cf. also* Renal Lesions
  ← anterior pituitary preparations 440
  → digitoxin *Table 126* 600
  → digitoxin ← spironolactone *Table 126* 600
  → dioxathion *Table 126* 600
  → dioxathion ← spironolactone *Table 126* 600
  → hexobarbital *Table 126* 600
  → hexobarbital ← spironolactone *Table 126* 600
  ← hypophysectomy 454
  → indomethacin *Table 126* 600
  → indomethacin ← spironolactone *Table 126* 600
  → mercury *Table 127* 624
  → mercury ← ureter ligature *Table 127* 624
pancreatectomy ← steroids **361**
PAS; *cf.* p-Aminosalicylic Acid
Pasteurella ← thyroid hormones 498
  pestis ← ACTH **415, 417**
    ← steroids 322, 323
    ← STH **430, 431**
Pb; *cf.* Lead
PCN → AAN *Table 73* 257
  → acetanilide *Table 24* 176
  → acrylamide *Table 25* 176
  → acrylonitrile *Table 26* 177
  → adrenal, weight *Table 140* 860
  → aminopyrine *Table 27* 179
  → barbital *Table 34* 198
  → barbiturates 198
  → bishydroxycoumarin *Table 28* 182
  → body weight *Table 140* 860
  → cadmium *Table 35* 200
  → caramiphen *Table 36* 201
  → carisoprodol *Table 37* 216
  → chlordiazepoxide *Table 38* 217

PCN → cinchophen *Table 39* 221
  → cocaine *Table 40* 221
  → F-COL *Tables 12, 13, 14* 133, 134
  → colchicine *Table 41* 222
  → DL-coniine *Table 42* 222
  → croton oil *Table 43* 223
  → cyclobarbital *Table 33* 198
  ← cycloheximide 78
  → cycloheximide *Tables 44, 45* 224
  → cyclophosphamide *Fig. 4 (B, D, F, J)* 225, 226, 227; *Table 46* 225
  → DHT *Table 117* 309
  → digitoxin *Tables 47, 48, 128* 228, 230, 630
  → digitoxin ← age *Table 50* 232
  → digitoxin ← parathyroidectomy, propylthiouracil, thyroidectomy *Table 124* 482
  → diisopropyl fluorophosphate *Tables 6, 7, 52* 89, 90, 234
  → dioxathion *Tables 91, 128* 280, 630
  → diphenylhydantoin *Table 53* 235
  → dipicrylamine *Table 54* 235
  → DOC *Table 15* 135
  → emetine *Table 55* 238
  → endotoxin *Table 123* 348
  → epinephrine *Table 23* 144
  → EPN *Table 99* 284
  → estradiol *Table 16* 135
  → ethion *Table 92* 281
  → ethylene glycol *Table 56* 243
  → ethylmorphine *Table 57* 244
  → flufenamic acid *Table 58* 245
  → fluphenazine *Table 59* 245
  → glutethimide *Table 63* 248
  → glycerol *Table 64* 249
  → guthion *Table 93* 281
  → hepatocytes, ultrastructural changes *Fig. 35* 732
  → heptachlor *Table 98* 283
  → hexamethonium *Table 61* 247
  → hexobarbital *Tables 6, 7, 9, 30, 32, 128* 89, 90, 96, 195, 197, 630
  → hexobarbital ← orchidectomy *Table 30* 195
  → hydroquinone *Table 65* 249
  → imipramine *Table 66* 250
  → indomethacin *Tables 67, 128* 250, 630
  → indomethacin ← age *Table 72* 254
  → kidney, weight *Table 140* 860
  → liver ← W-1372 *Figs. 18, 19* 310, 311
  → liver, weight *Table 140* 860
  → LSD *Table 74* 258
  → mechlorethamine *Table 75* 260
  → mephenesin *Table 76* 260
  → meprobamate *Table 77* 261
  → mercury *Table 78* 267
  → mersalyl *Table 80* 268

PCN → methadone *Table 82* 269
 → methylaniline *Table 83* 270
 → methyprylon *Table 84* 270
 → NaClO₄ *Table 90* 278
 → α-naphthylisothiocyanate *Table 85* 273
 → nicotine *Tables 86, 128* 274, 630
 → nikethamide *Table 87* 274
 → p-nitroanisole *Table 88* 275
 → OMPA *Table 94* 282
 → ovary, weight *Table 140* 860
 → pancuronium *Table 19* 136
 → parathion *Tables 6, 7, 95, 128* 89, 90, 282, 630
 → pentylenetetrazol *Table 89* 277
 → phenindione *Table 29* 183
 → phenyramidol *Table 100* 284
 → physostigmine *Table 101* 285
 → picrotoxin *Table 102* 286
 → piperidine *Table 103* 287
 → pralidoxime *Table 104* 288
 → preputial glands, weight *Table 140* 860
 → progesterone *Tables 6, 7, 9, 17, 128* 88, 90, 96, 136, 630
 → propionitrile *Table 105* 289
 → propylthiouracil *Tables 21, 22* 140, 141
repeated doses → dioxathion, hexobarbital, parathion, progesterone, zoxazolamine *Table 7* 90, 91
single dose → digitoxin, dioxathion, hexobarbital, indomethacin, nicotine, parathion, progesterone, zoxazolamine *Table 6* 88, 89
 → SKF 525-A *Table 106* 291
 → steroids 135
 → strychnine *Table 107* 292
 → T3 *Table 20* 140
 → TEA *Table 62* 248
 → theobromine *Table 108* 293
 → theophylline *Table 109* 293
 → thimerosal *Table 110* 294
 → thiopental *Table 31* 197
 → thymus, weight *Table 140* 860
 → thyroid, weight *Table 140* 860
 → triamcinolone *Table 18* 136
 → β-tribromoethanol *Table 111* 295
 → β-trichloroethanol *Table 112* 295
 → tri-o-cresyl phosphate *Table 113* 296
 → D-tubocurarine *Table 114* 296
 → tyramine *Table 115* 297
 → tyrosine *Fig. 13* 298; *Table 116* 299
 → uterus, weight *Table 140* 860
 → W-1372 *Figs. 18, 19* 310, 311; *Table 118* 309
 → zoxazolamine *Tables 6, 7, 9, 119, 128* 88, 90, 96, 315, 630
Pentachlorophenol (highly toxic herbicide)
 ← thyroid hormones 488

Pentobarbital ← anterior pituitary preparations **436**
 ← renal lesions 623
 → resistance 591
 ← sex 655
 ← steroids/mouse *Table 129* 677
 ← stressors 697
 ← thyroxine/mouse *Table 129* 677
Pentolinium ← steroids *Table 60 B* 246
Pentylenetetrazol (CNS stimulant, convulsive)
 ← ACTH 413
 ← epinephrine **533**, 539
 ← hepatic lesions **603**, 610
 ← histamine 556
 ← 5-HT **557**, 560
 ← norepinephrine **533**, 539
 ← oxandrolone *Table 89* 277
 ← pancreatic hormones 526
 ← phenobarbital *Diagram Table 139* 857; *Tables 89, 138* 277, 850
 ← posterior pituitary preparations 442
 ← renal lesions **622**, 623
 → resistance 585
 ← steroids **163**, 276; *Diagram Table 139* 857; *Tables 89, 138* 277, 850
 ← steroids/guinea pig, mouse **164**
 ← thyroid hormones **469**, 488
 ← thyroxine *Diagram Table 139* 857; *Tables 89, 138* 277, 850
Peptone ← epinephrine 539
 ← hepatic lesions 610
 ← pancreatic hormones 526
 ← parathyroids 517, 520
 ← steroids 277
 ← thyroid hormones 489, 514
Perchlorates ← parathyroids 517
 ← steroids **164**, 278
 ← stressors 694
 ← thyroid hormones 489
Perfusion of the liver, methods **19**, 22
"Perinatal pharmacology" 672
Peritonitis, appendical ← steroids 325
Permanganate ← parathyroids 517
 ← steroids 278
 ← stressors 694
Perphenazine (tranquilizer) ← thyroid hormones 489
Pesticides; *cf. also* Clinical Implications
 ← age **667**, 671
 ← barbiturates 577
 ← diet **592**, 593
 ← epinephrine 539
 ← genetic factors **675**, 680
 ← hepatic lesions **603**, 612
 → hepatic tissue **728**, 737
 ← hypophysectomy **446**, 452
 ← ionizing rays **683**

Pesticides ← norepinephrine 539
  ← pancreatic hormones 526
  → resistance **569**, 585
  ← sex **634**, 650
  ← species 680
  ← steroids **164**, 278
  ← stressors 694
  ← thyroid hormones **469**, 489
  toxicants 108, 109
Pethidine ← age 671
  ← pregnancy **661**, 663
Phalloidin ← hepatic lesions 612
Phanurane → steroids **122**, 124
Pharmacogenetics, experimental, monograph 655
Pharmacologic interactions between drugs **768**
Pharmacology, dose **93**
  general **53**
  route of administration **93**
  timing **82**
Pharmaco-pharmacologic interrelations, synopsis **768**
Phenaglycodol (sedative) ← hypophysectomy 452
  → resistance 586, 591
  ← SKF 525-A 62
Phenelzine **68**; *cf.* MAO-Inhibitors
Phenformin; *cf.* Pancreatic Hormones
Phenindione; *cf. also* Anticoagulants
  ← phenobarbital *Diagram Table 139* 857; *Tables 29, 138* 183, 850
  ← steroids *Diagram Table 139* 857; *Tables 29, 138* 183, 850
  ← thyroxine *Diagram Table 139* 857; *Tables 29, 138* 183, 850
Phenobarbital; *cf. also* Barbiturates
  → AAN *Diagram Table 139* 857; *Tables 73, 138* 257, 850
  → acetanilide *Diagram Table 139* 857; *Tables 24, 138* 176, 850
  → acrylamide *Diagram Table 139* 857; *Tables 25, 138* 176, 850
  → acrylonitrile *Table 26* 177
  → adrenal, weight *Table 140* 860
  → o-aminophenol *Diagram Table 139* 857; *Table 138* 850
  → aminopyrine *Diagram Table 139* 857; *Tables 27, 138* 179, 850
  → DL-amphetamine *Diagram Table 139* 857; *Table 138* 850
  → arsenic pentoxide *Diagram Table 139* 857; *Table 138* 850
  → barbital *Diagram Table 139* 857; *Tables 34, 138* 198, 850
  → bile-duct ligature *Diagram Table 139* 857
  → bishydroxycoumarin *Tables 28, 138* 182, 850

Phenobarbital → body weight *Table 140* 860
  → bromobenzene *Diagram Table 139* 857
  → brompheniramine *Diagram Table 139* 857
  → cadmium *Diagram Table 139* 857; *Tables 35, 138* 200, 850
  → caramiphen *Diagram Table 139* 857; *Tables 36, 138* 201, 850
  → carisoprodol *Diagram Table 139*, 857; *Tables 37, 138* 216, 850
  → chlordiazepoxide *Diagram Table 139* 857; *Tables 38, 138* 217, 850
  → cinchophen *Diagram Table 139* 857; *Tables 39, 138* 221, 850
  → cocaine *Diagram Table 139* 857; *Tables 40, 138* 221, 850
  → F-COL *Diagram Table 139* 857; *Tables 12, 13, 14, 137, 138* 133, 134, 848, 850
  → colchicine *Diagram Table 139* 857; *Tables 41, 138* 222, 850
  → DL-coniine *Diagram Table 139* 857; *Tables 42, 138* 222, 850
  → croton oil *Diagram Table 139* 857; *Tables 43, 138* 223, 850
  → cyclobarbital *Diagram Table 139* 857; *Tables 33, 138* 198, 850
  → cycloheximide *Diagram Table 139* 857; *Tables 44, 45, 138* 224, 850
  → cyclophosphamide *Diagram Table 139* 857; *Tables 46, 138* 225, 850
  → DDT *Diagram Table 139* 857; *Table 138* 850
  → DHT *Diagram Table 139* 857; *Tables 117, 137, 138* 848, 850
  → dicumarol *Diagram Table 139* 857
  → digitoxin *Diagram Table 139* 857; *Tables 47, 48, 128, 137, 138* 230, 630, 848, 850
  → diisopropyl fluorophosphate *Diagram Table 139* 857; *Tables 52, 138* 234, 850
  → dimercaprol *Diagram Table 139* 857
  → dinitrophenol *Diagram Table 139* 857
  → dioxathion *Diagram Table 139* 857; *Tables 91, 128, 137, 138* 280, 630, 848, 850
  → diphenylhydantoin *Diagram Table 139* 857; *Tables 53, 138* 235, 850
  → dipicrylamine *Diagram Table 139* 857; *Tables 54, 138* 235, 850
  → DOC *Diagram Table 139* 857; *Tables 15, 138* 135, 850
  → doxepin *Diagram Table 139* 857; *Table 138* 850
  → edrophonium *Diagram Table 139* 857
  → emetine *Diagram Table 139* 857; *Tables 55, 138* 238, 850

Phenobarbital → endotoxin *Diagram Table 139* 857; *Tables 123, 138* 348, 850
- → ephedrine *Diagram Table 139* 857; *Table 138* 850
- → epinephrine *Diagram Table 139* 857; *Tables 23, 138* 144, 850
- → EPN *Diagram Table 139* 857; *Table 99, 138* 284, 850
- → Escherichia coli *Table 138* 850
- → estradiol *Diagram Table 139* 857; *Tables 92, 138* 281, 850
- → ethion *Diagram Table 139* 857; *Tables 92, 138* 281, 850
- → ethyl alcohol *Diagram Table 139* 857; *Table 138* 850
- → ethylene chlorohydrin *Diagram Table 139* 857
- → ethylene glycol *Diagram Table 139* 857; *Tables 56, 138* 243, 850
- → ethylmorphine *Diagram Table 139* 857; *Tables 57, 138* 224, 850
- → fasting *Diagram Table 139* 857
- → flufenamic acid *Diagram Table 139* 857; *Tables 58, 138* 245, 850
- → fluphenazine *Diagram Table 139* 857; *Tables 59, 138* 245, 850
- → glutethimide *Diagram Table 139* 857; *Tables 63, 138* 248, 850
- → glycerol *Diagram Table 139* 857; *Tables 64, 138* 249, 850
- → griseofulvin *Diagram Table 139* 857; *Table 138* 850
- → guthion *Diagram Table 139* 857; *Tables 93, 138* 281, 850
- → haloperidol *Diagram Table 139* 857; *Table 138* 850
- → hepatic tissue 739
- → heptachlor *Diagram Table 139* 857; *Table 98, 138* 283, 850
- → hexamethonium *Diagram Table 139* 857; *Tables 61, 138* 247, 850
- → hexobarbital *Diagram Table 139* 857; *Tables 9, 32, 128, 137, 138* 96, 197, 630, 848, 850
- → hydrazine *Diagram Table 139* 857; *Table 65, 138* 249, 850
- → hydroquinone *Diagram Table 139* 857; *Tables 65, 138* 249, 850
- → imipramine *Diagram Table 139* 857; *Tables 66, 138* 250, 850
- → indium *Diagram Table 139* 857
- → indomethacin *Diagram Table 139* 857; *Tables 67, 128, 137, 138* 250, 630, 848, 850
- → kidney, weight *Table 140* 860
- → liver ← W-1372 *Fig. 19* 311
- → liver weight *Table 140* 860

Phenobarbital → LSD *Diagram Table 139* 857; *Tables 74, 138* 258, 850
- → mechlorethamine *Diagram Table 139* 857; *Tables 75, 138* 260, 850
- → mephenesin *Diagram Table 139* 857; *Tables 76, 138* 260, 850
- → meprobamate *Diagram Table 139* 857; *Tables 77, 138* 261, 850
- → mercury *Diagram Table 139* 857; *Tables 78, 138* 267, 850
- → mersalyl *Diagram Table 139* 857; *Tables 79, 138* 268, 850
- → methadone *Diagram Table 139* 857; *Tables 82, 138* 269, 850
- → methylaniline *Diagram Table 139* 857; *Tables 83, 138* 270, 850
- → methylphenidate *Diagram Table 139* 857; *Table 138* 850
- → methylsalicylate *Diagram Table 139* 857; *Table 138* 850
- → methyprylon *Diagram Table 139* 857; *Tables 84, 138* 270, 850
- → morphine *Diagram Table 139* 857; *Table 138* 850
- → $NaClO_4$ *Diagram Table 139* 857; *Tables 90, 138* 278, 850
- → α-naphthylisothiocyanate *Diagram Table 139* 857; *Tables 85, 138* 273, 850
- → neostigmine *Diagram Table 139* 857; *Table 138* 850
- → nephrectomy *Diagram Table 139* 857
- → nicotine *Diagram Table 139* 857; *Tables 86, 128, 137, 138* 274, 630, 848, 850
- → nikethamide *Diagram Table 139* 857; *Tables 87, 138* 274, 850
- → p-nitroanisole *Diagram Table 139* 857; *Tables 88, 138* 275, 850
- → OMPA *Diagram Table 139* 857; *Tables 94, 138* 282, 850
- → ovary, weight *Table 140* 860
- → pancuronium *Diagram Table 139* 857; *Tables 19, 138* 136, 850
- → parathion *Diagram Table 139* 857; *Tables 95, 128, 137, 138* 282, 630, 848, 850
- → pentylenetetrazol *Diagram Table 139* 857; *Tables 89, 138* 277, 850
- → phenindione *Diagram Table 139* 857; *Tables 29, 138* 183, 850
- → phenyl isothiocyanate *Diagram Table 139* 857; *Table 138* 850
- → phenyramidol *Diagram Table 139* 857; *Tables 100, 138* 284, 850
- → phosphorus, yellow *Diagram Table 139* 857

Phenobarbital → physostigmine *Diagram Table 139* 857; *Table 138* 850
→ picrotoxin *Diagram Table 139* 857; *Tables 104, 138* 288, 850
→ piperidine *Diagram Table 139* 857; *Tables 103, 138* 287, 850
→ pralidoxime *Diagram Table 139* 857; *Tables 104, 139* 288, 850
→ preputial glands, weight *Table 140* 860
→ progesterone *Diagram Table 139* 857; *Tables 9, 17, 128, 137, 138* 136, 630, 848, 850
prophylaxis by **855**
→ propionitrile *Diagram Table 139* 857; *Tables 105, 138* 289, 850
→ propylthiouracil *Diagram Table 139* 857; *Tables 21, 22, 138* 140, 141, 850
→ pyrilamine *Diagram Table 139* 857
repeated doses → dioxathion, hexobarbital, parathion, progesterone, zoxazolamine *Table 7* 90, 91
→ resistance 591
single dose → digitoxin, dioxathion, hexobarbital, indomethacin, nicotine, parathion, progesterone, zoxazolamine *Table 6* 88, 89
→ SKF 525-A *Diagram Table 139* 857; *Tables 106, 138* 291, 850
→ strychnine *Diagram Table 139* 857; *Tables 107, 138* 292, 850
→ T3 *Diagram Table 139* 857; *Tables 20, 138*, 140, 850
→ TEA *Diagram Table 139* 857; *Tables 62, 138* 248, 850
→ thallium *Diagram Table 139* 857
→ theobromine *Diagram Table 139* 857; *Tables 108, 138* 293, 850
→ theophylline *Diagram Table 139* 857; *Tables 109, 138* 293, 850
→ thimerosal *Diagram Table 139* 857; *Tables 110, 138* 294, 850
→ thioacetamide *Table 138* 850
→ thiopental *Diagram Table 139* 857; *Table 31, 138* 197, 850
→ thymus, weight *Table 140* 860
→ thyroid, weight *Table 140* 860
→ triamcinolone *Diagram Table 139* 857; *Tables 18, 138* 136, 850
→ tribromoethanol *Diagram Table 139* 857; *Tables 111, 138* 295, 850
→ trichloroethanol *Diagram Table 139* 857; *Tables 112, 138* 295, 850
→ tri-o-cresyl phosphate *Diagram Table 139* 857; *Table 113, 138* 296, 850
→ tremorine *Diagram Table 139* 857; *Table 138* 850

Phenobarbital → D-tubocurarine *Diagram Table 139* 857; *Tables 114, 138* 292, 850
→ tyramine *Diagram Table 139* 857; *Tables 115, 138* 297, 850
→ tyrosine *Diagram Table 139* 857; *Tables 116, 138* 299, 850
→ uterus, weight *Table 140* 860
→ W-1372 *Diagram Table 139* 857; *Fig. 19* 311; *Tables 118, 138* 309, 850
→ warfarin *Diagram Table 139* 857; *Table 138* 850
→ zoxazolamine *Diagram Table 139* 857; *Tables 9, 119, 128, 137, 138* 96, 313, 630, 848, 850
"Phenobarbital type", enzyme inducers 16
Phenol (antipruritic, cauterizing agent)
← steroids 282
← stressors 694
Phenothiazines → resistance **570**, 586
Phenoxybenzamine (adrenergic blocker, antihypertensive) ← steroids 282
Phentolamine → F-COL *Table 137* 848
→ DHT *Table 137* 848
→ digitoxin *Table 137* 848
→ dioxathion *Table 137* 848
→ hexobarbital *Table 137* 848
→ indomethacin *Table 137* 848
→ nicotine *Table 137* 848
→ parathion *Table 137* 848
→ progesterone *Table 137* 848
→ resistance 586
→ zoxazolamine *Table 137* 848
Phenylalanine (nutrient) ← steroids 284
← STH **426**, 428
Phenylbutazone ← age 671
← barbiturates 577
→ F-COL *Table 137* 848
→ DHT *Table 137* 848
→ digitoxin *Tables 128, 137* 630, 848
→ dioxathion *Tables 128, 137* 630, 848
→ hepatic microsomal drug metabolism in man **709**, 713
→ hepatic tissue 738
→ hexobarbital *Tables 128, 137* 630, 848
→ indomethacin *Tables 128, 137* 630, 848
→ nicotine *Tables 128, 137* 630, 848
→ parathion *Tables 128, 137* 630, 848
→ progesterone *Tables 128, 137* 630, 848
→ resistance **570**, 586, 591
← sex 652
→ zoxazolamine *Tables 128, 137* 630, 848
Phenyldiallylacetic acid ester of diethylaminoethanol; *cf.* CFT 1201
Phenyldione; *cf.* Anticoagulants
Phenylephrine → resistance 591
Phenylethylamine ← epinephrine 539

Phenyl isothiocyanate ← phenobarbital *Diagram Table 139* 857; *Table 138* 850
  ← steroids *Diagram Table 139* 857; *Table 138* 850
  ← thyroxine *Diagram Table 139* 857; *Table 138* 850
Phenyltoloxamine ← hypophysectomy 452
Phenyramidol ← phenobarbital *Diagram Table 139* 857; *Tables 100, 138* 284, 850
  ← steroids 284; *Diagram Table 139* 857; *Tables 100, 138* 284, 850
  ← thyroxine *Diagram Table 139* 857; *Table 138* 850
Phetharbital → F-COL *Table 137* 848
  → DHT *Table 137* 848
  → digitoxin *Table 137* 848
  → dioxathion *Table 137* 848
  → hexobarbital *Table 137* 848
  → indomethacin *Table 137* 848
  → nicotine *Table 137* 848
  → parathion *Table 137* 848
  → progesterone *Table 137* 848
  → zoxazolamine *Table 137* 848
Phlogogens ← hepatic lesions 612
Phlorhizin (obsolete antimalarial, causes glycosuria) ← steroids 284
Phosgene (war gas) ← posterior pituitary preparations 442
  ← steroids 284
Phosphatase ← corticoids 392
  ← hepatic lesions 621
Phosphates ← hypophysectomy 446, 452
  ← parathyroids 516, 517
  ← steroids 166, 284
  ← thyroid hormones 469, 490
Phosphorothioates; *cf.* Pesticides
Phosphorus ← steroids 166, 285
  ← thyroid hormones 490
  yellow ← phenobarbital *Diagram Table 139* 857
    ← steroids *Diagram Table 139* 857; *Table 138* 850
    ← thyroxine *Diagram Table 139* 857; *Table 138* 850
"Physiologic antagonisms" 15, 707
"Physiologic jaundice" 719
Physostigmine (parasympathomimetic, anticholinesterase) ← phenobarbital *Diagram Table 139* 857; *Tables 101, 138* 285, 850
  ← steroids 166, 285; *Diagram Table 139* 857; *Tables 101, 138* 285, 850
  ← thyroid hormones 469, 490
  ← thyroxine *Diagram Table 138* 857; *Tables 101, 138* 285, 850
Picrotoxin (CNS stimulant, antidote to barbiturates) ← barbiturates 577

Picrotoxin ← epinephrine 533, 539
  ← genetic factors 680
  ← 5-HT 557, 561
  ← parathyroids 517
  ← phenobarbital *Diagram Table 139* 857; *Tables 102, 138* 286, 850
  ← sex 652
  ← species 675
  ← steroids 167, 286; *Diagram Table 139* 857; *Tables 102, 138* 286, 850
  ← steroids/mouse 167; *Table 133* 680
  ← thyroid hormones 469, 490
  ← thyroxine *Diagram Table 139* 857; *Tables 102, 138* 286, 850
  ← thyroxine/mouse *Table 133* 680
Pigeon 172
Pilocarpine ← thyroid hormones 491
Pinealectomy → carcinogens 554
  → resistance 554
Piperidine (proposed as tranquilizer and muscle relaxant) ← phenobarbital *Diagram Table 139* 857; *Tables 103, 138* 287, 850
  ← steroids 167, 286; *Diagram Table 139* 857; *Tables 103, 138* 287, 850
  ← thyroxine *Diagram Table 139* 857; *Tables 103, 138* 287, 850
Pipradol (CNS stimulant) ← steroids 287; *Diagram Table 139* 857; *Table 138* 850
  ← thyroxine *Diagram Table 139* 857; *Table 138* 850
Pituitary extracts ← thyroid hormones 463
Placenta, extrahepatic conditioning 102
Plant extracts ← sex 652
  ← steroids 287
Plant poisons ← steroids 348
Plasmocid ← ACTH 413
  ← 5-HT 561
  ← norepinephrine 539
  ← pregnancy 665
  ← steroids 287
  ← STH 428
  ← stressors 694
Plasmodia ← sex 656
  ← steroids 330, 331
Plasmodium berghei 81, 82
  ← STH 430
  ← thymectomy 550, 551
"Pluricausal lesions" 7, 689
Pneumococci; *cf. also* Diplococcus Pneumoniae
  ← ACTH 415
  ← pancreatic hormones 527
  → resistance 595
  ← steroids 317, 328
  ← STH 430, 431
Poliomyelitis ← ACTH 415
  ← steroids 326, 328

Polyanetholsulfonate; *cf.* Anticoagulants
"Polycyclic hydrocarbon type", enzyme inducers 16
Polyoma virus ← thymectomy **549, 550**
Polyvinyl alcohol ← steroids 287
Porphyria **716**
Portal route of administration **31, 39**
Portal vein, occlusion of ← epinephrine, norepinephrine **545**
Posterior pituitary preparations → acetonitrile 441
 → anoxia **441**
 → bacteria **442**
 → bacterial toxins **441, 442**
 → barbiturates **441**
 → bromoethylamine hydrobromide **441**
 → carcinolytic agents **441**
 → chloral hydrate **441**
 → chlorpromazine **441**
 → cholesterol **441**
 → cold **441, 443**
 → digitalis **442**
 → drugs **441**
 → electric stimuli **441, 443**
 → ethanol **442**
 → folliculoids **441**
 → hemorrhage **441, 443**
 → histamine **441**
 → hormone-like substances **441**
 → hormones **441**
 → 5-HT **441**
 → hyperoxygenation **441, 443**
 → hypoxia **443**
 → infections **441**
 → ionizing rays **441, 443**
 → morphine **442**
 → paraphenylendiamine **442**
 → pentylenetetrazol **442**
 → phosgene **442**
 → potassium **442**
 → psychologic stress **443**
 → resistance **355**
 → sodium chloride **442**
 → steroids **441**
 ← steroids **138**
 → stress, psychologic **443**
 → strychnine **442**
 → suxamethonium **442**
 → trauma **443**
 → traumatic shock **441**
 → vitamin D, E **442**
 → water **442**
Potassium ← ACTH **413**
 ← epinephrine **540**
 ← parathyroids **517**
 ← posterior pituitary preparations **442, 652**
 ← steroids **166, 287**

Potassium ← stressors **694**
 ← thyroid hormones **491**
Pralidoxime (anticholinesterase inhibitor)
 ← cholesterol *Table 104* **288**
 ← phenobarbital *Diagram Table 139* **857**; *Tables 104, 138* **288, 850**
 ← steroids *Diagram Table 139* **857**; *Table 104, 138* **288, 850**
 ← thyroxine *Diagram Table 139* **857**; *Table 138* **850**
Prednisolone; *cf. also* Corticoids
 → AAN *Table 73* **257**
 → acetanilide *Table 24* **176**
 → acrylamide *Table 25* **176**
 → acrylonitrile *Table 26* **177**
 → adrenal, weight *Table 140* **860**
 → aminopyrine *Table 27* **179**
 anti-inflammatory activity *Table 122* **345**
 → barbital *Table 34* **198**
 → bishydroxycoumarin *Table 28* **182**
 → body weight *Table 140* **860**
 → cadmium *Table 25* **200**
 → caramiphen *Table 36* **201**
 → carisoprodol *Table 37* **216**
 → chlordiazepoxide *Table 38* **217**
 → cinchophen *Table 39* **221**
 → cocaine *Table 40* **221**
 → colchicine *Table 41* **222**
 → DL-coniine *Table 42* **222**
 → croton oil *Table 43* **223**
 → cyclobarbital *Table 33* **198**
 → cycloheximide *Tables 44, 45* **224**
 → cyclophosphamide *Table 46* **225**
 → DHT *Table 117* **309**
 → digitoxin *Tables 47, 48* **230**
 → digitoxin/mouse *Table 130* **677**
 → diisopropyl fluorophosphate *Table 52* **234**
 → dioxathion *Table 91* **280**
 → dioxathion/mouse *Table 132* **680**
 → diphenylhydantoin *Table 53* **235**
 → dipicrylamine *Table 54* **235**
 → DOC *Table 15* **135**
 → emetine *Table 55* **238**
 → endotoxin *Table 123* **348**
 → epinephrine *Table 23* **144**
 → EPN *Table 99* **284**
 → estradiol *Table 16* **135**
 → ethion *Table 92* **281**
 → ethylene glycol *Table 56* **243**
 → ethylmorphine *Table 57* **244**
 → flufenamic acid *Table 58* **245**
 → fluphenazine *Table 59* **245**
 → glutethimide *Table 63* **248**
 → glycerol *Table 64* **249**
 → guthion *Table 93* **281**
 → heptachlor *Table 98* **283**

Prednisolone → hexamethonium *Tables 60 A, B, 61* 246, 247
  → hexobarbital *Table 32* 197
  → hydroquinone *Table 65* 249
  → imipramine *Table 66* 250
  → indomethacin *Tables 67, 141* 250, 862
  → indomethacin/mouse *Table 131* 678
  → kidney, weight *Table 140* 860
  → lathyrogens *Fig. 9* 256
  → liver, weight *Table 140* 860
  → LSD *Table 74* 258
  → mechlorethamine *Table 75* 260
  → mephenesin *Table 76* 260
  → meprobamate *Table 77* 261
  → mercury *Tables 78, 81* 267, 269
  → mersalyl *Tables 79, 80* 268
  → methadone *Table 82* 269
  → methylaniline *Table 83* 270
  → methyprylon *Table 84* 270
  → $NaClO_4$ *Table 90* 278
  → α-naphthylisothiocyanate *Table 85* 273
  → nicotine *Table 86* 274
  → nikethamide *Table 87* 274
  → p-nitroanisole *Table 88* 275
  → OMPA *Table 94* 282
  → ovary, weight *Table 140* 860
  → pancuronium *Table 19* 136
  → parathion *Table 95* 282
  → pentobarbital/mouse *Table 129* 677
  → pentolinium *Table 60 B* 246
  → pentylenetetrazol *Table 89* 277
  → phenindione *Table 29* 183
  → phenyramidol *Table 100* 284
  → physostigmine *Table 101* 285
  → picrotoxin *Table 102* 286
  → piperidine *Table 103* 287
  → pralidoxime *Table 104* 288
  → preputial glands, weight *Table 140* 860
  → progesterone *Table 17* 136
  → propionitrile *Table 105* 289
  → propylthiouracil *Tables 21, 22* 140, 141
  repeated doses → dioxathion, hexobarbital, parathion, progesterone, zoxazolamine *Table 7* 90, 91
  → SKF 525-A *Table 106* 291
  ← SKF 525-A 61
  → strychnine *Table 107* 292
  → T3 *Table 20* 140
  → TEA *Tables 60 A, B, 62* 246, 248
  → theobromine *Table 108* 293
  → theophylline *Table 109* 293
  → thimerosal *Table 110* 294
  → thiopental *Table 31* 197
  → thymus, weight *Table 140* 860
  → thyroid, weight *Table 140* 860
  → triamcinolone *Table 18* 136
  → β-tribromoethanol *Table 111* 295

Prednisolone → β-trichloroethanol *Table 112* 295
  → tri-o-cresyl phosphate *Table 113* 296
  → D-tubocurarine *Table 114* 296
  → tyramine *Table 115* 297
  → tyrosine *Table 116* 299
  → uterus, weight *Table 140* 860
  → W-1372 *Table 118* 309
  → zoxazolamine *Table 119* 313
Prednisone; *cf. also* Corticoids
  anti-inflammatory activity *Table 122* 345
  → endotoxin *Table 120, 122* 344, 345
  → hexamethonium *Table 60 B* 246
  → mercury *Table 81* 269
  → pentolinium *Table 60 B* 246
  ← SKF 525-A 61
  → TEA *Table 60 B* 246
Pregnancy (abortifacient enzyme inducers) **722**
  → anaphylactoidogenic agents 661
  → anticoagulants 661
  → arsenic 661
  → bacteria 666
  → bacterial toxins 666
  → barbiturates **661**
  ← barbiturates 578
  → BCP 662
  → bile pigments 662
  → brucellosis **665**
  → cadmium 662
  → calcification, vascular ← DHT *Fig. 27* 664
  → carcinogens 662
  → catecholamines 661
  → CCl_4 662
  → cholesterol 663
  → choline 663
  → DHT **661**, 665; *Fig. 27* 664
  → diet 665
  → drugs **661**
  → dyes 663
  → endotoxins **665**
  → glucagon **660**
  → glucocorticoids 660
  → gluco-mineralocorticoids 660
  → 5-HT **660**, 661
  → hepatic enzymes 666
  → hepatic lesions 666
  ← hepatic lesions **619**, 620
  → hormone-like substances **660**
  → hyperbilirubinemia 720
  → ionizing rays 666
  → lathyrogens **661**, 663
  → meperidine **661**, 663
  → microorganisms **665**, 666
  → mineralocorticoids 660
  → morphine 663
  → nephrectomy **665**

Pregnancy → nonsteroidal hormones 660
    → pancreatic hormones 660
    → papain 663
    → parathyroid hormone 660
    → partial hepatectomy 665
    → pethidine 661, 663
    → plasmocid 665
    → progesterone 660
    → promazine 661, 665
    → renal lesions 666
    → resistance 659
    → steroids 660
    → stress 665, 666
    → TEA 665
    → thyroid hormones 660
    → thyroxine 660
    → vasopressin 661
    → viruses 666
    → vitamin D 661, 665
    → vitamin E 665
5β-Pregnane-3α-ol-20-one ← SKF 525-A 64
Pregnanedione; *cf. also* Luteoids
    → digitoxin ← spironolactone *Table 49* 231
Pregnenolone; *cf. also* Testoids
    → digitoxin ← spironolactone *Table 49* 231
    → steroids 133
Pregnenolone-16α-carbonitrile; *cf.* PCN
Preputial glands, weight ← phenobarbital *Table 140* 860
    ← steroids *Table 140* 860
    ← thyroxine *Table 140* 860
Prerequisites for the protective actions of hormones 770
Pretreatment, duration of, spironolactone → digitoxin *Table 4* 85
Primaquine (antimalarial) ← steroids 288
"Primary inducers" 73, 75
Primidone; *cf. also* Primaclone
    → resistance 591
Probenecid (uricosuric agent in gout) → resistance 587
Procaine (local anesthetic) ← CCl$_4$ 79
    ← enzymes, normal *Table 134* 759
    ← epinephrine 540
    ← sex 652
    ← SKF 525-A 61, 62
    ← steroids 288
"Progeria-like syndrome" 172, 174, 303, 654
Progestagenic steroids; *cf.* Luteoids
Progestational steroids; *cf.* Luteoids
Progesterone; *cf. also* Luteoids
    → AAN *Table 73* 257
    → acetanilide *Table 24* 176
    → acetylsalicylic acid *Table 137* 848
    → acrylamide *Table 25* 176
    → acrylonitrile *Table 26* 177
    → ACTH *Table 137* 848

Progesterone → adrenal, weight *Table 140* 860
    → aminopyrine *Table 27* 179
    ← anterior pituitary preparations **436**
    → barbital *Table 34* 198
    → barbiturates 197
    ← betamethasone *Table 128* 630
    ← bile duct ligature *Table 137* 848
    → bishydroxycoumarin *Table 28* 182
    → body weight *Table 140* 860
    → cadmium *Table 35* 200
    → caramiphen *Table 36* 201
    → carisoprodol *Table 37* 216
    → chlordiazepoxide *Table 38* 217
    → cholesterol 154
    → cinchophen *Table 39* 221
    → cocaine *Table 40* 221
    → F-COL *Tables 12, 13, 14* 133, 134
    → colchicine *Table 41* 222
    → DL-coniine *Table 42* 222
    → croton oil *Table 43* 223
    ← CS-1, repeated doses *Table 7* 90, 91
    ← CS-1, single dose *Table 6* 88, 89
    → cyclobarbital *Table 33* 198
    ← cycloheximide 78
    → cycloheximide *Tables 44, 45* 224
    → cyclophosphamide *Table 46* 225
    → DHT *Table 117* 390
    → digitoxin *Tables 47, 48, 137* 230, 848
    → digitoxin/mouse *Table 130* 677
    → digitoxin ← spironolactone *Table 49* 231
    → diisopropyl fluorophosphate *Table 52* 234
    → dioxathion *Table 91* 280
    → dioxathion/mouse *Table 132* 680
    → diphenylhydantoin *Table 53, 137* 235, 848
    → dipicrylamine *Table 54* 235
    → DOC *Table 15* 135
    → emetine *Table 55* 238
    → endotoxin *Table 123* 348
    → epinephrine *Table 23* 144
    → EPN *Table 99* 284
    → estradiol *Table 16* 135
    → ethion *Table 92* 281
    → ethylene glycol *Table 56* 243
    ← ethylestrenol *Table 128* 630
    → ethylmorphine *Table 57* 244
    → flufenamic acid *Table 58* 245
    → fluphenazine *Table 59* 245
    → glutethimide *Table 63* 248
    → glycerol *Table 64* 249
    → guthion *Table 93* 281
    → heptachlor *Table 98* 283
    → hexamethonium *Tables 60A, 61* 246, 247
    → hexobarbital *Tables 30, 32* 195, 197
    → hexobarbital ← orchidectomy *Table 30* 195
    → hydroquinone *Table 65* 249

Progesterone → imipramine *Table 66* 250
  → indomethacin *Table 67, 137* 250, 848
  → indomethacin/mouse *Table 131* 678
  → kidney, weight *Table 140* 860
  → liver ← W-1372 *Fig. 18* 310
  → liver, weight *Table 140* 860
  → LSD *Table 74* 258
  → mechlorethamine *Table 75* 260
  → mephenesin *Table 76* 260
  → meprobamate *Table 77* 261
  → mercury *Table 78* 267
  → mersalyl *Tables 79, 80* 268
  → methadone *Table 82* 269
  → methylaniline *Table 83* 270
  → methyprylon *Table 84* 270
  ← metyrapone *Table 125* 584
  → $NaClO_4$ *Table 90* 278
  → α-naphthylisothiocyanate *Table 85* 273
  → nicotine *Table 86, 137* 274, 848
  → nikethamide *Table 87* 274
  → p-nitroanisole *Table 88* 275
  → OMPA *Table 94* 282
  → ovary, weight *Table 140* 860
  ← pancreatic hormones **521**
  → pancreatic hormones **142**
  → pancuronium *Table 19* 136
  → parathion *Table 95* 282
  ← PCN *Table 128* 630
  ← PCN, repeated doses *Table 7* 90, 91
  ← PCN, single dose *Table 6* 88, 89
  → pentobarbital/mouse *Table 129* 677
  → pentylenetetrazol *Table 89* 277
  → phenindione *Table 29* 183
  ← phenobarbital *Diagram Table 139* 857; *Tables 9, 17, 128, 137, 138* 96, 136, 630, 848, 850
  ← phenobarbital, repeated doses *Table 7* 90, 91
  ← phenobarbital, single dose *Table 6* 88, 89
  ← phentolamine *Table 137* 848
  ← phenylbutazone *Table 128, 137* 630, 848
  → phenyramidol *Table 100* 284
  ← phetharbital *Table 137* 848
  → physostigmine *Table 101* 285
  → picrotoxin *Table 102* 286
  → piperidine *Table 103* 287
  → pralidoxime *Table 104* 288
  ← prednisolone, repeated doses *Table 7* 90, 91
  ← pregnancy 660
  → preputial glands, weight *Table 140* 860
  → propionitrile *Table 105* 289
  → propylthiouracil *Tables 21, 22* 140, 141
  → SKF 525-A *Table 106* 291
  ← salicylate *Table 137* 848
  ← spironolactone *Table 128* 630

Progesterone ← spironolactone, repeated doses *Table 7* 90, 91
  ← steroids *Diagram Table 139* 857; *Tables 9, 17, 136, 138* 96, 136, 836, 850
  ← STH *Table 137* 848
  → strychnine *Table 107* 292
  → T3 *Table 20* 140
  → TEA *Tables 60A, 62* 246, 248
  → theobromine *Table 108* 293
  → theophylline *Table 109* 293
  → thimerosal *Table 110* 294
  → thiopental *Table 31* 197
  → thymus, weight *Table 140* 860
  → thyroid, weight *Table 140* 860
  ← thyroxine *Diagram Table 139* 857; *Tables 17, 137, 138* 136, 848, 850
  ← tolbutamide *Table 137* 848
  → triamcinolone *Table 18* 136
  → β-tribromoethanol *Table 111* 295
  → β-trichloroethanol *Table 112* 295
  → tri-o-cresyl phosphate *Table 113* 296
  → D-tubocurarine *Table 114* 296
  → tyramine *Table 115* 297
  → tyrosine *Table 116* 299
  → uterus, weight *Table 140* 860
  ← vitamin A, C, D, E *Table 137* 848
  → W-1372 *Fig. 18* 310; *Table 118, 137* 309, 848
  → zoxazolamine *Table 119* 313
Promazine (tranquilizer) ← age 671
  ← pregnancy **661**, 665
  ← steroids 288
Prophylaxis by phenobarbital **855**
Propionitrile (has HCN-like toxicity) ← phenobarbital *Diagram Table 139* 857; *Tables 105, 138* 289, 850
  ← steroids 289; *Diagram Table 139* 857; *Tables 105, 138* 289, 850
  ← thyroid hormones 491
  ← thyroxine *Diagram Table 139* 851; *Tables 105, 138* 289, 850
Propylthiouracil; *cf. also* Thyroid and Thyroid Hormones
  → digitoxin ← PCN *Table 124* 428
  ← phenobarbital *Diagram Table 139* 857; *Tables 21, 22, 138* 140, 141, 850
  ← steroids *Diagram Table 139* 857; *Tables 21, 22, 138* 140, 141, 850
  ← thyroxine *Diagram Table 139* 857; *Tables 21, 22, 138* 140, 141, 850
  → tri-o-cresyl phosphate *Table 113* 296
Prostaglandin E_1 → resistance **563**, 564
Prostatic hypertrophy **716**
Protection against digitoxin **772**
  against indomethacin **772**

Protective actions of hormones, prerequisites 770
  indexes 771, 834
Protein deficiency ← steroids 313, 314
Protozoa ← steroids 330, 331
PSI (Protective Spectrum Index) 834
Psittacosis ← steroids 323
Psychologic stress ← posterior pituitary preparations 443
Purine oxidation 45
Puromycin (antimicrobial, antineoplastic) 75; *cf. also* Inhibitors *under* General Pharmacology
  aminonucleoside; *cf. also* Antibiotics
    ← ACTH 413
    → endotoxin ← cortisol *Table 121* 345
    ← hypophysectomy 446, 452
    ← parathyroids 517
    ← steroids 167, 289
    ← thyroid hormones 491
  → hepatectomy, partial 76
  → steroids 76
Pyloric ulcer ← indomethacin/rabbit *Fig. 28* 679
Pyribenzamine ← sex 653
  ← steroids 289
Pyridinolcarbamate → resistance 587
Pyrilamine (antihistaminic) ← steroids 289
Pyruvate ← ACTH 413
  ← phenobarbital *Diagram Table 139* 857
  ← steroids 290; *Diagram Table 139* 857; *Table 138* 850
  ← thyroid hormones 491; *Diagram Table 139* 857; *Table 138* 850

Rabbit 157, 158, 171, 174, 185, 203, 237, 240, 321, 335, 342, 350, 362, 364, 365, 369, 370, 372, 373, 377, 380, 415, 418, 419, 420, 474, 497, 505, 506, 508, 509, 558, 606, 633; *Fig. 28* 679; *Table 10* 99
Rabies ← ACTH 415
  ← steroids 326, 329
"Rail paper technique" VII
Rauscher virus ← splenectomy 553, 554
  ← thymectomy 550
"Rebound phenomenon" 318
Reductive detoxifying reactions 45
Regeneration, hepatic ← ionizing rays 684
  ← renal lesions 623, 624
  ← tumors 704
"Reid Hunt test" 460, 466
Renal; *cf. also* Kidney
  injury, standard 516
  interventions, methods 19, 23
  lesions ← ACTH 420, 421
    → barbiturates 622, 623, 624, 626
    ← calcitonin 520, 521

Renal lesions → digitoxin 626
  → digoxin 626
  → dioxathion 626
  ← gonadectomy 359, 361
  ← hepatic lesions 619
  → hepatic regeneration 624
  → hexobarbital 623, 626
  ← hypophysectomy 454, 455
  → indomethacin 626
  → mercury 623, 624, 626
  → parathyroid extract 623
  ← parathyroids 518, 519
  → pentobarbital 623
  → pentylenetetrazol 622, 623
  ← pregnancy 666
  → resistance 622
  ← sex 657
  ← steroids 359, 361
  ← STH 432, 433
  ← thyroid hormones 502, 503
  → tribromoethanol 623
Repeated breeding ← ACTH 422, 423
"Repression response" 399
Reproductive tract, extrahepatic conditioning 103
RES 82
  blockers ← ACTH 413
    → resistance 570, 587
    ← sex 653
    ← steroids 168, 290
  extrahepatic conditioning 102, 103
  theories 755
Reserpine (tranquilizer, sedative, hypotensive)
  ← histamine 556
  ← 5-HT 561
  ← hypophysectomy 452
  → resistance 588
  ← steroids 168, 290
  ← stressors 694
  ← thyroid hormones 469, 491
Resistance ← ACTH 405
  ← adrenochrome 571
  ← age 666
  ← allyl alcohol 571
  ← amiloride 567, 571
  ← amphenone 571
  ← amphetamine 591
  ← angiotensin 564
  ← anterior pituitary preparations 436, 439
  ← antibiotics 571
  ← anticoagulants 571
  ← antihistamines 571
  ← atropine 572, 591
  ← bacteria 595
  ← bacterial toxins 596
  ← barbiturates 567, 572
  ← benzydamine 578

Resistance ← bradykinin 564
 ← bromobenzene 579
 ← calcitonin **520**
 ← carcinogens 568, 579
 ← carisoprodol 591
 ← CCl$_4$ **568**
 ← cedar chips **569**, 579
 ← chlorcyclizine 591
 ← chlordane 591
 ← chloretone 591
 ← chlorpromazine 580, 591
 ← cholesterol 580
 ← cinchophen 580
 ← cobaltous chloride 580
 ← cortisone 591
 ← cycloheximide 580
 ← DDT 591
decrease **856**
 ← desipramine **569**, 580
 ← diazepam 591
 ← diet **592**
 ← digitalis 581
 ← diphenylhydantoin **569**, 581, 591
 ← disulfiram 581
 ← diurnal variations **704**, 705
 ← DMSO 581
 ← DOC 591
 ← drugs **567**
 ← drugs, review 591
effect of steroids upon **111**
 ← endotoxin 595
 ← epinephrine **531**, 533, 540, 591
 ← ergotamine 591
 ← erythropoietin **563**, 564
 ← ethanol 581
 ← ferric dextran 581
 ← genetic factors **673**
 ← glucose **569**, 581
 ← glutethimide 591
 ← hepatic extracts **564**, 565
 ← hepatic lesions **596**
 ← histamine **555**, 591
 ← hormones, nonsteroidal **405**
 ← 5-HT **556**, 557, 591
 ← hydrazine 581
 ← hypophysectomy **443**
 ← hypothalamic lesions **443**
 ← hypoxia **685**
 ← immune reactions **596**
 ← indomethacin 582
 ← iodine **569**, 582
 ← ionizing rays **682**
 ← iproniazid **569**
 ← isoproterenol 582
 ← kallikrein **563**
 ← lactone 582
 ← malaria (P. berghei) **595**

Resistance ← meprobamate 591
 ← mestranol 591
 ← methoxamine 591
 ← methoxyflurane 582
 ← 3-methylcholanthrene 591
 ← methylenedioxyphenyl compounds 582
 ← metyrapone **569**, 582
 ← microorganisms **595**
 ← nervous lesions **704**, 705
 ← nicotine 584
 ← nikethamide 584, 591
 ← nitrogen mustard **585**
 ← nonhormonal factors **567**
nonspecific **25**
 ← norepinephrine **531**, 540, 591
 ← norethynodrel 591
 ← pancreatic hormones **521**
 ← parabiosis **703**, 704
 ← parasites **595**
 ← parathyroids **515**
 ← pentobarbital 591
 ← pentylenetetrazol **585**
 ← pesticides **569**, 585
 ← phenaglycodol **586**, 591
 ← phenobarbital 591
 ← phenothiazines **570**, 586
 ← phentolamine 586
 ← phenylbutazone **570**, 586, 591
 ← phenylephrine 591
 ← pinealectomy **554**
 ← pneumococci **595**
 ← posterior pituitary preparations **355**
 ← pregnancy **659**
 ← primidone 591
 ← probenecid 587
 ← prostaglandin E$_1$ **563**, 564
 ← pyridinolcarbamate 587
 ← renal lesions **622**
 ← RES-blocking agents **570**, 587
 ← reserpine 588
 ← salicylic acid **570**, 588
 ← sex **626**
 ← sex, review 655
 ← SKF 525-A 591
 ← soterenol 588
 ← species **673**
 ← splenectomy **533**
 ← stressors **688**
 ← sucrose **570**, 588
 ← sulfur 589
 ← sulfur compounds **570**
 ← surgical interventions **554**
 ← surgical procedures, special **547**
 ← sympathectomy **554**
 ← temperature variations **686**
 ← tetrachloroethylene 590
 ← tetrahydrofurfuryl alcohol 591

Resistance ← thiopental 591
   ← threonine 590
   ← thymectomy 547
   ← thyroid hormones 460
   ← tissue extracts 564, 565
   ← "toxohormone" 563, 564
   ← triamterene 590
   ← triflupromazine 591
   ← tryptamine 590
   ← tumors 704, 705
   ← ultraviolet rays 685
   ← urethan 591
   ← vaccines 595
   ← vasopressin 591
   ← vitamin A 590
   ← vitamin B-12 590
   ← vitamin C 571, 598
   ← vitamin D 590
   ← vitamin E 571, 590
   ← W-1372 591
   ← xanthine 591
   ← yohimbine 591
Restraint; *cf. also* Stress
   → TEA *Table 60 C* 246
Reticuloendothelial system; *cf.* RES
Reversal of actions due to timing 83, 87
   of antagonist actions 84, 92
   of inducer actions 83, 87
   of substrate actions 84, 93
Reviews 1
   catatoxic steroids 3
   "drug effects on enzymes" 591
   drugs ← age 672
   enzyme induction 1, 3
   enzymes and adaptation 3
   enzymes ← corticoids 385
   hepatic lesions 739
   ionizing rays ← steroids 368
   resistance ← drugs 591
      ← sex 655
   steroid anesthesia 133
Ribosides synthesis 47
Rickettsia ← ACTH 415, 417
   ← steroids 323
RNA-polymerase ← corticoids 392
   ← stressors 699, 703
   theories 749
"Rotational shock" 545
Route of administration, portal 31, 39

Safrole ← sex 653
Salicylates; *cf. also* Sodium Salicylate
   → hepatic microsomal drug metabolism in man 713
   → hepatic tissue 728, 738
   ← pancreatic hormones 526
   ← parathyroids 517

Salicylates ← sex 653
   ← steroids 291
   ← stressors 695
   ← thyroid hormones 491
Salicylic acid → resistance 570, 588
Salinity tolerance ← ACTH 422
   ← anterior pituitary preparations 440
   ← steroids 383
   ← STH 433, 434
   ← thyroid hormones 514
Salmonella enteritidis ← steroids 323
   typhi ← steroids 323
      ← thyroid hormones 498
   typhimurium ← steroids 323
"Saprophytosis" 425
   ← ACTH 415, 417
   ← steroids 323
   ← STH 430
   syndrome 318
SC-5233 → barbiturates 197
   → steroids 133
SC-8109 → steroids 133
Sch 5705 66
Sch 5712 66
Schistosoma mansoni (bilharzia) ← steroids 330
Schistosomiasis ← steroids 332
Screening, first, of steroids protective potency 771
SDH ← pancreatic hormones 530
   (serine) ← corticoids 390
   ← thyroid hormones 514
"Secondary inducers" 73, 75
Secretin → bile flow/dog *Table 10* 99
Selenium ← sex 653
   ← steroids 291
Semicarbazide (reagent for ketones and aldehydes) ← thyroid hormones 491
SER in hepatocytes ← norbolethone *Fig. 33* 730
   ← spironolactone *Fig. 34* 731
SER, theories 747
Serine; *cf.* SDH *under* Influence of Steroids upon Enzymes
Serum proteins, extrahepatic conditioning 103
Sex → acetylcholine 635
   → ACTH 631
   → aminopterin 635
   → aminopyrine 635, 655
   → amphetamine 635
   → aniline 655
   → anoxia 657
   → antibiotics 635
   → arsenic 635
   → bacteria 656
   → bacterial toxins 656
   → barbiturates 632, 635, 655

Sex → barbiturates/dog, guinea pig, mouse, rabbit **633**, 635
→ BCP 640
→ benzene 640
→ burns 657
→ cadmium 641
→ caffeine 641
→ carbon monoxide 641
→ carcinogens **633**, 641
→ carcinolytics **633**, 643
→ carisoprodol 644, 655
→ catecholamines 631
→ CCl_4 **633**, 641
→ cerium 644
→ chloral hydrate 644
→ chloroform **634**, 644
→ cholesterol 644
→ choline **634**, 645
→ cold 657
→ cocaine 645
→ DHT **635**, 654
→ dibucaine 645
→ diet 659
differences 28, 34
→ digitalis **634**, 645
→ dinitrophenol 646
→ drugs **632**
→ dyes 646
→ electric stimuli 658
→ enzymes 657
→ epinephrine **631**
→ ergot 646
→ ergotamine **634**
→ EST 657
→ ether 646, 647
→ ethionine **634**, 646
→ ethyl alcohol 647
→ ethylene glycol **634**, 647
→ ethyl-0-ethylphenylurea 647
→ ethylmorphine 647
→ ethyl urethan 648
→ fluoride 648
→ glucuronidase 659
→ glycolic acid 648
→ hepatic enzymes 659
→ hepatic lesions **657**
→ hepatic tissue 739
→ hexachlorobenzene 648
→ hexaethyl tetraphosphate 648
→ hexamethonium 648
→ hexobarbital 655
→ histamine **631**, 632
→ hormone-like substances **631**
→ hormones, nonsteroidal **631**
→ hypoxia 658
→ immune reactions 657
→ indomethacin 648

Sex → insulin **631**
→ ionizing rays 657
→ isoproterenol 648
→ lathyrogens **634**, 648
→ lidocaine 648
→ lithium 648
→ magnesium 648
→ MAO-inhibitors 648
→ mepacrine 649
→ mercury 649
→ N-methylaniline 655
→ microorganisms **656**
→ monocrotaline 649
→ morphine 649
→ muscular performance **657**
→ neoprontosil 655
→ neotetrazolium 655
→ nickel sulfide 650
→ nicotine **634**, 650, 655
→ p-nitrobenzoate 655
→ nonsteroidal hormones **631**
→ OMPA 655
→ orotic acid **634**, 650
→ pancreatic hormones 632
→ parathyroid hormone 631
→ pentobarbital 655
→ pesticides **634**, 650
→ phenylbutazone 652
→ picrotoxin 652
→ plant extracts 652
→ plasmodia 656
→ potassium 652
→ procaine 652
→ pyribenzamine 653
→ renal lesions 657
→ RES-blocking agents 653
→ resistance **626**
→ safrole 653
→ salicylates 653
→ selenium 653
→ squill 653
→ steroids **627**
→ steroids/dog, frog, man, mouse 629, 630
→ stressors 658
→ strychnine **634**, 653, 655
→ sulfa drugs 654
→ tannic acid 654
→ temperature variations 658
→ thyroid hormones 632
→ thyroxine **631**
→ TKT 659
→ TPNH 655
→ trauma **657**
→ tumors **657**, 659
→ tyrosine **635**, 654
→ urethan 654
→ venoms 656

Sex → viruses **656**
  → vitamin B, C, K 654
  → vitamin D **635**, 654
  → zoxazolamine 655
Sexual cycle ← steroids **382, 383**
Sheep 344
Shigella ← thyroid hormones 498
Shock, hemorrhagic ← norepinephrine **545**
  "rotational" **545**
  tourniquet ← sympathectomy **554**
  traumatic ← thyroid hormones **512**
"Short-sleepers" **554, 675**
Silica; *cf. also* RES-blocking Agents
  ← hepatic lesions 612
Silicon; *cf.* RES
SKF 525-A (inhibitor of microsomal enzymes) 58
  → alanine 61
  → aminopyrine 60, 61
  → p-aminosalicylic acid 63
  → amphetamine 61
  → anticoagulants 63, 64
  → barbiturates 60, 61, 62, 63
  → carisoprodol 61
  → catatoxic steroids 63, 64
  → CCl_4 63
  → chloral hydrate 60
  → chlordiazepoxide 63
  → chloretone 62
  → chlorpromazine 62
  → cholesterol 61
  ← cholesterol *Table 106* 291
  → codeine 60, 61
  → cortisol 62
  → cyclophosphamide 62, 63
  → diazepam 63
  → 4-6-dienone, dethioacetylated 64
  → diphenylhydantoin 62, 63
  → DMBA 63
  → ephedrine 60
  → estradiol 62
  → estrone 63
  → p-ethoxyacetanilide 61
  → ethylestranol 63, 64
  → foreign compounds 61
  → glutethimide 62
  → hydroxydione 62
  → indocyanine green 63
  → lynestrenol 62
  → meperidine 60
  → mephenesin 61
  → meprobamate 62
  → mestranol 62
  → methadone 60
  → methorphinan 60
  → N-methylanaline 61
  → 3-methyl-4-monomethylaminoazobenzene 61

SKF 525-A → methyparafynol 60
  → monomethyl-4-aminoantipyrine 60, 61
  → morphine 60
  → narcotics 61
  → nikethamide 62
  → o-nitroanisole 61
  → phenaglycodol 62
  ← phenobarbital *Diagram Table 139* **857**; *Tables 106, 138* 291, 850
  → prednisolone 61
  → prednisone 61
  → 5β-pregnane-3α-ol-20-one 64
  → procaine 61, 62
  → resistance 591
  reversal of antagonist actions 84, 92
  → spironolactone 64
  → steroid hydroxylase 62
  ← steroids **168, 291**; *Diagram Table 139* **857**; *Tables 106, 138* 291, 850
  → strychnine 61, 62
  → substrates, naturally-occurring 61
  → succinylcholine 62
  → sulphacetamide 63
  → testosterone 62
  → thiophosphates 61
  ← thyroxine *Diagram Table 139* **857**; *Tables 106, 138* 291, 857
  → triflupromazine 62
  → urethan 62
Skim milk powder ← steroids 315
Smooth endoplasmic reticulum, history 40
  in hepatocytes, history **31**
Sodium ← steroids **168, 291**
  chloride ← thyroid hormones 491
    ← posterior pituitary preparations 442
  perchlorate; *cf.* $NaClO_4$
  salicylate → F-COL, DHT, digitoxin, dioxathion, hexobarbital, indomethacin, nicotine, parathion, progesterone, zoxazolamine *Table 137* 848
"Soil-factors" **863**
Solu-Cortef; *cf. also* Corticoids
  → endotoxin *Table 120* 344
Soman ← ethionine 79
Somatic growth ← steroids **382, 383**
Somatotrophic hormone; *cf.* STH
Soterenol → resistance 588
Sound ← 5-HT **558, 563**
  ← thyroid hormones **512, 513**
Sparteine (formerly used as antiarrhythmic and oxytocic) ← epinephrine **533, 540**
Species → acetonitrile **674, 675**
  → anticoagulants 675
  → bacterial toxins 681
  → barbiturates **675**
  → carisoprodol **675**, 678

Species → chloroform **675**
  → digitalis **678**
  → digitoxin **675**
  → drugs **674**
  → endotoxin **681**
  → hepatic enzymes **682**
  → hepatic lesions **682**
  → indomethacin **675, 679**
  → methyprylon **679**
  → pesticides **680**
  → picrotoxin **675, 680**
  → resistance **673**
  → steroids **673**
  → TKT **681, 682**
  → toxicants, nonpolar **681**
  → TPO **682**
Specific antagonisms, classification **17**
  detoxication **764**
  drug antagonisms **15**
  toxication **764**
Specificity of catatoxic steroid actions **855**
  of conditioning **95**
  of syntoxic steroid actions **855**
Spectrum index, protective **771**
Spermatogenic steroids **9**
Spinal cord lesion → TEA *Table 60 C* **246**
"Spironolactone bodies" **740**
Spironolactone → AAN *Table 73* **257**
  → acetanilide *Table 24* **176**
  → acrylamide *Table 25* **176**
  → acrylonitrile *Table 26* **177**
  ← actinomycin **75**
  → adrenal necrosis ← DMBA *Figs. 2, 3* **213, 214**
  → adrenal, weight *Table 140* **860**
  → aminopyrine *Table 27* **179**
  → barbital *Table 34* **198**
  → barbiturates **197**
  → bishydroxycoumarin *Table 28* **182**
  → body weight *Table 140* **860**
  → cadmium *Table 35* **200**
  → caramiphen *Table 36* **201**
  → cardiac necrosis, infarctoid ← F-COL *Fig. 1* **123**
  → cardiopathy ← digitoxin *Fig. 36* **733**
  → carisoprodol *Table 37* **216**
  → chlordiazepoxide *Table 38* **217**
  → cinchophen *Table 39* **221**
  → cocaine *Table 40* **221**
  → F-COL *Fig. 1* **123**; *Tables 12, 13, 14* **133, 134**
  → colchicine *Table 41* **222**
  → DL-coniine *Table 42* **222**
  → croton oil *Table 43* **223**
  → cyclobarbital *Table 33* **198**
  → cycloheximide *Tables 44, 45* **224**
  ← cycloheximide **77**

Spironolactone → cyclophosphamide *Table 46* **225**
  → DHT *Table 117* **309**
  → digitoxin *Tables 8, 47, 48, 126, 128* **94, 230, 600, 630**
  → digitoxin ← choledochus ligature *Table 126* **600**
  → digitoxin ← metyrapone *Table 51* **232**
  → digitoxin/mouse *Table 130* **677**
  → digitoxin ← partial hepatectomy *Table 126* **600**
  → digitoxin ← partial nephrectomy *Table 126* **600**
  → digitoxin ← steroids *Table 49* **231**
  → diisopropyl fluorophosphate *Table 52* **234**
  → dioxathion *Table 91, 126, 128* **280, 600, 630**
  → dioxathion ← choledochus ligature, partial hepatectomy, partial nephrectomy *Table 126* **600**
  → dioxathion/mouse *Table 132* **680**
  → diphenylhydantoin *Table 53* **235**
  → dipicrylamine *Table 54* **235**
  → DMBA *Figs. 2, 3* **213, 214**
  → DOC *Table 15* **135**
  duration of pretreatment → digitoxin *Table 4* **85**
  → emetine *Table 55* **238**
  → endotoxin *Table 123* **348**
  → epinephrine *Table 23* **144**
  → EPN *Table 99* **284**
  → estradiol *Table 16* **135**
  → ethion *Table 92* **281**
  → ethionine **79**
  → ethylene glycol *Table 56* **243**
  → ethylmorphine *Table 57* **244**
  → flufenamic acid *Table 58* **245**
  → fluphenazine *Table 59* **245**
  → glutethimide *Table 63* **248**
  → glycerol *Table 64* **249**
  → guthion *Table 93* **281**
  → heptachlor *Table 98* **283**
  → hexamethonium *Tables 60 A, 61* **246, 247**
  → hexobarbital *Tables 9, 32, 126, 128* **96, 197, 600, 630**
  → hexobarbital ← choledochus ligature, partial hepatectomy, partial nephrectomy *Table 126* **600**
  → hydroquinone *Table 65* **249**
  → imipramine *Table 66* **250**
  → indomethacin *Fig. 8* **251**; *Tables 67, 70, 71, 126, 128* **250, 253, 254, 600, 630**
  → indomethacin ← adrenalectomy + corticoids *Table 68, 69, 70, 71* **252, 253, 254**
  → indomethacin ← choledochus ligature, partial hepatectomy, partial nephrectomy *Table 126* **600**

Spironolactone → indomethacin ← metyrapone
  Table 51 232
  → indomethacin/mouse Table 131 678
  → kidney, weight Table 140 860
  → liver, weight Table 140 860
  → LSD Table 74 258
  → mechlorethamine Table 75 260
  → mephenesin Table 76 260
  → meprobamate Table 77 261
  → mercury Figs. 11, 12 263—266;
    Tables 78, 81 267, 269
  → mersalyl Tables 79, 80 268
  → methadone Table 82 269
  → methylaniline Table 83 270
  → methyprylon Table 84 270
  → NaClO₄ Table 90 278
  → α-naphthylisothiocyanate Table 85 273
  → nephrocalcinosis ← F-COL Fig. 1 123
  → nephrocalcinosis ← mercury Figs. 11, 12
    263
  → nicotine Tables 86, 128 274, 630
  → nikethamide Table 87 274
  → p-nitroanisole Table 88 275
  → OMPA Table 94 282
  → ovary, weight Table 140 860
  → pancuronium Table 19 136
  → parathion Tables 95, 128 282, 630
  → pentobarbital/mouse Table 129 677
  → pentylenetetrazol Table 89 277
  → phenindione Table 29 183
  → phenyramidol Table 100 284
  → physostigmine Table 101 285
  → picrotoxin Table 102 286
  → picrotoxin/mouse Table 133 680
  → piperidine Table 103 287
  → pralidoxime Table 104 288
  → preputial glands, weight Table 140 860
  → progesterone Tables 9, 17, 128 96, 136,
    630
  → propionitrile Table 105 289
  → propylthiouracil Tables 21, 22 140, 141
  ← puromycin 76
  repeated doses → dioxathion, hexobarbital,
    parathion, progesterone, zoxazolamine
    Table 7 90, 91
  → SER in hepatocytes Fig. 34 731
  ← SKF 525-A 64
  → SKF 525-A Table 106 291
  → steroids 121, 122
  → strychnine Table 107 292
  → T3 Table 20 140
  → TEA Tables 60 A, 62 246, 248
  → theobromine Table 108 293
  → theophylline Table 109 293
  → thimerosal Table 110 294
  → thiopental Table 31 197
  → thymus, weight Table 140 860

Spironolactone → thyroid,
    weight Table 140 860
  → triamcinolone Table 18 136
  → β-tribromoethanol Table 111 295
  → β-trichloroethanol Table 112 295
  → tri-o-cresyl phosphate Table 113 296
  → D-tubocurarine Table 114 296
  → tyramine Table 115 297
  → tyrosine Table 116 299
  → Tyzzer's disease 316, 319
  → ulcers, intestinal ← indomethacin Fig. 8
    251
  → uterus, weight Table 140 860
  → vitamin A/rat Fig. 14 301
  → W-1372 Table 118 309
  withdrawal → digitoxin Table 5 86
  → zoxazolamine Table 9, 119, 128 96, 313,
    630
Spiroxasone → mercury 162
  → steroids 122, 123
Spleen, extrahepatic conditioning 102, 103
Splenectomy → DMBA 553
  → drugs 553
  → hexobarbital 553
  → ionizing rays 553, 554
  → microorganisms 553
  → Moloney virus 553
  → p-nitroanisole 553
  → parathion 553
  → partial hepatectomy 553, 554
  → Rauscher virus 553, 554
  → resistance 553
  → vaccines 553
  → zoxazolamine 553
Squill (rodenticide) ← sex 653
  ← steroids 291
SSS steroid terminology 774
"Standard conditioners" VIII, IX, 180, 181,
    183, 234, 236, 240, 249, 279, 285, 287, 289, 361
"Standard renal injury" 516
Staphylococci ← ACTH 415, 417
  ← pancreatic hormones 527
  ← steroids 318, 324
  ← STH 430, 431
  ← thyroid hormones 498
Starvation 81
  ← acetanilide/mouse Table 3 81
  ← actinomycin 74
  → aminopyrine/mouse Table 3 81
  → chlorpromazine/mouse Table 3 81
  → hepatic microsomes Table 3 81
  → hexobarbital/mouse Table 3 81
  → neoprontosil/mouse Table 3 81
  → p-nitrobenzoic acid/mouse Table 3 81
  → toxicants/mouse Table 3 81
"Statistical evaluation" IX, 771

Steroid anesthesia, adaptation to 133
  anesthesia, review 133
  hormones, classification 16
  hydroxylase ← SKF 525-A 62
  -induced resistance, theories 763
  terminology, SSS 774
Steroidases (incl. bile acids, cholesterol); *cf.*
    also Cholesterol *under* Drugs
  in general, chemistry 49
  ← thyroid hormones 462
  ← tumors 704
Steroids 80; *cf. also* Catatoxic Steroids
  → AAN *Diagram Table 139* 857; *Table 138* 850
  → acetaldehyde 175
  → acetanilide 176; *Diagram Table 139* 857; *Table 138* 850
  → acetonitrile 175
  ← acetoxypregnenolone 133
  → acrylamide 176; *Diagram Table 139* 857; *Table 138* 850
  → acrylonitrile 176
  → ACTH 137
  ← ACTH 405
  → actinomycetes 316, 319
  activity index 863
  → adenovirus-12 325, 327
  ← adrenalectomy 127
  → adrenocortical hyperplasia with sexual anomalies 382, 383
  ← age 666, 668
  ← aldadiene (SC-9376) 122, 123
  → allyl alcohol 176
  → allylformiate 177
  → Ameba 330, 331
  → aminoglutethimide 177
  → 6-aminonicotinamide 177
  → o-aminophenol 177; *Diagram Table 139* 857; *Table 138* 850
  → aminopterin 177
  → aminopyrine 178; *Diagram Table 139* 857; *Table 138* 850
  → ammonium chloride 179
  → AMP (cyclic) 179
  → amphetamine 179; *Diagram Table 139* 857; *Table 138* 850
  → amyl nitrite 180
  ← anabolic steroids 114, 119
  → anaphylactoidogenic agents 148, 180
  → Ancylostoma caninum 330, 332
  → aniline 180
  → anterior lobe extracts 138
  → antibiotics 181
  → anticoagulants 148, 181
  anti-inflammatory activity *Table 122* 345
  ← antimineralocorticoids 121, 122
  → antipyrine 183

Steroids "antirachitic" 304
  ← antitestoids 126
  → arboviruses 325, 327
  → arsenic 183
  → arsenic pentoxide *Diagram Table 139* 857; *Table 138* 850
  → Bacillus anthracis 316, 319
  → Bacillus pertussis 316
  → Bacillus piliformis (Tyzzer's disease) 316, 319
  → bacteria 316; *Diagram Table 139* 857; *Table 138* 850
  → bacterial toxins 333, 337, 347
  → barbital 198; *Diagram Table 139* 857; *Table 138* 850
  ← barbiturates 574
  → barbiturates 149, 184
  → benzene 198
  → beryllium 199
  → Besnoitia 330, 331
  → bile duct ligature *Diagram Table 139* 857; *Table 138* 850
  → bilirubin 152, 199
  → bishydroxycoumarin *Table 138* 850
  → Bordetella pertussis 319
  → bromide 199
  → bromobenzene 200; *Diagram Table 139* 857; *Table 138* 850
  → brompheniramine *Diagram Table 139* 857; *Table 138* 850
  → bronchopulmonary aspergillosis 330
  → Brucella 316, 319
  → cadmium 200; *Diagram Table 139* 857; *Table 138* 850
  → caffeine 200
  → Candida albicans 329, 330
  → caramiphen 200; *Diagram Table 139* 857; *Table 138* 850
  → carbon monoxide 201
  → carcinogens 153, 213
  → carcinolytics 215
  → carisoprodol 215; *Diagram Table 139* 857; *Table 138* 850
  → casein 216
  → CCl_4 152, 201, 203
  → CCl_4/guinea pig, mouse, rabbit 203
  → cerium 216
  → chloral hydrate 216
  → chlordecone 216
  → chlordiazepoxide 153, 216; *Diagram Table 139* 857; *Table 138* 850
  → chloroform 153, 217
  → chloropicrin 217
  → chlorpromazine 217
  → chlortetracycline 218
  → chlorzoxazone 218
  → cholesterol 154, 218

Steroids → choline **154**
  → cinchophen **154**, 220; *Diagram Table 139* 857; *Table 138* 850
  → Clostridium tetani 319
  → Clostridium welchii **316**, 319
  → cocaine 221; *Diagram Table 139* 857; *Table 138* 850
  → codeine 222
  → F-COL *Diagram Table 139* 857; *Tables 136, 138* 836, 850
  → colchicine **155**, 222; *Diagram Table 139* 857; *Table 138* 850
  → Columbia-SK virus 327
  → DL-coniine 222; *Diagram Table 139* 857; *Table 138* 850
  → copper 222
  ← cortisone 133
  → Corynebacteria **317**, 319
  → Corynebacterium diphtheriae **317**
  → Coxsackie **325**, 327
  → croton oil 222; *Diagram Table 139* 857; *Table 138* 850
  ← CS-1 **122**, 124
  → curare 223
  → cyanides 223
  → cyclobarbital 198; *Diagram Table 139* 857; *Table 138* 850
  ← cycloheximide **77**
  → cycloheximide **155**, 223; *Diagram Table 139* 857; *Table 139* 850
  → cyclophosphamide **155**, 223; *Diagram Table 139* 857; *Table 139* 850
  → cyclopropane 224
  ← cyproterone 126
  → DDD 225
  → DDT **164**, 172; *Fig. 16* 305; *Diagram Table 139* 857; *Table 138* 850
dependent action **10**
determination of "protective spectrum" **834**
  → dexamphetamine 225
  → DHT *Diagram Table 139* 857; *Tables 136, 138* 836, 850
  → dicoumarol *Diagram Table 139* 857
  → diet **313**
  ← diet 592
  → diet, fat 315
  → diet, gallstone producing ration 315
  → diet, protein deficiency **313**, 314
  → diet, skim milk powder 315
  → diethylnitrosamine 228
  → digitalis **155**, 228, 234
  → digitalis/cat, dog, guinea pig, frog, hamster, mouse **155**, 232, 233
  → digitoxin 792; *Diagram Table 139* 857; *Tables 135, 135 B, 136, 138* 779, 807, 836, 850

Steroids → diisopropyl fluorophosphate (DFP) 234; *Diagram Table 139* 857; *Table 138* 850
  → dimercaprol 234; *Diagram Table 139* 857; *Table 138* 850
  → dinitrophenol 234; *Diagram Table 139* 857; *Table 138* 850
  → dioxathion **165**; *Diagram Table 139* 857; *Tables 136, 138* 836, 850
  → diphenylhydantoin 234; *Diagram Table 139* 857; *Table 138* 850
  → diphosphopyridine nucleotide (DPN) 235
  → dipicrylamine 235; *Diagram Table 139* 857; *Table 138* 850
  → Diplococcus pneumoniae 320
  → disulfiram 235
  → DMP **165**
  → DOC *Diagram Table 139* 857; *Table 138* 850
  → doxepin 236; *Diagram Table 139* 857; *Table 138* 850
  → drugs **148**
  → dyes **157**, 237, 238
  → dyes/chicken, dog, man, rabbit **157**, 238
  → edrophonium 238; *Diagram Table 139* 857; *Table 138* 850
  → EDTA (calcium disodium ethylenediaminetetraacetide) 238
effect upon resistance **111**
  → Eimeria mivati **330**, 331
  → electric stimuli **374**, 376
  → emetine 239; *Diagram Table 139* 857; *Table 138* 850
  → encephalomyelitis **325, 326**, 327
  → encephalomyocarditis **326**
  → endotoxin *Diagram Table 139* 857; *Tables 122, 138* 345, 850
  → enzymes **383**, 403
  → ephedrine 239; *Diagram Table 139* 857; *Table 138* 850
  ← epinephrine **531**; *Diagram Table 139* 857; *Table 138* 850
  → epinephrine **143**
  → EPN **165**; *Diagram Table 139* 857; *Table 138* 850
  ← 1,2α-epoxy-androstan-3,17-dione 133
  → ergot **157**, 239
  → Erysipelothrix rhusiopathiae **317**, 320
  → Escherichia coli **317**, 320; *Table 138* 850
  ← estradiol 133; *Diagram Table 139* 857; *Table 138* 850
  → ethanol/man, mouse, rabbit **158**, 239, 240
  → ether 240
  → ethion **165**; *Diagram Table 139* 857; *Table 138* 850
  → ethionine **158**

Steroids → ethyl alcohol *Diagram Table 139* 857; *Table 138* 850
→ ethylene chlorohydrin 241; *Diagram Table 139* 857; *Table 138* 850
→ ethylene glycol 241; *Fig. 7* 242; *Diagram Table 139* 857; *Table 138* 850
→ ethylmorphine **163**, 243; *Diagram Table 139* 857; *Table 138* 850
→ Fasciola hepatica **330, 332**
→ fasting **313**, 314; *Diagram Table 139* 857; *Table 138* 850
→ fencamfamine 244
→ flufenamic acid 244; *Diagram Table 139* 857; *Table 138* 850
→ fluoride 244
→ flurothyl 245
→ 5-fluorouracil 245
→ fluphenazine 245; *Diagram Table 139* 857; *Table 138* 850
← folliculoids **124**
→ food consumption **314**, 315
→ formaldehyde 245
→ fungi **329**
→ gallstone producing ration 315
→ ganglioplegics **159**, 245
→ ganglioplegics/guinea pig **159**
← genetic factors **673**
← glucocorticoids **111**, 112
← gluco-mineralocorticoids **113**
→ glutamic acid 247
→ glutethimide 247; *Diagram Table 139* 857; *Table 138* 850
→ glycerol 248; *Diagram Table 139* 857; *Table 138* 850
→ glycolic acid 248
→ gold 248
gonadal → ethionine 241
← gonadectomy **129**
→ griseofulvin *Diagram Table 139* 857; *Table 138* 850
→ guthion **165**; *Diagram Table 139* 857; *Table 138* 850
→ haloperidol *Diagram Table 139* 857; *Table 138* 850
→ hemorrhage/cat, dog, monkey, rabbit **369**, 370
→ hepatic lesions **354**, 358
← hepatic lesions **596**
→ hepatic microsomal drug metabolism in man 711
→ hepatic tissue **725**, 726, 728, 735
→ hepatitis virus **326, 327**
→ heptachlor *Diagram Table 139* 857; *Table 138* 850
→ hexadimethrine 248
→ hexamethonium *Diagram Table 139* 857; *Table 138* 850

Steroids → hexobarbital *Diagram Table 139* 857; *Tables 136, 138* 836, 850
→ histamine **145**
→ Histoplasma capsulatum **329**, 330
→ homatropine 249; *Diagram Table 139* 857; *Table 138* 850
→ hormone-like substances **137**
→ hormones, nonsteroidal **137**
→ 5-HT **146**
← 5-HT 558
→ hydrazine *Diagram Table 139* 857; *Table 138* 850
→ hydroquinone 249
→ Hymenolepis nana **330, 332**
→ hyperbilirubinemia **715**, 719
→ hyperoxygenation **370**
← hypophysectomy **444**
→ hypoxia **370**
→ immune reactions **325**, 349
→ imipramine 249; *Diagram Table 139* 857; *Table 138* 850
inactive → digitoxin *Table 135 A* 794
→ indomethacin *Table 135 A* 794
→ indium 249; *Diagram Table 139* 857; *Table 138* 850
→ indomethacin **159**, 250, **793**; *Diagram Table 139* 857; *Tables 135, 135 B, 136, 138* 779, 807, 836, 850
→ indomethacin/mouse **160**
→ infections 325
→ influenza **326**, 328
→ iodoacetate 254
→ ionizing rays **361**, 368
→ isoniazid 254
→ isoproterenol **160**, 255
→ Japanese encephalomyelitis **325**
→ Klebsiella pneumoniae 320
→ kutscheri **317**
→ lathyrogens **160**, 255
→ lathyrogens/chicken, mouse 258
→ lead 258
→ leptospira **317**, 320
→ lithium 258
→ local trauma **381**
→ LSD **161**, 258; *Diagram Table 139* 857; *Table 138* 850
← luteoids **120**
→ magnesium **161**, 259
→ malathion **165**
→ MAO-inhibitors 259
→ measles 328
→ mechlorethamine 259; *Diagram Table 139* 857; *Table 138* 850
→ meleagrimitis **330**
→ meperidine 259
→ mephenesin **161**, 260; *Diagram Table 139* 857; *Table 138* 850

Steroids → meprobamate **161**, 260; *Diagram Table 139* 857; *Table 138* 850
→ MER-25 261
→ mercury **162**, 267; *Diagram Table 139* 857; *Table 138* 850
→ mersalyl *Diagram Table 139* 857; *Table 138* 850
→ methadone 268; *Diagram Table 139* 857; *Table 138* 850
→ methanol 269
→ methylaniline 269; *Diagram Table 139* 857; *Table 138* 850
→ methylphenidate 269; *Diagram Table 139* 857; *Table 138* 850
→ methylsalicylate *Diagram Table 139* 857; *Table 138* 850
→ methyprylon **162**, 270; *Diagram Table 139* 857; *Table 138* 850
→ metyrapone 270
→ microorganisms **315**
← mineralocorticoids **113**
→ mitomycin 270
→ monocrotaline **162**, 271
→ morestan **165**
→ morphine **163**, 271; *Diagram Table 139* 857; *Table 138* 850
→ mumps 328
→ muscular dystrophy **382**, 383
→ mushrooms 349
→ mustard gas 272
→ mustard powder 272
→ Mycobacterium leprae 320
→ Mycobacterium lepraemurium **317**
→ Mycobacterium paratuberculosis (johnei) **317**, 321
→ Mycobacterium tuberculosis/guinea pig, mouse, rabbit **317**, 321, 322
→ mycoplasma 322
→ NaClO₄ *Diagram Table 139* 857; *Table 138* 850
→ naphthalene 272
→ α-naphthylisothiocyanate 273; *Diagram Table 139* 857; *Table 138* 850
→ Neisseria gonorrhoeae 322
→ neostigmine *Diagram Table 139* 857; *Table 138* 850
→ nephrectomy *Diagram Table 139* 857; *Table 138* 850
→ nickel sulfide 273
→ nicotine **163**, 273; *Diagram Table 139* 857; *Tables 136, 138* 836, 850
→ nicotinic acid 274
→ nikethamide 275; *Diagram Table 139* 857; *Table 138* 850
→ p-nitroanisole 275; *Diagram Table 139* 857; *Table 138* 850
→ nitrogen mustard 275

Steroids → nitrous oxide 275
→ Nocardia asteroides **317**, 322
→ nonsteroidal hormones **137**
← norepinephrine **531**
→ norepinephrine **143**
← norethandrolone **133**
→ nortriptyline 275
→ OMPA **165**; *Diagram Table 139* 857; *Table 138* 850
→ ornithosis 323
→ orotic acid 276
→ ozone 276
→ pancreatectomy, partial **361**
← pancreatic hormones **521**
→ pancreatic hormones **142**
→ pancuronium *Diagram Table 139* 857; *Table 138* 850
→ papain **163**, 276
→ parabromdylamine 276
→ parasites **315**, **330**
→ parathion **165**; *Diagram Table 139* 857; *Tables 136, 138* 836, 850
→ parathyroidectomy **361**
→ parathyroid hormones **141**
← parathyroids **515**
→ partial pancreatectomy **361**
→ Pasteurella pestis 322
→ Pasteurella tularensis 323
← PCN **135**
→ pentylenetetrazol **163**, 276; *Diagram Table 139* 857; *Table 138* 850
→ pentylenetetrazol/guinea pig, mouse **164**
→ peptone 277
→ perchlorates **164**, 278
→ peritonitis, appendical 325
→ permanganate 278
→ pesticides **164**, 278
← phanurane **122**, 124
→ phenindione *Diagram Table 139* 857; *Table 138* 850
→ phenol 282
→ phenoxybenzamine 282
→ phenylalanine 284
→ phenyl isothiocyanate *Diagram Table 139* 857; *Table 138* 850
→ phenyramidol 284; *Diagram Table 139* 857; *Table 138* 850
→ phlorhizin 284
→ phosgene 284
→ phosphates **166**, 284
→ phosphorus **166**, 285
→ phosphorus yellow *Diagram Table 139* 857; *Table 138* 850
→ physostigmine **166**, 285; *Diagram Table 139* 857; *Table 138* 850
→ picrotoxin **167**, 286; *Diagram Table 139* 857; *Table 138* 850

Steroids → picrotoxin/mouse **167**
  → piperidine **167**, 286; *Diagram Table 139* 857; *Table 138* 850
  → pipradol 287; *Diagram Table 139* 857; *Table 138* 850
  → plant extracts 287, **348**
  → plasmocid 287
  → Plasmodia **330**
  → Pneumococci **317**
  → pneumonia 328
  → poliomyelitis **326**, 328
  → polyvinyl alcohol 287
  → posterior pituitary hormones **318**
  ← posterior pituitary preparations 441
  → potassium **166**, 287
  → pralidoxime **167**, 288; *Diagram Table 139* 857; *Table 138* 850
  ← pregnancy **660**
  ← pregnenolone 133
  → primaquine 288
  → procaine 288
  → progesterone *Diagram Table 139* 857; *Tables 136, 138* 836, 850
  → promazine 288
  → propionitrile 289; *Diagram Table 139* 857; *Table 138* 850
  → propylthiouracil *Diagram Table 139* 857; *Table 138* 850
  protective potency **771**
    spectrum **771**
  → protein deficiency **313**, 314
  → protozoa **330**, 331
  → psittacosis 323
  → puromycin aminonucleoside (PAN) **167**, 289
  → pyribenzamine 289
  → pyrilamine 289; *Diagram Table 139* 857; *Table 138* 850
  → pyruvate 290
  → rabies **326**, 329
  "rachitogenic" 304
  → renal lesions **359**, 361
  → RES-blocking agents **168**, 290
  → reserpine **168**, 290
  → rickettsia 323
  → salicylates 291
  → salinity tolerance 383
  → Salmonella enteritidis 323
  → Salmonella typhi 323
  → Salmonella typhimurium 318, 323
  → "saprophytosis" 323
  ← SC-8109 133
  ← SC-5233 133
  → Schistosoma **330**, 332
  → selenium 291
  ← sex/dog, frog, man, mouse 627, 629, 630
  → sexual cycle **382**, 383

Steroids → SKF 525-A **168**, 291; *Diagram Table 139* 857; *Table 138* 850
  → skim milk powder 315
  → sodium **168**, 291
  → somatic growth **382**, 383
  → sound 383
  ← species **673**
  ← spironolactone **121**, 122
  ← spiroxazone **122**, 123
  → squill 291
  → staphylococci **318**, 324
  ← steroids 111, 115, **131**, 132, 133
  → STH **137**
  ← STH **424**
  ← stilbestrol 133
  → streptococci **318**, 324
  ← stressors **688**
  → strychnine **169**, 291; *Diagram Table 139* 857; *Table 138* 850
  → sulfa drugs 292
  → surgical procedures **361**
  syntoxic; *cf.* Syntoxic Steroids
  → T3 *Diagram Table 139* 857; *Table 138* 850
  → tannic acids 292
  → TEA *Diagram Table 139* 857; *Table 138* 850
  → temperature variations **372**, 374
  ← testoids **114**, 119
  ← testosterone 133
  → tetracaine 293
  → tetrahydronaphthylamine 293
  → thalidomide 293
  → thallium 293; *Diagram Table 139* 857; *Table 138* 850
  → theobromine 293; *Diagram Table 139* 857; *Table 138* 850
  → theophylline 293; *Diagram Table 139* 857; *Table 138* 850
  → thimerosal **169**, 294; *Diagram Table 139* 857; *Table 138* 850
  → thioacetamide **169**, 294; *Table 138* 850
  → thiopental *Diagram Table 139* 857; *Table 138* 850
  → thiourea 294
  → thyroid hormones **139**
  ← thyroid hormones **461**, 462
  → thyroid hormones/dog, guinea pig, man **139**
  → tissue extracts **147**
  ← TMACN **131**, 132
  toxicants **105**, 108
  → toxoplasma **330**, 332
  → trauma **376**, 378, 381
  → tremorine 294; *Diagram Table 139* 857; *Table 138* 850

Steroids → Treponema pallidum **318**, **325**
  → triamcinolone *Diagram Table 139* **857**; *Table 138* **850**
  → tribromoethanol **169**, **295**; *Diagram Table 139* **857**; *Table 138* **850**
  → Trichinella spiralis **330**, **332**
  → trichloroethanol **170**, **295**; *Diagram Table 139* **857**; *Table 138* **850**
  → trichloroethylene **295**
  → Trichophyton mentagrophytes **329**, **330**
  → Trichuris muris **330**, **332**
  → tri-o-cresyl phosphate **295**; *Diagram Table 139* **857**; *Table 138* **850**
  → Trypanosoma cruzi **331**
  → Trypanosomes **330**, **331**
  → trypsin **296**
  → tubocurarine **170**, **296**; *Diagram Table 139* **857**; *Table 138* **850**
  → tumors **382**
  → typhoid **318**
  → tyramine **296**; *Diagram Table 139* **857**; *Table 138* **850**
  → tyrosine **170**, **297**; *Diagram Table 139* **857**; *Table 138* **850**
  → ultraviolet rays **368**
  → uranium **297**
  → urethan **297**
  → vaccines **316**
  → vaccinia **326**, **329**
  → variola **326**, **329**
  → venoms **348**
  → venoms, spider, wasp **349**
  → viruses **325**
  → vitamin A **170**, **299**
  → vitamin A/rabbit, xenopus laevis **171**
  → vitamin B **172**, **301**
  → vitamin B/chicken, pigeon **172**
  → vitamin C **172**, **302**
  → vitamin C/guinea pig, mouse **172**
  → vitamin D **172**, **302**, **308**
  → vitamin E, K **309**
  → W-1372 **175**, **309**; *Diagram Table 139* **857**; *Table 138* **850**
  → warfarin *Diagram Table 139* **857**; *Table 138* **850**
  → water **310**
  → worms **330**, **332**
  → yeast **313**, **314**, **329**
  → yohimbine **312**
  → zoxazolamine **175**, **312**; *Diagram Table 139* **857**; *Tables 136, 138* **836**, **850**
STH → acrylonitrile **426**
  → aminopyrine **426**
  → anaphylactoidogenic agents **426**
  → anticoagulants **426**
  → bacteria **430**

STH → bacterial toxins **432**
  → barbiturates **426**
  → Candida albicans **430**
  → carcinogens **425**, **427**
  → CCl_4 **425**, **427**
  → choline **426**, **427**
  → chlorpromazine **427**
  → F-COL *Table 137* **848**
  → cold **432**
  → corticoids **425**
  → Corynebacteria **430**
  → DHT **426**, **428**; *Fig. 16* **305**; *Table 137* **848**
  → diet **430**
  → digitoxin *Table 137* **848**
  → dioxathion *Table 137* **848**
  → drugs **425**
  → "endotheliomyelosis" **430**
  → enzymes, hepatic **433**, **434**
  → enzymes, hepatic/mouse **433**
  → EST **433**, **434**
  → ethanol **427**
  → ethionine **427**
  → folliculoids **425**
  → fungi **432**
  ← glucocorticoids **137**
  → hepatic lesions **432**, **433**
  → hexobarbital *Table 137* **848**
  → immune reactions **432**, **433**
  → indomethacin *Table 137* **848**
  → influenza **430**
  → ionizing rays **432**, **434**
  → lathyrogens **426**, **427**
  → microorganisms **430**
  ← mineralocorticoids **137**
  → Mycobacterium tuberculosis **431**
  → nicotine *Table 137* **848**
  → nitrogen mustard **426**, **428**
  → parasites **430**, **432**
  → parathion *Table 137* **848**
  → Pasteurella pestis **430**, **431**
  → phenylalanine **426**, **428**
  → plasmocid **428**
  → Plasmodium berghei **430**
  → pneumococci **430**, **431**
  → progesterone *Table 137* **848**
  → renal lesions **432**, **433**
  → salinity tolerance **433**, **434**
  → "saprophytosis" **430**
  → staphylococci **430**, **431**
  ← steroids **137**
  → steroids **424**
  ← stressors **689**
  → stressors **432**, **434**
  → temperature variations **434**
  ← testoids **137**
  → Trypanosoma inopinatum **430**

STH → tryptophan **426**, 428
 → tuberculosis **430**
 → typhoid bacilli **430**, 431
 → typhoid endotoxin **430**
 → tyrosine **426**, 428
 → vaccines **430**
 → viruses **431**
 → vitamin A **426**, 428; *Fig. 21* **429**
 → vitamin C **428**
 → vitamin D **426**, 428
 → yeasts **432**
 → zinc **430**
 → zoxazolamine *Table 137* **848**
"Stiffness syndrome" **314**
Stilbestrol → barbiturates **196**
 → epinephrine **143**
 → pancreatic hormones **142**
 → steroids **133**
Streptococci ← ACTH **415**, 417
 ← pancreatic hormones **527**
 ← steroids **318**, 324
 ← thyroid hormones **499**
Stress ← actinomycin **74**
 → adrenocortical necrosis ← DMBA *Fig. 29* **693**
 → agar **689**, 690
 → aminopyrine **690**
 → amphetamine **689**, 690
 → anaphylactoidogenic agents **689**, 690
 → aniline **690**
 → antibiotics **689**
 → anticoagulants **689**, 690
 → bacteria **699**
 → bacterial endotoxins **698**
 → bacterial toxins **699**
 → barbiturates **689**, 690
 biologic **25**
 → bromides **692**
 → bromobenzene **692**
 → calcium **692**
 → carcinogens **692**
 → carrageenin **692**
 → catecholamines **688**
 → CCl$_4$ **692**
 → chloral hydrate **692**
 → chlorides **693**
 → chlorform **693**
 → chlorpromazine **697**
 → cholesterol **693**
 circulatory **377**
 → codeine **697**
 → corticoids **688**
 → defensive enzymes **698**
 → DHT *Figs. 31, 32* **696**, 697
 → diet, complex **698**
 → DMBA *Fig. 29* **693**
 → DNA-polymerase **699**, 703

Stress → drugs **689**
 → enzymes **703**
 → enzymes, defensive **698**
 → epinephrine **689**
 ← epinephrine **545**, 689
 → ethanol **693**
 → fatty acids **694**
 → formaldehyde **693**
 → ganglioplegics **693**; *Table 60* **246**
 → GOT **699**, 703
 → GPT **699**, 703
 → hepatic enzymes **700**
 → hexobarbital **697**
 → histamine **689**
 ← 5-HT **557**, 563
 → 5-HT **689**
 → hormone-like substances **688**
 ← hormone-like substances **563**
 → hyperoxygenation **700**
 → hypophyseal hormones **689**
 ← hypophysectomy **455**
 → hypoxia **700**
 → immune reactions **700**
 → indomethacin **694**
 → ionizing rays **698**, 700
 → isoproterenol **694**
 → lipids **694**
 → lysosomal hydrolases **699**, 702
 → magnesium **694**
 → meprobamate **697**
 → α-methyltyrosine **694**
 → microorganisms **698**, 699
 → morphine **694**
 → nicotine **694**
 → p-nitrobenzoic acid **697**
 "nonspecific" **452**
 → nonsteroidal hormones **688**
 ← norepinephrine **545**
 ← pancreatic hormones **528**
 → papain **694**; *Fig. 30* **695**
 → parasites **698**
 → parathyroid hormone **688**, 689
 ← parathyroids **519**
 → pentobarbital **697**
 → perchlorates **694**
 → permanganates **694**
 → pesticides **694**
 → phenol **694**
 → plasmocid **694**
 → potassium **694**
 ← pregnancy **665**, 666
 → reserpine **694**
 → resistance **688**
 → RNA-polymerase **699**, 703
 → salicylates **695**
 ← sex **658**
 → steroids **688**

Stress → STH 689
  ← STH 432, 434
  → TEA *Table 60 C* 246
  theories 760
  → thiouracil 688
  ← thyroid hormones 512
  → thyroid hormones 689
  → TKT 698, 700
  → TPO 698, 700
  → trypsin 703
  → tyrosine 695
  → venoms 698, 699, 700
  → vitamin A, D 697
  → zoxazolamine 697
Strychnine (CNS stimulant) ← age 667, 671
  ← barbiturates 577
  ← cholesterol *Table 107* 292
  ← epinephrine 533, 540
  ← genetic factors 675, 681
  ← hepatic lesions 603, 612
  ← 5-HT 557, 561
  ← norepinephrine 540
  ← parathyroids 517
  ← phenobarbital *Diagram Table 139* 857; *Tables 107, 138* 292, 850
  ← posterior pituitary preparations 442
  ← sex 634, 653, 655
  ← SKF 525-A 61, 62
  ← steroids 169, 291; *Diagram Table 139* 857; *Tables 107, 138* 292, 850
  ← thyroid hormones 491
  ← thyroxine *Diagram Table 139* 857; *Tables 107, 138* 292, 850
Style, analytico-synthetic V
  of this book V
Su 9055 ← ethionine 79
Su 10603 ← ethionine 79
Substrates, competition 70
  naturally-occurring ← SKF 525-A 61
  reversal of actions 84, 93
  type I and II, behavior 104
Subtotal hepatectomy; *cf. also* Hepatic Lesions
  methods 18, 20
Succinic acid derivatives; *cf.* Sch 5712, Sch 5705
Succinylcholine ← enzymes, normal *Table 134* 759
  ← SKF 525-A 62
Sucrose → resistance 570, 588
Sulfa compounds ← calcitonin 520
  drugs ← parathyroids 516, 517
    ← sex 654
    ← steroids 292
    ← thyroid hormones 492
Sulfonamide ← steroids 292

Sulfur → resistance 589
  compounds → resistance 570
Sulphacetamide ← SKF 525-A 63
Sulphuric acid esters 47
Summary 862
Surgical interventions → resistance 554
  interventions ← thyroid hormones 502
  methods 18, 19
  procedures; *cf. also* "Stress"
    special → resistance 547
    ← steroids 361
Suxamethonium ← posterior pituitary preparations 442
Sweat, extrahepatic conditioning 103
Sympathectomy → endotoxin 554
  → formaldehyde 554
  → histamine 554
  → resistance 554
  → tourniquet shock 554
Sympathetic nervous system, blockade of ← epinephrine 545
Synopsis of pharmaco-chemical interrelations 768
  of pharmaco-pharmacologic interrelations 768
Synoptic tables 771
"Syntoxic hormones" 6, 707
Syntoxic compounds 52, 862
  drugs 567
  steroids 9, 12
    classification 16
    clinical applications 863
    history 31, 40
    specificity of actions 855
Systemic trauma ← adrenalectomy 337, 380
  ← corticoids 376, 378
  ← corticoids/cat, dog, goat, man, mouse, rabbit 377, 380
  ← folliculoids 378, 381
  ← gonadectomy 378, 381
  ← luteoids 378, 381
  ← steroids 376, 378, 381
  ← testoids 378, 381

T 3; *cf. also* Thyroid and Thyroid Hormones
  ← phenobarbital *Diagram Table 139* 857; *Tables 20, 138* 140, 850
  ← steroids *Diagram Table 139* 857; *Tables 20, 138* 140, 850
  ← thyroxine *Diagram Table 139* 857; *Tables 20, 138* 140, 850
  → tri-o-cresyl phosphate *Table 113* 296
Table, diagram 772
Tables VIII
Tannic acid (astringent, styptic) ← ACTH 413
  ← sex 654
  ← steroids 292

TDH ← pancreatic hormones 530
   (threonine) ← corticoids 390
TEA ← ACTH *Table 60 C* 246
   ← bone fracture *Table 60 C* 246
   ← cold *Table 60 C* 246
   ← fasting *Table 60 C* 246
   ← formaldehyde *Table 60 C* 246
   ← hemorrhage *Table 60 C* 246
   ← phenobarbital *Diagram Table 139* 857;
      Tables 62, 138 248, 850
   ← pregnancy 665
   ← restraint *Table 60 C* 246
   ← spinal cord lesion *Table 60 C* 246
   ← steroids *Diagram Table 139* 857;
      Tables 60 A, B, C, 62, 138 246, 248, 850
   ← stressors *Table 60 C* 246
   ← thyroxine *Diagram Table 139* 857;
      Tables 62, 138 248, 850
Tears, extrahepatic conditioning 103
TEM; *cf.* Carcinolytics
Temperature variations ← ACTH 422
   ← ACTH/mouse 422
   ← adrenalectomy 373, 374
   → bacterial toxins 687
   → barbiturates 686
   → CCl₄ 686
   → chloral hydrate 687
   → cholesterol 687
   → dinitrophenol 687
   → drugs 686
   ← folliculoids 373, 374
   ← gonadectomy 373, 374
   ← gonadectomy/rabbit 373
   → hepatic enzymes 687
   ← hypophysectomy 456
   → immune reactions 687
   → magnesium 687
   → resistance 686
   ← sex 658
   ← steroids 372, 374
   ← STH 434
   ← testoids 373, 374
   ← thyroid hormones/fish, goat, guinea pig, hamster, mouse, rabbit 509, 510, 511
   → tyrosine 687
   → venoms 687
Terminology 5, 8
   anabolic steroids 9
   anesthetic steroids 9
   antimineralocorticoid 9
   catatoxic steroids 9, 13
   folliculoid 9
   glucocorticoid 9
   luteoid 9
   mineralocorticoid 9
   spermatogenic steroids 9
   syntoxic steroids 9, 12

Terminology, testoid 9
Testoids anabolics, "myotrophic" activity 313
Testoidases, chemistry 49
Testoids 9
   anabolics 54
   → bacterial toxins 337, 347
   → barbiturates 150, 187
   ← barbiturates 572
   → barbiturates/guinea pig, mouse 189
   → carcinogens 207
   → choline deficiency 219
   → DHT/rabbit 174
   → diet, choline deficient 219
   → electric stimuli 375, 376
   → enzymes 403
   → epinephrine 143, 144
   → folliculoids 115, 119
   → glucocorticoids 114, 115
   → gluco-mineralocorticoids 114, 118
   → hepatic lesions 354, 358
   → hepatic tissue 726, 734
   → hyperoxygenation 371, 372
   → hypoxia 371, 372
   → immune reactions 351, 353
   → ionizing rays/mouse, rabbit 362, 364, 365
   → lathyrogens 255
   → luteoids 114, 118
   → mercury 162, 261
   metabolism ← folliculoids *Graph* 125
      ← thyroid hormones *Graph* 125
   → mineralocorticoids 114, 118
   → norepinephrine 114
   → pancreatic hormones 142
   → renal lesions 359, 360
   → steroids 114, 119
   → STH 137
   → systemic trauma 378, 381
   → temperature variations 373, 374
   ← thyroid hormones 461, 462
   → vitamin D 174, 307
   → vitaminD/chicken 174
Testosterone; *cf. also* Testoids
   → barbiturates 197
   → digitoxin ← spironolactone *Table 49* 231
   "rachitogenic" 173
   ← SKF 525-A 62
   → steroids 133
Tetracaine (local anesthetic) ← ACTH 413
   ← steroids 293
Tetrachloroethylene → resistance 590
Tetraethylammonium; *cf.* TEA *and under* Ganglioplegics, Ganglionic-Blocking Agents
Tetraethylthiuram disulfide; *cf.* Disulfiram
Tetrahydrofurfuryl alcohol → resistance 591
Tetrahydronaphthylamine ← hepatic lesions 613

Tetrahydronaphthylamine ← steroids 293
 ← thyroid hormones 492
Thallium (rodenticide) ← phenobarbital
  Diagram Table 139 857
 ← steroids 293; *Diagram Table 139* 857;
  Table 138 850
 ← thymectomy 548, 549
 ← thyroid hormones 492
 ← thyroxine *Diagram Table 139* 857;
  Table 138 850
Theobromine ← phenobarbital *Diagram
  Table 139* 857; *Tables 108, 138*
  293, 850
 ← steroids 293; *Diagram Table 139* 857;
  Tables 108, 138 293, 850
 ← thyroxine *Diagram Table 139* 857;
  Tables 108, 138 293, 850
Theophylline ← phenobarbital *Diagram
  Table 139* 857; *Tables 109, 138* 293,
  850
 ← steroids 293; *Diagram Table 139* 857;
  Tables 109, 138 293, 850
 ← thyroid hormones 492
 ← thyroxine *Diagram Table 139* 857;
  Tables 109, 138 293, 850
Theories 743
 defense against "natural" vs. "foreign"
  compounds 758
 DNA 749
 "foreign" compounds 758
 hepatic enzymes 743
  glycogen 757
  participation 743
 homeostasis 763
 lysosomes 753
 microsomal enzymes 746
 microsomes 747
 "natural" vs. "foreign" compounds 758
 nonspecificity of steroid-induced resistance
  763
 reticulo-endothelial system (RES) 755
 RNA 749
 SER 747
 steroid-induced resistance 763
 stressors 760
 TKT 745
 TPO 745
 vitamin C 757
Thiadiazoles; *cf.* Sulfa Drugs
Thimerosal (antiseptic) ← phenobarbital
  Diagram Table 139 857; *Tables 110, 138*
  294, 850
 ← steroids 169, 294; *Diagram Table 139*
  857; *Table 110* 294
 ← thyroxine *Diagram Table 139* 857;
  Tables 110, 138 294, 850

Thioacetamide ← pancreatic hormones 526
 ← phenobarbital *Table 138* 850
 ← steroids 169, 294; *Table 138* 850
 ← thyroid hormones 492
 ← thyroxine *Table 138* 850
Thiodiazoles; *cf.* Sulfa Drugs
Thiopental; *cf. also* Barbiturates
 ← cholesterol *Table 31* 197
 ← phenobarbital *Diagram Table 139* 857;
  Tables 31, 138 197, 850
 → resistance 591
 ← steroids *Diagram Table 139* 857;
  Tables 31, 138 197, 850
 ← thyroxine *Diagram Table 139* 857;
  Tables 31, 138 197, 850
Thiophosphamide; *cf.* Carcinolytics
Thiophosphates ← SKF 525-A 61
"Thiosulfate serum" 589
Thiouracil ← pancreatic hormones 526
 ← stressors 688
Thiourea (toxic antithyroid agent) ← steroids
  294
 ← thyroid hormones 492
6-Thioxanthine ← enzymes, normal *Table 134*
  759
Thorium Dextrin; *cf.* RES-Blocking Agents
Thorotrast 81
"Three-Step Procedure" 18
Threonine (nutrient); *cf. also* TDH *under
  Influence of Steroids upon Enzymes*
 → resistance 590
Thrombin ← hepatic lesions 621
Thymectomy → adaptive enzyme formation
  552
 → adenovirus-12 551
 → bacteria 549, 550
 → bacterial toxins 551
 → *Candida albicans* 550
 → carcinogens 548
 → codeine 548
 → cold 553
 → curare 549
 → cytomegalic inclusion virus 551
 → drugs 547
 → *Eimeria tenella* 550, 551
 → endotoxins 550
 → enzyme formation, adaptive 552
 → extrahepatic conditioning 103
 → fungi 551
 → hepatic enzymes 553
 → hepatic lesions 552
 → heroin 548
 → histamine 547
 → hormone-like substances 547
 → hormones 547
 → immune reactions 551
 → ionizing rays 552

Thymectomy → lactate dehydrogenase virus 551
  → lymphocytic choriomeningitis 549, 550
  → microorganisms 549
  → Moloney virus 551
  → morphine 548, 549
  → parabiosis 552, 553
  → parasites 549, 551
  → parathyroid extract 547
  → Plasmodium berghei 550, 551
  → polyoma virus 549, 550
  → Rauscher virus 550
  → resistance 547
  → thallium 548, 549
  → thyroid 547
  → Trypanosoma lewisi 551
  → tumors 553
  → vaccines 550
  → viruses 549, 550
  → vitamin A, C, D 548, 549
  → yeasts 551
Thymus → chloroform 549
  extrahepatic conditioning 103
  weight ← phenobarbital *Table 140* 860
    ← steroids *Table 140* 860
    ← thyroxine *Table 140* 860
Thyroid ← epinephrine 531, 532
  history 26, 33
  hormones → acetaldehyde 470
    → acetonitrile/guinea pig, mouse 466, 470, 471
    → aconitine 471
    → adenosine diphosphate 471
    → allyl alcohol 471
    → allylformiate 471
    → p-aminosalicylate 471
    → amphetamine 466, 472
    → amphetamine/mouse 472
    → amyl nitrate 472
    → anaphylactoidogenic agents 467, 472
    → angiotensin 466
    → anticoagulants 473
    → antimony 473
    → arsenic 473
    → atropine 473
    → Bacillus anthracis 497
    → bacteria 496, 497
    → bacterial toxins 497, 500
    → barbiturates/ cat, frog, mouse, rabbit 467, 473, 474, 475
    → blood-vessel ligatures 504
    → Brucella melitensis 497
    → caffeine 475
    → carbon dioxide 475
    → carbon monoxide 467, 475
    → carcinogens 467, 476
    → catecholamines 463

Thyroid, hormones → CCl_4 467, 476
  → chloral hydrate 467, 477
  → chloralose 477
  → chlordiazepoxide 467, 477
  → chloroform 468, 478
  → chlorpromazine 478
  → cholesterol 468, 478
  → choline 477
  → clofibrate 478
  → cocaine 468, 478
  → codeine 479
  → colchicine 479
  → complex diets 495
  → compound MO-911 479
  → corticoids 461
  ← corticoids 139
  → curare 479
  → cyanide 479
  → cyano-compounds 468
  → cyclophosphamide 479
  → cystine 480
  → decamethonium 480
  → DHT 494
  → α-diaminobutyric acid 480
  → dibucaine 480
  → diets, complex 495
  → digitalis 468, 481
  → dihydroxyphenylalanine 481
  → diisopropylfluorophospate (DFP) 481
  → dinitrophenol 481
  → disulfiram 481
  → drugs 462, 466
  → dye 481
  → electric stimuli/guinea pig, mouse 511, 512
  → ephedrine 468, 482
  → epinephrine 465
  → ergot 482
  → ethanol 482
  → ether 483
  → fluoride 483
  → folliculoids 461, 462
  → folliculoids, metabolism *Graph* 125
  → α-GDPH 514
  → GPT 514
  → guanidine 483
  → halothane 483
  → hemorrhage 512, 513
  → hepatic enzymes 514
  → hepatic lesions 502, 503
  ← hepatic lesions 601
  → hepatic tissue 727, 736
  → heroin 483
  → histamine 464, 466
  → hormone-like substances 463
  → hormones, nonsteroidal 463
  → 5-HT 464, 466

Thyroid, hormones → hydroquinone 483
    → N-(p-hydroxyphenyl)glycine 483
    → hyperbilirubinemia 720
    → hyperoxygenation 508
    → hyperoxygenation/cat 508
    → hypophyseal hormones 464
    → hypoxia/dog, fish, guinea pig, mouse, rabbit 506, 507, 508
    → imipramine 468, 483
    → immune reactions 500
    → indomethacin 468, 484
    → interventions, surgical 502
    → iodides 484
    → ionizing rays/fish, goldfish, mouse, rabbit, toad 504, 505, 506
    → iproniazid 484
    → isoniazid 484
    → isoproterenol 484
    → Klebsiella pneumoniae 497
    → lathyrogens 468, 484
    → lathyrogens/duck 484
    → lead 485
    → magnesium 468, 485
    → meperidine 486
    → meprobamate 468, 486
    → methadone 468
    → methylphenidate 486
    → α-methyl-p-tyrosine 468
    → microorganisms 496
    → morphine 468, 486
    → muscular performance 512, 513
    → Mycobacterium tuberculosis/guinea pig, mouse, rabbit 497, 498
    → mycoplasma 498
    → neostigmine 487
    → nicotine 487
    → nitrogen dioxide 487
    → nitrogen mustard 488
    → nitrous oxide 488
    → nonsteroidal hormones 463
    → norepinephrine 465
    → nortriptyline 488
    → novocaine 488
    → oxalate 488
    → ozone 469, 488
    → pancreatic hormones 463, 464
    → paraldehyde 488
    → paraphenylenediamine 488
    → parasites 496, 499
    → parathyroid hormone 463, 464
    → pargyline 488
    → paroxypropionine 488
    → pasteurella 498
    → pentachlorophenol 488
    → pentylenetetrazol 469, 488
    → peptone 489, 514
    → perchlorates 489

Thyroid, hormones → perphenazine 489
    → pesticides 469, 489
    → phenol 490
    → phosphates 469, 490
    → physostigmine 469, 490
    → picrotoxin 469, 490
    → pilocarpine 491
    → pituitary extracts 463
    → potassium 491
    → pralidoxime 491
    ← pregnancy 660
    → propionitrile 491
    → puromycin aminonucleoside 491
    → pyruvate 491
    → quinine 491
    → renal lesions 502, 503
    → reserpine 469, 491
    → resistance 460
    → salicylates 491
    → salinity tolerance 514
    → Salmonella typhi 498
    → SDH 514
    → semicarbazide 491
    ← sex 631
    → shigella 498
    → shock, traumatic 512
    → sodium chloride 491
    → sound 512, 513
    → staphylococci 498
    → steroidases (incl. bile acids, cholesterol) 462
    → steroids 461, 462
    ← steroids/dog, guinea pig, man 139
    → streptococci 499
    → stressors 512
    ← stressors 689
    → strychnine 491
    → sulfa drugs 492
    → surgical interventions 502
    → temperature variations/cat, fish, goat, guinea pig, hamster, mouse, rabbit 509, 510, 511
    → testoids 461, 462
    → testoids, metabolism *Graph* 125
    → tetrahydronaphthylamine 492
    → thallium 492
    → theophylline 492
    → thioacetamide 492
    → thiourea 492
    ← thyroid hormones 464
    → thyroxine 463
    → TKT 514
    → TPO 514
    → trauma 512
    → traumatic shock 512
    → tribromoethanol 492
    → triton 493

Thyroid, hormones → trypan blue 514
   → tryptophan 493
   → tumors **513**
   → tyrosine **469**, 493
   → uranium 493
   → vaccines **496, 497**
   → venoms 500
   → viruses **496**, 499
   → vitamin A, B, C, D, E **469, 470**, 493, 494, 495
   → vitamins (pantothenic acid) 495
   → water 495
   → zoxazolamine **470**, 495
  → hyperbilirubinemia **715**
  morphology **740**
  ← norepinephrine **531, 532**
  ← pancreatic hormones **521**
  ← thymectomy **547**
  weight ← phenobarbital *Table 140* 860
   ← steroids *Table 140* 860
   ← thyroxine *Table 140* 860
Thyroidectomy → digitoxin ← PCN *Table 124* 482
Thyroxinase, chemistry 50
Thyroxine; *cf. also* Thyroid, Thyroid Hormones
  → AAN *Diagram Table 139* 857; *Tables 73, 138* 257, 850
  → acetanilide *Diagram Table 139* 857; *Tables 24, 138* 176, 850
  → acrylamide *Diagram Table 139* 857; *Tables 25, 138* 176, 850
  → acrylonitrile *Table 26* 177
  ← ACTH 406
  → adrenal, weight *Table 140* 860
  → o-aminophenol *Diagram Table 139* 857; *Table 138* 850
  → aminopyrine *Diagram Table 139* 857; *Tables 27, 138* 179, 850
  → DL-amphetamine *Diagram Table 139* 857; *Table 138* 850
  → arsenic pentoxide *Diagram Table 139* 857; *Table 138* 850
  → barbital *Diagram Table 139* 857; *Tables 34, 138* 198, 850
  → bile-duct ligature *Diagram Table 139* 857; *Table 138* 850
  → bishydroxycoumarin *Tables 28, 138* 182, 850
  → body weight *Table 140* 860
  → bromobenzene *Diagram Table 139* 857; *Table 138* 850
  → brompheniramine *Diagram Table 139* 857; *Table 138* 850
  → cadmium *Diagram Table 139* 857; *Tables 35, 138* 200, 850

Thyroxine → caramiphen *Diagram Table 139* 857; *Tables 36, 138* 201, 850
  → carisoprodol *Diagram Table 139* 857; *Tables 37, 138* 216, 850
  → chlordiazepoxide *Diagram Table 139* 857; *Tables 38, 138* 217, 850
  → cinchophen *Diagram Table 139* 857; *Tables 39, 138* 221, 850
  → cocaine *Diagram Table 139* 857; *Tables 40, 138* 221, 850
  → F-COL *Diagram Table 139* 857; *Tables 12, 13, 14, 137, 138* 133, 134, 848
  → colchicine *Diagram Table 139* 857; *Tables 41, 138* 222, 850
  → DL-coniine *Diagram Table 139* 857; *Tables 42, 138* 222, 850
  → croton oil *Diagram Table 139* 857; *Tables 43, 138* 223, 850
  → cyclobarbital *Diagram Table 139* 857; *Tables 33, 138* 198, 850
  → cycloheximide *Diagram Table 139* 857; *Tables 44, 45, 138* 224, 850
  → cyclophosphamide *Fig. 22* 480; *Diagram Table 139* 857; *Tables 46, 138* 225, 850
  → DDT *Diagram Table 139* 857; *Table 138* 850
  → DHT *Diagram Table 139* 857; *Tables 117, 137, 138* 309, 848, 850
  → dicumarol *Diagram Table 139* 857
  → digitoxin *Diagram Table 139* 857; *Tables 47, 48, 137, 138* 230, 848, 850
  → digitoxin/mouse *Table 130* 677
  → diisopropyl fluorophosphate *Diagram Table 139* 857; *Tables 52, 139* 234, 850
  → dimercaprol *Diagram Table 139* 857; *Table 138* 850
  → dinitrophenol *Diagram Table 139* 857; *Table 138* 850
  → dioxathion *Diagram Table 139* 857; *Table 91, 137, 138* 280, 848, 850
  → dioxathion/mouse *Table 132* 680
  → diphenylhydantoin *Diagram Table 139* 857; *Tables 53, 138* 235, 850
  → dipicrylamine *Diagram Table 139* 857; *Tables 54, 138* 235, 850
  → DOC *Diagram Table 139*, 857; *Tables 15, 138*, 135, 850
  → doxepin *Diagram Table 139* 857; *Table 138* 850
  → edrophonium *Diagram Table 139* 857; *Table 138* 850
  → emetine *Diagram Table 139* 857; *Tables 55, 138* 238, 850
  → endotoxin *Diagram Table 139* 857; *Tables 123, 138* 348, 850

Thyroxine → ephedrine *Diagram Table 139*
  857; *Table 138* 850
  → epinephrine *Diagram Table 139* 857;
    Tables 23, 138 144, 850
  → EPN *Diagram Table 139* 857;
    Tables 99, 138 284, 850
  → Escherichia coli *Table 138* 850
  → estradiol *Diagram Table 139* 857;
    Tables 16, 138 135, 850
  → ethion *Diagram Table 139* 857;
    Tables 92, 138 281, 850
  → ethyl alcohol *Diagram Table 139* 857;
    Table 138 850
  → ethylene chlorhydrin *Diagram Table 139*
    857; *Table 138* 850
  → ethylene glycol *Diagram Table 139* 857;
    Tables 56, 138 243, 850
  → ethylmorphine *Diagram Table 139* 857;
    Tables 57, 138 244, 850
  → fasting *Diagram Table 139* 857
  → flufenamic acid *Diagram Table 139* 857;
    Tables 58, 138 245, 850
  → fluphenazine *Diagram Table 139* 857;
    Tables 59, 138 245, 850
  → glutethimide *Diagram Table 139* 857;
    Tables 63, 138 248, 850
  → glycerol *Diagram Table 139* 857;
    Tables 64, 138 249, 850
  → griseofulvin *Diagram Table 139* 857;
    Table 138 850
  → guthion *Diagram Table 139* 857;
    Tables 93, 138 281, 850
  → haloperidol *Diagram Table 139* 857;
    Table 138 850
  ← hepatic lesions **599**
  → hepatic microsomal drug metabolism in
    man 714
  → heptachlor *Diagram Table 139* 857;
    Tables 98, 138 238, 850
  → hexamethonium *Diagram Table 139* 857;
    Tables 61, 138 247, 850
  → hexobarbital *Diagram Table 139* 857;
    Tables 32, 137, 138 197, 848, 850
  → homatropine *Diagram Table 139* 857;
    Table 138 850
  → hydrazine *Diagram Table 139* 857;
    Table 138 850
  → hydroquinone *Diagram Table 139* 857;
    Tables 65, 138 249, 850
  → imipramine *Diagram Table 139* 857;
    Tables 66, 138 250, 850
  → indium *Diagram Table 139* 857;
    Table 138 850
  → indomethacin *Diagram Table 139* 857;
    Tables 67, 137, 138 250, 848, 850
  → indomethacin/mouse *Table 131* 678
  → kidney, weight *Table 140* 860

Thyroxine → lathyrogens *Fig. 9* 256
  → liver, weight *Table 140* 860
  → LSD *Diagram Table 139* 857;
    Tables 74, 138 258, 850
  → mechlorethamine *Diagram Table 139*
    857; *Tables 75, 138* 260, 850
  → mephenesin *Diagram Table 139* 857;
    Tables 76, 138 260, 850
  → meprobamate *Diagram Table 139* 857;
    Tables 77, 138 261, 850
  → mercury *Diagram Table 139* 857;
    Tables 78, 138 267, 850
  → mersalyl *Diagram Table 139* 857;
    Tables 79, 80, 138 268, 850
  → methadone *Diagram Table 139* 857;
    Tables 82, 138 269, 850
  → methylaniline *Diagram Table 139* 857;
    Tables 83, 138 270, 850
  → methylphenidate *Diagram Table 139*
    857; *Table 138* 850
  → methylsalicylate *Diagram Table 139*
    857; *Table 138* 850
  → methyprylon *Diagram Table 139* 857;
    Tables 84, 138 270, 850
  → morphine *Diagram Table 139* 857;
    Table 138 850
  → NaClO$_4$ *Diagram Table 139* 857;
    Tables 90, 138 278, 850
  → α-naphthylisocyanate *Diagram Table 139*
    857; *Tables 85, 138* 273, 850
  → neostigmine *Diagram Table 139* 857;
    Table 138 850
  → nephrectomy *Diagram Table 139* 857;
    Table 138 850
  → nicotine *Diagram Table 139* 857;
    Tables 86, 137, 138 274, 848, 850
  → nikethamide *Diagram Table 139* 857;
    Tables 87, 138 274, 850
  → p-nitroanisole *Diagram Table 139* 857;
    Tables 88, 138 275, 850
  → OMPA *Diagram Table 139* 857;
    Tables 94, 138 282, 850
  → ovary, weight *Table 140* 860
  → pancuronium *Diagram Table 139* 857;
    Tables 19, 138 136, 850
  → parathion *Diagram Table 139* 857;
    Tables 95, 137, 138 282, 848, 850
  → pentobarbital/mouse *Table 129* 677
  → pentylenetetrazol *Diagram Table 139*
    857; *Table 89, 138* 277, 850
  → phenindione *Diagram Table 139* 857;
    Tables 29, 138 183, 850
  → phenyl isothiocyanate *Diagram Table
    139* 857; *Table 138* 850
  → phenyramidol *Diagram Table 139* 857;
    Tables 100, 138 284, 850

Thyroxine → phosphorus, yellow *Diagram Table 139* 857; *Table 138* 850
  → physostigmine *Diagram Table 139* 857; *Tables 101, 138* 285, 850
  → picrotoxin *Diagram Table 139* 857; *Tables 102, 138* 286, 850
  → picrotoxin/mouse *Table 133* 680
  → piperidine *Diagram Table 139* 857; *Tables 103, 138* 287, 850
  → pipradol *Diagram Table 139* 857; *Table 138* 850
  → pralidoxime *Diagram Table 139* 857; *Tables 104, 138* 288, 850
  ← pregnancy **660**
  → preputial glands, weight *Table 140* 860
  → progesterone *Diagram Table 139* 857; *Tables 17, 137, 138* 136, 848, 850
  → propionitrile *Diagram Table 139* 857; *Tables 105, 138* 289, 850
  → propylthiouracil *Diagram Table 139* 857; *Tables 21, 22, 138* 140, 141, 850
  → pyrilamine *Diagram Table 139* 857; *Table 138* 850
  ← sex **631**
  → SKF 525-A *Diagram Table 139* 857; *Tables 106, 138* 291, 850
  → strychnine *Diagram Table 139* 857; *Tables 107, 138* 292, 850
  → T 3 *Diagram Table 139* 857; *Tables 20, 138* 140, 850
  → TEA *Diagram Table 139* 857; *Tables 62, 138* 248, 850
  → thallium *Diagram Table 139* 857; *Table 138* 850
  → theobromine *Diagram Table 139* 857; *Tables 108, 138* 293, 850
  → theophylline *Diagram Table 139* 857; *Tables 109, 138* 293, 850
  → thimerosal *Diagram Table 139* 857; *Tables 110, 138* 294, 850
  → thioacetamide *Table 138* 850
  → thiopenthal *Diagram Table 139* 857; *Tables 31, 138* 197, 850
  → thymus, weight *Table 140* 860
  ← thyroid hormones **463**
  → thyroid, weight *Table 140* 860
  → tremorine *Diagram Table 139* 857; *Table 138* 850
  → triamcinolone *Diagram Table 139* 857; *Tables 18, 138* 136, 850
  → β-tribromoethanol *Diagram Table 139* 857; *Tables 111, 138* 295, 850
  → β-trichloroethanol *Diagram Table 139* 857; *Tables 112, 138* 295, 850
  → tri-o-cresyl phosphate *Diagram Table 139* 857; *Tables 113, 138* 296, 850

Thyroxine, → d-tubocurarine *Diagram Table 139* 857; *Tables 114, 138* 296, 850
  → tyramine *Diagram Table 139* 857; *Tables 115, 138* 297, 850
  → tyrosine *Diagram Table 139* 857; *Tables 116, 138* 299, 850
  → uterus, weight *Table 140* 860
  → W-1372 *Diagram Table 139* 857; *Tables 118, 138* 309, 850
  → warfarin *Diagram Table 139* 857; *Table 138* 850
  → zoxazolamine *Diagram Table 139* 857; *Tables 119, 137, 138* 848, 850
"Tigroid" necrosis ← papain + stress *Fig. 30* 695
Timing, pharmacology 82
Tissue extracts → resistance **564**, 565
  ← steroids 147
Tissues, morphology 740
"Tissue tranquilizers" **764**
TKT ← ACTH **423**, 424
  ← adrenalectomy 393
  ← age **667**, 672
  ← diurnal variations **704**
  ← genetic factors 682
  ← hepatic lesions 620
  ← hypophysectomy 457
  ← ionizing rays 684
  ← pancreatic hormones 530
  ← sex 659
  ← species **681**, 682
  ← stressors **698**, 700
  theories 745
  ← thyroid hormones 514
  ← tumors **704**
  (tyrosine) ← corticoids 385
    ← corticoids/mouse 389
TMACN → steroids **131**, 132
Toad **505**, 506
Tolbutamide; *cf. also* Pancreatic Hormones
  → F-COL *Table 137* 848
  → DHT *Table 137* 848
  → digitoxin *Table 137* 848
  → dioxathion *Table 137* 848
  → hexobarbital *Table 137* 848
  → indomethacin *Table 137* 848
  → nicotine *Table 137* 848
  → parathion *Table 137* 848
  → progesterone *Table 137* 848
  → zoxazolamine *Table 137* 848
Toluene diisocyanate ← pancreatic hormones 526
"Total overall protective index" 771
Tourniquet shock ← sympathectomy **554**
Toxicants, barbiturates 105, 109
  CCl₄ 108, 110
  (characteristics of typical substrates) **103**

Toxicants, cholesterol **105**
  digitalis compounds **105**, 108
  griseofulvin 110
  indomethacin **108**, 110
  mercury **108**, 110
  nicotine **108**, 110
  nonpolar ← species **681**
  pesticides **108**, 109
  ← starvation/mouse *Table 3* 81
  steroids **105**, 108
Toxication, nonspecific **764**
  specific **764**
"Toxohormone" **387, 699**
  → resistance **563**, 564
Toxoplasma ← steroids **330**, 332
TPNH ← sex **655**
TPO ← ACTH **423**, 424
  ← adrenalectomy **393**
  ← age **667**, 672
  ← genetic factors **682**
  ← hepatic lesions **620**
  ← hypophysectomy **457**
  ← ionizing rays **684**
  ← pancreatic hormones **530**
  ← species **682**
  ← stressors **698**, 700
  theories **745**
  ← thyroid hormones **514**
  (tryptophan) ← corticoids **385**
    ← corticoids/mouse **389**
  ← tumors **704**
Transsulfuration **48**
Tranylcypromine **68**; *cf.* MAO-Inhibitors
Trauma; *cf. also* Surgical Interventions
  ← ACTH **422**, 423
  ← epinephrine **545**
  local; *cf.* Local Trauma
  ← pancreatic hormones **529**
  ← posterior pituitary preparations **443**
  ← sex **657**
  systemic; *cf.* Systemic Trauma
  ← thyroid hormones **512**
Traumatic shock ← posterior pituitary preparations **441**
  ← thyroid hormones **512**
Tremorine (causes experimental Parkinsonism) ← epinephrine **540**
  ← 5-HT **561**
  ← norepinephrine **540**
  ← phenobarbital *Diagram Table 139* **857**; *Table 138* **850**
  ← steroids **294**; *Diagram Table 139* **857**; *Table 138* **850**
  ← thyroxine *Diagram Table 139* **857**; *Table 138* **850**
Treponema pallidum ← steroids **318**, 325

Triamcinolone; *cf. also* Corticoids
  → AAN *Table 73* **257**
  → acetanilide *Table 24* **176**
  → acrylamide *Table 25* **176**
  → acrylonitrile *Table 26* **177**
  → adrenal, weight *Table 140* **860**
  → aminopyrine *Table 27* **179**
  → barbital *Table 34* **198**
  → bishydroxycoumarin *Table 28* **182**
  → body weight *Table 140* **860**
  → cadmium *Table 35* **200**
  → caramiphen *Table 36* **201**
  → carisoprodol *Table 37* **216**
  → chlordiazepoxide *Table 38* **217**
  → cinchophen *Table 39* **221**
  → cocaine *Table 40* **221**
  → F-COL *Tables 12, 13, 14* **133, 134**
  → colchicine *Table 41* **222**
  → DL-coniine *Table 42* **222**
  → croton oil *Table 43* **223**
  → cyclobarbital *Table 33* **198**
  → cycloheximide *Tables 44, 45* **224**
  → cyclophosphamide *Table 46* **225**
  → DHT *Table 117* **309**
  → digitoxin *Tables 47, 48* **230**
  → digitoxin/mouse *Table 130* **677**
  → diisopropyl fluorophosphate *Table 52* **234**
  → dioxathion *Table 91* **280**
  → dioxathion/mouse *Table 132* **680**
  → diphenylhydantoin *Table 53* **235**
  → dipicrylamine *Table 54* **235**
  → DOC *Table 15* **135**
  → emetine *Table 55* **238**
  → endotoxin *Tables 120, 123* **344, 348**
  → epinephrine *Table 23* **144**
  → EPN *Table 99* **284**
  → estradiol *Table 16* **135**
  → ethion *Table 92* **281**
  → ethylaniline *Table 83* **270**
  → ethylene glycol *Fig. 7* **242**; *Table 56* **243**
  → ethylmorphine *Table 57* **244**
  → flufenamic acid *Table 58* **245**
  → fluphenazine *Table 59* **245**
  → glutethimide *Table 63* **248**
  → glycerol *Table 64* **249**
  → guthion *Table 93* **281**
  → heptachlor *Table 98* **283**
  → hexamethonium *Tables 60A, B, 61* **246, 247**
  → hexobarbital *Table 32* **197**
  → hydroquinone *Table 65* **249**
  → imipramine *Table 66* **250**
  → indomethacin *Tables 67, 141* **250, 862**
  → indomethacin/mouse *Table 131* **678**
  → kidney, weight *Table 140* **860**

Triamcinolone → liver, weight *Table 140* 860
→ LSD *Table 74* 258
→ mechlorethamine *Table 75* 260
→ mephenesin *Table 76* 260
→ meprobamate *Table 77* 261
→ mercury *Tables 78, 81* 267, 269
→ mersalyl *Tables 79, 80* 268
→ methadione *Table 82* 269
→ methyprylon *Table 84* 270
→ NaClO$_4$ *Table 90* 278
→ α-naphthylisothiocyanate *Table 85* 273
→ nicotine *Table 86* 274
→ nikethamide *Table 87* 274
→ p-nitroanisole *Table 88* 275
→ OMPA *Table 94* 282
→ ovary, weight *Table 140* 860
→ pancuronium *Table 19* 136
→ parathion *Table 95* 282
← PCN *Table 18* 136
→ pentobarbital/mouse *Table 129* 677
→ pentolinium *Table 60 B* 246
→ pentylenetetrazol *Table 89* 277
← phenobarbital *Diagram Table 139* 857; *Tables 18, 138* 136, 850
→ phenindione *Table 29* 183
→ phenyramidol *Table 100* 284
→ physostigmine *Table 101* 285
→ picrotoxin *Table 102* 286
→ picrotoxin/mouse *Table 133* 680
→ piperidine *Table 103* 287
→ pralidoxime *Table 104* 288
→ preputial glands, weight *Table 140* 860
→ progesterone *Table 17* 136
→ propionitrile *Table 105* 289
→ propylthiouracil *Tables 21, 22* 140,141
← puromycin 76
→ SKF 525-A *Table 106* 291
← steroids *Diagram Table 139* 857; *Tables 18, 138* 136, 850
→ strychnine *Table 107* 292
→ T 3 *Table 20* 140
→ TEA *Tables 60 (A + B), 62* 246, 248
→ theobromine *Table 108* 293
→ theophylline *Table 109* 293
→ thimerosal *Table 110* 294
→ thiopental *Table 31* 197
→ thymus, weight *Table 140* 860
→ thyroid, weight *Table 140* 860
← thyroxine *Diagram Table 139* 857; *Tables 18, 138* 136, 850
→ tribromoethanol *Table 111* 295
→ trichloroethanol *Table 112* 295
→ tri-o-cresyl phosphate *Table 113* 296
→ D-tubocurarine *Table 114* 296
→ tyramine *Table 115* 297
→ tyrosine *Table 116* 299
→ uterus, weight *Table 140* 860

Triamcinolone → W-1372 *Table 118* 309
→ zoxazolamine *Table 119* 313
Triamterene (potassium-sparing diuretic) → resistance 590
Tribromoethanol (basal anesthetic) ← phenobarbital *Diagram Table 139* 857; *Tables 111, 138* 295, 850
← renal lesions **623**
← steroids **169**, 295; *Diagram Table 139* 857; *Tables 111, 138* 295, 850
← thyroid hormones 492
← thyroxine *Diagram Table 139* 857; *Tables 111, 138* 295, 850
Trichinella spiralis ← ACTH **415**
← steroid **330, 332**
Trichloroethanol (basal anesthetic) ← phenobarbital *Diagram Table 139* 857; *Tables 112, 138* 295, 850
← steroids **170**, 295; *Diagram Table 139* 857; *Tables 112, 138* 295, 850
← thyroxine *Diagram Table 139* 857; *Tables 112, 138* 295, 850
Trichloroethylene (analgesic, anesthetic) ← steroids 295
Trichophyton mentagrophytes ← steroids **329**, 330
Trichuris muris ← steroids **330, 332**
Triflupromazine → resistance 591
← SKF 525-A 62
Tri-o-cresyl phosphate ← phenobarbital *Diagram Table 139* 857; *Tables 114, 138* 296, 850
← propylthiouracil *Table 113* 296
← steroids 295; *Diagram Table 139* 857 *Tables 113, 138* 296, 850
← T 3 *Table 113* 296
← thyroxine *Diagram Table 139* 857; *Tables 113, 138* 296, 850
Triton ← thyroid hormones 493
Trypan blue ← parathyroids 520
← thyroid hormones 514
Trypanosoma cruzi ← steroids 331
equiperdum ← pancreatic hormones 528
← steroids 331
inopinatum ← STH **430**
lewisi ← steroids 331
← thymectomy 551
Trypanosomes ← steroids **330**
Trypsin ← steroids 296
← stressors 703
Tryptamine → resistance 590
Tryptophan; *cf. also* TPO *under* Influence of Steroids upon Enzymes
← STH **426**, 428
← thyroid hormones 493
Tuberculosis ← hypophysectomy **453**
← STH **430**

Tubocurarine (skeletal muscle relaxant) ←
  phenobarbital *Diagram Table 139* 857;
  Tables 114, 138 296, 850
  ← steroids 170, 296; *Diagram Table 139*
    857; *Tables 114, 138* 296, 850
  ← thyroxine *Diagram Table 139* 857;
    Tables 114, 138 296, 850
Tumors; *cf. also* Carcinogens
  ← ACTH 423
  → aminopyrine-metabolizing enzymes 704
  ← hepatic lesions 618, 619
  → hepatic regeneration 704
  → hepatic tissue 739
  → hexobarbital-metabolizing enzymes 704
  ← hypophysectomy 457
  (in animals); *cf. also* Carcinogens *under*
    Drugs
  ← partial hepatectomy 704
  → regeneration, hepatic 704
  → resistance 704, 705
  ← sex 657, 659
  → steroidases 704
  ← steroids 382
  ← thymectomy 553
  ← thyroid hormones 513
  → TKT 704
  → TPO 704
Tumor transplants ← anterior pituitary
  preparations 440
  ← hypophysectomy 456
Tween 80 ← 5-HT 561
  ← norepinephrine 533, 540
Typhoid bacilli ← STH 430, 431
  endotoxin ← STH 430
  ← steroids 318
Tyramine (sympathomimetic) ← phenobarbital *Diagram Table 139* 857;
  Tables 115, 138 297, 850
  ← steroids 296; *Diagram Table 139* 857;
    Tables 115, 138 297, 850
  ← thyroxine *Diagram Table 139* 857;
    Tables 115, 138 297, 850
Tyrosine; *cf. also* TKT *under* Enzymes
  Influenced by Steroids
  ← actinomycin 74
  ← cholesterol *Table 116* 299
  ← PCN *Fig. 13* 298
  ← phenobarbital *Diagram Table 139* 857;
    Tables 116, 138 299, 850
  ← sex 635, 654
  ← steroids 170, 297; *Diagram Table 139*
    857; *Tables 116, 138* 299, 850
  ← STH 426, 428
  ← stressors 695
  ← temperature variations 687
  ← thyroid hormones 469, 493

Tyrosine ← thyroxine *Diagram Table 139* 857;
  Tables 116, 138 299, 850
Tyzzer's disease ← ACTH 416
  ← steroids 316, 319

UDP-ase ← corticoids 392
Ulcers, intestinal ← indomethacin +
  spironolactone *Fig. 8* 251
  pyloric ← indomethacin/rabbit *Fig. 28* 679
Ultrastructural changes in hepatocytes ←
  PCN *Fig. 35* 732
Ultraviolet rays → resistance 685
  ← steroids 368
Uranium ← pancreatic hormones 526
  ← parathyroids 516, 518
  ← steroids 297
  ← thyroid hormones 493
Urea-cycle enzymes ← corticoids 392
Ureter ligature; *cf. also* Renal Lesions
  temporary → mercury *Fig. 26* 625;
    Table 127 624
    → mercury ← partial nephrectomy
      Table 127 624
    → nephrocalcinosis ← mercury *Fig. 26*
      625
Urethan ← epinephrine 540
  ← hepatic lesions 613
  ← 5-HT 561
  ← norepinephrine 540
  → resistance 591
  ← sex 654
  ← SKF 525-A 62
  ← steroids 297
Uterus, morphology 740
  weight ← phenobarbital *Table 140* 860
    ← steroids *Table 140* 860
    ← thyroxine *Table 140* 860

Vaccines ← ACTH 415, 416
  ← epinephrine 541
  ← histamine 555, 556
  ← norepinephrine 541
  ← pancreatic hormones 527
  → resistance 595
  ← splenectomy 553
  ← steroids 316
  ← STH 430
  ← thymectomy 550
  ← thyroid hormones 496, 497
Vaccinia ← steroids 326, 329
Variola ← ACTH 415
  ← steroids 326, 329
Vasopressin ← hepatic lesions 601
  ← pregnancy 661
  → resistance 591

Venoms ← ACTH 416, 419
  cobra ← hypophysectomy 453
    ← sex 656
  ← epinephrine 541, 542
  ← hypophysectomy 453, 454
  ← norepinephrine 541
  ← sex 656
  snakes ← steroids 348
  spiders ← steroids 349
  ← steroids 348
  ← stressors 698, 699, 700
  ← temperature variations 687
  ← thyroid hormones 500
  wasp ← steroids 349
Virilizing steroids; cf. Testoids
Viruses ← ACTH 415, 417
  ← epinephrine 541
  ← norepinephrine 541
  ← pregnancy 666
  ← sex 656
  ← steroids 325
  ← STH 431
  ← thymectomy 549, 550
  ← thyroid hormones 496, 499
Virus hepatitis ← steroids 326, 327
Vitamin A ← anterior pituitary preparations 436, 439
  ← calcitonin 520, 521
  → F-COL Table 137 848
  → DHT Table 137 848
  → digitoxin Table 137 848
  → dioxathion Table 137 848
  → hexobarbital Table 137 848
  ← hypophysectomy 446, 452
  → indomethacin Table 137 848
  → nicotine Table 137 848
  → parathion Table 137 848
  → progesterone Table 137 848
  → resistance 590
  ← spironolactone/rat Fig. 14 301
  ← steroids/rabbit, xenopus laevis 170, 171
  ← STH 426, 428; Fig. 21 429
  ← stressors 697
  ← thymectomy 548, 549
  ← thyroid hormones 469, 493
  → zoxazolamine Table 137 848
Vitamin B; cf. also Aminopterin
  ← steroids 172, 301
  ← steroids/chicken, pigeon 172
  ← thyroid hormones 469, 494
Vitamin B complex ← sex 654
Vitamin B_1 ← pancreatic hormones 522, 526
Vitamin B-12 → resistance 590
Vitamin C ← ACTH 407, 414
  ← anterior pituitary preparations 439
  ← barbiturates 578

Vitamin C → F-COL Table 137 848
  → DHT Table 137 848
  → digitoxin Table 137 848
  → dioxathion Table 137 848
  → hexobarbital Table 137 848
  → indomethacin Table 137 848
  → nicotine Table 137 848
  → parathion Table 137 848
  ← parathyroids 518
  → progesterone Table 137 848
  ← resistance 571, 590
  ← sex 654
  ← steroids 172, 302
  ← steroids/guinea pig, mouse 172
  ← STH 428
  theories 757
  ← thymectomy 549
  ← thyroid hormones 470, 494
  → zoxazolamine Table 137 848
Vitamin D ← ACTH 408, 414
  ← adrenalectomy 173, 303
  ← barbiturates 578
  → F-COL Table 137 848
  → DHT Table 137 848
  → digitoxin Table 137 848
  → dioxathion Table 137 848
  ← epinephrine 533, 540
  ← folliculoids 173, 304
  ← glucocorticoids 302
  ← glucocorticoids/chicken, man, mouse 173
  ← gonadectomy 303
  ← hepatic lesions 604, 613
  → hexobarbital Table 137 848
  ← 5-HT 561
  ← hypophysectomy 452
  → indomethacin Table 137 848
  ← mineralocorticoids 303
  → nicotine Table 137 848
  ← norepinephrine 533
  ← pancreatic hormones 522, 526
  → parathion Table 137 848
  ← parathyroids 516, 518
  ← posterior pituitary preparations 442
  ← pregnancy 661, 665
  → progesterone Table 137 848
  → resistance 590
  ← sex 635, 654
  ← steroids 172, 302, 308
  ← STH 426, 428
  ← stressors 697
  ← testoids 174, 307
  ← testoids/chicken 174
  ← thymectomy 548, 549
  ← thyroid hormones 470, 494
  → zoxazolamine Table 137 848
Vitamin E → F-COL Table 137 848

Vitamin E → DHT *Table 137* 848
  → digitoxin *Table 137* 848
  → dioxathion *Table 137* 848
  → hexobarbital *Table 137* 848
  → indomethacin *Table 137* 848
  → nicotine *Table 137* 848
  → parathion *Table 137* 848
  ← posterior pituitary preparations 442
  ← pregnancy 665
  → progesterone *Table 137* 848
  → resistance **571**, 590
  ← steroids 309
  ← thyroid hormones **470**, 495
  → zoxazolamine *Table 137* 848
Vitamin K ← sex 654
  ← steroids 309
Vitamins (pantothenic acid) ← thyroid hormones 495

W-1372 → F-COL *Table 137* 848
  → DHT *Table 137* 848
  → digitoxin *Table 137* 848
  → dioxathion *Table 137* 848
  ← hepatic lesions 613
  → hexobarbital *Table 137* 848
  → indomethacin *Table 137* 848
  → liver *Figs. 18, 19* 310, 311
  → liver ← PCN *Figs. 18, 19* 310, 311
  → liver ← phenobarbital *Fig. 19* 311
  → liver ← progesterone *Fig. 18* 310
  → nicotine *Table 137* 848
  → parathion *Table 137* 848
  ← PCN *Figs. 18, 19* 310, 311; *Table 118* 309
  ← phenobarbital *Fig. 19* 311; *Diagram Table 139* 857; *Tables 118, 138* 309, 850
  ← progesterone *Fig. 18* 310
  → progesterone *Table 137* 848
  → resistance 591
  ← steroids **175**, 309; *Diagram Table 139* 857; *Tables 118, 138* 309, 850
  ← thyroxine *Diagram Table 139* 857; *Tables 118, 138* 309, 850
  → zoxazolamine *Table 137* 848
Warfarin; *cf. also* Anticoagulants
  ← phenobarbital *Diagram Table 139* 857; *Table 138* 850
  ← steroids *Diagram Table 139* 857; *Table 138* 850
  ← thyroxine *Diagram Table 139* 857; *Table 138* 850
Water ← posterior pituitary preparations 442
  ← steroids 310
  ← thyroid hormones 495
Welchia perfringens ← pancreatic hormones 527

Withdrawal, spironolactone → digitoxin *Table 5* 86
Worms ← steroids **330**, 332

Xanthine → resistance 591
"Xenobiotics" **59**, 759
Xenopus laevis 171
X-irradiation; *cf.* Ionizing Rays

"Yakriton" **564**
Yeast ← steroids **313**, 314, 329
  ← STH 432
  ← thymectomy 551
Yohimbine (adrenergic blocker, possibly aphrodisiac) ← epinephrine 540
  → resistance 591
  ← steroids 312

Zinc ← pancreatic hormones 526
  ← STH 430
Zn; *cf.* Zinc
Zoxazolamine (skeletal muscle relaxant) ← acetylsalicylic acid *Table 137* 848
  ← ACTH 414; *Table 137* 848
  ← betamethasone *Table 128* 630
  ← bile duct ligature *Table 137* 848
  ← CS-1 *Table 9* 96
  ← CS-1, repeated doses *Table 7* 90, 91
  ← CS-1, single dose *Table 6* 88, 89
  ← digitoxin *Table 137* 848
  ← diphenylhydantoin *Table 137* 848
  ← estradiol *Table 9* 96
  ← ethylestrenol *Tables 9, 128* 96, 630
  ← genetic factors **675**, 681
  ← hypophysectomy **447**, 453
  ← indomethacin *Table 137* 848
  ← nicotine *Table 137* 848
  ← norbolethone *Table 9* 96
  ← PCN *Tables 9, 128* 96, 630
  ← PCN, repeated doses *Table 7* 90, 91
  ← PCN, single dose *Table 6* 88, 89
  ← phenobarbital *Diagram Table 139* 857; *Tables 9, 119, 128, 137, 138* 96, 313, 630, 848, 850
  ← phenobarbital, repeated doses *Table 7* 90, 91
  ← phenobarbital, single dose *Table 6* 88, 89
  ← phentolamine *Table 137* 848
  ← phenylbutazone *Tables 128, 137* 630, 848
  ← phetharbital *Table 137* 848
  ← prednisolone, repeated doses *Table 7* 90, 91
  ← salicylate *Table 137* 848
  ← sex 655
  ← spironolactone *Tables 9, 128* 96, 630

Zoxazolamine ← spironolactone, repeated doses
  Table 7 90, 91
  ← splenectomy 553
  ← steroids **175**, **312**; *Diagram Table 139*
    857; *Tables 119, 136, 138* 313, 836, 850
  ← STH *Table 137* 848
  ← stressors 697

Zoxazolamine ← thyroid hormones **470**, **495**
  ← thyroxine *Diagram Table 139* 857;
    Tables 119, 137, 138 313, 848, 850
  ← tolbutamide *Table 137* 848
  ← vitamin A, C, D, E *Table 137* 848
  ← W-1372 *Table 137* 848

CPSIA information can be obtained at www.ICGtesting.com
Printed in the USA
LVOW05s0927040115

421371LV00007B/3/P